Maternity & Women's Health Care

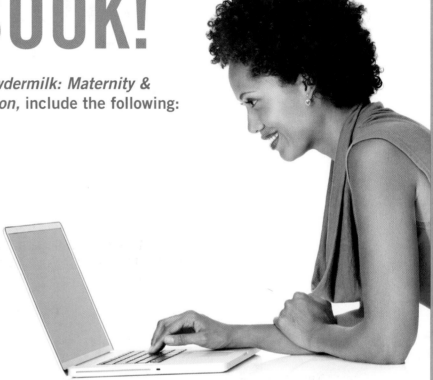

11th Edition

Maternity & Women's Health Care

Deitra Leonard Lowdermilk, RNC-E, PhD, FAAN
Clinical Professor Emerita, School of Nursing
University of North Carolina at Chapel Hill
Chapel Hill, North Carolina

Shannon E. Perry, RN, PhD, FAAN
Professor Emerita, School of Nursing
San Francisco State University
San Francisco, California

Kitty Cashion, RN-BC, MSN
Clinical Nurse Specialist, Department of Obstetrics and Gynecology, Division of Maternal-Fetal Medicine
University of Tennessee Health Science Center
Memphis, Tennessee

Kathryn Rhodes Alden, RN, MSN, EdD, IBCLC
Clinical Associate Professor, School of Nursing
University of North Carolina at Chapel Hill
Chapel Hill, North Carolina

Associate Editor

Ellen F. Olshansky, PhD, RN, WHNP-BC, NC-BC, FAAN
Professor, Program in Nursing Science
University of California, Irvine
Irvine, California

ELSEVIER

ELSEVIER

3251 Riverport Lane
St. Louis, MO 63043

MATERNITY & WOMEN'S HEALTH CARE, 11th ed ISBN: 978-0-323-16918-9

Notice

Knowledge and best practice in this field are constantly changing. As new research and experience broaden our understanding, changes in research methods, professional practices, or medical treatment may become necessary. Practitioners and researchers must always rely on their own experience and knowledge in evaluating and using any information, methods, compounds, or experiments described herein. In using such information or methods they should be mindful of their own safety and the safety of others, including parties for whom they have a professional responsibility.

With respect to any drug or pharmaceutical products identified, readers are advised to check the most current information provided (i) on procedures featured or (ii) by the manufacturer of each product to be administered, to verify the recommended dose or formula, the method and duration of administration, and contraindications. It is the responsibility of practitioners, relying on their own experience and knowledge of their patients, to make diagnoses, to determine dosages and the best treatment for each individual patient, and to take all appropriate safety precautions.

To the fullest extent of the law, neither the Publisher nor the authors, contributors, or editors, assume any liability for any injury and/or damage to persons or property as a matter of products liability, negligence or otherwise, or from any use or operation of any methods, products, instructions, or ideas contained in the material herein.

The Publisher

ISBN: 978-0-323-16918-9

Content Strategist: Sandra Clark
Content Development Manager: Laurie K. Gower
Senior Content Development Specialist: Heather Bays
Publishing Services Manager: Jeff Patterson
Senior Project Manager: Jeanne Genz
Designer: Ashley Miner

Printed in the U.S.A.

Last digit is the print number: 9 8 7 6 5 4 3 2 1

DEITRA LEONARD LOWDERMILK

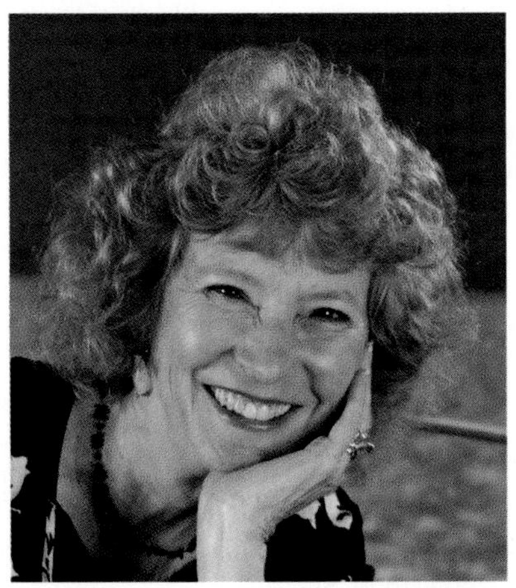

Deitra Leonard Lowdermilk is Clinical Professor Emerita, School of Nursing, University of North Carolina at Chapel Hill. She received her BSN from East Carolina University and her MEd and PhD in Education from UNC-CH. She is certified in In-Patient Obstetrics by the National Certification Corporation. She is a fellow in the American Academy of Nursing. In addition to being a nurse educator for more than 34 years, Dr. Lowdermilk has clinical experience as a public health nurse and as a staff nurse in labor and delivery, postpartum, and newborn units, and has worked in gynecologic surgery and cancer care units.

Dr. Lowdermilk has been recognized for her expertise in nursing education. She has repeatedly been selected as Classroom and Clinical Teacher of the Year by graduating seniors. She was a recipient of the Educator of the Year Award from both the District IV Association of Women's Health, Obstetric and Neonatal Nurses (AWHONN) and the North Carolina Nurses Association. She also received the 2005 AWHONN Excellence in Education Award.

She is active in AWHONN, having served as chair of the North Carolina Section of AWHONN and has served as chair and member of various committees in AWHONN at the national, district, state, and local levels. She has served as guest editor for the *Journal of Obstetric, Gynecologic and Neonatal Nursing* and served on editorial boards for other publications. Dr. Lowdermilk also is coauthor of *Maternity Nursing* (8th edition) and *Maternal Child Nursing Care* (5th edition).

Dr. Lowdermilk's most significant contribution to nursing has been to promote excellence in nursing practice and education in women's health through integration of knowledge into practice. In 2005 she received the first Distinguished Alumni Award from East Carolina University School of Nursing for her exemplary contributions to the nursing profession in the area of maternal-child care and the community. She was also Alumna of the Year for East Carolina University in 2005, and was selected as one of the 100 Incredible ECU Women in 2007 for Outstanding Leadership Among Women in the first 100 years of the university's founding.

In fall 2010, the East Carolina University College of Nursing named the Neonatal Intensive Care and Midwifery Laboratory in honor of Dr. Lowdermilk. In 2011 she was named one of the first 40 nurses inducted into the College of Nursing Hall of Fame.

SHANNON E. PERRY

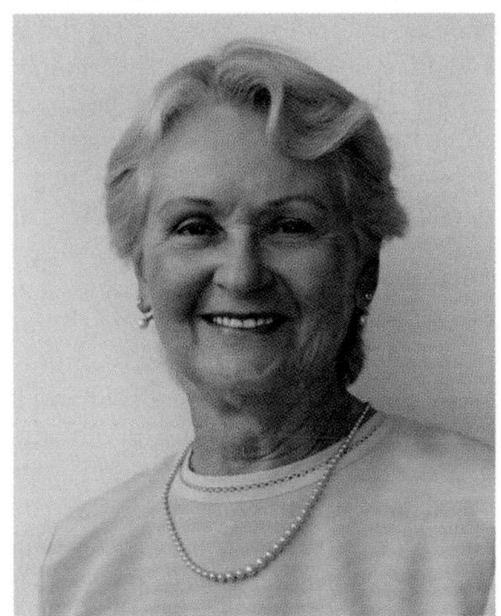

Shannon E. Perry is Professor Emerita, School of Nursing, San Francisco State University, San Francisco, California. She received her diploma in nursing from St. Joseph Hospital School of Nursing, Bloomington, Illinois; a baccalaureate in Nursing from Marquette University, an MSN from the University of Colorado Medical Center, and a PhD in Educational Psychology with a Specialization in Child Development from Arizona State University. She completed a 2-year postdoctoral fellowship in perinatal nursing at the University of California, San Francisco, as a Robert Wood Johnson Clinical Nurse Scholar.

Dr. Perry has had clinical experience as a staff nurse, head nurse, and supervisor in surgical nursing, obstetrics, pediatrics, gynecology, and neonatal nursing. She has served as an expert witness and legal consultant. She has taught in schools of nursing in several states for more than 30 years and was interim director and director of the School of Nursing and director of a Child and Adolescent Development baccalaureate program at SFSU. She was Marquette University College of Nursing Alumna of the Year in 1999, and was the University of Colorado School of Nursing Distinguished Alumna of the Year in 2000. She received the San Francisco State University Alumni Association Emeritus Faculty Award in 2005 and the Excellence in Education Award from the Beta Upsilon chapter of Sigma Theta Tau International (STTI) in 2012.

She is coauthor of *Maternity Nursing* (8th edition), *Maternal Child Nursing Care* (5th edition), and *Clinical Companion for Maternity & Newborn Nursing* (2nd edition) and has authored numerous chapters and articles on maternal-newborn topics and the legal aspects of nursing. She is a fellow in the American Academy of Nursing, a member of AWHONN, Arizona Nurses Association (AzNA), and National League for Nursing (NLN), first vice president of the American Association for the History of Nursing (AAHN), and a member of the AAHN Communications Committee and the STTI Foundation Fellows Committee. Dr. Perry's experience in international nursing includes teaching international nursing courses in the United Kingdom, Ireland, Italy, Thailand, Ghana, and China and participating in health missions in Ghana, Kenya, and Honduras. She is participating in establishing a school of nursing in Kenya, has supported the establishment of the library, and has had a wing of a dormitory named after her. For her "exemplary contributions to nursing, public service, and selfless commitment and passion in shaping the future of international health," she received the President's Award from the Global Caring Nurses Foundation, Inc., in 2008. In January 2012, she and 47 other women climbed Mt. Kilimanjaro, the highest mountain in Africa, to raise awareness of human trafficking and to raise funds to support projects to combat human trafficking.

KITTY CASHION

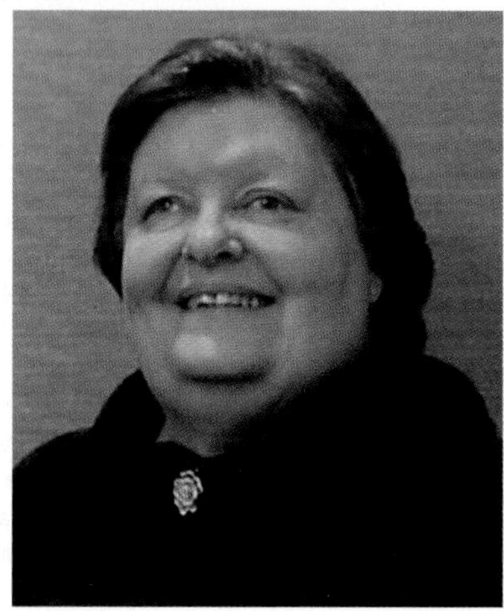

Kitty Cashion is a Clinical Nurse Specialist in the Maternal-Fetal Medicine Division, College of Medicine, Department of Obstetrics and Gynecology at the University of Tennessee Health Science Center in Memphis. She received her BSN from the University of Tennessee College of Nursing in Memphis and her MSN in Parent-Child Nursing from Vanderbilt University School of Nursing in Nashville, Tennessee. Ms. Cashion is certified as a high risk perinatal nurse through the American Nurses Credentialing Center (ANCC).

Ms. Cashion's job responsibilities at the University of Tennessee include providing education regarding low and high risk obstetrics to staff nurses in West Tennessee community hospitals. For more than 20 years Ms. Cashion has taught obstetric nursing in the clinical setting (mostly in Labor and Delivery) for students at Northwest Mississippi Community College in Senatobia, Mississippi, and Union University in Germantown, Tennessee.

Ms. Cashion has been an active AWHONN member, holding office at both the local and state levels. She also has served as an officer and board member of the Tennessee Perinatal Association and as an active volunteer for the Tennessee chapter, March of Dimes Birth Defects Foundation.

Ms. Cashion has contributed many chapters to maternity nursing textbooks over the years. She also coauthored a series of Virtual Clinical Excursions workbooks to accompany six obstetric nursing textbooks published by Elsevier. More recently she served as one of the authors for *Maternity & Women's Health Care* (10th edition), and *Clinical Companion for Maternity & Newborn Nursing* (2nd edition), and as an associate editor for *Maternal Child Nursing Care* (5th edition).

KATHRYN RHODES ALDEN

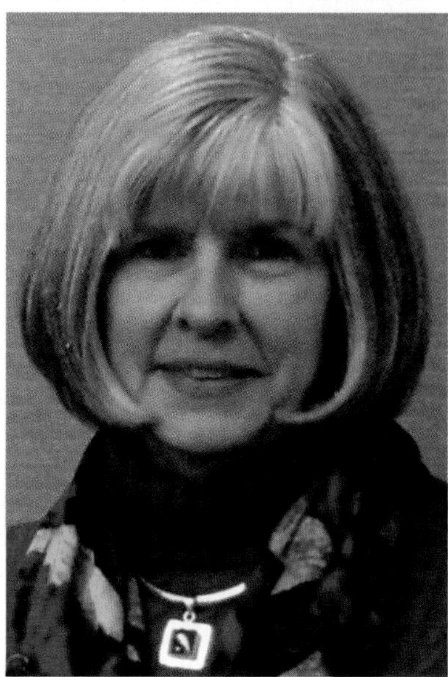

Kathryn Rhodes Alden is Clinical Associate Professor, University of North Carolina at Chapel Hill School of Nursing. She received a BSN from the University of North Carolina at Charlotte, an MSN from the University of North Carolina at Chapel Hill, and a doctorate in adult education from North Carolina State University.

Dr. Alden has extensive experience as a nursing educator, having served on the faculty at the University of North Carolina at Charlotte and the University of North Carolina at Chapel Hill. Dr. Alden has clinical experience in pediatrics, pediatric intensive care, and neonatal intensive care. She is also experienced in home health care, having provided nursing care to pediatric and obstetric clients. She has worked as a nursing administrator and coordinator of quality improvement. As a certified lactation consultant, Dr. Alden has provided inpatient and outpatient care for breastfeeding mothers and infants and she has taught prenatal breastfeeding classes to expectant parents. She has taught continuing education courses on breastfeeding throughout North Carolina.

For the past 25 years as an educator for baccalaureate nursing students at UNC-Chapel Hill School of Nursing, Dr. Alden has taught in maternal-newborn nursing courses, providing both classroom and clinical instruction. Dr. Alden coordinates and leads the academic counseling program, providing assistance to students and to faculty. She is actively involved in the leadership of the undergraduate nursing program as member and former chair of the Baccalaureate Executive Committee.

She has received numerous awards for excellence in nursing education at UNC, being recognized for clinical and classroom teaching expertise as well as for academic counseling. Dr. Alden was selected for the Great 100 Nurses in North Carolina in 2008.

Dr. Alden was an early adopter of high-fidelity simulation and has been instrumental in the use of this instructional strategy at UNC-Chapel Hill School of Nursing. She is actively involved in interprofessional collaboration with faculty from the UNC schools of Medicine and Pharmacy to offer obstetric and neonatal simulation learning activities to undergraduate nursing students, pharmacy students, and medical students in obstetrics and pediatrics. She has created numerous simulation scenarios including obstetric simulation cases for Elsevier. She has coauthored chapters on high-fidelity simulation and patient safety in publications by the Agency for Healthcare Research and Quality (AHRQ) and the NLN. Dr. Alden is an active member of AWHONN and the International Nursing Association for Clinical Simulation and Learning (INACSL).

Dr. Alden has authored numerous chapters on a variety of topics in maternity texts for Elsevier. She is associate editor for *Maternal Child Nursing Care* (5th edition) and *Maternity Nursing* (8th edition).

ELLEN F. OLSHANSKY

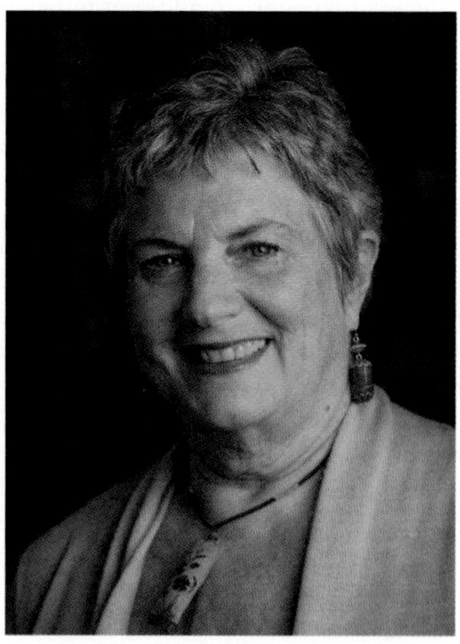

Ellen F. Olshansky is Professor in the Program in Nursing Science at the University of California, Irvine, and served as its founding director from 2007 to 2014. Under her leadership UC-Irvine initiated the BSN program, followed by the approval and initiation of both the MS and PhD degrees in nursing science. She is the founder of the UCI Nursing Science Center for the Advancement of Women's Health.

Dr. Olshansky earned a BA in Social Work from the University of California, Berkeley, and a BS, MS, and PhD from the University of California, San Francisco School of Nursing. She was a faculty member at the schools of nursing at the Oregon Health Sciences University, University of Washington, Duquesne University, and the University of Pittsburgh before taking her current position at the UC-Irvine. She is a fellow in the American Academy of Nursing, served as co-chair of its Expert Panel on Women's Health, and is a member of its Board of Directors. She is also a fellow in the Western Academy of Nursing.

Dr. Olshansky also serves as director of the Community Engagement Unit of the UC-Irvine Institute for Clinical and Translational Science, funded by a National Institutes of Health (NIH) Clinical Translational Science Award. Through this position she engages community members in community-based participatory research, encouraging collaborative research between university faculty and community organizations. She has expertise in qualitative research and community-based participatory research.

Dr. Olshansky is a women's health nurse practitioner, certified through the National Certification Corporation (WHNP-BC). Her research has focused on women's health across the life span, with a focus on reproductive health. Dr. Olshansky recently became a certified Integrative Nurse Wellness Coach, having completed the Integrative Nurse Coach Certification Program through the International Nurse Coach Association and successfully completing the certification exam through the American Holistic Nurses Credentialing Corporation (NC-BC). She is focused on working with people within their own communities to promote and maintain wellness. She is one of the founders of the Orange County Women's Health Project, which works in collaboration with the UCI Nursing Science Center for the Advancement of Women's Health. The purpose is to promote women's health and wellness in Orange County, California, including holding annual women's health policy summits.

She recently completed a 10-year term as editor of the *Journal of Professional Nursing,* the official journal of the American Association of Colleges of Nursing. She has published extensively in numerous nursing and other health-related journals as well as authored many book chapters and editorials.

CONTRIBUTORS

Jennifer T. Alderman, MSN, RNC-OB, CNL
Clinical Assistant Professor/Academic Counselor
School of Nursing
The University of North Carolina at Chapel Hill
Chapel Hill, North Carolina

Deborah Bambini, PhD, WHNP-BC, CNE, CHSE
Associate Professor
Kirkhof College of Nursing
Grand Valley State University
Grand Rapids, Michigan

Beth Perry Black, PhD, RN
Assistant Professor
School of Nursing
University of North Carolina at Chapel Hill
Chapel Hill, North Carolina

Dusty Dix, RN, MSN
Clinical Assistant Professor
School of Nursing
University of North Carolina at Chapel Hill
Chapel Hill, North Carolina

Noreen Esposito, EdD, WHNP-BC, PMHNP-BC, FNP-BC
Clinical Associate Professor
School of Nursing
University of North Carolina at Chapel Hill
Chapel Hill, North Carolina

Lisa L. Ferguson, DNP, RN, WHNP-BC
Adjunct Faculty
College of Nursing
Texas Woman's University
Dallas, Texas

Debbie Fraser, MN, RNC-NIC
Associate Professor
Director Nurse Practitioner Program
Faculty of Health Disciplines
Athabasca University;
Advanced Practice Nurse
NICU St. Boniface Hospital
Winnipeg, Manitoba

Pat Mahaffee Gingrich, MSN, WHNP-BC
Clinical Assistant Professor
School of Nursing
University of North Carolina at Chapel Hill
Chapel Hill, North Carolina

Jo M. Kendrick, WHNP- BC, CDE
Coordinator Perinatal Diabetes Program
Division of Maternal-Fetal Medicine
Department of Obstetrics and Gynecology
University of Tennessee Medical Center
Knoxville, Tennessee

Rhonda K. Lanning, RN, MSN, CNM, IBCLC
Clinical Assistant Professor
School of Nursing
University of North Carolina at Chapel Hill;
Program Coordinator
UNC Volunteer Doula Service
North Carolina Women's Hospital
Chapel Hill, North Carolina

Denise G. Link, PhD, WHNP-BC, CNE, FAAN, FAANP
Clinical Associate Professor
College of Nursing & Health Innovation
Arizona State University
Phoenix, Arizona

Peggy Mancuso, PhD, RN, CNM, CNE
Professor
College of Nursing
Texas Woman's University,
Dallas, Texas

Raquel Martinez-Campos, MSN, RN, FNP, WHNP-BC
Clinical Instructor
University of California-Irvine
Program in Nursing Science
Irvine, California

Diana McCarty, RNC-MNN, MSN
Teaching Assistant Professor
School of Nursing
West Virginia University
Morgantown, West Virginia

Susan A. McKenney, MSN, APRN, BC, OCN
Clinical Associate Professor
Department of Surgery;
Adjunct Associate Professor
School of Nursing
University of North Carolina at Chapel Hill
Chapel Hill, North Carolina

Kristen S. Montgomery, PhD, RN, SNM
Adjunct Faculty
School of Nursing & Health Sciences
Simmons College
Boston, Massachusetts

Mary Courtney Moore, RN, RD, PhD
Research Professor
Department of Molecular Physiology & Biophysics
Vanderbilt University School of Medicine
Nashville, Tennessee

Marcia Van Riper, PhD, RN, FAAN
Professor
School of Nursing;
Chair
Family Health Division
University of North Carolina at Chapel Hill
Chapel Hill, North Carolina

Jan Sherman, RN, NNP-BC, PhD
Associate Teaching Professor
Sinclair School of Nursing
University of Missouri-Columbia;
Adjunct Associate Professor
Department of Child Health
School of Medicine
University of Missouri-Columbia
Columbia, Missouri

Janet Tucker, MSN, RNC-OB
Program Director
Fetal Center
Le Bonheur Children's Hospital
Memphis, Tennessee

Deborah S. Walker, DNSc, CNM, WHNP-BC, FACNM, FAAN
Associate Professor
College of Nursing;
Graduate Director
Nurse-Midwife Concentration
Wayne State University
Detroit, Michigan

Cheryl R. Zauderer, PhD, CNM, NPP, IBCLC
Assistant Professor
Department of Nursing
New York Institute of Technology
New York, New York

Evolve Resources

NCLEX®-Style Review Questions

Daryle Wane, PhD, ARNP-BC
Professor of Nursing
Pasco-Hernando Community College
New Port Richey, Florida

PowerPoint Presentations

Meredith Milowski, RNC, MSN, CNM
Clinical Assistant Professor
College of Nursing and Health Innovation
Arizona State University
Phoenix, Arizona

TEACH for Nurses

Melanie Cole, MA
Freelance Editor
Community Treatment, Inc.
University of Missouri–St. Louis
St. Louis, Missouri

Test Bank

Barbara Pascoe, RN, BA, MA
Director
The Family Place
Concord Hospital
Concord, New Hampshire

REVIEWERS

Karen M. Bennett Gural, RN, MS
Faculty
College of Nursing
Crouse Hospital
Syracuse, New York

Kathleen Cerbin, MSN, RN
Lecturer
School of Nursing
Indiana University Northwest
Gary, Indiana

Robin Webb Corbett, PhD, RN
Associate Professor
College of Nursing
East Carolina University
Greenville, North Carolina

Janie D. Corbitt, RN, MLS
Instructor
Health Technology Core
Central Georgia Technical College
Milledgeville, Georgia

Amber Essman, MSN, RN, CNE
Assistant Professor
Chamberlain College of Nursing
Columbus, Ohio

Sara B. Forbus, RN, MSN, WHNP
Faculty
School of Nursing
Old Dominion University
Norfolk, Virginia

Margie Francisco, MSN, RN
Professor;
Second-Year Program Coordinator
Nursing
Illinois Valley Community College
Oglesby, Illinois

Marcella Gowan, MPH, CNM, NP, BSN
Assistant Professor
School of Nursing
George Fox University
Newberg, Oregon

Johnnetta Phillips Kelly, PhD, RN, CNE, FNP-BC
Associate Professor
Carr College of Nursing
Harding University
Searcy, Arkansas

Carolyn McCune, RN, MSN, CRNP, CEN
LPN Director
Columbiana County Career and Technical Center
Lisbon, Ohio

Meredith Milowski, BSN, MSN, RNC-OB, CNM
Clinical Assistant Professor
College of Nursing and Health Innovation
Arizona State University
Phoenix, Arizona

Cecile Oliver, RNC-OB/MNN, C-FM, MSN, CNS
Childbearing Health Lecture Leader
College of Nursing
Washington State University
Spokane, Washington

Janet Pinkelman, RNC, MSN
Professor
School of Nursing and Health Professions
Owens Community College
Toledo, Ohio

Joy A. Price, MSN, RN, CNE
Instructor
Associate Degree Nursing
Northeast Mississippi Community College
Booneville, Mississippi

Angela Schooley, RN, MSN
Assistant Professor
Department of Nursing
Purdue University North Central
Westville, Indiana

Jan Selliken, ND, RN
Associate Professor
School of Nursing
Linfield College
Portland, Oregon

Julie Symes, RN, MN, IBCLC
Instructor
Department of Nursing
University of South Dakota
Rapid City, South Dakota

Paulina Van, PhD, RN, CNE
Professor & Chair
Department of Nursing & Health Sciences
California State University, East Bay
Hayward, California

Daryle Wane, PhD, ARNP, FNP-BC
Professor of Nursing
Adult II/III Course Coordinator
Pasco-Hernando Community College
New Port Richey, Florida

Linda D. Ward, PhD, ARNP
Assistant Professor
College of Nursing
Washington State University
Spokane, Washington

Rebecca Weatherly, MSN, RN
Nursing Instructor and Course Coordinator
Maternal Newborn Nursing
College of Southern Nevada
Las Vegas, Nevada

Nancee Wozney, PhD, RN
Dean of Nursing/Allied Health;
Director of Nursing
Southeast Technical College
Winona, Minnesota

Evolve Resources

Donna Wilsker, MSN, RN
Assistant Professor
Dishman Department of Nursing
Lamar University
Beaumont, Texas

PREFACE

Women's health care encompasses reproductive health care and the unique physical, psychologic, and social needs of women throughout their life span. The specialties of women's health and maternity nursing offer challenges and opportunities. Nurses are challenged to assimilate knowledge and develop the technical and critical thinking skills needed to be reflective practitioners. Each woman, with her individual needs that must be identified and met, presents a challenge. However, the opportunities are sufficiently extraordinary to make this one of the most fulfilling specialties of nursing practice.

The goal of nursing education is to prepare today's students to meet the challenges of tomorrow. This preparation must extend beyond mastery of facts and skills. Nurses must be able to provide safe, quality, client-centered care through the combination of clinical reasoning skills, technical competence, and compassionate caring. They must address the physiologic as well as the psychosocial needs of their clients. They must look beyond the condition and see the woman as an individual with distinctive needs. Yet they must consider her needs in the context of family-centered care, realizing and acknowledging the influence and involvement of family members and significant others. Above all, nurses must strive to improve practice on the basis of sound evidence-based information. In a time of dwindling financial resources for health care, nurses can use evidence-based practice to produce measurable outcomes that can validate their unique and necessary role in the health care delivery system.

Maternity & Women's Health Care was designed to provide students with accurate and up-to-date information so that they can develop the knowledge and skills needed to become clinically competent, to think critically, and to attain the necessary sensitivity to become caring nurses. *Maternity & Women's Health Care* has been a leading maternity nursing text since it was first published in 1977. We are proud of the continued support this text has received. With this eleventh edition we have a responsibility to continue this leading tradition.

This edition has been revised and refined in response to comments and suggestions from educators, clinicians, and students. It includes the most accurate, current, and clinically relevant information available. We have had the assistance of expert faculty, nurse clinicians, and specialists from other health disciplines who authored, reviewed, and revised the text. Many exciting updates and additions will be noted throughout the book; they demonstrate the various dimensions of women's health care and areas of rapid and complex changes such as genetics, fetal assessment, and alternative therapies. However, we have retained the underlying philosophy that has been the strength of previous editions: our belief that pregnancy and childbirth and developmental changes in a woman's life are natural processes. We have also retained a base in physiology and a strong, integrated focus on the family and on evidence-based practice.

The text is also used as a reference for the practicing nurse. The most recent recommendations based on evidence from research and clinical experts have been included from professional organizations such as the Association of Women's Health, Obstetric and Neonatal Nurses; the National Association of Neonatal Nurses; the American College of Obstetricians and Gynecologists; the American Academy of Pediatrics; the American Diabetes Association; the Centers for Disease Control and Prevention; and the U.S. Preventive Health Services Task Force. The text can be used to prepare for certification courses and for review in graduate programs of study. The text and its electronic resources would be an excellent reference on the nursing unit.

Approach

Professional nursing practice continues to evolve and adapt to society's changing health priorities. The ever-changing health care delivery system offers new opportunities for nurses to alter the practice of maternity and women's health nursing and to improve the way care is given. Consumers of maternity and women's health care vary in age, ethnicity, culture, language, social status, marital status, sexual preference, and family configurations. They seek care from obstetricians, gynecologists, family practice physicians, nurse-midwives, nurse practitioners, nurses, and other health care providers in a variety of health care settings, including the home. Increasingly, many are self-treating, accessing web-based information, and using a variety of alternative and complementary therapies.

Nursing education must reflect these changes. Clinical education must be planned to offer students a variety of maternity and women's health care experiences in settings that include hospitals and birth centers, the home health setting, clinics and private physician offices, shelters for the homeless or women in need of protection, in prisons, and in other community-based settings. Advances in nursing education include the increased use of simulation learning activities. Simulation laboratories have emerged in schools of nursing and in health care institutions to provide students and staff with opportunities to engage in care of clients in focused, challenging situations while in the safety of a controlled environment. Simulation experiences offer students in maternity and women's health courses opportunities that are otherwise unavailable due to shrinking opportunities for clinical placements, decreased clinical time, and increased numbers of students in clinical rotations.

Today's nursing students are challenged to learn more than ever and often in less time than their predecessors. Students are diverse. They may be new high school graduates, college students, or older adults with families. They may be male or female. They may have college degrees in other fields and be interested in changing careers. They may represent various cultures; English may not be their first language. Students may be enrolled in associate degree or diploma programs, in baccalaureate or accelerated baccalaureate nursing programs, or in entry level master's programs. This eleventh edition, with its accompanying teaching and learning package, has been revised to meet these changing needs. Each chapter has been reviewed by a specialist to improve readability and comprehension, especially by a diverse student population. Focused content is presented in a clearly written and easily read manner while retaining the comprehensiveness of previous editions. The text can be used by all levels of nursing education, and in courses of varying lengths.

Health care today emphasizes *wellness* and *health promotion.* This focus is an integral part of our philosophy. Likewise the developmental changes a woman experiences throughout her life are considered natural and normal. In women's health care, the goal is promotion of wellness for the woman through knowledge of her body and its normal functioning throughout her life span, while developing an awareness of conditions that require professional intervention. The unit on women's health care emphasizes the wellness aspect of care but also includes information about common gynecologic problems as well as breast and gynecologic cancers. This unit has been placed before the units on pregnancy because many of the aspects of assessment and care can be applied to later chapters.

Pregnancy and birth are also part of a natural developmental process. We believe that students need to thoroughly understand and recognize the normal processes before they can identify complications and comprehend their implications for care. We present the entire normal childbearing cycle before discussing potential complications.

In this edition of *Maternity & Women's Health Care,* there is expanded and enhanced content related to the risks associated with obesity as it relates to women's health, pregnancy, and neonatal outcomes. In relevant chapters throughout the book, this content is addressed, based on the most current evidence-based information from the medical and nursing literature.

Readers will note that throughout the text, the authors use different terms to describe various racial and ethnic groups. Whenever statistical data are described, the terms in the reference are used, for instance, non-Hispanic black, non-Hispanic white, and Hispanic. When discussing individual clients or population groups and their health beliefs, the more commonly used terms are used, for instance, Latina or Hispanic, Caucasian, African-American, and Asian.

Features

The eleventh edition features a contemporary design and spacious presentation. Students will find that the logical, easy-to-follow headings and attractive full-color design highlight important content and increase visual appeal. More than 450 color photographs (many of them new) and drawings throughout the text illustrate important concepts and techniques to further enhance comprehension. Each chapter begins with a list of *Learning Objectives* designed to focus students' attention on the important content to be mastered. *Key Terms* that alert students to new vocabulary are in blue, defined within the chapter, and included in a glossary at the end of the book. Each chapter ends with *Key Points* that summarize important content. ***Community Activity*** exercises are included in most chapters to provide opportunities for students to increase their knowledge of community resources. ***Clinical Reasoning*** case studies are integrated to guide students in applying their knowledge and increasing their ability to think and reflect critically about maternity and women's health care issues. ***References*** have been updated significantly, with most citations being less than 5 years old and all chapters having citations within 1 year of publication. An expanded Table of Contents and Index make it easier for readers to locate exactly the information they are seeking. More of the additional outstanding features follow:

- ***Care Management*** is used as the consistent framework throughout nursing care chapters to discuss assessment, medical and surgical management, and more specifically, the nursing care related to each topic.
- ***Nursing Care Plans*** help students apply the nursing process in the clinical setting and use NANDA-approved nursing diagnoses, describe expected outcomes for client care, provide rationales for interventions, and include evaluation of care.
- ***Teaching for Self-Management*** boxes emphasize guidelines for the client to practice self-care and provide information to help students transfer learning from the hospital to the home setting.
- ***Emergency*** boxes alert students to the signs and symptoms of various emergency situations and provide interventions for immediate implementation.
- ***Signs of Potential Complications*** boxes alert students to signs and symptoms of potential problems and are included in chapters that cover uncomplicated pregnancy and birth.
- ***Nursing Alert*** and ***Safety Alert*** boxes and new ***Medication Alert*** boxes highlight critical information.
- ***Evidence-Based Practice*** is incorporated throughout in new boxes that integrate findings from several studies on selected clinical practices and changing practice; Quality and Safety Education for Nursing (QSEN) competencies are illustrated in these boxes. In addition, research findings summarized in *The Cochrane Pregnancy and Childbirth Database* and other resources for evidence-based practices that confirm effective practices or identify practices that have unknown, ineffective, or harmful effects are integrated throughout the text.
- ***Cultural Considerations*** boxes describe beliefs and practices about pregnancy, childbirth, parenting, and women's health concerns and the importance of understanding cultural variations when providing care.
- ***Legal Tips*** are integrated throughout to provide students with relevant information to deal with these important areas in the context of maternity and women's health nursing.
- ***Medication Guide*** boxes include key information about medications used in maternity and women's health care, including their indications, adverse effects, and nursing considerations.

Organization

The eleventh edition of *Maternity & Women's Health Care* comprises eight units organized to enhance understanding and learning and to facilitate easy retrieval of information.

Unit One, Introduction to *Maternity & Women's Health Care,* begins with an overview of contemporary issues in maternity and women's health nursing practice. Chapter 1 includes a section on historic milestones in maternity, women's health, and neonatal care and provides an overview of important therapies that can be used instead of or in addition to traditional techniques used in maternity and women's health care. Chapter

2 addresses the community as a unit of care, incorporating family theory, cultural aspects of care, and home care in relation to maternity and women's health nursing. Chapter 3 provides essential discussion about genetics in relation to maternity and women's health care.

Unit Two, Women's Health, is a thoroughly revised unit on women's health. Eight chapters discuss health promotion, screening, and physical assessment, and then present common reproductive concerns. The chapter on assessment and health promotion incorporates normal anatomy and physiology of the female reproductive system and integrates health promotion for common women's health problems. There are separate chapters on reproductive problems and concerns, sexually transmitted infections and other infections, contraception and abortion, infertility, violence, problems of the breast, and structural disorders and neoplasms of the female reproductive system.

Unit Three, Pregnancy, describes nursing care of the woman and her family from conception through preparation for birth. Nursing care during pregnancy includes both physiologic and psychologic aspects of care, as well as information on preparation for birth. A separate chapter on maternal and fetal nutrition emphasizes the important aspects of care, highlights cultural variations in diet, and stresses the importance of early recognition and management of nutritional problems.

Unit Four, Childbirth, focuses on collaborative care among physicians, nurse-midwives, nurses, and women and their families during the processes of labor and birth. Separate chapters deal with the nurse's role in maximizing comfort during labor and birth, and fetal monitoring, both of which have been updated significantly. All four chapters familiarize students with current childbirth practices and focus on evidence-based interventions to support and educate the woman and her family.

Unit Five, Postpartum, deals with a time of profound change for the entire family. Physiologic changes and nursing care based on the changes are addressed. The mother requires both physical and emotional support as she adjusts to her new role. The chapter on transition to parenthood discusses family dynamics in response to the birth of a child and describes ways nurses can facilitate parent-infant adjustment. Anticipatory guidance for the first few weeks at home and home follow-up care are addressed.

Unit Six, The Newborn, has been updated and addresses physiologic adaptations of the newborn and assessment and care of the newborn. Information on the nutritional needs of the newborn and nursing care associated with breastfeeding and formula feeding are highlighted in a separate chapter.

Unit Seven, Complications of Pregnancy, discusses conditions that place the woman, fetus, infant, and family at risk. This unit has been revised and updated and includes a chapter on assessment of the high risk pregnancy and eight other chapters covering specific pregnancy complications including hypertensive disorders, antepartal hemorrhagic disorders, endocrine and metabolic problems, medical-surgical problems, mental health problems and substance abuse, labor and birth complications, and postpartum complications. Care management focuses on achieving the best possible outcomes, as well as supporting the woman and family when expectations are not met.

Unit Eight, Newborn Complications, describes the nursing care for high risk newborns, emphasizing the care of the preterm infant. There is enhanced content on care of late preterm infants in this edition. It addresses the most common acquired conditions of the neonate as well as hematologic disorders and congenital anomalies. All chapters have been revised and updated. A separate chapter on loss and grief discusses care of the family experiencing a fetal or neonatal loss.

Teaching/Learning Package

Evolve, for Students: Evolve is an innovative website that provides a wealth of content, resources, and state-of-the-art information on maternity nursing. Learning resources for students include Case Studies, Content Updates, Printable Key Points, Nursing Skills, and NCLEX-Style Review Questions.

Simulation Learning System (SLS): The SLS is an online toolkit that helps instructors and facilitators effectively incorporate medium- to high-fidelity simulation into their nursing curriculum. Detailed patient scenarios promote and enhance the clinical decision-making skills of students at all levels. The SLS provides detailed instructions for preparation and implementation of the simulation experience, debriefing questions that encourage critical thinking, and learning resources to reinforce student comprehension. Each scenario in the SLS complements the textbook content and helps bridge the gap between lectures and clinical practice. The SLS provides the perfect environment for students to practice what they are learning in the text for a true-to-life, hands-on learning experience.

Study Guide: This comprehensive and challenging study aid presents a variety of questions to enhance learning of key concepts and content from the text. Multiple-choice and matching questions are included, as well as Critical Thinking Case Studies. Answers for all questions are included at the back of the study guide.

Virtual Clinical Excursions: Virtual Hospital and Workbook Companion: A Virtual Hospital and workbook package has been developed as a clinical experience to expand student opportunities for critical thinking. This package guides the student through a virtual clinical environment and helps the user apply textbook content to virtual clients in that environment. Case studies are presented that allow students to use this textbook as a reference to assess, diagnose, plan, implement, and evaluate "real" clients using clinical scenarios. The state-of-the-art technologies reflected in this virtual hospital demonstrate cutting-edge learning opportunities for students and facilitate knowledge retention of the information found in the textbook. The clinical simulations and workbook represent the next generation of research-based learning tools that promote critical thinking and meaningful learning.

Evolve, for Instructors includes these teaching resources:

- *Test Bank in ExamView format* contains more than 1000 NCLEX-style test items, including alternate format questions. An answer key with page references to the text, rationales, and NCLEX-style coding is included.
- *TEACH for Nurses* includes teaching strategies; in-class case studies; and links to animations, nursing skills, and nursing curriculum standards such as QSEN, concepts, and BSN Essentials.
- *Image Collection,* containing more than 700 full-color illustrations and photographs from the text, helps instructors develop presentations and explain key concepts.

- *PowerPoint slides,* with lecture notes for each chapter of the text, assist in presenting materials in the classroom. *Case Studies* and *Audience Response Questions* for i-clicker are included.
- A *Curriculum Guide* that includes a proposed class schedule and reading assignments for courses of varying lengths is provided. This gives educators suggestions for using the text in the most essential manner or in a more comprehensive way.

ACKNOWLEDGMENTS

The eleventh edition of *Maternity & Women's Health Care* would not have been possible without the contributions of many people. First, we want to thank the many nurse educators, clinicians, and nursing students in the United States, Canada, Australia, and Taiwan whose comments and suggestions about the manuscript led to this collaborative effort by an outstanding group of contributors. A special thanks goes to these people, many of whom are new to this edition, whose names appear in the list of Contributors. Their expertise and knowledge of current clinical practice and research have added to the relevancy and accuracy of the materials presented. We also thank Pat Gingrich for contributing to the Evidence-Based Practice boxes and Ed Lowdermilk for his assistance with Medication Guides and verification of other medication information. We are also appreciative of the critiques given by the reviewers, especially their attention to validating the accuracy of content and their challenge to present content differently and to include new ideas. These combined efforts have resulted in a revision that incorporates the most recent research and current information about the practice of maternity and women's health care.

We offer thanks for shared expertise and photographs to the staff of University of North Carolina Women's Hospital; University of North Carolina School of Nursing; Nurses Certificate Program in Interactive Imagery; and Polly Perez, Cutting Edge Press.

We also would like to thank the following photographers: Cheryl Briggs, RNC, Annapolis, MD; Michael S. Clement, MD, Mesa, AZ; Julie Perry Nelson, Loveland, CO; and Marjorie Pyle, RNC, Lifecircle, Costa Mesa, CA.

Thanks to the following individuals who allowed us to use their beautiful photos: Jennifer and Travis Alderman, Durham, NC; Freida Belding, Bird City, KS; Jodi Brackett, Phoenix, AZ; David A. Clarke, Philadelphia, PA; Thomas and Christie Coghill, Clayton, NC; Christina and Eva Gardner, Marion, AR; Kara and Casey George, Peoria, AZ; Patricia Hess, San Francisco, CA; Sharon Johnson, Petaluma, CA; Sara Kossuth, Los Angeles, CA; Mahesh Kotwal, MD, Phoenix, AZ; Paul Vincent Kuntz, Houston, TX; Wendy and Marwood Larson-Harris, Roanoke, VA; Lauren and Brian LiVecchi, Raleigh, NC; Ed Lowdermilk, Chapel Hill, NC; Norman L. Meyer, MD, PhD, Memphis, TN; Kim Molloy, Knoxville, IA; Amanda Politte, St. Louis, MO; Chris Rozales, San Francisco, CA; H. Gil Rushton, MD, Washington, DC; Brian and Mayannyn Sallee, Minot, ND; Shari Rivera Sharpe, Chapel Hill, NC; Margaret Spann, New Johnsonville, TN; Edward S. Tank, MD, Portland, OR; Danielle L. Tate, MD, Memphis, TN; Amy and Ken Turner, Cary, NC; Rebekah Vogel, Fort Collins, CO; Roni Wernik, Palo Alto, CA; and Randi and Jacob Wills, Clayton, NC.

Special words of gratitude are extended to Laurie Gower, Content Development Manager; Heather Bays, Senior Content Development Specialist; Jeff Patterson, Publishing Services Manager; Jeanne Genz, Senior Project Manager; and Ashley Miner, Book Designer, for their encouragement, inspiration, and assistance in preparing and producing this text. These talented and hardworking people helped change our manuscript into a beautiful book by editing the manuscript, designing an attractive format for our special features, and overseeing the production of the book from start to finish.

Deitra Leonard Lowdermilk
Shannon E. Perry
Kitty Cashion
Kathryn Rhodes Alden

CONTENTS

UNIT ONE Introduction To Maternity & Women's Health Care

UNIT FIVE Postpartum

UNIT EIGHT Newborn Complications

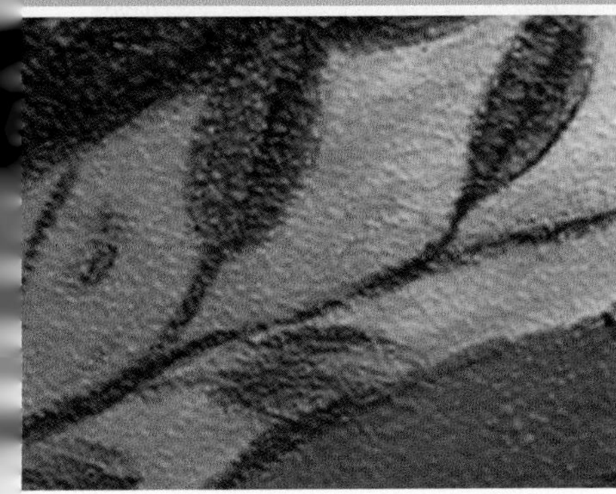

CHAPTER 1

21st Century Maternity and Women's Health Nursing

Shannon E. Perry

http://evolve.elsevier.com/Lowdermilk/MWHC/

LEARNING OBJECTIVES

- Describe the scope of maternity and women's health nursing.
- Evaluate contemporary issues and trends in maternity and women's health care.
- Examine social concerns in maternity nursing and women's health care.
- Integrate evidenced-based practice into care plans.
- Explain risk management and standards of practice in the delivery of nursing care.
- Discuss legal and ethical issues in perinatal nursing.
- Examine *Healthy People 2020* goals related to maternal and infant care.

Maternity nursing encompasses care of childbearing women and their families through all stages of pregnancy and childbirth and the first 4 weeks after birth. Throughout the prenatal period, nurses, nurse practitioners, and nurse-midwives provide care for women in clinics and physicians' offices and teach classes to help families prepare for childbirth. Nurses care for childbearing families during labor and birth in hospitals, in birthing centers (e.g., www.birthcenters.org), and in the home. Nurses with special training may provide intensive care for high risk neonates in special care units and for high risk mothers in antepartum units, in critical care obstetric units, or in the home. Maternity nurses teach about pregnancy; the process of labor, birth, and recovery; and parenting skills. They provide continuity of care throughout the childbearing cycle.

Women's health care focuses on the physical, psychologic, and social needs of women throughout their lives. In the care of women, their overall experience is emphasized: general physical and psychologic well-being, childbearing functions, and diseases. Women's health nurses specialize in and investigate conditions unique to women (such as reproductive malignancies and menopause) and sociocultural and occupational factors that are related to women's health problems (such as poverty, rape, incest, family violence, and human trafficking). They also provide care for women and their families during the childbearing cycle.

Nurses caring for women have helped make the health care system more responsive to women's needs. They have been critically important in developing strategies to improve the well-being of women and their infants and have led the efforts to implement clinical practice guidelines and to practice using an evidence-based approach. Through professional associations, nurses have a voice in setting standards and in influencing health policy by actively participating in the education of the public and of state and federal legislators (e.g., www.nursingworld.org; www.cannurses.ca; www.awhonn.org; www.capwhn.ca; www.nann.org; www.acnm.org). Some nurses hold elective office and influence policy directly. For example, Mary Wakefield, a nurse, is the administrator of the Health Resources and Services Administration (HRSA), the agency that oversees approximately 7000 community clinics that serve low-income and uninsured people.

ADVANCES IN THE CARE OF WOMEN AND INFANTS

Although tremendous advances have taken place in the care of mothers and their infants during the past 150 years (Box 1-1), serious problems exist in the United States related to the health and health care of mothers and infants. Lack of access to prepregnancy and pregnancy-related care for all women and the lack of reproductive health services for adolescents are major concerns. Sexually transmitted infections continue to affect reproduction adversely.

Racial and ethnic diversity is increasing within North America. It is estimated that by the year 2050, 46.6% of the population will be European-American, 27% Hispanic, 13% African-American, 7.7% Asian-American, 0.72% American Indians and Alaska Natives, and 0.22% native Hawaiian and other Pacific Islanders (U.S. Census Bureau, 2012). Significant disparity exists in health outcomes among people of various racial and ethnic groups despite the great strides in public health made by the United States.

In addition, people may have lifestyles, health needs, and health care preferences related to their ethnic or cultural backgrounds.

BOX 1-1 Historic Overview of Milestones in the Care of Mothers and Infants in the Western World from 1847

1847—James Young Simpson in Edinburgh, Scotland, used ether for an internal podalic version and birth; the first reported use of obstetric anesthesia
1861—Ignaz Semmelweis wrote *The Cause, Concept and Prophylaxis of Childbed Fever*
1906—First U.S. program for prenatal nursing care established
1908—Childbirth classes started by the American Red Cross
1908—Archibald Garrod pioneered work on inborn errors of metabolism
1909—First White House Conference on Children convened
1911—First milk bank in the United States established in Boston
1912—U.S. Children's Bureau established
1915—Radical mastectomy determined to be effective treatment for breast cancer
1916—Margaret Sanger established first American birth control clinic in Brooklyn, New York
1918—Condoms became legal in the United States
1923—First U.S. hospital center for premature infant care established at Sarah Morris Hospital in Chicago, Illinois
1929—The modern tampon (with an applicator) invented and patented
1933—Sodium pentothal used as anesthesia for childbirth; *Natural Childbirth* published by Grantly Dick-Read
1934—Dionne quintuplets born in Ontario, Canada, and survive partly due to donated breast milk
1935—Sulfonamides introduced as cure for puerperal fever
1941—Penicillin used as a treatment for infection
1941—Papanicolaou (Pap) tests introduced
1942—Premarin approved by the U.S. Food and Drug Administration (FDA) as treatment for menopausal symptoms
1953—Virginia Apgar, an anesthesiologist, published Apgar scoring system of neonatal assessment
1956—Oxygen determined to cause retrolental fibroplasia (now known as retinopathy of prematurity)
1958—Edward Hon reported on the recording of the fetal electrocardiogram (ECG) from the maternal abdomen (first commercial electronic fetal monitor produced in the late 1960s)
1958—Ian Donald, a Glasgow physician, was first to report clinical use of ultrasound to examine the fetus
1959—*Thank You, Dr. Lamaze* published by Marjorie Karmel
1959—Cytologic studies demonstrated that Down syndrome is associated with a particular form of nondisjunction now known as trisomy 21
1960—American Society for Psychoprophylaxis in Obstetrics (ASPO/Lamaze) formed
1960—International Childbirth Education Association founded
1960—Birth control pill introduced in the United States
1962—Thalidomide found to cause birth defects
1963—Title V of the Social Security Act amended to include comprehensive maternity and infant care for women who were low income and high risk
1965—Supreme Court ruled that married people have the right to use birth control
1967—Rh_0(D) immune globulin produced for treatment of Rh incompatibility
1967—Reva Rubin published article on Maternal Role Attainment
1968—Rubella vaccine became available
1969—Nurses Association of the American College of Obstetricians and Gynecologists (NAACOG) founded; renamed Association of Women's Health, Obstetric and Neonatal Nurses (AWHONN) and incorporated as a 501(c)3 organization in 1993
1969—Mammogram became available
1972—Special Supplemental Nutrition Program for Women, Infants, and Children (WIC) started
1973—Abortion legalized in United States
1974—First standards for obstetric, gynecologic, and neonatal nursing published by NAACOG
1975—The Pregnant Patient's Bill of Rights published by the International Childbirth Education Association
1976—First home pregnancy kits approved by FDA
1978—Louise Brown, first test-tube baby, born
1987—Safe Motherhood initiative launched by World Health Organization and other international agencies
1991—Society for Advancement of Women's Health Research founded
1992—USPHS recommended that pregnant women take folic acid to prevent neural tube defects
1992—Office of Research on Women's Health authorized by U.S. Congress
1993—Female condom approved by FDA
1993—Human embryos cloned at George Washington University
1993—Family and Medical Leave Act enacted
1994—DNA sequences of BRCA1 and BRCA2 identified
1994—Zidovudine guidelines to reduce mother-to-fetus transmission of HIV published
1996—FDA mandated folic acid fortification in all breads and grains sold in United States
1998—Newborns' and Mothers' Health Act went into effect
1998—COGNN becomes AWHONN Canada
1999—First emergency contraception pill for pregnancy prevention (Plan B) in women who had unprotected sex approved by FDA
2000—Working draft of sequence and analysis of human genome completed
2006—HPV vaccine available
2010—Centenary of the death of Florence Nightingale
2010—Patient Protection and Affordable Care Act signed into law by President Obama
2011—AWHONN Canada becomes the Canadian Association of Perinatal and Women's Health Nurses (CAPWHN)
2012—U.S. Supreme Court upheld individual mandate but not the Medicaid expansion provisions of the Patient Protection and Affordable Care Act
2012—Scientists reported findings of the ENCODE (Encyclopedia of DNA Elements) project showing that 80% of the human genome is active

HIV, Human immunodeficiency virus; *HPV,* human papillomavirus.

They may have dietary preferences and health practices that are not understood by caregivers. This presents a challenge for health care providers to provide culturally sensitive care.

The majority of nurses are Caucasian, about 78%, with 10.4% black and 5.1% Hispanic (AFL-CIO Department of Professional Employees, 2012). To meet the health care needs of a culturally diverse society, there must be increasing diversity of the nursing workforce.

EFFORTS TO REDUCE HEALTH DISPARITIES

Significant disparities in morbidity and mortality rates are experienced by African-Americans, Native Americans, Hispanics, Alaska Natives, and Asian/Pacific Islanders compared with Caucasians. Shorter life expectancy, higher infant and maternal mortality rates, more birth defects, and more sexually transmitted infections are found among these ethnic and racial minority groups. The disparities are thought to result from a complex interaction among biologic factors, environment, and health behaviors. Disparities in education and income are also associated with differences in morbidity and mortality.

The HRSA Health Disparities Collaboratives are part of a national effort with the goal of eliminating disparities and improving delivery systems of health care for everyone in the United States who is cared for in HRSA-supported health centers. More than 900 community health centers have implemented the collaboratives and are successful in improving quality of care (Chin, 2011). The National Institutes of Health has a commitment to improve the health of minorities and provides funding for research and training of minority researchers (www.nih.gov), and the National Institute of Nursing Research includes in its strategic plan support of research that promotes health equity and eliminates health disparities.

The Centers for Disease Control and Prevention (CDC) released the First Periodic Health Disparities and Inequalities Report—United States, 2011 (CDC, 2011). The report includes recent trends and variation in health disparities and inequalities in some social and health indicators and provides data against which to measure progress in eliminating disparities. Topics specific to perinatal nursing that are addressed are infant deaths, preterm births, and adolescent pregnancy and childbirth. Also in 2011 the U.S. Department of Health and Human Services (USDHHS) released the HHS Disparities Action Plan that provides a vision of "a nation free of disparities in health and health care" (USDHHS, 2011). Through this plan HHS promotes evidenced-based programs, integrated approaches, and best practices to reduce disparities. The plan complements the 2011 National Stakeholder Strategy for Achieving Health Equity prepared by the National Partnership for Action. This strategy proposes a comprehensive, community-driven approach to achieve health equity through collaboration and synergy (National Partnership for Action to End Health Disparities, 2011). The Affordable Care Act (ACA) addresses disparities in income. Through these initiatives the United States is making a concerted effort to eliminate health disparities.

This chapter presents a general overview of issues and trends related to the health and health care of women and infants.

CONTEMPORARY ISSUES AND TRENDS

Healthy People 2020 Goals

Healthy People provides science-based 10-year national objectives for improving the health of all Americans. It has four overarching goals: (1) attaining high-quality, longer lives free of preventable disease, disability, injury, and premature death; (2) achieving health equity, eliminating disparities, and improving the health of all groups; (3) creating social and physical environments that promote good health for all; and (4) promoting quality of life, healthy development, and healthy behaviors across all life stages (www.healthypeople.gov/2020/about/default.aspx). The goals of *Healthy People 2020* are based on assessments of major risks to health and wellness, changes in public health priorities, and issues related to the health preparedness and prevention of our nation. Of the approximately 1200 objectives of *Healthy People 2020*, 33 are related to maternal, infant, and child health (Box 1-2). Objectives in this topic area include to: (1) reduce the rate of fetal and infant deaths, (2) reduce the rate of maternal mortality, (3) reduce preterm births, and (4) reduce cesarean births among low risk women. (See www.healthypeople.gov/2020/topicsobjectives2020/objectiveslist.aspx?topicId+26 for a complete list of objectives.)

Millennium Development Goals

The United Nations Millennium Development Goals (MDGs) are eight goals to be achieved by 2015 that respond to the main development challenges in the world. The MDGs are drawn from the actions and targets contained in the Millennium Declaration that was adopted by 189 nations and signed by 147 heads of state and governments during the United Nations Millennium Summit in September 2000 (www.un.org/millenniumgoals). Goals three through five of the MDGs relate specifically to women and children (Box 1-3).

Interprofessional Education

Interprofessional education consists of faculty and students from two or more health professions who create and foster a collaborative learning environment. The underlying premise of interprofessional collaboration is that client care will improve when health professionals work together. Numerous organizations including the World Health Organization (WHO), the Institute of Medicine (IOM), the National Academies of Practice, and the American Public Health Association, have expressed support of interprofessional education (Buring, Bhushan, Broeseker, et al., 2009). The Interprofessional Education Collaborative published Core Competencies for Interprofessional Collaborative Practice (Interprofessional Education Collaborative Expert Panel, 2011). The interprofessional collaborative practice competency domains include: (1) values/ethics for interprofessional practice, (2) roles/responsibilities, (3) interprofessional communication, and (4) teams and teamwork.

Problems with the U.S. Health Care System

Structure of the Health Care Delivery System

The U.S. health care delivery system is often fragmented and expensive and is inaccessible to many. Opportunities exist for nurses to alter nursing practice and improve the way care is delivered through managed care, integrated delivery systems, and redefined roles. Information about health and health care is readily available on the Internet (e-health). Consumers use this information to participate in their own care and consult health care providers with a knowledge base previously difficult to access.

Reducing Medical Errors

Medical errors are a leading cause of death in the United States and result in as many as 98,000 deaths per year (Pham, Aswani, Rosen, et al., 2012). Since the IOM released its 1999 report, *To Err Is Human: Building a Safer Health System,* a concerted effort has been under way to analyze causes of errors and develop strategies to prevent them. Recognizing the multifaceted causes of medical errors, the Agency for Healthcare Research and Quality (AHRQ, 2000) prepared a fact sheet, "20 Tips to Help Prevent Medical Errors," for clients and the public. Clients are encouraged to be knowledgeable consumers of health care and to ask questions of providers, including physicians, midwives, nurses, and pharmacists.

BOX 1-2 *Healthy People 2020* Maternal, Infant, and Child Health Objectives

- Reduce the rate of fetal and infant deaths.
- Reduce the 1-year mortality rate for infants with Down syndrome.
- Reduce the rate of child deaths.
- Reduce the rate of adolescent and young adult deaths.
- Reduce the rate of maternal mortality.
- Reduce maternal illness and complications caused by pregnancy (complications during hospitalized labor and delivery).
- Reduce cesarean births among low-risk (full-term, singleton, vertex presentation) women.
- Reduce low birth weight (LBW) and very low birth weight (VLBW).
- Reduce preterm births.
- Increase the proportion of pregnant women who receive early and adequate prenatal care.
- Increase abstinence from alcohol, cigarettes, and illicit drugs in pregnant women.
- Increase the proportion of pregnant women who attend a series of prepared childbirth classes.
- Increase the proportion of mothers who achieve a recommended weight gain during their pregnancies.
- Increase the proportion of women of childbearing potential with intake of at least 400 mcg of folic acid from fortified foods or dietary supplements.
- Reduce the proportion of women of childbearing potential who have low red blood cell folate concentrations.
- Increase the proportion of women delivering a live birth; increase those who receive preconception care services and practice key recommended preconception health behaviors.
- Reduce the proportion of people ages 18 to 44 years who have impaired fecundity (i.e., a physical barrier preventing pregnancy or carrying a pregnancy to term).
- Decrease postpartum relapse of smoking in women who quit smoking during pregnancy.
- Increase the proportion of women giving birth who attend a postpartum care visit with a health worker.
- Increase the proportion of infants who are put to sleep on their backs.
- Increase the proportion of infants who are breastfed.
- Increase the proportion of employers who have worksite lactation programs.
- Reduce the proportion of breastfed newborns who receive formula supplementation within the first 2 days of life.
- Increase the proportion of live births that occur in facilities that provide recommended care for lactating mothers and their babies.
- Reduce the occurrence of fetal alcohol syndrome (FAS).
- Reduce the proportion of children diagnosed with a disorder through newborn blood spot screening who experience developmental delay requiring special education services.
- Reduce the proportion of children with cerebral palsy born as LBW infants (less than 2500 g).
- Reduce the occurrence of neural tube defects.
- Increase the proportion of young children with an autism spectrum disorder (ASD) and other developmental delays who are screened, evaluated, and enrolled in early intervention services in a timely manner.
- Increase the proportion of children, including those with special health care needs, who have access to a medical home.
- Increase the proportion of children with special health care needs who receive their care in family-centered, comprehensive, coordinated systems.
- Increase appropriate newborn blood-spot screening and follow-up testing.
- Increase the number of states, including the District of Columbia, that verify through linkage with vital records that all newborns are screened shortly after birth for conditions mandated by their state-sponsored screening program.
- Increase the proportion of screen-positive children who receive follow-up testing within the recommended time period.
- Increase the proportion of children with a diagnosed condition identified through newborn screening who have an annual assessment of services needed and received.
- Increase the proportion of VLBW infants born at level III hospitals or subspecialty perinatal centers.

Adapted from HealthyPeople.gov. (2012). Maternal, infant, and child health. www.healthypeople.gov/2020/topicsobjectives2020/objectiveslist.aspx?topicId=26

BOX 1-3 United Nations Millennium Development Goals

1. Eradicate extreme poverty and hunger.
2. Achieve universal primary education.
3. Promote gender equality and empower women.
4. Reduce child mortality.
5. Improve maternal health.
6. Combat HIV/AIDS, malaria, and other diseases.
7. Ensure environmental sustainability.
8. Develop a global partnership for development.

AIDS, Acquired immunodeficiency syndrome; *HIV,* human immunodeficiency virus.

BOX 1-4 National Quality Forum Serious Reportable Events Pertaining to Maternal and Child Health

- Maternal death or serious injury associated with labor or birth in a low-risk pregnancy while being cared for in a healthcare setting
- Death or serious injury of a neonate associated with labor or birth in a low-risk pregnancy
- Artificial insemination with the wrong donor sperm or wrong egg
- Abduction of a client/resident of any age

Data from National Quality Forum (NQF). (2011). *Serious reportable events in healthcare—2011 update: A consensus report.* Washington, DC: NQF.

In 2002 the National Quality Forum (NQF) published a list of Serious Reportable Events in Healthcare. The list was updated in 2006 and again in 2011, resulting in a total of 29 events. Of these 29 events, 3 pertain directly to maternity and newborn care (Box 1-4). The NQF also published *Safe Practices for Better Healthcare* and updated it in 2010 (www.qualityforum.org). The 34 safe practices included should be used in all applicable health care settings to reduce the risk of harm that results from processes, systems, and environments of care (NQF, 2010). In August 2007 the Centers for Medicare & Medicaid Services (CMS) issued a rule that became effective October 2008 that denies payment for eight hospital-acquired conditions. Five of the conditions are also on the NQF list. Almost 1300 U.S.

hospitals waive (do not bill for) costs associated with serious reportable events (O'Reilly, 2008).

High Cost of Health Care

Health care is one of the fastest growing sectors of the U.S. economy. Currently, 17.4% of the gross domestic product is spent on health care. Higher spending in the United States compared with 12 other industrialized countries is related to higher prices, readily accessible technology, and greater obesity (Squires, 2012). Most researchers agree that caring for the increased number of low-birth-weight (LBW) infants in neonatal intensive care units contributes significantly to overall health care costs. Nurse-midwifery care has helped contain some health care costs. However, not all insurance carriers reimburse nurse practitioners and clinical nurse specialists as direct care providers, nor do they reimburse for all services provided by nurse-midwives, a situation that continues to be a problem. Only 16 states and the District of Columbia allow nurse practitioners to practice to their fullest potential without physician involvement (American Academy of Nurse Practitioners, 2012). Nurse practitioners are among the health care providers included in the ACA.

Limited Access to Care

Barriers to access must be removed so pregnancy outcomes and care of children can be improved. The most significant barrier to access is the inability to pay. The number of uninsured people in the United States in 2011 was 48.6 million or 15.7% of the population (DeNavas-Walt, Proctor, & Smith, 2012). Lack of transportation and dependent child care are other barriers. In addition to a lack of insurance and high costs, a lack of providers for low-income women exists because many physicians either refuse to take Medicaid clients or take only a few such clients. This presents a serious problem because a significant proportion of births is to mothers who receive Medicaid.

Health Care Reform

In early 2010, President Obama signed into law the Patient Protection and Affordable Care Act (ACA). The act aims to make insurance affordable, contain costs, strengthen and improve Medicare and Medicaid, and reform the insurance market. There are provisions to promote prevention and improve public health; improve the quality of care for all Americans; reduce waste, fraud, and abuse; and reform the health delivery system. There are some immediate benefits, but implementation of the act will occur over the next several years.

The Association of Women's Health, Obstetric and Neonatal Nurses (AWHONN) advocated successfully for the inclusion in the ACA of contraceptive methods, services, and counseling, without any out-of-pocket costs to clients; preventive services such as mammograms, well-woman visits, and screening for gestational diabetes; and providing breastfeeding equipment and counseling for pregnant and nursing women in new insurance plans. Work continues on implementation. See Box 1-5 for resources for the ACA.

Accountable Care Organizations

In 2011, the CMS finalized new rules under the ACA to help health care providers and hospitals coordinate care better for Medicare clients through Accountable Care Organizations (ACOs). An ACO "agrees to be held accountable for improving the health and experience of care for individuals and improving the health of populations while reducing the rate of growth in health care spending" (USDHHS, CMS, 2012). These groups of health care providers and hospitals voluntarily come together to coordinate high-quality care, eliminate duplication of services, and prevent medical errors, which results in savings of health care dollars. As of December 2013, there are more than 360 ACOs (Medicare & Medicaid News, 2013).

BOX 1-5 Resources about the Affordable Care Act

www.HealthCare.gov (CuidadDeSalud.gov)
State-specific information
www.medscape.org/viewarticle/782776
CE module "What the Healthcare Marketplace Means for Practices and Patients"
Marketplace.cms.gov

Downloadable Educational Materials

www.hhs.gov/healthcare/facts/bystate/statebystate.html
Interactive map to show Americans how the ACA affects them; fact sheets

Social Media Resource

Facebook.com/HealthCare.gov (Facebook.com/CuidadoDeSalud.gov)
Twitter@HealthCareGov (Twitter@CuidadoDeSalud)

1-800-318-2596 (TTY: 1-855-889-4325)
Call center available 24/7 in 150 languages

Health Literacy

Health literacy involves a spectrum of abilities, ranging from reading an appointment slip to interpreting medication instructions. These skills must be assessed routinely to recognize a problem and accommodate clients with limited literacy skills. Most client education materials are written at too high a level for the average adult; e-health literacy has emerged as a concept. Individuals use the Internet for diagnosis, and more than half of these individuals seek the opinion of a medical professional rather than trying to care for themselves based on the information accessed (Dickens & Piano, 2013).

The CDC health literacy website (www.cdc.gov/healthliteracy) highlights implementation of goals and strategies of the National Action Plan to Improve Health Literacy (USDHHS, 2010b). Health literacy is part of the ACA.

As a result of the increasingly multicultural U.S. population, there is a more urgent need to address health literacy as a component of culturally and linguistically competent care. Older adults, racial or ethnic minorities, and those whose income is at or below the poverty level are most vulnerable. Lower health literacy is associated with adverse health outcomes (Dickens & Piano, 2013).

Health care providers contribute to health literacy by using simple, common words, avoiding jargon, and assessing whether the client understands the discussion. Speaking slowly and clearly and focusing on what is important will increase understanding.

BOX 1-6 Maternal/Infant Biostatistical Terminology

Abortus: An embryo or fetus that is removed or expelled from the uterus at 20 weeks of gestation or less, weighs 500 g or less, or measures 25 cm or less
Birth rate: Number of live births in 1 year per 1000 population
Fertility rate: Number of births per 1000 women between the ages of 15 and 44 years (inclusive), calculated on a yearly basis
Infant mortality rate: Number of deaths of infants younger than 1 year of age per 1000 live births
Maternal mortality rate: Number of maternal deaths from births and complications of pregnancy, childbirth, and puerperium (the first 42 days after end of the pregnancy) per 100,000 live births
Neonatal mortality rate: Number of deaths of infants younger than 28 days of age per 1000 live births
Perinatal mortality rate: Number of stillbirths and the number of neonatal deaths per 1000 live births
Stillbirth: An infant who, at birth, demonstrates no signs of life, such as breathing, heartbeat, or voluntary muscle movements

TRENDS IN FERTILITY AND BIRTH RATE

Fertility trends and birth rates reflect women's needs for health care. Box 1-6 defines biostatistical terminology useful in analyzing maternity health care. In 2012 the fertility rate, births per 1000 women from 15 to 44 years of age, was 63.0 (Martin, Hamilton, Osterman, et al., 2013). The highest birth rates occurred among women between 20 and 29 years of age. The birth rate, number of live births in 1 year per 1000 population, was 12.6 in 2012; the birth rate for teens 15 to 19 years was 29.4. In 2012 the percentage of births by unmarried women varied widely among racial groups in the United States: Hispanic, 72.6%; black, 62.6%; non-Hispanic white, 32.1%; and Asian or Pacific Islander, 22.9% (Martin et al.).

Low Birth Weight and Preterm Birth

The risks of morbidity and mortality increase for newborns weighing less than 2500 g (5 lb, 8 oz)—low-birth-weight (LBW) infants. In the United States in 2012, the LBW rate was 7.99 per 1000. Multiple births contribute to the incidence of LBW. The twin birth rate was 33.1 per 1000 in 2012. The downward trend in the birth rate of higher-order multiples (triplet, quadruplet, and greater) continued in 2012, with a rate of 124.4 per 100,000 (Martin et al., 2013).

Non-Hispanic black infants are almost twice as likely as non-Hispanic white infants to be of LBW and to die in the first year of life. For non-Hispanic black births, the incidence of LBW was 13.18%, whereas the rate was 6.97% for non-Hispanic white births and 6.96% for Hispanic births (Martin et al., 2013). Cigarette smoking is associated with LBW, prematurity, and intrauterine growth restriction. In 2010, 12.3% of pregnant women smoked, including 14.3% of non-Hispanic white women, 8.9% non-Hispanic black women, 3.4% of Hispanic women, 26% of American Indian/Alaska Native women, and 2.1% of Asian/Pacific Islander women (Tong et al., 2013).

The percentage of infants born preterm (i.e., born before 38 weeks of gestation) was 11.55% in 2012. There was variation in the percentage according to race and Hispanic origin: 18.46% for non-Hispanic black births, 11.58% for Hispanic births, and 10.29% for non-Hispanic white births (Martin et al., 2013). Multiple births accounted for 3.4% of births in 2012; most of the increase is associated with increased use of fertility drugs and older age at childbearing.

Infant Mortality in the United States

A common indicator of the adequacy of prenatal care and the health of a nation as a whole is the infant mortality rate. The U.S. infant mortality rate for 2010 was 6.14 (Mathews & MacDorman, 2013). The disparity in infant mortality rate between African-American infants and Caucasian infants has increased over time. The infant mortality rate continues to be higher for non-Hispanic black babies (11.46 per 1000) than for non-Hispanic whites (5.18 per 1000) and Hispanic (5.25 per 1000) babies (Mathews & MacDorman). Limited maternal education, young maternal age, unmarried status, poverty, lack of prenatal care, and smoking appear to be associated with higher infant mortality rates. Poor nutrition, alcohol use, and maternal conditions such as poor health or hypertension also are important contributors to infant mortality. To address the factors associated with infant mortality, a shift from the current emphasis on high-technology medical interventions to a focus on improving access to preventive care for low-income families must occur.

The leading cause of death in the neonatal period is congenital anomalies. Other causes of neonatal death include disorders related to short gestation and LBW, sudden infant death, respiratory distress syndrome, and the effects of maternal complications. Racial differences in the infant mortality rates continue to challenge public health experts. Increased rates of survival during the neonatal period have resulted largely from high-quality prenatal care and the improvement in perinatal services, including technologic advances in neonatal intensive care and obstetrics.

Commitment at national, state, and local levels is required to reduce the infant mortality rate. More research is needed to identify the extent to which financial, educational, sociocultural, and behavioral factors individually and collectively affect perinatal morbidity and mortality. Barriers to care must be removed and perinatal services modified to meet contemporary health care needs.

International Infant Mortality Trends

In 2008, the infant mortality rate of Canada (5.7/1000) ranked twenty-ninth, and that of the United States (6.6/1000) ranked thirty-first, when compared with those of other industrialized nations (Heisler, 2012). Decreases in the infant mortality rate in the United States do not keep pace with the rates of other industrialized countries. One reason for this is the high rate of LBW infants in the United States in contrast with the rates in other countries.

Maternal Mortality Trends

The United Nations estimated that 358,000 women died of problems related to pregnancy or childbirth in 2008, a decline from approximately 546,000 in 1990 (Wilmoth, Mizoguchi, Oestergaard, et al., 2012). In the United States in 2010, the annual maternal mortality rate (number of maternal deaths per 100,000 live births) was 21 (WHO, 2013). The CDC began working with national and international groups in 2001 to develop and implement programs to promote safe motherhood (Jones, 2008). Although the overall number of maternal deaths in the United States is small (548 in 2007), maternal mortality remains a significant problem because a high proportion of deaths are preventable, primarily through improving the access to and use of prenatal care services. In the United States, there is significant racial disparity in the rates of maternal death: non-Hispanic black women (28.4), non-Hispanic white women (10.5), and Hispanic women (8.9) (USDHHS, 2010a). The leading causes of maternal death attributable to pregnancy differ over the world. In general, three major causes have persisted for the past 50 years: hypertensive disorders, infection, and hemorrhage. The three leading causes of maternal mortality in the United States today are cardiovascular disease, infection/sepsis, and noncardiovascular diseases (CDC, 2013). Factors that are strongly related to maternal death include age (younger than 20 years and 35 years or older), lack of prenatal care, low educational attainment, unmarried status, and non-Caucasian race. The *Healthy People 2010* goal of 3.3 maternal deaths per 100,000 posed a significant challenge and was not achieved. Worldwide strategies to reduce maternal mortality rates include improving access to skilled attendants at birth, providing postabortion care, improving family planning services, and providing adolescents with better reproductive health services.

Maternal Morbidity

Although mortality is the traditional measure of maternal health and maternal health is often measured by neonatal outcomes, pregnancy complications are important. Currently no surveillance method is available to measure the incidence of maternal morbidity. It includes such conditions as acute renal failure, amniotic fluid embolism, cerebrovascular accident, eclampsia, pulmonary embolism, liver failure, obstetric shock, respiratory failure, septicemia, and complications of anesthesia (pulmonary, cardiac, central nervous system) (Berg, Mackay, Qin, et al., 2009). Maternal morbidity results in a high risk pregnancy. The diagnosis of high risk imposes a situational crisis on the family. The combined efforts of medical and nursing personnel are required to care for these clients, who often need the expertise of physicians and nurses trained in both critical care obstetrics and intensive care medicine or nursing.

Obesity

More than one third (36.2%) of women in the United States are obese (body mass index of 30 or greater); in Canada less than one fourth (23.9%) of women are obese. Obesity in women demonstrates significant racial disparities: in the United States 49.6% of non-Hispanic black women, 45.1% of Mexican-American women, and 33% of non-Hispanic white women ages 20 years and older are obese (Flegal, Carroll, Ogden, et al., 2010; Shields, Carroll, & Ogden, 2011). Approximately 20% of women who give birth in the United States are obese. The two most frequently reported maternal medical risk factors are hypertension associated with pregnancy and diabetes, both of which are associated with obesity. Decreased fertility, congenital anomalies, miscarriage, and fetal death are associated with obesity. Obesity in pregnancy is associated with the use of increased health care services and longer hospital stays.

REGIONALIZATION OF PERINATAL HEALTH CARE SERVICES

Not all facilities can develop and maintain the full spectrum of services required for high risk perinatal clients. A regionalized system focusing on integrated delivery of graded levels of hospital-based perinatal health care services is effective and results in improved outcomes for mothers and their newborns. This system of coordinated care can be extended to preconception and ambulatory prenatal care services. New guidelines for regionalization of maternal care are in preparation.

Ambulatory Prenatal Care

Guidelines have been established regarding the level of care that can be expected at any given facility. In ambulatory settings, providers must distinguish themselves by the level of care they provide. *Basic care* is provided by obstetricians, family physicians, certified nurse-midwives, and other advanced practice clinicians approved by local governance. Routine risk-oriented prenatal care, education, and support are provided. Providers offering *specialty care* are obstetricians who must provide fetal diagnostic testing and management of obstetric and medical complications in addition to basic care. *Subspecialty care* is provided by maternal-fetal medicine specialists and reproductive geneticists and includes the aforementioned in addition to genetic testing, advanced fetal therapies, and management of severe maternal and fetal complications. Collaboration among providers to meet the woman's needs is the key to reducing perinatal morbidity and mortality (American Academy of Pediatrics [AAP] & American College of Obstetricians and Gynecologists [ACOG], 2012).

HIGH-TECHNOLOGY CARE

Advances in scientific knowledge and the large number of high risk pregnancies have contributed to a health care system that emphasizes high-technology care. Maternity care has extended to preconception counseling, more and better scientific techniques to monitor the mother and fetus, more definitive tests for hypoxia and acidosis, and neonatal intensive care units. The labors of virtually all women who give birth in hospitals are monitored electronically despite the lack of evidence of efficacy of such monitoring. The numbers of assisted labors and births are increasing. Internet-based information is available to the public that enhances interactions among health care providers, families, and community providers. Point-of-care testing is available. Personal data assistants are used to enhance comprehensive care; the medical record is increasingly in electronic form.

Strides are being made in identifying genetic codes, and genetic engineering is taking place. Women's health has expanded to

BOX 1-7 Principles for Social Networking and the Nurse

- Nurses must not transmit or place online individually identifiable client information.
- Nurses must observe ethically prescribed professional client-nurse boundaries.
- Nurses should understand that clients, colleagues, institutions, and employers may view postings.
- Nurses should take advantage of privacy settings and seek to separate personal and professional information online.
- Nurses should bring content that could harm a client's privacy, rights, or welfare to the attention of appropriate authorities.
- Nurses should participate in developing institutional policies governing online contact.

From American Nurses Association. (2011). *Principles for social networking and the nurse: Guidance for the registered nurse*, Washington, DC: Author.

emphasize care of older women, new cancer-screening techniques, advances in the diagnosis and treatment of breast cancer, and work on an AIDS vaccine. In general, high-technology care has flourished, whereas "health" care has become relatively neglected. Nurses must use caution and prospective planning and assess the effect of the emerging technology.

Social Media

Social media uses Internet-based technologies to allow users to create their own content and participate in dialogue. The most common social media platforms are Facebook, Twitter, and LinkedIn (Duffy, 2011). Through use of these technologies, nurses can link with nurses with similar interests, share insights about client care, and advocate for clients (Saver, 2010). However, there are pitfalls for nurses using this technology. Client privacy and confidentiality can be violated, and institutions and colleagues can be cast in unfavorable lights with negative consequences for those posting the information. Nursing students have been expelled from school, and nurses have been fired or reprimanded by a board of nursing for injudicious posts. To help make nurses aware of their responsibilities when using social media, the American Nurses Association (ANA) published six principles for social networking and the nurse (Box 1-7). In addition, the National Council of State Boards of Nursing (NCSBN) issued *White Paper: A Nurse's Guide to the Use of Social Media* (NCSBN, 2011). The paper details issues of confidentiality and privacy, possible consequences of inappropriate use of social media, common myths and misunderstandings of social media, and tips on how to avoid problems.

COMMUNITY-BASED CARE

A shift in settings, from acute care institutions to ambulatory settings including the home, has occurred (see Chapter 2). Even childbearing women at high risk are cared for on an outpatient basis or in the home. Technology previously available only in the hospital is now found in the home. This has affected the organizational structure of care, the skills required in providing such care, and the costs to consumers. Nursing education curricula are increasingly community based.

CHILDBIRTH PRACTICES

Prenatal care can promote better pregnancy outcomes by providing early risk assessment and promoting healthy behaviors such as improved nutrition and smoking cessation. Prenatal care ideally begins before pregnancy because early decisions lay the foundation for the entire perinatal year. If at all possible, education continues in each trimester of pregnancy and extends through the early postpartum weeks. Some health care providers promote preconception care as an important component of perinatal services. Preconception or early pregnancy classes also emphasize health-promoting behavior as well as choices of care.

In the United States in 2012, 74.1% of all women received care in the first trimester. There is disparity in receiving prenatal care by race and ethnicity: 10% of non-Hispanic blacks, 7.5% of Hispanic women, and 4.3% of non-Hispanic whites received late or no prenatal care (CDC, 2012). In spite of these statistics, substantial gains have been made in the use of prenatal care since the early 1990s, which are attributed to the expansion in the 1980s of Medicaid coverage for pregnant women.

Women can choose physicians or nurse-midwives as primary care providers. In 2012, physicians attended 92% of all births and certified nurse-midwives attended 7.6% (Martin et al., 2013). Women who choose nurse-midwives as their primary providers participate more actively in childbirth decisions, receive fewer interventions during labor, and are less likely to give birth prematurely (Sandall, Soltani, Gates, et al., 2013). The rate of vaginal births after cesarean (VBACs) (10.2%) declined, whereas the cesarean birth rate of 32.8% of live births in the United States was unchanged in 2012 (Martin et al.; National Center for Health Statistics, 2012).

CLINICAL REASONING CASE STUDY

Safety and Efficacy of Midwifery Care

A group of nurse-midwives is setting up practice in your hometown. They are to collaborate with one of the groups of obstetricians in the same city. A letter to the editor appeared in the local newspaper stating that the presence of midwives will jeopardize the care of pregnant women in the community because midwives usually care for the poor and indigent, deliver babies at home, and therefore do not have the skills to work in hospitals and care for middle-class women who have insurance. The letter writer urged the community to boycott the midwives to ensure safe childbirth for women in the community.

1. Evidence—Is there sufficient evidence to document the qualifications of nurse-midwives and their safety record to write a response to this letter?
2. Assumptions—What assumptions can be made about midwifery care and the knowledge base of the public regarding that care?
3. What implications and priorities for nursing can be made at this time?
4. Does the evidence objectively support your conclusion?

With family-centered care, fathers, partners, grandparents, siblings, and friends may be present for labor and birth. Fathers or partners may be present for cesarean births and may participate in vaginal births by "catching the baby" or cutting the umbilical cord or both (Fig. 1-1). Doulas (i.e., trained and experienced female labor attendants) may be present to provide a

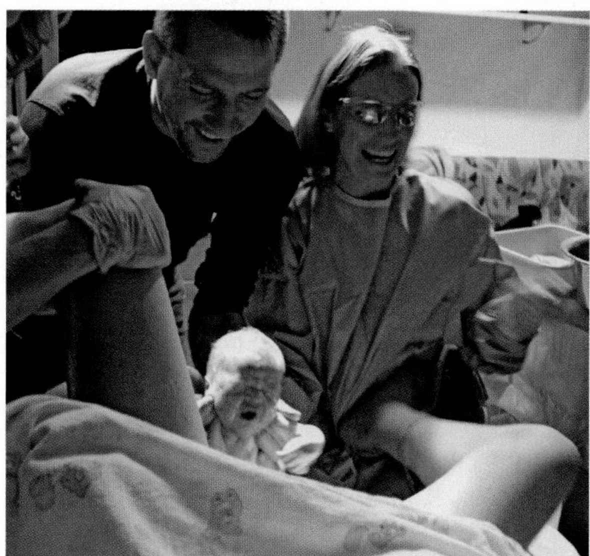

FIG 1-1 Father "catching" newborn daughter who cried before her lower body emerged following an unmedicated birth. (Courtesy Darren and Julie Nelson, Loveland, CO.)

continuous, one-on-one caring presence throughout the labor and birth. Ideally, newborns are placed skin-to-skin with the mother immediately after birth and are encouraged to breastfeed as soon as possible. Neonates often remain in the room with their parents and may never transfer to a newborn nursery. Parents actively participate in newborn care on mother/baby units, in nurseries, and in neonatal intensive care units.

Discharge of a mother and baby within 24 hours of birth has created a growing need for follow-up or home care. In some settings, discharge may occur as early as 6 hours after birth. Legislation has been enacted to ensure that mothers and babies are permitted to stay in the hospital for at least 48 hours after vaginal birth and 96 hours after cesarean birth, although they may choose to leave earlier. Focused and efficient teaching is necessary to enable the parents and infant to make the transition safely from the hospital to the home.

INVOLVING CONSUMERS AND PROMOTING SELF-MANAGEMENT

Self-management is appealing to clients as well as the health care system because of its potential to reduce health care costs. Maternity care is especially suited to self-management because childbearing is primarily health focused, women are usually well when they enter the system, and visits to health care providers can present the opportunity for health and illness interventions. Measures to improve health and reduce risks associated with poor pregnancy outcomes and illness can be addressed. Topics such as nutrition education, stress management, smoking cessation, alcohol and drug treatment, violence prevention, social support improvement, and parenting education are appropriate for such encounters.

INTERNATIONAL CONCERNS

Access to prenatal care and family planning education, care for women experiencing postpartum hemorrhage, obstructed labors with no access to hospital care or operative birth, fistulas due to obstructed labors, and HIV-positive parents are major international concerns. The high maternal and infant mortality in developing countries is a serious problem with limited resources to address the problems. Two concerns that nurses in the United States and Canada might encounter are female genital mutilation and human trafficking.

Female genital mutilation, infibulation (surgical closure of the labia majora), and *circumcision* are terms used to describe procedures in which part or all of the female external genitalia is removed for cultural or nontherapeutic reasons (WHO, 2013). Worldwide, many women undergo such procedures. The International Council of Nurses and other health professionals have spoken out against procedures that result in mutilation as harmful to women's health. In the United States, performing female genital mutilation on a person younger than 18 years is a crime (Sandy, 2011) (see Cultural Considerations: Female Genital Mutilation box in Chapter 4).

Human trafficking is a $32 billion business that exists in the United States and internationally (Dovydaitis, 2010). Trafficked individuals, mostly women and children, are forced into hard labor, sex work, and even organ donation (Budiani-Saberi, Raja, Findley, et al., 2014; Macy & Graham, 2012). Health care professionals may interact with victims who are in captivity. This provides an opportunity to identify victims, intervene to help them obtain necessary health services, and provide information about ways to escape from their situation (Fig. 1-2) (see Chapter 5). The National Human Trafficking Resource Center (1-888-373-7888) can provide assistance.

WOMEN'S HEALTH

Heart disease is the leading cause of death of women followed closely by malignant neoplasms including breast cancer. Symptoms of a heart attack in women are different from symptoms in men. Nurses providing care for women have opportunities for client education to ensure that their clients are aware of these differences (Longley, 2013). Early detection of breast cancer through mammography can reduce the mortality rate resulting from this type of cancer. However, because of lack of information or lack of insurance and access, many women never have mammograms. Wide disparity exists between Caucasian women and women of other races and between older and younger women in their rates of mammography, detection, and treatment of breast cancer, and in their survival rates (see Chapter 10). Cancer genetic predisposition testing is increasingly available. Women may approach providers of women's health services to request such testing (Mahon & Crecelius, 2013).

Various factors and conditions affect women's health. Race is a major factor: Caucasian women born in 2015 have a life expectancy at birth of 81.8 years, in contrast with 78.2 years for African-American women (Murphy, Xu, & Kochanek, 2012). The population has grown older: approximately 50 million women are older than 50 years of age; 51 is the median age for menopause. Hormone replacement therapy for menopausal women has been used for many years and has both benefits and risks (see Chapter 6).

Violence is a major factor affecting women (see Chapter 5). Violence includes battery, rape or other sexual assaults, and attacks with various weapons. Rates of reported intimate partner

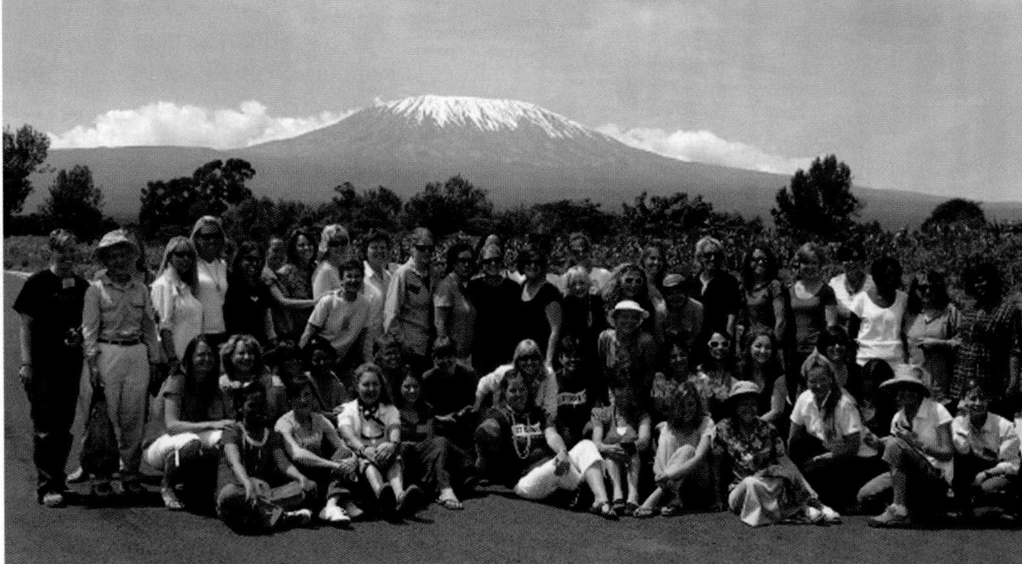

FIG 1-2 In January 2012, a group of 48 women participated in the Freedom Climb of Mt. Kilimanjaro, the tallest mountain in Africa. The women climbed to call attention to human trafficking and to raise funds to support projects to combat trafficking. The group raised more than $350,000, which went for projects such as prenatal care, education, safe houses, and micro loans for victims of trafficking in many countries served by Operation Mobilization (www.om.org). (Courtesy Shannon Perry, Phoenix, AZ.)

violence have increased, possibly because of better assessment and reporting mechanisms. Approximately 4% to 8% of pregnant women are battered; the incidence of battering increases during pregnancy. Violence is associated with complications of pregnancy such as bleeding. Alcoholism and substance abuse by the woman and her abuser are associated with violence and homelessness, which affect a growing number of women and children and place them at risk for a variety of health problems.

THE FUTURE OF NURSING

In 2008 the Robert Wood Johnson Foundation and the IOM initiated a 2-year process to meet the need to assess and transform the nursing profession. The IOM appointed a committee that developed four key messages: (1) nurses should practice to the full extent of their education and training; (2) nurses should achieve higher levels of education and training through an improved education system that promotes seamless academic progression; (3) nurses should be full partners with physicians and other health care professionals in redesigning health care in the United States; and (4) effective workforce planning and policymaking require better data collection and an improved information infrastructure (IOM, 2010). Throughout the United States individual states and nursing organizations are making concerted efforts to implement the recommendations of the report.

TRENDS IN NURSING PRACTICE

The increasing complexity of care for maternity and women's health clients has contributed to specialization of nurses working with these clients. This specialized knowledge is gained through experience, advanced degrees, and certification programs. Nurses in advanced practice (e.g., nurse practitioners and nurse-midwives) may provide primary care throughout a woman's life, including during the pregnancy cycle. In some settings the clinical nurse specialist and nurse practitioner roles are blended, and nurses deliver high-quality, comprehensive, and cost-effective care in a variety of settings. Lactation consultants provide services in the hospital setting, in clinics and physician offices, and during home visits.

Nursing Interventions Classification

When the IOM proposed that all client records be computerized by the year 2000, a need for a common language to describe the contributions of nurses to client care became evident. Nurses from the University of Iowa developed a comprehensive standardized language that describes interventions that are performed by generalist or specialist nurses. This language is included in the Nursing Interventions Classification (NIC) (Bulachek, Butcher, Dochterman, & Wagner, 2013). Examples of interventions for childbearing care to assist in the preparation for childbirth before, during, and after include breastfeeding assistance, childbirth preparation, circumcision care, electronic fetal monitoring, family planning, and kangaroo care.

Evidence-Based Practice

Evidence-based practice—providing care based on evidence gained through research and clinical trials—is increasingly emphasized. Although not all practice can be evidence based, practitioners must use the best available information on which to base their interventions. The AWHONN *Standards and Guidelines for Professional Nursing Practice in the Care of Women and Newborns* (AWHONN, 2009a) and the *Standards for Professional Perinatal Nursing Practice and Certification in Canada* (AWHONN, 2009b) include an evidence-based approach to practice. Discussion of nursing care and evidence-based practice boxes throughout this text provide examples of evidence-based practice in perinatal and women's health nursing (see Evidence-Based Practice box).

EVIDENCE-BASED PRACTICE

Seeking and Evaluating Evidence: A Necessary Competency for Quality and Safety

Throughout this text you will see Evidence-Based Practice boxes. These boxes provide examples of how a nurse might conduct an inquiry into an identified practice question. Curiosity and access to a virtual or real library are all the nurse needs to be confident that his or her practice has a sound foundation of evidence.

A literature search may reveal up to three levels of evidence. The first level consists of primary studies. The strongest of these are randomized controlled trials. Well-designed studies, even small ones, add another piece to the puzzle.

These primary studies may be combined into the second level of evidence. In systematic analyses such as those in the Cochrane Database, the researcher uses a methodology to identify all studies relevant to a particular question. If the data are similar enough, they can be pooled into a metaanalysis. If the evidence is strong, some analyses will form the basis for recommendations for practice and to guide further inquiry.

At the tertiary level professional organizations such as the Agency for Healthcare Research and Quality (AHRQ) (www.ahrq.gov) or the National Guidelines Clearinghouse (NGC) (guideline.gov) may decide to address a broad practice question by sorting through all the available primary and secondary evidence and consulting experienced clinicians. After thoughtful review, the committee of experts in the organization crafts its consensus statement. These recommendations for best practice stand on the shoulders of the systematic analysts, who stand on the many shoulders of the primary researchers.

Provided that the professional organization is well respected and the process is rigorous, these guidelines in the consensus statement carry enormous authority. Individuals and institutions may choose to adopt them with confidence. An example of this is the Association of Women's Health, Obstetric and Neonatal Nurses (AWHONN) (www.awhonn.org) Late Preterm Infant Initiative. This initiative began in 2005 in response to the confusion that surrounded the care of infants who do not qualify for neonatal intensive care unit (NICU) admission yet require extra vigilance. Nurseries can adapt these recommendations to their specific institutions, enabling nurses to become more effective at caring for the unique problems of this population of neonates. Like AWHONN, most of the professional organizations make their guidelines available free of charge on their websites.

To develop common language and goals for nursing education, the Quality and Safety Education for Nurses (QSEN) (www.qsen.org) project expert panel identified six competencies necessary to enable the new nurse to continually improve the health care system: client-centered care, teamwork and collaboration, evidence-based practice, quality improvement, safety, and informatics. Most nursing challenges require a combination of these competencies. Each competency is further defined as having targets for knowledge, skills, and attitude. The Evidence-Based Practice boxes in this textbook include examples that illustrate each of these targets specific to that competency. A mastery of QSEN competencies greatly enriches a nurse's ability to identify and improve client and health care–system problems and communicate within the interdisciplinary team.

Pat Mahaffee Gingrich

Cochrane Pregnancy and Childbirth Database

The Cochrane Pregnancy and Childbirth Database was first planned in 1976 with a small grant from the WHO to Dr. Iain Chalmers and colleagues at Oxford. In 1993, the Cochrane Collaboration was formed, and the Oxford Database of Perinatal Trials became known as the Cochrane Pregnancy and Childbirth Database. The Cochrane Collaboration oversees up-to-date, systematic reviews of randomized controlled trials of health care and disseminates these reviews. The premise of the project is that these types of studies provide the most reliable evidence about the effects of care.

The evidence from these studies should encourage practitioners to implement useful measures and to abandon those that are useless or harmless. Studies are ranked in six categories:

1. Beneficial forms of care
2. Forms of care that are likely to be beneficial
3. Forms of care with a trade-off between beneficial and adverse effects
4. Forms of care with unknown effectiveness
5. Forms of care that are unlikely to be beneficial
6. Forms of care that are likely to be ineffective or harmful

Joanna Briggs Institute

Established in 1996 as an initiative of the Royal Adelaide Hospital and the University of Adelaide in Australia, the Joanna Briggs Institute (JBI) uses a collaborative approach for evaluating evidence from a range of sources (www.joannabriggs.edu.au). The JBI has formed collaborations with a variety of universities and hospitals around the world including in the United States and Canada. The JBI uses the following grades of recommendation for evidence of feasibility, appropriateness, meaningfulness, and effectiveness: *A*, strong support that merits application; *B*, moderate support that warrants consideration of application; and *C*, not supported (JBI, 2013). The JBI provides another source for perinatal nurses to access information to support evidence-based practice.

Outcomes-Oriented Practice

Outcomes of care (that is, the effectiveness of interventions and quality of care) are receiving increased emphasis. Outcomes-oriented care measures effectiveness of care against benchmarks or standards. It is a measure of the value of nursing using quality indicators and answers the question, "Did the client benefit or not benefit from the care provided?" (Moorhead, Johnson, Maas, & Swanson, 2012). The Outcome and Assessment Information Set (OASIS) is an example of an outcomes system important for nursing. Its use is required by the CMS in all home health organizations that are Medicare accredited. The Nursing Outcomes Classification (NOC) is an effort to identify outcomes and related measures that can be used for evaluation of care of individuals, families, and communities across the care continuum (Moorhead et al.); for example, the scale for *Breastfeeding Establishment: Infant* ranges from Not Adequate to Totally Adequate. Indicators include proper alignment and latching, proper areolar grasp and compression, correct suck and tongue placement, and audible swallowing. Through this assessment, the nurse can determine whether the infant met the desired outcome of ingesting adequate nutrition.

A Global Perspective

Advances in medicine and nursing have resulted in increased knowledge and understanding in the care of mothers and infants and reduced perinatal morbidity and mortality rates. However, these advances have affected predominantly industrialized nations. For example, the majority of the 3.2 million children living with human immunodeficiency virus (HIV) or AIDS acquired the infection through perinatal transmission and live in sub-Saharan Africa. The State of the World's Mothers annual report from Save the Children is available at www.savethechildren.org/mothers.

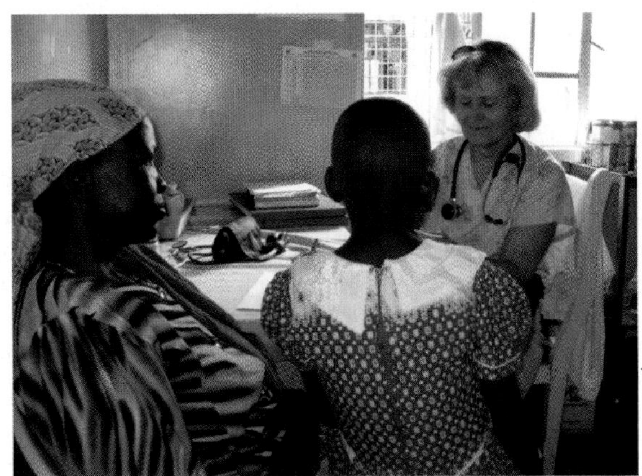

FIG 1-3 Nurse interviewing a young girl accompanied by her mother in a clinic in rural Kenya. (Courtesy Shannon Perry, Phoenix, AZ.)

As the world becomes smaller because of travel and communication technologies, nurses and other health care providers are gaining a global perspective and participating in activities to improve the health and health care of people worldwide. Nurses participate in medical outreach, providing obstetric, surgical, ophthalmologic, orthopedic, or other services (Fig. 1-3); attend international meetings; conduct research; and provide international consultation. International student and faculty exchanges occur. More articles about health and health care in various countries are appearing in nursing journals. Several schools of nursing in the United States are World Health Organization Collaborating Centers.

STANDARDS OF PRACTICE AND LEGAL ISSUES IN PROVISION OF CARE

Nursing standards of practice in perinatal and women's health nursing have been described by several organizations, including the ANA, which publishes standards for maternal-child health nursing; AWHONN, which publishes standards of practice and education for perinatal nurses (Box 1-8); ACNM, which publishes standards of practice for midwives; and the National Association of Neonatal Nurses (NANN), which

BOX 1-8 Standards of Care for Women and Newborns

Standards of Practice

Assessment
- Collects health data of the woman or newborn

Diagnosis
- Analyses data to determine nursing diagnosis

Outcome Identification
- Identifies expected outcomes that are individualized

Planning
- Develops a plan of care

Implementation
- Performs interventions for the plan of care
  - (a) *Coordination of Care.* Coordinated care delivery within her/his scope of practice
  - (b) *Health Teaching and Health Promotion.* Employs teaching strategies to promote, maintain, or restore health

Evaluation
- Evaluates effectiveness of interventions in relation to expected outcomes

Standards of Professional Performance

Quality of Practice
- Systematically evaluates and implements measures to improve quality, safety, and effectiveness of nursing practice

Education
- Acquires and maintains knowledge and competencies that reflect current evidence-based practice

Professional Practice Evaluation
- Evaluates own practice in relation to current evidence-based information, standards and guidelines, statutes, rules and regulations

Ethics
- Decisions and actions determined in an ethical manner and guided by a sound ethical decision-making process

Collegiality
- Interacts with and contributes to professional development of peers, colleagues, and other health care providers

Collaboration and Communication
- Collaborates and communicates with women, families, health care providers, and the community in the providing safe and effective care

Research
- Generates and/or integrates evidence to identify, examine, validate, and evaluate knowledge, theories, and approaches in providing care to clients

Resources and Technology
- Considers factors related to safety, effectiveness, technological advances, and costs in planning and delivering client care

Leadership
- Within appropriate roles, seeks to serve as a role model, change agent, consultant, and mentor to clients and other health care professionals

From Association of Women's Health, Obstetric and Neonatal Nurses (AWHONN). (2009). *Standards and guidelines for professional practice in the care of women and newborns* (ed. 7). Washington, DC: Author.

publishes standards of practice for neonatal nurses. These standards reflect current knowledge, represent levels of practice agreed on by leaders in the specialty, and can be used for clinical benchmarking.

In addition to these more formalized standards, agencies have their own policy and procedure books that outline standards to be followed in that setting. In legal terms, the standard of care is that level of practice that a reasonably prudent nurse would provide in the same or similar circumstances. In determining legal negligence, the care given is compared with the standard of care. If the standard was not met and harm resulted, negligence occurred. The number of legal suits in the perinatal area typically has been high. As a consequence, malpractice insurance costs are high for physicians, nurse-midwives, and nurses who work in labor and birth settings.

LEGAL TIP: Standard of Care

When you are uncertain about how to perform a procedure, consult the agency procedure book guidelines printed therein. These guidelines are the standard of care for that agency.

Risk Management

Risk management is an evolving process that identifies risks, establishes preventive practices, develops reporting mechanisms, and delineates procedures for managing lawsuits. Nurses should be familiar with concepts of risk management and their implications for nursing practice. These concepts can be viewed as systems of checks and balances that ensure high-quality client care from preconception until after birth. Effective risk management minimizes the risk of injury to clients and the number of lawsuits against nurses, doctors, and hospitals. Each facility or site develops site-specific risk management procedures based on accepted standards and guidelines. The procedures and guidelines must be reviewed periodically.

To decrease risk of errors in the administration of medications, The Joint Commission (TJC) (2009) developed a list of abbreviations, acronyms, and symbols *not* to use. In addition, each agency must develop its own list.

Sentinel Events

TJC describes a sentinel event as "an unexpected occurrence involving death or serious physical or psychological injury, or the risk thereof. Serious injury specifically includes loss of limb or function." These events are called *sentinel* because they signal a need for an immediate investigation and response. Reportable sentinel events in perinatal nursing include any maternal death related to the process of birth, any perinatal death unrelated to a congenital condition in an infant having a birth weight greater than 2500 g, severe neonatal hyperbilirubinemia (bilirubin greater than 30 mg/dl), and infant discharge to the wrong family (TJC, 2013). Other sentinel events that may occur in perinatal nursing include hemolytic transfusion reaction involving major blood group incompatibilities, leaving a foreign body (e.g., sponge or forceps) in a client after surgery, and falls that result in death or major permanent loss of function that is a direct result of the injuries caused by the fall. When a sentinel event occurs, there must be a root cause analysis and an action plan formulated that identifies strategies to reduce the risk of future similar events.

Failure to Rescue

Failure to rescue, that is, the failure to recognize or act on early signs of distress, was introduced in the 1990s in relation to the care of adult postsurgical clients (Beaulieu, 2009; Simpson, 2005). Mothers and babies are generally healthy, and complications leading to death in obstetrics are comparatively rare. When applying the concept of failure to rescue to the perinatal setting, Simpson proposed evaluating the ability of the perinatal team to decrease the risk of adverse outcomes by measuring processes involved in common complications and emergencies in obstetrics (Simpson, 2005, 2006). Key components of failure to rescue are (1) careful surveillance and identification of complications, and (2) quick action to initiate appropriate interventions and activate a team response. For the perinatal nurse, this involves careful surveillance, timely identification of complications, appropriate interventions, and activation of a team response to minimize client harm. The Fetal Safety Failure to Rescue Process Tool as adapted by Simpson from the AHRQ (2004) client safety indicators can be used for this purpose (Beaulieu). Maternal complications that are appropriate for process measurement are placental abruption, postpartum hemorrhage, uterine rupture, eclampsia, and amniotic fluid embolism (Simpson, 2005, 2006; Simpson, Knox, Martin, et al., 2011). Fetal complications include nonreassuring fetal heart rate and pattern, prolapsed umbilical cord, shoulder dystocia, and uterine hyperstimulation (Simpson, 2005, 2006; Simpson et al.). Perinatal nurses can use these complications to develop a list of expectations for monitoring, timely identification, interventions, and roles of team members. The list can be used to evaluate the perinatal team's response. Practicing emergency interventions as a team using simulation is important. Promoting a culture of safety, effective communication, and team building are important in providing safe care during labor and birth (Simpson et al.).

Quality and Safety Education for Nurses

Quality and Safety Education for Nurses (QSEN) is an effort to provide nurses with the competencies to improve the quality and safety of the systems of health care in which they practice (Cronenwett, Sherwood, Barnsteiner, et al., 2007). The competencies for nursing delineated by the IOM (2003) (Box 1-9) were adapted by QSEN faculty members and defined by describing essential features of a competent and respected nurse. They

BOX 1-9 Institute of Medicine QSEN Competencies for Nursing

Client-centered care
Teamwork
Collaboration
Evidence-based practice
Quality improvement
Safety
Informatics

Data from Institute of Medicine. (2003). *Health professions education: A bridge to quality*. Washington, DC: National Academies Press.

then developed knowledge, skills, and attitudes (KSAs) for each competency. Incorporation of these KSAs into prelicensure education for nurses helps faculty to plan learning experiences to prepare respected and qualified nurses. In this text, QSEN competencies are incorporated into the evidence-based practice boxes.

Teamwork and Communication

Situation, Background, Assessment, Recommendation

The situation, background, assessment, recommendation (SBAR) technique gives a specific framework for communication among health care providers about a client's condition. SBAR is an easy to remember, useful, concrete mechanism for communicating important information that requires a clinician's immediate attention (Kaiser Permanente of Colorado, 2014 (Table 1-1). Failure to communicate is one of the major reasons for errors in health care. The SBAR technique has the potential to serve as a means to reduce errors.

TeamSTEPPS

TeamSTEPPS (Team Strategies to Enhance Performance and Patient Safety) was developed by the Department of Defense's Patient Safety Program in collaboration with the AHRQ as a teamwork system for health professionals to provide higher quality, safer client care (AHRQ, n.d.). It provides an evidence base to improve communication and teamwork skills. Through this system medical teams use information, people, and resources to achieve the best possible clinical outcomes, increase team awareness and clarify roles and responsibilities of team members, resolve conflicts and improve sharing of information, and eliminate barriers to quality and safety.

The three phases of the TeamSTEPPS delivery system are to: (1) assess the need, (2) plan, train, and implement the TeamSTEPPS initiative, and (3) sustain the improvements in performance, processes, and outcomes that result from the initiative. Teams of trainers should include physicians, nurses, and support staff. Evaluation and revision of the plan as the needs change are built in to the system (AHRQ).

TABLE 1-1 Sample SBAR Report to Physician or Midwife about A Critical Situation

S	**Situation** I am calling about Mary Smith. I have just assessed her and she saturated a peripad in the last hour. Her blood pressure is 112/62, pulse 86, and respirations 18. I think she is bleeding excessively.
B	**Background** Mrs. Smith is 12 hours postpartum after giving birth vaginally to a 9 lb, 12 oz term infant after an uncomplicated pregnancy. She had a rapid labor, just over 4 hours, and had no analgesia. She plans to bottle-feed this baby. She had an IV with 10 units of Pitocin but it was completed and discontinued about 2 hours ago. This is her sixth birth. All were uncomplicated and she had an uneventful recovery from them.
A	**Assessment** Her fundus becomes firm after massage but relaxes again. She has voided and her bladder feels empty. I think she might have retained placenta and she needs to be examined.
R	**Recommendation** I would like you to come and examine her immediately. Do you want her IV restarted? Do you want her to have an Hb and HCT?

Hb, Hemoglobin; *HCT*, hematocrit; *IV*, intravenous.
The SBAR tool was developed by Kaiser Permanente. This example was prepared by Shannon Perry.

ETHICAL ISSUES IN PERINATAL NURSING AND WOMEN'S HEALTH CARE

Ethical concerns and debates have multiplied with the increased use of technology and with scientific advances. For example, with reproductive technology, pregnancy is now possible in women who thought they would never bear children, including some who are menopausal or postmenopausal. Should scarce resources be devoted to achieving pregnancies in older women? Is giving birth to a child at an older age worth the risks involved? Should older parents be encouraged to conceive a baby when they may not live to see the child reach adulthood? Should a woman who is HIV positive have access to assisted reproduction services? Should third-party payers assume the costs of reproductive technology such as the use of induced ovulation and in vitro fertilizations? With induced ovulation and in vitro fertilization, multiple pregnancies occur, and multifetal pregnancy reduction (selectively terminating one or more fetuses) may be considered.

Questions about informed consent and allocation of resources must be addressed with innovations such as intrauterine fetal surgery, fetoscopy, therapeutic insemination, genetic engineering, stem cell research, surrogate childbearing, surgery for infertility, "test tube" babies, fetal research, and treatment of very LBW (VLBW) babies.

The introduction of long-acting contraceptives has created moral choices and policy dilemmas for health care providers and legislators; that is, should some women (substance abusers, women with low incomes, or women who are HIV positive) be required to take these contraceptives? With the potential for great good that can come from fetal tissue transplantation, what research is ethical? What are the rights of the embryo? Should cloning of humans be permitted? Discussion and debate about these issues will continue for many years. Nurses and clients as well as scientists, physicians, attorneys, lawmakers, ethicists, and clergy must be involved in the discussions.

RESEARCH IN PERINATAL NURSING AND WOMEN'S HEALTH CARE

Research plays a vital role in establishing maternity and women's health science. It can validate that nursing care makes a difference. For example, although prenatal care is clearly associated with healthier infants, no one knows exactly which nursing interventions produce this outcome. The research into women's health must increase. In the past, medical researchers rarely included women in their studies, so more research in this area is crucial. Many possible areas of research exist in maternity and women's health care. The clinician can identify problems in the health and health care of women and infants. Through research, nurses can make a difference for these clients. Nurses should promote research funding and conduct research on maternity and women's health, especially concerning the effectiveness of nursing strategies for these clients.

Ethical Guidelines for Nursing Research

Research with perinatal clients may create ethical dilemmas for the nurse. For example, participating in research may cause additional stress to a woman concerned about outcomes of genetic testing or one who is waiting for an invasive procedure. Obtaining amniotic fluid samples or performing cordocentesis poses risks to the fetus. Nurses must protect the rights of human subjects (i.e., clients) in all of their research. For example, nurses can collect data on or care for clients who are participating in clinical trials. The nurse ensures that the participants are fully informed and aware of their rights as subjects. The nurse can be involved in determining whether the benefits of research outweigh the risks to the mother and the fetus. Following the ANA ethical guidelines in the conduct, dissemination, and implementation of nursing research helps nurses ensure that research is conducted ethically.

KEY POINTS

- Maternity nursing focuses on women and their infants and families during the childbearing cycle.
- Women's health nursing focuses on the special physical, psychologic, and social needs of women throughout their life spans.
- *Healthy People 2020* provides an update on goals for maternal and infant health.
- Nurses caring for women can play an active role in shaping health care systems to be responsive to the needs of contemporary women.
- Childbirth practices have changed to become more focused on the family and allow alternatives in care.
- A variety of factors, including race, age, violence, and human trafficking affect women's health.
- Canada ranks twenty-ninth and the United States ranks thirty-first among industrialized nations in infant mortality rates.
- Evidence-based practice and outcomes orientation are emphasized in current practice.
- Risk management and learning from sentinel events can improve quality of care.
- Research plays a vital role in establishing a scientific base for the care of women and infants.
- Ethical concerns have multiplied with the increasing use of technology and scientific advances.

REFERENCES

AFL-CIO Department of Professional Employees. (2012). *Fact sheet 2012. Nursing: A profile of the profession*. Available at www.dpeaflcio.org/wpcontent/uploads/Nursing-A-Profile-of-the-Profession-2012.pdf.

Agency for Healthcare Research and Quality (AHRQ). (2000). *20 Tips to help prevent medical errors. Patient fact sheet*. Available at www.ahqr.gov/patines-consumer/care-planning/errors/20tips/index.html.

Agency for Healthcare Research and Quality (AHRQ). (2004). *Patient safety indicators*. Available at www.qualityindicators.ahrq.gov.

Agency for Healthcare Research and Quality (AHRQ). (n.d.). *TeamSTEPPS: National implementation*. Available at http://teamstepps.ahrq.gov.

American Academy of Nurse Practitioners. (March 26, 2012). *Nurse practitioners: The key to accessible and cost-effective primary health care*. Press release. Available at www.aanp.org/component/content/article/28-press-room/2012-press-releases/1000-nps-the-key-to-accessible-and-cost-effective-primary-health-care.

American Academy of Pediatrics & American College of Obstetricians and Gynecologists.(2012). *Guidelines for perinatal care* (7th ed.). Washington, DC: AAP/ACOG.

American Nurses Association.(2001). *Code of ethics for nurses with interpretive statements*. Silver Spring, MD: Author.

Association of Women's Health, Obstetric and Neonatal Nurses (AWHONN). (2009a). *Standards and guidelines for professional nursing practice in the care of women and newborns* (7th ed.). Washington, DC: Author.

Association of Women's Health, Obstetric and Neonatal Nurses (AWHONN).(2009b). *Standards for professional perinatal nursing practice and certification in Canada* (2nd ed.). Washington, DC: Author.

Beaulieu, M. J. (2009). Failure to rescue as a process measure to evaluate fetal safety during labor. *MCN: The American Journal of Maternal/Child Nursing, 34*(1), 18–23.

Berg, C. J., Mackay, A. P., Qin, C., et al. (2009). Overview of maternal morbidity during hospitalization for labor and delivery in the United States: 1993-1997 and 2001-2005. *Obstetrics & Gynecology, 113*(5), 1075–1081.

Budiani-Saberi, D. A., Raja, K. R., Findley, K. C., et al. (2014). Human trafficking for organ removal in India: A victim-centered, evidence-based report. *Transplantation*. January 6 (Epub ahead of print).

Bulachek, B. M., Butcher, H. K., Dochterman, J. M., & Wagner, C. (2013). *Nursing interventions classification (NIC)* (6th ed.). St. Louis: Mosby.

Buring, S. M., Brushan, A., Broeseker, A., et al. (2009). Interprofessional education: Definitions, student competencies, and guidelines for implementation. *American Journal of Pharmaceutical Education, 73*(4), 1–8.

Centers for Disease Control and Prevention.(2011). CDC health disparities & inequalities report—United States, 2011. *MMWR Morbidity and Mortality Weekly Report, 60*(Suppl), 1–116.

Centers for Disease Control and Prevention. (2012). *User guide to the 2012 natality public use file*. Available at www.cdc.gov/pub/Health_Statistics/NCHS/Dataset_Documentation/DVS/natality/UserGuide.2012.pdf.

Centers for Disease Control and Prevention. (2013). *Pregnancy mortality surveillance system*. Available at www.dcd.gov/reproductivehealth/MaternalInfant-Health/PMSS.html.

Chin, M. H. (2011). Quality improvement implementation and disparities: The case of the health disparities collaborative. *Medical Care, 49*(Suppl), S65–S71.

Cronenwett, L., Sherwood, G., Barnsteiner, J., et al. (2007). Quality and safety education for nurses. *Nursing Outlook, 55*(3), 122–131.

DeNavas-Walt, C., Proctor, B., & Smith, J. (2012). *Income poverty, and health insurance coverage in the United States: 2011*. U.S. Census Bureau, current population reports, P60–240. Washington, DC: US Government Printing Office.

Dickens, C., & Piano, M. R. (2013). Health literacy and nursing: An update. *American Journal of Nursing, 113*(6), 51–58.

Dovydaitis, T. (2010). Human trafficking: The role of the health care provider. *Journal of Midwifery and Women's Health, 55*(5), 462–467.

Duffy, M. (2011). Facebook, Twitter, and LinkedIn, oh my! *American Journal of Nursing, 111*(4), 56–59.

Flegal, K. M., Carroll, M. D., Ogden, C. L., et al. (2010). Prevalence and trends in obesity among U.S. adults, 1999-2008. *Journal of the American Medical Association, 303*(3), 235–241.

Heisler, E. J. (2012). The U.S. infant mortality rate: International comparisons, underlying factors, and federal programs. *Congressional Research Service.* Available at www.fas.org/spg/crs/misc/R41278.pdf.

Institute of Medicine.(2003). *Health professions education: A bridge to quality.* Washington, DC: National Academies Press.

Institute of Medicine.2010). *The future of nursing: Leading change, advancing health.* Washington, DC: National Academy of Sciences.

Interprofessional Education Collaborative Expert Panel. (2011). *Core competencies for interprofessional collaborative practice: Report of an expert panel.* Washington, DC: Interprofessional Education Collaborative.

The Joanna Briggs Institute. (2013). *JBI grading of recommendations.* Available at http://joannabriggs.org/jbi-approach.html#tabbed-nav-Grades-of-Recommendation.

The Joint Commission. (2009). *Official "do not use" list.* Available at www.jointcommission.org/assets/1/18/Do_Not_Use_List.pdf.

The Joint Commission. (2013). *Sentinel event policy and procedures.* Available at www.jointcommission.org/Sentinel_Event_Policy_and_Procedures.

Jones, W. (2008). *At a glance. Safe motherhood. Promoting health for women before, during, and after pregnancy.* Available at www.cdc.gov/nccdphp/publications/aag/pdf/drh.pdf.

Kaiser Permanente of Colorado. (2014). *SBAR technique for communication: A situational briefing model.* Available at http://www.ihi.org/resources/Pages/Tools/SBARTechniqueforCommunicationASituationalBriefingModel.aspx.

Longley, R. (2013). *Women's heart attack symptoms are different from men's.* Available at usgovinfo.about.com/cs/healthmedical/a/womensami.htm.

Macy, R. J., & Graham, L. M. (2012). Identifying domestic and international sex-trafficking victims during human service provision. *Trauma, Violence, & Abuse, 13*(2), 59–76.

Mahon, S. M., & Crecelius, M. E. (2013). Practice considerations in providing cancer risk assessment and genetic testing in women's health. *Journal of Obstetric, Gynecologic, and Neonatal Nursing, 42*(3), 274–286.

Martin, J. A., Hamilton, B. E., Osterman, M. J. K., et al. (2013). Births: Final data for 2012. *National Vital Statistics Reports, 62*(9), 1–87.

Mathews, T. J., & MacDorman, M. F. (2013). Infant mortality statistics from the 2010 period linked birth/infant death data set. *National Vital Statistics Report, 62*(8), 1–53.

Medicare & Medicaid News. (2013). *Medicare's accountable care organizations continue growth as health care spending slows.* Available at www.seniorjournal.com/NEWS/Medicare/2013/20131223_Medicare's_Accountable_Care_Organizations_Grow_as_Health_Care_Spending_Slows.htm.

Moorhead, S., Johnson, M., Maas, M., & Swanson, E. (2012). *Nursing outcomes classification (NOC)* (5th ed.). St. Louis: Mosby.

Murphy, S. L., Xu, J., & Kochanek, K. (2012). Deaths: Preliminary data for 2010. *National Vital Statistics Reports, 60*(4), 1–51. Hyattsville, MD: National Center for Health Statistics.

National Center for Health Statistics. (2012). *User guide for the 2012 natality public use file.* Hyattsville, MD. Available from www.cdc.gov/nchs/data_access/Vitalstatsonline.htm.

National Council of State Boards of Nursing (NCBSN). (2011). *White paper: A nurse's guide to the use of social media.* Available at www.ncsbn.org/Social_Media.pdf.

National Partnership for Action to End Health Disparities. April, 2011). *National stakeholder strategy for achieving health equity.* Rockville, MD: U.S. Department of Health & Human Services, Office of Minority Health.

National Quality Forum (NQF).(2010). *Safe practices for better healthcare—2010 update: A consensus report.* Washington, DC: NQF.

O'Reilly, K. (2008). *No pay for "never event" errors becoming standard.* Available at www.ama-assn.org/amednews/2008/01/07/prsc0107.htm.

Pham, J. C., Aswani, M. S., Rosen, M., et al. (2012). Reducing medical errors and adverse events. *Annual Review of Medicine, 63,* 447–463.

Sandall, J., Soltani, H., Gates, S., et al. (2013). Midwife-led continuity models versus other models of care for childbearing women. *The Cochrane Collaboration.* CD004667.

Sandy, H. P. (2011). Female genital cutting: An overview. *American Journal of Nurse Practitioners, 15*(1/2), 53–59.

Saver, C. (2010). *Social responsibility: Social media opportunities and pitfalls.* 2010. Available at www.news.nurse.com/article/20100809/NATIONAL01/108090045/-1/frontpage.

Shields, M., Carroll, M. D., & Ogden, C. L. (2011). *Adult obesity prevalence in Canada and the United States, NCHS data brief, no 56.* Hyattsville, MD: National Center for Health Statistics.

Simpson, K. R. (2005). Failure to rescue in obstetrics. *MCN: The American Journal of Maternal/Child Nursing, 30*(1), 76.

Simpson, K. R. (2006). Measuring perinatal patient safety: Review of current methods. *Journal of Obstetric, Gynecologic, and Neonatal Nursing, 35*(3), 432–442.

Simpson, K. R., Knox, G. E., Martin, M., et al. (2011). Michigan Health & Hospital Association Keystone Obstetrics: A statewide collaborative for perinatal patient safety in Michigan. *Joint Commission Journal of Quality & Patient Safety, 37*(12), 544–552.

Squires, D. (May, 2012). Explaining high health care spending in the United States: An international comparison of supply, utilization, prices, and quality. *The Commonwealth Fund, 20.* Available at www.commonwealthfund.org/Publications/Issue-Briefs/2012/May/High-Health-Care-Spending.aspx.

Tong, V. T., Dietz, P. M., Morrow, B., et al. (2013). Trends in smoking before, during, and after pregnancy—Pregnancy risk assessment monitoring system, United States, 40 sites, 2000-2010. *MMWR Morbidity and Mortality Weekly Report, 62*(6), 1–19.

U.S. Census Bureau. (2012). *Table 6. Percent distribution of the projected population by race, and Hispanic origin for the United States: 2015 to 2060.* Available at www.census.gov/population/projections/data/national/2012/summarytables.html.

U.S. Department of Health and Human Services (USDHHS), Health Resources and Services Administration (HRSA), & Maternal and Child Health Bureau. (2010a). *Women's health USA 2010.* Rockville, MD: USDHHS.

U.S. Department of Health and Human Services, & Office of Disease Prevention and Health Promotion. (2010b). *National action plan to improve health literacy.* Washington, DC: Author.

U.S. Department of Health and Human Services. (2011). *HHS action plan to reduce racial and ethnic health disparities.* Available at www.minorityhealth.hhs.gov/npa/files/Plans/HHS/HHS_Plan_complete.pdf.

U.S. Department of Health and Human Services (HHS) & Centers for Medicare & Medicaid Services (CMS). (2012). *Summary of final rule provisions for accountable care organizations under the Medicare shared savings program.* Available at www.cms.gov/Medicare/Medicare-Fee-for-Service-Payment/sharedsavingsprogram/Downloads/ACO_Summary_Factsheet_ICN907404.pdf.

Wilmoth, J. R., Mizoguchi, N., Oestergaard, M. Z., et al. (2012). A new method for deriving global estimates of maternal mortality. *Statistics, Politics, and Policy, 3*(2). Article 3.

World Health Organization. (2013). *Female genital mutilation.* World Health Organization, Fact Sheet # 241. Available at www.who.int/mediacentre/factsheets/fs241/en.

World Health Organization. (2013). *United States of America: Health profile.* Available at www.who.int/hgo/countries/usa.pdf.

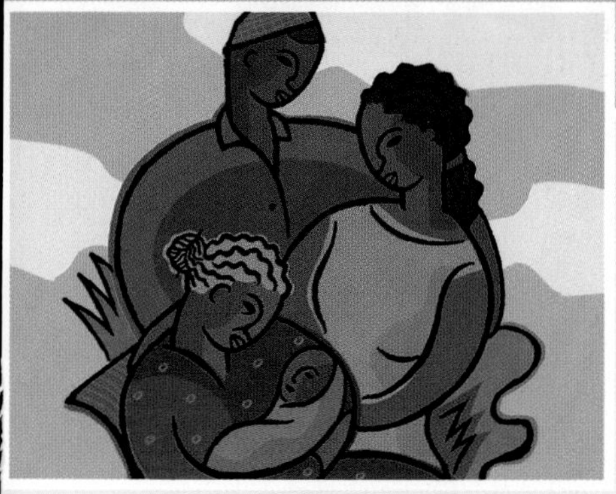

CHAPTER 2

Community Care: The Family and Culture

Raquel Martinez-Campos

http://evolve.elsevier.com/Lowdermilk/MWHC/

LEARNING OBJECTIVES

- Describe the main characteristics of contemporary family forms.
- Identify key factors influencing family health.
- Compare theoretic approaches for working with childbearing families.
- Relate the impact of culture on childbearing families.
- Discuss cultural competence in relation to one's own nursing practice.
- Identify key components of the community assessment process.
- List indicators of community health status and their relevance to perinatal health.
- Describe data sources and methods for obtaining information about community health status.
- Identify predisposing factors and characteristics of vulnerable populations.
- List the potential advantages and disadvantages of home visits.
- Explore telephonic nursing care options in perinatal nursing.
- Describe how home care fits into the maternity continuum of care.
- Describe the nurse's role in perinatal home care.

INTRODUCTION TO FAMILY, CULTURE, COMMUNITY, AND HOME CARE

The composition, structure, and function of the American family have changed dramatically in recent years, largely in response to economic, demographic, sociocultural, and technologic trends that influence family life and health. Despite current efforts to improve the overall health of the nation, there is widespread concern about family health and well-being as a reflection of individual, community, and national health status. Recent economic changes have further reduced the ability to access health care. The Patient Protection and Affordable Care Act (ACA) signed into law in 2010 aims to make insurance affordable, contain costs, strengthen and improve Medicare and Medicaid, and reform the insurance market. In addition to facing significant barriers in accessing needed services, women and families are faced with the challenge of overcoming discrimination in health care practices. It is critical to consider racial and ethnic differences and sexual orientation when addressing the health status of women. American women with a minority racial or ethnic affiliation share poorer outcomes in a wide variety of conditions. Lesbian women may conceal sexual orientation for fear of discrimination. As cultural diversity increases and demographics change, nurses must become culturally competent in order to recognize and reduce or eliminate health disparities (Freund, 2012).

Trends in maternal and infant health in the United States reveal that progress has been made in relation to reduced infant and fetal deaths and use of prenatal care (see Chapter 1). Although progress has been made, low-birth-weight, preterm birth, and infant mortality rates fell short of the *Healthy People 2010* target goals, therefore remaining as high priority areas for *Healthy People 2020*. Among the nation's most pressing challenges are reducing the rate of preterm births and reducing the infant death rate, which in 2011 remained higher than the infant death rate in 46 other countries (U.S. Department of Health and Human Services [HHS], 2013). Because many of these outcomes are preventable through access to prenatal care, the use of preventive health practices clearly demonstrates the need for comprehensive community-based care for mothers, infants, and families. As perinatal health trends emerge, nurses are assuming greater roles in assessing family health status and providing care across the perinatal continuum. This continuum begins with family planning and continues with the following categories of care: preconception (before pregnancy), prenatal, intrapartum, postpartum, newborn, interconception (between pregnancies), and the child from infancy to 1 year of age. In the community, health care ranges from individual care to group and community services and from primary prevention to tertiary care experiences and home health. Depending on the needs of the individual family unit, independent self-management, outpatient care, home care, low risk hospitalization, or specialized intensive care may be appropriate at different points along this continuum.

In community-based health care, both the population (group of people who may or may not interact with each other) and the aggregate (group of people within the larger population who possess some common characteristics) become the focus of intervention. Health professionals are required not only to determine health priorities but also develop successful plans of care to be delivered in the health clinic, the community health center, or the client's home (see Community Activity). This home- and community-based delivery system presents unique challenges for perinatal and maternity nurses.

COMMUNITY ACTIVITY

- Visit the Health Resources and Services Administration (HRSA) website at www.communityhealth.hrsa.gov. What is the definition of a health center by the HRSA? What populations do they serve? What are the different types of health centers?
- Locate a health center in your community at the HRSA website. What types of services do they provide? Do they provide primary and preventive maternal and women's health services? Is care provided regardless of a client's ability to pay?
- Visit your state center for health statistics (SCHS) website. Evaluate the health status of women and infants in your county. Vital statistics include live births, physician versus midwife attended births, out of wedlock births, cesarean births, low birth weight, maternal smoking, and fetal/infant mortality.

THE FAMILY IN CULTURAL AND COMMUNITY CONTEXT

The family and its cultural context play an important role in defining the work of maternity nurses. Despite modern stresses and strains, the family forms a social network that acts as a potent support system for its members. Family health-seeking behavior and relationships with providers are greatly influenced by culturally related health beliefs and values. Ultimately all of these factors have the power to affect maternal and child health outcomes. The current emphasis in working with families is on wellness and empowerment for families to achieve control over their lives. It is therefore essential that nurses become culturally competent in order to provide the most appropriate care possible.

Defining Family

The family has traditionally been viewed as the primary unit of socialization—the basic structural unit within a community. Being the oldest and most persistent of all social institutions, the family plays a pivotal role in health care, representing the primary target of health care delivery for maternal and newborn nurses. As one of society's most important institutions, the family represents a primary social group that influences and is influenced by other people and institutions. A variety of family configurations exist. Each of these is characterized by certain structural features.

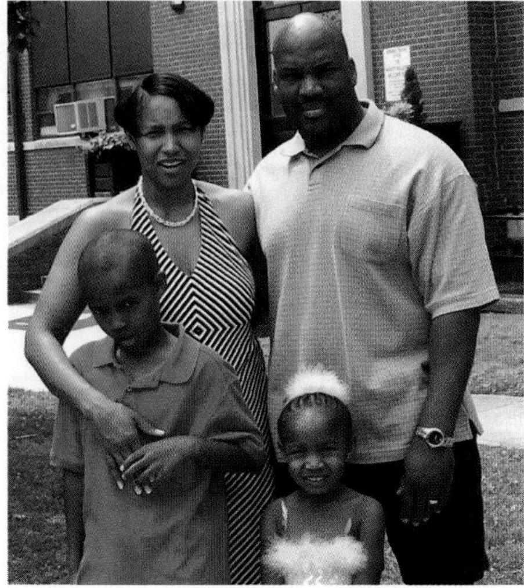

FIG 2-1 Nuclear family. (Courtesy Makeba Felton, Wake Forest, NC.)

Family Organization and Structure

The **nuclear family** has long represented the traditional American family in which husband, wife, and their children (either biologic or adopted) live as an independent unit, sharing roles, responsibilities, and economic resources (Fig. 2-1). Today the number of families living in a nuclear family structure is steadily decreasing in response to societal changes. By race and Hispanic origin, this family structure is represented as follows (Lofquist, Lugaila, O'Connell, M. & Feliz, 2012):

- Caucasian: 51.1%
- Hispanic: 50.1%
- African-American: 28.5%
- Asian: 59.7%
- American Indian and Alaska Native: 40.1%
- Native Hawaiian and Pacific Islander: 51.3%

According to the 2010 U.S. Vital and Health Statistics, 48.4% of children younger than the age of 18 live in a nuclear family. The percent distribution for non-Hispanic black children was 20.5%, 41% for Hispanic children, and 57.3% for non-Hispanic white children (Blackwell, 2010).

Many nuclear families have other relatives living in the same household. These extended family members include grandparents, aunts, uncles, or other people related by blood. Members of extended families can also live in close proximity to the nuclear family (Fig. 2-2). Due to societal changes, internet access, increased mobility, these families may also be a long-distance unit. For some groups, such as African-American and Hispanic-American, extended family is an important resource in terms of preventive health behavior. The **extended family** is becoming more common as American society ages. The extended family provides social, emotional, and financial support to one another. It is therefore important for nurses to recognize the desire for people of many cultures to include their family in making important decisions. This has implications for privacy and sharing individual health information under Health Insurance Portability and Accountability Act (HIPAA) rules.

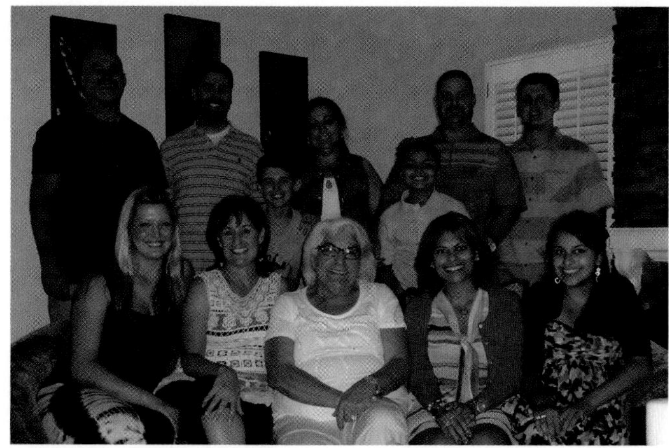

FIG 2-2 Extended family. (Courtesy Raquel Martinez-Campos, Lake Forest, CA.)

Multigenerational families consisting of three or more generations of relatives (grandparents, children, and grandchildren) are becoming increasingly common. In 2010 they made up 4.4% of all households (Lofquist et al., 2012). This type of arrangement can create stress for some because children must care for their parents as well as their own children. Other types of multigenerational families consist of grandparents supporting the children and grandchildren or as sole caregivers for the grandchildren.

No-parent families are those in which children live independently in foster or kinship care such as living with a grandparent. An estimated 5.4 million children in the United States live with a grandparent. Of these grandparents, 2.7 million are responsible for most of the basic needs (i.e., food, shelter, and clothing) of one or more grandchildren (U.S. Census Bureau, 2011a).

Married-blended families, those formed as a result of divorce and remarriage, consist of unrelated family members (stepparents, stepchildren, and stepsiblings) who join to create a new household. These family groups frequently involve a biologic or adoptive parent whose spouse may or may not have adopted the child.

Cohabiting-parent families are those in which children live with two unmarried biologic parents or two adoptive parents. Hispanic children are more than twice as likely as African-American children to live in cohabiting-parent families and about four times as likely as Caucasian children to live in this kind of family arrangement (Lofquist et al., 2012).

Single-parent families comprise an unmarried biologic or adoptive parent who may or may not be living with other adults. The single-parent family may result from the loss of a spouse by death, divorce, separation, or desertion; from either an unplanned or planned pregnancy; or from the adoption of a child by an unmarried woman or man. This family structure is continually on the rise. In 2012 according to the U.S. Census Bureau, 24% of children lived with only their mothers, 4% lived with only their fathers, and 4% lived with neither of their parents (America's Children, 2013).

The single-parent family tends to be vulnerable economically and socially, which can create an unstable and deprived environment for the growth of children. This is turn affects health status, school achievement, and high risk behaviors for these children (Scharte & Bolte, 2012). Alternatively some families become more stable with the absence of drugs, alcohol, and/or physical/emotional abuse.

Homosexual families (lesbian, gay, bisexual, and transgender [LGBT]) may live together with or without children. Usually formed by same-sex couples, they can also consist of single LGBT parents or multiple parenting figures. Children in LGBT families may be the offspring of previous heterosexual unions, conceived by one member of a lesbian couple through natural or therapeutic insemination, conceived by a gay couple using a surrogate, or adopted. Approximately 594,000 same-sex couple households lived in the United States in 2010, raising about 115,000 children ages less than 18 years. When these children are combined with LGBT parents who are raising children, almost 2 million children are being raised by LGBT parents in the United States (Siegel & Perrin, 2013).

The Family in Society

The social context for the family can be viewed in relation to social and demographic trends that define the population as a whole. Racial and ethnic diversity of the population has grown dramatically, necessitating consideration of such diversity in provision of health care. According to the 2010 U.S. Census, approximately 36.3% of the population belongs to a racial or ethnic minority group (Centers for Disease Control and Prevention [CDC], 2013a).

THEORETIC APPROACHES TO UNDERSTANDING FAMILIES

Family Nursing

Family plays a pivotal role in health care, representing the primary target of health care delivery for maternal and newborn nurses. It is crucial that nurses assist families as they incorporate new additions to their family (see Nursing Care Plan). When treating the woman and family with respect and dignity, health care providers listen to and honor perspectives and choices of the woman and family. They share information with families in ways that are positive, useful, timely, complete, and accurate. The family is supported in participating in the care and decision making at the level of their choice.

Because so many variables affect ways of relating, the nurse must be aware that family members may interact and communicate with each other in ways that are distinct from those of the nurse's own family of origin. Most families will hold some beliefs about health that are different from those of the nurse. Their beliefs can conflict with principles of health care management predominant in the Western health care system.

Family Theories

A family theory can be used to describe families and how the family unit responds to events both within and outside the family. Each family theory makes certain assumptions about the family and has inherent strengths and limitations. Most nurses use a combination of theories in their work with families. A brief synopsis of several theories useful in working with families is included in Table 2-1. Application of these concepts can guide assessment and interventions for the family.

NURSING CARE PLAN

Incorporating the Infant into the Family

NURSING DIAGNOSIS	EXPECTED OUTCOME	NURSING INTERVENTIONS	RATIONALES
Readiness for Enhanced Family Coping related to adaptation of family to new infant	Family members will verbalize that individual and family goals are met during a smooth transition of new family member into the home.	Assess type and amount of support available to family on daily basis during postpartum period.	To facilitate adaptation of family to situation of a new member
		Encourage family to use past successful coping mechanisms.	To enhance ability to cope with new situation and promote self-esteem
		Encourage mother to use family and other support or services.	To carry out daily household tasks to permit her to focus on herself and infant
		Suggest that woman take time to rest when infant sleeps.	To conserve energy for healing and limit responsibility to herself and infant
		Assess family structure and relationships, including culture.	To evaluate if longer period of adjustment may be expected
		Teach family about sensory needs and capabilities of infant.	To motivate family to meet infant's needs and set realistic expectations for infant's capabilities
		Refer to parent support group or community agencies, as needed.	To facilitate and validate ongoing positive adjustment of family to new family member
Ineffective Role Performance related to developmental challenge of addition of new family member	Each family member will verbalize realistic expectations regarding his or her role in the family and formulate a plan to incorporate the role into overall family goals.	Assess family structure, roles, and each member's perception of his or her role in family.	To evaluate impact of new member on structure and roles of family as perceived by members
		Evaluate individual's perception of goals and new roles during this transition.	To promote early intervention and correct any misinterpretation
		Encourage discussion of family members' thoughts and feelings regarding this transition.	To promote open communication and trust
		Provide positive reinforcement for family members' actions that promote positive environment for infant.	To increase self-esteem and provide encouragement
		Refer to community support groups.	To provide group reinforcement and further assistance
		Give information about sibling and grandparent classes and support groups as available.	To promote empowerment and self-esteem for significant others in family

Family Assessment

When selecting a family assessment framework, an appropriate model for a perinatal nurse is one that is a health-promoting rather than an illness-care model. The low risk family can be assisted in promoting a healthy pregnancy, childbirth, and integration of the newborn into the family. The high risk perinatal family has illness-care needs, and the nurse can help to meet those needs while also promoting the health of the childbearing family.

A family assessment tool such as the Calgary Family Assessment Model (CFAM) (Box 2-1) can be used as a guide for assessing aspects of the family. Such an assessment is based on "the nurse's personal and professional life experiences, beliefs, and relationships with those being interviewed" (Wright & Leahey, 2012) and is not "the truth" about the family but, rather, one perspective at one point in time.

The CFAM comprises three major categories: structural, developmental, and functional. Several subcategories are within each category. The three assessment categories and the many subcategories can be conceptualized as a branching diagram (Fig. 2-3). The categories and subcategories can be used to guide the assessment that will provide data to help the nurse better understand the family and formulate a nursing care plan. The nurse asks questions of family members about themselves to gain understanding of the structure, development, and function of the family at this point in time. Not all questions within the subcategories should be asked at the first interview, and some questions may not be appropriate for all families. Although individuals are the ones interviewed, the focus of the assessment is on interaction of individuals within the family.

Graphic Representations of Families

A family *genogram* (family tree format depicting relationships of family members over at least three generations) (Fig. 2-4) provides valuable information about a family and can be placed

TABLE 2-1 Theories and Models Relevant to Family Nursing Practice

THEORY	SYNOPSIS OF THEORY
Family Systems Theory (Wright & Leahey, 2012)	The family is viewed as a unit, and interactions among family members are studied rather than studying individuals. A family system is part of a larger suprasystem and is composed of many subsystems. The family as a whole is greater than the sum of its individual members. A change in one family member affects all family members. The family is able to create a balance between change and stability. Family members' behaviors are best understood from a view of circular rather than linear causality.
Family Life Cycle (Developmental) Theory (Carter & McGoldrick, 1999)	Families move through stages. The family life cycle is the context in which to examine the identity and development of the individual. Relationships among family members go through transitions. Although families have roles and functions, a family's main value is in relationships that are irreplaceable. The family involves different structures and cultures organized in various ways. Developmental stresses may disrupt the life cycle process.
Family Stress Theory (Boss, 1996)	How families react to stressful events is the focus. Family stress can be studied within the internal and external contexts in which the family is living. The internal context involves elements that a family can change or control, such as family structure, psychologic defenses, and philosophic values and beliefs. The external context consists of the time and place in which a particular family finds itself and over which the family has no control, such as the culture of the larger society, the time in history, the economic state of society, maturity of the individuals involved, success of the family in coping with stressors, and genetic inheritance.
McGill Model of Nursing (Allen, 1997; Gottlieb & Gottlieb, 2007)	Strength-based approach in clinical practice with families, as opposed to a deficit approach, is the focus. Identification of family strengths and resources, provision of feedback about strengths, and assistance given to family to develop and elicit strengths and use resources are key interventions.
Health Belief Model (Becker, 1974; Janz & Becker, 1984)	The goal of the model is to reduce cultural and environmental barriers that interfere with access to health care. Key elements of the Health Belief Model include the following: perceived susceptibility, perceived severity, perceived benefits, perceived barriers, cues to action, and confidence.
Human Developmental Ecology (Bronfenbrenner, 1979; 1989)	Behavior is a function of interaction of traits and abilities with the environment. Major concepts include ecosystem, niches (social roles), adaptive range, and ontogenetic development. Individuals are "embedded in a microsystem [role and relations], a mesosystem [interrelations between two or more settings], an exosystem [external settings that do not include the person], and a macrosystem [culture]" (Klein & White, 1996). Change over time is incorporated in the chronosystem.

BOX 2-1 Calgary Family Assessment Model

There are three major categories of the Calgary Family Assessment Model (CFAM): structural, developmental, and functional. Each category has several subcategories. In this box only the major categories are listed. A few sample questions are included.

Structural Assessment

Determine the members of the family, relationship among family members, and context of family.

Genograms and ecomaps (see Figs. 2-4; 2-5) are useful in outlining the internal and external structures of a family.

Sample Questions

- Who are the members of your family?
- Has anyone moved in or out lately?
- Are there any family members who don't live with you?

Developmental Assessment

Describe the life cycle—that is, the typical trajectory that most families experience.

Sample questions

- Is your family the size you wanted?
- When you think back, what do you most enjoy about your life?
- What do you regret about your life?
- Have you made plans for your care as your health declines?

Functional Assessment

Evaluate the way in which individuals behave in relation to each other in instrumental and expressive aspects. (Instrumental aspects are activities of daily living; expressive aspects include communication, problem solving, roles, etc.)

Sample questions

- Which one of the family is responsible for helping with the children while the mother is caring for the newborn?
- Whose turn is it to do the shopping and fix dinner for the family?
- How can we get more family involvement in care of the household?

Data from Wright, L.M., & Leahey, M. (2012). *Nurses and families: A guide to family assessment and intervention* (6th ed.). Philadelphia: F.A. Davis.

in the nursing care plan for easy access by care providers. An *ecomap,* a graphic portrayal of social relationships of the women and family, may also help the nurse understand the social environment of the family and identify support systems available to them (Fig. 2-5). Software is available to generate genograms and ecomaps (www.interpersonaluniverse.net).

THE FAMILY IN A CULTURAL CONTEXT

Cultural Factors Related to Family Health

The culture of an individual and a group is influenced by religion, environment, and historic events and plays a powerful role in the individual's and group's behavior and patterns of human interaction. Culture is not static; it is an ongoing process that influences a woman throughout her entire life, from birth to death. Culture is an essential element of what defines us as people.

Cultural knowledge includes beliefs and values about each facet of life and is passed from one generation to the next. Cultural beliefs and traditions relate to food, language, religion, art, health and healing practices, kinship relationships, and all other aspects of community, family, and individual life. Culture has also been shown to have a direct effect on health behaviors. Values, attitudes, and beliefs that are culturally acquired may influence perceptions of illness, as well as health care–seeking behavior and response to treatment. The political, social, and

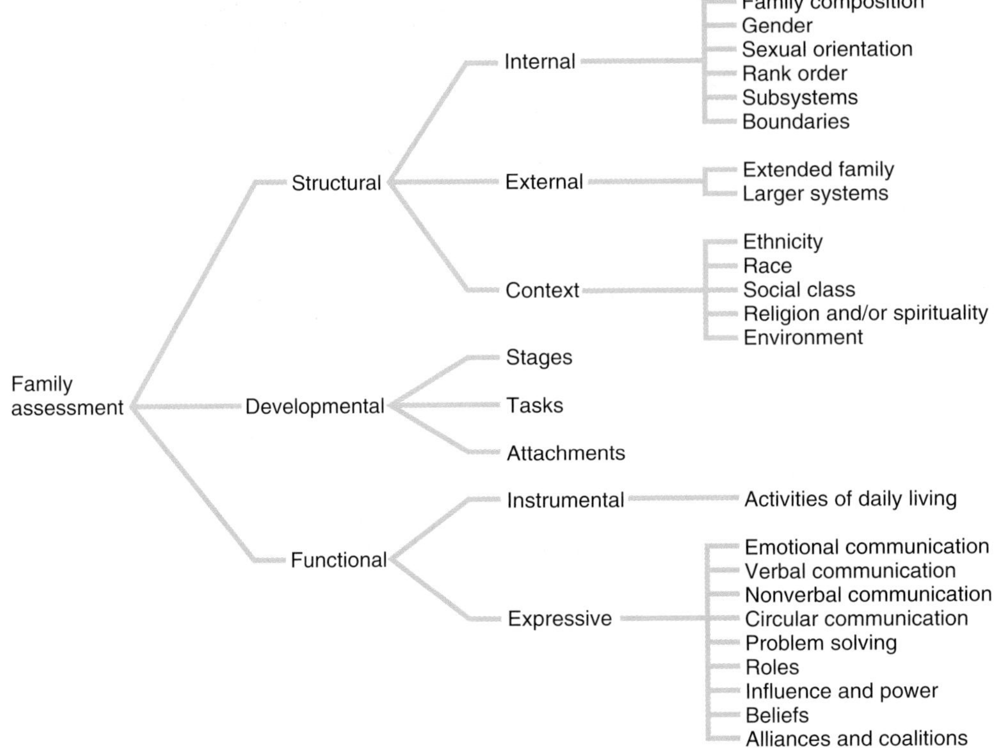

FIG 2-3 Branching diagram of Calgary Family Assessment Model (CFAM). (From Wright, L.M., & Leahey, M. [2012]. *Nurses and families: a guide to family assessment and intervention* [6th ed.]. Philadelphia: FA Davis).

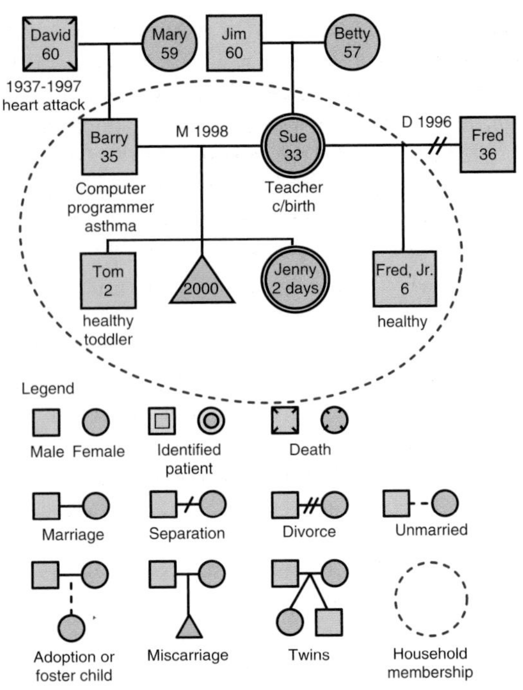

FIG 2-4 Example of a family genogram.

economic context of people's lives is also part of the cultural experience.

Culture, shared beliefs and values of a group, plays a powerful role in an individual's behavior, particularly when the individual is sick. Understanding a culture can provide insight into how a person reacts to illness, pain, and invasive medical procedures, as well as patterns of human interaction and expressions of emotion. The effect of these influences must be assessed by health care professionals in providing health care and developing effective intervention strategies.

Many subcultures may be found within each culture. **Subculture** refers to a group existing within a larger cultural system that retains its own characteristics. A subculture may be an ethnic group or a group organized in other ways. For example, in the United States and Canada, many ethnic subcultures such as African-Americans, Asian-Americans, Hispanic-Americans, and Native Americans exist. It is important to note that subcultures also exist within these groups. In addition, the Caucasian population in America has multiple subcultures of its own. Because every identified cultural group has subcultures and because it is impossible to study every subculture in depth, greater differences may exist among and between groups than is generally acknowledged. It is important to be familiar with common cultural practices within these subgroups. However, it is also important to avoid the generalization that every person practices every cultural belief within a group.

In a multicultural society, many groups can influence traditions and practices. As cultural groups come into contact with each other, acculturation and assimilation may occur.

Acculturation refers to the changes that occur within one group or among several groups when people from different cultures come into contact with one another. People may retain some of their own culture while adopting cultural practices of the dominant society. This familiarization among cultural groups results in overt behavioral similarity, especially in mannerisms, styles, and practices. Dress, language patterns,

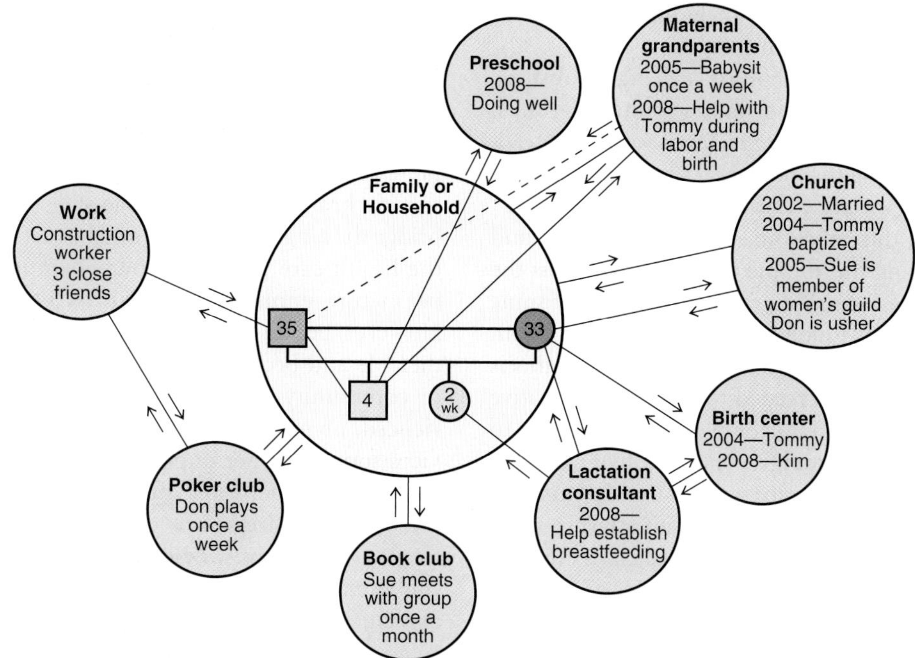

FIG 2-5 Example of an ecomap. An ecomap describes social relationships and depicts available supports.

food choices, and health practices are often much slower to adapt to the influence of acculturation. In the United States, second-generation Americans consider themselves to be fully American (Pew Research Center, 2013).

During times of family transitions such as childbearing, or during crisis or illness, a woman may rely on old cultural patterns even after becoming acculturated in many ways. This is consistent with the family developmental theory (Carter & McGoldrick, 1999) that states that during times of stress, people revert to practices and behaviors that are most comfortable and familiar.

Assimilation occurs when a cultural group loses its cultural identity and becomes part of the dominant culture. Assimilation is the process by which groups "melt" into the mainstream, thus accounting for the notion of a "melting pot," a phenomenon that has been said to occur in the United States. This is illustrated by individuals who identify themselves as being of Irish or German descent, without having any remaining cultural practices or values linked specifically to that culture such as food preparation techniques, style of dress, or proficiency in the language associated with their reported cultural heritage. Spector (2013) asserts that in the United States, the melting pot, with its dream of a common culture, is a myth. Instead, a mosaic phenomenon exists in which we must accept and appreciate the differences among people.

Implications for Nursing

As our society becomes more culturally diverse, it is essential that nurses become culturally competent. Nurses must examine their own beliefs so that they have a better appreciation and understanding of their clients' beliefs. Understanding the concepts of ethnocentrism and cultural relativism can help nurses care for families in a multicultural society.

Ethnocentrism is the view that one's own culture's way of doing things is best (Giger, 2013). Although the United States is a culturally diverse nation, the prevailing practice of health care is based on the beliefs and practices held by members of the dominant culture, primarily Caucasians of European descent. This practice is based on the biomedical model that focuses on curing disease states.

Pregnancy and childbirth, in this biomedical perspective, are viewed as processes with inherent risks that are most appropriately managed by using scientific knowledge and advanced technology. The medical perspective stands in direct contrast with the belief systems of many cultures. Among many women, birth is viewed as a completely normal process that can be managed with a minimum of involvement from health care practitioners. When encountering behavior in women unfamiliar with the biomedical model or those who reject it, the nurse may become frustrated and impatient and may label the women's behavior as inappropriate and believe that it conflicts with "good" health practices. If the Western health care system provides the nurse's only standard for judgment, the behavior of the nurse is ethnocentric.

Cultural relativism is the opposite of ethnocentrism. It refers to learning about and applying the standards of another's culture to activities within that culture. The nurse recognizes that people from different cultural backgrounds comprehend the same objects and situations differently. In other words, culture determines viewpoint. Cultural relativism does not require nurses to accept the beliefs and values of another culture. Instead, nurses recognize that the behavior of others can be based on a system of logic different from their own. Cultural relativism affirms the uniqueness and value of every culture.

Childbearing Beliefs and Practices

Nurses working with childbearing families care for families from many different cultures and ethnic groups. To provide culturally competent care the nurse must assess clients' beliefs and practices. When working with childbearing families, a nurse considers all aspects of culture, including communication, space, time orientation, and family roles.

Communication often creates the most challenging obstacle for nurses working with clients from diverse cultural groups. Communication is not merely the exchange of words. Instead, it involves (1) understanding the individual's language, including subtle variations in meaning and distinctive dialects; (2) appreciating individual differences in interpersonal style; and (3) accurately interpreting the volume of speech as well as the meanings of touch and gestures. For example, members of some cultural groups tend to speak loudly when they are excited, with great emotion and with vigorous and animated gestures; this is true whether their excitement is related to positive or negative events or emotions. It is important therefore for the nurse to avoid rushing to judgment regarding a person's intent when the client is speaking, especially in a language not understood by the nurse. Instead, the nurse should withhold an interpretation of what has been expressed until it is possible to clarify the client's intent. The nurse needs to enlist the assistance of a person who can help verify with the client the true intent and meaning of the communication (see Clinical Reasoning Case Study).

CLINICAL REASONING CASE STUDY

Providing Culturally Appropriate Care

Elisabeth, a 22-year-old first-generation Mexican-American, comes into your office for her initial prenatal visit. You are concerned because Elisabeth's fundal height is consistent with 32 weeks of gestation and this is her first prenatal visit. Elisabeth, who lives with her husband, four children (ages 6, 4, and 3 years and 15 months), her mother, her aunt, and her uncle, states that she has been doing well this pregnancy and did not start prenatal care in her previous pregnancies until she was almost ready to give birth. She also comments that all the babies were full term with uneventful labors and births. In obtaining the history you note the presence of a safety pin in Elisabeth's shirt and wonder what this is for. You want to provide culturally competent care to this woman and her family.

1. Evidence—Is there sufficient evidence to support the components of culturally competent care for Elisabeth?
2. Assumptions—Describe an underlying assumption about culturally competent care for Elisabeth in relation to these topics:
   a. The view of pregnancy in Elisabeth's culture
   b. The role of family in Elisabeth's culture
   c. The acceptability for women of Elisabeth's age to begin having children at such young ages
   d. The religious beliefs that Elisabeth may have that affect contraception
3. What implications and priorities for nursing care can be made at this time?
4. Does the evidence objectively support your conclusion?

Inconsistencies between the language of clients and the language of providers present a significant barrier to effective health care. For example, there are many dialects of Spanish that vary by geographic location. Because of the diversity of cultures and languages within the U.S. and Canadian populations, health care agencies are increasingly seeking the services of *interpreters* (of oral communication from one language to another) or *translators* (of written words from one language to another) to bridge these gaps and fulfill their obligation for culturally and linguistically appropriate health care (Box 2-2). Finding the best possible interpreter in the circumstance is critically important as well. Ideally, interpreters should have the same native language and be of the same religion or have the same country of origin as the client. Interpreters should have specific health-related language skills and experience and help bridge the language and cultural barriers between the client and the health care provider. The person interpreting also should be mature enough to be trusted with private information. However, because the nature of nursing care is not always predictable and because nursing care that is provided in a home or community setting does not always allow for expert, experienced, or mature adult interpreters, ideal interpretative services sometimes are impossible to find when they are needed. In crisis or emergency situations, or when family members are extremely stressed or emotionally upset, it may be necessary to use relatives, neighbors, or children as interpreters. If this situation occurs, the nurse must ensure that the client is in agreement and comfortable with using the available interpreter to assist. Having a man or a child interpret for a woman may create embarrassment and interfere with obtaining an accurate history or detail of symptoms.

When using an interpreter the nurse respects the family by creating an atmosphere of respect and privacy. Questions should be addressed to the woman and not to the interpreter. Even though an interpreter will of necessity be exposed to sensitive and privileged information about the family, the nurse should take care to ensure that confidentiality is maintained. A quiet location free from interruptions is ideal for interpretive services to take place. Culturally and linguistically appropriate educational materials that are easy to read, with appropriate text and graphics, should be available to assist the woman and her family in understanding health care information. To ensure understanding and avoid liability issues, it is important to make certain that the material has been translated by someone who is trained appropriately.

Personal Space

Cultural traditions define the appropriate personal space for various social interactions. Although the need for personal space varies from person to person and with the situation, the actual physical dimensions of comfort zones and taboos differ from culture to culture. Actions such as touching, placing the woman in proximity to others, taking away personal possessions, and making decisions for the woman can decrease personal security and heighten anxiety. Conversely, respecting the need for distance allows the woman to maintain control over personal space and support personal autonomy, thereby increasing her sense of security. Nurses must touch clients; however, they frequently do so without any awareness of the emotional distress they may be causing clients.

Time Orientation

Time orientation is a fundamental way in which culture affects health behaviors. People in cultural groups may be relatively more oriented to past, present, or future. Those who focus on the past strive to maintain tradition or the status quo and have little motivation for formulating goals. In contrast, individuals who focus primarily on the present neither plan for the future

BOX 2-2 Working with an Interpreter

Step 1: Before the interview

A. Outline your statements and questions. List the key pieces of information you want/need to know.

B. Learn something about the culture so that you can converse informally with the interpreter.

Step 2: Meeting with the interpreter

A. Introduce yourself to the interpreter and converse informally. This is the time to find out how well he or she speaks English. No matter how proficient or what age the interpreter is, be respectful. Some ways to show respect are to ask a cultural question to acknowledge that you can learn from the interpreter, or you could learn one word or phrase from the interpreter.

B. Emphasize that you do want the client to ask questions, because some cultures consider this inappropriate behavior.

C. Make sure the interpreter is comfortable with the technical terms you need to use. If not, take some time to explain them.

Step 3: During the interview

A. Ask your questions and explain your statements (see Step 1).

B. Make sure that the interpreter understands which parts of the interview are most important. You usually have limited time with the interpreter, and you want to have adequate time at the end for client questions.

C. Try to get a feel for how much is "getting through." No matter what the language is, if in relating information to the client, the interpreter uses far fewer or far more words than you do, something else is going on.

D. Stop every now and then and ask the interpreter, "How is it going?" You may not get a totally accurate answer, but you will have emphasized to the interpreter your strong desire to focus on the task at hand. If there are language problems (1) speak slowly; (2) use gestures (e.g., fingers to count or point to body parts); and (3) use pictures.

E. Ask the interpreter to elicit questions. This may be difficult, but it is worth the effort.

F. Identify cultural issues that may conflict with your requests or instructions.

G. Use the interpreter to help problem solve or at least give insight into possibilities for solutions.

Step 4: After the interview

A. Speak to the interpreter and try to get an idea of what went well and what could be improved. This will help you to be more effective in the future with this or another interpreter.

B. Make notes on what you learned for your future reference or to help a colleague.

Remember

Your interview is a *collaboration* between you and the interpreter. *Listen* as well as speak.

NOTES:

1. The interpreter may be a child, grandchild, or sibling of the client. Be sensitive to the fact that the child is playing an adult role.
2. Be sensitive to cultural and situational differences (e.g., an interview with someone from urban Germany will likely be different from an interview with someone from a transitional refugee camp).
3. Younger females telling older males what to do may be a problem for both a female nurse and a female interpreter. This is not the time to pioneer new gender relations. Be aware that in some cultures it is difficult for a woman to talk about some topics with a husband or a father present.

Courtesy Elizabeth Whalley, PhD, San Francisco State University.

nor consider the experiences of the past. These individuals do not necessarily adhere to strict schedules and are often described as "living for the moment," or "marching to their own drummer." Individuals oriented to the future maintain a focus on achieving long-term goals.

The time orientation of the childbearing family can affect nursing care. For example, talking to a family about bringing the infant to the clinic for follow-up examinations (events in the future) may be difficult for the family that is focused on the present concerns of day-to-day survival. Because a family with a future-oriented sense of time plans far in advance, thinking about the long-term consequences of present actions, they may be more likely to return as scheduled for follow-up visits. Despite the differences in time orientation, each family can be equally concerned for the well-being of its newborn.

Family Roles

Family roles involve the expectations and behaviors associated with a member's position in the larger family system (e.g., mother, father, grandparent). Social class and cultural norms also affect these roles, with distinct expectations for men and women clearly determined by social norms. For example, culture may influence whether a man actively participates in the pregnancy and childbirth, yet maternity care practitioners working in the Western health care system expect fathers to be involved. This can create a significant conflict between the nurse and the role expectations of very traditional Mexican or Arab families, who usually view the birthing experience as a female affair (see Cultural Considerations box). The way that health care practitioners manage such a family's care molds its experience and perception of the Western health care system.

CULTURAL CONSIDERATIONS

Questions to Ask to Elicit Cultural Expectations About Childbearing

1. What do you and your family think you should do to remain healthy during pregnancy?
2. What can you do to improve your health and the health of your baby?
3. What foods will help make a healthy baby?
4. Who do you want with you during your labor?
5. What can your labor support person do to help you be most comfortable during labor?
6. What actions are important for you and your family after the baby's birth?
7. What do you and your family expect from the nurse(s) caring for you?
8. How will family members participate in your pregnancy, childbirth, and parenting?

BOX 2-3 Strategies for Care Delivery and Providing Culturally Appropriate Care

Strategies for Care Delivery
- Break down the language barriers.
- Explain your rationale and reasons for suggestions.
- Integrate folk and Western treatments.
- Enlist the family caretaker and others.
- Get consent from the right person.
- Provide language-appropriate materials.

Providing Appropriate Care
- Ask about traditional beliefs, such as the role of hot and cold.
- Be sensitive regarding interpreters and language barriers.
- Ask about important dietary practices, particularly those related to events such as childbirth.
- Ask about group practices and beliefs.
- Ask about a woman's fears, and those of her family, regarding an unfamiliar care setting.

From Mattson, S. (2000). Providing culturally competent care: Strategies and approaches for perinatal clients, *AWHONN Lifelines*, *4*(5), 37-39.

In maternity nursing and women's health care, the nurse supports and nurtures the beliefs that promote physical or emotional adaptation to childbearing. However, if certain beliefs might be harmful, the nurse should carefully explore them with the woman and use them in the reeducation and modification process. Strategies for care delivery and providing appropriate care are presented in Box 2-3.

Table 2-2 provides examples of some cultural beliefs and practices surrounding childbearing.

The cultural beliefs and customs in this table are categorized on the basis of distinct cultural traditions and are not practiced by all members of the cultural group in every part of the country. Women from these cultural and ethnic groups may adhere to a few, all, or none of the practices listed. In using this table as a guide, the nurse should take care to avoid making stereotypic assumptions about any person based on sociocultural-spiritual affiliations. Nurses should exercise sensitivity in working with every family, being careful to assess the ways in which they apply their own mixture of cultural traditions.

TABLE 2-2 Traditional* Cultural Beliefs and Practices: Childbearing and Parenting

PREGNANCY	CHILDBIRTH	PARENTING
Hispanic (Based primarily on knowledge of Mexican-Americans; members of the Hispanic community have their origins in Spain, Cuba, Central and South America, Mexico, Puerto Rico, and other Spanish-speaking countries.)		
Pregnancy Pregnancy desired soon after marriage Late prenatal care Expectant mother influenced strongly by mother or mother-in-law Cool air in motion considered dangerous during pregnancy Unsatisfied food cravings thought to cause a birthmark Some pica observed in the eating of ashes or dirt (not common) Milk avoided because it causes large babies and difficult births Many predictions about sex of baby May be unacceptable and frightening to have pelvic examination by male health care provider Use of herbs to treat common complaints of pregnancy Drinking chamomile tea thought to ensure effective labor May wear ribbon or band around pregnant belly in belief that baby will be born healthy	***Labor*** Use of *partera* or lay midwife preferred in some places; may prefer presence of mother rather than husband After birth of baby, mother's legs brought together to prevent air from entering uterus Loud behavior in labor ***Postpartum*** Diet may be restricted after birth; for first 2 days only boiled milk and toasted tortillas permitted (special foods to restore warmth to body) Bed rest for 3 days after birth Keep warm Delay bathing Mother's head and feet protected from cold air; bathing permitted after 14 days Mother often cared for by her own mother Forty-day restriction on sexual intercourse Mother may want baby's first wet diaper to wipe her face in belief that it aids in making "mask of pregnancy" go away	***Newborn*** Breastfeeding begun after third day; colostrum may be considered "filthy" or "spoiled" or just not enough nourishment Olive oil or castor oil given to stimulate passage of meconium Male infant not circumcised Female infant's ears pierced Belly band used to prevent umbilical hernia Religious medal worn by mother during pregnancy; placed around infant's neck Infant protected from *mal de ojo* ("evil eye") Various remedies used to treat *mal de ojo* and fallen fontanel (depressed fontanel)
African-American (Members of the African-American community, many of whom are descendants of slaves, have different origins. Today a number of black Americans have immigrated from Africa, the West Indies, the Dominican Republic, Haiti, and Jamaica. There is much diversity among countries and tribes.)		
Pregnancy Acceptance of pregnancy depends on economic status Pregnancy thought to be state of "wellness," which is often the reason for delay in seeking prenatal care, especially by lower-income African-Americans Old-wives' tales include beliefs that having a picture taken during pregnancy will cause stillbirth and reaching up will cause cord to strangle baby Craving for certain foods, including chicken, greens, clay, starch, and dirt Pregnancy may be viewed by African-American men as a sign of their virility	***Labor*** Use of "Granny midwife" in certain parts of United States Varied emotional responses: some cry out, some display stoic behavior to avoid calling attention to selves Woman may arrive at hospital in far-advanced labor Emotional support often provided by other women, especially the woman's own mother ***Postpartum*** Vaginal bleeding seen as sign of sickness; tub baths and shampooing of hair prohibited Sassafras tea thought to have healing power Eating liver thought to cause heavier vaginal bleeding because of its high "blood" content	***Newborn*** Feeding very important: "good" baby thought to eat well Early introduction of solid foods May breastfeed or bottle-feed; breastfeeding may be considered embarrassing Parents fearful of spoiling baby Commonly call baby by nicknames May use excessive clothing to keep baby warm Belly band used to prevent umbilical hernia Abundant use of oil on baby's scalp and skin Strong feeling of family, community, and religion

TABLE 2-2 Traditional* Cultural Beliefs and Practices: Childbearing and Parenting—cont'd

Pregnancy	*Labor*	*Newborn*
Asian-American		
(Typically refers to groups from China, Korea, the Philippines, Japan, Southeast Asia [particularly Thailand], Indochina, and Vietnam)		
Pregnancy	***Labor***	***Newborn***
Pregnancy considered time when mother "has happiness in her body" Pregnancy seen as natural process Strong preference for female health care provider Belief in theory of hot and cold May omit soy sauce in diet to prevent dark-skinned baby Prefer soup made with ginseng root as general strength tonic Milk usually excluded from diet because it causes stomach distress Inactivity or sleeping late may cause difficult birth	Mother attended by other women, especially her own mother Father does not actively participate Labor in silence Cesarean birth not desired but cooperative if needed ***Postpartum*** Must protect self from *yin* (cold forces) for 30 days Ambulation limited Shower and bathing prohibited Warm room Diet: Warm fluids Some women are vegetarians Korean mother served seaweed soup with rice Chinese diet high in hot foods Chinese mother avoids fruits and vegetables	Concept of family important and valued Father is head of household; mother plays a subordinate role Birth of boy preferred May delay naming child Some groups (e.g., Vietnamese) believe colostrum is dirty; therefore, they may delay breastfeeding until milk comes in
European-American		
(Members of the European-American [Caucasian] community have their origins in countries such as Ireland, Great Britain, Germany, Italy, and France.)		
Pregnancy	***Labor***	***Newborn***
Pregnancy viewed as a condition that requires medical attention to ensure health Emphasis on early prenatal care Variety of childbirth education programs available, and participation encouraged Technology driven Emphasis on nutrition science Involvement of the father valued Written sources of information including online sources and DVDs valued	Birth is a public concern Technology dominated Birthing process in institutional setting valued Involvement of father expected Physician seen as head of team ***Postpartum*** Emphasis or focus on early bonding Medical interventions for dealing with discomfort Early ambulation and activity emphasized Self-management valued	Increased popularity of breastfeeding Breastfeeding begins as soon as possible after childbirth Facilitate bonding with "sacred hour after birth" ***Parenting*** Motherhood and transition to parenting seen as stressful time Nuclear family valued, although single-parenting and other forms of parenting more acceptable than in the past Women often deal with multiple roles Early return to pre-pregnancy activities
Native American		
(Many different tribes exist within the Native American culture; viewpoints vary according to tribal customs and beliefs.)		
Pregnancy	***Labor***	***Newborn***
Pregnancy considered a normal, natural process Late prenatal care Avoid heavy lifting Herbal teas encouraged	Prefers female attendant, although husband, mother, or father may assist with birth Birth may be attended by whole family Herbs may be used to promote uterine activity Birth may occur in squatting position ***Postpartum*** Herbal teas to stop bleeding	Infant not fed colostrum Use of herbs to increase flow of milk Use of cradle boards for infant Babies not handled often

NOTE: Most of these cultural beliefs and customs reflect the traditional culture and are not universally practiced. These lists are not intended to stereotype clients but rather to serve as guidelines while discussing meaningful cultural beliefs with a woman and her family.

*Variations in some beliefs and practices exist within subcultures of each group.

Data from Amaro, H. (1994). Women in the Mexican-American community: Religion, culture, and reproductive attitudes and experiences. *Journal of Comparative Psychology, 16*(1), 6-19; Bar-Yam, N. (1994). Learning about culture: A guide for birth practitioners. *International Journal of Childbirth Education, 9*(2), 8-10; Galanti, G. (1997). *Caring for patients from different cultures: Case studies from American hospitals* (2nd ed.). Philadelphia: University of Pennsylvania Press; D'Avanzo, C. (2008). *Mosby's pocket guide to cultural health assessment* (4th ed.). St. Louis: Mosby; Mattson, S. (1995). Culturally sensitive prenatal care for southeastern Asians. *Journal of Obstetric, Gynecologic and Neonatal Nursing, 24*(4), 335-341; Spector, R. (2013). *Cultural diversity in health and illness* (8th ed.). Upper Saddle River, NJ: Prentice-Hall; Williams, R. (1989). Issues in women's health care. In B. Johnson (Ed.), *Psychiatric mental health nursing: Adaptation and growth.* Philadelphia: JB Lippincott.

DEVELOPING CULTURAL COMPETENCE

Cultural competence has many names and definitions, all of which have subtle shades of difference but which are essentially the same: multiculturalism, cultural sensitivity, and intercultural effectiveness. Cultural competence involves acknowledging, respecting, and appreciating ethnic, cultural, and linguistic diversity. Culturally competent professionals act in ways that meet the needs of the client and are respectful of ways and traditions that may be very different from their own. In today's society it is of critical importance that nurses develop more than technical skill. At every level of preparation and throughout their professional lives, nurses must engage in a continual process of developing and refining attitudes and behaviors that will promote culturally competent care (Giger, 2013).

Key components of culturally competent care include:

- Recognizing that disparity exists between one's own culture and that of the client
- Educating and promoting healthy behaviors in a cultural context that has meaning for clients
- Taking abstract knowledge about other cultures and applying it in a practical way, so that the quality of service improves and policies are enacted that meet the needs of all clients
- Communicating respect for a wide range of differences, including client use of nontraditional healing practices and alternative therapies
- Recognizing the importance of culturally different communication styles, problem-solving techniques, concepts of space and time, and desires to be involved with care decisions
- Anticipating the need to address varying degrees of language ability and literacy, as well as barriers to care and compliance with treatment

In addition to issues of preserving and promoting human dignity, the development of cultural competence is of equal importance in terms of health outcomes. Nurses who relate effectively with clients are able to motivate them in the direction of health-promoting behaviors. Provider competence to address language barriers facilitates appropriate tailoring of health messages and preventive health teaching. Cross-cultural experiences also present an opportunity for the health care professional to expand cultural sensitivity, awareness, and skills.

COMMUNITY HEALTH PROMOTION

Best practices in community-based health initiatives involve understanding of community relationships and resources as well as participation of community leaders. The emphasis on community-based health promotion has grown in recent years, with recognition that many health issues require the collaborative efforts of a diverse community network to achieve public health goals. These efforts are particularly relevant in relation to maternal-newborn health, which is affected by multiple public health issues: lack of health insurance, undocumented status, recent economic challenges that include job loss, teen pregnancy, substance abuse, and the consequences of no or inadequate prenatal care.

Levels of Preventive Care

In community-based health promotion, three levels of prevention of disease exist. *Primary prevention* involves promoting healthy lifestyles through immunizations, encouraging exercise, and healthy nutrition. *Secondary prevention* involves targeting populations at risk for certain diseases. For example, women are encouraged to have mammograms; men are encouraged to have prostate screening. *Tertiary prevention* focuses on rehabilitation of an individual to health as optimal as is possible in the presence of a disease or injury. For example, a person who has experienced a stroke has an optimal expectation of being able to function at his or her fullest potential. As nurses we do what we can to ensure that this occurs.

During pregnancy, primary and secondary preventions are most relevant. The goal is to maintain a healthy pregnancy by preventing illness and screening those at risk for potential illnesses or complications that could arise during pregnancy. In pregnancy, primary prevention might involve providing influenza vaccine to women, whereas secondary prevention might involve performing an amniocentesis for a woman more than 35 years of age.

Promoting Family Health

Functioning within the social, cultural, environmental, and economic context of the community, the family becomes an integral component of community health-promotion efforts. For childbearing families, health promotion is focused primarily on early intervention through prenatal care and prevention of complications during the perinatal period. Often this early exposure to health information sets the stage for a successful birth and positive outcomes for mother, father, and baby. The nurse's role in this process is focused on collaboration with the family, identifying risk factors, and providing health information to facilitate positive health behaviors. Involving expectant mothers and fathers in identification of their learning needs is an essential first step to securing their participation in the health-promotion process.

A wide variety of strategies have been used to engage families and groups in health-promoting activities or community health programs. Some are more successful than others. Generally, participant engagement in the planning process and empowerment to create internal solutions are considered key factors in effective interventions. Many communities have organized coalitions to address specific health-promotion agendas related to sharing information, educating community members, or advocating for health policies around maternal and child health issues. The benefits of partnership with faith-based organizations for community health improvement have been demonstrated in health-promotion efforts aimed at lifestyle choices, health education, and maternal-child health outcomes.

Prepared childbirth classes are a well-established mechanism for increasing awareness of healthy behaviors during pregnancy and preparing parents for the care of themselves and their newborn during the postpartum period; these can occur through community hospitals and online courses. Mass media efforts such as those presented by the March of Dimes "Baby Your Baby," the Public Health Campaign "Safe to Sleep," and AWHONN's "40 Reasons to Go the Full 40 Weeks" are advertisements with clear consumer-friendly messages designed to reach a large target audience. Other venues include public health education in newspapers and magazines and health department programs such as the Special Supplemental Nutrition Program for Women, Infants, and Children (WIC), which offers a variety of health education and written information to mothers.

ASSESSING THE COMMUNITY

A community assessment is a tool that is used to assess the health and well-being of a community. One can define community either geographically or as having a common characteristic. For example, one can do a community assessment of clients who live in a particular neighborhood or of women who have developed preterm labor. In doing the community assessment, risk factors for certain diseases, patterns of illness, cultural beliefs, religious beliefs, transportation systems, and support systems are just a few factors that are assessed in order to determine how these components relate to certain patterns of illness.

In a community health assessment, data are collected, analyzed, and used to educate and mobilize communities, develop priorities, garner resources, and plan actions to improve public health. Many models and frameworks of community assessment are available, but the actual process often depends on the extent and nature of the assessment to be performed, the time and resources available, and the way the information is to be used (www.assesstoolkit.org).

Data Collection and Sources of Community Health Data

Important measures of community health, for example, are access to care, level of provider services available, availability of transportation, and family support. Consideration of a variety of these factors helps one to assess areas that may affect care so that nurses can introduce alternatives to meet clients' needs. For example, if a woman has to work Monday through Friday, from 8 AM to 5 PM, the nurse can facilitate an after-hours appointment. A community assessment model (Fig. 2-6) can be used to provide a comprehensive guide to data collection.

The most critical community indicators of perinatal health relate to access to care, maternal mortality, infant mortality, preterm birth, low birth weight, first-trimester prenatal care, and rates for mammography, Papanicolaou (Pap) smears, and other similar screening tests. Nurses can use these indicators as a reflection of access, quality, and continuity of health care in a community. For women and infants, access to a consistent source of care is critical. Those with a regular source of care are more likely to use preventive services and have more positive pregnancy outcomes, but many women lack access to a usual source of care or rely primarily on emergency services.

Access to health care relates not only to the *availability* of health department services, hospitals, public clinics, clinic hours, or other sources of care, but also to *accessibility* of care. In many areas where facilities and providers are available, geographic and transportation barriers render the care inaccessible for certain populations. This is particularly true in rural areas or other remote locations. Other barriers to care should also be evaluated including cultural and language barriers and lack

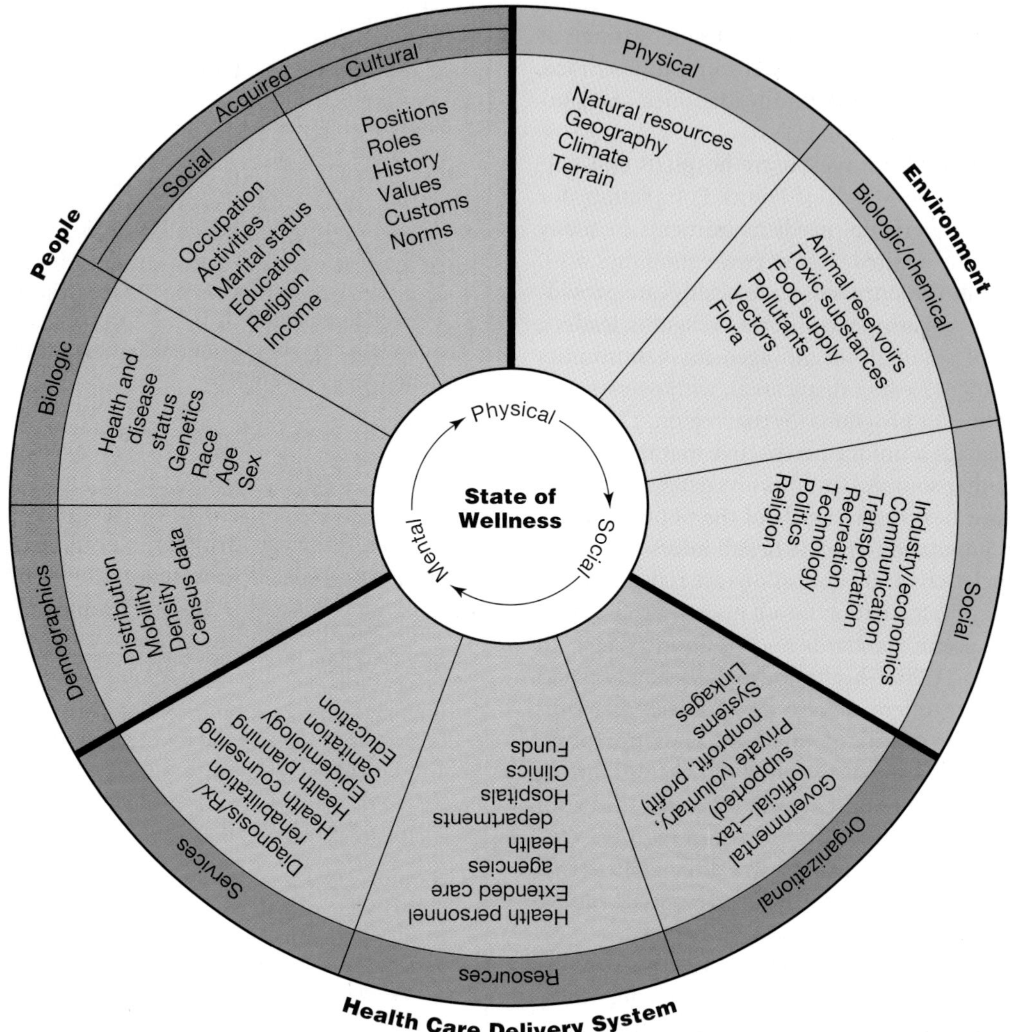

FIG 2-6 Community health assessment wheel. (From Clemen-Stone, S. [2002]. In S. Clemen-Stone, S. McGuire, & D. Eigsti. [Eds.], *Comprehensive community health nursing: Family, aggregate, & community practice* [6th ed.]. St. Louis: Mosby.)

of providers or specialty care. There is a growing trend in the United States to have walk-in clinics in grocery stores, an easily accessible location.

Health departments at the city, county, and state level are a valuable resource for annual reports of births and deaths. Local health departments also compile extensive statistics about the birth complications, causes of death, and leading causes of morbidity and mortality for each age group. Local and state health data are compiled and reported through the Centers for Disease Control and Prevention (CDC) (www.cdc.gov) to the National Center for Health Statistics (NCHS) (www.cdc.gov/nchs). The National Health Survey published annually from this source describes national health trends. However, national data are only as accurate and reliable as the local data on which they are based, so caution is needed in interpreting the data and applying it to specific population groups.

The U.S. census provides data on population size, age ranges, sex, racial and ethnic distribution, socioeconomic status, educational level, employment, and housing characteristics. Summary data are available for most large metropolitan areas, arranged by ZIP code and census tract, which usually corresponds to a neighborhood comprising approximately 3000 to 6000 people. Looking at individual census tracts within a community helps identify subpopulations or aggregates whose needs may differ from those of the larger community. For example, women at high risk for inadequate prenatal care according to age, race, and ethnic or cultural group can be readily identified and outreach activities appropriately targeted.

Other sources of useful information are hospitals and voluntary health agencies. The March of Dimes Foundation, for example, has supported perinatal needs assessments in many communities across the United States (www.modimes.org). Other community health resources include health care providers or administrators, government officials, religious leaders, and representatives of voluntary health agencies. Community or county health councils exist in many areas, with oversight of specific health initiatives or programs for that region. These **key informants** often provide a unique perspective that may not be accessible through other sources. Community gatekeepers who address the social and health care needs of the population are also critical links to population-specific health information.

Professional associations and publications are rich and readily accessible sources of information for all nurses. Professional associations publish useful standards and position papers. In addition to nursing and public health journals, behavioral and social science literature offers diverse perspectives on community health status for specific populations and subgroups. The Internet has increased the availability and accessibility of national, state, and local health data as well. However, the use of Internet-based resources for health information requires caution because data reliability and validity are difficult to verify. Guidelines for evaluation of Internet health resources can be found on the Health on the Net website (www.hon.ch).

Data collection methods may be either qualitative (e.g., by discussion, interview, observation) or quantitative (e.g., number, mean, standard deviation, percent of data collected) and may include visual surveys that can be completed by walking through a community, participant observation, interviews, focus groups, and analysis of existing data. Potential clients and health care consumers may be asked to participate in focus groups or community forums to present their views on needed community services and programs. Formal surveys, conducted by mail, telephone, the Internet, or face-to-face interviews, can be a valuable source of information not available from national databases or other secondary sources. Several drawbacks exist with this method: surveys are generally expensive to develop and time consuming to administer. In addition to the cost of such surveys, poor response rates often preclude a sufficiently representative response on which to base nursing interventions.

A **walking survey** is generally conducted by a walk-through observation of the community (Box 2-4), taking note of specific characteristics of the population, economic and social environment, transportation, health care services, and other resources. With this type of data collection, information is gathered based on what the data collector observes and is clearly objective data. **Participant observation** is another useful assessment method

BOX 2-4 Community Walk-Through

As you observe the community, take note of the following:

- **Physical environment**—Older neighborhood or newer subdivision? Sidewalks, streets, and buildings in good or poor repair? Billboards and signs? What are they advertising? Any health or safety promotion? Are lawns kept up? Is there trash in the streets? Parks or playgrounds? Parking lots? Empty lots? Industries?
- **People in the area**—Old, young, homeless, children; predominant ethnicity, language? Is the population homogeneous? What signs do you see of different cultural groups?
- **Stores and services available**—Restaurants: chain, local, ethnic? Grocery stores: neighborhood or chain? Department stores, gas stations, real estate or insurance offices, travel agencies, pawn shops, liquor stores, discount or thrift stores, newspaper stands?
- **Social**—Clubs, bars, fraternal organizations (e.g., Elks, American Legion), museums?
- **Religious**—Churches, synagogues, mosques? What denominations? Do you see evidence of their use other than on religious/holy days?
- **Health services**—Drugstores, doctors' offices, clinics, dentists, mental health services, veterinarians, urgent care facilities, hospitals, shelters, nursing homes, home health agencies, public health services, midwives, chiropractors, acupuncturists, traditional healers (e.g., herbalists, palmists)?
- **Transportation**—Cars, buses, taxis, light rail, sidewalks, bicycle paths, access for disabled persons?
- **Education**—Schools, before- and after-school sports or programs, extracurricular activities/clubs, child care, libraries, bookstores? What is the reputation of the schools?
- **Government**—What is the governance structure? Is there a mayor? City council? Are meetings open to the public? Are there signs of political activity (e.g., posters, campaign signs)?
- **Safety**—How safe is the community? What is the crime rate? What types of crimes are committed? Are police visible? Is there a fire station?
- **Evaluation of the community based on your observations**—What is your impression of the community? Is the environment pleasing? Are services and transportation adequate? How difficult is it for residents to obtain needed services, that is, how far do they have to travel? Would you want to live in this community? Why or why not?

in which the nurse actively participates in the community to understand the community more fully and to validate observations. As part of the assessment process, nurses working in multiethnic and multicultural groups need an in-depth assessment of culturally based health behaviors.

Analysis and synthesis of data obtained during the assessment process help to generate a comprehensive picture of the community's health status, needs, and problem areas, as well as its strengths and resources for addressing these concerns. The goal of this process is to assign priorities to community health needs and to develop a plan of action for correcting them. A comparison of community health data with state and national statistics can help identify appropriate target populations and develop interventions to improve health outcomes.

Vulnerable Populations in the Community

Assessment of population health includes indicators related to diverse groups and cultures, particularly disenfranchised or "vulnerable" community members. Vulnerability in terms of health status and health outcomes may take many forms, including sociocultural, economic, and environmental risk factors that contribute to disparities in health. Health disparities are conditions that disproportionately affect certain racial, ethnic, or other groups. African-Americans, Hispanic-Americans, Native Americans, Pacific Islanders, and Asian-Americans are all considered vulnerable populations because of the burden of preventable disease, death, and disability compared with nonminorities (CDC, 2013b).

Racial and ethnic disparities exist for a number of health conditions and services. According to the 2012 National Healthcare Disparities Report [AHRQ] (2013), our system of health care distributes services inefficiently and unevenly across populations. These disparities may occur for a variety of reasons, including differences in access to care, social determinants, provider biases, poor provider-client communication, and poor health literacy. A summary of the report described health care quality and access to be suboptimal, especially for minority and low-income groups. Overall quality of health care is improving and access is improving for some, however, disparities still exist. Urgent attention needs to be directed toward diabetes care, maternal and child health care, disparities in cancer care, and quality of care.

Women

Women make up 51% of the U.S. population, representing a very diverse, and largely at risk, group in relation to health (U.S. Census Bureau, 2011b). Although women assume leadership for health care decision making in most families, they also face significant challenges in accessing the health care system and meeting their own health needs and those of family members. Although there is no single contributing factor, the primary sources of health disparities for women fall into the areas of gender, socioeconomic status, and race or ethnicity. Significant gaps exist in the quality of care for women when compared with men.

The *National Report Card on Women's Health* describes significant deficiencies in women's health (National Women's Law Center [NWLC], 2010). States' performance in relation to 26 graded indicators was assessed; all but 3 were rated as *unsatisfactory* in relation to women's health status and policies influencing women's health. Key indicators focused on access to services, use of preventive health care and health promotion activities, the occurrence of certain health conditions, and an assessment of the community's effect on women's health. This report suggested that one of the primary factors compromising women's health is lack of access to acceptable-quality health care, which may manifest itself in many forms: lack of health insurance, living in a medically underserved area, or an inability to obtain needed services, particularly basic services such as prenatal care. With the enactment of the Patient Protection and Affordable Care Act, many of the policy goals will be realized as the act is implemented. By mid-April 2014, 7.5 million people had enrolled in the plan (Trumbull, 2014).

Although many women report that they are in good to excellent health, statistics reveal significant disparities in health status of women from all age groups and racial and ethnic backgrounds. Low levels of educational attainment (high school or lower) are also associated with lack of resources and difficulty navigating the health care system. This is particularly true of women of ethnic and racial minorities, whose limited English proficiency may compromise provider access and quality of care.

Racial and Ethnic Minorities

In addition to social, economic, and cultural barriers to optimal health, women who are in racial and ethnic minorities experience a disproportionate burden of disease, disability, and premature death. Significant health disparities continue to exist in the health of adult women and their infants. Although positive trends are evident, disparities persist among racial and ethnic groups in early prenatal care, an important factor in achieving healthy pregnancy outcomes.

Minority women, many of whom live in poverty, also have higher rates of chronic disease including heart disease, cancer, hepatitis, and acquired immunodeficiency syndrome (AIDS), as well as mental health issues. Women with underlying health conditions are at especially high risk for poor obstetric outcomes for themselves and their infants. They have high rates of preterm labor and gestational hypertension, and often have intrauterine growth restriction, resulting in the birth of infants who are small for gestational age. These are the women for whom the community-based perinatal nurse will be providing care, and their needs are complex, demanding high levels of expertise and skill.

Adolescent Girls

The adolescent population in the United States is generally considered healthy. However, adolescents participate in riskier behaviors and their health is often compromised as a result.

Although adolescents are concerned about becoming pregnant, they still engage in unprotected sex. They use a variety of sources for health information such as the media, friends, and sex education, yet they are misinformed, particularly about sexually transmitted infections (STIs) and human immunodeficiency virus (HIV) transmission. These findings have significant implications for perinatal outcomes and emphasize the importance of aggressive prevention programs and community outreach related to sexuality, teen pregnancy, and substance abuse.

It is crucial that nurses engage adolescents in health education programs that will encourage them to make informed decisions about their sexual health. It is also vital that nurses be a resource to these young women.

Older Women

Although women have a greater life expectancy than men, they are more likely to have chronic illnesses, less likely to use preventive services, and ultimately spend more on health care. As nurses, it is important that we engage this population at all levels of prevention, from primary to tertiary.

Incarcerated Women

The number of incarcerated women in the United States has continued to climb in recent years, increasing at a significantly greater rate than for men. In 2010, there were 113,000 women incarcerated in state and federal facilities, with the highest number of these being non-Hispanic black women (Sipes, 2012). Many of these women report a history of sexual and physical abuse.

Because their relationship histories are often unstable, and because they often lack the support of family, incarcerated women or those with a history of repeated incarceration frequently have difficulty providing emotional stability, secure housing, and health promotion role modeling for their children.

The lifestyle choices of this group, including risky sexual relationships, illicit drug use, and smoking, place them at high risk for STIs, HIV, and AIDS; other chronic and communicable diseases; and complicated pregnancies.

Immigrant, Refugee, and Migrant Women

As of 2010, nearly 40 million or 13% of the population in the United States was foreign born (Grieco, Acosta, de la Cruz, et al., 2012). This accounts for a rapidly growing diverse population for which nurses will be providing care.

An *immigrant* is an individual who moves from one country to another in an effort to take up legal residency, whereas a *refugee* is an individual who is forced to leave his or her home country, often in search of a safer and more stable living environment. Both populations are often challenged with not being able to easily access health care because they are not U.S. citizens. These women often do not seek medical care for fear of deportation. Access to care is further limited by health care policies that restrict Medicaid eligibility for these groups although a number of states provide some prenatal, birth, and postpartum care.

Along with their profound resilience and determination, refugees and immigrants have brought rich diversity to the United States in several important dimensions including cultural heritage and customs, economic productivity, and enhanced national vitality. In general, refugees are more likely to live in poverty than are immigrants. Over time, measures of health and well-being actually decline for the immigrant population as they become part of American society. Many of the conditions or illnesses that they acquire contribute to the persistence of disparities in maternal and neonatal health outcomes for both immigrants and refugees.

Migrant workers are those who work outside their home country or migrate within their own country seeking seasonal work. Migrant laborers and their families face many problems, including financial instability, child labor, poor housing, lack of education, language and cultural barriers, and limited access to health and social services. Poor dental health, diabetes, hypertension, malnutrition, tuberculosis, skin diseases, and parasitic infections are common health issues among migrant populations. Primary health care services are largely provided by a number of migrant health centers, of which there are more than 400 throughout the United States. In 2011 more than 862,000 seasonal and migrant farm workers and their families were served (HHS, 2011). Routine prenatal care and screening and treatment for hypertension and diabetes are provided. Community health nurses frequently encounter the challenges of providing culturally and linguistically appropriate care while facing numerous health issues.

Numerous reproductive health issues exist for migrant women, including less consistent use of contraception and increased rates of STIs. Migrants are less likely to receive early prenatal care and have a greater incidence of inadequate weight gain during pregnancy than do other poor women.

Rural Versus Urban Community Settings

Approximately 16% of the U.S. population lives in a rural area (Rural Assistance Center, 2011). Generally, rural residents are older, less educated, and generally in poorer health than their urban counterparts. Rural communities are disproportionately affected by poverty and poor access to health care services. Fewer physicians choosing to practice in rural areas and lack of insurance present additional factors contributing to poor health in rural areas.

Rural women are especially vulnerable to financial and transportation barriers to health care. Although women in rural counties report only *fair* to *poor* health, they pay considerably more for their health care. In rural communities women have less access to prenatal care, which contributes to higher rates of adverse pregnancy outcomes including higher rates of preterm birth, low birth weight, and infant mortality. The disproportionate distribution of poverty and of variations in race/ethnicity, age, education, and availability and access to medical resources may be the link to infant mortality in rural areas. The ACA is designed to reduce barriers to access.

Homeless Women

Homelessness among women is an increasing social and health issue in the United States. Although exact numbers are unknown because of the difficulty in tracking individuals without a permanent address, it is estimated that more than 636,000 people were homeless in 2011 (Homelessness in America, 2012). Single women make up 13% of the homeless population and are often on the street to escape domestic violence (Dray, 2012). Families with children make up the fastest-growing group of the homeless. In these families, one in five children experienced food insecurity (did not have enough to eat) in 2010 (National Coalition for the Homeless [NCH], 2011).

Health issues among the homeless are numerous and result primarily from a lack of preventive care and a lack of resources in general. Health problems include chronic illness, infectious diseases, asthma, circulatory problems, diabetes, substance abuse, and mental illness. Lifestyle factors and the vulnerability resulting from being homeless contribute to health problems. Women are at increased risk for illness and injury; many have been victims of domestic abuse, assault, and rape. Although little is known about pregnancy in this population, women do become pregnant while homeless. In addition to risk factors related to inadequate nutrition, inadequate weight gain, anemia, bleeding problems, and preterm birth, homeless women face multiple barriers to prenatal care: transportation, distance, and wait times. Most of these women underutilize available prenatal services. The unsafe environment and high risk lifestyles often result in adverse perinatal outcomes (American College of Obstetricians and Gynecologists [ACOG], 2010; Richards, Merrill, & Baksh, 2011). The United States has initiated programs to address these problems. For example, the U.S. Interagency Council on Homelessness and its 19 member agencies launched Opening Doors, the federal strategic plan to prevent and end homelessness in 2010 and updated it in 2011 (Opening Doors, 2012).

Implications for Nursing

Working in the community or in the home with the full spectrum of family organizational styles, vulnerable populations, and cultural groups presents challenges for nurses. Whether it involves perinatal care focused on women and their newborns or women's health care directed toward treatment and prevention of other health conditions such as communicable diseases and sexually transmitted infections, nursing must exhibit a high degree of professionalism. Cultural sensitivity, compassion, and a critical awareness of family dynamics and social stressors that will affect health-related decision making are critical components in developing an effective nursing care plan.

Although the long-term consequences of contemporary immigration for American society are unclear, the successful incorporation of immigrant families depends on the resources, benefits, and policies that ensure their healthy development and successful social adjustment. Culturally competent health care and involvement of the immigrant community in health care programs are recommended strategies for improving the access to and effectiveness of health care for this population.

The use of camp volunteers has been effective in assisting families living in migrant worker camps to obtain prenatal, postpartum, and infant care. Working in partnership with health professionals such as nurses, lay camp aides have been used effectively for outreach and health education; however, more strategies are needed to link traditional practices with the formal health care system. Guidance and information about other health resources are available to health care providers through the National Center for Farmworker Health, Inc. (www.ncfh.org) and the Migrant Clinicians Network (www.migrantclinician.org).

Nurses working with homeless women and families are challenged to treat them with dignity and respect to establish a therapeutic relationship. Case management is recommended to coordinate the services and disciplines that may be involved in meeting the complex needs of these families. Whenever possible, general screening and preventive health services must be provided when the woman seeks treatment because this may be the only opportunity to provide health information and intervention. Building on existing coping strategies and strengths, the health care provider helps the woman and her family reconnect with a social support system. Nurses also have an important role in advocating for funding to support health services for the homeless and improve access to preventive care for all homeless populations.

HOME CARE IN THE COMMUNITY

Modern home care nursing has its foundation in public health nursing, which provided comprehensive care to sick and well clients in their own homes. Specialized maternity home care nursing services began in the 1980s when public health maternity nursing services were limited and services had not kept pace with the changing practices of high risk obstetrics and emerging technology. Lengthy antepartum hospitalizations for such conditions as preterm labor and gestational hypertension created nursing care challenges for staff members of inpatient units.

Many women expressed their concern for the negative effect of antepartum hospitalizations on the family. Although clinical indications showed that a new nursing care approach was needed, home health care did not become a viable alternative until third-party payers (i.e., public or private organizations or employer groups that pay for health care) pushed for cost containment in maternity services.

In the current health care system, home care is an important component of health care delivery along the perinatal continuum of care (Fig. 2-7). The growing demand for home care is based on several factors:

- Interest in family birthing alternatives
- Shortened hospital stays
- New technologies that facilitate home-based assessments and treatments
- Reimbursement by third-party payers

As health care costs continue to rise, and because millions of American families lack health insurance, there is greater demand for innovative, cost-effective methods of health care delivery in the community. Large health care systems are developing clinically integrated health care delivery networks whose goals are: (1) improved coordination of care and care outcomes; (2) better communication among health care providers; (3) increased client, payer, and provider satisfaction; and (4) reduced cost. The integration of clinical services changes the focus of care to a continuum of services that are increasingly community based.

Communication and Technology Applications

As maternity care continues to consist of frequent and brief contacts with health care providers throughout the prenatal and postpartum periods, services that link maternity clients throughout the perinatal continuum of care have assumed increasing importance. These services include critical pathways, telephonic nursing assessments, discharge planning, specialized education programs, parent support groups, home visiting programs, nurse advice lines, and perinatal home care (Fig. 2-8). Hospitals may provide cross-training for hospital-based nurses to make postpartum home visits or to staff outpatient centers for postpartum follow-up.

Telephonic nursing through services such as warm lines, nurse advice lines, and telephonic nursing assessments is a valuable means of managing health care problems and bridging the gaps among acute, outpatient, and home care services. Providers use the Internet and Skype to communicate with clients. Newborns in distress in rural hospitals can be

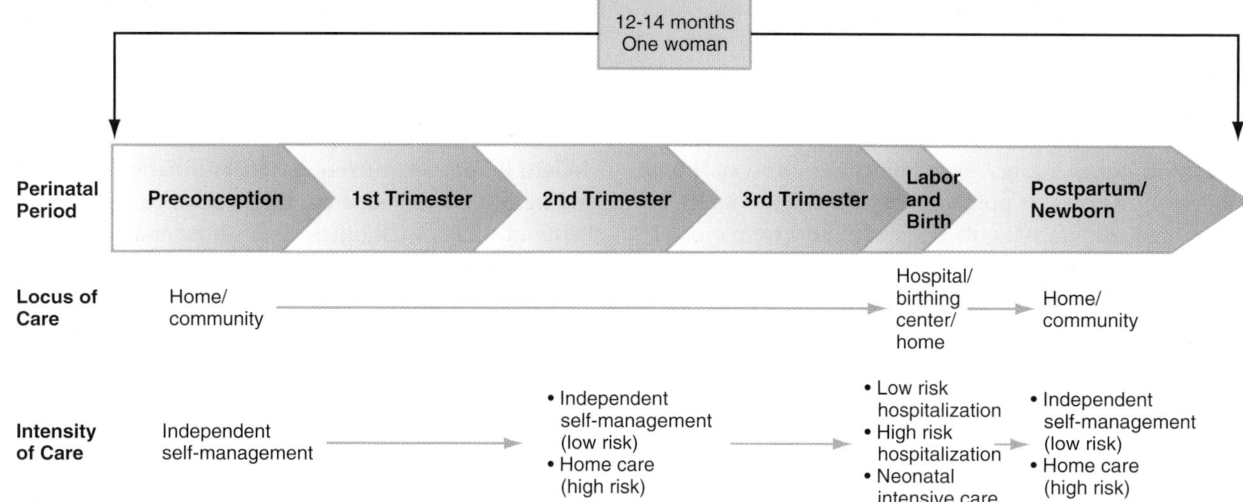

FIG 2-7 Perinatal continuum of care.

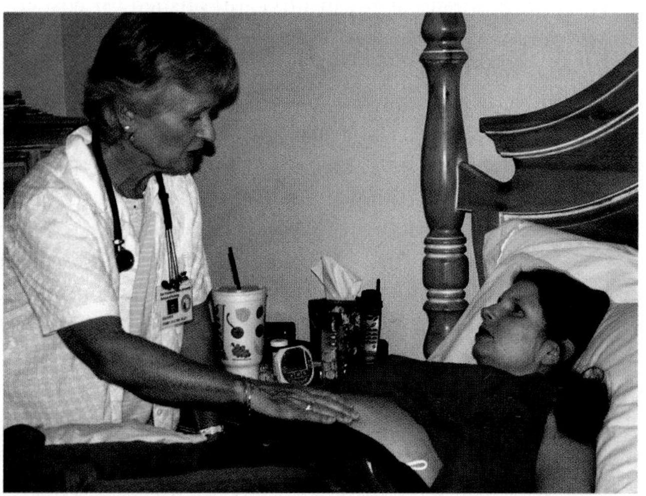

FIG 2-8 Home care nurse visits with a woman in preterm labor at home on bed rest. (Courtesy Shannon Perry, Phoenix, AZ.)

assessed by perinatologists using high-definition telemedicine robots. Nursing care that occurs by telephone is interactive and responsive to immediate health care questions about particular health care needs. Warm lines are telephone lines that are offered as a community service to provide new parents with support, encouragement, and basic parenting education. Nurse advice lines, or toll-free nurse consultation services, often are supported by third-party payers or health management organization/managed care organizations (HMO/MCOs) and are designed to provide answers to medical questions. Nurse care managers are prepared to guide callers through urgent health care situations, suggest treatment options, and provide health education. Telephonic nursing assessments, or nurse consultation, assessment, and health education that take place during a telephone conversation, can be added to the nursing care plan in conjunction with skilled nursing visits, or they may comprise a separate nursing contact for the woman. Telephonic nursing assessments are commonly used after a postpartum home care visit to reassess a woman's knowledge about the signs and symptoms of adequate hydration in breastfeeding or, after initiating home phototherapy, to assess the caregiver's knowledge regarding problems with equipment.

Guidelines for Nursing Practice

The Association of Women's Health, Obstetric and Neonatal Nurses (AWHONN, 2009) defines home care as the provision of technical, psychologic, and other therapeutic support in the woman's home rather than in an institution. The scope of nursing care delivered in the home is necessarily limited to practices deemed safe and appropriate to be carried out in an environment that is physically separated from a health care institution and its resources. Nursing practice at home is consistent with federal and state regulations that direct home care practice. The nurse demonstrates practice competence through formalized orientation and ongoing clinical education and performance evaluation in the respective home care agency. Standards for practice from key specialty organizations such as AWHONN, the National Association of Neonatal Nurses (NANN), ACNM, ACOG, the American Academy of Pediatrics (AAP), and the Intravenous Nursing Society (INS) provide the basis for clinical protocols and pathways and organizational programs in home care practice. The Joint Commission (www.jointcommission.org) provides criteria for home care operations based on Centers for Medicare & Medicaid Services (CMS) regulations (cms.hhs.gov).

A wide range of professional health care services and products can be delivered or used in the home by means of technology and telecommunication. For example, telehealth and telemedicine make it possible for clients in the home to be interviewed and assessed by a specialist located hundreds of miles away. Home health care can be viewed as an extension of in-hospital care.

Essentially the primary difference between health care in a hospital and home care is the absence of the continuous presence of professional health care providers in a client's home. Generally, but not always, home health care entails intermittent care by a professional who visits the client's home for a particular reason and/or provides care on site for fewer than

4 hours at a time. The home health care agency maintains on-call professional staff to assist home care clients who have questions about their care and for emergencies, such as equipment failure.

Perinatal Services

Home care perinatal services may be provided by hospital-based programs, independent proprietary (for-profit) agencies, or nonprofit home care agencies, and official or tax-supported agencies. Innovative programs may be supported by research grants for a period of years, but ultimately they must be sponsored by an agency with long-term funding. Home visits have advantages and disadvantages. The pregnant woman can maintain bed rest if indicated, and vulnerable neonates are not exposed to the weather or external sources of infection. The nurse can observe and interact with family members in their most natural and secure environment. Adequacy of resources and safety factors can be assessed. Teaching can be tailored to the actual home conditions, and other family members can be included. A home visit is less expensive than a day's hospitalization, but a 60- to 90-minute visit requires 2.5 to 3 hours of nursing time, including travel and documentation. Areas of challenge include limited availability of nurses with expertise in maternity care and concerns about the nurse's physical safety in the community. One alternative that is less expensive is contacting women via telephone.

Visits for outreach and health promotion are an integral part of community (or public) health nursing. In countries with national health systems, a nurse or midwife may see all women during pregnancy and after birth. In the United States, visits of this sort have been provided mainly to low-income families without health insurance and Medicaid recipients who use the clinics provided by local health departments. Until recently, private insurers did not reimburse for health promotion visits. MCOs now recognize that anticipatory guidance can be cost-effective, but home visitation programs for the most part still target specific, high risk populations, such as adolescents and women at risk for preterm labor.

Home care agencies are subject to regulation by governmental and professional organizations and provide interdisciplinary services including social work, nutrition, and occupational and physical therapy. Increasingly, their caseloads are made up of women who require high-technology care, such as infusions or home monitoring. Although the home health nurse develops the care plan, all care must be ordered by a physician. In addition, interventions must meet the insurer's criteria for reimbursement and services are limited to registered clients. Preconception care and low risk antepartum care can usually be provided more efficiently in offices. High-risk antepartum care can be provided by home care agencies; for example, women with hyperemesis gravidarum who require parenteral nutrition may be treated at home. Conditions requiring bed rest, such as preterm labor and hypertension, are other common indications for home care. Other conditions often managed with home care may include cardiac disease, substance abuse, and diabetes in pregnancy.

Insurers may reimburse for at least one postpartum visit to families after early discharge or in the presence of high risk factors. Many neonates who require long-term high-technology care are also managed with home care.

Client Selection and Referral

The office- or hospital-based nurse is often the key person in making effective referrals to home care. When considering a referral to home care, the following factors are evaluated:

- Health status of mother and fetus or infant: Is the condition serious enough to warrant home care, and is it stable enough for intermittent observation to be sufficient?
- Availability of professionals to provide the needed services within the woman's community.
- Family resources, including psychosocial, social, and economic resources: Will the family be able to provide care between nursing visits? Are relationships supportive? Is third-party reimbursement available, or can it be negotiated with the insurer? Could a voluntary or tax-supported community agency provide needed care without payment?
- Cost-effectiveness: Is it more reasonable for the woman to receive these services at home or to go to a local outpatient facility to receive them?

Community referrals should not be limited to women with physiologic complications of pregnancy that require medical treatment. Women at risk (e.g., young adolescents, families with a history of abuse, members of vulnerable population groups, developmentally disabled individuals) may need follow-up care at home. As we move more and more into an interdisciplinary health care society, it is crucial that nurses communicate with social workers to tap into valuable community resources that women can use in their own communities after being discharged.

Standardized forms simplify the referral process and ensure that all needed information will be forwarded to the home health agency. The nursing assessment should include the woman's physical and psychologic status, her level of knowledge about self-management activities, her willingness to learn, the availability of caregivers and social support in the home, and her level of comfort with home care. If the referral is for a mother-and-infant home care visit, the nursing assessment should include newborn data.

High-technology home care requires additional information to be collected from the chart, and consultation with the referring physician and other members of the health care team, before a home care referral is made. These additional data include the medical diagnosis, medical prognosis, prescribed therapies, medication history, drug-dosing information, potential ancillary supplies, type of infusion and access device, and the available systems of social support for the woman and family. The nursing assessment and therapy data provide baseline information for the home care nurse and other health care providers involved in the care plan.

Whenever a referral is called in to a home health care agency, a member of the nursing or admissions staff determines the agency's ability to accept the woman for service. The use of telecommunication modalities such as fax machines, cell phones, electronic files, and the Internet to transmit information has eliminated delays in initiating home care services, even in more remote rural areas.

CARE MANAGEMENT

Preparing for the Home Visit

The home care nurse reviews the available clinical data, demographic information, and completed care plan form and consults with the home care pharmacist or other health care team members who have previously contacted the woman to determine the goals of the visit. At this point the nurse uses the medical diagnosis and the location of the case on the perinatal continuum as a starting point to organize the woman's care. The nurse reviews agency policies and procedures, professional literature about diagnosis, and community resources as part of the previsit preparation work (Box 2-5).

First Home Care Visit

Making the first home care visit can be stressful for the nurse and the woman. The home care nurse is faced with an unknown environment controlled by the woman and her family. The woman and her family also experience feelings about the unknown, such as anxiety about the way the nurse will treat them or what the nurse will do during the visit. The challenge for the home care nurse is to establish a positive nurse-client

BOX 2-5 Protocol for Perinatal Home Visits

Previsit Interventions

1. Contact the family to arrange details for a home visit.
   a. Identify self, credentials, and agency role.
   b. Review purpose of home visit follow-up.
   c. Schedule convenient time for visit.
   d. Confirm address and route to family home.
2. Review and clarify appropriate data.
   a. Review all available assessment data for mother and fetus or infant (i.e., referral forms, hospital discharge summaries, identified learning needs of the family).
   b. Review records of any previous nursing contacts.
   c. Contact other professional caregivers as necessary to clarify data (i.e., obstetrician, nurse-midwife, pediatrician, referring nurse).
3. Identify community resources and teaching materials appropriate to meet those needs already identified.
4. Plan the visit, and prepare a bag with equipment, supplies, and materials necessary for assessments of mother and fetus or infant, actual care anticipated, and teaching.

In-Home Interventions: Establishing a Relationship

1. Reintroduce yourself and establish the purpose of the visit for mother, infant, and family; offer the family the opportunity to clarify their expectations of the contact.
2. Spend a brief time socially interacting with the family to become acquainted and establish a trusting relationship.

In-Home Interventions: Working with the Family

1. Conduct a systematic assessment of the mother and the fetus or newborn to determine their physiologic adjustment and any existing complications (Fig. 2-8).
2. Throughout visit, collect data to assess the emotional adjustment of individual family members to the pregnancy or birth and lifestyle changes. Note any evidence of family-newborn bonding and sibling rivalry; note relationships among mother, father, children, and grandparents.
3. Determine the adequacy of support system.
   a. To what extent does someone help with cooking, cleaning, and other home management tasks?
   b. To what extent is help being provided in caring for the newborn and any other children?
   c. Are support persons encouraging the new mother to care for herself and get adequate rest?
   d. Who is providing helpful information? Emotional support?
4. Throughout the visit observe the home environment for adequacy of resources.
   a. Space: privacy, safe play of children, sleeping
   b. Overall cleanliness and state of repair
   c. Number of steps pregnant woman/new mother must climb
   d. Adequacy of cooking arrangements
   e. Adequacy of refrigeration and other food storage areas
   f. Adequacy of bathing, toilet, and laundry facilities
   g. Arrangements in home for newborn: sleeping, bathing, formula preparation (if needed), layette items, and diapers
5. Throughout the visit observe the home environment for overall state of repair and existence of safety hazards.
   a. Storage of medications, household cleaners, and other substances hazardous to children
   b. Presence of peeling paint on furniture, walls, or pipes
   c. Factors that contribute to falls, such as dim lighting, broken steps, scatter rugs
   d. Presence of vermin
   e. Use of crib or playpen that fails to meet safety guidelines
   f. Existence of emergency plan in case of fire; fire alarm or extinguisher
6. Provide care to the mother, the newborn, or both as prescribed by their respective primary care provider or in accord with agency protocol.
7. Provide teaching on the basis of previously identified needs.
8. Refer the family to appropriate community agencies or resources, such as warm lines and support groups.
9. Ascertain that the woman knows potential problems to watch for and who to call if they occur.
10. Ensure that used disposable items have been handled appropriately and that reusable items are cleaned and repacked appropriately in the nurse's bag.

In-Home Interventions: Ending the Visit

1. Summarize the activities and main points of the visit.
2. Clarify future expectations, including the schedule of the next visit.
3. Review the teaching plan and provide major points in writing.
4. Provide information about reaching the nurse or agency if needed before the next scheduled visit.

Postvisit Interventions

1. Document the visit thoroughly, using the necessary agency forms to serve as a legal record of the visit and to allow third-party reimbursement, as possible.
2. Initiate the nursing care plan on which the next encounter with the woman and/or family will be based.
3. Communicate appropriately (by telephone, email, fax, letter, progress notes, or referral form) with the primary care provider, other health professionals, or referral agencies on behalf of the woman and family.

relationship and provide the prescribed home care services within the time provided for the initial home visit. One of the most important roles of the home care nurse is modeling health-related behaviors for the woman and others who are in the home during the visit.

Assessment and Nursing Diagnoses

The major areas of the assessment are demographics, medical history, general health history, medication history, psychosocial assessment (Box 2-6), home and community environment, and physical assessment. Information can be obtained from client records sent to the home care agency at the time of referral or from the previsit interview. These data will be used to develop and complete the nursing care plan, which is required for many licensed home health care agencies.

The nursing care plan is developed in collaboration with the woman, based on her health care needs. Home care nurses working in home health care agencies regulated by the CMS use a nursing care plan that includes client demographics, the health care provider's orders, home care goals, and the woman's level of functioning. This document is initiated at the time of referral to the home care agency and must be updated every 60 days or as specified by state regulations. The frequency of the skilled nursing visit may vary with the individual nursing care plan and reimbursement criteria established by the third-party payers.

BOX 2-6 Psychosocial Assessment

Language
- Identify the primary language spoken in the home.
- Assess whether there are any language barriers to receiving support.

Community Resources/Access to Care
- Identify primary and secondary means of transportation.
- Identify community agencies family uses for health care and support.
- Assess cultural and psychosocial barriers to receiving care.

Social Support
- Determine the people living with the pregnant woman.
- Identify who assists with household chores.
- Identify who assists with child care and parenting activities.
- Identify who the pregnant woman turns to for problems or during a crisis.

Interpersonal Relationships
- Identify the way decisions are made in the family.
- Identify the family's perception of the need for home care.
- Identify roles of adults in caring for family members.

Caregiver
- Identify the primary caregiver for home care treatments.
- Identify other caregivers and their roles.
- Assess the caregiver's knowledge of treatments and the care process.
- Identify potential strain from the caregiver role.
- Identify the level of satisfaction with the caregiver role.

Stress and Coping
- Identify what the woman perceives as lifestyle changes and their effect on her and her family.
- Identify the changes she and her family have made to adjust to her health condition and home health care treatments.

Nursing Considerations

There are several areas of concern when caring for a woman in the home. In home care the woman or family members are responsible for administration of medications in the absence of the nurse. A careful medication history should be obtained to see if the woman is taking her medications correctly and understands their desired action and potential side effects. It is important that women and caretakers have a clear understanding of medication regimens and are notified when medications change in any way.

Nurses have to be skilled at performing various procedures such as venipuncture and administration of intravenous medications or fluids. Nurses must be sure that women know how to respond in emergency situations. Women need to be able to have 24-hour access to resources in the community in emergency situations. Women and family members are also encouraged to learn how to perform cardiopulmonary resuscitation (CPR), especially for infants.

The homes of women using electronic home health care equipment, such as phototherapy equipment or infusion pumps, require physical inspection of any electrical outlets, electrical cords, and extension cords that will be used. Homes with faulty electrical wiring may place the woman at risk for being involved in an electrical fire; faulty wiring may require inspection and repair by a professional electrician before electronic devices are used. Findings from the assessment are incorporated into the nursing care plan.

Verbal explanations should be supplemented with clearly written instructions. General information to promote well-being, such as nutrition and common discomforts of pregnancy, should also be included. The need for preparation for childbirth can be addressed by using books or videos and supplemented by individual teaching at home. Coping with bed rest or other limitation of activity is a problem for many women with high risk pregnancies. The nurse can share strategies that others have used such as support groups for women on bed rest using Facebook or Skype, help with time management, and provide information about support services. Teaching about infant care or the special needs of the preterm infant may be appropriate during the prenatal period.

SAFETY ALERT

In caring for the home care client, Occupational Safety and Health Administration (OSHA) guidelines should be followed. The use of strict handwashing techniques, sharps containers, gloves, personal protective equipment (PPE), and proper equipment is essential in preventing the spread of disease to the care provider, the woman, and her family.

Use personal safety measures such as parking the car for access for a quick departure; never enter a home where guns are visible.

Clear documentation of assessments, problems identified, treatments and interventions performed, and the woman's response is essential. Third-party payers base reimbursement on the nurse's written record of providing skilled nursing care and assessments that support the woman's continuing need for those services. The nurse must promptly inform the health care provider by telephone, fax, or electronic file of any significant changes. When new orders are transmitted by telephone, a written copy must be sent for the physician's signature.

See the Nursing Care Plan for examples of nursing diagnoses related to home care and the community.

NURSING CARE PLAN

Community and Home Care

NURSING DIAGNOSIS	EXPECTED OUTCOME	NURSING INTERVENTIONS	RATIONALES
Readiness for Enhanced Family Coping related to family growth and development in new community	The family will identify at least three community groups that can serve as appropriate resources for an expectant family with small children.	Assess family structure and availability of significant others, friends, or family members to assist family with new baby and siblings.	To provide database for further interventions
		Encourage family to enlist assistance of individuals who are available to help family at birth of new baby.	To provide physical and emotional support
		Using therapeutic communication, assist family to assess coping strategies used in the past for new situations.	To provide clarification and promote empowerment of family in new situations
		Suggest strategies to find resources available in community.	To assist family during pregnancy, with new baby, and with small siblings
		Give information regarding community workshops, classes, or support groups.	To promote networking, community bonding, and support
Deficient Community Health related to resettlement of refugees in the community	The community will develop programs to meet the needs of new members of the community.	Conduct needs assessment of community.	To identify priority needs for new members of community
		Initiate health education programs based on topics identified in needs assessment.	To meet needs of members of community
		Prepare client education materials in a variety of languages.	To enhance understanding of community members
		Identify risks in community (e.g., environmental hazards, drug sales).	To provide target for community improvement
		With community leaders, develop plan to cope with and reduce environmental hazards.	To improve public health and safety
		Develop monitoring or surveillance system.	To ensure that progress will continue and new problems will be identified
Ineffective Community Coping related to presence of gangs and lack of community programs to redirect activities of youth	The health status of the community will improve.	Initiate health screening programs for community members.	To identify effects of environmental hazards in community
		Work with politicians and policymakers to develop community.	To provide safe environment with means of economic survival for community members
		Initiate programs such as Block Watch, Safe Houses, and Neighborhood Watch.	To enhance safety of environment
		Work with community leaders to develop or clean up playgrounds.	To provide safe place for children to play
		With community leaders and gang members, develop community grassroots initiatives for gang prevention.	To enable community members to take ownership in community
		Identify sites of lead exposure.	To decrease potential for lead poisoning in children
		Participate in immunization or vaccination clinics.	To reduce risk in community of infectious diseases
		Develop community education programs on drugs, alcohol, and tobacco.	To reduce exposure of young people to these products

KEY POINTS

- The family is a social network that acts as an important support system for its members.
- Family theories provide nurses with useful guidelines for understanding family function.
- Family socioeconomics, response to stress, and culture are key factors influencing family health.
- The economic, religious, kinship, and political structures are embedded in the reproductive beliefs and practices of a culture.
- Nurses must develop cultural competence and integrate it into the nursing care plan.
- Of necessity, most changes aimed at improving community health involve partnerships among community residents and health workers.
- Methods of collecting data useful to the nurse working in the community include walking surveys, analysis of existing data, informant interviews, and participant observation.
- Vulnerable populations are groups who are at higher risk for developing physical, mental, or social health problems.
- Social and economic factors affect the scope of perinatal nursing practice.
- Perinatal home care is a unique nursing practice that incorporates knowledge from community health nursing, acute care nursing, family therapy, health promotion, and client education.
- Telephonic nurse advice lines, telephonic nursing assessments, and warm lines are low-cost health care services that facilitate continuous client education, support, and health care decision making, even though health care is delivered in multiple sites.

REFERENCES

Agency for Healthcare Research and Quality (AHRQ). (2013). *National Healthcare Disparities Report, 2012*. Available at www.ahrq.gov/research/findings/nhqrdr/index.html.

Allen, F. (1997). Comparative theories of the expanded role in nursing and implications for nursing practice. *Nursing Papers, 9*(2), 38–45.

American College of Obstetricians and Gynecologists (ACOG).(2010). Health care for homeless women. ACOG Committee Opinion No. 454. *Obstetrics and Gynecology, 115*(2 pt 1), 396–399.

America's children. Key national indicators for well-being. (2013). Available at www.childstats.gov/americaschildren/famsoc1.asp.

Association of Women's Health, Obstetric and Neonatal Nurses (AWHONN). (2009). *Standards for professional nursing practice in the care of women and newborns* (7th ed.). Washington, DC: Author.

Becker, M. (1974). The health belief model and sick role behavior. *Health Education Monographs, 2*(4), 409–419.

Blackwell, D. L. (2010). Family structure and children's health in the United States: Findings from the National Health Interview Survey, 2001–2007. National Center for Health Statistics. *Vital Health Statistics, 10*(246), 1–166.

Boss, P. (1996). *Family stress management* (2nd ed.). Newbury Park, CA: Sage.

Bronfenbrenner, U. (1979). *The ecology of human development*. Cambridge, MA: Harvard University Press.

Bronfenbrenner, U. (1989). Ecological systems theory. In R. Vasta (Ed.), *Annals of child development* (vol. 6). Greenwich, CT: JAI.

Carter, B., & McGoldrick, M. (1999). *The expanded family life cycle: Individual, family, and social perspectives* (3rd ed.). Boston: Allyn & Bacon.

Centers for Disease Control and Prevention (CDC). (2013a). Office of Minority Health & Health Disparities (OMHD). *Racial & ethnic minority population*. Available at www.cdc.gov/omhd/populations.

Centers for Disease Control and Prevention (CDC). (2013b). *Minority health*. Available at www.cdc.gov/minority-health/populations/remp.html.

Dray, S. (2012). *What are the national statistics for homelessness?* Available at www.ehow.com/about_4597051_what-national-statistics-homelessness.html.

Freund, K. (2012). Health disparities among women. In L. Goldman, & A. Schafer (Eds.), *Goldman's Cecil medicine* (24th ed.). Available at www.mdconsult.com.

Gottlieb, L. N., & Gottlieb, B. (2007). The developmental/health framework within the McGill Model of Nursing: "Laws of Nature" guiding whole person care. *Advances in Nursing Science, 30*(1), E43–E57.

Giger, J. N. (2013). *Transcultural nursing: Assessment and intervention* (6th ed.). St. Louis: Mosby.

Grieco, E. M., Acosta, Y. D., de la Cruz, G. P., et al. (2012). *The foreign-born population in the United States: 2010*. Available at www.census.gov/prod/2012pubs/acs-19.pdf.

Homelessness in America.(2012). Available at www.homelessnessinamerica.com.

Janz, N., & Becker, M. (1984). The health belief model: A decade later. *Health Education Quarterly, 11*(1), 1–47.

Klein, D., & White, J. (1996). *Family theories: An introduction*. Newbury Park, CA: Sage.

Lofquist, D., Lugaila, T., O'Connell, M., & Feliz, S. (2012). *Households and families: 2010 census briefs* Available at www.census.gov/prod/cen2010/briefs/c2010br-14.pdf.

National Coalition for the Homeless (NCH). (2011). *Hunger and food insecurity* Available at www.nationalhomeless.org/fact-sheets/hunger.html.

National Women's Law Center (NWLC). (2010). *National report card on women's health*. Available at http://hrc.nwlc.org.

Opening Doors. (2012). *Federal strategic plan to prevent and end homelessness: Update 2011*. Available at www.usich.gov/resources/uploads/asset_library/USICH_FSPUpdate_2012_12312.pdf.

Pew Research Center. (2013). *Second-generation Americans. A portrait of the adult children of immigrants*. Washington, DC: Pew Research Center. Available at www.pewsocialtrends.org/files/2013/02/FINAL_immigrant_generations_report_2-7-13.pdf.

Richards, R., Merrill, R. M., & Baksh, L. (2011). Health behaviors and infant health outcomes in homeless pregnant women in the United States. *Pediatrics, 128*(3), 438–446.

Rural Assistance Center. (2011). *United States*. Available at www.raconline.org/states/unitedstates.php.

Scharte, M., & Bolte, G. (2012). Increased health risks of children with single mothers: The impact of socio-economic and environmental factors. *Journal of Public Health, 23*(3), 469–475.

Siegel, B. S., & Perrin, E. C. (2013). Policy statement: Promoting the well-being of children whose parents are gay or lesbian. *Pediatrics, 131*(4), 827–830.

Sipes, L. A. (2012). *Statistics on women offenders*. Available at www.corrections.com/news/article/30166-statistics-on-women-offenders.

Spector, R. (2013). *Cultural diversity in health and illness* (8th ed.). Upper Saddle River, NJ: Prentice-Hall.

Trumbull, M. (April 10, 2014). *Obamacare enrollment at 7.5 million. But how are exchanges really doing?*. Available at www.csmonitor.com/USA/DC-Decoder/2014/0410/Obamacare-enrollment-at-7.5-million.-But-how-are-exchanges-really-doing-video.

U.S. Census Bureau. (2011a). *Facts for features-grandparents day 2013*. Available at www.census.gov/newsroom/releases/archives/facts_for_features_special_editions/cb13-ff_18.html.

U.S. Census Bureau. (2011b). *Population estimates*. Available at www.census.gov/popest/data/national/asrh/2011/index.html.

U.S. Department of Health and Human Services (HHS). (2011). *Primary care: The health center program*. Available at http://bphc.hrsa.gov/about.

U.S. Department of Health and Human Services (HHS). (2013). Office of Disease Prevention & Health Promotion. *Maternal infant and child health*. Available at www.healthypeople.gov/2020/LHI/micHealth.

Wright, L., & Leahey, M. (2012). *Nurses and families: A guide to family assessment and intervention* (6th ed.). Philadelphia: F.A. Davis Co.

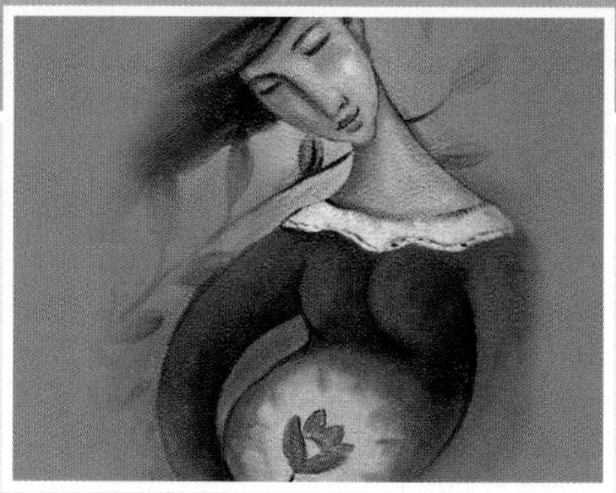

CHAPTER 3

Nursing and Genomics

Marcia Van Riper

http://evolve.elsevier.com/Lowdermilk/MWHC/

LEARNING OBJECTIVES

- Explore how recent advances in genetics have changed the field of health care.
- Discuss the essential competencies in genetics and genomics for all nurses.
- Describe expanded roles for nurses in genetics and genetic counseling.
- Discuss key findings of the Human Genome Project.
- Describe the different types of genetic testing.
- Identify genetic disorders commonly tested for in maternity and women's health nursing.
- Explore the possible benefits and risks of pharmacogenomics.
- Discuss the current status of gene therapy.
- Examine the ethical, legal, and social implications of the Human Genome Project.
- Explain the key concepts of basic human genetics.
- Discuss the education and counseling needs of individuals and families who undergo genetic testing.
- Explore the availability of genetic testing for individuals and families from diverse backgrounds.
- Describe the role of genomics in cancer care for women.
- Identify genetics resources for nurses and other health care professionals.

Remarkable advances in genomics and technology have revolutionized the field of health care and nursing practice by providing the tools needed to determine the hereditary component of many diseases, as well as improve our ability to predict susceptibility to disease, onset and progression of disease, and response to medications (Calzone, Jenkins, Nicoli, et al., 2013; Feero, Guttmacher, & Collins, 2010; Green & Guyer, 2011; McCarthy, McLeod, & Ginsburg, 2013). Since the human genome was sequenced, there has been a gradual shift from genetics to genomics. **Genetics** refers to the study of a particular gene, whereas **genomics** refers to the study of the entire genome. **Genes** are the basic physical units of inheritance that are passed from parents to offspring and contain the information needed to specify traits. The **genome** is the entire set of genetic instructions found in a cell. For these and other definitions of genetic terms, check out the *Talking Glossary of Genetic Terms* (www.genome.gov/Glossary).

With growing public interest in *personalized genomic information* (information about much or all of a person's genome), increasing development of practice guidelines, mounting commercial pressures, and ever-increasing opportunities for individuals, families, and communities to participate in the direction and design of their genomic health care, genetic services are rapidly becoming an integral part of routine health care (Guttmacher, McGuire, Ponder, & Stefansson, 2010; Manolio, Chisholm, Ozenberger, et al., 2013). Moreover, many individuals and families have participated in *direct-to-consumer genetic testing* (testing marketed directly to consumers through television, print advertisements, and websites for companies such as DNA Direct) (www.dnadirect.com) and 23 and Me (www.23andme.com). Although much of the information provided by direct-to-consumer testing companies is recreational (ancestry information, information about types of ear wax, and bitter taste perception), some of the information provided is health related and could be interpreted as diagnosis (Evans & Green, 2009). Because of this, direct-to-consumer testing that is provided without the involvement of competent health care professionals may be not only unhelpful, but also harmful (Beery, 2013; Guttmacher et al., 2010; McGuire & Burke, 2010).

Because of their frontline position in the health care system and their long-standing history of providing holistic family-centered care, nurses are likely to be one of the first health care professionals to whom individuals and families turn with questions about genetic risk and susceptibility and to seek guidance regarding the complexities of genetic testing and interpretation. Nowhere is this more apparent than in maternity and women's health care (Lewis, 2011). A growing number of maternity and women's health nurses provide information about the availability of genetics tests, answer question about them, and order and interpret genetic tests. Although most of these tests are used to determine a client's risk of having a child affected by a genetic condition such as Down syndrome, cystic fibrosis (CF), or sickle cell disease, the number of genetic tests used to determine the presence of, or susceptibility to, adult-onset disorders (e.g., hereditary colorectal cancer, hereditary breast and ovarian cancer, and Huntington's disease [HD]) continues to rise. Additionally, nurses working in maternity and women's health are caring for an increasing number of individuals and families who are dealing with complex ethical, legal, and social issues associated with genetic testing and the experience of living with someone who has a genetic condition (Sparbel & Tluczek, 2011; Sparbel & Williams, 2009; Van Riper, 2012; Van Riper & Choi, 2011; Wilke, Gallo, Yao, et al., 2013).

NURSING EXPERTISE IN GENETICS AND GENOMICS

Essential Competencies in Genetics and Genomics for All Nurses

Nearly 50 organizations, including the Association of Women's Health, Obstetric and Neonatal Nurses (AWHONN) and the National Association of Neonatal Nurses (NANN), have endorsed the *Essential Nursing Competencies and Curriculum Guidelines for Genetics and Genomics* (www.genome.gov/17517146). According to these guidelines, which were developed by an independent panel of nurse leaders from clinical, research, and academic settings and published by the American Nurses Association and the National Human Genome Research Institute of the National Institute of Health (Consensus Panel on Genetic/Genomic Nursing Competencies, 2009), all nurses need to have minimal competencies in genetics and genomics regardless of their academic preparation, practice setting, or specialty. Some of the competencies most relevant to nurses in the area of maternity and women's health include:

- Constructs a pedigree from collected family history information using standardized symbols and terminology
- Develops a plan of care that incorporates genetic and genomic assessment information
- Recognizes when one's own attitudes and values related to genetics and genomic science may affect care provided to clients
- Provides clients with credible, accurate, appropriate, and current genetic and genomic information, resources, services, and/or technologies that facilitate decision making
- Demonstrates in practice the importance of tailoring genetic and genomic information and services to clients based on their culture, religion, knowledge level, literacy, and preferred language
- Assesses clients' knowledge, perceptions, and responses to genetic and genomic information
- Facilitates referrals for specialized genetic and genomic services for clients as needed

Expanded Roles for Maternity and Women's Health Nurses

Expanded roles for nurses with expertise in genetics and genomics are developing in many areas of maternity and women's health nursing. These areas include but are not limited to prenatal screening and testing; carrier testing during pregnancy; newborn screening; palliative care for infants with life-threatening genetic conditions and their families; the identification and care of individuals with genetic conditions and their families; and the care of women with genetic conditions who require specialized care during pregnancy, such as women with neuromuscular disease, cystic fibrosis, and factor V Leiden (DeLuca, Zanni, Bonhomme, & Kemper, 2013; Frazer, Porter, & Goss, 2013; Johnson, Giarelli, Lewis, & Rice, 2013; Prows, Hopkin, Barnoy, & Van Riper, 2013; Sparbel & Tluczek, 2011; Sparbel & Williams, 2009; Van Riper, 2007, 2012; Weinstein, 2009; Wilke et al., 2013). The Oncology Nursing Society (ONS) (www.ons.org) has taken an active role in providing oncology nurses with the education and resources they need to integrate genetics and genomics into all phases of care for individuals and families affected by cancer, including information specifically related to cancers affecting women.

HUMAN GENOME PROJECT AND IMPLICATIONS FOR CLINICAL PRACTICE

Two key findings from the Human Genome Project (www.genome.gov/12011238) were that (1) all human beings are >99% identical at the deoxyribonucleic acid (DNA) level, and (2) there are probably about 20,500 genes in the human genome. The finding that human beings are >99% identical at the DNA level should help discourage the use of science as a justification for drawing biologically precise racial boundaries around certain groups of people. Originally, scientists had estimated that there were 50,000 to 140,000 genes in the human genome. It had been assumed that the main reason that humans are more evolved and more highly sophisticated than other species is that they have more genes. A new explanation for human complexity, given the relatively small number of genes, is that humans are more efficient with their genes. Humans are able to do much more with their genes than are other species. Instead of producing only one protein per gene, most human genes produce at least three proteins.

Importance of Family History

Completion of the Human Genome Project and the resultant identification of the inherited causes for many diseases has resulted in renewed interest in family history. Although it is easy to be impressed by the more than 3600 genetic tests currently available (www.ncbi.nlm.nih.gov/gtr), family history will most likely continue to be the single most cost-effective piece of genetic information. In 2008, Solomon, Jack, and Feero described a complete three-generation family history that includes ancestry information concerning both sides of family as the best genetic "test" applicable to preconception care. When nurses and other clinicians conduct a family history, they can gain not only valuable information about the structure of the family and diseases that affect various individuals in the family, but also a rich understanding of family relationships, social context, occupations, lifestyle, and health habits (American College of Obstetricians and Gynecologists [ACOG], 2011; De Sevo, 2009).

The process of collecting this information often facilitates the development of a relationship between the client/family and the clinician. In 2004, the U.S. Department of Health and Human Services launched the Family History Initiative by designating Thanksgiving Day as National Family History Day. The U.S. Surgeon General encouraged families to use their family gatherings as a time to talk about and collect important family health history. A number of family history tools are available free of charge online. One of the most widely used family history tools is the *My Family Health Portrait* (https://familyhistory.hhs.gov). Another helpful tool is the family health history tool, *Does it run in the family?* that was developed by the Genetic Alliance (www.doesitruninthefamily.org). The Centers for Disease Control and Prevention (CDC) also provides links to family history resources (www.cdc.gov/genomics/famhistory/famhist.htm).

The preconception period is an ideal time to review family history and provide personalized recommendations based on family history (ACOG, 2011). It is also one of the best times to counsel couples about carrier testing options that are based on known population-specific risks (Bodurtha & Strauss, 2012). Finally, the preconception period is an optimal time to refer couples, when appropriate, to specialists in high risk pregnancy and genetics.

Gene Identification and Testing

Initial efforts to sequence and analyze the human genome have proven invaluable in the identification of genes involved in disease and in the development of genetic tests. In an effort to bridge the transition from discovery to diagnostics and treatments, the National Institutes of Health launched the *Genetic Testing Registry* (GTR) in 2012. The GTR (www.ncbi.nlm.nih.gov/gtr) is a free online tool that can be used to obtain a list of available genetic tests. The GTR website also includes links to other resources such as *GeneReviews* and Online Mendelian Inheritance in Man (OMIM). *GeneReviews* is a collection of expert-authored, peer-reviewed disease descriptions presented in a standardized format and focused on clinically relevant and medically actionable information on the diagnosis, management, and genetic counseling of individuals and families with specific inherited conditions. OMIM is an online catalog of human genes and genetic disorders.

Genetic testing involves the analysis of human DNA, ribonucleic acid (RNA), which has a major role in protein synthesis, chromosomes (threadlike packages of genes and other DNA in the nucleus of a cell), or proteins to detect abnormalities related to an inherited condition. Genetic tests can be used to examine directly the DNA and RNA that make up a gene (direct or molecular testing), look at markers that are coinherited with a gene that causes a genetic condition (linkage analysis), examine the protein products of genes (biochemical testing), or examine chromosomes (cytogenetic testing). Cytogenetic analysis of malignant tissue has become a mainstay of oncology.

Most of the genetic tests now offered in clinical practice are tests for single-gene disorders in clients with clinical symptoms or who have a family history of a genetic disease (http://iml.dartmouth.edu/education/cme/Genetics). Some of these genetic tests are prenatal tests or tests used to identify the genetic status of a pregnancy at risk for a genetic condition. Current prenatal testing options include maternal serum screening (a blood test used to see if a pregnant woman is at increased risk for carrying a fetus with a neural tube defect or a chromosomal abnormality such as Down syndrome, trisomy 18 or trisomy 13), fetal ultrasound or sonogram (an imaging technique using high-frequency sound waves to produce images of the fetus inside the uterus), invasive procedures (chorionic villus sampling and amniocentesis), and noninvasive prenatal testing for fetal aneuploidy (a blood test that uses cell-free DNA from the plasma of pregnant women to screen for Down syndrome and, in some cases, trisomy 13 and trisomy18). The American College of Obstetricians and Gynecologists (ACOG) has recommended that all women, regardless of maternal age, be offered prenatal assessment for aneuploidy (an abnormal number of chromosomes within a cell) either by screening or invasive prenatal diagnosis. ACOG currently considers noninvasive prenatal testing for fetal aneuploidy as one option that can be used as a primary screening test in women considered to be at increased risk of aneuploidy, such as women with a history of a child affected by a trisomy or women who carry a balanced translocation. ACOG also considers this type of testing appropriate for follow-up testing for women with a positive prenatal screening test result from maternal serum screening. However, ACOG does not recommend the use of noninvasive prenatal testing for aneuploidy with low risk pregnant women or women with multiple gestations (ACOG, 2012).

Another type of genetic test is the carrier screening test used to identify individuals who have a gene mutation for a genetic condition but do not show symptoms of the condition because it is an autosomal recessive condition (e.g., CF, sickle cell disease, and Tay-Sachs disease). A third type of genetic testing is predictive testing, which is used to clarify the genetic status of asymptomatic family members. The two types of predictive testing are presymptomatic and predispositional. Mutation analysis for HD, a neurodegenerative disorder, is an example of presymptomatic testing. If the gene mutation for HD is present, symptoms of HD are certain to appear if the individual lives long enough. Testing for a BRCA1 gene mutation to determine breast cancer susceptibility is an example of predispositional testing. Predispositional testing differs from presymptomatic testing in that a positive result (indicating that a BRCA1 mutation is present) does not indicate a 100% risk of developing the condition (breast cancer).

In addition to using genetic tests to test for single-gene disorders in clients with clinical symptoms or who have a family history of a genetic disease, genetic tests are used for population-based screening. For example, each year in the United States, approximately 4 million infants undergo newborn screening (Bodurtha & Strauss, 2012; Guttmacher et al., 2010). Newborn screening is a mandatory, state-supported public health program. Initially, newborn screening in the United States was only concerned with a few conditions such as phenylketonuria (PKU). However, with the advent of tandem mass spectrometry, the number of conditions tested for during newborn screening grew rapidly (DeLuca et al., 2013). Currently, most states test newborns for 31 core disorders and 26 secondary disorders (McCarthy et al., 2013). A complete list of conditions tested for in each state is available on the National Newborn Screening and Genetics Resource website (http://genes-r-us.uthscsa.edu).

Another type of population-based screening is carrier screening for single-gene disorders such as CF, sickle cell disease, and Tay-Sachs disease either preconceptionally or prenatally. In 2001, the ACOG and the American College of Medical Genetics (ACMG) recommended that clinicians offer carrier screening for CF to individuals with a family history of CF, reproductive partners of individuals who have CF, and couples in whom one or both partners are Caucasian and are planning a pregnancy or seeking prenatal care (ACOG/ACMG, 2001). Recommendations for newborn screening for cystic fibrosis appeared in 2004, and soon after this many newborn screening programs in the United States began offering newborn screening for CF. One outcome of this broader carrier and newborn screening for CF is that more and more individuals are being informed they have a CF mutation. However the correlation between genotype (an individual's collection of genes) and phenotype (an individual's observable traits) is poor for many of the more than 1900 CF mutations identified to date. That is, whereas some CF mutations are associated with significant health problems (poor growth, greasy stools, and chronic respiratory problems), others are not. Because of this, the significance of many CF mutations is uncertain. As a result, nurses and other health care professionals are increasingly being asked to communicate results with uncertain significance to individuals and families during the preconception, prenatal, and newborn periods (Sparbel & Tluczek, 2011). In 2008 the National Human Genome Research Institute held a workshop to discuss lessons learned and new opportunities for population-based carrier screening (www.genome.gov/27026048). One of the main conclusions from this workshop was that a more coherent and systematic approach is needed for the introduction of new tests into population-based screening programs.

The use of genome sequencing (e.g., whole genome sequencing and next-generation sequencing), is entering the clinical setting (Conley, Biesecker, Gonsalves, et al., 2013; McCarthy et al., 2013; Wade, Tarini, & Wilfond, 2013). The cost of sequencing a human genome dropped from $100 million in 2001 to less than $10,000 in 2012. Current indications suggest that soon it may be possible to sequence a person's entire genome for around $1,000. The cost of sequencing has already dropped to the point that sequencing the whole genome may be cheaper and more efficient than testing a client who has a complex condition of unknown origin for a select group of genetic conditions.

Pharmacogenomics

One of the most promising clinical applications of the Human Genome Project has been pharmacogenomic testing (the use of genetic information to guide a client's drug therapy) (Ginsburg & Willard, 2009). Associations between genetic variation and drug effect have been observed for a number of commonly used drugs, including warfarin, an anticoagulant commonly used to reduce the risk of thromboembolic events in clients with a history of deep vein thrombosis, pulmonary embolism, myocardial infarction, or atrial fibrillation (McCarthy et al., 2013; Meckley, Gudgeon, Anderson, et al., 2010). Warfarin is a drug with a narrow therapeutic index; it can result in serious bleeding with supratherapeutic doses and thromboembolic events with subtherapeutic doses. Because of this and the fact that there is a great deal of inter- and intrapatient dose variation, warfarin is one of the most common causes of serious adverse drug reactions. There is mounting evidence that genotype-guided warfarin dosing may not only help reduce the serious adverse drug reactions commonly associated with warfarin, but also increase dosing accuracy, shorten the time to dose stabilization, and help identify individuals who may require more frequent monitoring. In August 2007, the U.S. Food and Drug Administration (FDA) approved updated labeling for warfarin. The updated labeling acknowledges that individuals with variations in their CYP2C9 and VKORC1 genes may require a lower initial dose of warfarin. However, there are not enough clinical data yet to recommend that this type of testing be mandatory.

Pharmacogenomic testing can also be used to target therapies. Trastuzumab (Herceptin), a monoclonal antibody that specifically targets HER2/neu overexpressing breast tumors, is an example of a drug for which an obligatory genetic test has been developed (McCarthy et al., 2013). The purpose of this obligatory genetic test is to identify the subset of women with breast cancer who overexpress HER2/neu. Women who overexpress HER2/neu are most likely the only breast cancer clients who will benefit from taking trastuzumab (www.herceptin.com/index.jsp).

Gene Therapy

In the early 1990s a great deal of optimism was felt about the possibility of using gene therapy to correct a long list of inherited diseases. Generally, **gene therapy** involves inserting a healthy copy of the defective gene into the **somatic cells** (any cell of the body except sperm and egg cells) of the affected individual. Although the early optimism about gene therapy was probably never fully justified, gene therapy has moved from preclinical to clinical studies for many diseases ranging from hemophilia and other single-gene disorders to complex disorders such as cancer, human immunodeficiency virus (HIV), and cardiovascular disorders (Gillet, Macadangdang, Fathke, et al., 2009). Early hype, failures, and tragic events, such as the death of Jesse Gelsinger (18-year-old male with an X-linked genetic liver disease who was the first person publicly identified as having died in a gene therapy clinical trial) have now largely been replaced by stepwise progress in carefully developed, scientifically precise clinical trials (Gillet et al; Kohn & Candotti, 2009). Major challenges to gene therapy include figuring out how to target the right gene to the right location in the right cells, expressing the transferred gene at the right time, and minimizing adverse reactions.

Ethical, Legal, and Social Implications

Before the beginning of the Human Genome Project, widespread concern about misuse of the information gained through genetics research resulted in 5% of the Human Genome Project budget being designated for the study of the **ethical, legal, and social implications (ELSIs)** of human genome research. Two large ELSI programs were created to identify, analyze, and address the ELSIs of human genome research at the same time that the basic science issues were being studied. Since 2004, issues of high priority for these programs have been privacy and fairness in the use and interpretation of genetic information; clinical integration of new genetics technologies; issues surrounding genetics research, such as possible discrimination and stigmatization; and education for professionals and the general public about genetics, genetics health care, and ELSI of human genome research. Both ELSI programs have excellent websites that include vast amounts of educational information, as well as links to other informative sites (www.genome.gov/10001618; www.ornl.gov/sci/techresources/Human_Genome/elsi/elsi.shtml).

The major risk associated with genetic testing concerns what happens with the information gained through testing: it may result in increased anxiety and altered family relationships; it may be difficult to keep confidential; and it may result in discrimination and stigmatization. More important, there is still a large gap between the ability to test for a genetic condition and the ability to treat the same condition. In addition, informed consent is difficult to ensure when some of the outcomes, benefits, and risks of genetic testing remain unknown. Also, many of the tests being used are as yet imperfect—few have a 100% detection rate. Individuals and families who receive false-positive results (the test results indicate that a person or fetus is affected by a genetic condition when he or she is not) may terminate an unaffected pregnancy or undergo unwarranted extreme measures such as bilateral prophylactic mastectomy. Individuals and families who receive false-negative results (the test results indicate that a person or fetus is not affected by a genetic condition when he or she is) may fail to follow surveillance strategies designed to improve their health outcomes because they have been falsely reassured that they are not at increased risk for a specific condition (see Community Activity).

COMMUNITY ACTIVITY

Select two web addresses for resources on genetics for parents. Access the sites.

- Compare and contrast the appearance, readability, and information contained in the sites.
- Is the information available for parents who do not read English?
- Do you agree that these sites are appropriate for parents?
- Is the information contained culturally relevant?
- How could you, as a nurse, use this information?
- Role play with a classmate, reviewing the information with a parent undergoing genetic testing.

Factors Influencing the Decision to Undergo Genetic Testing

The decision to undergo genetic testing is seldom an autonomous decision based solely on the needs and preferences of the individual being tested. Instead, it is often a decision based on feelings of responsibility and commitment to others (Van Riper, 2005). For example, a woman who is receiving treatment for breast cancer may undergo BRCA1/BRCA2 mutation testing not because she wants to find out if she carries a BRCA1 or BRCA2 mutation, but because her two unaffected sisters have asked her to be tested, and she feels a sense of responsibility and commitment to them. A female airline pilot with a family history of HD, who has no desire to find out if she has the gene mutation associated with HD, may undergo mutation analysis for HD because she feels she has an obligation to her family, her employer, and the people who fly with her.

Decisions about genetic testing are shaped, and in many instances constrained, by factors such as social norms, where care is received, and socioeconomic status. Most pregnant women in the United States now have at least one ultrasound examination, many undergo some type of multiple-marker screening, and a growing number undergo other types of prenatal testing. The range of prenatal testing options available to a pregnant woman and her family may vary significantly based on where the pregnant woman receives prenatal care and her socioeconomic status. Certain types of prenatal testing may not be available in smaller communities and rural settings (e.g., chorionic villus sampling and fluorescent in situ hybridization [FISH] analysis). In addition, certain types of genetic testing may not be offered in conservative medical communities (e.g., preimplantation genetic screening). Some types of genetic testing are expensive and typically not covered by health insurance. Because of this, these tests may be available only to a relatively small number of individuals and families: those who can afford to pay for them (Badzek, Henaghan, Turner, & Monsen, 2013).

Cultural and ethnic differences also have a significant effect on decisions about genetic testing. When prenatal diagnosis was first introduced, the principal constituency was a self-selected group of Caucasian, well-informed, middle- to upper-class women. Today the widespread use of genetic testing has introduced prenatal testing to new groups of women, women who had not previously considered genetic services. The fact that many of the women currently undergoing prenatal testing may not share mainstream U.S. views about the role of medicine and prenatal care, the meaning of disability, or how to respond to scientific risks and uncertainties further amplifies the complexity of ethical issues associated with prenatal testing.

The genetic testing experience raises fundamental questions about the mutual obligations of kin. Are individuals morally obligated to alert extended family members about inherited health risks? Conversely, do extended family members have a moral obligation to participate in research designed to determine genetic risk when unwanted information about them may be generated in the process? Another important question that must be considered is "Whose gene is it?" This question is likely to stimulate a great deal of debate, especially in the area of preimplantation genetic diagnosis (when one or both parents has a known genetic abnormality and testing is performed on an embryo to determine if it also carries a genetic abnormality).

CLINICAL GENETICS

Genetic Transmission

Human development is a complicated process that depends on the systematic unraveling of instructions found in the genetic material of the egg and the sperm. Development from conception to birth of a healthy, typically developing baby occurs without incident in most cases; however, the baseline risk of some type of birth defect is estimated to be 3% to 4% for all pregnancies.

Genes and Chromosomes

The hereditary material carried in the nucleus of each of the somatic cells determines an individual's characteristics. This material, called deoxribonucleic acid (DNA), forms threadlike strands known as *chromosomes*. Each chromosome is composed of the many smaller segments of DNA referred to as genes. Genes, or combinations of genes, contain coded information that determines an individual's unique characteristics. The "code" is found in the specific linear order of the molecules that combine to form the strands of DNA. Genes control both the types of proteins that are made and the rate at which they are produced. Genes never act in isolation; they always interact with other genes and the environment.

All normal human somatic cells contain 46 chromosomes arranged as 23 pairs of homologous (matched) chromosomes; one chromosome of each pair is inherited from each parent. There are 22 pairs of autosomes that control most traits in the body, and one pair of sex chromosomes. Whereas the Y chromosome is primarily concerned with sex determination, the X chromosome contains genes that are involved in much more than sex determination. The larger female chromosome is called the X; the smaller male chromosome is the Y. Generally the presence of a Y chromosome causes an embryo to develop as a male; in the absence of a Y chromosome, the individual develops as a female. Thus in a normal female, the homologous pair of sex chromosomes is XX, and in a normal male, the homologous pair is XY.

Homologous chromosomes (except the X and Y chromosomes in males) have the same number and arrangement of genes. In other words, if one chromosome has a gene for hair color, its partner chromosome also will have a gene for hair color, and these hair-color genes will have the same loci or be located in the same place on the two chromosomes. Although both genes code for hair color, they may not code for the same hair color. Genes at corresponding loci on homologous chromosomes that code for different forms or variations of the same trait are called alleles. An individual having two copies of the same allele for a given trait is said to be homozygous for that trait; with two different alleles, the person is heterozygous for the trait.

The term genotype typically is used to refer to the genetic makeup of an individual when discussing a specific gene pair, but at times, genotype is used to refer to an individual's entire genetic makeup or all the genes that the individual can pass on to future generations. Phenotype refers to the observable expression of an individual's genotype, such as physical features, a biochemical or molecular trait, and even a psychologic trait. A trait or disorder is considered dominant if it is expressed or phenotypically apparent when only one copy of an allele associated with the trait is present. It is considered recessive if it is expressed only when two copies of the alleles associated with the trait are present.

As more is learned about genetics and genomics, the concepts of dominance and recessivity have become more complex, especially in X-linked disorders. For example, traits considered to be recessive may be expressed even when only one copy of a gene located on the X chromosome is present. This occurs frequently in males because males have only one X chromosome; thus they have only one copy of the genes located on the X chromosome. Whichever gene is present on the one X chromosome determines which trait is expressed. Females, conversely, have two X chromosomes, so they have two copies of the genes located on the X chromosome. However, in any female somatic cell, only one X chromosome is functioning (otherwise, there would be inequality in gene dosage between males and females). This process, known as X-inactivation or the Lyon hypothesis, is generally a random occurrence. That is, there is a 50/50 chance as to whether the maternal X or the paternal X is inactivated. Occasionally the percentage of cells that have the X with an abnormal or mutant gene is very high. This helps explain why hemophilia, an X-linked recessive disorder, can clinically manifest itself in a female known to be a heterozygous carrier (a female who has only one copy of the gene mutation). It also helps explain why traditional methods of carrier detection are less effective for X-linked recessive disorders; the possible range for enzyme activity values can vary greatly, depending on which X chromosome is inactivated.

Chromosomal Abnormalities

Chromosomal abnormalities are a major cause of reproductive loss, congenital problems, and gynecologic disorders; the incidence is approximately 0.6% in newborns, 6% in stillbirths, and 60% in spontaneous abortions (Martin, 2008). Errors resulting in chromosomal abnormalities can occur during mitosis (cell division occurring in somatic cells that results in two identical daughter cells containing a diploid number of chromosomes) or meiosis (division of a sex cell into two and four haploid cells). These errors can occur in either the autosomes or the sex chromosomes. Even without the presence of obvious structural malformations, small deviations in chromosomes can cause problems in fetal development.

The pictorial analysis of the number, form, and size of an individual's chromosomes is known as a karyotype. Cells from any nucleated, replicating body tissue (not red blood cells, nerves, or muscles) can be used. The most commonly used tissues are white blood cells and fetal cells in amniotic fluid. The cells are grown in a culture and arrested when they are in metaphase (during metaphase, the chromosomes are condensed and visible with a light microscope), and then the cells are dropped onto a slide. This breaks the cell membranes and spreads the chromosomes, making them easier to visualize. Next the cells are stained with special stains (e.g., Giemsa stain) that create striping or "banding" patterns. These patterns aid in the analysis because they are consistent from person to person. Once the chromosome spreads are photographed or scanned by a computer, they are cut out and arranged in a specific numeric order according to their length and shape. The chromosomes are numbered from largest to smallest, 1 to 22, and the sex chromosomes are designated by the letter X or Y. Each chromosome is divided into two "arms" designated by p (short arm) and q (long arm). A female karyotype is designated as 46, XX and a male karyotype is designated as 46, XY. Figure 3-1 illustrates the chromosomes in a body cell.

Autosomal Abnormalities

Autosomal abnormalities involve differences in the number or structure of autosome chromosomes (pairs 1 to 22). They result from unequal distribution of genetic material during gamete (egg and sperm) formation.

Abnormalities of Chromosome Number. A euploid cell is a cell with the correct or normal number of chromosomes within the cell. Because most gametes are haploid (1N, 23 chromosomes) and most somatic cells are diploid (2N, 46 chromosomes), they are both considered euploid cells. Deviations from the correct number of chromosomes per cell can be one of two types: (1) polyploidy, in which the deviation is an exact multiple of the haploid number of chromosomes or one chromosome set (23 chromosomes); or (2) aneuploidy, in which the numerical deviation is not an exact multiple of the haploid set. A triploid (3N) cell is an example of a polyploidy. It has 69 chromosomes. A tetraploid (4N) cell, also an example of a polyploidy, has 92 chromosomes.

Aneuploidy is the most commonly identified chromosome abnormality in humans and the leading genetic cause of intellectual disability. A monosomy is the product of the union between a normal gamete and a gamete that is missing a chromosome. Monosomic individuals have only 45 chromosomes in each of their cells. The product of the union of a normal gamete with a gamete containing an extra chromosome is a trisomy. The most common autosomal aneuploid conditions involve trisomies. Trisomic individuals have 47 chromosomes in most or all their cells.

The vast majority of trisomies occurs during oogenesis (the process by which a premeiotic female germ cell divides into a mature egg) and the incidence of these types of chromosomal errors increases exponentially with advancing maternal age

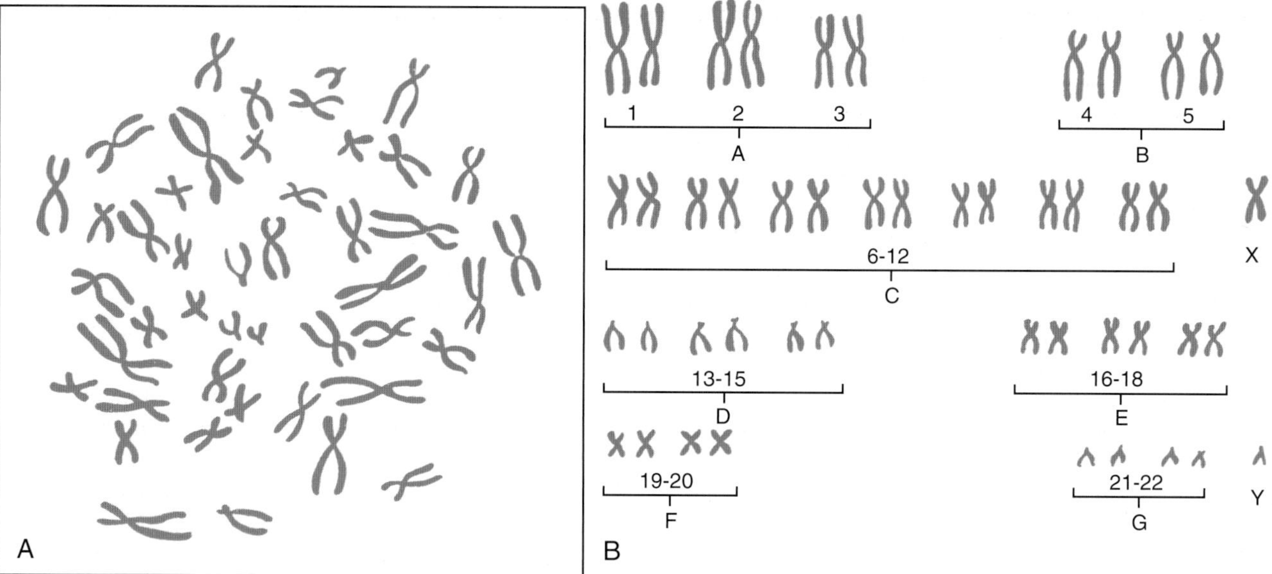

FIG 3-1 Chromosomes during cell division. **A,** Example of photomicrograph. **B,** Chromosomes arranged in karyotype; female and male sex-determining chromosomes.

(Hassold & Hunt, 2009; Hunt & Hassold, 2008). Although variation exists among trisomies with regard to the parent and stage of origin of the extra chromosome, most trisomies are maternal meiosis I (MI) errors. This means that most trisomies are caused by nondisjunction during the first meiotic division. The first meiotic division involves the segregation of homologous or similar chromosomes. One pair of chromosomes fails to separate. One resulting cell contains both chromosomes, and the other contains none. The fact that most trisomies are maternal MI errors is not that surprising, because maternal MI occurs over a long time span. It is initiated in precursor cells during fetal development, but it is not completed until the time those cells undergo ovulation after menarche.

The most common trisomal abnormality is Down syndrome (DS). In the United States, approximately 1 in every 691 newborns has DS, and it is estimated that there are more than 400,000 individuals with DS living in the United States (Prows et al., 2013; www.cdc.gov/ncbddd/birthdefects/DownSyndrome.html; http://ndsccenter.org; www.ndss.org). Current estimates suggest there are around 6 million people with DS in the world. Approximately 95% of individuals with DS have trisomy 21 or an extra chromosome 21 (47, XX +21, female with DS; or 47, XY +21, male with DS). Another type of DS, translocation, occurs when extra chromosome 21 material is present in every cell of the individual but it is attached to another chromosome. This type of DS affects approximately 3% to 4% of individuals with DS. In the third type of DS, mosaicism, extra chromosome 21 material is found in some but not all of the cells. Only 1% to 2% of individuals with DS have mosaicism.

Although the clinical presentation of DS is complex and variable (Bull & Committee on Genetics, 2011; Ivan & Cromwell 2013a), all individuals with DS have some level of intellectual disability. Common characteristics seen in individuals with Down syndrome are as follows:

- Oblique palpebral fissures or an upward slant to the eyes
- Epicanthal folds or small skinfolds on the inner corners of the eyes
- Small, white, crescent-shaped spots on the irises called Brushfield spots
- A flat facial profile that usually includes a somewhat depressed nasal bridge and a small nose
- Enlargement of the tongue in relationship to size of the mouth
- Small ears, which may be abnormally shaped or abnormally rotated
- Short, broad hands with a fifth finger that has one flexion crease instead of two
- A single deep crease across the center of the palm, often referred to as a simian crease
- Excessive space between the large and second toes
- Hyperflexibility, an excessive ability to extend the joints
- Muscle hypotonia or low muscle tone

Some individuals with DS have all of these characteristics, but others have only a few. Figure 3-2 is a picture of an infant with DS who has some of the characteristics commonly associated with that syndrome (see Nursing Care Plan).

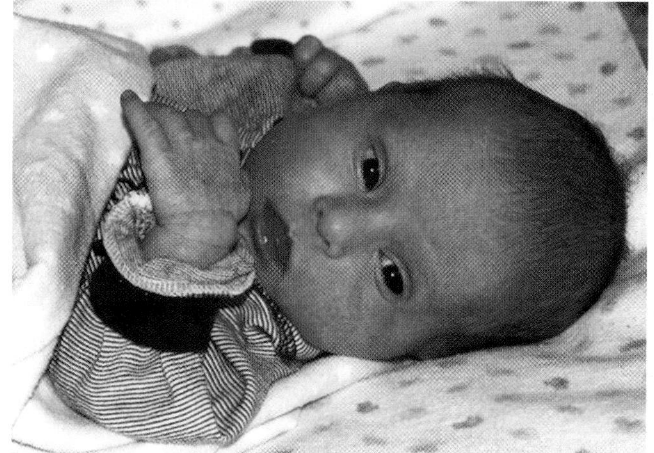

FIG 3-2 Infant with Down syndrome. Note upward slant to eyes, flat nasal bridge, slightly protruding tongue, and mottled skin. (Courtesy Thomas and Christie Coghill, Clayton, NC.)

NURSING CARE PLAN

The Family Living with a Neonate with Down Syndrome

NURSING DIAGNOSIS	EXPECTED OUTCOME	NURSING INTERVENTIONS	RATIONALES
Interrupted Family Processes related to birth of a neonate with Down syndrome	The couple will verbalize accurate information about Down syndrome, including implications for future pregnancies.	Assess knowledge base of couple regarding the clinical signs and symptoms of Down syndrome.	To correct any misconceptions and establish basis for teaching plan
		Provide information throughout the genetic evaluation regarding risk status and clinical signs and symptoms of Down syndrome.	To give couple a realistic picture of neonate's defects and assist with decision making for future pregnancies
		Use therapeutic communication during discussions with the couple.	To provide opportunity for expression of concern
		Refer to support groups, social services, or counseling.	To assist family with cohesive actions and decision making
		Refer to child development specialist.	To provide family with realistic expectations regarding cognitive and behavioral abilities of child with Down syndrome
Situational Low Self-Esteem related to diagnosis of Down syndrome as evidenced by parents' statements of guilt and shame	The parents will express an increased number of positive statements regarding their neonate with Down syndrome.	Assist parents to list strengths and coping strategies that have been helpful in past situations.	To use appropriate strategies during this situational crisis
		Encourage expression of feelings using therapeutic communication.	To provide clarification and emotional support
		Clarify and provide information regarding Down syndrome.	To decrease feelings of guilt and gradually increase feelings of positive self-esteem
		Refer for further counseling as needed.	To provide more in-depth and ongoing support
Risk for Impaired Parenting related to birth of neonate with Down syndrome	Parents will bond with and provide appropriate care for the infant.	Assist parents to see and describe normal aspects of infant.	To promote bonding
		Encourage and assist with breastfeeding if that is parents' choice of feeding method.	To facilitate closeness with infant and provide benefits of breast milk
		Assure parents that information regarding the neonate will remain confidential.	To assist the parents to maintain some situational control and allow for time to work through their feelings
		Discuss and role-play with parents ways of informing family and friends of infant's diagnosis and prognosis.	To promote positive aspects of infant and decrease potential isolation from social interactions
		Provide anticipatory guidance about what to expect as infant develops.	To assist family to provide appropriate stimulation to enhance development
Spiritual Distress related to situational crisis of child born with Down syndrome	Parents will seek appropriate support persons (family members, priest, minister, rabbi) for assistance.	Listen for cues indicative of parents' feelings ("Why did God do this to us?").	To identify messages indicating spiritual distress
		Acknowledge parents' spiritual concerns and encourage expression of feelings.	To help build a therapeutic relationship
		Facilitate visits from clergy and provide privacy during visits.	To demonstrate respect for parents' relationship with clergy
		Encourage parents to discuss concerns with clergy.	To use expert spiritual care resources to help the parents
		Facilitate interaction with family members and other support persons.	To encourage expressions of concern and seek comfort
Social Isolation related to full-time caretaking responsibilities for a neonate with Down syndrome	Parents will describe a plan to use resources to prevent social isolation.	Provide opportunity for parents to express feelings about caring for a neonate with Down syndrome.	To facilitate effective communication and trust
		Discuss with parents their expectations about caring for the neonate.	To identify potential areas of concern
		Assist parents to identify potential caregiving resources	To permit parents to return to a routine at home
		Identify appropriate referrals for home care.	To provide continuity of care

Although the risk of having a child with Down syndrome increases with maternal age, children with Down syndrome can be born to mothers of any age: 80% of children with Down syndrome are born to mothers younger than 35 years (National Down Syndrome Society, 2013). The risk of a mother having a second child with Down syndrome is about 1% when the cause of the Down syndrome is trisomy 21 (see also Chapter 36).

Other autosomal trisomies that maternity and newborn nurses may see in practice are trisomy 18 and trisomy 13. Trisomy 18 (Edward syndrome) is more common than trisomy 13 (Patau syndrome); it occurs in about 1 out of every 3000 live births versus 1 out of every 10,000 live births for trisomy 13. Infants with trisomy 18 may exhibit more than 130 different anomalies, but some of the major phenotypic features and medical complications are small for gestational age or low birth weight; craniofacial abnormalities including cleft lip and/or palate, small mouth, and small jaw; weak cry; feeding difficulties; cardiac malformations; central nervous system manifestations including hypertonia, seizures, and apnea; and extremity malformations such as small fingernails and toenails, clenched fist with index finger overlapping the third finger, and rocker-bottom feet (http://trisomy.org; www.hopefortrisomy13and18.org; www.trisomy18.org/site/PageServer?pagename=homepage).

As with trisomy 18, infants with trisomy 13 have numerous abnormalities, the most common of which are central nervous system anomalies, visual abnormalities, microcephaly (small head), absent nasal bridge, cleft lip and palate, holoprosencephaly (one large eyelike structure in the center of the face due to fusion of the developing eyes), capillary hemangiomas, cardiac defects, extremity deformities including polydactyly (extra fingers or toes), renal abnormalities, and genital abnormalities (http://trisomy.org; http://www.hopefortrisomy13and18.org).

Infants with trisomy 18 and trisomy 13 usually have severe to profound intellectual disabilities. Although both conditions have a poor prognosis, with the vast majority of affected infants dying before they reach their first birthday, a growing number of infants with these trisomies are living longer and a small number are actually living into their 20s and 30s.

Nondisjunction also can occur during mitosis. If this occurs early in development when cell lines are forming, the individual has a mixture of cells, some with a normal number of chromosomes and others either missing a chromosome or containing an extra chromosome. This condition is known as mosaicism. The most common form of mosaicism in autosomes is mosaic Down syndrome.

Depending on when the nondisjunction occurs during development, different body tissues will have different numbers of chromosomes. The clinical characteristics of Down syndrome may be mild or with varying degrees of severity, depending on the number and location of the abnormal cells. An individual with mosaic Down syndrome may have normal intelligence. Mosaicism of both trisomy 18 and trisomy 13 has been reported. Both situations usually lead to a partial clinical expression of the phenotype. Infants who have mosaic trisomy 18 or trisomy 13 usually have a longer life span than infants with these disorders who are not mosaic.

Abnormalities of Chromosome Structure. Structural abnormalities can occur in any chromosome. Types of structural abnormalities include translocation, duplication, deletion, microdeletion, and inversion. Translocation results when there is an exchange of chromosomal material between two chromosomes. Exposure to certain drugs, viruses, and radiation can cause translocations, but often they arise for no apparent reason. The two major types of translocations are reciprocal and robertsonian. Reciprocal translocations are the most common. In a reciprocal translocation, either the parts of the two chromosomes are exchanged equally (balanced translocation) or a part of a chromosome is transferred to a different chromosome, creating an unbalanced translocation because there is extra chromosomal material—extra of one chromosome but the correct or deficient amount of the other chromosome. In a balanced translocation the individual is phenotypically normal because there is no extra chromosome material; it is just rearranged. In an unbalanced translocation, the individual will be both genotypically and phenotypically abnormal.

In a *robertsonian translocation,* the short arms (p arms) of two different acrocentric chromosomes (chromosomes with very short p arms) break, leaving sticky ends that then cause the two long arms (q arms) to stick together. This forms a new, large chromosome that is made of the two long arms. The individual with a balanced robertsonian translocation has 45 chromosomes. Because the short arm of acrocentric chromosomes contains genes for ribosomal RNA and these genes are represented elsewhere, the individual usually does not show any symptoms. The individual may produce an unbalanced gamete (sperm or egg with too many or two few genes). This can lead to reproductive difficulties such as miscarriages or birth defects. Of all cases of Down syndrome, 3% to 4% occur because one parent has a balanced robertsonian translocation, a translocation between chromosomes 21 and 14. The child with this type of Down syndrome has an unbalanced translocation because there is an extra part of chromosome 21. The second most common robertsonian translocation occurs between chromosomes 13 and 14.

Deletions result in the loss of chromosomal material and partial monosomy for the chromosome involved. Loss of chromosomal material at the end of a chromosome is referred to as a terminal deletion. In contrast, loss of chromosomal material anywhere else in the chromosome is called an interstitial deletion. The resulting clinical phenotype of either a terminal or an interstitial deletion will depend on how much of the chromosome has been lost and the number and function of the genes contained in the missing segment. Microdeletions are deletions too small to be detected by standard cytogenetic techniques. These deletions can be identified with FISH analysis. FISH technology uses a single-stranded piece of DNA with a fluorescent label that will adhere to its complementary piece of DNA in the chromosome being investigated.

Whenever a portion of a chromosome is deleted from one chromosome and added to another, the gamete produced may have either extra copies of genes or too few copies. The clinical effects produced can be mild or severe, depending on the amount of genetic material involved. Two of the more common conditions are the deletion of the short arm of chromosome 5 *(cri du chat syndrome)* and the deletion of the long arm of chromosome 18. Cri du chat syndrome, so named after the typical mewing cry of the affected infant, causes severe intellectual disability with microcephaly and unusual facial appearance. Deletion of the long arm of chromosome 18 causes severe psychomotor delay with multiple organ malformations. *Velocardiofacial syndrome,* characterized by cardiac and craniofacial abnormalities, is an example of a microdeletion. In this syndrome, a very small piece of the long arm of chromosome 22 is missing. Microdeletions in the Y chromosome have been found in men with infertility problems.

Inversions are deviations in which a portion of the chromosome has been rearranged in reverse order. Few birth defects have been attributed to the presence of inversions, but it is suspected that inversions may be responsible for problems with infertility and miscarriages. Some inversions can be detected prenatally. Inversions do not appear to occur randomly; it is estimated that more than 40% of all inversions involve chromosome 9.

Sex Chromosome Abnormalities

Several sex chromosome abnormalities are caused by nondisjunction during gametogenesis in either parent. The most common deviation in females is *Turner syndrome* or monosomy X (45, X). The affected female is missing an X chromosome. She usually exhibits juvenile external genitalia with undeveloped ovaries. She is short and often has webbing of the neck, a low hairline in the back, low-set ears, and lymphedema of her hands and feet. Intelligence may be impaired (www.turnersyndrome.org; www.genetic.org). Most affected embryos miscarry spontaneously. In most cases of Turner syndrome, it is the paternal X or Y that is lost.

The most common deviation in males is *Klinefelter syndrome,* or trisomy XXY. The affected male has an extra X chromosome and exhibits poorly developed secondary sexual characteristics and small testes. He is infertile, usually tall, and may be slow to learn (www.genetic.org). Males who have mosaic Klinefelter syndrome may be fertile.

Patterns of Genetic Transmission

Heritable characteristics are those that can be passed on to offspring. The patterns by which genetic material is transmitted to the next generation are affected by the number of genes involved in the expression of the trait. Many phenotypic characteristics result from two or more genes on different chromosomes acting together (referred to as multifactorial inheritance); others are controlled by a single gene (referred to as unifactorial inheritance). Specialists in genetics (e.g., geneticists, genetic counselors, and nurses with advanced expertise in genetics and genomics) predict the probability of the presence of an abnormal gene from the known occurrence of the trait in the individual's family and the known patterns by which the trait is inherited.

Multifactorial Inheritance

Most common congenital malformations result from multifactorial inheritance, a combination of genetic and environmental factors. Examples are cleft lip, cleft palate, congenital heart disease, neural tube defects, and pyloric stenosis. Each malformation may range from mild to severe, depending on the number of genes for the defect present or the amount of environmental influence. A neural tube defect may range from spina bifida, a bony defect in the lumbar region of the vertebrae with little or no neurologic impairment, to anencephaly, absence of brain development, which is always fatal. Some malformations occur more often in one sex. For example, pyloric stenosis and cleft lip are more common in males, and cleft palate is more common in females.

Unifactorial Inheritance

If a single gene controls a particular trait or disorder, its pattern of inheritance is referred to as *unifactorial mendelian,* or single-gene inheritance. The number of single-gene disorders far exceeds the number of chromosomal abnormalities. Potential patterns of inheritance for single-gene disorders include autosomal dominant, autosomal recessive, and X-linked dominant and recessive modes of inheritance.

Autosomal Dominant Inheritance. Autosomal dominant inheritance disorders are those in which only one copy of a variant allele is needed for phenotypic expression. The variant allele may be a result of a mutation, a spontaneous and permanent change in the normal gene structure, in which case the disorder occurs for the first time in the family. Usually an affected individual comes from multiple generations having the disorder. An affected parent who is heterozygous for the trait has a 50% chance of passing the variant allele to each offspring (Fig. 3-3, *B* and *C*). There is a vertical pattern of inheritance (there is no skipping of generations; if an individual has an autosomal dominant disorder such as HD, so must one of his or her parents). Males and females are equally affected.

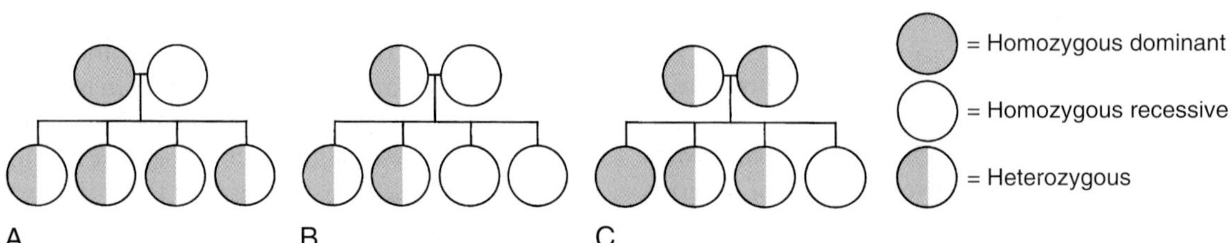

FIG 3-3 Possible offspring in three types of matings. **A,** Homozygous-dominant parent and homozygous-recessive parent. Children all heterozygous, displaying dominant trait. **B,** Heterozygous parent and homozygous-recessive parent. Children 50% heterozygous, displaying dominant trait; 50% homozygous, displaying recessive trait. **C,** Both parents heterozygous. Children 25% homozygous, displaying dominant trait; 25% homozygous, displaying recessive trait; 50% heterozygous, displaying dominant trait.

Autosomal dominant disorders are not always expressed with the same severity of symptoms. For example, a woman who has an autosomal dominant disorder may show few symptoms and may not become aware of her diagnosis until after she gives birth to a severely affected child. Predicting whether an offspring will have a minor or severe abnormality is not possible. Sometimes an individual can acquire a de novo mutation (new mutation that spontaneously occurred in a gene carried by an individual germ cell) that can result in an autosomal dominant disorder (Prows et al., 2013). Examples of autosomal dominant disorders are HD, Marfan syndrome, neurofibromatosis, myotonic dystrophy, Stickler syndrome, Treacher Collins syndrome, and achondroplasia (dwarfism).

Neurofibromatosis (NF) is a progressive disorder of the nervous system that causes tumors to form on nerves anywhere in the body. NF affects all races, all ethnic groups, and both sexes equally. Half of the cases of NF result from a spontaneous genetic mutation, whereas the other half of cases are inherited in an autosomal dominant manner. Individuals with NF due to a spontaneous mutation have a 50% chance of transmitting the variant allele to the next generation with each pregnancy. Two genetically distinct forms of NF include NF1, the most common type, with an incidence of 1 in 3000 (Prows et al., 2013) and NF2, with an incidence of 1 in 40,000 (Clarke, 2009). The most distinctive features of NF1 are multiple neurofibromas (benign, soft tumors), freckles in the axilla or groin, and patches of skin pigmentation called café-au-lait spots (www.understandingnf1.org). Generally, symptoms of NF1 are mild and affected individuals are able to live healthy, productive lives. Individuals with NF2 typically develop bilateral vestibular schwannomas (tumors on the eighth cranial nerves, which are hearing and balance nerves); these tumors often cause pressure damage to nearby nerves that may result in the individual with NF2 experiencing headaches, facial pain, and facial numbness. Other symptoms typically experienced by individuals with NF2 include tinnitus (ringing noise in the ear) and poor balance. Some individuals with NF2 experience hearing loss in their teen years.

NF1 is inherited in an autosomal dominant manner with almost complete penetrance by age 5 years. Penetrance is defined as the proportion of heterozygotes for a dominant trait who express a trait, even mildly. Expression of NF1 is very variable. Affected members of the same family can look strikingly different as far as disease severity is concerned. The NF2 gene has been mapped to chromosome 22. The gene product, merlin, is thought to be a cytoskeleton protein that acts as a tumor suppressor. No treatment for NF is available, other than the surgical removal of the tumors. Once removed, the tumors may grow back.

Factor V Leiden (FVL) is the most common inherited risk factor for primary and recurrent venous thromboembolisms (Moll, 2009; www.fvleiden.org). It is an autosomal dominant disorder that markedly increases an individual's risk for deep vein thrombosis (blood clots in the large veins of the legs) and pulmonary emboli (blood clots that travel through the bloodstream and become embedded in the lungs), especially if the individual is a woman who (a) uses oral contraceptives, (b) is pregnant, or (c) is on hormone replacement therapy during menopause. FVL is due to a mutation in the factor V gene, which leads to activated protein C (APC) resistance. If a woman is heterozygous (has inherited one copy of the FVL mutation), she has a 4- to 8-fold increase in her chance of developing venous blood clots, but her risk increases by a factor as high as 75- to 80-fold if she is homozygous (has inherited two copies of the FVL mutation) (National Institutes of Health, 2010). Women who carry the FVL mutation should not take oral contraceptives. In addition, if they become pregnant and they have a history of blood clots, it is recommended that they receive prophylactic anticoagulation (with low-molecular-weight heparin) during their pregnancy and for 6 weeks postpartum (Marik & Plante, 2008).

FVL can be accurately detected with genetic testing, but the most cost-effective way to screen for FVL is taking a careful individual and family history. Women with a personal or close family history of venous blood clots, pulmonary emboli, early onset and recurrent preeclampsia, recurrent fetal growth restriction, recurrent pregnancy loss and stillbirth, or placental abruption should be screened for FVL.

Autosomal Recessive Inheritance. Autosomal recessive inheritance disorders are those in which both genes of a pair are forms associated with the disorder to be expressed. Heterozygous individuals have only one variant allele and are unaffected clinically because their normal gene (wild-type allele) overshadows the variant allele. They are known as carriers of the recessive trait. Because these recessive traits are inherited by generations of the same family, an increased incidence of the disorder occurs in consanguineous matings (closely related parents). For the trait to be expressed, two carriers must each contribute a variant allele to the offspring (see Fig. 3-3, *C*). The chance of the trait occurring in each child is 25%. A clinically normal offspring may be a carrier of the gene. Autosomal recessive disorders have a horizontal pattern of inheritance rather than the vertical pattern seen with autosomal dominant disorders. That is, autosomal recessive disorders are usually observed in one or more siblings, but not in earlier generations. Males and females are equally affected. Most recessive disorders tend to have severe clinical manifestations, and affected offspring may not be able to, or choose not to, reproduce. If they do, all their offspring will at least be carriers for the disorder. Most inborn errors of metabolism (IEMs), such as PKU, galactosemia, maple syrup urine disease, Tay-Sachs disease, sickle cell anemia, and CF, are autosomal recessive inherited disorders.

Inborn Errors of Metabolism. More than 350 inborn errors of metabolism have been recognized (Jorde, Carey, & Bamshad, 2010). Individually, IEMs are relatively rare, but collectively, they are common (1 in 5000 live births). Archibald Garrod first used the term "*inborn errors of metabolism*" in 1908 when he described variants of metabolism. Garrod recognized that IEMs illustrate our "chemical individualities." As noted, most IEMs are inherited in an autosomal recessive pattern. IEMs occur when a gene mutation reduces the efficiency of encoded enzymes to a level at which normal metabolism cannot occur. Defective enzyme action interrupts the normal series of chemical reactions from the affected point onward. The result may be an accumulation of a damaging product, such as phenylalanine in

PKU, or the absence of a necessary product, such as the lack of melanin in albinism caused by lack of tyrosinase. Diagnostic and carrier testing is available for a growing number of IEMs. In addition, many U.S. states have started screening for specific IEMs as part of their expanded newborn screening programs using tandem mass spectrometry. However, many of the deaths caused by IEMs are due to enzyme variants not currently screened for in many of the newborn screening programs (Jorde et al.).

Phenylketonuria is a relatively uncommon autosomal recessive disorder. A deficiency in the liver enzyme phenylalanine hydroxylase results in failure to metabolize the amino acid phenylalanine, allowing its metabolites to accumulate in the blood. The incidence of this disorder is 1 in every 10,000 to 20,000 births. The highest incidence is found in Caucasians (from northern Europe and the United States). It is rarely seen in Jewish, African, or Japanese populations. Screening for PKU is routinely performed as part of state-mandated newborn screening in the United States.

Tay-Sachs disease is a lipid-storage disease that occurs more commonly in Ashkenazi Jews and French-Canadians from Quebec. It results from a deficiency in hexosaminidase. Until age 4 to 6 months, infants with Tay-Sachs disease appear normal; their facial features are considered very beautiful. Then the clinical symptoms appear: apathy and regression in motor and social development and decreased vision. Death occurs between ages 3 and 4 years. No treatment exists for Tay-Sachs disease.

X-Linked Dominant Inheritance. X-linked dominant inheritance mimics autosomal dominant inheritance, except that male-to-male transmission cannot occur unless the father has Klinefelter syndrome due to XY disomy. X-linked dominant inheritance disorders occur in males and heterozygous females, but because of X inactivation, affected females are usually less severely affected than affected males and they are more likely to transmit the abnormal gene (variant allele) to their offspring. Heterozygous females (females who have one wild-type allele and one variant allele) have a 50% chance of transmitting the abnormal gene (variant allele) to each offspring. Mating of an affected male and an unaffected female is uncommon as a result of the tendency for the variant allele to be lethal in affected males because they have no normal gene (wild-type allele). Relatively few X-linked dominant disorders have been identified. Two examples are vitamin D–resistant rickets and Rett syndrome.

X-Linked Recessive Inheritance. Abnormal genes for X-linked recessive inheritance disorders are carried on the X chromosome. Females may be heterozygous or homozygous for traits carried on the X chromosome because they have two X chromosomes. Males are hemizygous because they have only one X chromosome, which carries genes with no alleles on the Y chromosome. Therefore, X-linked recessive disorders are most commonly manifested in the male, with the abnormal gene on his single X chromosome. Hemophilia, color blindness, and Duchenne muscular dystrophy are X-linked recessive disorders.

The male with an X-linked recessive disorder receives the disease-associated allele from his carrier mother on her affected X chromosome. Female carriers (those heterozygous for the trait) have a 50% probability of transmitting the disease-associated allele to each offspring. An affected male can pass the disease–associated allele to his daughters but not to his sons. The daughters will be carriers of the trait if they receive a normal gene on the X chromosome from their mother. They will be affected only if they receive a disease-associated allele on the X chromosome from both their mother and their father.

Fragile X syndrome (FXS), the leading monogenic cause of intellectual disability and autism, is an X-linked disorder that has a complex pattern of inheritance (Bagni & Oostra, 2013). FXS is almost exclusively caused by a trinucleotide repeat expansion (CGG) at a "fragile site" on the long arm of the X chromosome. Most people have 5 to 40 CGG repeats. Individuals with FXS have more than 200 CGG repeats. The abnormally expanded CGG segment inactivates or silences the FMR1 (fragile X intellectual disability) gene, which prevents the gene from producing a protein called fragile X intellectual disability protein. Loss of this protein leads to the characteristic physical features (large ears, long face, prominent forehead, protruding ears, hypermobile joints, and macroorchidism or increased testicular volume in postpubertal males) and behavior problems (poor eye contact, hyperactivity, social avoidance, repetitive speech, and self-injurious behavior) associated with FXS (Jorde et al., 2010; Schneider, Hagerman, & Hessl, 2009). Males and females can be affected by FXS, but because males have only one X chromosome, a CGG repeat expansion on one X is likely to affect males more severely than females. Also the degree of intellectual disability tends to be milder and more variable in females than in males. Unlike Down syndrome, FXS is not generally detectable through a physical examination at birth. Delays and behavioral abnormalities gradually become apparent during the first 2 years of life, but ultimately the diagnosis of FXS can be verified only through DNA testing.

Individuals with more than 55 but fewer than 200 CGG repeats are said to be permutation carriers. These individuals were originally thought to be unaffected, but research has shown that about 20% of adult carrier females may develop premature ovarian failure (cessation of menses before 40 years of age). Elderly male permutation carriers may manifest fragile X–associated tremor/ataxia syndrome (FXTAS), which consists of parkinsonism, intention tremors, autonomic dysfunction, peripheral neuropathy, weakness in the legs, cognitive decline, and cerebellar ataxia (www.fragilex.org).

CANCER GENOMICS

Gene Mutations That Can Lead to Cancer

There are three main ways that people acquire gene mutations that can lead to cancer. The first is from the environment. Known factors in the environment that cause cancer are ultraviolet (UV) light (skin cancer) and tobacco smoke (lung cancer). The second way that people acquire mutations is by chance. Normal metabolic processes can generate chemicals that damage DNA. Third, people inherit mutations from their parents; hereditary mutations are thought to be a major factor in about 5% to 10% of all cancers.

The two main types of genes that have been recognized as playing a critical role in the development of cancer are *oncogenes* and *tumor suppressor genes* (American Cancer Society [ACS],

2013). Oncogenes are mutated forms of proto-oncogenes. The main functions of proto-oncogenes are to encourage and promote normal growth and development. When proto-oncogenes mutate to become carcinogenic oncogenes, the result is excessive cell multiplication. The activation of oncogenes has been compared to a jammed accelerator in a car. Most mutations of proto-oncogenes are acquired mutations, such as mutations in the *KIT* gene which are thought to cause most cases of gastrointestinal stromal tumor (GIST). This type of cancer can be treated with drugs that target the KIT gene, such as imatinib (Gleevec). Two examples of inherited mutations of proto-oncogenes are ERBB2, located on chromosome 13, and KRAS2, located on chromosome 12. ERBB2 is involved in breast, ovarian, lung, gastric, and salivary gland cancers. KRAS2 is involved in breast, pancreatic, thyroid, colorectal, bladder, and lung cancers, as well as acute myeloid leukemia.

Tumor suppressor genes normally function to inhibit or "put the brakes on" the cell growth and division cycle. They function to prevent the development of tumors. Mutations in tumor suppressor genes cause the cell to ignore one or more of the components of the network of inhibitory signals, removing the brakes from the cell cycle. This results in a higher rate of uncontrolled growth: cancer. Acquired mutations of the tumor protein p53 gene appear in a wide range of cancers, including lung, colorectal, and breast cancer. Examples of inherited tumor suppressor genes include APC, located on chromosome 5 and involved with familial adenomatous polyposis of the colon (FAP); BRCA1, located on chromosome 17 and associated with hereditary breast cancer and ovarian cancer; and RB1, found on chromosome 13 and involved with familial retinoblastoma.

Hereditary Breast and Ovarian Cancer (HBOC)

Breast cancer is a common disease and a central concern in women's health. In the United States, breast cancer is the most common form of cancer for women and the second most common cause of death. Hereditary mutations are considered to be a key factor in approximately 5% to 10% of all breast and ovarian cancers. Another 15% to 20% of female breast cancers occur in women who have a family history of breast and ovarian cancer but do not carry a mutation in one of the genes that are known to be strongly associated with breast and ovarian cancer susceptibility.

BRCA1 and BRCA2 mutations account for approximately 20% to 25% of hereditary breast cancers and about 5% to 10% of all breast cancers (National Cancer Institute, 2013). These mutations are inherited in an autosomal dominant pattern, thus each offspring of an individual found to carry a BRCA mutation has a 50% chance of inheriting the same mutation. According to estimates of lifetime risk, approximately 12% of women in the general population will develop breast cancer sometime during their lifetime, compared to about 55% to 65% women who have inherited a deleterious mutation in their BRAC1 or BRCA2 gene. Another way of saying this is that a woman with a deleterious BRCA1 or BRCA2 mutation is about five times more likely to develop breast cancer than a woman who does not carry a deleterious BRCA1 or BRCA2 mutation. Even though only about 6% of the men who carry a BRCA mutation develop breast cancer, men who carry a BRCA mutation have a 50% chance of passing the mutation on to their offspring. As far as lifetime risk estimates for ovarian cancer, about 1.4% of women in the general population will be diagnosed with ovarian cancer during their lifetime, compared with 39% of women who have a deleterious BRCA1 or BRCA2 mutation. Carriers of BRCA1 mutations may also be at increased risk for pancreatic, prostate, peritoneal, and uterine tube cancer.

Genetic testing for HBOC has been commercially available in the United States since 1995. The cost for testing usually ranges from several hundred to several thousand dollars. Although some insurance policies cover the cost of this type of genetic testing, others do not. Individuals who are considering undergoing BRCA1 and BRCA2 testing are encouraged to check their insurance coverage prior to undergoing testing. Women newly diagnosed with breast cancer are increasingly being asked to consider undergoing BRCA1 and BRCA2 testing before they make decisions about their treatment options because there is growing evidence that a woman's short-term risk of developing a second breast cancer is substantially affected by whether she carries a BRCA1 or BRCA2 mutation, and prophylactic surgery has been found to decrease the risk of breast and ovarian cancer by more than 90%. The main advantage to offering BRCA1 and BRCA2 testing before the onset of treatment is that it gives women who are found to carry a deleterious mutation the option of choosing risk-reduction surgery concurrent with therapeutic surgical treatment.

Colon Cancer

Colon cancer is the third most common cancer in women and the third cause of cancer-related deaths in women. Only 10% of colon cancer cases are likely to involve a mutation in one of several predisposing genes. Two examples of predisposing genes are mutations in the APC tumor suppressor gene and mutations in a mismatch repair gene. Mutations in the APC tumor suppressor gene have been associated with FAP, a rare, autosomal dominant syndrome that accounts for about 1% of all colon cancer. It is typically diagnosed clinically. Affected individuals have 100 to 1000 polyps in their colon by the time they are 20 to 30 years old. Genetic testing is greater than 80% sensitive. Identification of high risk individuals guides surveillance strategies and the timing of a prophylactic colectomy. Low risk individuals can stop the increased surveillance.

Hereditary nonpolyposis colon cancer (HNPCC) results from mutations in one of many mismatch repair (MMR) genes. Mutations in two of these MMR genes (i.e., MSH2 and MLH1) account for 50% to 60% of HNPCC. Families at high risk for HNPCC often have three or more relatives with colorectal cancer; colorectal cancer present in at least two generations; and a diagnosis of colorectal cancer before age 50 years in at least one case. HNPCC is characterized by an increased risk of colon cancer and other cancers that include cancers of the ovary, endometrium, stomach, small intestine, upper urinary tract, hepatobiliary tract, brain, and skin. The lifetime risk of colon cancer for individuals with HNPCC is approximately 80%. The majority of these cancers occurs in the proximal colon. Genetic tests are available to test for MSH2 and MLH1. Testing should be done first on the affected family member. At-risk clients should be offered a prophylactic colectomy. Women may be offered a total abdominal hysterectomy with a salpingo-oophorectomy to decrease cancer risk. If colon cancer develops, a total colectomy is recommended.

GENETIC COUNSELING

Genetic counseling is a service that grew out of a need for professionals who could provide genetics information, education, and support to individuals and families with ongoing or potential genetic health concerns. In 2014, there were 32 accredited genetic counseling programs in the United States and 3 in Canada. At the same time, there were more than 3000 American Board of Genetic Counseling (ABGC)–certified genetic counselors. The National Society of Genetic Counselors was formed in 1979 (www.nsgc.org) and the International Society of Nurses in Genetics (ISONG) was formed in 1988 (www.isong.org/index.php). The number of nursing programs offering courses in genetics and genomics is growing rapidly. A small number of graduate nursing programs offer advanced practice courses and/or specialty options in genetics and genomics. Examples of these are the University of California, San Francisco, School of Nursing and the University of Pittsburgh School of Nursing.

Definition of Genetic Counseling

In 2006, the Genetic Counseling Definition Task Force of the National Society of Genetic Counselors developed the following definition of genetic counseling. According to this definition:

"Genetic counseling is the process of helping people understand and adapt to the medical, psychological and familial implications of genetic contributions to disease. This process integrates:

- Interpretation of family and medical histories to assess the chance of disease occurrence or recurrence;
- Education about inheritance, testing, management, prevention, resources and research; and
- Counseling to promote informed choices and adaptation to the risk or condition" (Resta, Biesecker, Bennett, et al., 2006).

Access and Referral to Genetic Counseling

Genetic counseling is typically provided by a team of genetics specialists that includes clinical geneticists (physicians with an MD or DO), medical geneticists with a PhD, genetics fellows, genetics counselors, and, in a growing number of cases, advanced practice genetics nurse specialists. Cytogeneticists, biochemical geneticists, and molecular geneticists support the clinical genetics team by providing laboratory expertise that helps with the diagnosis and management of individuals and families affected by genetic conditions.

Until recently most individuals and families interested in receiving genetic counseling went to regional genetics centers or major medical centers. Genetic counseling also was provided in outreach or satellite genetics clinics, public health clinics, and some community hospitals. Now that genetics is entering the mainstream of health care, genetic counseling is being offered in a wide variety of other settings. These include, but are not limited to, managed health care organizations, commercial facilities, and private practices. A number of specialized groups provide genetics education and counseling for individuals and families affected by specific genetic disorders, such as Down syndrome, CF, diabetes, muscular dystrophy, HD, and cancer. Genetic counseling also is offered over the Internet.

Individuals and families seek out, or are referred for, genetic counseling for a wide variety of reasons and at all stages of their lives. Some seek preconception or prenatal information; others are referred after the birth of a child with a birth defect or a suspected genetic condition; still others seek information because they have a family history of a genetic condition. Regardless of the setting or the individual and family's stage of life, genetic counseling should be offered and available to all individuals and families who have questions about genetics and their health. However, there is a shortage of appropriately trained genetics professionals who can provide genetic counseling. This means that many individuals and families will not be offered genetic counseling when they undergo genetic testing. Moreover, some of the genetics education and counseling that is provided will be less than adequate.

It may take years before a sufficient number of health care professionals feel comfortable and are proficient in providing genetics, genomics, and genetic counseling (Calzone, Jenkins, Yates, et al., 2012). Until then it is imperative that all health care professionals become familiar with existing genetics resources, such as the CDC (www.cdc.gov/genomics/default.htm), the Genetic Alliance (www.geneticalliance.org), the Jackson Laboratory (www.jax.org), Genetics Program for Nursing Faculty Cincinnati Children's Hospital Medical Center (www.cincinnatichildrens.org/ed/clinical/gpnf/default.htm), National Human Genome Research Institute Education (www.genome.gov/Education), and GenomeTV (www.genome.gov/genometv).

Estimation of Risk

Most families with a history of genetic disease want an answer to the following: What is the chance that our future children will have this disease? Because the answer to this question may have profound implications for individual family members and the family as a whole, health care professionals must be able to answer as accurately as they can in a timely manner. In some cases, estimation of risk is rather straightforward; in other cases, it becomes rather complicated. Because of this, health care professionals should be prepared to refer families with a history of genetic disease to genetics professionals if they are at all unsure. Again, the answer to this question can have profound implications for individual family members and the family as a whole, so health care professionals must do their best to ensure that the answer is accurate.

If a couple has not yet had children but they are known to be at risk for having children with a genetic disease, they will be given an occurrence risk. Once the mating of a couple has produced one or more children with a genetic disease, the couple will be given a recurrence risk. Both occurrence and recurrence risks are determined by the mode of inheritance for the genetic disease in question. For genetic diseases caused by a factor that segregates during cell division (genes and chromosomes), risk can be estimated with a high degree of accuracy by application of the mendelian principles.

In an autosomal dominant disorder, both the occurrence and recurrence risk is 50%, or one in two, when one parent is affected and the other is not. The recurrence risk for autosomal recessive disorders is 25%, or one in four, if both parents are carriers (they each have one recessive disease gene and one normal gene). Occasionally an individual homozygous for a recessive disease gene mates with an individual who is a carrier of the same recessive gene. In this case the recurrence risk is 50%, or one in two. If two individuals affected by an autosomal recessive disorder mate, all of their children will be affected. For X-linked disorders, recurrence risk is related to the sex of the child. Translocation disorders have a high risk of recurrence.

A number of autosomal disorders display fairly complex patterns of inheritance, making estimation of risk somewhat difficult. For example, if a child is born with a genetic disease and there has been no history of the disease in the family, the disease may have been caused by a new mutation (this is more likely if the disease in question is an autosomal dominant disorder, such as achondroplasia). If the child's genetic disease has been caused by a new mutation, the recurrence risk for the parents' subsequent children is low (1% to 2%), but it is not as low as that for the general population. Offspring of the affected child may have a substantially elevated occurrence risk.

The risk of recurrence for multifactorial conditions can be estimated empirically. An empiric risk is based not on genetics theory but rather on experience and observation of the disorder in other families. Recurrence risks are determined by applying the frequency of a similar disorder in other families to the case under consideration.

An important concept to be emphasized to individuals and families during a genetic counseling session is that *each pregnancy is an independent event.* For example, in monogenic disorders in which the risk factor is one in four that the child will be affected, the risk remains the same no matter how many affected children are already in the family. Families may maintain the erroneous assumption that the presence of one affected child ensures that the next three will be free of the disorder. However, "chance has no memory." The risk is one in four for each pregnancy. Conversely, in a family with a child who has a disorder with multifactorial causes, the risk increases with each subsequent child born with the disorder.

Interpretation of Risk

The guiding principle for genetics counselors has traditionally been nondirectiveness. According to the principle of nondirectiveness, the individual who is providing genetic counseling respects the right of the individual or family being counseled to make autonomous decisions. Counselors using a nondirective approach avoid making recommendations, and they try to communicate genetics information in an unbiased manner. The first step in providing nondirective counseling is becoming aware of one's own values and beliefs. Another important step is recognizing how one's values and beliefs can influence or interfere with the communication of genetics information.

If the individual who is providing genetic counseling has difficulty being nonjudgmental and objective, he or she may either intentionally or unintentionally influence the decision-making process. Individuals and families also may pressure the counselor to make decisions for them with questions such as, "What would you do if you were me?" Families and individuals need education, guidance, and support throughout the counseling process. They should be given the facts and possible consequences, as well as all of the assistance they need in problem solving, but the final decision regarding a course of action must be their own.

CLINICAL REASONING CASE STUDY

Counseling About Genetic Risk

Camille has presented for her routine yearly physical examination and tells you she and her husband are planning to become pregnant within the next year. She confides in you that several infants have been born into her family with serious anomalies. She is interested in finding out more about her risks of having a baby with an anomaly and wants to know whom she should consult for that information.

1. Evidence—Is there sufficient evidence to provide Camille with answers to her questions about her risks of having a baby with an anomaly?
2. Assumptions—What assumptions can be made about estimating and interpreting risk?
   a. The appropriate person to provide this information
   b. The accuracy of this information
   c. The benefits of this information
3. What implications and priorities for nursing can be made at this time?
4. Does the evidence objectively support your conclusion?

Multiple Roles for Nurses in Genetics

Nurses play many roles in genetics. Some nurses play a key role in identifying families in need of genetic counseling, and they collaborate with other health care professionals to make referrals to genetics specialists. Other nurses take a more active role in genetic counseling: they might provide appropriate genetics information before, during, and after the initial genetics counseling session; construct family pedigrees of three or more generations; clarify the genetics information that family members receive during counseling sessions or from other sources such as the public library, the Internet, or support groups; help families manage the ongoing challenges associated with living with a genetic disorder; make referrals to support groups and national organizations; and provide long-term follow-up of families affected by genetic conditions.

Probably the most important of all nursing functions is to provide emotional support during all aspects of the counseling process. Feelings that are generated under the real or imagined threat posed by a genetic disorder are as varied as the people being counseled. Responses may include a variety of stress reactions, such as apathy, denial, anger, hostility, fear, embarrassment, grief, and loss of self-esteem. Guilt and self-blame are universal reactions. Many look on the disorder as a stigma, especially if the disorder is visible to others. Old-wives' tales, superstitions, and long-held misconceptions may influence a family's reaction to a genetic disorder.

FUTURE PROMISE OF GENETICS

Overall, the Human Genome Project and other sequencing efforts have been a huge success. Our understanding of the human genome, as well as other genomes, has grown exponentially in recent years. The increased availability of genetic testing and other genetics services gives individuals and families unprecedented opportunities to learn whether they have heightened risk for certain diseases or the potential to transmit gene mutations to their offspring. Awareness of genetic risk also can facilitate informed health care decisions and, in some cases, can promote risk reduction behaviors that have the potential to reduce morbidity and mortality. Ultimately it is hoped that advances in molecular biology and genomics will make it possible to offer diagnostic, preventive, and treatment options not only for genetic diseases but also for common diseases such as cancer, atherosclerosis, diabetes, and Alzheimer's disease.

Advances made possible through the Human Genome Project have been remarkable, but our ability to offer treatment options, even for single-gene disorders, remains very limited. Progress in the acquisition of genetics information and the development of genetics technology continue to outpace the development of therapeutic interventions. For most genetic conditions, therapeutic interventions are nonexistent or disappointingly limited. Consequently the most useful means of reducing the incidence of genetic disorders now is preventing transmission. Only three reproductive options exist for individuals at risk for transmitting a genetic disorder: the avoidance of pregnancy; genetic diagnosis during an ongoing pregnancy; and prevention of transmission of an altered gene or genes through preimplantation genetics. For many families none of these options is viewed as acceptable.

Dialogue among pregnant women, expectant families, health care professionals, and disability advocates concerning prenatal testing for Down syndrome and other genetic disorders is urgently needed. Clinical and technical information must be complemented by social understanding of the experience of disability in contemporary society. The picture of life with a disability should be more balanced than that currently portrayed. It is critical that the voices of individuals and families living with disabilities be heard.

Nurses are in an ideal position to help individuals and families maximize the benefits of the genetics revolution, but first, nurses need (1) a working knowledge of human genetics, (2) an awareness of recent advances in genetics and genomics, and (3) an understanding of the potential effects of genomic discoveries on individual and family well-being. More research is needed concerning the family experience of genetic testing. Nurses must understand why individuals and families decide to undergo genetic testing. Nurses also need to be aware of how individuals and families define and manage ethical, legal, and social issues that emerge during the genetic testing experience.

KEY POINTS

- Advances in molecular biology and genomics have revolutionized the field of health care by providing the tools needed to determine the hereditary component of many diseases.
- Increasingly, nurses from all specialty areas, as well as all practice settings, are expected to have competencies in genetics and genomics.
- The major force behind the genetics revolution has been the Human Genome Project.
- All humans are >99% identical at the DNA level.
- Approximately 20,000 to 25,000 genes are found in the human genome.
- Most of the genetic tests being offered in clinical practice are tests for single-gene disorders.
- Pharmacogenomics will probably be the most immediate clinical application of the Human Genome Project.
- The decision to undergo genetic testing is often based on feelings of responsibility and commitment to others.
- Genes are the basic units of heredity responsible for all human characteristics. They comprise 23 pairs of chromosomes: 22 pairs of autosomes and 1 pair of sex chromosomes.
- Chromosomal abnormalities occur in both autosomes and sex chromosomes.
- Multifactorial inheritance includes genetic and environmental contributions.
- Advances in genetics have complex ethical, legal, and social implications.
- Cancer genetics is an important emerging field.

REFERENCES

American Cancer Society. (2013). *Oncogenes, tumor suppressor genes and cancer*. Available at www.cancer.org/docroot/ETO/content/ETO_1_4x_oncogenes_and_tumor_suppressor_genes.asp.

American College of Obstetricians and Gynecologists. (2012). Committee opinion no. 545; Noninvasive prenatal testing for fetal aneuploidy. *Obstetrics & Gynecology, 120*(6), 1532–1534.

American College of Obstetricians and Gynecologists Committee on Genetics. (2011). Committee opinion no. 478. Family history as a risk assessment tool. *Obstetrics & Gynecology, 117*(3), 747–750.

American College of Obstetricians and Gynecologists/American College of Medical Genetics.(2001). *Preconception and prenatal carrier screening for cystic fibrosis: Clinical and laboratory guidelines*. Washington, DC: Author.

Badzek, L., Henaghan, M., Turner, M., & Monsen, R. (2013). Ethical, legal, and social issues in the translation of genomics into health care. *Journal of Nursing Scholarship, 45*(1), 15–24.

Bagni, C., & Oostra, B. (2013). Fragile x syndrome: From protein to therapy. *American Journal of Medical Genetics Part A, 161*(11), 2809–2821.

Beery, T. (2013). Genetic and genomic testing in clinical practice: What you need to know. *Rehabilitation Nursing, 39*(2), 1–6.

Bodurtha, J., & Strauss, J. F. (2012). Genomics and perinatal care. *Genomics Medicine, 366*(1), 64–73.

Bull, M. J., & Committee on Genetics (2011). Clinical report—Health supervision for children with Down syndrome. *Pediatrics, 128*(2), 393–406.

Calzone, K. A., Jenkins, J., Nicoli, N., et al. (2013). Relevance of genomics to healthcare and nursing practice. *Journal of Nursing Scholarship, 45*(1), 1–2.

Calzone, K. A., Jenkins, J., Yates, J., et al. (2012). Survey of nursing integration of genomics into nursing practice. *Journal of Nursing Scholarship, 44*(4), 428–436.

Clarke, L. (2009). Neurofibromatosis 2: A family's journey. *Canadian Journal of Neuroscience Nursing, 31*(4), 7–14.

Conley, Y., Biesecker, L. G., Gonsalves, S., et al. (2013). Current and emerging technology approaches in genomics. *Journal of Nursing Scholarship, 45*(1), 5–14.

Consensus Panel on Genetic/Genomic Nursing Competencies.(2009). *Essentials of genetic and genomic nursing: Competencies, curricula guidelines, and outcome indicators* (2nd ed.). Silver Spring, MD: American Nurses Association.

DeLuca, J., Zanni, K. L., Bonhomme, N., & Kemper, A. R. (2013). Implications of newborn screening for nurses. *Journal of Nursing Scholarship, 45*(1), 25–33.

De Sevo, M. R. (2009). Unlocking the clues of family health history: The importance of creating a pedigree. *Nursing for Women's Health, 13*(2), 122–131.

Evans, J., & Green, R. (2009). Direct to consumer genetic testing: Avoiding a culture war. *Genetics in Medicine, 11*(8), 568–569.

Feero, W. G., Guttmacher, A. E., & Collins, F. (2010). Genomic medicine—An updated primer. *New England Journal of Medicine, 362*(21), 2001–2007.

Frazer, K., Porter, S., & Goss, C. (2013). The genetics and implications of neuromuscular diseases in pregnancy. *Journal of Perinatal & Neonatal Nursing, 27*(3), 205–214.

Gillet, J. P., Macadangdang, B., Fathke, R. L., et al. (2009). The development of gene therapy: From monogenic recessive disorders to complex diseases such as cancer. *Methods in Molecular Biology, 542*, 5–54.

Ginsburg, G., & Willard, H. (2009). Genomic and personalized medicine: Foundations and applications. *Translational Research, 154*(6), 277–287.

Green, E. D., & Guyer, M. S. (2011). Charting a course for genomic medicine from base pairs to bedside. *Nature, 470*(7333), 204–213.

Guttmacher, A. E., McGuire, A., Ponder, B., & Stefansson, K. (2010). Personalized genomic information: Preparing for the future of genetic medicine. *Nature Reviews Genetics*. Published online 12 January 2010.

Hassold, T., & Hunt, P. (2009). Maternal age and chromosomally abnormal pregnancies: What we know and what we wish we knew. *Current Opinion in Pediatrics, 21*(6), 703–708.

Hunt, P. A., & Hassold, T. J. (2008). Human female meiosis: What makes a good egg go bad. *Trends in Genetics, 24*(2), 86–93.

Ivan, D. L., & Cromwell, P. (2013a). Clinical practice guidelines for management of children with Down syndrome: Part 1. *Journal of Pediatric Health Care (Epub ahead of print)*.

Johnson, N. L., Giarelli, E., Lewis, C., & Rice, C. E. (2013). Genomics and autism spectrum disorder. *Journal of Nursing Scholarship, 45*(1), 69–78.

Jorde, L., Carey, J., & Bamshad, M. (2010). *Medical genetics* (4th ed.). St. Louis: Mosby.

Kohn, D. B., & Candotti, F. (2009). Gene therapy fulfilling its promise. *New England Journal of Medicine, 360*, 518–521.

Lewis, J. A. (2011). Genetics and genomics: Impact on perinatal nursing. *Journal of Perinatal and Neonatal Nursing, 25*(2), 144–147.

Manolio, T. A., Chisholm, R. L., Ozenberger, B., et al. (2013). Implementing genomic medicine in the clinic: The future is here. *Genetics in Medicine, 15*(4), 258–267.

Marik, P. E., & Plante, L. A. (2008). Venous thromboembolic disease. *New England Journal of Medicine, 359*(19), 2025–2033.

Martin, R. (2008). Meiotic errors in human oogenesis and spermatogenesis. *Reproductive BioMedicine Online, 16*(4), 523–531.

McCarthy, J. J., McLeod, H. L., & Ginsburg, G. S. (2013). Genomic medicine: A decade of successes, challenges, and opportunities. *Translational Medicine, 5*(189), 1–17.

McGuire, A. L., & Burke, W. (2010). An unwelcome side effect of direct-to-consumer personal genome testing. *JAMA, 300*(22), 2669–2671.

Meckley, L. M., Gudgeon, J. M., Anderson, J. L., et al. (2010). A policy model to evaluate the benefits, risks, and costs of warfarin pharmacogenetic testing. *Pharmacogenomics, 28*(1), 61–74.

Moll, S. (2009). Thrombophilia: 2009 update. *Current Treatment Options in Cardiovascular Medicine, 11*(2), 114–128.

National Cancer Institute.(2013). *BRCA1 and BRCA2; cancer risk and genetic testing*. Available at www.cancer.gov/cancertopics/factsheet/Risk/BRCA.

National Down Syndrome Society. (2013). *Down syndrome facts*. Available at www.ndss.org/Down-Syndrome/Down-Syndrome-Facts.

National Institutes of Health. (2010). *Learning about factor v Leiden thrombophilia*. Available at www.genome.gov/15015167.

Prows, C. A., Hopkin, R. J., Barnoy, S., & Van Riper, M. (2013). An update of childhood genetic disorders. *Journal of Nursing Scholarship, 45*(1), 34–42.

Resta, R., Biesecker, B. B., Bennett, R. L., et al. (2006). A new definition of genetic counseling: National Society of Genetic Counselors' Task Force report. *Journal of Genetic Counseling, 15*(2), 77–83.

Schneider, A., Hagerman, R. J., & Hessl, D. (2009). Fragile X syndrome—From genes to cognition. *Developmental Disabilities Research Reviews, 15*(4), 333–342.

Sparbel, K. J., & Tluczek, A. (2011). Patient and family issues regarding genetic testing for cystic fibrosis: A review of prenatal carrier testing and newborn screening. *Annual Review of Nursing Research, 29*(1), 303–329.

Sparbel, K. J., & Williams, J. K. (2009). Pregnancy as foreground in cystic fibrosis carrier testing decisions in primary care. *Genetic Testing and Molecular Biomarkers, 13*(1), 133–142.

Van Riper, M. (2005). Genetic testing and the family. *Journal of Midwifery & Women's Health, 50*(3), 227–233.

Van Riper, M. (2007). Families of children with Down syndrome: Responding to a "change of plans" with resilience. *Journal of Pediatric Nursing, 22*(2), 116–128.

Van Riper, M. (2012). Changing landscape of prenatal testing: Ethical and social implications for families. *MCN: The American Journal of Maternal/Child Nursing, 37*(3), 143.

Van Riper, M., & Choi, H. (2011). Family-provider interactions surrounding the diagnosis of Down syndrome. *Genetic Medicine, 13*(8), 714–716.

Wade, C. H., Tarini, B. A., & Wilfond, B. S. (2013). Growing up in the genomic era: Implications of whole-genome sequencing for children, families, and pediatric practice. *Annual Review of Genomics and Human Genetics, 14*, 535–555.

Weinstein, S. M. (2009). Factor V Leiden: Impact on infusion nursing practice. *Journal of Infusion Nursing, 32*(4), 219–223.

Wilke, D. J., Gallo, A. M., Yao, Y., et al. (2013). Reproductive health choices for young adults with sickle cell disease or trait: Randomized controlled trial immediate posttest effects. *Nursing Research, 62*(5), 352–361.

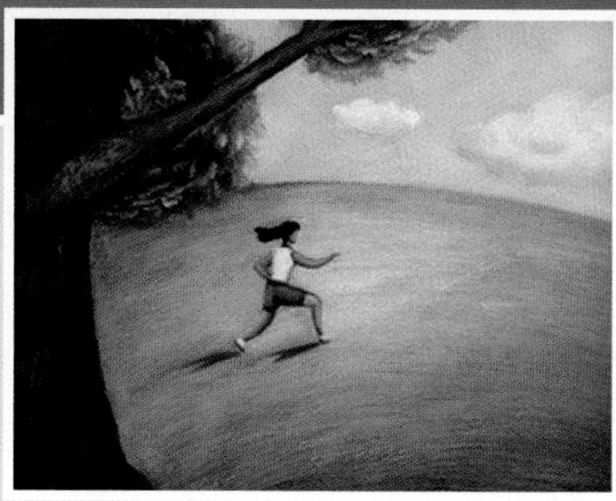

CHAPTER 4

Assessment and Health Promotion

Ellen Frances Olshansky

http://evolve.elsevier.com/Lowdermilk/MWHC/

LEARNING OBJECTIVES

- Identify the structures and functions of the female reproductive system.
- Describe the menstrual cycle in relation to hormonal, ovarian, and endometrial response.
- Identify the phases of the sexual response cycle.
- Describe common reasons that women enter the health care system.
- Analyze barriers that may affect a woman's decision to seek health care.
- Describe risk factors for women's health in the childbearing years.
- Describe the components of the history and physical examination.
- Describe how to adapt the history and physical examination for women with special needs.
- Describe how to screen for signs of abuse and how to refer to community agencies.
- Identify the steps for assisting with and collecting specimens for Papanicolaou (Pap) testing.
- Outline the health-screening and immunization recommendations for women across the life span.
- Describe anticipatory guidance that prevents disease and promotes health and self-management.

Care of the well woman is focused on health promotion and illness prevention, recognizing that a woman is a biopsychosocial-spiritual being, requiring a holistic approach to nursing care. To encourage appropriate health-promotion activities, it is important to conduct systematic health assessments and screenings. This chapter presents an overview of the nurse's role in encouraging health promotion and illness prevention in women. It provides guidelines for how to conduct a complete history and physical examination. This chapter also includes a schedule of screening tests recommended for women at different stages of their lives. As background to understanding assessment, a review of female anatomy and physiology as well as the menstrual cycle is presented. Barriers that women encounter when they try to enter the health care system and risk factors for women's health during the childbearing years are described. Anticipatory guidance suggestions, including nutrition, exercise, and stress management, are included. Examples of health-promotion efforts in the community are presented in an effort to emphasize community health approaches to care, especially because much of well-woman care occurs in the community.

FEMALE REPRODUCTIVE SYSTEM

The female reproductive system consists of external structures visible from the pubis to the perineum and internal structures located in the pelvic cavity. The external and internal female reproductive structures develop and mature in response to estrogen and progesterone. This process starts in fetal life and continues through puberty and the childbearing years. Reproductive structures atrophy with age or in response to a decrease in ovarian hormone production. A complex nerve and blood supply supports the functions of these structures. The appearance of the external genitalia varies greatly among women. Heredity, age, race, and the number of children a woman has borne influence the size, shape, and color of her external organs.

External Structures

The external genital organs, or *vulva*, include all structures visible externally from the pubis to the perineum. These include the *mons pubis, labia majora, labia minora*, clitoris, vestibular glands, vaginal vestibule, vaginal orifice, and urethral opening. The external genital organs are illustrated in Figure 4-1.

The mons pubis is a fatty pad that lies over the anterior surface of the symphysis pubis. In the postpubertal female the mons is covered with coarse, curly hair. The labia majora are two rounded folds of fatty tissue covered with skin that extend downward and backward from the mons pubis. The labia are highly vascular structures that develop hair on the outer surfaces after puberty. They protect the inner vulvar structures. The labia minora are two flat, reddish folds of tissue visible when the labia majora are separated. There are no hair follicles on the labia

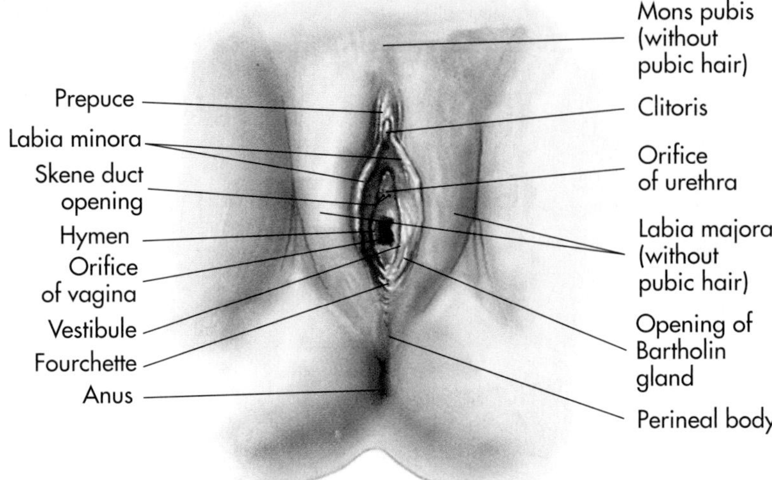

FIG 4-1 External female genitalia.

minora, but many sebaceous follicles and a few sweat glands are present. The interior of the labia minora comprises connective tissue and smooth muscle and is supplied with extremely sensitive nerve endings. Anteriorly, the labia minora fuse to form the *prepuce* (the hoodlike covering of the clitoris) and the *frenulum* (the fold of tissue under the clitoris). The labia minora join to form a thin, flat tissue called the *fourchette* underneath the vaginal opening at midline. The clitoris is located underneath the prepuce. It is a small structure composed of erectile tissue with numerous sensory nerve endings. During sexual arousal, the clitoris increases in size.

The vaginal *vestibule* is an almond-shaped area enclosed by the labia minora that contains openings to the urethra, Skene glands, vagina, and Bartholin glands. The urethra is not a reproductive organ but is discussed here because of its location. It usually is found about 2.5 cm below the clitoris. Skene glands are located on each side of the urethra and produce mucus, which aids in lubrication of the vagina. The vaginal opening is in the lower portion of the vestibule and varies in shape and size. The hymen, a connective tissue membrane that surrounds the vaginal opening, can be perforated during strenuous exercise, insertion of tampons, masturbation, and vaginal intercourse. Bartholin glands lie under the constrictor muscles of the vagina and are located posteriorly on the sides of the vaginal opening, although the ductal opening usually is not visible. During sexual arousal, the glands secrete clear mucus to lubricate the vaginal introitus.

The area between the fourchette and the anus is the perineum, a skin-covered muscular area that covers the pelvic structures. The perineum forms the base of the perineal body, a wedge-shaped mass that serves as an anchor for the muscles, fascia, and ligaments of the pelvis. The muscles and ligaments form a sling that supports the pelvic organs.

Internal Structures

The internal structures include the vagina, uterus, uterine tubes, and ovaries. The description of these structures follows.

The vagina is a fibromuscular, collapsible tubular structure that lies between the bladder and rectum and extends from the vulva to the uterus. During the reproductive years the mucosal lining is arranged in transverse folds called *rugae.* These rugae allow the vagina to expand during childbirth. Estrogen deprivation that occurs after childbirth, during lactation, and at menopause causes dryness and thinning of the vaginal walls and smoothing of the rugae. The vagina, particularly the lower segment, has few sensory nerve endings. Vaginal secretions are slightly acidic (pH 4 to 5) so that vaginal susceptibility to infections is limited. The vagina serves as a passageway for menstrual flow, as a female organ of copulation, and as a part of the birth canal for vaginal childbirth. The uterine cervix projects into a blind vault at the upper end of the vagina. Anterior, posterior, and lateral pockets called fornices (singular: *fornix*) surround the cervix. The internal pelvic organs can be palpated through the thin walls of these fornices.

The *uterus* is a muscular organ shaped like an upside-down pear that sits midline in the pelvic cavity between the bladder and rectum and above the vagina. Four pairs of ligaments support the uterus: cardinal, uterosacral, round, and broad. Single anterior and posterior ligaments also support the uterus. The cul-de-sac of Douglas is a deep pouch, or recess, posterior to the cervix formed by the posterior ligament.

The uterus is divided into two major parts: an upper triangular portion called the *corpus* and a lower cylindric portion called the *cervix* (Fig. 4-2). The *fundus* is the dome-shaped top of the uterus and is the site at which the uterine tubes (fallopian tubes) enter the uterus. The isthmus, or lower uterine segment, is a short, constricted portion that separates the corpus from the cervix.

The uterus serves for reception, implantation, retention, and nutrition of the fertilized ovum and later of the fetus during pregnancy and for expulsion of the fetus during childbirth. It is also responsible for cyclic menstruation.

The uterine wall is made up of three layers: the endometrium, the myometrium, and part of the peritoneum. The endometrium is a highly vascular lining made up of three layers, the outer two of which are shed during menstruation. The myometrium is made up of layers of smooth muscles that extend in three different directions (longitudinal, transverse, and oblique) (Fig. 4-3). Longitudinal fibers of the outer myometrial

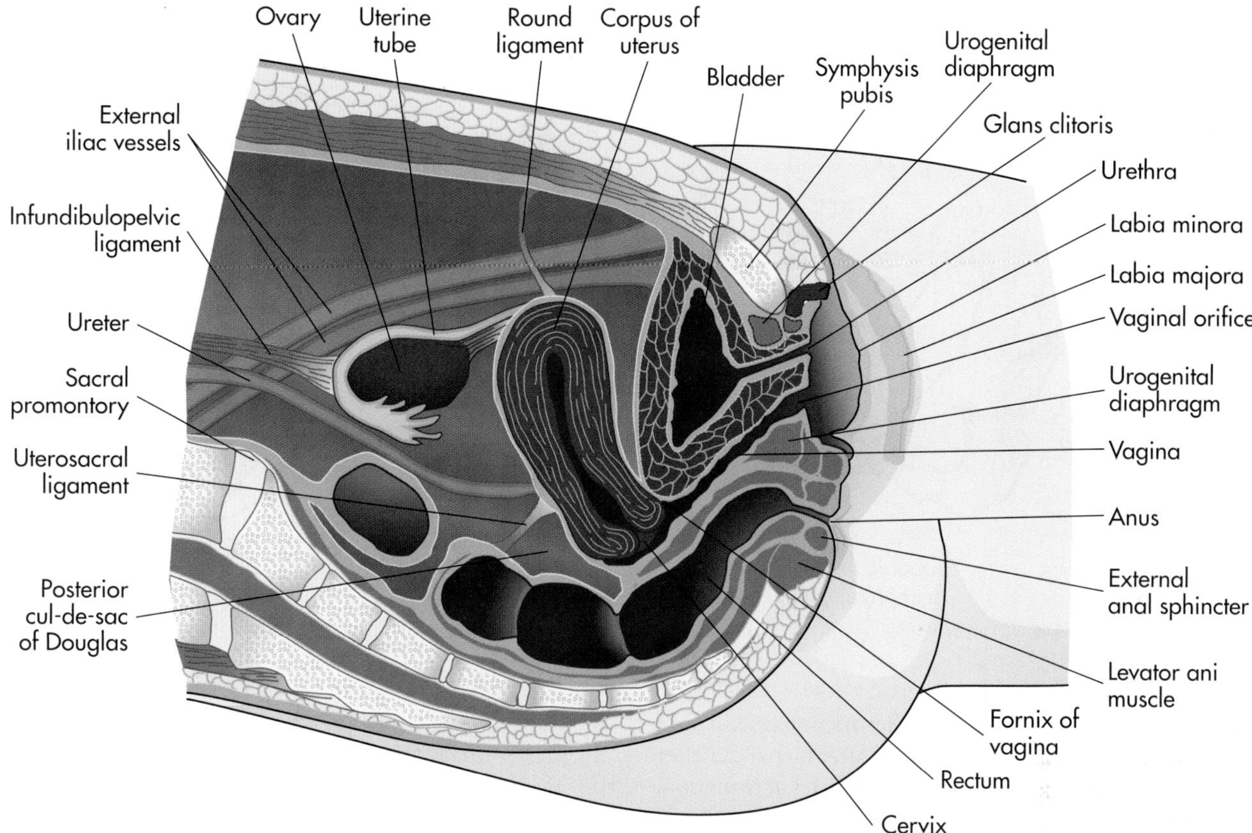

FIG 4-2 Midsagittal view of female pelvic organs with woman lying supine.

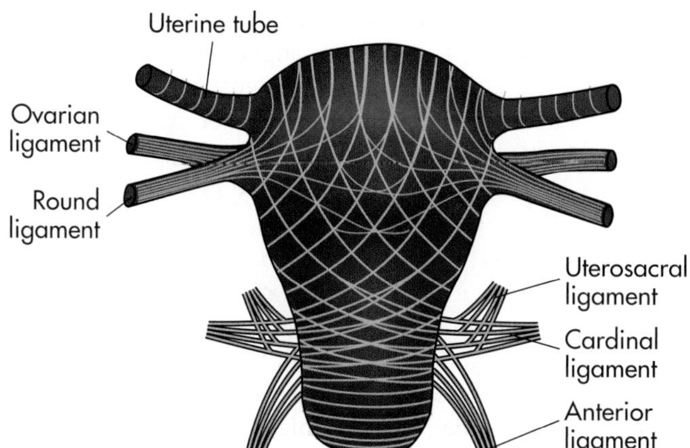

FIG 4-3 Schematic arrangement of directions of muscle fibers. Note that uterine muscle fibers are continuous with supportive ligaments of uterus.

layer are found mostly in the fundus, and this arrangement assists in expelling the fetus during the birth process. The middle layer contains fibers from all three directions, which form a figure-eight pattern encircling large blood vessels. These fibers assist in ligating blood vessels after childbirth and control blood loss. Most of the circular fibers of the inner myometrial layer are around the site where the uterine tubes enter the uterus and around the internal cervical os (opening). These fibers help keep the cervix closed during pregnancy and prevent menstrual blood from flowing back into the uterine tubes during menstruation.

The cervix is made up of mostly fibrous connective tissues and elastic tissue, making it possible for the cervix to stretch during vaginal childbirth. The opening between the uterine cavity and the canal that connects the uterine cavity to the vagina (endocervical canal) is the internal os. The narrowed opening between the endocervix and the vagina is the external os, a small circular opening in women who have never been pregnant. The cervix feels firm (like the end of a nose) with a dimple in the center that marks the external os.

The outer cervix is covered with a layer of squamous epithelium. The mucosa of the cervical canal is covered with columnar epithelium and contains numerous glands that secrete mucus in response to ovarian hormones. The squamocolumnar junction, where the two types of cells meet, is usually located just inside the cervical os. This junction is also called the *transformation zone* and is the most common site for neoplastic changes. Cells from this site are scraped for the Papanicolaou (Pap) test (see later discussion).

The *uterine tubes* attach to the uterine fundus. The tubes are supported by the broad ligaments and range from 8 to 14 cm in length. The tubes are divided into four sections: the interstitial portion is closest to the uterus; the isthmus and the ampulla are the middle portions; and the infundibulum is closest to the ovary. The uterine tubes provide a passage between the ovaries and the uterus for the movement of the ovum. The infundibulum has fimbriated (fringed) ends, which pull the ovum into the tube. The ovum is pushed along the tubes to the uterus by rhythmic contractions of muscles of the tubes and by the current produced by the movement of the cilia that line the tubes. The ovum is usually fertilized by the sperm in the ampulla portion of one of the tubes.

The *ovaries* are almond-shaped organs located on each side of the uterus below and behind the uterine tubes. During the reproductive years they are approximately 3 cm long, 2 cm wide,

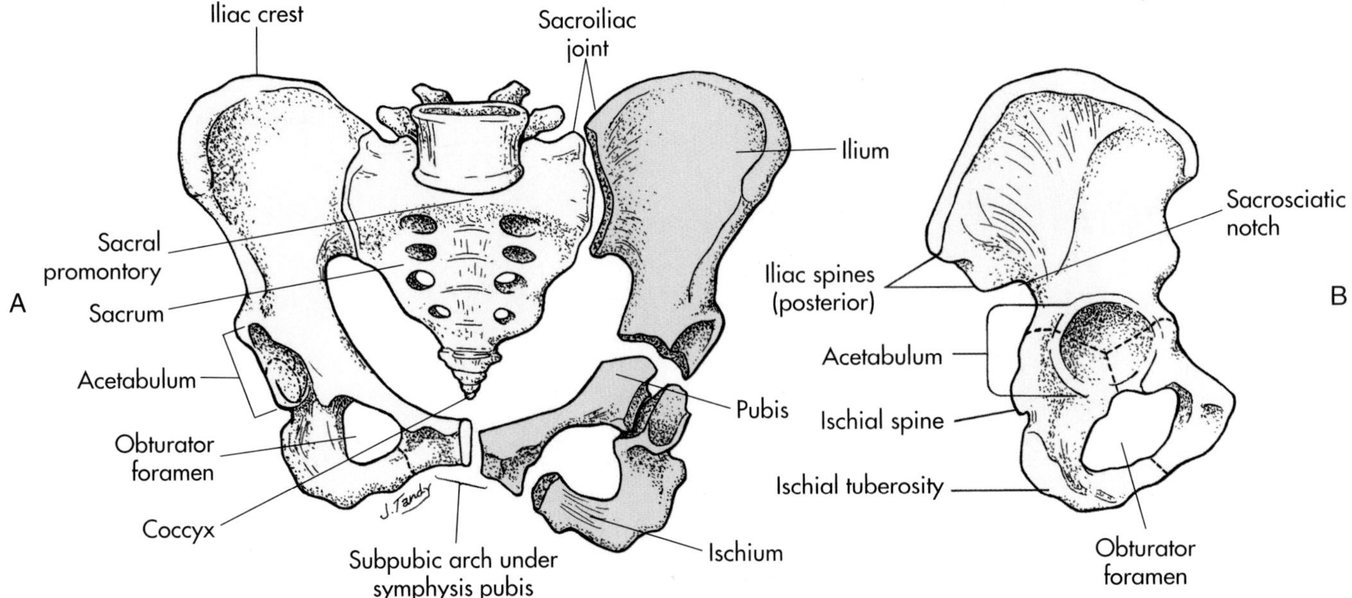

FIG 4-4 Adult female pelvis. **A,** Anterior view. **B,** External view of innominate bone (fused).

and 1 cm thick; they diminish in size after menopause. Before menarche, each ovary has a smooth surface; after menarche, they are nodular because of repeated ruptures of follicles at ovulation. The two functions of the ovaries are ovulation and hormone production. Ovulation is the release of a mature ovum from the ovary at intervals (usually monthly). Estrogen, progesterone, and androgen are the hormones produced by the ovaries.

The Bony Pelvis

The bony pelvis serves three primary purposes: protection of the pelvic structures, accommodation of the growing fetus during pregnancy, and anchorage of the pelvic support structures. The two innominate (hip) bones (consisting of ilium, ischium, and pubis), the sacrum, and the coccyx make up the four bones of the pelvis (Fig. 4-4). Cartilage and ligaments form the symphysis pubis, sacrococcygeal joint, and two sacroiliac joints that separate the pelvic bones.

The pelvis is divided into two parts: the false pelvis and the true pelvis (Fig. 4-5). The false pelvis is the upper portion above the pelvic brim or inlet. The true pelvis is the lower, curved, bony canal, which includes the inlet, the cavity, and the outlet through which the fetus passes during vaginal birth. The upper portion of the outlet is at the level of the ischial spines, and the lower portion is at the level of the ischial tuberosities and the pubic arch. Variations that occur in the size and shape of the pelvis are usually related to age, race, and sex. Pelvic ossification is complete at about 20 years of age.

Breasts

The breasts are paired mammary glands located between the second and sixth ribs (Fig. 4-6). About two thirds of the breast overlies the pectoralis muscle, between the sternum and midaxillary line, with an extension to the *tail of Spence*. The lower one third of the breast overlies the serratus anterior muscle. The breasts are attached to the muscles by connective tissue or fascia.

The breasts of the healthy, mature woman are approximately equal in size and shape but often are not absolutely symmetric. The size and shape vary with the woman's age, heredity, and nutrition. However, the contour should be smooth with no retractions, dimpling, or masses. Estrogen stimulates growth of the breast by inducing fat deposition in the breasts, development of stromal tissue (i.e., increase in its amount and elasticity), and growth of the extensive ductile system. Estrogen also increases the vascularity of breast tissue.

Once ovulation begins in puberty, progesterone levels increase. The increase in progesterone causes maturation of mammary gland tissue, specifically the lobules and acinar structures. During adolescence fat deposition and growth of fibrous tissue contribute to the increase in the size of the glands. Full development of the breasts is not achieved until after the end of the first pregnancy or in the early period of lactation.

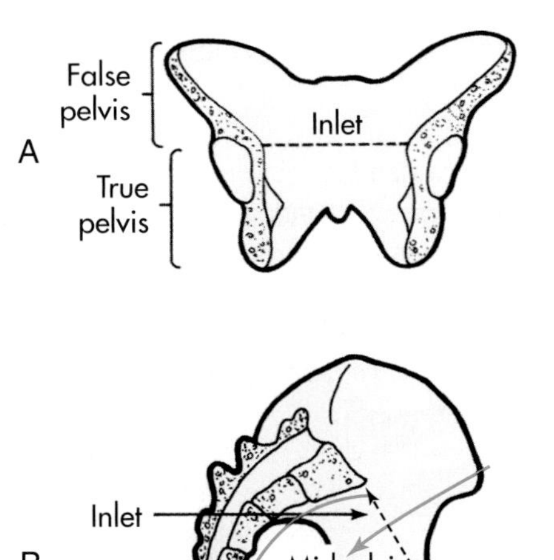

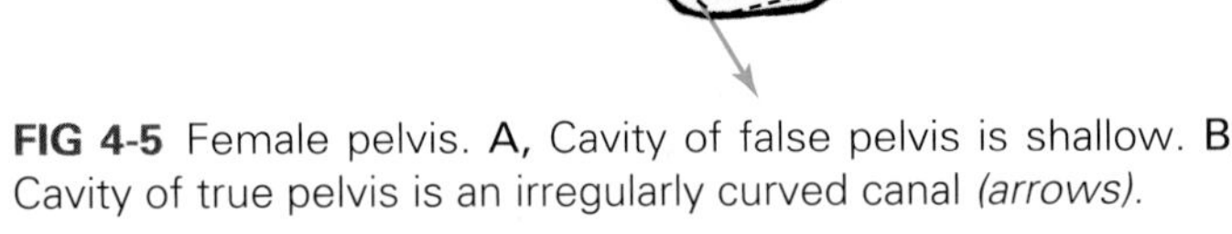

FIG 4-5 Female pelvis. **A,** Cavity of false pelvis is shallow. **B,** Cavity of true pelvis is an irregularly curved canal *(arrows)*.

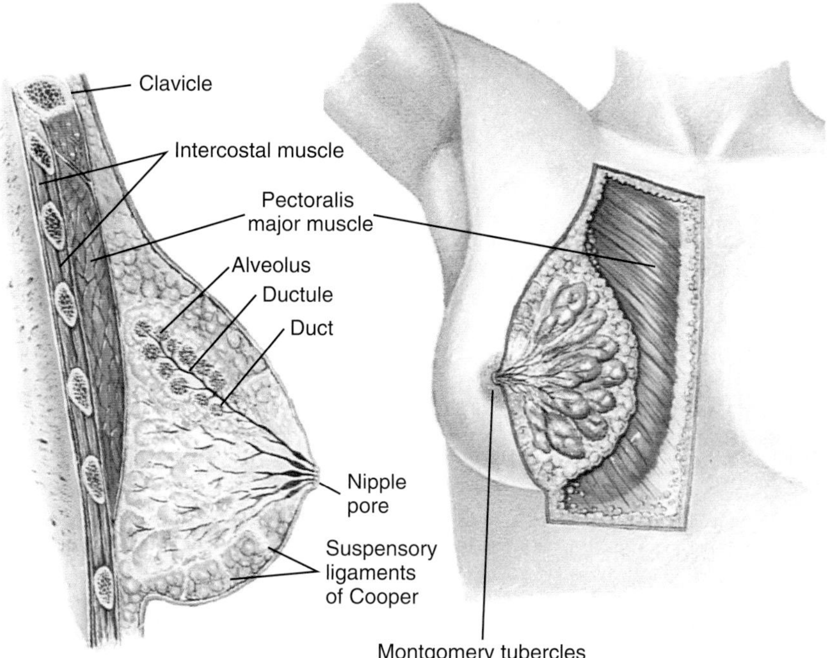

FIG 4-6 Anatomy of the breast, showing position and major structures. (Adapted from Seidel, H., et al. [2011]. *Mosby's guide to physical examination* [7th ed.]. St. Louis: Mosby.)

Each mammary gland is made of a number of lobes that are divided into lobules. Lobules are clusters of acini. An acinus is a saclike terminal part of a compound gland emptying through a narrow lumen or duct. The acini are lined with epithelial cells that secrete colostrum and milk. Just below the epithelium is the myoepithelium (*myo*, or muscle), which contracts to expel milk from the acini.

The ducts from the clusters of acini that form the lobules merge to form larger ducts draining the lobes. Ducts from the lobes converge in a single nipple (mammary papilla) surrounded by an areola. The anatomy of the ducts is similar for each breast but varies among women. Protective fatty tissue surrounds the glandular structures and ducts. *Cooper ligaments,* or fibrous suspensory ligaments, separate and support the glandular structures and ducts. Cooper ligaments provide support to the mammary glands while permitting their mobility on the chest wall (see Fig. 4-6). The round nipple is usually slightly elevated above the breast. On each breast the nipple projects slightly upward and laterally. It contains 4 to 20 openings from the milk ducts. The nipple is surrounded by fibromuscular tissue and covered by wrinkled skin (the areola). Except during pregnancy and lactation, there is usually no discharge from the nipple.

The nipple and surrounding areola are usually more deeply pigmented than the skin of the breast. The rough appearance of the areola is caused by sebaceous glands, *Montgomery tubercles,* directly beneath the skin. These glands secrete a fatty substance thought to lubricate the nipple. Smooth muscle fibers in the areola contract to stiffen the nipple to make it easier for the breastfeeding infant to grasp.

The vascular supply to the mammary gland is abundant. In the nonpregnant state there is no obvious vascular pattern in the skin. The normal skin is smooth without tightness or shininess. The skin covering the breasts contains an extensive superficial lymphatic network that serves the entire chest wall and is continuous with the superficial lymphatics of the neck and abdomen. The lymphatics form a rich network in the deeper portions of the breasts. The primary deep lymphatic pathway drains laterally toward the axillae.

Besides their function of lactation, breasts function as organs for sexual arousal in the mature adult female. The breasts change in size and nodularity in response to cyclic ovarian changes throughout reproductive life. Increasing levels of both estrogen and progesterone in the 3 to 4 days before menstruation increase the vascularity of the breasts, induce growth of the ducts and acini, and promote water retention. The epithelial cells lining the ducts proliferate in number, the ducts dilate, and the lobules distend. The acini become enlarged and secretory, and lipid (fat) is deposited within their epithelial cell lining. As a result, breast swelling, tenderness, and discomfort are common symptoms just before the onset of menstruation. After menstruation, cellular proliferation begins to regress, acini begin to decrease in size, and retained water is lost. After breasts have undergone changes numerous times in response to the ovarian cycle, the proliferation and involution (regression) are not uniform throughout the breast. In time, after repeated hormonal stimulation, small, persistent areas of nodulations may develop. This normal physiologic change must be remembered when breast tissue is examined. Nodules may develop just before and during menstruation, when the breast is most active. The physiologic alternations in breast size and activity reach their minimum level about 5 to 7 days after menstruation stops. Therefore, **breast self-examination (BSE)** (systematic palpation of breasts to detect signs of breast cancer or other changes) is best carried out during this phase of the menstrual cycle (see Evidence-Based Practice box). Although monthly BSE used to be recommended to all women, the current guidelines recommend BSE as an option (American Cancer Society [ACS], 2013a), mostly because the

EVIDENCE-BASED PRACTICE

Teaching Women Breast Self-Examination: Is It Worthwhile?

Ask the Question

Does teaching women breast self-examination actually result in fewer deaths from breast cancer?

Search for the Evidence

Search Strategies Professional organization guidelines, meta-analyses, systematic reviews, randomized controlled trials, nonrandomized prospective studies, and retrospective studies since 2011.

Databases Used CINAHL, Cochrane, MEDLINE, National Guideline Clearinghouse, and websites for the Association for Women's Health, Obstetric and Neonatal Nurses, American Cancer Society (ACS), and National Cancer Institute

Critical Appraisal of the Evidence

The ideal screening test for breast cancer would have a high sensitivity for breast cancer in an early, curable stage, thus decreasing mortality. Moreover, it would have a high specificity, meaning few false positives and thus few unnecessary diagnostic tests. Screening for breast cancer has conventionally consisted of breast self-examination monthly, clinical breast examination (CBE) yearly, and screening mammogram every 1 to 2 years after 40 years of age. Although a screening mammogram has been considered the gold standard, believed to be responsible for a 15% decrease in mortality, a review (Gotzche & Jorgensen, 2013) concluded that because of the large incidence of overdiagnosis and overtreatment, estimated to be 30%, over a 10-year period, for every 2000 women screened, 1 will actually avoid death from breast cancer and 10 healthy women will be treated unnecessarily.

Mammograms are usually accompanied by a CBE by a trained examiner. Since the 1970s, women were also routinely taught to do breast self-examination (BSE). The assumption was the BSE was a low-tech screening tool for women to detect tumors in the early, more treatable stages. This theory was challenged by a classic metaanalysis of two randomized controlled trials that involved 388,535 women in Russia and Shanghai, which found no difference in cancer mortality between groups taught BSE and control groups without BSE education (Kosters & Gotzsche, 2003; updated 2007). In fact, the BSE group was twice as likely to undergo unnecessary biopsy with benign results as the control group. The authors noted the poor compliance with BSE, but also acknowledged that it was possible that BSE may have decreased mortality in some countries. The ACS noted that all women should be informed about the benefits as well as the limitations of BSE so that even if BSE alone does not save lives, women learn what normal breasts feel like and may detect any changes. Also, breastcancer.org continues to recommend that women do BSE.

Apply the Evidence: Nursing Implications

BSE is a low-tech, low-cost technique that can empower some women to discover breast changes earlier. It is not clear that this will decrease mortality. BSE and CBE also may result in unnecessary testing. Organizations such as the Susan G. Komen Foundation (2013) emphasize "understanding breast cancer," which includes having regular screening tests. Nurses should offer to teach the technique of BSE to women who wish to learn. However, some women are not comfortable examining their breasts or find it frightening. All women should be taught to follow the recommended guidelines for CBE yearly and mammograms based on age and personal history.

Quality and Safety Competencies: Evidence-Based Practice*

Knowledge

Nurses must be up to date on the current evidence that supports or does not support the efficacy of BSE and especially must be able to synthesize conflicting evidence.

Skills

Nurses must continue to be able to teach BSE to women and must be able to explain why BSE may be something that a woman would choose to do.

Attitudes

Nurses must be able to help women understand their breasts, including what breasts feel and look like, creating an attitude of comfort with their own bodies, helping them to be able to notice any changes.

References

American Cancer Society. (2013). *Breast cancer: Early detection* Available at www.cancer.org/cancer/breastcancer/moreinformation/breastcancerearlydetection/breast-cancer-early-detection-acs-recs.

breastcancer.org. (2012). *Breast self-exam* Available at www.breastcancer.org/symptoms/testing/types/self_exam.

Gotzsche, P. C., & Jorgensen, K. (2013). Screening for breast cancer with mammography. *The Cochrane Database of Systematic Reviews, 6*, CD001877.

Komen, S. G. (2013). *Understanding breast cancer: Early detection and screening* Available at www.komen.org/breastcancer/earlydetectionampscreening.html.

Kosters, J. (2003). *The Cochrane Database of Systematic Reviews 2003*(2). CD003373.

*Adapted from QSEN at www.qsen.org.

ACS believes that many unnecessary biopsies and other procedures result. However, breastcancer.org (2012) continues to recommend that all women perform BSE monthly (see Teaching for Self-Management box).

MENSTRUATION AND MENOPAUSE

Menarche and Puberty

Although young girls secrete small, rather constant amounts of estrogen, a marked increase occurs between 8 and 11 years of age. The term menarche denotes first menstruation. Puberty is a broader term that denotes the entire transitional stage between childhood and sexual maturity. Increasing amounts and variations in gonadotropin and estrogen secretion develop into a cyclic pattern at least a year before menarche. In North America this occurs in most girls at about 13 years of age.

Initially, menstrual periods are irregular, unpredictable, painless, and *anovulatory* (no ovum is released from the ovary). After 1 or more years, a hypothalamic-pituitary rhythm develops and the ovary produces adequate cyclic estrogen to make a mature ovum. *Ovulatory* (ovum released from the ovary)

TEACHING FOR SELF-MANAGEMENT

Breast Self-Examination

If you choose to perform a breast self-examination, the best time is when breasts are not tender or swollen.

How to examine your breasts:

1. Lie down and put a pillow under your right shoulder. Place your right arm behind your head (Fig. 1).

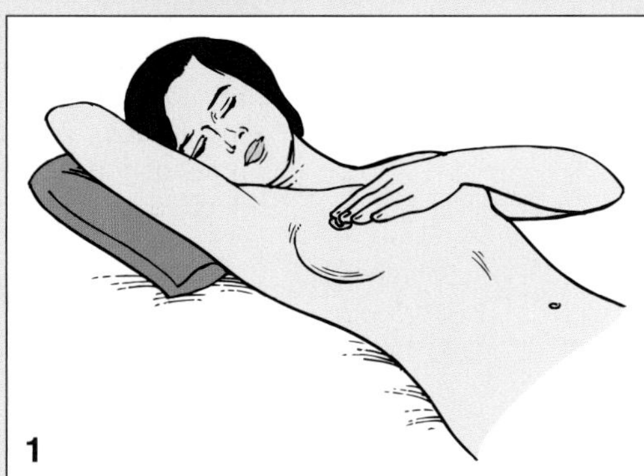

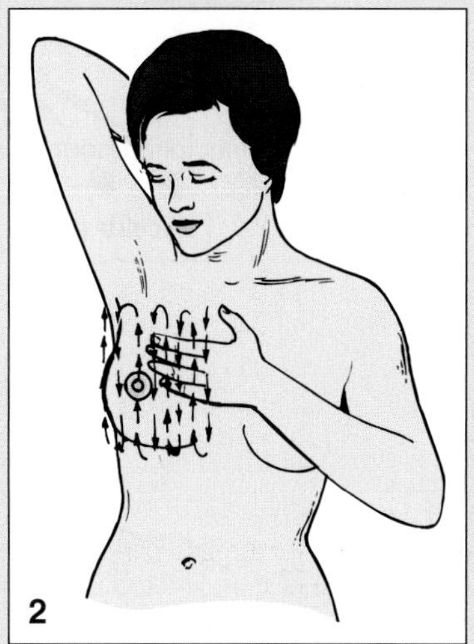

2. Use the finger pads of your three middle fingers on your left hand to feel for lumps or thickening. Your finger pads are the top third of each finger. Use circular motions of the finger pads to feel the breast tissue.
3. Press firmly enough to know how your breast feels. Use light pressure to feel the tissue just under the skin, medium pressure for a little deeper, and firm pressure to feel the breast tissue close to the chest and ribs. A firm ridge in the lower curve of the breast is normal.
4. Move around the breast in a set way, such as using an up-and-down or vertical line pattern (Fig. 2). Go up to the collar bone and down to the ribs and from your underarm on the side to the middle of your chest. Use the same technique every time. It will help you to make sure that you have gone over the entire breast area and to remember how your breast feels.
5. Now examine your left breast. Put a pillow under your left shoulder. Place your right arm behind your head and use your finger pads of your right hand, similar to the description in Step 2.
6. You may want to check your breasts while standing in front of a mirror. See if there are any changes in the way your breasts look: dimpling of the skin, changes in the nipple, or redness or swelling.
7. Checking the area between the breast and the underarm and the underarm itself is important. Examine the area above the breast to the collarbone and to the shoulder while you are standing or sitting up with your arms lightly raised.
8. If you find any changes, see your health care provider right away.

Adapted from American Cancer Society: Breast awareness and self-exam, 2014, www.cancer.org.

periods tend to be regular, with estrogen dominating the first half of the cycle and progesterone dominating the second half.

Although pregnancy can occur in exceptional cases of true precocious puberty, most pregnancies in young girls occur after the normally timed menarche. All young adolescents of both sexes would benefit from knowing that pregnancy can occur at any time after the onset of menses.

Menstrual Cycle

Menstruation is the periodic uterine bleeding that begins approximately 14 days after ovulation. It is controlled by a feedback system of three cycles: endometrial, hypothalamic-pituitary, and ovarian. The average length of a menstrual cycle is 28 days, but variations are normal. The first day of bleeding is designated as day 1 of the menstrual cycle, or menses (Fig. 4-7). The average duration of menstrual flow is 5 days (with a range of 3 to 6 days) and the average blood loss is 50 ml (with a range of 20 to 80 ml), but this duration of flow and blood loss vary greatly. For about 50% of women, menstrual blood does not appear to clot. The menstrual blood clots within the uterus, but the clot usually liquefies before being discharged from the uterus. Uterine discharge includes mucus and epithelial cells in addition to blood.

The menstrual cycle is a complex interplay of events that occur simultaneously in the endometrium, the hypothalamus, the pituitary glands, and the ovaries. The menstrual cycle prepares the uterus for pregnancy. When pregnancy does not occur, menstruation follows. A woman's age, physical and emotional status, and environment influence the regularity of her menstrual cycles.

Hypothalamic-Pituitary Cycle

Toward the end of the normal menstrual cycle, blood levels of estrogen and progesterone decrease. Low blood levels of these ovarian hormones stimulate the hypothalamus to secrete gonadotropin-releasing hormone (GnRH). In turn, GnRH stimulates anterior pituitary secretion of follicle-stimulating hormone (FSH). FSH stimulates development of ovarian graafian follicles and their production of estrogen. Estrogen levels begin to decrease, and hypothalamic GnRH triggers the anterior pituitary to release luteinizing hormone (LH). A marked surge of LH and a smaller peak of estrogen (day 12) (see Fig. 4-7) precede the expulsion of the ovum from the graafian follicle by about 24 to 36 hours. LH peaks at about day 13 or 14 of a 28-day cycle. If fertilization and implantation of the ovum have not occurred by this time, regression of the corpus luteum follows. Levels of

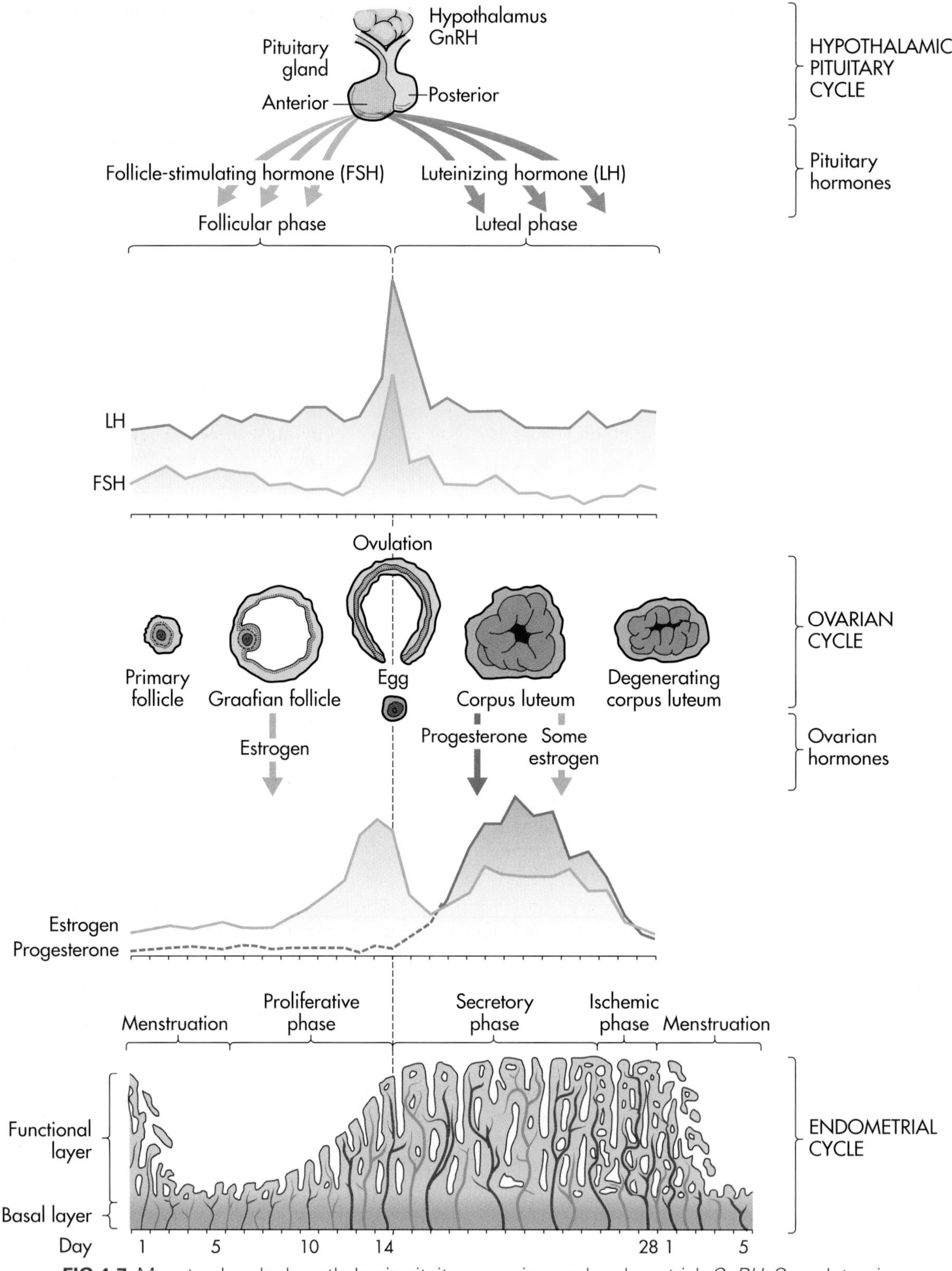

FIG 4-7 Menstrual cycle: hypothalamic-pituitary, ovarian, and endometrial. *GnRH,* Gonadotropin-releasing hormone.

progesterone and estrogen decline, menstruation occurs, and the hypothalamus is once again stimulated to secrete GnRH. This process is called the *hypothalamic-pituitary cycle.*

Ovarian Cycle

The primitive graafian follicles contain immature oocytes (primordial ova). Before ovulation, from 1 to 30 follicles begin to mature in each ovary under the influence of FSH and estrogen. The preovulatory surge of LH affects a selected follicle. The oocyte matures, ovulation occurs, and the empty follicle begins its transformation into the corpus luteum. This follicular phase (preovulatory phase) (see Fig. 4-7) of the ovarian cycle varies in length from woman to woman. Almost all variations in ovarian cycle length are the result of variations in the length of the follicular phase. On rare occasions (i.e., 1 in 100 menstrual cycles), more than one follicle is selected and more than one oocyte matures and undergoes ovulation.

After ovulation, estrogen levels drop. For 90% of women, only a small amount of withdrawal bleeding occurs, and it goes unnoticed. In 10% of women, there is sufficient bleeding for it to be visible, resulting in what is termed *midcycle bleeding.*

The luteal phase begins immediately after ovulation and ends with the start of menstruation. This postovulatory phase of the ovarian cycle usually requires 14 days (range 13 to 15 days). The corpus luteum reaches its peak of functional activity 8 days after ovulation, secreting the steroids *estrogen* and *progesterone.* Coincident with this time of peak luteal functioning, the fertilized ovum is implanted in the endometrium. If no implantation occurs, the corpus luteum regresses and steroid levels drop. Two weeks after ovulation, if fertilization and implantation do not occur, the functional layer of the uterine endometrium is shed through menstruation.

Endometrial Cycle

The four phases of the endometrial cycle are: (1) the menstrual phase, (2) the proliferative phase, (3) the secretory phase, and (4) the ischemic phase (see Fig. 4-7). During the menstrual phase shedding of the functional two thirds of the endometrium (the compact and spongy layers) is initiated by periodic vasoconstriction in the upper layers of the endometrium. The basal layer is always retained, and regeneration begins near the end of the cycle from cells derived from the remaining glandular remnants or stromal cells in this layer.

The proliferative phase is a period of rapid growth lasting from about the fifth day to the time of ovulation. The endometrial surface is completely restored in approximately 4 days, or slightly before bleeding ceases. From this point on, an 8- to 10-fold thickening occurs, with a leveling off of growth at ovulation. The proliferative phase depends on estrogen stimulation derived from ovarian follicles.

The secretory phase extends from the day of ovulation to about 3 days before the next menstrual period. After ovulation, large amounts of progesterone are produced. An edematous, vascular, functional endometrium is now apparent. At the end of the secretory phase, the fully matured secretory endometrium reaches the thickness of heavy, soft velvet. It becomes luxuriant with blood and glandular secretions, creating a suitable protective and nutritive bed for a fertilized ovum.

Implantation of the fertilized ovum generally occurs about 7 to 10 days after ovulation. If fertilization and implantation do not occur, the corpus luteum, which secretes estrogen and progesterone, regresses. With the rapid decrease in progesterone and estrogen levels, the spiral arteries go into spasm. During the ischemic phase, the blood supply to the functional endometrium is blocked and necrosis develops. The functional layer separates from the basal layer, and menstrual bleeding begins, marking day 1 of the next cycle (see Fig. 4-7).

Other Cyclic Changes

When the hypothalamic-pituitary-ovarian axis functions properly, other tissues undergo predictable responses. Before ovulation a woman's basal body temperature is often less than 37° C (98.6° F); after ovulation, with increasing progesterone levels, her basal body temperature rises. Changes in the cervix and cervical mucus follow a generally predictable pattern. Preovulatory and postovulatory mucus is viscous (thick) so that sperm penetration is discouraged. At the time of ovulation, cervical mucus is thin and clear. It looks, feels, and stretches like egg white. This stretchable quality is termed *spinnbarkeit.* Some women have localized lower abdominal pain called *mittelschmerz* that coincides with ovulation. Some spotting may occur.

Prostaglandins

Prostaglandins (PGs) are oxygenated fatty acids classified as hormones. The different kinds of PGs are distinguished by letters (PGE and PGF), numbers (PGE_2), and letters of the Greek alphabet ($PGF_{2\alpha}$).

PGs are produced in most organs of the body, including the uterus. Menstrual blood is a potent PG source. PGs are metabolized quickly by most tissues. They are biologically active in minute amounts in the cardiovascular, gastrointestinal, respiratory, urogenital, and nervous systems. They also exert a marked effect on metabolism, particularly on glycolysis. PGs play an important role in many physiologic, pathologic, and pharmacologic reactions. $PGF_{2\alpha}$, PGE_4, and PGE_2 are most commonly used in reproductive medicine.

PGs affect smooth muscle contractility and modulation of hormonal activity. Indirect evidence indicates that PGs have an effect on ovulation, fertility, changes in the cervix, and cervical mucus that affect receptivity to sperm, tubal and uterine motility, sloughing of endometrium (menstruation), onset of miscarriage and induced abortion, and onset of labor (term and preterm). After exerting biologic actions, newly synthesized PGs are rapidly metabolized by tissues in such organs as the lungs, kidneys, and liver.

PGs may play a key role in ovulation. If PG levels do not rise along with the surge of LH, the ovum remains trapped within the graafian follicle. After ovulation, PGs may influence production of estrogen and progesterone by the corpus luteum.

The introduction of PGs into the vagina or the uterine cavity (from ejaculated semen) increases the motility of uterine musculature, which may assist the transport of sperm through the uterus and into the oviduct.

PGs produced by a woman cause regression of the corpus luteum and regression and sloughing of the endometrium, resulting in menstruation. PGs increase myometrial response to oxytocic stimulation, enhance uterine contractions, and cause cervical dilation. They may be a factor in the initiation of labor, the maintenance of labor, or both. They may also be involved in dysmenorrhea (see Chapter 6) and preeclampsia/eclampsia (see Chapter 27).

Climacteric and Menopause

The climacteric is a transitional phase during which ovarian function and hormone production decline. This phase spans the years from the onset of premenopausal ovarian decline to the postmenopausal time when symptoms stop. Menopause (from Latin *mensis,* month, and Greek *pauses,* to cease) refers only to the last menstrual period. However, unlike menarche, menopause can be dated with certainty only 1 year after menstruation ceases. The average age at natural menopause is 51.4 years, with an age range of 35 to 60 years. Perimenopause is a period preceding menopause that lasts about 4 years. During this time ovarian function declines. Ova slowly diminish, and menstrual cycles may be anovulatory, resulting in irregular bleeding. The ovary stops producing estrogen, and eventually menses no longer occur.

SEXUAL RESPONSE

The hypothalamus and anterior pituitary glands in females regulate the production of FSH and LH. The target tissue for these hormones is the ovary, which produces ova and secretes estrogen and progesterone. A feedback mechanism that consists of hormone secretion from the ovaries, hypothalamus, and anterior pituitary controls the production of sex cells and steroid sex hormone secretion.

Although the first outward appearance of maturing sexual development occurs at an earlier age in females, both females and males achieve physical maturity at approximately 17 years of age; however, individual development varies greatly. Anatomic and reproductive differences notwithstanding, women and men are more alike than different in their physiologic response to sexual excitement and orgasm. For example, the glans clitoris and the glans penis are embryonic homologs. Little difference exists between female and male sexual response; the physical response is essentially the same whether stimulated by coitus, fantasy, or masturbation. Physiologic sexual response can be analyzed in terms of two processes: vasocongestion and myotonia.

Sexual stimulation results in increase in circulation to circumvaginal blood vessels (lubrication in the female), causing engorgement and distention of the genitals. Venous congestion is localized primarily in the genitalia, but it also occurs to a lesser degree in the breasts and other parts of the body. Arousal is characterized by myotonia (increased muscular tension), resulting in voluntary and involuntary rhythmic contractions. Examples of sexually stimulated myotonia are pelvic thrusting, facial grimacing, and spasms of the hands and feet (carpopedal spasms).

The **sexual response cycle** is classically divided into four phases: excitement, plateau, orgasmic, and resolution, according to the seminal work of Masters and Johnson (1966). The four phases occur progressively, with no sharp dividing line between any two phases. The time, intensity, and duration for cyclic completion also vary for individuals and situations. Other researchers have suggested different models to explain sexual response. Leeman and Rogers (2012) emphasized the need to address sexuality and possible sexual difficulties with women in the postpartum period. Specific issues related to this period (and prior procedures such as episiotomy) must be considered in counseling to promote healthy sexuality during the postpartum period. Despite these alternate models of sexual response, it is still common to describe the classic four stages in which specific body changes take place in sequence, and this description is useful in educating and talking with women who may have concerns about possible sexual dysfunction. Table 4-1 compares male and female body changes during each of the four phases of the sexual response cycle.

REASONS FOR ENTERING THE HEALTH CARE SYSTEM

Women enter the health care system for myriad reasons, including those specifically related to women's reproductive health, but also for general well-woman care. Nurses play a key role in working with women who enter the health system (Box 4-1). The following section describes common reasons that women enter the health care system.

TABLE 4-1 Four Phases of Sexual Response

REACTIONS COMMON TO BOTH SEXES	FEMALE REACTIONS	MALE REACTIONS
Excitement Phase		
Heart rate and blood pressure increase. Nipples become erect. Myotonia begins.	Clitoris increases in diameter and swells. External genitalia become congested and darken. Vaginal lubrication occurs; upper two thirds of vagina lengthens and extends. Cervix and uterus pull upward. Breast size increases.	Erection of the penis begins; penis increases in length and diameter. Scrotal skin becomes congested and thickens. Testes begin to increase in size and elevate toward the body.
Plateau Phase		
Heart rate and blood pressure continue to increase. Respirations increase. Myotonia becomes pronounced; grimacing occurs.	Clitoral head retracts under the clitoral hood. Lower one third of vagina becomes engorged. Skin color changes occur—flush may be observed across breasts, abdomen, or other surfaces.	Head of penis may enlarge slightly. Scrotum continues to grow tense and thicken. Testes continue to elevate and enlarge. Preorgasmic emission of two or three drops of fluid appears on the head of the penis.
Orgasmic Phase		
Heart rate, blood pressure, and respirations increase to maximum levels. Involuntary muscle spasms occur. External rectal sphincter contracts.	Strong rhythmic contractions are felt in the clitoris, vagina, and uterus. Sensations of warmth spread through the pelvic area.	Testes elevate to maximum level. Point of "inevitability" occurs just before ejaculation and an awareness of fluid in the urethra. Rhythmic contractions occur in the penis. Ejaculation of semen occurs.
Resolution Phase		
Heart rate, blood pressure, and respirations return to normal. Nipple erection subsides. Myotonia subsides.	Engorgement in external genitalia and vagina resolves. Uterus descends to normal position. Cervix dips into seminal pool. Breast size decreases. Skin flush disappears. Women do not have a refractory period before they can have another orgasm.	Fifty percent of erection is lost immediately with ejaculation; penis gradually returns to normal size. Testes and scrotum return to normal size. Refractory period (time needed for erection to occur again) varies according to age and general physical condition.

Preconception Counseling and Care

Preconception health promotion provides women and their partners with information that is needed to make decisions about their reproductive future. Preconception counseling and care guide couples on how to avoid unintended pregnancies, identify and manage risk factors in their lives and their environment, and identify healthy behaviors that promote the well-being of the woman and her potential fetus. Approximately half of all pregnancies in the United States are unintended (Guttmacher Institute, 2012a). Preconception care targets all women of reproductive age, from menarche to menopausal transition. It has been estimated that 31% of pregnant women experience some complications of pregnancy, including mental health issues (mostly depression) and factors that lead to the need for cesarean birth (HealthyPeople.gov, 2012b). In addition, 12% of births result in preterm infants and 8.2% result in low-birth-weight (LBW) infants (HealthyPeople.gov, 2012a).

Activities that promote healthy mothers and babies must be initiated before the period of critical fetal organ development, which is between 17 and 56 days after fertilization. By the end of the eighth week after conception and certainly by the end of the first trimester, any major structural anomalies in the fetus are already present. Because many women do not realize that they are pregnant and do not seek prenatal care until well into the first trimester, the rapidly growing fetus may be exposed to many types of intrauterine environmental hazards during this most vulnerable developmental phase. These hazards include drugs, viruses, and chemicals. In many instances, counseling can promote behavior modification before damage is done or the woman can make an informed decision about her willingness to accept potential hazards.

Preconception care is important for women who have had a problem with a previous pregnancy (e.g., miscarriage or preterm birth). Although causes are not always identifiable, in many cases problems can be discovered and treated and do not recur in subsequent pregnancies. Preconception care is also important to minimize fetal malformations. For example, the offspring of women who have type 1 diabetes mellitus have significantly more congenital anomalies than do children of mothers without diabetes. The rate of malformation is greatly reduced when the insulin-dependent woman with diabetes has excellent blood glucose control at the time she becomes pregnant and maintains euglycemia (normal blood sugar level) throughout the period of organ development in the fetus. The incidence of neural tube defects such as spina bifida and anencephaly is decreased significantly with the intake of 600 mcg of supplemental folic acid.

The components of preconception care such as health promotion, risk assessment, and interventions are outlined in Box 4-2.

BOX 4-1 Role of Nurses in Women's Health Promotion and Illness Prevention

Registered nurses work with women to promote wellness by:
- Integrating various modalities of care ("integrative nurse coaching")
- Collaborating with other health care practitioners
- Providing care in the community; working with individuals, families, communities
- Working to influence health policy

Advanced practice nurses work with women to promote wellness by:
- Providing comprehensive primary care
- Coordinating care in communities (from hospitals to home to communities)
- Working with social service resources for clients in the community; influencing health policy

BOX 4-2 Components of Preconception Care

Health Promotion: General Teaching
- Nutrition
  - Healthy diet, including folic acid
  - Optimal weight
- Exercise and rest
- Avoidance of substance abuse (tobacco, alcohol, "recreational" drugs)
- Use of risk-reducing sex practices
- Attending to family and social needs

Risk Factor Assessment
- Chronic diseases
  - Diabetes, heart disease, hypertension, asthma, thyroid disease, kidney disease, anemia, mental illness
- Infectious diseases
  - HIV/AIDS, other sexually transmitted infections, vaccine-preventable diseases (e.g., rubella, hepatitis B)
- Reproductive history
  - Contraception
  - Pregnancies—unplanned pregnancy, pregnancy outcomes
  - Infertility
- Genetic or inherited conditions (e.g., sickle cell anemia, Down syndrome, cystic fibrosis)
- Medications and medical treatment
  - Prescription medications (especially those contraindicated in pregnancy), over-the-counter medication use, radiation exposure
- Personal behaviors and exposures
  - Smoking, alcohol consumption, illicit drug use
  - Overweight or underweight; eating disorders
  - Folic acid supplement use
  - Spouse or partner and family situation, including intimate partner violence
  - Availability of family or other support systems
  - Readiness for pregnancy (e.g., age, life goals, stress)
  - Environmental (home, workplace) conditions
  - Safety hazards
  - Toxic chemicals
  - Radiation

Interventions
- Anticipatory guidance or teaching
  - Treatment of relevant medical conditions
  - Medications
  - Cessation or reduction in substance use and abuse
  - Immunizations (e.g., rubella, hepatitis)
- Nutrition, diet, weight management
- Exercise
- Referral for genetic counseling
- Referral to and use of:
  - Family planning services
  - Family and social needs management

AIDS, Acquired immunodeficiency syndrome; *HIV,* human immunodeficiency virus.

BOX 4-3 Major Goals of Prenatal Care

- Define health status of the mother and fetus.
- Determine the gestational age of the fetus, and monitor fetal development.
- Identify the woman at risk for complications, and minimize the risk whenever possible.
- Provide appropriate education and counseling.

Pregnancy

A woman's entry into the health care system is often associated with pregnancy, for either diagnosis or actual prenatal care. Early entry into prenatal care (i.e., within the first 12 weeks) allows for identification of the woman at risk for complications and initiation of measures to prevent problems or treat them if they arise. The U.S. Department of Health and Human Services (HHS, 2012) has emphasized the importance of early and consistent prenatal care to improve outcomes for both mother and infant. Major goals of prenatal care are listed in Box 4-3 and should be addressed in the first visit. Extensive discussion of pregnancy is found in Chapter 15.

Well-Woman Care

Current trends in women's health care have expanded beyond a reproductive focus. A holistic approach to women's health care includes a woman's health needs throughout her lifetime. This view goes beyond simply her reproductive needs. This restructuring places women's health within the primary health care delivery system. Women's health assessment and screening focus on a multisystem evaluation emphasizing the maintenance and enhancement of wellness.

Health care needs vary with culture, religion, age, and personal differences. The changing responsibilities and roles of women, their socioeconomic status, and their personal lifestyles also contribute to differences in the health and behavior of women. Employment outside of the home, physical disability, inadequate or no health insurance, divorce, single parenthood, and sexual orientation also can affect women's ability to seek and receive health care in clinical settings. As women age, many continue to address their primary health care needs within their established gynecologic care setting; therefore, well-women's health care should include a complete history, physical examination, age-appropriate screening, and health promotion.

Fertility Control and Infertility

As noted, almost half of the pregnancies in the United States each year are unintended (Guttmacher Institute, 2012a), and the majority of these occurs in women who either do not use contraception or who experienced a contraceptive failure. Education is the key to encouraging women to make family planning choices based on preference and actual benefit-to-risk ratios. Providers can influence the user's motivation and ability to use the method correctly.

The concept of health promotion applies to contraception, as can be seen in Box 4-4. The nurse can influence women positively regarding the need for child spacing, methods of family planning that are consistent with religious and personal preferences, noncontraceptive benefits of certain methods, the appropriate use of methods selected, and the protection of future fertility when so desired.

BOX 4-4 Contraceptive Health Promotion

- Child spacing and quality maternity care improve perinatal outcomes and health in general of mother and children.
- Achieving desired family size enables a better sharing of all resources, with attendant increases in education, health care, and other positive societal parameters
- Contraceptives themselves may positively affect future health. For example, use of condoms may prevent acquisition of HIV infection; combined OCs may provide some protection against later development of cancer of ovary and endometrium; barrier methods decrease transmission of STIs, which can develop into pelvic inflammatory disease with resultant infertility or sterility and thus affect future childbearing capacity.

HIV, Human immunodeficiency virus; *OCs,* oral contraceptives; *STIs,* sexually transmitted infections.

Women also enter the health care system because of their desire to become pregnant. Approximately 15% of couples in the United States have some degree of infertility. Many couples have delayed starting their families until they are in their 30s or 40s, which allows more time to be exposed to factors that affect fertility negatively (including age-related infertility for the woman). In addition, STIs, which can predispose to decreased fertility, are becoming more common and many women and men are in workplaces and home settings, where they may be exposed to reproductive environmental hazards.

Infertility can cause emotional pain for many couples, and the inability to produce offspring sometimes results in feelings of failure and places inordinate stress on the couple's relationship. Much time, money, and emotional investment can be used for testing and treatment in efforts to build a family.

Steps toward prevention of infertility should be undertaken as part of ongoing routine health care, and information about how women may prevent some causes of infertility is especially appropriate in preconception counseling. Primary care providers can undertake initial evaluation and counseling before couples are referred to specialists. (For additional information about infertility, see Chapter 9.)

Menstrual Problems

Irregularities or problems with the menstrual period are among the most common concerns of women and often cause them to seek help from the health care system. Common menstrual disorders include amenorrhea, dysmenorrhea, premenstrual syndrome, endometriosis, and menorrhagia or metrorrhagia. Simple explanation and counseling may handle the concern; however, history and examination must be completed, as well as laboratory or diagnostic tests, if indicated. Questions should never be considered inconsequential, and age-specific reading materials are recommended, especially for teenagers. (See Chapter 6 for an in-depth discussion of menstrual problems.)

Perimenopause

The body responds to this natural transition in a number of ways, most of which are caused by the decrease in estrogen.

Most women seeking health care during the perimenopausal period do so because of irregular bleeding. Others are concerned about vasomotor symptoms (hot flashes and flushes). Although fertility is greatly reduced during this period, women are urged to maintain some method of birth control because pregnancies still can occur. All women need to have factual information, the dispelling of myths, a thorough examination, and periodic health screenings thereafter. (See Chapter 6 for an in-depth discussion of perimenopausal problems.)

BARRIERS TO ENTERING THE HEALTH CARE SYSTEM

Access to care varies greatly, depending on type and size of the system, source of payment for services, private versus public programs, availability of and accessibility to providers, individual preferences, and insurance coverage or ability to pay. The existing system continues to be oriented to treatment of acute or episodic conditions rather than to the promotion of health and comprehensive care, despite the fact that people are discharged earlier from hospitals, requiring more care in homes and community settings. With a greater focus on preventive health care services and with 32,000,000 formerly uninsured clients having access to health care, nurses, advanced practice nurses, including nurse practitioners, nurse-midwives, and clinical nurse specialists, are critical to the provision of high-quality, safe, effective, and accessible health care (see Box 4-1).

Financial Issues

In the United States, disparity among races and socioeconomic classes affects many facets of life including health. Limited finances are associated with lack of access to care, delay in seeking care, few prevention activities, and little accurate information about health and the health care system. Women use health care services more often than men but are more likely than men to have difficulty in financing the services. Many poor women have traditionally been underinsured or uninsured, but rules about health insurance and who and what are covered are undergoing a transition with the Affordable Care Act (healthcare.gov, 2012). People will not be denied insurance because of preexisting conditions, and various preventive health services will be covered under health insurance. However, this legislation is far from decided, and its effect on the American people will not be known for years.

Cultural Issues

We live in a multicultural society with constantly changing demographics, and for nursing care of women to be optimal, cultural differences must be addressed with great sensitivity and competency. Nurses are in excellent positions to be responsible for providing culturally sensitive and competent health care (Escallier, Fullerton, & Messina, 2011). A variety of reasons are given to explain some of the differences in accessing care when financial barriers are adjusted. Some women experience racial discrimination or disrespectful, disillusioning, or discouraging encounters with community service providers such as social services and health care providers. Many women do not seek care from the health care system because of lack of trust (Yang, Matthews, & Hillemeier, 2011). A lack of cross-cultural communication also presents problems. Desired health outcomes are best achieved when the health care provider has knowledge of and understanding about the culture, language, values, priorities, and health beliefs of those in various ethnic groups. Conversely, members of these various groups should understand the health goals to be achieved and the methods proposed to do so. Language differences can produce profound barriers between clients and providers. Even with an interpreter, misinformation can occur on both sides of the communication.

Providers must consider culturally based differences that could affect the treatment of diverse groups of women, and the women themselves must share practices and beliefs that could influence their responses to treatment or willingness to adhere to treatment. For example, women in some cultures value privacy to such an extent that they are reluctant to disrobe and, as a result, avoid physical examination unless absolutely necessary. Other women rely on their husbands to make major decisions, including those affecting the woman's health. Religious beliefs may dictate a plan of care, as with birth control measures or blood transfusions. Some cultural groups prefer folk medicine, homeopathy, or prayer to traditional Western medicine, and others attempt combinations of some or all practices. Nurses can integrate into their own practice various holistic approaches to care, in accordance with Dossey's (2013) *Theory of Integral Nursing*. It is critically important to be sensitive to cultural differences and at the same time not stereotype and assume that a woman has certain beliefs because of her ethnic background. Although the amount of health information on the Internet is increasing, information in languages other than English is limited and not all information on the Internet is accurate, making health literacy an important issue in culturally competent care.

Gender Issues

Gender influences provider-client communication and may influence access to health care in general. Researchers have reported significant male-female differences in receipt of major diagnostic and therapeutic interventions, especially with cardiac and kidney problems. Women tend to use primary care services more often than do men and, some believe, more effectively. The gender of the provider plays a role. The concept of "gender concordance," in which the client's gender matches the health care provider's gender, was found to be important for women seeking Pap tests (McAlearney, Oliveri, Post, et al., 2011). McAlearney and associates found that women were more comfortable having a Pap test performed by a female physician and having a female nurse present.

Sexual orientation may produce another barrier. Nurses need to understand the specific health care needs and issues related to sexual orientation (Brennan, Barnsteiner, de Leon Siantz, et al., 2012). Some lesbians may not disclose their sexual orientation to health care providers because they feel they may be at risk for hostility, inadequate health care, or breach of confidentiality. In many health care settings, heterosexuality is assumed, and the setting may be one in which the woman does not feel welcome (magazines, brochures, and environment reflect heterosexual couples, or the health care provider shows discomfort interacting with the woman). Lesbians themselves may hold beliefs that are incorrect (e.g., that they have immunity to human immunodeficiency virus [HIV], sexually transmitted infections [STIs], and certain cancers [e.g., cervical]). The perceived lack of risk can result in lesbians avoiding health care, as well as in health care providers giving incorrect advice or not providing appropriate screening for these women. Not all gynecologic cancers are related to sexual activity; lesbians who have never had children may still be at risk for breast, ovarian, and endometrial cancer. Their risk for heart disease, cancer of the lung, and colon cancer is not different from that of the heterosexual woman. To offset stereotypes, it is necessary for providers to develop an approach that does not assume that all clients are heterosexual. More content related to this issue needs to be included in nursing curricula.

HEALTH RISKS TO WOMEN

Maintaining optimal health is a goal for all women. Essential components of health maintenance are the identification of unrecognized problems and potential risks and the education and health promotion needed to reduce them. Current trends in women's health care have expanded beyond a reproductive focus. A holistic approach to women's health care goes beyond simple reproductive needs and includes a woman's health needs throughout her lifetime, with attention to physical, mental/emotional, social, and spiritual health. Women's health is considered to be part of the primary health care delivery system with assessment and screening focusing on a multisystem evaluation that emphasizes the maintenance and enhancement of wellness. Prevention of cardiovascular disease, promotion of mental health, and prevention of cancers beyond just reproductive-related cancers are all components of well-woman care. It is important to consider all aspects of women's health, particularly in light of the fact that the leading causes of death in women in the United States include more than just reproductive health conditions (Box 4-5).

Even when focusing on reproductive health, it is critical to take a holistic approach to the health of women. This is especially important for women in their childbearing years because conditions that increase a woman's health risks are related not only to her well-being but also the well-being of both mother and baby in the event of a pregnancy. Prenatal care is an example of prevention that is practiced after conception. However, prevention and health maintenance are needed before conception because many of the mother's risks can be identified and eliminated, or at least modified.

As a female progresses through developmental ages and stages, she is faced with conditions that are age related. An overview of conditions and circumstances that increase health risks in women across the life span is presented in the next section. In a later section, tips for promoting health and preventing illness are presented.

BOX 4-5 Top 10 Leading Causes of Death in Women in the United States

1. Heart disease
2. Malignant neoplasm (cancer)
3. Cardiovascular disease (stroke)
4. Chronic lower respiratory disease
5. Alzheimer's disease
6. Unintentional injury
7. Diabetes mellitus
8. Influenza and pneumonia
9. Nephritis
10. Septicemia

Data from U.S. Department of Health and Human Services, Health Resources and Services Administration, Maternal and Child Health Bureau. (2011). *Women's health USA*. Rockville, MD; U.S. Department of Health and Human Services. (2013). *Leading causes of death in females, United States, 2009*. Available at www.cdc.gov/women/lcod/2009/index.htm; mchb.hrsa.gov/whusa11.

Age

Adolescence

All teens undergo progressive development of sex characteristics. They experience the developmental tasks of adolescence such as establishing identity and sexual orientation, emancipating from family, and establishing career goals. Some of these processes can produce great stress for the adolescent, and the health care provider should treat her very carefully. Female teenagers who enter the health care system usually do so for screening or because of a problem such as episodic illness or accidents. Previous guidelines recommended that young women should be screened with Pap tests at age 18 or when they become sexually active. Guidelines now suggest that Pap tests begin at age 21, but controversy exists about the evidence to support these new guidelines, with some health care providers providing evidence for earlier testing (Zhao, Kalpos-Novak, & Austin, 2011). Gynecologic problems are often associated with menses (either bleeding irregularities or dysmenorrhea), vaginitis or leukorrhea, STIs, contraception, or pregnancy. The adolescent is also at risk for use of street drugs, for eating disorders, and for stress, depression, and anxiety.

Many women first enter the health care delivery system for a Pap test or for contraception. Visits to the nurse may be their only contact with the system unless they become ill. Some women postpone examination until a specific need arises such as pregnancy, infertility, pain, abnormal bleeding, or vaginal discharge. The availability of the human papillomavirus (HPV) vaccine has created another reason for young women to enter the health care system (Saraiya, Rosser, & Cooper, 2012).

Teenage Pregnancy. Most young women begin having sex in their mid- to late teens. At age 15, 13% of teens have had sex, but by age 19, 70% of teens have had sexual intercourse (Guttmacher Institute, 2012b). A sexually active teen who does not use contraception has a 90% chance of pregnancy within 1 year. The United States has the highest teen pregnancy rate in the industrialized world. By age 20, one third of all American girls get pregnant; most of these pregnancies are unintended (Centers for Disease Control and Prevention [CDC], 2012a).

Effective educational programs about sex and family life are imperative to control the rate of teen pregnancy and STIs. The nurse can provide information regarding methods of family planning that are consistent with religious and personal preferences, noncontraceptive benefits of certain methods, the appropriate use of methods selected, the need for child spacing, and the protection of future fertility when so desired.

Pregnancy in the teenager who is 16 years of age or younger often introduces additional stress into an already stressful developmental period. The emotional level of such teens is commonly characterized by impulsiveness and self-centered behavior, and they often place primary importance on the beliefs and actions of their peers. In attempts to establish a personal and independent identity, many teens do not realize the consequence of their behavior; their thinking processes do not include planning for the future.

Teenagers usually lack the financial resources to support a pregnancy and may not have the maturity to avoid teratogens or have prenatal care and instruction or follow-up care. Children of teen mothers may be at risk for abuse or neglect because of the teen's inadequate knowledge of growth, development, and parenting. Implementation of specialized adolescent programs in schools, communities, and health care systems is demonstrating continued success in reducing the birth rate in teens.

Young and Middle Adulthood

Because women ages 20 to 40 years have a need for contraception, pelvic and breast screening, and pregnancy care, they may prefer to use their gynecologic or obstetric provider as their primary care provider. During these years the woman may be juggling family, home, and career responsibilities, with resulting increases in stress-related conditions. Health maintenance includes not only pelvic and breast screening but also promotion of a healthy lifestyle (i.e., good nutrition, regular exercise, no smoking, moderate or no alcohol consumption, sufficient rest, stress reduction, and referral for medical conditions and other specific problems). Common conditions requiring well-woman care include vaginitis, urinary tract infections, menstrual variations, obesity, sexual and relationship issues, and pregnancy.

Parenthood After Age 35. The woman older than 35 years does not have a different physical response to a pregnancy per se but, rather, may have health status changes as a result of time and the normal aging process. These changes may be responsible for age-related pregnancy conditions. For example, a woman with type 2 diabetes may not have had expression of her diabetes at age 22 but may have the full-blown disease at age 38. Other chronic or debilitating diseases or conditions increase in severity with time, and these in turn may predispose to increased risks during pregnancy. Of significance to women in this age group is the risk for certain genetic anomalies (e.g., Down syndrome). The opportunity for genetic counseling should be available to all (see Chapter 3).

Late Reproductive Age

Women of later reproductive age are often experiencing change and reordering personal priorities. In general, the goals of education, career, marriage, and family have been achieved and now the woman has increased time and opportunity for new interests and activities. Divorce rates are high at this age, and children leaving home may produce an "empty nest syndrome," resulting in increased levels of depression. Chronic diseases also become more apparent. Most problems for the well woman are associated with perimenopause (e.g., bleeding irregularities and vasomotor symptoms). Health maintenance screening continues to be of importance because some conditions such as breast disease or ovarian cancer occur more often during this stage.

Social, Cultural, Economic, and Genetic Factors

Differences exist among people from different socioeconomic levels and ethnic groups with respect to risk for illness and distribution of disease and death. Some diseases are more common among people of selected ethnicity (e.g., sickle cell anemia in African-Americans, Tay-Sachs disease in Ashkenazi Jews, adult lactase deficiency in Chinese, beta thalassemia in Mediterranean people, and cystic fibrosis in northern Europeans). Cultural and religious influences also increase health risks because the woman and her family may have life and societal values and a view of health and illness that dictate practices different from those expected in the Judeo-Christian Western model. These may include food taboos or frequencies, methods of hygiene, effects of climate, care-seeking behaviors, willingness to undergo screening and diagnostic procedures, and conflicts in values.

Socioeconomic status affects birth outcomes. The rates of perinatal and maternal deaths, preterm births, and LBW babies are considerably higher in disadvantaged populations (Hogue & Silver, 2011). Social consequences for poor women as single parents are great because many mothers with few skills are caught in the bind of insufficient income to afford child care. These families generate fewer and fewer resources and increase their risks for health problems. Multiple roles for women in general produce overload, conflict, and stress, resulting in higher risks for psychologic illness.

Substance Use and Abuse

Use of illicit drugs and inappropriate use of prescription drugs continue to increase and are found in all ages, races, ethnic groups, and socioeconomic strata. Addiction to substances is seen as a biopsychosocial disease, with several factors contributing to risk. These include biogenetic predisposition, lack of resilience to stressful life experiences, and poor social support. Women are less likely than men to abuse drugs, but the rate in women is increasing significantly. Substance-abusing pregnant women create severe problems for themselves and their offspring, including interference with optimal growth and development and addiction. In many instances, the use of substances is identified through screening programs in prenatal clinics and obstetric units.

COMMUNITY ACTIVITY

- Visit the National Women's Health Resource Center website at www.healthywomen.org. Go to the conditions and treatments link and select a condition. Review the client information sections about diagnosis, treatment, prevention, facts to know, questions to ask, and lifestyle tips.
- Visit the WomensHealth.gov and go to the various women's health topics and publications. Review the information to see what areas of women's health might be of interest to you, including how you might advocate in the community on behalf of a women's health issue.
- Visit the smokefree.gov website to learn about smoking in your state. How does your state rank compared to other states?
- Visit the Office of Women's Health Research website at http://orwh.od.nih.gov and view the various research that is being conducted in women's health.

Smoking

Tobacco use is the leading cause of preventable death and illness. Smoking is linked to cardiovascular disease, various types of cancers (especially lung and cervical), chronic lung disease, and negative pregnancy outcomes. Premature death is estimated to occur in 443,000 people annually because of either smoking or being exposed to secondhand smoke, and 8.6 million people are estimated to be seriously ill as a result of smoking. However, it is also estimated that 46.6 million adults in the United States smoke; 17.3% of women are smokers (CDC, 2011). The American Cancer Society (ACS, 2013b) notes that women who smoke decrease their life span by 14.5 years compared with nonsmokers. Tobacco contains nicotine, which is an addictive substance that creates physical and psychologic dependence. Smoking in pregnancy is known to cause a decrease in placental perfusion and is one cause of LBW in infants. During pregnancy, women seem to be highly motivated to stop or at least to limit smoking. If a pregnant woman is able to stop smoking during the first trimester, she decreases the chance of having a LBW baby (ACS, 2013b). (Chapter 31 discusses other aspects of smoking.)

Cigarette smoking impairs fertility in both women and men, may reduce the age for menopause, and increases the risk for osteoporosis after menopause. Passive, or secondhand, smoke (environmental tobacco smoke) contains similar hazards and presents additional problems for the smoker and harm for the nonsmoker.

Alcohol Consumption

Women ages 35 to 49 have the highest rates of chronic alcoholism, but women ages 21 to 34 have the highest rates of specific alcohol-related problems. About one third of alcoholics are women, and many relate the onset of their drinking problem to stressful events. Women who are problem drinkers are often depressed, have more motor vehicle injuries, and have a higher incidence of attempted suicide than do women in the general population. They are also at risk for alcohol-related liver damage. Early case finding and treatment are important in alcoholism for both the ill individual and family members. (Additional discussion about alcohol consumption is included in Chapter 31.)

Prenatal alcohol exposure has been found to increase the chance of birth defects significantly, with one study reporting a fourfold increase (O'Leary, Nassar, Kurinczuk, et al., 2011). Although fetal alcohol syndrome (FAS) is a known consequence of prenatal alcohol intake, studies also indicate that other consequences include increased risk for miscarriage, stillbirth, preterm birth, and sudden infant death syndrome (SIDS). Clearly, alcohol consumption during pregnancy has wide-reaching effects (Bailey & Sokol, 2011). A 2020 national health objective is to have 98.3% of pregnant women abstain from alcohol use (HealthyPeople.gov, 2012c).

Alcohol use during pregnancy can lead to fetal alcohol spectrum disorder (FASD), which includes FAS, fetal alcohol effects, and alcohol-related neurologic developmental disabilities. Approximately 40,000 babies per year are born with FASD; however, recent research reveals that multivitamin supplement use during pregnancy may lessen the effects of prenatal alcohol exposure in the children of women who are unable or unwilling to curtail their alcohol abuse when pregnant (Avalos, Kaskutas, Block, et al., 2011). LBW, intellectual disability, behavior problems, and learning and physical problems are some of the symptoms of FAS babies (see Chapter 35). Severe facial deformities of FAS occur at day 20 of conception when women may not even suspect that they are pregnant.

Caffeine

Caffeine is found in society's most popular drinks: coffee, tea, and soft drinks. It is a stimulant that can affect mood and interrupt body functions by producing anxiety and sleep interruptions. Heart dysrhythmias may be made worse by caffeine, and there can be interactions with certain medications such as lithium. Birth defects have not been related to caffeine consumption; however, high intake has been related to a slight decrease in birth weight and may also increase risk for miscarriage. The March of Dimes (2013) recommends that pregnant women, or women who are trying to conceive, limit their caffeine intake to no more than 200 mg/day, which is the equivalent of one 12-ounce cup of coffee.

Prescription Drug Use

Psychotherapeutic medications such as stimulants, sleeping pills, tranquilizers, and pain relievers are used by an estimated 2% of American women. Such medications can bring relief from undesirable conditions such as insomnia, anxiety, and pain. Because the medications have mind-altering capacity, misuse can produce psychologic and physical dependency in the same manner as illicit drugs. Risk-to-benefit ratios should be considered when such medications are used for more than a very short period. Depression and anxiety are the most common mental health problems in women (depression used to be considered the most common, but recently it has been noted that depression occurs comorbidly with anxiety). Many kinds of medications are used to treat depression and anxiety. All of these psychotherapeutic drugs can have some effect on the fetus and must be monitored very carefully.

Illicit Drugs

Illicit drugs are taken for unlawful purposes. When they are unprescribed they are usually obtained on the street for the purpose of getting high or for their body-mind-altering characteristics. Almost any drug can be abused or even illegal if taken in excess, including alcohol and prescription medication. See Chapter 31 for further discussion of substance abuse.

Nutritional Deficiencies

Good nutrition is essential for optimal health. A well-balanced diet helps prevent illness and treat certain health problems. Conversely, poor eating habits, eating disorders, and obesity are linked to disease and debility. Environmental factors play an important role in nutrition. Dubowitz, Ghosh-Dastidar, Eibner, and colleagues (2012) presented data from the Women's Health Initiative (WHI) clinical trial that indicated availability of healthy food was correlated with decreased obesity in women. These data suggest that social conditions and access to nutritious food are important contributors to women's health.

Overt disease caused by a lack of certain nutrients is rarely seen in the United States. However, insufficient amounts or imbalanced nutrients do pose problems for individuals and families. Overweight or underweight status, malabsorption, listlessness, fatigue, frequent colds and other minor infections, constipation, dull hair and nails, and dental caries are examples of problems that can be related to nutrition and indicate the need for further nutritional assessment. Poor nutrition, especially related to obesity and high fat and cholesterol intake, may lead to more serious conditions in later life, which supports the need to ensure healthy nutrition as a preventive measure. The Academy of Nutrition and Dietetics (2012) noted that five of the eight most common causes of death in adults ages 65 and older are related to nutritional problems.

Obesity

During the past 20 years, obesity has increased dramatically in the United States. More than one third of women in the United States are obese (body mass index [BMI] of 30 or greater), with adults ages 40 to 59 having the highest prevalence. The BMI is defined as a measure of an adult's weight in relation to his or her height, specifically the adult's weight in kilograms divided by the square of his or her height in meters (see Chapter 14). It is estimated that one third of adults and one sixth of children and adolescents are in the obese range (HealthyPeople.gov, 2012b). Overweight and obesity are known risk factors for premature death, diabetes, heart disease, stroke, hypertension, type 2 diabetes, gallbladder disease, diverticular disease, some anemias, oral disease, constipation, osteoarthritis, gout, osteoporosis, respiratory dysfunction, sleep apnea, and some types of cancer (uterine, breast, colorectal, kidney, and gallbladder) (ACS, 2013c). In addition, obesity is associated with high cholesterol, menstrual irregularities, hirsutism (excess body/facial hair), stress incontinence, depression, complications of pregnancy, increased surgical risk, and shortened life span. Pregnant women who are morbidly obese are at increased risk for hypertension, diabetes, gallbladder disease, postterm pregnancy, musculoskeletal problems, intrauterine growth restriction, and intrauterine fetal demise (American College of Obstetricians and Gynecologists [ACOG], 2013).

Other Considerations: Eating Disorders

Anorexia nervosa and bulimia are two forms of eating disorders, although there are additional forms, such as subclinical eating disorders. Some women, especially adolescents, do not have symptoms that lend themselves to a diagnosis of anorexia nervosa or bulimia. These women are diagnosed as having a subclinical eating disorder, which is usually associated with disorders of mood and anxiety and requires accurate diagnosis and prompt treatment (Touchette, Henegar, Godart, et al., 2011). Research suggests that eating disorders are often associated with difficulties in intimate relationships, and interpersonal psychotherapy has been considered as an approach to treatment of women with eating disorders (Murphy, Straebler, Basden, et al., 2012).

It is important to assess for and treat women with eating disorders early because they are at increased risk for serious physical problems as well as diminished quality of life (Vallance, Latner, & Gleaves, 2011). Eating disorders during pregnancy are also associated with increased risk to the pregnant woman and her fetus (Pasternak, Weintraub, Shoham-Vardi, et al., 2012).

Anorexia Nervosa. Some women have a distorted view of their bodies and, no matter what their weight, perceive themselves to be much too heavy. As a result, they undertake strict and severe diets and rigorous extreme exercise. This chronic eating disorder is known as anorexia nervosa. Women can carry this condition to the point of starvation, with resulting endocrine and metabolic abnormalities. If not corrected, significant complications of dysrhythmias, amenorrhea, cardiomyopathy, and congestive heart failure occur and, in the extreme, can lead to death. The condition commonly begins during adolescence in young women who have some degree of personality disorder. They gradually lose weight over several months, have amenorrhea, and are abnormally concerned with body image. A coexisting depression usually accompanies anorexia.

There are no specific tests to diagnose anorexia nervosa. A medical history, physical examination, and screening tests help identify women at risk for eating disorders. Several tools are available to use in primary care settings. The SCOFF questionnaire, developed by Morgan, Reid, and Lacey (1999) is easy to administer and can help the nurse decide whether an eating disorder is likely and whether the woman needs further assessment and possibly psychiatric and medical intervention. More recently Hautala, Junnila, Alin and colleagues (2009) provided further evidence for the validity and usefulness of the SCOFF. See Box 4-6 for a description of the SCOFF.

Bulimia Nervosa. Bulimia refers to secret, uncontrolled binge eating alternating with methods to prevent weight gain: self-induced vomiting, laxatives or diuretics, strict diets, fasting, and rigorous exercise. During a binge episode, a large number of calories are consumed, usually consisting of sweets and junk foods. Binges occur at least twice per week. Bulimia usually begins in early adulthood (ages 18 to 25 years) and is found primarily in females. Complications can include dehydration and electrolyte imbalance, gastrointestinal abnormalities, and cardiac dysrhythmias. Bulimia is somewhat similar to anorexia in that it is an eating disorder and usually involves some degree of depression (Skinner, Haines, Austin, et al., 2012). Unlike those with anorexia, individuals with bulimia may feel shame or disgust about their disorder and tend to seek help earlier. The SCOFF screening assessment also can be used to assess clients with bulimia (see Box 4-6).

Binge-Eating Disorder. The hallmark of binge-eating disorder is eating large amounts of food in a short period (a couple of hours) and not being able to stop eating. The woman may eat when she's not hungry or until uncomfortably full. She may choose to eat alone because she is embarrassed about how much she eats. Binge-eating disorder involves bingeing

BOX 4-6 Screening for Eating Disorders

SCOFF Questions

Each question scores 1 point. A score of 2 or more indicates the person may have anorexia nervosa or bulimia.

1. Do you make yourself **S**ick (i.e., induce vomiting) because you feel too full?
2. Do you worry about loss of **C**ontrol over the amount you eat?
3. Have you recently lost more than **O**ne stone (6.4 kg [14 lb]) in a 3-month period?
4. Do you think you are too **F**at even if others think you are too thin?
5. Does **F**ood dominate your life?

From Morgan, J.F., & Lacey, J. (1999). The SCOFF questionnaire: Assessment of a new screening tool for eating disorders. *BMJ, 319*(7223), 1467-1468.

that alternates with a restricted dietary intake. An associated syndrome called *night eating syndrome* is when limited food is eaten early in the day and most of the day's food intake is consumed after the evening meal. Over time, obesity and related complications of being overweight can develop. Common personality traits found in those with binge-eating disorder include excessive concern about body size and shape and low self-esteem. Depression and anxiety commonly occur along with binge eating, which makes treatment and recovery more difficult. Binge eating is not associated with anorexia nervosa or bulimia nervosa.

Lack of Exercise

Lack of adequate exercise is an important risk factor to women's health. Exercise contributes to good health by lowering risks for a variety of conditions that are influenced by obesity and a sedentary lifestyle. It is effective in the prevention of cardiovascular disease and in the management of chronic conditions such as hypertension, arthritis, diabetes, respiratory disorders, and osteoporosis. Exercise also contributes to stress reduction and weight maintenance. Women report that engaging in regular exercise improves their body image and self-esteem and acts as a mood enhancer. Aerobic exercise produces cardiovascular involvement because an increased amount of oxygen is delivered to working muscles. Anaerobic exercise such as weight training improves individual muscle mass without stress on the cardiovascular system. Because women are concerned about both cardiovascular and bone health, weight-bearing aerobic exercises such as walking, running, racquet sports, and dancing are preferred. However, excessive or strenuous exercise can lead to hormone imbalances, resulting in amenorrhea and its consequences. Physical injury is also a potential risk.

SAFETY ALERT

Before beginning any planned physical activity program, a woman should see her primary care nurse practitioner (NP) or physician for a thorough medical evaluation to prevent potential injuries or harm.

Stress

The modern woman faces increasing levels of stress and, as a result, is prone to a variety of stress-induced complaints and illnesses. Stress often occurs because of multiple roles in which coping with job and financial responsibilities conflicts with parenting and duties at home. To add to this burden, women are socialized to be caregivers, which is emotionally draining, creating additional stress. They also may find themselves in positions of minimal power that do not allow them control over their everyday environments. Some stress is normal and contributes to positive outcomes. Many women thrive in busy surroundings. However, excessive or high levels of ongoing stress trigger physical reactions such as rapid heart rate, elevated blood pressure, slowed digestion, release of additional neurotransmitters and hormones, muscle tenseness, and a weakened immune system. Consequently, constant stress can contribute to clinical illnesses such as flare-ups of arthritis or asthma, frequent colds or infections, gastrointestinal upsets, cardiovascular problems, and infertility. Box 4-7 lists symptoms that may be related to chronic or extreme stress. Psychologic symptoms such as anxiety, irritability, eating disorders, depression, insomnia, and substance abuse have also been associated with stress.

Depression, Anxiety, and Other Mental Health Conditions

Women experience depression and/or anxiety frequently. In addition, depression is sometimes described as a co-traveler because it is exists comorbidly with other physical conditions. Depression and/or anxiety create difficulties for quality of life and, at the extreme, create a risk for suicide. Research (Berecki-Gisolf, McKenzie, Dobson, et al., 2012) suggests that women with comorbid anxiety and depression are at greater risk for developing cardiac disease. In addition to depression and anxiety, women experience other mental health disorders, such as bipolar disease (see Chapter 31).

BOX 4-7 Stress Symptoms

Physical
- Perspiration/sweaty hands
- Increased heart rate
- Trembling
- Nervous tics
- Dryness of throat and mouth
- Tiring easily
- Urinating frequently
- Sleeping problems
- Diarrhea, indigestion, vomiting
- Butterflies in stomach
- Headaches
- Premenstrual tension
- Pain in the neck and lower back
- Loss of appetite or overeating
- Susceptibility to illness

Behavior
- Stuttering and other speech difficulties
- Crying for no apparent reason
- Acting impulsively
- Startling easily
- Laughing in a high-pitched and nervous tone of voice
- Grinding teeth
- Increased smoking
- Increased use of drugs and alcohol
- Being accident-prone
- Losing appetite or overeating

Psychologic
- Feeling anxious
- Feeling scared
- Feeling irritable
- Feeling moody
- Low self-esteem
- Fear of failure
- Inability to concentrate
- Embarrassed easily
- Worrying about the future
- Preoccupation with thoughts or tasks
- Forgetfulness

Adapted from State University of New York Counseling Center. (2002). *Stress management*. University of Buffalo, NY: State University of New York.

Sleep Disorders

Many women suffer from sleep disorders, including difficulty initiating sleep or staying asleep and experiencing nonrestorative sleep. Restless leg syndrome may be a cause of sleep disorders or a comorbid condition. Sleep disorders are correlated with physical and mental health problems, including depression, pain, and fibromyalgia. Mong, Baker, Mahoney and associates (2011) presented a review of studies conducted on gender differences related to sleep, suggesting that, although further research is needed, women experience insomnia significantly more than do men. It is important that the nurse talk with the woman about her sleep patterns and discuss ways to improve sleep, such as avoiding alcohol before going to sleep and sleeping in a regular pattern.

Environmental and Workplace Hazards

Environmental hazards in the home, the workplace, and the community can contribute to poor health at all ages. Categories and examples of health-damaging hazards include the following: (1) pathogenic agents (viruses, bacteria, fungi, parasites); (2) natural and synthetic chemicals (natural toxins from animals, insects, and plants; consumer and industrial products such as pesticides and hydrocarbon gases; medical and diagnostic devices; tobacco; fuels; and drugs and alcohol); (3) radiation (radon, heat waves, sound waves); (4) food substances (added components that are not necessary for nutrition); and (5) physical objects (moving vehicles, machinery, weapons, water, and building materials).

Environmental hazards can affect fertility, fetal development, live birth, and the child's future mental and physical development. Children are at special risk for poisoning from lead found in paint and soil. Everyone is at risk from air pollutants such as tobacco smoke, carbon monoxide, smog, suspended particles (dust, ash, and asbestos), and cleaning solvents; noise pollution; pesticides; chemical additives; and poor food preparation. Workers also face safety and health risks caused by ergonomically poor work stations and stress. It is important that risk assessments continue to be in effect to identify and understand environmental problems in public health. The March of Dimes (2011) has published a helpful resource that summarizes the various risks posed in the environment to pregnant women and their fetuses.

Sexual Practices

Potential risks related to sexual activity include undesired pregnancy and STIs. The risks are particularly high for adolescents and young adults who engage in sexual intercourse at earlier and earlier ages. Adolescents report many reasons for wanting to be sexually active: peer pressure, desire to love and be loved, experimentation, to enhance self-esteem, and to have fun. However, many teens do not have the decision-making or values-clarification skills needed to take this important step. They may also lack knowledge about contraception and STIs. Many do not believe that becoming pregnant or getting an STI will happen to them.

Although some STIs can be cured with antibiotics, many cause significant problems. Possible sequelae include infertility, ectopic pregnancy, neonatal morbidity and mortality, genital cancers, acquired immunodeficiency syndrome (AIDS), and even death. The incidence of STIs is increasing rapidly and reaching epidemic proportion. Choice of contraception has an effect on the risk for contracting an STI. No method of contraception offers complete protection. (See Chapter 7 for a discussion of STIs and Chapter 8 for a discussion of contraception.)

Prevention of STIs is predicated on the reduction of high risk behaviors by educating toward a behavioral change. Behaviors of concern include multiple and casual sexual partners and unsafe sexual practices. The abuse of alcohol and drugs is a high risk behavior, resulting in impaired judgment and thoughtless acts. Behavioral changes must come from within; therefore, the nurse must provide sufficient information for the individual or group to "buy into" the need for change. Education is a powerful tool in health promotion and prevention of STIs and pregnancy. However, it works best when delivered in a way that considers the language, culture, and lifestyle of the intended listener.

! NURSING ALERT

A comprehensive sexual assessment should be integrated into all health histories.

Medical Conditions

Most women of reproductive age are relatively healthy. Heart disease; lung, breast, colon, and other nongynecologic cancers; chronic lung disease; and diabetes are all concerns for adult women because they are among the leading causes of death in women. Certain medical conditions present during pregnancy can have deleterious effects on both the woman and the fetus. Of particular concern are risks from all forms of diabetes, urinary tract disorders, thyroid disease, hypertensive disorders of pregnancy, cardiac disease, and seizure disorders. Effects on the fetus vary and include intrauterine growth restriction, macrosomia, anemia, prematurity, immaturity, and stillbirth. Effects on the woman also can be severe. These conditions are discussed in later chapters. See Clinical Reasoning Case Study on cardiovascular disease in women.

CLINICAL REASONING CASE STUDY

Cardiovascular Disease—The Leading Cause of Death in Women

Selena is a 56-year-old Hispanic menopausal client who presents for her annual well-woman examination. She is a nonsmoker and nondrinker who lives a sedentary lifestyle. She does not exercise. Her mother died of a heart attack at age 60.

Body mass index (BMI) at today's visit is 33, blood pressure (BP) 150/100, high-density lipoprotein (HDL) 25.

She says she knows that she is overweight and should probably exercise and lose weight. How would you respond to her statement?

1. Evidence—Is there evidence that supports how the nurse should respond?
2. Assumptions—What assumptions can be made about the following issues?
   a. Effects of primary and secondary cardiovascular risk factors
   b. Elevated blood pressure
   c. Low HDL
   d. Role of her culture
3. What implications and priorities for nursing care can be made at this time?
4. Does the evidence objectively support your conclusion?

Gynecologic Conditions

Women are at risk throughout their reproductive years for pelvic inflammatory disease, endometriosis, STIs and other vaginal infections (see Chapter 7), uterine fibroids, uterine deformities such as bicornuate uterus, ovarian cysts, interstitial cystitis, and urinary incontinence related to pelvic relaxation. These gynecologic conditions may contribute negatively to pregnancy by causing infertility, miscarriage, preterm labor, and fetal and neonatal problems. Gynecologic cancers also affect women's health, although the risk for most cancers is low in pregnancy. Risk factors depend on the type of cancer. The impact of developing a gynecologic problem or cancer on women and their families is shaped by a number of factors, including the specific type of problem or cancer, the implications of the diagnosis for the woman and her family, and the timing of the occurrence in the woman's and the family's lives. These conditions are discussed in Chapter 11.

Female Genital Mutilation

Female genital mutilation is practiced in more than 45 countries, the majority of which are in Africa. As emigrants from these countries arrive in North America, nurses in the United States and Canada will see clients who have had such procedures performed (see the Culture box).

CULTURAL CONSIDERATIONS

Female Genital Mutilation

Defined by the World Health Organization (WHO, 2013), female genital mutilation (FGM) is "all procedures that involve partial or total removal of the external female genitalia, or other injury to the female genital organs for non-medical reasons" (2013). It is a recognized violation of girls and women and is something that is done intentionally to alter or cause injury to female genital organs. There are no medical reasons for this procedure and it can have many untoward consequences, including severe pain, shock, hemorrhage (bleeding), tetanus or sepsis (bacterial infection), urine retention, open sores in the genital region, and injury to nearby genital tissue. Long-term consequences include bladder and urinary tract infections, cysts, infertility, and increased risk for complications of childbirth and newborn death.

It is an attempt to control women through controlling their sexuality. FGM is supposed to remove sexual desire so that the girl will not become sexually active until married.

FGM is illegal in the United States and punishable by fines, prison, and deportation. An obstetrician may incise the closed labia to allow for a vaginal birth, or remove cysts, but may not sew the labia back to its previous state of reinfibulation. If performed on a minor, FGM is considered child abuse in the United States. "The practice also violates the rights to health, security and physical integrity of the person, the right to be free from torture and cruel, inhuman or degrading treatment, and the right to life when the procedure results in death" (WHO).

Nurses are providing care to a growing number of women who have emigrated from the Middle East, Asia, and Africa, where female circumcision is more common. Nurses must be sensitive to the unique needs of these clients, especially if these women have concerns about maintaining or restoring the intactness of the circumcision after childbirth.

Data from World Health Organization. (2013). *Female genital mutilation.* World Health Organization, Fact Sheet # 241. Available at www.who.int/mediacentre/factsheets/fs241/en.

Violence Against Women

Intimate partner violence (IPV) is the most common form of violence experienced by women worldwide, with a reported incidence of 1 of every 6 women having been a victim of domestic violence. In the United States, IPV is a significant social problem and a major health care problem that affects millions of women and men each year and costs millions of dollars in annual medical costs. Statistics from the U.S. Department of Justice, Office of Violence Against Women (2012) reported that 1 in 4 women in the United States has experienced severe physical violence by a current or former intimate partner. In addition, 5.2 million women were victimized by stalkers. It is estimated that 1.3 million women are raped in the United States annually.

Women of all races and of all ethnic, educational, religious, and socioeconomic backgrounds are affected. Pregnancy is often a time when violence begins or escalates. The magnitude of the problem is far greater than the statistics indicate because violent crimes against women are the most underreported data as a result of fear, lack of understanding, and stigma surrounding violent situations. Maternity and women's health nurses, by the very nature of their practice, are in a unique position to conduct case finding, provide sensitive care to women experiencing abusive situations, engage in prevention activities, and influence health care and public policy toward decreasing the violence. For further discussion of violence against women, see Chapter 5.

HEALTH ASSESSMENT

Trends in women's health have expanded beyond a reproductive focus to include a holistic approach to health care across the life span and place women's health within the scope of primary care. Women's health assessment and screening focus on a systems evaluation that begins with a careful history and physical examination. During assessment and evaluation, the responsibility for self-care and management, health promotion, and enhancement of wellness is emphasized. Nursing care includes assessment, planning, education, counseling, and referral as needed, as well as commendations for good self-care that the woman has practiced. This enables women to make informed decisions about their own health care.

In a market-driven system such as managed care, specific guidelines may be provided for health screening by the insurer or the managed care organization. A nurse often takes the history, orders diagnostic tests, interprets test results, makes referrals, coordinates care, and directs attention to problems requiring medical intervention. Advanced practice nurses who have specialized in women's health, such as nurse practitioners, clinical nurse specialists, and nurse-midwives, perform complete physical examinations, including gynecologic examinations.

Interview

Contact with the woman usually begins with an interview, which is an integral part of the history. This interview should be conducted in a private, comfortable, and relaxed setting (Fig. 4-8). The nurse is seated and makes sure that the woman is comfortable. The woman is addressed by her title and name (e.g., Mrs. Martinez), and the nurse introduces herself or himself using name and title. It is important to phrase questions in a sensitive and nonjudgmental manner. Body language should match oral communication. The nurse is aware of a woman's vulnerability and assures her of strict confidentiality. For many women, fear, anxiety, and modesty make the examination a dreaded and stressful experience. Many women are uninformed, misguided by myths, or afraid they will appear ignorant by asking questions about sexual or reproductive functioning. The woman is assured that no question is irrelevant. Cultural considerations must be addressed in the interview process (see Culture box).

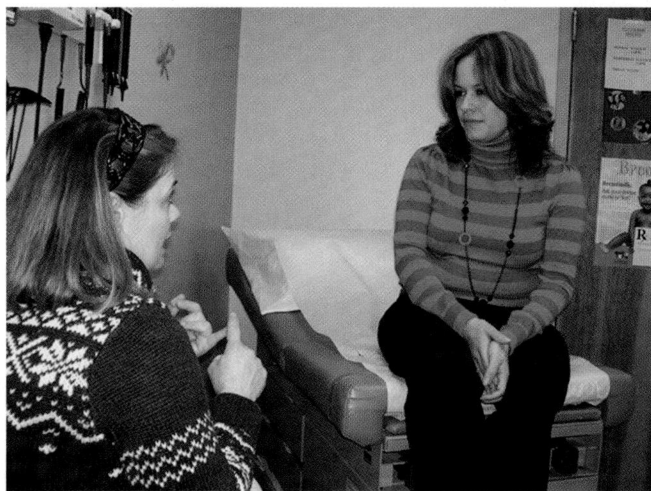

FIG 4-8 Nurse interviews woman as part of history-taking prior to physical examination. (Courtesy Ed Lowdermilk, Chapel Hill, NC.)

CULTURAL CONSIDERATIONS

Communication Variations

- Conversational style and pacing: Silence may show respect or acknowledgment that the listener has heard. In cultures in which a direct "no" is considered rude, silence may mean no. Repetition or loudness may mean emphasis or anger.
- Personal space: Cultural conceptions of personal space differ. Based on one's culture, for example, someone may be perceived as distant for backing off when approached, or aggressive for standing too close.
- Eye contact: Eye contact varies among cultures from intense to fleeting. Consistent with the effort to refrain from invading personal space, avoiding direct eye contact may be a sign of respect.
- Touch: The norms about how people should touch each other vary among cultures. In some cultures, physical contact with the same sex (embracing, walking hand in hand) is more appropriate than that with an unrelated person of the opposite sex.
- Time orientation: In some cultures involvement with people is more valued than being "on time." In other cultures, life is scheduled and paced according to clock time, which is valued over personal time.

Data from Galanti, G. (2008). *Caring for patients from different cultures* (4th ed.). Philadelphia: University of Pennsylvania Press; Mattson, S. (2000). Striving for cultural competence: Providing care in the changing face of the U.S. *AWHONN Lifelines, 4*(3), 48-52.

The history begins with an open-ended question such as "What brings you into the office/clinic/hospital today?" and is furthered by other questions such as "Anything else?" and "Tell me about it." Additional ways to encourage women to share information include:

- **Facilitation:** Using a word or posture that communicates interest such as leaning forward, making eye contact, or saying "Mm-hmmm" or "Go on"
- **Reflection:** Repeating a word or phrase that a woman has used
- **Clarification:** Asking the woman what is meant by a stated word or phrase
- **Empathic responses:** Acknowledging the feelings of a woman by statements such as "That must have been frightening"
- **Confrontation:** Identifying something about the woman's behavior or feelings not expressed verbally or apparently inconsistent with her history
- **Interpretation:** Putting into words what you infer about the woman's feelings or about the meaning of her symptoms, events, or other matters

Direct questions may be necessary to elicit specific details. These should be worded in language that is understandable to the woman and expressed neutrally so that the woman will not be led into a specific response. The nurse asks about one item at a time and proceeds from the general to the specific (Seidel, Ball, Dains, et al., 2011).

Nurses need to develop rapport and trust with their clients as they take a history; because communication within a caring context is core to nursing practice, nurses are well suited to taking a comprehensive client history. Nurses should ask questions incrementally to build a comprehensive understanding. They should also share insights with the woman by eliciting her concerns or thoughts as well as offering clarification (Fawcett & Rhynas, 2012).

Cultural Considerations

Recognizing signs and symptoms of disease and deciding when to seek treatment are influenced by cultural perceptions. It is essential that a nurse have respect for the rich and unique qualities that cultural diversity brings to individuals. In recognizing the value of these differences, the nurse can modify the plan of care to meet the needs of each woman.

To understand the woman's point of view, it is important to ask the right questions. Galanti (2008) suggests the use of the 4 C's of Cultural Competence. These include:

1. Call—What do you call your problem?
2. Cause—What do you think caused your problem?
3. Cope—How do you cope with your condition?
4. Concerns—What are your concerns regarding your condition?

Using the 4 C's of Cultural Competence along with cultural proficiency, biomedical values, and evidence-based practice allows the nurse to individualize care with a client-focused approach. Trust that the woman is the expert on her life, culture, and experiences. If the nurse asks with respect and a genuine desire to learn, the woman will tell the nurse how to care for her.

Modifications may be necessary for the physical examination. In some cultures it may be considered inappropriate for the woman to disrobe completely for the physical examination. In many cultures a female examiner is preferred. Communication

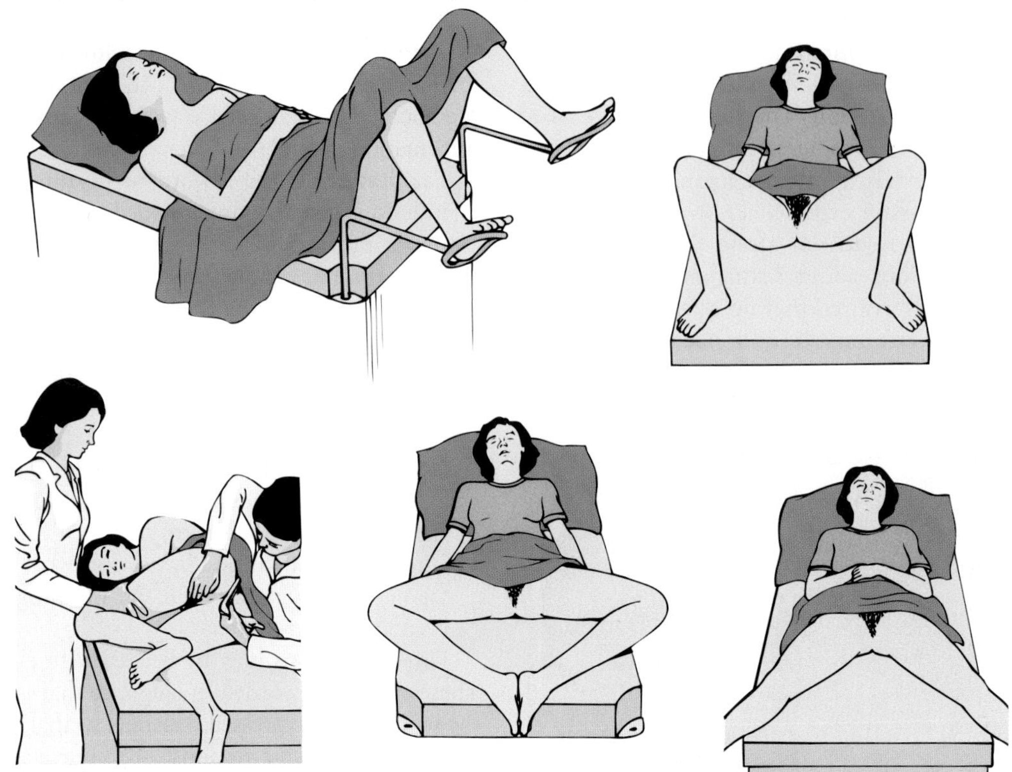

FIG 4-9 Lithotomy and variable positions for women who have a disability.

may be hindered by different beliefs even when the nurse and woman speak the same language (see Cultural Considerations: Strategies for Care Delivery and Providing Cultural Appropriate Care in Chapter 2, Box 2-3).

Women with Special Needs

Women with Disabilities

Women with emotional or physical disorders have special needs. Women who have vision, hearing, emotional, or physical disabilities should be respected and involved in the assessment and physical examination to the full extent of their abilities. The nurse should communicate openly and directly with sensitivity. It is often helpful to learn about the disability directly from the woman while maintaining eye contact (if eye contact is culturally appropriate). Family and significant others should be relied on only when absolutely necessary. The assessment and physical examination can be adapted to each woman's individual needs.

Communication with a woman who is hearing impaired can be accomplished without difficulty. Most of these women read lips, write, or both; thus an interviewer who speaks and enunciates each word slowly and in full view may be easily understood. If a woman is not comfortable with lip reading, she may use an interpreter. In this case it is important to continue to address the woman directly, avoiding the temptation to speak directly with the interpreter.

The visually impaired woman needs to be oriented to the examination room and may have her guide dog with her. As with all women, the visually impaired woman needs a full explanation of what the examination entails before proceeding. Before touching her, the nurse explains, "Now I am going to take your blood pressure. I am going to place the cuff on your right arm." The woman can be asked if she would like to touch each of the items that will be used in the examination.

Many women with physical disabilities cannot comfortably lie in the lithotomy position for the pelvic examination. Several alternative positions may be used, including a lateral (side-lying) position, a V-shaped position, a diamond-shaped position, and an M-shaped position (Piotrowski & Snell, 2007) (Fig. 4-9). The woman can be asked what has worked best for her previously. If she has never had a pelvic examination, or has never had a comfortable pelvic examination, the nurse proceeds by showing her a picture of various positions and asking her which one she prefers. The nurse's support and reassurance can help the woman relax, which will make the examination go more smoothly.

Abused Women

Nurses should screen all women entering the health care system for potential abuse. Nelson, Bougatsos, and Blazina (2012), representing the U.S. Preventive Services Task Force, recommended that screening women for potential abuse can have beneficial consequences with minimal negative outcomes. Help for the woman may depend on the sensitivity with which the nurse screens for abuse, the discovery of abuse, and subsequent intervention. The nurse must be familiar with the laws governing abuse in the state in which she or he practices.

Pocket cards listing emergency numbers (abuse counseling, legal protection, and emergency shelter) may be available from the local police department, a women's shelter, or an emergency department. It is helpful to have these on hand in the setting where screening is done. An abuse-assessment screen (Fig. 4-10) can be used as part of the interview or written history.

ABUSE ASSESSMENT SCREEN

- Are you with a spouse or partner who threatens or physically hurts you?
  - Yes ______ No ______
- Are you with a spouse or partner who emotionally hurts you?
  - Yes ______ No ______
- Within the past year or in this pregnancy (if the woman is pregnant) has anyone hit, slapped, kicked, or otherwise hurt you?
  - Yes ______ No ______
  - If yes, by whom ________________
  - Number of times ________________
  - Mark the area of injury on the body map.
- Has anyone forced you to have sexual activities that made you uncomfortable?
  - Yes ______ No ______
  - If yes, by whom ________________
  - Number of times ________________
- Are you afraid of your partner or anyone you listed above?
  - Yes ______ No ______

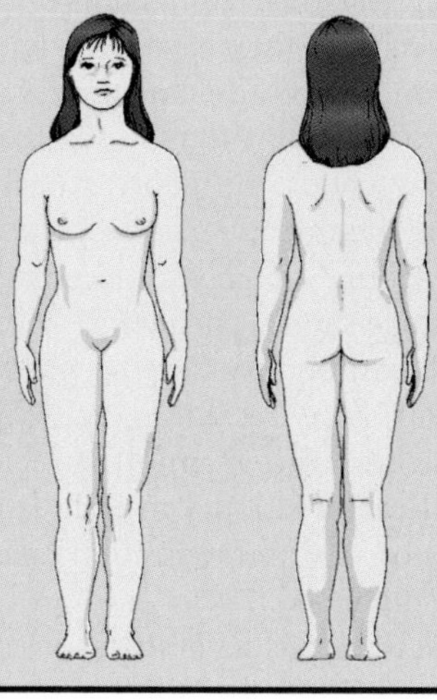

FIG 4-10 Abuse assessment screen. Screening for Intimate Partner Violence. (Adapted from American College of Obstetricians and Gynecologists [ACOG], 2012). *Are you being abused? Screening tools for domestic violence.* Available at www.acog.org/About_ACOG/ACOG_Departments/Violence_Against_Women/Are_you_Being_Abused.)

If a male partner is present, he should be asked to leave the room because the woman may not disclose experiences of abuse in his presence, or he may try to answer questions for her to protect himself. The same procedure would apply for partners of lesbians, parents of teens, or adult children of older women.

Fear, guilt, and embarrassment may keep many women from giving information about family violence. Clues in the history and evidence of injuries on physical examination should give a high index of suspicion. The areas most commonly injured in women are the head, the neck, the chest, the abdomen, the breasts, and the upper extremities. Burns and bruises in patterns resembling hands, belts, cords, or other weapons may be seen as well as multiple traumatic injuries. Attention should be given to women who repeatedly seek treatment for somatic complaints such as headaches, insomnia, choking sensation, hyperventilation, gastrointestinal symptoms, and pain in the chest, back, and pelvis. During pregnancy the nurse should assess for injuries to the breasts, the abdomen, and the genitals. (See Chapter 5 for further discussion of violence.)

Adolescents (Ages 13 to 19 Years)

As a young woman matures, she should be asked the same questions that are included in any history. Particular attention should be paid to hints about risky behaviors, eating disorders, and depression. Do not assume that a teenager is not sexually active. After rapport has been established, it is best to talk to a teen with the parent (partner or friend) out of the room. Questions should be asked with sensitivity and in a gentle and nonjudgmental manner (Seidel et al., 2011).

A teen's first speculum examination is the most important because she will develop perceptions that will remain with her for future examinations. What the examination entails should be discussed with the teen while she is dressed. Models or illustrations can be used to show exactly what will happen. All of the necessary equipment should be assembled so that there are no interruptions. Pediatric speculums that are 1 to 1.5 cm wide can be inserted with minimal discomfort. If the teen is sexually active, a small adult speculum may be used.

Injury prevention should be a part of the counseling at routine health examinations, with special attention to seat belts, helmets, firearms, recreational hazards, and sports involvement. The use of drugs and alcohol and the nonuse of seat belts contribute to motor vehicle injuries, accounting for the greatest proportion of accidental deaths in women. Contraceptive use and STI prevention information may be needed for teens who are sexually active.

To provide developmentally appropriate care, it is important to review the major tasks for women in this stage of life. Major tasks for teens include values assessment; education and work goal setting; formation of peer relationships that focus on love, commitment, and becoming comfortable with sexuality; and separation from parents. Individuality may be reflected in areas such as sexuality, politics, and career choices. Conflict exists between making and keeping commitments to keep options open. The teen is egocentric as she progresses rapidly through emotional and physical changes. Her feelings of invulnerability may lead to serious misconceptions, such as that unprotected sexual intercourse will not lead to pregnancy.

Midlife and Older Women (Ages 50 Years and Older)

The assessment of women ages 50 and older presents unique challenges. Women may be experiencing major lifestyle changes, such as children leaving home, caring for their aging parents, job change, retirement, separation, divorce or death of a partner, and aging-related changes and health problems. The nurse uses reflection and empathy to communicate in an open and caring manner. It may be necessary to schedule a longer appointment time because older women have longer histories or have a need to talk. Some women may fail to report symptoms because they fear their complaints will be attributed to old age, or they feel that they have lived with a chronic condition (e.g., incontinence, dyspareunia, interstitial cystitis, decreased libido, depression) for so long that nothing can be done. Women may choose to ignore a problem if they have symptoms that are life threatening (e.g., chest pain or a breast lump) because they traditionally put the needs of others first. As a result, the nurse should encourage the woman to express her concerns and fears and reassure her that her problems are important and will be addressed. Exercise, hormone therapy, diet, vitamins, calcium with vitamin D supplementation, daily aspirin, breast self-examination, Pap and mammogram recommendations, colonoscopy, immunization updates, and sun protection should be discussed.

Functional assessment is included as part of the history in women older than 70 years and those with disabilities. In the review of systems, the nurse should ask about self-management activities such as walking, getting to the bathroom, bathing, hair combing, dressing, and eating. Questions about driving, using public transportation, using the telephone or the Internet, hanging up clothes, buying groceries, taking medications, and meal preparation should be included.

Sexual assessment continues to be important in women 50 and older. Unless directly asked, women may omit mention of sexual concerns. Questions asked with sensitivity may invite responses regarding changes in sexual desire or response or physical issues that challenge her sexual enjoyment. Open and reflective questions also affirm a woman's right to sexual enjoyment throughout the life span.

Women older than 50 years commonly experience menopause and have physical changes associated with decreased estrogen. A decrease in estrogen causes numerous cytologic and structural changes of the vagina, vulva, and lower urinary tract. Estrogen deficiency leads to a narrowing and shortening of the vagina and thinning of the vaginal walls. This can result in vaginal dryness, itching, burning, and dyspareunia. Estrogen loss also causes reduced smooth muscle relaxation, decreased vaginal blood flow and decreased vaginal secretions. Estrogen plays a role in the formation of bone matrix, and a decrease may lead to osteoporosis. The risk for heart disease increases because of changes in lipid metabolism related to declining estrogen levels. Decreases in estrogen can cause a relaxation of ligaments and connective tissue, which affects the support of the bladder and uterus. Decreases in estrogen affect the hypothalamus, causing hot flashes, which are disturbing to most women (see Chapter 6).

Physical changes can result in increased discomfort during the pelvic examination. It is important to be both gentle and thorough during the examination. A small adult speculum may be used to view the cervix. The uterus in a menopausal woman is small and firm, and the ovaries are nonpalpable. In postmenopausal women the specimen from the vaginal pool may be useful to detect endometrial cells. A woman with palpable adnexal masses or vaginal bleeding after menopause needs immediate gynecologic referral.

A respectful and reassuring approach toward caring for women ages 50 and older will ensure their continued participation in seeking health care. Because the risk of breast, ovarian, uterine, cervical, colon, and skin cancers increases with age, the nurse has the opportunity to educate women about the importance of preventive screening. It is the nurse's responsibility to ensure a positive health care experience that encourages future visits for prevention and chronic and acute care.

Advance directives can be introduced on any entry into a health care system. It is a good idea to have a formal statement in the medical record regarding a woman's wishes in the event of accident or illness regarding life-maintaining measures or organ donation. Most states have laws formalizing such statements in writing. A woman can designate the durable power of attorney for health care authority to a trusted relative or friend.

Many women find that spirituality is helpful in maintaining wellness as well as coping with illness. Spirituality refers to the essence of our being and humanity, reflected in a connection to a Sacred Source. The concept of Sacred Source is experienced in different ways, with some experiencing it as a person, some as a presence, and some as a nondescribable mystery (Burkhardt & Nagai-Jacobson, 2013). The idea of connection is important, and experiencing this connection in a sacred space is central to spirituality. Spirituality may be experienced within a context of organized religion. Nurses, taking a holistic approach to women's wellness, must be sensitive and nonjudgmental to the spiritual aspect of their clients. In an optimal healing approach to care, nurses can facilitate and encourage the client to express her spirituality in a way that is comfortable for her. Box 4-8 presents a spiritual wellness self-assessment guide.

BOX 4-8 Spiritual Wellness Self-Assessment

1. How do you describe your purpose in life?
2. What activities do you do regularly that bring you joy?
3. What goals do you have for 6 months from now?
4. What goals do you have for 2 years from now?
5. What activities make you feel nourished?
6. What kinds of things do you do for yourself every day?
7. What do you hope for in the future?
8. Are there people you can reach out to?
9. On whom can you count for encouragement and/or support?
10. Are there others to whom you give encouragement and/or support?
11. Who loves you?
12. Whom do you love or care about?
13. In what areas are you growing?
14. How do you go about forgiving yourself?
15. How do you go about forgiving others?
16. To whom do you confide your hopes, dreams, and pain?
17. Do you believe in some kind of higher power?
18. What do you hope for in the future?
19. When do you reach out to people?
20. Do you look forward to getting up in the morning?
21. Would you like to live to be 100?

The more questions you answer in the positive, the higher the level of spiritual wellness.

Adapted from Condon, M. (2004). *Women's health: Body, mind, spirit: An integrated approach to wellness and illness.* Upper Saddle River, NJ: Prentice-Hall.

Healthy Aging

Women in the United States can expect on average to live to be 80 years old and may spend one third of their lives as postmenopausal women. With a healthy lifestyle, many women are living to be 100 years old or older. Proper nutrition, exercise, and mental and social stimulation are critical to keeping the body healthy and the mind active and alert into old age. Menopause is a time in which women can integrate wisdom and become wise women as they look toward the future (McCloskey, 2012).

History

At a woman's first visit, she is often expected to fill out a form with biographic and historical data before meeting with the examiner. This form aids the health care provider in completing the history during the interview. Most forms include information about these categories:

- Biographic data
- Reason for seeking care
- Present health or history of present illness
- Past health
- Family history
- Screening for abuse
- Review of systems
- Functional assessment (activities of daily living)

Box 4-9 describes a complete health history.

Physical Examination

In preparation for the physical examination, the woman is instructed to undress and is given a gown to wear during the examination. She is usually given the opportunity to undress privately. Objective data are recorded by system or location. A general statement of overall health status is a good way to start. Findings are described in detail.

- General appearance: age, race, sex, state of health, posture, height, weight, development, dress, hygiene, affect, alertness, orientation, cooperativeness, and communication skills
- Vital signs: temperature, pulse, respiration, blood pressure
- Skin: color; integrity; texture; hydration; temperature; edema; excessive perspiration; unusual odor; presence and description of lesions; hair texture and distribution; nail configuration, color, texture, and condition; presence of nail clubbing
- Head: size, shape, trauma, masses, scars, rashes, or scaling; facial symmetry; presence of edema or puffiness
- Eyes: pupil size, shape, reactivity, conjunctival injection, scleral icterus, fundal papilledema, hemorrhage, lids, extraocular movements, visual fields and acuity
- Ears: shape and symmetry, tenderness, discharge, external canal, and tympanic membranes; hearing—Weber should be midline (loudness of sound equal in both ears) and Rinne negative (no conductive or sensorineural hearing loss); should be able to hear whisper at 3 feet
- Nose: symmetry, tenderness, discharge, mucosa, turbinate inflammation, frontal or maxillary sinus tenderness; discrimination of odors
- Mouth and throat: hygiene; condition of teeth; dentures; appearance of lips, tongue, buccal and oral mucosa; erythema; edema; exudate; tonsillar enlargement; palate; uvula; gag reflex; ulcers
- Neck: mobility, masses, range of motion, tracheal deviation, thyroid size, carotid bruits
- Lymphatic: cervical, intraclavicular, axillary, trochlear, or inguinal adenopathy; size, shape, tenderness, and consistency
- Breasts: skin changes, dimpling, symmetry, scars, tenderness, discharge, masses; characteristics of nipples and areolae
- Heart: rate, rhythm, murmurs, rubs, gallops, clicks, heaves, or precordial movements
- Peripheral vascular: jugular vein distention, bruits, edema, swelling, vein distention, Homans sign, or tenderness of extremities
- Lungs: chest symmetry with respirations, wheezes, crackles, rhonchi, vocal fremitus, whispered pectoriloquy, percussion, and diaphragmatic excursion; breath sounds equal and clear bilaterally
- Abdomen: shape, scars, bowel sounds, consistency, tenderness, rebound, masses, guarding, organomegaly, liver span, percussion (tympany, shifting, dullness), or costovertebral angle tenderness
- Extremities: edema, ulceration, tenderness, varicosities, erythema, tremor, or deformity
- Genitourinary: external genitalia, perineum, vaginal mucosa, cervix; inflammation, tenderness, discharge, bleeding, ulcers, nodules, or masses; internal vaginal support, bimanual and rectovaginal palpation of cervix, uterus, and adnexa
- Rectal: sphincter tone, masses, hemorrhoids, rectal wall contour, tenderness, and stool for occult blood
- Musculoskeletal: posture, symmetry of muscle mass, muscle atrophy, weakness, appearance of joints, tenderness or crepitus, joint range of motion, instability, redness, swelling, or spinal deviation
- Neurologic: mental status, orientation, memory, mood, speech clarity and comprehension, cranial nerves II to XII, sensation, strength, deep tendon and superficial reflexes, gait, balance, and coordination with rapid alternating motions

Table 4-2 highlights physical assessment findings that differ in women across the life span.

Pelvic Examination

Many women fear the gynecologic portion of the physical examination. The nurse can be instrumental in allaying these fears by providing information and assisting the woman to express her feelings to the examiner (Box 4-10).

The woman is assisted into the lithotomy position (see Fig. 4-9) for the pelvic examination. When she is in the lithotomy position, her hips and knees are flexed, with buttocks at the edge of the table, and her feet are supported by heel or knee stirrups.

Some women prefer to keep their shoes or socks on, especially if the stirrups are not padded. Many women express feelings of vulnerability and strangeness when in the lithotomy position. During the procedure the nurse assists the woman with relaxation techniques.

Many women find it distressing to attempt to converse in the lithotomy position. Most women appreciate an explanation of the procedure as it unfolds, as well as coaching for the types of sensations they may expect. Generally, however, women prefer not to have to respond to questions until they are again upright and at eye level with the examiner. Being asked questions during

BOX 4-9 Health History and Review of Systems

Identifying data: Name, age, race, sex, marital status, occupation, religion, and ethnicity

Reason for seeking care: A response to the question, "What problem or symptom brought you here today?" If the woman lists more than one reason, focus on the one she thinks is most important.

Present health: Current health status is described with attention to the following:

- *Use of safety measures:* seat belts, bicycle helmets, designated driver
- *Exercise and leisure activities:* regularity
- *Sleep patterns:* length and quality
- *Sexuality:* Is she sexually active? With men, women, or both? Risk-reducing sex practices?
- *Diet, including beverages:* 24-hour dietary recall; caffeine: coffee, tea, cola, or chocolate intake
- *Nicotine, alcohol, illicit or recreational drug use:* type, amount, frequency, duration, and reactions
- *Environmental and chemical hazards:* home, school, work, and leisure setting; exposure to extreme heat or cold, noise, industrial toxins such as asbestos or lead, pesticides, diethylstilbestrol (DES), radiation, cat feces, or cigarette smoke

History of present illness: A chronologic narrative that includes the onset of the problem, the setting in which it developed, its manifestations, and any treatments received are noted. The woman's state of health before the onset of the present problem is determined. If the problem is long standing, the reason for seeking attention at this time is elicited. The principal symptoms should be described with respect to the following:

- Location
- Quality or character
- Quantity or severity
- Timing (onset, duration, frequency)
- Setting
- Factors that aggravate or relieve
- Associated factors
- Woman's perception of the meaning of the symptom

Past health:

- *Infectious diseases:* measles, mumps, rubella, whooping cough, chickenpox, rheumatic fever, scarlet fever, diphtheria, polio, tuberculosis (TB), hepatitis
- *Chronic disease and system disorders:* arthritis, cancer, diabetes, heart, lung, kidney, seizures, thyroid, stroke, ulcers, sickle cell anemia
- *Adult injuries, accidents*
- *Hospitalizations, operations, blood transfusions*
- *Obstetric history*
- *Allergies:* medications, previous transfusion reactions, environmental allergies
- *Immunizations:* diphtheria, pertussis, tetanus, polio, hepatitis B, varicella, influenza, pneumococcal vaccine, last TB skin test, measles, mumps, rubella (MMR)
- *Last date of screening tests:* Pap test, mammogram, stool for occult blood, sigmoidoscopy or colonoscopy, hematocrit, hemoglobin, rubella titer, urinalysis, cholesterol test; electrocardiogram; last vision, dental, hearing examination
- *Current medications:* name, dose, frequency, duration, reason for taking, and compliance with prescription medications; home remedies, over-the-counter drugs, vitamin and mineral or herbal supplements used over a 24-hour period

Family history: Information about the ages and health of family members may be presented in narrative form or as a family tree or genogram: age, health or death of parents, siblings, spouse, children. Check for history of diabetes; heart disease; hypertension; stroke; respiratory, renal, or thyroid problems; cancer; bleeding disorders; hepatitis; allergies; asthma; arthritis; TB; epilepsy; mental illness; human immunodeficiency virus infection; or other disorders.

Screen for abuse: Has she ever been hit, kicked, slapped, or forced to have sex against her wishes? Has she been verbally or emotionally abused? Does she have a history of childhood sexual abuse? If yes, has she received counseling or does she need referral?

Review of systems: It is probable that all questions in each system will not be included every time a history is taken. Some questions regarding each system should be included in every history. The essential areas to be explored are listed in the following head-to-toe sequence. If a woman gives a positive response to a question about an essential area, more detailed questions should be asked.

- *General:* weight change, fatigue, weakness, fever, chills, or night sweats
- *Skin:* skin, hair, and nail change; itching, bruising, bleeding, rashes, sores, lumps, or moles
- *Lymph nodes:* enlargement, inflammation, pain, suppuration (pus), or drainage
- *Head:* trauma, vertigo (dizziness), convulsive disorder, syncope (fainting); headache: location, frequency, pain type, nausea and vomiting, or visual symptoms present
- *Eyes:* glasses, contact lenses, blurriness, tearing, itching, photophobia, diplopia, inflammation, trauma, cataracts, glaucoma, or acute visual loss
- *Ears:* hearing loss, tinnitus (ringing), vertigo, discharge, pain, fullness, recurrent infections, or mastoiditis
- *Nose and sinuses:* trauma, rhinitis, nasal discharge, epistaxis, obstruction, sneezing, itching, allergy, or smelling impairment
- *Mouth, throat, and neck:* hoarseness, voice changes, soreness, ulcers, bleeding gums, goiter, swelling, or enlarged nodes
- *Breasts:* masses, pain, lumps, dimpling, nipple discharge, fibrocystic changes, or implants; breast self-examination practice
- *Respiratory:* shortness of breath, wheezing, cough, sputum, hemoptysis, pneumonia, pleurisy, asthma, bronchitis, emphysema, or TB; date of last chest x-ray
- *Cardiovascular:* hypertension, rheumatic fever, murmurs, angina, palpitations, dyspnea, tachycardia, orthopnea, edema, chest pain, cough, cyanosis, cold extremities, ascites, intermittent claudication (leg pain caused by poor circulation to the leg muscles), phlebitis, or skin color changes
- *Gastrointestinal:* appetite, nausea, vomiting, indigestion, dysphagia, abdominal pain, ulcers, hematochezia (bleeding with stools), melena (black, tarry stools), bowel-habit changes, diarrhea, constipation, bowel movement frequency, food intolerance, hemorrhoids, jaundice, or hepatitis; sigmoidoscopy, colonoscopy, barium enema, ultrasound
- *Genitourinary:* frequency, hesitancy, urgency, polyuria, dysuria, hematuria, nocturia, incontinence, stones, infection, or urethral discharge; menstrual history (e.g., age at menarche, length and flow of menses, last menstrual period [LMP], dysmenorrhea, intermenstrual bleeding, age at menopause or signs of menopause), dyspareunia, discharge, sores, itching
- *Sexual health and sexual activity:* with men, women, or both; contraceptive use; sexually transmitted infections
- *Peripheral vascular:* coldness, numbness and tingling, leg edema, claudication, varicose veins, thromboses, or emboli
- *Endocrine:* heat and cold intolerance, dry skin, excessive sweating, polyuria, polydipsia, polyphagia, thyroid problems, diabetes, or secondary sex characteristic changes
- *Hematologic:* anemia, easy bruising, bleeding, petechiae, purpura, or transfusions
- *Musculoskeletal:* muscle weakness, pain, joint stiffness, scoliosis, lordosis, kyphosis, range-of-motion instability, redness, swelling, arthritis, or gout
- *Neurologic:* loss of sensation, numbness, tingling, tremors, weakness, vertigo, paralysis, fainting, twitching, blackouts, seizures, convulsions, loss of consciousness or memory
- *Mental status:* moodiness, depression, anxiety, obsessions, delusions, illusions, or hallucinations
- *Functional assessment:* ability to care for self

TABLE 4-2 Female Reproductive Physical Assessment Across the Life Cycle

	ADOLESCENT	ADULT	POSTMENOPAUSAL
Breasts	Tender when developing; buds appear; small, firm; one side may grow faster; areola diameter increases; nipples more erect	Grow to full shape in early adulthood; nipples and areola become pinker and darker	Become stringy, irregular, pendulous, and nodular; borders less well delineated; may shrink, become flatter, elongated, and less elastic; ligaments weaken; nipples are positioned lower
Vagina	Vagina lengthens; epithelial layers thicken; secretions become acidic	Growth complete by age 20	Introitus constricts; vagina narrows, shortens, loses rugation; mucosa is pale, thin, and dry; walls may lose structural integrity
Uterus	Musculature and vasculature increase; lining thickens	Growth complete by age 20	Size decreases; endometrial lining thins
Ovaries	Increase in size and weight; menarche occurs between 8 and 16 years of age; ovulation occurs monthly	Growth complete by age 20	Size decreases to 1 to 2 cm; follicles disappear; surface convolutes; ovarian function ceases between 40 and 55 years of age
Labia majora	Become more prominent; hair develops	Growth complete by age 20	Labia become smaller and flatter; pubic hair sparse and gray
Labia minora	Become more vascular	Growth complete by age 20	Become shinier and drier
Uterine tubes	Increase in size	Growth complete by age 20	Decrease in size

BOX 4-10 Procedure: Assisting with Pelvic Examination

1. Wash hands. Assemble equipment (see below).

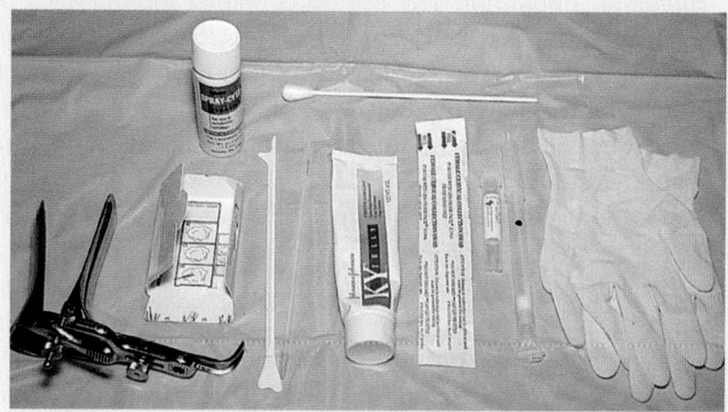

Equipment used for pelvic examination. (Courtesy Michael S. Clement, MD, Mesa, AZ.)

2. Ask the woman to empty her bladder before the examination (obtain clean-catch urine specimen as needed).
3. Assist with relaxation techniques. Have the woman place her hands on her chest at about the level of the diaphragm and breathe deeply and slowly.
4. Encourage the woman to become involved with the examination if she shows interest. For example, a mirror can be placed so that she can see the area being examined.
5. Assess for and treat signs of problems such as supine hypotension.
6. Warm the speculum in warm water if a prewarmed one is not available.
7. Instruct the woman to bear down when the speculum is being inserted.
8. Apply gloves and assist the examiner with collection of specimens for cytologic examination, such as a Pap test. After handling specimens, remove gloves and wash hands.
9. Put gloves on. Lubricate the examiner's fingers with water or water-soluble lubricant before bimanual examination.
10. Assist the woman at completion of the examination to a sitting position and then a standing position.
11. Provide tissues to wipe lubricant from perineum.
12. Provide privacy for the woman while she is dressing.

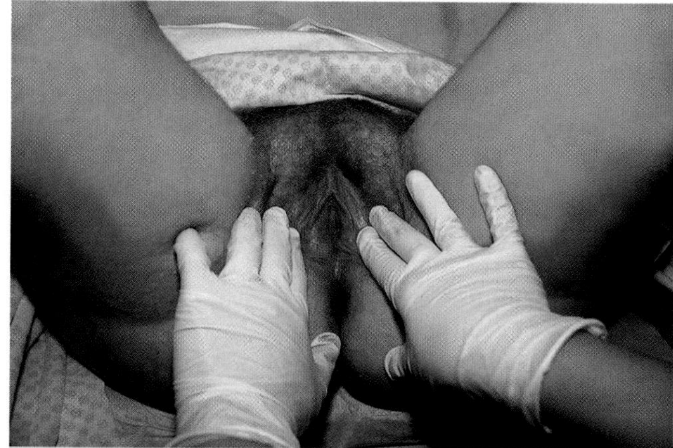

FIG 4-11 External examination: separation of the labia. (From Wilson, S., & Giddens, J. [2013]. *Health assessment for nursing practice* [5th ed.]. St. Louis: Mosby.)

the procedure, especially if they cannot see their questioner's eyes, may make women tense.

External Inspection. The examiner wears gloves and sits at the foot of the table for the inspection of the external genitalia and the speculum examination. In good lighting, the external genitalia: clitoris, labia, and perineum, are examined and inspected for sexual maturity, and lesions indicative of STIs are noted. After childbirth or other trauma, healed scars may be present.

External Palpation. Before touching the woman, the examiner explains what is going to be done and what the woman should expect to feel (e.g., pressure). The examiner may touch the woman in a less sensitive area such as the inner thigh to alert her that the genitalia examination is beginning. This gesture may put the woman more at ease. The labia are spread apart to expose the structures in the vestibule: urinary meatus, Skene glands, vaginal orifice, and Bartholin glands (Fig. 4-11). To assess Skene glands, the examiner inserts one finger into the vagina and "milks" the area of the urethra. Any exudate from the urethra or the Skene glands is cultured. Masses and erythema of either structure are assessed further. Ordinarily the openings to the Skene glands are not visible; prominent openings may be seen if the glands are infected (e.g., with gonorrhea). During the examination the examiner keeps in mind the data from the review of systems such as history of burning on urination.

The vaginal orifice is examined. Hymenal tags are normal findings. With one finger still in the vagina, the examiner repositions the index finger near the posterior part of the orifice. With the thumb outside the posterior part of the labia majora, the examiner compresses the area of Bartholin glands located at the 8 o'clock and 4 o'clock positions and looks for swelling, discharge, and pain.

The support of the anterior and posterior vaginal wall is assessed. The examiner spreads the labia with the index and middle finger and asks the woman to strain down. Any bulge from the anterior wall (urethrocele or cystocele) or posterior wall (rectocele) is noted and compared with the history, such as difficulty starting the stream of urine or constipation.

The perineum (area between the vagina and anus) is assessed for scars from old lacerations or episiotomies, thinning, fistulas, masses, lesions, and inflammation. The anus is assessed for hemorrhoids, hemorrhoidal tags, and integrity of the anal sphincter. The anal area is also assessed for lesions, masses, abscesses, and tumors. If there is a history of STI, the examiner may want to obtain a culture specimen from the anal canal at this time. Throughout the genital examination the examiner notes any odor, which may indicate infection or poor hygiene.

Vulvar Self-Examination. The pelvic examination provides a good opportunity for the practitioner to emphasize the need for regular vulvar self-examination (VSE) and to teach this procedure. Because there has been a dramatic increase in cancerous and precancerous conditions of the vulva, VSE should be an integral part of preventive health care for all women who are sexually active or 18 years of age or older. VSE should be performed monthly between menses or more often if there are symptoms or a history of serious vulvar disease. Most lesions, including malignancy, condyloma acuminatum (wartlike growth), and Bartholin cysts, can be seen or palpated and are easily treated if diagnosed early.

The VSE can be performed by the practitioner and woman together by using a mirror. A simple diagram of the anatomy of the vulva can be given to the woman, with instructions to perform the examination herself that evening to reinforce what she has learned. She does the examination in a sitting position with adequate lighting, holding a mirror in one hand and using the other hand to expose the tissues surrounding the vaginal introitus. She then systematically examines the mons pubis, clitoris, urethra, labia majora, perineum, and perianal area and palpates the vulva, noting any changes in appearance or abnormalities such as ulcers, lumps, warts, and changes in pigmentation.

Internal Examination. A vaginal speculum consists of two blades and a handle. Specula come in a variety of types and styles. A vaginal speculum is used to view the vaginal vault and cervix. The speculum is gently placed into the vagina and inserted to the back of the vaginal vault. The blades are opened to reveal the cervix and are locked into the open position. The cervix is inspected for position and appearance of the os: color, lesions, bleeding, and discharge (Fig. 4-12, *A-D*). Cervical findings that are not within normal limits include ulcerations, masses, inflammation, and excessive protrusion into the vaginal vault. Anomalies such as a cockscomb (a protrusion over the cervix that looks like a rooster's comb), a hooded or collared cervix (seen in diethylstilbestrol [DES] daughters), or polyps are noted.

Collection of Specimens. The collection of specimens for cytologic examination is an important part of the gynecologic examination. Infection can be diagnosed by examination of specimens collected during the pelvic examination. These infections include candidiasis, trichomoniasis, bacterial vaginosis, group B streptococcus, gonorrhea, chlamydia, and herpes simplex virus. Once the diagnoses have been made, treatment can be instituted.

Papanicolaou Test. Carcinogenic conditions, whether potential or actual, can be determined by examination of cells from the cervix collected during the pelvic examination (i.e., a Pap test) (Box 4-11).

Vaginal Wall Examination. After the specimens are obtained, the vagina is viewed when the speculum is rotated. The speculum blades are unlocked and partially closed. As the speculum is withdrawn, it is rotated; the vaginal walls are inspected for color, lesions, rugae, fistulas, and bulging.

Bimanual Palpation. The examiner stands for this part of the examination. A small amount of lubricant is placed on the first and second fingers of the gloved hand for the internal examination. To avoid tissue trauma and contamination, the thumb is abducted, and the ring and little fingers are flexed into the palm (Fig. 4-13).

The vagina is palpated for distensibility, lesions, and tenderness. The cervix is examined for position, shape, consistency, motility, and lesions. The fornix around the cervix is palpated.

The other hand is placed on the abdomen halfway between the umbilicus and symphysis pubis and exerts pressure downward toward the pelvic hand. Upward pressure from the pelvic hand traps reproductive structures for assessment by palpation. The uterus is assessed for position, size, shape, consistency, regularity, motility, masses, and tenderness.

With the abdominal hand moving to the right lower quadrant and the fingers of the pelvic hand in the right lateral fornix, the adnexa is assessed for position, size, tenderness, and masses. The examination is repeated on the woman's left side.

Just before the intravaginal fingers are withdrawn, the woman is asked to tighten her vagina around the fingers as much as she can. If the muscle response is weak, the woman is assessed for her knowledge about Kegel exercises.

Rectovaginal Palpation. To prevent contamination of the rectum from organisms in the vagina (e.g., *Neisseria gonorrhoeae*), it is necessary to change gloves, add fresh lubricant, and then reinsert the index finger into the vagina and the middle finger into the rectum (Fig. 4-14). Insertion is facilitated if the woman strains down. The maneuvers of the abdominovaginal examination are repeated. The rectovaginal examination permits assessment of the rectovaginal septum, the posterior surface of the uterus, and the region behind the cervix and the adnexa. The vaginal finger is removed and folded into the palm, leaving the middle finger free to rotate 360 degrees. The rectum is palpated for rectal tenderness and masses.

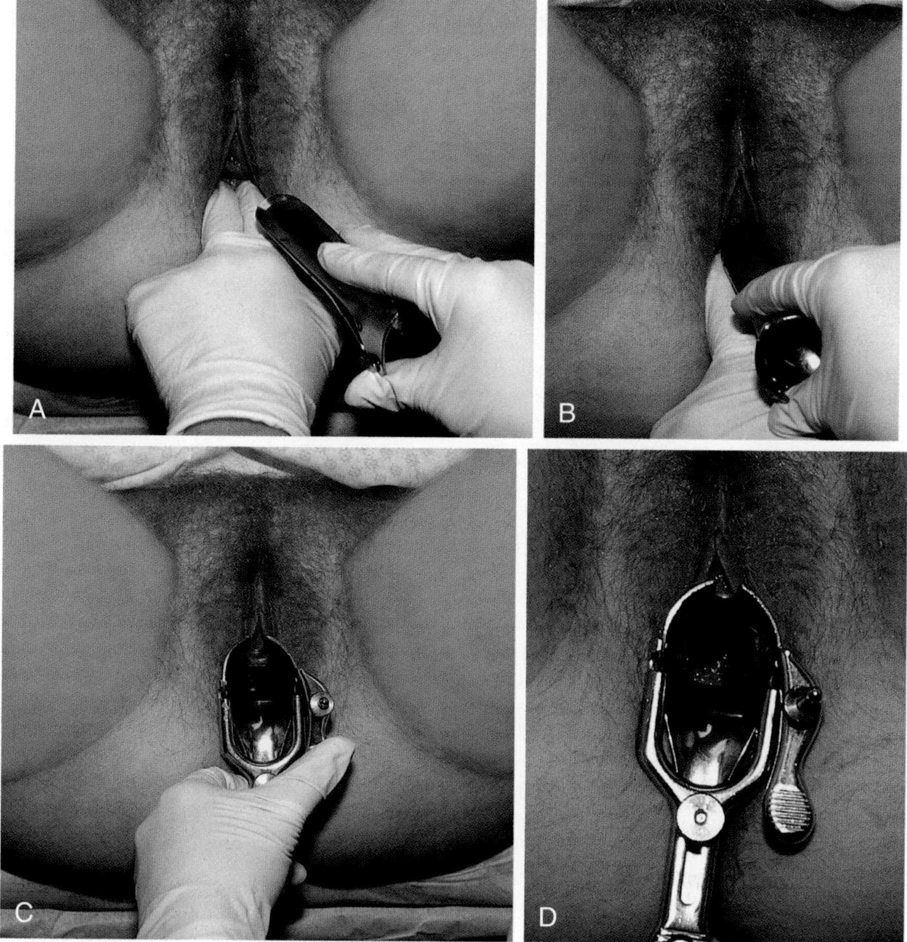

FIG 4-12 Insertion of speculum for vaginal examination. **A,** Opening of the introitus. **B,** Oblique insertion of the speculum. **C,** Final insertion of the speculum. **D,** Opening of the speculum blades. (From Wilson, S., & Giddens, J. [2013]. *Health assessment for nursing practice* [5th ed.]. St. Louis: Mosby.)

After the rectal examination the woman is assisted into a sitting position, given tissues or wipes to cleanse herself, and afforded privacy to dress. The examiner returns after the woman is dressed to discuss findings and the plan of care.

Pelvic Examination During Pregnancy

The pelvic examination during pregnancy is done in the same way as it is during a routine examination on a nonpregnant woman. Pelvic measurements are completed, and uterine size is estimated. A Pap test may be done initially and cytologic specimens collected to test for gonorrhea, chlamydia, human papillomavirus, herpes simplex virus, and group B streptococcus. As the pregnancy progresses, the nurse inspects the woman's abdomen, palpates fetal size and position, auscultates fetal heart tones, and measures fundal height at each visit.

While the pregnant woman is in lithotomy position, the nurse must watch for supine hypotension (decrease in blood pressure) caused by the weight of the uterus pressing on the vena cava and aorta. Symptoms of supine hypotension include pallor, dizziness, faintness, breathlessness, tachycardia, nausea, clammy skin, and sweating. The woman should be positioned on her side until symptoms resolve and vital signs stabilize. The vaginal examination can be done with the woman in lateral position.

Pelvic Examination After Hysterectomy

The pelvic examination after hysterectomy is done much as it is done on a woman with a uterus. Vaginal screening using the Pap test is not recommended in women who have had a total hysterectomy with removal of the cervix for benign disease. Because of the epidemic of human papillomavirus, which causes vaginal intraepithelial neoplasia, sampling of the vaginal walls after hysterectomy may still be practiced, with schedules varying from every year to every 2 to 3 years.

Laboratory and Diagnostic Procedures

The following laboratory and diagnostic procedures are ordered at the discretion of the clinician, considering the client and family history: hemoglobin, fasting blood glucose, total blood cholesterol, lipid profile, urinalysis, syphilis serology (Venereal Disease Research Laboratories [VDRL] or rapid plasma reagent [RPR]) and other screening tests for STIs, mammogram, tuberculosis skin testing, hearing, visual acuity, electrocardiogram, chest x-ray, pulmonary function, fecal occult blood, flexible sigmoidoscopy, and bone mineral density (dual energy x-ray absorptiometry [DEXA] scan). Results of these tests may be reported in person, by phone call, or by letter. Tests for HIV, hepatitis B, and drug screening may be offered with informed consent in high risk populations. These test results are usually

BOX 4-11 Procedure: Papanicoloau Test

- In preparation, make sure the woman has not douched, used vaginal medications, or had sexual intercourse for 24 to 48 hours before the procedure. Reschedule the test if the woman is menstruating. Midcycle is the best time for the test.
- Explain to the woman the purpose of the test and what sensations she will feel as the specimen is obtained (e.g., pressure but not pain).
- The woman is assisted into a lithotomy position. A speculum is inserted into the vagina.
- The cytologic specimen is obtained before any digital examination of the vagina is made or endocervical bacteriologic specimens are taken. A cotton swab may be used to remove excess cervical discharge before the specimen is collected.
- The specimen is obtained by using an endocervical sampling device (Cytobrush, Cervex-brush, spatula, or broom) (see Fig. *A* and *B*). If the two-sample method of obtaining cells is used, the Cytobrush is inserted into the canal and rotated 90 to 180 degrees, followed by a gentle smear of the entire transformation zone by using a spatula. Broom devices are inserted and rotated 360 degrees five times. They obtain endocervical and ectocervical samples at the same time. If the woman has had a hysterectomy, the vaginal cuff is sampled. Areas that appear abnormal on visualization will require colposcopy and biopsy. If using a one-slide technique, the spatula sample is smeared first. This is followed by applying the Cytobrush sample (rolling the brush in the opposite direction from which it was obtained), which is less subject to drying artifact; then the slide is sprayed with preservative within 5 seconds.
- The ThinPrep or SurePath Pap test is a liquid-based method of preserving cells that reduces blood, mucus, and inflammation. The Pap specimen is obtained in the manner described above except that the cervix is not swabbed before collection of the sample. The collection device (brush, spatula, or broom) is rinsed in a vial of preserving solution that is provided by the laboratory. The sealed vial with solution is sent off to the appropriate laboratory. A special processing device filters the contents, and a thin layer of cervical cells is deposited on a slide, which is then examined microscopically. The AutoPap and Papnet tests are similar to the ThinPrep test. If cytology is abnormal, liquid-based methods allow follow-up testing for human papillomavirus (HPV) DNA with the same sample.
- Label the slides or vial with the woman's name and site. Include on the form to accompany the specimens the woman's name, age, parity, and chief complaint or reason for taking the cytologic specimens.
- Send specimens to the pathology laboratory promptly for staining, evaluation, and a written report, with special reference to abnormal elements, including cancer cells.
- Advise the woman that repeated tests may be necessary if the specimen is not adequate.
- Instruct the woman concerning routine checkups for cervical and vaginal cancer. Women vaccinated against HPV should follow the same screening guidelines as unvaccinated women. Current recommendations of the U.S. Preventive Services Task Force (USPSTF, 2012) and the American Cancer Society (ACS, 2013d) for Pap tests are that women ages 21 through 65 be screened every 3 years, or for women ages 30 through 65 every 5 years (if they had a Pap test plus HPV test that were both negative). These guidelines recommend no screening in women younger than 21, although if a girl becomes sexually active, the guidelines recommend that she get a Pap test within 3 years of initiating sexual activity or at age 21—whichever comes first. Women with high risk factors such as exposure to diethylstilbestrol (DES) in utero, those treated for cervical intraepithelial neoplasia (CIN) 2, CIN 3, cervical cancer, or human immunodeficiency virus (HIV) may need more frequent screening.
- Young women who have been treated with excisional procedures for dysplasia have an increase in premature births. A large majority of the cervical dysplasias in adolescents caused by HPV resolve on their own without treatment. It is important to avoid unnecessary instrumentation and procedures that negatively affect the cervix. Women who have had a complete hysterectomy for noncancerous reasons who have no history of high-grade CIN may have routine cervical cytology testing discontinued. Women who are older than 65 years who have not had serious cervical precancer or cancer in the past 20 years may discontinue cervical cancer screening (ACS, 2014).
- Record the examination date on the woman's record.
- Communicate findings to the woman per agency protocol.

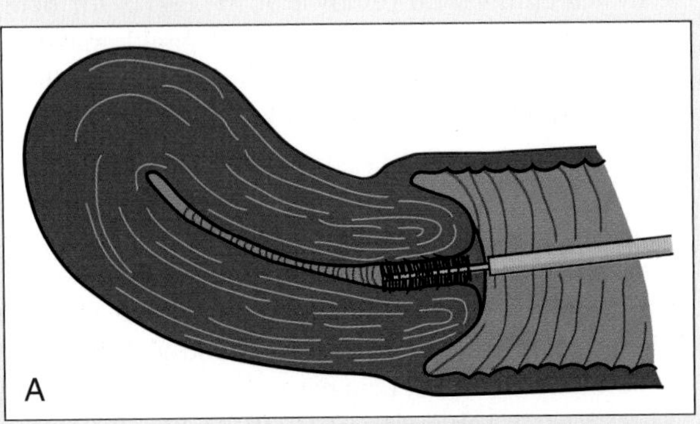

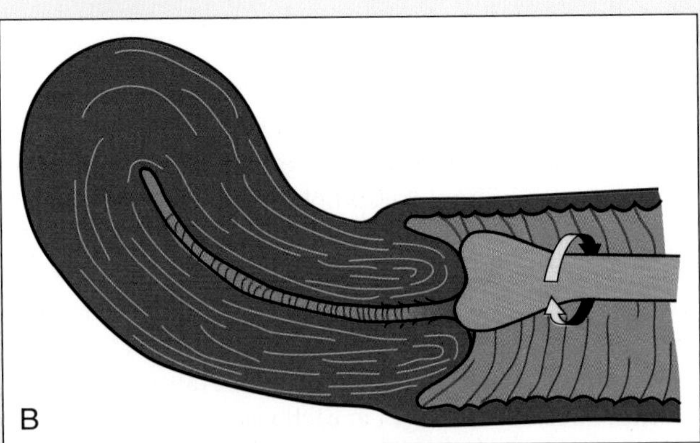

(From Lentz, G.M., Lobo, R.A., Gershenson D.M., Katz, V. (2012). *Comprehensive gynecology* (ed. 6). St. Louis: Mosby.)

Adapted from American Cancer Society. (2012). *Chronological history of ACS recommendations for early detection of cancer in asymptomatic people.* Available at www.cancer.org; American Cancer Society. (2013). *Early detection: Facts and figures.* Available at www.cancer.org/research/cancerfactsfigures/cancerpreventionearlydetectionfactsfigures/cancer-prevention-early-detection-facts-figures; American Cancer Society. (2013). *Guidelines for the early detection of cancer.* Available at www.cancer.org/healthy/findcancerearly/cancerscreeningguidelines/american-cancer-society-guidelines-for-the-early-detection-of-cancer; American College of Obstetricians and Gynecologists (2013). *New guidelines for cervical cancer screening.* Available at http://www.acog.org/For_Patients/Search_FAQs/documents/New_Guidelines_for_Cervical_Cancer_Screening/Announcements/New%20Cervical%20Cancer%20Screening%20Recommendations.aspx; U.S. Preventive Services Task Force. (2012). *Screening for cervical cancer.* Available at www.preventiveservicestaskforce.org/uspstf/uspscerv.htm.

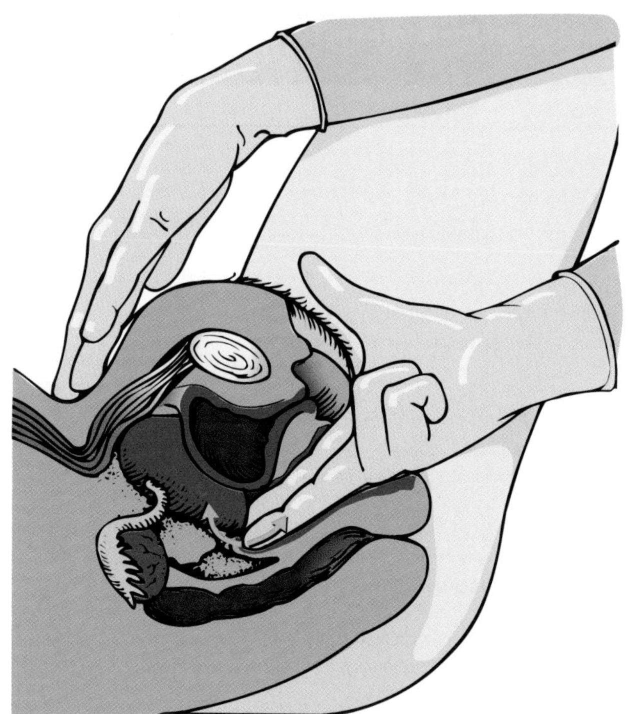

FIG 4-13 Bimanual palpation of the uterus. (From Seidel, H., Ball, J., Dains, J., et al. [2011]. *Mosby's guide to physical examination* [7th ed.]. St. Louis: Mosby.)

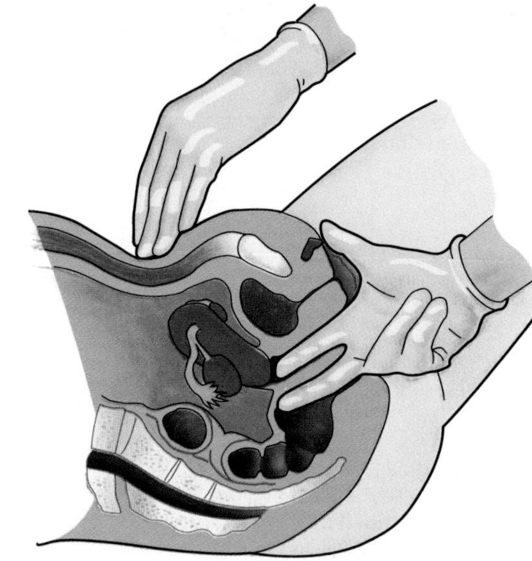

FIG 4-14 Rectovaginal examination. (From Seidel, H., Ball, J., Dains, J., et al. [2011]. *Mosby's guide to physical examination* [7th ed.]. St. Louis: Mosby.)

reported in person. The CDC (2012b) has developed new guidelines that recommend testing people who were born in 1945 through 1965 for hepatitis C.

To promote wellness and prevent illness, it is imperative that women adhere to specific screening guidelines to detect conditions that, if found early, are amenable to treatment and/or cure. Table 4-3 summarizes the screening procedures for women across the life span.

ANTICIPATORY GUIDANCE FOR HEALTH PROMOTION AND ILLNESS PREVENTION

Over the past several decades women have made tremendous strides in education, careers, policymaking, and overall participation in today's complex society. There have been costs for these advances, and although women are living longer, they may not be living better.

As a result, the health care system must pay greater attention to the health consequences for women. In addition, women must be active participants in their own health promotion and illness prevention. Health promotion is the motivation to increase well-being and actualize health potential. Illness prevention is the desire to avoid illness, detect it early, or maintain optimal functioning when illness is present.

Nurses have a major opportunity and responsibility to help women understand risk factors and to motivate them to adopt healthy lifestyles that prevent disease. Lifestyle factors that affect health over which the woman has some control include diet; tobacco, alcohol, and substance use; exercise; sunlight exposure; stress management; and sexual practices. Other influences, such as genetic and environmental factors, may be beyond the woman's control, although some opportunities for prevention exist (e.g., through environmental legislation activism or genetic counseling services).

Knowledge alone is not enough to bring about healthy behaviors. The woman must be convinced that she has some control over her life and that healthy life habits, including periodic health examinations, are a sound investment. She must believe in the efficacy of prevention, early detection, and therapy and in her ability to perform self-management practices, such as BSE. Many people believe that they have little control over their health, or they become immobilized by fear and anxiety in the face of life-threatening illnesses, such as cancer, so they delay seeking treatment. The nurse must explore the reality of each woman's perceptions about health behaviors and individualize teaching if it is to be effective. In an earlier section of this chapter, risk factors to women's health were described. The following section describes actions that women can take to promote their health and prevent illness, along with the nurse's role in facilitating such actions.

Nutrition

Dietary Guidelines for Americans (U.S. Department of Agriculture, 2010) provides evidence-based recommendations to promote health and reduce risks for chronic diseases through diet and physical activity. This guide, published by the U.S. government, contains resources for health professionals and consumers on dietary guidelines. New guidelines will be issued after the Department of Health and Human Services in collaboration with the Department of Agriculture have established the 2015 Dietary Guidelines Advisory Committee (DGAC). They convened an initial meeting in June 2013, but the guidelines have not yet been made public (www.health.gov/DietaryGuidelines). The Food Guide Pyramid has been replaced by MyPlate (myplate.gov), a guide to healthy eating recommended by the *Dietary Guidelines for Americans* (HealthyPeople.gov, 2012b).

TABLE 4-3 Health Screening Guidelines and Immunization Recommendations for Women Ages 18 Years and Older

ASSESSMENT	RECOMMENDATION*
Physical Examination	
Blood pressure	Every visit, but at least every 2 years
Height and weight	Every visit, but at least every 2 years
Pelvic examination	Annually until age 70; recommended for any woman who has ever been sexually active
Breast Examination	
Clinical examination	Every 3 years, ages 20 to 39; after age 40 with periodic examination, preferably annually
High risk	Annually after age 18 with history of premenopausal breast cancer in first-degree relative
Risk Groups	
Skin examination	Family history of skin cancer or increased exposure to sunlight every 3 years between ages 20 and 40; annually after age 40; monthly mole self-examinations also recommended
Oral cavity examination	History of mouth lesions or exposure to tobacco or excessive alcohol at least annually
Laboratory and Diagnostic Tests	
Blood cholesterol (fasting lipoprotein analysis)	Between ages 20 and 45 only if high risk; beginning at age 45 if level is within normal limits, every 5 years; more often if abnormal levels or have risk factors for coronary artery disease
Papanicolaou (Pap) test	Between ages 21 and 65—every 3 years with Pap test done Between ages 30 and 65—every 5 years if Pap test plus human papillomavirus (HPV) test done After age 65 and 3 negative tests and no risks and after total hysterectomy for benign disease—women may choose to stop screening
Mammography†	Every 1 to 2 years between ages 40 and 49 or earlier if at high risk Annually after age 40 Annually after age 50 Biennially, ages 50 to 74 After age 75, discuss with your health care provider
Colon cancer screening	Use 1 of these 3 methods: • Fecal occult blood test annually ages 50 to 74 • Flexible sigmoidoscopy every 5 years ages 50 to 74 • Colonoscopy every 10 years ages 50 to 74 Screen more often if family history of colon cancer or polyps After age 75, discuss with your health care provider
Hearing screen	Starting at age 18, then every 10 years until 49 Every 3 years after age 50 Annually with exposure to excessive noise or when loss is suspected
Vision screen	At least once between ages 20 and 29; at least twice between ages 30 and 39 Every 2 to 4 years between ages 40 and 64; every 1 to 2 years after age 65
Risk Groups	
Fasting blood sugar	Annually with family history of diabetes or gestational diabetes or if significantly obese; every 3 to 5 years for all women older than 45 years
Thyroid-stimulating hormone (TSH) test	As determined by the health care provider
Sexually transmitted infection test (e.g., gonorrhea, syphilis, herpes)	As needed if sexually active with multiple partners and engaging in risky sexual behaviors
Chlamydia test	If sexually active, yearly until age 25; after age 25, test as needed when sexually active with new or multiple partners
Human immunodeficiency virus (HIV) test	At least once between ages 18 and 64 to determine HIV status; test if there is a high risk for HIV infection
Tuberculin skin test	Annually with exposure to persons with tuberculosis or in risk categories for close contact with the disease
Endometrial biopsy	At menopause for women at risk for endometrial cancer; repeat as needed
Bone mineral density testing	All women ages 65 and older at least once; repeat testing as needed; younger women with risk for osteoporosis may need periodic screenings
Hepatitis C testing	All people born between 1945 and 1965, one test
Immunizations	
Tetanus-diphtheria-pertussis (Td/Tdap)	Tdap vaccine once, then booster is given every 10 years
Measles, mumps, rubella	Once if born after 1956 and no evidence of immunity
Hepatitis A	Primary series of two injections for all who are in risk categories
Hepatitis B	Primary series of three injections for all who are in risk categories
Influenza	Annually

TABLE 4-3 Health Screening Guidelines and Immunization Recommendations for Women Ages 18 Years and Older—cont'd

ASSESSMENT	RECOMMENDATION*
Pneumococcal	1 or 2 doses between ages 19 and 64; 1 dose after age 65
Herpes zoster (shingles)	One dose at age 65
Human papillomavirus (HPV) vaccine	Primary series of three injections for girls ages 9 to women 26 years old; intended for those not previously exposed to HPV

*The information in this table is only a guide; health care providers will individualize the timing of tests and immunizations for each woman.

†Note: No consensus has been reached regarding mammograms for women between 40 and 49 years of age; therefore, various recommendations are listed. Women are urged to discuss circumstances with their health care providers.

Data from American Cancer Society (ACS). (2013). *Cancer prevention and early detection facts and figures.* Available at www.cancer.org/research/cancerfactsfigures/cancerpreventionearlydetectionfactsfigures/cancer-prevention-early-detection-facts-figures-2013; Centers for Disease Control and Prevention (CDC), Advisory Committee on Immunization Practices. (2012). *Recommended adult immunization schedule, United States.* Available at www.cdc.gov/vaccines; CDC. (2012). *Hepatitis C testing for anyone born during 1945-1965: New CDC recommendations.* Available at www.cdc.gov/features/hepatitisctesting; American College of Obstetricians and Gynecologists (ACOG). (2012). *New cervical screening recommendations from the U.S. Preventive Services Task Force and the American Cancer Society/American Society for Colposcopy and Cervical Pathology/American Society for Clinical Pathology.* Washington, D.C. Available at www.acog.org/About%20ACOG/Announcements/New%20Cervical%20Cancer%20Screening%20Recommendations.aspx; Centers for Disease Control and Prevention. (2010). Sexually transmitted diseases treatment guidelines. *MMWR Recommendations and Reports, 59*(RR12), 1-109; National Women's Health Information Center. (2012). *Screenings tests for women.* Available at www.womenshealth.gov; U.S. Preventive Services Task Force. (2012). *Screening for cervical cancer.* Available at www.preventiveservicestaskforce.org/uspstf/uspscerv.htm.

These guidelines recommend that half of the plate be filled with fruits and vegetables, one quarter with grains, and one quarter with protein.

Folic acid helps reduce high levels of homocysteine, an amino acid that damages the heart and blood vessels and increases the risk of heart disease, stroke, and dementia. Folic acid is present in citrus fruits, broccoli, spinach, asparagus, peas, lettuce, beans, whole grains, and orange juice. It is in many fortified grains and pasta or can be taken as a daily vitamin supplement (USDHHS, 2010).

Antioxidants are thought to be effective in helping to prevent oxidative damage in the body such as cancer, heart disease, and stroke; however, more research is needed in this area. Vitamins C and E, selenium (a mineral), and a group known as beta-carotenes (carotenoids) can be found in a diet containing fruits, vegetables, and whole grains.

Most women do not recognize the importance of calcium to health, and their diets are insufficient in calcium. Women who are unlikely to have enough calcium in the diet may need calcium supplements in the form of calcium carbonate with vitamin D, which contains more elemental calcium than do other preparations. Although calcium and vitamin D are still recommended for women's health, research has raised some concerns about the efficacy of its preventive effect of fractures in premenopausal women (Moyer for the U.S. Preventive Services Task Force, 2013). Nestle and Nesheim (2013), also working with the U.S. Preventive Services Task Force, suggested that insufficient evidence exists for the currently recommended doses of vitamin D and calcium to be effective in preventing fractures, and further stated that there is a small risk of developing renal stones due to these recommended dosages.

The diet can be assessed by using a standard assessment form—a 24-hour recall is adequate and quick—and then food likes and dislikes, including cultural variations and typical food portions and dietary habits should be discussed and incorporated into counseling (see Chapter 14).

Exercise

Physical activity and exercise counseling for persons of all ages should be undertaken at schools, worksites, and primary care settings. Specific recommendations include 150 minutes per week of moderate exercise or 75 minutes per week of vigorous exercise. For moderate exercise, this can be practically achieved through 30 minutes a day, five times a week. The American Heart Association (AHA) notes that dividing the 30 minutes per day into two or three segments of 10 to 15 minutes each is also beneficial (AHA, 2013). Few Americans exercise this often, and physical inactivity increases with age, especially during adolescence and early adulthood. Even small increases in activity can be beneficial. The nurse should stress the importance of daily exercise throughout life for weight management and health promotion, suggesting exercises that are enjoyable to the individual (Fig. 4-15). Physical activity builds healthy bones, muscles, and joints and reduces the risk of colon and breast cancer. It also reduces feelings of depression and anxiety and improves mood and promotes a feeling of well-being.

During pregnancy, an ongoing exercise regimen can be continued but intensity and duration should be decreased. Sedentary women should obtain medical clearance to initiate exercise during pregnancy and should begin with low-intensity and low-impact workouts.

Activities do not need to be strenuous to bring health benefits. What is important is to include activities as part of a regular health routine. Activities that are especially beneficial when performed regularly include brisk walking, hiking, stair climbing, aerobic exercise, jogging, running, bicycling, rowing, swimming, soccer, and basketball. Before beginning any planned activity program, a woman should see her primary care nurse practitioner (NP) or physician for a thorough medical evaluation to prevent potential injuries or harm.

For women who are sedentary or are not able to exercise vigorously, even moderate- and low-intensity activities, when performed daily, can have long-term health benefits such as

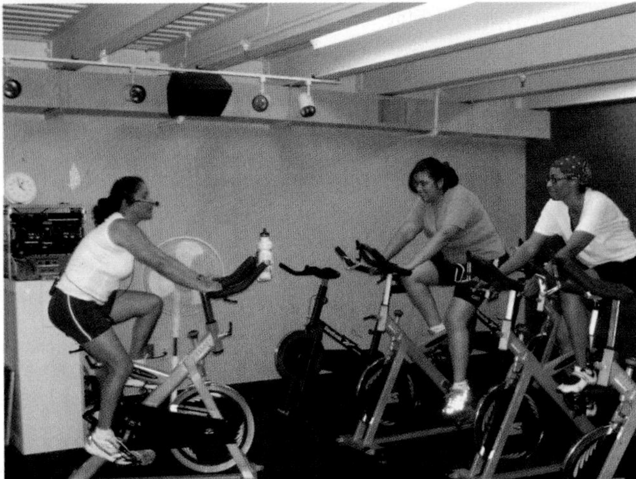

FIG 4-15 Exercise should be a part of one's regular health routine. A cycle class is fun and provides moderate to vigorous exercise. (Courtesy Shari Rivera Sharpe, Chapel Hill, NC.)

lowering the risk of cardiovascular disease. Regular physical activity can reduce or eliminate some of these risk factors by lowering blood pressure, maintaining a reasonable weight or facilitating weight loss, and lowering cholesterol levels to less than 200 mg/dl.

Home maintenance, yard work, and gardening are other activities that promote health and a sense of well-being, especially for older adults. Attention to safety factors and wearing clothing and shoes appropriate to each activity are advised. Care should be taken not to aggravate existing conditions or create muscle and joint discomfort by an overly aggressive approach to exercise.

Kegel Exercises

Kegel exercises, or pelvic muscle exercises, were developed to strengthen the supportive pelvic floor muscles to control or reduce incontinent urine loss. These exercises also are beneficial during pregnancy and postpartum. They strengthen the muscles of the pelvic floor, providing support for the pelvic organs and control of the muscles surrounding the vagina and urethra. Educational strategies for teaching women how to perform Kegel exercises (compiled by nurse researchers who conducted a research utilization project for the Association of Women's Health, Obstetric and Neonatal Nurses [AWHONN]) are described in the Teaching for Self-Management box).

Stress Management

Because it is neither possible nor desirable to avoid all stress, women must learn how to manage it. The nurse should assess each woman for signs of stress, using therapeutic communication skills to determine risk factors and the woman's ability to function. Box 4-5 lists symptoms of stress. Some women must be referred for counseling or other mental health therapy. Women are twice as likely as men to suffer from depression, anxiety, or panic attacks (WebMD, 2012, 2013). Nurses must be alert to the symptoms of serious mental disorders such as depression and anxiety and make referrals to mental health practitioners when necessary. Women experiencing major life changes such as separation and divorce, bereavement, serious illness, and unemployment also need special attention.

For many women, the nurse is able to provide comfort, reassurance, and advice concerning helping resources, such as support groups. Many centers offer support groups to help women prevent or manage stress. Social support and good coping skills can improve a woman's self-esteem and give her a sense of mastery. Anticipatory guidance for developmental or expected situational crises can help her plan strategies for dealing with potentially stressful events. Role playing, relaxation techniques, biofeedback, meditation, desensitization, imagery, assertiveness

TEACHING FOR SELF-MANAGEMENT

Kegel Exercises

Description and Rationale

Kegel exercises, or pelvic muscle exercise, is a technique used to strengthen the muscles that support the pelvic floor. This exercise involves regularly tightening (contracting) and relaxing the muscles that support the bladder and urethra. By strengthening these pelvic muscles a woman can prevent or reduce accidental urine loss.

Technique

The woman needs to learn how to target the muscles for training and how to contract them correctly. One suggestion for teaching is to have the woman pretend she is trying to prevent the passage of intestinal gas. Have her use this tightening motion on the muscles around her vagina and the upper pelvis. She should feel these muscles drawing inward and upward. Other suggested techniques are to have the woman pretend she is trying to stop the flow of urine in midstream or to have her think about how her vagina is able to contract around and move up the length of the penis during intercourse.

The woman should avoid straining or bearing-down motions while performing the exercise. She should be taught how bearing down feels by having her take a breath, hold it, and push down with her abdominal muscles as though she were trying to have a bowel movement. Then the woman can be taught how to avoid straining down by exhaling gently and keeping her mouth open each time she contracts her pelvic muscles.

Specific Instructions

1. Each contraction should be as intense as possible without contracting the abdomen, thighs, or buttocks.
2. Contractions should be held for at least 10 seconds. The woman may have to start with as little as 2 seconds per contraction until her muscles get stronger.
3. The woman should rest for 10 seconds or more between contractions so that the muscles have time to recover and each contraction can be as strong as she can make it.
4. The woman should feel the pulling up over the three muscle layers so that the contraction reaches the highest level of her pelvis.

Data from Sampselle, C. (2003). Behavior interventions in young and middle-aged women: Simple interventions to combat a complex problem. *American Journal of Nursing, 103*(Suppl), 9-19; Sampselle, C. (2000). Behavioral interventions for urinary incontinence in women: Evidence for practice. *Journal of Midwifery & Women's Health, 45*(2), 94-103; Sampselle, C., Wyman, J., Thomas, K., et al. (2000). Continence for women: A test of AWHONN's evidence-based protocol. *Journal of Obstetric, Gynecologic, and Neonatal Nursing, 29*(1), 312-317.

BOX 4-12 Interventions for Smoking Cessation: the Five A's

Ask
- What was her age when she started smoking?
- How many cigarettes does she smoke a day? When was her last cigarette?
- Has she tried to quit?
- Does she want to quit?

Assess
- What were her reasons for not being able to quit before, or what made her start again?
- Does she have anyone who can help her?
- Does anyone else smoke at home?
- Does she have friends or family who have quit successfully?

Advise
- Give her information about the effects of smoking on pregnancy and her fetus, on her own health, and on the members of her household.

Assist
- Provide support; give self-help materials.
- Encourage her to set a quit date.
- Refer to a smoking cessation program, or provide information about nicotine replacement products (not recommended during pregnancy) if she is interested.
- Teach and encourage use of stress-reduction activities.
- Provide for follow-up with a phone call, letter, or clinic visit.

Arrange follow-up
- Arrange to follow the woman to find out about her smoking-cessation status.
- Make a phone call around the time of her quit date. Assess her status at every prenatal visit.
- Congratulate her on her success, or provide support for her if she relapses.
- Referral to intensive treatment may be necessary.

From Fiore, M.C., Jaen, C.R., Baker, T.B., Bailey, W.C., Benowitz, N.L., Curry, S.J., et al (2008). *Treating tobacco use and dependence: 2008 update. Clinical Practice Guideline.* Rockville, MD: U.S. Department of Health and Human Services, Public Health Service. Available at http://www.surgeongeneral.gov/tobacco/treating_tobacco_use08.pdf.

training, yoga, diet, exercise, and weight control are all techniques nurses can include in their repertoire of helping skills. Some women must be referred for counseling or other mental health therapy. Careful follow-up of all women experiencing difficulty in dealing with stress is important.

Substance Use Cessation

All women of all ages will receive substantial and immediate benefits from smoking cessation. However, this task is not easy, and most people stop several times before they accomplish their goal. Many are never able to do so. Box 4-12 describes an intervention, referred to as the Five A's to encourage smoking cessation. Those who wish to stop smoking can also be referred to a smoking-cessation program where individualized methods can be implemented. At the very least, individuals should be guided to self-help materials available from the March of Dimes, the American Lung Association, and the ACS.

New approaches to increase cessation among smokers and to discourage smoking among young women—especially in adolescence and during pregnancy—are needed. Health care providers can have a positive effect on smoking behavior and should attempt to motivate smokers to stop.

Counseling women who appear to be drinking alcohol excessively or using drugs may include promoting strategies to increase self-esteem and teaching new coping skills to resist and maintain resistance to alcohol abuse and drug use. Appropriate referrals should be made, with the health care provider arranging the contact and then following up to be sure that appointments are kept. General referral to sources of support also should be provided. National groups that provide information and support for those who are chemically dependent have local branches or contacts that can be found on the internet.

Anticipatory guidance includes teaching about the health and safety risks of alcohol and mind-altering substances and discouraging drug experimentation among preteen and high school students, because the use of drugs at an early age tends to be a predictor of greater involvement later.

Sexual Practices That Reduce Risk

Prevention of STIs has been discussed earlier in this chapter. The nurse plays an important role in educating women about how to practice safer sex. Chapter 7 includes more detail related to STI prevention. In addition to the prevention of STIs, women of childbearing years need information regarding contraception and family planning (see Chapter 8). A comprehensive sexual assessment should be integrated into all health histories. Women and girls also will benefit from being encouraged to be vaccinated with the HPV series of three vaccinations to prevent cervical cancer.

Health Screening Schedule

Periodic health screening includes history, physical examination, education, counseling, immunizations, and selected diagnostic and laboratory tests. This regimen provides the basis for overall health promotion, prevention of illness, early diagnosis of problems, and referral for appropriate management. Such screening should be customized according to a woman's age and risk factors. In most instances it is completed in health care offices, clinics, or hospitals; however, portions of the screening are now being carried out at events such as community health fairs. An overview of health screening recommendations and immunizations for women 18 years and older is provided in Table 4-3.

Health Risk Prevention

Simple safety factors often are forgotten or perceived not to be important, yet injuries continue to have a major effect on the health status of all age groups. Being aware of hazards and implementing safety guidelines will reduce risks. The nurse should frequently reinforce the following commonsense concepts that will protect the individual:

- Wear seat belts at all times in a moving vehicle.
- Wear safety helmets when riding a motorcycle, bicycle, or inline skates.
- Follow driving "rules of the road."
- Place smoke alarms throughout the home and workplace. Avoid secondhand smoke.
- Lock doors and windows to ensure personal safety.

- Reduce noise pollution or safeguard against hearing loss.
- Protect skin and eyes from ultraviolet light with the use of sunscreen, protective clothing, sunglasses, and hats.
- Practice water safety.
- Never walk or run alone, especially at night.
- Consider storing personal health information (PHI) in a digital database that can be accessed from anywhere you travel.
- Never share computer passwords with strangers, to safeguard financial, personal, and health data.
- Take precautions and avoid dangerous situations.

Health Protection

Nurses can make a difference in stopping violence against women and preventing further injury. Educating women that abuse is a violation of their rights and facilitating their access to protective and legal services constitutes a first step. Encouraging health care institutions to implement appropriate domestic violence screening programs also is of great value (see Chapter 5). Other helpful measures for women to discourage their entry into abusive relationships include promoting assertiveness and self-defense courses; suggesting support and self-help groups that encourage positive self-regard, confidence, and empowerment; and recommending educational and skills development classes that will enhance independence and self-care.

Numerous national and local organizations provide information and assistance for women in abusive situations. All nurses who work in women's health care should become familiar with local services and legal options.

KEY POINTS

- Normal feedback regulation of the menstrual cycle depends on an intact hypothalamic-pituitary-gonadal mechanism.
- The female's reproductive tract structures and breasts respond predictably to changing levels of sex steroids across her life span.
- The myometrium of the uterus is uniquely designed to expel the fetus and promote hemostasis after birth.
- The changing status and roles of women affect their health, needs, and ability to cope with problems.
- Anticipatory guidance is enhanced in a private, safe environment in which the interaction is culturally competent, nonjudgmental, and confidential.
- Culture, religion, socioeconomic status, personal circumstances, the uniqueness of the individual, and the stage of development influence a person's recognition of need for care and the response to the health care system and therapy.
- Preconception counseling allows identification and possible remediation of potentially harmful personal and social conditions, medical and psychologic conditions, environmental conditions, and barriers to care before pregnancy occurs.
- Conditions that increase a woman's health risks also increase risks for her offspring.
- Effective educational programs about sex and family life are imperative to control the rate of teen pregnancy and STIs.
- Health promotion and prevention of illness assist women to actualize health potential by increasing motivation, providing information, and suggesting how to access specific resources.
- IPV against women is a major social and health care problem in the United States and includes physical, sexual, emotional, psychologic, and economic abuse.
- Periodic health screening, including history, physical examination, and diagnostic and laboratory tests, provides the basis for overall health promotion, prevention of illness, early diagnosis of problems, and referral for management.

REFERENCES

Academy of Nutrition and Dietetics. (2012). Position of the American Academy of Nutrition and Dietetics: Food and nutrition for older adults: Promoting health and wellness. *Journal of the Academy of Nutrition and Dietetics*, *112*(8), 1255–1277.

American Cancer Society. (2013a). *Breast awareness and self exam*. Available at www.cancer.org/cancer/breastcancer/moreinformation/breastcancerearlydetection/breast-cancer-early-detection-acs-recs-bse.

American Cancer Society. (2013b). *Women and smoking*. Available at www.cancer.org/cancer/cancercauses/tobaccocancer/womenandsmoking/women-and-smoking-toc.

American Cancer Society. (2013c). *Body weight and cancer risk*. Available at www.cancer.org/cancer/cancercauses/dietandphysicalactivity/bodyweightand-cancerrisk/body-weight-and-cancer-toc.

American Cancer Society. (2013d). *Guidelines for the early detection of cancer*. Available at www.cancer.org/healthy/findcancerearly/cancerscreeningguidelines/american-cancer-society-guidelines-for-the-early-detection-of-cancer.

American College of Obstetricians and Gynecologists. (2013). Obesity and pregnancy. *Committee Opinion, 549*. Available at www.acog.org/Resources%20And%20Publications/Committee%20Opinions/Committee%20on%20Obstetric%20Practice/Obesity%20in%20Pregnancy.aspx.

American Heart Association. (2013). *American Heart Association recommendations for physical activity in adults*. Available at http:///www.heart.org/HEARTORG/GettingHealthy/PhysicalActivity/StartWalking/American-Heart-Association-Guidelines_UCM_307976_Article.jsp.

Avalos, L. A., Kaskutas, L., Block, G., et al. (2011). Does lack of multinutrient supplementation during early pregnancy increase vulnerability to alcohol-related preterm or small-for-gestational-age births? *Maternal and Child Health Journal*, *15*(8), 1324–1332.

Bailey, B. A., & Sokol, R. J. (2011). Prenatal alcohol exposure and miscarriage, stillbirth, preterm delivery, and sudden infant death syndrome. *Alcohol Research and Health, 34*(1), 86–91.

Berecki-Gisolf, J., McKenzie, S. J., Dobson, A. J., et al. (2012). A history of co-morbid depression and anxiety predicts new onset of heart disease. *Journal of Behavioral Medicine* (epub ahead of print).

breastcancer.org. (2012). *Breast self-exam.* Available at www.breastcancer.org/symptoms/testing/types/self_exam.

Brennan, A. M. W., Barnsteiner, J., de Leon Siantz, M. L., et al. (2012). Lesbian, gay, bisexual, transgendered, or intersexed content for nursing curricula. *Journal of Professional Nursing, 28*(2), 96–104.

Burkhardt, M. A., & Nagai-Jacobson, M. G. (2012). Spirituality and health. In B. M. Dossey, & L. Keegan (Eds.), *Holistic nursing: A handbook for practice* (6th ed.). Burlington, MA: Jones and Bartlett.

Centers for Disease Control and Prevention. (2011). *Chronic disease prevention and health promotion: Tobacco use.* Available at www.cdc.gov/chronicdisease/resources/publications/aag/osh.htm.

Centers for Disease Control and Prevention. 2012a). Prepregnancy contraceptive use among teens with unintended pregnancies resulting in live birth: Pregnancy risk assessment monitoring system (PRAMS), 2004-2008. *MMWR Morbidity and Mortality Weekly Report, 61*(02), 25–29.

Centers for Disease Control and Prevention. (2012b). *Hepatitis C testing for anyone born during 1945-1965: New CDC recommendations.* Available at www.cdc.gov-/features/hepatitisctesting.

Dossey, B. M. (2013). Integral and holistic nursing: Local to global. In B. M. Dossey, & L. Keegan (Eds.), *A handbook for practice* (6th ed.). Burlington, MA: Jones and Bartlett.

Dubowitz, T., Ghosh-Dastidar, M., Eibner, C., et al. (2012). The women's health initiative: The food environment, neighborhood socioeconomic status, BMI, and blood pressure. *Obesity, 20*(4), 862–871.

Escallier, L. A., Fullerton, J. T., & Messina, B. A. M. (2011). Cultural competence outcomes assessment: A strategy and model. *International Journal of Nursing and Midwifery, 3*(3), 35–42.

Fawcet, T., & Rhynas, S. (2012). Taking a patient history: The role of the nurse. *Nursing Standard, 26*(24), 41–46.

Galanti, G. (2008). *Caring for patients from different cultures* (4th ed.). Philadelphia: University of Pennsylvania Press.

Guttmacher Institute. (2012a). *Facts on unintended pregnancy in the United States.* Available at www.guttmacher.org/pubs/FB-Unintended-Pregnancy-US.html.

Guttmacher Institute. (2012b). *Facts on American teens sexual and reproductive health.* New York: NY. Available at www.guttmacher.org/pubs/FB-ATSRH.html.

Hautala, L., Junnila, J., Alin, J., et al. (2009). Uncovering hidden eating disorders using the SCOFF questionnaire: Cross-sectional survey of adolescents and comparison with nurse assessments. *International Journal of Nursing Studies, 46*(11), 1439–1447.

Healthcare.gov. (2012). *Women and the affordable care act.* Available at www.healthcare.gov/news/factsheets/2011/08/women.html.

HealthyPeople.gov. (2012a). *Maternal, infant, and child health.* Available at www.healthypeople.gov/2020/LHI/micHealth.aspx.

HealthyPeople.gov. (2012b). *Nutrition, physical activity, and obesity.* Available at http://healthypeople.gov/2020/LHI/nutrition.aspx.

HealthyPeople.gov. (2012c). *Pregnancy health and behaviors.* Available at www.healthypeople.gov/2020/topicsobjectives2020/objectiveslist.aspx?topicid=26.

Hogue, C. J. R., & Silver, R. M. (2011). Racial and ethnic disparities in the United States: Stillbirth rates: Trends, risk factors, and research needs. *Seminars in Perinatology, 35*(4), 221–233.

Leeman, L. M., & Rogers, R. C. (2012). Sex after childbirth: Postpartum sexual function. *Obstetrics and Gynecology, 119*(3), 647–655.

March of Dimes. (2011). *Environmental risks and pregnancy.* Available at www.marchofdimes.com/pregnancy/stayingsafe_indepth.html.

March of Dimes. (2013). *Eating and nutrition.* Available at www.marchofdimes.com/pregnancy/caffeine-in-pregnancy.aspx.

Masters, W., & Johnson, V. (1996). *Human sexual response.* New York: Bantam Books.

McAlearney, A. S., Oliveri, J. M., Post, D. M., et al. (2011). Trust and distrust among Appalachian women regarding cervical cancer screening: A qualitative study. *Patient Education and Counseling, 86*(1), 120–126.

McCloskey, C. R. (2012). Changing focus: Women's perinatal journey. *Health Care for Women International, 33*(6).

Mong, J. A., Baker, F. C., Mahoney, M. M., et al. (2011). Sleep, rhythms, and the endocrine brain: Influence of sex and gonadal hormones. *Journal of Neuroscience, 31*(45), 16107–16116.

Morgan, J., Reid, F., & Lacey, J. (1999). The SCOFF questionnaire: Assessment of a new screening tool for eating disorders. *BMJ, 319*(7223), 1467–1468.

Moyer, V. A., LeFevre, M. L., Siu, A. L., et al. (2013). Vitamin D and calcium supplementation to prevent fractures in adults: U.S. Preventive Services Task Force Recommendation abuse. *Annals of Internal Medicine, 158*(9), 691–696.

Murphy, R., Straebler, S., Basden, S., et al. (2012). Interpersonal psychotherapy for eating disorders. *Clinical Psychology & Psychotherapy, 19*(2), 150–158.

Nelson, H. D., Bougatsos, C., & Blazina, I. (2012). *Screening women for intimate partner violence: A systematic review to update the U.S. Preventive Services Task Force Recommendation.* Available at www.uspreventiveservicestaskforce.org/uspstf12/ipvelder/ipvelderart.htm.

Nestle, M., & Nesheim, M. C. (2013). To supplement or not to supplement: The U.S. Preventive Services Task Force recommendations on calcium and vitamin D. *Annals of Internal Medicine, 158*(9), 701–702.

O'Leary, C., Nassar, N., Kurinczuk, J. J., et al. (2011). Prenatal alcohol exposure and risk of birth defects. *Obstetrical & Gynecological Survey, 66*(2), 88–90.

Pasternak, Y., Weintraub, A. Y., Shoham-Vardi, I., et al. (2012). Obstetric and perinatal outcomes in women with eating disorders. *Journal of Women's Health, 21*(1), 61–65.

Piotrowski, K., & Snell, L. (2007). Health needs of women with disabilities across the lifespan. *Journal of Obstetric, Gynecologic, and Neonatal Nursing, 36*(1), 79–87.

Saraiya, M., Rosser, J. I., & Cooper, C. P. (2012). Cancers that U.S. physicians believe the HPV vaccine prevents: Findings from a physician survey, 2009. *Journal of Women's Health, 21*(2), 111–117.

Seidel, H., Ball, J., Dains, J., et al. (2011). *Mosby's guide to physical examination* (7th ed.). St. Louis: Mosby.

Skinner, H. H., Haines, J., Austin, B., et al. (2012). A prospective study of overeating, binge eating, and depressive symptoms among adolescent and young adult women. *Journal of Adolescent Health, 50*(5), 478–483.

Touchette, E., Henegar, A., Godart, N. T., et al. (2011). Subclinical eating disorders and their comorbidity with mood and anxiety disorders in adolescent girls. *Psychiatry Research, 185*(1), 185–192.

U.S. Department of Agriculture, Center for Nutrition and Policy Promotion. (2010). *Dietary guidelines for Americans.* Available at www.cnpp.usda.gov/DietaryGuidelines.htm.

U.S. Department of Health and Human Services. (2010). *Dietary guidelines for Americans 2010.* Available at http://www.health.gov/dietaryguidelines.

U.S. Department of Health and Human Services. (2012). *Performance indicators.1.C.3.* Available at www.hhs.gov/secretary/about/appendixb_goal1.html.

U.S. Department of Justice. (2012). *Office on violence against women.* Available at www.ovw.usdoj.gov.

U.S. Preventive Services Task Force. (2013). *Final recommendation statement screening for intimate partner violence of elderly and vulnerable adults.* Available at www.uspreventiveservicestaskforce.org/uspstf12/ipvelder/ipvelderfinalrs.htm.

Vallance, J. K., Latner, J. D., & Gleaves, D. H. (2011). The relationship between eating disorder psychopathology and health-related quality of life within a community sample. *Quality of Life Research, 20*(5), 675–682.

WebMD. (2012). *Anxiety and panic disorders health center.* Available at www.webmd.com/anxiety-panic/guide/panic-attack-symptoms.

WebMD. (2013). *Depression health center.* Available at www.webmd.com/depression/guide/depression-women.

World Health Organization. (2013). *Female genital mutilation. World Health Organization, Fact Sheet #241.* Available at www.who.int/mediacentre/factsheets/fs241/en.

Yang, T. S., Matthews, S. A., & Hillemeier, M. M. (2011). Effect of health care system distrust on breast and cervical cancer screening in Philadelphia, Pennsylvania. *American Journal of Public Health, 101*(7), 1297–1305.

Zhao, C., Kalpos-Novak, P., & Austin, M. (2011). Follow-up findings in young females with high-grade squamous intraepithelial lesion Papanicolaou test results. *Archives of Pathology & Laboratory Medicine, 135*(3), 361–364.

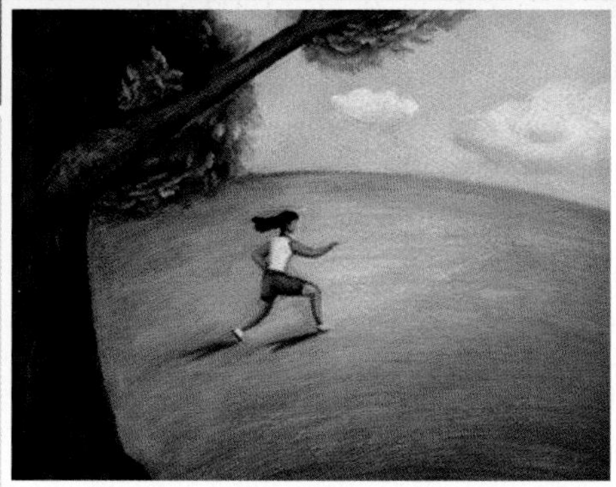

CHAPTER 5

Violence Against Women

Noreen Esposito

http://evolve.elsevier.com/Lowdermilk/MWHC/

LEARNING OBJECTIVES

- Describe the beliefs and practices that historically have perpetuated violence against women.
- Examine the prevalence and effects of intimate partner violence.
- Contrast the theoretic premises underlying the victimization of women.
- Discuss theories of violence and how they can be used in assessment and intervention for women who are abused.
- Develop a nursing care plan for a woman who is experiencing intimate partner violence.
- Review the dynamics of sexual assault.
- Describe the rape-trauma syndrome.
- Develop a nursing care plan for a woman in the acute phase of rape-trauma syndrome.
- Evaluate resources available to women experiencing abuse.
- Describe human sex trafficking and implications for health care providers.

Violence against women (VAW) is a public health problem that exists worldwide. It has been more than twenty years since the United Nations defined VAW as "any act of gender-based violence that results in or is likely to result in physical, sexual, or mental harm or suffering to women including threats of such acts, coercion, or arbitrary deprivation of liberty whether occurring in public or private" (Blanchfield, 2008; United Nations, 1993). Since then research efforts have increased what is known about the various dimensions of VAW. Around the globe VAW takes many different forms including, but not limited to, intimate partner violence, sexual assault, marital rape, dowry-related violence, sexual trafficking and exploitation, and female genital mutilation. This chapter focuses on intimate partner violence, sexual assault, and trafficking of women.

INTIMATE PARTNER VIOLENCE

Intimate partner violence (IPV) is the most common form of VAW, with a reported global prevalence of 30% and rates ranging from 36% in poorer regions such as Africa, Central and South America, and Southeast Asia to 23% in higher-income regions such as Australia, Canada, the United States, and developed countries of Western Europe (World Health Organization [WHO], 2013a). The National Violence Against Women Survey (NVAWS) defines IPV as "the actual or threatened physical, sexual, psychologic, or emotional abuse by a spouse, ex-spouse, boyfriend, girlfriend, ex-boyfriend, ex-girlfriend, date, or cohabiting partner" (Tjaden & Thoennes, 2006). The National Intimate Partner and Sexual Violence Survey (NISVS) expanded on that work with an ongoing telephone survey that focuses on five types of IPV: sexual violence, physical violence, stalking, psychologic aggression, and control of reproductive or sexual health (Black, Basile, Breiding, et al., 2011). The survey added stalking and IPV among same-sex partners, information that was not tracked in the past. IPV can be thought of as "a continuum ranging from one hit that may or may not impact the victim to chronic, severe battering" (Centers for Disease Control and Prevention [CDC], 2010a). Other terms such as partner abuse and domestic or family violence are common. Older terms such as wife battering or spouse battering are generally not used. Battery has been used in the past to refer to physical contact with another with the intent of harm, but the World Health Organization (WHO) has an updated definition of battery to refer to an escalation of violence with increasing threats and increasing terror. IPV is the preferred term in that it encompasses not only physical contact but also emotional and other forms of violence previously ignored (WHO, 2012).

IPV is a complex, stigmatizing problem involving issues of emotional distress, personal safety, and social isolation. In many places in the United States and abroad IPV has been socially tolerated or ignored. Lack of reporting and inconsistent definitions have made it difficult to get an accurate count of the number of victims, as there are wide ranges of estimates.

In the United States the prevalence of some form of IPV (rape, physical violence, and/or stalking) during a woman's lifetime is estimated to be 35.6% (Black et al., 2011). In a prospective survey of 2737 urban public hospital emergency department

(ED) clients, 548 (20%) identified themselves as victims of IPV. Greater victim-perceived danger was associated with lower physical and mental health functioning in the 216 of those who returned for follow-up (Straus, Cerulli, McNutt, et al., 2009). Throughout the world more than one third of female homicides occur at the hands of an intimate partner (Stockl, Devries, Rotskein, et al., 2013). In 2010, there were 1095 women murdered by an intimate partner in the United States (U.S. Department of Justice, 2011).

Abusive relationships exist in couples who are dating, living together, or married. The abuse, which may be physical, sexual, psychologic, or financial, can continue after the relationship ends. One partner behaves in a way that injures, intimidates, humiliates, frightens, or terrorizes the other partner. These behaviors can be insidious, slowly happening over time. Emotional abuse may include name calling, acting in a jealous or possessive manner, trying to isolate the woman from her family or friends, putting her down in front of others, threatening her children or alienating her children from her, not wanting her to go out or go to work, or insisting that she account for every minute she is away from home. Physical violence may never be used, or used rarely, but threats can be as effective as actual violence. If the abuser becomes physically violent, the threat of recurrence always exists.

CLINICAL REASONING CASE STUDY

Intimate Partner Violence

Elena, a 17-year-old Hispanic client, is in the clinic for her fifth month prenatal visit. She missed her last two appointments. She is accompanied by her boyfriend, with whom she lives. The nurse suggests that he wait outside while she asks intake questions about Elena's health. Elena looks down and says quietly, "It's fine if he stays, really it is." The nurse notices that he is very attentive to Elena, is very nice to the nurse, and answers for Elena most of the time she is asked a question. You explain that the clinic has a policy that the interviews are done in private. He reluctantly leaves the room. After some routine questions about her general health since her last prenatal visit, the nurse asks her about intimate partner violence and safety. "Have you been hit, slapped, kicked, or in other ways physically hurt by someone?" Elena shakes her head and says, "No" in a quiet voice. The nurse notices Elena glance at a small bruise on the inner part of her arm. The nurse asks Elena if she is being physically hurt or threatened in her relationship. She gets teary but says, "No." What is the nurse's responsibility in this instance regarding confidentiality, questioning Elena about intimate partner violence, and risks to Elena if she discloses that she has been hurt by her boyfriend? What is the nurse's responsibility to report the incident to the police?

1. Evidence—Is there sufficient evidence to draw conclusions about Elena as a woman experiencing abuse?
2. Assumptions—What assumptions can be made about the following?
   a. Characteristic behaviors of a woman in an abusive relationship
   b. Cultural considerations
   c. Pregnancy and abuse
   d. Relationship expectations—adolescents and abuse
3. What implications and priorities for nursing care can be made at this time?
4. Does the evidence objectively support your conclusion?

IPV may begin in pregnancy or may have already begun before the pregnancy. If it already exists, IPV may increase, decrease, or stay the same during the pregnancy (Macy, Martin, Kupper, et al., 2007; Taylor & Nabors, 2009) (see later discussion in section Intimate Partner Violence in Pregnancy.)

The consequences of IPV are profound. Approximately 28% of women in the NISVS linked the experience of IPV with some type of negative consequence including fear (26%), safety concerns (22%), posttraumatic stress disorder (PTSD) symptoms (22%), an injury (15%), the need for medical care (8%), lack of housing (2.4%), legal services (7.6%), missed days at work or school (10%), pregnancy (1.7%), or contracting a sexually transmitted infection (1.5%) (Black et al., 2011). In a study comparing abused women with never abused women, abused women had a higher incidence of social and family problems, substance abuse, menstrual and other reproductive disorders, sexually transmitted infections (STIs), musculoskeletal and gastrointestinal (GI) disorders, chest pain, abdominal pain, urinary tract infections (UTIs), and headaches (Bonomi, Anderson, Reid, et al., 2009). Prolonged exposure to acute or chronic stress like IPV is linked with structural changes in the brain now associated with mental health problems, emotion regulation, and cognitive problems. In one study abused women with PTSD who were shown angry faces and angry male faces during functional magnetic resonance imaging (*f*MRI) had hyperresponsiveness in the amygdala and the entire limbic system compared with women who had no abuse history (Fonzo, Simmons, Thorp, et al., 2010). Based on a review of multiple large population-based surveys, the WHO developed pathways suggesting links between exposures to violence and adverse health effects of IPV (WHO, 2013a).

Medical costs alone in the United States for interpersonal violence are estimated to be $2.7 to $7 billion for the first 12 months after victimization, and annual medical costs for any past intimate partner victimization, not limited to the last year, range from $25 to $59 billion (Brown, Finkelstein, & Mercy, 2008). These figures do not include the cost of police and court costs, shelters, foster care, sick leave, and non-productivity. Reducing the rates of IPV and sexual violence are *Healthy People 2020* sub-objectives under the main objective of violence prevention (U.S. Department of Health and Human Services [USDHHS], 2013).

Historical Perspective

Women have been treated inhumanely throughout history. In ancient Rome, wives were divorced or killed by husbands for adultery, public drunkenness, or attending public games, whereas men could engage in these activities daily. In the 1700s, under English common law, the "rule of thumb" gave men permission to chastise their wives physically as long as the implement they used was no wider than their thumbs. In the late 1600s, Pilgrims and Puritans directed male heads of the family to use force when needed to maintain conduct of their wives. Although American law prohibited beating wives, the Puritans supported physical force by husbands as legitimate. In the 1800s men gradually lost the right to beat their wives. Slow progress was made in the early 20th century. There was little awareness from both health care professionals and the legal and justice systems to the plight of women in intimate relationships. As late as the 1960s, it was believed that violence in the family was rare and committed only by the mentally ill.

The first shelter for women opened in London in 1971, and books and articles on domestic violence began to appear in the 1970s. Battered woman syndrome was described by Lenore Walker in 1979 and battered women programs emerged in the 1980s. In the 1990s the American Nurses Association issued a position statement against VAW, the American Medical Association declared that physicians were liable if they did not recognize IPV, and The Joint Commission issued standards to identify and manage IPV clients. The National Domestic Violence Hotline was established in 1996. The CDC promotes the phrase intimate partner violence over domestic violence (CDC, 2013). Health care providers, law enforcement, the legal system, and the general public are slowly acknowledging IPV, but power imbalances, persistent beliefs that family problems are private matters, the victim's feelings of shame, and fear continue to keep women from disclosing abuse.

Conceptual and Theoretic Perspectives

In the late 1970s little was known about IPV. Lenore Walker, a pioneer in the field, interviewed 120 victims, from which she generated the phrase "battered woman syndrome," which identified victim characteristics such as learned helplessness and abuser characteristics such as mental health problems. At the time Walker proposed a model of how IPV might appear in some families. The model, referred to as the *cycle of violence,* described three phases in an IPV relationship: tension building, acute battering, and the honeymoon phase. In her proposed model, violence was neither random nor constant but occurred in repeated cycles. Her continued research led to modifications in her early interpretations. Ongoing research from different disciplines has expanded today's understanding of IPV. Current thought does not support the general applicability of the cycle of violence.

IPV is heterogeneous. Not all batterers are alike, not all victims are alike, and not all relationships and patterns of abuse are alike. In some relationships physical and psychologic abuse happen on a regular basis. In other relationships, physical abuse or the threat of abuse may happen rarely, but emotional abuse is more persistent. In some relationships abuse happens after stressful events or pregnancy. Walker's work was an important first step and helped raise awareness and concern. Because the cycle of violence was the only available explanation for IPV, the model became a core part of IPV training for health professionals, social workers, law enforcement officers, and judges. Despite limited evidence of its usefulness many professionals still believe that the cycle of violence explains IPV (Dutton, 2009).

There is a growing body of literature about the characteristics and dynamics of IPV. Along with feminist ideologies that play a critical role in gender-based violence, theories from biology, psychology, and sociology all help to partially explain various aspects of violence against women. No single theory can completely explain this complex problem. Following is a brief discussion of some of these theoretic perspectives.

Biologic Factors

A complete explanation of the biologic perspective is beyond the scope of this chapter, but evidence indicates that neurobiologic and hormonal factors influence aggression in men. Areas in the brain believed to play a role in aggressive behavior are the limbic system, the frontal lobes, and the hypothalamus. Changes in structural functioning of the limbic system, such as occur with brain lesions, substance use, epilepsy, and head injuries, affect the emotional experience and behavior of the individual and thus can increase or decrease the potential for aggressive behavior (Stuart & Hamolia, 2009).

Neurochemical factors also can play a role in aggressive behavior so that dysfunction or dysregulation of certain neurotransmitters can result in aggression. Increased levels of norepinephrine and L-dopa foster aggressive behavior. Reducing the levels of serotonin in animals causes aggressive behavior. The amino acid gamma-aminobutyric acid (GABA) inhibits aggressive behavior. The occurrence of violence in neurologic disorders also is reported, especially when violent reactions are out of proportion to the provoking events (Stuart & Hamolia, 2009).

In animal studies, aggression is associated with abnormally high levels of testosterone. Soler, Vinayak, & Quadagno (2000) reported higher testosterone levels in abusive male subjects and suggested that heritability is an issue that warrants the inclusion of this variable in future studies of violent behavior. There is no conclusive evidence in biologic theory, except perhaps in instances of neurologic damage, that it is impossible to control aggressive behavior.

Psychologic Perspective

Psychology, the study of emotion and behavior, places responsibility for behaviors such as aggression on the individual. Early psychoanalytic theory suggested that aggression is a basic instinctual drive leading to mastery and accomplishment. In men aggression was seen as a positive force that connoted boldness, forcefulness, energy, and enterprise. Thus early psychologic theory saw aggression in men as normal. Early psychoanalytic theory promoted gender-stereotypic expectations for women to be caring and nurturing; aggression in women was and still is viewed negatively, and aggressive women are often labeled as hostile and belligerent.

The myth that abuse is committed by people who have some type of mental illness perpetuates the notion that violence occurs among people who are not "normal." Mental illness accounts for a very small percentage of IPV. Men who batter vary from having modest personality dysfunction to having significant personality pathology such as borderline and antisocial personality disorders (Capaldi & Kim, 2007). Population-based Canadian studies suggest demographic risk factors include a partner who is underemployed, low income, or alcohol or substance abuse (Stewart, MacMillan, & Wathen, 2013). Although a diagnosis of alcohol abuse is frequently found in abusers, it should not be misconstrued as the cause of violence. There is some evidence that alcohol may increase the risk of violent behavior because survivors of violence often report substance abuse by the abuser (Torres & Han, 2003). There is no diagnostic profile of an abuser, but Box 5-1 provides some characteristics of men who batter that nurses may consider when assessing clients' relationships.

Women with severe and persistent mental illness are likely to be more vulnerable to being involved in controlling and violent

BOX 5-1 Characteristics of a Potential Male Batterer

- Low self-esteem
- Problems with abandonment, loss, helplessness, dependency, insecurity, and intimacy
- Inadequate verbal skills, especially difficulty expressing feelings
- Deficits in assertiveness
- Personality disorders frequently diagnosed
- Low frustration tolerance (loses temper easily)
- Higher incidence of growing up in an abusive or violent home
- Denies, minimizes, blames, and lies about own actions
- Violence is consistent with his view of himself and the world; it is an acceptable way of dealing with everyday life
- Inability to empathize with others
- Rigidity in male and female behaviors (sex-role stereotypes)
- Perception of self as "special" and deserving special attention for being the provider, protector
- Substance abuse problems are common
- Displays of an unusual amount of jealousy (e.g., expects partner to spend all of her time with him or to keep him informed of her whereabouts)

relationships. However, numerous mental health problems (such as depression, psychophysiologic illnesses, substance abuse, eating disorders, PTSD, and anxiety reactions) experienced by women with abusive partners are more likely to be consequences of long-term abuse rather than causes (WHO, 2013a). Relationship violence differs by severity and frequency, the individual's characteristics, and whether it is confined to the family or occurs outside the family. Not all victims see their violence experiences in the same way; different women experience violence differently. Women with dependent personality traits as well as independent women have been victims of IPV. Although there may be shared characteristics, each person's experience and response is individual (Nurius & Macy, 2008).

Newer studies in psychology are exploring the unique differences among individuals who are in violent relationships. We know that men who are involved in relationship violence are not all alike. Heterogeneity is seen in the characteristics of the men, in their partners, and in the relationship dynamics. When trying to understand some types of violence, there is growing interest in considering both members of a relationship. In one conceptual model Capaldi and Kim (2007) explored the typologies of couples experiencing violence. They offered a dynamic systems model that considers what each person brings to a relationship. For example, personal characteristics such as depression or antisocial behavior might be combined with a person's emotional development to create a unique individual. Individuals come together to create a pattern of interactions, and these interactions occur in the context of various social stresses such as substance use, financial stress, or separation. The dynamics can lead to some type of incident that is potentially or actually violent. Viewed this way, this dynamic model provides many potential areas for intervention. Research is needed to further explore the possibilities of this approach.

Sociologic Perspective

The social structure and conditions in Western society provide the basis for many of the prevailing attitudes toward violent behavior. U.S. history is filled with examples of violence, such as war, as a means of social control. Social acceptance and promotion of violence in men are double standards because women are expected to be nonviolent. Thus psychologic theories of gender-based behaviors can influence social beliefs and responses to particular behaviors. Because men are socially expected to be aggressive, their violence is sometimes treated with more leniency and less stigma than violence in women, particularly in the justice system. The use of physical force in normal societal encounters can lead to the acceptance of violence in society.

Family dynamics in which there are certain roles assumed within the family, the amount of time spent together, the degree of privacy, emotional involvement, and stress and conflict may all contribute to violence. Power and violence, or even the threat of physical force, contribute to the persistent patriarchal view of a woman's place in the home and in the rest of society. Gender inequality, in both economic opportunities and physical strength, serves to perpetuate the power imbalance in relationships.

Another family issue is the multigenerational transmission of violence; some perpetrators of violence and some victims learn about violence in families of origin by either witnessing or experiencing violence while growing up (Cannon, Bonomi, Anderson, & Rivara, 2009). In families in which violence occurs, both the lack of emotional support experienced by children and the awareness that people who love each other can be violent are important factors. Children in these environments do not have role models to help them develop mental models of healthy family dynamics. Abuse as a child, however, does not consistently determine later violent behavior because many children who were abused grow up to avoid violent behavior.

Feminist Perspective

One contemporary view of violence is derived from feminist theory. This view, with the primary theme of male dominance and coercive control, enhances our understanding of all forms of violence against women, including IPV, stranger and acquaintance rape, incest, and sexual harassment in the workplace. A gender and power perspective is taken as a way to understand the victimization that occurred. In numerous cases, power and control tactics were central events leading to the violence. The power and control wheel developed by the Duluth, Minnesota, Domestic Abuse Intervention Project identifies ways that men may exercise the power and control that underlie many types of IPV and has been used to help women, men, and care providers understand violence (Fig. 5-1).

As our understanding of the complexity of violence against women has evolved over time, so has the need for an evolving feminist viewpoint. Using frontline workers' perspectives of current feminist thought, one study proposed an integrative feminist model. Keeping gender and other forms of oppression as the roots of IPV, an integrative model offers flexibility in exploring multiple additional models emerging in violence research (McPhail, Busch, Kulkarni, & Rice, 2007).

Ecologic Model

An ecologic model is a useful tool when trying to understand a complex social issue like IPV. Ecologic models help make apparent the dynamic relationship between the individual and the environment. Bronfenbrenner (1979, 2005) explained how

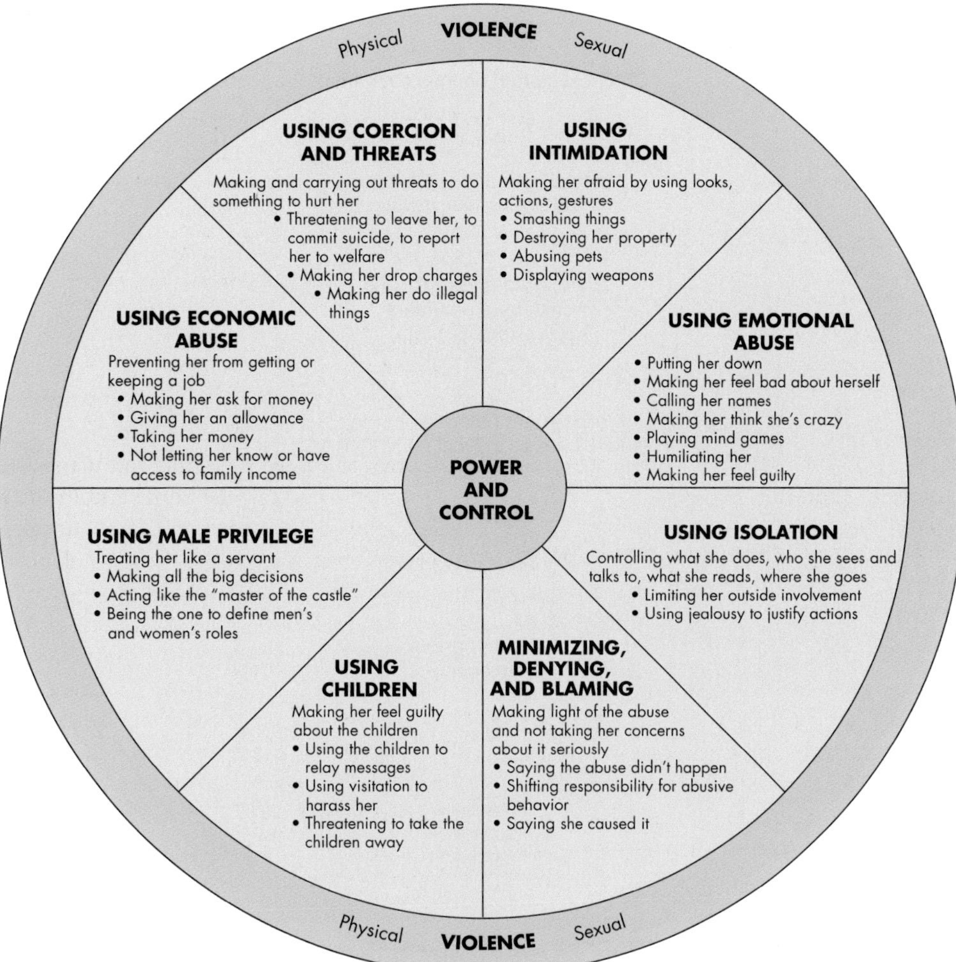

FIG 5-1 Model of how power and control issues perpetuate battering. (Developed by the Duluth Domestic Abuse Intervention Project, Duluth, MN.)

an ecologic model might explain child development. An ecologic model is sometimes drawn as nested circles that represent characteristics of the individual and the factors in that person's immediate and larger environment that influence the phenomenon of concern. The model has been adapted and used to understand a variety of health behaviors and social issues. The WHO (2010) uses an ecologic model to examine and understand various communities. Heise (1998) adapted one for IPV and Campbell, Dworkin, & Cabral (2009) developed a similar model for sexual assault.

Figure 5-2 is an ecologic model of IPV. The individual woman is at the center of the model. Her unique characteristics, such as age, life experience, race/ethnicity, social class, education, personality, emotional well-being, finances, and others influence who she is and how she is in the world. In her immediate environment is her intimate partner, his characteristics, and the characteristics of their relationship. At the next level *(microsystem)* are her children, family, friends, and the people, such as her neighbors, employer, or coworkers, and activities in her daily life that are important. Surrounding the social network are community resources such as women's groups, violence prevention programs, and local resources *(mesosystem)*. The *exosystem* refers to organizations and formal agencies, health care systems, and providers such as nurses, the police, and the legal system, all of which are influenced by the larger sociocultural beliefs, myths, and media *(macrosystem)*. Finally, the *chronosystem* represents the influence of events over time.

For example, a woman (individual) experiencing IPV over time may develop chronic depression and hopelessness, finding it more difficult to mount the energy needed to change or leave the relationship. Her partner interactions may have pushed away her friends, and her emotional state makes it difficult to rebuild relationships. Perhaps her family or friends are influenced by social or cultural expectations not to interfere in someone else's marriage, express disbelief, or blame the woman (Sylaska & Edwards, 2014). The woman is socially isolated. She may hear about IPV issues from a local women's group, helping to destigmatize her perception of the issue. If she risks disclosing her experience to a nurse and receives validation and support, she may be more likely to seek help again in the future, perhaps with the health care system, or with another social agency. The nurse who interacted with the woman is also influenced by that experience in providing support to a victim of IPV. All facets of the model are influenced by one another, and those influences change over time.

Women Experiencing Intimate Partner Violence

Characteristics of Women in Abusive Relationships

Every segment of society has people experiencing abuse. Race, religion, social background, age, and educational level do not

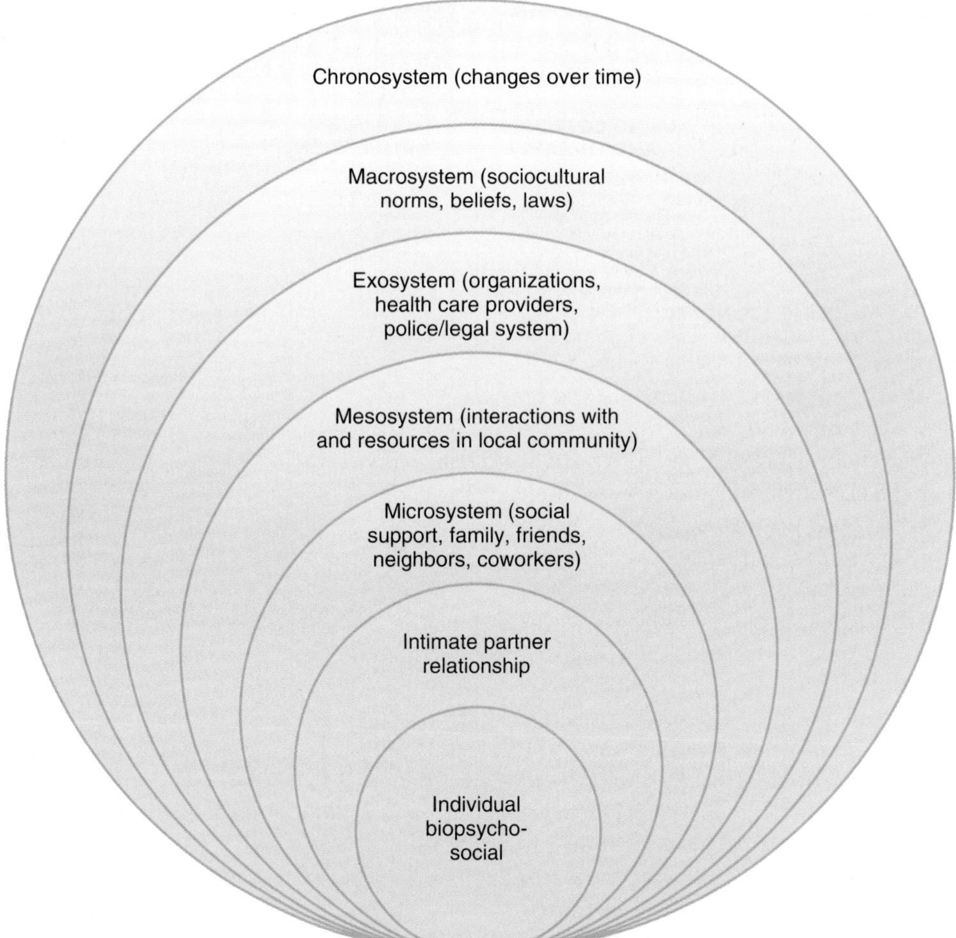

FIG 5-2 Ecologic framework for intimate partner violence. (Adapted from Bronfenbrenner, U. [1979]. *The ecology of human development: Experiments by nature and design.* Cambridge, MA: Harvard University Press; Bronfenbrenner, U. [2005]. *Making human beings human: Bioecological perspectives on human development.* Thousand Oaks, CA: Sage; Heise, L. [1998]. Violence against women: An integrated, ecological framework. *Violence Against Women, 4*[3], 262-290; Campbell, R., Dworkin, E., & Cabral, G. [2009]. An ecological model of the impact of sexual assault on women's mental health. *Trauma Violence and Abuse, 10*[3], 225-246.)

differentiate women at risk. Poor and uneducated women tend to be disproportionately represented because they are seen in EDs, are financially more dependent, have fewer resources and support systems, and may have fewer problem-solving skills. Women with educational or financial resources have been hidden from public awareness but can just as easily be victims (Thompson, Bonomi, Anderson, et al., 2006). They may be disadvantaged in other ways in that they do not fit the stereotype of an abused woman and find it difficult to come to terms with the idea that they are in an abusive relationship (Steiner, 2009). Health care providers may even dismiss this possibility.

The value women place on their social roles may have some influence in IPV. Traditional feminine characteristics such as compassion, sympathy, and yielding often result in greater tolerance of male dominance and more acceptance of partner violence. In contrast the traits of assertiveness, independence, and willingness to take a stand have been viewed as more characteristic in women who are in nonviolent relationships (Faramarzi, Esmailzadeh, & Mosavi, 2005.) There is little research that tells us how these characteristics might change if independent, assertive women found themselves in abusive relationships. Although women who are in abusive relationships may appear passive or even helpless to an outside observer, their behaviors can represent attempts to reduce the risk of violence as they survive day to day (Dutton, 2009). It is important therefore not to attach causation to traditional feminine characteristics.

Survivors of IPV may believe they are to blame for their situations because they are "not good enough, not efficient enough, not pretty enough." The woman may blame herself for bringing on the violent behavior in her relationship because she believes she must try harder to please the abuser. In many cases, a traumatic bonding with the man hinges on loyalty, fear, and terror. Some women have low self-esteem. Some may have histories of domestic violence in their families of origin. Often abused women are socially isolated. This may be the result of stigma, fear, restrictions placed on them by their partners, or partner behaviors that discourage others from being involved.

Based on the self-appraisal of 448 victims who filed police reports, Nurius and Macy (2008) identified five subgroups of victims. Each group varied in their feelings of vulnerability, sense of power, symptoms of depression, social relationships with others, type and duration of exposure to violence, and physical health. The largest group was composed of women who felt vulnerable to continued abuse and had high depression scores. The second group included women struggling with depression but with a low sense of vulnerability. A third group felt vulnerable to violence or abuse but were otherwise healthy with low rates of depression and strong social relationships. The fourth group included women with multiple resources including good health, low depression scores, lower sense of being vulnerable, and high social support. The last group included women with high rates of vulnerability, physical injury, depression, and negative social relationships. Some survivors of IPV may be formally diagnosed as having PTSD if their symptoms meet the criteria in the *Diagnostic and Statistical Manual of Mental Disorders* (American Psychiatric Association [APA], 2013).

Some characteristics of PSTD sufferers include a re-experiencing of the traumatic event through dreams, flashbacks, or recollections. They also may have a distorted sense of self-blame or blame of others, become estranged from others, have diminished interest in activities, difficulty sleeping, or being aggressive, reckless, or engage in self-destructive behavior (APA, 2013).

Leaving an abusive relationship is extremely difficult and the most dangerous time because most homicides occur shortly after separation (Campbell, 2004b). Most women report IPV to at least one person in their social network, often a family member or friend. They disclose less frequently to health professionals. In a study on disclosure, women found that the most helpful reactions were emotional support, allowing the woman to talk, giving helpful advice and providing useful or practical support. Negative responses included encouraging the woman to leave the abuser, giving unhelpful advice or minimizing the problem, avoiding the victim, or showing annoyance when the woman did not leave or take advice, or being angry at the abuser (Sylaska & Edwards, 2013).

Health professionals can also become frustrated by women they see repeatedly who have numerous signs of abuse but seem unable to liberate themselves from the battering relationships. As with other human dynamics that are not easily explained, health professionals and others may rationalize the woman's behaviors to justify their own lack of involvement. A number of misconceptions are used to account for the woman's perceived self-destructive behavior. If nurses and other professionals believe these misconceptions, they may become judgmental (such as blaming the victim) or respond in unhelpful ways, rather than being empathic and empowering women to take control over their lives (Westbrook, 2009). Empowerment is built on respect for the woman. Providing supportive empathy, validation, and information that can be lifesaving is empowering behavior. Table 5-1 lists some myths and facts about IPV.

TABLE 5-1 Myths and Facts about Intimate Partner Violence

MYTHS	FACTS
Intimate partner violence (IPV) occurs in a small percentage of the population.	One fourth of all women experience IPV.
Being pregnant protects a woman from IPV.	From 4% to 8% of all women who experience violence experience it during pregnancy. IPV frequently begins or escalates in frequency and intensity during pregnancy. Pregnancy may be the result of forced sex or of the man's control of contraception.
IPV occurs only in "problem" or lower-class families.	IPV can occur in any family. Although lower-class families have a higher reported incidence of IPV, it also occurs in middle- and upper-income families. Incidence is not really known because of the tendency of middle- and upper-income families to hide their IPV.
IPV women like to be beaten and deliberately provoke the attack. They are masochistic.	Women are terrified of their assailants and go to great lengths to avoid a confrontation. In some cases the woman may provoke her partner to release tension that if left unchecked might lead to a more severe beating and possible death.
Only men with psychologic problems abuse women.	Many batterers are successful professionals, including politicians, ministers, physicians, and lawyers. Research indicates that only a small number of abusers have psychologic problems.
Only people who come from abusive families end up in abusive relationships.	Most abused women report that their partner was the first person to abuse them.
Alcohol and drug abuse cause IPV.	Although alcohol may be involved in abusive incidents, it is not the cause. Many batterers use alcohol as an excuse to be violent, and shift the blame to the alcohol.
Women would leave the relationship if the abuse were really that bad.	Those women who stay in the relationship do so out of fear and financial dependence. Shelters have long waiting lists.
Victims and perpetrators of IPV cannot change.	Counseling may effectively help both victims and abusers of women.

Data from Gelles, R. (1997). *Intimate violence in families* (3rd ed.). Thousand Oaks, CA: Sage; National Institute on Alcohol Abuse and Alcoholism. (1997). Alcohol, violence, and aggression. *Alcohol Alert, 38,* 1-6; Office of Women's Health, U.S. Department of Health and Human Services. (2011). *Violence against women.* Available at www.womanshealth.gov/violence-against-women/index.html

Reporting rates may not reflect the magnitude of the problem because many women do not disclose violence out of fear or embarrassment or because they are not asked about IPV by their health care providers.

Since 1994 there has been a growing official acknowledgment of IPV across the globe. In 1994 the United States enacted the Violence Against Women Act (VAWA), followed by Guatemala and El Salvador in 1996, China in 1997, Colombia in 2000, and Japan in 2001. Mexico passed its first law in 2007 (Montalvo-Liendo, 2009). Women from almost all cultures identify fear as a common factor in IPV.

An important cultural consideration relates to refugees and immigrants. Immigrant women face unique challenges related

Cultural Considerations

IPV is seen in all countries, cultures, races, ethnicities, religions, and socioeconomic backgrounds (Breiding, Ziembroski, & Black, 2009; WHO, 2013a). In the United States, Caucasian women report less IPV than do non-Caucasians. Native American and Alaska Native women report significantly more instances of IPV than do women of any other racial background; Asian women report significantly less IPV than do other racial groups (Montalvo-Liendo, 2009; Tjaden & Thoennes, 2006).

to their noncitizen status as well as their unfamiliarity with the health care and legal systems. The objectification of women and power inequalities in human social arrangements support the abuse of women. These are especially apparent in any social or cultural system of oppression. The cross-cultural meaning of violence is difficult to ascertain because cultures also differ in their perceptions and definitions of abuse. Finding accurate data about the incidence and prevalence of violence in ethnic groups has been challenging because the groups are infrequently represented in research studies, and violence may be underreported as a result of cultural norms. For example, groups that distrust police or immigration officials may not report abuse because they fear repercussions.

Nurses must be sensitive to immigrant women and their intimate partners because acculturation is gradual, and cultural expectations from their birth countries may heavily influence beliefs and behaviors. Nurses must consider all forces that shape a woman's identity—ethnicity, race, class, language, citizenship, religion, and culture—while recognizing that abuse is against the law and injurious to the health and well-being of women and children (and men). Becoming familiar with the client's cultural influences and increasing the numbers of nurses from various ethnic groups will increase the opportunity to provide culturally appropriate care. The following paragraphs describe some of the cultural variations, but this must be understood with caution in that not all members of a cultural group conform to the general norms of that group. In other words, it is important to understand and respect cultural differences, while also recognizing that there can be individual variation within a group.

African-American Culture. The African-American culture supports unity among humans, nature, and the spiritual world, and social connectedness and relatedness as important norms. African-American men are more likely to be psychologically, socially, and economically oppressed and discriminated against. Violence may occur more frequently as a result of anger generated by environmental stresses and limited resources (Campbell, D., Sharps, Gary, et al., 2002). Respondents to the NISVS reported 43.7% lifetime prevalence of rape, physical violence, and/or stalking by an intimate partner (Black, Basile, & Breiding, et al., 2011). The devalued status of the female survivor, racial stereotype, and fear of putting another African-American man in jail, may be barriers to African-American women seeking and receiving help (Morrison, Luchok, Richter, & Parra-Medina, 2006). In a study of 431 women of African descent, the severity of abuse was significantly associated with mental health problems but not associated with the use of mental health services (Sabri, Bolyard, McFadgion, et al., 2013).

Hispanic (and Latino) Cultures. Hispanic (or Latino) describes someone whose country of origin is Mexico, the largest group at 63%, followed by Puerto Rico, Cuba, Spanish-speaking Central and South American countries, or other Spanish cultures (U.S. Census Bureau, 2011). Thus Hispanics range from newly immigrated and strongly influenced by their native culture to second-generation or later Americans steeped in U.S. popular culture. It is difficult to generalize on culture among these groups. When data are collected, Americans who are of Hispanic descent may be grouped with those born in other countries. Despite the rapidly changing Hispanic population in the United States there have been few studies of IPV differences based on Hispanic country of origin (Cummings, Gonzalez-Guarda, & Sandoval, 2013; Kantor, Jasinski, & Aldarondo, 1994). In a study of South and Central American women, Colombian women reported less IPV than other Central or South American countries (Gonzalez-Guarda, Vermeesch, Florom-Smith, et al., 2013).

Hispanics as a group are described as family oriented with a strong family network in which unity, cooperation, respect, and loyalty are important. Traditional families, as with most immigrant groups, are very hierarchic, with authority often given to older adults, parents, and men. Sex roles are clearly delineated. Employment, higher income, being retired, and marriage are consistently found to be protective factors against IPV in Hispanics (Caetano, Ramisetty-Mikler, & Harris, 2010). Hispanics in the United States have been found to have a slightly higher prevalence of IPV (37%) than non-Hispanic white women (34.6%) (Black et al., 2011). In one study, researchers found that they had significantly more mental health issues than non-Hispanic women who experienced IPV (Bonomi, Anderson, Cannon, et al., 2009). Another difference is in the characteristics of the abusive relationship. In one study the partners of Hispanic women were more likely to have alcohol problems and to force sex but less likely to own a gun, use illegal drugs, or threaten suicide than non-Hispanics in abusive relationships (Glass, Perrin, Hanson, et al., 2009).

Native American Culture. Empiric evidence about abuse in the Native American culture is limited (Duran, Oetzel, Parker, et al., 2009). Native American and Alaska Native women report the highest rates of IPV in the United States with the prevalence of physical violence by an intimate partner at 46%. Rape and stalking were not reported by this group (Black et al., 2011). Research indicates the IPV occurs within the context of complex racial and unique sociocultural factors. Oetzel and Duran (2004) proposed an ecologic framework to guide health care providers in understanding the causes and possible areas for intervention with Native Americans and Alaska Natives.

Asian Culture. Asian women in the United States have the lowest prevalence of IPV at 19.6% (Black et al., 2011). In contrast, the international rates are significantly higher. The prevalence of IPV in Southeast Asia is the highest in the world at 37.7% (WHO, 2013a). It is likely that the lower rate is a function of underreporting. One challenge in the United States is that Asian women are often artificially grouped into one homogeneous group despite their vast and varied cultures. The reasons for not disclosing IPV vary across cultures. Women from South Asia, including Afghanistan, Bangladesh, Bhutan, Sri Lanka, India, the Maldives, Nepal, and Pakistan, were reported to be worried about immigrant laws, were concerned about family honor, and believed that men had the right to abuse. Urban women from Bangladesh were fearful of being killed, felt helpless, and were worried about community retaliation and judgment (Naved, Azim, Bhuiya, & Persson, 2006). Jordanian women expressed fear, shame, religious beliefs, and lack of social support as reasons for not disclosing. The majority of Jordanian men and women deny the problem of wife abuse and oppose discussions of it in society, a reflection of this patriarchal society (Btoush & Haj-Yahia, 2008). Chinese women reported they were worried that they would be criticized and were fearful of not saving face and disappointing relatives. Japanese women reported feeling shame, fearful of escalating violence, and victim blaming (Yoshihama, 2002). Vietnamese women put the needs of the family before their individual needs and kept the woman's role subordinate to men to maintain harmony in the family (Shiu-Thornton, Senturia, & Sullivan, 2005).

Intimate Partner Violence During Pregnancy

IPV has serious consequences for the health of the mother and fetus. The prevalence of IPV during pregnancy is unclear, but the CDC (2012) estimates that 324,000 pregnant women experience it annually and may be more common than the conditions for which pregnant women are normally screened, such as gestational diabetes and preeclampsia. Daoud, Urquia, O'Campo, et al., (2012) estimated that there was a prevalence of 6% of abuse in pregnant women. Women who are abused before pregnancy may continue to be abused during the pregnancy.

Some clinicians believe that abuse may begin or escalate with pregnancy, but some studies suggest that both lethal and nonlethal abuse can actually decrease during pregnancy in some couples (Taylor & Nabors, 2009). In a small longitudinal study, Macy, Martin, Kupper, Casanueva, & Guo (2007) found that rates of physical abuse among women with a history of recent abuse peaked during the first 3 months of pregnancy, then declined, whereas women without a recent history of abuse had low rates of abuse during pregnancy. Thus pregnancy may be protective for some women. In the same study, rates of psychologic abuse were highest in the first month after the birth, as was sexual abuse. Rates of IPV in pregnancy vary by country, from 1% in Japan to 28% in Peru (WHO, 2011).

It is clear that IPV has negative effects on pregnancy. Maternal complications of depression, suicide, low weight gain, infections, and substance abuse have been related to being in an abusive relationship (Campbell, J., Jones, Dienemann, et al., 2002; Plichta, 2004). GI symptoms may occur from chronic stress, as may hypertension and chest pain. Other conditions are gynecologic problems such as STIs, bleeding, UTIs, chronic pelvic pain, and genital trauma. A history of abuse prior to the pregnancy is associated with a higher risk of postpartum depression (Records & Rice, 2009).

Homicide is the leading cause of trauma death in pregnancy and postpartum (Chang, Berg, Saltzman, & Herndon, 2005; Horon & Cheng, 2005). Estimates are that 16% to 66% of pregnancy-related murders are by intimate partners. IPV may be a risk factor for suicide attempts in pregnancy (Martin, Macy, Sullivan, & Magee, 2007).

Not only is physical abuse harmful to the mother, the risk of fetal injury also is very high. Trauma can result in low birth weight, preterm birth, fetal demise, premature separation of placenta, hemorrhage, infections, and other injuries (Morland, Leskin, Block, et al., 2008; Shah & Shah, 2010). Higher rates of IPV at 6 months postpartum have been associated with more depression in mothers at 15 months and subsequent harsh parenting at 24 months (Gustafsson & Cox, 2012).

Pregnant adolescents may be abused at higher rates than are adult women, so they should be considered at higher risk. There is a greater likelihood of unintended pregnancy in adolescents who often delay prenatal care (Plichta, 2004). Physical abuse and pregnancy in teenagers constitute a particularly difficult situation. Adolescents may be more trapped in the abusive relationship than adult women because of their inexperience. They may ignore the violence because the jealous and controlling behavior is interpreted as love and devotion. Because pregnancy in adolescent girls is frequently the result of sexual abuse, feelings about the pregnancy should be assessed. Teens report abuse from partners, former partners, and family members (Renker, 2002). Many who had been abused throughout the pregnancy also were abused afterward, and others who were not abused during pregnancy reported initial abuse after giving birth (Harrykissoon, Rickert, & Wiemann, 2002). Adolescents have been found to be at very high risk for abuse in the postpartum period. Quinlivan and Evans (2005) found that IPV and drug abuse in adolescents affected maternal attachment and infant temperament.

CARE MANAGEMENT

The nurse has an important role in assisting victims and survivors of IPV. Preparation for that role begins with the nurse's own self-assessment. Dienemann, Glass, & Hyman (2005) found that women want health care providers who provide documentation, protection, and immediate response; give options; and be there for the survivor later. They also want to be treated with respect and concern. An exploration of attitudes toward women in abusive situations, awareness of thoughts and emotions that can lead to unhelpful communication, and knowledge about the many aspects of IPV are preparations for care. One challenge for health care providers such as nurses is the tension between wanting to make things better and the reality that IPV is complex and not easily fixed (Williston & Lafreniere, 2013).

Exactly what drives a woman to seek assistance is not clear. Women who belong to any of the following three groups are more likely to seek assistance: (1) those who are beaten frequently and severely; (2) those who have not experienced or witnessed family violence in their family of origin; and (3) those who see an alternative to life in an abusive relationship, specifically women with jobs. Sometimes women seek help after their children have been hurt or when their children start imitating the abuser's behavior.

Women experiencing IPV may be reluctant to seek help for various reasons, including the need to avoid the stigma associated with the nature of the family violence; the fear that they will not be believed; the fear of reprisal from their husbands or partners; and in some states in which battering is a reportable crime, the desire to avoid involvement with police.

Assessment

Clients in any women's health care setting may be at risk for abuse. Nurses are encouraged to assess for abuse in all women entering the health care system (McFarlane, Campbell, Sharps, & Watson, 2002). Health care providers may be the first and only contact that a socially isolated woman makes with someone outside the relationship (ACOG, 2012). Failure to identify IPV and to recognize the risk of serious injury or even death further endangers the lives of women and their children.

LEGAL TIP: Mandatory Reporting of Domestic Violence

Domestic violence is considered a crime in all states, but it varies between being categorized a misdemeanor and a felony, the majority calling it a misdemeanor. Mandatory reporting of domestic violence is controversial. Mandatory reporting is considered appropriate in child abuse because a minor is unable to make an informed decision about his or her own safety. In domestic violence situations involving adults, mandatory reporting takes away a woman's right to make informed decisions and may put her in danger. The Association of Women's Health, Obstetric and Neonatal Nurses (AWHONN) and the American College of Obstetricians and Gynecologists (ACOG) oppose mandatory reporting (ACOG, 2012; AWHONN Board of Directors, 2007). Few states have mandatory reporting for domestic violence of any kind. Forty states and the District of Columbia have laws that mandate reporting by health care providers only in situations in which the woman has an injury that may be caused by a deadly weapon. Some states also require reports when there is a reason to believe that the woman's injury may have resulted from an illegal act or an act of violence. California has the strongest reporting law. Colorado, New Mexico, and Kentucky mandate that health care providers report injuries resulting from IPV to law enforcement or public welfare. Ohio mandates that IPV be documented in the medical record. Rhode Island requires that domestic violence injuries be reported for statistical purposes only. Texas mandates that IPV be documented and that clients be informed that IPV is against the law and be offered shelter referral.

Because of the wide variation from state to state in mandatory reporting, nurses must be knowledgeable about the reporting requirements of the state in which they practice. The website www.futureswithoutviolence.org can be a useful resource for nurses.

A woman suspected of being emotionally abused or physically threatened or abused should be examined and interviewed in private. Some women with male partners may feel safer with a female health care provider. Nurses should *never* ask about abuse with a partner present because this may place the woman in danger and decrease the likelihood for disclosure. When one is taking a psychosocial history, the following information provides clues to violence or potential for violence: does the woman feel safe at home with her partner, how do the woman and her partner resolve conflict, what happens when the woman's partner becomes angry, does fighting occur during disagreements, and if fighting occurs, does it ever escalate to restraining or physical means. It may help the woman to disclose information if these events are normalized by the nurse stating, "Many people [families] have difficulty in expressing anger or dealing with conflict. What is that like for you and your partner?" The nurse listens for any evidence of power and control in the relationship. While inquiring about abuse, trauma, or injuries, the nurse should ask directly if the woman has been injured by her husband or intimate partner. Have you ever been physically abused by your partner or someone important to you? Confusion can occur when vague terms like "he disrespects me" or even labels like "domestic violence" or "abuse" are used. The following are examples of direct questions the nurse can ask:

- Has your partner hit, slapped, kicked, or otherwise hurt you?
- Do you (or did you) feel controlled or isolated by your partner?
- Do you feel safe in your relationship? Do you ever feel afraid of your partner?
- Has your partner or anyone forced you to have sexual activities that made you uncomfortable?

Women who are safe in a current relationship may still carry the physical and emotional consequences of previous trauma.

- Has any of this happened to you in previous relationships?

These questions give a woman permission to disclose sensitive information (Chamberlain & Levenson, 2010).

The Center for Research on Women with Disabilities (2002) recommends the following additional questions for women with disabilities:

- Has anyone ever prevented you from using a wheelchair, cane, or other devices you need?
- Has your partner refused to help you or threatened to not help you with important personal needs like taking medicine, getting dressed, getting food, or other personal needs?

Assessment tools such as the one in Figure 4-10 in Chapter 4 give the nurse useful information and are an important part of the interview. Patterns of violence in relationships can change over time and reports show an increase in the identification of victims of domestic violence when the nurse inquires at each visit whether a woman has been hit or threatened since her last visit (Macy et al., 2007; Walton-Moss & Campbell, 2002). Cues to abuse are delay in seeking medical assistance (hours or days), missed appointments, vague explanation of injuries, nonspecific somatic complaints, social isolation, lack of eye contact, a husband or partner who does not want to leave the woman alone with the primary health care provider, and substance abuse.

For some abused women, day-to-day survival is exhausting. They may cope by denying to the nurse the probabilities of impending abuse, severity of injury, future recurrence, and death. Women may be embarrassed about their abusive relationships and believe the abuse is caused by their inadequacies. Other abused women may cope by denying to themselves that their partner's violent behavior will happen again. By asking a woman directly about abuse, telling her that similar injuries are common in women who have been abused, and pointing out that she is not responsible for another's violent behavior, the nurse may help her to disclose the violence she is experiencing.

In the United States a pregnant woman may be accompanied by her husband to the antepartum appointment. This is especially true if the woman does not speak English and the husband does. The use of an interpreter is preferred over the partner, child, or other person accompanying the woman; it may be useful for the interpreter to be a woman and important that the interpreter communicate the nurse's sensitivity and concern accurately. All women should be seen for some part of the visit without the partner or children present.

During pregnancy the nurse should assess for abuse at each prenatal visit and on admission to labor, although it is not appropriate to ask questions during active labor. Assessment for abuse continues after birth because abuse may begin or escalate then; well-baby clinics and pediatric settings may be important settings for screening women for abuse (Cruz, Cruz, Weirich, et al., 2013; Martin, Macy, Sullivan, & Magee, 2007).

Assessment techniques are straightforward but do require the nurse to be comfortable asking about this socially stigmatized issue. Of utmost importance for women who disclose that they are experiencing or have experienced IPV (or sexual assault, another hidden trauma) is to validate that they have been heard. The nurse might say something like, "What you have just told me is very important, I'm glad you have shared this with me; no one has the right to hurt you this way." It can be demoralizing when, despite taking the risk to disclose, the health care provider does not acknowledge the importance of what has just been said. The next important step is to establish the woman's safety at the moment and in the future. Psychosocial assessment findings may indicate symptoms of anxiety, insomnia, self-directed abuse, depression, smoking, and drug or alcohol abuse (Downs & Rindels, 2004; Gerber, Gantz, Lichter, et al., 2005; WHO, 2013b). During the physical examination, the woman should be observed for injuries to the face, breasts, abdomen, and buttocks. These injuries may be old or new and may range from minor bruising to serious. Other physical signs include fractures that required significant force or that would rarely occur by accident; multiple injuries at various stages of healing; and patterns left by whatever might inflict injury, such as teeth, utensils, fists, or hot objects.

Nursing Interventions

A therapeutic relationship and skillful interviewing help women disclose and describe their abuse. Language is important when talking with women. A major factor in addressing abuse is to identify the woman as a survivor, not a victim. Victim connotes someone who is harmed, is made to suffer, and may have little or no control. Survivor is an empowering term that connotes coping and decision making in relation to taking control of one's life. The nurse might ask the woman how she sees herself. Women who have identified their abuse may appear passive, hostile, anxious, depressed, or hysterical because they may think they are at the mercy of the man's temper. In addition, they may be embarrassed, afraid, angry, sad, or shocked. Transitioning to a different self-image takes time, persistence, and support. A tool that provides a framework for sensitive nursing interventions is the *ABCDES* of caring for the abused woman (Campbell & Furniss, 2002):

- *A* is reassuring the woman that she is not *alone.* The isolation and denigration by the abuser keep her from knowing that others are in the same situation and that health care providers can help.
- *B* is expressing the *belief* that violence against the woman is not acceptable in any situation and that it is not her fault; no one deserves to be hurt or mistreated. This may be the first step in empowering her to think about self-protection and acceptable boundaries.
- *C* is *confidentiality* of the information being shared, particularly because the woman may believe that if the abuse is reported, the perpetrator will retaliate (and in reality, this may happen). Explain the mandatory reporting laws, when applicable.
- *D* is for descriptive *documentation* and includes the following: (1) the woman's quoted statement, "My husband punched me," a clear statement by the woman about the abuse. It should not include her subjective opinion, such as "I provoked the abusive behavior"; (2) accurate descriptions of injuries and a history of the first, worst, and most recent incident of violence may be included; and (3) with the woman's consent, evidence, or photographs (Box 5-2).
- *E* is for *education,* especially that violence is likely to recur and escalate. Education about options including community resources such as where a woman can be referred for help and information about local shelters; for example, National Domestic Violence/Abuse Hotline—800-799-SAFE. Ask if she knows how to obtain a restraining order.
- *S* is for *safety,* the most significant part of the intervention because one of the most dangerous times for a woman is when she decides to leave. Tell the woman to call 911 if she is in imminent danger, and to consider alerting neighbors to call the police if they hear or see signs of conflict. A safety plan should be developed. The safety plan will be adapted based on whether the woman chooses to stay in the relationship or leave. The woman may be conflicted and need support as she goes through a decision-making process (Glass, Eden, Bloom, & Perrin, 2009). The woman can be offered a telephone to call the shelter if she chooses. If she chooses to go back to the abuser, a safety plan includes necessities for a quick escape: a bag packed with personal items for an overnight stay (can be hidden or left with a neighbor), money or a checkbook, an extra set of car keys, and any legal documents to use for identification. Legal

BOX 5-2 Documenting Abuse

Documentation can be useful to women later in court should they choose to press charges or obtain child support, custody, or alimony. Medical records are most helpful if the examiner:

- Takes photographs of the injuries known or believed to have been caused by domestic violence
- Writes clearly
- Sets off the woman's words in quotation marks and uses such phrases as "client states" to indicate the information recorded reflected the woman's words. Describes the offender and the event in the words of the woman, for example, the client said, "My husband kicked me in the stomach."
- Avoids such legalistic phrases as "woman claims" or "woman alleges" that cast doubt about the truth of the statements. Avoids terms such as "alleged perpetrator." If the health care provider's observations differ from the woman's account of the victimization, states the reason for the difference.
- Does not summarize a client's report in conclusive terms that lack the supporting factual information, for example, "the client is a battered woman" because it will render the report inadmissible. In the same theme, does not place the term "domestic violence" in the diagnosis section of the medical record because it does not convey factual information and is not medical terminology.
- Describes the woman's demeanor, whether she is crying, shaking, angry, calm, laughing, or sad, even if it belies the evidence of abuse
- Records the time of day of the examination and indicates whenever possible how much time has passed since the abuse

NURSING CARE PLAN

The Woman Experiencing Intimate Partner Violence

NURSING DIAGNOSIS	EXPECTED OUTCOME	NURSING INTERVENTIONS	RATIONALES
Risk for Self-Directed Violence related to history of abuse by partner as evidenced by physical injuries	Woman will identify dynamics of violence in her unique relationship and develop plan for safety	Provide opportunity to verbalize feelings in a nonthreatening atmosphere.	To give emotional support
		Be alert for cues indicative of abuse.	To provide database for interventions
		Provide information on options available to women experiencing intimate partner violence (IPV) (e.g., counseling, shelters, legal assistance).	To provide information in developing a plan for safety for herself and any children
		Refer to social services and support groups.	To give further information and share experiences
Social Isolation related to stigma of abuse as evidenced by behaviors of withdrawal	Woman will demonstrate an increase in social contacts	Provide private opportunity to express feelings of aloneness.	To initiate and maintain a therapeutic relationship
		Support opportunities for social interaction.	To increase feelings of self-worth and self-confidence
		Encourage interaction with groups for socialization and support.	To increase number of social contacts
Compromised Family Coping related to situational crisis	Family will identify feelings and the need for support during this situational crisis	Provide an appropriate time and place for therapeutic communication.	To promote trust and allow expression of feelings
		Identify effective coping mechanisms.	To provide the family with a foundation of familiar interventions
		List support systems available.	To assist the family to use outside resources
		Refer the woman and family to counseling and social services.	To provide ongoing support

options, such as those for restraining orders or arrest of the perpetrator, also are important aspects of the safety plan. A restraining order can be obtained 24 hours a day from the county court or police department. Many communities have battered women's hotlines where they can get counseling. Pennell and Francis (2005) identified safety conferencing as a means of building the individual and collective strength to assist women to reshape connections, make sound choices, and promote their safety (see Nursing Care Plan).

One part of safety planning is trying to sort out the potential danger in a relationship. A validated danger assessment tool (Fig. 5-3) was designed to assess the level of violence in a relationship and to identify abused women who are at risk of being murdered (Campbell, 2004a; Campbell, Webster, & Glass, 2009). The nurse and the abused woman can go through the tool collaboratively. Online training and permission to use the tool are available at www.dangerassessment.com.

If the woman is pregnant, collaboration with maternity nurses who will be involved in her care during the pregnancy may be helpful. Each nurse can plan care that will point out the woman's strengths and increase her self-esteem. The husband or partner may attend prenatal visits and classes and is included in other ways if the woman chooses to stay with him. The first days after birth are particularly crucial because the mother is physically and emotionally vulnerable and usually tired, and the baby's crying may be intolerable to both the father and the mother. The danger of abuse to mother and child is acute during this time. Facilitating the woman's establishment of a support network of maternity and pediatric staff, community health nurses, and shelter and parental crisis center personnel is important during this crucial period. Referral to resources and provision for follow-up examination by health care providers also should be part of the nursing intervention.

Nurses sometimes become frustrated when a woman returns to a previously abusive situation (Davis, Park, Kaups, et al., 2003; Williston & Lafreniere, 2013). It is important to remember that many women have been abused for a long time, which may make it difficult for them to seek and accept help. Women in repeatedly abusive situations may have lost their ability to perceive the possibility of success and may have become very passive. In addition to understanding the many reasons women stay in abusive relationships, recognizing that the most dangerous period for a woman is when she is in the process of leaving may help nurses to be less judgmental about the woman's dilemma.

A woman may indicate her readiness to leave the relationship when she believes that she is capable of planning for herself, investing in herself, and recognizing that the abuse is part

DANGER ASSESSMENT

Jacquelyn C. Campbell, Ph.D., R.N.
Copyright, 2003; www.dangerassessment.com

Several risk factors have been associated with increased risk of homicides (murders) of women and men in violent relationships. We cannot predict what will happen in your case, but we would like you to be aware of the danger of homicide in situations of abuse and for you to see how many of the risk factors apply to your situation.

Using a calendar, please mark the approximate dates during the past year when you were abused by your partner or ex-partner. Write on that date how bad the incident was according to the following scale:

1. Slapping, pushing; no injuries and/or lasting pain
2. Punching, kicking; bruises, cuts, and/or continuing pain
3. "Beating up"; severe contusions, burns, broken bones
4. Threat to use weapon; head injury, internal injury, permanent injury
5. Use of weapon; wounds from weapon

(If **any** of the descriptions for the higher number apply, use the higher number.)

Mark **Yes** or **No** for each of the following. ("He" refers to your husband, partner, ex-husband, ex-partner, or whoever is currently physically hurting you.)

________ 1. Has the physical violence increased in severity or frequency over the past year?
________ 2. Does he own a gun?
________ 3. Have you left him after living together during the past year?
3a. (If you have *never* lived with him, check here________)
________ 4. Is he unemployed?
________ 5. Has he ever used a weapon against you or threatened you with a lethal weapon?
(If yes, was the weapon a gun?________)
________ 6. Does he threaten to kill you?
________ 7. Has he avoided being arrested for domestic violence?
________ 8. Do you have a child that is not his?
________ 9. Has he ever forced you to have sex when you did not wish to do so?
________ 10. Does he ever try to choke you?
________ 11. Does he use illegal drugs? By drugs, I mean "uppers" or amphetamines, "meth", speed, angel dust, cocaine, "crack", street drugs or mixtures.
________ 12. Is he an alcoholic or problem drinker?
________ 13. Does he control most or all of your daily activities? For instance: does he tell you who you can be friends with, when you can see your family, how much money you can use, or when you can take the car? (If he tries, but you do not let him, check here:________)
________ 14. Is he violently and constantly jealous of you? (For instance, does he say "If I can't have you, no one can.")
________ 15. Have you ever been beaten by him while you were pregnant? (If you have never been pregnant by him, check here:________)
________ 16. Has he ever threatened or tried to commit suicide?
________ 17. Does he threaten to harm your children?
________ 18. Do you believe he is capable of killing you?
________ 19. Does he follow or spy on you, leave threatening notes or messages on answering machine, destroy your property, or call you when you don't want him to?
________ 20. Have you ever threatened or tried to commit suicide?

________ Total "Yes" Answers

Thank you. Please talk to your nurse, advocate or counselor about what the Danger Assessment means in terms of your situation.

FIG 5-3 Danger assessment tool. (From Campbell, J. [2004]. *Danger assessment.* Available at www.dangerassessment.org; Campbell, J., Webster, D., & Glass, N. [2009]. The danger assessment: Validation of a lethality risk assessment instrument for intimate partner femicide. *Journal of Interpersonal Violence, 24*(4), 653-674.)

of a continuing pattern. She also needs to believe that she will have economic and other resources to "make it" on her own. Going to a shelter may be an option; however, shelter stays are typically limited to 30 to 90 days, and therefore a long-term plan must be in place. Also, her being in a shelter may make the husband or partner angrier. Nurses can be helpful in directing women to sources of information, continuing to be expert listeners, and offering encouragement as women struggle in their decision-making process toward freedom and control in their lives.

Prevention

Screening is a common approach to preventing the progression of health problems. Currently because research is limited and screening studies were not paired with interventions, there is insufficient evidence to say that universal screening prevents further incidents of IPV in asymptomatic women (ACOG, 2012; MacMillan, Wathen, Jamieson, et al., 2009; Moyer & Force, 2013; WHO, 2013a). Nevertheless, major health care organizations including the U.S. Preventive Services Task Force recommend universal screening of all women (ACOG, 2012; Moyer & Force). Screening alone is not enough, but assessment with adequate intervention can be useful in improving outcomes (Klevens & Saltzman, 2009). Because IPV has been linked to many other health problems such as headaches, GI problems, chronic pain, arthritis, STIs, pelvic pain, substance abuse, depression, PTSD and suicide, women with any of these symptoms should be carefully assessed.

Nurses can make a difference in stopping the violence and preventing further injury. Educating women that abuse is a violation of their rights and facilitating their access to protective and legal services constitute a first step. Other measures that may help women to discourage the risk of abusive relationships are promoting assertiveness and self-defense courses; suggesting support and self-help groups that encourage positive self-regard, confidence, and empowerment; and recommending educational and skills development classes that will enhance independence or at least the ability to take care of oneself (Pennell & Francis, 2005). Classes for learning English can be particularly helpful to immigrant women. Nurses can offer information on local classes. Preventive education with children encourages and teaches them androgynous gender roles: men and women are equal; both can be nurturing; and neither needs to dominate the other or to engage in violent behavior to have needs met. Helping children to gain problem-solving and conflict management skills may eliminate the need for violent solutions to life stresses. Encouraging schoolchildren to form Students Against Violence Everywhere (SAVE) groups (http://nationalsave.org), which is a nationwide pro-peace effort that promotes justice, respect, and love, gives them an appreciation for these qualities in all facets of life. Adolescents benefit from discussion about sex roles, their relationships, and the consequences of the "macho" concept. School nurses can be instrumental in developing and implementing informational activities for adolescents (Walton-Moss & Campbell, 2002). Other means of prevention are to advocate against violence in all arenas and to participate actively in promoting legislation and policies toward stopping violent acts.

SEXUAL VIOLENCE

Sexual violence is a broad term that encompasses a wide range of sexual victimization including sexual harassment, sexual assault, and rape. *Sexual harassment* includes unwelcome degrading sexual remarks, contact, or behavior such as exhibitionism that makes the work or other environment uncomfortable or difficult. Sexual assault refers to intentional unwanted completed or attempted touching of the victim's genitals, anus, groin, or breasts, directly or through clothing as well as by voyeurism (Basile, Chen, Black, & Saltzman, 2007). It also includes exhibitionism, exposing someone to pornography, or displays of images taken of the victim in a private context (CDC, 2014). Rape is a legal term that is defined differently by each state. It usually refers to forced sexual intercourse or penetration of the mouth, anus, or vagina by a body part or object without consent; it may or may not include the use of a weapon. It involves the use of force, threats, or a victim who is incapable of giving consent. The term is a legal and not a medical one. *Molestation* consists of noncoital sexual activity between a child and an adolescent or adult. *Statutory rape* involves penetration as described above by a person who is 18 years or older of a person younger than the age of consent, and the specifics vary from state to state.

The National Intimate Partner and Sexual Violence Survey reported almost 1 of 5 women experienced rape at some time in their lives, and about 1 in 20 women experienced sexual assault other than rape (Black et al., 2011). Based on another national survey of 5000 women, researchers estimated that more than 1 million women from diverse ethnic and social backgrounds are raped each year in the United States (Kilpatrick, Resnick, Ruggiero, et al., 2007). McCauley, Amstadter, Danielson, et al. (2009) reported that almost one third of all sexual assault victims were adolescents when the assault occurred. Rape may occur within intimate, casual, or work relationships. Rapists may be intimate partners or spouses. They may be family members or acquaintances such as friends, neighbors, or dates. Or they may be strangers, police, prison guards, or soldiers. Rape occurs in the general population, in institutional settings such as colleges, in the military, and in prisons.

Why Do Some Men Rape?

Multiple theories exist on the causes of sexual violence from the perspective of the perpetrator (Stinson, Sales, Becker, & American Psychological Association, 2008). Some risk factors for perpetrators include having themselves been sexually abused in childhood; seeing women as sex objects and viewing them negatively, with hostility, or as dangerous; supporting beliefs that justify rape such as male entitlement to sex or that a woman is asking or deserving to be raped because she dresses provocatively. Some perpetrators are conditioned to become aroused to forced sexual violence. Using violent pornography may normalize preexisting sexually aggressive impulses (Casey & Lindhorst, 2009).

Acquaintance rape involves persons who know one another such as friend, neighbor, family member, classmate, date, or acquaintance. If there is a relationship, then trust is violated. Victims may fear retaliation from the assailant or harassment from family or friends who know the person (Rape, Abuse, and Incest National Network [RAINN], 2009).

Stranger rape is the least common type of rape. The assailant may be a total stranger who suddenly attacks the victim in a public place or in the home. Other stranger rapes occur when the assailant has brief contact with the victim prior to the assault, for example, engaging the victim in conversation to earn trust at a bar or party. Women are more likely to report stranger rape than acquaintance rape (Jones, Wynn, Kroeze, et al., 2004).

Sexual assault and rape are considered forcible when there is threat or actual use of force on an unwilling victim. An incapacitated sexual assault or rape occurs when the victim is under the influence of alcohol or drugs, rendering the person unconscious or otherwise unable to give consent. Estimates are that more than half of rapes involve alcohol—as many as half of reported rapes are either drug facilitated or the result of self-induced intoxication. Alcohol is the most common drug associated with sexual assault (Hindmarch, El Sohly, Gambles, & Salamone, 2001; McCauley, Kilpatrick, Walsh, & Resnick, 2013). Alcohol makes it more difficult for women to identify potentially dangerous situations and to resist unwanted sexual advances. A drug-facilitated sexual assault occurs when alcohol and/or drugs are taken unwillingly or unknowingly. The use of date rape drugs such as flunitrazepam (Rohypnol, or "roofies"), gamma-hydroxybutyrate (GHB), ketamine, and carisoprodol (Soma) incapacitate the victim and may produce amnesia. These drugs are potentiated by alcohol, and the combination can be lethal. The frequency with which these drugs are used can be underestimated because they are rapidly excreted, and lab testing has to be done within a few hours of ingestion (Crawford, Wright, & Birchmeier, 2008). Signs indicating that a woman may have been drugged include having no recall after taking a drink laced with the drug, feeling as if sex has occurred but not having any memory of the incident, feeling more intoxicated than what would be a usual response to the amount of alcohol consumed, or feeling fuzzy on awakening.

Not all women report sexual assault to police. Kilpatrick and coworkers (2007) found that only 16% of victims reported. Many factors deter a woman from reporting the crime, so data regarding sexual assaults may underestimate the magnitude of the problem. Women do not report rape because of the associated stigma; embarrassment; guilt that in some way they provoked the assault; fear of retribution from the rapist or his friends; dread of being humiliated and figuratively "raped" again by the criminal justice system publicly; distrust of law enforcement; involvement in illegal substance use; and discouragement generated by the dismally small number of convictions. Rape survivors often fear the reactions of husbands, lovers, friends, family, and children and prefer to suffer alone.

Mental Health Consequences of Sexual Assault

Rape produces long-term mental health consequences similar to those experienced by combat veterans. Most sexual assaults result in minor physical injuries; genital trauma may or may not be apparent. However, the psychologic effect can be severe. Sexual assault and rape are associated with depression, rape-trauma syndrome (RTS) and PTSD, substance abuse, suicidality, and a host of physical disorders including chronic pelvic pain and sexual dysfunction. One third of women seek counseling as a direct result of their sexual assault (Tjaden & Thoennes, 2006).

Why is rape so traumatic? Victims may have been threatened by a weapon, pushed, shoved, overpowered, or coerced. The assailant may have threatened to return and kill the victim if the incident is reported to anyone. In the aftermath victims can be frightened, angry, embarrassed, or ashamed. They can feel betrayed if there was a preexisting relationship with the assailant. Some may withdraw, feeling socially isolated, unable to tell the people closest to them, fearful of being judged or rejected. Some victims are afraid to return to their homes, workplace, or wherever the assault happened. The emotional suffering can take over women's lives and whereas some seek support from family, friends, health care professionals, or police, others may carry this experience silently, never telling anyone (Esposito, 2005).

Rape-Trauma

When humans experience fear, horror, or helplessness after a life-threatening traumatic event such as rape or combat, there is an intense initial stress response. In the first few hours and days an initial neurobiologic dysregulation in the brain interferes with learning new information, making memories, responding to stress, and regulating the level of arousal. In some survivors this dysregulation and other neurobiologic changes persist (Heim & Nemeroff, 2009). For example, in most trauma survivors cortisol levels in the brain rise in response to stress. Emerging research suggests that in people who then develop PTSD, brain cortisol levels, rather than being elevated during stressful events, are low. Some theories suggest that the brain may become oversensitive to cortisol, and minor stress events may cause the person to overreact and major traumas may produce an underreaction (Wheeler, 2008). Variations in brain function and structure are important in understanding the trauma-related symptoms seen in some but not all rape victims. Why do some victims not recover? Suggested possibilities include genetic differences, neuroanatomic differences, sex differences, personality styles, past exposures to stress, and the characteristics and context of the specific trauma and subsequent experiences. Researchers are working on finding specific neurobiopsychologic strategies such as medications and/or therapies that can prevent and treat trauma sequelae like PTSD.

The neurobiologic changes that occur produce an array of symptoms. In the 1970s RTS was identified as a cluster of characteristic symptoms and related behaviors seen in the weeks and months after a rape (Burgess & Holmstrom, 2000). These researchers described three phases (see following). Understanding the pattern of responses that victims may experience is crucial in helping the nurse provide woman-centered supportive and responsive care.

Acute Phase: Disorganization

According to Burgess and Holmstrom (2000) the assault itself marks the beginning of the acute phase of RTS, which can last for several days or up to 3 weeks. Reactions such as shock, denial, and disbelief are common. The rape survivor feels embarrassed, degraded, fearful, angry, and vengeful, and she can blame herself. The victim can feel unclean and want to bathe and douche, although this can destroy evidence. Fear is the primary feeling. Observable reactions can be controlled, expressed, or disoriented. In *controlled emotions* the survivor hides her emotions; has a subdued, calm demeanor; and seems to act as if nothing happened. She may answer questions and interact in a matter-of-fact way. Her affect seems incongruent with what she has just experienced. The second type of acute phase reaction is *expressed emotions.* Here the survivor can appear agitated or hysterical. She can be restless, crying, tense, or anxiously smiling. Her affect can change rapidly from crying to being calm and controlled. She relives the scene over and over in her mind and considers things she "should have done." *Shocked disbelief* or *disorientation* marks the third type of reaction. The victim can feel disoriented, have difficulty concentrating or making decisions, and can have poor recall of the event. Memory can be fragmented and intrusive thoughts can provide bits and pieces of information (Campbell, 2012). Physiologically she can be uncomfortable, experiencing skeletal muscle pain or tension, GI irritability, sighing, hyperventilation, and flushing.

Outward Adjustment Phase

During the adjustment phase the survivor may appear to have resolved her crisis. She may return to a job or to maintaining a household, or both, but she is denying and suppressing her thoughts and feelings. She needs this time to regain some control in her life. She may move, change jobs, buy a weapon to protect herself, or install an alarm system in her home. She may not be able to stop talking about the assault, letting it dominate her life, or she may minimize or suppress the event, refusing to discuss it, acting as if it did not happen. She may try to analyze the details of how it happened, trying to explain how it happened and what the rapist was thinking. She may seek safety by fleeing her job, her home, or making other radical changes. She may experience fear, anxiety, phobias, mood swings, anger and rage, depression, insomnia, hypervigilance, and continued flashbacks. She may withdraw from support systems and be afraid to leave her home or go to certain places. She may develop sexual problems.

Long-Term Process: Reorganization Phase

The third phase is reorganization. Denial and suppression are difficult to maintain. Disclosing personal thoughts and feelings has a profound effect on improving health and reducing stress. As a rape survivor's suppression of feelings and emotions starts to deteriorate, she becomes depressed and anxious. Her own healthy spirit pressures her to discuss the rape with someone. Because she is losing her control of denial, her fears start to surface; she may be afraid to be alone or in a crowd or may fear being attacked from behind. Nightmares and eating disorders are common in these last two phases.

The recovery process can take years and can be difficult and painful. The victim has progressed through recovery when the physical distress and the constant memories of the rape have diminished. She no longer blames herself for what happened and can truly call herself a survivor. These phases are not necessarily linear and survivors can move back and forth between the phases. RTS can meet the criteria for PTSD and be formally diagnosed.

CARE MANAGEMENT

Nurses in women's health care and EDs are most likely to see rape victims in the acute phase. However, all women who manifest any of the signs of other phases should be assessed for posttraumatic experiences (Esposito, 2006). It is important to remember that sexual assault acute care has a dual purpose. First and foremost is to address the health care needs of the woman. The second purpose is to facilitate the collection of evidence and documentation of findings for use by the justice system. Health care is the nurse's first priority.

Facilities that provide initial treatment for rape victims vary in protocols and resources. In its 1992 guidelines, The Joint Commission (TJC) required EDs and ambulatory care departments to have protocols on physical assault; rape or sexual assault; and domestic abuse of older adults, spouses, partners, and children. These protocols must address client consent, examination, and treatment guidelines and the health care facility's responsibility for collecting evidence, photographing injuries, and releasing evidence to law enforcement officials. In addition, the EDs and ambulatory care departments must provide to victims a referral list of community-based and private service agencies dealing with family violence. The nurse interacting with the sexual assault client should be guided by the particular treatment center's protocol. The *National Protocol for Sexual Assault Medical Forensic Exams, Adults/Adolescents*, identifies the unique roles of the many different professionals including sexual assault nurse examiners (SANEs), physicians, police, forensic specialists, prosecutors, and counseling advocacy in the aftercare of a sexual trauma victim (U.S. Department of Justice & Office of Violence Against Women, 2013). Agency or state recommendations for care are continually evolving as new research and forensic techniques emerge.

Many treatment centers have initiated the use of SANEs as described in the above protocols. A SANE is educated in the specialty of forensic nursing and is prepared to examine clients; recognize, collect, and preserve evidence; counsel the client; link the client with vital community resources; follow up cases; and, if necessary, testify in court. When cared for by a SANE, victims receive better quality care, appropriate prophylaxis for infection and pregnancy, and are more satisfied than when cared for in settings without SANEs (Campbell, 2008). Information on becoming a SANE, which currently requires a 40-hour course, is available at www.iafn.org. If a SANE is not available in a particular facility, TJC member organizations must implement a plan for educating an appropriate staff member about identifying, treating, and referring abuse victims. Additional resources can include a social worker who is called when a woman who has been raped is admitted. A local rape crisis center may have volunteers on call who can provide emotional support; provide transportation; help the woman interact with her family, friends, and various authorities; inform her of RTS; and find other resources for her as needed. Male volunteers may counsel male members of the victim's family and her male friends.

Psychologic First Aid

When victims seek help from people in their social network, from the police or from health care settings, the response they get is critical to their healing process. The goal of supportive care is to help victims feel less threatened, feel safer, and have lower levels of anxiety. We do not know which victims will go on to develop PTSD but we do know that negative experiences in the law enforcement and health care system are associated with an increase in PTSD. Research indicates that victims who report and have negative experiences have worse mental health outcomes. The neurobiology of trauma can create for victims a flood of intrusive thoughts. Interviewers, whether law enforcement or health care providers may try to clarify the victim's fragmented story that comes out in bits and pieces. Repeated retelling as well as negative or judgmental feedback has a powerful impact on survivors, and can be experienced as secondary victimization (Campbell, 2008, 2012).

The nurse may be one of the first people to talk with a victim of sexual trauma. Initial distress is not abnormal and most sexual assault victims are able to recover. Even though there is limited evidence for specific treatments to prevent PTSD in sexual assault victims, trauma experts suggest that one promising approach is Psychological First Aid (Litz, 2008). Psychological First Aid has eight core goals that are consistent with and can be easily adapted to nursing practice. They are to: (1) respond when a survivor reaches out to you or when you initiate contact with the survivor, in a nonintrusive, compassionate, and helpful manner; (2) enhance the survivor's safety and provide physical and emotional comfort; (3) stabilize by calming and orienting the survivor if she is emotionally overwhelmed; (4) identify immediate needs and concerns and gather information; (5) offer practical help in addressing needs; (6) offer to help establish contact with personal supports; (7) provide information about stress and coping responses to sexual assault; and (8) link the survivor with community and other services (National Child Traumatic Stress Network and National Center for PTSD, 2006; Ruzek, Brymer, Jacobs, et al., 2007). Nurses who understand postassault experiences can influence the responses of their nursing units, hospital, or institution and community.

The Sexual Assault Examination

Because sexual assault is a crime, the first nurse to see the sexually assaulted client must consider the need to preserve evidence. However, the preservation of evidence should not overshadow a survivor's rights to be treated as a human being with respect, courtesy, and dignity. Client-centered care takes into consideration the psychologic needs of the victim, and the nurse adapts the examination accordingly. There are short- and long-term physical, emotional, and legal implications of this examination. Details are described in the National Protocol for Sexual Assault Medical Forensic Exams, Adults and Adolescents. The following discussion is an overview of the protocol.

LEGAL TIP: Collector of Evidence

Consent forms must be signed before evidence can be collected and released to the police and before photographs can be taken. If the victim is a minor (see individual state laws for age cutoff) a pediatric SANE, or a child sexual assault pediatrician is notified. Child sexual assault is beyond the scope of this chapter. A parent or guardian is required to sign the consent forms. A children's protective service may need to be called to facilitate consent.

Any health care and/or evidence collection is done only with the permission of the woman. She should be informed of all the steps involved in the sexual assault examination, treatment, and follow-up care. Written informed consent for medical care and human immunodeficiency virus (HIV) testing must be obtained. In addition, consent must be obtained for collection and storage of sexual offense evidence, including forensic photography. A signed consent for release of evidence must be obtained. Unless there is a court order, medical records are confidential. The woman can choose to stop her care or the evidence examination at any time. Informed consent includes information on what will happen during the examination, what tests will be done, what treatments can be offered, what risks occur without treatment, and what evidence collection may provide. It is important for the nurse to remember that the examination cannot determine if an assault (nonconsensual sexual encounter) has happened. That is a legal determination that happens in court. The examination provides information that may or may not be consistent with sexual contact. Not all sexual assaults produce trauma, and not all sexual trauma is nonconsensual.

History. History taking is an important step in early care. History includes a statement of the traumatic event whether or not evidence will be collected. The woman needs privacy but should not be left alone. It is important to tell the woman that she is safe, that the incident is not her fault, and that she is not alone in what she has experienced. She also needs assurance of confidentiality and may need a great deal of support and patience in verbalizing the offender's acts. For example, giving the woman permission to describe the situation however she chooses and restating what the client has said (without minimizing) tells the woman she has been heard and ensures that what the nurse documents accurately reflects what she said. It also is important to obtain sexual, gynecologic, and obstetric histories (see Chapter 4).

The medicolegal record in a sexual assault case is likely to be used in court. A key feature used in court to establish rape is the absence of consent. The victim who is developmentally delayed, who is unconscious or otherwise physically unable to move, who has been drugged without her knowledge, or who is a minor (statutory rape) is not capable of giving consent. Bribery, threat, or coercion implies the lack of consent. The nurse's documentation is an important part of the medicolegal record. The wording of the history should reflect the woman's report, and her exact words should be used as often as possible (New York State Department of Health, 2008). When documenting, it is important for the nurse to remember that care is provided to the woman without judgment. Thus nurses should avoid using legal terms or words that suggest value judgments when documenting or referring to the woman. For example use of the term "alleged" or "claims" suggests that the nurse questions the woman's report. It is not the role of the nurse to determine whether a sexual assault occurred but to treat the woman as any other trauma victim. The court must prove absence of consent.

LEGAL TIP: Documentation

Clear, legible, accurate documentation is imperative. The woman's name should be on each page, and date, times, and signatures should be legible. Document an interpreter's name if one was used.

Physical Examination and Laboratory Tests. The nurse can assist with or, if trained, perform the physical examination, which is conducted after the procedure is explained to the woman and consent is obtained. Some victims may view the examination as a second traumatic event. Preservation of the woman's dignity is of utmost importance during the examination. The woman can choose a female attendant, rape counselor, or other person to remain with her during the examination. The room will require standard examination equipment, comfort supplies for the woman, a sexual assault evidence collection kit, a method to dry evidence, a camera, lab testing supplies, a light source, and an anoscope. Some settings also have a colposcope, a microscope, and toluidine blue dye (U.S. Department of Justice &

Office of Violence Against Women, 2013). The physician, nurse practitioner, or SANE informs her of every step of the procedure. The content of the examination is based on the history. For example, if there was oral penetration but no removal of clothing and genital contact, a speculum exam may not be appropriate. However many victims do not recall what happened during parts or all of the assault, and examination of all orifices is suggested. A standardized sexual assault evidence collection kit is used to obtain and package specimens. The kit gives detailed instructions on how to collect and package specimens and other evidence.

If the woman needs to urinate or defecate prior to the examination, the nurse should ask her to avoid wiping away vaginal or other secretions until after evidence is collected. Collect the first voided specimen for possible drug-facilitated sexual assault testing and document the time it was collected. If the woman has a tampon, panty liner, or contraceptive device in the vagina, she should not remove or discard them. The woman remains clothed while her vital signs and blood pressure are determined, and her clothing is inspected for stains, tears, and foreign material. Clothing is handled only by the woman and if pertinent to the assault may be collected, allowed to air dry, and sealed in a bag to be checked for evidence. She is assisted to undress and is draped for the physical examination. Her body is inspected for bruises, swelling, scratches, lacerations, or other wounds. A head-to-toe examination is performed as indicated. Victims can have injuries to other parts of their body including the head, face, and neck. An ultraviolet light (Wood's lamp) is used to find dried secretions on the victim's skin. External genitals, thighs, buttocks, and lower abdomen are assessed, and if there are injuries, bruises, or marks, photographs can be taken or drawings made. Pubic and scalp hair is combed for collection. Perianal, oral, and vaginal swabs are collected. If the victim scratched her attacker, her nails are scraped to obtain material that can aid in identification.

A speculum examination, often using magnification, is performed gently to detect tears or bruises and to collect appropriate specimens. Many victims have some type of genital injury, even if it is asymptomatic. A bimanual pelvic examination is not usually performed for evidence collection if a SANE is doing the examination. Internal pelvic assessment may be done by the nurse practitioner or physician if internal injury is suspected.

Laboratory tests can include oral swabs for the victim's deoxyribonucleic acid (DNA) to distinguish her DNA from the suspect's DNA; a urine or blood pregnancy test; blood tests for hepatitis B virus; and oral or blood tests for HIV (CDC, 2010b). A preexisting pregnancy will affect treatment decisions for possible HIV prophylaxis. Testing for HIV is a typical part of the sexual assault exam; however, HIV status should be checked within 72 hours if the assault was high risk. Cultures for gonorrhea, chlamydia, and syphilis are not recommended because women are treated prophylactically, test results will not change treatment, and testing can have negative consequences in court (Lewis-O'Connor, Franz, & Zuniga, 2005; New York State Department of Health, 2008; U.S. Department of Justice & Office of Violence Against Women, 2013).

During the examination, the woman's emotional status is assessed, and findings are recorded: what reactions she exhibits to the assault; her orientation to time and place; and her attention span, affect, and verbal description and feelings about the assault. The availability of family or peer-support systems is assessed. She is asked about her plans to report the crime to the police. After the examination, the woman should be allowed to shower and offered fresh clothes or a gown. She can be given time to rest and to talk with the nurse, rape crisis counselor, family, or friends.

It is important that the chain of custody be maintained. *Chain of custody* is a legal term that refers to the continual guarding of evidence and describes evidence from the moment that it is first collected until it appears in court. All items of evidence are individually labeled with the name of examiner, client, date, and source. The evidence is never left unattended or with the family, woman, or support person such as an advocate. During the examination chain of custody is the responsibility of the examiner. When evidence is turned over to the next custodian, each person signs that the evidence was given and received. Signing indicates that no one touched or tampered with the evidence during that person's watch. This ensures that the evidence can be used in court.

Immediate Care. Nursing diagnoses for the rape victim during the immediate and later posttrauma period are listed in Box 5-3. Consent is needed for treatment and medical management that includes (1) treating the physical injuries, including tetanus toxoid booster if indicated; (2) providing prophylactic antibiotic therapy for STIs (e.g., chlamydia, gonorrhea); and (3) providing prophylaxis for pregnancy if the woman is not pregnant. If physical trauma is life threatening, appropriate intervention takes precedence over collecting evidence. A pregnancy test

BOX 5-3 Nursing Diagnoses for the Rape Victim During the Immediate and Later Posttrauma Periods

Immediate Posttrauma Period

- *Anxiety/fear* related to:
  —Rape-trauma experience
  —Interactions with police and caregivers
  —Physical examination to assess injury and collect evidence
- *Acute pain* related to:
  —Physical injury from rape
  —Examination
- *Disturbed body image* related to:
  —The rape
- *Rape-trauma* related to:
  —Aftermath of being sexually assaulted
  —Feelings of being unclean and humiliated
  —Silent reaction of being unable to discuss the rape
- *Decisional conflict* related to:
  —Discussing rape with family
  —Possible pregnancy

Later Posttrauma Period

- *Risk for infection* related to:
  —Sexually transmitted infections
  —Sexual assault by an assailant of unknown sexual history
- *Impaired social interaction* related to:
  —The rape
  —Strained relationships with family, friends, intimate partners

should be done on all women at risk for pregnancy (with their consent). Most pregnancy tests are sensitive by 9 days after conception. If the woman is at risk for pregnancy and the pregnancy test is negative, emergency contraception should be offered to her. Emergency contraception (see Table 8-2, Chapter 8) is most effective if used within 120 hours after intercourse. The earlier it is taken, the more effective. The woman should be advised that emergency contraception does not guarantee pregnancy prevention, and that she should repeat the pregnancy test if she has not had a menstrual period within 3 to 4 weeks. She is apprised of the availability of abortion or menstrual extraction as a backup measure. If the woman is pregnant at the time of the assault, she should be observed for several hours for uterine contractility.

The woman can be provided with prophylactic antibiotic therapy to prevent STIs, hepatitis B postexposure prophylaxis (PEP), and if there is a high risk of exposure, for example, if the assailant is known to be infected with HIV, the PEP for HIV may be offered.

Discharge. The woman is discharged with medications and printed instructions about their use, printed instructions for self-care, and names and telephone numbers of resource people if she requires assistance. Money and transportation to wherever she is staying (an alternative place may be found for her) add to the woman's comfort and perception of being in control. A medical follow-up examination in the gynecology or pediatric clinic is scheduled in 1 to 2 weeks for cultures for gonorrhea and other STIs; at 6 weeks for assessment of healing injuries; and at 6, 12, and 24 weeks for repeated serology tests for syphilis and HIV infection if initial test results were negative. The woman and her counselor determine whether there is a need for an additional medical or psychologic follow-up examination between the scheduled visits. The woman has a choice of site for follow-up testing. Some women choose to continue with the health care provider who first performed the examination, some prefer their primary health care provider, and others need referral to a clinic in the area (city, state) in which they live.

Nurses must be aware that responses to sexual assault are variable. Self-blame and humiliation can alternate with anger and fear. The woman needs to be reassured again before she leaves that her feelings are normal and that she is not alone. The initial care of a woman will affect her recovery and her decision to return for follow-up care. Nurses can assist women through an examination that is as nontraumatic as possible, with kindness, skill, and empathy.

After Discharge. Because of the phases of recovery, telephone contact by the health care provider to whomever the woman is referred is continued until the woman has no further need for such help. Education in prevention strategies is often offered by community agencies or rape-awareness groups. The focus of the classes is usually on increasing women's awareness of situations that put them at high risk for rape or sexual assault. Other courses teach self-defense methods or how to change personal behaviors to reduce the risk of being victimized, such as avoiding being alone in isolated places and being alert to unusual activities or persons in one's environment. Still other courses focus on changing societal attitudes about rape. Nurses can play a role in preventive education by offering courses or participating in courses offered by community or health care groups. Nurses must be knowledgeable about the epidemiology of sexual assault, reporting requirements, and services available in their community for victims, and should screen all women for a history of assault and any sequelae.

SEX TRAFFICKING

Human trafficking is a $32 billion business in the United States and internationally (Dovydaitis, 2010). Although the number of U.S. victims is unknown, it is estimated that 14,000 to 50,000 individuals are trafficked each year (ACOG, 2011; National Human Trafficking Resource Center [NHTRC], 2012). Trafficked individuals, mostly women and children, are forced into hard labor, sex work, and even organ donation (Budiani-Saberi, Raja, Findley, et al., 2014; Macy & Graham, 2012). Human sex trafficking is a serious and understudied phenomenon. It is actually the most prevalent form of what is referred to as "modern-day slavery" (USDHHS, 2012; Walker-Rodriguez & Hill, 2011). Sex trafficking refers to a commercial sex act, which is defined as a sex act that is performed under coercion and in exchange for the promise of something of value, such as a job, or if the person is less than 18 years old. Coercion can be psychologic or physical and includes human bondage and threats of serious harm (USDHHS).

Although victims of sex trafficking can be male or female, the vast majority are women and girls, who are lured by false promises, such as a job or a marriage, or are sold by parents or kidnapped by traffickers. Often, once they are enslaved by the traffickers, many of them begin to experience what is referred to as the "Stockholm Syndrome" in which the slaves become attached to their enslavers (De Fabrique, Romano, Vecchi, & Van Hasselt, 2007). It is important to understand that these sex slaves are usually isolated and may not even know where they are (e.g. what city).

The traffickers are often people involved in organized crime internationally but also in the United States (Walker-Rodriguez & Hill, 2011). The three primary sex trafficking U.S. networks are Asian, Latino, and domestic (U.S. citizen) networks (NHTRC, 2012). Sex trafficking can occur in one's neighborhood without neighbors' awareness.

Health care professionals may interact with victims who are in captivity. This provides an opportunity to identify victims, intervene to help them obtain necessary health services, and provide information about ways to escape from their situation. The nurse or other health care provider must be alert to signs and symptoms, such as being accompanied to the visit by another person who appears very controlling, showing signs of being fearful, not being comfortable with answering questions, difficulty communicating, presenting with signs of abuse, and lacking documentation of citizenship (Crane & Moreno, 2011). Victims of sex trafficking also may be younger than 18 years of age and report multiple sex partners, and multiple episodes of STIs, or have evidence of sexual abuse (ACOG, 2011).

The nurse is challenged to create an opportunity to assess for victimization and establish a trusting climate while also

COMMUNITY ACTIVITY

- Research the laws regarding intimate partner violence in your state. Is it considered a misdemeanor or felony crime? Is mandatory reporting of domestic violence by health care providers required? What is the definition of statutory rape in your state? Visit www.futureswithoutviolence.org for information on state statutes and policies on domestic violence.
- What are the resources for victims of intimate partner violence in your community?
- Visit http://nhtrc.polarisproject.org. Find out about the National Human Trafficking Resource Center and the resources and services that may be available in your community.

speaking with the client alone. In 2000 the U.S. government enacted the Trafficking Victims Protection Act, which makes trafficking, including sex trafficking, a federal crime. Health care providers play a critical role in identifying perpetrators and victims of this crime. The NHTRC (1-888-373-7888) can provide assistance.

KEY POINTS

- Violence against women is a major social and health care problem in the United States, costing thousands of lives and billions of dollars in direct and indirect health care costs.
- IPV includes physical, sexual, emotional, psychologic, and economic abuse.
- To provide effective care, nurses must increase awareness of their own beliefs and values regarding victimization of women.
- Theoretic frameworks—psychologic, sociologic, biologic, and feminist perspectives—provide the foundation for understanding the complexity of the victimization of women.
- Cultural influences regarding violent behaviors and relationships sensitize the nurse to the special needs of women from various ethnic groups.
- IPV affects young, middle-aged, and older women of all races; all socioeconomic, educational, and religious groups; and pregnant women.
- All states have mandatory reporting of the abuse of children and older adults; some states have initiated mandatory reporting of domestic abuse. Mandatory reporting is controversial and takes away the right for women to choose.
- Rape is a legal term defined by each state differently but usually refers to penetration of an orifice against someone's will.
- Nurses in all professional areas should respond with sensitivity and caring to women who experience abuse and victimization.
- Follow-up and collaborative care are important in all instances of abuse.
- Nurses should be knowledgeable about reporting requirements and available community services for women who have been sexually assaulted.
- Health care professionals may have an opportunity to identify victims of human sex trafficking, intervene to help them obtain necessary health services, and provide information about ways to escape from their situation.

REFERENCES

American College of Obstetricians and Gynecologists. (2011). ACOG Committee Opinion No. 507: Human trafficking. *Obstetrics and Gynecology, 118*(3), 767–770.

American College of Obstetricians and Gynecologists. (2012). ACOG Committee Opinion No. 518: Intimate partner violence. *Obstetrics and Gynecology, 119* (2 Pt 1), 412–417.

American Psychiatric Association. (2013). *Diagnostic and statistical manual of mental disorders* (5th ed.). Arlington, VA: American Psychiatric Association.

Association of Women's Health, Obstetric and Neonatal Nurses (AWHONN) Board of Directors. (2007). *Mandatory reporting of intimate partner violence.* Available at www.awhonn.org/awhonn/content.do?name=07_PressRoom/07_PositionStatements.htm.

Basile, K., Chen, J., Black, M., & Saltzman, L. (2007). Prevalence and characteristics of sexual violence victimization among U.S. adults, 2001-2003. *Violence and Victims, 22*(4), 437–448.

Black, M. C., Basile, K. C., Breiding, M. J., et al. (2011). *The National Intimate Partner and Sexual Violence Survey (NISVS).* Atlanta: National Center for Injury Prevention and Control, Centers for Disease Control and Prevention.

Blanchfield, L. (2008). *United Nations system efforts to address violence against women.* Available at http:fpc.state.gov/documents/organization/109495.pdf.

Bonomi, A., Anderson, M., Cannon, E., et al. (2009). Intimate partner violence in Latina and non-Latina women. *American Journal of Preventive Medicine, 36*(1), 43–48.

Bonomi, A., Anderson, M., Reid, R., et al. (2009). Medical and psychosocial diagnoses in women with a history of intimate partner violence. *Archives of Internal Medicine, 169*(18), 1692–1697.

Breiding, M., Ziembroski, J., & Black, M. (2009). Prevalence of rural intimate partner violence in 16 US states, 2005. *Journal of Rural Health, 25*(3), 240–246.

Bronfenbrenner, U. (1979). *The ecology of human development: Experiments by nature and design.* Cambridge, MA: Harvard University Press.

Bronfenbrenner, U. (2005). *Making human beings human: Bioecological perspectives on human development.* Thousand Oaks, CA: Sage Publications.

Brown, D., Finkelstein, E., & Mercy, J. (2008). Methods for estimating medical expenditures attributable to intimate partner violence. *Journal of Interpersonal Violence, 23*(12), 1747–1766.

Btoush, R., & Haj-Yahia, M. (2008). Attitudes of Jordanian society toward wife abuse. *Journal of Interpersonal Violence, 23*(11), 1531–1554.

Budiani-Saberi, D. A., Raja, K. R., Findley, K. C., et al. (2014). Human trafficking for organ removal in India: A victim-centered, evidence-based report. *Transplantation* (epubl ahead of print). Available at www.ncbi.nlm.nih.gov/pubmed/24398855.

Burgess, A., & Holmstrom, L. (2000). Rape trauma syndrome. In A. Burgess (Ed.), *Violence through a forensic lens*. King of Prussia, PA: Nursing Spectrum.

Caetano, R., Ramisetty-Mikler, S., & Harris, T. R. (2010). Neighborhood characteristics as predictors of male to female and female to male partner violence. *Journal of Interpersonal Violence, 25*(11), 1986–2009.

Campbell, D., Sharps, P., Gary, F., et al. (2002). Intimate partner violence in African-American women. *Online Journal of Issues in Nursing, 7*(1), 5.

Campbell, J. (2004a). Danger assessment. Available at www.dangerassessment.org.

Campbell, J. (2004b). Helping women understand their risk in situations of intimate partner violence. *Journal of Interpersonal Violence, 19*(12), 1464–1477.

Campbell, J., & Furniss, K. (2002). *Violence against women: Identification, screening and management of intimate partner violence*. Washington, DC: Association of Women's Health, Obstetric and Neonatal Nurses.

Campbell, J., Jones, A., Dienemann, J., et al. (2002). Intimate partner violence and physical health consequences. *Archives of Internal Medicine, 162*(10), 1157–1163.

Campbell, J., Webster, D., & Glass, N. (2009). The danger assessment: Validation of a lethality risk assessment instrument for intimate partner femicide. *Journal of Interpersonal Violence, 24*(4), 653–674.

Campbell, R. (2008). The psychological impact of rape victims. *American Psychologist, 63*(8), 702–717.

Campbell, R. (2012, December 3). *The neurobiology of sexual assault*. Available at http://nij.gov/multimedia/presenter/presenter-campbell/pages/presenter-campbell-transcript.aspx.

Campbell, R., Dworkin, E., & Cabral, G. (2009). An ecological model of the impact of sexual assault on women's mental health. *Trauma, Violence, & Abuse, 10*(3), 225–246.

Cannon, E., Bonomi, A., Anderson, M., & Rivara, F. (2009). The intergenerational transmission of witnessing intimate partner violence. *Archives of Pediatric and Adolescent Medicine, 163*(8), 706–708.

Capaldi, D., & Kim, H. (2007). Typological approaches to violence in couples: A critique and alternative conceptual approach. *Clinical Psychology Review, 27*(3), 253–265.

Casey, E., & Lindhorst, T. (2009). Toward a multi-level, ecological approach to the primary prevention of sexual assault: Prevention in peer and community contexts. *Trauma, Violence, & Abuse, 10*(2), 91–114.

Center for Research on Women with Disabilities. (2002). *Development of the abuse assessment screen-disability (AAS-D).Violence against women with physical disabilities: Final report submitted to the Centers for Diease Control and Prevention*. Houston: Baylor College of Medicine. Available at www.bcm.edu/crowd/index.cfm?pmid=2137.

Centers for Disease Control and Prevention. (2010a). *Intimate partner violence definitions*. Available at www.cdc.gov/ViolencePrevention/intimatepartnerviolence/definitions.html.

Centers for Disease Control and Prevention (CDC). (2010b). Sexually transmitted diseases treatment guidelines 2010. *MMWR Morbidity and Mortality Weekly Report, 59*(RR12), 1–109.

Centers for Disease Control and Prevention. (2012). *Intimate partner violence during pregnancy: A guide for clinicians*. Available at www.cdc.gov/reproductivehealth/violence/intimatepartnerviolence/sld001.htm.

Centers for Disease Control and Prevention. (2013). *Definitions: Intimate partner violence. Injury prevention and control*. Available at www.cdc.gov/violenceprevention/intimatepartnerviolence/definitions.html.

Centers for Disease Control and Prevention. (2014). *Sexual violence: Definitions*. Available at www.cdc.gov/violenceprevention/sexualviolence/definitions.html.

Chamberlain, L., & Levenson, R. (2010). *Reproductive health and partner violence guidelines: An integrated response to intimate partner violence and reproductive coercion*. San Francisco: Family Violence Prevention Fund.

Chang, J., Berg, C., Saltzman, L., & Herndon, J. (2005). Homicide: A leading cause of injury deaths among pregnant and postpartum women in the United States, 1991-1999. *American Journal of Public Health, 95*(3), 471–477.

Crane, P. A., & Moreno, M. (2011). Human trafficking: What is the role of the health care provider? *Journal of Applied Research on Children: Informing Policy for Children at Risk, 2*(1). Article 7. Available at http://digitalcommons.library.tmc.edu/childrenatrisk/vol2/iss1/7.

Crawford, E., Wright, M., & Birchmeier, Z. (2008). Drug-facilitated sexual assault: College women's risk perception and behavioral choices. *Journal of American College Health, 57*(3), 261–272.

Cruz, M., Cruz, P. B., Weirich, C., et al. (2013). Referral patterns and service utilization in a pediatric hospital-wide intimate partner violence program. *Child Abuse and Neglect, 37*(8), 511–519.

Cummings, A. M., Gonzalez-Guarda, R. M., & Sandoval, M. F. (2013). Intimate partner violence among Hispanics: A review of the literature. *Journal of Family Violence, 28*(2), 153–171.

Daoud, N., Urquia, M. L., O'Campo, P., et al. (2012). Prevalence of abuse and violence before, during, and after pregnancy in a national sample of Canadian women. *American Journal of Public Health, 102*(10), 1893–1901.

Davis, J., Park, S., Kaups, K., et al. (2003). Victims of domestic violence on the trauma service: Unrecognized and underreported. *Journal of Trauma, 54*(2), 352–355.

De Fabrique, N., Romano, S. J., Vecchi, G. M., & Van Hasselt, V. B. (2007). Understanding Stockholm syndrome. *FBI Law Enforcement Bulletin, 76*(7), 11–15.

Dienemann, J., Glass, N., & Hyman, R. (2005). Survivor preferences for response to IPV disclosure. *Clinical Nursing Research, 14*(3), 215–233.

Dovydaitis, T. (2010). Human trafficking: The role of the health care provider. *Journal of Midwifery and Women's Health, 55*(5), 462–467.

Downs, W., & Rindels, B. (2004). Adulthood depression, anxiety, and trauma symptoms: A comparison of women with nonabusive, abusive, and absent father figures in childhood. *Violence and Victims, 19*(6), 659–671.

Duran, B., Oetzel, J., Parker, T., et al. (2009). Intimate partner violence and alcohol, drug, and mental disorders among American Indian women in primary care. *American Indian Alaskan Native Mental Health Research, 16*(2), 11–27.

Dutton, M. (2009). *Update of the "battered woman syndrome" critique*. Available at www.vawnet.org.

Esposito, N. (2005). Manifestations of enduring during interviews with sexual assault victims. *Qualitative Health Research, 15*(7), 912–927.

Esposito, N. (2006). Women with a history of sexual assault. Health care visits can be reminders of a sexual assault. *American Journal of Nursing, 106*(3), 69-71, 73.

Faramarzi, M., Esmailzadeh, S., & Mosavi, S. (2005). A comparison of abused and non-abused women's definitions of domestic violence and attitudes to acceptance of male dominance. *European Journal of Obstetrics, Gynecology, and Reproductive Biology, 122*(2), 225–231.

Fonzo, G. A., Simmons, A. N., Thorp, S. R., et al. (2010). Exaggerated and disconnected insular-amygdalar blood oxygenation level-dependent response to threat-related emotional faces in women with intimate-partner violence posttraumatic stress disorder. *Biological Psychiatry, 68*(5), 433–441.

Gerber, M., Gantz, M., Lichter, E., et al. (2005). Adverse health behaviors and the detection of partner violence by clinicians. *Archives of Internal Medicine, 165*(9), 1016–1021.

Glass, N., Eden, K., Bloom, T., & Perrin, N. (2009). Computerized aid improves safety decision process for survivors of intimate partner violence. *Journal of Interpersonal Violence, 25*(11), 1947–1964.

Glass, N., Perrin, N., Hanson, G., et al. (2009). Patterns of partners' abusive behaviors as reported by Latina and non-Latina survivors. *Journal of Community Psychology, 37*(2), 156–170.

Gonzalez-Guarda, R. M., Vermeesch, A. L., Florom-Smith, A. L., et al. (2013). Birthplace, culture, self-esteem, and intimate partner violence among community-dwelling Hispanic women. *Violence Against Women, 19*(1), 6–23.

Gustafsson, H. C., & Cox, M. J. (2012). Relations among intimate partner violence, maternal depressive symptoms, and maternal parenting behaviors. *Journal of Marriage and the Family, 74*(5), 1005–1020.

Harrykissoon, S., Rickert, V., & Wiemann, C. (2002). Prevalence and patterns of intimate partner violence among adolescent mothers during the postpartum period. *Archives of Pediatric and Adolescent Medicine, 156*(4), 325–330.

Heim, C., & Nemeroff, C. (2009). Neurobiology of posttraumatic stress disorder. *CNS Spectrums, 14*(1 Suppl 1), 13–24.

Heise, L. (1998). Violence against women: An integrated, ecological framework. *Violence Against Women, 4*(3), 262–290.

Hindmarch, I., El Sohly, M., Gambles, J., & Salamone, S. (2001). Forensic urinalysis of drug use in cases of alleged sexual assault. *Journal of Clinical Forensic Medicine, 8*(4), 197–205.

Horon, I., & Cheng, D. (2005). Underreporting of pregnancy-associated deaths. *American Journal of Public Health, 95*(11), 1879–1880.

Jones, J., Wynn, B., Kroeze, B., et al. (2004). Comparison of sexual assaults by strangers versus known assailants in a community-based population. *American Journal of Emergency Medicine, 22*(6), 454–459.

Kantor, G. K., Jasinski, J. L., & Aldarondo, E. (1994). Sociocultural status and incidence of marital violence in Hispanic families. *Violence and Victims, 9*(3), 207–222.

Kilpatrick, D., Resnick, H., Ruggiero, K., et al. (2007). *Drug-facilitated, incapacitated and forcible rape: A national study (No. 219181)*. Charleston, SC: Medical University of South Carolina, National Crime Victims Research and Treatment Center.

Klevens, J., & Saltzman, L. E. (2009). The controversy on screening for intimate partner violence: A question of semantics? *Journal of Women's Health (Larchmont), 18*(2), 143–145.

Lewis-O'Connor, A., Franz, H., & Zuniga, L. (2005). Limitations of the national protocol for sexual assault medical forensic examinations. *Journal of Emergency Nursing, 31*(3), 267–270.

Litz, B. (2008). Early intervention for trauma: Where are we and where do we need to go? A commentary. *Journal of Traumatic Stress, 21*(6), 503–506.

MacMillan, H., Wathen, C., Jamieson, E., et al. (2009). Screening for intimate partner violence in health care settings: A randomized trial. *Journal of the American Medical Association, 302*(5), 493–501.

Macy, R. J., & Graham, L. M. (2012). Identifying domestic and international sex-trafficking victims during human service provision. *Trauma, Violence, & Abuse, 13*(2), 59–76.

Macy, R., Martin, S., Kupper, L., et al. (2007). Partner violence among women before, during, and after pregnancy: Multiple opportunities for intervention. *Women's Health Issues, 17*(5), 290–299.

Martin, S., Macy, R., Sullivan, K., & Magee, M. (2007). Pregnancy-associated violent deaths: The role of intimate partner violence. *Trauma, Violence, & Abuse, 8*(2), 135–148.

McCauley, J., Amstadter, A., Danielson, C., et al. (2009). Mental health and rape history in relation to non-medical use of prescription drugs in a national sample of women. *Addictive Behaviors, 34*(8), 641–648.

McCauley, J. L., Kilpatrick, D. G., Walsh, K., & Resnick, H. S. (2013). Substance use among women receiving post-rape medical care, associated post-assault concerns and current substance abuse: Results from a national telephone household probability sample. *Addictive Behavior, 38*(4), 1952–1957.

McFarlane, L., Campbell, J., Sharps, P., & Watson, K. (2002). Abuse during pregnancy and femicide: Urgent implications for women's health. *Obstetrics and Gynecology, 100*(1), 27–35.

McPhail, B., Busch, N., Kulkarni, S., & Rice, G. (2007). An integrative feminist model: The evolving feminist perspective on intimate partner violence. *Violence Against Women, 13*(8), 817–841.

Montalvo-Liendo, N. (2009). Cross-cultural factors in disclosure of intimate partner violence: An integrated review. *Journal of Advanced Nursing, 65*(1), 20–34.

Morland, L., Leskin, G., Block, C., et al. (2008). Intimate partner violence and miscarriage: Examination of the role of physical and psychological abuse and posttraumatic stress disorder. *Journal of Interpersonal Violence, 23*(5), 652–669.

Morrison, K., Luchok, K., Richter, D., & Parra-Medina, D. (2006). Factors influencing help-seeking from informal networks among African American victims of intimate partner violence. *Journal of Interpersonal Violence, 21*(11), 1493–1511.

Moyer, V. A., & U.S. Preventive Services Task Force. (2013). Screening for intimate partner violence and abuse of elderly and vulnerable adults: U.S. Preventive Services Task Force recommendation statement. *Annals of Internal Medicine, 158*(6), 478–486.

Naved, R., Azim, S., Bhuiya, A., & Persson, L. (2006). Physical violence by husbands: Magnitude, disclosure and help-seeking behavior of women in Bangladesh. *Social Science Medicine, 62*(12), 2917–2929.

National Child Traumatic Stress Network and National Center for PTSD. (2006). Psychological first aid: Field operations guide. Available at www.vdh.virginia.gov/mrc/WTMRC/documents/pdf/PSY1STAID-v2.pdf.

National Human Trafficking Resource Center. (2012). Sex trafficking in the U.S. Available at www.polarisproject.org/human-trafficking/sex-trafficking-in-the-us.

New York State Department of Health. (2008). *State of New York protocol for the acute care of the adult patient reporting sexual assault.* October 2008. Available at www.nyhealth.gov/professionals/protocols_guideline/sexual_assault.

Nurius, P., & Macy, R. (2008). Heterogeneity among violence-exposed women: Applying person-oriented research methods. *Journal of Interpersonal Violence, 23*(3), 389–415.

Oetzel, J., & Duran, B. (2004). Intimate partner violence in American Indian and/or Alaska Native communities: A social ecological framework of determinants and interventions. *American Indian Alaskan Native Mental Health Research, 11*(3), 49–68.

Pennell, J., & Francis, S. (2005). Safety conferencing: Toward a coordinated and inclusive response to safeguard women and children. *Violence Against Women, 11*(5), 666–692.

Plichta, S. (2004). Intimate partner violence and physical health consequences. *Journal of Interpersonal Violence, 19*(11), 1296–1323.

Rape, Abuse, and Incest National Network (RAINN). (2009). Acquaintance rape. Available at www.rainn.org/get-information/types-of-sexual-assault/acquaintance-rape.

Records, K., & Rice, M. J. (2009). Lifetime physical and sexual abuse and the risk for depression symptom in the first 8 months after birth. *Journal of Psychosomatic Obstetrics and Gynaecology, 30*(3), 181–190.

Renker, P. (2002). "Keep a blank face. I need to tell you what has been happening to me." Teens' stories of abuse and violence before and during pregnancy. *MCN: The American Journal of Maternal/Child Nursing, 27*(2), 109–116.

Ruzek, J., Brymer, J., Jacobs, A., et al. (2007). Psychological first aid. *Journal of Mental Health Counseling, 29*(1), 17–49.

Sabri, B., Bolyard, R., McFadgion, A. L., et al. (2013). Intimate partner violence, depression, PTSD, and use of mental health resources among ethnically diverse black women. *Social Work in Health Care, 52*(4), 351–369.

Shah, P. S., & Shah, J. (2010). Maternal exposure to domestic violence and pregnancy and birth outcomes: A systematic review and meta-analyses. *Journal of Women's Health, 19*(11), 2017–2031.

Shiu-Thornton, S., Senturia, K., & Sullivan, M. (2005). "Like a bird in a cage": Vietnamese women survivors talk about domestic violence. *Journal of Interpersonal Violence, 20*(8), 959–976.

Soler, H., Vinayak, P., & Quadagno, D. (2000). Biosocial aspects of domestic violence. *Psychoneuroendocrinology, 25*(7), 721–739.

Steiner, L. (2009). *Crazy love: A memoir.* New York: St. Martin's Press.

Stewart, D. E., MacMillan, H., & Wathen, N. (2013). Intimate partner violence. Canadian Journal of Psychiatry. *Revue canadienne de psychiatrie, 58*(6) Insert 1-15.

Stinson, J., Sales, B., Becker, J American Psychological Association (2008). *Sex offending: Causal theories to inform research, prevention, and treatment.* Washington, DC: American Psychological Association.

Stockl, H., Devries, K., Rotstein, A., et al. (2013). The global prevalence of intimate partner homicide: A systematic review. *Lancet, 382*(9895), 859–865.

Straus, H., Cerulli, C., McNutt, L., et al. (2009). Intimate partner violence and functional health status: Associations with severity, danger, and self-advocacy behaviors. *Journal of Women's Health (Larchmont), 18*(5), 625–631.

Stuart, G., & Hamolia, C. (2009). Preventing and managing aggressive behavior. In G. Stuart (Ed.), *Principles and practice of psychiatric nursing* (9th ed.). St. Louis: Mosby.

Sylaska, K. M., & Edwards, K. M. (2014). Disclosure of intimate partner violence to informal social support network members: A review of the literature. *Trauma, Violence, & Abuse, 15*(1), 3–21.

Taylor, R., & Nabors, E. (2009). Pink or blue...black and blue? Examining pregnancy as a predictor of intimate partner violence and femicide. *Violence Against Women, 15*(11), 1273–1293.

Thompson, R., Bonomi, A., Anderson, M., et al. (2006). Intimate partner violence: Prevalence, types, and chronicity in adult women. *American Journal of Preventive Medicine, 30*(6), 447–457.

Tjaden, P., & Thoennes, N. (2006). *Extent, nature and consequences of rape victimization: Findings from the National Violence Against Women Survey.* Available at www.ojp.usdoj.gov/nij/pubs-sum/210346.htm.

Torres, S., & Han, H. (2003). Women's perceptions of their male batterers' characteristics and level of violence. *Issues in Mental Health Nursing, 24*(6), 667–673.

U.S. Census Bureau. (2011). *the Hispanic Profile, 2010.* Available at www.census.gov/PROD/cen2010/briefs/c2010br-04.pdf.

U.S. Department of Health and Human Services. (2012). *Fact sheet: Sex trafficking.* Available at www.acf.hhs.gov/programs/orr/resource/fact-sheet-sex-trafficking-english.

U.S. Department of Health and Human Services. (2013). *Healthy People 2020 objectives.* Available at http://healthypeople.gov/HP2020/default.asp.

U.S. Department of Justice. (2011). *Crime in the United States, 2010. Federal Bureau of Investigation, Uniform Crime Reports.* Washington, DC: U.S. Department of Justice.

U.S. Department of Justice, & Office of Violence Against Women. (2013). *A National Protocol for Sexual Assault Medical Forensic Examinations Adults/Adolescents* (2nd ed.). Washington DC: U.S. Department of Justice, & Office of Violence Against Women.

United Nations. (December 20, 1993). *Declaration of the elimination of violence against women.* Available at www2.ohchr.org/english/law/eliminationvaw.htm.

Walker-Rodriguez, A., & Hill, R. (2011). Human sex trafficking. *FBI Law Enforcement Bulletin, 8*(3). Available at www.fbi.gov.

Walton-Moss, B., & Campbell, J. (2002). Intimate partner violence: Implications for nursing. *Online Journal of Issues in Nursing, 7*(1), 6.

Westbrook, L. (2009). Information myths and intimate partner violence: Sources, contexts, and consequences. *Journal of the American Society for Information Science and Technology, 60*(4), 826–836.

Wheeler, K. (2008). *Psychotherapy for the advanced practice psychiatric nurse.* St. Louis: Mosby.

Williston, C. J., & Lafreniere, K. D. (2013). "Holy cow, does that ever open up a can of worms": health care providers' experiences of inquiring about intimate partner violence. *Health Care Women International, 34*(9), 814–831.

World Health Organization. (2011). *Intimate partner violence during pregnancy. Information Sheet.* Available at www.who.int/entity/reproductivehealth/publications/violence/rhr_11_35/en.

World Health Organization. (2012). *Intimate partner violence. Understanding and addressing violence against women.* Available at http://apps.who.int/iris/bitstream/10665/77432/1/WHO_RHR_12.36_eng.pdf.

World Health Organization. (2013a). *Global and regional estimates of violence against women: Prevalence and health effects of intimate partner violence and non-partner sexual violence.* Geneva: World Health Organization.

World Health Organization. (2013b). *Responding to intimate partner violence and sexual violence against women: WHO clinical and policy guidelines.* Geneva, Switzerland: World Health Organization.

Yoshihama, M. (2002). Breaking the web of abuse and silence: Voices of battered women in Japan. *Social Work, 47*(4), 389–400.

6 CHAPTER

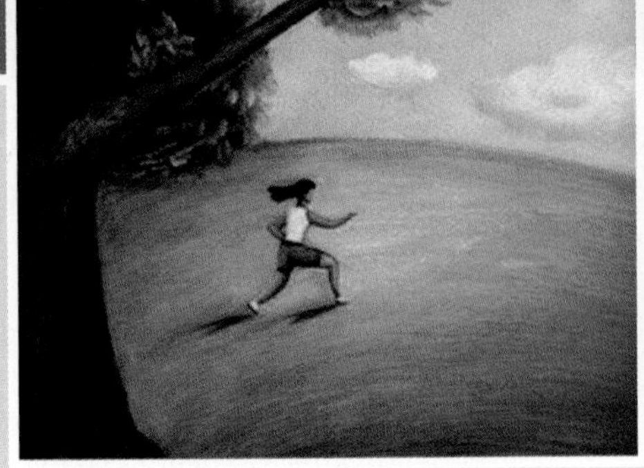

Reproductive System Concerns

Ellen Frances Olshansky

http://evolve.elsevier.com/Lowdermilk/MWHC/

LEARNING OBJECTIVES

- Describe and differentiate signs and symptoms of common menstrual disorders.
- Develop a nursing care plan for a woman with primary dysmenorrhea.
- Describe premenstrual syndrome (PMS) and premenstrual dysphoric disorder (PMDD).
- Relate the symptoms of endometriosis to the associated pathophysiology.
- Develop a nursing care plan for a woman with endometriosis.
- Summarize the therapies for menstrual disorders and menopausal symptoms, including risks and benefits.
- Differentiate the various causes of abnormal uterine bleeding.
- Identify health risks of perimenopausal women.
- Describe the common signs and symptoms of perimenopause.
- Develop a teaching plan for managing symptoms in menopausal women.
- Examine the risks and benefits of menopausal hormone therapy.
- Summarize client teaching strategies for prevention of osteoporosis.

Problems may occur at any point in the menstrual cycle. In addition, many factors, including anatomic abnormalities, physiologic imbalances, and lifestyle, can affect the menstrual cycle. Many women seek out nurses as advisers, counselors, and health care providers for information about menstrual cycle experiences, concerns, or disorders. If they are to meet their clients' needs, nurses must have accurate, up-to-date information. This chapter provides information on menstrual cycle experiences, including menarche through postmenopause; common menstrual disorders; abnormal bleeding problems; and problems associated with perimenopause and postmenopause.

Knowledge of the normal parameters of menstruation is essential to the assessment of menstrual cycle experiences and disorders. The menstrual cycle is a result of a complex interplay among the reproductive, neurologic, and endocrine systems. The hypothalamus produces gonadotropin-releasing hormone (GnRH), which stimulates the pituitary gland to produce follicle-stimulating hormone (FSH) and luteinizing hormone (LH). In turn, FSH and LH stimulate the ovaries to produce first estrogen and then progesterone. In response to the hormones, the endometrium, or lining of the uterus, proliferates and then sheds. Chapter 4 provides additional information on the menstrual cycle and endocrine physiology.

Normal menstrual patterns are averages based on observations and reports from large groups of healthy women. When counseling an individual woman, remember that these values are averages only. Generally a woman's menstrual frequency stabilizes at every 28 days within 1 to 2 years after puberty, with a range from 26 to 34 days (Blackburn, 2013). Although no woman's cycle is exactly the same length every month, the typical month-to-month variation in an individual's cycle is usually plus or minus 2 days. However, greater but still normal variations are noted frequently.

During her reproductive years a woman may have more than one physiologic variation in her menstrual cycle. It is essential that nurses understand the physiologic variations that occur in several age groups. Menstrual cycle length is most irregular at the extremes of the reproductive years including the 2 years after menarche and the 5 years before menopause, when anovulatory cycles are most common. Irregular bleeding, both in length of cycle and amount, is the rule rather than the exception in early adolescence. It takes approximately 15 months for completion of the first 10 cycles and an average of 20 cycles before ovulation occurs regularly. Cycle lengths of 15 to 45 days are not unusual, and during the first 2 years after menarche intervals of 3 to 6 months between menses can be normal.

Women's knowledge and understanding of the menstrual cycle may be limited and are often influenced by myths and misunderstandings. Women typically have menstrual cycles for about 40 years. Once the irregular nature of menses in the first 1 to 2 years after menarche subsides and a cyclic, predictable pattern of monthly bleeding is established, women may worry about any deviation from that pattern, or from what they have been told is normal for all menstruating women. A woman may be concerned about her ability to conceive and bear children or she may believe that she is not really a woman without monthly evidence. A sign such as amenorrhea or excess menstrual bleeding can be a source of severe distress and concern for women.

COMMON MENSTRUAL DISORDERS

Amenorrhea

Amenorrhea, the absence of menstrual flow, is a clinical sign of a variety of disorders. Although these criteria for a clinical problem of amenorrhea are not universal, these circumstances should generally be evaluated: (1) the absence of both menarche and secondary sexual characteristics by age 14 years; (2) absence of menses by age 16, regardless of presence of normal growth and development (primary amenorrhea); or (3) a 3- to 6-month absence of menses after a period of menstruation (secondary amenorrhea) (Fritz & Speroff, 2011; Lobo, 2012d).

A moderately obese girl (20% to 30% above ideal weight) may have early-onset menstruation, whereas delay of onset is known to be related to malnutrition (starvation such as that with anorexia). Girls who exercise strenuously before menarche can have delayed onset of menstruation until about age 18 (Lobo, 2012d).

Although amenorrhea is not a disease, it is often the sign of one. Still, most commonly and most benignly, amenorrhea is a result of pregnancy. It also can result from anatomic abnormalities such as outflow tract obstruction, anterior pituitary disorders, other endocrine disorders such as polycystic ovary syndrome, hypothyroidism or hyperthyroidism, chronic diseases such as type 1 diabetes, medications such as phenytoin (Dilantin), drug abuse (alcohol, tranquilizers, opiates, marijuana, cocaine), or oral contraceptive use.

Hypogonadotropic amenorrhea reflects a problem in the central hypothalamic-pituitary axis. In rare instances a pituitary lesion or genetic inability to produce FSH and LH is at fault. More commonly it results from hypothalamic suppression as a result of two principal influences: stress (in the home, school, or workplace) or a sudden and severe weight loss, eating disorders, strenuous exercise, or mental illness (Wambach & Alexander, 2012). Research has demonstrated a biologic basis for the relationship of stress to physiologic processes. Amenorrhea is one of the classic signs of anorexia nervosa, and the interrelatedness of disordered eating, amenorrhea, and altered bone mineral density has been described as the female athlete triad (American College of Sports Medicine [ACSM], 2011; Mencias, Noon, & Hoch, 2012). Calcium loss from bone, comparable to that seen in postmenopausal women, may occur with this type of amenorrhea.

Exercise-associated amenorrhea can occur in women undergoing vigorous physical and athletic training. The pathophysiology is complex and is thought to be associated with many factors, including body composition (height, weight, and percentage of body fat); type, intensity, and frequency of exercise; nutritional status; and the presence of emotional or physical stressors (Lobo, 2012d). In addition, it is probably due to diminished secretion of GnRH. Women who participate in sports emphasizing low body weight are at greatest risk (Quinn, 2011), including the following (Bonci, Bonci, Granger, et al., 2008):

- Sports in which performance is subjectively scored (e.g., distance running, cycling)
- Endurance sports favoring participants with low body weight (e.g., distance running, cycling)
- Sports in which body contour–revealing clothing is worn (e.g., swimming, diving, volleyball)
- Sports with weight categories for participation (e.g., rowing, martial arts)
- Sports in which prepubertal body shape favors success (e.g., gymnastics, figure skating)

Assessment of amenorrhea begins with a thorough history and physical examination. An important initial step, often overlooked, is to be sure that the woman is not pregnant. Specific components of the assessment process depend on a client's age—adolescent, young adult, or perimenopausal—and whether she has previously menstruated.

Once pregnancy has been ruled out by a β-human chorionic gonadotropin (β-hCG) pregnancy test, diagnostic tests can include FSH level, thyroid-stimulating hormone (TSH) and prolactin levels, radiographic or computed tomography scan of the sella turcica, and a progestational challenge (Lobo, 2012d).

Management

When amenorrhea is a result of hypothalamic disturbances, the nurse is an ideal health professional to assist women because many of the causes are potentially reversible (e.g., stress, weight loss for nonorganic reasons). Counseling and education are primary interventions and appropriate nursing roles. When a stressor known to predispose a client to hypothalamic amenorrhea is identified, initial management involves addressing the stressor. Together the woman and the nurse plan how the woman can decrease or discontinue medications known to affect menstruation, correct weight loss, deal more effectively with psychologic stress, address emotional distress, and alter her exercise routine (Vorvick, Storck, & Zieve, 2012).

The nurse works with the woman to help her identify, cope with, and possibly resolve sources of stress in her life. Deep-breathing exercises and relaxation techniques are simple yet effective stress-reduction measures. Referral for biofeedback or massage therapy also may be useful. In some instances, referrals for psychotherapy may be indicated.

If a woman's exercise program is thought to contribute to her amenorrhea, several options exist for management. The American College of Sports Medicine (ACSM) recommends increasing nutritional intake to increase energy availability and reducing exercise energy expenditure as the first line of treatment (Quinn, 2011). Therefore, the woman may decide to decrease the intensity or duration of her training if possible or to gain 2% to 3% in body weight. Coming to accept this alternative may be difficult for one who is committed to a strenuous exercise regimen, and the nurse and the client may have several sessions before the woman elects to try exercise reduction. Many young female athletes may not understand the consequences of low bone density or osteoporosis; nurses can point out the connection between low bone density and stress fractures. The nurse and the woman also should investigate other factors that may be contributing to the amenorrhea and develop plans for altering lifestyle and decreasing stress.

Although research on effectiveness is inconclusive, a daily calcium intake of 1200 to 1500 mg plus 400 to 800 International Units of vitamin D and 60 to 90 mg of potassium are recommended for women experiencing amenorrhea associated with the female athlete triad. Oral contraceptives have a positive effect on bone density in amenorrheic women but are usually not used in young women with amenorrhea associated with female athlete triad unless the woman is not willing to comply with dietary and exercise recommendations or she continues to be amenorrheic even with compliance (Joy, 2012).

Cyclic Perimenstrual Pain and Discomfort

Cyclic perimenstrual pain and discomfort (CPPD) is a useful concept to describe women's experiences of discomfort during the menstrual cycle and therefore the literature has been updated to reflect the relevance of CPPD (Association of Women's Health, Obstetric and Neonatal Nurses [AWHONN], 2013). This concept includes dysmenorrhea, premenstrual syndrome (PMS), and premenstrual dysphoric disorder (PMDD) as well as symptom clusters that occur before and after the menstrual flow starts. Symptoms occur cyclically and can include mood swings as well as pelvic pain and physical discomforts. These symptoms can range from mild to severe and can last a day or two or up to 2 weeks (Marshall & Jones, 2011). CPPD is a health problem that can have a significant effect on a woman's quality of life. The following discussion focuses on the three main conditions of CPPD.

Dysmenorrhea

Dysmenorrhea, pain during or shortly before menstruation, is one of the most common gynecologic problems in women of all ages. Many adolescents have dysmenorrhea in the first 3 years after menarche. Young adult women ages 17 to 24 are most likely to report painful menses. Approximately 75% of women report some level of discomfort associated with menses, and approximately 15% report severe dysmenorrhea (Lentz, 2012); however, the amount of disruption in women's lives is difficult to determine. Researchers have estimated that as many as 10% of women with dysmenorrhea have severe enough pain to interfere with their functioning for 1 to 3 days a month. Menstrual problems, including dysmenorrhea, are relatively more common in women who smoke and are obese. Severe dysmenorrhea is also associated with early menarche, nulliparity, and stress (Lentz). Traditionally dysmenorrhea is differentiated as primary or secondary. Symptoms usually begin with menstruation, although some women have discomfort several hours before onset of flow. The range and severity of symptoms are different from woman to woman and from cycle to cycle in the same woman. Symptoms of dysmenorrhea may last several hours or several days.

Pain is usually located in the suprapubic area or lower abdomen. Women describe the pain as sharp, cramping, or gripping or as a steady dull ache. For some women pain radiates to the lower back or upper thighs.

Primary Dysmenorrhea

Primary dysmenorrhea is a condition associated with ovulatory cycles. Research has shown that primary dysmenorrhea has a biochemical basis and arises from the release of prostaglandins with menses. During the luteal phase and subsequent menstrual flow, prostaglandin F_2-alpha ($PGF_{2\alpha}$) is secreted. Excessive release of $PGF_{2\alpha}$ increases the amplitude and frequency of uterine contractions and causes vasospasm of the uterine arterioles, resulting in ischemia and cyclic lower abdominal cramps. Systemic responses to $PGF_{2\alpha}$ include backache, weakness, sweats, gastrointestinal symptoms (anorexia, nausea, vomiting, and diarrhea), and central nervous system symptoms (dizziness, syncope, headache, and poor concentration). Pain usually begins at the onset of menstruation and lasts 8 to 48 hours (Lentz, 2012).

Primary dysmenorrhea usually appears 6 to 12 months after menarche when ovulation is established. Anovulatory bleeding, common in the few months or years after menarche, is painless. Because both estrogen and progesterone are necessary for primary dysmenorrhea to occur, it is experienced only with ovulatory cycles. This problem is more common among women in their late teens and early 20s than in women in older age groups; the incidence declines with age. Psychogenic factors may influence symptoms, but symptoms are definitely related to ovulation and do not occur when ovulation is suppressed.

Management. Management of primary dysmenorrhea depends on the severity of the problem and an individual woman's response to various treatments. Important components of nursing care are information and support. Because menstruation is so closely linked to reproduction and sexuality, menstrual problems such as dysmenorrhea can have a negative influence on sexuality and self-worth. Nurses can correct myths and misinformation about menstruation and dysmenorrhea by providing facts about what is normal. Nurses must support their clients' feelings of positive sexuality and self-worth.

Often more than one alternative for alleviating menstrual discomfort and dysmenorrhea can be offered. Women can then try options and decide which ones work best for them. Heat (heating pad or hot bath) minimizes cramping by increasing vasodilation and muscle relaxation and minimizing uterine ischemia. Massaging the lower back can reduce pain by relaxing paravertebral muscles and increasing the pelvic blood supply. Soft, rhythmic rubbing of the abdomen (effleurage) is useful because it provides a distraction and an alternative focal point. Biofeedback, transcutaneous electrical nerve stimulation (TENS), progressive relaxation, Hatha yoga, acupuncture, and meditation are also used to decrease menstrual discomfort, although evidence is insufficient to determine their effectiveness (Lentz, 2012). Research findings from Chien Change, and Liu (2013) concluded that an 8-week yoga intervention decreased serum homocysteine levels, alleviating dysmenorrhea in women with primary dysmenorrhea.

Exercise helps relieve menstrual discomfort through increased vasodilation and subsequent decreased ischemia. It also releases endogenous opiates (specifically beta-endorphins), suppresses prostaglandins, and shunts blood flow away from the viscera, resulting in reduced pelvic congestion. One specific exercise that nurses can suggest is pelvic rocking.

In addition to maintaining good nutrition at all times, specific dietary changes are helpful in decreasing some of the systemic symptoms associated with dysmenorrhea. Decreased salt and refined sugar intake 7 to 10 days before expected menses may reduce fluid retention. Natural diuretics such as asparagus, cranberry juice, peaches, parsley, or watermelon may help reduce edema and related discomforts. A low-fat vegetarian diet may also help minimize dysmenorrheal symptoms (Lentz, 2012).

A major role of the nurse is to assist the client in managing her menstrual discomfort. The Clinical Reasoning Case Study provides an example of how a nurse can help the woman.

Medications used to treat primary dysmenorrhea in women not desiring contraception include prostaglandin synthesis inhibitors, primarily nonsteroidal antiinflammatory drugs (NSAIDs) (Lentz, 2012) (Table 6-1). NSAIDs are effective if begun 2 to 3 days before menses or with the sign of first bleeding; this regimen decreases the possibility of a woman taking these drugs early in pregnancy (Fritz & Speroff, 2011). All NSAIDs have potential gastrointestinal side effects, including nausea, vomiting, and indigestion. All women taking NSAIDs should be warned to report dark-colored stools because this may be an indication of gastrointestinal bleeding.

CLINICAL REASONING CASE STUDY

Management of Dysmenorrhea

Cheri, 16, has come to the adolescent health clinic for a checkup. She reports that she has "really bad cramps" for the first 2 days of her period. She has been taking Midol Menstrual Complete but says that it does not help "a lot." She wants to know if anything else can be done to relieve her pain. How should the nurse respond?

1. Evidence—Is evidence sufficient to draw conclusions about what advice the nurse should give?
2. Assumptions—Describe underlying assumptions about the following issues:
   a. Causes and symptoms of primary dysmenorrhea
   b. Cyclic perimenstrual pain and discomfort
   c. Self-help strategies (e.g., comfort measures, medications)
3. What implications and priorities for nursing care can be drawn at this time?
4. Does the evidence objectively support your conclusion?

TABLE 6-1 Nonsteroidal Antiinflammatory Agents Used to Treat Dysmenorrhea

DRUG	BRAND NAME AND STATUS	RECOMMENDED DOSAGE (ORAL)*	COMMON SIDE EFFECTS†	COMMENTS	CONTRAINDICATIONS
Diclofenac	Cataflam Rx	50 mg tid or 100 mg initially, then 50 mg tid up to 150 mg/day	Nausea, diarrhea, constipation, abdominal distress, dyspepsia, heartburn, flatulence, dizziness, tinnitus, itching, rash	Enteric coated; immediate release	For all NSAIDs: Do not give if woman has hemophilia or bleeding ulcers; do not give if woman has had an allergic or anaphylactic reaction to aspirin or another NSAID; do not give if woman is taking anticoagulant medication
Ibuprofen	Motrin Rx, Advil OTC, Nuprin OTC, Motrin IB OTC	400 mg q6-8h, 200 mg q4-6h up to 1200 mg/day	See *diclofenac*	If GI upset occurs, take with food, milk, or antacids; avoid alcoholic beverages; do not take with aspirin; stop taking and call care provider if rash occurs	
Ketoprofen	Orudis Rx	25-50 mg q6-8h up to 300 mg/day	See *diclofenac*	See *ibuprofen*	
	Orudis KT OTC, Actron OTC	12.5 mg q6-8h up to 75 mg/day			
Meclofenamate	Meclomen Rx	100 mg tid up to 300 mg	See *diclofenac*	See *ibuprofen*	
Mefenamic acid	Ponstel Rx	500 mg initially, then 250 mg q6h up to 1000 mg/day	See *diclofenac*	Very potent and effective prostaglandin-synthesis inhibitor; antagonizes already formed prostaglandins; increased incidence of adverse GI side effects	
Naproxen	Naprosyn Rx	500 mg initially, then 250 mg q6-8h up to 1250 mg/day	See *diclofenac*	See *ibuprofen*	
Naproxen sodium	Anaprox Rx	550 mg initially, then 275 mg q6-8h or 550 mg q12h up to 1375 mg/day	See *diclofenac*	See *ibuprofen*	
	Aleve OTC	440 mg initially, then 220 mg q6-8h up to 660 mg/day			
Celecoxib	Celebrex	400 mg initially, then 200 mg bid	See *diclofenac*	See *ibuprofen*	

*Dosages are current recommendations and should be verified before use. Recommended doses for over-the-counter preparations are generally less than recommendations for therapeutic doses. As-needed dosing is recommended by manufacturer; scheduled dosing may be more effective.

†Risk with all NSAIDs is gastrointestinal ulceration, possible bleeding, and prolonged bleeding time. Incidence of side effects is dose related. Reported incidence, 1% to 10%.

GI, Gastrointestinal; *NSAID*, nonsteroidal antiinflammatory drug; *OTC*, over the counter.

Data from Facts and Comparisons. (2012). *Nonsteroidal antiinflammatory drugs*. Available at www.factsandcomparisons.com; Lentz, G.M. (2012). Primary and secondary dysmenorrhea, premenstrual syndrome, and premenstrual dysphoric disorder: Etiology, diagnosis, and management. In G.M. Lentz, R.A. Lobo, D.M. Gershenson, et al. (Eds.), *Comprehensive gynecology* (6th ed.). Philadelphia: Mosby; U.S. Department of Health and Human Services, U.S. Food and Drug Administration. (2008). *Medication guide for nonsteroidal antiinflammatory drugs (NSAIDs)*. Available at www.fda.gov/CDER/drug/infopage/COX2/NSAIDmedguide.htm.

MEDICATION ALERT

If one NSAID is ineffective, a different one may often be effective. If the second drug is unsuccessful after a 6-month trial, combined oral contraceptive pills (OCPs) may be used. Women with a history of aspirin sensitivity or allergy should avoid all NSAIDs.

OCPs are a reasonable choice for women who want to use a contraceptive agent. The benefits of their use are attributed to decreased prostaglandin synthesis associated with an atrophic decidualized endometrium (Lentz, 2012). OCPs are effective in relieving symptoms of primary dysmenorrhea for approximately 90% of women. No single OCP has been shown to be superior to another for the relief of primary dysmenorrhea, including low-dose and extended-cycle OCPs (Lentz). OCPs are a particularly good choice for therapy because they combine contraception with a positive effect on dysmenorrhea, menstrual flow, and menstrual irregularities. Adolescents may benefit from use of the long-acting injectable contraceptive (depot medroxyprogesterone), but more research is needed. Because OCPs have side effects, women may not wish to use them for dysmenorrhea. They may be contraindicated for some women. (See Chapter 8 for a complete discussion of OCPs.)

Over-the-counter (OTC) preparations that are indicated for primary dysmenorrhea include the same active ingredients (e.g., ibuprofen, naproxen sodium) as prescription preparations; however, the labeled recommended dose may be subtherapeutic. Preparations containing acetaminophen are less effective because acetaminophen does not have the antiprostaglandin properties of NSAIDs.

If dysmenorrhea is not relieved by one of the NSAIDs, further investigation into the cause of the symptoms is necessary. Conditions associated with dysmenorrhea include müllerian duct anomalies, endometriosis, and pelvic inflammatory disease.

Alternative and complementary therapies are increasingly popular and used in developed countries. Chinese medicine, including herbal preparations, have been used in Western integrative medicine, an approach that combines complementary and allopathic approaches (Dobos & Tao, 2011). Therapies such as acupuncture, acupressure, biofeedback, desensitization, hypnosis, massage, Reiki, relaxation exercises, and therapeutic touch have been used to treat pelvic pain. Herbal preparations have long been used for management of menstrual problems including dysmenorrhea (Table 6-2). Herbal medicines may be valuable in treating dysmenorrhea; however, it is essential that women understand that these therapies are not without potential toxicity and may cause drug interactions. Additional study is needed to generate the evidence for the use of these various alternative methods (Smith & Kaunitz, 2013).

NURSING ALERT

Nurses must routinely ask women about use of herbal and other alternative therapies and document their use.

Secondary Dysmenorrhea

Secondary dysmenorrhea is acquired menstrual pain that develops later in life than primary dysmenorrhea, typically after age 25 years. This condition is associated with pelvic pathology, such as adenomyosis, endometriosis, pelvic inflammatory disease, endometrial polyps, or submucous or interstitial myomas (fibroids). Women with secondary dysmenorrhea often have other symptoms that may suggest an underlying cause. For example, heavy menstrual flow with dysmenorrhea suggests a diagnosis of leiomyomata, adenomyosis, or endometrial polyps. Pain associated with endometriosis often begins a few days before menses, but can be present at ovulation and continue through the first days of menses or start after menstrual flow has begun. In contrast to primary dysmenorrhea, the pain of secondary dysmenorrhea is often characterized by dull, lower abdominal aching radiating to the back or thighs. Often women experience feelings of bloating or pelvic fullness. In addition to a physical examination with a careful pelvic examination, diagnosis may be assisted by ultrasound examination, dilation and curettage, endometrial biopsy, or laparoscopy. Treatment is directed toward removing the underlying pathology. Many of the measures described for pain relief of primary dysmenorrhea also are helpful for women with secondary dysmenorrhea.

Premenstrual Syndrome and Premenstrual Dysphoric Disorder

Approximately 30% to 80% of women experience mood or somatic symptoms (or both) that occur with their menstrual cycles (Lentz, 2012). Establishing a universal definition of

TABLE 6-2 Herbal Medicinals Taken Orally for Menstrual Disorders

SYMPTOMS OR INDICATIONS	HERBAL THERAPY*	ACTION
Menstrual cramping, dysmenorrhea	Black haw	Uterine antispasmodic
	Fennel	Uterotonic
	Catnip	Uterine antispasmodic
	Dong quai	Uterotonic; antiinflammatory
	Ginger	Antiinflammatory
	Motherwort	Uterotonic
	Wild yam	Uterine antispasmodic
	Valerian	Uterine antispasmodic
Premenstrual discomfort, tension	Black cohosh root	Estrogen-like luteinizing hormone suppressant; binds to estrogen receptors
	Chamomile	Antispasmodic
Breast pain	Chaste tree fruit	Decreases prolactin levels
	Bugleweed	Antigonadotropic; decreases prolactin levels
Menorrhea, metrorrhagia	Lady's mantle	Uterotonic
	Raspberry	Uterotonic
	Shepherd's purse	Uterotonic

*Many herbs do not have rigorous scientific studies backing their use; most uses and properties of herbs have not been validated by the U.S. Food and Drug Administration.

Data from Annie's Remedy. (2012). *Herbal remedies for dysmenorrhea.* Available at www.anniesremedy.com; National Center for Complementary and Alternative Medicine. (2010). *Herbs at a glance.* Available at www.nccam.nih.gov.

premenstrual syndrome (PMS) is difficult, given that so many symptoms have been associated with the condition, and at least two different syndromes have been recognized: PMS and premenstrual dysphoric disorder (PMDD).

PMS is a complex, poorly understood condition that includes one or more of a large number (more than 100) of physical and psychologic symptoms beginning in the luteal phase of the menstrual cycle, occurring to such a degree that lifestyle or work is affected, and followed by a symptom-free period. Symptoms include fluid retention (abdominal bloating, pelvic fullness, edema of the lower extremities, breast tenderness, and weight gain); behavioral or emotional changes (depression, crying spells, irritability, panic attacks, and impaired ability to concentrate); premenstrual cravings (sweets, salt, increased appetite, and food binges); and headache, fatigue, and backache.

All age groups are affected, with women in their 20s and 30s most frequently reporting symptoms. Ovarian function is necessary for the condition to occur because it does not occur before puberty, after menopause, or during pregnancy. The condition is not dependent on the presence of monthly menses: women who have had a hysterectomy without bilateral salpingo-oophorectomy (BSO) still can have cyclic symptoms.

The American College of Obstetricians and Gynecologists (ACOG 2011) has noted that a diagnosis of PMS must include:

- A pattern in which the woman's symptoms are present in the 5 days before menses begins
- This pattern must occur for at least three menstrual cycles in a row
- Symptoms must end within 4 days after menses begins
- This pattern is cyclic
- Symptoms must interfere with some of her normal activities

PMDD is a more severe variant of PMS in which 3% to 8% of women have marked irritability, dysphoria, mood lability, anxiety, fatigue, appetite changes, and a sense of feeling overwhelmed (Lentz, 2012). The most common symptoms are those associated with mood disturbances. Gallenberg (2012) notes that extreme mood shifts associated with PMDD can be disruptive in work and relationships.

PMDD is included as a diagnosis in the American Psychiatric Association [APA] Diagnostic and Statistical Manual (DSM). This is important because it recognizes that women do experience some specific symptoms that coincide with the week before onset of menses, with a decrease in such symptoms within a few days after onset of menses (American Psychiatric Association [APA], 2013). Symptoms can be related to mood or physical changes, with the key factor being the cyclical nature of the symptoms.

The actual diagnosis of PMDD requires that a woman notes at least five specific symptoms (derived from a list of symptoms) and that one of those is related to mood state. These symptoms include (Storck, 2012):

- No interest in daily activities and relationships
- Fatigue or low energy
- Feelings of sadness or hopelessness, possible suicidal thoughts
- Feelings of tension or anxiety
- Feeling out of control
- Food cravings or binge eating
- Mood swings with periods of crying
- Panic attacks
- Irritability or anger that affects other people
- Physical symptoms, such as bloating, breast tenderness, headaches, and joint or muscle pain
- Problems sleeping
- Trouble concentrating

The causes of PMS and PMDD are not known, but there is general agreement that they are distinct psychiatric and medical syndromes rather than an exacerbation of an underlying psychiatric disorder. They do not occur if there is no ovarian function. A number of biologic and neuroendocrine etiologies have been suggested; however, none has been conclusively substantiated as the causative factor. It is likely that biologic, psychosocial, and sociocultural factors contribute to PMS and PMDD (Lentz, 2012).

Management

There is little agreement on management. A careful, detailed history and daily log of symptoms and mood fluctuations spanning several cycles may give direction to a plan of management. Any changes that assist a woman with PMS to exert control over her life have a positive effect. For this reason, lifestyle changes are often effective in the treatment of PMS.

Education is an important component of the management of PMS. Nurses can advise women that self-help modalities often result in significant symptom improvement. Women have found a number of complementary and alternative therapies to be useful in managing the symptoms of PMS. Nurses can suggest that women:

- Not smoke and limit their consumption of refined sugar (less than 5 tablespoons/day), salt (less than 3 g/day), red meat (up to 3 ounces/day), alcohol (less than 1 ounce/day), and caffeinated beverages
- Include whole grains, legumes, seeds, nuts, vegetables, fruits, and vegetable oils in their diet
- Eat three small to moderate-sized meals and three small snacks a day that are rich in complex carbohydrates and fiber (ACOG, 2011; Lentz, 2012)
- Use natural diuretics (see section on dysmenorrhea management on earlier in the chapter) to help reduce fluid retention

Nutritional supplements may assist in symptom relief. Calcium (1200 mg daily) and vitamin B_6 have been shown to be moderately effective in relieving symptoms, to have few side effects, and to be safe. Daily supplements of evening primrose oil are reportedly useful in relieving breast symptoms with minimal side effects, but research reports are conflicting (Biggs & Demuth, 2011; Lentz, 2012). The Mayo Clinic (2013) noted that evening primrose oil changes the balance of fatty acids, which may explain why it alleviates breast pain. Other herbal therapies have long been used to treat PMS; however, research on effectiveness is lacking, or studies are flawed (Dante & Facchinetti, 2011).

Regular exercise (aerobic exercise three or four times a week), especially in the luteal phase, is widely recommended for relief of PMS symptoms (Lentz, 2012). A monthly program that varies in intensity and type of exercise according to PMS symptoms is best. Women who exercise regularly seem to have less premenstrual anxiety than do nonathletic women. Researchers believe aerobic exercise increases beta-endorphin levels to offset symptoms of depression and elevate mood.

Yoga, acupuncture, hypnosis, light therapy, chiropractic therapy, and massage therapy have all been reported to have a beneficial effect on PMS. Further research is needed to determine the effectiveness of these suggested therapies.

Nurses can explain the relation between cyclic estrogen fluctuation and changes in serotonin levels, that serotonin is one of the brain chemicals that assist in coping with normal life stresses, and the ways in which the different recommended management strategies help maintain serotonin levels. Support groups or individual or couples counseling may be helpful. Stress reduction techniques also may assist with symptom management (Lentz, 2012).

If these strategies do not provide significant symptom relief in 1 to 2 months, medication is often added. Many medications have been used in treatment of PMS, but no single medication alleviates all PMS symptoms. Medications often used in the treatment of PMS include diuretics, prostaglandin inhibitors (NSAIDs), progesterone, and OCPs. These have been used mainly for the physical symptoms. Studies of progesterone have not shown that it is an effective treatment (Ford, Lethaby, Roberts, & Mol, 2012). Serotonergic-activating agents, including the selective serotonin reuptake inhibitors (SSRIs) such as fluoxetine (Prozac or Sarafem), sertraline (Zoloft), citalopram (Celexa), escitalopram (Lexapro), and paroxetine (Paxil CR) are approved by the U.S. Food and Drug Administration (FDA) as agents for PMS and are first-line pharmacologic therapy. Use of these medications during the luteal phase of the menstrual cycle results in a decrease in emotional premenstrual symptoms, especially depression (Biggs & Demuth, 2011; Lentz, 2012). Common side effects are headaches, sleep disturbances, dizziness, weight gain, dry mouth, and decreased libido (see Nursing Care Plan).

Endometriosis

Endometriosis is characterized by the presence and growth of endometrial glands and stroma outside of the uterus. The tissue may be implanted on the ovaries; the anterior and posterior cul-de-sac; the broad, uterosacral, and round ligaments; the uterine tubes; the rectovaginal septum; the sigmoid colon; the appendix; the pelvic peritoneum; the cervix; and the inguinal area (Fig. 6-1). Endometrial lesions have been found in the vagina and on surgical scars, as well as on the vulva, the perineum, and the bladder, and sites far from the pelvic area such as the thoracic cavity, the gallbladder, and the heart. A chocolate cyst is a cystic area of endometriosis in the ovary. Old blood causes the dark coloring of the cyst's contents.

Endometrial tissue contains glands and stroma and responds to cyclic hormonal stimulation in the same way that the uterine endometrium does. During the proliferative and secretory phases of the cycle, the endometrial tissue grows. During or

NURSING CARE PLAN

Premenstrual Syndrome

NURSING DIAGNOSIS	EXPECTED OUTCOME	NURSING INTERVENTIONS	RATIONALES
Acute Pain related to cyclic breast changes as evidenced by woman's report	Woman will report a decrease in the intensity of pain or discomfort after interventions.	Assess timing and intensity of pain or discomfort.	To validate relation to cyclic changes
		Counsel woman to take medications if prescribed.	
		Suggest that woman wear a supportive bra.	To minimize breast tenderness
Situational Low Self-esteem related to cyclic hormonal changes as evidenced by woman's verbal report	Woman will report increased number of feelings of self-worth.	Provide therapeutic communication.	To validate feelings of depression and mood swings
		Encourage woman to limit caffeine and eat small, frequent meals.	To lessen irritability aggravated by caffeine and hypoglycemia
		Refer woman to support groups.	To encourage the sharing of experiences, feelings, and self-help tips
Excess Fluid Volume related to cyclic hormonal influences as evidenced by weight gain before start of menstrual period	Woman will report no significant changes in body weight before start of menstrual period.	Encourage woman to limit intake of salt and sodium-containing foods.	To decrease fluid retention
		Counsel woman to take diuretics as prescribed.	To facilitate fluid excretion
		Encourage consumption of natural diuretic foods.	To encourage fluid excretion
Anxiety related to anticipation of cyclic pain	Woman will report a decrease in anxiety level.	Teach woman to recognize anxiety.	To prompt early preventive interventions in order to decrease anxiety
		Identify relaxation techniques.	
		Encourage woman to attend support groups.	To encourage expression of feelings and self-help interventions

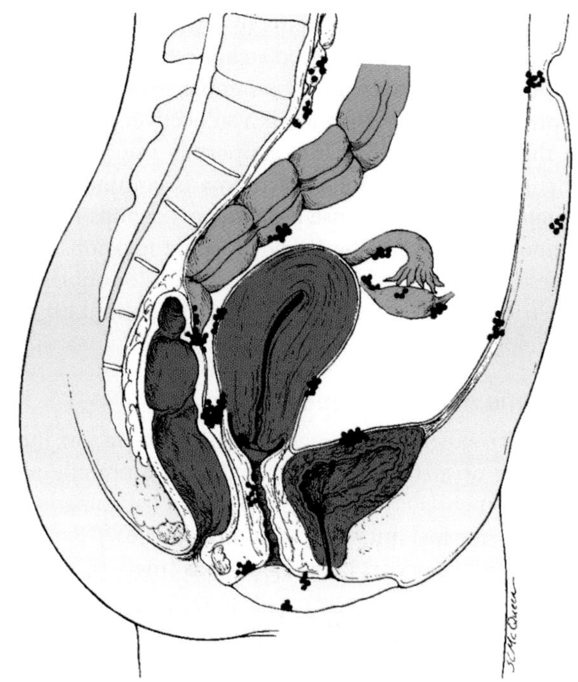

FIG 6-1 Common sites of endometriosis. (From Lentz, G.M., Lobo, R.A., Gershenson, D.M., et al. [Eds.]. (2012). *Comprehensive gynecology* [6th ed.]. Philadelphia: Elsevier.)

immediately after menstruation, the tissue bleeds, resulting in an inflammatory response with subsequent fibrosis and adhesion to adjacent organs.

The overall incidence of endometriosis is 5% to 15% in reproductive-age women, 30% to 45% in infertile women, and 33% in women with chronic pelvic pain (Lobo, 2012b). Although the condition usually develops in the third or fourth decade of life, endometriosis has been found in adolescents with disabling pelvic pain or abnormal vaginal bleeding (Steenberg, Tanbo, & Qvigstad, 2013). Endometriosis may worsen with repeated cycles, or it may remain asymptomatic and undiagnosed, eventually disappearing after menopause. However, it has been reported to occur in about 5% of postmenopausal women receiving menopausal hormone therapy. There appears to be a familial tendency to develop endometriosis; the condition is seven times more prevalent in women who have a first-degree relative with endometriosis as compared with the general population (Lobo).

Several theories concerning the cause of endometriosis have been suggested. However, the etiology and pathology of this condition continue to be poorly understood. One of the most widely accepted theories is transplantation or retrograde menstruation. According to this theory endometrial tissue is refluxed through the uterine tubes during menstruation into the peritoneal cavity, where it implants on the ovaries and other organs. Retrograde menstruation has been documented in a number of surgical studies and is estimated to occur in 90% of menstruating women. For most women endometrial tissue outside the uterus is disintegrated before it can implant or seed in the peritoneal cavity or elsewhere. Other theories include genetic disposition, immunologic changes, and hormonal influences (Lobo, 2012b).

Symptoms vary among women, from nonexistent to incapacitating. Severity of symptoms can change over time and may be disproportionate to the extent of the disease. The major symptoms of endometriosis are pelvic pain, dysmenorrhea, dyspareunia (painful intercourse), abnormal menstrual bleeding, and infertility. Women also may experience chronic noncyclic pelvic pain, pelvic heaviness, or pain radiating to the thighs. Many women report bowel symptoms such as diarrhea, pain with defecation, and constipation caused by avoiding defecation because of the pain. Less common symptoms include abnormal bleeding (hypermenorrhea, menorrhagia, or premenstrual staining) and pain during exercise as a result of adhesions (Lobo, 2012b).

Women, especially adolescents, who have endometriosis often have other comorbid conditions, including pain, mood disorders, and asthma (Smorgick, Marsh, As-Sanie, et al., 2013).

Impaired fertility may result from adhesions around the uterus that pull the uterus into a fixed, retroverted position. Adhesions around the uterine tubes may block the fimbriated ends or prevent the spontaneous movement that carries the ovum to the uterus.

Management

Treatment is based on the severity of symptoms and the goals of the woman or couple. Women without pain who do not want to become pregnant need no treatment. In women with mild pain who may desire a future pregnancy, treatment may be limited to use of NSAIDs during menstruation (see earlier discussion of these medications).

Suppression of endogenous estrogen production and subsequent endometrial lesion growth is the cornerstone of management of the disease. Two main classes of medications are used to suppress endogenous estrogen levels: GnRH agonists and androgen derivatives. GnRH agonist therapy (leuprolide [Lupron], nafarelin acetate [Synarel], goserelin acetate [Zoladex]) acts by suppressing pituitary gonadotropin secretion. FSH and LH stimulation of the ovary declines markedly, and ovarian function decreases significantly. A medically induced menopause develops, resulting in anovulation and amenorrhea. Shrinkage of already established endometrial tissue, significant pain relief, and interruption in further lesion development follow. The hypoestrogenism results in hot flashes in almost all women. Trabecular bone loss is common, although most loss is reversible within 12 to 24 months after the medication is stopped (Lobo, 2012b).

Leuprolide (3.75 mg intramuscular injection given once a month for up to 6 months), nafarelin (200 mg administered twice daily by nasal spray for up to 6 months), and goserelin 3.6 mg every 28 days for up to 6 months by subcutaneous implant are effective and well tolerated. These medications reduce endometrial lesions and pelvic pain associated with endometriosis and have posttreatment pregnancy rates similar to that of danazol (Danocrine) therapy (Lobo, 2012b). Common side effects of these drugs are those of natural menopause—hot flashes and vaginal dryness. Occasionally women report headaches and muscle aches. Treatment is usually limited to 6 months to minimize bone loss. Although unlikely, it is possible for a woman to become pregnant while taking a GnRH agonist. Because the potential teratogenicity of this drug is unclear, women should use a barrier contraceptive during treatment.

Danazol, a mildly androgenic synthetic steroid, suppresses FSH and LH secretion, thus producing anovulation and hypogonadotropism. This results in decreased secretion of estrogen and progesterone and regression of endometrial tissue. Danazol can produce side effects severe enough to cause a woman to discontinue the drug, including masculinizing traits (weight gain, edema, decreased breast size, oily skin, hirsutism, and deepening of the voice), all of which often disappear when treatment is discontinued. Other side effects are amenorrhea, hot flashes, vaginal dryness, insomnia, and decreased libido. Migraine headaches, dizziness, fatigue, and depression are also reported. Danazol treatment has been reported to adversely affect lipids, with a decrease in high-density lipoprotein levels and an increase in low-density lipoprotein levels. Danazol should never be prescribed when pregnancy is suspected, and barrier contraception should be used with it because ovulation may not be suppressed. Danazol can produce pseudohermaphroditism in female fetuses. The medication is contraindicated in women with liver disease and should be used with caution in women with cardiac and renal disease. Danazol is used less frequently to treat endometriosis than other medical therapies (Lobo, 2012b).

Women who have early symptomatic disease and who can postpone pregnancy may be treated with continuous OCPs that have a low estrogen-to-progestin ratio to shrink endometrial tissue. Any low-dose OCPs can be used if taken for 15 weeks, followed by 1 week of withdrawal. This therapy is associated with minimal side effects and can be taken for extended periods (Lobo, 2012b). Limited data exist on the effectiveness of progestagen-only medications for treating pain related to endometriosis (Brown, Kives, & Akhtar, 2012).

Continuous combined hormone therapy (OCPs, estrogen/progestin patch, estrogen/progestin vaginal ring) for menstrual suppression and administration of NSAIDs is the usual treatment for adolescents younger than the age of 16 who have endometriosis. GnRH agonist therapy for severe symptoms may have possible adverse effects on bone mineralization in adolescents, and bone mineral density should be carefully monitored (Laufer, 2008).

Fritz and Speroff (2011) described an "add-back therapy" with low-dose estrogen-progestin combinations as leading to a normal bone mineral density while on GnRH agonist therapy.

Surgical intervention is often needed for severe, acute, or incapacitating symptoms. Decisions regarding the extent and type of surgery are influenced by a woman's age, desire for children, and location of the disease. For women who do not want to preserve their ability to have children, the only definite cure is total abdominal hysterectomy with BSO (TAH with BSO). In women in their childbearing years who want children and in whom the disease does not prevent bearing children, reproductive capacity should be retained through careful removal by laparoscopic surgery or laser therapy (coagulation, vaporization, or resection) of all endometrial tissue possible with retention of ovarian function (Lobo, 2012b).

Regardless of the type of treatment (short of TAH with BSO), endometriosis recurs in approximately 40% of women. Thus for many women endometriosis is a chronic disease with conditions such as chronic pain or infertility. Counseling and education are critical components of nursing care for women with endometriosis. Women need an honest discussion of treatment options, with review of the potential risks and benefits of each option. Because pelvic pain is a subjective, personal experience that can be frightening, support is important. Sexual dysfunction resulting from dyspareunia is common and may necessitate referral for counseling. Support groups for women with endometriosis may be found in some locations. Resolve (www.resolve.org), an organization for infertile couples, or the Endometriosis Association (www.ivf.com/endohtml.html) may also be helpful (see Nursing Care Plan).

Alterations in Cyclic Bleeding

Women often experience changes in amount, duration, interval, or regularity of menstrual cycle bleeding. Commonly women worry about menstruation that is infrequent (oligomenorrhea), is scanty at normal intervals (hypomenorrhea), is excessive (menorrhagia), or occurs between periods (metrorrhagia).

Oligomenorrhea/Hypomenorrhea

The term oligomenorrhea often is used to describe decreased menstruation, either in amount, time, or both. However, oligomenorrhea more correctly refers to infrequent menstrual periods characterized by intervals of 40 to 45 days or longer, and hypomenorrhea to scanty bleeding at normal intervals. The causes of oligomenorrhea are often abnormalities of hypothalamic, pituitary, or ovarian function. Oligomenorrhea also can be physiologic, or part of a woman's normal pattern for the first few years after menarche or for several years before menopause.

Treatment is aimed at reversing the underlying cause, if possible. Hormonal therapy using progestins, with or without estrogens, also may be used to prevent complications of unopposed estrogen production (endometrial hyperplasia or carcinoma) or of absent estrogen (vaginal dryness, hot flashes or flushes, or osteoporosis).

Women with menstruation characterized by prolonged intervals between cycles need education and counseling. The cause of the condition and the rationale for a specific treatment should be discussed, as should advantages and disadvantages of hormonal therapy. If a woman chooses medical intervention, she should be provided with written instructions, taught how to take the medications, and made aware of their side effects. Teaching and counseling should emphasize the importance of the woman keeping careful records of her vaginal bleeding.

One of the most common causes of scanty menstrual flow is OCPs. If a woman is considering OCPs for contraception, it is important to explain in advance that the use of OCPs can decrease menstrual flow by as much as two thirds. This effect is caused by the continuous action of the progestin component, which produces a decidualized endometrium with atrophic glands.

Hypomenorrhea also may be caused by structural abnormalities of the endometrium or the uterus that result in partial disintegration of the endometrium. These conditions include Asherman syndrome, in which adhesions resulting from curettage or infection obliterate the endometrial cavity, and congenital partial obstruction of the vagina.

NURSING CARE PLAN

Endometriosis

NURSING DIAGNOSIS	EXPECTED OUTCOMES	NURSING INTERVENTIONS	RATIONALES
Acute Pain related to menstruation secondary to endometriosis	Woman will verbalize a decrease in intensity and frequency of pain during each menstrual cycle.	Assess location, type, and duration of pain and history of discomfort.	To determine severity of dysmenorrhea
		Administer analgesics.	To assist with pain relief
		Administer hormone-altering medications if ordered.	To suppress ovulation
		Provide nonpharmacologic methods such as heat.	To increase blood flow to the pelvic region
Deficient Knowledge related to unfamiliarity with treatment, as evidenced by woman's statements	Woman will verbalize correct understanding of the use of self-care methods and prescribed therapies.	Assess woman's current understanding of the disorder and related therapies.	To validate the accuracy of knowledge base
		Give information to woman regarding the disorder and treatment regimen.	To empower the client to become a partner in her own care
Situational Low Self-esteem related to infertility as evidenced by woman's statements of decreased self-worth	Woman will verbalize positive feelings of self-worth.	Provide therapeutic communication.	To validate feelings and provide support
		Refer to support group.	To enhance feelings of self-worth through group communication
Anxiety related to possible invasive surgical procedure as evidenced by woman's verbal report	Woman will report a decreased number of anxious feelings.	Provide opportunity to discuss feelings.	To identify source of anxiety
		Reinforce information provided.	To keep expectations realistic and dispel myths or inaccuracies
		Provide emotional support.	To encourage verbalization of feelings
Risk for Injury related to disease progression	Woman will report any changes in health status to health care provider.	Teach woman to report any changes in health status.	To initiate prompt treatment
		Review side effects of medications.	To recognize possible causes for changes in health status
		Encourage ongoing communication.	To promote trust and comfort

Metrorrhagia

Metrorrhagia, or intermenstrual bleeding, refers to any episode of bleeding, whether spotting, menses, or hemorrhage, that occurs at a time other than the normal menses. *Mittlestaining,* also referred to as *mittelschmerz,* a small amount of bleeding or spotting that occurs at the time of ovulation (14 days before onset of the next menses), is considered normal. The cause of mittlestaining is not known; however, its common occurrence can be documented by its repetition in the menstrual cycle.

Women taking OCPs may have midcycle bleeding or spotting. (See Chapter 8 for a discussion of the side effects of OCPs.) If the OCP does not maintain a sufficiently hypoplastic endometrium, the endometrium will begin to shed, usually in small amounts at a time, a process termed *breakthrough bleeding,* which is most common in the first three cycles of OCPs. The reduced potency of OCPs (resulting in increased safety) has decreased the amount of available hormones, making it more important that blood levels be kept constant. Taking the pill at exactly the same time each day may alleviate the woman's problem. If the spotting continues, a different formulation of the OCP that increases either the estrogen or progestin component of the pill can be tried.

Progestin-only contraceptive methods (oral and injectable) also may cause midcycle bleeding, especially in the first several cycles. Women should be advised of this and counseled to report continuation of breakthrough bleeding after the first three to six cycles to their health care provider.

Women with an intrauterine device (IUD) may have spotting between their periods and possibly heavier menstrual flow.

The causes of intermenstrual bleeding are varied (Table 6-3). It is important that the nurse always consider the possibility

TABLE 6-3 Causes of Intermenstrual Bleeding

REPRODUCTIVE DISORDER	PREGNANCY PROBLEMS	INFECTIONS
Functional ovarian cyst	Pregnancy implantation	Endometritis
Cervical erosion	Miscarriage	Sexually transmitted infections
Leiomyoma	Ectopic pregnancy	
Polyps, uterine or endocervical	Molar pregnancy	
Trauma	Retained placenta, miscarriage, or induced abortion	
Foreign body	Retained placenta, birth	
Malignancy of reproductive tract		

EVIDENCE-BASED PRACTICE

Treatments for Heavy Menstrual Bleeding

Ask the Question

For young women with heavy menstrual bleeding, what are the safest and most beneficial medical and surgical interventions?

Search for the Evidence

Search Strategies English language research-based publications since 2011 on dysfunctional uterine bleeding, heavy menstrual bleeding, and menorrhagia were included.

Databases Used Cochrane Database of Systematic Reviews, National Guideline Clearinghouse (AHRQ), CINAHL, PubMed, UpToDate, and the professional websites for ACOG and AWHONN.

Critical Appraisal of the Evidence

Heavy menstrual bleeding (HMB) can occur from reproductive hormonal imbalance, local uterine pathology, or clotting disorders. HMB may be linked to the inflammatory processes of the menstrual cycle, in which endometrial immune cells facilitate tissue breakdown, repair, and remodeling for menstruation (Berbic & Fraser, 2013).

- First-line treatment for HMB is nonsurgical. The most effective nonsurgical treatments, in order of efficacy, are:
  1. levonorgestrel-releasing intrauterine system (LNR-IUS), an intrauterine device (IUD) placed to deliver progestogen locally to the endometrium
  2. danazol, an oral progestogen derivative that shortens bleeding duration but can cause significant masculinizing side effects
  3. antifibrinolytic (tranexamic acid)
  4. nonsteroidal antiinflammatories (Lethaby, Duckitt, & Farquhar, 2013; Matteson, Rahn, Wheeler, et al., 2013)
- If medical therapy does not stop the bleeding, surgical interventions become necessary. Hysterectomy is the most effective but involves costly hospitalization and risk for surgical complications.
- Women who do not desire any more children can be offered an outpatient procedure in which the uterine lining is ablated (destroyed) to stop the bleeding.
- Direct visualization of the uterine lining, using a hysteroscope through the cervix, has been the gold standard technique for endometrial ablation. This requires a skilled practitioner. The endometrial lining is cauterized using
  - Laser
  - Rollerball electrocautery
  - Loop electrocautery (also called transcervical resection)
- Several newer techniques that do not require a hysteroscope include thermal ablation using a heated balloon, radiofrequency, or microwave. These are easier, shorter, and less likely to perforate or damage local tissue. However, technical difficulties with equipment erase any clear advantage the newer techniques offer women (Lethaby, Penninx, Hickey, et al., 2013).
- Endometrial ablation is best done when the endometrium is 4 mm or less. To facilitate endometrial thinning and ease of surgery, women may be prescribed one of the following
  - Gonadotropin-releasing hormone analogue (GnRHa), which competes for natural GnRH receptor sites, decreasing estrogen production, or danazol (Tan & Lethaby, 2013)

Apply the Evidence: Nursing Implications

- HMB negatively affects quality of life: women report physical, social, and sexual distress; pain; and anemia. The woman and her family may feel isolated and embarrassed. They may be fearful of serious disease, such as cancer.
- Nonsurgical treatments are frequently ineffective. This can be very frustrating and discouraging to women whose activities of daily living such as work, school, travel, and social activities may become restricted.
- Surgical interventions that ablate the endometrium result in loss of ability to become pregnant. For women who do not desire future pregnancy, the resulting amenorrhea can be a great relief. For women who planned future pregnancies, this alteration in their life plan is a life-altering loss, requiring sensitivity.
- Couples and significant others, such as parents, may benefit from grief counseling and group support. See Chapter 9 for more information about the psychologic implications of infertility.

Quality and Safety Competencies: Evidence-Based Practice*

Knowledge

Demonstrate comprehensive understanding of the concepts of pain and suffering, including physiologic models of pain and comfort.

The nurse should ask the woman and her family what meaning this disorder and its treatment have for them.

Skills

Initiate effective treatments to relieve pain and suffering in light of client values, preferences, and expressed needs.

Explaining the treatments and answering questions can help the family understand and cope with disease and life change.

Attitudes

Recognize that women's expectations influence outcomes in management of pain or suffering.

Collaborative decision making requires that the woman and her family expectations and goals be addressed in all aspects of care.

References

Berbic, M., & Fraser, I. S. (2013). Immunology of normal and abnormal menstruation. *Women's Health (London)*, *9*(4), 387–395.

Lethaby, A., Duckitt, K., & Farquhar, C. (2013). Non-steroidal anti-inflammatory drugs for heavy menstrual bleeding. *The Cochrane Database of Systematic Reviews*, 1. Chichester, UK: John Wiley & Sons.

Lethaby, A., Penninx, J., Hickey, M., et al. (2013). Endometrial resection and ablation techniques for heavy menstrual bleeding. *The Cochrane Database of Systematic Reviews*, 8. Chichester, UK: John Wiley & Sons.

Matteson, K. A., Rahn, D. D., Wheeler, T. L., et al. (2013). Nonsurgical management of heavy menstrual bleeding: A systematic review. *Obstetrics and Gynecology*, *121*(3), 632–643.

Tan, Y. H., & Lethaby, A. (2013). Pre-operative endometrial thinning agents before endometrial destruction for heavy menstrual bleeding. *The Cochrane Database of Systematic Reviews*. Chichester, UK: John Wiley & Sons.

Pat Mahaffee Gingrich

*Adapted from QSEN at www.qsen.org.

that any woman who has not undergone menopause and who seeks care for intermenstrual bleeding is or recently has been pregnant.

Treatment of intermenstrual bleeding depends on the cause and may include reassurance and education concerning mittlestaining, observation of three menstrual cycles for suspected functional ovarian cyst, adjustment of an OCP, removal of foreign bodies, and treatment for vaginal infections. More complex treatment may consist of removal of polyps; evaluation and treatment of an abnormal Papanicolaou (Pap) test, including colposcopy, biopsy, cautery, cryosurgery, or conization; and surgery, chemotherapy, or radiation treatment for malignancy. Important nursing roles include reassurance, counseling, education, and support.

Menorrhagia

Menorrhagia (hypermenorrhea) is defined as excessive menstrual bleeding, in either duration or amount. The causes of heavy menstrual bleeding are many, including hormonal disturbances, systemic disease, benign and malignant neoplasms, infection, and contraception (IUDs). A single episode of heavy bleeding may occur, or a woman may have regular flooding as a pattern in which she changes tampons or pads every few hours for several days.

> **! NURSING ALERT**
>
> If the woman herself considers the amount or duration of bleeding to be excessive, the problem should be investigated.

Hemoglobin and hematocrit provide objective indicators to actual blood loss and should always be assessed.

A single episode of heavy bleeding may signal an early pregnancy loss. This type of bleeding is often thought to be a period that is heavier than usual, perhaps delayed, and is associated with abdominal pain or pelvic discomfort. When early pregnancy loss is suspected, a hematocrit and serum β-hCG pregnancy test should be done.

Infectious and inflammatory processes such as acute or chronic endometritis and salpingitis may cause heavy menstrual bleeding. Although rare, systemic diseases of nonreproductive origin such as blood dyscrasias, hypothyroidism, and lupus erythematosus also can cause hypermenorrhea. In obese women anovulation caused by increased peripheral conversion of androstenedione to estrogen may develop and manifest as menorrhagia. Medications also may cause abnormal bleeding. Chemotherapy, anticoagulants, neuroleptics, and steroid hormone therapy all have been associated with excessive flow.

Uterine *leiomyomata* (fibroids or myomas) are a common cause of menorrhagia. Fibroids are benign tumors of the smooth muscle of the uterus, the etiology of which is unknown. Fibroids are estrogen sensitive and commonly develop during the reproductive years and shrink after menopause. Other uterine growths ranging from endometrial polyps to adenocarcinoma and endometrial cancer are common causes of heavy menstrual bleeding, as well as of intermenstrual bleeding.

Treatment for menorrhagia depends on the cause of the bleeding. If the bleeding is related to the contraceptive method, the nurse provides factual information and reassurance and discusses other contraceptive options. If bleeding is related to the presence of fibroids, the degree of disability and discomfort associated with the fibroids and the woman's plans for childbearing will influence treatment decisions. Treatment options include medical and surgical management. Most fibroids can be monitored by frequent examinations to judge growth, if any, and correction of anemia, if present. Women with menorrhagia should be warned not to use aspirin because of its tendency to increase bleeding. Medical treatment depends on the cause, client preferences, possibility of pregnancy, and future desire to have children (UpToDate, 2012). This reduction in bleeding is often accomplished with the use of a GnRH agonist. If the woman wishes to retain childbearing potential, a myomectomy may be done. Myomectomy, or removal of the tumors only, is particularly difficult if multiple myomas must be removed. If the woman does not want to preserve her childbearing function, or if she has severe symptoms (severe anemia, severe pain, considerable disruption of lifestyle), hysterectomy or endometrial ablation (laser surgery or electrocoagulation) may be done (see Chapter 11). Uterine artery embolization, based on the assumption that control of arterial blood flow to the fibroid will control symptoms, has been reported to result in reduced menorrhagia, less dysmenorrhea, and reduced pelvic pressure and urinary symptoms. This method of treatment is used for women who have completed their childbearing because there is a risk for loss of fertility (see Chapter 11).

Dysfunctional Uterine Bleeding

Abnormal uterine bleeding (AUB) is any form of uterine bleeding that is irregular in amount, duration, or timing and not related to regular menstrual bleeding. Box 6-1 lists possible causes of AUB. Although often used interchangeably, the terms AUB and dysfunctional uterine bleeding (DUB) are not synonymous. DUB is a subset of AUB defined as "excessive uterine bleeding with no demonstrable organic cause, genital or extragenital" (Lobo, 2012a). DUB is most frequently caused by anovulation. When there is no surge of LH, or if insufficient progesterone is produced by the corpus luteum to support the endometrium, it will begin to involute and shed. This process most often occurs at the extremes of a woman's reproductive years—when the menstrual cycle is just becoming established at menarche or when it draws to a close at menopause. DUB also can be found with any condition that gives rise to chronic anovulation associated with continuous estrogen production. Such conditions include obesity, hyperthyroidism and hypothyroidism, polycystic ovary syndrome, and any of the endocrine conditions discussed in the sections on amenorrhea and oligomenorrhea. A diagnosis of DUB is made only after ruling out all other causes of abnormal menstrual bleeding (Lobo).

When uterine bleeding is profuse and a woman's hemoglobin level is less than 8 g/dL (hematocrit of 23% or 24%), the woman may be hospitalized and given conjugated estrogens (e.g., Premarin), 25 mg intravenously. The dose may be repeated every 4 to 6 hours until bleeding stops or slows significantly (Estephan

BOX 6-1 Possible Causes of Abnormal Uterine Bleeding

Pregnancy-Related Conditions
- Threatened or spontaneous miscarriage
- Retained products of conception after elective abortion
- Ectopic pregnancy
- Placenta previa/placenta abruptio
- Trophoblastic disease

Lower Reproductive Tract Infections
- Cervicitis
- Endometritis
- Myometritis
- Salpingitis

Benign Anatomic Abnormalities
- Adenomyosis
- Leiomyomata
- Polyps of the cervix or endometrium

Neoplasms
- Endometrial hyperplasia
- Cancer of cervix and endometrium
- Hormonally active tumors (rare)
- Vaginal tumors (rare)

Malignant Lesions
- Cervical squamous cell carcinoma
- Endometrial adenocarcinoma
- Estrogen-producing ovarian tumors
- Testosterone-producing ovarian tumors
- Leiomyosarcoma

Trauma
- Genital injury (accidental, coital trauma, sexual abuse)
- Foreign body
- Lacerations

Systemic Conditions
- Adrenal hyperplasia and Cushing disease
- Blood dyscrasias
- Coagulopathies
- Hypothalamic suppression (from stress, weight loss, excessive exercise)
- Polycystic ovary disease
- Thyroid disease
- Pituitary adenoma or hyperprolactinemia
- Severe organ disease (renal or liver failure)

Iatrogenic Conditions
- Medications with estrogenic activity
- Anticoagulants
- Exogenous hormone use (oral contraceptives, menopausal hormone therapy)
- Selective serotonin reuptake inhibitors
- Tamoxifen
- Intrauterine devices
- Herbal preparation (ginseng)

Modified from Albers, J.R., Hull, S.K., & Wesley, R.M. (2004). Abnormal uterine bleeding. *American Family Physician, 69,* 1915-1926; 1931-1932.

& Sinert, 2012). If the bleeding has not stopped in 12 to 24 hours, dilation and curettage (D&C) may be done to control severe bleeding and hemorrhage. An endometrial biopsy may be collected at the same time to evaluate endometrial tissue or rule out endometrial cancer. After this treatment, oral conjugated estrogen, 2.5 mg, is given daily, followed by the addition of progesterone (e.g., medroxyprogesterone [Provera], 10 mg by mouth), given in the final 10 days of therapy to initiate withdrawal bleeding. Alternatively, a combined OCP is given for 21 days after intravenous therapy. Once the acute phase has passed, the woman is maintained on cyclic low-dose OCPs for 3 to 6 months. Such long-term treatment helps prevent recurrence of the pattern of DUB and hemorrhage. If the woman wants contraception, she should continue to take OCPs. If the woman has no need for contraception, the treatment may be stopped to assess her bleeding pattern. If menstruation does not resume, a progesterone regimen (e.g., medroxyprogesterone, 10 mg/day for 10 days before the expected date of her menstrual period) may be prescribed after ruling out pregnancy. This is done to prevent persistent anovulation with chronic unopposed endogenous estrogen hyperstimulation of the endometrium, which can result in eventual atypical tissue changes (Lobo, 2012a).

If the recurrent, heavy bleeding is not controlled by hormonal therapy or D&C, ablation of the endometrium through laser treatment may be performed. Nursing roles include counseling and educating women about their options as needed and referring women to the appropriate specialists and health care services.

CARE MANAGEMENT

Medical and nursing management has been discussed with each menstrual problem. It is important that the health care provider completes a systematic assessment, including a thorough menstrual, obstetric, sexual, and contraceptive history; the woman's perceptions of her condition; and cultural, ethnic, and lifestyle influences and patterns of coping. Assessment also involves evaluating the amount of pain or bleeding and noting ways the woman tries to alleviate pain and/or bleeding, including home remedies and prescriptions. It is helpful to ask the woman to keep a diary of her symptoms and ways that she alleviates those symptoms. Nursing care involves accepting the woman's symptoms as valid, correlating data from the daily diary of emotional status, subjective feelings, and physical state with physiologic changes, encouraging the woman to express her feelings about her symptoms, providing information about therapeutic options she chooses, and providing information about local support groups.

MENOPAUSE

With the increasing life span of American women, most can expect to live one third of their lives after their reproductive years. As women age many experience transitions that present challenges and require adaptation such as changing health, work, or marital status. Nowhere is this more true than with the changes associated with menopause. In the United States, menopause usually occurs during the late 40s and early 50s, with the median age being 51 to 52 years (Lobo, 2012c). The average age for the onset of the perimenopausal transition is 46 years; 95% of women experience the onset between ages 39 and 51. The average duration of the perimenopause period is 4 to 5 years, with 95% of women postmenopausal by age 58 (Lobo). Cigarette smoking and a history of short intermenstrual intervals seem to decrease the age at onset of menopause. African-American and Hispanic women in the United States experience menopause earlier than Caucasian women. However, heredity is the major determinant of age at menopause; genetics may explain most of the variation in menopause age (Lobo).

Perimenopause is the period that encompasses the transition from normal ovulatory cycles to cessation of menses and is marked by irregular menstrual cycles. Another term used to signal the period when a woman moves from the reproductive stage of life through the perimenopausal transition and menopause to the postmenopausal years is the climacteric. Menopause refers to the complete cessation of menses and is a single physiologic event said to occur when women have not had menstrual flow or spotting for 1 year, and it can be identified only in retrospect. Surgical menopause occurs with hysterectomy and bilateral oophorectomy. Postmenopause is the time after menopause.

Although all women have similar hormonal changes with menopause, the experience of each woman is influenced by her age, cultural background, health, type of menopause (spontaneous or surgical), childbearing desires, and relationships. Women may view menopause as a major change in their lives—either positive, such as freedom from troublesome dysmenorrhea and the need for contraception, or negative, such as feeling "old" or losing childbearing possibilities.

Physiologic Characteristics

Knowledge of the normal changes that occur during perimenopause is essential in assessing menopausal experiences and problems. Natural menopause is a gradual process with progressive increases in anovulatory cycles and eventual cessation of menses. In the 2 to 8 years preceding menopause, subtle hormonal changes eventually lead to altered menstrual function and later to amenorrhea. When women are in their 40s, anovulation occurs more often, menstrual cycles increase in length, and ovarian follicles become less sensitive to hormonal stimulation from FSH and LH. Because of these changes, a follicle is stimulated to the point that an ovum grows to maturity and is released in some months, whereas in other months, no ovulation takes place. Without ovulation and release of an ovum, progesterone is not produced by the corpus luteum. The lining continues to grow until it lacks a sufficient blood supply, at which point it bleeds. During this time a woman's cycle becomes more irregular. She may skip or miss periods; have shorter or lighter periods or longer, heavier periods; and have clotting. FSH levels become elevated, reflecting an attempt to stimulate a follicle to produce estrogen.

Physical Changes During the Perimenopausal Period

Bleeding

During the perimenopausal years, women may have longer menstrual periods that differ in the type of bleeding. They may have 2 to 3 days of spotting followed by 1 to 2 days of heavy bleeding, or they may have regular menses followed by 2 to 3 days of spotting. Such symptoms are characteristic of degenerating corpus luteum function. After menopause women continue to have small amounts of circulating estrogen. Although the ovaries do not produce estrogen, androgens (androstenedione and testosterone) are produced for some time after menopause. Androgens produced by the adrenal glands are converted to estrone, a form of estrogen, in the liver and fat cells. With advanced age the ovaries stop producing androstenedione, which further limits the amount of estrone in the body. Obese women are more likely to have dysfunctional uterine bleeding and endometrial hyperplasia because women with more body fat have higher circulating levels of estrone. This occurs because the estrogen that is stored in the body's fat cells is converted into a form of estrogen (estrone) that is available to the estrogen receptors within the endometrium.

Genital Changes

The vagina and urethra are estrogen-sensitive tissues, and low levels of estrogen can cause atrophy of both. Age-related vaginal changes not affected by estrogen also occur. Through both processes the vaginal membranes thin, hold less moisture, and lubricate more slowly. However, not all women have symptoms of genital atrophy. Women who are sexually active have less vaginal atrophy and fewer problems related to intercourse. Thin women are more likely to have more symptoms related to reduced estrogen levels such as vaginal dryness because of lack of adipose tissue and thus stored estrogen. Additionally, vaginal pH increases, lactobacillus growth can be depressed, and other bacteria tend to multiply. This combination of factors can lead to vaginitis.

Dyspareunia (painful intercourse) can occur because the vagina becomes smaller, the vaginal walls become thinner and drier, and lubrication during sexual stimulation takes longer. Intercourse becomes painful and may result in postcoital bleeding. Some women decide to forgo intercourse altogether.

In some women the shrinking of the uterus, the vulva, and the distal portion of the urethra associated with aging leads to disturbing symptoms, including urinary frequency, dysuria, uterine prolapse, and stress incontinence. Vaginal relaxation with cystocele, rectocele, and uterine prolapse is not caused by reduced estrogen levels but may be a delayed result of childbearing or other cause of weakness of pelvic support structures. Urinary frequency sometimes occurs after menopause because the distal portion of the urethra, which has the same embryologic origin as the reproductive organs, shortens and shrinks. Irritants have easier access to the urinary tract with its short urethra and may cause frequency and urinary tract infections.

Urinary incontinence and uterine displacement are two other common age-related rather than menopause-related findings in the postmenopausal period. These conditions are discussed in Chapter 11.

Vasomotor Instability

Investigators have devoted significant attention to identifying ovarian, hypothalamic, and pituitary hormonal mechanisms that produce symptoms related to menopause. Two symptoms appear to increase in incidence as women progress through menopause: hot flashes and night sweats. Many of the other changes commonly associated with menopause, such as decrease in size of genital structures, skin changes, and changes in breast size, are more correctly attributed to aging.

Vasomotor instability in the form of hot flashes or flushes is a result of fluctuating estrogen levels and is the most common disturbance of the perimenopausal years, occurring in up to 75% of women having natural menopause and 90% of women who have a surgical menopause. In the United States, Hispanic and African-American women report a higher incidence of these symptoms than Caucasian women; Asian women have the lowest incidence (Lobo, 2012c). Vasomotor instability occurs most frequently in the first 2 postmenopausal years; the number of episodes decreases over time. However, some women have hot flashes before menopause and continue to have them for 10 or more years afterward. During this time women experience changeable vasodilation and vasoconstriction as a hot flush (visible red flush of skin and perspiration) or hot flash (sudden warm sensation in neck, head, and chest) and night sweats. For some women hot flashes may be an infrequent, possibly pleasant, sensation of warmth; for others, they may be an intensely unpleasant sensation of heat or warmth that may occur 20 to 50 times a day, create intense anxiety, and significantly decrease quality of life. Several factors can precipitate or aggravate an episode, including crowded or warm rooms, alcohol, hot drinks, spicy foods, proximity to a heat source, and stress.

Night sweats, characterized by profuse perspiration and heat radiating from the body during the night, are another form of vasomotor instability experienced by many women. Sleep may be interrupted nightly because nightclothes and bed linens are soaked. Women may find that they are not able to go back to sleep. Sleep deprivation is a primary complaint of women experiencing hot flashes (Lobo, 2012c). Other problems associated with perimenopausal fluctuations of vasoconstriction or vascular spasms include dizziness, numbness and tingling in fingers and toes, and headaches.

Mood and Behavioral Responses

The tendency to associate hormonal changes with psychologic symptoms in midlife that has been prevalent in medical literature for decades and continues today was fueled by a belief that postmenopausal women have "estrogen deficiency." However, there is no concrete evidence that menopause has a deleterious effect on mental health of midlife women. Reviews of epidemiologic studies on menopause and depression found no causal association between menopause and depression (Lobo, 2012c). Women with hot flashes and night sweats do report insomnia, fatigue from loss of sleep, and depressed mood. They complain of feeling more emotionally labile, nervous, or agitated, with less control of their emotions. However, the interaction of psychologic, biologic, and sociocultural factors is so complex that it is difficult to determine whether a woman's reported mood shifts are the result of hormonal changes, normal aging, or cultural conditioning. Most likely a woman's psychologic makeup, cultural background, intercurrent stresses, and changing life roles and circumstances are more important than estrogen levels. Dealing with teenage children; having teenagers leave home; helping aging parents; becoming widowed or divorced; the onset of a major illness or disability (even death) in a spouse, relative, or friend; grieving for friends and family who are ill or dying; retirement; and financial insecurity are among the many stresses of women in their 40s and 50s.

Cultural messages also influence a woman's perception of menopause. Experiences with menopause are not universal and vary among cultural groups. Women do not find symptoms to be a cause for concern; however, they do report that symptoms are bothersome. Many women have accepted childbearing and childrearing as their major role in life, and the inability to bear children is a significant loss. Others see menopause as the first step to old age and associate it with a loss of attractiveness, physical ability, and energy. Western culture values youth and physical attractiveness; the wisdom gained from life experience is not valued, and older adults have a loss of status, function, and role. No rituals give older women a special place and function. In cultures in which postmenopausal women gain status, such as India, the Far East, and the South Pacific islands, depression among menopausal women is not observed. Western women, however, may have little to compensate for their losses.

For other women, menopause is not a loss or a symbol of losses, but a relief. For some, menopause is a relief from the fear of pregnancy, the discomfort and bother of menstruation, and the inconveniences of contraception.

The ability to cope with any stress involves three factors: the person's perception or understanding of the event, the support system, and coping mechanisms. Nurses counseling a woman in the perimenopausal years must therefore assess her understanding of perimenopausal changes, her perceptions of stressful experiences, her support systems, and her coping skills.

Health Risks of Perimenopausal Women

Osteoporosis and coronary heart disease are the major health risks of perimenopausal women and the focus of the following discussion.

Osteoporosis

Aging is associated with a progressive decrease in bone density in men and women. Osteoporosis is a generalized, metabolic disease characterized by decreased bone mass and increased incidence of bone fractures. Normally there is a dynamic balance between bone formation (osteoblastic activity) and bone resorption (osteoclastic activity). Because one of the functions of estrogen is to stimulate the osteoblasts, the postmenopausal decrease in estrogen levels causes an imbalance between bone formation and resorption. Old bone deteriorates faster than new bone is formed, resulting in a slow thinning of the bones. Estrogen also is required for the conversion of vitamin D into calcitonin, which is essential in the absorption of calcium by the intestine. Reduced calcium absorption from the gut, in addition to the thinning of the bones, places postmenopausal women at risk for problems associated with osteoporosis.

Osteoporosis is a major health problem in the United States, affecting more than 9 million people, the majority of whom are women (National Osteoporosis Foundation [NOF], 2013). Osteoporosis, is one of the key diseases that predominantly affect women. In fact, half of all women ages 50 and older will break a bone due to osteoporosis in their lifetime and 2 million bone breaks are caused by osteoporosis every year. Approximately 50% of U.S. women have some degree of osteoporosis, making women who are older than 50 at particular risk in their lifetimes for breaking a bone as a result of osteoporosis (NOF). One in two Caucasian women will have changes severe enough to predispose them to fractures. In the United States, the incidence of osteoporosis-related fractures has increased.

It has been estimated that 5.75% of older women who suffer hip fractures will die during the first 3 months following the fracture, with 1-year mortality rates ranging from 12% to 37% (Walker, 2013). During the first 5 to 6 years after menopause, women lose bone six times more rapidly than men. By age 65, one third of women have had a vertebral fracture; by age 81, one third have had a hip fracture. By the time women reach age 80, they have lost 47% of their trabecular bone, concentrated in the vertebrae, the pelvis and other flat bones, and the epiphyses. The most well-defined risk factor for osteoporosis is the loss of the protective effect of estrogen associated with cessation of ovarian function, particularly at menopause. Women at risk are likely to be Caucasian or Asian, small boned, and thin. Obese women have higher estrogen levels resulting from the conversion of androgens in adipose tissue; mechanical stress from extra weight also helps preserve bone mass. A family history of the disease is common. Much more research needs to be done to determine genetic testing for those at higher risk for osteoporosis (Fritz & Speroff, 2011).

Inadequate calcium intake is a risk factor, particularly during adolescence and into the third and fourth decades, when peak bone mass is attained. An excessive caffeine intake increases calcium excretion, causing a systemic acidosis that stimulates bone resorption. Vitamin D deficiency can affect the physiologic regulation and stimulation of intestinal absorption of calcium (NOF, 2010). Smoking is associated with earlier and greater bone loss and decreases estrogen production. Excessive alcohol intake interferes with calcium absorption and depresses bone formation. A greater phosphorus than calcium intake, which occurs with soft drink consumption, may be a risk factor. Other risk factors include steroid therapy and disorders such as hypogonadism, hyperthyroidism, and diabetes mellitus.

The first sign of osteoporosis is often loss of height resulting from vertebral fracture and collapse (Fig. 6-2). Back pain, especially in the lower back, may or may not be present. Later signs include "dowager's hump," in which the vertebrae can no longer support the upper body in an upright position, and fractured hip, in which the fracture often precedes a fall. Damage to the vertebrae usually precedes bone loss in the hip by an average of 10 years. Osteoporosis cannot be detected by radiographic examination until 30% to 50% of the bone mass has been lost; thus routine screening is not warranted in women younger than age 65. However, bone density testing is recommended for women who are age 65 and older or in younger women who are at a risk that is equal to or greater than a 65-year-old Caucasian woman without additional risk factors (U.S. Preventive Health Services Task Force, 2011).

COMMUNITY ACTIVITY

- Visit the Office of Women's Health website at www.WomensHealth.gov. Select menopause from the list of topics on women's health issues to understand better the resources available to women who have questions about menopause.
- Visit the National Osteoporosis Foundation website at www.nof.org. Review the client information regarding osteoporosis, prevention, management, and finding a doctor. What are the resources for women with osteoporosis in your community?
- Visit the North American Menopause Society (NAMS) website at www.menopause.org. Review Memo Note and the Menopause Guidebook. How can this information help you in teaching your clients about how to manage menopausal symptoms?

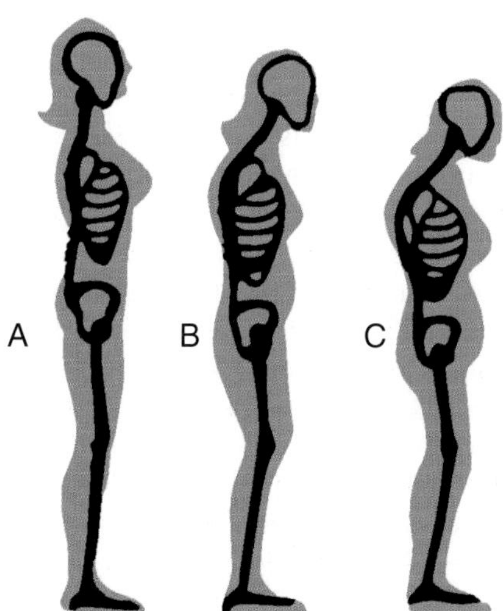

FIG 6-2 Skeletal changes secondary to osteoporosis assessed by height and body shape at **A**, age 55 years; **B**, age 65 years; and **C**, age 75 years.

Coronary Heart Disease

A woman's risk of developing and dying of cardiovascular disease increases after menopause. Diseases of the heart are the leading cause of death for U.S. women. The lifetime risk is 31% versus 3% for breast cancer in postmenopausal women. Known risk factors for coronary heart disease include obesity, cigarette smoking, elevated cholesterol and blood pressure levels, diabetes mellitus, family history of cardiac disease, alcohol abuse, and the effects of aging on the cardiovascular system (Lobo, 2012c). Estrogen has a favorable effect on circulating lipids, decreasing low-density lipoprotein (LDL) and total cholesterol and increasing high-density lipoprotein (HDL), and has a direct antiatherosclerotic effect on arteries. Postmenopausal women are at risk for coronary artery disease because of changes in lipid metabolism: a decline in serum levels of HDL cholesterol and an increase in LDL levels (Lobo). These changes can be favorably reduced by diet and exercise.

Menopausal Hormonal Therapy

Until 2002 **menopausal hormonal therapy (MHT)**—either as *estrogen replacement therapy (ERT)* or *estrogen therapy*

(ET), in which a woman takes only estrogen, or *hormonal replacement therapy (HRT)* or *hormonal therapy (HT)*, in which she takes both estrogen and progestins—was widely prescribed for discomforts associated with the perimenopausal years, including hot flashes and vaginal and urinary tract atrophy. Further, MHT was aggressively used for therapeutic and preventive management. At the same time its use remained highly controversial in women's health. Some authorities recommended HT or ET for all women; these proponents viewed the perimenopause as a disease or deficiency state. Others insisted that the use of hormones was never indicated for menopausal symptoms. The middle-ground approach advocated the use of MRT for women who have specific discomforts (therapeutic management) and for women in certain high risk groups (preventive management). Research studies challenged these beliefs in the preventive and beneficial effects of HT. Findings from the Women's Health Initiative (WHI), a study by the National Institutes of Health (NIH), documented an increase in heart disease with use of continuous combined estrogen plus progestin (NIH, 2010). There is also an increased risk for breast cancer in women taking hormone therapy, although that risk returns to normal 3 years after discontinuation of hormonal therapy (American Cancer Society [ACS], 2013a). These findings changed the way MHT is used. Many women stopped taking MHT and sought alternative therapies to treat their menopausal symptoms. Others chose to continue with the MHT but had questions about the available regimens and associated risks.

The North American Menopause Society (NAMS, 2012) supports the use of estrogen therapy beyond 3 to 5 years for menopausal women to prevent osteoporosis, but they do not support this long-term use of estrogen-progesterone therapy because of its correlation with increased risk for breast cancer. Chen, Chou, and Chang (2013), however, disagree with the recommendations of NAMS.

The U.S. Preventive Services Task Force (2013) recommends against using hormone therapy (combined estrogen and progestin) for postmenopausal women for the prevention of chronic conditions, and against the use of estrogen to prevent chronic conditions in postmenopausal women who have had a hysterectomy.

Recommendations from ACOG (2014) continue to support the use of MHT, but encourages greater use of nonhormonal alternatives, such as SSRI as well as selective serotonin and norepinephrine reuptake inhibitors. The recommendations also mention newer combined estrogen drugs, referred to as selective estrogen receptor modulators. Specifically mentioned are two new drugs: bazedoxifine for hot flashes and osteoporosis. The other is ospemifene for vaginal dryness and atrophy. The report recommends against the use of progestin by itself as well as testosterone, and it indicates that more research is needed regarding the use of bioidentical hormones. (See later discussion on bioidentical hormones.)

Decision to Use Hormone Therapy

All women considering ET or HT must understand that studies on MHT are ongoing, and there is still much to be learned. Nurses can provide information and counseling to assist women to make decisions regarding MHT use. Important teaching points include the following:

- For women taking MHT for short-term (1 to 3 years) relief of menopausal discomforts and who do not have increased risks for cardiovascular disease, the benefits may outweigh the risks. The decision to use MRT should be made between a woman and her health care provider.
- If used, MHT should be taken at the lowest effective dose for the shortest possible duration.
- When a woman decides to stop MHT, a recurrence of symptoms will occur whether the medication is tapered or discontinued abruptly. NAMS makes no recommendation on how to discontinue the medication, although some clinicians recommend a gradual withdrawal.
- Older women who are taking or considering MHT only for the prevention of cardiovascular disease should be counseled on other methods to reduce their risks of cardiovascular disease.
- Alternatively there may be beneficial cardiovascular effects associated with MHT for younger, more recently menopausal women, but more research is needed in this area.
- Women who are taking MHT only for prevention of osteoporosis or other chronic conditions should be counseled regarding their personal risks and benefits for continuing the therapy because there are conflicting recommendations (Chen, Chou, & Chang, 2013; NAMS, 2012; U.S. Preventive Services Task Force, 2013). These women should be reassured that there are effective alternatives for long-term prevention. Bone density studies also may be indicated to determine the degree of risk in an individual woman (U.S. Preventive Health Services Task Force, 2011).
- Women with a high risk for breast cancer or who have had breast cancer should be informed of the current research that links MHT to breast cancer (ACS, 2013a).
- Conjugated estrogens are associated with an increased incidence of gallbladder disease, and women with a known history of gallbladder disease should not use MHT (MacReady, 2013).

Side Effects

Side effects associated with estrogen use include headaches, nausea and vomiting, bloating, ankle and foot swelling, weight gain, breast soreness, brown spots on the skin, eye irritation with contact lenses, and depression. The type of estrogen used for postmenopausal hormonal therapy is much less potent than ethinyl estradiol used in OCPs and has fewer serious side effects. Side effects that occur with MHT may disappear with a change in estrogen preparation or a decrease in the dose prescribed.

Treatment Guidelines

Research in MHT continues; however, nurses who counsel women about MHT must understand what is available and teach women who choose to continue MHT how to take the medications correctly. Thus the following discussion about the different regimens of MHT is included.

Many different estrogen preparations, natural and synthetic, and ways of administering them—oral tablets, topical creams, transdermal preparations, suppositories, and vaginal rings—are available (Table 6-4).

There are multiple dosing regimen options for combining progesterone with estrogen for women who have a uterus.

TABLE 6-4 Hormone Medications for Menopausal Symptoms

MEDICATION NAME	COMPOSITION	AVAILABLE DOSES
Estrogens		
Oral		
Premarin	Conjugated estrogens	0.3 mg; 0.45 mg; 0.625 mg; 0.9 mg; 1.25 mg
Cenestin, Congest, C.E.S., PMS-Conjugated	Synthetic conjugated estrogens, A	0.3 mg; 045 mg; 0.625 mg; 0.9 mg; 1.25 mg; 0.3 mg; 0.625 mg; 0.9 mg, 1.25 mg, 2.5 mg; 0.3 mg, 0.625 mg, 0.9 mg, 1.25 mg; 0.3 mg, 0.625 mg, 0.9 mg, 1.25 mg
Enjuvia	Synthetic conjugated estrogens, B	0.3 mg; 0.45 mg; 0.625 mg; 0.9 mg; 1.25 mg
Estrace, various generics	Micronized estradiol	0.5 mg; 1 mg; 2 mg
Menest	Esterified estrogens	0.3 mg; 0.625 mg; 1.25 mg; 2.5 mg
Femtrace	Estradiol acetate	0.45 mg; 0.9 mg; 1.8 mg
Ortho-Est	Estropipate	0.625 mg; 1.25 mg; 2.5 mg
Transdermal		
Estraderm	Estradiol reservoir patch	0.05 mg; 0.1 mg twice weekly
Climera, Esclim, Estradot	Estradiol matrix patch	0.025 mg; 0.0375 mg; 0.05 mg; 0.075 mg; 0.1 mg once weekly
Vivelle	Estradiol matrix patch	0.05 mg; 0.1 mg twice weekly
Vivelle-Dot	Estradiol matrix patch	0.025 mg; 0.0375 mg; 0.05 mg; 0.1 mg twice weekly
Menostar	Estradiol matrix patch	0.014 mg once weekly
Alora	Estradiol matrix patch	0.0025 mg; 0.05 mg; 0.075 mg; 0.1 mg twice weekly
Divigel	Estradiol gel 0.1%	0.003 mg; 0.009 mg; 0.027 mg daily
EstroGel	Estradiol gel 0.06%	0.035 mg daily
Elestrin	Estradiol gel 0.06%	0.0125 mg daily
Evamist	Estradiol spray	0.021 mg per spray daily; may increase to 2 or 3 sprays daily
Estrasorb	Estradiol emulsion	0.05 mg/2 packets daily
Vaginal		
Premarin cream	Conjugated estrogens	0.5 g to 2 g/day (0.0625 mg/g)
Estrace cream	Estradiol	1 g/day (0.1 mg/g)
Femring vaginal ring	Estradiol acetate	12.4 mg or 24.8 mg; releases 0.05 mg/day or 0.10 mg/day for 90 days
Estring vaginal ring	Estradiol	2 mg; releases 7.5 mcg daily for 90 days
Vagifem vaginal tablet	Estradiol hemihydrate	25-mcg tablet twice a week
Progestogens		
Oral		
Provera	Medroxyprogesterone acetate	2.5 mg; 5 mg; 10 mg
Aygestin	Norethindrone acetate	5 mg
Micronor	Norethindrone	0.35 mg
Norgestrel	Ovrette	0.075 mg
Progesterone capsule (in peanut oil)	Prometrium	100 mg; 200 mg
Intrauterine		
Levonorgestrel	Mirena	Approximately 20 mcg/day
Vaginal		
Progesterone gel	Prochieve 4%	45 mg/applicator
Combination Estrogen-Progestin		
Oral		
Premphase	Conjugated estrogens (E)	0.625 mg E daily for 28 days
	Medroxyprogesterone acetate (P)	5 mg P on day 14 through day 28
Prempro	Conjugated estrogens (E)	0.0625 mg E plus 2.5 or 5 P daily
	Medroxyprogesterone acetate (P)	0.3 mg or 0.45 mg E plus 1.5 P daily
Activella	Estradiol (E) and norethindrone acetate (NETA)	1 mg E plus 0.5 mg NETA daily
Femhrt	Ethinyl estradiol and norethindrone acetate (NETA)	2.5 mcg E plus 0.5 mg NETA daily
Transdermal		
CombiPatch	Estradiol/norethindrone acetate (NETA)	0.05 mg estradiol/0.14 mg NETA or 0.05 mg estradiol/0.25 mg NETA twice weekly
Climera Pro	Estradiol and levonorgestrel	0.045 mg/0.015 mg weekly

Modified from North American Menopause Society. (2012). *Hormone products for postmenopausal use in the United States and Canada*. Available at www.menopause.org/docs/professional/htcharts.pdf?sfvrsn=6. Copyright © The North American Menopause Society, November 19, 2012.

According to NAMS, estrogen therapy is the treatment of choice for vulvar and vaginal atrophy, and low-dose local vaginal estrogen therapy is best if the woman is only experiencing vaginal symptoms. In addition, NAMS (2012) recommends transdermal or low-dose estrogen for women at risk for venous thromboembolism or stroke, although this recommendation is given with caution because there is still not enough research. There is evidence to recommend keeping exposure to progesterone at a minimum. An oral continual-cyclic regimen that is most commonly prescribed is estrogen on days 1 to 28 and a progestogen (e.g., medroxyprogesterone) on days 14 to 28. Women usually do not have cyclic bleeding with this regimen and are less likely to have progestin side effects.

There are also multiple regimen options for ET for women who have had a hysterectomy. The transdermal estrogen patch is applied once or twice a week to a hairless area of skin. Transdermal gels and sprays are applied daily. Any site on the trunk or upper arms provides adequate absorption. Sites should be rotated. The patches should not be placed on the breasts because of their sensitivity. Some women report minor skin irritation and reddening at the patch site. Generally transdermal estrogen offers the same relief of menopausal symptoms as the oral preparation. The transdermal method of delivery of estrogen does not have the same side effects such as breast tenderness and fluid retention. Oral progestin therapy can be used with transdermal ET. Combined estrogen-progestin transdermal patches also are available.

Vaginal creams and tablets are inserted daily or twice a week. Usually these local administrations of low-dose estrogen are used for vaginal symptoms of dryness and atrophy. Vaginal rings are inserted and left in place for 90 days. Although minimal systemic absorption is possible, there are no reports of adverse effects when a low dose is used (NAMS, 2012).

Bioidentical and Custom-Compounded Hormones

Bioidentical hormones, sometimes referred to as natural hormones, are structurally identical to those produced by the ovary. Bioidentical hormone preparations are available as government-approved, well-tested brand-name prescription medications. Others are made at compounding pharmacies. Custom-compounded hormones are custom mixes of one or more hormones in varying amounts. These mixes can provide individualized doses and mixtures of hormones that are not available commercially. They also include ingredients that are nonhormonal (e.g., dyes, preservatives). The risks are that these mixtures have not been studied to confirm whether appropriate absorption occurs or if predictable levels can be detected in blood and tissue (NAMS, 2012). Preparations may vary from one pharmacy to another, meaning that a woman may not get consistent amounts of medication. These preparations are not approved by any regulatory agency (NAMS). Although these hormones may relieve menopausal symptoms, more research is needed to determine their effects on the body. Women who choose to take these hormones need to understand and accept the potential risks. Expense is also an issue because these drugs often are more expensive and are not covered by third-party payers.

Controversy continues in regard to the use of herbal preparations and bioidentical hormone therapy for menopause. ACOG's (2012) Committee Opinion concluded that there is not enough evidence to support the efficacy and safety of compounded bioidentical hormones as better than conventional hormone therapy, and customized preparations are too variable (i.e., lacking standardization), creating greater risks and difficulty determining correct dosage.

Alternative Therapies

Many complementary and alternative therapies are useful for relieving some of the changes associated with altered estrogen levels. Homeopathy, acupuncture, and herbs have been used with varying degrees of success for menopausal problems such as heavy bleeding, hot flashes, irritability, and headaches.

Homeopathy views menopausal symptoms as the body's efforts to heal itself from the hormonal changes it is experiencing. Examples of remedies commonly prescribed during menopause by homeopaths are sepia, made from the inky juice of the cuttlefish, to relieve symptoms such as dry mouth, eyes, and vagina; nux vomica, derived from the poison nut, to relieve backaches, constipation, and frequent awakenings; and pulsatilla, made from the windflower, to relieve severe menstrual symptoms and hot flashes. Homeopathic remedies are subject to regulation by the U.S. Food and Drug Administration (FDA), although the FDA does not require proof of effectiveness. More study is needed to determine the effectiveness of homeopathic remedies.

Acupuncturists also treat hot flashes, but it is important that women evaluate their acupuncturists carefully. The American Association of Acupuncturists and Oriental Medicine will supply a list of acupuncturists in a given state. Questions to ask are: Is the acupuncturist certified by the National Commission for the Certification of Acupuncture? Is the acupuncturist certified in the state in which he or she practices? Does the acupuncturist carry malpractice insurance? Hendrick (2011) reported on a study of 53 menopausal women, comparing those who received acupuncture with those who received a sham acupuncture. The women who received acupuncture experienced fewer hot flashes as well as a lessening of other symptoms. More research is necessary in this area.

Herbal therapy also has been used to treat menopausal discomforts. Herbs can be ingested as teas or tinctures. Many herbal preparations also are available in capsule form. It is important that women understand mechanisms of action, contraindications, and potential side effects of each herb.

SAFETY ALERT

Most herbal preparations have not undergone long-term testing for safety and efficacy. Benefits and risks are not completely known. Women should always consult with their health care provider before beginning herbal therapy. Questions regarding the use of herbal therapy and other supplements must be a component of a client history.

In addition to resolving physical symptoms, herbs also are used to combat mood swings and depression. Ginseng has been claimed to be helpful in alleviating hot flashes, although research studies have not supported this assertion. Women should be advised against prolonged use of ginseng in high doses because it can increase blood pressure. Oriental herbal teas composed of licorice, ginseng, coptis, red raspberry leaf, and Chinese rhubarb may be of some help in relieving hot flashes.

Dong quai has been recognized as possibly helping to alleviate menopausal symptoms, although research has not provided evidence for a safe and effective dose (Mayo Clinic, 2012). Black cohosh, too, has been recognized as possibly being effective to treat menopausal symptoms, but evidence is lacking to justify its use without further systematic clinical trials (Leach & Moore, 2012).

Some plant foods contain phytoestrogens (isoflavones) and are capable of interacting with estrogen receptors in the body. These foods include red clover, wild yams, dandelion greens, cherries, alfalfa sprouts, black beans, and soybeans. Use of soy-rich foods as an alternative to traditional hormonal therapy for menopause has been studied. NAMS (2011), in a report on the role of isoflavones in menopause, concluded that more study is needed to demonstrate evidence for beneficial effects on menopausal symptoms.

For women who want to add soy to their diets, tofu, roasted soy nuts, and soy milk are good sources. Foods should be added gradually because some women have gastrointestinal discomfort from the high fiber content of these foods. Spreading out the daily intake over several meals may be the best way to include soy products in the diet.

Vitamin E is a popular alternative among women who do not take MHT. Nihira (2012) reviewed a variety of treatments for hot flashes, and included vitamin E as a possible treatment. Vitamin E is found in a variety of foods, including spinach, peanuts, wheat germ, vegetable oils, and soybeans, or it may be taken as a supplement. Dosage varies widely, from 400 to 800 International Units per day.

Layered clothing, ice packs, ice water, and fans may offer symptomatic relief from hot flashes (see Teaching for Self-Management box). Women can be counseled to avoid hot curries and other spicy foods. Reassurance that hot flashes will not last forever may be of comfort even if duration of the problem cannot be predicted accurately. Many women find that hot flashes lessen in frequency and intensity or disappear within 4 to 6 years after menopause.

Nurses should be aware of the availability of natural remedies for menopausal symptoms and be knowledgeable about the indications for complementary and alternative therapies so clients can be counseled appropriately.

CARE MANAGEMENT

Most women know little about menopause, and misinformation can cause anxiety. They need to know what to expect, why it happens, and what measures will help make them more comfortable. Women appreciate the opportunity to discuss what they are experiencing. They need to know that their discomforts have a normal physiologic basis and that other women experience similar discomforts.

Planning for nursing care requires knowledge of the perimenopausal period and great sensitivity. Treatment must be individualized for the specific woman. A thorough health history, physical examination, and laboratory tests are essential to distinguish pathologic conditions from the normal perimenopausal experiences. Informed consent regarding MHT, weight-bearing exercise, and calcium supplements is a major concern because treatment may involve tests, inconvenience, and side effects. Menopause clinics are needed where research

TEACHING FOR SELF-MANAGEMENT

Comfort Measures for Menopausal Symptoms

Hot Flashes/Flushes

During the Day

- Wear layered clothing so you can take things off if you get warm.
- Avoid "triggers" that bring on a flash/flush; these include vigorous exercise on hot days and eating spicy foods, caffeine, hot beverages, and alcohol.
- Splash your face with cool water, drink ice water, or take a cool shower if you get warm.
- Try slow, deep breathing.

At Night

- Sleep in cotton clothes, use cotton sheets, and keep room cool.
- Avoid heavy blankets that make you too warm at night.
- Keep a thermos of water by the bed.

Insomnia

- Avoid caffeine, alcohol, or tobacco in the evening.
- Avoid liquids after dinner.
- Exercise regularly but limit exercise to the daytime and early evening.
- Develop a bedtime routine.
- Establish a regular time to go to bed.
- Try drinking warm milk or taking a hot bath.
- Use your bed only for sleeping or sexual activity; don't watch TV, read, etc.
- Encourage your body's circadian rhythm.
- If you can't sleep, get up and do something until you feel tired.
- Avoid naps during the day.
- Sprinkle lavender oil on the pillow.
- Drink chamomile tea (do not use if allergic to ragweed or chrysanthemums).

Headaches

- Try to avoid stress and get plenty of rest.
- Eat or drink foods that contain natural diuretics (parsley).

Urogenital Symptoms

- Drink lots of water (i.e., at least 8 glasses a day), and empty bladder frequently.
- Practice Kegel exercises daily.
- Wear cotton underwear and avoid wearing wet bathing suits for a prolonged time.
- Use water-soluble lubricants for vaginal dryness.

Nervousness, Irritability

- Practice yoga or other meditation.
- Do relaxation or deep-breathing exercises.
- Practice guided imagery.

Data from Woods, N., & Mitchell, E. (2008). Mid-life women's health. In C. Fogel & N. Woods (Eds.), *Women's health care in advanced practice nursing.* New York: Springer.

on the effects of various treatments can be developed and evaluated and where care by the various specialty groups involved, such as endocrinology, radiology, psychosocial resources, exercise physiology, and nutrition, can be effectively coordinated. Women's support groups also are needed. Sexual counseling, nutrition, exercise, and support are topics that are included for further discussion.

Sexual Counseling

Sexuality is a lifelong behavior, and contrary to common stereotypes, sex does not end with menopause. Many women remain sexually active throughout their entire lives. However, women and their partners may change their expression of sexuality during and after menopause, depending on physical changes, changes in the partner, and cultural myths and messages. Some women report decreases in interest and desire. These decreases in sexuality with aging are influenced more by culture and attitudes than by nature and physiology (hormones). Although some women report that it takes longer to reach orgasm and that the orgasm is not so intense, the capacity for orgasm is not decreased. There is no way to prevent the inevitable aging process that the body undergoes. For people who see aging as loss, sexuality may become difficult to incorporate into what they perceive to be a less attractive identity. The fear of rejection may be present.

Changes in a male partner may influence whether he continues to want to engage in sexual activity. As men age, they, too, take longer to reach orgasm; erections take longer to occur and are less firm. Men may believe they are becoming impotent or ill and give up sexual activity, viewing it as too frustrating. Women may believe their partners are losing interest in them. Couples may need counseling to understand these changes. Although women tend to outlive men, that is not always the case, and some men may lack available female partners.

The two most important influences on older women's sexual activity are the strength of a relationship and the physical condition of each partner. The lack of available male partners can have a negative effect on sexual expression for many midlife and older women. Women outlive men, and older widowed and divorced women frequently have fewer opportunities to develop relationships because they are less sought after. In counseling older women who do engage in intercourse, the nurse cannot assume that new or nonmonogamous partners are free of sexually transmitted infections (STIs) and should inform women of their risk for human immunodeficiency virus infection (HIV) and other STIs and the need to use condoms.

As long as women are able to bear children, some accept intercourse as part of their responsibility as wives. When menopause frees them from this duty, they may choose to forgo intercourse. For other women, libido may increase without the fuss of contraception, fear of pregnancy, or interruption from menses.

Older lesbian women largely have been a silent group whose sexual needs and special social circumstances have not been acknowledged or recognized. Although lesbian women in midlife and in later years do not face the problem of a lack of available male partners, they are faced with negative attitudes accompanying being old, female, and lesbian—all of which can adversely affect sexuality and sexual expression.

Nurses must give accurate information on matters such as appropriate contraception, sexuality, and the physiology of menopause and should offer support and nonjudgmental guidance. Women need advice about contraception because ovulation may not cease for a year after the last menstrual cycle, and menopausal women can still become pregnant. The nurse's attitude toward sex and the older woman is important. Negative attitudes can reinforce the woman's misgivings about maintaining an active and satisfying sex life. The nurse can reassure the woman grieving over lost youth and attractiveness that the desire for sex into old age is a natural one and that the body has the capacity for sexual satisfaction. Only minor adjustments may be required.

Muscle tone around the reproductive organs decreases after menopause. Kegel exercises (see Chapter 4 for more detailed information) strengthen these muscles, improve tone, and, if practiced regularly, help prevent prolapsed uterus and stress incontinence. This is a low-cost, effective, noninvasive intervention to control symptoms. However, symptoms return if exercises are discontinued.

Lubricating jelly (e.g., K-Y, Femglide, Aqualube) is a water-soluble lubricant that provides relief from painful intercourse. It may be applied directly to the vulva and the penis. Vaginal moisturizers may be water based but also contain other products such as vitamin E and aloe (e.g., K-Y Longlasting, Replens, Astroglide). They are inserted into the vagina using a prefilled applicator. Oil-based lubricants such as petroleum jelly (Vaseline) should not be used because they clog vaginal glands, which can then be sites for bacterial infection.

Prolonged hospitalization of an older adult partner may have a significant effect on the couple's sexual relationship. They may have difficulty renewing sexual activity when the separation is over and may need counseling or referral. In the event that a couple is admitted to a nursing home, the nurse should encourage placement of the couple together. With the aging of the American population and changing attitudes about the appropriateness of lifelong sexual expression, long-term care, extended care, and full-time care facilities are more receptive to providing opportunities for sexual activity between marital partners.

The nurse can refer couples to a counselor or physician for problems beyond the scope of nursing practice.

Nutrition

Obesity and osteoporosis are common health problems of midlife and older women. As women move out of their childbearing years, they may need to change their diets. Because metabolic rates decrease with age and many women exercise less, fewer calories are needed for weight maintenance as women age. In general, foods chosen should be high in nutrients, fiber, and calcium but moderate in calories and low in fat to allow adequate nutritional intake while maintaining body weight. Nurses can suggest that women substitute skim for whole milk or chicken without skin for steak. Excessive protein should be avoided. Fat-free milk and yogurt are good sources of calcium and vitamin D. Women should avoid excessive intake of alcohol, soft drinks, and caffeinated coffee.

Calcium is an essential part of any therapeutic regimen for women with osteoporosis and those who want to prevent osteoporosis. The best source of calcium is food; however, it is difficult to eat other foods that contain calcium (sesame seeds, spinach, greens, broccoli, and seaweed) in quantities sufficient to meet daily requirements. Calcium supplements are recommended when a woman's diet does not supply recommended amounts of calcium. Although calcium cannot reverse loss of bone mass or prevent fractures, calcium supplementation may retard the development of osteoporosis after menopause. Menopausal women without contraindications to calcium supplementation (history of kidney stones, kidney failure, hypercalcemia) should be encouraged to consume a diet that has 1200 to 1500 mg of calcium a day or to add an amount of calcium supplementation that will increase their daily intake to this level. Calcium supplements are best taken in divided doses and with meals because of the increase in acid secretions and extended time in the stomach. At least 8 ounces of water to increase solubility is recommended. Calcium supplements should not be taken with caffeinated beverages. Calcium is most commonly available as calcium carbonate, calcium lactate, and calcium phosphate.

The *Osteoporosis Report* (Feb 2011) states that the Institute of Medicine (IOM) recommends 600 International Units of vitamin D for healthy adults up to age 70 and 800 International Units for those who are 71 and older. NOF (2013), however, recommends that women younger than 50 take 400 to 800 International Units daily and those older than age 50 take vitamin D 800 to 1000 International Units daily. Sources of vitamin D include sunlight, food (e.g., fortified dairy products, fatty fish, liver, egg yolks), and supplements. Usually a supplement is needed to get the required daily dose. A combination of vitamin D and calcium is available, and most multivitamins contain some vitamin D.

Exercise

All too often midlife women are sedentary—the demands of family and work constraints increase, and energy levels decrease. Unfortunately little or no exercise predisposes women to weight gain and does not help prevent cardiac disease or osteoporosis. Exercise alone cannot prevent or reverse osteoporosis, but data indicate that weight-bearing exercise, such as walking and stair climbing, may delay bone loss and increase bone mass at any age. Aerobics and strength training have positive effects on midlife women's health, including cardiorespiratory function, weight, bone density, and quality of life (Mishra, Mishra, & Devanshi, 2011). Mishra and colleagues recommended that women exercise 2 hours and 30 minutes per week, doing moderate aerobic exercise.

Water aerobics is excellent for cardiovascular fitness and is a good choice for older women who may be unable to engage in weight-bearing exercises. The nurse can help women plan an exercise program. Examples of exercises are available from the NOF (Fig. 6-3).

Medications for Osteoporosis

In addition to calcium and exercise, there are a number of FDA-approved medications for preventing and treating osteoporosis (Box 6-2). The medications assist in delaying bone loss, increasing bone mass, and preventing fractures. These include salmon calcitonin (Miacalcin); bisphosphonates (alendronate sodium [Fosamax], risedronate sodium [Actonel]),

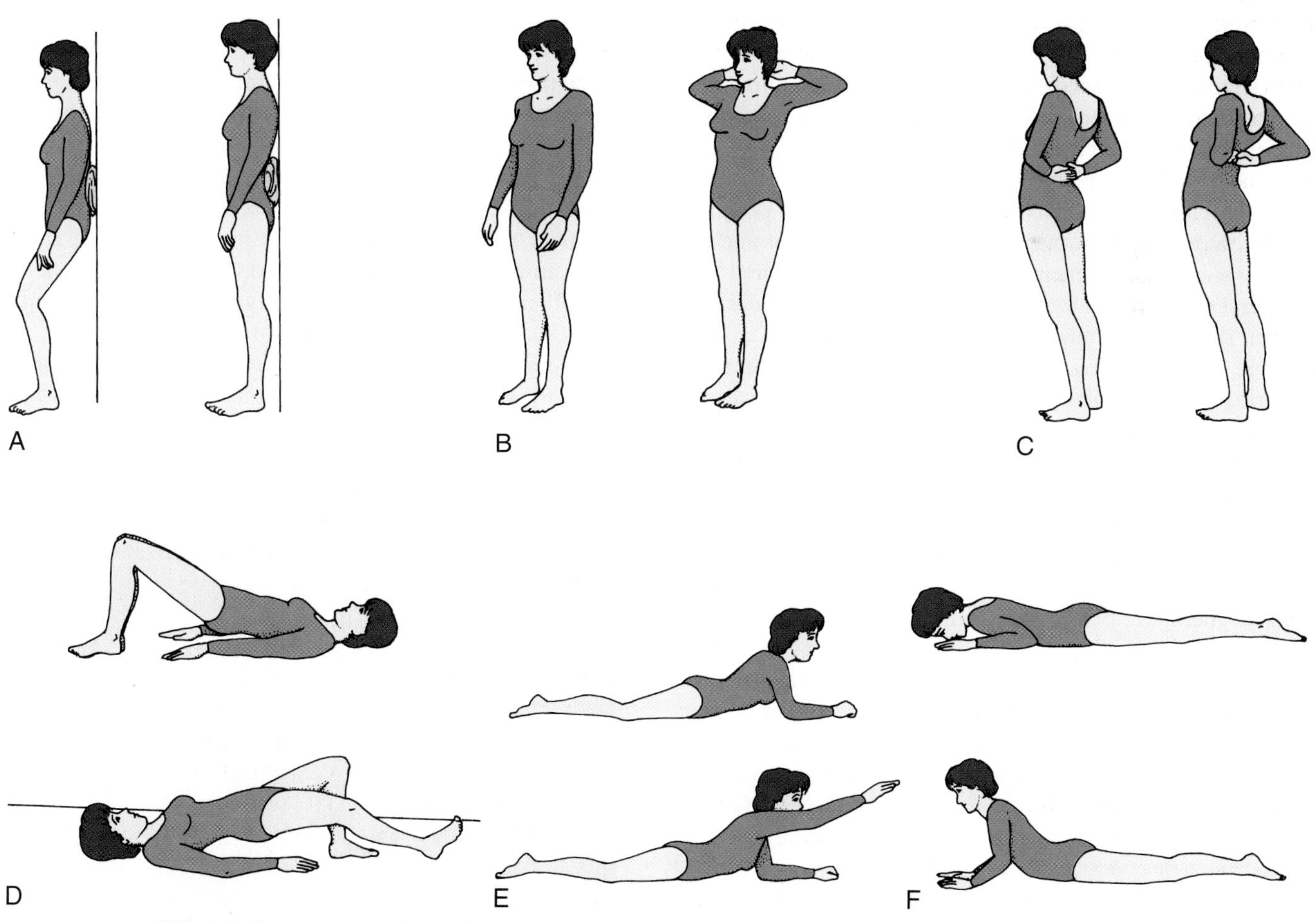

FIG 6-3 Posture exercises. **A,** Wall standing and pelvic tilt. **B,** Isometric posture correction. **C,** Standing back bend. **D,** The bridge. **E,** The elbow prop. **F,** Prone press-ups with deep breathing. (From *Boning Up on Osteoporosis.* Courtesy the National Osteoporosis Foundation.)

BOX 6-2 Prevention of Osteoporosis

- All postmenopausal women should be evaluated clinically for risk for osteoporosis and to determine the need for bone mineral density (BMD) testing.
- A BMD test is the only way to diagnose osteoporosis and determine risk for future fracture. The U.S. Preventive Services Task Force and the National Osteoporosis Foundation recommend testing for postmenopausal women and all women ages 65 and older.
- To protect bone health it is important that all individuals have a nutritionally balanced diet, which includes calcium-rich foods and vitamin D. Adults 50 and older need 1200 mg of calcium and 800 to 1000 International Units of vitamin D daily. Adults younger than 50 need 1000 mg of calcium and 400 to 800 International Units of vitamin D daily.
- A program of regular weight-bearing and muscle-strengthening exercises further helps promote bone health. Weight-bearing exercises may increase bone density and weight-bearing exercise and muscle strengthening can increase balance and agility and reduce the risk of falls and fractures. Eliminating environmental hazards in the home can decrease the risk of falls.
- Avoidance of excessive alcohol intake and tobacco smoking is advised.
- U.S. Food and Drug Administration (FDA)–approved medications for the prevention and/or treatment of osteoporosis include:
  - Bisphosphonates: alendronate, alendronate plus D; risedronate, risedronate with 500 mg calcium; ibandronate; zoledronic acid (prevention and treatment)
  - Calcitonin (treatment)
  - Estrogens (estrogen or hormone therapy) (prevention)
  - Estrogen agonist-antagonist (prevention and treatment)
  - Parathyroid hormone (treatment)

ibandronate [Boniva], zoledronic acid [Reclast]); estrogen agonist/antagonists such as raloxifene (Evista), parathyroid hormone (teriparatide [Fortéo]), and ET or HT (NOF, 2014).

Calcitonin reduces the rate of bone turnover and stabilizes bone mass in women with osteoporosis and may have some analgesic effects. Although calcitonin can reduce the incidence of spinal fractures, no data are available about its use to protect against hip fractures. Calcitonin may be used with women who are at least 5 years postmenopausal and in whom estrogen is contraindicated or not tolerated. The drug usually is administered intranasally on a daily basis; subcutaneous administration is also available. The medication is considered safe; however, side effects of nausea, vomiting, anorexia, and rhinitis (if used intranasally) have been reported (NOF, 2010).

Bisphosphonates are approved for prevention and treatment of osteoporosis, especially in reducing the incidence of spinal fractures. Side effects include gastrointestinal problems such as difficulty swallowing, inflammation of the esophagus, and gastric ulcer. Depending on the medication used, the oral drugs may be taken daily or monthly. Some formulations contain vitamin D (NOF, 2010). Alendronate is available in the United States in a generic preparation. Ibandronate is available as an intravenous injection every 3 months; zoledronic acid is given intravenously yearly for treatment of osteoporosis and every 2 years for prevention (NOF).

Raloxifene is approved by the FDA for osteoporosis prevention and treatment in postmenopausal women only. This medication seemingly preserves the beneficial effects of estrogen, including protection against cardiovascular diseases and osteoporosis, without stimulating breast and uterine tissues. Studies have shown that raloxifene may lower the relative risk of breast cancer by 40% (ACS, 2013b). The medication modestly increases bone density. Calcium supplements up to 1500 mg should be taken if dietary intake is inadequate.

MEDICATION ALERT

Because food and certain minerals reduce the absorption of bisphosphonates, women must take alendronate sodium and risedronate sodium on an empty stomach with 6 to 8 ounces of plain water only, at least 30 minutes before eating or drinking to improve absorption; remaining upright for these 30 minutes also is recommended (NOF, 2010).

Parathyroid hormone is approved for the treatment of osteoporosis in postmenopausal women at high risk for fractures. It is administered by daily subcutaneous injection. It can be used for a maximum of 2 years. The drug is well tolerated although some women report dizziness and leg cramps (NOF, 2010).

Estrogen/hormone therapy is approved for the prevention of osteoporosis. It should be used in the lowest effective doses for the shortest treatment time. The FDA recommends that it should not be used solely for the prevention of osteoporosis until after approved nonestrogen treatments are tried (NOF, 2010).

Midlife Support Groups

Nurses should be familiar with local resources and direct women to classes that supply appropriate information and support. They can encourage women to develop a supportive network with other women with whom they can share their concerns (Fig. 6-4).

Women's centers and clinics may have support groups and classes for women who want to discuss menopause and other midlife events. If no group or class is available in the community, nurses should consider starting one.

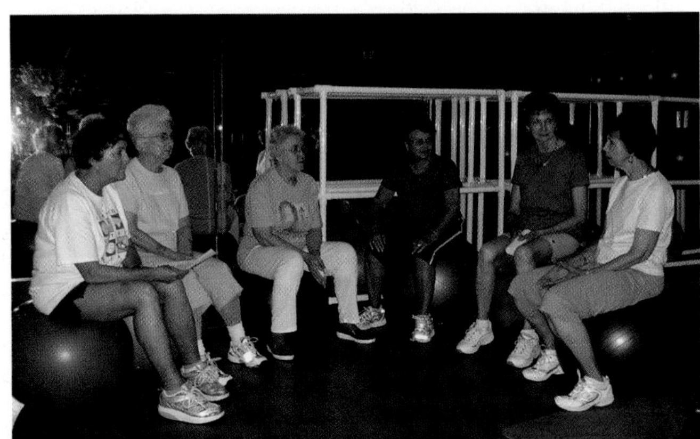

FIG 6-4 Midlife women can develop a supportive network. (Courtesy Dee Lowdermilk, Chapel Hill, NC.)

KEY POINTS

- Menstrual disorders diminish the quality of life for affected women and their families.
- Amenorrhea is most commonly a result of pregnancy.
- Dysmenorrhea is one of the most common gynecologic problems in women.
- PMS is a disorder with symptoms that begin in the luteal phase of the menstrual cycle and end with the onset of menses.
- Endometriosis is characterized by secondary amenorrhea, dyspareunia, abnormal uterine bleeding, and infertility.
- Perimenopause is a normal developmental phase during which a woman passes from the reproductive to the nonreproductive stage.
- During perimenopause women seek care for symptoms that arise from bleeding irregularities, vasomotor instability, fatigue, genital changes, and changes related to sexuality.
- Menopausal hormonal therapy, if used, should be taken at the lowest effective dose for the shortest possible time.
- Alternative therapies are beneficial in relieving discomforts associated with menstrual disorders and menopause.
- Osteoporosis, a progressive loss of bone mass that results from decreasing levels of estrogen after menopause, can be prevented or minimized with lifestyle changes and medication.
- Postmenopausal women are at increased risk for coronary artery disease because of changes in lipid metabolism.
- Sexuality and the capacity for sexual expression continue after menopause.

REFERENCES

American Cancer Society (ACS). (2013a). *Menopausal therapy and cancer risk.* Available at www.cancer.org/cancer/cancercauses/othercarcinogens/medicaltreatments/menopausal-hormone-replacement-therapy-and-cancer-risk.

American Cancer Society (ACS). (2013b). *Medicines to reduce the risk of breast cancer: Tamoxifen and raloxifene.* Available at www.cancer.org/cancer/breastcancer/moreinformation/medicinestoreducebreastcancer/medicines-to-reduce-breast-cancer-risk-tamoxifen.

American College of Obstetricians and Gynecologists (ACOG). (2011). *Frequently asked questions—Premenstrual syndrome FAQ057.* Available at www.acog.org.

American College of Obstetricians and Gynecologists (ACOG). (2012). *Committee on opinion: Compounded bioidentical menopausal hormone therapy.* Available at www.acog.org/Resources%20And%20Publications/Committee%20Opinions/Committee%20on%20Gynecologic%20Practice/Compounded%20Bioidentical%20Menopausal%20Hormone%20Therapy.aspx.

American College of Obstetricians and Gynecologists (ACOG). (2014). Practice Bulletin #141: Management of Menopausal Symptoms. *Journal of Obstretrics and Gynecology, 123*(1), 202–216.

American College of Sports Medicine. (2011). *The female athlete triad.* Available at www.acsm.org/docs/brochures/the-female-athlete-triad.pdf.

American Psychiatric Association. (2013). Depressive disorders. In *Diagnostic and statistical manual of mental disorders* (5th ed.). Arlington, VA: American Psychiatric Publishing.

Association of Women's Health, Obstetric and Neonatal Nurses (AWHONN). (2013). *Research-based practice: Cyclic pelvic pain and discomfort management* Available at www.awhonn.org/awhonn/content.do?name=03_JournalsPubsResearch/3G5_CyclicPelvicPain.htm.

Biggs, W. S., & Demuth, R. H. (2011). Premenstrual syndrome and premenstrual dysphoric disorder. *American Family Physician, 84*(8), 918–924.

Blackburn, S. (2013). *Maternal, fetal, & neonatal physiology: A clinical perspective* (4th ed.). Maryland Heights, MO: Elsevier.

Bonci, C., Bonci, L., Granger, L., et al. (2008). National Athletic Trainers' Association position statement: Preventing, detecting, and managing disordered eating in athletes. *Journal of Athletic Training, 43*(1), 808–820.

Brown, J., Kives, S., & Akhtar, M. (2012). Progestogens and anti-progestogens for pain associated with endometriosis. *The Cochrane Database of Systematic Reviews, 3*, CD002122.

Chien, L.-W., Chang, H.-C., & Liu, C.-F. (2013). Effect of yoga on serum homocysteine and nitric oxide levels in adolescent women with and without dysmenorrhea. *Journal of Complementary and Alternative Medicine, 19*(1), 20–23.

Chen, R. J., Chou, C. H., & Chang, T. C. (2013). We do not agree with the 2012 statement's recommendation of long-duration HT use that may last until the age of 51 years (or longer) if needed for symptom management. *Menopause, 20*(5), 587.

Dante, G., & Facchinetti, F. (2011). Herbal treatments for alleviating premenstrual symptoms: A systematic review. *Journal of Psychosomatic Obstetrics and Gynaecology, 32*(1), 42–51.

Dobos, G., & Tao, I. (2011). The model of western integrative medicine: The role of Chinese medicine. *Chinese Journal of Integrative Medicine, 17*(1), 11–20.

Estephan, A., & Sinert, R. H. (2012). Dysfunctional uterine bleeding in emergency medicine treatment and management. *Medscape Emedicine.* Available at http://emedicine.medscape.com/article/795587-treatment.

Ford, O., Lethaby, A., Roberts, H., & Mol, B. W. J. (2012). Progesterone for premenstrual syndrome. *The Cochrane Database of Systematic Reviews, 3*, CD003415.

Fritz, M., & Speroff, L. (2011). *Clinical gynecologic endocrinology and infertility* (8th ed.). Philadelphia: Lippincott Williams & Wilkins.

Gallenberg, M. (2012). Premenstrual syndrome. *Mayo Clinic Newsletter.* Available at www.mayoclinic.com/health/pmdd/AN01372.

Hendrick, B. (2011). *Menopausal Health Center, Web MDAcupuncture may ease hot flashes.* Available at www.webmd.com/menopause/news/20110307/acupuncture-may-ease-hot-flashes.

Joy, E. (2012). Invited commentary: Is the pill the answer for patients with female athlete triad? *Current Sports Medicine Report, 11*(2), 54–55.

Laufer, M. R. (2008). Current approaches to optimizing the treatment of endometriosis in adolescents. *Gynecologic Obstetric Investigation, 66*(Suppl 1), 19–27.

Leach, M. J., & Moore, V. (2012). Black cohosh *(Cimicifuga spp.)* for menopausal symptoms. *The Cochrane Database of Systematic Reviews, 9*, CD007244.

Lentz, G. (2012). Primary and secondary dysmenorrhea, premenstrual syndrome, and premenstrual dysphoric disorder: Etiology, diagnosis, and management. In G. M. Lentz, R. Lobo, D. Gershenson, & V. Katz (Eds.), *Comprehensive gynecology* (6th ed.). Philadelphia: Elsevier.

Lobo, R. (2012a). Abnormal uterine bleeding: Ovulatory and anovulatory dysfunctional uterine bleeding: Management of acute and chronic excessive bleeding. In G. M. Lentz, R. Lobo, D. Gershenson, & V. Katz (Eds.), *Comprehensive gynecology* (6th ed). Philadelphia: Elsevier.

Lobo, R. (2012b). Endometriosis: Etiology, pathology, diagnosis, management. In G. M. Lentz, R. Lobo, D. Gershenson, & V. Katz (Eds.), *Comprehensive gynecology* (6th ed.). Philadelphia: Elsevier.

Lobo, R. (2012c). Menopause: Endocrinology, consequences of estrogen deficiency, effects of hormone replacement therapy, treatment regimens. In G. M. Lentz, R. Lobo, D. Gershenson, & V. Katz (Eds.), *Comprehensive gynecology* (6th ed.). Philadelphia: Elsevier.

Lobo, R. (2012d). Primary and secondary amenorrhea and precocious puberty. In G. M. Lentz, R. Lobo, D. Gershenson, & V. Katz (Eds.), *Comprehensive gynecology* (6th ed.). Philadelphia: Elsevier.

MacReady, N. (2013). *Menopausal hormone therapy may raise risk for gallstones.* Available at www.medscape.com/viewarticle/780938.

Marshall, S., & Jones, K. (2011). *Female pelvic pain.* Available at www.webmd.com/hw-popup/chronic-female-pelvic-pain.

Mayo Clinic. (2012). *Dong quai (Angelica sinensus).* Available at www.mayoclinic.com/health/dong-quai/NS_patient-Dongquai/DSECTION=dosing.

Mayo Clinic. (2013). *Breast pain: Alternative medicine.* Available at www.mayoclinic.com/health/breast-pain/DS00760/DSECTION=alternative-medicine.

Mencias, T., Noon, M., & Hoch, A. (2012). Female athlete triad screening in National Collegiate Athletic Association division I athletes: Is the pre-participation evaluation form effective? *Clinical Journal of Sport Medicine, 22*(2), 122–125.

Mishra, N., Mishra, V. N., & Devanshi (2011). Exercise beyond menopause: Do's and don'ts. *Journal of Midlife Health, 2*(2), 51–56.

National Institutes of Health. (2010). *WHI study data confirm short-term heart disease risks of combination hormone therapy for postmenopausal women.* Available at www.nih.gov/news/health/feb2010/nhlbi-15.htm.

National Osteoporosis Foundation (NOF). (2013). *Clinician's guide to the prevention and treatment of osteoporosis.* Washington, DC.

National Osteoporosis Foundation (NOF). (2013). *NOF encourages women to break free from osteoporosis in honor of women's health week.* Available at www.nof.org/news/1107.

National Osteoporosis Foundation (NOF). (2010). Vitamin D and bone health. http://nof.org/files/nof/public/content/file/78/upload/52.pdf Retrieved 07-27-14.

National Osteoporois Foundation (2014). Clinician's guide to prevention and treatment of osteoporosis. http://nof.org/files/nof/public/content/file/2791/upload/919.pdf, retrieved 07027014.

Nihira, M. A. (2012). *Menopause and hot flashes.* Available at www.webmd.com/menopause/guide/hot-flashes.

North American Menopause Society. (2011). The role of soy isoflavones in menopausal health: Report of the North American Menopause Society/Wulf H. Utian Translational Science Symposium in Chicago, IL (2010). *Menopause: The Journal of the North American Menopause Society, 18*(7), 732–753.

North American Menopause Society. (2012). The 2012 hormone therapy position statement of the North American Menopause Society. *Menopause, 19*(3), 257–271.

Osteoporosis Report. (2011). Institute of Medicine (IOM) updates vitamin D recommendations. *Osteoporosis Report, 26*(1). Available at www.nof.org/files/nof/public/content/file/703/upload/283.pdf.

Quinn, E. (2011). Amenorrhea in athletes. *About.com Sports Medicine.* Available at http://sportsmedicine.about.com/od/women/a/Amenorrhea.htm.

Smith, R. P., & Kaunitz, A. M. (2013). Patient information: Painful menstrual periods (dysmenorrhea) and beyond. Available at www.uptodate.com/contents/painful-menstrual-periods-dysmenorrhea-beyond-the-basics.

Smorgick, N., Marsh, C. A., As-Sanie, S., et al. (2013). Prevalence of pain syndromes, mood conditions, and asthma in adolescents and young women with endometriosis. *Journal of Pediatric Adolescent Gynecology, 26*(3), 171–175.

Steenberg, C. K., Tanbo, T. G., & Qvigstad, E. (2013). Endometrosis in adolescences: Predictive markers and management. *Acta Obstetrica et Gynecologica Scandinavica, 92*(5), 491–495.

Storck, S. (2012). Premenstrual dysphoric disorder. *Medline Plus Medline Encyclopedia.* Available at http://www.nlm.nih.gov/medlineplus/ency/article/007193.htm.

U.S. Preventive Health Services Task Force. (2011). *Screening for osteoporosis: Recommendation statement.* Available at www.uspreventiveservicestaskforce.org/uspstf10/osteoporosis/osteors.htm.

U.S. Preventive Services Task Force. (2013). *Menopausal therapy for the primary prevention of chronic conditions.* Available at www.uspreventiveservicestaskforce.org/uspstf/uspspmho.htm.

UpToDate. (2012). *Medical treatment for menorrhagia.* Available at www.uptodate.com/contents/menorrhagia-excessive-menstrual-bleeding-beyond-the-basics.

Vorvick, L. J., Storck, S., & Zieve, D. (2012). *Amenorrhea*: Available at www.nlm.nih.gov/medlineplus/ency/article/001218.htm.

Walker, K. M. (2013). Hip fractures in adults. Available at www.uptodate.com/contents/hip-fractures-in-adults.

Wambach, C. M., & Alexander, C. J. (2012). Menstrual disorders. In P. J. Disaia, G. Chaudhuri, L. C. Guidice, et al. (Eds.), *Women's health review: A clinical update in obstetrics-gynecology.* Philadelphia: Elsevier.

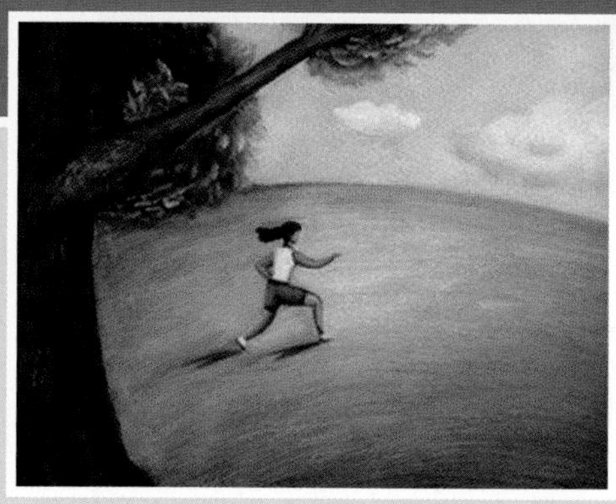

CHAPTER 7

Sexually Transmitted and Other Infections

Deitra Leonard Lowdermilk

http://evolve.elsevier.com/Lowdermilk/MWHC/

LEARNING OBJECTIVES

- Describe prevention of sexually transmitted infections in women, including risk reduction measures.
- Differentiate signs, symptoms, diagnosis, and management of nonpregnant and pregnant women with selected sexually transmitted bacterial infections (chlamydia, gonorrhea, syphilis).
- Examine the care of nonpregnant and pregnant women with selected sexually transmitted viral infections (human immunodeficiency virus [HIV]; hepatitis A, B, and C; human papillomavirus; genital herpes).
- Compare and contrast signs, symptoms, and management of selected vaginal infections in nonpregnant and pregnant women.
- Discuss the effect of group B streptococci (GBS) on pregnancy and management of pregnant women with GBS.
- Identify the effects of TORCH infections on pregnancy and the fetus.
- Describe the health consequences (e.g., ectopic pregnancy, infertility) for women who are infected with reproductive tract infections.
- Develop a nursing care plan for a woman who is 12 weeks pregnant and has been diagnosed with HIV.
- Review principles of infection control for HIV and blood-borne pathogens.

Reproductive tract infection is a term that encompasses both sexually transmitted infections and other common genital tract infections (Marrazzo & Cates, 2011). **Sexually transmitted infections (STIs)** include more than 30 organisms that cause infections or infectious disease syndromes primarily transmitted by close, intimate contact (World Health Organization [WHO], 2013b) (Box 7-1). Caused by a wide spectrum of bacteria, viruses, protozoa, and ectoparasites (organisms that live on the outside of the body, such as a louse), STIs are a direct cause of tremendous human suffering, place heavy demands on health care services, and cost society hundreds of millions of dollars to treat. Despite the U.S. Surgeon General's targeting STIs as a priority for prevention and control efforts, STIs are among the most common health problems in the United States, especially for young people. The Centers for Disease Control and Prevention (CDC) estimate that almost 20 million Americans are infected with STIs every year; almost half of those infected are between the ages of 15 and 24. About 51% of infections for this age group are in young women who, if untreated, could face serious long-term consequences, specifically infertility (CDC, 2013d).

The most common STIs in women are chlamydia, gonorrhea, human papillomavirus, herpes simplex virus type 2, syphilis, and human immunodeficiency virus (HIV) infection; these are discussed in this chapter. Common vaginal infections are also discussed. Neonatal effects of STIs are discussed in Chapter 35.

PREVENTION

Preventing infection (primary prevention) is the most effective way of reducing the adverse consequences of STIs for women and for society. With the advent of serious and potentially lethal STIs that are not readily cured or are incurable, primary prevention becomes critical. Prompt diagnosis and treatment of current infections (secondary prevention) also can prevent personal complications and transmission to others.

Preventing the spread of STIs requires that women at risk for transmitting or acquiring infections change their behavior. A critical first step is for the nurse to include questions about a woman's sexual history, risky sexual behaviors, and drug-related risky behaviors as a part of her assessment. The Five P's—Partners, Prevention of Pregnancy, Protection from STIs, Practices, and Past History of STIs—approach to obtaining a sexual history is an example of an effective strategy for eliciting information concerning five key areas of interest (CDC, 2010c) (Box 7-2). Techniques that are effective in providing prevention counseling include using open-ended questions, using understandable language, and reassuring the woman that treatment

BOX 7-1 Selected Sexually Transmitted Infections

Bacteria
- Chlamydia
- Gonorrhea
- Syphilis
- Chancroid
- Lymphogranuloma venereum

Viruses
- Human immunodeficiency virus
- Herpes simplex virus, types 1 and 2
- Cytomegalovirus
- Viral hepatitis, types A and B
- Human papillomavirus

Protozoa
- Trichomoniasis

Parasites
- Pediculosis
- Scabies

Data from Planned Parenthood. (2013). *Sexually transmitted diseases (STDs)*. Available at www.plannedparenthood.org/health-topic/stds-hiv-safer-sex-101.htm; World Health Organization. (2013). *Sexually transmitted infections (STIs)*. Available at www.who.int/mediacentre/factsheets/fs110/en/index.html.

will be provided regardless of factors such as ability to pay, language spoken, or lifestyle (Marrazzo & Cates, 2011). Prevention messages should include descriptions of specific actions to be taken to avoid acquiring or transmitting STIs (e.g., refraining from sexual activity when STI-related symptoms are present) and should be individualized for each woman, giving attention to her specific risk factors.

To be motivated to take preventive actions, a woman must believe that acquiring a disease will be serious for her and that she is at risk for infection. However, most individuals tend to underestimate their personal risk of infection in a given situation; thus many women, and especially adolescents, may not perceive themselves as being at risk for contracting an STI. Telling them that they should carry condoms may not be well received. Although levels of awareness of STIs are generally high, widespread misconceptions or specific gaps in knowledge also exist. Therefore, nurses have a responsibility to ensure that their clients have accurate, complete knowledge about transmission and symptoms of STIs and behaviors that place them at risk for contracting an infection.

Primary preventive measures are individual activities aimed at deterring infection. Risk-free options include complete abstinence from sexual activities that transmit semen, blood, or other body fluids or that allow skin-to-skin contact (Marrazzo & Cates, 2011). Alternatively, involvement in a mutually monogamous relationship with an uninfected partner also eliminates risk of contracting STIs. When neither of these options is realistic for a woman, however, the nurse and woman must focus on other, more feasible measures.

Risk-Reduction Measures

An essential component of primary prevention is counseling women regarding risk-reduction practices, including knowledge of her partner, reduction of the number of partners, low risk sex, avoiding the exchange of body fluids, and vaccination (CDC, 2010c).

No aspect of prevention is more important than knowing one's partner. Reducing the number of partners and avoiding partners who have had many sexual partners decreases a woman's chance of contracting an STI. Deciding not to have sexual contact with casual acquaintances also may be helpful. Discussing each new partner's previous sexual history and exposure to STIs augments other efforts to reduce risk; however, sexual partners may not always be truthful about their sexual history. Women must be informed that practicing risk-reduction measures is always advisable, even when partners insist otherwise. Critically important is whether male partners resist or accept wearing condoms. This is crucial when women are not sure about their partners' history. Women should be cautioned

BOX 7-2 Assessing Sexually Transmitted Infections and HIV Risk Behaviors Using the 5 P'S

The Five P's: Partners, Prevention of Pregnancy, Protection from Sexually Transmitted Infections (STIs), Practices, and Past History of STIs

1. Partners
- Do you have sex with men, women, or both?
- In the past 2 months, how many partners have you had sex with?
- In the past 12 months, how many partners have you had sex with?
- Is it possible that any of your sex partners in the past 12 months had sex with someone else while they were still in a sexual relationship with you?

2. Prevention of Pregnancy
- What are you doing to prevent pregnancy?

3. Protection from STIs
- What do you do to protect yourself from STIs and human immunodeficiency virus (HIV)?

4. Practices
- To understand your risks for STIs, I need to understand the kind of sex you have had recently.
- Have you had vaginal sex, meaning 'penis in vagina sex'? If yes, "do you use condoms: never, sometimes, or always?
- Have you had anal sex, meaning 'penis in rectum/anus sex'? If yes, "do you use condoms: never, sometimes, or always?
- Have you had oral sex, meaning "mouth on penis/vagina"?

For condom answers:
- If "never", why don't you use condoms?
- If "sometimes", in what situations (or with whom) do you not use condoms?

5. Past History of STIs
- Have you ever had an STI?
- Have any of your partners had an STI?

Additional questions to identify HIV and viral hepatitis risk include:
- Have you or any of your partners ever injected drugs?
- Have any of your partners exchanged money or drugs for sex?
- Is there anything else about your sexual practices that I need to know about?

From Centers for Disease Control and Prevention (CDC). (2010). Sexually transmitted diseases treatment guidelines 2010. *MMWR Morbidity and Mortality Weekly Report, 59*(RR-12), 1-109.

TABLE 7-1 Risk-Reduction Practices

SAFEST	LOW BUT POTENTIAL RISK	HIGH RISK (UNSAFE)
Abstinence Self-masturbation Monogamous (both partners and no high risk activities) and tested negative for HIV and other STIs Hugging, massage, touching (assuming no break in skin) Dry kissing Mutual masturbation without contact with semen or vaginal secretions and no broken skin Drug abstinence Sexual fantasy Erotic conversation, books, movies Erotic bathing, showering Eroticizing feet, fingers, buttocks, abdomen, ears	Wet kissing* Vaginal intercourse with condom; anal intercourse with condom Monogamous (both partners and no high risk activities) but not tested for HIV or other STIs Oral sex with woman wearing female condom Oral sex with man wearing condom Mutual masturbation without contact with semen or vaginal secretions; healthy intact skin or use of latex or plastic barrier Urine contact with intact skin	Unprotected anal intercourse; unprotected vaginal intercourse Oral-anal contact Multiple sexual partners, no HIV or STI testing Any sex (fisting, rough vaginal or anal intercourse, rape) that causes tissue damage or bleeding Oral sex on man or woman without a latex or plastic barrier Sharing sex toys, douche equipment Sharing needles Blood contact, including menstrual blood

*Assumes no breaks in skin.

HIV, Human immunodeficiency virus; *STI,* sexually transmitted infection.

Data from Centers for Disease Control and Prevention. (2010). Sexually transmitted diseases treatment guidelines, 2010. *MMWR Morbidity and Mortality Weekly Report, 59*(RR-12), 1-109; Marrazzo, J.M., & Cates, W. (2011). Reproductive tract infections, including HIV and sexually transmitted infections. In R. Hatcher, J. Trussell, A. Nelson, et al. (Eds.), *Contraceptive technology* (20th ed.). New York: Ardent Media.

against making decisions about a partner's sexual and other behaviors based on appearances and unfounded assumptions such as the following (Marrazzo & Cates, 2011):

- Single people have many partners and risky practices.
- Older people have few partners and infrequent sexual encounters.
- Sexually experienced people know how to use risk-reduction measures.
- Married people are heterosexual, low risk, and monogamous.
- People who look healthy are healthy.
- People with good jobs do not use drugs.

Sexually active people also may benefit from carefully examining a partner for lesions, sores, ulcerations, rashes, redness, discharge, swelling, and odor before initiating sexual activity. Teach women about low risk sexual practices and which sexual practices to avoid (Table 7-1).

The physical barrier promoted for the prevention of sexual transmission of HIV and other STIs is the condom (male and female). Nurses can help motivate clients to use condoms by initiating a discussion with them. This gives women permission to discuss any concerns, misconceptions, or hesitations they may have about using condoms. Information to be discussed includes the importance of using latex or plastic male condoms rather than natural skin condoms for STI protection. The nurse should remind women to use a condom with every sexual encounter, to use each one only once, to use a condom with a current expiration date, and to handle it carefully to avoid damaging it with fingernails, teeth, or other sharp objects. Condoms should be stored away from high heat. Although it is not ideal, women may choose to safely carry condoms in wallets, shoes, or inside a bra. Women can be taught the differences among condoms: price ranges, sizes, and where they can be purchased. Explicit instructions for how to apply a male condom are included in Box 8-3.

The female condom—a lubricated polyurethane sheath with a ring on each end, one that is inserted into the vagina and the other covering the labia (see Figure 8-7)—has been shown in laboratory studies to be an effective mechanical barrier to viruses, including HIV. Although no clinical studies have been completed to evaluate the efficacy of female condoms in protecting against STIs, laboratory studies have demonstrated that polyurethane can block smaller viruses such as the herpesvirus and HIV (Cates & Harwood, 2011). The CDC (2010c) stated that when used correctly and consistently, the female condom may reduce STI risk and recommended its use when a male condom cannot be used properly. What is important and should be stressed by nurses is the consistent use of condoms for every act of sexual intimacy when there is the possibility of transmission of disease.

Despite concern about the potential for cervicovaginal epithelial disruption with nonoxynol-9 (N-9)–based spermicides, interest in vaginally applied chemical barriers that provide dual contraceptive and protection against bacterial STIs remains. Evidence has shown, however, that vaginal spermicides do not protect against certain STIs such as cervical gonorrhea and chlamydia and are not effective in preventing HIV infection. Condoms lubricated with N-9 are not recommended for prevention of HIV and STIs (CDC, 2010c).

A key issue in condom use as a preventive strategy is to stress to women that in sexual encounters men must comply with a woman's suggestion or request that they use a condom. Moreover, condom use must be renegotiated with every sexual contact, and women must address the issue of control of sexual decision making every time they request a male partner to use a condom. Women may fear that their partner would be offended if a condom were introduced. Some women may fear rejection and abandonment, conflict, potential violence, or loss of economic support if they suggest the use of condoms to prevent STI transmission. For many individuals, condoms are symbols of extra-relationship activity. Introduction of a condom into a long-term relationship in which one has not been used previously threatens the trust assumed in most long-term relationships.

Nurses must suggest strategies to enhance a woman's condom negotiation and communication skills. It can be suggested that she talk with her partner about condom use at a time removed from sexual activity, which may make it easier to bring up the subject. Role-playing possible partner reactions with a woman and her alternative responses can be helpful. Asking a woman who appears particularly uncomfortable to rehearse how she might approach the topic is useful, particularly when a woman fears her partner may be resistant. The nurse might suggest the woman begin by saying, "I need to talk with you about something that is important to both of us. It's hard for me, and I feel embarrassed, but I think we need to talk about reducing risk during sex." If women are able to sort out their feelings and fears before talking with their partners, they may feel more comfortable and in control of the situation. Women can be reassured that it is natural to be uncomfortable and that the hardest part is getting started. Nurses should help their clients clarify what they will and will not do sexually because it will be easier to discuss their concerns with their partners if they have thought about what to say. Women can be reminded that their partner may need time to think about what they have said and that they must pay attention to their partner's response.

Many women do not anticipate or prepare for sexual activity in advance; embarrassment or discomfort in purchasing condoms may prevent some women from using them. Cultural barriers also may impede the use of condoms; for example, Hispanic gender roles may make it difficult for Hispanic women to suggest using condoms to a partner. In general, suggesting condom use implies that a woman is sexually active, that she is "available" for sex, and that she is "seeking" sex; these are messages that many women are uncomfortable conveying, given the prevailing mores of our country. In a society that commonly

TABLE 7-2 Sexually Transmitted Infections and Drug Therapies for Women*

DISEASE	NONPREGNANT WOMEN (13-17 yr)	NONPREGNANT WOMEN (>18 yr)	PREGNANT WOMEN	LACTATING WOMEN†
Chlamydia	*Recommended:* azithromycin, 1 g orally once *or* doxycycline, 100 mg orally bid for 7 days	*Recommended:* azithromycin, 1 g orally once *or* doxycycline, 100 mg orally bid for 7 days	*Recommended:* azithromycin, 1 g orally once *or* amoxicillin, 500 mg orally tid for 7 days	*Recommended:* azithromycin, 1 g orally once *or* amoxicillin, 500 mg orally tid for 7 days
Gonorrhea	*Recommended:* ceftriaxone, 125 mg IM once (adolescents who weigh >45 kg can be treated with any regimen recommended for adults), plus treatment for chlamydia as above	*Recommended:* ceftriaxone, 250 mg IM once, plus treatment for chlamydia as above	*Recommended:* ceftriaxone, 250 mg IM once, plus treatment for chlamydia as above	*Recommended:* ceftriaxone, 250 mg IM once, plus treatment for chlamydia as above
Syphilis	**Primary, secondary, early latent disease:** *Recommended:* benzathine penicillin G, 2.4 million units IM once **Late-latent or unknown-duration disease:** *Recommended:* benzathine penicillin G, 7.2 million units total, administered as three doses, 2.4 million units each, at 1-wk intervals Penicillin allergy: doxycycline, 100 mg orally qid for 14 days *or* tetracycline, 500 mg orally qid for 14 days	**Primary, secondary, early latent disease:** *Recommended:* benzathine penicillin G, 2.4 million units IM once **Late-latent or unknown-duration disease:** *Recommended:* benzathine penicillin G, 7.2 million units total, administered as three doses, 2.4 million units each, at 1-wk intervals **Penicillin allergy:** doxycycline, 100 mg orally qid for 14 days *or* tetracycline, 500 mg orally qid for 14 days	**Primary, secondary, early latent disease:** *Recommended:* benzathine penicillin G, 2.4 million units IM once (some experts recommend a second dose of benzathine penicillin, 2.4 million units, 1 wk later) **Late-latent or unknown-duration disease:** *Recommended:* benzathine penicillin G, 7.2 million units total, administered as three doses, 2.4 million units each, at 1-wk intervals No proven alternatives to penicillin in pregnancy Pregnant women who have a history of allergy to penicillin should be desensitized and treated with penicillin.	**Primary, secondary, early latent disease:** *Recommended:* benzathine penicillin G, 2.4 million units IM once
Human papillomavirus	*Recommended for external genital warts:* **Client applied:** podofilox, 0.5% solution, or gel to wart bid for 3 days followed by 4-day rest for ≤4 cycles *or* imiquimod, 5% cream, at bedtime 3 times a week for ≤16 wk *or* sinecatechins 15% oint tid for ≤16 wk **Provider applied:** cryotherapy with liquid nitrogen or cryoprobe *or* podophyllin resin, 10%-25% in tincture of benzoin compound weekly (wash off in 1-4 hr). Repeat weekly as necessary *or* trichloroacetic acid (TCA) or bichloroacetic acid (BCA) 80%-90% weekly	*Recommended for external genital warts:* **Client applied:** podofilox, 0.5% solution, or gel to wart bid for 3 days followed by 4-day rest for ≤4 cycles *or* imiquimod, 5% cream, at bedtime 3 times a week for ≤16 wk *or* sinecatechins 15% oint tid for ≤16 wk **Provider applied:** cryotherapy with liquid nitrogen or cryoprobe *or* podophyllin resin, 10%-25% in tincture of benzoin compound weekly (wash off in 1-4 hr). Repeat weekly as necessary *or* TCA or BCA 80%-90% weekly	*Recommended for external genital warts:* **Provider applied:** cryotherapy with liquid nitrogen or cryoprobe *or* trichloroacetic acid (TCA) or bichloroacetic acid (BCA) 80%-90% weekly imiquimod, podophyllin (Podocon-25), sinecatechins, and podofilox should not be used in pregnancy	*Recommended for external genital warts:* **Provider applied:** cryotherapy with liquid nitrogen or cryoprobe *or* TCA or BCA 80%-90% weekly imiquimod, podophyllin, sinecatechins, and podofilox should not be used during lactation

TABLE 7-2 **Sexually Transmitted Infections and Drug Therapies for Women*—cont'd**

DISEASE	NONPREGNANT WOMEN (13-17 yr)	NONPREGNANT WOMEN (>18 yr)	PREGNANT WOMEN	LACTATING WOMEN†
Genital herpes simplex virus (HSV-1 *or* HSV-2)	**Primary infection:** acyclovir, 400 mg orally tid for 7-10 days *or* acyclovir, 200 mg orally 5 times a day for 7-10 days *or* famciclovir, 250 mg orally tid for 7-10 days *or* valacyclovir, 1 g orally bid for 7-10 days **Recurrent infection:** acyclovir, 400 mg orally tid for 5 days *or* acyclovir, 800 mg orally bid for 5 days *or* acyclovir, 800 mg orally tid for 2 days *or* famciclovir, 125 mg orally bid for 5 days *or* famciclovir 1000 mg orally bid for 1 day *or* famciclovir, 500 mg once, then 250 mg bid for 2 days *or* valacyclovir, 500 mg orally bid for 3 days *or* valacyclovir, 1 g orally once a day for 5 days **Suppression therapy:** Take daily for 1 year or more: acyclovir, 400 mg orally bid *or* famciclovir, 250 mg orally bid *or* valacyclovir, 500 mg orally once a day *or* valacyclovir, 1 g orally once a day	**Primary infection:** acyclovir, 400 mg orally tid for 7-10 days *or* acyclovir, 200 mg orally 5 times a day for 7-10 days *or* famciclovir, 250 mg orally tid for 7-10 days *or* valacyclovir, 1 g orally bid for 7-10 days **Recurrent infection:** acyclovir, 400 mg orally tid for 5 days *or* acyclovir, 800 mg orally bid for 5 days *or* acyclovir, 800 mg orally tid for 2 days *or* famciclovir, 125 mg orally bid for 5 days *or* famciclovir, 1000 mg orally bid for 1 day *or* famciclovir 500 mg once, then 250 mg bid for 2 days *or* valacyclovir, 500 mg orally bid for 3 days *or* valacyclovir, 1 g orally once a day for 5 days **Suppression therapy:** Take daily for 1 year or more: acyclovir, 400 mg orally bid *or* famciclovir, 250 mg orally bid *or* valacyclovir, 500 mg orally once a day *or* valacyclovir, 1 g orally once a day	No increase in birth defects beyond the general population has been found with acyclovir use in pregnancy. Acyclovir, 400 mg orally tid for 7 days for first episode or severe recurrent infection; may be given IV if infection is severe Suppression therapy 4 wk before the birth for women with recurrent infections can reduce the need for a cesarean birth	Acyclovir usually is considered compatible with breastfeeding. Acyclovir, 400 mg orally tid for 7 days

*List is not inclusive of all drugs that may be used as alternatives.
†These medications are usually compatible with breastfeeding.
bid, Twice daily; *HSV,* herpes simplex virus; *IM,* intramuscular; *IV,* intravenous; *qid,* four times daily; *tid,* three times daily.
Data from American Academy of Pediatrics Committee on Drugs. (2002). The transfer of drugs and other chemicals into human milk. *Pediatrics, 108*(3), 776-789; Centers for Disease Control and Prevention (CDC). (2010). Sexually transmitted diseases treatment guidelines, 2010. *MMWR Morbidity and Mortality Weekly Report, 59*(RR-12), 1-109; CDC. (2012). Update to CDC's sexually transmitted diseases treatment guidelines, 2010: Oral cephalosporins no longer recommended for gonococcal infections. *MMWR Morbidity and Mortality Weekly Report, 61*(31), 590-594.

views a woman who carries a condom as overprepared, possibly oversexed, and willing to have sex with any man, expecting her to insist on the use of condoms in a sexual encounter is somewhat optimistic at best and unrealistic at worst.

Finally, women should be counseled to watch out for situations that make it hard to talk about and to practice safer sex. These include romantic times when condoms are not available and when alcohol or drugs make it impossible to make wise decisions about safer sex.

Preexposure vaccination is an effective method for the prevention of some STIs such as hepatitis B and human papillomavirus (HPV). Hepatitis B vaccine is recommended for women at high risk for STIs (CDC, 2010c). Two HPV vaccines are available for females aged 9 to 26 years to prevent cervical precancer and cancer: the quadrivalent (HPV types 6, 11, 16, and 18) HPV vaccine (Gardasil) and the bivalent (HPV types 16 and 18) HPV vaccine (Cervarix). Gardasil also prevents genital warts. Routine vaccination of females ages 11 or 12 years is recommended with either vaccine, as is catch-up vaccination for females ages 13 to 26 years (CDC, 2012c) . It is also approved for males ages 9 to 26. (See later discussion).

SEXUALLY TRANSMITTED BACTERIAL INFECTIONS

Chlamydia

Chlamydia trachomatis is the most commonly reported STI in American women. In 2011 there were more than 1.4 million cases reported; the rate of infection was more than 2½ times the rate for men (CDC, 2012e). These infections are often silent and highly destructive; their sequelae and complications can be very serious. In women, chlamydial infections are difficult to diagnose; the symptoms, if present, are nonspecific, and the organism is expensive to culture.

Early identification of *C. trachomatis* is important because untreated infection often leads to acute salpingitis or pelvic inflammatory disease. Pelvic inflammatory disease (PID) is the most serious complication of chlamydial infections, and past chlamydial infections are associated with an increased risk of ectopic pregnancy and tubal factor infertility. Furthermore, chlamydial infection of the cervix causes inflammation, resulting in microscopic cervical ulcerations, and thus may increase the risk of acquiring HIV infection. More than half of infants born to mothers with chlamydia will develop conjunctivitis or pneumonia after perinatal exposure to the mother's infected cervix. *C. trachomatis* is the most common infectious cause of ophthalmia neonatorum. Neonatal ocular prophylaxis with silver nitrate solution or antibiotic ointment does not prevent perinatal transmission from mother to infant, nor does it adequately treat chlamydial infection (see Chapter 35).

Sexually active women ages 15 to 24 have the highest rates of infection, with women ages 18 to 20 years having the highest rates. In 2011, the rates were highest in black women at more than 7 times the rate of white women. American Indian, Alaska Native, and Hispanic women also had higher rates than white women (CDC, 2012e). Women older than 30 years have the lowest rate of infection. Risky behaviors, including multiple partners and nonuse of barrier methods of birth control, increase a woman's risk of chlamydial infection. Lower socioeconomic status may be a risk factor, especially with respect to treatment-seeking behaviors.

Screening and Diagnosis

In addition to obtaining information regarding the presence of risk factors, the nurse should inquire about the presence of any symptoms. The CDC (2010c) strongly recommends screening of asymptomatic women at high risk in whom infection would otherwise go undetected (see www.cdc.org). CDC guidelines recommend yearly screening of all sexually active adolescents, women between ages 20 and 25 years, and women older than 25 years who are at high risk (e.g., those with new or multiple partners). In addition, whenever possible, all women with two or more of the risk factors for chlamydia should be cultured. All pregnant women should have cervical cultures for chlamydia at the first prenatal visit. Screening late in the third trimester (36 weeks) may be carried out if the woman was positive previously, or if she is younger than 25 years, has a new sex partner, or has multiple sex partners.

Although chlamydial infections are usually asymptomatic, some women may experience spotting or postcoital bleeding, mucoid or purulent cervical discharge, or dysuria. Bleeding results from inflammation and erosion of the cervical columnar epithelium.

Laboratory diagnosis of chlamydia is by culture (expensive and labor intensive), deoxyribonucleic acid (DNA) probe (relatively less expensive but less sensitive), enzyme immunoassay (also relatively less expensive but less sensitive), and nucleic acid amplification tests (NAATs) (expensive but has relatively higher sensitivity) (CDC, 2010c; Fantasia, Fontenot, Sutherland, & Harris, 2011). Special culture media and proper handling of specimens are important, so the nurse should always know what is required in his or her individual practice site. Chlamydial culture testing is not always available, primarily because of expense.

Management

The CDC recommendations for treatment of urethral, cervical, and rectal chlamydial infections are azithromycin or doxycycline (CDC, 2010c) (see Table 7-2). Azithromycin is often prescribed when compliance may be a problem, because only one dose is needed; however, expense is a concern with this medication. If the woman is pregnant, azithromycin or amoxicillin is used. Pregnant women should be retested in 3 weeks to determine if treatment was effective; if at high risk for reinfection, the pregnant woman should be retested in the third trimester (Ruhl, 2013). Women who have a chlamydial infection and also are infected with HIV should be treated with the same regimen as those who are not infected with HIV.

Because chlamydia is often asymptomatic, the woman should be cautioned to take all medication prescribed. All exposed sexual partners should be treated.

Gonorrhea

Gonorrhea is probably the oldest communicable disease in the United States and second to chlamydia in reported cases. In 2012, a total of 334,826 cases of gonorrhea was reported in the United States (CDC, 2014). The incidence of drug-resistant cases of gonorrhea, in particular, penicillinase-producing *Neisseria gonorrhoeae* (PPNG), is increasing dramatically in the United States. Only a single class of antibiotics now meets CDC's standard for treatment—the cephalosporins (CDC, 2012e).

Gonorrhea is caused by the aerobic gram-negative diplococcus, *N. gonorrhoeae*. Gonorrhea is almost exclusively transmitted by sexual contact. The principal means of communication is genital-to-genital contact; however, it also is spread by oral-to-genital and anal-to-genital contact. There also is evidence that infection can spread in females from vagina to rectum. Age is probably the most important risk factor associated with gonorrhea. In the United States the highest reported rates of infection are among sexually active teenagers, young adults, and blacks. In 2012, the highest rates were in young women ages 15 to 24 and the rate in blacks was 15 times higher than for whites. American Indian, Alaska Native, and Hispanic rates were also higher than the rate for whites (CDC, 2014). Women are often asymptomatic, with one third of infections in adolescent women going unnoticed. When symptoms are present they are often less specific than are the symptoms in men. Women may have a purulent endocervical discharge, but discharge is usually minimal or absent. Menstrual irregularities may be the presenting symptom, or women may complain of pain—chronic or acute severe pelvic or lower abdominal pain or longer, more painful menses. Infrequently, dysuria, vague abdominal pain, or low backache prompts a woman to seek care. Gonococcal rectal infection may occur in women after anal intercourse. Individuals with rectal gonorrhea may be completely asymptomatic or, conversely, have severe symptoms with profuse purulent anal discharge, rectal pain, and blood in the stool. Rectal itching, fullness, pressure, and pain also are common symptoms, as is diarrhea. A diffuse vaginitis with vulvitis is the most common form of gonococcal infection in prepubertal girls. There may be few signs of infection, or vaginal discharge, dysuria, and swollen, reddened labia may be present.

Gonococcal infections in pregnancy can affect mother and fetus. In women with cervical gonorrhea, salpingitis may develop in the first trimester. Perinatal complications of gonococcal infection include premature rupture of membranes, preterm birth, chorioamnionitis, neonatal sepsis, intrauterine growth restriction, and maternal postpartum sepsis. Amniotic infection syndrome manifested by placental, fetal, and umbilical cord inflammation after premature rupture of the membranes may result from gonorrheal infections during pregnancy. Ophthalmia neonatorum, the most common manifestation of neonatal gonococcal infections, is highly contagious and, if untreated, may lead to blindness of the newborn (see Chapter 35).

Screening and Diagnosis

Because gonococcal infections in women often are asymptomatic, the CDC recommend screening all women at risk for gonorrhea (CDC, 2010c). All pregnant women should be screened at the first prenatal visit, and infected women and those not infected but identified with risky behaviors should be rescreened at 36 weeks of gestation. Gonococcal infection cannot be diagnosed reliably by clinical signs and symptoms alone. Individuals may have "classic" symptoms, vague symptoms that can be attributed to a number of conditions, or no symptoms at all. Cultures with selective media are considered the gold standard for diagnosis of gonorrhea.

Specific diagnosis of infection with *N. gonorrhoeae* can be performed by testing endocervical, vaginal, or urine specimens. Culture and nonculture tests (nucleic acid hybridization tests and NAATs) are available for the detection of genitourinary infection with *N. gonorrhoeae.* Cultures should be obtained from the endocervix, the rectum, and when indicated, the pharynx. Thayer-Martin cultures are recommended to diagnose gonorrhea in women. NAATs allow testing of the widest variety of specimen types including endocervical swabs, vaginal swabs, and urine (CDC, 2010c). Because coinfection is common, any woman suspected of having gonorrhea should have a chlamydial culture and serologic test for syphilis if one has not been done in the past 2 months.

Management

Management of gonorrhea is straightforward, and the cure is usually rapid with appropriate antibiotic therapy (see Table 7-2). Single-dose efficacy is a major consideration in selecting an antibiotic regimen for women with gonorrhea. Another important consideration is the high percentage of women with coexisting chlamydial infections. The treatment of choice for uncomplicated urethral, endocervical, and rectal infections in pregnant and nonpregnant women is ceftriaxone (CDC, 2012f). The CDC recommends concomitant treatment for chlamydia (CDC, 2010c). A test of cure in 3 to 4 weeks after treatment is not recommended for pregnant women (Ruhl, 2013). All women with both gonorrhea and syphilis should be treated for syphilis according to CDC guidelines (see discussion of syphilis in this chapter).

Gonorrhea is a highly communicable disease. It is important to notify partners if a woman is diagnosed with a gonorrheal infection. Recent (past 30 days) sexual partners should be examined, cultured, and treated with appropriate regimens. Most treatment failures result from reinfection. The woman must be informed of this, as well as of the consequences of reinfection in terms of chronicity, complications, and potential infertility. Women are counseled to use condoms. All clients with gonorrhea should be offered confidential counseling and testing for HIV infection.

> **LEGAL TIP: Reporting Communicable Diseases**
>
> Gonorrhea is a reportable communicable disease. Health care providers are legally responsible for reporting all cases to the health authorities, usually the local health department in the client's county of residence. Women should be informed that the case will be reported, told why, and informed of the possibility of being contacted by a health department epidemiologist.

Syphilis

Syphilis, one of the earliest described STIs, is caused by *Treponema pallidum,* a motile spirochete. Transmission is thought to be by entry in the subcutaneous tissue through microscopic abrasions that can occur during sexual intercourse. The disease also can be transmitted through kissing, biting, or oral-genital sex. Transplacental transmission can occur at any time during pregnancy; the degree of risk is related to the quantity of spirochetes in the maternal bloodstream.

In 2012, a total of 49,903 cases of syphilis were reported in the United States; this number included 15,667 cases of primary and secondary syphilis (CDC, 2014). The rates of primary and secondary syphilis were highest among women ages 20 to 24 years. The rates were highest in black women (CDC, 2014).

Syphilis is a complex disease that can lead to serious systemic disease and even death when untreated. Infection manifests itself in distinct stages with different symptoms and clinical manifestations. *Primary* syphilis is characterized by a primary lesion, the chancre, that appears 5 to 90 days after infection. This lesion often begins as a painless papule at the site of inoculation and then erodes to form a nontender, shallow, indurated, clean ulcer several millimeters to centimeters in size (Fig. 7-1, *A*). *Secondary* syphilis occurs 6 weeks to 6 months after the appearance of the chancre and is characterized by a widespread, symmetric maculopapular rash on the palms and soles and generalized lymphadenopathy. The infected individual also may experience fever, headache, and malaise. Condylomata lata (broad, painless, pink-gray wartlike infectious lesions) may develop on the vulva, the perineum, or the anus (see Fig. 7-1, *B*). If the woman is untreated, she enters a latent phase that is asymptomatic for the majority of individuals. Latent infections are those that lack clinical manifestations but are detected by serologic testing. If the infection was acquired in the preceding year, the infection is termed an *early latent* infection. If it is left untreated, tertiary syphilis will develop in about one third of these women. Neurologic, cardiovascular, musculoskeletal, or multiorgan system complications can develop in the third stage.

Screening and Diagnosis

All women who are diagnosed with another STI or with HIV should be screened for syphilis. All pregnant women should be screened for syphilis at the first prenatal visit and again early in the third trimester and at the time of giving birth if high risk (CDC, 2010c). Diagnosis is dependent on microscopic examination of primary and secondary lesion tissue and serology during latency and late infection. A test

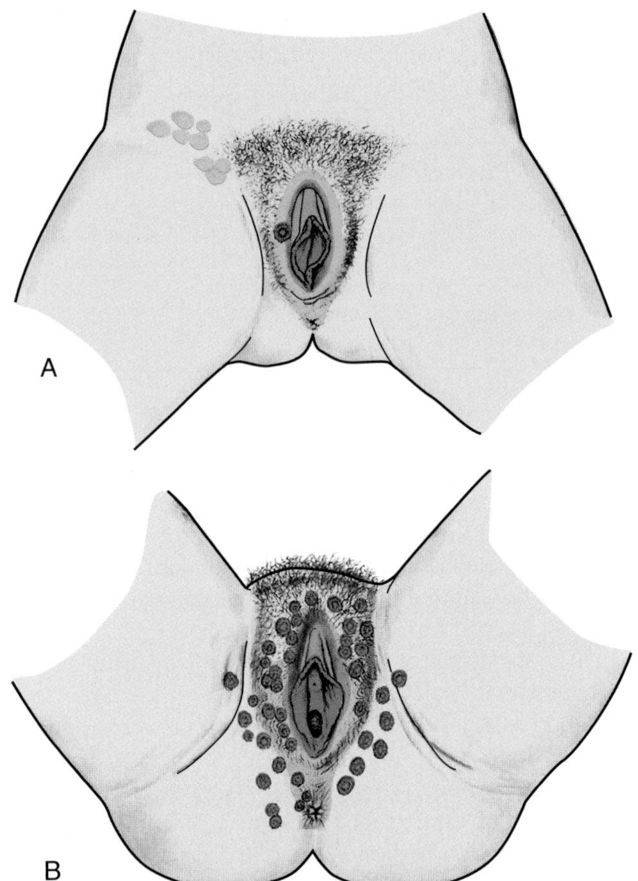

FIG 7-1 Syphilis. **A,** Primary stage: chancre with inguinal adenopathy. **B,** Secondary stage: condylomata lata.

for antibodies may not be reactive in the presence of active infection because it takes time for the body's immune system to develop antibodies to any antigens. Up to one third of people with early primary syphilis may have nonreactive serologic tests. Two types of serologic tests are used: nontreponemal and treponemal. Nontreponemal antibody tests such as the Venereal Disease Research Laboratories (VDRL) or rapid plasma reagin (RPR) are used as screening tests. False-positive results are not unusual, particularly when acute infection, autoimmune disorders, malignancy, pregnancy, and drug addiction exist and after immunization or vaccination. The treponemal tests, fluorescent treponemal antibody-absorbed (FTA-ABS), and microhemagglutination assays for antibody to *T. pallidum* (MHA-TP), are used to confirm positive results. Test results in clients with early primary or incubating syphilis can be negative. Seroconversion usually takes place 6 to 8 weeks after exposure, so testing should be repeated in 1 to 2 months when a suggestive genital lesion exists. Tests for concomitant STIs (e.g., chlamydia and gonorrhea) should be done (e.g., wet preps and cultures) and HIV testing offered if indicated.

Management

Penicillin G is the preferred drug for treating clients with syphilis (see Table 7-2). It is the only proven therapy that has been widely used for clients with neurosyphilis, congenital syphilis, or syphilis during pregnancy. Intramuscular benzathine penicillin G is used to treat primary, secondary, and early latent syphilis. Although doxycycline, tetracycline, and erythromycin are alternative treatments for penicillin-allergic clients, both tetracycline and doxycycline are contraindicated in pregnancy, and erythromycin is unlikely to cure a fetal infection. Therefore, pregnant women should, if necessary, receive skin testing and be treated with penicillin or be desensitized (CDC, 2010c). Specific protocols are recommended by the CDC.

MEDICATION ALERT

Clients treated for syphilis with penicillin may experience a Jarisch-Herxheimer reaction. This acute febrile reaction is often accompanied by headache, myalgias, and arthralgias that develop within the first 24 hours of treatment. The reaction can be treated symptomatically with analgesics and antipyretics. If the treatment precipitates this reaction in the second half of pregnancy, women are at risk for preterm labor and birth. They should be advised to contact their health care provider if they notice any change in fetal movement or have any contractions.

Monthly follow-up is mandatory so that repeated treatment may be given if needed. The nurse should emphasize the necessity of long-term serologic testing even in the absence of symptoms. The woman should be advised to practice sexual abstinence until treatment is completed, all evidence of primary and secondary syphilis is gone, and serologic evidence of a cure is demonstrated. Women should be told to notify all partners who may have been exposed. They should be informed that the disease is reportable. Preventive measures should be discussed.

CLINICAL REASONING CASE STUDY

Sexually Transmitted Infection Counseling in Pregnancy

Shawanda is an 18-year-old African-American, gravida 1 para 0, who has come to the prenatal clinic for her first visit. She has a history of drug use (marijuana). She says her current boyfriend is her support person but he is not the father of the baby. Shawanda is unemployed and living with her mother. She has been given an explanation of the prenatal laboratory tests that will be done during her examination. She says that she does not see why she has to have the tests for sexually transmitted infections (STIs) because she has not had these infections.

1. Evidence—Is there sufficient evidence to draw conclusions about what advice the nurse should give?
2. Assumptions—Describe underlying assumptions about the following issues:
   a. STI effects on pregnancy and the fetus
   b. STI risk factors
   c. Risk-reduction measures to prevent transmission of STIs
   d. Prevention of maternal-fetal transmission of human immunodeficiency virus (HIV)
3. What implications and priorities for nursing care can be drawn at this time?
4. Does the evidence objectively support your conclusion?

Pelvic Inflammatory Disease

Pelvic inflammatory disease (PID) is an infectious process that most commonly involves the uterine (fallopian) tubes (salpingitis), uterus (endometritis), and more rarely, the ovaries and peritoneal surfaces. Multiple organisms have been found to cause PID, and most cases are associated with more than one organism. In the past, the most common causative agent was thought to be *N. gonorrhoeae;* however, *C. trachomatis* is now estimated to cause half of all cases of PID. In addition to gonorrhea and chlamydia, a wide variety of anaerobic and aerobic bacteria are recognized to cause PID. PID encompasses a wide variety of pathologic processes; the infection can either be acute, subacute, or chronic and can have a wide range of symptoms.

Most PID results from ascending spread of microorganisms from the vagina and endocervix to the upper genital tract. This spread most frequently happens at the end of or just after menses following reception of an infectious agent. During the menstrual period several factors facilitate the development of an infection: the cervical os is slightly open, the cervical mucus barrier is absent, and menstrual blood is an excellent medium for growth. PID also can develop after a miscarriage or an induced abortion, pelvic surgery, or childbirth.

Risk factors for acquiring PID are those associated with the risk of contracting an STI, including young age (most cases of acute PID are in women younger than age 25), nulliparity, multiple partners, high rate of new partners, and a history of STIs and PID. Women who use intrauterine devices (IUDs) may be at increased risk for PID up to 3 weeks after insertion (Eckert & Lentz, 2012). PID tends to recur.

Women who have had PID are at increased risk for ectopic pregnancy, infertility, and chronic pelvic pain. After a single episode of PID, a woman's risk for ectopic pregnancy increases sevenfold compared with the risk for women who have never had PID. Other problems associated with PID include dyspareunia (painful intercourse), pyosalpinx (pus in the uterine tubes), tuboovarian abscess, and pelvic adhesions.

The symptoms of PID vary, depending on whether the infection is acute, subacute, or chronic; however, pain is common to all types of infections. It may be dull, cramping, and intermittent (subacute) or severe, persistent, and incapacitating (acute). Women may also report one or more of the following: fever, chills, nausea and vomiting, increased vaginal discharge, symptoms of a urinary tract infection, and irregular bleeding. Abdominal pain is usually present (Eckert & Lentz, 2012).

Screening and Diagnosis

PID is difficult to diagnose because of the accompanying wide variety of symptoms. The CDC recommends treatment for PID in all sexually active young women and others at risk for STIs if the following criteria are present and no other cause or causes of the illness are found: lower abdominal tenderness, bilateral adnexal tenderness, and cervical motion tenderness. Other criteria for diagnosing PID include an oral temperature of 38.3° C or above, abnormal cervical or vaginal discharge, elevated erythrocyte sedimentation rate, elevated C-reactive protein, and laboratory documentation of cervical infection with *N. gonorrhoeae* or *C. trachomatis* (CDC, 2010c).

Management

Perhaps the most important nursing intervention is prevention. Primary prevention includes education about preventing the acquisition of STIs, and secondary prevention involves preventing a lower genital tract infection from ascending to the upper genital tract. Instructing women in self-protective behaviors such as practicing risk-reduction measures and using barrier methods is critical. Also important is the detection of asymptomatic gonorrheal and chlamydial infections through routine screening of women with risky behaviors or specific risk factors such as age.

TABLE 7-3 Treatment of Pelvic Inflammatory Disease

PARENTERAL TREATMENT	ORAL TREATMENT
Regimen A **Cefotetan,** 2 g IV q12h *OR* **cefoxitin,** 2 g IV q6h for at least 24 hours after improvement *PLUS* **doxycycline,** 100 mg orally or IV q12h for 14 days **Regimen B** **Clindamycin,** 900 mg IV q8h *PLUS* **Gentamicin,** loading dose IV or IM (2 mg/kg of body weight), followed by maintenance dose (1.5 mg/kg) q8h. Single daily dosing may be substituted. Parenteral therapy can be discontinued 24 hours after clinical improvement; ongoing oral therapy should consist of **doxycycline** 100 mg orally twice a day, or **clindamycin** 450 mg orally four times a day to complete a total of 14 days of therapy.	**Ceftriaxone** 250 mg IM in a single dose *PLUS* **Doxycycline** 100 mg orally twice a day for 14 days *WITH or WITHOUT* **Metronidazole** 500 mg orally twice a day for 14 days *OR* **Cefoxitin** 2 g IM in a single dose and **probenecid,** 1 g orally administered concurrently in a single dose *PLUS* **Doxycycline** 100 mg orally twice a day for 14 days *WITH or WITHOUT* **Metronidazole** 500 mg orally twice a day for 14 days *OR* **Other parenteral third-generation cephalosporin** (e.g., ceftizoxime or cefotaxime) *PLUS* **Doxycycline** 100 mg orally twice a day for 14 days *WITH or WITHOUT* **Metronidazole** 500 mg orally twice a day for 14 days

IM, Intramuscular; *IV,* intravenous.

Data from Centers for Disease Control and Prevention. (2010). Sexually transmitted diseases treatment guidelines, 2010. *MMWR Morbidity and Mortality Weekly Report, 59*(RR-12), 1-109; Marrazzo, J.M., & Cates, W. (2011). Reproductive tract infections, including HIV and other sexually transmitted infections. In R. Hatcher, J. Trussell, A. Nelson, et al. (Eds.), *Contraceptive technology* (20th ed.). New York: Ardent Media.

Although treatment regimens vary with the infecting organism, a broad-spectrum antibiotic is generally used (Table 7-3). Treatment for mild to moderately severe PID may be oral, or a combination of oral and parenteral, and regimens can be administered in inpatient or outpatient settings (CDC, 2010c; Marrazzo & Cates, 2011). The woman with acute PID should be on bed rest in a semi-Fowler position. Comfort measures include analgesics for pain and all other nursing measures applicable to a woman confined to bed. The woman should have as few pelvic examinations as possible during the acute phase of the disease. During the recovery phase the woman should restrict her activity and make every effort to get adequate rest and a nutritionally sound diet. Follow-up laboratory work after treatment should include endocervical cultures for a test of cure.

Health education is central to effective management of PID. Explain to women the nature of their disease, and encourage them to comply with all therapy and prevention recommendations, emphasizing the necessity of taking all medication, even if symptoms disappear. Counsel women to refrain from sexual intercourse until their treatment is completed. Provide contraceptive counseling. Suggest that the woman select a barrier method such as condoms, contraceptive sponge, or a diaphragm. A woman with a history of PID may choose an IUD as her contraceptive method: however, the rate of treatment failure and recurrent PID in women continuing to use an IUD is unknown. There are no data regarding treatment outcomes by type of IUD (e.g., copper or levonorgestrel) (CDC, 2010c).

The potential or actual loss of reproductive capabilities can be devastating and can adversely affect a woman's self-concept. The woman may need help in adjusting her self-concept to fit reality and accept alterations in a way that promotes health. Because PID is so closely tied to sexuality, body image, and self-concept, the woman diagnosed with it will need supportive care. She should be encouraged to discuss her feelings. Referral to a support group or for counseling may be appropriate.

SEXUALLY TRANSMITTED VIRAL INFECTIONS

Human Papillomavirus

Human papillomavirus (HPV) infections, also known as *condylomata acuminata,* or *genital warts,* is the most common viral STI seen in ambulatory health care settings. An estimated 79 million Americans are infected with HPV, and about 14.1 million new infections occur every year (CDC, 2013b). The CDC estimates that 50% of sexually active women will become infected in their lifetimes. The highest rate of HPV infections occurs in women ages 20 to 24 years (CDC, 2013b).

HPV, a double-stranded DNA virus, has more than 40 serotypes that can be sexually transmitted, 5 of which are known to cause genital wart formation, and 8 of which are thought to have oncogenic potential (CDC, 2013b). HPV infection, types 16 and 18 are responsible for almost all cervical cancers (American Cancer Society [ACS], 2014).

HPV lesions in women are most commonly seen in the posterior part of the introitus; however, lesions also are found on the buttocks, the vulva, the vagina, the anus, and the cervix (Fig. 7-2). Typically the lesions are small—2 to 3 mm in diameter and 10 to 15 mm in height—soft, papillary swellings occurring singly or in clusters on the genital and anorectal region. Infections of long duration may appear as a cauliflower-like mass. In moist areas such as the vaginal introitus, the lesions may appear to have multiple, fine finger-like projections. Vaginal lesions are often multiple. Flat-topped papules, 1 to 4 mm in diameter, are seen most often on the cervix and often are visualized only under magnification. Warts are usually flesh colored or slightly darker on Caucasian women, black on African-American women, and brownish on Asian women. The lesions are often painless but may be uncomfortable, particularly when very large, inflamed, or ulcerated. Chronic vaginal discharge, pruritus, or dyspareunia can occur.

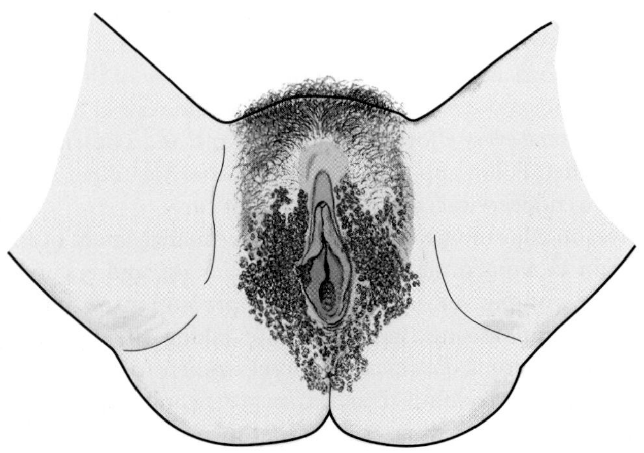

FIG 7-2 Human papillomavirus infection. Genital warts or condylomata acuminata.

HPV infections are thought to be more frequent in pregnant than in nonpregnant women, with an increase in incidence from the first trimester to the third. Furthermore, a significant proportion of preexisting HPV lesions enlarge greatly during pregnancy, a proliferation presumably resulting from the relative state of immunosuppression present during pregnancy. Lesions can become so large during pregnancy that they affect urination, defecation, mobility, and fetal descent, and can obstruct the birth canal, necessitating a cesarean birth (Marrazzo & Cates , 2011). HPV infection may be acquired by the neonate during birth; the frequency of such transmission is unknown. The preventive value of cesarean birth is unknown, and it is not recommended solely to prevent transmission of HPV infection to newborns (Marrazzo & Cates).

Screening and Diagnosis

A woman with HPV lesions may complain of symptoms such as a profuse irritating vaginal discharge, itching, dyspareunia, or postcoital bleeding. She also may report "bumps" on her vulva or labia. History of a known exposure is important; however, because of the potentially long latency period and the possibility of subclinical infections in men, the lack of a history of known exposure cannot be used to exclude a diagnosis of HPV infection.

Physical inspection of the vulva, the perineum, the anus, the vagina, and the cervix is essential whenever HPV lesions are suspected or seen in one area. Because speculum examination of the vagina may block some lesions, it is important to rotate the speculum blades until all areas are visualized. When lesions are visible, the characteristic appearance previously described is considered diagnostic. However, in many instances, cervical lesions are not visible, and some vaginal or vulvar lesions also may be unobservable to the naked eye. Because of the potential spread of vulvar or vaginal lesions to the anus, gloves should be changed between vaginal and rectal examinations.

Viral screening and typing for HPV are available but not standard practice. History, evaluation of signs and symptoms, Papanicolaou (Pap) test, and physical examination are used in making a diagnosis. The HPV-DNA test can be used in women older than age 30 in combination with the Pap test to screen for types of HPV that are likely to cause cancer or in women with abnormal Pap test results (ACS, 2014). The only definitive diagnostic test for the presence of HPV is histologic evaluation of a biopsy specimen.

HPV lesions must be differentiated from molluscum contagiosum and condylomata lata. Molluscum contagiosum lesions are half-domed, smooth, flesh-colored to pearly white papules with depressed centers. Condylomata lata are a form of secondary syphilis and generally flatter and wider than genital warts. A serologic test for syphilis confirms the diagnosis of secondary syphilis.

EVIDENCE-BASED PRACTICE

Age-Based Cervical Screening Recommendations Using Cytology and/or Human Papillomavirus Typing

Ask the Question

How does cytology screening (conventional or liquid-based) compare to human papillomavirus (HPV) typing in sensitivity and specificity for detection and treatment of cervical cancer? Does age make a difference in recommendations?

Search for the Evidence

Search Strategies English language reviews, systematic reviews, metaanalyses, and Practice Guidelines on cervical cytology and HPV typing were included.

Databases Used Cochrane Database of Systematic Reviews, National Guideline Clearinghouse (AHRQ), PubMed, UpToDate, CINAHL, and the professional website for AWHONN

Critical Appraisal of the Evidence

Whitlock, Vesco, Eder, et al. (2011):

- Cervical abnormalities that may progress to cervical cancer are caused by certain high risk oncogenic HPV types.
- Cervical screening includes conventional Papanicolaou (Pap) slide preparation, liquid-based cytology (LBC), and HPV typing.
- Conventional cytology is equal to LBC for sensitivity and specificity for cervical intraepithelial neoplasia (CIN), but LBC is superior for adequate cell capture.
- HPV typing is a trade-off: It is more sensitive at detecting cervical abnormality, but its lower specificity means more false positives, and therefore more overdiagnosis and possible overtreatment. All studies lack data on harm from overuse of colposcopy and treatment procedures.
- Using HPV typing first, with follow-up cytology for high risk HPV results, enhances the detection of severe precancerous cervical changes (CIN 3).
- The major benefit from using HPV typing as the primary screen may be a longer screening interval for a low risk population.
- Ongoing research in HPV subtypes, markers, and clinical history can further focus screening targets.

Schwaiger, Aruda, LaCoursiere, & Rubin (2012):

- HPV is very commonly found in women younger than 30 years of age, yet 90% resolve within 2 years; progression to cervical cancer is rare in this age group.

ACOG Committee on Practice Bulletins (2012): Women with normal immune systems and no history of risk factors are tested based on the following guidelines, regardless of HPV vaccine status:

- Cytology screening alone is recommended every 3 years for women 21 to 29 years old.
- For women ages 30 to 65, cytology and HPV typing are recommended every 5 years. Alternately, cytology alone every 3 years is acceptable.
- In the presence of hysterectomy and no history of CIN 2 or higher, screening may be discontinued.
- Screening may be discontinued for women after age 65, if adequate testing has been negative for 10 years.

Apply the Evidence: Nursing Implications

Schwaiger, Aruda, LaCoursiere, & Rubin (2012):

- Nurses can help update textbooks and protocols to reflect the targeted use of HPV typing and the change away from routine yearly Pap testing.
- The appropriate cancer prevention focus for adolescents is sexually transmitted infection (STI) protection and HPV vaccination.
- Women's health exams are an ideal time to educate clients about the risks of smoking and substance abuse in increasing HPV morbidity, as well as prevention of concurrent STIs, including human immunodeficiency virus (HIV).

Quality and Safety Competencies: Evidence-Based Practice*

Knowledge

Explain the role of evidence in determining best clinical practice.

Describe targeted cervical screening recommendations that result from research on the sensitivity and specificity of HPV typing.

Skills

Participate in structuring the work environment to facilitate integration of new evidence into standards of practice.

Educate clients about best practices for screening and prevention of HPV and cervical cancer.

Attitudes

Value the need for continuous improvement in clinical practice based on new knowledge.

Keep up with changes in recommendations as further research on targeting HPV subtypes, markers, and risk factors is published.

References

American College of Obstetricians and Gynecologists (ACOG) Committee on Practice Bulletins. (2012). Practice bulletin number 131: Screening for cervical cancer. *Obstetrics and Gynecology, 120*(5), 1222–1238.

Schwaiger, C., Aruda, M., LaCoursiere, S., & Rubin, R. (2012). Current guidelines for cervical cancer screening. *Journal of American Academy of Nurse Practitioners, 24*(7), 417–424.

Whitlock, E. P., Vesco, K. K., Eder, M., et al. (2011). Liquid-based cytology and human papillomavirus testing to screen for cervical cancer: A systematic review for the U.S. Preventive Services Task Force. *Annals of Internal Medicine, 155*(10), 687–697.

Pat Mahaffee Gingrich

*Adapted from QSEN at www.qsen.org.

Management

Untreated HPV infection resolves spontaneously in young women because their immune systems may be strong enough to fight the HPV infection. However, if the virus persists, depending on the type of virus, genital warts or cancer can develop months or years after the person has been infected with HPV (CDC, 2013b). No therapy has been shown to eradicate HPV. The goal of treatment for genital warts is removal of warts and relief of signs and symptoms. Treatment for cervical cancer is discussed in Chapter 11.

Treatment of genital warts should be guided by preference of the woman, available resources, and experience of the health care provider. The woman often must make multiple office visits, and many different treatment modalities will be used. None of the treatments is superior to all other treatments, and no one treatment is ideal for all warts (CDC, 2010c).

Available treatments are outlined in Table 7-2. Imiquimod, podophyllin, podofilox, and sinecatechins should not be used during pregnancy (CDC, 2010c; Fantasia, 2012). Because the lesions can proliferate and become friable during pregnancy, many experts recommend their removal by using cryotherapy or various surgical techniques during pregnancy (CDC).

Women with discomfort associated with genital warts may find that bathing with an oatmeal solution and drying the area with a cool hair dryer provides some relief. Keeping the area clean and dry also decreases growth of the warts. Cotton underwear and loose-fitting clothes that decrease friction and irritation also may decrease discomfort. Women should be advised to maintain a healthy lifestyle to aid the immune system; women can be counseled regarding diet, rest, stress reduction, and exercise.

Royer and Falk (2012) found that young women tend to have misconceptions about HPV. Client counseling is essential to reducing the prevalence of HPV and in improving the management of HPV in women who are infected. Women need to know that HPV infection is very common, and in most cases, will clear up spontaneously. Some infections will progress to genital warts, precancerous lesions, or cancers. Women must understand how the virus is transmitted, that no immunity is conferred with infection, and that reacquisition of the infection is likely with repeated contact. Because HPV is highly contagious, the majority of partners of women with HPV will be infected even if they are asymptomatic. All sexually active women with multiple partners or a history of HPV should be encouraged to use latex condoms for intercourse to decrease the risk of acquisition or transmission of genital HPV.

Instructions for all medications and treatments must be detailed. Women should be told that treatments are for the conditions caused by the virus but not HPV itself. Women should be informed before treatment of the possibility of posttreatment pain associated with specific therapies. The importance of thorough treatment of concurrent vaginitis or STI should be emphasized. The link between cervical cancer and some HPV infections and the need for close follow-up should be discussed. Annual health examinations are recommended to assess disease recurrence and screening for cervical cancer. Women should be counseled to have regular Pap screening, as recommended for women without genital warts (CDC, 2010c). Preventive strategies such as those presented in the following section should also be discussed.

Prevention

Preventive strategies include abstinence from all sexual activity, staying in a long-term monogamous relationship, limiting the number of sexual partners, and prophylactic vaccination (CDC, 2010c, 2013b).

Two vaccines, Cervarix and Gardasil, are available and other vaccines continue to be investigated. The two vaccines are recommended for 11- and 12-year-old girls and boys and are safe and effective in protecting against some of the most common types of HPV that can lead to genital warts and cancers. Cervarix protects against types 16 and 18 HPV infections while Gardasil protects against types 6, 11, 16, and 18. The vaccines are most effective if given before the woman has her first sexual contact (CDC, 2012c). The vaccines can be given to girls as early as 9 years of age and can also be given to young women ages 13 to 26 years if they did not receive the vaccine previously. The vaccine is given in three doses over a 6-month period (CDC, 2012c).

Genital Herpes Simplex Virus

Unknown until the middle of the 20th century, genital herpes simplex virus (HSV) infection is now widespread in the United States. HSV infection results in painful recurrent genital ulcers and is caused by two different antigen subtypes of herpes simplex virus: herpes simplex virus 1 (HSV-1) and herpes simplex virus 2 (HSV-2). HSV-2 is usually transmitted sexually, and HSV-1, nonsexually. Although HSV-1 is more commonly associated with gingivostomatitis and oral labial ulcers (fever blisters; cold sores) and HSV-2 with genital lesions, neither type is exclusively associated with the respective sites.

Although HSV infection is not a reportable disease, it is estimated that about 50 million people or about 1 in 6 people ages 14 to 49 years in the United States are infected with genital herpes (CDC, 2010c). Genital HSV is more common in women: approximately 1 in 5 women ages 14 to 49 are infected (CDC, 2013a). Non-Hispanic black women have the highest rates of any racial group. Women between the ages of 15 and 34 are most likely to become infected, especially if they have multiple sex partners.

Many persons infected with HSV-2 are asymptomatic and therefore undiagnosed. They can transmit the infection unaware that they are infected.

An initial HSV genital infection is characterized by multiple painful lesions, fever, chills, malaise, and severe dysuria and may last 2 to 3 weeks. Women generally have a more severe clinical course than men. Women with primary genital herpes have many lesions that progress from macules to papules, then forming vesicles, pustules, and ulcers that crust and heal without scarring (Fig. 7-3). These ulcers are extremely tender, and primary infections may be bilateral. Women also can have itching, inguinal tenderness, and lymphadenopathy. Severe vulvar edema may develop, and women may have difficulty sitting. HSV cervicitis also is common with initial HSV-2 infections. The cervix may appear normal or be friable, reddened, ulcerated, or necrotic. A heavy watery-to-purulent vaginal discharge is common. Extragenital lesions may be present because of autoinoculation. Urinary retention and dysuria may occur secondary to autonomic involvement of the sacral nerve root.

Women with recurrent episodes of HSV infections commonly have only local symptoms that are usually less severe than those associated with the initial infection. Systemic symptoms are usually absent, although the characteristic prodromal genital tingling is common. Recurrent lesions are unilateral, less severe, and usually last 5 to 7 days. Lesions begin as vesicles and

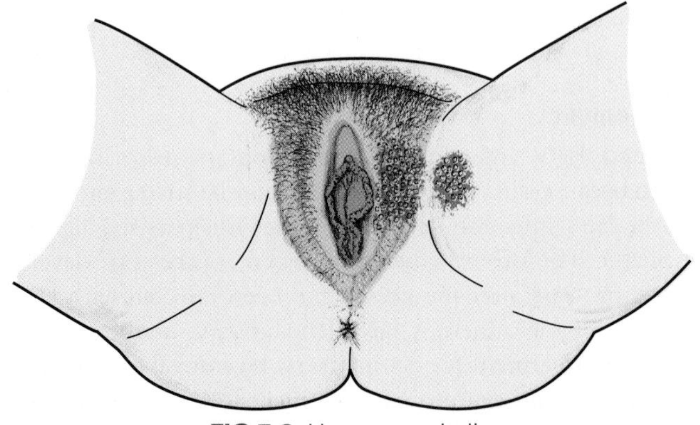

FIG 7-3 Herpes genitalis.

progress rapidly to ulcers. Few women with recurrent disease have cervicitis.

During pregnancy, maternal infection with HSV-2 can have adverse effects on both the mother and fetus. Viremia occurs during the primary infection, and congenital infection is possible, though rare. Primary infections during the first trimester have been associated with increased miscarriage rates (CDC, 2010c). The most severe complication of HSV infection is neonatal herpes, a potentially fatal or severely disabling disease occurring in 1 in 2000 to 1 in 10,000 live births. Most mothers of infants who contract neonatal herpes lack histories of clinically evident genital herpes. Risk of neonatal infection is highest among women with primary herpes infection who are near term and is low among women with recurrent herpes (CDC 2010c).

Screening and Diagnosis

A history provides much information when making a diagnosis of herpes. A history of exposure to an infected person is important, although infection from an asymptomatic individual is possible. A history of having viral symptoms such as malaise, headache, fever, or myalgia is suggestive. Local symptoms such as vulvar pain, dysuria, itching or burning at the site of infection, and painful genital lesions that heal spontaneously also are highly suggestive of HSV infections. The nurse should ask about a history of a primary infection, prodromal symptoms, vaginal discharge, and dyspareunia. Women should be asked whether they or their partner(s) have had genital lesions.

During the physical examination the nurse should assess for inguinal and generalized lymphadenopathy and elevated temperature. The entire vulvar, perineal, vaginal, and cervical areas should be carefully inspected for vesicles or ulcerated or crusted areas. A speculum examination may be very difficult for the woman because of the extreme tenderness often associated with herpes infections. Any suggestive or recurrent lesions found during pregnancy should be cultured to verify HSV. Although a diagnosis of herpes infection may be suspected from the history and physical, it is confirmed by laboratory studies. A viral culture is obtained by swabbing exudate during the vesicular stage of the disease. Type-specific serologic tests for HSV-2 antibodies are also available (CDC, 2010c).

Management

Genital herpes is a chronic and recurring disease for which there is no known cure. Management is directed toward specific treatment during primary and recurrent infections, prevention, self-help measures, and psychologic support.

Systemic antiviral medications partially control the symptoms and signs of HSV infections when used for the primary or recurrent episodes or when used as daily suppressive therapy. However, these medications do not eradicate the infection nor do they alter subsequent risk or frequency of recurrences after the medication is stopped. Three antiviral medications provide clinical benefit: acyclovir, valacyclovir, and famciclovir. Treatment recommendations are given in Table 7-2. The safety of acyclovir, valacyclovir, and famciclovir therapy during pregnancy has not been established; however, acyclovir may be used to reduce the symptoms of HSV if the benefits to the woman outweigh the potential harm to the fetus (CDC, 2010c). Continued investigation of HSV therapy with these medications in pregnancy is needed.

Cleaning lesions twice a day with saline helps prevent secondary infection. Bacterial infection must be treated with appropriate antibiotics. Measures that may increase comfort for women when lesions are active include warm sitz baths with baking soda; keeping lesions dry by blowing the area dry with a hair dryer set on cool or patting dry with a soft towel; wearing cotton underwear and loose clothing; using drying aids such as hydrogen peroxide, Burow solution, or oatmeal baths; applying cool, wet, black tea bags to lesions; and applying compresses with an infusion of cloves or peppermint oil and clove oil to lesions.

Oral analgesics such as aspirin, acetaminophen, or ibuprofen may be used to relieve pain and systemic symptoms associated with initial infections. Because the mucous membranes affected by herpes are extremely sensitive, any topical agents should be used with caution. Nonantiviral ointments, especially those containing cortisone, should be avoided. A thin layer of lidocaine ointment or an antiseptic spray may be applied to decrease discomfort, especially if walking is painful.

Counseling and education are critical components of the nursing care of women with herpes infections. Information regarding the etiology, signs and symptoms, transmission, and treatment should be provided. The nurse should explain that each woman is unique in her response to herpes and emphasize the variability of symptoms. Women should be helped to understand when viral shedding and thus transmission to a partner are most likely. They should be counseled to refrain from sexual contact from the onset of prodrome until complete healing of lesions. Suppressive therapy may be an option because it can decrease the risk of transmission to partners (CDC, 2010c).

Some authorities recommend consistent use of condoms for all persons with genital herpes. Condoms may not prevent transmission, particularly male-to-female transmission; however, this does not mean that the partners should avoid all intimacy. Women can be encouraged to maintain close contact with their partners while avoiding contact with lesions. They should be taught how to look for herpetic lesions using a mirror and good light source and a wet cloth or finger covered with a finger cot to rub lightly over the labia. The nurse should ensure that women understand that when lesions are active, sharing intimate articles (e.g., washcloths or wet towels) that come into contact with the lesions should be avoided. Only plain soap and water are needed to clean hands that have come into contact with herpetic lesions; isolation is neither necessary nor appropriate.

Stress, menstruation, trauma, febrile illnesses, chronic illnesses, and ultraviolet light have all been found to trigger genital herpes. Women may wish to keep a diary to identify stressors that seem to be associated with recurrent herpes attacks so that they can then avoid these stressors when possible. The role of exercise in reducing stress can be discussed. Referral for stress-reduction therapy, yoga, or meditation classes may be indicated. Avoiding excessive heat and sun and hot baths and using a lubricant during sexual intercourse to reduce friction also may be helpful. Women in their childbearing years should be counseled regarding the risk of herpes infection during pregnancy. They should be instructed to use condoms if there is any risk of contracting an STI from a sexual partner. If they become pregnant while taking acyclovir, the risk of birth defects does not appear to be higher than for the general population; however, continued use should be based on whether the benefits for the woman outweigh the possible risks to the fetus. Acyclovir does enter breast milk but the amount of medication ingested during breastfeeding is very low and is usually not a health concern (Weiner & Buhimschi, 2009).

Because neonatal HSV infection is such a devastating disease, prevention is critical. Recommendations include carefully examining and questioning all women about symptoms at onset of labor. If visible lesions are not present at onset of labor, vaginal birth is acceptable. Cesarean birth is recommended if visible lesions are present (CDC, 2010c). Infants who are born through an infected vagina should be carefully observed and cultured (see Chapter 35).

The emotional effect of contracting an incurable STI such as herpes is considerable. At diagnosis, many emotions may surface—helplessness, anger, denial, guilt, anxiety, shame, or inadequacy. Women need the opportunity to discuss their feelings and help in learning to live with the disease. Herpes can affect a woman's sexuality, her sexual practices, and her current and future relationships. She may need help in raising the issue with her partner or with future partners.

Viral Hepatitis

Five different viruses (hepatitis viruses A, B, C, D, and E) account for almost all cases of viral hepatitis in humans. Hepatitis viruses A, B, and C are discussed. Hepatitis D and E viruses, common among users of intravenous (IV) drugs and recipients of multiple blood transfusions, are not included in this discussion.

> **COMMUNITY ACTIVITY**
>
> Visit the Centers for Disease Control and Prevention website at www.cdc.gov. Select a sexually transmitted infection. What is the prevalence of the disease in your state? Evaluate the rank, number of cases, rate per 100,000 population, and cumulative percent. Review the client information about facts and treatment, including concerns and treatment during pregnancy. Locate an STI treatment clinic in your area. Is the location easily accessible by public transportation? Are the hours convenient for clients who are not available in the daytime? What is included in the appointment? What, if any, are the costs of care?

Hepatitis A

Hepatitis A virus (HAV) infection is acquired primarily through a fecal-oral route by ingestion of contaminated food, particularly milk, shellfish, or polluted water, or person-to-person contact (CDC, 2012a). Women living in the western United States, Native Americans, Alaska Natives, and children and employees in daycare centers are at high risk. Hepatitis A, like other enteric infections, can be transmitted during sexual activity.

HAV infection is characterized by flulike symptoms with malaise, fatigue, anorexia, nausea, pruritus, fever, and right upper quadrant pain. Serologic testing to detect the immunoglobulin M (IgM) antibody is done to confirm acute infections. The IgM antibody is detectable 5 to 10 days after exposure and can remain positive for up to 6 months. Because HAV infection is self-limited and does not result in chronic infection or chronic liver disease, treatment is usually supportive. Women who become dehydrated from nausea and vomiting or who have fulminating hepatitis A may need to be hospitalized. Medications and other ingested substances that might cause liver damage or that are metabolized in the liver (e.g., acetaminophen, ethyl alcohol) should be avoided. A well-balanced diet is recommended. Hepatitis A vaccine (two doses) is recommended for women at high risk for being exposed to HAV infection. The safety of the vaccine has not been established in pregnancy; therefore, immune globulin (gamma globulin) or immune-specific globulin is indicated for a pregnant woman exposed to HAV. All household contacts of the woman also should receive gamma globulin (CDC, 2010c).

Hepatitis B

Hepatitis B virus (HBV) is the virus most threatening to the fetus and neonate. It is caused by a large DNA virus and is associated with three antigens and their antibodies: hepatitis B surface antigen (HBsAg), HBV antigen (HBeAg), HBV core antigen (HBcAg), antibody to HBsAg (anti-HBs), antibody to HBeAg (anti-HBe), and antibody to HBcAg (anti-HBc). Screening for active or chronic disease or disease immunity is based on testing for these antigens and their antibodies.

Populations at risk include women of Asian, Pacific Island (Polynesian, Micronesian, Melanesian), or Alaskan-Inuit descent and women born in Haiti or Sub-Saharan Africa. Women who have a history of acute or chronic liver disease, who work or receive treatment in a dialysis unit, or who have household or sexual contact with a hemodialysis client are at greater risk. Women who work or live in institutions for the mentally challenged are considered to be at risk, as are women with a history of multiple blood transfusions. Health care workers and public safety workers exposed to blood in the workplace are at risk. Behaviors such as having multiple sexual partners and a history of IV drug use increase the risk of contracting HBV infections.

HBsAg has been found in blood, saliva, sweat, tears, vaginal secretions, and semen. Drug abusers who share needles are at risk, as are health care workers who are exposed to blood and needlesticks. Perinatal transmission most often occurs in infants of mothers who have acute hepatitis infection late in the third trimester or during the intrapartum or postpartum period from exposure to HBsAg-positive vaginal secretions, blood, amniotic fluid, saliva, and breast milk. HBV has also been transmitted by artificial insemination. Although HBV can be transmitted via blood transfusion, the incidence of such infections has decreased significantly since testing of blood for HBsAg became routine.

HBV infection is a disease of the liver and is often a silent infection. In an adult the course can be sudden and severe, and the outcome fatal. Symptoms of HBV infection are similar to those of hepatitis A: arthralgias, arthritis, lassitude, anorexia, nausea, vomiting, headache, fever, and mild abdominal pain. Later the woman may have clay-colored stools, dark urine, increased abdominal pain, and jaundice. Between 5% and 10% of individuals with HBV have persistence of HBsAg and become chronic hepatitis B carriers.

Screening and Diagnosis. All women at high risk for contracting HBV should be screened regularly. However, screening only individuals at high risk may not identify up to 50% of HBsAg-positive women. Screening for the presence of HBsAg is recommended on all pregnant women at the first prenatal visit, regardless of whether they have been tested previously; screening should be done on admission for labor and birth for women at high risk for infection who were not tested in pregnancy or if prenatal test results are not available (CDC, 2012a).

The HBsAg screening test is usually performed, given that a rise in HBsAg occurs at the onset of clinical symptoms and usually indicates an active infection. If HBsAg persists in the blood, the woman is identified as a carrier. If the HBsAg test result is positive, further laboratory studies may be ordered: anti-HBe, anti-HBc, serum glutamic-oxaloacetic transaminase (SGOT), alkaline phosphatase, and liver panel.

Management. There is no specific treatment for hepatitis B. Recovery is usually spontaneous in 3 to 16 weeks. Pregnancies complicated by acute viral hepatitis are managed on an outpatient basis. Women should be advised to increase rest periods; eat a high-protein, low-fat diet; and increase their fluid intake. They should avoid medications metabolized in the liver, and alcohol. Pregnant women with a definite exposure to HBV should be given hepatitis B immune globulin and should begin the hepatitis B vaccine series within 14 days of the most recent contact to prevent infection (CDC, 2010a). Vaccination during pregnancy is not thought to pose risks to the fetus.

All nonimmune women at high or moderate risk of hepatitis should be informed of the availability of hepatitis B vaccine. Vaccination is recommended for all individuals who have had multiple sex partners within the past 6 months (CDC, 2010c). In addition, IV drug users, residents of correctional or long-term care facilities, people seeking care for an STI, prostitutes, women whose partners are IV drug users or bisexual, and women whose occupation exposes them to high risk should be vaccinated. The vaccine is given in a series of three (four if rapid protection is needed) doses over a 6-month period, with the first two doses given at least 1 month apart. The vaccine is given in the deltoid muscle (CDC).

Client education includes explaining the meaning of hepatitis B infection, including transmission, state of infectivity, and sequelae. The nurse also should explain the need for immunoprophylaxis for household members and sexual contacts. To decrease transmission of the virus, women with hepatitis B or who test positive for HBV should be advised to maintain a high level of personal hygiene (e.g., wash hands after using the toilet; carefully dispose of tampons, pads, and bandages in plastic bags; do not share razor blades, toothbrushes, needles, or manicure implements; have male partner use a condom if unvaccinated and without hepatitis; avoid sharing saliva through kissing, or sharing of silverware or dishes; and wipe up blood spills immediately with soap and water). They should inform all health care providers of their carrier state. Postpartum women should be reassured that breastfeeding is not contraindicated if their infants received prophylaxis at birth and are currently on the immunization schedule.

Hepatitis C

Hepatitis C virus (HCV) infection has become an important health problem as increasing numbers of persons acquire the disease. The CDC estimates that individuals born between 1945 and 1965 make up about 75% of all HCV infections. Hepatitis C is responsible for nearly 50% of the cases of chronic viral hepatitis. Risk factors include having STIs such as HBV and HIV, multiple sexual partners, history of blood transfusions, and history of IV drug use. HCV is readily transmitted through exposure to blood and much less efficiently via semen, saliva, or urine (CDC, 2012a).

Most clients with HCV are asymptomatic or have general influenza-like symptoms similar to those of HAV. Previously HCV testing was done on people based on known risk factors and clinical manifestations. In August 2012, the CDC recommended that one-time testing of adults born between 1945 and 1965 be instituted without prior determination of HCV risk factors (CDC, 2012d). HCV infection is confirmed by the presence of anti-C antibody during laboratory testing.

Interferon alfa alone or with ribavirin for 6 to 12 months is the main therapy for chronic HCV-related liver disease, although effectiveness of this treatment varies (CDC, 2010c). Currently, no vaccine is available for HCV. Transmission of HCV through breastfeeding has not been reported.

Human Immunodeficiency Virus

Approximately 47,500 new HIV infections occur in the United States each year. An estimated 20% of these new infections occur in women. Black women are estimated to have 64% of these infections, white women are estimated to have 18%, Hispanic women, 15%, and American Indian women less than 1% (CDC, 2013c).

Severe depression of the cellular immune system associated with HIV infection characterizes acquired immunodeficiency syndrome (AIDS). Although behaviors that place women at risk have been well documented, all women should be assessed for the possibility of HIV exposure. The most commonly reported opportunistic diseases are *Pneumocystis (jirovecii)* pneumonia (PCP), *Candida* esophagitis, and wasting syndrome. Other viral infections such as HSV and cytomegalovirus infections seem to be more prevalent in women than men (CDC, 2010c). PID is often more severe in HIV-infected women than in the general population, and rates of HPV and cervical dysplasia are sometimes higher in non–HIV-infected women (Eckert & Lentz, 2012). The clinical course of HPV infection in women with HIV infection is accelerated, and recurrence is more frequent in non–HIV-infected women.

Once HIV enters the body, seroconversion to HIV positivity usually occurs within 6 to 12 weeks. Although HIV seroconversion may be totally asymptomatic, it usually is accompanied by a viremic influenza-like response. Symptoms include fever, headache, night sweats, malaise, generalized lymphadenopathy, myalgias, nausea, diarrhea, weight loss, sore throat, and rash.

Laboratory studies may reveal leukopenia, thrombocytopenia, anemia, and an elevated erythrocyte sedimentation rate. HIV has a strong affinity for surface-marker proteins on T lymphocytes. This affinity leads to significant T-cell destruction. Both clinical and epidemiologic studies have shown that declining CD4 levels are strongly associated with increased incidence of AIDS-related diseases and death in many different groups of HIV-infected people.

Transmission of the virus from mother to child can occur throughout the perinatal period. Exposure may occur to the fetus through the maternal circulation as early as the first trimester of pregnancy, to the infant during labor and birth by inoculation or ingestion of maternal blood and other infected fluids, or to the infant through breast milk (CDC, 2013f).

Screening and Diagnosis

Screening, teaching, and counseling regarding HIV risk factors, indications for being tested, and testing are major roles for nurses caring for women today. A number of behaviors place women at risk for HIV infection, including IV drug use, high risk sexual partners, multiple sex partners, and a history of multiple STIs. HIV infection is usually diagnosed by using HIV-1 and HIV-2 antibody tests. Antibody testing is first done with a sensitive screening test such as the enzyme immunoassay (EIA). Reactive screening tests must be confirmed by an additional test, such as the Western blot or an immunofluorescence assay. If a positive antibody test is confirmed by a supplemental test, it means that a woman is infected with HIV and is capable of infecting others. HIV antibodies are detectable in at least 95% of individuals within 3 months after infection. Although a negative antibody test usually indicates that a person is not infected, antibody tests cannot exclude recent infection. Although HIV antibody crosses the placenta, definitive diagnosis of HIV in children younger than 18 months is based on laboratory evidence of HIV in blood or tissues by culture, nucleic acid, or antigen detection (CDC, 2010c).

The U.S. Food and Drug Administration (FDA) (2008) approves six rapid HIV antibody screening tests for clinical use. These tests use a blood sample obtained by fingerstick or venipuncture, an oral fluid sample, or a urine sample to provide test results within 20 minutes, with sensitivity and specificity rates of more than 99%. If the results are reactive, further testing is necessary (CDC, 2010c). Quicker results mean that clients do not have to make extra visits for follow-up standard tests, and the oral test provides an option for clients who do not want to have a blood test.

The CDC (2010c) recommends offering HIV testing to all women whose behavior places them at risk for HIV infection. It may be useful to allow women to self-select for HIV testing. On entry to the health care system, a woman can be handed written information about the risk factors for HIV and asked to inform the nurse if she believes she is at risk. She should be told that she does not have to say why she may be at risk, only that she thinks she might be.

All pregnant women in the United States should be tested for HIV infection as early during pregnancy as possible. The woman should first be informed that she will be tested for HIV as part of the panel of prenatal tests, unless she declines, or opts-out of, screening. For women who decline, providers should continue to encourage testing and address her concerns about testing (CDC, 2010c).

Counseling for HIV Testing

Counseling before and after HIV testing is standard nursing practice today. It is a nursing responsibility to assess a woman's understanding of the information such a test would provide and to be sure the woman thoroughly understands the emotional, legal, and medical implications of a positive or negative result before she is ready to take an HIV test.

> **! NURSING ALERT**
>
> Counseling associated with HIV testing has two components: pretest and posttest. During pretest counseling, a personalized risk assessment is conducted, the meaning of positive and negative test results is explained, informed consent for HIV testing is obtained, and women are helped to develop a realistic plan for reducing risk and preventing infection. Posttest counseling includes informing the woman of the test results, reviewing the meaning of the results, and reinforcing prevention messages. It is important to document all pretest and posttest counseling.

Given the strong social stigma attached to HIV infection, nurses must consider the issue of confidentiality and documentation before providing counseling and offering HIV testing to clients.

> **LEGAL TIP: HIV Testing**
>
> If HIV test results are placed in the client's chart—the appropriate place for all health information—they are available to all who have access to the chart. Inform the woman of this availability before testing. Informed consent must be obtained before an HIV test is performed. In some states, written consent is mandated. In many states, HIV testing is performed unless women decline (i.e., opt-out). Nurses must know what procedures are being used for informed consent in their facility.

Unless rapid testing is done, there is generally a 1- to 3-week waiting period after testing for HIV, which can be a very anxious time for the woman. It is helpful if the nurse informs her that this time period between blood drawing and test results is routine. Test results, whatever they are, always must be communicated in person, and women need to be informed in advance that such is the procedure. Whenever possible, the person who provided the pretest counseling also should tell the woman her test results.

When some women are informed of negative results, they may escalate their risk behaviors because of equating negativity with immunity. Others may believe that negative means "bad" and positive means "good." Women's reactions to a negative test should be explored, such as by asking, "How do you feel?" HIV-negative result counseling sessions are another opportunity to provide education. Emphasis can be placed on ways in which a woman can remain HIV free. She should be reminded that if she has been exposed to HIV in the past 6 months, she should be retested, and that if she continues high risk behaviors, she should have ongoing testing.

In posttest counseling to an HIV-positive woman, privacy with no interruptions is essential. Adequate time for the counseling sessions should be provided. The nurse must make sure that the woman understands what a positive test means and review the reliability of the test results. Risk-reduction practices should be reemphasized. Referral for appropriate medical evaluation and follow-up should be made, and the need or desire for psychosocial or psychiatric referrals should be assessed.

It's important to stress early medical evaluation so that a baseline assessment can be made and prophylactic medication begun. If possible, the nurse should make a referral or appointment for the woman at the posttest counseling session.

Management

During the initial contact with an HIV-infected woman, the nurse should establish what the woman knows about HIV infection and that she is being cared for by a medical practitioner or facility with expertise in caring for people with HIV infections, including AIDS. Psychologic referral also may be indicated. Resources such as counseling for financial assistance, legal advocacy, suicide prevention, and death and dying may be appropriate. All women who are drug users should be referred to a substance-abuse program. A major focus of counseling is prevention of HIV transmission to partners.

Nurses counseling seropositive women wishing contraceptive information can recommend oral contraceptives, hormonal implants, and latex condoms or tubal sterilization or vasectomy and latex condoms. Injectable progestins may be used for the HIV-positive woman, but there is not enough evidence to recommend use by women at high risk for HIV (WHO, 2013a). Female condoms or abstinence can be used by women whose male partners refuse to use condoms. Women should be reminded that of these methods suggested, only condoms offer protection from HIV and other STIs.

No cure is available for HIV infections. Rare and unusual diseases are characteristic of HIV infections. Opportunistic infections and concurrent diseases are managed vigorously with treatment specific to the infection or disease. Routine gynecologic care for HIV-positive women should include a pelvic examination every 6 months. Thorough Pap screening is essential because of the greatly increased incidence of abnormal findings on examination (CDC, 2010c). In addition, HIV-positive women should be screened for syphilis, gonorrhea, chlamydia, and other vaginal infections and treated if infections are present. General prevention strategies are an important part of care (e.g., smoking cessation, sound nutrition) as is antiretro viral therapy. Discussion of the medical care of HIV-positive women or women with AIDS is beyond the scope of this chapter because of the rapidly changing recommendations. The reader is referred to the CDC (www.cdc.gov), CDC National AIDS hotline (800-342-2437), and Internet websites such as HIV/AIDS Treatment Information Service (www.hivatis.org) for current information and recommendations.

HIV and Pregnancy

HIV counseling and testing should be offered to all women at their initial prenatal care visit as part of routine prenatal testing unless the woman opts-out of the screening (CDC, 2010c). Universal testing is recommended versus selective testing for maternal HIV because it results in a greater number of women being screened and treated and can reduce the likelihood of perinatal transmission and maintain women's health (CDC). The CDC also recommends retesting in the third trimester for women known to be at high risk for HIV and rapid HIV testing in labor for women with unknown HIV status.

Perinatal transmission of HIV has decreased significantly since 2004 because of the administration of antiretroviral prophylaxis (e.g., zidovudine) to pregnant women in the prenatal and the perinatal periods. Treatment of HIV-infected women with the triple-drug antiretroviral therapy (ART) or highly active antiretroviral therapy (HAART) during pregnancy has been reported to decrease the mother-to-child transmission to 1% to 2% (CDC, 2010c). All HIV-infected women should be treated with a combination of ART during pregnancy, regardless of their CD4 cell counts (Panel on Treatment of HIV-Infected Pregnant Women and Prevention of Perinatal Transmission [The Panel], 2012). Data are insufficient to support or refute the teratogenic risk of antiretroviral medications given for prophylaxis in the first 10 weeks of pregnancy. Research does not support major teratogenic effects for most of the antiretroviral agents (The Panel). Women who are infected with HIV and need treatment for their own health should start the therapy as soon as possible, even in the first trimester; women who are taking the therapy as prophylaxis usually start therapy after the first trimester (The Panel).

ART is administered orally and continued throughout pregnancy. The major side effect of this therapy is bone marrow suppression. Periodic hematocrit, white blood cell count, and platelet count assessments should be performed (The Panel, 2012). Women who are HIV positive should also be vaccinated against hepatitis B, pneumococcal infection, *Haemophilus influenzae* type B, and viral influenza. To support any pregnant woman's immune system, appropriate counseling is provided about optimal nutrition, sleep, rest, exercise, and stress reduction. Condom use is encouraged to minimize further exposure to HIV from a sexual partner who may be a source.

In the intrapartum period ART and cesarean birth are recommended to prevent vertical transmission of HIV (The Panel, 2012). The Panel recommends a scheduled cesarean birth at 38 weeks of gestation for women with a viral load of more than 1000 copies/ml. A vaginal birth may be an option for HIV-infected women who have a viral load of fewer than 1000 copies/ml at 36 weeks, if a woman has ruptured membranes and labor is progressing rapidly, or if she declines a cesarean birth. IV zidovudine is recommended during the intrapartum period for HIV-infected pregnant women with viral loads of more than 400 copies/ml or unknown HIV status (The Panel). The drug is administered 3 hours before a scheduled cesarean birth and continued until the baby is born. It should be given during labor if the woman is having a vaginal birth (The Panel). Artificial rupture of membranes, fetal scalp electrode, and scalp pH sampling should be avoided because these procedures may result in inoculation of the fetus with the virus. Similarly the use of forceps or vacuum extractor should be avoided when possible (The Panel). Infants should receive oral zidovudine for 6 weeks after birth. Avoidance of breastfeeding is recommended in the United States and most developed countries (CDC, 2010; The Panel).

Women who have HIV but who are without symptoms may have an unremarkable postpartum course. Immunosuppressed women with symptoms may be at increased risk for postpartum urinary tract infections (UTIs), vaginitis, postpartum endometritis, and poor wound healing. Good perineal hygiene should be stressed. Women who are HIV positive but who were not on antiretroviral drugs before pregnancy should be tested in the postpartum period to determine whether therapy that was initiated in pregnancy should be continued (The Panel, 2012). After the initial bath the newborn may be with the mother. In planning for discharge, comprehensive care and support services need to be arranged. After discharge the woman and her infant are referred to physicians who are experienced in treating HIV and AIDS and associated conditions for intensive monitoring and follow-up (The Panel).

VAGINAL INFECTIONS

Vaginal discharge and itching of the vulva and vagina are among the most frequent reasons a woman seeks help from a health care provider. More women complain of vaginal discharge than of any other gynecologic symptom. Vaginal discharge resulting from infection must be distinguished from normal secretions. Women who have adequate endogenous or exogenous estrogen will have vaginal secretions. Normal vaginal secretions, or leukorrhea, are clear to cloudy and may turn yellow after drying; the discharge is slightly slimy, is nonirritating, and has a mild, inoffensive odor. Normal vaginal secretions are acidic, with a pH of 4 to 5. Normal vaginal secretions contain lactobacilli and epithelial cells. The amount of leukorrhea differs with phases of the menstrual cycle, with greater amounts occurring at ovulation and just before menses. Leukorrhea also is increased during pregnancy.

Vaginitis or abnormal vaginal discharge is an infection caused by a microorganism. The most common vaginal infections are bacterial vaginosis, candidiasis, and trichomoniasis. Although streptococcus B is considered normal vaginal flora, it may also cause infection. Vulvovaginitis, or inflammation of the vulva and vagina, may be caused by vaginal infection or copious amounts of leukorrhea, which can cause tissue maceration. Chemical irritants, allergens, and foreign bodies that produce inflammatory reactions can also cause vulvovaginitis.

Bacterial Vaginosis

Bacterial vaginosis (BV), formerly called nonspecific vaginitis, *Haemophilus vaginitis,* or *Gardnerella,* is the most common cause of vaginal symptoms today (Eckert & Lentz, 2012). The prevalence is most common in women of childbearing age—ages 14 to 49 in the United States. Non-white women (blacks and Hispanics) have higher rates than white women CDC, 2010a). Women with new or multiple sexual partners are at higher risk for infection. BV can increase susceptibility to STIs such as chlamydia, gonorrhea, genital herpes, and HIV (CDC). BV is associated with preterm labor and birth. The exact etiology of BV is unknown. It is a syndrome in which normal H_2O_2-producing lactobacilli are replaced with high concentrations of anaerobic bacteria (*Gardnerella* and *Mobiluncus*). With the increased amount of anaerobes, the level of vaginal amines is increased, and the normal acidic pH of the vagina is altered. Epithelial cells slough, and numerous bacteria attach to their surfaces (clue cells). When the amines are volatilized, the characteristic odor of BV occurs.

Many women with BV complain of the characteristic "fishy odor." The odor may be noticed by the woman or her partner after heterosexual intercourse because semen releases the vaginal amines. When present, the BV discharge usually appears profuse, thin, and white or gray, or milky. Some women also may experience mild irritation or pruritus.

Screening and Diagnosis

A focused history may help distinguish BV from other vaginal infections if the woman is symptomatic. Reports of fishy odor and increased thin vaginal discharge are most significant, and a report of increased odor after intercourse is also suggestive of BV.

TABLE 7-4 Wet Smear Tests for Vaginal Infections

INFECTION	TEST	POSITIVE FINDINGS
Trichomoniasis	Saline wet smear (vaginal secretions mixed with normal saline on a glass slide)	Presence of many white blood cell protozoa
Candidiasis	Potassium hydroxide (KOH) prep (vaginal secretions mixed with KOH on a glass slide)	Presence of hyphae and pseudohyphae (buds and branches of yeast cells)
Bacterial vaginosis	Normal saline smear	Presence of clue cells (vaginal epithelial cells coated with bacteria)
	Whiff test (vaginal secretions mixed with KOH)	Release of fishy odor

Microscopic examination of vaginal secretions is always performed (Table 7-4). Both normal saline and 10% potassium hydroxide (KOH) smears are made. The presence of more than 20% clue cells (vaginal epithelial cells coated with bacteria) on wet saline smear is highly diagnostic because the phenomenon is specific to BV. Vaginal secretions are tested for pH and amine odor. Nitrazine paper is sensitive enough to detect a pH of 4.5 or greater. The fishy odor of BV will be released when KOH is added to vaginal secretions on the lip of the withdrawn speculum (Eckert & Lentz, 2012).

Management

Treating bacterial vaginosis with oral metronidazole (Flagyl) is most effective (CDC, 2010c). Table 7-5 outlines treatment guidelines. Side effects of metronidazole are numerous, including sharp, unpleasant metallic taste in the mouth; furry tongue; central nervous system reactions; and urinary tract disturbances. When oral metronidazole is taken, the woman is advised not to drink alcoholic beverages or she will experience the severe side effects of abdominal distress, nausea, vomiting, and headache. Gastrointestinal symptoms are common but less severe if alcohol is not consumed. Treating sexual partners is not recommended routinely (CDC, 2010c).

Metronidazole is not recommended if the woman is breastfeeding. However, if it is necessary to prescribe it, the woman can suspend breastfeeding (pump and discard to maintain milk supply) during treatment and for 12 to 24 hours after the last dose to reduce the infant's exposure to metronidazole (CDC, 2010c).

Candidiasis

Vulvovaginal candidiasis (VVC), or yeast infection, is the second most common type of vaginal infection in the United States. Although vaginal candidiasis infections are common in healthy women, those seen in women with HIV infection are often more severe and persistent. Genital candidiasis lesions may be painful coalescing ulcerations necessitating continuous prophylactic therapy.

TABLE 7-5 Vaginal Infections and Drug Therapies for Women

DISEASE	NONPREGNANT WOMEN (13-17 yr)	NONPREGNANT WOMEN (>18 yr)	PREGNANT WOMEN	LACTATING WOMEN
Bacterial vaginosis	*Recommended:* metronidazole, 500 mg bid for 7 days (no alcohol) *or* metronidazole gel 0.75%, 5 g intravaginally bid for 7 days *or* clindamycin cream 2%, 5 g intravaginally at bedtime for 7 days (less effective)	*Recommended:* metronidazole, 500 mg bid for 7 days (no alcohol) *or* metronidazole gel 0.75%, 5 g intravaginally bid for 7 days *or* clindamycin cream 2%, 5 g intravaginally at bedtime for 7 days (less effective)	High risk asymptomatic or symptomatic women *Recommended:* metronidazole, 500 mg orally bid for 7 days (no alcohol) *or* metronidazole, 250 mg orally tid for 7 days *or* clindamycin, 300 mg orally bid for 7 days	*Recommended:* clindamycin cream or ovules
Trichomoniasis	*Recommended:* metronidazole, 2 g orally once *or* tinidazole, 2 g orally once	*Recommended:* metronidazole, 2 g orally once	*Recommended:* metronidazole, 2 g orally once	Metronidazole not recommended during lactation; stop breastfeeding treat, resume breastfeeding in 12-24 hours after drug completed Tinidazoles: Stop breastfeeding and resume 3 days after treatment Pump and discard milk to maintain supply
Candidiasis	Numerous OTC intravaginal agents: butoconazole, clotrimazole, miconazole, tioconazole, terconazole; treatment with "azole" drugs more effective than nystatin Dose varies by agent from one dose a day to one dose for 3 to 7 days *Oral agent:* fluconazole 150-mg oral tablet once	Numerous OTC intravaginal agents: butoconazole, clotrimazole, miconazole, tioconazole, terconazole; treatment with "azole" drugs more effective than nystatin Dose varies by agent from one dose a day to one dose for 3 to 7 days *Oral agent:* fluconazole 150-mg oral tablet once	OTC "azole" intravaginal agents: butoconazole, clotrimazole, miconazole, terconazole Use for 3 to 7 days Oral agents not recommended	OTC "azole" intravaginal agents: butoconazole, clotrimazole, miconazole, terconazole Use for 3 to 7 days

OTC, Over the counter.
Data from Centers for Disease Control and Prevention. (2010). Sexually transmitted diseases treatment guidelines 2010. *MMWR Morbidity and Mortality Weekly Report, 59*(RR-12), 1-109.

The most common organism is *Candida albicans;* estimates indicate that more than 90% of the yeast infections in women are caused by this organism. However, since 2004, the incidence of non–*C. albicans* infections has risen steadily. Women with chronic or recurrent infections often are infected with these organisms (Eckert & Lentz, 2012).

Numerous factors have been identified as predisposing a woman to yeast infections, including antibiotic therapy, particularly broad-spectrum antibiotics such as ampicillin, tetracycline, cephalosporins, and metronidazole; diabetes, especially when uncontrolled; pregnancy; obesity; diets high in refined sugars or artificial sweeteners; use of corticosteroids and exogenous hormones; and immunosuppressed states. Clinical observations and research have suggested that tight-fitting clothing and underwear or pantyhose made of nonabsorbent materials create an environment in which a vaginal fungus can grow.

The most common symptom of yeast infections is vulvar and possibly vaginal pruritus. The itching can be mild or intense, interfere with rest and activities, and may occur during or after intercourse. Some women report a feeling of dryness. Others may experience painful urination as the urine flows over the vulva, which usually occurs in women who have excoriations resulting from scratching. Most often the discharge has a thick, white, lumpy, and cottage cheese–like consistency. The discharge may be found in patches on the vaginal walls, cervix, and labia. Commonly, the vulva is red and swollen, as are the labial folds, vagina, and cervix. Although there is not a characteristic odor with yeast infections, sometimes a yeasty or musty smell is noted.

Screening and Diagnosis

In addition to a complete history of the woman's symptoms, their onset, and course, the history is a valuable screening tool for identifying predisposing risk factors. Physical examination should include a thorough inspection of the vulva and vagina. A speculum examination is always done. Commonly health care practitioners will obtain saline and KOH wet smears and check vaginal pH (see Table 7-4). Vaginal pH is normal with a yeast infection; if the pH is greater than 4.5, trichomoniasis or BV should be suspected. The characteristic pseudohyphae (bud or branching of a fungus) may be seen on a wet smear done with normal saline; however, they may be confused with other cells and artifacts (CDC, 2010c).

Management

A number of antifungal preparations are available for the treatment of *C. albicans.* Many of these medications (e.g., miconazole [Monistat] and clotrimazole [Gyne-Lotrimin]) are available as over-the-counter (OTC) agents. Exogenous lactobacillus (in the form of dairy products [yogurt] or powder, tablet, capsule, or suppository supplements) and garlic have been suggested for prevention and treatment of vulvovaginal candidiasis, but research is inconclusive, and no recommendations have been developed for use in practice (Eckert & Lentz, 2012). The first time a woman suspects that she may have a yeast infection she should see a health care provider for confirmation of the diagnosis and treatment recommendations. If she has another infection, she may wish to purchase an OTC preparation and self-treat. If she elects to do this, she should always be counseled to seek care for numerous recurrent or chronic yeast infections. If vaginal discharge is extremely thick and copious, vaginal debridement with a cotton swab followed by application of vaginal medication may be effective.

Women who have extensive irritation, swelling, and discomfort of the labia and vulva may find sitz baths helpful in decreasing inflammation and increasing comfort. Adding colloidal oatmeal powder to the bath may also increase the woman's comfort. Not wearing underpants to bed may help decrease symptoms and prevent recurrences. Completing the full course of treatment prescribed is essential to removing the pathogen. Instruct women to continue the medication even during menstruation. Explain that they should avoid using tampons during menses because the tampon will readily absorb the medication. If possible, women should avoid intercourse during treatment; if abstinence is not feasible, the woman's partner should use a condom to prevent the introduction of more organisms (see Teaching for Self-Management box).

TEACHING FOR SELF-MANAGEMENT

Prevention of Genital Tract Infections

- Practice genital hygiene.
- Choose underwear or hosiery with a cotton crotch.
- Avoid tight-fitting clothing (especially tight jeans).
- Select cloth car seat covers instead of vinyl.
- Limit time spent in damp exercise clothes (especially swimsuits, leotards, and tights).
- Limit exposure to bath salts or bubble bath.
- Avoid colored or scented toilet tissue.
- If sensitive, discontinue use of feminine deodorant sprays.
- Use condoms.
- Void before and after intercourse.
- Decrease dietary sugar.
- Drink yeast-active milk and eat yogurt (with lactobacilli).
- Do not douche.

Trichomoniasis

Trichomonas vaginalis is almost always an STI and is also a common cause of vaginal infection (5% to 50% of all vaginitis) and discharge (Eckert & Lentz, 2012).

Trichomoniasis is caused by *T. vaginalis,* an anaerobic one-celled protozoan with characteristic flagellae. Although trichomoniasis may be asymptomatic, commonly women have characteristically yellowish to greenish, frothy, mucopurulent, copious, malodorous discharge. Inflammation of the vulva, the vagina, or both may be present, and the woman may complain of irritation and pruritus. Dysuria and dyspareunia are often present. Typically the discharge worsens during and after menstruation. Often the cervix and the vaginal walls will demonstrate the characteristic "strawberry spots" or tiny petechiae, and the cervix may bleed on contact. In severe infections, the vaginal walls, the cervix, and occasionally the vulva may be acutely inflamed.

Screening and Diagnosis

In addition to obtaining a history of current symptoms, a careful sexual history should be obtained. Any history of similar symptoms in the past and treatment used should be noted. The nurse should determine whether the woman's partner(s) was treated and if she has had subsequent relations with new partners.

A speculum examination is always done, even though it may be very uncomfortable for the woman; relaxation techniques and breathing exercises may help the woman with the procedure. Any of the classic signs can be present on physical examination. The typical one-celled flagellate trichomonads are easily distinguished on a normal saline wet prep. Trichomoniasis also can be identified on Pap tests. Because trichomoniasis is an STI, once diagnosis is confirmed, appropriate laboratory studies for other STIs should be carried out.

Management

The recommended treatment is metronidazole or tinidazole orally in a single dose (CDC, 2010c) (see Table 7-5). Although the male partner is usually asymptomatic, it is recommended that he receive treatment also because he often harbors the trichomonads in the urethra or prostate. It is important that nurses discuss the importance of partner treatment with their clients, because if they are not treated it is likely that the infection will recur.

Women with trichomoniasis need to understand the sexual transmission of this disease. The woman must know that the organism may be present without symptoms being present, perhaps for several months, and that it is not possible to determine when she became infected. Women should be informed of the necessity for treating all sexual partners and helped with ways to raise the issue with their partner(s).

Group B Streptococcus

Group B streptococcus (GBS) may be considered a part of the normal vaginal flora in a woman who is not pregnant and is present in about 25% of healthy pregnant women (CDC, 2012b). GBS infection has been associated with poor pregnancy outcomes. These infections are an important factor in neonatal morbidity and mortality, usually resulting from vertical transmission from the birth canal of the infected mother to the infant during birth (Cunningham, Leveno, Bloom, et al., 2014).

Risk factors for neonatal GBS infection include positive prenatal culture for GBS in the current pregnancy; preterm birth of less than 37 weeks of gestation; premature rupture of membranes for a duration of 18 hours or more; intrapartum maternal fever higher than 38° C; and a positive history for early-onset neonatal GBS (Cunningham et al., 2014).

To decrease the risk of neonatal GBS infection, it is recommended that all women be screened at 35 to 37 weeks of gestation for GBS using a rectovaginal culture, and that IV antibiotic prophylaxis (IAP) be offered during labor to all who test positive. If a culture is not available at onset of labor or if a risk factor is present, IAP is also offered. IAP is not recommended before a cesarean birth if labor or rupture of membranes has not occurred. The recommended treatment is penicillin G, 5 million units IV loading dose, and then 2.5 million units IV every 4 hours during labor. Ampicillin, 2 g IV loading dose, followed by 1 g IV every 4 hours, is an alternative therapy (CDC, 2010b).

MATERNAL AND FETAL EFFECTS OF SEXUALLY TRANSMITTED INFECTIONS

Sexually transmitted infections in pregnancy are responsible for significant morbidity and mortality. Some consequences of maternal infection, such as infertility and sterility, last a lifetime. Congenitally acquired infection may affect a child's length and quality of life. Table 7-6 describes the effects of several common STIs on the pregnant woman and the fetus. It is difficult to predict these effects with certainty. Factors such as coinfection with other STIs and when in pregnancy the infection was acquired and treated can affect outcomes.

TORCH Infections

*T*oxoplasmosis, *o*ther infections (e.g., hepatitis), *r*ubella virus, *c*ytomegalovirus (CMV), and *h*erpes simplex virus, known collectively as **TORCH infections,** form a group of organisms capable of crossing the placenta. TORCH infections can affect a pregnant woman and her fetus. Generally, all TORCH infections produce influenza-like symptoms in the mother, but fetal and neonatal effects are more serious. TORCH infections and their maternal and fetal effects are shown in Table 7-7. Neonatal effects are discussed in Chapter 35

TABLE 7-6 Maternal and Fetal Effects of Common Sexually Transmitted Infections

INFECTION	MATERNAL EFFECTS	FETAL EFFECTS
Chlamydia	Premature rupture of membranes Preterm labor Postpartum endometritis	Low birth weight
Gonorrhea	Miscarriage Preterm labor Premature rupture of membranes Amniotic infection syndrome Chorioamnionitis Postpartum endometritis Postpartum sepsis	Preterm birth IUGR
Group B streptococci	Urinary tract infection Chorioamnionitis Postpartum endometritis Sepsis Meningitis (rare)	Preterm birth
Herpes simplex virus	Intrauterine infection (rare)	Congenital infection (rare)
Human papillomavirus (HPV)	Dystocia from large lesions Excessive bleeding from lesions after birth trauma	None known
Syphilis	Miscarriage Preterm labor	IUGR Preterm birth Stillbirth Congenital infection

IUGR, Intrauterine growth restriction.
Data from Gilbert, E. (2011). *Manual of high risk pregnancy & delivery* (5th ed.). St. Louis: Mosby; Duff, P., Sweet, R., & Edwards, R. (2009). Maternal and fetal infections. In R. Creasy, R. Resnik, J. Iams, et al. (Eds.), *Creasy and Resnik's maternal-fetal medicine: Principles and practice* (6th ed.). Philadelphia: Saunders.

CARE MANAGEMENT

Women may delay seeking care for STIs and other infections because they fear social stigma, have little accessibility to health care services, are asymptomatic, or are unaware that they have an infection. A comprehensive assessment focuses on lifestyle issues that are often personal or sensitive. A culturally sensitive, nonjudgmental approach is essential to facilitate accurate data collection. Throughout this chapter the discussion for each STI has included essential areas of assessment including signs and symptoms of the current problem, history (medical, personal, and social, and lifestyle behaviors), diagnostic tests, and physical examination.

Nursing diagnoses are derived from assessment data. The following nursing diagnoses are representative of those used in a plan of care for a woman with an STI and/or other vaginal infection:

Anxiety/Situational Low Self-Esteem/Disturbed Body Image related to:
- Perceived effects on sexual relationships and family processes
- Possible effects on pregnancy or fetus
- Long-term sequelae of infection

Deficient Knowledge related to:
- Transmission/prevention of infection/reinfection
- Behaviors that reduce risk for STIs
- Management of infection

Acute Pain/Impaired Tissue Integrity related to:
- Effects of infection process
- Scratching (excoriation) of pruritic areas
- Hygiene practices

Sexual Dysfunction related to:
- Effects of infection process

Social Isolation and Impaired Social Interaction related to:
- Perceived effects on relationships with others if STI status is unknown

Expected outcomes of care focus on physical and psychologic needs and include that the woman will:
- Be free of infection or, in the case of viral infection, have remission or stabilization of the infection
- Identify and be able to discuss the etiology, management, and expected course of the infection and its prevention
- Be able to identify her risky behaviors and discuss plans for decreasing her risk for infection

Management of the care for the woman with an STI has been discussed with each infection (see Nursing Care Plan). The Teaching for Self-Management box summarizes the important points of teaching about STIs.

TABLE 7-7 **TORCH Infection: Maternal and Fetal**

INFECTION	MATERNAL EFFECTS	FETAL EFFECTS	COUNSELING: PREVENTION, IDENTIFICATION, AND MANAGEMENT
***T**oxoplasmosis (protozoa)*	Most infections asymptomatic Acute infection similar to mononucleosis Woman immune after first episode (except in immunocompromised clients)	Congenital infection is most likely to occur when maternal infection develops during the third trimester. The risk of fetal injury, however, is greatest when maternal infection occurs during the first trimester.	Good handwashing technique should be used. Eating raw or rare meat and exposure to litter used by infected cats should be avoided; toxoplasma titer should be checked if there are cats in the house. If titer is rising during early pregnancy, therapeutic abortion may be considered an option.
***O**ther infections*			
Hepatitis A (infectious hepatitis) (virus)	Liver failure (extremely rare) Low-grade fever, malaise, poor appetite, right upper quadrant pain and tenderness, jaundice, and light-colored stools	Perinatal transmission virtually never occurs.	Spread by fecal-oral contact especially by culinary workers; gamma globulin can be given as prophylaxis for hepatitis A. Hepatitis A vaccine is available.
Hepatitis B (serum hepatitis) (virus)	May be transmitted sexually Approximately 10% of clients become chronic carriers. Some people with chronic hepatitis B eventually develop severe chronic liver disease, such as cirrhosis or hepatocellular carcinoma.	Infection occurs during birth. Maternal vaccination during pregnancy should present no risk for fetus; however, data are not available.	Generally passed by contaminated needles, syringes, or blood transfusions; also can be transmitted orally or by coitus (but incubation period is longer); hepatitis B immune globulin can be given prophylactically after exposure. Hepatitis B vaccine recommended for populations at risk
Rubella (3-day or German measles) (virus)	Rash, fever, mild symptoms such as headache, malaise, myalgias, and arthralgias; postauricular lymph nodes may be swollen; mild conjunctivitis	Approximately 50%-80% of fetuses exposed to the virus within 12 weeks after conception will show signs of congenital infection. Very few fetuses are affected if infection occurs after 18 weeks of gestation. The most common fetal anomalies associated with congenital rubella syndrome are deafness, eye defects (e.g., cataracts or retinopathy), central nervous system defects, and cardiac defects.	Vaccination of pregnant women is contraindicated; non-immune women should be vaccinated in the early postpartum period; pregnancy should be prevented for 1 month after vaccination. Women may breastfeed after vaccination and the vaccine can be administered along with immunoglobulin preparations such as Rh immune globulin.
Cytomegalovirus (CMV) (a herpes-virus)	Most adults are asymptomatic or have only mild influenza-like symptoms. The presence of CMV antibodies does not totally prevent reinfection.	The fetus can be infected transplacentally. Infection is much more likely with a primary maternal infection. The most common indications of congenital infection include hepatosplenomegaly, intracranial calcifications, jaundice, growth restriction, microcephaly, chorioretinitis, hearing loss, thrombocytopenia, hyperbilirubinemia, and hepatitis.	The virus is transmitted by transplantation of an infected organ, transfusion of infected blood, sexual contact, or contact with contaminated saliva or urine. Virus may be reactivated and cause disease in utero or during birth in subsequent pregnancies; fetal infection may occur during passage through infected birth canal. Prevention includes use of CMV-negative blood products if transfusion of pregnant women is necessary and teaching all women to wash hands carefully after handling infant diapers and toys.
Herpes genitalis (herpes simplex virus, type 1 or type 2 [HSV-1 or HSV-2])	Primary infection with painful blisters, tender inguinal lymph nodes, fever, viral meningitis (rare) Recurrent infections are much milder and shorter.	Transplacental infection resulting in congenital infection is rare and usually occurs with primary maternal infection. The risk mainly exists with infection late in pregnancy.	As many as two thirds of women with HSV-2 antibodies acquired the infection asymptomatically; however, asymptomatic women can give birth to seriously infected neonates. Risk of transmission is greatest during vaginal birth if woman has active lesions; thus cesarean birth is recommended Acyclovir can be used to treat recurrent outbreaks during pregnancy or as suppressive therapy late in pregnancy to prevent an outbreak during labor and birth.

Data from Duff, P., Sweet, R., & Edwards, R. (2009). Maternal and fetal infections. In R. Creasy, R. Resnik, J. Iams, et al. (Eds.), *Creasy and Resnik's maternal-fetal medicine: Principles and practice* (6th ed.). Philadelphia: Saunders.

INFECTION CONTROL

Interrupting the transmission of infection is crucial to STI control. Many STIs are reportable; all states require that the five traditional STIs—gonorrhea, syphilis, chancroid, lymphogranuloma venereum, and granuloma inguinale—be reported to public health officials. Many other states require that other STIs such as chlamydial infections, genital herpes, and genital warts be reported. In addition, all states require that AIDS cases be reported. In 2013, 32 state laboratories were required to report viral load and CD4 data for people who have HIV infections (CDC, 2013e).

NURSING CARE PLAN

Sexually Transmitted Infections

NURSING DIAGNOSIS	EXPECTED OUTCOME	NURSING INTERVENTIONS	RATIONALES
Ineffective Health Maintenance related to practicing prevention of sexually transmitted infections (STIs) as evidenced by client positive diagnosis of STI	Woman will verbalize which health practices directly led to positive diagnosis of an STI.	Inquire about woman's sexual history and sexual health practices.	To provide database for current problem
		Use therapeutic communication for private, nonjudgmental discussion.	To facilitate learning and promote self-esteem
		Provide emotional support.	To indicate awareness of woman's feelings about this sensitive topic
		Provide information about transmission of disease, including cause, symptoms, and treatment for both partners.	To enhance woman's knowledge base and correct any misinformation
		Discuss the use and importance of safe sexual practices.	To raise woman's awareness and motivation to avoid future risk-taking behaviors
		Instruct woman and sexual partner to complete medication regimen.	To completely eradicate transmitted organism
Impaired Social Interaction related to diagnosis of STI as evidenced by client verbal report	Woman will report increased incidences of social interaction.	Provide nonjudgmental, confidential therapeutic communication.	To increase woman's feelings of self-worth
		Refer to support groups.	To provide group interaction, discussion, and information
Impaired Tissue Integrity related to effects of disease process as evidenced by client report of itching and vaginal discharge	Woman's tissue integrity will be restored.	Assess, monitor, and document characteristics of the damaged skin area, including color, lesions, drainage, and edema.	To provide database
		Instruct woman in correct genital hygiene practices.	To prevent further infection of damaged tissues with other organisms
		Provide warm soaks or sitz baths.	To promote comfort, circulation, and healing
		Administer prescribed medications.	To promote comfort and eradication of organism
		Provide written self-help materials and pamphlets.	To prevent further skin integrity loss
		Teach woman to perform vulvar self-examination.	To encourage participation in self-care
Anxiety related to diagnosis of STI	Woman will report decreased level of anxiety.	Provide opportunity for therapeutic communication.	To promote trust and expression of feelings
		Assist woman to identify effective coping mechanisms.	To decrease anxiety
		Refer to support groups.	To share feelings and common effective strategies

TEACHING FOR SELF-MANAGEMENT

Sexually Transmitted Infections

- Take your medication as directed.
- Use comfort measures for symptom relief as suggested by your health care provider.
- Keep your appointment for repeat cultures or checkups after your treatment to make sure your infection is cured.
- Inform your sexual partner(s) of the need to be tested and treated, if necessary.
- Abstain from sexual intercourse until your treatment is completed or for as long as you are advised by your health care provider.
- Use sex practices that decrease risk when sexual intercourse is resumed.
- Call your health care provider immediately if you notice bumps, sores, rashes, or discharges.
- Keep all future appointments with your health care provider, even if things appear normal.

Infection-control measures are essential to protect care providers and to prevent health personnel–related infection of clients, regardless of the infectious agent. The risk for occupational transmission varies with the disease. Even when the risk is low, as with HIV, the existence of any risk warrants reasonable precautions. Precautions against airborne disease transmission are available in all health care agencies. Standard Precautions (to use for infection control when caring for everyone) and additional precautions for labor and birth settings are listed in Box 7-3.

LEGAL TIP: Sexually Transmitted Infection Reporting

The primary health care provider is legally responsible for reporting all cases of those diseases identified as reportable and should know what the requirements are in the state in which she or he practices. The woman must be informed when a case will be reported and be told why. Failure to inform the woman that the case will be reported is a serious breach of professional ethics.

BOX 7-3 Standard Precautions

Medical history and examination cannot reliably identify everyone infected with human immunodeficiency virus (HIV) or other bloodborne pathogens. Standard Precautions should therefore be used consistently in the care of all clients. These precautions apply to blood, body fluids, and all secretions and excretions, except sweat, nonintact skin, and mucous membranes. The following infection-control practices should be applied during the delivery of health care to reduce the risk of transmission of microorganisms from known and unknown sources of infection:

1. *Hand hygiene.* During the delivery of health care, avoid unnecessary touching of surfaces in close proximity to the client to prevent both contamination of clean hands from environmental surfaces and transmission of pathogens from contaminated hands to surfaces. Wash dirty or contaminated hands with either a nonantimicrobial or an antimicrobial soap and water. If hands are not visibly soiled, decontaminate hands with an alcohol-based handrub, or hands may be washed with an antimicrobial soap and water. Perform hand hygiene: (1) before having direct contact with clients; (2) after contact with blood, body fluids, or excretions, mucous membranes, nonintact skin, or wound dressings; (3) after contact with a client's intact skin (e.g., when taking a pulse or blood pressure or lifting a client); (4) if hands will be moving from a contaminated body site to a clean body site during client care; (5) after contact with inanimate objects (including medical equipment) in the immediate vicinity of the client; and (6) after removing gloves. Wash hands with nonantimicrobial or antimicrobial soap and water if contact with spores (e.g., *Clostridium difficile* or *Bacillus anthracis*) is likely to have occurred. The physical action of washing and rinsing hands under such circumstances is recommended because alcohols, chlorhexidine, iodophors, and other antiseptic agents have poor activity against spores. Do not wear artificial fingernails or extenders if duties include direct contact with clients at high risk for infection and associated adverse outcomes.
2. *Personal protective equipment (PPE).* Observe the following principles of use:
   - *Gloves.* Wear gloves when a reasonable possibility exists for contact with blood or other potentially infectious materials, mucous membranes, nonintact skin, or potentially contaminated intact skin (e.g., of a client incontinent of stool or urine). Gloves should be worn during infant eye prophylaxis, care of the umbilical cord, circumcision site, parenteral procedures, diaper changes, contact with colostrum, and postpartum assessments. Wear gloves with fit and durability appropriate to the task. Remove gloves after contact with a client or the surrounding environment (including medical equipment) using proper technique to prevent hand contamination. Do not wear the same pair of gloves for the care of more than one client. Change gloves during client care if the hands will move from a contaminated body site (e.g., perineal area) to a clean body site (e.g., face).
   - *Gowns.* Wear a gown that is appropriate to the task to protect the skin and prevent soiling or contamination of clothing during procedures and client-care activities when contact with blood, body fluids, secretions, or excretions is anticipated. Remove the gown and perform hand hygiene before leaving the client's environment. Do not reuse gowns, even for repeated contacts with the same client. Routine donning of gowns on entrance into a high risk unit (e.g., intensive care unit [ICU], neonatal intensive care unit [NICU]) is not indicated.
   - *Mouth, nose, eye protection.* Use PPE to protect the mucous membranes of the eyes, nose, and mouth during procedures and client-care activities that are likely to generate splashes or sprays of blood, body fluids, secretions, and excretions. Select masks, goggles, face shields, and combinations of each according to the need anticipated by the task performed.
3. *Respiratory hygiene and cough etiquette.* Post signs at entrances and in strategic places (e.g., elevators, cafeterias) within ambulatory and inpatient settings with instructions to clients and others with symptoms of a respiratory infection to cover their mouth and nose when coughing or sneezing, use and dispose of tissues, and perform hand hygiene after hands have been in contact with respiratory secretions. Provide tissues and no-touch receptacles (e.g., foot pedal–operated lid or open, plastic-lined wastebasket) for disposal of tissues. Provide resources and instructions for performing hand hygiene in or near waiting areas in ambulatory and inpatient settings; provide conveniently located dispensers of alcohol-based handrubs and, where sinks are available, supplies for handwashing. During periods of increased respiratory infections in the community, offer masks to coughing clients and other symptomatic individuals (e.g., people who accompany ill clients) on entry into the facility, and encourage them to maintain special separation, ideally a distance of at least 3 feet, from others in common waiting areas.
4. *Safe injection practices.* The following recommendations apply to the use of needles, cannulas that replace needles, and, where applicable, intravenous delivery systems:
   - Use aseptic technique to prevent contamination of sterile injection equipment. Needles, cannulas, and syringes are sterile, single-use items; they should not be reused for another client. Use fluid infusion and administration sets (i.e., intravenous bags, tubing, and connectors) for one client only, and dispose appropriately after use. Use single-dose vials for parenteral medications whenever possible. If multidose vials must be used, both the needle (or cannula) and the syringe used to access the multidose vial must be sterile. Do not keep multidose vials in the immediate client treatment area, and store in accordance with the manufacturer's recommendations; discard if sterility is compromised or questionable.

Modified from Siegel, J.D., Rhinehart, E., Jackson, M., et al. (2007). *Guideline for isolation precautions: Preventing transmission of infectious agents in healthcare settings.* Available at www.cdc.gov/ncidod/dhqp/pdf/isolation2007.pdf.

KEY POINTS

- Reproductive tract infections include STIs and common genital tract infections.
- Young, sexually active women who do not practice risk-reducing sexual behaviors and have multiple partners are at greatest risk for STIs and HIV.
- Risk-reduction sexual practices are key STI-prevention strategies.
- STIs are responsible for substantial morbidity and mortality, great personal suffering, and heavy economic burden in the United States.
- HIV is transmitted through body fluids, primarily blood, semen, and vaginal secretions.
- Prevention of mother-to-newborn HIV transmission is most effective when the woman receives antiretroviral drugs during pregnancy and labor and birth, and the infant receives the drugs after birth.
- STIs and vaginitis are biologic events for which all individuals have a right to expect objective, compassionate, and effective health care.
- Pregnancy confers no immunity against infection, and both mother and fetus must be considered when the pregnant woman contracts an infection.
- HPV is the most common viral STI.
- Syphilis has reemerged as a common STI, affecting black women more than any other ethnic or racial group.
- Because history and examination cannot reliably identify everyone with HIV or other blood-borne pathogens, blood and body-fluid precautions should be used consistently for everyone all the time.
- Chlamydia is the most common STI in women in the United States and the most common cause of PID.
- Viral hepatitis has several forms of transmission; HBV infections carry the greatest risk.

REFERENCES

American Cancer Society (ACS). (2014). *Cancer facts and figures 2014.* Atlanta: Author.

Cates, W., & Harwood, B. (2011). Vaginal barriers and spermicides. In R. Hatcher, J. Trussell, A. Nelson, et al. (Eds.), *Contraceptive technology* (20th ed.). New York: Ardent Media.

Centers for Disease Control and Prevention (CDC). (2010a). *Bacterial vaginosis (BV) statistics* Available at www.cdc.gov/std/bv/stats/htm.

Centers for Disease Control and Prevention (CDC). (2010b). 2010 guidelines for the prevention of perinatal group B streptococcal disease. *MMWR Morbidity and Mortality Weekly Report, 59*(RR10), 1–32.

Centers for Disease Control and Prevention (CDC). (2010c). Sexually transmitted diseases treatment guidelines 2010. *MMWR Morbidity and Mortality Weekly Report, 59*(RR-12), 1–109.

Centers for Disease Control and Prevention (CDC). (2012a). *ABC's of hepatitis.* Available at www.cdc.gov/hepatits/resources/professionals/PDFs/ABCTable-bw.pdf.

Centers for Disease Control and Prevention (CDC). (2012b). *CDC fast facts and statistics on GBS-group B strep.* Available at www.cdc.gov/groupbstrep/about/fast-facts.html.

Centers for Disease Control and Prevention (CDC). (2012c). *HPV vaccination information for clinicians-fact sheet.* Available at www.cdc.gov/std/hpv/STDFact-HPV-vaccine-hcp.htm.

Centers for Disease Control and Prevention (CDC). (2012d). Recommendations for the identification of chronic hepatitis C virus infection among persons born during 1945-1965. *MMWR Morbidity and Mortality Weekly Report, 61*(RR04), 1–18.

Centers for Disease Control and Prevention (CDC). (2012e). Update to CDC's *sexually transmitted diseases treatment guidelines, 2010*: Oral cephalosporins no longer a recommended treatment for gonococcal infections. *MMWR Morbidity and Mortality Weekly Report, 61*(31), 590–594.

Centers for Disease Control and Prevention (CDC). (2013a). *Genital herpes—CDC fact sheet.* Available at www.cdc.gov/STD/hpv/stdfact-hpv.htm.

Centers for Disease Control and Prevention (CDC). (2013b). *Genital HPV infection—CDC fact sheet.* Available at www.cdc.gov/STD/hpv/stdfact-hpv.htm.

Centers for Disease Control and Prevention (CDC). (2013d). *HIV among women.* Available at www.cdc.gov/hiv/risks/gender/women/facts/index.htm.

Centers for Disease Control and Prevention (CDC). (2013d). *Incidence, prevalence, and costs of sexually transmitted infections in the United States.* Available at www.cdc.gov/stats/STI-Estimates-Fact-Sheet-Feb-2013.pdf.

Centers for Disease Control and Prevention (CDC). (2013e). *State laboratory reporting laws: Viral load and CD4 requirements.* Available at www.cdc.gov/hiv/law/states/laboratory.htm.

Centers for Disease Control and Prevention (CDC). (2013f). *STDs and pregnancy.* Available at www.cdc.gov/std/pregnancy/STDFact-pregnancy.htm.

Centers for Disease Control and Prevention (CDC). (2014). *Sexually transmitted disease surveillance, 2012.* Atlanta: U.S. Department of Health and Human Services.

Cunningham, F., Leveno, K., Bloom, S., et al. (2014). *Williams obstetrics* (24th ed.). New York: McGraw-Hill.

Eckert, L. O., & Lentz, G. M. (2012). Infections of the lower and upper genital tract. In G. Lentz, R. Lobo, D. Gershenson, & V. Katz (Eds.), *Comprehensive gynecology* (6th ed.). Philadelphia: Mosby.

Fantasia, H. C. (2012). Sinecatechins ointment 15% for the treatment of external genital warts. *Nursing for Women's Health, 16*(5), 418–422.

Fantasia, H. C., Fontenot, H. B., Sutherland, M., & Harris, A. L. (2011). Sexually transmitted infections in women. *Nursing for Women's Health, 15*(1), 47–57.

Marrazzo, J. M., & Cates, W. (2011). Reproductive tract infections, including HIV and other sexually transmitted infections. In R. Hatcher, J. Trussell, A. Nelson, et al. (Eds.), *Contraceptive technology* (20th ed.). New York: Ardent Media.

Panel on Treatment of HIV-Infected Pregnant Women and Prevention of Perinatal Transmission. (2012). *Recommendations for use of antiretroviral drugs in pregnant HIV-1-infected women for maternal health and interventions to reduce perinatal HIV transmission in the United States. July 31, 2012.* Available at http://aidsinfo.nih.gov/ContentFiles/lvguidelines/PerinatalGL.pdf.

Royer, H. R., & Falk, E. C. (2012). Young women's beliefs regarding human papillomavirus. *Journal of Obstetric, Gynecologic and Neonatal Nursing, 4*(1), 92–102.

Ruhl, C. (2013). Update on chlamydia and gonorrhea screening during pregnancy. *Nursing for Women's Health, 17*(2), 143–146.

U.S. Food and Drug Administration (FDA). (2008). *HIV testing*. Available at www.fda.gov/oashi/aidstest.html.

Weiner, C., & Buhimschi, C. (2009). *Drugs for pregnant and lactating women* (2nd ed.). Philadelphia: Saunders.

World Health Organization. (2013a). *Hormonal contraception and HIV*. Available at www.who.int/reproductivehealth/topics/family_planning/hc_hiv/en.

World Health Organization. (2013b). *Sexually transmitted infection (STIs)*. Available at www.who.int/mediacentre/factsheets/fs110/en/index.html.

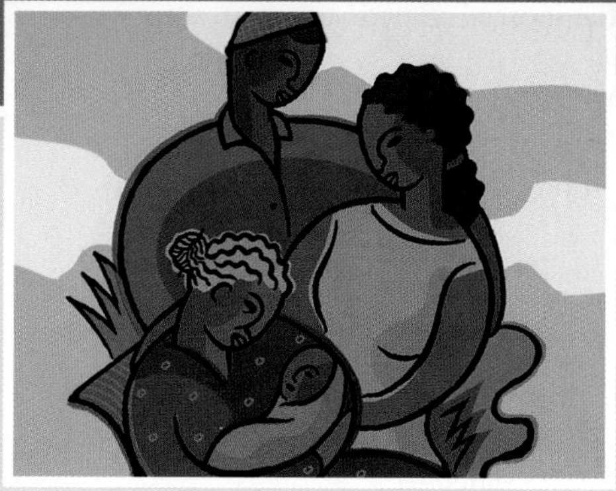

CHAPTER 8

Contraception and Abortion

Lisa L. Ferguson and Peggy Mancuso

http://evolve.elsevier.com/Lowdermilk/MWHC/

LEARNING OBJECTIVES

- Compare various methods of contraception.
- Identify the advantages and disadvantages of commonly used methods of contraception.
- Explain the common nursing interventions that facilitate contraceptive use.
- Examine the various ethical, legal, cultural, and religious considerations of contraception.
- Describe the techniques used for medical and surgical interruption of pregnancy.
- Discuss the various ethical and legal considerations of elective abortion.
- Outline a plan of care for a woman who needs emergency contraception.

CONTRACEPTION

The Centers for Disease Control and Prevention (CDC) noted that the capability of Americans to engage in effective family planning as a result of the modern era of contraception was one of the 10 greatest public health achievements of the 20th century. Nevertheless, nearly half of all U.S. pregnancies are not planned (Woodhams & Gilliam, 2012; Finer & Zolna, 2011). Among adolescent women, approximately 80% of those who became pregnant did not intend to do so (Epidemiology and Efficacy; Fritz & Speroff, 2011b). The nurse can play a vital role in prevention of unwanted pregnancy through counseling and education regarding family planning, contraception, and effective birth control.

Family planning is the conscious decision on when to conceive or to avoid pregnancy throughout the reproductive years. **Contraception** is defined as the intentional prevention of pregnancy during sexual intercourse. **Birth control** is the device and/or practice used to decrease the risk of conceiving or bearing offspring.

With the wide assortment of birth control options available, it is possible for a woman to use several different contraceptive methods at various stages throughout her fertile years. Nurses interact with the individual as well as the couple to compare and contrast available contraceptive options. Factors to consider include reliability, relative cost of the method, any protection from sexually transmitted infections (STIs), the individual's comfort level with the method, and the partner's willingness to use a particular birth control method. Those who use contraception can still be at risk for pregnancy if their choice of contraceptive method results in one that is not used correctly or if it is not as reliable as other methods. Expanding access to contraception, especially long-acting reversible methods, and improving accurate and reliable use of birth control methods can decrease the chance of unintended pregnancy (CDC, 2013).

COMMUNITY ACTIVITY

Nurses provide discharge planning after childbirth; they commonly staff family planning clinics and provide contraceptive information to those clients and others in the community. Education concerning contraceptive use in the postpartum period is a common component of discharge planning in many countries, with wide variation among health care delivery systems. Education at this time assumes women's receptiveness to information about contraception and that education or receptiveness to such information could be less at a later period. However, clinical trials have not demonstrated that education in the immediate postpartum period is effective. Contact a clinic in your community to see if you can talk with one of the nurses about their procedures in caring for postpartum women, focusing on what the nurses do related to education about family planning.

CARE MANAGEMENT

A multidisciplinary approach may assist a woman in choosing and correctly using an appropriate contraceptive method. Nurses, nurse-midwives, nurse practitioners, and other advanced practice nurses as well as physicians have the knowledge and expertise to assist a woman in making decisions about contraception that will satisfy her personal, social, cultural, and interpersonal needs.

Family, friends, media, partner or partners, religious affiliation, and health care professionals influence a woman's perception of contraceptive choices. These external influences form a woman's unique view. The nurse assists in supporting the woman's decision based on her individual situation.

Evaluation of the couple desiring contraception involves assessing the woman's reproductive history (menstrual, obstetric, gynecologic, contraceptive), physical examination, and, sometimes, current laboratory tests. The nurse must determine the woman's knowledge about reproduction, contraception, and STIs, as well as her sexual partner's commitment to any particular method. Religious and cultural factors may influence a couple's choice regarding a particular contraceptive method. The couple may believe in certain reproductive myths. For example, 30% of all adolescent pregnancies were in women who engaged in unprotected intercourse because of the perception that they could not get pregnant at the time of intercourse. Unbiased client teaching is fundamental to initiating and maintaining any form of contraception

Assessment of the client begins with the following appraisals:

- Determining the woman's knowledge about contraception and her sexual partner's commitment to any particular method
- Collecting data about the frequency of coitus, the number of sexual partners, the level of contraceptive involvement, and her or her partner's objections to any methods
- Assessing the woman's level of comfort and willingness to touch her genitals and cervical mucus
- Identifying any misconceptions, as well as religious and cultural factors, and paying close attention to the woman's verbal and nonverbal responses to hearing about the various available methods
- Considering the woman's reproductive life plan
- Completing a history (including menstrual, contraceptive, and obstetric), physical examination (including pelvic examination), and laboratory tests (as needed for identifying presence of STIs).

Informed consent is a vital component in educating a client about contraception or sterilization. The nurse often has the responsibility of documenting information provided and the understanding of that information by the client. The mnemonic BRAIDED may be useful (see Legal Tip).

Once the assessment is complete, nursing diagnoses can be identified to help develop the nursing care plan and interventions. Nursing diagnoses related to contraception include the following:

- *Decisional Conflict* related to
  - Contraceptive alternatives; partner's willingness to agree on contraceptive method.
- *Fear* related to
  - Contraceptive method side effects.
- *Risk for Infection* related to
  - Unprotected sexual intercourse; use of contraceptive method; broken skin or mucous membrane after surgery or intrauterine device (IUD) insertion.
- *Ineffective Sexuality Patterns* related to
  - Fear of pregnancy.
- *Acute Pain* related to
  - Postoperative recovery after sterilization.
- *Risk for Spiritual Distress* related to
  - Discrepancy between religious or cultural beliefs and choice of contraceptive method.

Education is the cornerstone of the nursing care plan and planned interventions. Developing applicable interventions increases client understanding that leads to improved adherence to the contraceptive plan and increased client satisfaction. The nurse should teach about the specific contraceptive used. Following the teaching-learning session, the nurse should ask the woman to perform a return demonstration of how a device is used, if appropriate, and assess her understanding of this contraceptive method. The nurse should also provide the woman and her partner with written instructions about the contraceptive method and with contact information in case she has questions later. If a woman has difficulty understanding written instructions, offer her (and her partner, if available) graphic material and contact information (telephone number, email) for questions of the clinic if necessary, and let her know that she may return to the clinic for further instruction if needed. It is very important to provide the woman and her partner additional information about backup methods of birth control and emergency contraception.

A private setting should be provided for contraceptive counseling. The woman should feel safe and free to communicate with the nurse. Distractions should be minimized, and samples of birth control devices for interactive teaching should be available. The nurse counters myths with facts, clarifies misinformation, and fills in gaps of knowledge. The ideal contraceptive should be safe, easily available, economical, acceptable, simple to use, and promptly reversible. Although no method may ever achieve all these objectives, new contraceptive technologies are being developed, and couples have more choices available to them now than ever before (Lessard, Karasek, Ma, et al., 2012).

Contraceptive failure rate refers to the percentage of contraceptive users expected to have an unplanned pregnancy during the first year of use, even when they use a method consistently and correctly. Contraceptive effectiveness varies from couple to couple and depends on the properties of the method and the characteristics of the user (Box 8-1). Effectiveness of a method can be expressed as theoretic effectiveness, or how effective the method is with perfect use, and as typical effectiveness, or how effective the method is with typical use. Failure rates decrease over time, either because a user gains experience and uses a method more appropriately or because the less effective users

LEGAL TIP: Informed Consent

- B—Benefits: information about advantages and success rates
- R—Risks: information about disadvantages and failure rates
- A—Alternatives: information about other available methods
- I—Inquiries: opportunity to ask questions
- D—Decisions: opportunity to decide or to change her mind
- E—Explanations: information about method and how it is used
- D—Documentation: information given and client's understanding

BOX 8-1 Factors Affecting Contraceptive Method Effectiveness

- Frequency of intercourse
- Motivation to prevent pregnancy
- Understanding of how to use the method
- Adherence to method
- Provision of short- or long-term protection
- Likelihood of pregnancy for the individual woman
- Consistent use of method

stop using the method. Safety of a method may be affected by a woman's medical history (e.g., thromboembolic problems and contraceptive methods containing estrogen). In most instances, pregnancy would be more dangerous to the woman with medical problems than a particular contraceptive method, but thromboembolic problems is an example of why a certain type of contraception should be avoided. On the other hand, the use of many contraceptive methods is associated with health promotion effects. For example, barrier methods, such as the male condom, offer some protection from acquiring STIs, and oral contraceptives lower the incidence of ovarian and endometrial cancer.

SAFETY ALERT

Make sure the woman has a backup method of birth control and contraceptive pills (CPs) readily available during the initial learning phase when she uses a new method of contraception to help prevent an unintentional conception.

CLINICAL REASONING CASE STUDY

Contraception for Adolescents

Maria is a 16-year-old Hispanic client who comes to the family planning clinic seeking contraception. She has recently become sexually active and tells the nurse that she is concerned that her mother will find out. She also has many questions about the type of contraception to use. She seeks the nurse's advice to help in her decision making.

1. Evidence—Is there sufficient evidence to draw conclusions about what advice to give Maria?
2. Assumptions—What assumptions can be made about contraception for adolescents:
   a. Types of contraception
   b. Legal issues
   c. Implications of culture on choice
3. What implications and priorities for nursing care can be drawn at this time?
4. Does the evidence objectively support your conclusion?

Methods of Contraception

The following discussion of contraceptive methods provides the nurse with information needed for client teaching. After implementing the appropriate teaching for contraceptive use, the nurse supervises return demonstrations and practice to assess client understanding (Fig. 8-1).

The most effective contraceptive methods at preventing pregnancy are the long-acting, reversible contraceptive (LARC) methods (e.g., contraceptive implants, intrauterine contraception). With these methods, theoretic and typical pregnancy rates are the same because the method requires no user intervention after correct insertion. Other effective methods include those that prevent pregnancy through exogenous hormones (estrogen and/or progestins), such as contraceptive injections, oral contraceptive pills, contraceptive patches, and vaginal rings. Each of these methods involves user interventions, so typical use pregnancy rates are higher than pregnancy rates with perfect use. The least effective contraceptive methods include the barrier methods and natural family planning. Examples include condoms, diaphragms, cervical caps, spermicides, withdrawal, and periodic abstinence during perceived ovulation. Effectiveness rates for these methods vary from user to user, depending on correct application of the method and consistency of use.

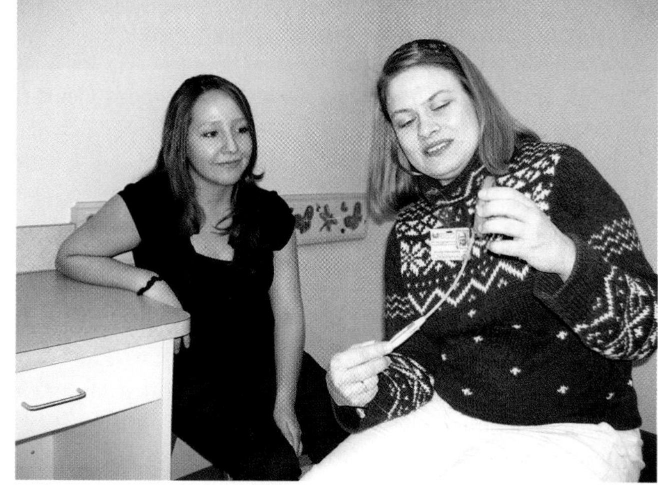

FIG 8-1 Nurse counseling woman about contraceptive methods. (Courtesy Dee Lowdermilk, Chapel Hill, NC.)

Coitus Interruptus

Coitus interruptus (withdrawal) involves the male partner withdrawing the penis from the woman's vagina before he ejaculates. Although coitus interruptus is one of the least effective methods of contraception, it is a good choice for couples who do not have another contraceptive available (Kowal, 2011). Effectiveness is similar to barrier methods and depends on the man's ability to withdraw his penis before ejaculation. The percentage of women who will experience an unintended pregnancy within the first year of typical use (failure rate) of withdrawal is about 22% (Trussell, 2011). Coitus interruptus does not protect against STIs or human immunodeficiency virus (HIV) infection.

Fertility Awareness–Based Methods (Natural Family Planning)

Fertility awareness–based (FAB) methods of contraception, also known as periodic abstinence or natural family planning (NFP), depend on identifying the beginning and end of the fertile period of the menstrual cycle. These methods provide contraception by relying on avoidance of intercourse during fertile periods. Natural family planning methods are the only contraceptive practices acceptable to the Roman Catholic Church.

BOX 8-2 Potential Pitfalls of Using Fertility Awareness Methods of Contraception

Potential pitfalls of using fertility awareness methods include the five R's:
- Restriction on sexual spontaneity
- Rigorous daily monitoring
- Required training
- Risk of pregnancy during prolonged training period
- Risk of pregnancy high on unsafe days

From Zieman, M., Hatcher, R., Cwiak, C., et al. (2012). *A pocket guide to managing contraception.* Tiger, GA: Bridging the Gap Foundation.

When women who want to use FABs are educated about the menstrual cycle, three phases are identified:
1. Infertile phase: before ovulation
2. Fertile phase: about 5 to 7 days around the middle of the cycle, including several days before and during ovulation and the day afterward
3. Infertile phase: after ovulation

The human ovum can be fertilized no later than 12 to 24 hours after ovulation (Cunningham, Leveno, Bloom, et al., 2014; Schulman, 2011). Motile sperm have been recovered from the uterus and the oviducts as long as 60 hours after coitus, but their ability to fertilize the ovum probably lasts no longer than 24 to 48 hours. One problem with FABs is that the exact time of ovulation cannot be predicted accurately, and couples may find it difficult to exercise restraint for several days before and after ovulation. In addition, women with irregular menstrual periods have the greatest risk of failure with FABs.

Although ovulation can be unpredictable in many women, teaching the woman about how she can directly observe her fertility patterns is an empowering tool. There are nearly a dozen categories of FABs. To prevent pregnancy, each one uses a combination of charts, records, calculations, tools, observations, and either abstinence or barrier methods of birth control during the fertile period in the menstrual cycle (Jennings & Burke, 2011). The charts and calculations associated with these methods can also be used to increase the likelihood of detecting the optimal timing of intercourse to achieve conception. Signs and symptoms of fertility awareness most commonly used with abstinence are menstrual bleeding, cervical mucus, and basal body temperature, as described later in the chapter (Jennings & Burke).

Advantages of these methods include low to no cost, heightened awareness and understanding of personal fertility, increased self-reliance, absence of chemicals, instant availability, increased involvement and intimacy with partner, and the ability of the couple to follow religious/cultural traditions. In addition, these methods can be used to establish fertile days for conception in the couple who wants to achieve pregnancy. Disadvantages of FABs include difficulty with adherence to strict record-keeping, requirement of male partner support, lower typical effectiveness than other regimens, decreased effectiveness in women with irregular cycles (particularly adolescents who have not established regular ovulatory patterns), decreased spontaneity of coitus, and no protection from STIs including HIV infection. (Association of Reproductive Health Professionals [ARHP], 2011; Fehring, Schneider, Barron, & Pruzy, 2013; Jennings & Burke, 2011) (Box 8-2). The typical failure rate for most FABs is 24% during the first year of use (Trussell, 2011).

FABs involve several techniques to identify fertile days. The following discussion includes the most common techniques as well as some promising techniques for the future.

Calendar-Based Methods

Calendar Rhythm Method. Practice of the calendar rhythm method is based on the number of days in each cycle, counting from the first day of menses. With this method the fertile period is determined after accurately recording the lengths of menstrual cycles for at least 6 months. Increased reliability can be obtained with 8 to 12 months of menstrual data (Planned Parenthood, 2013). The beginning of the fertile period is estimated by subtracting 18 days from the length of the shortest cycle. The end of the fertile period is determined by subtracting 11 days from the length of the longest cycle (Jennings & Burke, 2011). If the shortest cycle is 24 days and the longest is 30 days, application of the formula to calculate the fertile period is as follows:

Shortest cycle: 24 − 18 = sixth day
Longest cycle: 30 − 11 = nineteenth day

To avoid conception the couple would abstain during the fertile period—days 6 through 19. If the woman has very regular cycles of 28 days each, the formula indicates the fertile days to be as follows:

Shortest cycle: 28 − 18 = tenth day
Longest cycle: 28 − 11 = seventeenth day

To avoid pregnancy the couple abstains from days 10 through 17 because ovulation occurs on day 14 plus or minus 2 days. A major drawback of the calendar method is that one is trying to predict future events with past data. The unpredictability of the menstrual cycle also is not taken into consideration. The calendar rhythm method is most useful as an adjunct to the basal body temperature or the cervical mucus method.

Standard Days Method. The Standard Days Method (SDM) is essentially a modified form of the calendar rhythm method that has a "fixed" number of days of fertility for each cycle—that is, days 8 to 19 (ARHP, 2011). A CycleBeads necklace—a color-coded string of beads—can be purchased as a concrete tool to track fertility (Fig. 8-2). Day 1 of the menstrual flow is the first day to begin counting. Women who use this device are taught to avoid unprotected intercourse on days 8 to 19 (white beads on CycleBeads necklace). Although this method is useful to women whose cycles are regular and occur at 26- to 32-day intervals, the SDM is unreliable for those who have longer or shorter cycles. Factors that may make this method less effective include the use of hormonal contraception (including emergency contraception), IUDs, breastfeeding, or a recent pregnancy (Planned Parenthood, 2013). The typical failure rate for the SDM is 12% during the first year of use (Jennings & Burke, 2011).

Symptoms-Based Methods

TwoDay Method. The TwoDay Method is based on the monitoring and recording of cervical secretions (ARHP, 2011). Unlike other methods that rely on this indicator, such as the ovulation mucus method or the symptothermal method, it does not involve analyzing the characteristics of the secretions (e.g., amount, color, consistency, slipperiness, stretchability, or viscosity) (Contracept.org, 2013). Each day the woman asks herself, (1) "Did I note secretions today?" and (2) "Did I note secretions yesterday?" If the answer to either question is

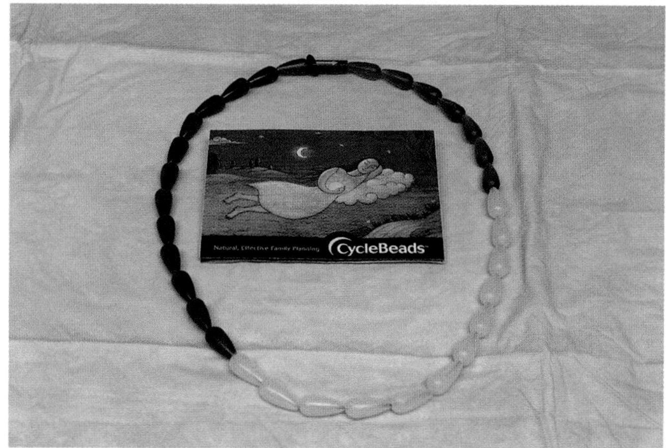

FIG 8-2 CycleBeads. Red bead marks the first day of the menstrual cycle. White beads mark days that are likely to be fertile days; therefore, unprotected intercourse should be avoided. Brown beads are days when pregnancy is unlikely and unprotected intercourse is permitted. (Courtesy Dee Lowdermilk, Chapel Hill, NC.)

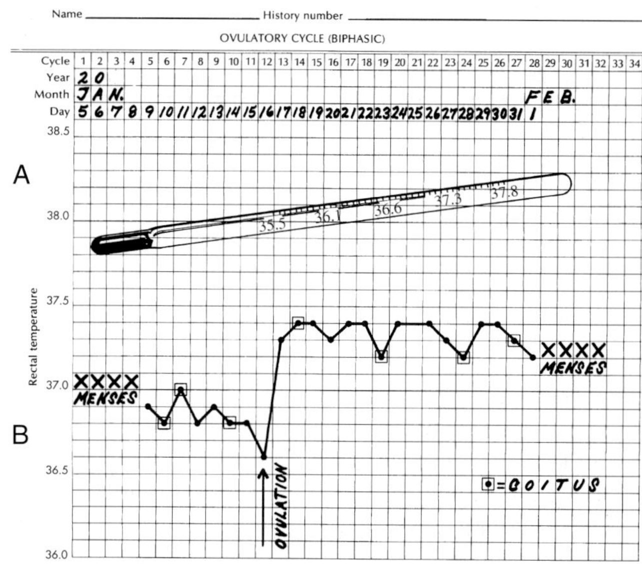

FIG 8-3 A, Special thermometer for recording basal body temperature, marked in tenths to enable person to read more easily. B, Basal temperature record shows drop and sharp rise at time of ovulation. Biphasic curve indicates ovulatory cycle.

yes, she should avoid coitus or use a backup method of birth control. If the answer to both questions is no, her probability of getting pregnant is very low. After 2 days without secretions, the woman may resume unprotected intercourse. The TwoDay Method appears to be simpler to teach, learn, and use than other natural methods. Results suggest that the method can be an effective alternative for low-literacy populations or for programs that find current natural family planning methods too time consuming or otherwise not feasible to incorporate into their services. Studies have found the typical failure rate of the TwoDay Method to be 24% (ARHP). This method could affect Third World fertility planning. For a more global perspective on these implications, see Institute for Reproductive Health at http://irh.org/?q=content/twoday-method.

Cervical Mucus Ovulation Detection Method. The cervical mucus ovulation detection method (i.e., Billings method or Creighton model ovulation method) requires that the woman recognize and interpret the cyclic changes in the amount and consistency of cervical mucus that characterize her own unique pattern of changes at the time of ovulation. Cervical mucus transforms prior to and during ovulation in order to facilitate and promote the viability and motility of sperm. Without adequate cervical mucus, coitus does not result in conception. This method requires that a woman check the quantity and character of mucus on the vulva or introitus with her fingers or tissue paper each day for several months and evaluate the mucus for cloudiness, tackiness, and slipperiness. This way she can learn how her cervical mucus responds to ovulation during her menstrual cycles. To ensure an accurate assessment of changes, the cervical mucus should be free from semen, contraceptive gels or foams, and blood or discharge from vaginal infections for at least one full cycle. Other factors that create difficulty in identifying mucus changes include douches and vaginal deodorants, being in a sexually aroused state (which thins the mucus), and taking medications such as antihistamines (which dry the mucus). Intercourse is considered safe without restriction beginning the fourth day after the last day of wet, clear, slippery mucus, which would indicate that ovulation has occurred 2 to 3 days previously (Jennings & Burke, 2011).

Some women find this method unacceptable if they are uncomfortable touching their genitals. Whether or not a woman wants to use this method for contraception, it is to her advantage to learn to recognize mucus characteristics at ovulation (see Teaching for Self-Management). Self-evaluation of cervical mucus can be highly accurate and useful diagnostically for any of the following purposes:

- To alert the couple to the reestablishment of ovulation while breastfeeding and after discontinuation of oral contraception
- To note anovulatory cycles at any time and at the beginning of menopause
- To assist couples in planning a pregnancy

Basal Body Temperature Method. The basal body temperature (BBT) is the lowest body temperature of a healthy person, taken immediately after waking and before getting out of bed. The BBT usually varies from 36.2° to 36.3° C during menses and for approximately 5 to 7 days afterward (Fig. 8-3).

About the time of ovulation a slight drop in temperature (approximately 0.5° C) may occur in some women just prior to ovulation, but other women may have no decrease at all. After ovulation, in concert with the increasing progesterone levels of the early luteal phase of the cycle, the BBT increases slightly (approximately 0.4° to 0.8° C). Before ovulation, 96° to 98° F is normal in many women. After ovulation, temperature increases to 97° to 99° F. The temperature remains on an elevated plateau until 2 to 4 days before menstruation. Then BBT decreases to the low levels recorded during the previous cycle unless pregnancy has occurred. In pregnant women the temperature remains elevated. If ovulation fails to occur, the pattern of lower body temperature continues throughout the cycle.

To use this method, the fertile period is defined as the day of first temperature drop, or first elevation, through 3 consecutive days of elevated temperature. Abstinence begins the first day of menstrual bleeding and lasts through 3 consecutive days of sustained temperature rise (at least 0.2° C). The decrease and subsequent increase in temperature are referred

TEACHING FOR SELF-MANAGEMENT

Cervical Mucus Characteristics

Setting the Stage

- Show charts of menstrual cycle along with changes in the cervical mucus.
- Have the woman practice with raw egg white.
- Supply her with a basal body temperature log and graph if she does not already have one.
- Explain that assessment of cervical mucus characteristics is best when mucus is not mixed with semen, contraceptive jellies or foams, or discharge from infections. Tell her to refrain from douching before the assessment.

Content Related to Cervical Mucus

- Explain to the woman (couple) how cervical mucus changes throughout the menstrual cycle.
  - Postmenstrual mucus: scant
  - Preovulation mucus: cloudy, yellow or white, sticky
  - Ovulation mucus: clear, wet, sticky, slippery
  - Postovulation fertile mucus: thick, cloudy, sticky
  - Postovulation, postfertile mucus: scant
- Right before ovulation, the watery, thin, clear mucus becomes more abundant and thick (Fig. A). It feels similar to a lubricant and can be stretched 5+ cm between the thumb and forefinger; this quality of mucus is called spinnbarkeit (Fig. B), and its presence indicates the period of maximal fertility. Sperm deposited in this type of mucus can survive until ovulation occurs.

Assessment Technique

- Stress that good handwashing is imperative to begin and end all self-assessments.
- Start observation from last day of menstrual flow.
- Assess cervical mucus several times a day for several cycles. Mucus can be obtained from vaginal opening; reaching into the vagina to the cervix is unnecessary.
- Record the findings on the same record on which the basal body temperature is entered.

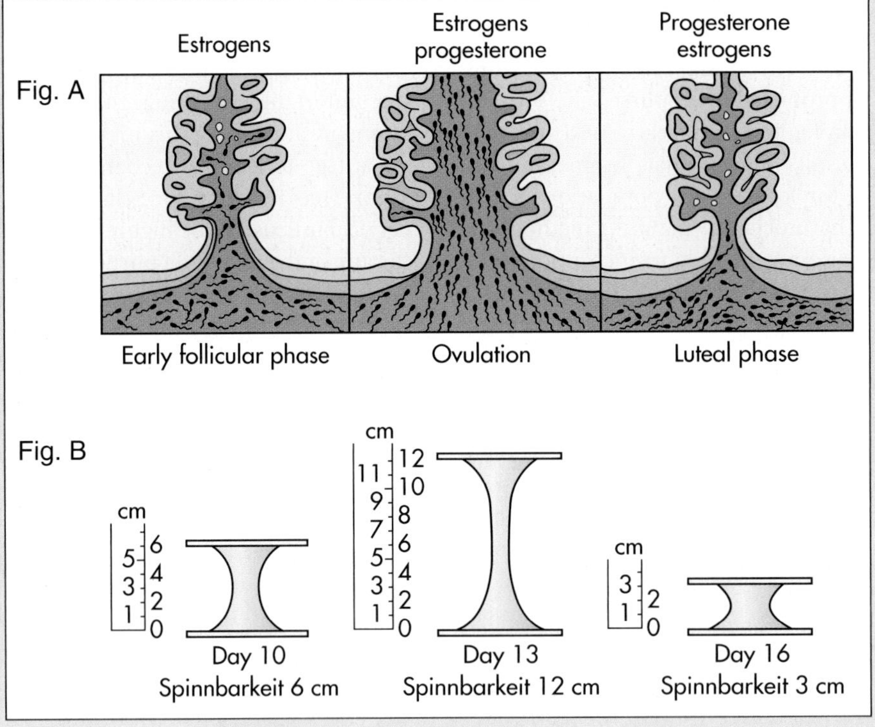

to as the *thermal shift.* When the entire month's temperatures are recorded on a graph, the pattern described is more apparent. It is more difficult to perceive day-to-day variations without the entire picture (see Teaching for Self-Management). Either a glass mercury thermometer or a digital thermometer may be used for BBT, but the thermometer must measure the temperature within 0.1 degree. The glass mercury thermometer needs no batteries but is fragile and can break. A digital thermometer will require batteries but may have a history recall function and an audible beep when the temperature assessment is finished. Digital thermometers that monitor temperature throughout the day combined with an accelerometer to monitor movement have been cleared for use by the U.S. Food and Drug Administration (FDA). These devices can be wirelessly uploaded to a computer through a companion device. Their use in FABs needs further research.

Infection, fatigue, less than 3 hours of sleep per night, awakening late, and anxiety may cause temperature fluctuations and alter the expected pattern. If a new BBT thermometer is purchased, this fact is noted on the chart because the readings may vary slightly. Jet lag, alcohol taken the evening before, or sleeping in a heated waterbed must also be noted on the chart because each affects the BBT. Therefore, the BBT alone is not a reliable method of predicting ovulation.

TEACHING FOR SELF-MANAGEMENT

Basal Body Temperature

- Discuss basal body temperature (BBT) with the woman.
- Show the woman a diagram depicting the phases of the menstrual cycle.
- Discuss the hormones in the woman's body that are responsible for her menstrual cycle and ovulation. Leave time for questions.
- Show the woman a sample BBT graph (see Fig. 8-4) and the biphasic line seen in ovulatory cycles.
- Show the woman the BBT thermometer and how it is calibrated.
- Provide a demonstration.
- Encourage the woman to demonstrate taking and reading the thermometer and graphing the temperature while the nurse watches.
- Encourage the woman to start a log to keep track of any other activity that might interfere with her true BBT.

Symptothermal Method. The symptothermal method combines the BBT and cervical mucus methods with awareness of secondary phase–related signs and symptoms of the menstrual cycle. The woman gains fertility awareness as she learns the psychologic and physiologic signs and symptoms that mark the phases of her cycle. Secondary signs and symptoms include increased libido, midcycle spotting, mittelschmerz (cramplike pain prior to ovulation), pelvic fullness or tenderness, and vulvar fullness.

The woman is taught to palpate her cervix to assess for changes indicating ovulation: the cervical os dilates slightly, the cervix softens and rises in the vagina, and cervical mucus is copious and slippery. The woman notes days on which coitus, changes in routine, illness, and other changes that might affect BBT have occurred (Fig. 8-4). Calendar calculations and cervical mucus changes are used to estimate the onset of the fertile period; changes in cervical mucus or the BBT are used to estimate the end of the fertile period.

Biologic Marker Methods

Home Predictor Test Kits for Ovulation. Although the methods previously discussed are characteristic of ovulation, they do not prove that ovulation actually occurred or indicate the exact timing. The urine predictor test for ovulation is a major addition to the NFP and fertility-awareness methods to help women who want to plan the time of their pregnancies and for those who are trying to conceive (Fig. 8-5). The urine predictor test for ovulation detects the sudden surge of luteinizing hormone (LH) that occurs approximately 12 to 24 hours before ovulation. Unlike BBT, this test is not affected by illness, emotions, or physical activity. For home use, a test kit contains sufficient material for several days' testing during each cycle. A positive response indicating an LH surge is noted by a color change that is easy to interpret. Directions for use of urine predictor test kits vary with the manufacturer.

The Marquette Model. The Marquette Model (MM) is a natural family planning method that was developed through the Marquette University College of Nursing Institute for Natural Family Planning (Fehring, Schneider, & Barron, 2008). The MM uses cervical monitoring along with the ClearPlan Easy Fertility Monitor. The ClearPlan monitor is a handheld device that uses test strips to measure urinary metabolites of estrogen and LH. The monitor provides the user with "low," "high," and "peak" fertility readings. The MM incorporates the use of the monitor as an aid to learning NFP and fertility awareness. The MM is currently being tested at different sites in the United States for its effectiveness in helping couples avoid pregnancy. One study has shown a typical use failure rate of 10.6% (Fehring et al.).

Spermicides and Barrier Methods

Barrier contraceptives have gained in popularity not only as a contraceptive method but also as protection against the spread of STIs such as human papillomavirus and herpes simplex virus (HSV). Some male condoms and female vaginal methods provide a physical barrier to several STIs, and some male condoms provide protection against HIV (Cates & Harwood, 2011). Spermicides serve as chemical barriers against semen and inhibit the ability of sperm to fertilize the ovum.

The nurse should remember that any user of a barrier method of contraception must also be aware of emergency contraception options in case there is a failure of the method. An example of a barrier method failure would be if a condom broke during intercourse. In this instance, emergency contraception would be indicated to prevent unplanned pregnancy.

Spermicides. Spermicides such as nonoxynol-9 (N-9) work by reducing the sperm's mobility. The chemicals attack the sperm flagella and body, thereby preventing the sperm from reaching the cervical os. N-9, the most commonly used spermicidal chemical in the United States, is a surfactant that destroys the sperm cell membrane. Results from data analyses suggest that frequent use (more than two times a day) of N-9 or the use of N-9 as a lubricant during anal intercourse may increase the transmission of HIV and can cause lesions (Cates & Harwood, 2011). There is no evidence that the addition of spermicides to male condoms decreases the risk of subsequent pregnancy. Women with high risk behaviors that increase their likelihood of contracting HIV and other STIs are advised to avoid the use of spermicidal products containing N-9, including lubricated condoms, diaphragms, and cervical caps to which N-9 is added (CDC, 2010).

Intravaginal spermicides are marketed and sold without prescriptions as aerosol foams, tablets, suppositories, creams, films, and gels (Fig. 8-6). Preloaded, single-dose applicators small enough to be carried in a small purse are available. Effectiveness of spermicides depends on consistent and accurate use. Clients should be cautioned against misunderstanding terms: contraceptive gel differs from fruit jelly, and cosmetics or hair products containing the nonspermicidal forms of nonoxynol are not adequate substitutes for contraception. The spermicide should be inserted high into the vagina so that it makes contact with the cervix. Some spermicide should be inserted at least 15 minutes before, and no longer than 1 hour before, sexual intercourse. Spermicide must be reapplied for each additional act of intercourse, even if a barrier method is used. Studies have shown varying effectiveness rates for spermicidal use alone. Typical failure rate in the first year of spermicidal use alone is 28% (Trussell, 2011). Some female barrier methods (e.g., diaphragm, cervical caps) offer more effective protection against pregnancy with the addition of spermicides.

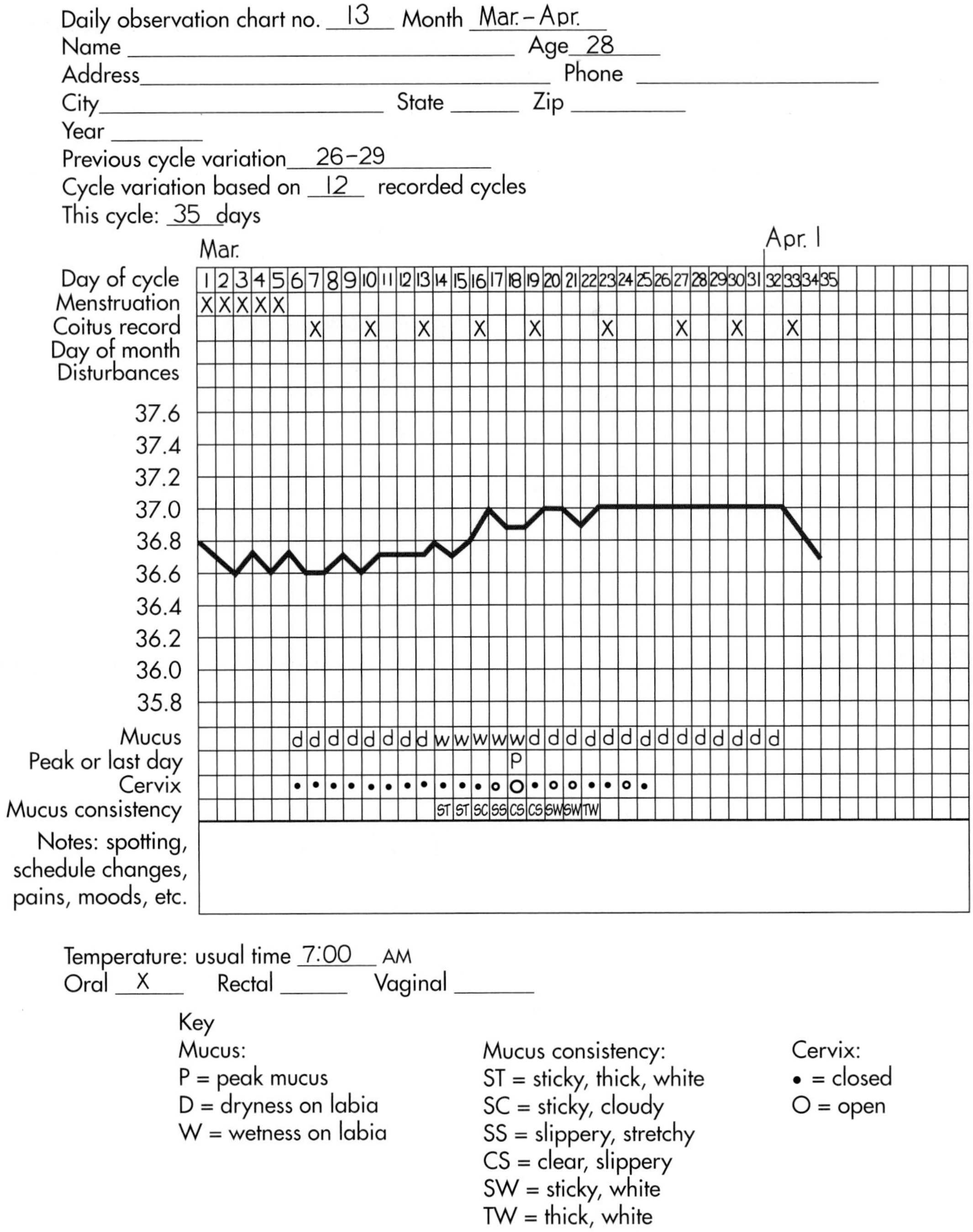

Daily observation chart no. 13 Month Mar.–Apr.
Name ______ Age 28
Address ______ Phone ______
City ______ State ______ Zip ______
Year ______
Previous cycle variation 26–29
Cycle variation based on 12 recorded cycles
This cycle: 35 days

Mar. Apr. 1

Temperature scale: 37.6, 37.4, 37.2, 37.0, 36.8, 36.6, 36.4, 36.2, 36.0, 35.8

Day of cycle	Menstruation	Coitus record	Day of month	Disturbances	Mucus	Peak or last day	Cervix	Mucus consistency
1	X							
2	X							
3	X							
4	X							
5	X							
6					d		•	
7		X			d		•	
8					d		•	
9					d		•	
10		X			d		•	
11					d		•	
12					d		•	
13		X			d		•	
14					w		•	ST
15					w		•	ST
16		X			w		•	SC
17					w		o	SS
18					w	P	O	CS
19		X			d		•	CS
20					d		o	SW
21					d		o	SW
22					d		•	TW
23		X			d		•	
24					d		o	
25					d		•	
26					d			
27		X			d			
28					d			
29					d			
30		X			d			
31					d			
32					d			
33		X						
34								
35								

Notes: spotting, schedule changes, pains, moods, etc.

Temperature: usual time 7:00 AM
Oral X Rectal ______ Vaginal ______

Key

Mucus:
P = peak mucus
D = dryness on labia
W = wetness on labia

Mucus consistency:
ST = sticky, thick, white
SC = sticky, cloudy
SS = slippery, stretchy
CS = clear, slippery
SW = sticky, white
TW = thick, white

Cervix:
• = closed
O = open

FIG 8-4 Example of a completed symptothermal chart.

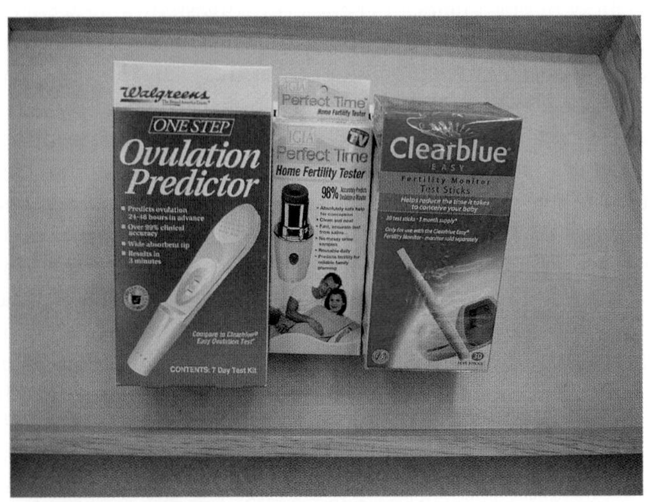

FIG 8-5 Examples of ovulation prediction tests. (Courtesy Shannon Perry, Phoenix, AZ.)

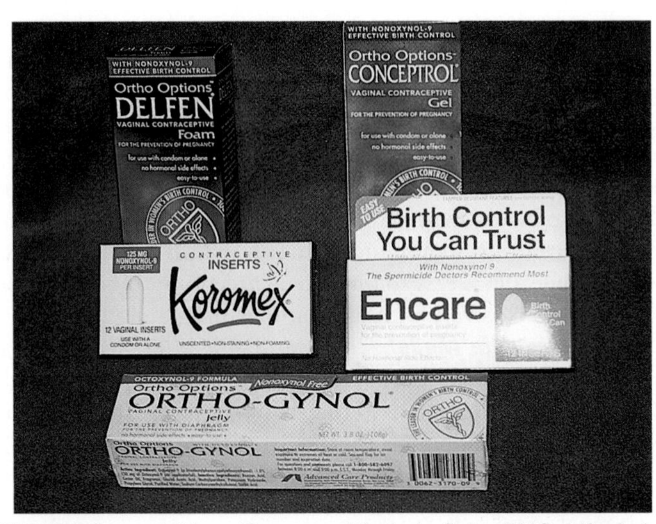

FIG 8-6 Spermicides. (Courtesy Marjorie Pyle, RNC, Lifecircle, Costa Mesa, CA.)

Condoms. The male condom is a thin, stretchable sheath that covers the penis before genital, oral, or anal contact and is removed when the penis is withdrawn from the partner's orifice after ejaculation. Condoms are made of latex rubber, which provides a barrier to sperm and STIs (including HIV); polyurethane (strong, thin plastic); or natural membranes (animal tissue). In addition to providing a physical barrier for sperm, nonspermicidal latex condoms also provide a barrier for STIs (particularly gonorrhea, chlamydia, and trichomoniasis) and HIV transmission (CDC, 2010). Condoms lubricated with N-9 are not recommended for preventing STIs or HIV and do not increase protection against pregnancy. Latex condoms break down with oil-based lubricants (e.g., petroleum jelly and suntan oil) and should be used only with water-based or silicone lubricants (Warner & Steiner, 2011). Because of the growing number of people with latex allergies, condom manufacturers have begun using polyurethane, which is thinner and stronger than latex.

SAFETY ALERT

All clients should be questioned about the potential for latex allergy. Latex condom use is contraindicated for clients with latex sensitivity.

Although polyurethane condoms are as effective for STI prevention as latex condoms, they are more likely to slip or lose contour when compared with latex condoms. With perfect use, therefore, latex condoms offer better protection against pregnancy. Polyurethane condoms do offer equivalent pregnancy protection as most barrier products. A small percentage of condoms are made from lamb cecum (natural skin). Natural skin condoms do not provide the same protection against STIs and HIV infection as latex condoms. Natural skin condoms contain small pores that could allow passage of viruses such as hepatitis B, HSV, and HIV and are not recommended generally.

A functional difference in condom shape is the presence or absence of a sperm reservoir tip. To enhance vaginal stimulation, some condoms are contoured and rippled or have ribbed or roughened surfaces. Thinner construction increases heat transmission and sensitivity. A wet jelly or dry powder lubricates some condoms. Condoms must be discarded after each single use. They are available without a prescription and from a variety of sources, including vending machines. Typical failure rate for the first year of use of the male condom is 18% (Trussell, 2011). To prevent unintended pregnancy and the spread of STIs, it is essential that condoms be used consistently and correctly. Instructions, such as those listed in Box 8-3, can be used

BOX 8-3 Male Condoms

Mechanism of Action
- Sheath is applied over the erect penis before insertion or loss of preejaculatory drops of semen. Used correctly, condoms prevent sperm from entering the cervix. Spermicide-coated condoms cause ejaculated sperm to be immobilized rapidly, thus increasing contraceptive effectiveness.

Failure Rate
- Typical users: 18%
- Correct and consistent users: 2%

Advantages
- Safe
- No side effects
- Readily available
- Premalignant changes in cervix can be prevented or ameliorated in women whose partners use condoms
- Method of male nonsurgical contraception

Disadvantages
- Must interrupt lovemaking to apply sheath
- Sensation may be altered
- If used improperly, spillage of sperm can result in pregnancy
- Condoms occasionally may tear during intercourse

STI Protection
- If a condom is used throughout the act of intercourse and there is no unprotected contact with female genitals, a latex rubber condom, which is impermeable to viruses, can act as a protective measure against STIs.

Nursing Considerations

Teaching should include the following instructions:
- Use a new condom (check expiration date) for each act of sexual intercourse or other acts between partners that involve contact with the penis.
- Place condom after penis is erect and before intimate contact.
- Place condom on head of penis (Fig. A) and unroll it all the way to the base (Fig. B).

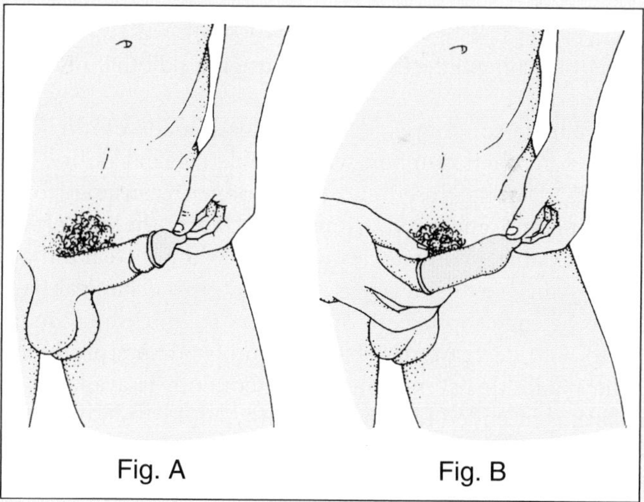
Fig. A Fig. B

- Leave an empty space at the tip (Fig. A); remove any air remaining in the tip by gently pressing air out toward the base of the penis.
- If a lubricant is desired, use water-based products such as K-Y lubricating jelly. Do *not* use petroleum-based products because they can cause the condom to break.
- After ejaculation, carefully withdraw the still-erect penis from the vagina, holding on to condom rim; remove and discard the condom.
- Store unused condoms in cool, dry place.
- Do not use condoms that are sticky, brittle, or obviously damaged.

STIs, Sexually transmitted infections.

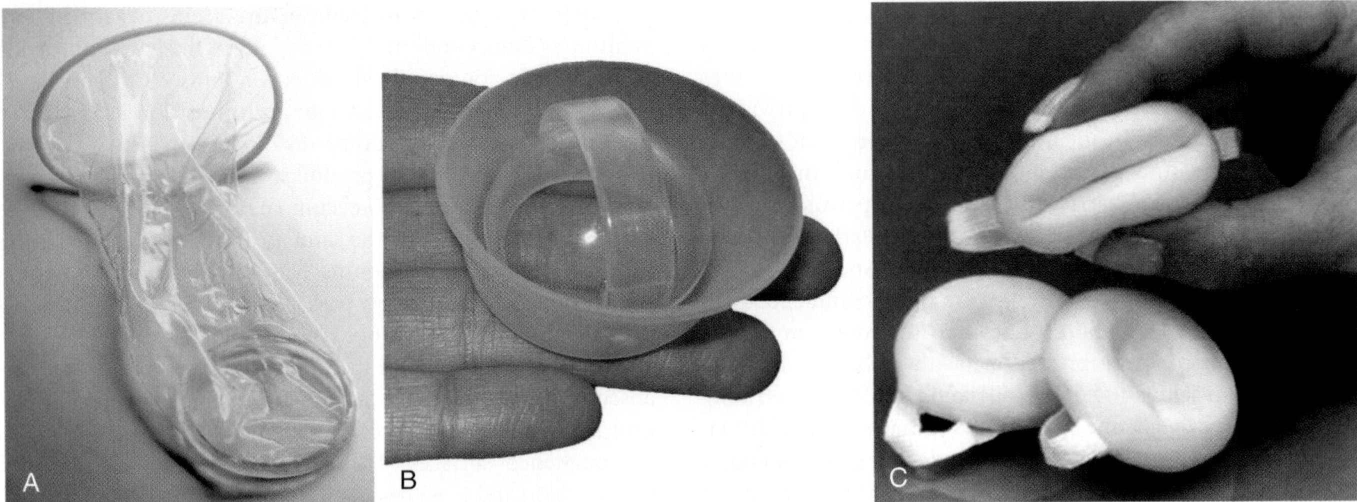

FIG 8-7 Barrier methods. **A**, Female condom (FC2). **B**, FemCap. **C**, Contraceptive sponge. (**A**, Courtesy The Female Health Company, Chicago; **B**, courtesy FemCap, Del Mar, CA; **C**, Today® vaginal contraceptive sponge. Courtesy Mayer Laboratories, Inc., 2014.)

SAFETY ALERT

It is a false assumption that everyone knows how to use condoms. To prevent unintended pregnancy and the spread of STIs, it is essential for condoms to be used correctly. Proper instruction in use must be provided. The sheath is applied over the erect penis before insertion and before the loss of preejaculatory drops of semen. All types of condoms must be discarded after each single use.

for client teaching. Effective condom use is a skill that must be taught.

The female condom is a vaginal sheath made of nitrile, a non-latex synthetic rubber, with flexible rings at both ends (Fig. 8-7, *A*). The closed end of the pouch is inserted into the vagina and anchored around the cervix; the open ring covers the labia. Women whose partner will not wear a male condom can use this device as a protective mechanical barrier. Rewetting drops or oil- or water-based lubricants can be used to help decrease the distracting noise that is produced during penile thrusting. The female condom is available in one size, is intended for single use only, and is sold over the counter. Male condoms should not be used concurrently because the friction from both sheaths can increase the likelihood of either or both tearing (Cates & Harwood, 2011). Typical failure rate in the first year of female condom use is 21% (Trussell, 2011).

Diaphragms. The contraceptive diaphragm is a shallow dome-shaped latex or silicone device with a flexible rim that covers the cervix. There are four types of diaphragms: coil spring, arcing spring, flat spring, and wide seal rim. Available in many sizes, the diaphragm should be the largest size the woman can wear without her being aware of its presence. The typical failure rate of the diaphragm combined with spermicide is 12% in the first year of use (Trussell, 2011). Effectiveness of the diaphragm is less when used without spermicide. Women at high risk for HIV should avoid use of N-9 spermicides with the diaphragm (AIDS.gov, 2012).

The woman is informed that she needs an annual gynecologic examination to assess the fit of the diaphragm. The device should be inspected before every use, replaced every 2 years, and may have to be refitted for a 20% weight fluctuation, after any abdominal or pelvic surgery, and after every pregnancy (World Health Organization Department of Reproductive Health & Research [WHO/RHR] & Johns Hopkins Bloomberg School of Public Health/Center for Communications Programs [CCP], 2011). Because various types of diaphragms are on the market, the nurse should use the package insert for teaching a woman how to use and care for the diaphragm (see Teaching for Self-Management box).

Disadvantages of diaphragm use include the reluctance of some women to insert and remove it. Although it can be inserted up to 6 hours before intercourse, a cold diaphragm and a cold gel temporarily reduce vaginal response to sexual stimulation if insertion of the diaphragm occurs immediately before intercourse. Some women or couples object to the messiness of the spermicide. These annoyances of diaphragm use, along with failure to insert the device once foreplay has begun, are the most common reasons for failures of this method. Side effects may include irritation of tissues related to contact with spermicides. The diaphragm is not a good option for women with poor vaginal muscle tone or recurrent urinary tract infections. For proper placement the diaphragm must rest behind the pubic symphysis and completely cover the cervix. To decrease the chance of exerting urethral pressure, the woman should be reminded to empty her bladder before diaphragm insertion and immediately after intercourse. Diaphragms are contraindicated for women with pelvic relaxation (uterine prolapse) or a large cystocele. Women with a latex allergy should not use latex diaphragms.

Toxic shock syndrome (TSS), although reported in very small numbers, can occur in association with the use of the contraceptive diaphragm and cervical caps (Cates & Harwood, 2011). The nurse should instruct the woman about ways to reduce her risk for TSS. These measures include prompt removal 6 to 8 hours after intercourse, not using the diaphragm or cervical caps during menses, and learning and watching for danger signs of TSS.

> **SAFETY ALERT**
>
> The nurse should inform the woman who uses a diaphragm or cervical cap as a contraceptive method to be alert for signs of TSS. The most common signs include a sunburn type of rash, diarrhea, dizziness, faintness, weakness, sore throat, aching muscles and joints, sudden high fever, and vomiting (WHO/RHR & CCP, 2011).

Cervical Caps. The FemCap (see Fig. 8-7, *B*) is the only type of cervical cap available in the United States. It comes in three sizes and is made of silicone rubber. The cap fits snugly around the base of the cervix close to the junction of the cervix and vaginal fornices. It is recommended that the cap remain in place no less than 6 hours and not more than 48 hours at a time. It is left in place at least 6 hours after the last act of intercourse. The seal provides a physical barrier to sperm: spermicide inside the cap adds a chemical barrier. The extended period of wear may be an added convenience for women.

Instructions for the actual insertion and use of the cervical cap closely resemble those for a contraceptive diaphragm. Some of the differences are that the cervical cap can be inserted hours before sexual intercourse without a later need for additional spermicide, the cervical cap requires less spermicide than the diaphragm when initially inserted, and no additional spermicide is required for repeated acts of intercourse. Effectiveness of the first-generation FemCap has been found to be less than the diaphragm (Fritz & Speroff, 2011a).

The angle of the uterus, the vaginal muscle tone, and the shape of the cervix may interfere with the cervical cap's ease of fitting and use. Correct fitting requires time, effort, and skill from both the woman and the clinician. The woman must check the cap's position before and after each act of intercourse.

Because of the potential risk of TSS associated with the use of the cervical cap, another form of birth control is recommended for use during menstrual bleeding and up to at least 6 weeks postpartum. The cap should be refitted after any gynecologic surgery or birth and after major weight losses or gains. Otherwise the size should be checked at least once a year.

Women who are not good candidates for wearing the cervical cap include those with abnormal Papanicolaou (Pap) test results, those who cannot be fitted properly with the existing cap sizes, those who find the insertion and removal of the device too difficult, those with a history of TSS, those with vaginal or cervical infections, and those who experience allergic responses to the latex cap or spermicide. Failure rates the first year of use are 16% in nulliparous and 32% in multiparous women (WHO/RHR & CCP, 2011).

Contraceptive Sponge. The vaginal sponge is a small, round polyurethane sponge that contains N-9 spermicide (see previous discussion of N-9) (see Fig. 8-7, *C*). It is designed to fit over the cervix (one size fits all). The side that is placed next to the cervix is concave for better fit. The opposite side has a woven polyester loop to be used for removal of the sponge.

The sponge must be moistened with water before it is inserted. It provides protection for up to 24 hours and for repeated instances of sexual intercourse. The sponge should be left in place for at least 6 hours after the last act of intercourse. Wearing it longer than 24 to 30 hours may put the woman at risk for TSS (Cates & Harwood, 2011). The typical failure rate in the first year of use is 24% for parous women and 12% for nulliparous women (Trussell, 2011).

TABLE 8-1 Hormonal Contraception

COMPOSITION	ROUTE OF ADMINISTRATION	DURATION OF EFFECT
Combination estrogen and progestin (synthetic estrogens and progestins in varying doses and formulations)	Oral	24 hours; extended cycle—12 weeks
	Transdermal	7 days
	Vaginal ring insertion	3 weeks
Progestin only		
Norethindrone, norgestrel	Oral	24 hours
Medroxyprogesterone acetate	Intramuscular injection; subcutaneous injection	3 months
Progestin, etonogestrel	Subdermal implant	Up to 3 years
Levonorgestrel	Intrauterine device	Up to 5 years

Hormonal Methods

More than 30 different hormonal contraceptive formulations are available in the United States. General classes are described in Table 8-1. Because of the wide variety of preparations available, the woman and the nurse must read the package insert for information about specific products prescribed. Formulations include combined estrogen-progestin medications and progestational agents. The formulations are administered orally, transdermally, vaginally, by implantation, by injection, or by intrauterine insertion.

Combined Estrogen-Progestin Contraceptives

Oral Contraceptives. The normal menstrual cycle is maintained by a feedback mechanism. Follicle-stimulating hormone (FSH) and LH are secreted in response to fluctuating levels of ovarian estrogen and progesterone. Regular ingestion of combined oral contraceptive pills (COCs) suppresses the action of the hypothalamus and anterior pituitary, leading to insufficient secretion of FSH and LH; therefore, follicles do not mature, and ovulation is inhibited.

Other contraceptive effects are induced by the combined steroids. Maturation of the endometrium is altered, making it a less favorable site for implantation. COCs also have a direct effect on the endometrium, so that from 1 to 4 days after the last COC is taken, the endometrium sloughs and bleeds as a result of hormone withdrawal. The withdrawal bleeding is usually less profuse than that of normal menstruation and may last only 2 to 3 days. Some women have no bleeding at all. The cervical mucus remains thick from the effect of the progestin (Nelson & Cwiak, 2011).

Cervical mucus under the effect of progesterone does not provide as suitable an environment for sperm penetration as does the thin, watery mucus at ovulation. The possible effect, if any, of altered tubal and uterine motility induced by COCs is not clear.

Monophasic pills provide fixed dosages of estrogen and progestin. Multiphasic pills (e.g., biphasic and triphasic oral contraceptives) alter the amount of progestin and sometimes the amount of estrogen within each cycle. These preparations reduce the total dosage of hormones in a single cycle without sacrificing contraceptive efficacy (Nelson & Cwiak, 2011). To maintain adequate hormonal levels for contraception and enhance compliance, COCs should be taken at the same time each day.

Advantages. Because taking the pill does not relate directly to the sexual act, its acceptability may be increased. Improvement in sexual response may occur once the possibility of pregnancy is not an issue. For some women it is convenient to know when to expect the next menstrual flow.

TEACHING FOR SELF-MANAGEMENT

Use and Care of the Diaphragm

Inspection of the Diaphragm

You must inspect your diaphragm carefully before each use. The best way to perform this inspection is as follows:

- Hold the diaphragm up to a light source. Carefully stretch the diaphragm at the area of the rim, on all sides, making sure there are no holes. Remember, sharp fingernails can puncture the diaphragm.
- Another way to check for pinholes is to fill the diaphragm with water carefully. If any problem develops, you will see it immediately.
- A diaphragm that is puckered, especially near the rim, could mean thin spots.
- If you see any of these problems, do not use the diaphragm; avoid sexual intercourse or use another method of birth control; consult your health care provider about replacing the diaphragm.

Preparation of the Diaphragm

Rinse off the cornstarch. Your diaphragm must always be used with a spermicidal lubricant to be effective. Pregnancy cannot be prevented effectively by the diaphragm alone.

Always empty your bladder before inserting the diaphragm. Place approximately 2 teaspoons of contraceptive jelly or contraceptive cream on the side of the diaphragm that will rest against the cervix (or whichever way you have been instructed). Spread it around to coat the surface and the rim. This measure aids in insertion and offers a more complete seal. Many women also spread some jelly or cream on the other side of the diaphragm (Fig. A).

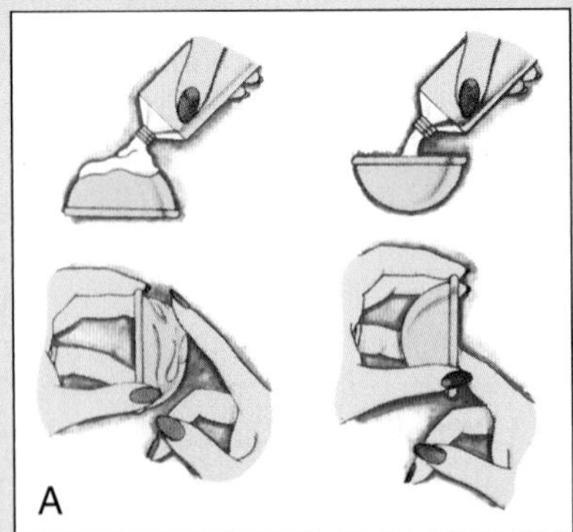

Positions for Insertion of the Diaphragm

Squatting: Squatting is the most commonly used position, and most women find it satisfactory.

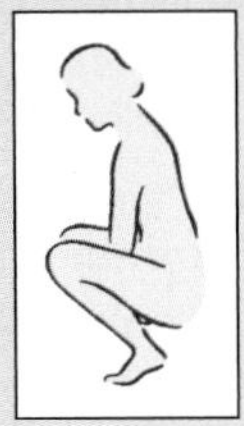

Leg-up method: Another position is to raise the left foot (if right hand is used for insertion) on a low stool, and, while in a bending position, insert the diaphragm.

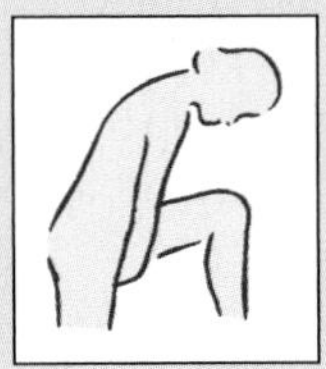

Chair method: Another practical method for diaphragm insertion is to sit far forward on the edge of a chair.

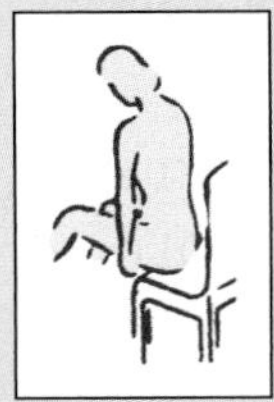

Reclining: You may prefer to insert the diaphragm while in a semi-reclining position in bed.

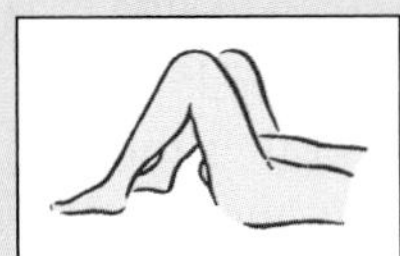

Insertion of the Diaphragm

1. The diaphragm can be inserted up to 6 hours before intercourse. Hold the diaphragm between your thumb and fingers. The dome can be either up or down, as directed by your health care provider. Place your index finger on the outer rim of the compressed diaphragm (Fig. B).

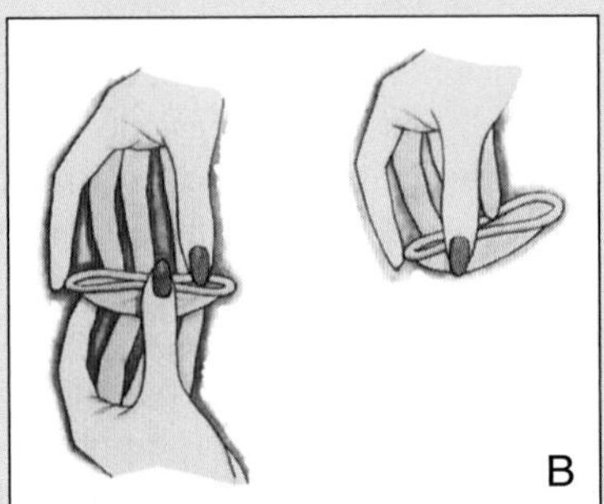

2. Use the fingers of the other hand to spread the labia (lips of the vagina). This action will assist in guiding the diaphragm into place.

Noncontraceptive benefits of low-dose oral contraceptives (less than 35 mg estrogen) have been well demonstrated (Schindler, 2013). The noncontraceptive health benefits of COCs include decreased menstrual blood loss and decreased iron deficiency anemia, regulation of menorrhagia and irregular cycles, and reduced incidence of dysmenorrhea and premenstrual syndrome (PMS). Oral contraceptives also offer protection against endometrial cancer and ovarian cancer, reduce the incidence of benign breast disease, improve acne, protect against the development of functional ovarian cysts and salpingitis, and decrease

TEACHING FOR SELF-MANAGEMENT—cont'd

Use and Care of the Diaphragm

3. Insert the diaphragm into the vagina. Direct it inward and downward as far as it will go to the space behind and below the cervix (Fig. C).

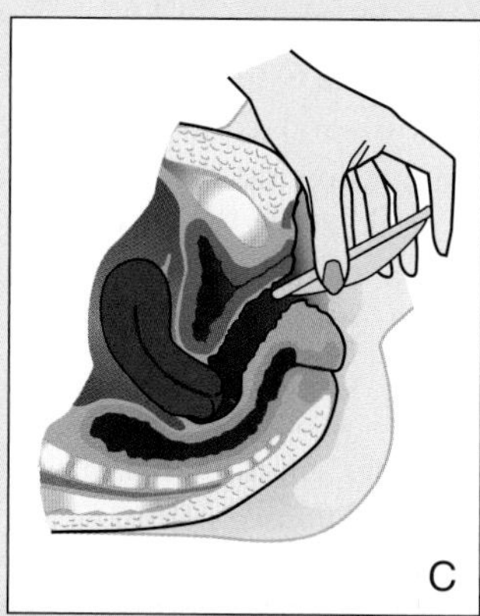

4. Tuck the front of the rim of the diaphragm behind the pubic bone so that the rubber hugs the front wall of the vagina (Fig. D).

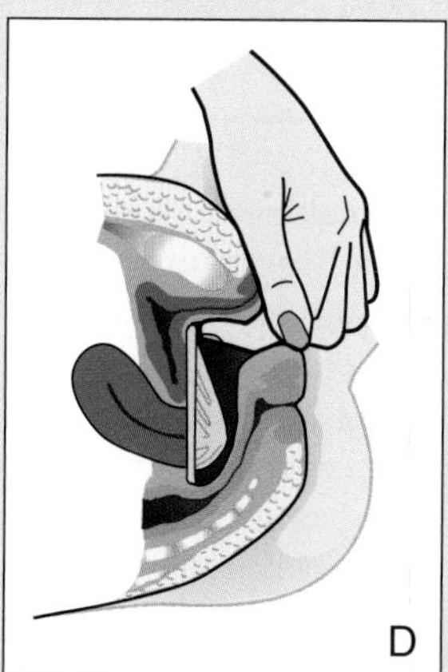

5. Feel for your cervix through the diaphragm to be certain it is properly placed and securely covered by the rubber dome (Fig. E).

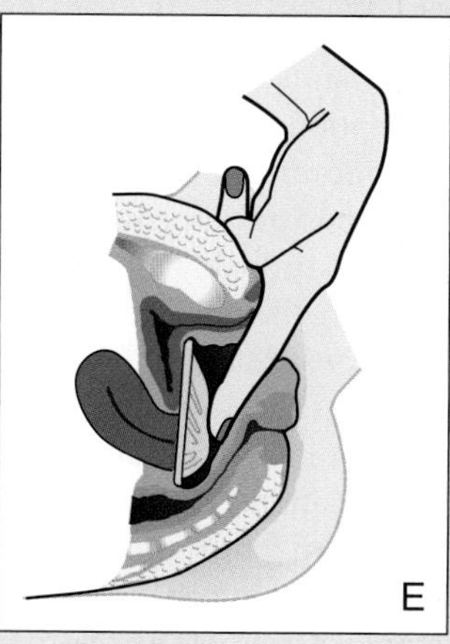

General Information

Regardless of the time of the month, you must use your diaphragm every time intercourse takes place. The cervix moves its position throughout the month, requiring that the angle of insertion of the diaphragm will change slightly. Your diaphragm must be left in place for at least 6 hours after the last intercourse. If you remove your diaphragm before the 6-hour period, you will greatly increase your chance of becoming pregnant. If you have repeated intercourse, you must add more spermicide for each act of intercourse.

Removal of the Diaphragm

The only proper way to remove the diaphragm is to insert your forefinger up and over the top side of the diaphragm and slightly to the side.

Next, turn the palm of your hand downward and backward, hooking the forefinger firmly on top of the inside of the upper rim of the diaphragm, breaking the suction.

Pull the diaphragm down and out. This technique prevents tearing the diaphragm with the fingernails. You should not remove the diaphragm by trying to catch the rim from below the dome (Fig. F).

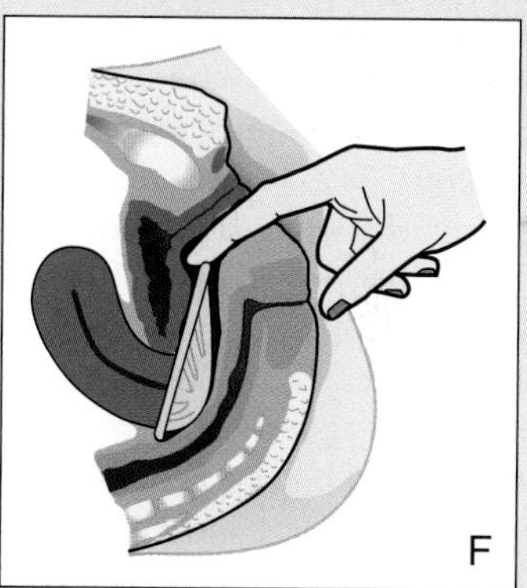

Care of the Diaphragm

When using a vaginal diaphragm, avoid using oil-based products, such as certain body lubricants, mineral oil, baby oil, vaginal lubricants, or vaginitis preparations. These products can weaken the rubber.

A little care means longer wear for your diaphragm. After each use wash the diaphragm in warm water and mild soap. Do not use detergent soaps, cold-cream soaps, deodorant soaps, and soaps containing oil products because they can weaken the rubber.

After washing, dry the diaphragm thoroughly. Remove all water and moisture with a towel. Then dust the diaphragm with cornstarch. Do not use scented talc, body powder, baby powder, or similar products because they can weaken the rubber.

To clean the introducer (if one is used), wash with mild soap and warm water, rinse, and dry thoroughly.

Place the diaphragm back in the plastic case for storage. Do not store it near a radiator or heat source or in a location that is exposed to light for an extended period.

the risk of ectopic pregnancy. Oral contraceptives are considered a safe option for nonsmoking women until menopause. Perimenopausal women can benefit from regular bleeding cycles, a regular hormonal pattern, and the noncontraceptive health benefits of oral contraceptives (Nelson & Cwiak, 2011).

A pelvic examination and Pap test are not necessary before initiating COCs (WHO/RHR & CCP, 2011). If STI screening is indicated, a urine-based test can be used for some infections (e.g., chlamydia, gonorrhea); others require a pelvic examination and cultures of vaginal or cervical secretions or blood tests (Planned Parenthood, 2013). Most health care providers assess the woman 3 months after beginning COCs to detect any complications.

Use of oral hormonal contraceptives is initiated on one of the first days of the menstrual cycle (day 1 of the cycle is the first day of menses) or after childbirth or abortion. With a "Sunday start," women begin taking pills on the first Sunday after the start of their menstrual period. If contraceptives are to be started at any time other than during normal menses or within 4 weeks after birth, miscarriage, or induced abortion, another method of contraception should be used throughout the first week to avoid the risk of pregnancy (Nelson & Cwiak, 2011). Taken exactly as directed, oral contraceptives prevent ovulation, and pregnancy cannot occur; the overall effectiveness rate is almost 100%. Almost all failures (i.e., pregnancy occurs) are caused by omission of one or more pills during the regimen. The typical failure rate of COCs due to omission is 9% (Trussell, 2011).

Disadvantages and Side Effects. Since hormonal contraceptives have come into use, the amount of estrogen and progestational agent contained in each tablet has been reduced considerably. This is important because adverse effects are, to a degree, dose related.

Women must be screened for conditions that present absolute or relative contraindications to oral contraceptive use. Contraindications for COC use include a history of thromboembolic disorders, cerebrovascular or coronary artery disease, breast cancer, gallbladder disease, jaundice with prior pill use, estrogen-dependent tumors, pregnancy, severe cirrhosis, liver tumor, lactation less than 6 weeks postpartum, smoking if older than 35 years, headaches with focal neurologic symptoms, surgery with prolonged immobilization or any surgery on the legs, hypertension (140/90 mm Hg), and diabetes mellitus (of more than 20 years' duration) with vascular disease (Curtis & Peterson, 2011; Nelson & Cwiak, 2011; WHO/RHR & CCP, 2011).

Certain side effects of COCs are attributable to estrogen, progestin, or both. Serious adverse effects documented with high doses of estrogen and progesterone include stroke, myocardial infarction, thromboembolism, hypertension, gallbladder disease, and liver tumors (Nelson & Cwiak, 2011). Common side effects of estrogen excess include nausea, breast tenderness, fluid retention, and chloasma. Side effects of estrogen deficiency include early spotting (days 1 to 14), hypomenorrhea, nervousness, and atrophic vaginitis leading to painful intercourse (dyspareunia). Side effects of progestin excess include increased appetite, tiredness, depression, breast tenderness, vaginal yeast infection, oily skin and scalp, hirsutism, and postpill amenorrhea. Side effects of progestin deficiency include late spotting and breakthrough bleeding (days 15 to 21), heavy flow with clots, and decreased breast size. One of the most common side effects of combined COCs is bleeding irregularities (Nelson & Cwiak).

In the presence of side effects, especially those that are bothersome to a woman, another product, a different drug content, or another method of contraception may be required. The "right" product for a woman contains the lowest dose of hormones that prevents ovulation and that has the fewest and least harmful side effects. There is no way to predict the right dosage for any particular woman. Issues to consider in prescribing oral contraceptives include history of oral contraceptive use, side effects during past use, menstrual history, and drug interactions (Nelson & Cwiak, 2011).

Large prospective studies have not shown a relationship between use of oral contraceptives available and diabetes or glucose intolerance (Nelson & Cwiak, 2011). The risks and benefits should be assessed before prescribing oral contraceptives for women who have diabetes with vascular problems.

The effectiveness of oral contraceptives can be negatively influenced when the following medications are taken concurrently (Nelson & Cwiak, 2011; WHO/RHR & CCP, 2011):

- *Anticonvulsants:* barbiturates, oxcarbazepine, phenytoin, phenobarbital, felbamate, carbamazepine, primidone, and topiramate
- *Systemic antifungals:* griseofulvin
- *Antituberculosis drugs:* rifampicin and rifabutin
- *Anti-HIV protease inhibitors:* nelfinavir, amprenavir

MEDICATION ALERT

Over-the-counter medications, as well as some herbal supplements (such as St. John's wort) can alter the effectiveness of COCs. Women should be asked about their use when COCs are being considered for contraception.

No strong pharmacokinetic evidence exists that shows a relation between broad-spectrum antibiotic use and altered hormonal levels among oral contraceptive users, although potential antibiotic interaction can occur. Studies on the incidence of breast cancer have not found a significant increase of breast cancer in women who use COCs (Nelson & Cwiak, 2011).

After discontinuing oral contraception, return to fertility usually happens quickly (Nelson & Cwiak, 2011). Many women ovulate the next month after stopping oral contraceptives, although it may take longer for ovulation to occur in some women. Women who discontinue oral contraception for a planned pregnancy commonly ask whether they should wait before attempting to conceive. Studies indicate that these infants have no greater chance of being born with any type of birth defect than do infants born to women in the general population, even if conception occurred in the first month after the medication was discontinued. Little evidence suggests that oral contraceptives cause postpill amenorrhea. Amenorrhea after oral contraceptive use is probably related to the woman's menstrual cycle before taking the pill (Nelson & Cwiak).

Nursing Interventions. Many different preparations of oral hormonal contraceptives are available. The nurse reviews the prescribing information in the package insert with the woman. Because of the wide variations, each woman must be clear about the unique dosage regimen for the preparation prescribed for her. Directions for care after missing one or two pills also vary. Figure 8-8 depicts an example of a simple way to manage missed pills.

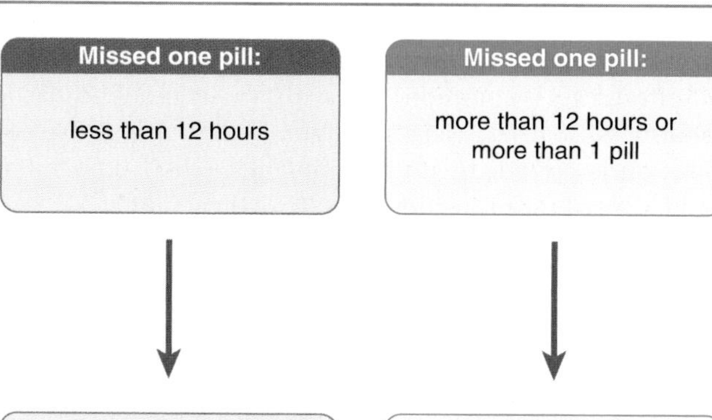

Take pill immediately and take rest of pack at the usual time

- No backup method needed
- No EC needed

Take pill as soon as remembered and continue rest of pack at usual time

- Use EC if had unprotected intercourse in the past 7 days
- Use condoms or abstinence for next 7 days

FIG 8-8 Simplified management for missed active contraceptive pills. *EC,* Emergency contraception. (Data from Nelson, A.L., & Cwiak, C. [2011]. In R. Hatcher, J. Trussell, A. Nelson, et al. [Eds.], *Contraceptive technology* [20th rev. ed.]. New York: Ardent Media.)

Withdrawal bleeding tends to be short and scanty when some combination pills are taken. A woman may see no fresh blood at all. A drop of blood or a brown smudge on a tampon or the underwear counts as a menstrual period.

Only about 67% of women who start taking oral contraceptives continue to take them after 1 year (Trussell, 2011). All women choosing to use oral contraceptives should be provided with a second method of birth control and be instructed in and comfortable with this backup method. Most women stop taking oral contraceptives for nonmedical reasons.

The nurse also reviews the signs of potential complications associated with the use of oral contraceptives (see Signs of Potential Complications). Oral contraceptives do not protect a woman against STIs or HIV. A barrier method such as condoms and spermicide should be used for protection.

SIGNS OF POTENTIAL COMPLICATIONS

Oral Contraceptives

Before oral contraceptives are prescribed and periodically throughout hormone therapy, alert the woman to stop taking the pill and to report any of the following symptoms to the health care provider immediately. Use the mnemonic ACHES to help remember this list:

A—Abdominal pain may indicate a problem with the liver or gallbladder.

C—Chest pain or shortness of breath may indicate possible clot problem within the lungs or heart.

H—Headaches (sudden or persistent) may be caused by cardiovascular accident or hypertension.

E—Eye problems may indicate vascular accident or hypertension.

S—Severe leg pain may indicate a thromboembolic process.

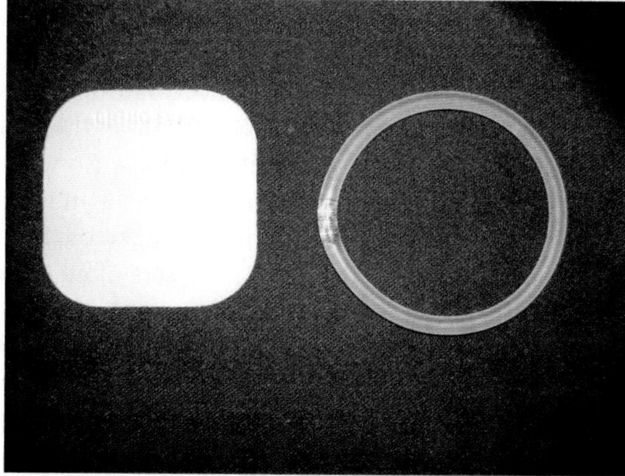

FIG 8-9 Hormonal contraceptive transdermal patch and vaginal ring. (Courtesy Dee Lowdermilk, Chapel Hill, NC.)

Oral Contraceptive 91-Day Regimen. Some women prefer to take COCs in 3-month cycles and have fewer menstrual periods. Levonorgestrel/ethinyl estradiol (Seasonale), FDA approved for extended cycle use, contains both estrogen and progestin and is taken in 3-month cycles of 12 weeks of active pills followed by 1 week of inactive pills. Menstrual periods occur during the thirteenth week of the cycle. There is no protection from STIs, and risks are similar to COCs. Other monophasic COCs may be prescribed for extended cycle use and must be taken on a daily schedule, regardless of the frequency of intercourse (Nelson & Cwiak, 2011; WHO/RHR & CCP, 2011).

Transdermal Contraceptive System. Available by prescription only, the contraceptive transdermal patch delivers continuous levels of norelgestromin (progestin) and ethinyl estradiol. The patch can be applied to intact skin of the upper outer arm, the upper torso (front and back, excluding the breasts), the lower abdomen, or the buttocks (Fig. 8-9). Application is on the same day once a week for 3 weeks, followed by a week without the patch. Withdrawal bleeding occurs during the "no-patch" week. Mechanism of action, efficacy, contraindications, skin reactions, and side effects are similar to those of COCs. The typical failure rate during the first year of use is less than 9% in women weighing less than 198 pounds (90 kg) (Trussell, 2011).

Vaginal Contraceptive Ring. Available only with a prescription, the vaginal contraceptive ring is a flexible ring (made of ethylene vinyl acetate copolymer) worn in the vagina to deliver continuous levels of etonogestrel (progestin) and ethinyl estradiol (see Fig. 8-9). One vaginal ring remains in the vagina for 3 weeks, followed by a week without the ring. The ring is inserted by the woman and does not have to be fitted. Some wearers may experience vaginitis, leukorrhea, and vaginal discomfort (Nanda, 2011). Withdrawal bleeding occurs during the "no-ring" week. If the woman or partner notices discomfort during coitus, the ring can be removed from the vagina, but only up to 3 hours to still be effective when reinserted. Mechanism of action, efficacy, contraindications, and side effects are similar to those of COCs. The typical failure rate of the vaginal contraceptive ring is reportedly less than 9% during the first year of use (Trussell, 2011).

Progestin-Only Contraceptives. Progestin-only methods impair fertility by inhibiting ovulation, thickening and decreasing the amount of cervical mucus, thinning the endometrium, and altering cilia in the uterine tubes (Fritz & Speroff, 2011d).

Oral Progestins (Minipill). The failure rate of progestin-only pills for typical users is about 1% to 10% in the first year of use (WHO/RHR & CCP, 2011). Effectiveness is increased if minipills are taken correctly. Because minipills contain such a low dose of progestin, the minipill must be taken at the same time every day (Fritz & Speroff, 2011d). Users often complain of irregular vaginal bleeding.

Injectable Progestins. Depot medroxyprogesterone acetate (DMPA or Depo-Provera), 150 mg, is given intramuscularly in the deltoid or the gluteus maximus muscle. A 21- to 23-gauge needle, 2.5 to 4 cm long, should be used. DMPA should be initiated during the first 5 days of the menstrual cycle and administered every 11 to 13 weeks. A subcutaneous injection is also available (Fritz & Speroff, 2011c).

MEDICATION ALERT

When administering an intramuscular injection of progestin (e.g., Depo-Provera), do not massage the site after the injection because this action can hasten the absorption and shorten the period of effectiveness.

Advantages of DMPA include a contraceptive effectiveness comparable to that of perfect use of COCs, long-lasting effects, requirement of injections only four times a year, and the improbability of lactation being impaired. Side effects at the end of a year include decreased bone mineral density, weight gain, irregular vaginal spotting, and breast changes (Bartz & Goldberg, 2011). Other disadvantages include no protection against STIs (including HIV). Return to fertility may be delayed as long as up to 18 months after discontinuing DMPA. The typical failure rate is 6% in the first year of use (Trussell, 2011).

MEDICATION ALERT

Women who use DMPA may lose significant bone mineral density with increasing duration of use. This bone loss can be regained within 2 to 4 years after discontinuation (Fritz & Speroff, 2011c). It is unknown if use of DMPA during adolescence or early adulthood, a critical period of bone accretion, will reduce peak bone mass and increase the risk of osteoporotic fracture in later life. Women who receive DMPA should be counseled about calcium intake and exercise (Bartz & Goldberg, 2011).

Implantable Progestins. Contraceptive implants consist of one or more nonbiodegradable flexible tubes or rods that are inserted under the skin of a woman's arm. These implants contain a progestin hormone and are effective for contraception for at least 3 years. They must be removed at the end of the recommended time. The FDA has approved two devices for use in the United States: a two-rod subdermal levonorgestrel implant (Jadelle) and a single-rod etonogestrel implant (Implanon, Nexplanon) that is effective for up to 3 years and is the only implant available in the United States. Implants will prevent some, but not all, ovulatory cycles and will thicken cervical mucus. Other advantages include reversibility and long-term continuous contraception that is not related to frequency of coitus. Irregular menstrual bleeding is the most common side effect. Less common side effects include headaches, nervousness, nausea, skin changes, and vertigo. No STI protection is provided with the implant method, so condoms should be used for protection (Fritz & Speroff, 2011c).

Emergency Contraception. Emergency contraception (EC) is available in more than 100 countries, and in about one third of these countries it is available without a prescription. In the United States, Plan B has been the only EC method available without a prescription and only in limited pharmacies and clinics in pharmacy access states. States where legislation has been passed to allow this practice include Alaska, Arkansas, California, Colorado, Connecticut, Hawaii, Illinois, Maine, Massachusetts, Minnesota, New Hampshire, New Jersey, New Mexico, New York, Oregon, South Carolina, Texas, Utah, Vermont, Washington, and Wisconsin and the District of Columbia. These states have enacted legislation requiring hospitals or health care facilities to provide information about and/or initiate emergency contraception therapy to women who have been sexually assaulted (National Conference of State Legislators, 2012).

Plan B One-Step (a single 1500-mcg levonorgestrel pill) replaced the two-tablet Plan B in 2009. At the same time a generic form of Plan B was authorized for use. The following year, the FDA approved 30-mg ulipristal acetate, marketed as ella, for use as emergency contraception. On June 20, 2013, the federal government announced that Plan B One-Step can be sold over the counter in the family planning aisle of pharmacies. Anyone, regardless of age or gender, is allowed to purchase this morning-after pill at the local pharmacy (FDA, 2013). Other options that the FDA has determined to be safe for emergency contraception include high doses of oral estrogen or COCs (ECPs) and insertion of a copper IUD (Trussell & Schwarz, 2011). These options continue to be available by prescription only.

Emergency contraception should be taken by a woman as soon as possible but within 72 hours of unprotected intercourse, or birth control mishap (broken condom, dislodged ring or cervical cap, missed oral contraceptive pills, late for injection, and so on) to prevent unintended pregnancy (Trussell & Schwartz, 2011; WHO/RHR & CCP, 2011). If taken before ovulation, emergency contraception prevents ovulation by inhibiting follicular development. If taken after ovulation occurs, there is little effect on ovarian hormone production or the endometrium. Oral medication regimens with ECPs are presented in Table 8-2. To minimize the side effect of nausea that occurs with high doses of estrogen and progestin, the woman can be advised to take an over-the-counter antiemetic 1 hour before each dose. Women with contraindications for estrogen use should use progestin-only emergency contraception. No medical contraindications for emergency contraception exist, except pregnancy and undiagnosed abnormal vaginal bleeding. If the woman does not begin menstruation within 21 days after taking the pills, she should be evaluated for pregnancy. Emergency contraception is ineffective if the woman is pregnant because the pills do not disturb an implanted pregnancy. Risk of pregnancy is reduced by as much as 75% (estrogen-progestin) and 89% (progestin only) if the woman takes ECPs (Trussell & Schwarz, 2011).

MEDICATION ALERT

Emergency contraception will not protect a woman against pregnancy if she engages in unprotected intercourse in the days or weeks that follow treatment. Because ingestion of emergency contraceptive pills may delay ovulation, caution the woman that she needs to establish a reliable form of birth control in order to prevent unintended pregnancy (Trussell & Schwarz, 2011). Information about emergency contraception method options and access to providers is available at www.NOT-2-LATE.com or by calling 1-888-NOT-2-LATE.

IUDs containing copper (see later discussion) provide another emergency contraception option. The IUD should be inserted within 5 days of unprotected intercourse (Trussell & Schwarz, 2011). This method is suggested only for women who wish to have the benefit of long-term contraception. The risk of pregnancy is reduced by as much as 99% with emergency insertion of the copper-releasing IUD.

TABLE 8-2 Oral Emergency Contraceptives

BRAND NAMES	DOSE (WITHIN 120 hr)
Antiprogestin	**One Dose Only**
ella	1 white pill
Progestin-Only Levonorgestrel 1.5 mg/Dose	**One Dose Only**
Plan B One-Step	1 white pill
My Way	1 white pill
Next Choice One Dose	1 peach pill
Combined Progestin and Estrogen Pills (100 to 120 mcg Ethyl Estradiol and Levonorgestrel 0.50 to 0.60 mg/Dose)*	**Take 2 Doses 12 Hours Apart**
Ogestrel	2 white pills
Cryselle	4 white pills
Jolessa	4 pink pills
Portia	4 pink pills
Seasonale	4 pink pills
Altavera	4 peach pills
Lo/Ovral	4 white pills
Amethia	4 white pills
Low-Ogestrel	4 white pills
Enpresse	4 orange pills
Nordette	4 light orange pills
Levora	4 white pills
Quasense	4 white pills
Trivora	4 yellow pills
Seasonique	4 light blue-green pills
Camrese	4 light blue-green pills
Lessina	5 pink pills
CamreseLo	5 orange pills
Aviane	5 orange pills
LoSeasonique	5 orange pills
Syronx	5 white pills
Lutera	5 white pills
Lybel	6 yellow pills
Amethyst	6 white pills

*Antinausea medications needed for any of the combined oral contraceptives.
Data from American College of Obstetricians and Gynecologists. (2010). Emergency contraception: ACOG Practice Bulletin No. 112. *Obstetrics and Gynecology, 115*(5), 1100-1109; Office of Population Research and Association of Reproductive Health Professionals. (2013). *Types of emergency contraception.* Available at http://ec.princeton.edu.

Contraceptive counseling should be provided to all women requesting emergency contraception, including a discussion of modification of risky sexual behaviors to prevent STIs and unwanted pregnancy.

Intrauterine Devices

An IUD is a small T-shaped device with bendable arms for insertion through the cervix (Fig. 8-10). Once the trained health care provider inserts the IUD against the uterine fundus, the arms open near the fallopian tubes to maintain position of the device and to adversely affect the sperm motility and irritate the lining of the uterus. Two strings hang from the base of the stem through the cervix and protrude into the vagina for the woman to feel for assurance that the device has not been dislodged (Dean & Schwarz, 2011). The woman should have had a negative pregnancy test, treatment for dysplasia if present, cervical cultures to rule out STIs, and a consent form signed before IUD insertion. Advantages to choosing this method of contraception include long-term protection from pregnancy and immediate return to fertility when removed. Disadvantages include increased risk of pelvic inflammatory disease (PID) shortly after placement, unintentional expulsion of the device, infection, and possible uterine perforation. IUDs offer no protection against HIV or other STIs. Therefore, women who are in mutually monogamous relationships are the best candidates for this device.

There are three FDA-approved IUDs: the ParaGard Copper T 380A and the hormonal intrauterine systems Mirena and Skyla. The ParaGard Copper T 380A is made of radiopaque polyethylene and fine solid copper and is approved for 10 years of use. The copper primarily serves as a spermicide and inflames the endometrium, preventing fertilization (Dean & Schwarz, 2011). Sometimes women experience more bleeding and cramping within the first year after insertion, but nonsteroidal, antiinflammatory drugs (NSAIDs) can be taken for pain relief. The typical failure rate in the first year of use of the copper IUD is less than 1% (Trussell, 2011).

Mirena and Skyla release levonorgestrel from their vertical reservoirs. Effective for up to 5 years for Mirena and 3 years for Skyla, they impair sperm motility, thicken cervical mucus, decrease the lining of the uterus, and have some anovulatory effects (Dean & Schwarz, 2011; www.skyla-us.com). Uterine cramping and bleeding are usually decreased with these devices, although irregular spotting is common in the first few months following insertion. The typical failure rate in the first year of use is less than 1% (Skyla-US, 2013; Trussell, 2011).

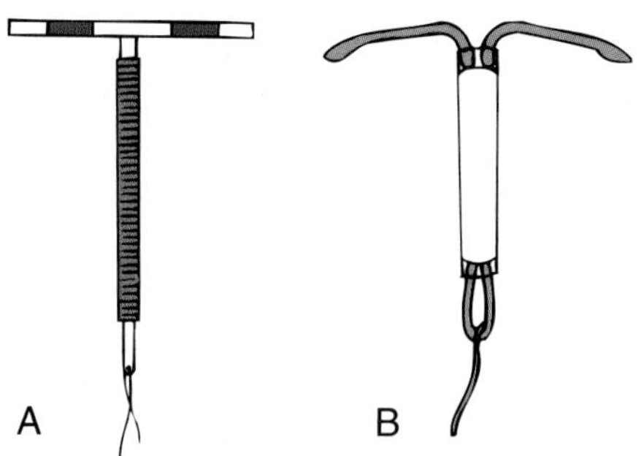

FIG 8-10 Intrauterine devices (IUDs). **A**, Copper T 380A. **B**, Levonorgestrel-releasing IUD.

EVIDENCE-BASED PRACTICE BOX

Emergency Contraception and Obesity

Ask the Question

What is the best emergency contraception for overweight and obese women?

Search for the Evidence

Search Strategies English language research–based publications since 2011 on emergency contraception, overweight, and obesity were included.

Databases Used Cochrane Collaborative Database, National Guideline Clearinghouse (AHRQ), CINAHL, PubMed, UpToDate, and the professional websites for ACOG and AWHONN

Critical Appraisal of the Evidence

One out of nine sexually active women in the United States has used a form of emergency contraception (EC) during their reproductive years. About half of these used EC because their primary method failed (Daniels, Jones, & Abma, 2013). Three options for emergency contraception are:

- Levonorgestrel (LNG-EC), a progestin commonly used in oral contraceptives, causes a delay in ovulation when taken at a higher dose (e.g., Plan B). It is most effective when taken as soon as possible after unprotected intercourse (UPIC), and can still prevent pregnancy when taken up to 96 hours.
- Ulipristal acetate (UPA) is a progesterone receptor modulator, which interrupts the action of endogenous progesterone that is necessary to ovulate and maintain pregnancy (e.g., ella). It can delay ovulation when taken up to 120 hours after intercourse. Metaanalysis of outcomes of women in the United States, United Kingdom, and Ireland have revealed that UPA is more effective than LNG-EC, particularly in obese women (Glasier, Cameron, Blithe, et al., 2011).
- Both oral ECs cause thinning of the endometrium, but research has not established whether this inhibits implantation (Moreau & Trussell, 2012). Neither LNG-EC nor UPA will disrupt an already implanted pregnancy.
- Copper intrauterine device (Cu IUD, Paragard) insertion within 5 days post intercourse disrupts uterine readiness for implantation. It is the only method of the three that provides ongoing contraception. It requires a skilled health care provider for insertion. Being overweight and obese negatively affects the ability of oral EC to prevent pregnancy.
- The risk for pregnancy after taking oral EC goes up 1.5 times for overweight (body mass index [BMI] 26-29) women and 2 to 4 times for obese (BMI 30+) women, over normal- or low-weight women (Glasier et al., 2013; Moreau & Trussell, 2012).
- In absolute weight, LNG-EG was no longer effective at preventing pregnancy at 154 pounds (70 kg), and UPA became no longer effective at 194 pounds (88 kg) (Glasier et al., 2011).

Apply the Evidence: Nursing Implications

- Oral EC is most effective at preventing pregnancy when taken early. A systematic analysis of 17 studies reveals that having a supply on hand results in 2 to 7 times greater use of EC, although pregnancy reduction was not demonstrated (Rodrigues, Curtis, Gaffield, et al., 2013).
- Male partners tend to know and approve of emergency contraception, although only a minority discuss it with their partners (Marcell, Waks, Rutlow, et al., 2012). Involving partners in any education may provide support and uptake of EC.
- The first choice EC for obese women would be a Cu IUD insertion, when available and acceptable to the women. Women should be informed that it acts to prevent implantation. If oral EC is preferred, UPA is a better choice than LNG-EC.
- Because oral EC merely delays ovulation, the other most significant factor for pregnancy is subsequent UPIC during the rest of that cycle (Glasier et al., 2011; Moreau & Trussell, 2013). Women should be provided with highly reliable contraception immediately, and cautioned that EC offers no subsequent protection against pregnancy.

Quality and Safety Competencies: Evidence-Based Practice (EBP)*

Knowledge

Describe how the strength and relevance of available evidence influences the choice of interventions in provision of client-centered care.

Use of high-level evidence to provide women in need of emergency contraception with individualized care

Skills

Locate evidence reports related to clinical practice topics and guidelines.

Relevant systematic reviews and professional guidelines provide recommendations for improving pregnancy prevention outcomes.

Attitudes

Value the concept of EBP as integral to determining best clinical practices.

EBP guides practice and fosters client confidence and efficacy.

References

Daniels, K., Jones, J., & Abma, J. (2013). Use of emergency contraception among women aged 15-44: United States, 2006-2010. *NCHS Data Brief, 2013*(112). Available at www.cdc.gov/nchs/data/databriefs/db112.pdf.

Glasier, A., Cameron, S. T., Blithe, D., et al. (2011). Can we identify women at risk of pregnancy despite using emergency contraception? Data from randomized trials of ulipristal acetate and levonorgestrel. *Contraception, 84*(4), 363–367.

Marcel, A. V., Waks, A. B., Rutlow, L., et al. (2012). What do we know about males and emergency contraception? A synthesis of literature. *Perspectives on Sexual and Reproductive Health, 44*(3), 184–193.

Moreau, C., & Trussell, J. (2012). Results from pooled phase III studies of ulipristal acetate for emergency contraception. *Contraception, 86*(6), 673–680.

Rodriguez, M. I., Curtis, K. M., Gaffield, M. L., et al. (2013). Advance supply of emergency contraception: A systematic review. *Contraception, 87*(5), 590–601.

Pat Mahaffee Gingrich

*Adapted from QSEN at www.qsen.org.

Nursing Interventions. The woman should be taught to check for the presence of the IUD strings after menstruation to rule out expulsion of the device. If pregnancy occurs with the IUD in place, an ultrasound should confirm that it is not ectopic. Early removal of the IUD helps decrease the risk of spontaneous miscarriage or preterm labor (Dean & Schwarz, 2011). In some women who are allergic to copper, a rash develops, necessitating the removal of the copper-bearing IUD. Signs of potential complications to be taught to the woman are listed in the Signs of Potential Complications box.

SIGNS OF POTENTIAL COMPLICATIONS

Intrauterine Devices (IUDs)

Signs of potential complications related to IUDs can be remembered in the following manner:

P—Period late, abnormal spotting or bleeding
A—Abdominal pain, pain with intercourse
I—Infection exposure, abnormal vaginal discharge
N—Not feeling well, fever, or chills
S—String missing; shorter or longer

Data from Zieman, M., Hatcher, R., Cwiak, C., et al. (2012). *A pocket guide to managing contraception.* Tiger, GA: Bridging the Gap Foundation.

Sterilization

Sterilization refers to surgical procedures intended to render a person infertile. Most procedures involve the occlusion of the passageways for the ova and sperm (Fig. 8-11). For the woman, the oviducts (uterine tubes) are occluded; for the man, the sperm ducts (vas deferens) are occluded. Only surgical removal of the ovaries (oophorectomy) or uterus (hysterectomy) or both will result in absolute sterility for the woman. All other sterilization procedures have a small but definite failure rate; that is, pregnancy may result.

Female Sterilization. Female sterilization (bilateral tubal ligation [BTL]) may be done immediately after childbirth (within 24 to 48 hours), concomitant with induced abortion, or as an interval procedure (during any phase of the menstrual cycle). If sterilization is performed as an interval procedure, the health care provider must be certain that the woman is not pregnant. Half of all female sterilization procedures are performed immediately after a pregnancy (Roncari & Hou, 2011). Sterilization procedures can be safely done on an outpatient basis.

Tubal Occlusion. A laparoscopic approach or a minilaparotomy can be used for tubal ligation (Fig. 8-12), tubal electrocoagulation, or the application of bands or clips. Electrocoagulation and ligation are considered to be permanent methods. Use of the bands or clips has the theoretic advantage of possible removal and return of tubal patency.

For the minilaparotomy, the woman is admitted the morning of surgery, having received nothing by mouth since midnight. Preoperative sedation is given. The procedure can be carried out with a local anesthetic, but a regional or general anesthetic can also be used. A small incision is made in the abdominal wall below the umbilicus. The woman may experience sensations of tugging, but no pain, and the operation is completed within 20 minutes. She may be discharged several hours later if she has recovered from anesthesia or next day if done postpartum. Any abdominal discomfort usually can be controlled with a mild analgesic (e.g., acetaminophen). Within days the scar is almost invisible (see Teaching for Self-Management). As with any surgery, there is always a possibility of complications of anesthesia, infection, hemorrhage, and trauma to other organs.

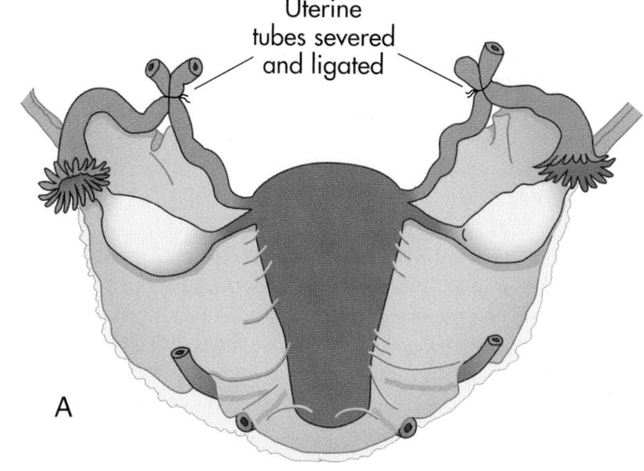

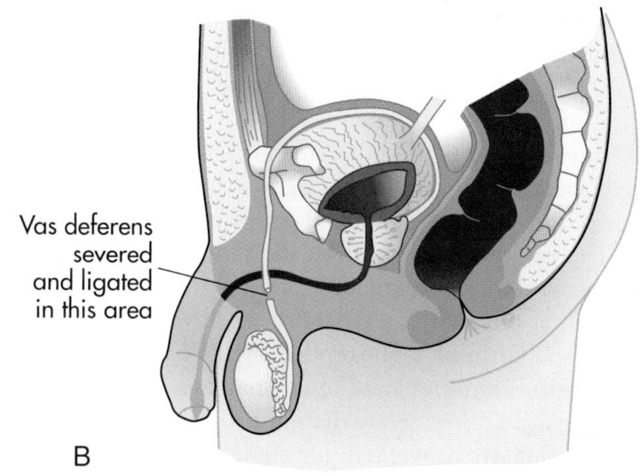

FIG 8-11 Sterilization. **A,** Uterine tubes severed and ligated (tubal ligation). **B,** Sperm duct severed and ligated (vasectomy).

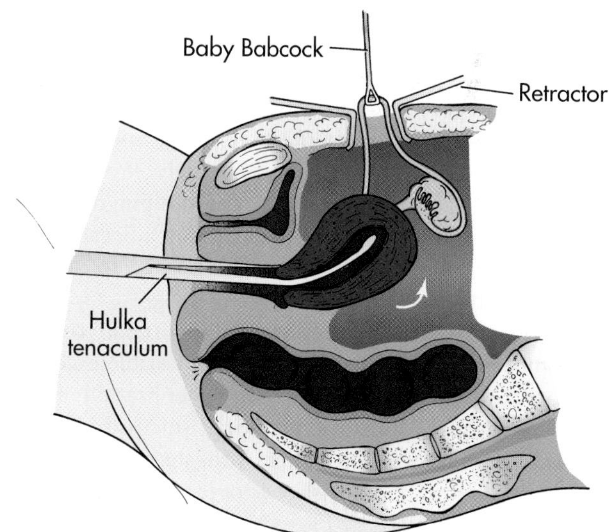

FIG 8-12 Use of minilaparotomy to gain access to uterine tubes for occlusion procedures. Tenaculum is used to lift uterus *(arrow)* toward incision.

TEACHING FOR SELF-MANAGEMENT

What to Expect After Tubal Ligation

- You should expect no change in hormones and their influence.
- Your menstrual period will be about the same as before the sterilization.
- You may feel pain at ovulation.
- The ovum disintegrates within the abdominal cavity.
- It is highly unlikely that you will become pregnant.
- You should not have a change in sexual functioning; you may enjoy sexual relations more because you will not be concerned about becoming pregnant.
- Sterilization offers no protection against sexually transmitted infections (STIs); therefore, you may need to use condoms.

Transcervical Sterilization. Hysteroscopic techniques can be used to inject occlusion agents into the uterine tubes. One FDA-approved device is the Essure system, an interval sterilization method (not intended for the postpartum period). The Essure device contains polyester fibers within a metal coil. A trained health care professional inserts a small catheter holding the device through the vagina and cervix and into the fallopian tubes. The device works by stimulating the woman's own scar tissue formation to occlude the uterine tubes and prevent conception (Fritz & Speroff, 2011b). An advantage is that the nonhormonal form of contraception can be inserted during an office procedure without anesthesia. Analgesia is recommended to decrease mild to moderate discomfort associated with tubal spasm. Particularly convenient for obese women or those with abdominal adhesions, the transcervical approach eliminates the need for abdominal surgery. Because the procedure is not immediately effective, it is essential that the woman and her partner use another form of contraception until tubal blockage is proven. It may take up to 3 months for tubal occlusion to fully occur, and success must be confirmed by hysterosalpingogram. Other disadvantages include possible expulsion and perforation. Providers do become more effective at placing the device correctly with experience, and approximately 96% of women have occluded tubes confirmed by hysterosalpingogram. The 1-year pregnancy rate is 1.1% (Fritz & Speroff). Because Essure is relatively new, more research may be needed to determine potential side effects.

Tubal Reconstruction. Restoration of tubal continuity (reanastomosis) and function is technically feasible except after laparoscopic tubal electrocoagulation. Sterilization reversal, however, is costly, difficult (requiring microsurgery), and uncertain. The success rate varies with the extent of tubal destruction and removal. The risk of ectopic pregnancy after tubal reanastomosis is increased by 1% to 7% (Roncari & Hou, 2011).

Male Sterilization. *Vasectomy* is the sealing, tying, or cutting of a man's vas deferens so that the sperm cannot travel from the testes to the penis (Roncari & Hou, 2011). It is considered the easiest and most commonly used operation for male sterilization. Vasectomy can be carried out with local anesthesia on an outpatient basis. Pain, bleeding, infection, and other postsurgical complications are considered the disadvantages to the surgical procedure. It is considered a permanent method of sterilization because reversal is generally unsuccessful.

Two methods are used for scrotal entry: conventional (scalpel incision) and no-scalpel (small puncture) vasectomy. The surgeon identifies and immobilizes the vas deferens through the scrotum. Then the vas is ligated or cauterized (see Fig. 8-11, *B*). Surgeons vary in their techniques to occlude the vas deferens: ligation with sutures, division, cautery, application of clips, excision of a segment of the vas, fascial interposition, or some combination of these methods (Roncari & Hou, 2011).

The man is instructed in self-care to promote a safe return to routine activities. To reduce swelling and relieve discomfort, ice packs are applied to the scrotum intermittently for a few hours after surgery. A scrotal support may be applied to decrease discomfort. Moderate inactivity for about 2 days is advisable because of local scrotal tenderness. The skin suture can be removed 5 to 7 days after surgery. Sexual intercourse may be resumed as desired; however, sterility is not immediate. Some sperm will remain in the proximal portions of the sperm ducts after vasectomy. One week to several months are required to clear the ducts of sperm; therefore, some form of contraception is needed until the sperm count in the ejaculate on two consecutive tests is down to zero (Roncari & Hou, 2011).

Vasectomy has no effect on potency (ability to achieve and maintain erection) or volume of ejaculate. Endocrine production of testosterone continues, so secondary sex characteristics are not affected. Sperm production continues, but sperm are unable to leave the epididymis and are lysed by the immune system. Less common are painful granulomas from accumulation of sperm (Roncari & Hou, 2011).

Complications after bilateral vasectomy are uncommon and usually not serious. They include bleeding (usually external), suture reaction, and reaction to anesthetic agent. The failure rate for male sterilization is 0.15% (Trussell, 2011).

Tubal Reconstruction. Microsurgery to reanastomose (restoration of tubal continuity) the sperm ducts can be accomplished successfully in more than 90% of cases (i.e., sperm in the ejaculate); however, the fertility rate varies widely from 38% to 89% (Roncari & Hou, 2011). The rate of success decreases as the time since the procedure increases. The vasectomy may result in permanent changes in the testes that leave men unable to father children. The changes are those ordinarily seen only in older adults (e.g., interstitial fibrosis [scar tissue between the seminiferous tubules]). In some men, antibodies develop against their own sperm (autoimmunization). The role of antisperm antibodies in fertility after vasectomy reversal has not been completely determined. Additional research is needed to explore a possible link between vasectomy and prostate cancer.

Laws and Regulations. All states have strict regulations for informed consent. Many states permit voluntary sterilization of any mature, rational woman without reference to her marital or pregnancy status. Although the partner's consent is not required by law, the man or woman is encouraged to discuss the situation with the partner, and health care providers may request the partner's consent. Sterilization of minors or mentally incompetent individuals is restricted by most states and often requires the approval of a board of eugenicists or other court-appointed individuals (see Legal Tip).

LEGAL TIP: Sterilization

If federal funds are used for female or male sterilization:

- The person must be age 21 years or older.
- Informed consent must include an explanation of the risks, benefits, and alternatives; a statement that describes sterilization as a permanent, irreversible method of birth control; and a statement that mandates a 30-day waiting period between giving consent and the sterilization.
- Informed consent must be in the man's or woman's native language, or an interpreter must be provided to read the consent form to the man or woman.

Nursing Interventions. The nurse plays an important role in assisting people with decision making so all requirements for informed consent are met. The nurse also provides information about alternatives to sterilization, such as contraception. The nurse acts as a "sounding board" for people who are exploring the possibility of choosing sterilization and their feelings about and motivation for this choice. The nurse records this information, which may be the basis for referral to a family planning clinic, a psychiatric social worker, or another professional health care provider.

Information must be given about what is entailed in various procedures, how much discomfort or pain can be expected, and what type of care is needed. Many individuals fear sterilization procedures because of the imagined effect on their sex life. They need reassurance concerning the hormonal and psychologic basis for sexual function and that uterine tube occlusion or vasectomy has no biologic sequelae in terms of sexual adequacy (Roncari & Hou, 2011). Preoperative care consists of health assessment, which includes a psychologic assessment, physical examination, and laboratory tests. The nurse assists with the health assessment, answers questions, and confirms the client's understanding of printed instructions (e.g., nothing by mouth after midnight). Ambivalence and extreme fear of the procedure are reported to the physician.

Postoperative care depends on the procedure performed (e.g., laparoscopy, laparotomy for tubal occlusion, or vasectomy). General care includes recovery after anesthesia, monitoring of vital signs and fluid and electrolyte balance (intake and output, laboratory values), prevention of or early identification and treatment for infection or hemorrhage, control of discomfort, and assessment of emotional response to the procedure and recovery.

Discharge planning depends on the type of procedure performed. In general, the client is given written instructions about observing for and reporting symptoms and signs of complications, the type of recovery to be expected, and the date and time for a follow-up appointment.

Breastfeeding: Lactational Amenorrhea Method

The *lactational amenorrhea method (LAM)* can be a highly effective, *temporary* method of birth control. It is more popular in underdeveloped countries and traditional societies, where breastfeeding is used to prolong birth intervals. The method has seen limited use in the United States because most American women do not establish breastfeeding patterns that provide maximum protection against pregnancy (Kennedy & Trussell, 2011).

When the infant suckles at the mother's breast, a surge of prolactin hormone is released, which inhibits estrogen production and suppresses ovulation and the return of menses. LAM works best if the mother is exclusively or almost exclusively breastfeeding, if the woman has not had a menstrual flow since giving birth, and if the infant is younger than 6 months of age. Effectiveness is enhanced by frequent feedings at intervals of less than 4 hours during the day and no more than 6 hours during the night, long duration of each feeding, and no bottle supplementation or limited supplementation by spoon or cup. The woman should be counseled that disruption of the breastfeeding pattern or supplementation can increase the risk of pregnancy. The typical failure rate is 1% to 2% (Kennedy & Trussell, 2011).

Future Trends

Contraceptive options are more limited in the United States and Canada than in some other industrialized countries. Lack of funding for research, governmental regulations, conflicting values about contraception, and high costs of liability coverage for contraception have been cited as blocks to new and improved methods. Existing methods of contraception are being improved, however, and a variety of new methods are being developed.

Lower-dose COCs (15 mcg of ethinyl estradiol) are available in Europe. Female barrier methods (new female condoms, client-fitted diaphragms, and new vaginal sponges) are being tested. Vaginal delivery systems including progestin-only vaginal rings and progesterone daily suppositories are under investigation. Two new IUDs and spermicidal microbicides are being evaluated. Male hormonal methods are also being investigated, including hormonal injections (testosterone and progestin), targeted gene therapy, gonadotropin-releasing hormone antagonists, antisperm compounds, vas occlusion, vas muscle inhibitor, botanicals, immunologic methods, ultrasonic massage, internal/external heat, and contraceptive vaccines (Male Contraceptives.org, 2011; Schwartz & Gabelnick, 2011).

INDUCED ABORTION

Induced abortion is the purposeful interruption of a pregnancy before 20 weeks of gestation. (Spontaneous abortion or miscarriage is discussed in Chapter 28). If the abortion is performed at the woman's request, the term elective abortion is usually used; if performed for reasons of maternal or fetal health or disease, the term therapeutic abortion applies. Many factors contribute to a woman's decision to have an abortion. Indications include: (1) preservation of the life or health of the mother, (2) genetic disorders of the fetus, (3) rape or incest, and (4) the pregnant woman's request. The control of birth, dealing as it does with human sexuality and the question of life and death, is one of the most emotional components of health care. It has been the most controversial social issue in the last half of the 20th century and the beginning of the 21st century. Regulations exist to protect the mother from the complications of abortion.

Abortion is regulated in most countries, including the United States. Before 1970 legal abortion was not widely available in the United States. However, in January 1973, the U.S.

Supreme Court set aside previous antiabortion laws and legalized abortion as a result of the Roe versus Wade decision (U.S. Reports, 1973). This decision established a trimester approach to abortion. In the first trimester, abortion is permissible, the decision is between the woman and her health care provider, and a state has little right to interfere (Paul & Stein, 2011). In the second trimester, abortion is left to the discretion of the individual states to regulate procedures as long as they are reasonably related to the woman's health. In the third trimester, abortions may be limited or even prohibited by state regulation unless the restriction interferes with the life or health of the pregnant woman (Paul & Stein, 2011).

Currently 39 states legislate that abortion be performed by a licensed physician. Nurse practitioners can perform abortions (if the practice is within their scope of practice) in the states of California, Montana, Vermont, New Hampshire, and Rhode Island. Congress has legislated that Medicaid funds can only be used to pay for abortion when a woman's life is endangered. States vary on the financing of abortion, with 17 states using their own funds to pay for abortions, depending on the circumstances surrounding the procedure. States also vary regarding parental notification if a minor is requesting an abortion and/or consent regarding abortion, with 37 states providing legislation for some type parental involvement in the abortion of a fetus. Individual health care providers may refuse to participate in abortion in 46 states (Guttmacher Institute, 2013b).

In 1992, the U.S. Supreme Court made another landmark ruling, this time allowing states to restrict early abortion services as long as the restrictions did not place an "undue burden" on the woman's ability to choose abortion. Since then many bills have been introduced to limit access and funds for women seeking abortion. The Supreme Court will again play a major role in deciding the future of abortions as states introduce bills to limit or ban access to abortions.

LEGAL TIP: Induced Abortion

It is important for nurses to know the laws regarding abortion in their country or state of practice before they offer abortion counseling or nursing care to a woman choosing an abortion. Many states enforce a mandatory delay or state-directed counseling before a woman may legally obtain an abortion.

Incidence

In 2008 in the United States there were approximately 6.5 million pregnancies, and approximately 19% of these pregnancies were terminated (Sedgh, Singh, Shah, et al., 2012). The numbers of abortions in the United States have decreased from 1.31 million abortions in 2000 to 1.21 million abortions in 2008 to 784,507 in 2009 (Guttmacher Institute, 2013a; Pazol, Andreea, Creanga, et al., 2012). Most terminations were performed in women who were unmarried (84%). Non-Hispanic Causcasian women comprised 36% of those who experienced elective abortion; non-Hispanic African American women comprised 30% of those who experienced elective abortions, Hispanic women comprised 25%, and women of other races accounted for 9% of abortions (Guttmacher Institute). Most abortions occur in women who already have children, and abortion rates tend to be higher in women whose income is below the poverty level.

The Decision to Have an Abortion

Rates of biologic complications after abortions such as ectopic pregnancy, infection, or hemorrhage tend to be low if the woman aborts during the first trimester. Psychologic sequelae of induced abortion are uncommon and may be related to circumstances and support systems surrounding the pregnant woman, such as the attitudes reflected by friends, family, and health care workers. The woman facing an abortion is pregnant and will exhibit the emotional responses shared by all pregnant women, including the possibility of depression.

Nurses and other health care providers often struggle with the same values and moral convictions as those of the pregnant woman. The conflicts and doubts of the nurse can be readily communicated to women who are already anxious. Regardless of personal views on abortion, nurses who provide care to women seeking abortion have an ethical responsibility to counsel women about their options and to make appropriate referrals.

The Association of Women's Health, Obstetric and Neonatal Nurses (AWHONN, 2009) continues to support a nurse's right to choose whether to participate in abortion procedures in keeping with his or her "personal, moral, ethical, or religious beliefs." AWHONN also advocates that "nurses have a professional obligation to inform their employers, at the time of employment, of any attitudes and beliefs that may interfere with essential job functions."

LEGAL TIP: Institutional Policies for Nurses' Rights and Responsibilities Related to Abortion

Nurses' rights and responsibilities related to caring for abortion clients should be protected through policies that describe how the institution will accommodate the nurse's ethical or moral beliefs and what the nurse should do to avoid client abandonment in such situations. Nurses should know what policies are in place in their institutions and encourage such policies to be written.

CARE MANAGEMENT

A thorough assessment is conducted through history, physical examination, and laboratory tests. The length of pregnancy and the condition of the woman must be determined to select the appropriate type of abortion procedure. An ultrasound examination should be performed before a second-trimester abortion is done. If the woman is Rh negative, she is a candidate for prophylaxis against Rh isoimmunization. She should receive $Rh_o(D)$ immune globulin within 72 hours after the abortion if she is D negative and if Coombs' test results are negative (if the woman is unsensitized or isoimmunization has not developed).

The woman's understanding of alternatives, the types of abortions, and expected recovery are assessed. Misinformation and gaps in knowledge are identified and corrected. The record is reviewed for the signed informed consent, and the woman's understanding is verified. General preoperative, operative, and postoperative assessments are performed.

Analysis of data leads to identification of the appropriate nursing diagnoses for the woman undergoing elective abortion. Potential nursing diagnoses are listed in Box 8-4.

BOX 8-4 Selected Nursing Diagnoses for Women Having Elective Abortion

- *Decisional Conflict* related to
  - Value system
- *Fear* related to
  - Abortion procedure
  - Potential complications
  - Implications for future pregnancies
  - What others might think
- *Anticipatory Grieving* related to
  - Distress at loss or feelings of guilt
- *Risk for Infection* related to
  - Effects of the procedure
  - Lack of understanding of preoperative and postoperative self-care
- *Acute Pain* related to
  - Effects of the procedure or postoperative events

Counseling about abortion includes help for the woman in identifying how she perceives the pregnancy, information about the choices available (i.e., having an abortion or carrying the pregnancy to term and then either keeping the infant or placing the baby for adoption), and information about the types of abortion procedures.

CLINICAL REASONING CASE STUDY

Termination of Pregnancy

Angelica is a 19-year-old single client whose contraceptive method failed. An examination determines that she is 6 weeks pregnant and is seeking termination of the pregnancy. She has many questions for the nurse in the family planning clinic: Which procedure is most likely to be chosen at this gestation? What are the risks associated with the procedure? Should her boyfriend be involved in the decision to terminate the pregnancy?

1. Evidence—Is there sufficient evidence to draw conclusions about what information the nurse should provide Angelica?
2. Assumptions—What assumptions can be made about Angelica's reaction to termination of the pregnancy?
   a. Psychologic/emotional reaction and sequelae
   b. Physical response
   c. Future childbearing
   d. Relationship with her boyfriend
3. What implications and priorities for nursing care can be drawn at this time?
4. Does the evidence objectively support your conclusion?

First-Trimester Abortion

Methods for performing early abortion (less than 9 weeks of gestation) include surgical (aspiration) and medical methods (mifepristone with misoprostol and methotrexate with misoprostol).

Aspiration

Aspiration (vacuum or suction curettage) is the most common procedure in the first trimester, with slightly more than 74% of all procedures being performed by this method (Pazol et al., 2012). Aspiration abortion is usually performed under local anesthesia in the physician's office, the clinic, or the hospital. The suction procedure for performing an early elective abortion (ideal time is 8 to 12 weeks since the last menstrual period) usually requires less than 5 minutes.

A bimanual examination is done before the procedure to assess uterine size and position. A speculum is inserted and the cervix is anesthetized with a local anesthetic agent. The cervix is dilated if necessary and a cannula connected to suction is inserted into the uterine cavity. The products of conception are evacuated from the uterus.

During the procedure the nurse or physician keeps the woman informed about what to expect next (e.g., menstrual-like cramping, sounds of the suction machine). The nurse assesses the woman's vital signs. The aspirated uterine contents must be carefully inspected to ascertain whether all fetal parts and adequate placental tissue have been evacuated. After the abortion the woman rests on the table until she is ready to stand. She remains in the recovery area or waiting room for 1 to 3 hours for detection of excessive cramping or bleeding; then she is discharged.

Bleeding after the operation is normally about the equivalent of a heavy menstrual period, and cramps are rarely severe. Excessive vaginal bleeding and infection, such as endometritis or salpingitis, are the most common complications of elective abortion. Retained products of conception are the primary cause of vaginal bleeding. Evacuation of the uterus, uterine massage, and administration of oxytocin or methylergonovine (Methergine) or both may be necessary. Prophylactic antibiotics to decrease the risk of infection are commonly prescribed (Paul & Stein, 2011). Postabortion pain may be relieved with NSAIDs such as ibuprofen.

Postabortion instructions differ among health care providers (e.g., tampons should not be used for at least 3 days or should be avoided for up to 3 weeks, and resumption of sexual intercourse may be permitted within 1 week or discouraged for 2 weeks). The woman may shower daily. Instruction is given to watch for excessive bleeding and other signs of complications and to avoid douches of any type.

SAFETY ALERT

The woman who has an induced abortion should be given clear instructions to return immediately to the health care facility or emergency department for any of the following symptoms:

- Fever greater than 38° C (100.4° F)
- Chills
- Bleeding greater than two saturated pads in 2 hours or heavy bleeding lasting a few days
- Foul-smelling vaginal discharge
- Severe abdominal pain, cramping, or backache
- Abdominal tenderness (when pressure applied)

The woman may expect her menstrual period to resume 4 to 6 weeks from the day of the procedure. Information about the birth control method the woman prefers is offered, if this has not been done previously during the counseling interview that usually precedes the decision to have an abortion. Some methods can be initiated immediately such as an IUD insertion. Hormonal methods may be started immediately or within a week (Paul & Stein, 2011). The woman must be strongly encouraged to return for her follow-up visit so complications can be detected. A pregnancy test may also be performed at that time to determine whether the pregnancy was successfully terminated.

Medical Abortion

Early medical abortion has been popular in Canada and Europe for more than 15 years, but it is a relatively new procedure in the United States. Medical abortions are available for use in the United States for up to 9 weeks after the last menstrual period. Methotrexate, misoprostol, and mifepristone are the drugs used in the current regimens to induce early abortion. About 16.5% of all reported abortion procedures in the United States in 2009 were medical procedures (Pazol et al., 2012).

Methotrexate is a cytotoxic drug that causes early abortion by blocking folic acid in fetal cells so that they cannot divide. Misoprostol (Cytotec) is a prostaglandin analog that acts directly on the cervix to soften and dilate and on the uterine muscle to stimulate contractions. Mifepristone, formerly known as RU 486, was approved by the FDA in 2000. It works by binding to progesterone receptors and blocking the action of progesterone, which is necessary for maintaining pregnancy (Paul & Stein, 2011).

Methotrexate and Misoprostol. There is no standard protocol, but methotrexate is given intramuscularly or orally (usually mixed with orange juice). Vaginal placement of misoprostol follows in 3 to 7 days. The woman returns for a follow-up visit in 1 week to confirm the abortion is complete. If not, the woman is offered an additional dose of misoprostol or vacuum aspiration is performed (Paul & Stein, 2011).

Mifepristone and Misoprostol. Mifepristone can be given up to 7 weeks after the last menstrual period. The FDA-approved regimen is that the woman takes 600 mg of mifepristone orally; 48 hours later she returns to the office and takes 400 mcg of misoprostol orally (unless abortion has already occurred and been confirmed). Two weeks after the administration of mifepristone, the woman must return to the office for a clinical examination or ultrasound to confirm that the pregnancy has been terminated. In 4% to 6% of cases, the drugs do not work, and surgical abortion (aspiration) is needed (Paul & Stein, 2011).

Research has demonstrated a more effective regimen that has fewer side effects. This regimen can be given up to 9 weeks after the last menstrual period and includes administration of 200 mg mifepristone orally followed by misoprostol 800 mcg vaginally in 24 to 48 hours. This vaginal insertion can be done at home by the woman. A follow-up visit is in 4 to 8 days (Paul & Stein, 2011).

With any medical abortion regimen, the woman usually will experience bleeding and cramping. Side effects of the medications include nausea, vomiting, diarrhea, headache, dizziness, fever, and chills. These are attributed to misoprostol and usually subside in a few hours after administration (Paul & Stein, 2011).

Second-Trimester Abortion

Second-trimester abortion is associated with more complications and costs than first-trimester abortions. Dilation and evacuation (D&E) accounts for almost all procedures performed in the second trimester in the United States. Induction of uterine contractions with hypertonic solutions (e.g., saline, urea) injected directly into the uterus and uterotonic agents (e.g., misoprostol, dinoprostone) account for only about 0.5% of all abortions (Pazol et al., 2012).

Dilation and Evacuation

D&E can be performed at any point up to 20 weeks of gestation although this procedure is more commonly performed between 13 and 16 weeks of gestation. The cervix requires more dilation because the products of conception are larger. Often, osmotic dilators (e.g., laminaria) are inserted several hours or several days before the procedure, or misoprostol can be applied to the cervix. The procedure is similar to vaginal aspiration except a larger cannula is used and other instruments may be needed to remove the fetus and placenta. Nursing care includes monitoring vital signs, providing emotional support, administering analgesics, and postoperative monitoring. Disadvantages of D&E may include possible long-term harmful effects to the cervix.

Nursing Interventions

The woman will need help exploring the meaning of the various alternatives and consequences to herself and her significant others. It is often difficult for a woman to express her true feelings (e.g., what having an abortion means to her now, how she may feel about her decision in the future, and what support or regret her friends and peers may demonstrate). A calm, matter-of-fact approach on the part of the nurse can be helpful (e.g., "Yes, I know you are pregnant. I am here to help. Let's talk about alternatives"). Listening to what the woman has to say and encouraging her to speak are essential. Neutral responses such as "Oh," "Uh-huh," and "Umm," and nonverbal encouragement such as nodding, maintaining eye contact, and use of touch are helpful in setting an open, accepting environment. Clarifying, restating, and reflecting statements, open-ended questions, and feedback are communication techniques that can be used to maintain a realistic focus on the situation and bring the woman's concerns into the open.

Information about alternatives to abortion such as referral to adoption agencies or to support services if the woman chooses to keep her baby should be provided. If a decision is made to have an abortion, the woman must be assured of continued support. Information about what is entailed in various procedures, how much discomfort or pain can be expected, and what type of care is needed must be given. A discussion of the various feelings including depression, guilt, regret, and relief that the woman might experience after the abortion is needed. Information about community resources for postabortion counseling may be needed (Paul & Stein, 2011). If family or friends cannot be involved, scheduling time for nursing personnel to give the necessary support is an essential component of the plan for care.

After an abortion, studies have indicated that most women report relief, but some have temporary distress or mixed emotions. A systematic review of the literature found no difference in the long-term mental health outcomes of women who had abortions and women who did not have abortions (Charles, Polis, Sridhara, & Blum, 2008). Because symptoms can vary among women who have had abortions, nurses must assess women for grief reactions and facilitate the grieving process through active listening and nonjudgmental support and care.

NURSING CARE PLAN

Sexual Activity and Contraception

NURSING DIAGNOSIS	EXPECTED OUTCOME	NURSING INTERVENTIONS	RATIONALES
Decisional Conflict related to contraceptive alternatives	Woman and partner will verbalize understanding of different methods of contraception and will choose the method best suited for their needs.	Provide information regarding reliability, use, indications, contraindications, and side effects of different methods of contraception.	To facilitate the decision-making process
		Use privacy and therapeutic communication during discussion of sexual activity and methods of contraception.	To provide clarification of information and client trust of caregiver
Risk for Infection related to ongoing sexual activity as evidenced by client history	Woman and her partner will remain free of sexually transmitted infections.	Provide information regarding sex practices to reduce risk of STIs and use of barrier methods.	To raise client awareness of methods to prevent infection
Ineffective Health Maintenance related to unfamiliarity with contraceptive method	Woman and partner will verbalize intent to use chosen contraception correctly.	Review information given regarding use, reliability, and side effects of chosen contraceptive method.	To ensure woman's and partner's understanding
		Provide list of informational resources.	To promote consistency of use of chosen method
		Encourage ongoing effective communication with health care provider.	To promote trust

STIs, Sexually transmitted infections.

KEY POINTS

- A variety of contraceptive methods are available with various effectiveness rates, advantages, and disadvantages.
- Women and their partners should choose the contraceptive method or methods best suited to them.
- Effective contraceptives are available through prescription and nonprescription sources.
- A variety of techniques are available to enhance the effectiveness of periodic abstinence in motivated couples who prefer this natural method.
- Hormonal contraception includes both precoital and postcoital prevention through various modalities and requires thorough client education.
- The barrier methods of diaphragm and cervical cap provide safe and effective contraception for women or couples motivated to use them consistently and correctly.
- Intrauterine devices can provide long-term (5 to 10 years) protection.
- Emergency contraception should be taken as soon as possible after unprotected intercourse, but no later than 120 hours.
- Proper, concurrent use of spermicides and latex condoms provides protection against STIs.
- Tubal ligations and vasectomies are permanent sterilization methods used by increasing numbers of women and men.
- Induced abortion performed in the first trimester is safer than an abortion performed in the second trimester.
- The most common complications of induced abortion include infection, retained products of conception, and excessive vaginal bleeding.
- Major psychologic sequelae of induced abortion are rare.

REFERENCES

AIDS.gov. (2012). *Sexual risk factors.* Available at http://aids.gov/hiv-aids-basics/prevention/reduce-your-risk/sexual-risk-factors.

Association of Reproductive Health Professionals. (2011). *Choosing a birth control method: Fertility awareness.* Available at www.arhp.org/Publications-and-Resources/Quick-Reference-Guide-for-Clinicians/choosing/Fertility-awareness.

Association of Women's Health, Obstetric and Neonatal Nurses. (2009). *AWHONN position statement. Ethical decision making in the clinical setting: Nurses' rights and responsibilities.* Available at www.awhonn.org/awhonn/binary.content.do?name=Resources/Documents/pdf/5_Ethics.pdf.

Bartz, D., & Goldberg, A. (2011). Injectable contraceptives. In R. Hatcher, J. Trussell, A. Nelson, et al. (Eds.), *Contraceptive technology* (20th rev. ed.). New York: Ardent Media.

Cates, W., & Harwood, B. (2011). Vaginal barriers and spermicides. In R. Hatcher, J. Trussell, A. Nelson, et al. (Eds.), *Contraceptive technology* (20th rev. ed.). New York: Ardent Media.

Centers for Disease Control and Prevention (CDC). (2010). Sexually transmitted diseases treatment guidelines. *MMWR Morbidity and Mortality Weekly Report, 59*(RR-12), 1–110.

Centers for Disease Control and Prevention (CDC). (2013). *Reproductive health: Unintended pregnancy prevention.* Available at www.cdc.gov/reproductivehealth/unintendedpregnancy.

Charles, V., Polis, C., Sridhara, S., & Blum, R. (2008). Abortion and long-term mental health outcomes: A systematic review of the evidence. *Contraception, 78*(6), 436–450.

Contracept.org. (2013). *Fertility awareness methods: The TwoDay method.* Available at www.contracept.org/twoday-method.php.

Cunningham, F., Leveno, K., Bloom, S., Spong, C.Y., Dashe, J. (2014). *Williams obstetrics* (24th ed.). New York: McGraw-Hill.

Curtis, K., Peterson, H., & U.S. medical eligibility criteria. (2011). In R. Hatcher, J. Trussell, A. Nelson, et al. (Eds.), *Contraceptive technology* (20th rev. ed.). New York: Ardent Media.

Dean, G., & Schwarz, E. (2011). Intrauterine contraceptives (IUCs). In R. Hatcher, J. Trussell, A. Nelson, et al. (Eds.), *Contraceptive technology* (20th rev. ed.). New York: Ardent Media.

Fehring, R., Schneider, M., & Barron, M. (2008). Efficacy of the Marquette method of natural family planning. *MCN The American Journal of Maternal/Child Nursing, 33*(6), 348–354.

Fehring, R., Schneider, M., Barron, M., & Pruzy, J. (2013). Influence of motivation on the efficacy of natural family planning. *MCN The American Journal of Maternal/Child Nursing, 38*(6), 352–358.

Finer, L., & Zolna, M. (2011). Unintended pregnancy in the United States: Incidents and disparities, 2006. *Contraception, 84*(5), 478–485.

Fritz, M., & Speroff, L. (2011a). Barrier methods of contraception and withdrawal. In M. Fritz, & L. Speroff (Eds.), *Clinical gynecologic endocrinology and infertility* (8th ed.). Philadelphia: Lippincott Williams & Wilkins (LWW).

Fritz, M., & Speroff, L. (2011b). Family planning, sterilization, and abortion. In M. Fritz, & L. Speroff (Eds.), *Clinical gynecologic endocrinology and infertility* (8th ed.). Philadelphia: Lippincott Williams & Wilkins (LWW).

Fritz, M., & Speroff, L. (2011c). Long-acting methods of contraception. In M. Fritz, & L. Speroff (Eds.), *Clinical gynecologic endocrinology and infertility* (8th ed.). Philadelphia: Lippincott Williams & Wilkins (LWW).

Fritz, M., & Speroff, L. (2011d). Oral contraception. In M. Fritz, & L. Speroff (Eds.), *Clinical gynecologic endocrinology and infertility* (8th ed.). Philadelphia: Lippincott Williams & Wilkins (LWW).

Glasier, A., Cameron, S. T., Blithe, D., et al. (2011). Can we identify women at risk of pregnancy despite using emergency contraception? Data from randomized trials of ulipristal acetate and levonorgestrel. *Contraception, 84*(4), 363–367.

Guttmacher Institute. (2013a). *In brief: Fact sheet. Facts on induced abortion in the United States.* Available at www.guttmacher.org/pubs/fb_induced_abortion.html.

Guttmacher Institute. (2013b). *State policies in brief: An overview of abortion laws.* Available at www.guttmacher.org/statecenter/spibs/spib_OAL.pdf.

Jennings, V., & Burke, A. (2011). Fertility awareness-based methods. In R. Hatcher, J. Trussell, A. Nelson, et al. (Eds.), *Contraceptive technology* (20th rev. ed.). New York: Ardent Media.

Kennedy, K., & Trussell, J. (2011). Postpartum contraception and lactation. In R. Hatcher, J. Trussell, A. Nelson, et al. (Eds.), *Contraceptive technology* (20th rev. ed.). New York: Ardent Media.

Kowal, D. (2011). Coitus interruptus (withdrawal). In R. Hatcher, J. Trussell, A. Nelson, et al. (Eds.), *Contraceptive technology* (20th rev. ed.). New York: Ardent Media.

Lessard, L. N., Karasek, D., Ma, S., et al. (2012). Contraceptive features preferred by women at high risk of unintended pregnancy. *Perspectives on Sexual & Reproductive Health, 44*(3), 194–200.

Male contraceptives.org. (2011). *What are experimental male contraceptives?* Available at http://malecontraceptives.org/methods/index.php.

Moreau, C., & Turssell, J. (2013). Results from pooled phase III studies of ulipristal acetate for emergency contraception. *Contraception, 86*(6), 673–680.

Nanda, K. (2011). Contraceptive patch and vaginal contraceptive ring. In R. Hatcher, J. Trussell, A. Nelson, et al. (Eds.), *Contraceptive technology* (20th rev. ed.). New York: Ardent Media.

National Conference of State Legislators. (2012). *Emergency contraception state laws.* Available at www.ncsl.org/issues-research/health/emergency-contraception-state-laws.aspx.

Nelson, A., & Cwiak, C. (2011). Combined oral contraceptives (COCs). In R. Hatcher, J. Trussell, A. Nelson, et al. (Eds.), *Contraceptive technology* (20th rev. ed.). New York: Ardent Media.

Paul, M., & Stein, T. (2011). Abortion. In R. Hatcher, J. Trussell, A. Nelson, et al. (Eds.), *Contraceptive technology* (20th rev. ed.). New York: Ardent Media.

Pazol, K., Gamble, S., Parker, W., et al. (2012). Abortion surveillance, United States, 2009. *MMWR Morbidity and Mortality Weekly Report, 61*(SS 08), 1–44.

Planned Parenthood. (2013). *Health info & services: STD testing, treatment & vaccines in Denton, TX.* Available at www.plannedparenthood.org/health-center/centerDetails.asp?f=2190&;a=91620&v=details#!-service=std-testing-treatment.

Roncari, D., & Hou, M. (2011). Female and male sterilization. In R. Hatcher, J. Trussell, A. Nelson, et al. (Eds.), *Contraceptive technology* (20th rev. ed.). New York: Ardent Media.

Schindler, A. (2013). Non-contraceptive benefits of oral hormonal contraceptives. *International Journal of Endocrinology & Metabolism, 11*(1), 41–47.

Schwartz, J., & Gabelnick, H. (2011). Contraceptive research and development. In R. Hatcher, J. Trussell, A. Nelson, et al. (Eds.), *Contraceptive technology* (20th rev. ed.). New York: Ardent Media.

Sedgh, G., Shah, S., Åhman, E., et al. (2012). Induced abortion: Incidence and trends worldwide from 1995 to 2008. *Lancet, 279*(9816), 625–632.

Shulman, L. (2011). The menstrual cycle. In R. Hatcher, J. Trussell, A. Nelson, et al. (Eds.), *Contraceptive technology* (20th rev. ed.). New York: Ardent Media.

www.skyla-us.com/what-is-skyla.php. (2013). What is Skyla?

Trussell, J. (2011). Contraceptive efficacy. In R. Hatcher, J. Trussell, A. Nelson, et al. (Eds.), *Contraceptive technology* (20th rev. ed.). New York: Ardent Media.

Trussell, J., & Schwarz, E. (2011). Emergency contraception. In R. Hatcher, J. Trussell, A. Nelson, et al. (Eds.), *Contraceptive technology* (20th rev. ed.). New York: Ardent Media.

U.S. Food and Drug Administration. (2013). *FDA approves Plan B One-Step emergency contraceptive for use without a prescription for all women of child-bearing potential.* Available at www.fda.gov/NewsEvents/Newsroom/PressAnnouncements/ucm358082.htm.

U.S. Reports (1973). Roe v Wade, 401 U.S. 113.

Warner, L., & Steiner, M. (2011). Male condoms. In R. Hatcher, J. Trussell, A. Nelson, et al. (Eds.), *Contraceptive technology* (20th rev. ed.). New York: Ardent Media.

Woodhams, E. J., & Gilliam, M. (2012). Epidemiology and efficacy. In Cotton, D., Taichman, D., & Williams, S. (Eds.) In the Clinic Contraception. *Annals of Internal Medicine 157*(7), p. ITC4-2.

World Health Organization Department of Reproductive Health & Research (WHO/RHR) and Johns Hopkins Bloomberg School of Public Health/Center for Communication Programs (CCP). (2011). *Family planning: A global handbook for providers.* Baltimore & Geneva: WHO & CCP.

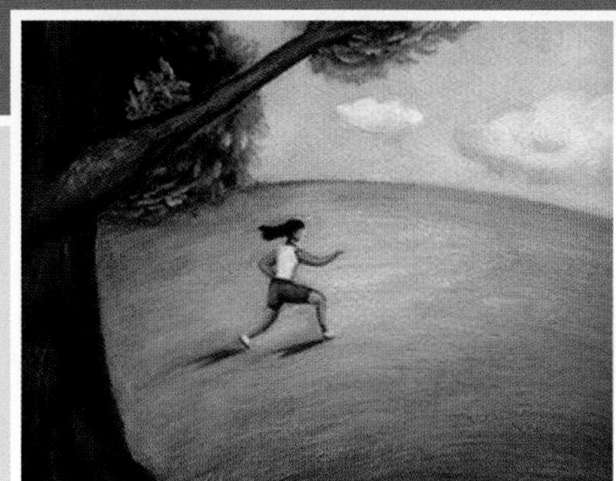

CHAPTER 9

Infertility

Pat Mahaffee Gingrich

http://evolve.elsevier.com/Lowdermilk/MWHC/

LEARNING OBJECTIVES

- List common causes of infertility.
- Discuss the psychosocial impact of infertility.
- Identify common diagnoses and treatments for infertility.
- Identify reproductive and nonreproductive alternatives for infertile couples.
- Examine the various ethical and legal considerations of assisted reproductive therapies for infertility.

This chapter addresses infertility, associated tests, and common therapies. The available alternatives and the psychosocial implications of infertility are discussed.

INCIDENCE

Infertility is a serious medical concern that affects quality of life for approximately 15% of reproductive-age couples (American Society for Reproductive Medicine [ASRM], 2011). The term *infertility* implies subfertility, a prolonged time to conceive, as opposed to *sterility*, which means inability to conceive. Normally a fertile couple has approximately a 20% chance of conception in each ovulatory cycle. If a couple does not achieve pregnancy after a year of unprotected intercourse, they are normally advised to seek specialized fertility evaluation. This evaluation is recommended sooner, after 6 months of attempting pregnancy, for women older than 35, or who have a known risk factor such as endometriosis or male subfertility (ASRM, 2012a). Primary infertility refers to difficulty conceiving when there has never been a pregnancy; secondary infertility refers to difficulty conceiving after having had a pregnancy, regardless of the outcome.

Many factors, both male and female, contribute to infertility. In general, about 10% to 20% of couples will have idiopathic (unexplained) infertility. Among the 80% of couples who have an identifiable cause of infertility, about 40% are related to factors in the female partner, 40% are related to factors in the male partner, and 20% are related to factors in both partners. The prevalence of female infertility is relatively stable among the overall population, but increases with age, accelerating after age 35 (ASRM, 2011). Boxes 9-1 and 9-2 list factors affecting female and male infertility.

FACTORS ASSOCIATED WITH INFERTILITY

A normally developed reproductive tract in both the male and female partner is essential for fertility. Normal functioning of an intact hypothalamic-pituitary-gonadal axis supports gametogenesis—the formation of sperm and ova. The life spans of the sperm and the ovum are short. Although sperm remain viable in the female's reproductive tract for 48 hours or more, only a few retain fertilization potential for more than 24 hours. Ova remain viable for about 24 hours. Infertility also may be caused by something as simple as poor timing or inadequate frequency of intercourse or lack of penile penetration. The couple should be taught about the menstrual cycle and the ways to detect ovulation (see Chapters 4 and 8). Basal body temperature can be assessed to help determine ovulation (see Teaching for Self-Management: Basal Body Temperature, Chapter 8).

Probable causes include the trend toward delaying pregnancy until later in life, when fertility decreases naturally due to ovulatory dysfunction, and the cumulative reproductive organ damage from toxins and diseases such as endometriosis and tubal infection (ASRM, 2012a). Male infertility can result from unfavorable sperm production due to physical or endocrine dysfunction, cumulative metabolic disease, or toxins (ASRM, 2012b).

Female Infertility Causes

Hormonal and Ovulatory Factors

Anovulation may be primary or secondary (see Chapter 6). Primary anovulation may be caused by a pituitary or hypothalamic hormone disorder or an adrenal gland disorder, such as congenital adrenal hyperplasia. It is usually seen in adolescents. Secondary anovulation, usually seen in young to midlife women, is relatively common and is caused by the disruption of the hypothalamic-pituitary-ovarian axis. Besides aging, common causes of ovulatory dysfunction include obesity, polycystic ovary syndrome, strenuous exercise, thyroid dysfunction, and hyperprolactinemia (ASRM, 2012a).

Although relatively rare, amenorrhea after the discontinuation of hormonal contraceptives is seen more frequently in women with a history of menstrual dysfunction. Because most women resume menstruating within 6 months, any workup should be delayed until that time, in the absence of other symptoms.

BOX 9-1 Factors Affecting Female Fertility

Ovarian Factors
Developmental anomalies
Anovulation, primary or secondary
Pituitary or hypothalamic hormone disorder
Adrenal gland disorder
Congenital adrenal hyperplasia
Disruption of hypothalamic-pituitary-ovarian axis
Amenorrhea after discontinuing oral contraceptive pills
Premature ovarian failure
Increased prolactin levels

Uterine, Tubal, and Peritoneal Factors
Developmental anomalies
Tubal motility reduced
Inflammation within the tube
Tubal adhesions
Endometrial and myometrial tumors
Asherman syndrome (uterine adhesions or scar tissue)
Endometriosis
Chronic cervicitis
Hostile or inadequate cervical mucus

Other Factors
Nutritional deficiencies (e.g., anemia)
Obesity
Substance abuse
Thyroid dysfunction
Genetic disorders (e.g., Turner syndrome)
Anxiety

BOX 9-2 Factors Affecting Male Fertility

Poor Sperm Quality
Substance abuse, especially tobacco
Age
Sexually transmitted infections
Exposure to workplace hazards such as radiation or toxic substances
Exposure of scrotum to high temperatures
Nutritional deficiencies
Obesity
Antisperm antibodies

Structural or Hormonal Disorders
Undescended testes
Hypospadias
Varicocele
Obstructive lesions of the vas deferens or epididymis
Low testosterone levels
Hypopituitarism
Endocrine disorders
Testicular damage caused by mumps
Retrograde ejaculation

Other Factors
Genetic disorders (e.g., Klinefelter syndrome)
Decrease in libido—heroin, methadone, selective serotonin reuptake inhibitors (SSRIs), and barbiturates
Impotence—alcohol, antihypertensive medications

Occasionally women experience menopause before they are 40 years old. In a vast majority of cases of early menopause, the ovaries do not respond to ovulation-inducing drugs. Nutritional deficits, such as eating disorders or a diet low in vegetables or high in animal protein, can also contribute to ovulatory dysfunction (Sharma, Beidenharn, Fedor, & Agarwal, 2013). Cancer treatments involving radiation and chemotherapy can decrease or halt ovarian function. Smoking, even passive exposure, is significantly associated with early menopause, infertility, and poor pregnancy outcomes (ASRM, 2012e). Environmental exposure to air pollution, heavy metals, and insecticide is associated with decreased fertility (Sharma et al.).

An increased prolactin level may cause anovulation and amenorrhea in the same way it does during lactation. Hyperprolactinemia can be a side effect of drugs, such as phenothiazine, opiates, diazepam, reserpine, methyldopa, and tricyclic antidepressants. Prolactin also may be elevated as a result of physical stressors such as surgery, cranial lesions or injury, or severe emotional stress. Benign pituitary adenoma may also cause hyperprolactinemia.

The decline in fertility rate in women accelerates after age 35 (Kimberly, Case, Cheung, et al., 2012). Decreased *ovarian reserve,* or total number and quality of follicles, is thought to be the primary reason for age-associated infertility (ASRM, 2012a).

Progesterone, produced by the ovarian corpus luteum, is necessary to mature and maintain the uterine lining. Exogenous progesterone has not been found to improve pregnancy outcomes in women with luteal phase defect, threatened miscarriage, or a history of pregnancy loss. However, synthetic progesterone is beneficial as adjunct therapy to improve the uterine lining after stimulated ovulation or when donor oocytes are used (see later discussion of assisted reproductive technology) (Ozlu, Gungor, Donmez, & Duran, 2012).

Tubal and Peritoneal Factors

Tubal factors account for up to 25% to 35% of female infertility (ASRM, 2012d). Impaired tubal patency and motility result from infections, adhesions, scarring, tumors, or intentional sterilization. In rare instances, one tube may be congenitally absent. One tube may be relatively shorter than the other, which is often associated with an abnormally developed uterus.

Women who have used contraception (barrier methods such as condoms) are more likely to conceive than those who did not, presumably because of the protective effects against tubal damage from sexually transmitted infections (STIs), especially chlamydia (Sharma et al., 2013). Inflammation of the tube or the fimbriated ends resulting from pelvic infections may impair fertility. When infection with purulent discharge heals, scar tissue adhesions form. In the process, the tube can be blocked or kinked anywhere along its length. Adhesions may permit the tiny sperm to pass through the tube, but then prevent a larger fertilized egg from completing the journey into the intrauterine cavity. This results in an ectopic pregnancy, which can completely destroy the tube and be life threatening if untreated.

Endometriosis is the inflammatory peritoneal damage caused by endometrial tissue that has migrated out of the uterus and implanted on pelvic organs or connective tissue (see Chapter 6). Endometriosis is found in less than 5% of fertile women, but in 25% to 50% of infertile women (ASRM, 2012c; Harb, Gallos, Chu, et al., 2013). Risk factors for endometriosis include low body mass index (BMI), alcohol and tobacco use, and Caucasian race.

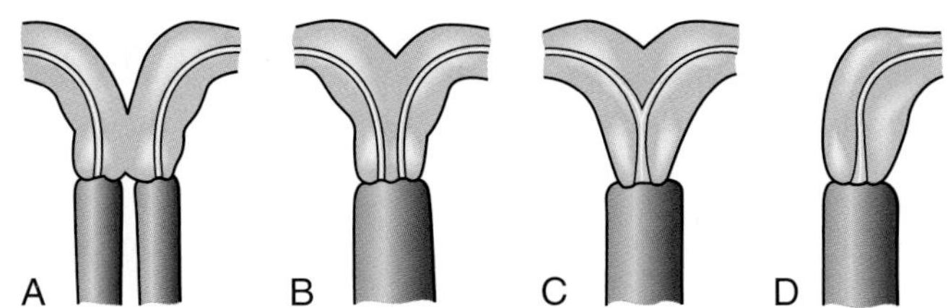

FIG 9-1 Abnormal uterus. **A,** Complete bicornuate uterus with vagina divided by a septum. **B,** Complete bicornuate uterus with normal vagina. **C,** Partial bicornuate uterus with normal vagina. **D,** Unicornuate uterus.

Adhesions can result in pelvic distortion. Inflammatory changes can impair ovarian function and tubal transport (ASRM).

Uterine Factors

Minor developmental anomalies of the uterus are fairly common; major anomalies occur rarely. Müllerian malformations of the uterine cavity, such as bicornuate or septate uterus (Fig. 9-1) or tumors of the endometrium and myometrium (e.g., polyps or myomas), can impair implantation and normal fetal growth. If a functional uterus can be reconstructed, pregnancy may be possible.

Asherman syndrome (uterine adhesions or scar tissue) is characterized by hypomenorrhea. The adhesions prevent normal cyclic endometrial proliferation necessary for implantation. This can result from endometriosis or surgical interventions such as too-vigorous curettage (scraping) after an elective abortion or miscarriage.

Endometritis (inflammation of the endometrium) may result from the same organisms that cause infection of the cervix or uterine tubes (e.g., chlamydia).

Vaginal-Cervical Factors

Vaginal fluid is acidic (pH 4 to 5), which is not favorable for long-term sperm survival. The more alkaline cervical mucus (pH of 7 or more) helps support sperm and permits their ascending transportation. Endocervical mucus normally obstructs or plugs the cervix, acting as a barrier against infection, until increasing estrogen levels cause the mucus to become clear, thin, and nutritionally supportive of sperm. This change occurs around the time of ovulation and lasts approximately 48 to 72 hours (see Teaching for Self-Management: Cervical Mucus Characteristics, Chapter 8).

Inflammation and white blood cells from vaginal or cervical infections often destroy or dramatically reduce the number of viable motile sperm before they enter the cervical canal. The amount of mucus and its physical changes are influenced by the presence of blood, pathogenic bacteria, and irritants such as an intrauterine device (IUD) or a polyp. Severe emotional stress, antibiotic therapy, and diseases such as diabetes mellitus diminish the supportive alkalinity of the cervical mucus.

Some infertile women develop sperm antibodies. Sperm may be immobilized or agglutinated within the cervical mucus, rendering them incapable of migration into the uterus.

Male Infertility Causes

Male infertility can be caused by structural or hormonal disorders such as undescended testes, hypospadias, varicocele (varicose veins on the spermatic vein in the groin), low testosterone levels, or previous vasectomy, all of which can cause *azoospermia* (no sperm cells produced) or *oligospermia* (few sperm cells produced). A low sperm count may occur when spermatic fluid is ejaculated backward, or *retrograde,* into the bladder. Mumps, especially after adolescence, can result in permanent damage to the testes. Testicular cancer or pituitary tumors may present as infertility (ASRM, 2012b).

Male infertility also may be caused by some of the same health issues that affect women, such as nutritional problems, endocrine disorders, genetic disorders, psychologic disorders, and STIs. Male obesity can lead to decreased semen quality. Exposure to hazards in the workplace such as radiation, heavy metals, air pollution, or insecticides also can affect sperm production (Sharma et al., 2013). Exposure of the scrotum to high temperatures can cause a decrease in sperm production as well as abnormal sperm production. Cancer treatments can decrease production or quality of sperm.

Substance abuse can be a major factor in male infertility. Alcohol consumption can cause erectile dysfunction (impotence). Cigarette smoking has been associated with a decrease in number and quality of sperm as well as chromosomal damage (ASRM, 2012e). Recreational drugs decrease sperm quality. Heroin, methadone, selective serotonin reuptake inhibitors (SSRIs), and barbiturates decrease libido. Monoamine oxidase inhibitors (MAOIs), a class of antidepressants, adversely affect spermatogenesis. In addition, some antihypertensives may cause impotence.

Male fertility declines slowly after age 40 (Sharma et al., 2013); however, no cessation of sperm production occurs analogous to menopause in women. Advanced paternal age (greater than 40 years old) is associated with a slightly increased risk for some autosomal dominant conditions, autism spectrum disorder, and schizophrenia in their offspring (Kimberly, Casey, Cheung, et al., 2012).

CARE MANAGEMENT

The nurse begins assessment by obtaining data relevant to fertility through interview and assisting in physical examination. The database must include information to identify whether infertility is primary or secondary. Religious, cultural, and ethnic data are noted (Box 9-3). Many couples have already visited various health care providers and have read extensively on the subject. Their previous infertility experiences and knowledge should be explored and recorded.

Much of the data needed to investigate impaired fertility is of a sensitive, personal nature. Obtaining these data may be viewed as an invasion of privacy. The tests and examinations are occasionally painful and intrusive. Couples may experience some difficulty abstaining from intercourse for 2 to 4 days before expected ovulation. Timed intercourse can take the romance out of lovemaking. The medical investigation requires time (3 to 4 months) and considerable financial expense. It can cause emotional distress and strain on the couple's relationship. A high level of motivation from both partners is needed to the investigation. Preparatory and concurrent counseling support is recommended. Further discussion on psychosocial issues is presented later in this chapter.

Investigation of impaired fertility begins for the woman and the man with a complete history and physical examination. A complete general physical examination is followed by a specific assessment of the reproductive tract and laboratory data. The nurse can alleviate some of the anxiety associated with diagnostic testing by explaining to clients the timing and rationale for

BOX 9-3 Religious and Cultural Considerations of Fertility

Religious Considerations

- Civil laws and religious proscriptions about sex must always be kept in mind by the health care provider.
- Conservative and reform Jewish couples are accepting of most infertility treatment; however, the Orthodox Jewish husband and wife may face problems with infertility investigation and management because of religious laws that govern marital relations. For example, according to Jewish law, the Orthodox couple may not engage in marital relations during menstruation and through the following 7 "preparatory days." The wife then is immersed in a ritual bath *(mikvah)* before relations can resume. Fertility problems can arise when the woman has a short cycle (i.e., a cycle of 24 days or fewer; when ovulation would occur on day 10 or earlier).
- The Roman Catholic Church regards the embryo as a human being from the first moment of existence and regards as unacceptable technical procedures such as in vitro fertilization (IVF), masturbation to collect semen for husband/partner or therapeutic donor insemination, and freezing of embryos.
- Other religious groups may have ethical concerns about infertility tests and treatments. For example, most Protestant denominations and Muslims usually support infertility management as long as IVF is done with the husband's sperm, there is no reduction of fetuses, and insemination is done with the husband's sperm. These groups are less supportive of surrogacy and use of donor sperm and eggs. Christian Scientists do not permit surgical procedures or IVF but do permit insemination with husband and donor sperm.
- Care providers should seek to understand the woman's spirituality and how it affects her perception of health care, especially in relation to infertility. Women may wish to seek infertility treatment but have questions about proposed diagnostic and therapeutic procedures because of religious proscriptions. These women are encouraged to consult their minister, rabbi, priest, or other spiritual leader for advice.

Cultural Considerations

- Worldwide cultures continue to use symbols and rites that celebrate fertility. One fertility rite that persists today is the custom of throwing rice at the bride and groom.
- In many cultures the responsibility for infertility is usually attributed to the woman. A woman's inability to conceive may be a result of her sins, of evil spirits, or of the fact that she is an inadequate person. The virility of a man in some cultures remains in question until he demonstrates his ability to reproduce by having at least one child.

Modified from D'Avanzo, C. (2008). *Mosby's pocket guide to cultural health assessment* (4th ed.). St. Louis: Mosby.

TABLE 9-1 Tests for Impaired Fertility

TEST OR EXAMINATION	TIMING (MENSTRUAL CYCLE DAYS)	RATIONALE
Hysterosalpingogram	7-10	Late follicular, early proliferative phase; will not disrupt a fertilized ovum; may open uterine tubes before time of ovulation
Sonohysterogram	7-10	Same as hysterosalpingogram
Basal body temperature	Chart entire cycle	Elevation occurs in response to progesterone, documents ovulation
Ovulation detection kit	Begin on day 11 of 28-day cycle	Detects luteinizing hormone surge, 12-36 hours prior to ovulation
Assessment of cervical mucus	Variable, ovulation	Cervical mucus should have low viscosity, high spinnbarkeit
Ultrasound diagnosis of follicular collapse	Ovulation	Collapsed follicle is seen after ovulation
Serum assay of plasma progesterone	20-25	Midluteal midsecretory phase; check adequacy of corpus luteal production of progesterone
Endometrial biopsy	21-27	Late luteal, late secretory phase; check endometrial response to progesterone and adequacy of luteal phase. Not done if chance of pregnancy. Not recommended as a routine test.
Hysteroscopy	Variable	Direct visualization of inside of uterus, via cervix
Laparoscopy	Variable	Direct visualization of outside of uterus, ovaries, and tubes, via abdomen

each test (Table 9-1). Test findings that are favorable to fertility are summarized in Box 9-4.

Couples should be cautioned that all tests can be normal and conception still may not occur. Conversely, pregnancy can occur despite poor test results.

Assessment of Female Infertility

Fertility data for the woman include evaluation of the cervix, uterus, tubes, and peritoneum; detection of ovulation; assessment of immunologic compatibility; and evaluation of

CLINICAL REASONING CASE STUDY

Infertility

Diane is a 39-year-old accountant who has recently married for the first time. Charles is 41 and has two children from a previous marriage. Diane has a history of amenorrhea when she was in college and a member of the track team. Currently her menstrual periods are irregular. She wants to have a baby "before it's too late," and she and Charles have been having unprotected sex for almost a year. They have come to the fertility clinic today for an evaluation. Diane tells the nurse that she has heard a lot about the success of in vitro fertilization (IVF) and wants to know if she will be able to have it performed. How should the nurse respond to Diane's comments and questions?

1. Evidence—Is evidence sufficient to draw conclusions about what response the nurse should give?
2. Assumptions—Describe underlying assumptions about the following issues:
   a. Age and fertility
   b. Infertility as a major life stressor
   c. Success rates for IVF pregnancy and birth
   d. Causes of female infertility
3. What implications and priorities for nursing care can be drawn at this time?
4. Does the evidence objectively support your conclusion?

BOX 9-4 Summary of Findings Favorable to Fertility

1. Follicular development, ovulation, and luteal development are supportive of pregnancy:
   a. Basal body temperature (presumptive evidence of ovulatory cycles) is biphasic, with temperature elevation that persists for 12 to 14 days before menstruation.
   b. Cervical mucus characteristics change appropriately during phases of the menstrual cycle.
   c. Days 3 to 10 follicle-stimulating hormone (FSH) levels are low enough to verify presence of adequate ovarian follicles.
   d. Day 3 estradiol levels are low enough to verify presence of adequate ovarian follicles.
   e. Woman reports a history of regular, predictable menses with consistent premenstrual and menstrual symptoms.
2. The luteal phase is supportive of pregnancy:
   a. Levels of plasma progesterone are adequate to indicate ovulation.
   b. Luteal phase of menstrual cycle is of sufficient duration to support pregnancy.
3. Cervical factors are receptive to sperm during expected time of ovulation:
   a. Cervical os is open.
   b. Cervical mucus is clear, watery, abundant, and slippery and demonstrates good spinnbarkeit and arborization (fern pattern) at time of ovulation.
   c. Cervical examination reveals no lesions or infections.
4. The uterus and uterine tubes support pregnancy:
   a. Uterine and tubal patency are documented by (1) spillage of dye into the peritoneal cavity, and (2) outlines of uterine and tubal cavities of adequate size and shape with no abnormalities.
   b. Laparoscopic examination verifies normal development of internal genitals and absence of adhesions, infections, endometriosis, and other lesions.
5. The male partner's reproductive structures are normal:
   a. There is no evidence of developmental anomalies of penis, testicular atrophy, or varicocele (varicose veins on the spermatic vein in the groin).
   b. There is no evidence of infection in the prostate, seminal vesicles, and urethra.
   c. Testes are more than 4 cm in largest diameter.
6. Semen is supportive of pregnancy:*
   a. Sperm (number per milliliter) are adequate in the ejaculate (at least 15 mil/ml).
   b. Most sperm show normal morphology.
   c. Most sperm are motile and forward moving.
   d. No autoimmunity exists.
   e. Seminal fluid is normal (volume is at least 1.5 ml).

*World Health Organization. (2010). *Laboratory manual for the examination of human semen* (5th ed.). Geneva: WHO.

psychogenic factors. See the Clinical Reasoning box to explore how to assist women using evidence and best practices.

Detection of Ovulation

All infertile women should have ovulatory function assessed, because a history of monthly menstruation is inadequate to conclude that ovulation is occurring and is optimal for conception.

Documentation of time of ovulation is important in the investigation of impaired fertility. Direct proof of ovulation is pregnancy or the retrieval of an ovum from the uterine tube. Indirect or presumptive proof can be provided by over-the-counter ovulation detection kits, which test the urine for the luteinizing hormone surge at 24 to 36 hours prior to ovulation (ASRM, 2012a). When drawn at 1 week prior to the expected onset of the next menses, an elevated serum progesterone level gives reliable presumptive evidence of ovulation. Other indirect detections of ovulation include assessment of basal body temperature (BBT) and cervical mucus characteristics, as well as ultrasound imaging, described later. Occurrence of mittelschmerz and midcycle spotting provides unreliable presumptive evidence of ovulation.

Endometrial biopsy is no longer recommended as a routine test for ovulation or luteal phase endometrial development (ASRM, 2012a).

Hormone Analysis

Hormone analysis is performed to assess endocrine function of the hypothalamic-pituitary-ovarian axis when menstrual cycles are absent or irregular or to assess the woman's ovarian reserve. Determination of blood levels of prolactin and the thyroid hormones may be necessary to diagnose the cause of irregular or absent menstrual cycles. A serum progesterone level in the latter half of the cycle verifies sufficient amounts to maintain pregnancy.

If assisted reproductive technology is anticipated, ovarian reserve is established to predict response to ovarian stimulants. Serum follicle-stimulating hormone (FSH) and estradiol (E2) are drawn on day 3 of the cycle. High FSH and low estradiol may indicate ovarian failure. Ovarian stimulation is attempted using a clomiphene citrate challenge test (CCCT). Ovarian follicle development is subsequently assessed visually using transvaginal ultrasound or via a blood test for antimüllerian hormone (AMH), produced by developing follicles (ASRM, 2012a). Poor ovarian reserve may indicate the need for donor eggs.

Ultrasonography

Transvaginal ultrasound is used to assess pelvic structures (Fig. 9-2) for abnormalities such as fibroid tumors and ovarian cysts; to verify follicular development and maturity; and to assess thickness of the endometrium around the time of ovulation. *Sonohysterography* uses fluid infused into the uterus through the cervix to help define the uterine cavity and the depth of the uterine lining, using vaginal ultrasound (ASRM, 2012a).

Hysterosalpingography

Hysterosalpinography, a radiographic (x-ray) film examination allows visualization of the uterine cavity and tubes after the instillation of radiopaque contrast material through the cervix (Fig. 9-3). The contrast material or dye is gently pushed through the uterus and out into the uterine tubes, where it can sometimes have the therapeutic effect of opening a blocked tube (ASRM, 2012a).

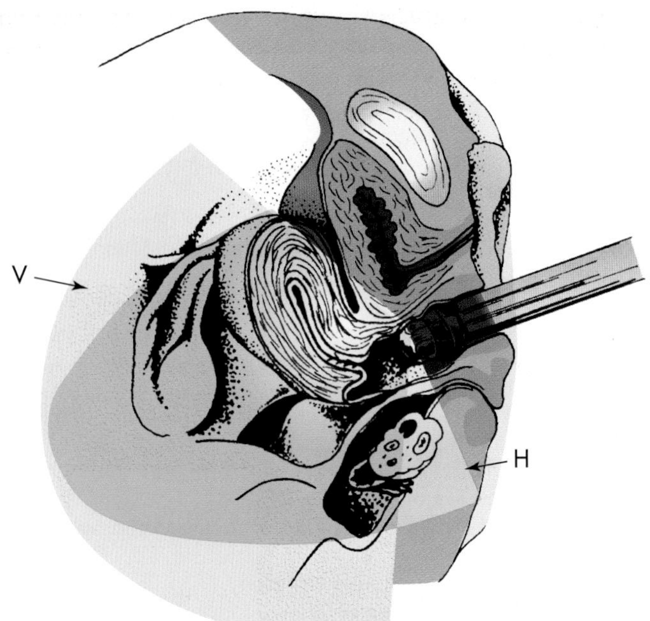

FIG 9-2 Vaginal ultrasonography. Major scanning planes of transducer. *H,* Horizontal; *V,* vertical.

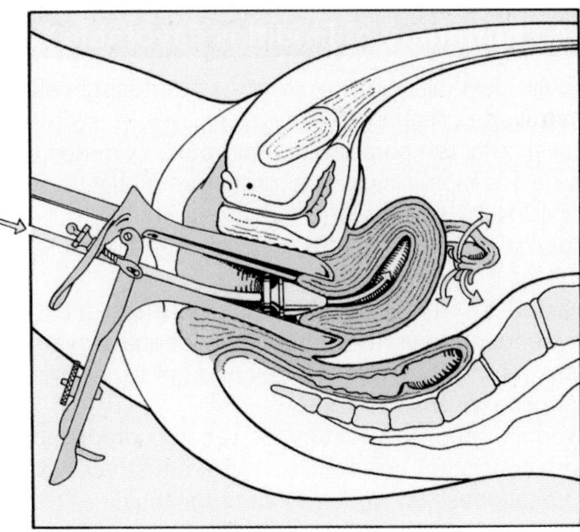

FIG 9-3 Hysterosalpingography. Note that contrast medium flows through an intrauterine cannula and out through the uterine tubes.

Hysterosalpingography is scheduled 2 to 5 days after menstruation to avoid flushing a potential fertilized ovum out through a uterine tube into the peritoneal cavity. Endometrial blood vessels are closed at this time, and all menstrual debris has been discharged. This decreases the risk of embolism or of forcing menstrual debris into the peritoneal cavity.

! NURSING TIP

Referred shoulder pain may occur during a hysterosalpingogram. The referred pain is indicative of subphrenic irritation from the contrast media if it is spilled out of the patent uterine tubes. The discomfort can be managed with position change and mild analgesics. Pain usually subsides within 12 to 14 hours. Women with blocked tubes may have cramping for up to 48 hours.

Hysteroscopy

Hysteroscopy uses a flexible scope threaded through the cervix to directly view the uterine cavity. This is the definitive method for evaluation of leiomyomas (fibroids) and adhesions that might impair implantation. It is also the most expensive and invasive, so it is not a first-line assessment method (ASRM, 2012a).

Laparoscopy

Laparoscopy is useful to view the pelvic structures intraperitoneally, outside the uterus, which may reveal endometriosis, pelvic adhesions, tubal occlusion, leiomyomas, or polycystic ovaries. It is indicated for women with symptoms, and possibly to rule out endometriosis in long-term infertility of unknown reason (ASRM, 2012a). Performed early in the menstrual cycle, under either general or local anesthesia, a small endoscope is inserted through a small incision in the anterior abdominal wall. Cold fiberoptic light sources allow superior visualization of the internal pelvic structures

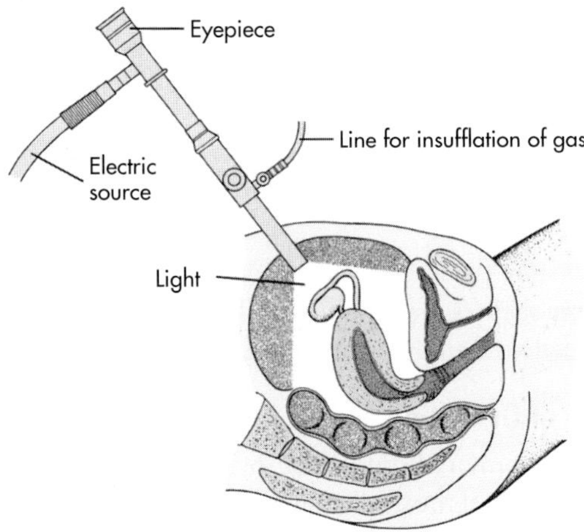

FIG 9-4 Laparoscopy.

(Fig. 9-4). A needle is inserted, and carbon dioxide gas is pumped into the peritoneum to elevate the abdominal wall from the organs, thereby creating an empty space that permits visualization and exploration with the laparoscope. If tubal patency is being assessed, a cannula is used to instill a dye contrast medium through the cervix.

After surgery, deflation of most gas is done by direct expression. Trocar and needle sites are closed with a single absorbable suture or skin clip, and an adhesive bandage is applied. Referred shoulder pain or subcostal discomfort usually lasts only 24 hours and is relieved with a mild analgesic.

Assessment of Male Infertility

Fertility data in the man include evaluation of general health, penis, meatus, testes, scrotum, prostate, hair distribution and breast development; semen analysis; assessment of immunologic compatibility; endocrine evaluations; imaging, as indicated; genetic screening; and evaluation of psychogenic factors.

Semen Analysis

The most basic test of male fertility, the complete semen analysis, assesses sperm number, morphology, and motility (see Box 9-4). Semen is collected by ejaculation into a clean container or a plastic sheath that does not contain a spermicidal agent. The specimen is usually collected by masturbation after 2 to 5 days of abstinence from ejaculation. The semen is kept at room or body temperature and taken to the laboratory in a sealed container within 1 hour of ejaculation (ASRM, 2012b). If results are in the fertile range, no further sperm evaluation is necessary. Poor sperm morphology predicts a poor prognosis for assisted reproductive technology using in vitro fertilization (IVF) or intrauterine insemination, discussed later.

Semen analysis may reveal leukocytes from genital tract infection or agglutination from antisperm antibodies of the male (ASRM, 2012b).

Ultrasonography

Scrotal ultrasound is used to examine the testes for the presence of varicocele and to identify abnormalities in the scrotum and spermatic cord. Transrectal ultrasound can be used to evaluate the ejaculatory ducts, seminal vesicles, and vas deferens for obstruction.

Other Tests

Seminal deficiency can be attributable to one or more of a variety of factors. The male is assessed for these factors: hypopituitarism; nutritional deficiency; debilitating or chronic disease, including obesity and metabolic disease; trauma; exposure to environmental hazards such as radiation and toxic substances; use of tobacco, alcohol, recreational drugs, or anabolic steroids; and gonadotropic inadequacy.

Genetic testing may reveal other reproductive problems. Hormone analyses are done for testosterone, gonadotropin, FSH, and luteinizing hormone (LH). In the presence of a mass, testicular biopsy may be warranted.

Interventions

The management of clients with infertility problems includes psychosocial, nonmedical, medical, and surgical interventions. Assisted reproductive therapies may be indicated. Nursing interventions are an important aspect of care (see Nursing Care Plan).

Psychosocial

Couples frequently refer to their experience with infertility as a "roller coaster" of emotions. Infertility is recognized as a major life stressor that can affect self-esteem, relationships, and careers. Complex feelings may stem from myths, superstitions, misinformation, or magical thinking about the causes of infertility. Individuals experiencing infertility are at risk for distress, anger, isolation, marital dysfunction, and grief. The stress of

NURSING CARE PLAN

Infertility

NURSING DIAGNOSIS	EXPECTED OUTCOME	NURSING INTERVENTIONS	RATIONALES
Deficient Knowledge related to lack of understanding of the reproductive process with regard to conception	Woman and partner will verbalize understanding of the components of the reproductive process, common problems leading to infertility, usual infertility testing, and the importance of completing testing in a timely manner.	Assess woman's current level of understanding of the factors promoting conception.	To identify gaps or misconceptions in knowledge base
		Provide information in a supportive manner regarding factors promoting conception, including common factors leading to infertility of either partner.	To raise woman's awareness and promote trust in caregiver
		Identify and describe the basic infertility tests and the rationale for precise scheduling.	To enhance completion of the diagnostic phase of the infertility workup
Ineffective Individual Coping related to inability to conceive	Woman and partner will identify situational stressors and positive coping methods to deal with testing and unknown outcomes.	Provide opportunities through therapeutic communication to discuss feelings and concerns.	To identify common feelings and perceived stressors
		Evaluate couple's support system, including support of each other during this process.	To identify any barriers to effective coping
		Identify support groups and refer as needed.	To enhance coping by sharing experiences with other couples experiencing similar problems
Hopelessness related to inability to conceive	Woman and partner will verbalize a realistic plan to decrease feelings of hopelessness.	Provide support for couple while grieving for loss of fertility.	To allow couple to work through feelings
		Assess for behaviors indicating possible depression, anger, and frustration.	To prevent impending crisis
		Refer to support groups.	To promote a common bond with other couples during expression of feelings and concerns

infertility and its treatment can exacerbate preexisting anxiety or depression. Conversely, stress can be a cause of infertility for men and women, making it difficult to identify cause and effect (Sharma et al., 2013; Vellani, Colasante, Mamzza, et al., 2013). Table 9-2 discusses some therapeutic nursing actions in response to emotional behaviors associated with impaired fertility.

Men as well as women can experience emotional vulnerability. However, women may have more stress from tests and treatments, and often place greater importance on having children. In contrast, men more frequently express distress in their partner's suffering and the resulting changes in their partnership and sexual relationship. Either partner may exhibit grief behaviors associated with loss. The loss of one's genetic continuity with the generations to come leads to a loss of self-esteem, to a sense of inadequacy as a woman or a man, and to a loss of control over one's destiny. The investigative process leads to a loss of spontaneity and control over the couple's marital relationship and sometimes to a loss of control over progress toward career and life goals.

Same-sex couples desire pregnancy and parenthood for the same reasons as do heterosexual couples, but may feel unaccepted and marginalized in health care settings (Corbett, Frecker, Shapiro, & Yudin, 2013). This can add to the stress of fertility treatments.

Couples often need assistance in separating and reframing their concepts of success and failure related to fertility treatment. Couples making the difficult decision to undergo infertility treatments benefit significantly from instruction in stress management and coping skills (Monach, 2013; Sharma et al., 2013). Health team members must respect affected individuals' and couples' desires in choosing to stop treatment and to select other alternatives, such as adoption.

Psychologic responses to a diagnosis of infertility may tax a couple's giving and receiving of physical and sexual closeness. Sexual dysfunction can manifest as dyspareunia, decreased libido, unrealistic or rigid routines, decreased body image, depression, and ambivalence. Couples sometimes report orgasmic dysfunction or erectile disorders around the time of presumed ovulation.

To be able to deal comfortably with a couple's sexuality, nurses must be comfortable with their own sexuality so that they can better help couples understand why the private act of lovemaking must be shared with health care professionals. Nurses need up-to-date factual knowledge about human sexual practices and must be accepting and nonjudgmental of the preferences and activities of others (including same-sex couples). They need skills in interviewing and in therapeutic use of self, sensitivity to the nonverbal cues of others, and knowledge regarding each couple's sociocultural and religious beliefs. Gender-neutral and inclusive language, as well as pictures and brochures depicting all types of families, including same-sex couples, establishes a tone of respect and safety in the health care setting (Corbett, Frecker, Shapiro, & Yudin, 2013).

The support systems of the couple with impaired fertility must be explored. It is important to identify support available from family and friends, support groups, and their greater spiritual community. Individuals undergoing infertility evaluation and treatment should be encouraged to share their infertility experiences with all other providers of health care, including mental health practitioners.

If the couple conceives, the nurse must be aware that previously infertile couples may continue to experience concerns, including anxiety. Many couples are overjoyed with the pregnancy; however, some are not. Some couples have rearranged their lives, sense of selves, and personal goals within their acceptance of their infertile state, only to be shocked to find that they feel resentment of impending parenthood. Pregnancy, once a cherished dream, now necessitates another change in goals, aspirations, and identities. Reactions of couples range from feeling overwhelmed, to worrying about miscarriage, to thinking about choosing to abort the pregnancy. The couple may need extra preparation to adjust to realities of pregnancy, labor, and parenthood because they may have idealized childbearing when they thought it was beyond their reach. A history of impaired fertility is considered to be a risk factor for pregnancy. A higher level of anxiety, noted in women with assisted pregnancies, could be a risk factor for postpartum depression; therefore, ongoing supportive psychologic therapy should be encouraged.

If the couple does not conceive, they are assessed regarding their desire to be referred for help with adoption, therapeutic intrauterine insemination, other reproductive alternatives, or choosing a child-free state. The couple may find a list of agencies, support groups, and other resources in their community helpful such as ASRM (www.asrm.org) and RESOLVE (www.resolve.org).

Nonmedical Therapy

Simple changes in lifestyle may be effective in the treatment of subfertile men. High scrotal temperatures can be caused by daily hot-tub bathing or saunas or some sports in which the testes are kept at temperatures too high for efficient spermatogenesis. Loose clothing may improve sperm count. Many commonly used lubricants can diminish sperm motility and quality. Cell phones worn at the belt or hip have been linked to decreased sperm quality (Sharma et al., 2013).

Changes in nutrition and habits may increase fertility for men and women. A well-balanced plant-based diet, exercise, stress management, decreased alcohol intake, and avoidance of smoking or recreational drugs can increase fertility for both partners (Sharma et al., 2013). Women who are overweight or obese have a reduced chance of pregnancy following IVF and a significantly greater risk of spontaneous abortion following infertility treatment as compared with women of normal weight. Even modest weight loss (5% to 10%) can be sufficient to increase their chances of achieving a successful pregnancy.

Counseling couples on optimal timing of intercourse can also help. Encouraging intercourse a day before ovulation and the day of ovulation will maximize chances of pregnancy. Sexual counseling may help couples if there is a question of sexual dysfunction that is affecting penile penetration (e.g., vaginismus, obesity).

Complementary and Alternative Measures

Most herbal remedies have not been proven clinically to promote fertility or to be safe in early pregnancy. Women should

TABLE 9-2 Nursing Actions in Response to Behavior Associated with Impaired Fertility

BEHAVIORAL CHARACTERISTIC	NURSING ACTION
Surprise: Each person assumes she or he is fertile and that pregnancy is an option.	Point out resemblance to grieving process—a normal, expected reaction to loss. Refer to support group. Prepare clients for length of time it may take to grieve and for types of feelings (psychologic, somatic) to expect. Encourage and allow time to talk of past and present feelings of sexuality, self-image, and self-esteem.
Denial: "It can't happen to me!"	Allow time for denial, because it gives the body and mind time to adjust a little at a time. Do not feed into the client's denial; instead say, "It must be hard to believe such a devastating report."
Anger: Toward others (perhaps even the nurse) or themselves	Explain that the reaction to loss of control and to a feeling of helplessness is often anger, which can easily be projected onto another person. Anger is a natural feeling. Allow time to express anger at losing sense of control over bodies and destinies. A helpful approach may be, "It's OK to be angry . . . at those who are pregnant, at people who want abortions, at self, at mate, at caregivers," and so forth.
Bargaining: "If I get pregnant, I'll dedicate the child to God."	Accept bargaining statements without comment.
Depression: Isolation: Personal	Allow time for both woman and man to talk about how it feels whenever a sight, event, or word serves as a reminder of his or her own state of impaired fertility. Develop role-playing situations to practice interactions with others under various circumstances to increase the couple's ability to cope and to solve problems (increases their self-confidence). The nurse may say, "You must feel so terribly alone sometimes."
Guilt or unworthiness	Allow time to identify feelings that may be related to earlier behaviors (such as abortion, premarital sex, contact with sexually transmitted infections [STIs]).
Acceptance (resolution)	Couple or person comes to the realization that "unworthiness" and impaired fertility are unrelated. Clients need to know that grief feelings are never laid away forever; they may be activated by special reminders (such as anniversaries).

Adapted from Resolve. (2013). *Emotional aspects of infertility.* Available at www.resolve.org/support-and-services/Managing-Infertility-Stress/emotional-aspects.html.

take these only when prescribed by a physician, nurse-midwife, or nurse practitioner who has expertise in herbology. Relaxation, osteopathy, stress management (e.g., aromatherapy, yoga), and nutritional and exercise counseling have increased pregnancy rates in some women. Integrative mind-body-spirit programs for teaching attitudes of kindness, flexibility, curiosity, acceptance, and openness effectively decrease stress and anxiety related to infertility in women (Chan, Chan, Ng, et al., 2012; Galhardo, Cunha, & Pinto-Gouveia, 2013). Antioxidant vitamins E and C, selenium, zinc, coenzyme Q10, and ginseng have shown beneficial effects for male infertility (Clark, Will, Moravek, & Fisseha, 2013; Sharma et al., 2013).

Acupuncture can decrease anxiety and improve live birth rates for women undergoing IVF. Ovulation induction therapy may have better outcomes when supplemented by black cohosh, progesterone, or phytoestrogens (Clark et al., 2013).

Medical Therapy

Correcting Preexisting Factors. For women, pretreatment or surgery may be indicated to optimize conditions for conception. Infections are treated with appropriate antimicrobial formulations. Surgery or hysterosalpingogram may be necessary to correct tubal blockage or pelvic distortion. Uterine fibroids may need removal via laparotomy, laparoscopy, or hysteroscopy (accessed via the cervix) (Bosteels, Kasius, Weyers, et al., 2013). Laparoscopic removal of endometrial adhesions and implants, and draining of hydrosalpinges (endometrial fluid pockets) can normalize reproductive function (ASRM, 2012d). Weight normalization and optimal nutritional and blood sugar maintenance maximize the chance of pregnancy, especially for women with polycystic ovary syndrome.

Drug therapy may be indicated for male infertility. Problems with the thyroid or adrenal glands are corrected with appropriate medications. Infections are identified and treated promptly with antimicrobials. Surgery may be needed to correct varicoceles, blockages, or tumors. FSH, gonadotropins, and clomiphene may be used to stimulate spermatogenesis in men with hypogonadism. Other health issues, such as weight or smoking, may need to be addressed through counseling.

The primary care provider is responsible for informing clients fully about the prescribed medications. However, the nurse must be ready to answer clients' questions and to confirm their understanding of the drug, its administration, potential side effects, and expected outcomes.

Ovarian Stimulation. If the ovarian reserve is determined to be sufficient, pharmacologic therapy is often directed at stimulating the ovary to produce follicles. The most common ovarian stimulants include the selective estrogen receptor modulator (clomiphene citrate) or gonadotropin (FSH, LH). Clomiphene is an oral medication taken on set days early in the cycle, whereas gonadatropins are injected daily. However, if the ovarian reserve is low, interventions center on using donor eggs and IVF (see following discussion of Assisted Reproductive Technology).

Drugs supporting ovulation include metformin (an insulin sensitizing agent) or dexamethasone (a steroid) to potentiate clomiphene for anovulatory cycling women who have polycystic ovary disease (Misso, Teede, Hart, et al., 2012); bromocriptine to treat anovulation associated with hyperprolactinemia; and TSH (Synthroid) for hypothyroidism. Women with polycystic ovary syndrome, a history of recurrent miscarriage, or who have experienced oocyte retrieval may have insufficient progesterone to maintain an early pregnancy. Exogenous progesterone or human chorionic gonadotropin may be given to support early pregnancy until placental production is sufficient (Shah & Nagarajan, 2013). Commonly used medications are summarized in the Medication Guide.

MEDICATION GUIDE

Infertility Medications

DRUG	INDICATION	MECHANISM OF ACTION	DOSAGE	COMMON SIDE EFFECTS
Clomiphene citrate	Ovulation induction, treatment of luteal phase inadequacy	Thought to bind to estrogen receptors in the pituitary, blocking them from detecting estrogen	Tablets, starting with 50 mg/day by mouth for 5 days beginning on fifth day of menses; if ovulation does not occur, may increase dose next cycle-variable dosage	Vasomotor flushes, abdominal discomfort, nausea and vomiting, breast tenderness, ovarian enlargement
Menotropins (human menopausal gonadotropins [hMG])	Ovarian follicular growth and maturation	LH and FSH in 1:1 ratio, direct stimulation of ovarian follicle; given sequentially with human chorionic gonadotropin (hCG) to induce ovulation	IM or subcutaneous injections, dosage regimen variable based on ovarian response. Initial dose is 75 International Units of FSH and 75 International Units of LH (1 ampule) daily for 7-12 days followed by 10,000 International Units hCG	Ovarian enlargement, ovarian hyperstimulation, local irritation at injection site, multifetal gestations
Follitropins (purified FSH)	Treatment of polycystic ovary syndrome (PCOS); follicle stimulation for assisted reproductive techniques	Direct action on ovarian follicle	Subcutaneous or IM injections, dosage regimen variable	Ovarian enlargement, ovarian hyperstimulation, local irritation at injection site, multifetal gestations
Human chorionic gonadotropin (hCG)	Ovulation induction	Direct action on ovarian follicle to stimulate meiosis and rupture of the follicle	5000-10,000 International Units IM 1 day after last dose of menotropins; dosage regimen variable	Local irritation at injection site; headaches, irritability, edema, depression, fatigue
Exogenous progesterone	Treatment of luteal phase inadequacy	Direct stimulation of endometrium	Vaginal gel 8%, 1 prefilled applicator per day; after ovulation induction, continue through 10-12 weeks of pregnancy	Breast tenderness, local irritation, headaches
GnRH antagonists (ganirelix acetate, cetrorelix acetate)	Controlled ovarian stimulation for infertility treatment	Suppress gonadotropin secretion; inhibit premature LH surges in women undergoing ovarian hyperstimulation	250 mcg daily subcutaneously usually in the early to midfollicular phase of the menstrual cycle; usually followed by hCG administration	Abdominal pain, headache, vaginal bleeding, irritation at the injection site
Metformin (off-label use)	Restores cyclic ovulation and menses in many women with PCOS	Induces ovulation through reducing insulin resistance and thus affecting gonadotropins and androgens; stimulates the ovary	Initial dose is 500 mg/day and titrated up over several weeks to 1500 mg/day. Administered orally	Nausea, vomiting, diarrhea, lactic acidosis, liver dysfunction
Letrozole (off-label use)	Ovulation induction	Aromatase inhibitor that inhibits E_2 production, which causes an increase in LH:FSH ratio	2.5- to 5-mg tablets Administered orally for 5 days beginning on day 3 to 5 of menses	Hot flashes, headaches, breast tenderness, may increase risk of congenital anomalies

FSH, Follicle-stimulating hormone; *IM,* intramuscular; *LH,* luteinizing hormone.

Data from American Society for Reproductive Medicine (ASRM). (2012). *Medications for inducing ovulation: A patient guide.* Available at www.asrm.org/Factsheetsandbooklets; Facts and Comparisons (2013). *A to Z drug facts.* Available at www.factsandcomparisons.com; Lobo, R. (2012). Infertility: Etiology, diagnostic evaluation, management, prognosis. In G. Lentz, R. Lobo, D. Gershenson, & V. Katz (Eds.), *Comprehensive gynecology.* Philadelphia: Mosby.

Assisted Reproductive Technology

The Centers for Disease Control and Prevention (CDC) (2014) define assisted reproductive technology (ART) as fertility treatments in which both eggs and sperm are handled. In general, these treatments involve removing the eggs from the woman, fertilizing the eggs in the laboratory, and returning the embryo or embryos to the woman or surrogate carrier. Although vital for some patients, IVF and similar treatments account for less than 3% of infertility services (ASRM, 2013). The following discussion describes the commonly used ARTs.

Intrauterine Insemination. Ovarian stimulation therapy is then followed with timed intercourse. If sperm quality is low or female factors such as unfavorable cervical mucus, semen allergy, or endometriosis is suspected, the sperm can be introduced directly into the uterus using *intrauterine insemination* (IUI) (Veltman-Verhulst, Cohlen, Hughes, & Heineman, 2012). This is also the preferred technique for introducing donor sperm, or sperm that needs to be washed.

In Vitro Fertilization. *In vitro fertilization–embryo transfer* (IVF-ET) is used when blockage or inflammatory changes of endometriosis are suspected to impair fertilization or tubal transport or in the case of male subfertility (Pandian, Gibreel, & Bhattacharya, 2012). Ovarian follicles are monitored via ultrasound and removed at maturity through intravaginal needle aspiration or laparoscopic procedure. Fertilization with sperm occurs in a dish. If sperm are not available via ejaculation, they can be retrieved via needle from the testicle, epididymis, or vas deferens.

A micromanipulation technique of the follicle called *intracytoplasmic sperm injection* (ICSI) makes it possible to achieve fertilization even with few or poor-quality sperm by introducing sperm beneath the zona pellucida directly into the egg. ICSI offers the opportunity to enhance the chances of fertilization in cases of a severe male factor (i.e., poor sperm quality). Another micromanipulation option is *assisted hatching*. In some instances, the zona pellucida is thick or tough and the embryo cannot break through, or "hatch," through this coating in the blastocystic phase of development. An infrared laser is used to create a hole in the zona pellucida so that the embryo can break through and implant.

Preimplantation genetic diagnosis (PGD) can be done on a single cell removed from each embryo after 3 to 4 days. PGD is a form of early genetic testing designed to screen for inherited diseases. Developing embryos without the gene associated with the disease are transferred to the uterus. Couples must be counseled about their options and choices, when genetic analysis is considered.

With the availability of extended culture medium, embryos transferred at the blastocyst stage (day 5) have a significantly better chance of live birth than the older practice of transferring the embryo at the cleavage stage (day 3) (ASRM, 2013a). Because of this improvement, the ASRM recommends no more than two embryo transfers at a time, except in women with poor fertility prognosis (ASRM, 2013b). See the Community Activity Box, which has some suggestions for further exploration about IVF.

COMMUNITY ACTIVITY

Visit the Attain IVF website (www.attainfertility.com). Research what an Attain IVF program is. Review the client information about Attain IVF programs using the woman's own eggs and those using donor eggs. Compare success rates and costs of these programs. Use this website to find the availability of a fertility clinic in your area that offers the Attain IVF program. Is the location accessible to public transportation and are the clinic hours convenient for clients? Review the clinic information regarding treatment options, success rates, financial considerations, client support, and other client resources. Is the information written so that it can be easily understood by a client with no medical background? Do you have suggestions for other information that could be included?

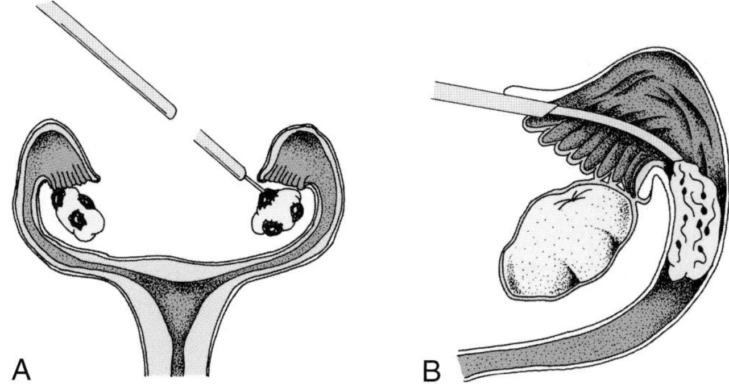

FIG 9-5 Gamete intrafallopian transfer. **A,** Through laparoscopy, a ripe follicle is located and fluid containing the egg is removed. **B,** The sperm and egg are placed separately in the uterine tube, where fertilization occurs.

Gamete Intrafallopian Transfer and Zygote Intrafallopian Transfer. *Gamete intrafallopian transfer* (GIFT) is similar to IVF-ET. GIFT requires women to have at least one normal uterine tube. Ovulation is induced as in IVF-ET, and the oocytes are aspirated from follicles via laparoscopy (Fig. 9-5, *A*). Semen is collected before laparoscopy. The ova and sperm are then transferred to one uterine tube (see Fig. 9-5, *B*), permitting natural fertilization and cleavage. *Zygote intrafallopian transfer* (ZIFT) is similar to GIFT except fertilization occurs in vitro, and then the zygote is placed in the uterine tube. Less than 1% of all ARTs use intrafallopian transfer (ASRM, 2011).

Legal Tip: Cryopreservation

Sperm, ovarian tissue, oocytes, or embryos can be cryopreserved for later use. Couples who have excess embryos frozen for later transfer must be fully informed before consenting to the procedure, to make decisions regarding the disposal of embryos in the event of (1) death, (2) divorce, or (3) the decision that the couple no longer wants the embryos. Embryos can be frozen for prolonged periods, and live births have occurred from embryos frozen for 20 years (ASRM, 2011).

Oocyte Donation. Women who have ovarian failure or oophorectomy, who have a genetic defect, or who fail to achieve pregnancy with their own oocytes may be eligible for the use of *donor oocytes* (eggs). Oocyte donation is usually done by women who are younger than 35 years and healthy, and who are recruited and paid to undergo ovarian stimulation and oocyte retrieval. The donor eggs are then fertilized in the laboratory with the male partner's sperm. The recipient woman undergoes hormonal stimulation to allow development of the uterine lining. Embryos are then transferred. The psychosocial issues are similar to those in therapeutic donor insemination. Historically, the courts have upheld the gestational mother as the legal mother. Sometimes the gestational mother is also a surrogate mother (see later discussion), however, which could complicate the legal aspects. It is expected that the egg donor will have no rights or responsibilities in relation to the offspring.

Embryo Donation. On occasion a couple decides that they do not want their frozen embryos, and they release these for "adoption" by other infertile couples. Infertility centers are struggling to develop guidelines and protocols to address the various legal and ethical issues associated with these procedures. Extensive medical testing of both partners who wish to release the embryos is required as well.

Surrogate Mothers and Embryo Hosts. Surrogate motherhood can be achieved by two methods. The first is for the surrogate mother to be inseminated with semen from the infertile woman's partner and to carry the baby until the birth. The baby is then formally adopted by the infertile couple. A less common method is to retrieve an ovum from the infertile woman, fertilize it with her partner's sperm, and place it into the uterus of a surrogate, who becomes an embryo host or gestational carrier. These interventions raise considerable legal and ethical issues that require extensive counseling of couples and the women who choose to become surrogates.

Therapeutic Donor Insemination. *Therapeutic donor insemination* (TDI), previously referred to as artificial insemination by donor, is used when the male partner has no sperm or a very low sperm count (less than 20 million motile sperm/ml), the couple has a genetic defect, or the male partner has antisperm antibodies. Couples need to be counseled extensively regarding the mutuality of their decision, their ability (particularly of the male partner) to grieve the loss of a biologic child, and long-term issues relating to parenting the child conceived through TDI. Couples also must be aware of the legal status of TDI in their state.

Table 9-3 summarizes ART procedures and their possible indications.

Success Rates and Costs of Assisted Reproductive Technology

Although remarkable developments have occurred in reproductive medicine, ARTs account for about 1% of all U.S. births (CDC, 2014). They are associated with many ethical and legal issues (Box 9-5). The lack of information or misleading information about success rates and the risks and benefits of treatment alternatives create difficulties for couples in making informed decisions.

BOX 9-5 Issues to Be Addressed by Infertile Couples Before Treatment

- Risks of multiple gestation
- Possible need for multifetal reduction
- Possible need for donor oocytes, sperm, or embryos, or for gestational carrier (surrogate mother)
- Whether to or how to disclose facts of conception to offspring
- Freezing embryos for later use
- Possible risks of long-term effects of medications and treatment on women, children, and families
- Stress management techniques and recommendation for ongoing psychologic and couples counseling

TABLE 9-3 Assisted Reproductive Technologies

PROCEDURE	DEFINITION	INDICATION
Intrauterine insemination	Prepared sperm is placed in uterus at ovulation.	Male subfertility; cervical factor; vaginal factors
In vitro fertilization–embryo transfer (IVF-ET)	A woman's eggs are collected from her ovaries, fertilized in the laboratory with sperm, and transferred to her uterus after normal embryo development has occurred.	Tubal disease or blockage; severe male infertility; endometriosis; unexplained infertility; cervical factor; immunologic infertility
Intracytoplasmic sperm injection	Selection of one sperm cell that is injected directly into the egg to achieve fertilization. Used with IVF-ET.	Male partner is azoospermic or has a very low sperm count; couple has a genetic defect; male partner has antisperm antibodies.
Assisted hatching	The zona pellucida is penetrated chemically or manually to create an opening for the dividing embryo to hatch and implant into uterine wall. Used with IVF-ET.	Recurrent miscarriages; to improve implantation rate in women with previously unsuccessful IVF attempts; advanced age
Gamete intrafallopian transfer (GIFT)	Oocytes are retrieved from the ovary, placed in a catheter with washed motile sperm, and immediately transferred into the fimbriated end of the uterine tube. Fertilization occurs in the uterine tube.	Same as for IVF-ET, except there must be normal tubal anatomy, patency, and absence of previous tubal disease in at least one uterine tube
Zygote intrafallopian transfer (ZIFT)	This process is similar to IVF-ET; after in vitro fertilization the ova are placed in one uterine tube during the zygote stage.	Same as for GIFT
Donor oocyte	Eggs are donated by an IVF procedure, and the donated eggs are inseminated. The embryos are transferred into the recipient's uterus, which is hormonally prepared with estrogen/progesterone therapy.	Early menopause; surgical removal of ovaries; congenitally absent ovaries; autosomal or sex-linked disorders; lack of fertilization in repeated IVF attempts because of subtle oocyte abnormalities or defects in oocyte-spermatozoa interaction
Donor embryo (embryo adoption)	A donated embryo is transferred to the uterus of an infertile woman at the appropriate time (normal or induced) of the menstrual cycle.	Infertility not resolved by less aggressive forms of therapy; absence of ovaries; male partner is azoospermic or is severely compromised
Gestational carrier (embryo host); surrogate mother	Gestational carrier: A couple undertakes an IVF cycle, and the embryo(s) is transferred to the uterus of another woman (the carrier) who has contracted with the couple to carry the baby to term. The carrier has no genetic investment in the child. Surrogate motherhood is a process by which a woman is inseminated with semen and then carries the fetus until birth.	Congenital absence or surgical removal of uterus; a reproductively impaired uterus, myomas, uterine adhesions, or other congenital abnormalities; a medical condition that might be life threatening during pregnancy, such as diabetes, immunologic problems, or severe heart, kidney, or liver disease; or gay male couple seeking genetic offspring
Therapeutic donor insemination (TDI)	Donor sperm are used to inseminate the female partner. Can be used with IUI, IVF-ET, GIFT or ZIFT	Male partner is azoospermic or has a very low sperm count; couple has a genetic defect; male partner has antisperm antibodies; lesbian couple

Data from American Society for Reproductive Medicine. (2011). *Assisted reproductive technologies.* Available at www.asrm.org.

Nurses can provide information so that couples have an accurate understanding of their chances for a successful pregnancy and live birth. In 2011, the success rate for live birth with ART transfer procedures ranged from 46% for women younger than 35 years, to 9% for women more than 42 years (Society for Assisted Reproductive Technology [SART], 2013). Nurses also can provide anticipatory guidance about the moral and ethical dilemmas regarding the use of ARTs.

Success rates for pregnancy and for live births vary widely from center to center. Each couple's physical status, age, whether the embryos are fresh or frozen, and from eggs of the woman or a donor all factor into their individual chances for pregnancy. Costs vary by treatment and by region of the country: one cycle of IVF-ET averages $12,400 (ASRM, 2011).

Risks of Assisted Reproductive Technology

ART carries the established risks associated with ovarian stimulation, such as nausea, fluid retention, or ovarian hyperstimulation; invasive procedures; psychologic stress; and general anesthesia (ASRM, 2011). The more common transvaginal needle aspiration requires only local or intravenous analgesia. Evidence of increased risk of congenital malformations associated with ART is mixed: the anomalies can be related to the underlying cause of infertility. In addition, the underlying cause of infertility, such as severe male infertility factor, can be passed on to the offspring. Infertility treatment increases the risk of placental problems and miscarriage. Multiple gestations are more likely and are associated with increased risks for both the mother and fetuses. Ectopic pregnancies occur more often, and these carry a significant maternal risk.

Adoption

Couples may choose to build their family through adoption of children who are not their own biologically. With increased availability of birth control and abortion and increasing numbers of single mothers keeping their babies, however, the adoption of Caucasian infants is extremely limited. Minority infants and infants with special needs, older children, and foreign adoptions are other options (Fig. 9-6).

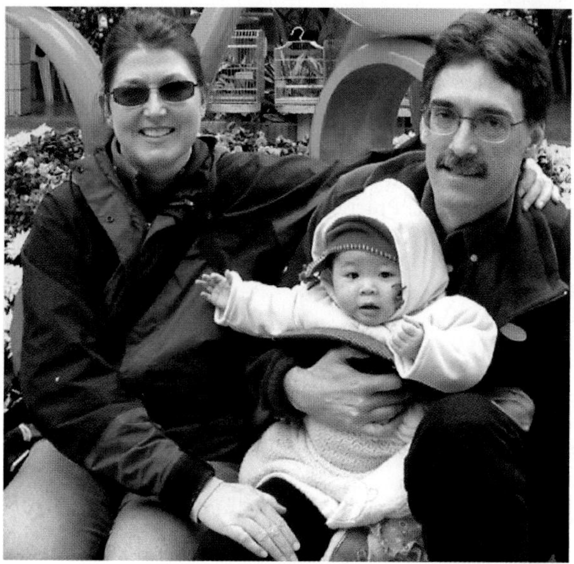

FIG 9-6 After two miscarriages, this couple chose foreign adoption. (Courtesy Shannon Perry, Phoenix, AZ.)

Most adults assume that they will be able to have children of their own. The discovery that they are unable to do so is often accompanied by feelings of guilt or blame. These feelings and frustrations, combined with the anxiety of waiting for pregnancies, feelings of loss, and the multiple medical procedures to investigate infertility, plus the legal uncertainties and potential financial considerations surrounding adoption, create many challenges for the adoptive couple preparing for parenthood.

Couples who decide to adopt a child have decided that being a parent and having a child is more important than the actual process of birthing the baby. The birth process is a very small aspect of becoming a parent. Prospective parents can become so focused on attempting to become pregnant with their own genetic child that they don't see alternate ways of creating a family and parenting a child. The question for potential adoptive couples to ponder is, "What is important to you—that you become parents or that you go through the experience of pregnancy and birth?" Nurses should have information on options for adoption available for couples or refer them to community resources for further assistance.

Some couples, after undergoing infertility treatments to no avail, will decide to live without children. Although this was not a choice initially, it does become a choice for some couples as they resolve their infertility (not physically, but psychologically).

KEY POINTS

- Infertility is the inability to conceive and carry a child to term gestation when the couple has chosen to do so.
- Infertility affects approximately 15% of otherwise healthy adults. Infertility increases as the woman ages, especially after age 40.
- In the United States, about 20% of infertility causes are unexplained. Of that 80% in which causative factors are known, about 40% are related to female causes, 40% are related to male causes, and 20% are attributable to both male and female causes.
- Common etiologic factors of infertility include decreased sperm production, ovulation disorders, tubal occlusion, and endometriosis. Obesity or smoking in either partner is receiving increasing attention as a cause of infertility.
- The investigation of infertility is conducted systematically and simultaneously for male and female partners.
- The couple's relationship dynamics, sexuality, and ability to cope with the psychologic and emotional effects caused by diagnostic procedures and treatment of infertility must be considered in the plan of care. Ongoing support is recommended.
- Most infertility cases are treated with conventional medical and surgical therapies.
- Reproductive alternatives for family building include ovarian stimulation, followed by IUI, IVF-ET, GIFT, or ZIFT, oocyte donation, embryo donation, TDI, gestational or surrogate motherhood, and adoption.

REFERENCES

American Society for Reproductive Medicine (ASRM). (2011). *Assisted reproductive technologies: A guide for patients*. Available at www.asrm.org.

American Society for Reproductive Medicine (ASRM) Practice Committee. (2012a). Diagnostic evaluation of the infertile female: A committee opinion. *Fertility and Sterility, 98*(2), 302–307.

American Society for Reproductive Medicine (ASRM) Practice Committee. (2012b). Diagnostic evaluation of the infertile male: A committee opinion. *Fertility and Sterility, 98*(2), 302–307.

American Society for Reproductive Medicine (ASRM) Practice Committee. (2012c). Endometriosis and infertility: A committee opinion. *Fertility and Sterility, 98*(3), 591–598.

American Society for Reproductive Medicine (ASRM) Practice Committee. (2012d). Committee opinion: Role of tubal surgery in the era of assisted reproductive technology. *Fertility and Sterility, 97*(3), 539–545.

American Society for Reproductive Medicine (ASRM) Practice Committee. (2012e). Smoking and infertility: A committee opinion. *Fertility and Sterility, 98*(6), 1400–1406.

American Society for Reproductive Medicine (ASRM). (2013). *Frequently asked questions about infertility*. Available at www.asrm.org/awards/index.aspx?id=3012.

American Society for Reproductive Medicine (ASRM) & Society for Assisted Reproductive Technology (SART) Practice Committees. (2013a). Blastocyst culture and transfer in clinical-assisted reproduction: A committee opinion. *Fertility and Sterility, 99*(3), 667–672.

American Society for Reproductive Medicine (ASRM) & Society for Assisted Reproductive Technology (SART) Practice Committees. (2013b). Criteria for number of embryos to transfer: A committee opinion. *Fertility and Sterility, 99*(1), 44–46.

Bosteels, J., Kasius, J., Weyers, S., et al. (2013). Hysteroscopy for treating subfertility associated with suspected major uterine cavity abnormalities. In *The Cochrane Database of Systematic Reviews 2013, 1*, CD009461.

Centers for Disease Control and Prevention. (2014). *What is assistive reproductive technology?* Available at www.cdc.gov/art.

Chan, C. H., Chan, C. L., Ng, E. H., et al. (2012). Incorporating spirituality in psychosocial group intervention for women undergoing in vitro fertilization: A prospective randomized controlled study. *Psychology & Psychotherapy, 85*(4), 356–373.

Clark, N. A., Will, M., Moravek, M. B., & Fisseha, S. (2013). A systematic review of the evidence for complementary and alternative medicine in infertility. *International Journal of Gynecology and Obstetrics, 122*(3), 202–206.

Corbett, S. L., Frecker, H. M., Shapiro, H. M., & Yudin, M. H. (2013). Access to fertility services for lesbian women in Canada. *Fertility & Sterility, 100*(4), 1077–1080.

Galhardo, A., Cunha, M., & Pinto-Gouveia, J. (2013). Mindfulness-based program for infertility: Efficacy study. *Fertility & Sterility, 100*(4), 1059–1067.

Harb, H., Gallos, I., Chu, J., et al. (2013). The effect of endometriosis on in vitro fertilization outcome: A systematic review and meta-analysis. *British Journal of Obstetrics and Gynaecology, 120*(11), 1308–1320.

Kimberly, L., Case, A., Cheung, A. P., et al. (2012). Advanced reproductive age and fertility. *International Journal of Gynecology & Obstetrics, 117*(1), 95–102.

Monach, J. (2013). Developments in infertility counselling and its accreditation. *Human Fertility (Cambridge,), 16*(1), 68–72.

Misso, M. L., Teede, H. J., Hart, R., et al. (2012). Status of clomiphene citrate and metformin for fertility in PCOS. *Trends in Endocrinology & Metabolism, 23*(10), 533–543.

Ozlu, T., Gungor, A. C., Donmez, M. E., & Duran, B. (2012). Use of progestogens in pregnant and infertile patients. *Archives of Gynecology and Obstetrics, 286*(2), 495–503.

Pandian, Z., Gibreel, A., & Bhattacharya, S. (2012). In vitro fertilization for unexplained subfertility. In *The Cochrane Database of Systematic Reviews 2012, 4*, CD003357.

Shah, D., & Nagarajan, N. (2013). Luteal insufficiency in first trimester. *Indian Journal of Endocrinology & Metabolism, 17*(1), 44–49.

Sharma, R., Biedenharm, K. R., Fedor, J. M., & Agarwal, A. (2013). Lifestyle factors and reproductive health: Taking control of your fertility. *Reproductive Biology & Endocrinology, 11*, 66, 1–15.

Society for Assisted Reproductive Technology. (2013). *Clinic summary report 2011—All SART member clinics*. Available at www.sartcorsonline.com/rptCSR_PublicMultYear.aspx?ClinicPKID=0.

Vellani, E., Colasante, A., Mamzza, L., et al. (2013). Association of state and trait anxiety to semen quality of in vitro fertilization patients: A controlled study. *Fertility & Sterility, 99*(6), 1565–1572.

Veltman-Verhulst, S. M., Cohlen, B. J., Hughes, E., & Heineman, M. J. (2012). Intra-uterine insemination for unexplained subfertility. In *The Cochrane Database of Systematic Reviews 2012, 9*, CD001838.

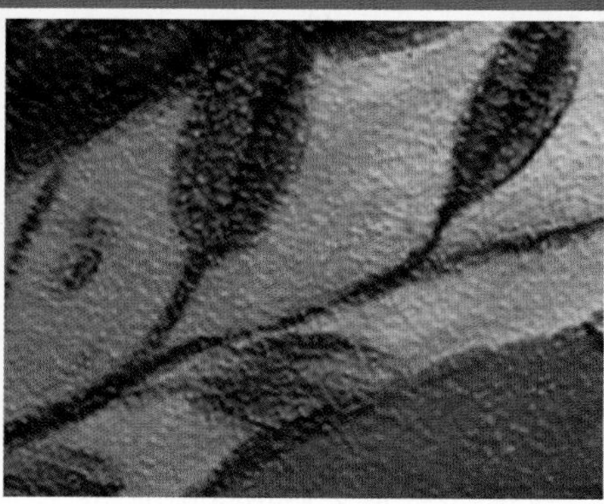

CHAPTER 10

Problems of the Breast

Susan McKenney

http://evolve.elsevier.com/Lowdermilk/MWHC/

LEARNING OBJECTIVES

- Discuss the pathophysiology of both benign and malignant breast disease affecting women through the life cycle.
- Design a nursing plan of care for the woman with a benign breast disorder.
- Understand the relevance and application of assessing risk for the development of breast cancer.
- Evaluate treatment alternatives for women with breast cancer.
- Integrate critical elements for teaching clients who have undergone medical-surgical management of malignant neoplasms of the breast.
- Examine survivorship issues for the woman and her family after treatment for breast cancer.

Problems of the breast affect women throughout most of their lives; starting at early ages with variances in breast development, through the naturally occurring changes related to aging, gaining weight, or becoming pregnant. These changes continue through menopause. Variables that can affect these changes include certain foods or hormones, both endogenous and exogenous. There are variations in the presentation and management of benign breast diseases. Understanding breast disease, along with understanding how to recognize and address risk factors, is not only critical for a woman's care, but also vital in ensuring that adequate breast cancer prevention strategies are used.

This chapter explores breast conditions, including benign and malignant breast diseases, and how breast cancer diagnosis and treatment affect women of all age groups. The unique complexities of the very young and the recent changes to care of older women are addressed. Relevant survivorship issues are discussed with implications for primary women's health care.

Nurses, as important advocates in the health care team, provide expertise through education, support, and advocacy. They teach women about breast disease and cancer. They provide support and advocacy through the actual nursing care delivered, which includes holistic attention to all biopsychosocial and spiritual issues in helping women achieve quality outcomes.

BENIGN CONDITIONS OF THE BREAST

Anatomy and physiology of the normal breast is discussed in Chapter 4. The following text focuses on the normal variations of the breasts and the most common benign breast conditions.

Anatomic Variances

Micromastia and Macromastia

Micromastia, or underdevelopment of breast tissue, is a congenital condition that can affect a woman's self-esteem. Augmentation may be done to correct the variant in development, but usually it is not done until breast development is complete. Because this procedure usually is considered to be cosmetic, it may not be covered by all insurance companies. However, if there is documentation of a congenital abnormality, it might be covered.

Macromastia, or breast hyperplasia, is a condition in which women have very large, heavy, and pendulous breasts. Like the former condition, it is not usually corrected by a plastic surgeon until after complete breast development and then only if the woman chooses to have this procedure. If done too early, the breast can continue to grow after reduction. Breast reduction mammoplasty can relieve a woman of pain in the neck and shoulders. It should be noted that if reduction is done, breast feeding later in life might be difficult due to potential damage to milk-producing ducts, and there can be decreased sensations and pain secondary to scar tissue.

Developmental Anomalies

Asymmetric breast development is often seen in adolescent women and is a normal variation unless a palpable abnormality is detected (Katz & Dotters, 2012). A teenager may choose a prosthetic to achieve symmetry until she is fully matured, at which point she can decide if she still needs the prosthesis.

Supernumerary nipples or breasts are fairly common anomalies that are found along the breast or milk lines that go from the axilla to the groin area. Usually there is no treatment recommended, but if the extra nipples or breast tissue is bothersome, it can be removed surgically (Katz & Dotters, 2012).

Pathophysiology of Benign Breast Disease

In defining breast disorders from a pathologic standpoint, they are best understood as a heterogeneous group of lesions that may represent a palpable mass, a nonpalpable abnormality on imaging, or an incidental microscopic finding discovered during surgery. The two goals in the pathologic evaluation of a breast biopsy are to distinguish benign from malignant in situ or invasive tumors of the breast and to assess the risk of subsequent breast cancer associated with the lesion.

Nonproliferative lesions, including cysts, papillary apocrine change, epithelial calcifications (on mammography), or hyperplasia of the usual type, do not increase risk for breast cancer (Katz & Dotters, 2012). Proliferative lesions without atypia include intraductal papilloma, moderate hyperplasia, sclerosing adenosis, radial scar, and fibroadenomas. The estimated elevated risk is 1.5 to 2 times that of women who do not have these lesions (Katz & Dotters). Atypical hyperplasias are defined as proliferative lesions that possess some, but not all the features of carcinoma in situ. Atypical ductal hyperplasia (ADH) and atypical lobular hyperplasia (ALH) are the two most common, with a risk factor 4 to 5 times greater for developing breast cancer (Katz & Dotters).

Cystic Masses

Fibrocystic Changes

The most common benign breast problem is fibrocystic change, found in varying degrees in healthy women's breasts. Fibrocystic changes are characterized by lumpiness, with or without tenderness, in both breasts (Katz & Dotters, 2012). Fibrocystic breast condition involves the glandular breast tissue. The sole known biologic function of these glands is the production and secretion of milk. Except for proliferative change known as hyperplasia, which is associated with a slightly elevated risk of breast cancer, or atypical hyperplasia, which is associated with a moderately increased risk of breast cancer, the histologic findings associated with fibrocystic changes are part of the spectrum of normal involutional patterns of the breast (Katz & Dotters).

Etiology. Fibrocystic changes tend to appear most commonly in women in their second and third decades of life. The most significant contributing factor to fibrocystic breast condition is a woman's normal hormonal variation during her monthly cycle. Many hormonal changes occur as a woman's body prepares each month for a possible pregnancy. The most important of these hormones are estrogen and progesterone, which directly affect the breast tissues by causing cells to proliferate. Other hormones, however, also play an important role in fibrocystic changes. Prolactin, growth factor, insulin, and thyroid hormones can affect cell growth within the breast tissue.

Clinical Manifestations and Diagnosis. The usual clinical presentation of fibrocystic change is lumpiness in both breasts; however, single simple cysts also can occur. Symptoms usually develop about a week before menstruation begins and subside about a week after menstruation ends. They include dull, heavy pain and a sense of fullness and tenderness, often in the upper outer quadrants of the breasts, that increases in the premenstrual period. Physical examination may reveal excessive nodularity. Women in their 20s report the most severe pain. Women in their 30s have premenstrual pain and tenderness; small multiple nodules are usually present. Women in their 40s usually do not report severe pain, but cysts will be tender and often regress in size. The woman with fibrocystic change can form cysts that manifest as painful enlarging lumps in her breasts. Cysts are common in premenopausal women who are not receiving estrogen therapy. The cysts are soft on palpation, well differentiated, and movable. Deeper cysts, especially aggregations of cysts, are indistinguishable by palpation from carcinomas, which are malignant growths that infiltrate surrounding tissue.

A first step in the workup of a breast lump is ultrasonography to determine if it is fluid filled or solid. Fluid-filled cysts are aspirated, and the woman is monitored on a routine basis for development of other cysts. If the lump is solid and the woman is older than 35 years, mammography is obtained. A fine-needle aspiration (FNA) is performed, regardless of the woman's age, to determine the nature of the lump. In some cases, a core biopsy may be necessary after FNA to harvest adequate amounts of tissue for pathologic examination (Katz & Dotters, 2012).

Therapeutic Management. Treatment for fibrocystic changes is usually conservative. Management can depend on the severity of the symptoms. Dietary changes and vitamin supplements are one management approach. Although research findings are contradictory, some practitioners advocate reducing consumption of or eliminating methylxanthines (i.e., colas, coffee, tea, chocolate) (Katz & Dotters, 2012). Some symptom relief may be achieved by refraining from both smoking and consuming alcohol. Recommended pain relief measures include analgesics or nonsteroidal antiinflammatory drugs (NSAIDs) such as ibuprofen, wearing a supportive bra, and applying heat to the breasts.

Taking vitamin E and B_6 supplements and decreasing sodium intake or taking mild diuretics before menses have been reported to reduce symptoms. Some women report relief while taking oral contraceptives, but others report worsening of symptoms. Danazol, bromocriptine, and tamoxifen have also been used with varying degrees of success (Katz & Dotters, 2012). Evening primrose oil can be effective for some women, although adequate evidence is lacking. It is important to stress that women may need to try several approaches for a number of months before noting improvement (Katz & Dotters).

Surgical removal of nodules is attempted only in rare cases. In the presence of multiple nodules, the surgical approach involves multiple incisions and tissue manipulation and may not prevent the development of more nodules.

Breast Pain (Mastalgia)

Breast pain occurs in many women at some time in their reproductive years, especially the perimenopausal years. The symptom of breast pain commonly is associated with fibrocystic changes that were previously discussed. Breast pain is unusual in breast cancer and, if it is present, is more likely (though uncommon) only in a locally advanced breast cancer. This is important information because many women fear that their breast pain is a symptom of cancer. The character and pattern of breast pain are important in understanding how to manage this symptom. It is important to distinguish between cyclic versus noncyclic, and diffuse versus focal. Patterns can clue one into whether or not the pain is hormonal or related to a specific etiology—a cyst or trauma from external injury or surgery (Katz & Dotters, 2012).

Diagnostic procedures may include serologic tests for prolactin and human chorionic gonadotropin (hCG) levels in premenopausal women, ultrasound, mammography, and aspiration and biopsy for cysts. Treatment depends on the cause of the pain and may include the measures described for pain related to fibrocystic changes. Idiopathic pain is usually treated with NSAIDs (Katz & Dotters, 2012).

Solid Masses

A benign solid mass in contrast to a cystic mass has no fluid component. It is generally described as a smooth, round, mobile, painless lesion that is discrete on palpation. It is a pseudoencapsulated or multilobulated lesion that originates in the stroma of the breast. Solid benign masses in this category with no associated increased risk for breast cancer include fibroadenomas, radial scar, granular cell tumor, fibromatosis, pseudoangiomatous stromal hyperplasia (PASH), and hamartoma. Lipoma, a fatty tumor, is also common, whereas hemangiomas or vascular lesions are less common.

Fibroadenoma

The most common solid mass of the breast is a fibroadenoma. It is the single most common type of tumor seen in the adolescent population, although it can also occur in women in their 20s and 30s. Fibroadenomas are discrete, usually solitary lumps less than 3 cm in diameter (Katz & Dotters, 2012). Occasionally the woman with a fibroadenoma experiences tenderness in the tumor during the menstrual cycle. Fibroadenomas do not increase in size in response to the menstrual cycle (in contrast to fibrocystic cysts). The mass tends to remain the same size or increase in size slowly over time. Fibroadenomas increase in size during pregnancy and decrease in size as a woman ages. Diagnosis is made by a review of the client history and physical examination. Mammography, ultrasonography, or magnetic resonance imaging (MRI) may be used to determine the type of lesion, and FNA may be used to determine the underlying disorder. Surgical excision may be necessary if the lump is suspicious or if the symptoms are severe. Fibroadenomas do not respond to either dietary changes or hormonal therapy. Periodic observation of masses by professional physical examination or mammography may be all that is necessary for those masses not requiring surgical intervention (Katz & Dotters).

Reactive Inflammatory Lesions

Mammary duct ectasia or periductal mastitis is the most common benign lesion in this category. Granulomatous mastitis is a rare cause for inflammation. It is characterized by granuloma and abscess formation and is more common in women ages 40 to 60 (Katz & Dotters, 2012). Other reactive inflammatory lesions include fat necrosis, which results from trauma to the fatty tissue of the breast; Mondor disease, which is phlebitis secondary to trauma; and diabetic mastopathy, which is an autoimmune, painful fibrotic mass commonly seen in women who are insulin dependent.

Mammary Duct Ectasia

Mammary duct ectasia characterized by dilated ducts and nipple inversion (acquired; not congenital) most commonly presents during middle age, usually in women who are still menstruating. It is not common in postmenopausal years. The incidence is higher in women who smoke or who have diabetes. Pathologically, the ducts are dilated with thick walls. There is fibrotic stroma, rupture, and leakage of secretion into surrounding tissue that results in inflammation and fat necrosis. Characteristic signs include pain, redness of the skin, nipple inversion, and greenish nipple discharge. Fever can be present or absent. The breast tissue is thickened and inflamed, suggestive of mastitis, but abscess formation is also possible. Management includes pain medication and antibiotics. Applying heat to the breast, wearing a supportive bra, using a breast pad for leaking, and sleeping on the unaffected side may provide comfort. A surgical incision and drainage are usually performed for abscess. Recurrence rates are higher in women who smoke (Mayo Foundation for Medical Education and Research, 2012).

Nipple Discharge

Nipple discharge is a common occurrence that concerns many women. Though most nipple discharge is physiologic, each woman who presents with this problem must be evaluated carefully because in a small percentage of women, nipple discharge can be related to a serious endocrine disorder or malignancy. Bilateral serous discharge from multiple ducts, expressed during nipple stimulation, can be considered a normal finding. Spontaneous discharge, bloody discharge, or discharge from only one or two ducts must be evaluated (Katz & Dotters, 2012).

One form of nipple discharge not related to malignancy is galactorrhea, a bilaterally spontaneous, milky, sticky discharge. It is a normal finding in pregnancy. Galactorrhea can also occur as the result of elevated prolactin levels. Increased prolactin levels can be a result of a thyroid disorder, pituitary tumor, coitus, eating, stress, trauma, or chest wall surgery. Obtaining a complete medical history on each woman is essential. Certain medications may precipitate galactorrhea. Some tranquilizers (i.e., tricyclic antidepressants), narcotics, and antihypertensive medications, as well as oral contraceptives, can precipitate galactorrhea (Lobo, 2012). Diagnostic tests include a prolactin level, a microscopic analysis of the discharge from each breast, a thyroid profile, a pregnancy test, and a mammogram. Ideally, prolactin levels should not be drawn directly after a breast examination, sexual activity, or exercise because these activities may increase the levels above the normal range (Lobo).

Nipple discharge ranges from milky white to bloody and can be green and brown. If blood is suspected, Hemoccult testing should be done because bloody discharge may be related to malignancy (Katz & Dotters, 2012).

Intraductal Papilloma

Intraductal papilloma is a relatively rare, benign condition that develops in the terminal nipple ducts. The cause is unknown. It usually occurs in women between ages 30 and 50. Papillomas are usually too small to be palpated (less than 0.5 cm), and present with the characteristic sign of serous, serosanguineous, or bloody nipple discharge. The discharge is unilateral and spontaneous. A ductogram (imaging technique to evaluate lesions causing nipple discharge) is a common way of making the diagnosis, along with mammography and core biopsy. After the possibility of malignancy is eliminated, treatment for papillomas includes excision of the affected segments of the ducts and breasts (Katz & Dotters, 2012).

TABLE 10-1 Comparison of Common Manifestations of Benign Breast Masses

FIBROCYSTIC CHANGES	FIBROADENOMA		INTRADUCTAL PAPILLOMA	MAMMARY DUCT ECTASIA
Multiple lumps	Single lump	Single lump	Nonpalpable	Mass behind nipple
Nodular	Well delineated	Well defined	Not well delineated	Not well delineated
Palpable	Palpable	Palpable	Nonpalpable	Palpable
Movable	Movable	Movable	Nonmobile	Nonmobile
Round, smooth	Round, lobular	Round, lobular	Small, sometimes multiple	Irregular
Firm or soft	Firm	Soft	Firm or soft	Firm
Tenderness influenced by menstrual cycle	Usually asymptomatic	Nontender	Usually nontender	Painful, burning, itching
Bilateral	Unilateral	Unilateral	Unilateral	Unilateral
May or may not have nipple discharge	No nipple discharge	No nipple discharge	Serous or bloody nipple discharge	Thick, sticky nipple discharge

Table 10-1 compares common manifestations of benign breast masses.

Infections of the Breast

Cellulitis with and without abscess formation is very common in women in most age groups but uncommon in younger developing girls. The at-risk population has some shared characteristics such as obesity, large breasts, previous surgeries, radiation, sebaceous cysts of the chest and axillae, smoking, and diabetes. Nipple piercing has been associated with infection and abscess formation (Katz & Dotters, 2012). The most common pathogen is *Staphylococcus aureus;* however, methicillin-resistant *Staphylococcus aureus* (MRSA) is becoming prevalent. Cellulitis of the breast presents as painful, red inflamed skin that is usually thickened. It feels warm or hot to touch. Abscess is present when there is a ballotable mass associated with these symptoms. Imaging studies identify a mixed fluid collection on ultrasound. If abscess is present, it can be managed by percutaneous ultrasound aspiration or, if large enough, incision and drainage. Treatment for cellulitis usually includes antibiotics.

Lactational infections are similar to cellulitis, except they occur during pregnancy and postpartum. Mastitis is discussed in Chapters 25 and 33.

CLINICAL REASONING CASE STUDY

Breast Cancer Treatment Options

Susan is a 36-year-old with stage I breast cancer. Her family history includes her mother being diagnosed with breast cancer at age 55 and her maternal aunt diagnosed with ovarian cancer at age 48. Both succumbed to their diseases. Her menstrual periods started at age 11. She has one sibling, a sister, age 40, who has had no breast health issues. Susan is divorced, has two young children, both in elementary school, and is employed full-time as a dental assistant. She states that she is scared and doesn't want to have a mastectomy but thinks she should because she has heard that is the best treatment for long-term survival. How would you respond to this statement?

1. Evidence—Is there sufficient evidence to draw conclusions about what the nurse should say?
2. Assumptions—What assumptions can be made about the following issues?
   a. Differences between breast-conserving surgery and mastectomy for stage I cancer
   b. Genetic and family risk factors
   c. Psychosocial and socioeconomic needs of single parent facing breast cancer treatment
3. What implications and priorities for nursing care can be made at this time?
4. Does the evidence objectively support your conclusion?

CARE MANAGEMENT FOR WOMEN WITH BENIGN BREAST CONDITIONS

Assessment of the woman with a benign breast condition should include a careful history and physical examination. The history should focus on the woman's risk factors for breast diseases, events related to the breast mass, and health maintenance practices. (Risk factors for breast cancer are discussed later in this chapter.) Information related to the breast symptoms should include how, when, and by whom the symptoms were discovered. The interval between discovery and seeking care is crucial. The following client information is documented: presence of pain, whether symptoms increase with menses, dietary habits, smoking habits, use of oral contraceptives or hormone replacement therapy, personal history of breast cancer, family history of breast cancer, regularity of breast self-examination (BSE), and the examination technique used. It is important to note, however, that in regard to BSE, as mentioned later in this chapter, the American Cancer Society (2013) no longer recommends this as a monthly screening, but they do recommend clinical breast exam by a clinician. The woman's emotional status, including her stress level, fears, and concerns, and her ability to cope also should be assessed.

Physical examination may include assessment of the breasts for symmetry, masses (size, number, consistency, mobility), and nipple discharge.

Nursing actions might include the following:

- Discuss the intervals for and facets of breast screening, including professional examination and mammography (see Table 10-3). Women with breast implants may need special views (called push backs) of the breast, and precautions taken not to rupture the implant during mammography.
- Provide written educational materials.
- Encourage the verbalization of fears and concerns about treatment and prognosis.
- Provide specific information regarding the woman's condition and treatment, including dietary changes, drug therapy, comfort measures, complementary and alternative therapies, stress management, and surgery.
- Demonstrate correct BSE technique if a woman desires to practice it (see Teaching for Self-Management: Breast Self-Examination in Chapter 4).
- Describe pain-relieving strategies in detail, and collaborate with the primary health care provider to ensure effective pain control.
- Encourage discussion of feelings about body image.
- Refer to a stress management resource if needed to cope with long-term consequences of benign breast conditions.

MALIGNANT CONDITIONS OF THE BREAST

Breast cancer remains the second leading cause of cancer death in women ages 45 to 55, with 232,670 new cases estimated in 2013 (American Cancer Society [ACS], 2013a). Non-Hispanic white women have a higher incidence than other racial/ethnic groups, but mortality rates are higher among black women. The incidence has decreased since the year 2000, and is now stable at 1:8 women at risk for breast cancer. This is most likely due to adherence of American Cancer Society (ACS) screening and better targeted therapies for treatment. Statistics suggest that about 79% of breast cancers are found in women over the age of 50. There are 2.9 million survivors of breast cancer, with statistics indicating a survival rate of 83% at 10 years after diagnosis (ACS 2013a), which has implications for women's primary health care and prevention of second malignancies. Although the exact cause for breast cancer remains unknown, at least 15% are related to a genetic mutation.

Etiology of Breast Cancer and Risk Factors

The risk factors are considered a mosaic of statistical data points that, when put together and used correctly, can help one understand what groups of women need more heightened surveillance in high risk clinics or referral to a genetic counselor for genetic testing. Some risk factors cannot change, such as gender, age, the time of menarche, menopause, and time of first live birth. The length of time on unopposed estrogen is a significant risk factor. Having a personal history of breast cancer is a constant risk factor, leading to a risk for developing a second malignancy. Breast cancer affects predominantly women, but 1% of all breast cancers occur in men. Geographic differences are related to breast cancer risk. For instance, when women from Japan, where there is one of the lowest rates of breast cancer, move to Western countries, their risk equalizes to that of the native population. Whether this is due to diet or other environmental exposure is not yet clear but may be a combination of the two. Experiencing a first pregnancy after age 40 is another risk factor. Having fibrocystic disease with any of the previously discussed proliferative diseases with atypia increases one's risk fourfold. Higher breast density may make interpretation of mammography more difficult. Legislation has mandated that radiologists need to communicate this information to women, probably more as a liability protection.

Relative factors such as maintaining one's ideal body weight is important in that heavier women have higher circulating estrogens and that regular exercise reduces risk by about 20%. Dietary risk factors include high saturated fats and moderate to high alcohol consumption. The use of exogenous hormones such as oral contraception or hormone replacement for postmenopausal support becomes a risk factor when used for more than 10 years. Diethylstilbestrol (DES), a drug used years ago to maintain pregnancy, is slightly correlated with elevated risk.

Genetic Considerations

Having a genetic mutation, either BRCA1 or BRCA2, may create an 85% chance of developing breast cancer in a woman's lifetime. There are other mutations such as the Li-Fraumeni syndrome and Cowden syndrome, which have different family pedigrees. Genetic testing is complex and it is very important that this be done in conjunction with genetic counseling. Not all women with family history of cancer are at risk, and there are statistical models that help determine the risk-benefit ratio of testing for a genetic mutation. Also if the estimated risk determines that there is probability for a mutation, it is suggested that the living family member with breast cancer be tested first. This helps validate whether additional testing is needed in the family. After testing, if the result is negative, the genetics team can determine the tested family members' estimated risk for subsequent development of breast cancer. This information uniquely tailors surveillance for women who remain at greater than a 20% risk. Women and men who carry a mutation have choices to make in how they manage their lives. They can be followed in a dedicated high risk clinic with biannual clinical breast examinations by an expert, along with imaging that alternates between diagnostic mammography at one visit and breast MRI at the other visit.

BOX 10-1 Risk Factors Included in the Breast Cancer Risk Assessment Tool

- Woman's age
- Number of first-degree relatives affected
- Age of woman at menarche
- Age of woman at first live birth
- Number of breast biopsies
- History of atypical hyperplasia in biopsy specimens

The Breast Cancer Risk Assessment Tool (Gail Model), a risk calculator used in the first- and second-generation national prevention trials, can quantify risk for development of breast cancer at 5 years and then a lifetime risk (up to age 90). (Risk factors are listed in Box 10-1; the tool is available at www.nci.nih.gov/bcrisktool.)

Chemoprevention

Some drugs are used for prevention of breast cancer, although research is ongoing to test their efficacy. Chemoprevention can be approached with either tamoxifen or raloxifene, both U.S. Food and Drug Administration (FDA) approved to prevent invasive cancers (Mayo Clinic, 2011). Both these drugs are taken once daily, but have very different side effect profiles. Tamoxifen can cause hot flashes, weight gain, cataracts, chemical hepatitis, and blood clots and carries a small risk for uterine cancer. Raloxifene can contribute to heart disease or stroke. Raloxifene is a good choice for healthier women who might be at risk for osteopenia. Tamoxifen is available for pre- and postmenopausal women, whereas raloxifene is available only for postmenopausal women. (See Medication Guides later in this chapter.) Providing comprehensive information on these drugs helps women to make informed decisions, empowering them to take charge of their lives.

Pathophysiology of Malignant Breast Disease

Although breast cancer presents within the breast, it is, in fact, considered to be a systemic disease because as it is growing in the breast, invasive tumors have the capability of traveling elsewhere in the body (Redig & McAllister, 2013). There are more than 20 types of breast cancers that can be identified and they all act and behave differently. Genetic alterations, either inherited or spontaneous, are found in the epithelial cells, compromising ductal or lobular tissue. Researchers are investigating which oncogenes (potentially cancer-inducing genes) may cause breast cancer or change its growth pattern and how the process can be stopped.

Breast cancer begins in the epithelial cells lining the mammary ducts of the breast. The rate of breast cancer growth depends on the effects of estrogen and progesterone and other prognostic factors such as its grade, Ki67 score (a proliferative marker), human epidermal growth factor receptor 2 (HER2)/neu receptor status, and other variables. These cancers can be either invasive (infiltrating) or noninvasive/nonspreading (in situ). Invasive or infiltrating breast cancers can grow into the wall of the mammary duct and into the surrounding tissues.

Generally breast cancer is either ductal or lobular. By far the most frequently occurring cancer of the breast is invasive ductal carcinoma. Ductal carcinoma originates in the lactiferous ducts and invades surrounding breast structures. The tumor is usually unilateral, not well delineated, solid, nonmobile, and nontender.

Lobular carcinoma originates in the lobules of the breasts. This type of breast cancer can be nonpalpable and appear smaller on imaging studies than its actual size.

Nipple carcinoma (Paget disease) originates in the nipple. It usually occurs with invasive ductal carcinoma and can cause bleeding, oozing, and crusting of the nipple.

A rarer form of breast cancer is known as inflammatory breast cancer, which is diagnosed by the appearance of a rash or reddish skin of the breast. It can be misdiagnosed as mastitis. A skin punch biopsy is performed, and the pathology report will state that there are breast cancer cells in the dermal lymphatic channels. It is usually aggressive and is classified as stage II breast cancer from its onset. There are also other types of less common forms of breast cancers such as mucinous and malignant phyllodes tumors.

Breast cancer can invade surrounding tissues in such a way that the primary tumor can have tentacle-like projections (referred to as being a spiculated mass). This invasive growth pattern can result in the irregular tumor border felt on palpation. As the tumor grows, fibrosis develops around it and can shorten Cooper ligaments, which result in the characteristic peau d'orange (orange peel–like skin) changes and edema associated with some breast cancers. If the breast cancer invades the lymphatic channels, tumors can develop in the regional lymph nodes, often occupying the axillary lymph nodes. The tumor may invade the outer layers of skin, creating ulcerations. Figure 10-1 indicates the portions of the breast where most breast cancers originate.

Metastasis results from seeding of the breast cancer cells into the blood and lymph systems, leading to tumor development in the bones, the lungs, the brain, and the liver. Breast cancer can be small or large—the size doesn't always equate with aggressiveness. Some aggressive small tumors spread quickly and some large tumors spread very slowly.

Clinical Manifestations and Diagnosis

When breast cancer is detected either as a palpable lump or ill-defined thickening in the breast, it is usually painless. One might see nipple retraction, skin dimpling or skin changes to the nipple, or redness with edema and pitting of the skin, which is suggestive of a locally advanced and aggressive form of breast cancer. Lymph nodes are always clinically examined to determine extent of the clinical stage. Clinical staging helps to understand the parameters of the breast problem and whether lymph node involvement is suspected. The clinical stage is what helps providers decide on how to proceed with treatment. This is referred to as the TNM system (National Cancer Institute, 2013) (Table 10-2). It sorts stage by size of *t*umor, lymph *n*ode, and whether *m*etastasis is involved. It is the pathologic stage, which is determined after

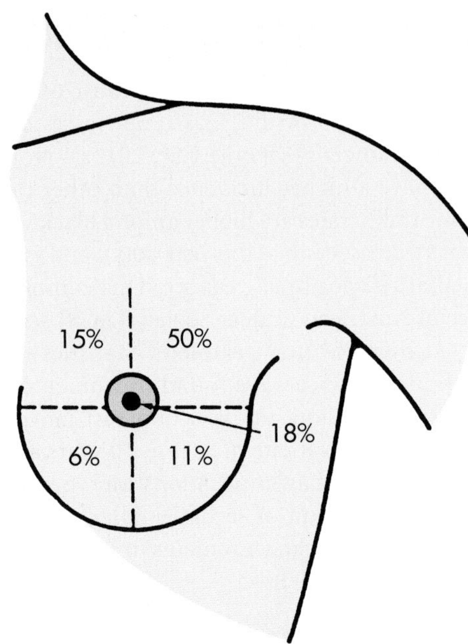

FIG 10-1 Relative location of malignant lesions of the breast. (Modified from DiSaia, P., & Creasman, W. [2007]. *Clinical gynecologic oncology* [7th ed.]. St. Louis: Mosby.)

TABLE 10-2 Staging of Breast Cancer*

STAGE	DEFINITION
Stage 0	Carcinoma in situ (intraductal carcinoma, lobular carcinoma, Paget disease) (Tis-N0-M0)
Stage I	Tumor <2 cm with negative nodes (T1-N0-M0) (includes microinvasive T1, <0.1 cm)
Stage IIA	Tumor 0 to 2 cm with positive nodes (including micrometastasis N1, or <0.2 cm), or 2 to 5 cm with negative nodes (T0-N1, T1-N1, T2-N0, all M0)
Stage IIB	Tumor 2 to 5 cm with positive nodes or >5 cm with negative nodes (T2-N1, T3-N0, all M0)
Stage IIIA	No evidence of primary tumor or tumor <2 cm with involved fixed lymph nodes, or tumor >5 cm with involved movable or nonmovable nodes (T0-N2, T1-N2, T2-N2, T3-N1, T3-N2, all M0)
Stage IIIB	Tumor of any size with direct extension to chest wall or skin, with or without involved lymph nodes, or any size tumor with involved internal mammary lymph nodes (T4-any N, any T-N3, all M0)
Stage IV	Any distant metastasis (includes ipsilateral supraclavicular nodes) (any T, any N, all M1)

*Breast cancer is most frequently staged according to the TNM classification system, which evaluates the tumor size (T), involvement of regional lymph nodes (N), and distant spread of the disease or metastases (M).

From National Cancer Institute. (2012). *What you need to know about breast cancer—Stages.* Available at www.cancer.gov/cancertopics/wyntk/breast.

TABLE 10-3 Screening Guidelines for Early Breast Cancer Detection

AGE (YR)	EXAMINATION	FREQUENCY
Average Risk for Asymptomatic Women		
20-39	Breast self-examination (BSE)	Not specified; inform women about the benefits and limitations of BSE, offer instructions; women may choose to perform regularly, irregularly, or not at all
	Clinical breast examination	At least every 3 years
40 and older	BSE	Not specified; inform women about the benefits and limitations of BSE, offer instructions; women may choose to perform regularly, irregularly, or not at all
	Clinical breast examination	Yearly
	Mammography	Yearly
High Risk Women (>20% Lifetime Risk)		
30 and older*	Clinical breast examnation MRI and mammogram	Yearly

MRI, Magnetic resonance imaging.
*The best age to start should be decided between physician and woman after looking at her individual status.
Modified from American Cancer Society. (2013a). *Breast cancer facts and figures 2013-2014.* Atlanta, GA: Author. Available at http://www.cancer.org/acs/groups/content/@research/documents/document/acspc-040951.pdf.

surgery, that really correlates with overall prognosis and one's risk for recurrence at 2, 5, or 10 years.

Screening

Guidelines for breast cancer screening continue to evolve as new evidence is generated. BSE, once standard, has been scrutinized for its benefit in early detection and overall survival and is no longer recommended as a monthly examination (ACS, 2013). Clinical breast examinations are omitted by many clinicians, evidenced by lack of documentation in medical records and by client reports that this is not part of an annual examination. These two factors are significant in that women are often referred to breast clinics prematurely by their health care providers because there is a lack of understanding of normal variation versus real disease. Guidelines for screening mammography have changed. The U.S. Preventive Services Task Force (2009) recommends baseline mammography in average risk women at age 50, with mammograms every 2 years after that. The ACS (2013), however, continues to recommend baseline mammography at age 40 with annual mammograms after that.

Screening guidelines based on risk are outlined in Table 10-3. Nurses are key to educating women about screening. There is growing evidence among geriatric oncologists of the need to comprehensively assess older women. Women with multiple comorbidities may opt out of screening earlier, but all these decisions are individually based on discussions between the woman and her health care provider.

When caring for a woman with breast cancer, as in all situations, her cultural and ethnic background must be taken into account (see Cultural Considerations).

CULTURAL CONSIDERATIONS

Breast Screening Practices

Certain minority women tend to have low compliance rates in the use of early screening methods for breast cancer. Many factors play a role in influencing the screening practices of these women. African-American women reported not participating in early breast cancer screening because of discomfort with impersonal care from providers, lack of health care insurance, lack of funds to pay for mammograms, lack of awareness of community assistance within the health care system, lack of access to transportation, and feelings of fatalism, fear, helplessness, and powerlessness. Hispanic women cited lack of a regular physician, lack of health insurance coverage, inaccessibility of screening facilities, lack of access to transportation, and being unable to obtain time off from work. Asian women cited unawareness of mammography tests, gender and modesty concerns unique to their cultural beliefs, and fear resulting from a sense of vulnerability to breast cancer.

Interventions that will encourage minority women to participate in early breast cancer screening practices begin with the development of culturally sensitive community education programs designed to help women overcome barriers to reaching optimal levels of health. Programs should be designed to educate small groups of women about risk factors of breast cancer, prevention strategies, and early detection methods. Recruitment of women may be communicated through fliers in neighborhoods, women's groups, churches, clubs, and organizations. Use of incentives to reward participation may be helpful. Nurses and guest speakers of similar ethnicity as the attending group who are breast cancer survivors are valuable in providing meaningful information and support, and providing past, present, and future perspective to the educational content.

Data from Ansell, D., Grabler, P., Whitman, S., et al. (2009). A community effort to reduce the black/white breast cancer mortality disparity in Chicago. *Cancer Causes & Control, 20*(9), 1681-1688; Han, H., Lee, J., Kim, J., et al. (2009). A meta-analysis of interventions to promote mammography among ethnic minority women. *Nursing Research, 58*(4), 246-254; Sim, H., Seah, M., & Tan, M. (2009). Breast cancer knowledge and screening practices: A survey of 1,000 Asian women. *Singapore Medical Journal, 50*(2), 132-138.

Mammography

Mammography remains the gold standard for breast cancer screening and early detection. New technologies that are considered for breast cancer screening must equal or exceed the performance of screen-film mammography to be accepted as screening tools. In other words, these technologies must demonstrate identification of more breast cancers that are missed by mammography, such as a higher fraction of early-stage cancers (stages 0 and I), and be cost-effective, noninvasive, and available and acceptable to clients. Full-field digital mammography (FFDM) is much like standard film mammography in that x-rays are used to produce an image of the breast. Film mammography is captured on x-ray film, however, and digital mammography is recorded with a computer.

Digital mammography is often recommended for women less than 50 years old, for women with high-density breasts, or for women who are not yet menopausal or have been in menopause for less than a year. For women in these groups, digital mammography detects more abnormalities that would otherwise go undetected, and both digital and standard mammography have the same rate of false-positive findings (WebMD, 2012). These images enable the radiologist to enlarge the image as well as lighten and darken the background contrast and to find abnormalities that may go undetected with film mammography. An additional method to assist radiologists with reading mammograms, which can be important for facilities that do not have dedicated breast imaging radiologists, is computer-aided detection and diagnosis (CAD). For nearly two decades this device has been in use to help radiologists find suspicious changes on mammography studies. This can be especially important for film mammography evaluation. CAD electronically scans the mammogram first. It can detect tumors or other breast abnormalities and flag them for the radiologist to further investigate (ACS, 2013b).

A screening mammogram (Fig. 10-2) is performed on women who do not have any signs or symptoms of a breast abnormality. Diagnostic mammograms are performed when a screening mammogram identifies something warranting further inspection or if the woman or her physician or nurse finds a sign such as a lump, nipple discharge, or other breast symptom that is new.

One of the most valuable uses of mammography is the identification of calcifications within the breast. Though most are benign, some can be an early sign of breast cancer. There are two types of calcifications:

- Macrocalcifications—mineral deposits that are most likely changes in the breast caused by aging of the breast arteries, old injuries, or inflammation. They appear as large white dots or dashes. These deposits are related to noncancerous conditions and do not require a biopsy. These types of calcifications are found in about half of women older than age 50 and in 1 in 10 women younger than 50.
- Microcalcifications—fine white specks of calcium in the breast. They may be alone or in clusters and resemble grains of sand or salt. These can be more concerning depending on their pattern and shape. Those that are tightly clustered together and have irregular edges can be a sign of ductal carcinoma in situ (DCIS) or early stage I breast cancer and warrant biopsy.

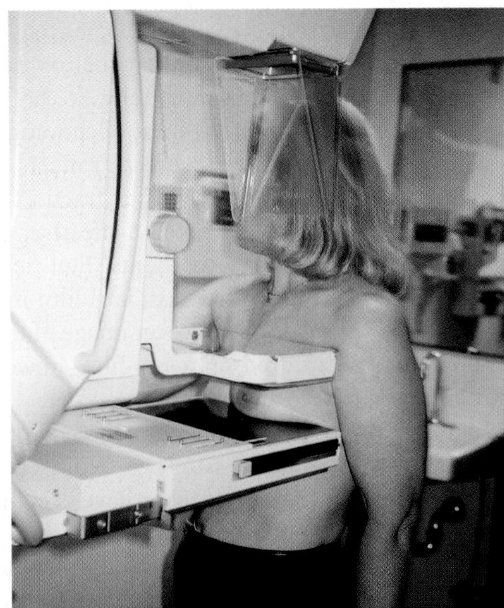

FIG 10-2 Mammography. (Courtesy Shannon Perry, Phoenix, AZ.)

Mammography does have its limitations. It has not proven helpful in screening younger women due to the high breast density associated with youth. Roughly 78% of breast cancer can be identified through mammography, although this number is increased to 83% among women older than age 50 (Komen Foundation, 2013a). Ultrasound has become a valuable screening adjunct to mammography, especially for women with significant breast density. It is cost-effective, noninvasive, and widely available. Ultrasound has been helpful in distinguishing between fluid-filled masses (cysts) and solid masses (benign and malignant). It uses high-frequency sound waves to assess the breast tissue and axillae. The test is painless and noninvasive and requires no exposure to radiation. It has also been useful in performing image-guided biopsies (ACS, 2013a).

Magnetic Resonance Imaging

MRI has become a valuable screening adjunct to mammography and ultrasound. It may be useful in women with difficult-to-find masses, sometimes referred to as occult breast cancers (Komen Foundation, 2013b). There is growing popularity to use it for women diagnosed with breast cancer to rule out the presence of multicentric disease and determine the size of tumors (such as invasive lobular carcinomas), and it has been used increasingly for high risk women (such as those who carry a BRCA gene mutation). It is not, however, without drawbacks. One concern with MRI is that although it helps find small, difficult-to-detect abnormalities, it has been found to lead to more unnecessary mastectomies instead of lumpectomies with radiation (Komen, 2013b).

Positron emission tomography (PET) scans, which are based on glucose uptake metabolism, can help determine if breast cancer has spread to other parts of the body, identifying metastatic disease. Newer technologies for breast cancer screening are under development.

Biopsy

When a suspicious finding on a mammogram is noted or a lump is detected, diagnosis is confirmed by core needle biopsy (stereotactically or ultrasound-guided core) or by needle localization biopsy (Fig. 10-3). The latter procedure requires the collaborative efforts of both the radiologist and the surgeon. This often requires that the procedure take place in two different environments (radiology and surgery), so women need specific information regarding procedures, duration, and outcomes. In most facilities, core biopsies can be performed and the pathology results known the following day, providing the woman with

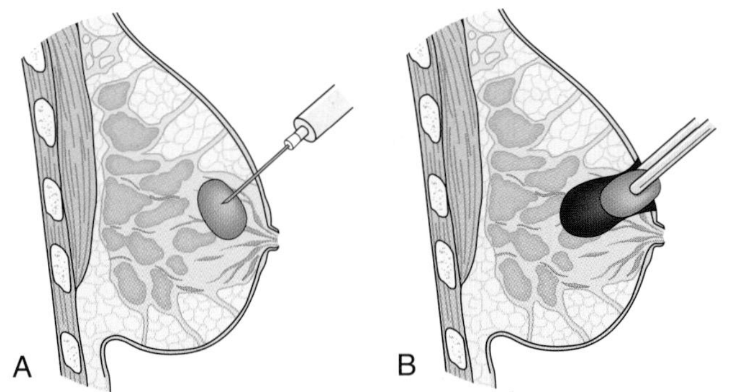

FIG 10-3 Diagnosis. **A,** Needle aspiration. **B,** Open biopsy.

rapid results. This is especially important because women are often highly anxious while waiting for biopsy results.

Prognosis

Nodal involvement and tumor size remain the most significant prognostic criteria for long-term survival (Fig. 10-4). Certain biologic factors include estrogen receptor assay, progesterone receptor assay, tumor *ploidy* (the amount of deoxyribonucleic acid (DNA) in a tumor cell compared with that in a normal cell), S-phase index or growth rate (the percentage of cells in the S phase of cellular division done by flow cytometric determinations of the S-phase fraction), Ki67 (another proliferation marker), and histologic or nuclear grade (Shockney & Tsangaris, 2008). Estrogen and progesterone receptors are proteins in the cell cytoplasm and surface of some breast cancer cells. When these receptors are present, they bind to estrogen or progesterone, which promotes cancer cell growth. A breast cancer can have estrogen or progesterone receptors (ERs, PRs) or both. It is valuable to know the ER status of the cancer to predict which women will respond to hormone therapy (Nelson, Fu, Griffin, et al., 2009). Molecular and biologic factors are valuable indicators for prognosis and treatment of breast cancer. HER2, which is associated with cell growth, is overexpressed in 30% of all breast cancers and is associated with loss of cell regulation and uncontrolled cell proliferation. Thus a positive HER2 status is associated with aggressive tumors, poor prognosis, and resistance to certain chemotherapeutic drugs (ACS, 2013a). Luminal A or B tumors are receptor-positive tumors and are for the most part less aggressive. Tumors expressing H2NU can be more aggressive. Tumors referred to as basal types are tumors that have no receptors. The basal tumors are more aggressive and there are limited therapies, usually chemotherapy based.

CARE MANAGEMENT FOR WOMEN WITH BREAST CANCER

Breast cancer is treated in a variety of ways, using one or a combination of the following approaches: surgery, radiation, systemic therapies, and plastic surgical reconstruction. The specific treatment approach depends on the size of the abnormality and whether there is palpable lymph node involved.

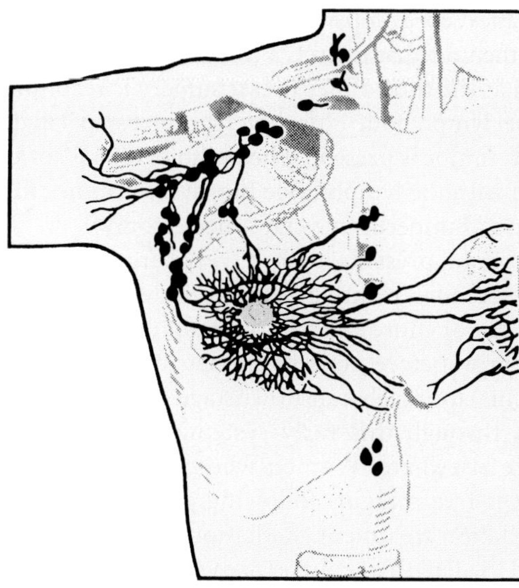

FIG 10-4 Lymphatic spread of breast cancer.

Breast reconstruction, immediately with surgery or delayed, is usually an option for women with mastectomy. Delayed reconstruction is the preferred course for women with locally advanced disease that will most likely need radiation after mastectomy and those with a high chance of local recurrence. Immediate reconstruction is best suited to those women with noninvasive tumors or lymph node–negative disease.

Surgery

Surgical approaches for the treatment of breast cancer include breast-conserving surgeries (BCS) and mastectomy. BCS include lumpectomy (see Fig 10-5, *A*), which involves the removal of the small tumor and a rim of healthy tissue around it, to ensure clear margins; segmental mastectomy (also called partial mastectomy) (see Fig. 10-5, *B*), which includes *wide excision* and/or *quadrantectomy* and involves removal of the tumor, which may be larger, along with a rim of healthy tissue around it, to ensure clear margins.

BCS are used for the primary treatment of women with early-stage (I or II) breast cancer The criteria for recommending BCS are as follows: a tumor that is relatively small compared to breast volume; no previous breast radiation; no previous mantle field radiation (area includes neck, chest, and underarm lymph nodes) as a youth; and no evidence of multicentric disease (ACS, 2013a).

Mastectomy is the removal of the breast, including the nipple and areola. Women who are advised to have mastectomy instead of BCS are women who have:

- Had radiation to the breast
- Multiple tumors in the breast occupying several quadrants of the breast
- Invasive or extensive DCIS that occupies a large area of the breast tissue
- A large tumor compared to breast volume

There are several different types of mastectomies. These include:

- *Total simple mastectomy* (see Fig. 10-5, *C*): This is removal of the breast, nipple, and areola. No lymph nodes from the axillae are taken. Recovery from this procedure, if no reconstruction is done at the same time, is usually 1 to 2 weeks. Hospitalization varies; for some it may be an outpatient procedure, whereas other women may require an overnight stay.
- *Modified radical mastectomy*: This procedure is removal of the breast, nipple, and areola as well as axillary node dissection. Recovery, when surgery is done without reconstruction, is usually 2 to 3 weeks.
- *Skin-sparing mastectomy*: This is the removal of the breast, nipple, and areola, keeping the outer skin of the breast intact. It is a special method of performing a mastectomy that allows for a good cosmetic outcome when combined with a reconstruction done at the same time. A tissue expander may also be placed as a space holder for later reconstruction.
- *Nipple-sparing mastectomy*: This kind of mastectomy is reserved for a smaller number of women with tumors that are not near the nipple areola area. The surgeon makes an incision on the outer side of the breast or around the edge of the areola and hollows out the breast, removing the areola

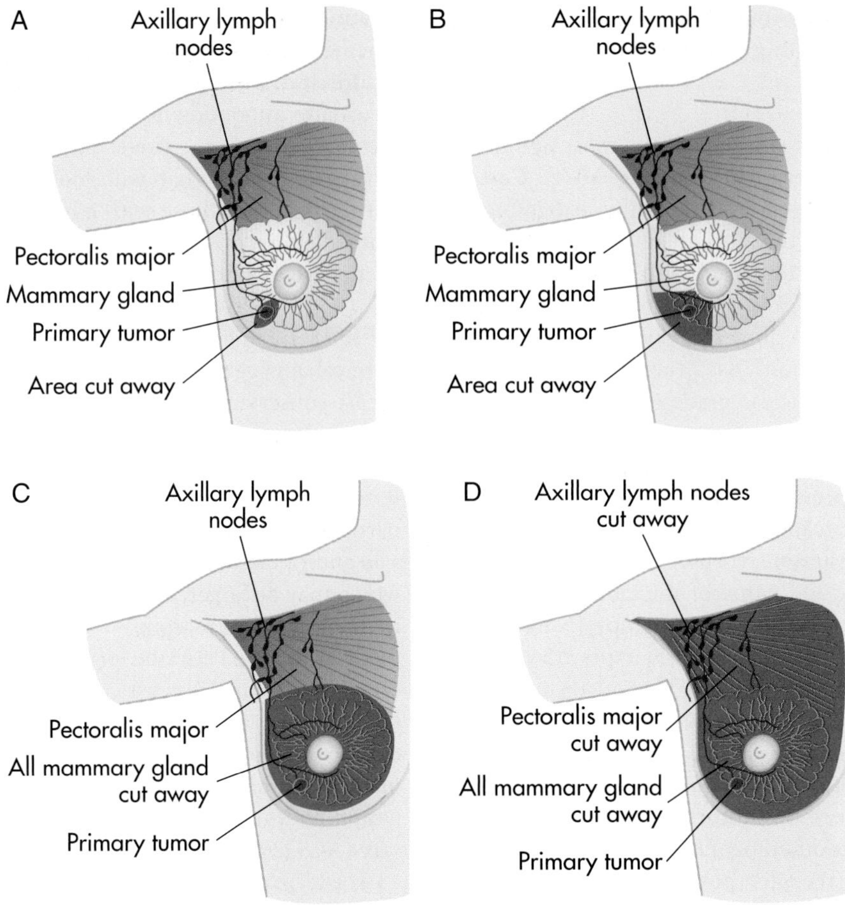

FIG 10-5 Surgical alternatives for breast cancer. **A,** Lumpectomy. **B,** Segmental mastectomy. **C,** Total (simple) mastectomy. **D,** Radical mastectomy.

and keeping the nipple intact. Sometimes the completed reconstruction is performed at the same time, and in other cases a tissue expander is inserted as a space holder for later reconstruction.

- *Preventive/prophylactic mastectomy*: Prophylactic mastectomy is designed to remove one or both breasts in order to dramatically reduce the risk of developing breast cancer. Women who test positive for certain genetic mutations like BRCA1 and BRCA2, or who have a strong family history of breast cancer, may elect this kind of surgery. When this type of mastectomy is performed, no lymph nodes need to be removed because there is no evidence of cancer present. It is necessary to have a mammogram within 90 days before the procedure to ensure that it is healthy breast tissue being removed for preventive purposes.

If there is only one area of concern that has been biopsy-proven, and it is not so large that it occupies more than 50% of a woman's breast, then a BCS is an option. For tumors greater than 50% or multiple tumors that occupy other quadrants, total mastectomy is recommended. If the tumor is invasive with no palpable lymph nodes, there is a 10% chance of having lymph node involvement, and a sentinel lymph node procedure is recommended. The sentinel node is the first node that receives lymphatic drainage from the tumor, and is identified by injecting vital blue dye and radioactive dye in the area surrounding the tumor. A small incision in the axilla allows for identification of the blue-stained lymphatic channel leading to the blue sentinel node, both visually and by gamma probe. This node can then be removed and examined for the presence of tumor cells, as opposed to an entire axillary dissection. It is helpful to indicate whether nodes are positive for metastatic cells in determining the need for adjuvant systemic treatment. A study of more than 1000 cases of sentinel node biopsy has found an accuracy rate in detecting cancer cells of between 97% and 98.3% (Fancellu, Cottu, Feo, et al., 2012).

For women who have a palpable lymph node that is suspected of malignancy, core biopsy of the lymph node confirms the histology. If the node has cancer, a traditional axillary lymph node dissection at the time of her breast surgery is recommended. If the sentinel lymph node is positive, the next step will depend on how much tumor is present. The pathologic stage of the tumor combined with the lymph node biopsy determines the surgical options (e.g., lumpectomy versus mastectomy).

If a woman presents with a very large palpable, locally advanced tumor, positive lymph node, or medium-sized tumor (3 cm or more) and BCS would deform her, then systemic therapy before surgery or neoadjuvant therapy is an option. This approach can downstage the tumor before surgery and, through this early systemic therapy, can prevent recurrence elsewhere. Women who choose BCS will have to have cancer-free margins following surgery, before proceeding to radiation treatment. Radiation treatments are 5 days a week, and the length of courses are variable (discussed in more detail later).

Ductal carcinoma in situ (DCIS) is an early form of noninvasive breast cancer. Although DCIS does not spread, it does require management. The surgical approach is usually a BCS (e.g., lumpectomy) followed by radiation. In invasive or extensive DCIS, segmental mastectomy with radiation or mastectomy may be recommended. If the actual tumor is small on mammogram, there is no need for lymph node assessment; if it is large, the woman may be advised to have sentinel lymph node biopsy because this procedure must be done before mastectomy. If an invasive tumor is found and no sentinel was done, then she would be committed to an axillary lymph node dissection.

Breast Reconstruction

The goals of surgical breast reconstruction are achievement of symmetry and preservation of body image. Surgical reconstruction can be done immediately or at a later date. Immediate reconstruction at the time of mastectomy does not change survival rates or interfere with therapy or the treatment of recurrent disease. It is important that women be aware of this. Women choosing surgical reconstruction offer the following rationale for reconstructive surgery: to feel complete again, to avoid using an external prosthesis, to achieve symmetry, to decrease self-consciousness about appearance, and to enhance femininity.

Major achievements have been made in breast reconstruction following mastectomy surgery. No longer do women need to face long, jagged scars that affect their self-image. Instead, advanced techniques have given plastic surgeons the tools to rebuild a woman's breast in such a way that her silhouette is once again whole.

Women with breast cancer have two main considerations regarding reconstructive surgery—when to have surgery and what type of surgery to have. The options for when to have reconstruction are (Table 10-4):

- *Simultaneous reconstruction*: Women have the option to have immediate reconstruction of their breast(s) at the same time as their mastectomy. This is a reasonable option for women who do not need breast irradiation.
- *Delayed reconstruction*: A woman may opt for delayed reconstruction if, after her mastectomy, a plastic surgeon was not involved. Many women who did not know their options at the time of mastectomy fall into this category. More and more these women are discovering that surgically re-creating their breasts is possible and is required to be covered by insurance as a result of a federal law passed in 1998. Delayed reconstruction is preferred medically, if the pathologic stage requires postmastectomy radiation.

The types of surgical options for breast reconstruction include implants and flap procedures. Implants are made out of silicone or saline or a combination of both and can be inserted at the same time as a mastectomy or later. They are placed underneath the chest muscle versus on top of it, as in the case of breast augmentation. Silicone implants have been deemed safe and are an option for women having breast reconstruction following mastectomy.

Flap procedures are done by plastic and reconstructive surgeons who specialize in microsurgery. During flap reconstruction a breast is created using tissue taken from other parts of the body, such as the abdomen, back, buttocks, or thighs, which is then transplanted to the chest by reconnecting the blood vessels to new ones in the chest region. Due to the high level of skill required for microsurgery, as well as the equipment and staff needed, these techniques are available only at specialized centers. Thus, most breast centers are still using "old fashioned" techniques—transverse rectus abdominis myocutaneous (TRAM) flaps and latissimus dorsi flaps—which result in the woman sacrificing either her abdominal muscles or her upper back muscles. Although these procedures were the best options decades ago, they result in a higher risk of hernia, weakness, abdominal bulging, and limits on physical activity.

After a woman has recovered from initial reconstructive surgery, she may choose to have nipple and areolar reconstruction. Nipple reconstruction is achieved by using an autologous skin graft to construct a nipple, either from tissue from the remaining nipple or from a donor site. Tiny flaps from the new breast itself also may be used. This outpatient procedure requires local anesthesia, intravenous sedation, or a combination of both, depending on how much sensation has returned to the breast. The procedure lasts about an hour. Following this procedure, a woman may choose to have a tattoo to create an areola and match the color of the natural nipple (Breastcancer.org, 2013b).

Radiation

Radiation to the breast destroys tumor cells remaining after manipulation and handling of the tumor during surgery. The total recommended radiation dose is 45 to 60 Gy in 1.8- to 2-Gy fractions over several weeks (Advanced Radiation Center, 2013). The risk of local recurrence depends on extent of breast resection, tumor margins, technical details of radiation therapy, and use of adjuvant systemic therapy. Although radiation after lumpectomy surgery is standard protocol, some large breast tumors (due to the disease being locally advanced) may be irradiated before surgery to facilitate easier surgical removal. Side effects of radiation therapy include swelling and heaviness in the breast, sunburn-like skin changes in the treated area, and fatigue. Changes to the breast tissue and skin usually, but not always, resolve in 6 to 12 months. The breast may become smaller and firmer after radiation therapy. Radiation therapy in the area of the axilla can cause lymphedema of the arm on the affected side. Close medical follow-up is important after conservative surgery and radiation. Recommended guidelines include a breast physical examination every 4 to 6 months for 5 years and then yearly. A mammogram is recommended 6 months after radiation and then annually (National Comprehensive Cancer Network [NCCN], 2012).

A variety of radiation methods are widely used. These include accelerated therapy and brachytherapy.

- *Accelerated breast radiation.* External beam radiation for 6 weeks, 5 days a week, can be inconvenient for a woman. Research has been conducted to develop ways to shorten this time frame and still deliver the therapy needed to prevent recurrence of this disease. Accelerated radiation was created with this goal in mind and delivers a slightly larger dose of radiation over a 3-week period. Skin changes (resembling sunburn) can be slightly more prevalent because of the more intense period of time and corresponding dosage.
- *Brachytherapy.* Initially created for other types of cancer, like prostate, this form of radiation enables the client to complete her radiation in an even shorter time and is not delivered via external beam. Instead a deflated balloon is inserted into the

space left by the lumpectomy and is filled with saline. The balloon is left in place until the margins are confirmed as clear. The balloon is removed and replaced with another balloon specifically created to allow radiation to be inserted within it. Radiation rods or seeds are inserted into the balloon each day for 5 days, and the radiation is completed, at which time the balloon is removed. This enables partial breast radiation to be delivered, recognizing that most local recurrences happen at or near the location of the original cancer.

- *Partial breast radiation.* Intraoperative radiation done at the time of surgery in the operating room. Indications are for small less aggressive tumors. This technique is still not yet standard of care.

Adjuvant Systemic Therapy

Chemotherapy administered soon after surgical removal of the tumor is referred to as **adjuvant chemotherapy.** The role of adjuvant chemotherapy (chemotherapy and endocrine therapy)

TABLE 10-4 Reconstructive Breast Surgery Options

NAME OF OPTION	BRIEF DESCRIPTION	ADVANTAGES	DISADVANTAGES
Simultaneous reconstruction	Reconstruction of the breast done at the same time as surgery to remove the cancer	• The woman wakes up with a breast mound already in place, having been spared the experience of seeing herself with no breast at all. • The process is done in the shortest time possible and is not a series of complex surgeries over a length of time.	• If there is a recurrence of the cancer, the reconstruction may need to be modified. • If there are postsurgery complications, the woman may need to have more surgeries. • Small revision surgeries or matching procedures on the opposing breast may be required. • Rarely it is determined that a woman will need radiation, which can compromise reconstructed breast tissue.
Staged reconstruction	This reconstruction involves placement of a temporary tissue expander at time of mastectomy. The expander gradually stretches the muscle and skin in preparation for either an implant or flap reconstruction.	• The surgeon creates a natural "pocket" in which a permanent implant or a tissue flap may be placed. • The overall result is more symmetric, natural, and aesthetically pleasing. • It allows a woman to complete radiation treatment while having a "placeholder" implanted. • It allows enough time to make sure all of the cancer has been treated.	• It takes longer to "complete" the breast cancer process. • During the time of temporary tissue expansion, the breasts do not look natural. • Small revision surgeries or matching procedures on the opposing breast may be required.
Delayed reconstruction	This reconstruction happens after all of the recommended treatment is completed.	• Some women aren't comfortable weighing all the options at once when they are struggling with a diagnosis of cancer. • Some women need time to come to terms with losing their breast(s). • Some women who are overweight, smokers, or who have high blood pressure may be advised to wait. • It allows enough time to make sure all of the cancer has been treated.	• It takes longer to "complete" the breast cancer treatment. • Women may not feel whole without their breast(s).
Implant	A breast implant is a silicone shell filled with either silicone gel or a saltwater solution known as saline.	• The recovery from the initial expander placement surgery and from the permanent implant placement surgery is usually quicker than flap surgery. • It may be easier to control the final size of the reconstructed breast with implant reconstruction. • There are no additional scars on the woman's body other than those on the breasts. • For women without excess fatty tissue and who do not require radiation treatment, implants are a good choice, one with good final results.	• Because most women require placement of an expander first followed by secondary replacement of the expander with an implant, this type of reconstruction almost always requires at least two surgical stages and multiple visits to the plastic surgeon's office between these stages for tissue expansion. • It is important to realize that for women who are having a unilateral (one-sided) mastectomy, matching the other natural breast with an implant can be difficult. The shape and feel of an implant are not exactly like that of a natural breast. • In the short term, implants can become infected or malpositioned and require surgery to correct these problems. • Implant-based reconstruction is not generally recommended if women require radiation, due to the risk of complications. In the longer term, implants can develop capsular contracture (tightening of the soft tissues around the implant), implant malposition, and implant rupture. • In the case of complications, secondary procedures may be required.

TABLE 10-4 **Reconstructive Breast Surgery Options—cont'd**

NAME OF OPTION	BRIEF DESCRIPTION	ADVANTAGES	DISADVANTAGES
Deep inferior epigastric perforator (DIEP) flap, superficial inferior epigastric artery (SIEA) flap, bilateral simultaneous superior gluteal artery perforator (SGAP) flap	The DIEP flap is the technique in which skin and tissue (no muscle) are taken from the abdomen in order to re-create the breast. Other flap techniques, called the SIEA flap and the SGAP flap, take tissue from the lower abdomen or lateral buttock regions.	• Because the reconstruction involves using the woman's own tissues, the risks of implant reconstruction are avoided, particularly in the case of radiation. • Most women have less postoperative pain than after a TRAM flap and are therefore able to leave the hospital sooner and return to normal activities more quickly than after a TRAM flap. • Because the abdominal muscle is not removed as in the TRAM flap, women have much less risk of developing hernias, bulges, and core weakness at the site where the flap is removed. This advantage is much greater in bilateral (both sides) reconstruction. • It is typically easier to match the contralateral natural breast with the woman's own tissue when compared with implant reconstruction. • Women essentially end up with a "tummy tuck," "bottom lift," or other cosmetic benefits at the same time as the breast reconstruction.	• DIEP/SIEA/SGAP flap reconstruction generally requires a longer and more challenging surgery at the first stage when compared with implants or TRAM flaps. • Women will have a scar across the lower abdomen or the upper part of the buttock where the flap is obtained. However, this does not differ from the TRAM flap as the abdominal scars are equivalent. • Small revision surgeries or matching procedures on the opposing breast or donor site may be required. • Women who smoke, are obese, or who have diabetes are not ideal candidates for this type of surgery.
Transverse rectus abdominis myocutaneous (TRAM) flap	In a pedicle TRAM flap, the tissue remains attached to its original site, retaining its blood supply. The flap, consisting of the skin, fat, and muscle with its blood supply, is tunneled beneath the skin to the chest, creating a pocket for an implant or, in some cases, creating the breast mound itself, without need for an implant. The free TRAM flap involves less muscle.	• Shorter and less complex surgery than the other flaps	• This was state of the art decades ago and has since been replaced by other, more advanced procedures. • The woman may have more postoperative pain and longer hospital stays. • There is a risk of abdominal bulge or hernias, and as a result there might be a limit to how much weight the woman can lift. • Other newer procedures may offer more natural results.

Data from Shockney, L., & Tsangaris, T. (2008). *Johns Hopkins breast cancer handbook for health care professionals.* Sudbury, MA: Jones and Bartlett.

in treating breast cancer is either to eradicate or impede the growth of micrometastatic (microscopic cell metastasis) disease. Often it is not possible to detect the presence of micrometastasis at the time of initial treatment, and when it is present, mutations can occur in the tumor cells. These mutations make tumor cells resistant to the effects of chemotherapeutic agents despite tumor sensitivity to drug therapy being greatest when the tumor burden is small. Consequently the prediction cannot be made with confidence that all tumors of 1 cm or less can be cured with initial local and regional treatment. The early introduction of systemic adjuvant therapy, as determined by the estimated risk of tumor recurrence in certain subsets of women with node-negative disease, is a prudent course of treatment. Adjuvant therapy may help to destroy undetected cancers that were not surgically removed (ACS, 2013a). For women diagnosed with early-stage breast cancer and favorable prognostic factors (hormone receptor positive and HER2/neu negative), a special pathology test may help determine the woman's risk of recurrence. This test, called Oncotype DX, provides a score that represents the likelihood of her specific cancer recurring. Such information can be useful for a woman whose known benefit for receiving chemotherapy may be minimal based on her prognostic factors from the tumor itself. For women with a low score, commonly only hormonal therapy is recommended, and for those with a high score, chemotherapy is strongly considered.

Neoadjuvant therapy is systemic treatment given before surgery; the goal is to reduce tumor burden, making breast-conserving treatment an option.

Hormonal Therapy. To determine whether a woman is a candidate for hormonal therapy, a receptor assay is done. After the entire tumor or a portion is removed by biopsy or excision, a pathologist examines the cancer cells for ERs and PRs.

The presence of a receptor on the cell wall indicates that the woman is positive for that type of hormone receptor. If these receptors are present, the growth of the woman's breast cancer can be influenced by estrogen, progesterone, or both. It is unknown exactly how these hormones affect breast cancer growth. Bilateral oophorectomy may benefit women diagnosed with their first breast cancer before age 50 by reducing exposure to endogenous estrogen. Studies indicate that among women with a BRCA1 mutation and no previous breast cancer, the risk of developing breast cancer was 14% for those who chose prophylactic salpingo-oophorectomy compared with a 20% risk among women who did not choose this surgery. The risk of developing breast cancer was 7% in women with BRCA2 mutation and no previous breast cancer who chose to have a prophylactic salpingo-oophorectomy as compared to a 23% risk in those women who did not choose this surgery (Komen Foundation, 2013c). Thus oophorectomy may be an option that helps decrease the odds of recurrence and improve length of survival. In addition to or instead of oophorectomy, medications may be given to stop tumor growth that is influenced by hormones. Ovarian suppression may also be recommended by a medical oncologist as part of the hormonal therapy treatment.

There are several hormonal therapy drugs. Tamoxifen, the oldest and used the longest, is an oral antiestrogen medication that mimics progesterone and estrogen. Tamoxifen attaches to the hormone receptors on cancer cells and prevents natural hormones from attaching to the receptors. When tamoxifen fits into the receptors, the cell is unable to grow. Tamoxifen has been shown to decrease the risk of recurrence of breast cancer by 40% to 50% in postmenopausal women and by 30% to 50% in premenopausal women; and it reduces by 50% the development of a new cancer in the other breast (Breastcancer.org, 2013c). Adjuvant hormonal therapy with tamoxifen is recommended for most premenopausal women with breast cancer whose tumors are hormone receptor positive. In this age group, adjuvant tamoxifen therapy improves disease-free survival and, in some cases, length of survival. Use of hormonal therapy for 5 years in premenopausal women with breast cancer significantly reduces recurrence and mortality rates (see Medication Guide: Tamoxifen).

MEDICATION GUIDE

Tamoxifen (Nolvadex)

Action

A selective estrogen receptor modulator that exerts antiestrogenic effects; attaches to hormone receptors on cancer cells and prevents natural hormones from attaching to the receptors

Indications

For treatment of advanced-stage or metastatic breast cancer; treatment of early-stage breast cancer after breast cancer surgery and radiation therapy; to reduce the incidence of breast cancer in women at high risk

Dosage and Route

20 mg orally, daily, but can vary depending on the reason for taking tamoxifen

Adverse Reactions

Common side effects include hot flashes, night sweats, nausea, vaginal discharge, mood swings, weight gain, and cataracts. Hair loss is an uncommon effect. Serious side effects include deep vein thrombosis, increased risk of endometrial cancer, and stroke. Symptoms include abnormal vaginal bleeding, leg swelling or tenderness, chest pain, shortness of breath, weakness or numbness of extremities, sudden severe headache, and chemical hepatitis.

Nursing Considerations

The medication may be taken on an empty stomach or with food. Missed doses should be taken as soon as possible, but taking two doses at once is not recommended. A barrier or nonhormonal form of contraception is recommended in premenopausal women because tamoxifen may be harmful to the fetus if pregnancy should occur. Client counseling should concentrate on annual Pap smear (if no hysterectomy, annual eye exam, bone density every 3 years, and liver function tests (LFTs) every 6 months.

The National Cancer Comprehensive Network (NCCN) guidelines (2012) recommend adjuvant hormonal therapy for women with hormone receptor–positive breast cancer regardless of menopause status, age, or HER2/neu status, with the exception of women with lymph node–negative cancers less than or equal to 0.5 cm or 0.6 to 1 cm in diameter with favorable prognostic features. Women treated with hormonal therapy should receive therapy for at least 5 years for chemoprevention. Length of time for invasive disease may extend to 10 years if prognostically indicated (Gray, Rea, Handley, et al., 2013).

Raloxifene is an oral selective ER modulator. It is used to prevent osteoporosis in menopausal women. It was also used in a second-generation National Cancer Institute (NCI) prevention trial. It demonstrated the same 50% risk reduction in invasive breast cancer in postmenopausal women with a high risk for breast cancer with fewer thromboembolic events and lower risk of uterine cancer when compared with the use of tamoxifen (see Medication Guide: Raloxifene Hydrochloride).

Aromatase inhibitors (AIs) are a classification of hormonal therapy in use. They suppress plasma estrogen levels in postmenopausal women by inhibiting or inactivating aromatase, the enzyme responsible for synthesizing estrogens from androgens (Breastcancer.org, 2013a). AIs such as anastrozole, letrozole, and exemestane are effective agents in hormonal therapy

MEDICATION GUIDE

Raloxifene Hydrochloride (Evista)

Action

A selective estrogen receptor modulator, serving as an agonist and antagonist to estrogen receptor sites

Indications

Treatment and prevention of osteoporosis; reduction in the risk of invasive breast cancer in postmenopausal women with osteoporosis; and reduction of risk of invasive breast cancer in postmenopausal women at high risk for invasive breast cancer

Dosage and Route

60 mg orally, daily

Adverse Reactions

Common side effects include hot flashes, nausea, peripheral edema, joint pain, leg cramps, flulike symptoms, sweating. Serious and life-threatening side effects can occur from existing condition. Women who have had a heart attack or are at risk for a heart attack have increased risk of dying from a stroke. There is an increased risk of blood clots in the legs and lungs. Raloxifene is contraindicated in women with an active or past history of venous thromboembolism.

Nursing Considerations

The medication may be taken on an empty stomach or with food. Missed doses should be taken as soon as possible, but taking two doses at once is not recommended. Counsel woman to contact her physician if leg pain or feeling of warmth in lower legs, swelling of hands and feet, sudden chest pain or shortness of breath, or sudden changes in vision occur. Calcium 1500 mg plus vitamin D 400 to 800 International Units daily is recommended.

for breast cancer. Clinical trials indicate that letrozole is convincingly better than tamoxifen in treating advanced disease in postmenopausal women, and anastrozole is at least as good. In early-stage breast cancer, adjuvant therapy with anastrozole appears to be superior to adjuvant therapy with tamoxifen in reducing recurrence in postmenopausal women. AIs appear to be well tolerated with lower incidence of adverse effects as compared with tamoxifen. AIs are more commonly given to postmenopausal women whose tumors are hormone receptor positive (Ito, Blinder, & Elkin, 2012) (see Medication Guide: Letrozole).

MEDICATION GUIDE

Letrozole (Femara)

Action
An aromatase inhibitor; inhibits the conversion of androgens to estrogen

Indications
For adjuvant treatment of early breast cancer in postmenopausal women who have received 5 years of tamoxifen therapy; first-line treatment of postmenopausal women with hormone receptor–positive or hormone receptor–unknown locally advanced or metastatic cancer; adjuvant treatment of postmenopausal women with hormone receptor–positive early breast cancer

Dosage and Route
2.5 mg once a day by mouth

Adverse Reactions
Common side effects include hot flashes, nausea, increased sweating, joint or muscle pain, fluid retention, vaginal dryness, constipation, dizziness, fatigue, headache. Severe side effects include serious allergic reactions (e.g., rash, hives, difficulty breathing), vomiting, chest pain, intense bone pain, and calf pain or tenderness.

Nursing Considerations
The medication may be taken on an empty stomach or with food. Missed doses should be taken as soon as possible, but taking two doses at once is not recommended. The woman should use caution if driving or using machinery because this medication may cause drowsiness or dizziness. Women who are not postmenopausal should not take letrozole.

Chemotherapy. Chemotherapy drugs are most often given in combination regimens, which have been shown to improve or increase the disease-free survival time after therapy. The most common chemotherapy regimens used for adjuvant treatment of node-positive and node-negative tumors are listed in Box 10-2.

Adjuvant chemotherapy has been most useful in premenopausal women who have breast cancer with positive nodes, regardless of hormone receptor status. It is postulated that younger women often have tumors with a higher S-phase fraction and proliferative rate, which makes the tumors more sensitive to chemotherapy. Although adjuvant chemotherapy effectively decreases the risks for recurrence and mortality in premenopausal women with node-positive disease, postmenopausal women can also be offered chemotherapy, depending on the cancer size, nodal involvement, and morphologic and biologic factors or markers of the particular cancer (Shockney & Tsangaris, 2008).

BOX 10-2 Common Chemotherapy Regimens for Adjuvant Treatment of Breast Cancer

- CAF: cyclophosphamide, doxorubicin (Adriamycin), fluorouracil
- TAC: docetaxel, doxorubicin, and cyclophosphamide
- AC → T: doxorubicin and cyclophosphamide followed by paclitaxel or docetaxel (Herceptin may be given with the paclitaxel or docetaxel for HER2/neu-positive tumors.)
- FEC: fluorouracil, epirubicin, and cyclophosphamide (this may be followed by docetaxel)
- TC: docetaxel and cyclophosphamide
- TCH: docetaxel, carboplatin, and Herceptin for HER2/neu-positive tumors
- Less common regimens include:
  - CMF: cyclophosphamide, methotrexate, fluorouracil
  - AC: doxorubicin, cyclophosphamide
  - EC: epirubicin, cyclophosphamide
  - A → CMF: doxorubicin followed by CMF

American Cancer Society. (2013). Chemotherapy for breast cancer. Available at www.cancer.org/cancer/breastcancer/detailedguide/breast-cancer-treating-chemotherapy.

Chemotherapy with multiple drug combinations is used in the treatment of recurrent and advanced breast cancer with positive results. First-line single agents for women with locally advanced or metastatic breast cancer include paclitaxel, docetaxel, epirubicin, doxorubicin, pegylated liposomal doxorubicin, capecitabine, vinorelbine, and gemcitabine. Combination regimens and sequential single agents can be used (NCCN, 2012). The use of herceptin and bevacizumab has advanced response rates and lowered recurrences. Because chemotherapy drugs kill rapidly reproducing cells, treatment also affects normal body cells that rapidly reproduce (red and white blood cells, gastric mucosa, and hair). Thus chemotherapy can cause leukopenia, neutropenia, thrombocytopenia, anemia, gastrointestinal side effects (nausea, vomiting, anorexia, mucositis), and partial or full hair loss.

Chemotherapy treatments are usually administered in ambulatory care settings once or twice per month. During the informed consent process, before the treatment is selected, the woman and her family members should be educated about the names of the medications, routes of administration, treatment schedule, timing and ordering of medications, length of time of administration, reimbursed and unreimbursed costs of therapy, potential side effects, management of side effects, possible changes in body image (e.g., full or partial hair loss), recovery time after treatment (necessitating lost work time), and need for a caregiver to transport the woman to treatment and care for her afterward. Depending on the medications used, the treatments can include intravenous, subcutaneous, and oral administration. Often a long-term central venous catheter is inserted when the women will be receiving chemotherapy for an extended period or when she will receive medications that may damage the vein. Presence of a central venous catheter, hair loss, loss of part or all of her breast, menopause, and possible infertility all have the potential to cause a change in body image and increase emotional distress.

Treatment with chemotherapy, hormonal therapy, or a combination of the two often causes changes in reproductive function. The premenopausal woman may experience these changes along with symptoms of menopause and possible infertility. It is not known whether hormonal therapy to ease the effects of menopause is safe for women with breast cancer; therefore, it is not recommended. For this reason the nurse must use other measures to help the woman cope with menopause (see Chapter 6).

Women receiving chemotherapy and their partners must understand that chemotherapy can be teratogenic, that is, chemotherapy agents can cause congenital birth defects. Any woman who is of childbearing age and receiving chemotherapy, even though no longer menstruating, must use birth control. Although a woman may not be menstruating, she may still be able to become pregnant.

Birth control pills are not recommended because they contain hormones that may assist in the growth of cancer. A birth control method must be chosen with the assistance of a gynecologist and a medical oncologist, and it must be used before chemotherapy begins and continue to be used until the medical oncologist and gynecologist believe it is safe to discontinue.

Special Groups

Young Women. Of the new diagnosed breast cancers, approximately 12% will affect women younger than age 40. The diagnosis of concomitant pregnancy and breast cancer is estimated at about 1 in 3000. Although the basic treatment modalities for breast cancer are used, the unique importance in this age population requires careful consideration of their developmental tasks. Nurses can identify developmental tasks and help young women cope with their disease.

In identifying special surgical concerns for young women diagnosed with breast cancer, one would have to address the timing and extent of the surgery offered. A younger woman is more likely than not to harbor a mutation, and therefore genetic testing may be an important aspect in deciding a surgical plan. She may in fact want to use the genetic results to decide on whether to consider bilateral mastectomies. If chemotherapy is planned, a neoadjuvant approach would allow enough time for surgical decision making while still actively receiving treatment. Choosing a breast-conserving approach requires a careful discussion because it leaves the woman with a higher chance for recurrence.

Systemic therapy, whether adjuvant or neoadjuvant, will affect fertility. Depending on the specific type of chemotherapeutic agent and the age of the women, the rate of premature ovarian failure ranges from 30% to 80% (Rosenberg & Partridge, 2013). It is important to include a consult to a reproductive gynecologist early after diagnosis to discuss preserving fertility.

Chapter 11 presents information about young women who are diagnosed with breast cancer during pregnancy. This is an important area for nurses to understand.

Young women with breast cancer face different challenges than do the majority of older diagnosed women. The biology of their tumors together with the genetic implications suggests a more threatening outcome. The defining difference, however, is the time of life at which the disease strikes. Independence, autonomy, integration into society, and fusion in the family are the foundations on which nursing interventions should focus in achieving the best outcomes for quality of life and survivorship.

The future might also appear different for these women. Although the risk of recurrence plagues all women with breast cancer, younger women with this disease face the possibility of second or third malignancies if they survive long term. The consideration of undergoing prophylactic surgery can be an overwhelming decision for these young women. Successful survivorship will be defined by their ability to move beyond treatments, continue to work productively, have their families, and find meaning in their lives.

Women Ages 65 and Older. Although the occurrence of breast cancer is declining, the incidence of women being diagnosed with breast cancer at age 65 and older is increasing (ACS, 2013a). Women who are 65 years of age are expected to live another 20 years. The same standard of care in treating breast cancer applies as in treating younger women (American Society of Clinical Oncology [ASCO], 2013). There are, however, developments in which treatment for breast cancer can be modified for this aging population. The variations in treatment are largely based on comorbidities. Other variables include the woman's functional disability, socioeconomic resources, difficulties with access and transportation to health care, resulting in not having an annual clinical breast examination or mammogram (Schapira & Muss, 2013). The majority of older woman diagnosed with breast cancer will likely be estrogen receptor positive and demonstrate less aggressive forms of disease. Geriatric oncology is an emerging specialty, and the American Society of Clinical Oncology (ASCO) has supported endocrine therapy with an aromatase inhibitor, either initially adjuvantly or sequenced after tamoxifen; the optimal timing and duration remain unresolved. There is also evidence for use of an aromatase inhibitor alone as primary therapy (Balakrishnan & Ravichandran, 2011).

The overall success in treating older women is based largely on integrating geriatrics with oncology. There are available tools through ASCO and NCCN that can help with providing geriatric assessments. Older women are faced with treatment decisions based on many factors, with quality of life being a major one.

Survivorship Issues

Because women are living longer after treatment for breast cancer, survivorship issues have become very important in relation to quality of life. In the 1990s ASCO developed evidence-based guidelines that standardize surveillance and include history and physical examination every 3 to 6 months during the first 3 years, every 6 to 12 months during years 4 and 5, and annually thereafter. At that point women can be transitioned into primary care. In addition, mammography is annual, with the first at 6 months postradiation to establish a new baseline. It is recommended that women who carry a genetic mutation have MRI added to their surveillance. Routine gynecologic care is suggested. Many women suffer from many sequelae of cancer treatment, including vasomotor symptoms, sexual dysfunction, infertility, osteoporosis, musculoskeletal pain, weight gain, cognitive changes, fatigue, neuropathy, and congestive heart failure. Whether a woman is in a specialty clinic or primary care, the ability to recognize and treat these problems is critical for optimum health.

Vasomotor symptoms occur in many women treated for breast cancer, partly due to hormonal treatments. Lifestyle changes such as keeping room temperatures down, avoiding spicy food and caffeine, and dressing in layers can be useful. Hormone replacement therapy is contraindicated. Some pharmacologic agents, including antidepressants such as paroxetine, fluoxetine, citalopram, and venlafaxine, as well as anticonvulsants such as gabapentin and the antihypertensive clonidine have been used with varying success (Stan, Loprinzi, & Ruddy, 2013).

Sexual dysfunction may be related to the endocrine changes that result from systemic therapy. The most common reported issue for women is decreased libido, followed by decreased arousal or lubrication, dyspareunia, and body image. Helping women overcome these problems requires the nurse to discuss such symptoms openly with their clients.

Osteoporosis caused by systemic chemotherapy or antiestrogen therapies is a potential major comorbidity of breast cancer treatment. The incidence of bone fractures in this population is five times higher than in the general population (Stan, Loprinzi, & Ruddy 2013). With this in mind, screening for osteoporosis with dual-energy x-ray absorptiometry (DEXA) scans every 1 to 2 years is recommended in survivors 65 years or older (60 to 64 for those women deemed at risk or on AI therapy). They should be given additional counseling for weight-bearing exercises, supplemental vitamin D and calcium, smoking cessation, and avoidance of excessive alcohol intake. Bisphosphonates can treat or prevent osteoporosis in breast cancer survivors.

Weight gain is common in women treated for breast cancer. Chemotherapy causes sarcopenic obesity, characterized by lean mass loss and fat gain. Decreased physical activity caused by fatigue and to a lesser degree overeating are considered factors (Stan, Loprinzi, & Ruddy, 2013). Most women who are actively being treated are encouraged to exercise to combat fatigue and improve symptoms. The ACS recommends strength training at least twice per week and 150 minutes of aerobic exercise per week.

Studies have demonstrated a 15% to 75% occurrence of cognitive changes associated with breast cancer treatments, including problems with concentration, attention, and memory (Afiles, Root, & Ryan, 2012). Although most of the literature suggests chemotherapy as a causative agent, data suggest pretreatment factors and hormonal therapy with tamoxifen should be included. Older women and those with lower cognitive reserve are more vulnerable to the treatment effects.

Cancer-related fatigue (CRF) is a persistent feeling of emotional, physical, and cognitive exhaustion associated with cancer diagnosis and treatment that is out of proportion to the average population. It is reported as one of the most common side effects associated with treatment and has a great effect on quality of life. The prevalence varies between 15% and 90% (NCCN, 2012). NCCN recommends routine screening for this symptom. It has long been known that radiation causes fatigue, but the combination of chemotherapy and other systemic therapies is considered synergistic.

Cardiotoxicity is well recognized as a side effect of breast cancer treatment. The most common cause is anthracycline-based regimens; however, with the addition of taxanes, this incidence has increased. Women who are on either anthracyclines or taxanes need regular heart function monitoring and dose modifications, along with cardiac management. Neuropathies, another side effect of taxanes, are chronic and may require dose modifications. Long-term drug therapy is required to manage side effects (Stan, Loprinzi, & Ruddy, 2013).

Nursing Interventions

Nursing care of a woman with breast cancer depends on the treatment chosen. Data that guide the care include a client history, a physical examination, laboratory and diagnostic test results, and psychosocial assessment.

Emotional Support After Diagnosis. When a woman is diagnosed with cancer, she confronts mortality and potential bodily changes. The emotional reaction to the diagnosis varies with each woman, but is often intense, and the many disruptions caused by the disease challenge the woman's and family's ability to cope. Disruptions may be caused by costs of treatment, loss of role function, lack of stress-relieving activities, spouse's or child's reaction to the diagnosis, change in body image and sexual function, disability, and pain. The woman may feel despair, fear, and shame. Sexuality issues related to breast cancer include a change in body image, changes in sexual function (such as decreased vaginal lubrication caused by hormonal therapy), and relational distress. Health care providers are responsible for discussing the influence of breast cancer on the woman's life and in assisting her and her family to cope effectively.

Women and their families often undergo a period of distress after the diagnosis of cancer. It is difficult to accept the diagnosis when the woman may feel and look well. This period may be characterized by anguish and shock followed by disbelief and denial. During this time absorbing information and education can be difficult, and the nurse should be sensitive as to how this may affect decision-making abilities. Flexibility is the key to sensitive nursing care. As the woman and family begin to accept her diagnosis, more and more information can be shared, and care planning with full client participation can take place, including the following:

- Validate and reinforce accurate information processing by the woman and her family.
- Assist in client decision making and arrange for the woman to speak with breast cancer survivors who have chosen a variety of treatment options (Box 10-3).
- Suggest approaches the woman might take to deal with the sexual concerns of her significant other.

BOX 10-3 Decision-Making Questions to Ask

1. What kind of breast cancer is it (invasive or noninvasive)?
2. What is the stage of the cancer (i.e., how extensive is the spread)?
3. What further tests are recommended (e.g., estrogen receptor assay, HER2 status)?
4. What are the treatment options (pros and cons of each, including side effects)?
5. If surgery is recommended, what will the scar look like?
6. If a mastectomy is done, can breast reconstruction be done (at the time of surgery or later)?
7. How long will the woman be in the hospital? What kind of postoperative care will she need?
8. How long will treatment last if radiation or chemotherapy is recommended? What effects can the woman expect from these treatments?
9. What community resources are available for support?

Data from American Cancer Society. (2013). *Questions to ask my doctor about breast cancer.* Available at www.cancer.org/acs/groups/cid/documents/webcontent/003284-pdf.pdf.

- Discuss the application of alternative therapies to alleviate stress and promote healing, such as exercise, guided imagery, meditation, and progressive muscle relaxation.
- Refer the woman to the ACS's Reach to Recovery program or other resources that provide trained survivor volunteers for one-on-one support (Box 10-4).
- Refer the woman to a cancer rehabilitation program, such as Encore, an exercise program run by the YWCA.

The NCCN (www.nccn.org) and the ACS (www.cancer.org) provide specific, up-to-date recommendations on breast cancer treatments on the Internet. These are invaluable resources for women to learn about scientifically tested treatment protocols for each stage of breast cancer.

BOX 10-4 Internet Resources for Information on Breast Cancer

Susan B. Komen Breast Cancer Foundation: www.ww5.komen.org
National Ovarian Cancer Coalition: www.ovarian.org
National Breast Cancer Foundation: www.nationalbreastcancer.org
National Alliance of Breast Cancer Organizations: www.nabco.org
Reach to Recovery International: www.reachtorecoveryinternational.org
American Cancer Society: www.cancer.org
Association of Cancer Online Resources: www.acor.org
Breast Cancer National Cancer Institute: www.cancer.gov/cancertopics/types/breast
National Breast Cancer Awareness Month: www.nbcam.org
Breast Cancer Alliance: www.breastcanceralliance.org/category/patient-information-resources/

COMMUNITY ACTIVITY

Research the availability of rehabilitation programs for breast cancer survivors in your community such as the American Cancer Society (ACS)'s Reach to Recovery program. Contact the agency (e.g., local ACS agency) to identify the services provided by the program and the requirements for becoming a volunteer. How are the resources and programs promoted in the community (e.g., brochures in waiting areas of clinics, newspaper ads)? Are nurses in the community involved and if so, how? Do women who use the services provide evaluation about their experiences, and if so, how is it collected and used?

After assisting the woman with accepting the diagnosis and obtaining support, consider nursing care in the preoperative, postoperative, and convalescent periods. The discussion that follows describes nursing care at each of these periods for a woman having a **modified radical mastectomy** (see Nursing Care Plan).

NURSING CARE PLAN

The Woman Having Breast-Conserving Surgery and Axillary Node Dissection

NURSING DIAGNOSIS	EXPECTED OUTCOME	NURSING INTERVENTIONS	RATIONALES
Acute Pain related to surgical incision and surgical drains, as evidenced by client verbalizations	Woman will report minimal intensity and decreased number of painful episodes.	Use pain scale to assess type and intensity of pain.	To provide accurate database
		Administer analgesics as ordered.	To decrease perception of pain
		Teach and reinforce use of relaxation techniques.	To reduce anxiety and provide distraction that may decrease the perception of pain
		Reposition woman with affected arm elevated.	To promote comfort and lymphatic channel return
Risk for Infection related to disruption of skin integrity and removal of lymph nodes	Woman will experience no clinical manifestations of infection.	Assess clinical manifestations of infection at the incision and drain sites that may include redness, swelling, localized heat, fever, increasing pain, and foul-smelling drainage.	To facilitate prompt treatment
		Demonstrate the procedure for emptying and recording the amount of drainage from the Jackson-Pratt drain(s).	To provide information to the surgeon as to the appropriate removal time of drains. Drains are usually removed when drainage is less than 30 ml of fluid in 24 hours.
		Explain the need to avoid trauma or irritation to the affected arm.	To reinforce to the woman that alterations in sensation and removal of some lymph nodes may affect ability to sense irritation or prevent infection
		Reinforce to the woman the need to protect the arm from injury and to avoid blood drawing or blood pressures to be taken on the affected arm.	To avoid trauma and infection because decreased sensation may be present as well as decreased lymphatic return

NURSING CARE PLAN—cont'd

The Woman Having Breast-Conserving Surgery and Axillary Node Dissection

NURSING DIAGNOSIS	EXPECTED OUTCOME	NURSING INTERVENTIONS	RATIONALES
		Explain the importance of reporting any clinical manifestations of infection to the caregiver as soon as possible.	To provide identification and treatment of problem
Disturbed Body Image related to loss of all or part of a breast as evidenced by client statements	Woman will report acceptance of herself as she is and regain a positive body image.	Provide opportunity through therapeutic communication to express feelings about body image changes.	To clarify and validate feelings
		Refer to support groups.	To facilitate verbalization of feelings with women who have similar concerns
Impaired Physical Mobility related to pain and tissue trauma	Woman will return to her preoperative level of mobility.	Encourage woman to do hand, arm, and wrist exercises that can be performed in the immediate postoperative period.	To enhance fluid return and prevent muscle atrophy
		Encourage woman to perform activities of daily living as much as possible.	To encourage woman to focus on her strengths rather than her limitations
		Teach woman exercises to be performed after the drains are removed.	To promote range of motion in the arm that had the axillary nodes dissected
		Teach woman to do exercises slowly and gently.	To prevent injury and pain
		Caution woman not to lift anything heavier than 10 pounds for 4 to 6 weeks.	To avoid exerting strain on affected arm

Preoperative Care. General preoperative teaching and care are given, including expectations regarding physical appearance, pain management, equipment to be used (e.g., intravenous therapy, drains), and emotional support. Some emotional support may be obtained by arranging for a visit from a member of an organization such as Reach to Recovery. The woman is reminded that when she awakens after surgery, her arm on the affected side will feel tight.

Immediate Postoperative Care. After recovery from anesthesia, the woman is returned to her room. Special precautions must be observed to prevent or to minimize lymphedema of the affected arm.

! NURSING ALERT

When vital signs are taken, never apply the blood pressure cuff to the arm affected by the axillary lymph node dissection.

The affected arm is elevated with pillows above the level of the right atrium. Blood is not drawn from this arm, and this arm is not used for intravenous therapy or any injections. Early arm movement is encouraged. Any increase in the circumference of that arm is reported immediately.

Nursing care of the wound involves observing for signs of hemorrhage (dressing, drainage tubes, and Hemovac or Jackson-Pratt drainage reservoirs are emptied at least every 8 hours and more frequently as needed), shock, and infection. Dressings are reinforced as necessary. The woman is asked to turn (alternating between unaffected side and back), cough (while the nurse or the woman applies support to the chest), and deep breathe every 2 hours. Breath sounds are auscultated every 4 hours. Active range-of-motion (ROM) exercise of legs is encouraged. Parenteral fluids are given until adequate oral intake is possible. Emotional support is continued.

Care given during the immediate postoperative period is continued as necessary. Most women who undergo lumpectomy have surgery as ambulatory clients and return home a few hours after surgery. Women are discharged 24 hours or less after mastectomy without reconstruction. Women having a mastectomy with tissue expander placement will be in the hospital for 24 hours. Those having flap reconstruction at the same time will be hospitalized for 3 to 5 days. Because of the generally short time spent in the hospital, thorough teaching is important. It is best to do as much teaching as possible before surgery if the outcome is known. If this is not possible, discharge teaching should be done with the woman's caregiver present. This is to acknowledge the possibility that emotional stress or recovery from anesthesia may cause the woman to forget some of the discharge instructions. Printed information also should be provided for the woman and family to refer to at home.

Women who have had breast cancer surgery are usually seen by their surgeon within 5 to 7 days of surgery. This follow-up visit is important because it allows the physician to assess the outcome of surgical treatment as well as provide reinforcement of education and emotional support. A woman having simultaneous reconstruction will also be seen by her plastic surgeon within a week postoperatively.

Early ambulation is encouraged to improve circulation and ventilation and to prevent loss of bone calcium. The psychologic benefits of early mobility include resumption of self-care and activities of daily living that serve to reinforce the woman's control over her life and help her move from a sick role to the role of breast cancer survivor.

Arm exercises are encouraged at least four times daily (Box 10-5). Exercise is increased as tolerated and is stopped at the point of pain. Initially the woman alternately clenches and extends her fingers and then progresses to wrist and elbow exercises, gradually abducting her arm and raising it to and over her head. She is encouraged to exercise by assisting with her care—washing her face, brushing her teeth, and eating with her hand and arm on the affected side. Physical therapy may be prescribed to improve strength and mobility of the affected arm. Women having a sentinel node biopsy only should have full ROM back within a few days. A woman having axillary dissections will need to work more vigorously at restoring ROM. She should have returned to her baseline ROM by the end of the third week postoperatively.

It is important to discuss the appearance of the woman's breast if dressings have not been removed before discharge. Some women may not want to view their surgical site, but it is important to give them the opportunity to do so and to provide emotional support at that time. The woman should be encouraged to express her emotions and verbalize her feelings. She needs to know that it will take time to become accustomed to her change of appearance. A woman who has undergone reconstruction at the same time should be encouraged to look at herself as a work in progress—swelling, positioning of tissue expanders, appearance of flaps, and presence of multiple drains initially can be difficult to accept. Over time, when drains are out and swelling subsides, she will begin to see her new silhouette take shape.

An option for restoring body image is choosing an external prosthesis to replace the lost breast or portion of breast

BOX 10-5 Arm Exercises After Lymph Node Dissection

Exercises After Breast Surgery

It is important that the woman talk to her physician before starting any exercises. A physical therapist or occupational therapist can help design an exercise program for the woman.

Exercises in Lying Position

These exercises should be performed on a bed or the floor while lying on your back with your knees and hips bent, feet flat.

Wand Exercise

This exercise helps increase the forward motion of the shoulders. You will need a broom handle, yardstick, or other similar object to perform this exercise.

- Hold the wand in both hands with palms facing up.
- Lift the wand up over your head (as far as you can) using your unaffected arm to help lift the wand, until you feel a stretch in your affected arm.
- Hold for 5 seconds.
- Lower arms and repeat 5 to 7 times.

Elbow Winging

This exercise helps increase the mobility of the front of your chest and shoulder. It may take several weeks of regular exercise before your elbows will get close to the bed (or floor).

- Clasp your hands behind your neck with your elbows pointing toward the ceiling.
- Move your elbows apart and down toward the bed (or floor).
- Repeat 5 to 7 times

Exercises in Sitting Position

Shoulder Blade Stretch

This exercise helps increase the mobility of the shoulder blades.

- Sit in a chair very close to a table with your back against the chair back.
- Place the unaffected arm on the table with your elbow bent and palm down. Do not move this arm during the exercise.
- Place the affected arm on the table, palm down with your elbow straight.
- Without moving your trunk, slide the affected arm toward the opposite side of the table. You should feel your shoulder blade move as you do this.
- Relax your arm and repeat 5 to 7 times.

Shoulder Blade Squeeze

This exercise also helps increase the mobility of the shoulder blade.

- Facing straight ahead, sit in a chair in front of a mirror without resting on the back of the chair.
- Arms should be at your sides with elbows bent.
- Squeeze shoulder blades together, bringing your elbows behind you. Keep your shoulders level as you do this exercise. Do not lift your shoulders up toward your ears.
- Return to the starting position and repeat 5 to 7 times.

Side Bending

This exercise helps increase the mobility of the trunk/body.

- Clasp your hands together in front of you and lift your arms slowly over your head, straightening your arms.
- When your arms are over your head, bend your trunk to the right while bending at the waist and keeping your arms overhead.
- Return to the starting position and bend to the left.
- Repeat 5 to 7 times.

Exercises in Standing Position

Chest Wall Stretch

This exercise helps stretch the chest wall.

- Stand facing a corner with toes approximately 8 to 10 inches from the corner.
- Bend your elbows and place forearms on the wall, one on each side of the corner. Your elbows should be as close to shoulder height as possible.
- Keep your arms and feet in position and move your chest toward the corner. You will feel a stretch across your chest and shoulders.
- Return to starting position and repeat 5 to 7 times.

Shoulder Stretch

This exercise helps increase the mobility in the shoulder.

- Stand facing the wall with your toes approximately 8 to 10 inches from the wall.
- Place your hands on the wall. Use your fingers to "climb the wall," reaching as high as you can until you feel a stretch.
- Return to starting position and repeat 5 to 7 times.

Modified from American Cancer Society. (2013). *Exercises after breast surgery.* Available at www.cancer.org/cancer/breastcancer/moreinformation/exercises-after-breast-surgery.

tissue for a client who has a mastectomy without reconstruction. The external prosthesis is inserted into a mastectomy bra. Women who choose to use a partial external prosthesis after BCS or full external prosthesis after mastectomy need information about where to obtain prostheses and an appropriate bra. Usually a temporary prosthesis is worn for the first 3 months before the woman is fitted for a permanent one. Women should be advised on how to submit the cost of the prosthesis to their insurance company. Volunteers of the Reach to Recovery program are able to provide this information, as well as a list of sources for prostheses, bathing suits, and lingerie. They can offer helpful hints and suggestions for coping with prostheses and wearing apparel. Some women find that an external prosthesis does not restore body image and seek surgical reconstruction of the missing or disfigured breast (see earlier discussion). It is also important to note that some women may choose to forgo a prosthesis as well as surgical reconstruction.

Discharge Planning and Follow-up Care. Before discharge, considerable time should be spent counseling the woman and her family about self-management. These instructions are summarized in the Teaching for Self-Management box. Printed instructions should be given to the woman and her family. A referral for home nursing care may be made if the woman needs assistance caring for her incision.

Teaching Needs for the Client and Family Undergoing Adjuvant Therapies. It is important that the woman and her family be given thorough instructions regarding side effects and avoidance of possible complications of adjuvant treatment. A common side effect of radiation therapy is skin irritation and breakdown. The woman should avoid using lotions, powders, or ointments on the skin at the radiation site unless instructed by the radiologist. The skin should be cleansed gently with mild soap and water, rinsed thoroughly, and patted dry. Skin markings that direct the placement of the radiation beam should not be removed. Soft, nonirritating clothing should be worn over the site, and the skin protected from exposure to sun and heat.

Common side effects of chemotherapy include alopecia, fatigue, nausea, vomiting, mouth sores, and immunosuppression. The woman receiving chemotherapy that produces hair loss should be encouraged to obtain a wig matching her own hair color and style before beginning treatments so that she is prepared when hair loss begins. Of course, some women may choose not to wear a wig or a scarf. The local ACS can assist in obtaining a wig and head coverings designed for women experiencing hair loss from chemotherapy. The woman should be taught the importance of rest periods when fatigue occurs. She and her family will need to know that work and family schedules may need adjustment to accommodate needed rest. Exercise

TEACHING FOR SELF-MANAGEMENT

After a Mastectomy Without Reconstruction

- Wash hands well before and after touching incision area or drains.
- Empty surgical drains twice a day and as needed, recording the date, time, drain sites (if more than one drain is present), and amount of drainage in milliliters in the diary you will take to each surgical checkup until your drains are removed. (Before discharge, you may receive a graduated container for emptying drains and measuring drainage.)
- Avoid driving, lifting more than 10 pounds, or reaching above your head until given permission by the surgeon.
- Take medications for pain as soon as pain begins.
- Perform arm exercises as directed.
- Call your physician if inflammation of incision or swelling of the incision or the arm occurs.
- Avoid tight clothing, tight jewelry, and other causes of decreased circulation in the affected arm.
- Until drains are removed, wear loose-fitting underwear (camisole or half-slip) and clothes, pinning surgical drains inside of clothing. (You will be taught how to do this safely.)
- After drains are removed and surgical sites are healing and still tender, wear a mastectomy bra or camisole with a cotton-filled, muslin temporary prosthesis. Temporary prostheses of this type are often available from Reach to Recovery.
- Avoid depilatory creams, strong deodorants, and shaving of affected chest area, axilla, and arm.
- Sponge bathe for the first 48 hours; then you may shower. Thoroughly dry yourself afterward and reapply fresh dressings.
- Return to the surgeon's office for incision check, drain inspection, and possible drain removal as directed.
- Contact Reach to Recovery or a breast center nursing staff member for assistance in obtaining external prosthesis and lingerie when dressings, drains, and staples are removed and wound is healing and nontender.
- Contact insurance company for information about coverage of prosthesis and wig if needed. Obtain prescriptions for prosthesis and wig to submit with receipts of purchase for these items to the insurance company. If insurance does not pay for these items, contact the hospital or agency social worker or local American Cancer Society for assistance.
- Practice breast self-examination (BSE) of unaffected side and affected surgical site and axilla.
- Keep follow-up visits for professional examination, mammography, and testing to detect recurrent breast cancer.
- Expect decreased sensation and tingling at incision sites and in the affected arm for weeks to months after surgery.
- Resume sexual activities as desired.
- Participate in breast cancer survivor support group if desired.
- Encourage mother, sisters, and daughters (if applicable) to learn and practice BSE and to have annual professional breast examinations and mammography (if appropriate).

Additional Nursing Care for Women Undergoing Mastectomy with Reconstruction

- No tight compression of the reconstructed breasts until approved by her plastic surgeon.
- Wear loose-fitting garments for first 3 to 4 weeks.
- Emphasize to the woman that her surgery is still a work in progress and that final cosmetic result of reconstruction takes many weeks.
- Assess the skin for potential of poor peripheral circulation that may cause skin necrosis, and report any skin changes immediately.
- See drain care instructions under axillary dissection section.

may help in increasing energy and decreasing fatigue. Nausea and vomiting should be reported to the physician and are treated with antiemetics. Mouth sores may be very painful, and the woman should be instructed to maintain good oral hygiene and avoid trauma to the oral mucosa by using a soft toothbrush. The mouth should be rinsed frequently with water or saline, and mouthwashes containing alcohol or glycerin should be avoided as well as spicy or irritating foods (see Box 11-4 for other suggestions). Topical anesthetic medications may be prescribed by the physician. The woman with immunosuppression should be instructed to use frequent handwashing and avoid crowds and other large gatherings of people, especially during cold and flu season. She should be taught to avoid eating raw fruits and vegetables (low-bacteria diet), maintain strict personal hygiene, and recognize the signs and symptoms of infection and report them to the health care provider immediately.

KEY POINTS

- The most common benign breast problems are fibrocystic changes and fibroadenomas.
- The development of breast neoplasms, whether benign or malignant, can have a significant physical and emotional effect on a woman and her family.
- The risk of American women developing cancer of the breast is 1 in 8.
- An estimated 90% of all breast lumps are detected by the woman.
- Clinical breast examinations by a health care provider (starting in one's 20s), and routine screening mammograms (after age 40) are recommended by the ACS for early detection of breast cancer.
- Digital mammography is superior to traditional analog mammography.
- The primary therapy for most women with stage I or stage II breast cancer is breast-conserving surgery followed by radiation therapy.
- Adjuvant chemotherapy is most helpful to premenopausal women with breast cancer that has spread to the lymph nodes.
- Tamoxifen, along with raloxifene and anastrozole, provides the first real hope in preventing breast cancer.
- The emotional diagnosis of breast cancer is always intense, and the many disruptions caused by the disease challenge the woman and her family's ability to cope.
- There are more reconstruction options today than ever before.
- 85% of women diagnosed today with breast cancer will be long-term survivors.

REFERENCES

Advanced Radiation Center. (2013). *Radiation therapy dosage. Medical News.* Available at www.news-medical.net/health/Radiation-Therapy-Dosage.aspx.

Afiles, T. A., Root, J. C., & Ryan, E. L. (2012). Cancer and cancer treatment—Associated cognitive change: An update on the state of the science. *Journal of Clinical Oncology, 30*(30), 3675–3686.

American Cancer Society. (2013a). *Breast cancer facts and figures 2013-2014.* Atlanta, GA: Author. http://www.cancer.org/acs/groups/content/@research/documents/document/acspc-042725.pdf.

American Cancer Society (ACS). (2013b). *Mammograms and other imaging tests.* Available at www.cancer.org/treatment/understandingdiagnosis/examsandtestdescriptions/mammogramsandotherbreastimaging-procedures/index.

American Society of Clinical Oncology. (2013). New studies highlight ASCO's innovative programs to improve the quality of cancer patient care. Available at www.asco.org.

Balakrishnan, A., & Ravichandran, D. (2011). Early operable breast cancer in elderly women treated with an aromatase inhibitor letrozole as sole therapy. *British Journal of Cancer, 105*(12), 1825–1829.

Breastcancer.org. (2013a). *Aromatase inhibitors.* Available at www.breastcancer.org/treatment/hormonal/aromatase_inhibitors.

Breastcancer.org. (2013b). Nipple reconstruction. *Types of breast reconstruction.* Available at www.breastcancer.org/treatment/surgery/reconstruction/types/nipple.

Breastcancer.org. (2013c). *Tamoxifen in pill form (brand name: Nolvadex).* Available at www.breastcancer.org/treatment/hormonal/serms/tamoxifen.

Fancellu, A., Cottu, P., Feo, C. F., et al. (2012). Sentinel node biopsy in early breast cancer: Lessons learned from more than 1,000 cases at a single institution. *Tumori, 98*(4), 413–420.

Gray, R.G., Rea, D., Handley, K., et al., aTTom (2013). Long-term effects of continuing adjuvant tamoxifen to 10 years versus stopping in 5 in 6,953 women with early breast cancer. aTTom presented at ASCO 2013. *Journal of Clinical Oncology, 31*(18), suppl, abstract 5.

Ito, K., Blinder, V. S., & Elkin, E. B. (2012). Cost effectiveness of fracture prevention in postmenopausal women who received aromatase inhibitors for early breast cancer. *Journal of Clinical Oncology, 30*(13), 1468–1475.

Katz, V., & Dotters, D. (2012). Breast disease: Diagnosis and treatment of benign and malignant disease. In G. Lentz, R. Lobo, D. Gershenson, & V. Katz (Eds.), *Comprehensive gynecology* (6th ed.). Philadelphia: Mosby.

Komen Foundation. (2013a). Accuracy of mammograms. *Early detection and screening.* Available at ww5.komen.org/BreastCancer/Accuracy-ofMammograms.html.

Komen Foundation. (2013b). Breast magnetic resonance imaging. *Emerging areas in diagnosis.* Available at ww5.komen.org/Content.aspx-?id=6946&terms=MRI.

Komen Foundation. (2013c). Preventive surgery reduces breast cancer risk in women with BRCA1 or BRCA2 mutations. *Understanding breast cancer.* Available at ww5.komen.org/KomenNewsArticle.aspx?id=6442452462.

Lobo, R. (2012). Hyperprolactinemia, galactorrhea, and pituitary adenomas: Etiology, differential diagnosis, natural history, management. In G. Lentz, R. Lobo, D. Gershenson, & V. Katz (Eds.), *Comprehensive gynecology* (6th ed.). Philadelphia: Mosby.

Mayo Clinic. (2011). *Breast cancer chemoprevention: Medicines that reduce breast cancer risk.* Available at www.mayoclinic.com/health/breast-cancer/WO00092.

Mayo Foundation for Medical Education and Research. (2012). *Mammary duct ectasia.* Available at www.mayoclinic.com/health/mammary-duct-ectasia.

National Cancer Institute. (2013). *Breast cancer treatment.* Available at www.cancer.gov/cancertopics/pdq/treatment/breast/healthprofessional/page3.

National Comprehensive Cancer Network (NCCN). (2012). *Breast cancer treatment guidelines for patients (online)*. Available at www.nccn.org/treatment-summaries.aspx.

Nelson, H., Fu, R., Griffin, J., et al. (2009). Systematic review: Comparative effectiveness of medications to reduce risk for primary breast cancer. *Annals of Internal Medicine*, *17*(10), 703–715.

Redig, A. J., & McAllister, S. S. (2013). Breast cancer as a systemic disease: A view of metastasis. *Journal of Internal Medicine*, *274*(2), 113–126.

Rosenberg, S. M., & Partridge, A. H. (2013). Premature menopause in young breast cancer: Effects on quality of life and treatment interventions. *Journal of Thoracic Disease (Special Supplement: Breast Cancer in Young Women)*, *5*(1), SS55–61.

Schapira, L., & Muss, H. (2013). Issues in treating older women with breast cancer. 35th Annual San Antonio Breast Cancer Symposium (SABCS), March 29, 2013.

Shockney, L., & Tsangaris, T. (2008). *Johns Hopkins breast cancer handbook for health care professionals*. Sudbury, MA: Jones and Bartlett.

Stan, D., Loprinzi, C. L., & Ruddy, K. J. (2013). Breast cancer survivorship issues. *Hematology Oncology Clinics of North America*, *27*(4), 805–827.

U.S. Preventive Services Task Force. (2009). *Screening for breast cancer: Recommendation statement* Available at www.uspreventiveservicestaskforce.org/uspstf09/breastcancer/brcanrs.htm.

WebMD. (2012). *Digital mammograms: A clearer picture* (reviewed by Arnold Wax, MD, June 26, 2012). Breast Cancer Health Center. Available at www.webmd.com/breast-cancer/digital-mammograms-a-clearer-picture?page=2.

11 CHAPTER

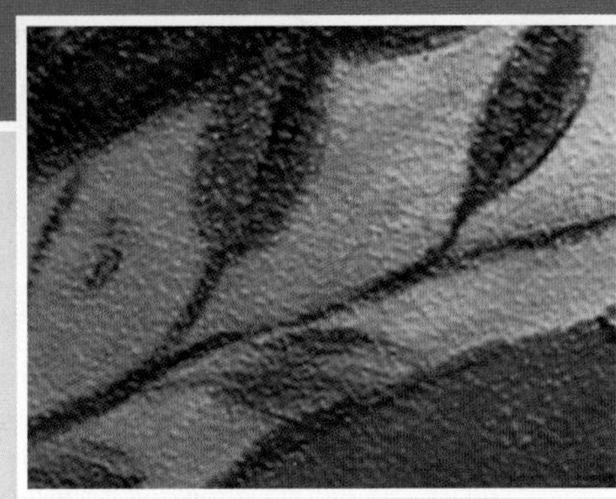

Structural Disorders and Neoplasms of the Reproductive System

Deitra Leonard Lowdermilk

http://evolve.elsevier.com/Lowdermilk/MWHC/

LEARNING OBJECTIVES

- Describe the various structural disorders of the uterus and vagina.
- Discuss the pathophysiology of selected benign and malignant neoplasms of the female reproductive tract.
- Compare the common medical and surgical therapies for selected benign gynecologic conditions.
- Explain diagnostic procedures in client-centered terms.
- Examine the emotional effects of benign and malignant neoplasms.
- Develop a nursing care plan for a woman with endometrial cancer who has had a hysterectomy.
- Differentiate treatments for preinvasive and invasive conditions.
- Identify critical elements for teaching clients with selected benign or malignant neoplasms.
- Investigate health-promoting behaviors that reduce cancer risk.
- Assess the effects of and treatments for malignant neoplasms during pregnancy.
- Discuss the development and sequelae of gestational trophoblastic neoplasia.

Women are at risk for structural disorders and neoplastic diseases of the reproductive system from the age of menarche through menopause and the older years. Problems may include structural disorders of the uterus and vagina related to pelvic relaxation and urinary incontinence and chronic pain related to vulvodynia. Benign neoplasms of the reproductive organs, such as fibroids and cysts, and malignant neoplasms of the reproductive system also may occur. Benign tumors usually do not endanger life, tend to grow slowly, and are not invasive. Malignant tumors (cancers) grow rapidly in a disorganized manner and invade surrounding tissues. The development of structural disorders and benign or malignant neoplasms can have far-reaching effects for the woman and her family. Beyond the obvious physiologic alterations, the woman also experiences threats to her self-concept and her ability to cope. A woman's concept of herself as a sexual being can be affected by the condition and its treatments. A woman's family also is challenged in the way it responds to her diagnosis. When cancer occurs with pregnancy, it adds to the complexity of physical and emotional responses to childbearing, with increased fears related to pregnancy and the fetus.

Nurses have important roles in teaching women about early detection and treatment and in providing supportive care to women and their families. This chapter presents information that will assist the nurse in assessing and identifying issues associated with structural problems or benign or malignant reproductive neoplasms. Nursing care concepts related to early detection, treatment methods, and education are included.

STRUCTURAL DISORDERS OF THE UTERUS AND VAGINA

Alterations in Pelvic Support

Alterations in pelvic support include uterine displacement and prolapse, cystoceles and rectoceles, urinary incontinence, and genital fistulas. Research by Wu, Hundley, Fulton, & Myers (2009) suggested that the prevalence of these disorders will increase by as much as 55% in the United States by the year 2050 as the numbers of older women increase.

Uterine Displacement and Prolapse

The round ligaments normally hold the uterus in anteversion, and the uterosacral ligaments pull the cervix backward and upward (see Fig. 4-3). **Uterine displacement** is a variation of this normal placement. The most common type of displacement is posterior displacement, or retroversion, in which the uterus is tilted posteriorly, and the cervix rotates anteriorly. Other variations include retroflexion and anteflexion (Fig. 11-1).

By 2 months postpartum the ligaments should return to normal length, but in about a third of women, the uterus remains retroverted. This condition is rarely symptomatic, but subsequent conception may be difficult because the cervix points

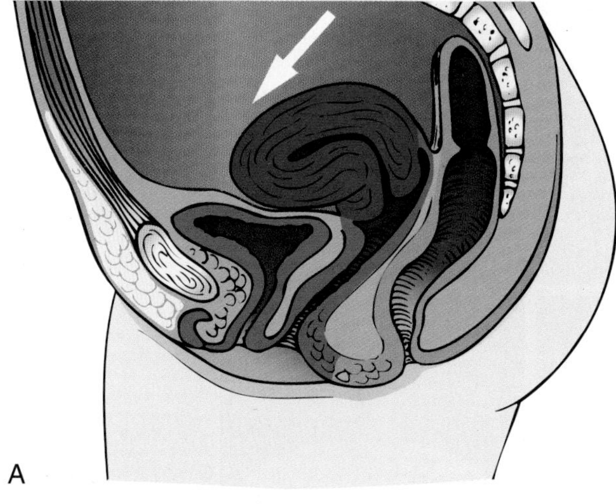

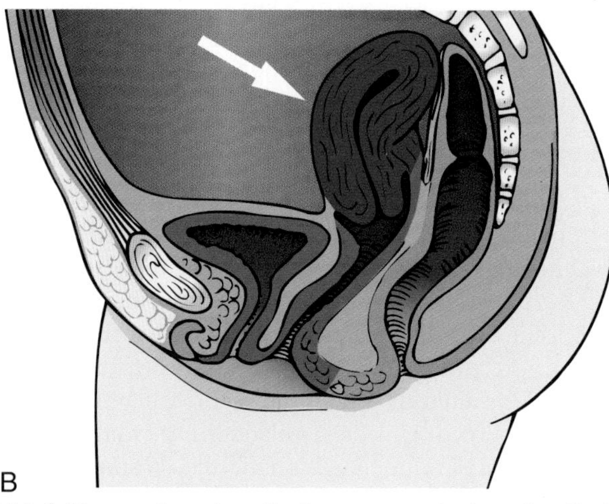

FIG 11-1 Types of uterine displacements. **A**, Anterior displacement. **B**, Retroversion (backward displacement of the uterus).

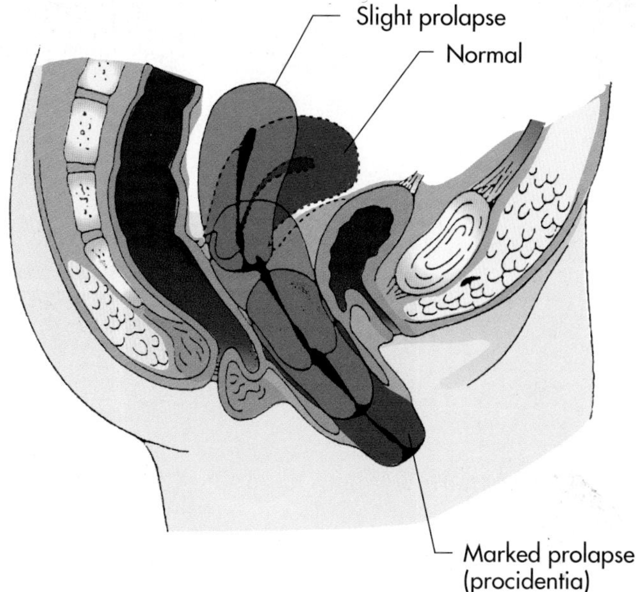

FIG 11-2 Prolapse of uterus.

toward the anterior vaginal wall and away from the posterior fornix, where seminal fluid pools after coitus. If symptoms occur, they may include pelvic and low back pain, dyspareunia, and exaggeration of premenstrual symptoms.

Uterine prolapse is a more serious type of displacement. The degree of prolapse can vary from mild to complete. In complete prolapse, the cervix and body of the uterus protrude through the vagina, and the vagina is inverted (Fig. 11-2).

Uterine displacement and prolapse can be caused by congenital or acquired weakness of the pelvic support structures (often called pelvic relaxation). In many cases problems can be a result of vaginal childbirth–related injury. Although extensive damage may be noted and repaired shortly after birth, symptoms related to pelvic relaxation most often appear during the perimenopausal period, when the effects of ovarian hormones on pelvic tissues are lost and atrophic changes begin. Pelvic trauma, stress and strain, and the aging process also are contributing factors. Other causes of pelvic relaxation include obesity, reproductive surgery, and pelvic radiation (Lentz, 2012b).

Clinical Manifestations. Symptoms of pelvic relaxation generally relate to the structure involved: urethra, bladder, uterus, vagina, cul-de-sac, or rectum. The most common complaints are pulling and dragging sensations, pressure, protrusions, fatigue, and low backache. Symptoms may be worse after prolonged standing or deep penile penetration during intercourse. Urinary incontinence can be present.

Medical and Surgical Management. If discomfort related to uterine displacement is a problem, several interventions can be implemented to treat this condition. Kegel exercises (see Teaching for Self Managment box: Kegel Exercises in Chapter 4) can be performed several times a day to increase muscular strength. A knee-chest position performed for a few minutes several times a day can correct a mildly retroverted uterus. A fitted pessary to support the uterus and hold it in the correct position may be inserted into the vagina (Fig. 11-3). Usually a pessary is used for only a short time because it can lead to pressure necrosis and vaginitis. After a period of treatment, most women are free of symptoms and do not require the pessary. Surgical correction is rarely indicated.

Treatment for uterine prolapse depends on the degree of prolapse. Pessaries can be useful in mild prolapse and are recommended by many health care providers as the first-line management of uterine prolapse (Bugge, Adams, Gopinath, & Reid, 2013). Estrogen therapy may be used in the older woman to improve tissue tone. If these conservative treatments do not correct the problem or the degree of prolapse is significant, vaginal hysterectomy with a vaginal vault suspension (see later discussion) is usually recommended (Lentz, 2012b).

Nursing Interventions. Nurses can educate women on how to perform Kegel exercises and use a pessary. Good hygiene is important when using a pessary. Some women are taught to remove the pessary at night, cleanse it, and replace it in the morning. If the pessary is always left in place, regular douching with commercially prepared solutions or weak vinegar solutions (e.g., 1 tbsp to 1 qt of water) to remove increased secretions and keep the vaginal pH at 4.0 to 4.5 can be suggested.

Cystocele and Rectocele

Cystocele and rectocele almost always accompany uterine prolapse, causing the uterus to sag even farther backward and downward into the vagina. Cystocele (Fig. 11-4, *A*) is the protrusion of the bladder downward into the vagina that develops

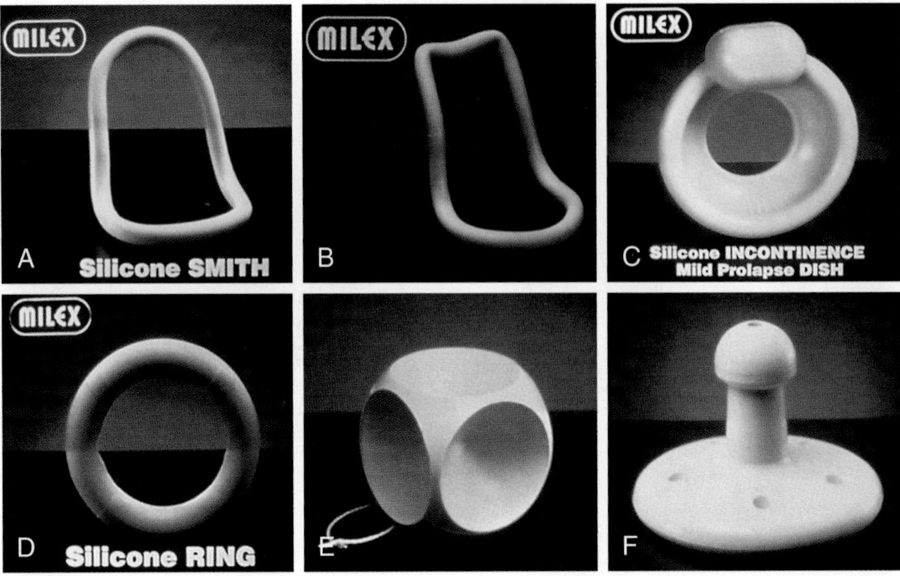

FIG 11-3 Examples of pessaries. **A,** Smith. **B,** Hodge without support. **C,** Incontinence dish without support. **D,** Ring without support. **E,** Cube. **F,** Gellhorn. (Courtesy Milex Products, Inc., a division of CooperSurgical, Trumbull, CT.)

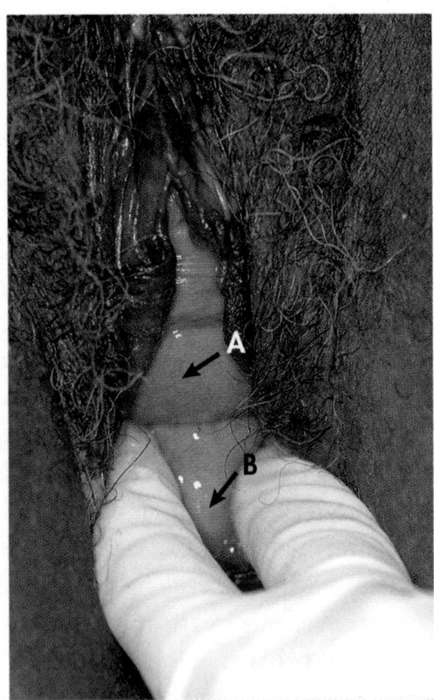

FIG 11-4 **A,** Cystocele. **B,** Rectocele. (From Seidel, H., Ball, J., Dains, J., Flynn, J., Solomon, B., & Stewart, R. [2011]. *Mosby's guide to physical examination* [7th ed.]. St. Louis: Mosby.)

when supporting structures in the vesicovaginal septum are injured. Anterior wall relaxation gradually develops over time as a result of congenital defects of support structures, childbearing, obesity, or advanced age. When the woman stands, the weakened anterior vaginal wall cannot support the weight of the urine in the bladder; the vesicovaginal septum is forced downward, and the bladder is stretched, resulting in an increase in capacity. With time the cystocele enlarges until it protrudes into the vagina. Complete emptying of the bladder is difficult because the cystocele sags below the bladder neck.

Rectocele is the herniation of the anterior rectal wall through the relaxed or ruptured vaginal fascia and rectovaginal septum; it appears as a large bulge that may be seen through the relaxed introitus (see Fig. 11-4, *B*).

Clinical Manifestations. Cystoceles and rectoceles often are asymptomatic. If symptoms of cystocele are present, they include complaints of a bearing-down sensation or that "something is in my vagina." Other symptoms include urinary frequency, retention, and incontinence, as well as possible recurrent cystitis and urinary tract infections (UTIs). Pelvic examination reveals a bulging of the anterior wall of the vagina when the woman is asked to bear down. Unless the bladder neck and urethra are damaged, urinary continence is unaffected. Women with large cystoceles complain of having to push upward on the sagging anterior vaginal wall to be able to void.

Rectoceles may be small and produce few symptoms, but some are so large that they protrude outside of the vagina when the woman stands. Symptoms are absent when the woman is lying down. A rectocele causes a disturbance in bowel function, the sensation of bearing down, or the sensation that the pelvic organs are falling out. With a very large rectocele it may be difficult to have a bowel movement. Each time the woman strains during bowel evacuation, the feces are forced against the thinned rectovaginal wall, stretching it more. Some women facilitate evacuation by applying digital pressure vaginally to hold up the rectal pouch.

Medical and Surgical Management. Treatment for a cystocele includes use of a vaginal pessary or surgical repair. An anterior repair (colporrhaphy) is the surgical procedure usually done for large symptomatic cystoceles. This involves a surgical shortening of pelvic muscles to provide better support for the bladder. An anterior repair is often combined with a vaginal hysterectomy. Use of Kegel exercises helps strengthen pelvic floor muscles and may relieve some of the symptoms of pressure caused by the cystocele (Lentz, 2012b).

Small rectoceles may not need treatment. The woman with mild symptoms may get relief from a high-fiber (e.g., 25 g) diet and adequate fluid intake, stool softeners, or mild laxatives. Vaginal pessaries and Kegel exercises may be useful. Large rectoceles that are causing significant symptoms are usually repaired surgically. A posterior repair (colporrhaphy) is

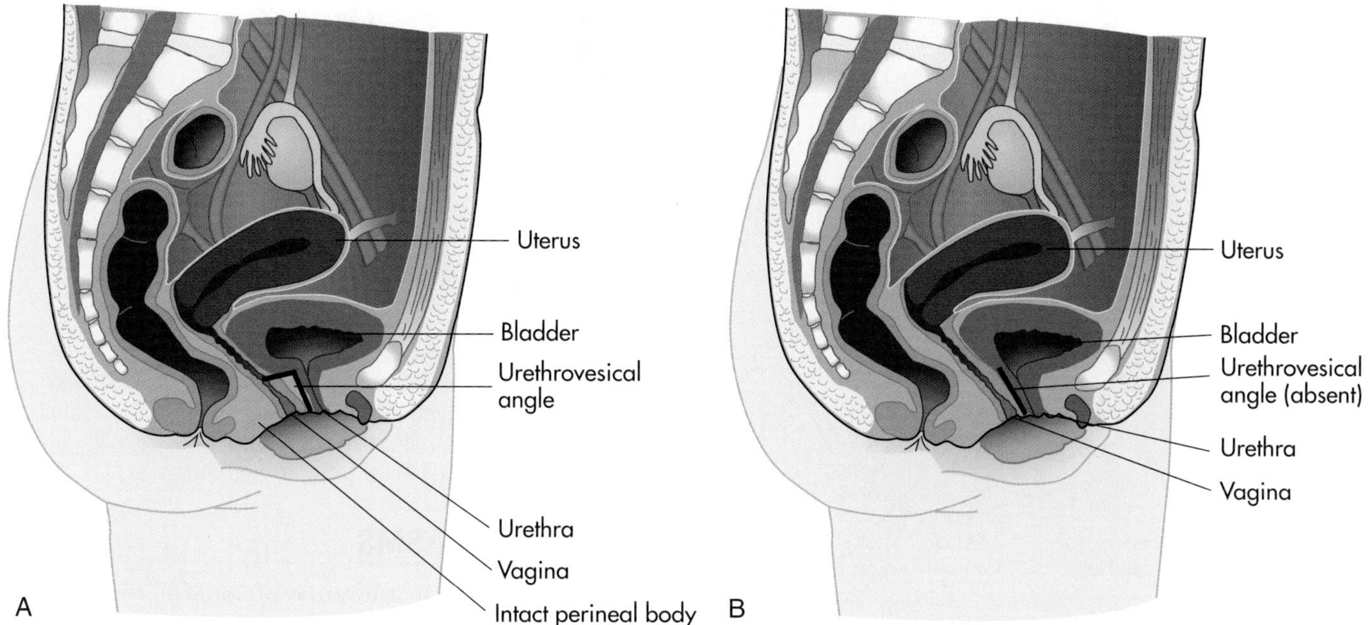

FIG 11-5 Urethrovesical angle. **A,** Normal angle. **B,** Widening (absence) of angle.

the usual procedure. This surgery is performed vaginally and involves shortening the pelvic muscles to provide better support for the rectum. Anterior and posterior repairs can be performed at the same time and with vaginal hysterectomy. Even though the surgery corrects the anatomic position, the woman may still have problems with defecation (Lentz, 2012b).

Genital Fistulas

Genital fistulas are perforations between genital tract organs. Most occur between the bladder and the genital tract (e.g., vesicovaginal); between the urethra and the vagina (urethrovaginal); and between the rectum or sigmoid colon and the vagina (rectovaginal) (Fig. 11-5). Genital fistulas may be a result of a congenital anomaly, gynecologic surgery, obstetric trauma, cancer, radiation therapy, gynecologic trauma, or infection (e.g., in the episiotomy).

Clinical Manifestations. Signs and symptoms of vaginal fistulas depend on the site but can include presence of urine, flatus, or feces in the vagina; odors of urine or feces in the vagina; and irritation of vaginal tissues.

Medical and Surgical Management. Management of genital fistulas depends on the location. Surgical repair is the usual treatment; however, it may not be successful.

Nursing Interventions. Nursing interventions for women with a mild cystocele or rectocele are similar to those suggested for women with uterine prolapse. However, nursing care of the woman with a rectocele or genital fistula requires great sensitivity because the woman's reactions are often intense. She can become withdrawn or hostile because of embarrassment about odors and soiling of her clothing that are beyond her control. Her sexuality is threatened; her partner may refuse sexual intimacy.

The nurse can suggest hygiene practices that reduce odor. Commercial deodorizing douches are available, or noncommercial solutions such as diluted chlorine (e.g., 1 tsp chlorine household bleach to 1 qt water) may be used. The chlorine solution is also useful for external perineal irrigation. Sitz baths and thorough washing of the genitalia with unscented, mild soap and warm water are helpful. Sparse dusting with deodorizing powders can be useful.

If a rectovaginal fistula is present, enemas given before leaving the house may provide temporary relief from oozing of fecal material until corrective surgery is performed. Irritated skin and tissues may benefit from use of a heat lamp or application of an emollient. Hygienic care is time consuming and may need to be repeated frequently throughout the day; protective pads or pants may need to be worn. All of these activities can be demoralizing to the woman and frustrating to her and her family.

Urinary Incontinence

Urinary incontinence (UI) affects women of all ages, with the prevalence increasing as the woman ages. Although nulliparous women can have UI, the incidence is higher in women who have given birth and increases with parity. Women who are overweight and those who smoke also are at increased risk (Lentz, 2012a). There are conflicting data about ethnicity and race as contributing factors, although Caucasian women reportedly are at higher risk than women of other races (Mitchell & Woods, 2013). Conditions that disturb urinary control include stress incontinence due to sudden increases in intra-abdominal pressure (such as sneezing or coughing); urge incontinence, caused by disorders of the bladder and urethra, such as urethritis and urethral stricture, trigonitis, and cystitis; neuropathies, such as multiple sclerosis, diabetic neuritis, and pathologic conditions of the spinal cord; and congenital and acquired urinary tract abnormalities.

Stress incontinence may follow injury to bladder neck structures. A sphincter mechanism at the bladder neck compresses the upper urethra, pulls it upward behind the symphysis, and forms an acute angle at the junction of the posterior urethral wall and the base of the bladder (urethrovesical angle) (Fig. 11-6). To empty the bladder the sphincter complex relaxes, and the trigone contracts to open

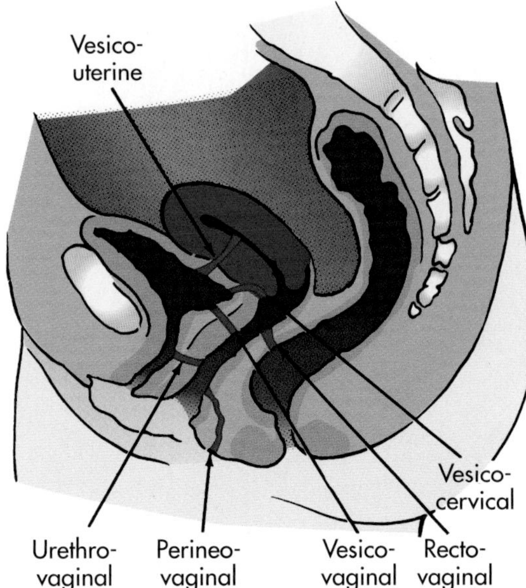

FIG 11-6 Types of fistulas that may develop in the vagina, uterus, or rectum. (From Monahan F., Sands, J.K., Neighbors, M., et al. [2007]. *Phipps' medical-surgical nursing: Health and illness perspectives* [8th ed.]. St. Louis: Mosby.)

the internal urethral orifice and pull the contracting bladder wall upward, forcing urine out. The angle between the urethra and the base of the bladder is lost or increased if the supporting pubococcygeus muscle is injured; this change, coupled with urethrocele, causes incontinence. Urine spurts out when the woman is asked to bear down or cough when she is in the lithotomy position.

Clinical Manifestations. Involuntary leaking of urine is the main sign. Episodes of leaking are common during coughing, laughing, and exercise.

Medical Management. Mild to moderate UI can be significantly decreased or relieved in many women by bladder training and pelvic muscle (Kegel) exercises (Hay-Smith, Herderschee, Dumoulin, & Herbison, 2012; Hersh & Salzman, 2013). Other management strategies include pelvic flow support devices (i.e., pessaries), vaginal estrogen therapy, serotonin-norepinephrine reuptake inhibitors, electrical stimulation, insertion of an artificial urethral sphincter, and surgery (e.g., anterior repair) (Hersh & Salzman; Tarnay & Bhatia, 2010).

Nursing Interventions. Nursing care for a woman with UI can include education about bladder training and pelvic muscle exercises and guidance in lifestyle changes (e.g., losing weight, smoking cessation). Women may need to be assessed for depression that can result from decreased quality of life and functional status.

In summary, nurses working with women who have UI or other pelvic structural problem can provide information and self-care education to prevent problems, to manage or reduce symptoms, to promote comfort and hygiene if symptoms are already present, and to recognize when further intervention is needed. This information can be part of all postpartum discharge teaching or can be provided at postpartum follow-up visits in clinics or physician/nurse-midwife/nurse practitioner offices, during postpartum home visits, or during gynecologic health examinations.

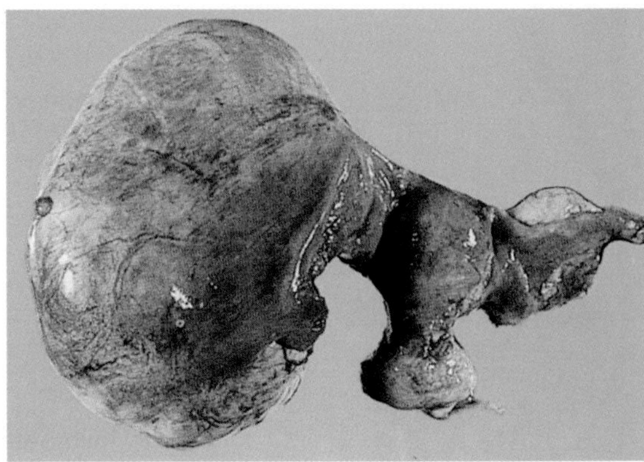

FIG 11-7 Ovarian cyst. (From Seidel, H., Ball, J., Dains, J., Flynn, J., Solomon, B., & Stewart, R. [2011]. *Mosby's guide to physical examination* [7th ed.]. St. Louis: Mosby.)

BENIGN NEOPLASMS

Benign neoplasms include a variety of nonmalignant cysts and tumors of the ovaries, the uterus, the vulva, and other organs of the reproductive system.

Ovarian Cysts

Functional ovarian cysts (Fig. 11-7) are dependent on hormonal influences associated with the menstrual cycle. These cysts may be classified as follicular cysts, corpus luteum cysts, theca-lutein cysts, endometrial cysts, and polycystic ovary syndrome (PCOS). Other benign ovarian neoplasms include dermoid cysts and ovarian fibromas.

Follicular Cysts

Follicular cysts develop most commonly in normal ovaries of young women as a result of the mature graafian follicle failing to rupture, or when an immature follicle does not resorb fluid after ovulation. A cyst is usually asymptomatic unless it ruptures, in which case it causes severe pelvic pain. If the cyst does not rupture, it usually shrinks after two or three menstrual cycles.

Corpus Luteum Cysts

Corpus luteum cysts occur after ovulation and are possibly caused by an increased secretion of progesterone that results in an increase of fluid in the corpus luteum. Clinical manifestations associated with a corpus luteum cyst include pain, tenderness over the ovary, delayed menses, and irregular or prolonged menstrual flow. A rupture can cause intraperitoneal hemorrhage. Corpus luteum cysts usually disappear without treatment within one or two menstrual cycles.

Theca-Lutein Cysts

Theca-lutein cysts are uncommon—up to 50% of cases are associated with hydatidiform mole (see Chapter 28). Theca-lutein cysts develop as a result of prolonged stimulation of the ovaries by human chorionic gonadotropin (hCG). They also can occur if the woman has taken ovulation induction drugs; if she is pregnant and a large placenta is present, such as in the presence of a multiple gestation; or if she has diabetes (Katz, 2012). The cysts are almost always bilateral. The woman may note a feeling of pelvic fullness if the ovary is enlarged, but most women are asymptomatic.

Medical and Surgical Management. A variety of interventions can be implemented for the woman with a functional cyst. If expectant management is the treatment, the woman is advised to keep appointments for pelvic examinations to monitor the changes in size of the cyst (enlarging or shrinking). Pharmacologic interventions such as analgesics may be prescribed for pain management. Oral contraceptives may be ordered for several months to suppress ovulation for functional cysts. Large cysts (greater than 8 cm) or cysts that do not shrink may be removed surgically (cystectomy). Corpus luteum cysts are treated similarly. Theca-lutein cysts are usually managed conservatively (they often regress without treatment) or by removal of the hydatidiform mole (Katz, 2012).

Nursing Interventions. Nursing care focuses on educating the woman regarding treatment options as well as pain management with analgesics or comfort measures such as heat to the abdomen or relaxation techniques. If surgery is performed, the nurse provides preoperative and postoperative care. Discharge teaching includes signs of infection, postoperative incision care, the possibility of recurrence, and advice regarding follow-up appointments.

Polycystic Ovary Syndrome

Polycystic ovary syndrome (PCOS) occurs when an endocrine imbalance results in high levels of estrogen, testosterone, and luteinizing hormone (LH) and decreased secretion of follicle-stimulating hormone (FSH). This syndrome is associated with a variety of problems in the hypothalamic-pituitary-ovarian axis and with androgen-producing tumors. The condition can be transmitted as an X-linked dominant or autosomal dominant trait (Stein-Leventhal syndrome). Multiple follicular cysts develop on one or both ovaries and produce excess estrogen. The ovaries often double in size.

Clinical Manifestations. Clinical manifestations include obesity, hirsutism (excessive hair growth), irregular menses or amenorrhea, and infertility. Impaired glucose tolerance and hyperinsulinemia occur in about 40% of women with PCOS (Lobo, 2012). Affected women are at high risk for developing type 2 diabetes mellitus, nonalcoholic fatty liver disease, and possibly cardiovascular disease (Huang & Coviello, 2012). PCOS is often diagnosed in adolescence when menstrual irregularities and other symptoms appear (Lobo).

Medical Management. The treatment for PCOS depends on what symptoms are of greatest concern to the woman. Lifestyle modifications (e.g., losing weight) and management of presenting symptoms such as infertility, irregular menses, and hirsutism are the focus. Oral contraceptives (OCs) are the usual treatment for irregular menses, if pregnancy is not desired, because they inhibit LH and decrease testosterone levels. OCs can also lessen acne to some degree. Spironolactone, an antiandrogen, is frequently used with an OC. In severe cases, gonadotropin-releasing hormone (GnRH) analogs may be used to treat hirsutism if OCs aren't effective. If pregnancy is desired, ovulation-inducing medications are given (Lobo, 2012). Metformin and other insulin medications for type 2 diabetes also are used to lower insulin, testosterone, and glucose levels, which in turn can reduce acne, hirsutism, abdominal obesity, amenorrhea, and other PCOS symptoms (Lobo).

Nursing Interventions. Nurses can provide information and counseling for women with PCOS. Information may be needed about the syndrome or about its long-term effects on the woman's health. Research has shown that women report symptoms of psychologic distress including depression, anxiety, and social fears (Benson, Hahn, Tan, et al., 2010). They may need to discuss their feelings about the physical manifestations of PCOS and may need emotional support if they have self-image problems related to the symptoms. Teaching about lifestyle modifications such as exercise and diet may be needed as well as education about the medications that are prescribed. Information about finding a support group or information on the Internet may be useful.

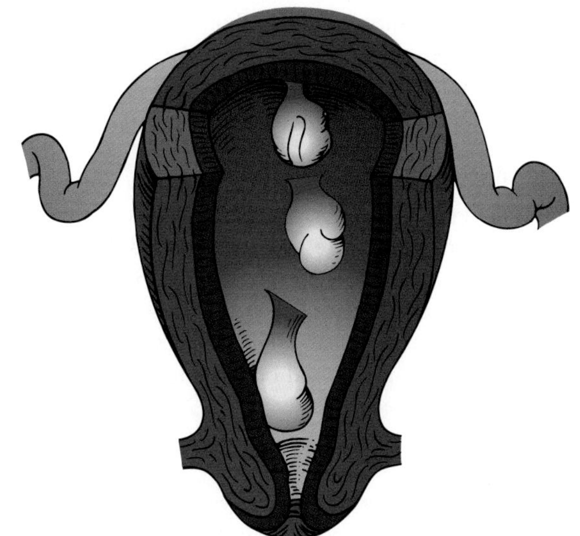

FIG 11-8 Endometrial polyps.

Other Benign Ovarian Cysts and Neoplasms

Two other ovarian neoplasms are dermoid cysts and ovarian fibromas. Dermoid cysts are germ cell tumors, usually occurring in childhood. These cysts contain substances such as hair, teeth, sebaceous secretions, and bones. Unless the cyst is large enough to put pressure on other organs, it is usually asymptomatic. Dermoid cysts may develop bilaterally and are often attached to the ovary. Treatment is usually surgical removal.

Ovarian fibromas are solid ovarian neoplasms developing from connective tissue, and most often occurring after menopause. Fibromas range in size from small nodules to large masses weighing more than 23 kg. Most fibromas are unilateral. They are usually asymptomatic, but if large enough, they may cause ascites, feelings of pelvic pressure, or abdominal enlargement. Treatment is usually surgical removal.

Nursing care of women who have surgery for the removal of dermoid cysts and ovarian fibromas is similar to that described for functional ovarian cysts.

Uterine Polyps

Uterine polyps may be endometrial or cervical in origin. They are tumors that are on pedicles (stalks) arising from the mucosa (Fig. 11-8). The etiology is unknown, although they may develop in response to hormonal stimulus or be the result of inflammation. Polyps are the most common benign lesions of the cervix and endometrium that occur during the reproductive years. These polyps may be single or multiple. Endocervical polyps are most common in multiparous women older than 40 years. The woman may be asymptomatic or she may have premenstrual or postmenstrual staining, menorrhagia, postmenstrual spotting, or postcoital bleeding (Katz, 2012).

Surgical Management

Clinical management of endometrial polyps is by surgical removal. Cervical polyps are usually removed in an office or clinic procedure without anesthesia. The polyp is grasped with a clamp and twisted or cut off. All polyps should be sent for pathologic examination. Endometrial sampling (which may require local anesthesia) should be done to determine if other pathologic conditions are present (Katz, 2012).

Nursing Interventions

Nursing care includes preparing the woman for what to expect during the removal procedure, encouraging relaxation and breathing exercises, and providing support during the procedure. After the procedure the woman is advised to avoid using tampons, having sexual intercourse, and douching for up to 1 week or until the site is healed. She is taught how to identify signs of infection and to notify her health care provider if she experiences heavy bleeding (more than one pad in 1 hour).

Leiomyomas

Leiomyomas, also known as fibroid tumors, fibromas, myomas, or fibromyomas, are slow-growing benign tumors arising from the muscle tissue of the uterus (Katz, 2012). They are the most common benign tumors of the reproductive system, occurring most often after age 50. They tend to occur more often in African-American women and women who have never been pregnant. Fibroids also occur more often in women who are overweight (Katz). They rarely become malignant. Because their growth is influenced by ovarian hormones, these benign tumors can become quite large when the woman is pregnant or taking hormone therapy. They often spontaneously shrink after menopause when circulating ovarian hormones diminish (Katz).

Clinical Manifestations

The cause of leiomyomas remains unknown, although genetic factors may be involved. Most of the tumors are found in the body of the uterus. Leiomyomas are classified according to the location in the uterine wall. *Subserous* leiomyomas (Fig. 11-9, *A*) develop beneath the peritoneal surface of the uterus and appear as small or large masses that protrude from the outer uterine surface. *Intramural* leiomyomas (Fig. 11-9, *B*) are tumors that develop within the wall of the uterus. *Submucosal* leiomyomas (Fig. 11-9, *C*) are the least common tumors, but often cause the most symptoms; they develop in the endometrium and protrude into the uterine cavity. Leiomyomas can develop in the cervix and on the broad ligaments (Fig. 11-9, *D*). They can grow on pedicles or stalks (Fig. 11-9, *E*). Occasionally these break off the pedicle and attach to other tissues (become parasitic).

Most women are asymptomatic; abnormal uterine bleeding is the most common symptom of fibroids. If the tumor is very large, pelvic circulation may be compromised, and surrounding viscera may be displaced. A woman may complain of backache, low abdominal pressure, constipation, urinary incontinence, or dysmenorrhea (painful menstruation). Nausea and vomiting may occur if the tumor obstructs the intestines. The woman also may notice an abdominal mass if the tumor is large. Anemia can occur if the woman has excessive bleeding. Pedunculated tumors can twist and become necrotic, causing pain (Katz, 2012).

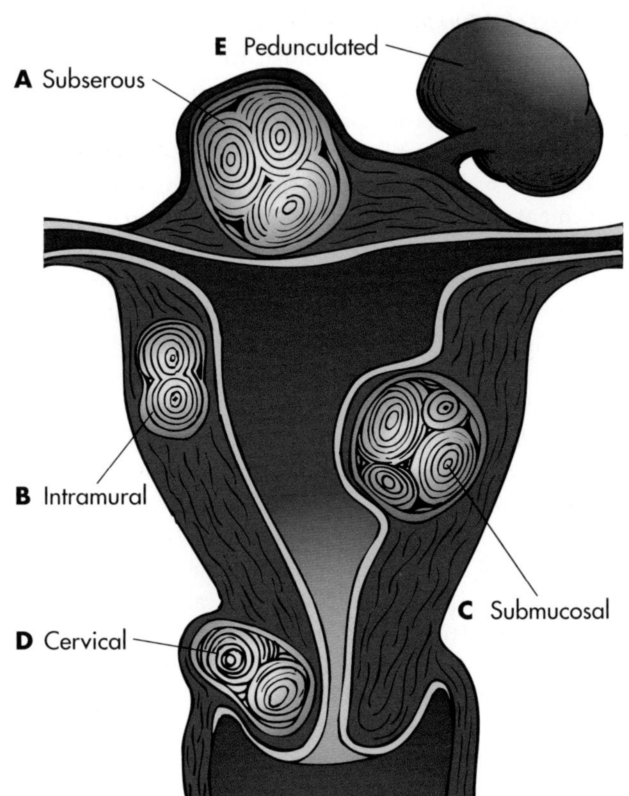

FIG 11-9 Types of leiomyomas. **A,** Subserous. **B,** Intramural. **C,** Submucosal. **D,** Cervical. **E,** Pedunculated.

The tumors appear to be influenced by the presence of estrogen. Fibroids can affect implantation and maintenance of pregnancy. During pregnancy the tumors can produce complications such as preterm labor, miscarriage, or dystocia (difficult labor). The severity of the symptoms seems to be directly related to the size and location of the tumors.

CARE MANAGEMENT

Assessment should include a history of symptoms (which might include abnormal bleeding, abdominal pain, dysmenorrhea, pelvic fullness or heaviness, or problems with elimination) and a pelvic examination. Diagnosis is usually accomplished by a process of elimination. A pelvic examination usually identifies the presence of uterine enlargement. Negative pregnancy tests rule out pregnancy as the cause of the symptoms. Laparoscopy may be used to differentiate ovarian masses from uterine masses. Ultrasound examination can differentiate between inflammatory masses or endometriosis and subserous fibroids.

Possible nursing diagnoses for a woman with a leiomyoma include the following:

- *Anxiety* related to
  - –Uncertain diagnosis
  - –Fear of malignancy
  - –Potential surgical treatment

- *Acute or chronic pain* related to
  –Leiomyomas
- *Sexual dysfunction* related to
  –Dyspareunia

Knowledge of the medical-surgical management of leiomyomas is essential in planning nursing care. This knowledge enables the nurse to work collaboratively with other health care providers and to meet the woman's informational and emotional needs. Clinical management of benign tumors of the uterus depends on the severity of the symptoms, the age of the woman, and her desire to preserve childbearing potential.

Medical Management

Medications. If symptoms are mild, regular checkups may suffice to observe for growth or changes in size. Nonsteroidal antiinflammatory drugs (NSAIDs) may be prescribed for pain; OCs inhibit ovulation and may relieve symptoms. Medical management is based on using medications to reduce circulating levels of estrogen and progesterone. GnRH agonists may be prescribed to reduce the size of the leiomyoma. Other medications include medroxyprogesterone acetate (Depo-Provera), danazol (Danocrine), antiprogesterone (mifepristone), selective estrogen receptor modulators (SERMs), and aromatase inhibitors (Katz, 2012; Sabry & Al-Hendy, 2012). The ideal medical therapy for treating fibroids has not been found, and research in this area continues. Two oral agents that show promise as treatment options for prevention of fibroids are vitamin D and green tea extract (Sabry & Al-Hendy, 2012).

Nursing Interventions. The woman who prefers medication for treatment will need information about the various medications, their actions and side effects, and routes of administration. A woman who is receiving GnRH agonists to decrease the size of the fibroid must understand that regrowth will occur after the treatment is stopped. She also must know that a small loss in bone mass and changes in lipid levels can occur; therefore, long-term use is not recommended. Amenorrhea may occur; however, women who wish to avoid pregnancy should use a nonhormonal or barrier method of contraception. A discussion of administration methods for GnRH agonists, including subcutaneous and intramuscular injections, intranasal administration, and subcutaneous implantation, will assist the woman in making a decision about her preferred method of administration (see Medication Guide: Infertility Medications in Chapter 9).

Uterine Artery Embolization. Uterine artery embolization (UAE) is a treatment during which polyvinyl alcohol (PVA) pellets or other embolic materials are injected into selected blood vessels to block the blood supply to the fibroid and cause shrinkage and resolution of symptoms (Katz, 2012). The procedure is done under local anesthesia and conscious sedation and can be done as an outpatient procedure, although some women will have the procedure in the hospital setting and remain overnight or be discharged within 4 to 6 hours (Katz). An incision is made into the groin, and a catheter is threaded into the femoral artery to the uterine artery. An arteriogram identifies the vessels supplying the fibroid. Most fibroids are reduced in size by 50% within 3 months. Temporary amenorrhea or early menopause can occur in some women. Although symptom improvement occurs for most women, data are lacking about the effects on future fertility and pregnancy outcomes. Preterm birth, intrauterine growth restriction, and miscarriage have been reported. Complications are usually minor and of short duration (Katz; van der Kooij, Ankum, & Hehenkamp, 2012). There is an increase in the likelihood that further surgical intervention will be needed within 2 to 5 years of the initial procedure (Gupta, Sinha, Lumsden, & Hickey, 2012).

Nursing Interventions. Preoperative teaching includes advising the woman not to drink alcohol or smoke and not to take aspirin or anticoagulant medications 24 hours before the procedure. If the procedure is done on an outpatient basis, the woman will usually need to take acid-suppressing medications, NSAIDs, and antihistaminic drugs as well as laxatives beginning the day before the procedure (Pisco, Bilhim, Duarte, & Santos, 2009). She is told to expect cramping during injection of the PVA pellets. Explanations about what to expect postoperatively include pelvic pain, fever, malaise, and nausea and vomiting that may be caused by acute fibroid degeneration. Pain can be controlled with NSAIDs or narcotic analgesics if needed. Postoperative nursing assessments include checking for bleeding in the groin, taking vital signs, assessing pain level, and checking the pedal pulse and neurovascular condition of the affected leg. Discharge teaching includes signs of possible complications and when to notify the physician, self-care instructions, and follow-up advice (see Teaching for Self-Management).

TEACHING FOR SELF-MANAGEMENT

Care After Uterine Artery Embolization

- Take prescribed medications as ordered.
- Call your physician if you have any of the following symptoms:
  - Bleeding
  - Pain
  - Swelling or hematoma at the puncture site
  - Fever of 39° C (102.2° F)
  - Urinary retention
  - Abnormal vaginal drainage (foul odor, brown color, tissue)
- Eat a normal diet including fluids and fiber.
- Do not use tampons, douche, or have vaginal intercourse for at least 4 weeks.
- Avoid straining during bowel movements.
- Keep your follow-up appointment.

Surgical Management

In addition to the surgical options of hysterectomy and myomectomy, other techniques have been developed to treat leiomyomas. These include laparoscopic techniques; hysteroscopic techniques; myolysis by heat, cold, and laser; and magnetic resonance–guided focused ultrasound surgery. Not all of these techniques are suitable for every woman nor are all of them universally available.

Laser Surgery. Laser surgery or electrocauterization can be used to destroy small fibroids through a laparoscopic (abdominal) or hysteroscopic (vaginal) approach. Hysteroscopic uterine *ablation* (vaporization of tissues) can be performed under local or general anesthesia, usually as an outpatient procedure. Medical therapy using GnRH agonists to control bleeding temporarily and to suppress endometrial tissue may be given for 8 to 12 weeks before surgery. Although the uterus remains in place, the vaporization process can cause scarring and adhesions in the uterine cavity, affecting future fertility. Therefore, this procedure is for women who wish to retain their uterus but no longer desire childbearing potential (Nelson & Gambone, 2010). Risks of the procedure include uterine perforation, cervical injury, and fluid overload (caused by the leaking into blood vessels of fluid used to expand the uterus during surgery). The woman may experience postoperative cramping and a slight vaginal discharge for a few days. Before discharge the following information is given:

- Analgesics or NSAIDs can be used for pain relief as needed.
- Normal activities can be resumed within several days.
- Vaginal discharge is to be expected for 4 to 6 weeks.
- Use of tampons or vaginal intercourse should be avoided for 2 weeks.
- The next menstrual period may be irregular.
- The woman should be reminded about the effects of ablation on her fertility, if appropriate.
- The physician should be called if the woman has heavy bleeding or signs of infection.

Myomectomy. If the tumor is near the outer wall of the uterus, the uterine size is no larger than the equivalent of 12 to 14 weeks of gestation, and symptoms are significant, myomectomy (removal of the tumor) may be performed (Katz, 2012). Myomectomy can be performed through a laparoscopic or abdominal incision approach or a vaginal (hysteroscopic) approach. Myomectomy leaves the uterine muscle walls relatively intact, thereby preserving the uterus and allowing the possibility of future pregnancies. It is usually performed in the proliferative phase of the menstrual cycle to avoid interrupting a possible pregnancy. GnRH therapy may be given before surgery to reduce the size of the fibroid. Fibroids can recur after myomectomy; further treatment may be needed (Nelson & Gambone, 2010).

Hysterectomy. A total hysterectomy (removal of the entire uterus) is the treatment of choice if bleeding is severe or if the fibroid is obstructing normal function of other organs. An abdominal or vaginal surgical approach depends on the size and location of the tumors. For example, abdominal hysterectomy is usually performed for leiomyomas larger than a uterus would be at 12 to 14 weeks of gestation or for multiple leiomyomas. The uterus is removed through either a vertical or transverse incision. In some circumstances the cervix is not removed, although there is a lack of evidence about the benefits of leaving the cervix over total hysterectomy for benign disease (Kives, Lefebvre, Wolfman, et al., 2010). Vaginal approaches can be used for smaller tumors. In both abdominal and vaginal approaches, the uterus is removed from the supporting ligaments (broad, round, and uterosacral). These ligaments are then attached to the vaginal cuff, allowing maintenance of normal depth of the vagina (Fig. 11-10). Alternatives to these procedures are the *laparoscopic assisted vaginal hysterectomy (LAVH)* and the *laparoscopic assisted supracervical hysterectomy (LASH)*. LAVH converts an abdominal procedure to a vaginal one by using a laparoscope in the abdomen to assist with removal of the uterus. LASH allows the cervix to remain. Both are associated with a quicker recovery and fewer postoperative complications (Guo, Tian, & Wang, 2013).

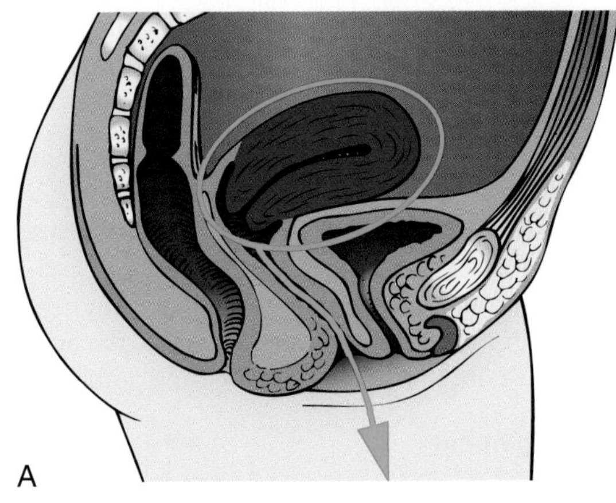

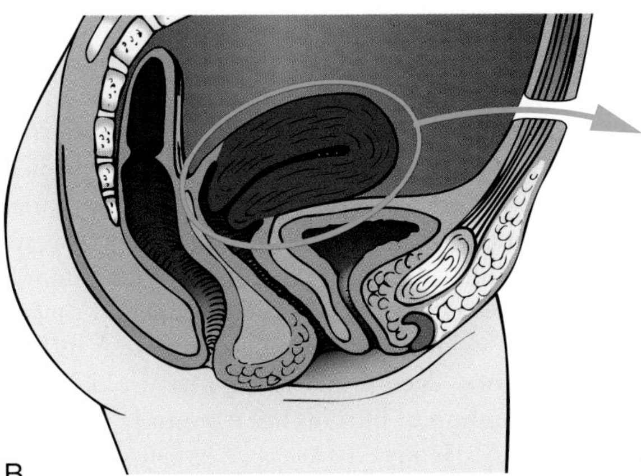

FIG 11-10 Hysterectomy. **A,** Vaginal. **B,** Abdominal.

BOX 11-1 Questions for a Woman to Ask to Ensure Informed Consent

- Why is this procedure proposed for my condition/problem?
- What are the risks/benefits of the proposed surgery?
- Are there alternatives to this surgery? If so, what are the risks and benefits of these alternatives?
- How many times have you performed this surgery?
- How long will I be hospitalized? Can the procedure be done in an outpatient setting? How long will it take to recover?
- What types of anesthesia can be used?
- What hospital and surgical procedures can I expect?
- How will the surgery affect me (e.g., any changes in physical function, sexual function, or childbearing ability)?

From Wade, J., Pletsch, P., Morgan, S., & Menting, S. (2000). Hysterectomy: What do women need and want to know? *Journal of Obstetric, Gynecologic, and Neonatal Nursing, 29*(1), 33-42.

Preoperative Nursing Interventions. Assessments needed before surgery include the woman's knowledge of treatment options, her desire for future fertility if she is premenopausal, the benefits and risks of each procedure, preoperative and postoperative procedures (Boxes 11-1 and 11-2), and the recovery process. If the woman demonstrates understanding of this information, she can make an informed decision about treatment and feel a sense of control over the surgical experience. Resources on helping women to make decisions about treatment can be found at the website for the Fibroid Treatment Collective at www.fibroid.org.

BOX 11-2 Preoperative Procedures for Hysterectomy

- Vaginal examination or physical examination
- Laboratory tests
  - Complete blood count, type, and crossmatch
  - Urinalysis
- Chest radiograph
- Electrocardiogram
- Teaching for postoperative routines
  - Turning, coughing, deep breathing
  - Passive and active leg exercises
  - Need for early ambulation
  - Pain relief options
- Nothing by mouth after midnight or as ordered
- Enema if ordered
- Douche if ordered
- Abdominal: mons or perineal shave if ordered
- Removal of makeup, nail polish
- Removal of glasses, contact lenses, dentures, etc.
- Identification band in place
- Signed consent form in chart
- Have woman empty bladder immediately before surgery

CLINICAL REASONING CASE STUDY

Informed Decision Making for Treatment of Leiomyoma

Selena, a 41-year-old married Hispanic (non–English speaking) client, has just been diagnosed with a uterine leiomyoma. She has expressed concern about the treatment because she does not want to have a hysterectomy and her friends have told her that she will probably have to have one. What response by the nurse would be appropriate?

1. Evidence—Is there sufficient evidence to draw conclusions about what the nurse should say?
2. Assumptions—What assumptions can be made about the following issues?
   a. Medical therapy and observation for leiomyomas
   b. Differences between myomectomy and hysterectomy for leiomyoma treatment
   c. Uterine artery embolization as a treatment option for leiomyomas
   d. Cultural implications for Selena in making a decision
3. What implications and priorities for nursing care can be made at this time?
4. Does the evidence objectively support your conclusion?

Psychologic assessment is essential, particularly for a woman who is scheduled for a hysterectomy. Areas to be explored include the significance of the loss of the uterus for the woman, misconceptions about effects of surgery, and adequacy of her support system. Women who have not completed their childbearing, who believe that their self-concept is related to having a uterus (to be a complete woman), who feel that sexual functioning is related to having a uterus, or who have too little or too much anxiety about the surgery may be at risk for postoperative emotional reactions (Pauls, 2010). Yen, Chen, Long and associates, et al. (2008) found that postoperatively most women reported positive feelings about femininity and their body image, less anxiety and depression, but still reported a worsening of sexual functioning.

Postoperative Nursing Interventions. Postoperative assessments and care after myomectomy and abdominal

BOX 11-3 Postoperative Care after Hysterectomy

- Monitor vital signs every 15 minutes until stable, then every 4 hours for 48 hours
- Maintain unobstructed airway
- Remind client to turn, cough, deep breathe every 2 hours for 24 hours
  - Assist her to splint incision with hands or pillow
- Incentive spirometry if ordered
- Leg exercises every 2 to 4 hours until ambulatory
- Assess Homans sign
- Assess bleeding
  - Abdominal: assess dressing or incision
  - Vaginal: perineal pad count (one saturated pad in less than 1 hour is excessive; vaginal bleeding is usually minimal)
- Check laboratory values, especially hematocrit
- Assess lung sounds
- Assess bowel sounds and monitor bowel function
- Monitor intake and output
  - Foley catheter may be in place for 24 hours after abdominal surgery
  - After vaginal hysterectomy, urinary retention may occur because of manipulation of the urethra during surgery
- Assess abdominal incision or vagina for signs of infection
- Observe for signs of complications
  - Abdominal hysterectomy: assess for signs of wound evisceration, pulmonary embolism, thrombophlebitis, pneumonia, bowel obstruction, bleeding (incisional or vaginal)
  - Vaginal hysterectomy: assess for signs of urinary tract infection, urinary retention, wound infection, vaginal bleeding
- Pain relief
  - Pharmacologic measures: patient-controlled analgesia (PCA) or epidural narcotics may be ordered for the first 24 hours, followed by oral analgesics and nonsteroidal antiinflammatory drugs (NSAIDs)
  - Nonpharmacologic measures: breathing and relaxation exercises, position changes, guided imagery, application of heat to the abdomen (abdominal hysterectomy), and sitz baths or ice packs for the perineum (vaginal hysterectomy); ambulation may relieve gas pains
- Psychologic assessments
  - Assess for depression or other emotional reactions
  - Assess support systems
  - Assess sexual concerns

hysterectomy are similar to those for other abdominal surgery (Box 11-3). Specific to abdominal and vaginal hysterectomy are assessments for vaginal bleeding (one perineal pad saturated in less than 1 hour is excessive), urinary retention (especially after vaginal hysterectomy), perineal pain after vaginal hysterectomy, and psychologic assessments (e.g., depression).

Discharge Planning and Teaching. Discharge planning and teaching are similar for myomectomy and hysterectomy (see Teaching for Self-Management). Myomectomy and vaginal hysterectomy may be performed in an ambulatory setting, and women may be discharged the evening of the surgery. Women who have an abdominal hysterectomy may have a 1- to 2-day stay in the hospital before being discharged.

If a hysterectomy was performed, the woman is reminded that she will experience cessation of menses. If the woman is premenopausal, she will not experience menopause at this time unless her ovaries also were removed. If the ovaries were not removed, there will be no reason for her to consider hormone

TEACHING FOR SELF-MANAGEMENT

Care After Myomectomy or Hysterectomy

- Eat foods high in protein, iron, and vitamin C to aid in tissue healing; include foods with high fiber content; and drink six to eight 8-ounce glasses of water daily.
- Rest when tired; resume activities as comfort level permits. Avoid vigorous exercise and heavy lifting for 6 weeks. Avoid sitting for long periods. Resume driving when comfort allows or on advice from health care provider.
- Avoid tub baths, intercourse (vaginal rest), and douching until after the follow-up examination.
- When vaginal intercourse is resumed, water-soluble lubricants may decrease discomfort.
- Report the following symptoms to your health care provider: vaginal bleeding, gastrointestinal changes, persistent postoperative symptoms (cramping, distention, change in bowel habits), and signs of wound infection (redness, swelling, heat, or pain at incision site).
- Keep your follow-up appointment with your health care provider.

replacement therapy. If the ovaries are removed, the woman will need the most current information on the risks and benefits of hormone replacement therapy (see Chapter 6). Other symptoms include pain, sleep disturbance, fatigue, anxiety, and depression.

Vaginal intercourse may be uncomfortable at first, especially after vaginal procedures. Water-soluble lubricants, relaxation exercises, and positions that control penile penetration may be beneficial. Women can be assured that this discomfort will decrease over time.

The schedule for follow-up care depends on the procedure performed, but usually a postoperative visit is scheduled within a week. Vaginal screening with cytology or Papanicolaou (Pap) test after total hysterectomy for a nonmalignant reason is not recommended (American Cancer Society [ACS], 2014a). (See Table 4-3 for Pap test recommendations.)

Vulvar Problems

Bartholin Cysts

Bartholin cysts are the most common benign lesions of the vulva. They arise from obstruction of the Bartholin duct, which causes it to enlarge. Small cysts often are asymptomatic; however, large cysts or infected cysts cause symptoms such as vulvar pain, dyspareunia (painful intercourse), and a feeling of a mass in the vulvar area (Eckert & Lentz, 2012).

Medical and Surgical Management. If the woman is asymptomatic no treatment is necessary. If the cyst is symptomatic or infected, surgical incision and drainage may provide temporary relief. Cysts tend to recur; therefore, a permanent opening for drainage may be recommended. This procedure is called *marsupialization* and is the formation of a new duct opening for drainage (Eckert & Lentz, 2012).

Nursing Interventions. Nursing care after surgery includes teaching the woman about pain-relief measures such as sitz baths, heat lamps to the perineum, and use of analgesics. The woman is taught to assess the incision site for signs of healing and infection and to take antibiotics, if prescribed, to prevent infection.

Vulvodynia

Vulvar pain is a common gynecologic problem. Vulvodynia, also called *vulvar pain syndrome* or *vulvovestibulitis,* is reportedly experienced by about 15% of women. The incidence is thought to be the same for women of all races and ethnicities (Katz, 2012; Reed, Harlow, Sen, et al., 2012).

Vulvodynia is a complex condition thought to be a chronic pain disorder of the vulvar area. The term *vulvodynia* is used if pain is present with no visible abnormality or no identified neurologic diagnosis. Pain can be described as provoked (e.g., by inserting a tampon or having vaginal intercourse) or unprovoked and localized to the vestibule or generalized over the vulvar area (Katz, 2012).

Etiology has not been established although psychologic and biologic theories have been proposed. The most common theory is that vulvodynia is caused by a chronic neuropathic pain syndrome. Inflammation may also be a causative factor and continues to be investigated (Katz, 2012).

A feature of neuropathic pain is *allodynia,* which is a painful sensation that is from something not supposed to be painful. It commonly occurs in women with vulvodynia. Several triggers that reportedly cause allodynia in the vulvar area include use of OCs; presence of candidiasis or human papillomavirus; wearing tight-fitting underwear and pants, especially synthetic materials; sexual activity; and tampon use (Katz, 2012). However, with all these triggers, research evidence is conflicting and the search for scientific evidence is ongoing.

Assessment of a woman with possible vulvodynia includes a health history including a mental health history, specifically inquiring about anxiety or depression. A thorough pain assessment is essential. Questions about provoking and palliative factors, the quality of pain, radiation of the pain, strength of the pain, and the timing of pain occurrence are included. A history may elicit complaints about burning, stinging, or irritation in the vulvar area, and reports of how the woman thinks her symptoms affect her physical activities and ability for sexual intimacy.

A thorough pelvic examination is recommended to rule out other causes of pain such as infection or trauma. The vulva should be inspected for erythema, ulcerations, and hyperpigmentation (Katz, 2012). A cotton swab is used to identify areas of pain on pressure to confirm presence of allodynia. A systematic assessment (e.g., using positions of the face of a clock) is suggested, and pain should be rated as mild, moderate, or severe. A speculum (a pediatric size is recommended) is used to examine the vagina for redness, erosions, and dryness. A swab of vaginal secretions is obtained and can be tested for yeast, increased white blood cells, and pH. Cultures for *Candida* and bacteria can be obtained. A bimanual examination may be performed (Katz).

Management strategies are individualized to the woman. Often a series of therapies or a combination of therapies is implemented to find the best treatment. There is little evidence to support one therapy over another. Oral medications include gabapentin and tricyclic antidepressants (Katz, 2012; Ventolini, 2011). Topical therapies include the use of lidocaine 5% ointment that can be applied nightly or prophylactically (i.e., before sexual intercourse) (Katz).

Other therapeutic measures that are reportedly helpful for symptoms include pelvic floor exercises, biofeedback, vaginal dilator training, hypnosis, and cognitive-behavioral therapy (Katz, 2012; Ventolini, 2011).

Hygienic measures include wearing white cotton underwear, using 100% cotton menstrual pads, using soaps and detergents for sensitive skin, avoiding wearing tight clothing over the vulvar area, avoiding lubricants that contain propylene glycol, and using natural oils such as olive oil for lubricants (Ventolini, 2011).

Surgery is usually not recommended until other measures have proven to be ineffective. The surgical procedure is a vestibulectomy, a difficult procedure that removes the vestibule and hymen and has a high rate of complications (Katz, 2012). Success rates are reported to be between 65% and 90% (Ventolini, 2011). Laser ablation of the vulvar epithelium may also be an option, and response rates are reported to be similar to that of vestibulectomy (Ventolini).

Client information about vulvodynia including how to locate support groups is available on various websites including:

- International Society for the Study of Vulvovaginal Disease: www.issvd.org
- National Vulvodynia Association: www.nva.org
- Vulvar Pain Society: www.vulvarpainsociety.org

MALIGNANT NEOPLASMS

Malignant neoplasms of the reproductive system include cancers of the endometrium, the cervix, the ovary, the vulva, the vagina, and the uterine tubes. In 2014 an estimated 94,990 women in the United States were diagnosed with a gynecologic cancer; an estimated 228,790 women died from having endometrial cancer (ACS, 2014a). Overweight and obesity are associated with increased risk for developing many cancers, including cancers of the endometrium, ovary, and cervix. Evidence also suggests that being overweight increases the risk for cancer recurrence and decreases the likelihood of survival for these cancers (ACS).

Cancer of the Endometrium

Incidence and Etiology

Endometrial cancer is the most common malignancy of the reproductive system (ACS, 2014a). It is most commonly seen in perimenopausal and postmenopausal women between ages 50 and 65. Certain risk factors have been associated with the development of endometrial cancer, including obesity (especially upper body fat localization), nulliparity, infertility, late onset of menopause, diabetes mellitus, hypertension, PCOS, and family history of ovarian or breast disease (ACS; Creasman & Miller 2012). There appears to be an increased risk for endometrial cancer in families with hereditary nonpolyposis colorectal cancer (HNPCC). Hormone imbalance, however, seems to be the most significant risk factor. Numerous studies have correlated the use of exogenous estrogens (unopposed stimulation, i.e., absence of progesterone) in postmenopausal women with an increased incidence of uterine cancer. Tamoxifen taken by women for breast cancer also has been related to a slight increase in endometrial cancer (Creasman & Miller). Pregnancy and use of low-dose oral contraceptive pills appear to offer some protection (ACS). The incidence of endometrial cancer among Caucasian women is higher than that among African-American and Hispanic women; however, the mortality rates are higher in African-American women (ACS).

Endometrial cancer is slow growing and for that reason has a good prognosis if diagnosed at a localized stage. Most endometrial cancers are adenocarcinomas that develop from endometrial hyperplasia. The tumor usually develops in the fundus of the uterus and can spread directly to the myometrium and cervix, as well as to other reproductive organs. Metastasis (spread of cancer from its original site) is through the lymphatic system in the pelvis and through the blood to the liver, the lungs, and the brain.

CARE MANAGEMENT

Clinical Manifestations and Diagnoses

Assessment includes a history of physical symptoms. The cardinal sign of endometrial cancer is abnormal uterine bleeding (e.g., postmenopausal bleeding and premenopausal recurrent metrorrhagia). Thirty percent of postmenopausal bleeding is caused by carcinoma. Late signs include a mucosanguineous vaginal discharge, low back pain, or low pelvic pain. A pelvic examination may reveal the presence of a uterine enlargement or mass.

! NURSING ALERT

Women can be informed that they can identify their own risk for developing endometrial as well as ovarian, cervical, and breast cancers by filling out a confidential cancer risk assessment survey that is available at the American Cancer Society (ACS) website—www.cancer.org.

Histologic examination is used for diagnosis. A Pap test of cellular material obtained by aspiration of the endocervix identifies only one third to one half of cases. Endometrial biopsy or fractional curettage yields the most accurate results. Fractional curettage involves scraping the endocervix and endometrium for histologic evaluation to determine the grade of neoplasm and its stage (extent). Perforation of the uterus is a possible complication of this procedure. Endometrial biopsy is more commonly performed and identifies about 90% of cases (Creasman & Miller, 2012). It is usually done on an outpatient basis under local anesthesia. A suction-type curette is used to remove tissue for sampling. It is recommended that women at risk for HNPCC have an annual biopsy or transvaginal ultrasound beginning at age 35 (ACS, 2014a). Tests to determine the spread of cancer include liver function tests, renal function tests, chest x-ray, intravenous pyelography (IVP), barium enema, computed tomography (CT), magnetic resonance imaging (MRI), bone scans, and biopsy of suspicious tissues. The International Federation of Gynecology and Obstetrics (FIGO) classification system is used to describe the stages of endometrial carcinoma (Table 11-1).

Medical and Surgical Management

Collaborative efforts from various health disciplines are needed to work with the woman with endometrial cancer. All must have an understanding of the treatments that may be used.

For stage I adenocarcinoma of the endometrium limited to the uterus, total abdominal hysterectomy (TAH) and bilateral salpingo-oophorectomy (BSO) is the usual treatment

TABLE 11-1 2009 FIGO Classification of Endometrial Carcinoma

STAGE	DESCRIPTION
I (Includes grades 1, 2, or 3)	Tumor limited to corpus uteri
IA	No or less than half myometrial invasion
IB	Invasion equal to or more than half of the myometrium
II	Cervical stromal invasion, not extending beyond the uterus
III (Includes grades 1, 2, or 3)	Local and regional spread of tumor
IIIA	Tumor invades the serosa of the corpus uteri and/or adnexas
IIIB	Vaginal and/or parametrial involvement
IIIC	Metastases to pelvic and/or paraaortic lymph nodes IIIC1 Positive pelvic nodes IIIC2 Positive paraaortic lymph nodes with or without positive pelvic lymph nodes
IV (Includes grades 1, 2, or 3)	Tumor invasion of bladder and/or bowel mucosa and/or distant metastasis
IVA	Tumor invasion of bladder and/or bowel mucosa
IVB	Distant metastases, including intraabdominal metastasis and/or inguinal lymph nodes

From Creasman, W.T., & Miller, D.S. (2012). Adenocarcinoma of the uterine corpus. In P.J. DiSaia, W.T. Creasman, R.S. Mannel, & D.S. Mutch (Eds.), *Clinical gynecologic oncology* (8th ed.). Philadelphia: Saunders.

(Creasman & Miller, 2012). Radiation use in stage I continues to be studied; it can reduce the risk of recurrence, but evidence does not demonstrate improved survival rates or reduced metastasis to distant sites. It can be used when the woman is a poor surgical risk (Soliman & Lu, 2012). A radical hysterectomy (abdominal hysterectomy with wide excision of parametrial tissue laterally and uterosacral ligaments posteriorly), BSO, and pelvic node dissection usually are performed for stage II endometrial cancer. If nodes are positive or if there is extensive uterine disease or metastasis outside the uterus, external pelvic radiation (see "External Therapy" later in chapter) is usually done postoperatively. Internal radiation therapy or brachytherapy (placement of an applicator loaded with a radiation source into the uterine cavity) (see "Internal Therapy" later in chapter) also may be used before surgery or combined with external radiation. Treatment of advanced stages is individualized but usually includes a TAH-BSO plus chemotherapy or radiation, or both (Soliman & Lu).

Chemotherapy is used to treat advanced and recurrent disease, although no effective treatment regimen has been established (Soliman & Lu, 2012).

Progestational therapy—use of medroxyprogesterone (Depo-Provera) and megestrol (Megace)—may be effective for recurrent cancers, especially those that are estrogen receptor positive. These drugs usually do not cause acute side effects. Tamoxifen and raloxifene (see Medication Guide Guides: Tamoxifen and Raloxifene Hydrochloride: in Chapter 10) are antiestrogens that have shown some effectiveness against recurrent endometrial cancer (Creasman & Miller, 2012; Soliman & Lu, 2012).

Nursing Interventions

Nursing care is individualized to the woman and her specific situation and diagnosis. Interventions for the woman having surgery are directed by assessing her perception of the anticipated surgery, her knowledge of what to expect after surgery, and any preoperative special procedures, such as cleansing enemas or douches. In today's practice of short hospital stays even for radical surgery, many of these preoperative procedures are performed at home before admission, so assessment of understanding becomes a critical nursing action (see Cultural Considerations). Nursing care for the woman having a TAH-BSO is similar to the care for a woman having a hysterectomy for leiomyoma described earlier. The following section focuses on care of the woman having a radical hysterectomy (see Nursing Care Plan).

CULTURAL CONSIDERATIONS

Meaning of Cancer

A woman's culture influences the meaning she attaches to cancer screening and diagnosis of cancer. Some women may be reluctant to be screened because of language barriers, lack of knowledge about the risks of gynecologic cancers, or belief that they are not at risk. Some women do not believe that care providers are sensitive to their values of modesty. A woman's response to a cancer diagnosis also must be appropriate to her cultural context for it to be acceptable to her. For example, body image issues (e.g., loss of uterus), the meaning of death, and pain responses (e.g., stoic or expressive) are influenced by cultural beliefs and values. In making assessments about these issues, the nurse takes into account the influence of culture before developing a plan of care.

Guimond, M.E., & Salman, K. (2013). Modesty matters: Cultural sensitivity and cervical cancer prevention in Muslim women in the United States. *Nursing for Women's Health, 17*(3), 210-217.

Preoperative Care. The nurse working with the woman preparing for a radical hysterectomy and pelvic node dissection should explain any preoperative procedures (see Box 11-2). Additional teaching is needed for the woman having a radical hysterectomy regarding possible postsurgical events (e.g., a suprapubic drain often remains in place for several days to a week).

Postoperative Care. Assessment of vital signs usually follows a postanesthesia protocol, gradually decreasing in frequency to two to four times a day. Intravenous fluids are maintained at a rate rapid enough to maintain hydration and electrolyte balance and are usually discontinued when the woman is taking oral fluids well and has no elevated temperature. A regular diet is resumed as tolerated. Intake and output are monitored. The Foley catheter is usually removed the morning after surgery and the first few voidings are measured.

The woman should turn and take deep breaths with assistance as needed. Breath sounds are assessed, and any deviations from normal are reported immediately. The most significant single cause of morbidity and prolonged hospitalization after major procedures is respiratory complications. Anesthesia and surgery alter breathing patterns and ability to cough. Atelectasis, pneumonia, and pulmonary embolus may occur.

To promote venous return and prevent deep vein thrombosis, the woman may wear antiembolic stockings or wear pneumonic pressure devices (i.e., boots) while she is in bed. Leg exercises and early ambulation are beneficial. Most women are encouraged to get out of bed the evening of or the day after surgery. Assistance in getting up and walking may be needed.

NURSING CARE PLAN

Hysterectomy for Endometrial Cancer

NURSING DIAGNOSIS	EXPECTED OUTCOME	NURSING INTERVENTIONS	RATIONALES
Anxiety related to lack of understanding of diagnosis, treatment, and prognosis of endometrial cancer as evidenced by woman's questions and concerns	Woman will identify source of anxiety and verbalize understanding of diagnosis, effects of hysterectomy, and prognosis.	Assess woman's level of understanding of procedure and its effects.	To correct any misunderstanding, provide clarification, and identify starting point for further information
		Provide information about cancer of the endometrium, individualizing information to the woman's situation.	To provide clarification concerning treatment regimen
		Provide preoperative and postoperative teaching.	To give anticipatory guidance and rationales for upcoming events
Fear related to diagnosis of endometrial cancer as evidenced by woman's questions and concerns	Woman will be able to verbalize that fears have diminished after the procedure.	Through therapeutic communication, encourage verbalization of fears.	To provide clarification and validation of feelings
		Encourage woman to identify support system.	To have resources readily available as needed
Acute Pain related to surgical procedure as evidenced by woman's verbal and nonverbal behaviors	Woman will verbalize decrease in intensity and number of painful episodes after interventions.	Assess the location and intensity of pain by using a pain scale.	To use appropriate treatment
		Administer prescribed analgesics.	To decrease perception of pain
		Use nonpharmacologic techniques such as distraction, relaxation, position changes, and heat.	To decrease perception of pain
		Monitor effectiveness of interventions.	To modify interventions if needed
Risk for Infection related to surgical incision and impaired skin integrity	Woman will experience no infection after the procedure.	Assess for clinical manifestations of infection: fever, drainage, redness, swelling at the incision site.	To provide prompt treatment
		Encourage a diet high in protein, vitamin C, and calories.	To promote wound healing
		Teach woman to maintain aseptic technique when performing dressing changes, such as good handwashing.	To decrease chance of introducing microorganisms at the incision site
Disturbed Body Image related to loss of uterus as evidenced by woman's statements of fears or concerns	Woman will maintain a positive body image.	Encourage expression of feelings through therapeutic communication.	To provide clarification of and validity of feelings
		Encourage woman to share feelings with significant other.	To obtain emotional support
		Assist woman to identify support systems.	To be available in case she needs to ventilate feelings
Sexual Dysfunction related to perceived loss of femininity	Woman will resume sexual relationship with partner.	Encourage verbalization of feelings related to sexuality.	To provide clarification
		Provide opportunity for role-playing.	To alleviate fears about interactions with partner
		Encourage communication with partner.	To address concerns about resumption of sexual relations
		Refer to sexual counselor.	To provide in-depth intervention as needed

Hemorrhage is always a possible complication after surgery. The wound drainage tube is emptied as needed or every 4 hours, and the amount and character of drainage are recorded. Drainage from any tube is assessed for bleeding. Vaginal drainage, if any, should be serosanguineous. Hematuria is noted and recorded. The primary health care provider is kept apprised of any deviations from normal expectations.

Paralytic ileus may occur after surgery in which the intestines have been manipulated. Use of a nasogastric tube, limiting oral fluids, and early ambulation all support the return of gastrointestinal function. An enema or suppository may bring relief of flatus and stimulate the return of bowel function. Oral laxatives should not be given until lower bowel function has returned.

Narcotic analgesics and NSAIDs are used for postoperative pain. Nursing measures such as massages, repositioning, and emotional support are all helpful adjuncts to pharmacologic control of discomfort.

Because the in-hospital convalescent period is generally short, close observation by the nurse and attention to detail

BOX 11-4 Nutritional Management for Common Problems Related to Gynecologic Cancer or Treatment

Altered Taste
- Rinse mouth with baking soda solution
- 1 teaspoon salt, 1 teaspoon baking soda to 1 quart (liter) water
- Use extra seasoning, spices
- Use sauces and marinades for meats
- Eat fish or chicken instead of red meat
- Eat tart foods to stimulate taste buds
- Try sugar-free mints, gum, hard sour candy

Anorexia
- Eat with family, friends
- Eat favorite foods any time
- Try new foods, recipes
- Use smaller servings
- Eat high-calorie, high-protein snacks
- Drink nutritional supplements
- Exercise before meals to stimulate appetite

Nausea and Vomiting
- Drink clear liquids
- Avoid carbonated fluids
- Avoid sweet, rich, fatty foods
- Eat cool foods rather than hot or warm foods
- Eat six to eight small meals a day
- Consume a high-calorie, high-protein diet
- Eat toast, bland foods
- Avoid lying down at least 1 hour after eating
- Take antiemetics before meals

Stomatitis
- Eat small meals
- Eat soft, bland foods
- Avoid rough-textured foods (e.g., chips, crackers)
- Drink 8 to 10 cups of fluids a day
- Avoid citrus fruits, spicy foods
- Avoid alcohol
- Avoid very hot or very cold foods
- Drink nutritional supplements, milkshakes
- Drink through a straw if mouth is sore
- Rinse mouth frequently with baking soda solution or prescribed mouthwash
- Eat liquid or pureed foods as needed

Constipation
- Increase fiber (bran, fresh fruits, and vegetables)
- Drink 8 to 10 cups of fluids a day (2 to 2.4 L/day)
- Eat natural laxative foods (prunes, apples)
- Avoid cheese products
- Drink warm drinks with breakfast

Diarrhea
- Limit milk to 2 cups a day (500 ml)
- Avoid high-fiber, spicy, fatty foods
- Eat foods high in potassium
- Increase fluid intake (3 L/day) (12.5 cups); avoid caffeine and carbonated fluids
- Add nutmeg to food to decrease gastric motility
- Eat a high-protein, high-carbohydrate diet
- Eat small meals and snacks

Postoperative Recovery
- Eat food high in iron
- Eat high-protein foods
- Eat foods high in vitamins C, B complex, and K
- Drink 6 to 8 glasses of fluids a day (1.5 to 2 L/day)

Data from American Cancer Society. (2013). *Managing eating problems caused by surgery, radiation, and chemotherapy*. Available at www.cancer.org.

are critical. Nursing actions appropriate to this period include monitoring for urinary retention after the catheter is removed, monitoring the woman's appetite and diet, monitoring bowel function, and encouraging progressive ambulation and self-care.

Discharge Planning and Teaching. Discharge planning and teaching are done throughout the preoperative and postoperative phases and culminate during the convalescent phase. Discharge teaching topics for the woman with a radical hysterectomy are similar to those that can be found in the Teaching for Self-Management box: Care After Myomectomy or Hysterectomy.

Care for the woman who has had external or internal radiation therapy is the same as that described for the woman with cervical cancer (see later discussion).

Nursing care for the woman undergoing chemotherapy depends on the type of drug given. If alopecia is likely, the nurse can suggest wigs, scarves, or other kinds of head coverings. If the therapy affects the appetite or causes gastrointestinal side effects, suggestions such as those in Box 11-4 may be useful.

After discharge the woman may require continued nursing care or monitoring of her physical status or advice for managing the treatment effects of the cancer. The family is likely to provide much of the woman's care. Nurses must identify what families see as their greatest need so that interventions are planned that best use the family's resources.

Psychologic care for the woman with endometrial cancer is essential. A woman needs to be able to discuss her concerns about having cancer and the potential for recurrence. She may have fears of death, permanent disfigurement, and change in functioning; altered feelings of self as a woman; and concerns regarding her femininity, sexuality, and loss of reproductive capacity. She may have questions arising from things she has heard about posthysterectomy changes, radiation therapy, or chemotherapy. Significant others should be encouraged to express their questions and concerns as well. The client and her significant others may benefit from a referral to a community cancer support group (see the ACS website, www.cancer.org).

Cancer of the Ovary

Incidence and Etiology

Ovarian cancer is the second most frequently occurring reproductive cancer and causes more deaths than any other female genital tract cancer (ACS, 2014a). Because the symptoms of this type of cancer are vague and definitive screening tests do not exist, ovarian cancer is often diagnosed in an advanced stage. The 5-year survival rate for cancer diagnosed at a localized stage is about 92%; however, only about 15% of all ovarian cancers are found at this stage. For advanced stages, the rate is about 27% (ACS). Malignant neoplasia of the ovaries occurs at all ages, including in infants and children. However, cancer of the ovary is seen primarily in women older than age 50, with the greatest number of cases found in women ages 60 to 64 years (Eisenhauer, Salani, & Copeland, 2012).

Major histologic cell types occur in different age groups, with malignant germ cell tumors most common in women between 20 and 40 years of age and epithelial cancers occurring in the perimenopausal age groups. The spread of ovarian cancer is by direct extension to adjacent organs, but distal spread can occur through the lymph system to the liver and the lungs.

The cause of ovarian cancer is unknown; however, a number of risk factors have been identified. These factors include nulliparity, infertility, previous breast cancer, family history of ovarian or breast cancer, and history of HNPCC. Inherited BRCA1 and BRCA2 mutations increase the risk, but 90% of women do not have inherited ovarian cancer (Coleman, Ramirez, & Gershenson, 2012; Eisenhauer, 2012). Women of North American or northern European descent have the highest incidence of ovarian cancers. Pregnancy and use of oral contraceptives seem to have some protective benefits against ovarian cancer, whereas use of postmenopausal estrogen may increase the risk. Research has shown that preventive removal of the ovaries and uterine tubes can decrease the risk (ACS, 2014a). Genital exposure to talc, a diet high in fat, lactose intolerance, and use of fertility drugs have been suggested as risk factors, but research findings are inconclusive (Coleman et al.; Eisenhauer et al).

Clinical Manifestations and Diagnosis

Ovarian cancer was once called a silent disease because early warning symptoms that would send a woman to her health care provider are absent (e.g., no bleeding or other discharge and no pain). However research has shown that some women experience symptoms that are associated with early ovarian cancer. These include abdominal bloating, noticeable increase in abdominal girth, pelvic or abdominal pain, difficulty eating or feeling full quickly, and urinary urgency or frequency (ACS, 2014a; Eisenhauer et al., 2012). The increase in abdominal girth (caused by ovarian enlargement or ascites) is usually attributed to an increase in weight or a shift in weight that is seen commonly in women entering their middle years. An ovary enlarged 5 cm or more than normal that is found during routine examination requires careful diagnostic workup. Pelvic pain, anemia, and general weakness and malnutrition are signs of late-stage disease.

Early diagnosis of ovarian cancer is uncommon. Attempts at early detection have not proven to be reliable. Taking a family history is important because it may reveal cancer of the uterus or breast. Transvaginal ultrasound, CA-125 antigen (a tumor-associated antigen) testing, and frequent pelvic examinations have all been used without a great deal of success. Research continues on the use of proteomics (study of proteins in blood) to identify ovarian cancer in its earlier stages (Eisenhauer et al., 2012).

Transvaginal ultrasound and CA-125 screening currently are not recommended for routine screening in the general population but are recommended for women who are at high risk (e.g., BRCA1 mutation carriers) (ACS, 2014a). Routine pelvic examination continues to be the only practical screening method for detecting early disease, even though few cancers are detected in women without symptoms. Any ovarian enlargement should be considered highly suggestive and needs further evaluation by laparoscopy or laparotomy. Responsibility for diagnosis rests with the pathologist. The size of the tumor is not indicative of the severity of disease. Clinical staging is done surgically and gives direction to treatment and prognosis (Eisenhauer et al., 2012).

Medical and Surgical Management

Treatment is dictated by the stage of the disease at the time of initial diagnosis. Surgical removal of as much of the tumor as possible is the first step in therapy for all stages. This may involve just the removal of one ovary and tube (if the cancer is limited to one ovary and childbearing is desired) or the radical excision of the uterus, ovaries, tubes, and omentum. Cytoreductive surgery (the debulking of the poorly vascularized larger tumors) also is done. The smaller the volume of tumor remaining, the better the response to adjuvant therapy. Because about three quarters of women are in stage II, III, or IV disease at the time of diagnosis, surgical cure is not possible; therefore, after tumor reduction surgery is performed, women with epithelial cell carcinoma will receive chemotherapy.

A platinum-based combination of antineoplastic drugs such as carboplatin and paclitaxel is recommended for most women with advanced disease (Eisenhauer et al., 2012).

Second-look surgery is used to determine the response of the disease to chemotherapy and whether treatment should be continued; however, this procedure usually is not done unless it is part of a research protocol (Eisenhauer et al., 2012).

Radiation has been used to treat early-stage disease, and some women have had long-term survival after debulking surgery followed by radiation therapy. It has also been used as a palliative measure in advanced disease (Coleman et al., 2012).

Nursing Interventions

Awareness of the symptoms of and risk factors for ovarian cancer are low in the general population. Therefore, nurses need to be involved in raising the awareness of these risks and symptoms with the public and with women who are seeking care in health care settings such as clinics and physician offices.

The woman diagnosed with ovarian cancer has concerns similar to those described for the woman with endometrial and cervical cancer. Nursing interventions for the woman having surgery, chemotherapy, or external radiation therapy for ovarian cancer are described in other sections of this chapter.

Women with advanced ovarian cancer have a significant rate of recurrence. Follow-up for 5 years must be intensive. When a cure or remission cannot be achieved, palliative measures are initiated that alleviate symptoms of the progressing disease and provide comfort and maximal function. As the disease progresses, nutritional support, including enteral feedings and parenteral hyperalimentation, may be needed because of the effects on the gastrointestinal tract of both the disease and the treatments. The goal of nursing care is assisting the woman to maintain quality of life and to remain at home with her family as much as possible.

Because the period between a focus on cure and a focus on palliation is often prolonged, the woman with ovarian cancer is apt to experience most of the grief stages described by Kübler-Ross and to need support and encouragement through each stage. After diagnosis the woman often experiences denial and then anger. As treatment begins, she may "bargain" for a cure. If treatment is successful and death is forestalled by remission or cure, the process of adjustment to dying ceases, and the woman again focuses on life and its challenges but may continue to have uncertainty about her diagnosis . When treatment fails to secure a cure or remission ends, the woman must turn again to the task of adjustment (see Legal Tip).

LEGAL TIP: Advance Directives

Nurses who work with clients in hospitals with federal funding must know that because of the Patient Self-Determination Act, all clients must be asked if they have knowledge of advance directives and be provided with the information if desired. This is important to nurses working in gynecology-oncology settings, where decisions about living wills and "no codes" may be issues.

Family and friends also have diverse feelings. When grieving is prolonged, as it often is when the woman has cancer, the stress can be enormous and can interfere with other interpersonal relationships. If the woman is hospitalized, the environment may further intrude on relationships, limiting privacy and access to the woman and hindering opportunities for caring gestures. The nurse can assist the woman and her family to share their feelings with each other and help them develop a support network. Referral to a cancer support group may be useful (e.g., National Ovarian Cancer Coalition, www.ovarian.org; Ovarian Cancer National Alliance, www.ovariancancer.org).

Cancer of the Cervix

Incidence and Etiology

Cervical cancer is the third most common reproductive cancer. The accessible location of the cervix to both cell and tissue study and direct examination have led to a refinement of diagnostic techniques, contributing to improved diagnosis and management of these disorders. The incidence of invasive cancer has decreased since the 1980s, reducing mortality rates (ACS, 2014a).

Cancer of the cervix begins as neoplastic changes in the cervical epithelium. Terms that have been used to describe these epithelial changes or preinvasive lesions include dysplasia and cervical intraepithelial neoplasia (CIN), the term currently used. CIN 1 refers to abnormal cellular proliferation in the lower one third of the epithelium; this change tends to be self-limiting and generally regresses to normal. CIN 2 involves the lower two thirds of the epithelium and may progress to carcinoma in situ. CIN 3 involves the full thickness of the epithelium and often progresses to carcinoma in situ. Carcinoma in situ (CIS) is diagnosed when the full thickness of epithelium is replaced with abnormal cells (Creasman, 2012) (Fig. 11-11).

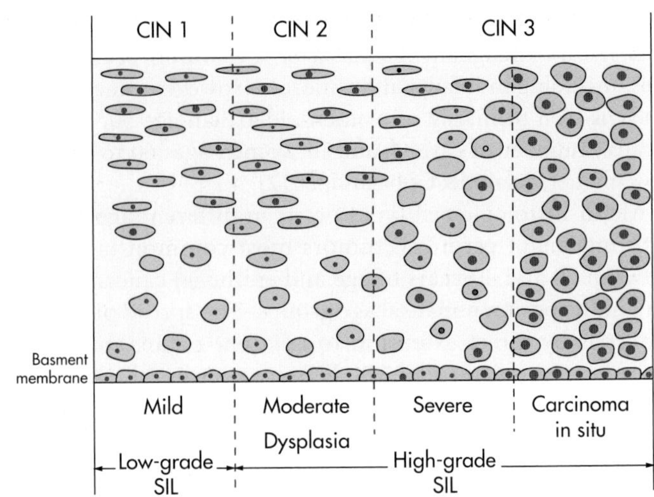

FIG 11-11 Diagram of cervical epithelium showing progressive changes and various terminology. *CIN,* Cervical intraepithelial neoplasia; *SIL,* squamous intraepithelial lesion.

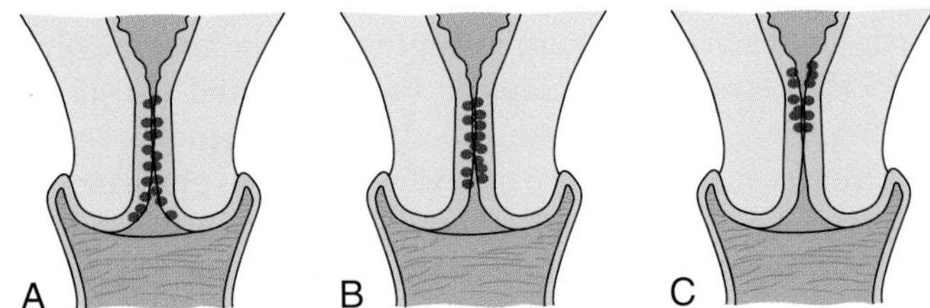

FIG 11-12 Location of squamocolumnar junction according to age. The location where the endocervical glands meet the squamous epithelium becomes progressively higher with age. **A,** Puberty. **B,** Reproductive years. **C,** Postmenopausal.

Terms used to describe neoplastic changes in abnormal cervical cytology reports are low-grade and high-grade squamous intraepithelial lesions (SILs); however, CIN continues to be a common term used in clinical practice.

Preinvasive lesions are limited to the cervix and usually originate in the squamocolumnar junction or transformation zone (Fig. 11-12). Intensive study of the cervix and the cellular changes that take place has shown that most cervical tumors have a gradual onset rather than an explosive one. Preinvasive conditions may exist for years before the development of invasive disease. These preinvasive conditions are highly treatable in many cases.

Invasive carcinoma is the diagnosis when abnormal cells penetrate the basement membrane and invade the stroma. There are two types of invasive carcinomas of the cervix: microinvasive and invasive. Microinvasive carcinoma is defined as one or more lesions that penetrate no more than 3 mm into the stroma below the basement membrane with no areas of lymphatic or vascular invasion (Creasman, 2012). Invasive carcinoma describes invasion that goes beyond these parameters. The staging of invasive carcinoma extends from CIS to distant metastasis or disease outside the true pelvis.

Approximately 90% of cervical malignancies are squamous cell carcinomas; 10% are adenocarcinomas. Squamous cell carcinomas can spread by direct extension to the vaginal mucosa, the pelvic wall, the bowels, and the bladder. Metastasis usually occurs in the pelvis, but it can occur in the lungs and the brain through the lymphatic system.

The average age range for the occurrence of cervical cancer is 40 to 50 years; however, preinvasive conditions may exist for 10 to 15 years before the development of an invasive carcinoma. About 70% to 80% of cervical cancers are caused by human papillomavirus (HPV) (Creasman, 2012). A strong link has been established between HPV types 16 and 18 and cervical neoplasia (see Chapter 7 for a discussion of HPV including preventive vaccines). Risk factors for persistent HPV infections include early age at first coitus (younger than 20 years), multiple sexual partners (more than two), a sexual partner with a history of multiple sexual partners, high parity, and belonging to a lower socioeconomic group. Potential factors include long-term use of OCs, cigarette smoking, and intrauterine exposure to diethylstilbestrol (DES) (ACS, 2014a; Creasman; Tewari & Monk, 2012). Low levels of beta-carotene, vitamin C, and folate are being investigated as potential risk factors (Tewari & Monk).

The incidence of cervical cancer in the United States is highest in Hispanic women and lowest in Native-American women, whereas the highest mortality occurs in African-American women (ACS, 2014a). Factors that may influence cervical screening behaviors for these groups include lack of a health promotion or disease prevention perspective, lack of knowledge about Pap tests and availability of services, financial barriers, and failure of health care providers to recommend screening (ACS). There also is a high rate of CIN in human immunodeficiency virus–positive women, suggesting that altered immune status is a risk factor (Creasman, 2012).

COMMUNITY ACTIVITY

- Visit the website www.cdc.gov/cancer/cervical/what_cdc_is_doing/amigas.htm.
- What is AMIGAS? What is a *promotora*? Why is this program important for the health of Hispanic women? How does this program promote cervical cancer screening among Hispanic women? What are the components of this educational model?
- Find out if there is an AMIGAS program in your community. If so, what is its effect?

Clinical Manifestations and Diagnosis

Preinvasive cancer of the cervix is often asymptomatic. Abnormal bleeding, especially postcoital bleeding, is the classic symptom of invasive cancer. Other late symptoms include rectal bleeding, hematuria, back pain, leg pain, and anemia. Diagnosis includes taking a history that includes menstrual and sexual activity information, particularly sexually transmitted infections and abnormal bleeding episodes (Creasman, 2012). A pelvic examination usually is normal except in late-stage cancer.

The most widely used method to detect preinvasive cancer is the Pap test, which can detect 90% of early cervical changes. According to the ACS, the American Society for Colposcopy and Cervical Pathology, and the American Society for Clinical Pathology, cervical cancer screening should begin at age 21. For women ages 21 to 29, screening should be done every 3 years with conventional or liquid-based Pap tests. For women ages 30 to 65, screening should be done every 5 years with both the HPV test and the Pap test (preferred method), or every 3 years with the Pap test alone (acceptable). Women who are 65 years or older who have had 3 or more consecutive negative Pap tests or more than 2 consecutive negative HPV and Pap tests within the past 10 years, with the most recent test occurring within 5 years, and women who have had a total hysterectomy can stop cervical cancer screening (ACS, 2014a; Moyer and U.S. Preventive Services Task Force, 2012; Saslow, Soloman, Lawson, et al., 2012). Women in high risk categories should have more frequent Pap tests.

BOX 11-5 2001 Bethesda System for Reporting Cervical Cytology Results

Results/Interpretations

Negative for Intraepithelial Malignancy

- Organisms (e.g., evidence of infections)
- Other nonneoplastic findings (e.g., inflammation, radiation changes, atrophy)
- Glandular cells status posthysterectomy
- Atrophy

Epithelial Cell Abnormalities

- Squamous cells
  - Atypical squamous cell (ASC)
  - Of undetermined significance (ASC-US)
  - Cannot exclude high-grade squamous intraepithelial lesion (HSIL) (ASC-H)
- Low-grade squamous intraepithelial lesion (LSIL)
  - Human papillomavirus (HPV), cervical intraepithelial neoplasia (CIN) 1
- HSIL
  - CIN 2, CIN 3
- Squamous cell carcinoma

Glandular Cell

- Atypical cells including endocervical, endometrial, and glandular or not otherwise specified
- Atypical cells including endocervical or glandular, suggestive of neoplasia (endocervical or not otherwise specified)
- Endocervical adenocarcinoma in situ
- Adenocarcinoma (endocervical, endometrial, extrauterine, or not otherwise specified)

Data from Creasman, W. (2012). Preinvasive disease of the cervix. In P.J. DiSaia, W.T. Creasman, R.S. Mannel, & D.S. Mutch (Eds.), *Clinical gynecologic oncology* (8th ed.). Philadelphia: Saunders.

Pap test results have been recorded by using several different classification systems. The reporting system most often used today is the Bethesda system, which reports on gynecologic cytology as well as histology of cervical lesions (Box 11-5). Changes secondary to inflammation, treatment (e.g., radiation), and contraceptive devices can be reported, as well as changes caused by infections. Epithelial cell abnormalities are described in three categories: atypias, or atypical squamous cells (ASC); low-grade squamous intraepithelial lesions (LSILs); and high-grade squamous intraepithelial lesions (HSILs).

Several options for follow-up of a finding of ASC of undetermined significance (ASC-US) are suggested. These include immediate colposcopy, repeating cytology at 6 months and 12 months, or HPV testing and referral for colposcopy if the test is positive. Colposcopy is recommended for evaluation of LSIL except in adolescents; teens can be followed with cytology tests at 6 and 12 months. Follow-up for a report of HSIL includes colposcopy or loop electrosurgical excision (Creasman, 2012).

Colposcopy is the examination of the cervix with a stereoscopic binocular microscope that magnifies the view of the cervix. Usually a solution of 3% acetic acid is applied to the cervix for better visualization of the epithelium and to identify areas for biopsy. Colposcopy is not an invasive procedure and is usually well tolerated. However, a woman who is scheduled for colposcopy because of an abnormal Pap test may be anxious and may need explanations or written information about what to expect during the procedure.

Biopsy is the removal of cervical tissue for study; several techniques can be used. An endocervical curettage is an effective diagnostic tool in about 90% of cases. It can be performed as an outpatient procedure with little or no anesthesia. It may be uncomfortable, and interventions to help the woman relax and cope with the pain may be needed.

Conization and loop electrosurgical excision procedure (LEEP) (see later discussion) can be done as outpatient procedures, although neither is usually performed unless the biopsy is positive or the results of the colposcopy are unsatisfactory. Conization involves removal of a cone of tissue from the exocervix and endocervix (Fig. 11-13). It can be a cold knife procedure, a laser excision, or an electrosurgical excision (Fig. 11-14) (see later discussion). There are two advantages to a cone biopsy. It can be used (1) to establish the diagnosis and (2) to effect a cure. If CIS is diagnosed, and if the woman wishes to retain her childbearing capacity, conization removes the abnormal tissue; further treatment (e.g., hysterectomy) is unnecessary. The woman is monitored with Pap tests and colposcopy when indicated.

If invasive cancer is diagnosed, other diagnostic tests can assess the extent of spread (see earlier discussion under endometrial cancer). Once the extent of the cancer is known, treatment begins.

CARE MANAGEMENT

For the woman diagnosed with invasive carcinoma of the cervix, pretherapy assessment includes physical, psychologic, and educational components, regardless of whether surgery or radiation is the method of treatment. Physical assessment includes a review of current medications because medications for other medical problems may have to be continued. Skin is assessed to identify potential pressure points; respiratory and gastrointestinal status and state of nutrition are important factors to assess. Urinalysis and complete blood count also are commonly performed. An electrocardiogram and a chest x-ray examination

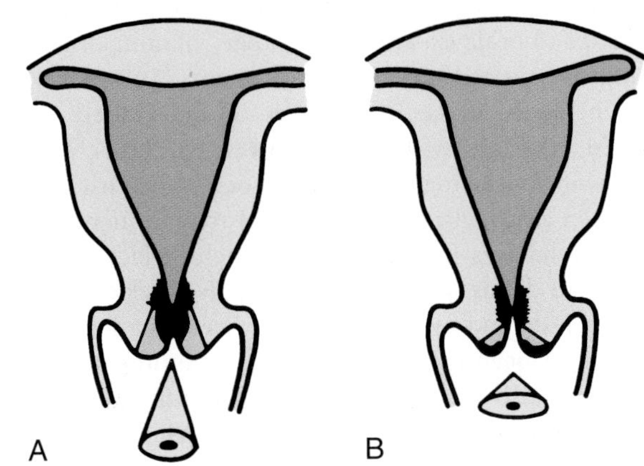

FIG 11-13 **A,** Cone biopsy for endocervical disease. Limits of lesion were not seen colposcopically. **B,** Cone biopsy for cervical intraepithelial neoplasia of the exocervix. Limits of lesion were identified colposcopically. (From Creasman, W. [2007]. Preinvasive disease of the cervix. In P.J. DiSaia, W.T. Creasman, R.S. Mannel, & D.S. Mutch [Eds.], *Clinical gynecologic oncology* [8th ed.]. Philadelphia: Saunders.)

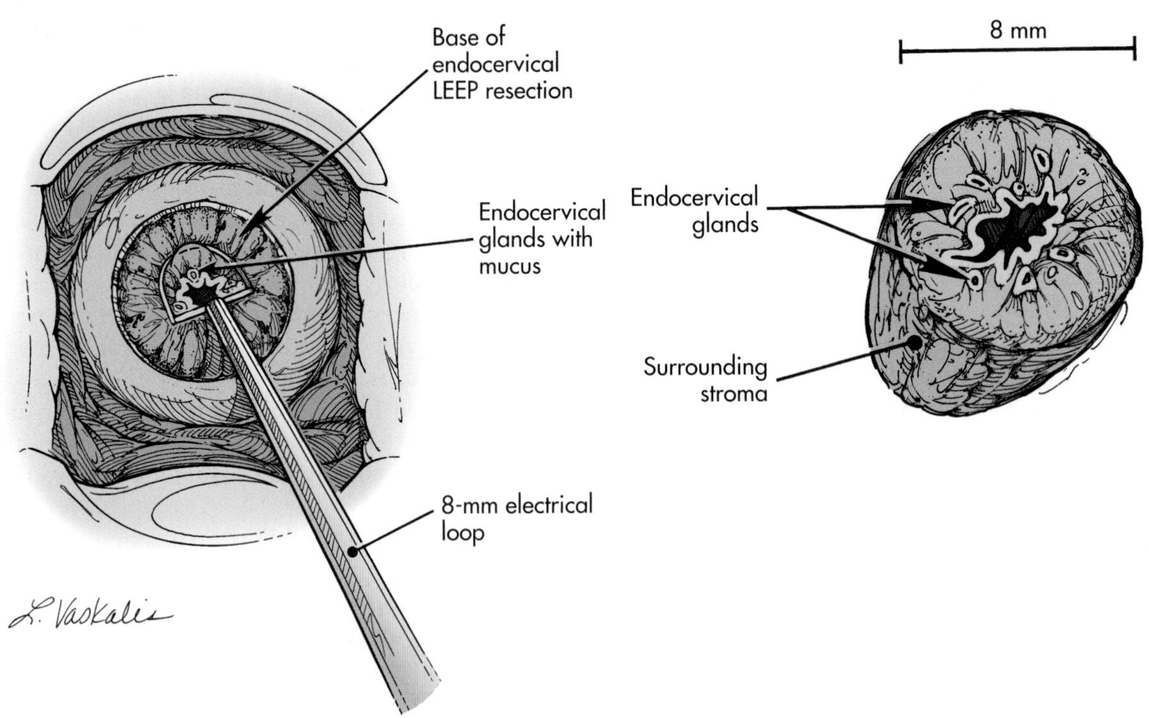

FIG 11-14 Electrosurgical excision. The electric loop vaporizes quickly and removes cone of tissue. *LEEP,* Loop electrosurgical excision procedure. (From Nichols, D., & Clark-Pearson, D. [2000]. *Gynecologic, obstetric, and related surgery* [2nd ed.]. St. Louis: Mosby.)

may be done if use of a general anesthetic is anticipated for surgery or placement of internal applicators.

Psychologic assessment is important because frequently these women are emotionally distressed about the diagnosis and anticipated treatment (i.e., fear of being radioactive and fear of surgery and pain) and fear that family or significant others will become distant.

Educational assessment involves identifying the woman's current knowledge base regarding the diagnosis and proposed therapeutic regimen.

Nursing diagnoses for the woman having surgery for cervical cancer are similar to those identified for the woman having a hysterectomy for endometrial cancer (see Nursing Care Plan: Hysterectomy for Endometrial Cancer). Nursing diagnoses for a woman having external or internal radiation therapy are listed in Box 11-6.

Medical and Surgical Management

Once a diagnosis has been identified, a course of treatment is planned. For preinvasive lesions, several techniques are used. As stated, because many preinvasive conditions are detected in younger women who may wish to continue childbearing, treatment is geared toward eradicating abnormal cells while attempting to preserve the structure of the cervix. The techniques available for preinvasive lesions are cryotherapy, laser therapy, and LEEP, all of which have comparable success rates in treating CIN (Creasman, 2012) (Box 11-7). Five-year survival rates are more than 91% when the cancer is localized (ACS, 2014a).

Treatment for invasive cancer includes surgery, radiation therapy, and chemotherapy. Once the cancer is staged, treatment is begun. Microinvasive cancer is usually treated with conization, but a hysterectomy is often done if childbearing is not desired. The choice of treatment for early-stage invasive cancer is hysterectomy or chemoradiation therapy (Tewari & Monk, 2012). A radical hysterectomy (see previous discussion) is performed if the cancer has extended beyond the cervix but not to the pelvic wall. Locally advanced stages of cervical cancer usually are treated with radiation therapy, both external and internal, and chemotherapy. Late stages are usually treated with radiation and chemotherapy.

Radiation Therapy. Radiation may be delivered by internal radium applications to the cervix or external radiation therapy that includes lymphatics of the pelvic side wall. In preparation for radiation therapy the woman must maintain good nutritional status and a high-protein, high-vitamin, and high-calorie diet. Anemia, if present, should be corrected before initiating radiotherapy.

External radiation therapy and internal radiation therapy are given in various combinations for the best results and are tailored to each woman and her particular lesion. For example, external radiation may be given first to treat regional pelvic nodes and to shrink the tumor. External radiation is usually an outpatient procedure given 5 days a week for 4 to 6 weeks. Internal radiation therapy consists of one or two intracavitary treatments at least 2 weeks apart (Tewari & Monk, 2012).

External radiation is provided by megavoltage machines such as cobalt, and supervoltage machines such as linear accelerators and betatron, all of which have the distinct advantage

BOX 11-6 Nursing Diagnoses for the Woman Having Radiation Therapy

Deficient Knowledge related to:
- Treatment procedures

Fear/Anxiety related to:
- Diagnosis
- Anticipated pain
- Concerns about radioactivity
- The response of the significant other or family

Disturbed Sensory Perception related to:
- Internal radiation therapy
- Restricted contact with visitors and nursing staff

Risk for Impaired Skin Integrity related to:
- External radiation exposure
- Immobility and bed rest (internal radiation therapy)

Risk for Injury related to:
- Dislodgment of internal radiation source

Acute Pain related to:
- Internal applicators

Sexual Dysfunction related to:
- Treatment or concerns of significant other

BOX 11-7 Surgical Alternatives for Preinvasive Cancer of the Cervix

Cryosurgery
- A technique to freeze abnormal cells is used, and when sloughing occurs, normal tissue is regenerated.
- Side effects occurring after treatment are usually few and not serious. A profuse watery discharge can persist for 2 to 4 weeks.
- Endocervical cells are thought to regenerate, leaving a normal cervical canal in most instances.
- Surveillance with frequent Pap tests and colposcopic examination must continue indefinitely after this type of conservative therapy.

Laser Ablation
- A laser mounted on a colposcope that allows precise direction of a beam of light (heat) is used to remove diseased tissue.
- For treatment of the cervix (relatively insensitive tissue), little or no anesthesia may be needed, although a burning or cramping sensation may be noticed.
- The cervix treated with CO_2 laser will show epithelial regrowth beginning by 2 days afterward. The site is usually healed in 4 to 6 weeks. The original architecture of the cervix is preserved, and the squamocolumnar junction remains visible; however, there can be more damage to normal tissues than with other treatments.
- Women usually have less vaginal discharge than with cryosurgery, but can have more discomfort after the procedure (Noller, 2012).

LEEP (Loop Electrosurgical Excision Procedure)
- A standard treatment for cervical intraepithelial neoplasia in the United States that uses a wire loop electrode that can excise and cauterize with minimal tissue damage (see Fig. 11-14)
- Healing is rapid, and there is only a mild discharge afterward.
- Possible complications include bleeding, cervical stenosis, infertility, and loss of cervical mucus.

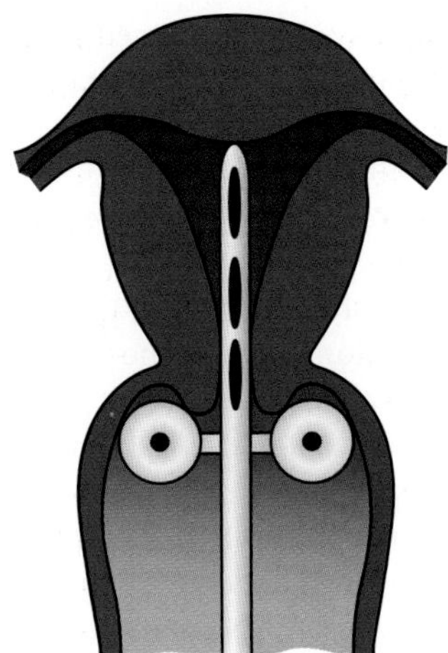

FIG 11-15 Intracavitary implant. Applicator in place in uterus is loaded with radium source.

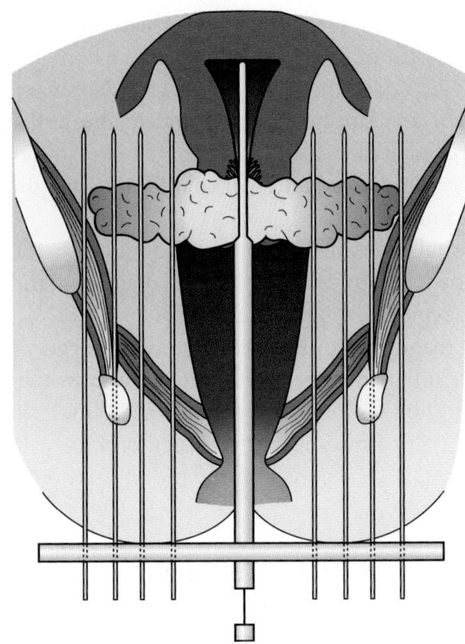

FIG 11-16 Interstitial-intracavitary implant.

of providing a more homogeneous dose to the pelvis. Before treatment begins, a localization procedure is done to determine the best way to deliver the treatments. Markings or small tattoos may be placed on the body to make sure the woman is positioned correctly to receive treatment (Workman, 2013).

For internal radiation therapy the woman may be treated in the hospital or in a special outpatient unit. If treatment is done in the hospital, she is taken to the operating room, and while she is under general or spinal anesthesia, a specially designed applicator is placed into her vagina and cervix. X-rays are taken to make sure the applicator is correctly placed. The woman is returned to her room, where the radioactive source is placed into the applicator (Fig. 11-15). The source remains in place from 12 hours to 3 days. If treatment is in the outpatient setting, the applicator is inserted into the uterus in a treatment room; use of high-dose implants shortens the treatment time and is being used more frequently than low-dose implants because no hospital stay is required (Tewari & Monk, 2012; Workman, 2013).

In advanced carcinoma of the cervix, conventional intracavitary applicators are not applicable. Interstitial therapy uses a template to guide the transperineal insertion of a group of 18-gauge hollow steel needles into the lesion (Fig. 11-16). After the needles are placed, the iridium wires are inserted when the woman is returned to her room.

Nursing Interventions. Nursing actions for external and internal radiation differ, so they are discussed separately.

External Therapy. Before external radiation therapy the woman's anxiety may be so high that information given by the radiologist may not be processed. The nurse should reinforce or fill in gaps, especially related to the following: the equipment, which is similar to that used for x-ray examination except larger; the hyperbaric oxygen chamber, which may be used to increase cellular oxygen and thus make tumor cells more radiosensitive; the radiotherapist, who will be behind a shield, but still close by and in communication with her; the position she will be put in and asked to maintain for some minutes; and the therapy, which is painless.

During the course of therapy, the woman is counseled regarding maintaining general good health. To maintain good skin care the woman is taught to assess her skin often; avoid soaps, ointments, cosmetics, and deodorants if the axilla is being irradiated because these may contain metals that alter the dose she receives and could lead to skin breakdown; wear loose clothing over the area and cotton underwear (or no underwear); use an air mattress or cover the mattress with foam pads or sheepskin; avoid exposing the irradiated areas to temperature extremes (e.g., hot tubs); and especially avoid removing the markings made by the radiologist. If her skin becomes red or itchy she can treat it with remedies recommended by the radiologist (e.g., aloe vera lotion, Aquaphor, or warm sitz baths). To treat skin that is broken or desquamating, the woman is shown how to use remedies prescribed by the radiologist (e.g., irrigation with warm water, application of antibiotic or lanolin ointment, exposure to air, and application of a loose dressing). The use of adhesive (or any) tape directly on the target area of skin should be avoided (Workman, 2013).

To maintain good nutrition the woman is reminded to keep a daily record of weight; use high-protein supplements; eat small, attractive, appetizing meals that are more bland than spicy; and keep the environment light, airy, clean, and quiet (especially before and after meals). A dietitian consult may be needed to help the woman and her family plan to meet her nutritional needs. If she is ill enough to be hospitalized, she may need total parenteral nutrition or tube feedings. Nausea interferes with adequate intake; therefore, the woman may take antiemetics, as necessary. High daily fluid intake (2 to 3 L) should be suggested if not contraindicated. To increase her comfort, minimize infection, and promote adequate food intake, she is encouraged to perform frequent oral hygiene. Box 11-4 provides other suggestions for nutritional problems associated with radiation treatment.

The nurse explains, as necessary, the need for routine blood studies to monitor the white blood cell count (to determine degree of immunosuppression). The woman and her family will need information about neutropenia, thrombocytopenia, and anemia and precautions to be taken. Because she is more vulnerable to infection, she is reminded of general measures to avoid infection (e.g., practice good hygiene, avoid people with infection, avoid large crowds, keep environment clean).

After the radiation treatment is completed, the woman needs information for self-care (see Teaching for Self-Management). She should also be informed that side effects of the treatment, especially fatigue and altered taste sensations, can continue for weeks after the therapy is completed.

TEACHING FOR SELF-MANAGEMENT

Care After External Radiation Therapy

- Avoid infection and report symptoms of infection to the health care provider immediately.
- Maintain good nutrition and fluid intake.
- Anticipate possible effects of radiation for 10 to 14 days after the last treatment.
- Expect signs of healing to occur in about 3 weeks.
- Maintain good skin and mouth care to support a sense of well-being and prevent infection.
- Report the following symptoms to your health care provider:
  - Continued gastrointestinal symptoms (nausea, vomiting, anorexia, diarrhea)
  - Increasing skin irritation at the site of therapy (redness, swelling, pain, pruritus)
- Take medications as prescribed, and avoid any medications not prescribed or approved by the health care provider.

Internal Therapy. Internal radiation therapy may require hospitalization or may be done in a special outpatient unit. Radiation safety officers determine the precautions to be observed in each situation. This discussion focuses on treatment in the hospital setting, but similar precautions are used in the outpatient setting. Printed instruction sheets are usually available, stating precautions to be followed for each type of radiation substance used. A precaution sign is placed on the door of the woman's room.

SAFETY ALERT

Personnel who come into direct contact with anyone receiving radiation therapy should wear a film badge or other device to monitor the amount of exposure received.

Nurses must protect themselves from overexposure to radiation. Precautions include the following (Workman, 2013):

- Careful isolation techniques: wearing gloves while handling bodily fluids and observing good handwashing technique. These behaviors reflect knowledge that alpha and beta rays cannot pass through skin but may be in body fluids and excrement.
- Careful planning of nursing activity to limit time (to 30 minutes or less per 8 hours) spent in proximity to the woman to avoid exposure to gamma rays, which can penetrate several inches of lead.

Exposure to radiation is controlled in three ways: distance, time, and shielding (with lead). For the woman with sealed radiotherapy, a movable lead screen can be placed between the area in which the therapeutic applicator is located and the personnel. The lead screen also is used to protect visitors from radiation. Increasing the distance from the source also decreases exposure (Workman, 2013).

Familiarity with applicators is a must for all nurses working with people receiving radiotherapy so that if a "strange object" is found in the linen or on the floor, it is not touched. Today most hospital protocols include having a lead container and forceps in the room for use if a radioactive implant is dislodged.

The woman is prepared for insertion with the following care, which is accompanied by an explanation for each activity. To reduce the need for attention to bowel elimination for a few days, the gastrointestinal tract is usually prepared by using low-residue diet, enemas, and sometimes bowel sedation. The vaginal vault is usually prepared with an antiseptic douche, such as povidone-iodine.

An indwelling urinary catheter is inserted, as ordered, to prevent bladder distention that could dislodge the applicator. Food and fluids are withheld for a specified time before the procedure in anticipation of using general anesthesia. Preoperative medications may be ordered for the morning of the procedure. Deep-breathing exercises, range-of-motion (ROM) exercises, and positioning are all demonstrated before the procedure to minimize the effects of immobilization afterward. An intravenous (IV) solution will probably be started before the procedure, and IV therapy may be continued if nausea prevents good intake of oral fluids. The woman is assured that pain will be managed.

Explanations about restricted visitation of personnel and visitors also are given in the preinsertion phase. Women are often encouraged to bring books, magazines, electronic readers, laptop computers, iPods, or other devices or materials to the hospital to combat the boredom that isolation imposes on them. In addition, many units are equipped with televisions and CD and DVD players.

The applicator is inserted into the woman's vaginal vault during surgery, and after the usual postanesthesia recovery care, the woman is returned to her room, where the applicators are loaded with the radioactive substance.

A lead shield is placed next to the bed in line with the woman's pelvic area to protect the caregivers and visitors. Vital signs are monitored every 4 hours. Active ROM and deep-breathing exercises are encouraged every 2 hours; the woman is positioned on her back and may not be permitted to turn from side to side, although log-rolling may be done occasionally to relieve back pressure. The head of the bed may or may not be elevated slightly.

The woman's diet is changed from clear liquid to low residue, as ordered. Many individuals have difficulty eating while lying flat or even if the bed is elevated slightly. The nurse arranges the food so that it is easy to reach. Finger foods or liquids are generally more manageable. Parenteral or oral fluids are given, up to 3 L daily.

The urinary catheter remains in the bladder while the implant is in place. However, no perineal or catheter care is given. Intake and output are measured. The woman is given a partial bath, washing only above her waist. Massage is restricted to her shoulders and neck. Linen is changed only as absolutely necessary. Any linen or equipment used is retained in the room until therapy is complete to prevent loss of an applicator or seed. If vaginal or rectal bleeding or hematuria occurs, the physician is notified immediately.

Emotional support is provided by planning to be with the woman for short periods, encouraging her to verbalize concerns and needs, and encouraging family members, clergy, or others to visit for short periods daily or to communicate by telephone. Pregnant women and children are not permitted to visit.

Many women undergoing internal radiation treatment are given medication to prevent complications and to promote comfort during the procedure. Such medications might include antibiotics to prevent bladder infections, heparin injections to prevent thrombophlebitis, sedatives for relaxation, antiemetics for nausea, and narcotics for pain. The woman is considered radioactive during the time the internal sources are in place (Workman, 2013).

After the radium is removed the Foley catheter is removed, and the woman is assisted in getting out of bed the first time. She is usually discharged the same day. Discharge teaching can be found in the Teaching for Self-Management box: Care After Internal Radiation Therapy. The woman and her family are reassured that she is not radioactive after the treatment.

TEACHING FOR SELF-MANAGEMENT

Care After Internal Radiation Therapy

- Eat three balanced meals a day, and increase fluid to 3 L daily.
- Rest when tired, and resume normal activities as comfort permits.
- Maintain good hygiene (e.g., daily showers and daily douches until discharge stops).
- Use a vaginal dilator if needed for vaginal stenosis. Sexual intercourse may be resumed in 7 to 10 days or as recommended by your physician.
- Understand that sterility and cessation of menstruation usually occur with this procedure if you are premenopausal.
- Report any of the following to your health care provider: bleeding (vaginal, rectal, or in the urine), foul-smelling vaginal discharge, fever, abdominal distention, or pain.
- Take any prescribed medications as directed.
- Call your health care provider or clinic if there are concerns or problems.
- Keep scheduled follow-up visits to determine emotional as well as physical recovery.

Posttreatment complications range from those arising from immobilization, such as thrombophlebitis, pulmonary embolism, and pneumonia, to those arising from the treatment itself, such as hemorrhage, skin reactions (rashes or inflammation), diarrhea, cramping, dysuria, and vaginal stenosis. The woman is assessed for any of these complications before discharge.

The woman may experience altered patterns of sexuality related to treatment side effects. A decrease in vaginal secretions and sensation may occur, as well as vaginal stenosis. These can contribute to decreased sexual desire, because pain and discomfort during intercourse can affect the desire to resume sexual activities. The nurse can initiate a discussion with the woman and her partner, offer information about the effects of radiation on the ability to have sexual intercourse, and offer suggestions for specific problems, such as using a water-based lubricant for vaginal dryness and using a vaginal dilator as directed by her health care provider. If necessary, the couple can be referred to other resources.

Complications of Radiation Therapy. Morbidity as a direct result from properly conducted therapy is usually minimal. Some of the morbidity seen may be caused by the uncontrolled tumor and not by the therapy. Acute treatment complications occurring during or shortly after therapy include irritation of the rectum, the small bowel, and the bladder; reactions in the skinfolds; and mild bone marrow suppression. Dysuria and frequency may occur. Late complications, although not common, include genital fistulas and necrosis (Yashar, 2012).

Recurrent and Advanced Cancer of the Cervix

Approximately one third of women with invasive cervical cancer have recurrent or persistent disease after therapy. The 1-year survival rate is between 10% and 15% (Terwari & Monk, 2012). Irradiation of metastatic areas is commonly successful in providing local control and symptomatic relief.

Pelvic Exenteration. The woman who has recurrence only within the pelvis may be considered for pelvic exenteration if a cure is thought to be possible. A total exenteration involves removal of the perineum, the pelvic floor, the levator muscles, and all reproductive organs. Additionally, pelvic lymph nodes, rectum, sigmoid colon, urinary bladder, and distal ureters are removed, and a colostomy and ileal conduit are constructed (Tewari & Monk, 2012) (Fig. 11-17, *A*). In select cases the procedure can be modified to either an anterior or a posterior exenteration. In anterior pelvic exenteration all of the previously mentioned pelvic viscera are removed except the rectosigmoid, which is preserved. Urine is rerouted through an ileal conduit (see Fig. 11-17, *B*). In the posterior pelvic exenteration procedure, all pelvic viscera with the exception of the bladder are removed. The feces are rerouted through a colostomy (see Fig. 11-17, *C*). A neovagina (new vagina) may be constructed.

Women are carefully selected for this procedure; 5-year survival rates range from 20% to 62% (Tewari & Monk, 2012). Many of the complications that follow this surgery are those that follow any form of major surgery, for example, pulmonary embolism, pulmonary edema, myocardial infarction, and cerebrovascular accident. These complications are seen immediately after surgery. Infection originating in the pelvic cavity usually occurs later, if it occurs.

Nursing Interventions. Nursing care of the woman having a pelvic exenteration depends on what is removed. General preoperative considerations include assessments similar to those for a woman having a radical hysterectomy. Additionally, a thorough sexual assessment is needed because of the dramatic changes involved. The woman needs information about the construction of a neovagina if that is an option. She will need to be assessed for stoma site selection and information about management of colostomy or ileal conduit if appropriate. Extensive preoperative bowel preparation is needed before surgery. Pain management is discussed, as is what to expect postoperatively (e.g., nasogastric tubes, arterial catheters). Significant others should be included in preoperative discussions when possible because their postoperative support is essential.

Postoperative care usually begins in an intensive care unit until the woman's condition is stable. She is monitored for shock, hemorrhage, pulmonary embolus and other pulmonary

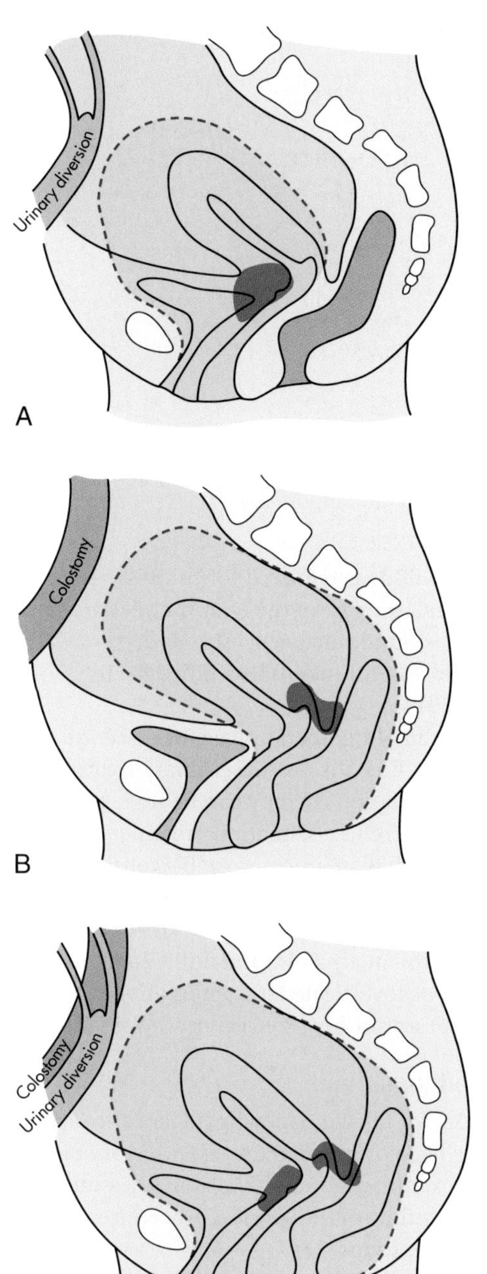

FIG 11-17 Pelvic exenteration procedures. **A,** Anterior exenteration. **B,** Posterior exenteration. **C,** Total exenteration.

complications, fluid and electrolyte imbalance, and urinary complications (Tewari & Monk, 2012). Nursing care continues after the woman is stabilized and moved back to her room. Wound care consists of irrigation with half-strength normal saline, followed by drying of the area with either a hair dryer on cool setting or a heat lamp placed at least 12 inches from the perineal area. The woman is taught how to care for her colostomy or ileal conduit when she is able to begin self-care. Assessment for psychologic reactions is important. The woman will probably experience a grief reaction over her mutilated body. She may become depressed during the long convalescence.

The woman may be discharged to a long-term care facility or to her home. She will need assistance in her physical care for at least 6 months. Teaching needed for home care includes colostomy or ureterostomy care; dietary needs for healing; perineal care, including use of perineal pads to protect clothing from discharge; ROM exercises and physical activities permitted by her health care provider; and signs of complication, especially infection and bowel obstruction.

Because she will have sexual disruption and possibly be unable to have vaginal intercourse (if the vagina is not reconstructed), counseling about sexual activity is needed. Usually even with a vaginal reconstruction, vaginal intercourse is not advised until healing has taken place, usually in 12 to 18 months. Women with neovaginas may complain of decreased vaginal sensations or chronic discharge or that the vagina is too short or too long. Women with colostomies or ureterostomies may worry about leakage or odors during sexual activities or may be concerned about their change in appearance. They may need counseling about alternative activities for sexual expression for themselves and their partners. The woman and her partner may need referral for further sexual counseling.

Chemotherapy. Chemotherapy may be used in advanced cancer of the cervix to reduce tumor size before surgery or as adjuvant therapy for poor-prognosis tumors. In general, no long-term benefits are derived with chemotherapy, although chemotherapy concurrent with radiation therapy can improve survival (Tewari & Monk, 2012). Cisplatin is the most effective; other chemotherapeutic agents used in combination with cisplatin include carboplatin, cyclophosphamide, ifosfamide, methotrexate, mitomycin C, bleomycin, paclitaxel, topotecan, and hydroxyurea (Chu & Rubin, 2012).

Cancer of the Vulva

Incidence and Etiology

Vulvar carcinoma accounts for about 4% of all female genital malignancies and is the fourth most commonly occurring gynecologic cancer. It appears most frequently in women in their middle 60s to 70s (Schilder & Stehman, 2012). Vulvar cancers in older women do not appear to be caused by HPV infection. The incidence of vulvar cancer, specifically vulvar intraepithelial neoplasia (VIN), is increasing in younger women. Almost 20% of vulvar cancers occur in women younger than 50 years of age, and most women are in their 20s. HPV infection is thought to be responsible for most of these cancers (ACS, 2014b). Women who have a history of genital warts (condylomata acuminata) and who smoke have an increased risk of developing VIN (ACS).

By far the majority (90%) of vulvar carcinoma is squamous cell; other vulvar neoplasms are attributed to Paget disease, adenocarcinoma of Bartholin glands, fibrosarcoma and melanoma, and basal cell carcinoma. VIN is the first neoplastic change, progressing over time to CIS and then to invasive cancer. Metastasis is by direct extension and lymphatic spread (Schilder & Stehman, 2012).

Prognosis depends on the size of the lesion and the tumor grade at the time of diagnosis; 50% of women have symptoms for 2 to 16 months before seeking treatment. Fortunately vulvar cancer grows slowly, extends slowly, and metastasizes fairly late. Even with a pattern of delayed diagnosis, survival rates are approximately 90% if nodes are negative. Survival rates drop to 40% to 50%, however, if lymph node metastasis has occurred (Schilder & Stehman, 2012).

Clinical Manifestations and Diagnosis

Itching is the most common symptom of VIN; a lump or lesion is more common with invasive cancer (Schilder & Stehman, 2012). The most common site for vulvar lesions is on the labia majora. The vulvar lesion is usually asymptomatic until it is 1 to 2 cm in diameter. When it is symptomatic, women may complain of vulvar pruritus, burning, or pain. Necrosis and infection of the lesion result in ulceration with bleeding or watery discharge.

VINs are usually multifocal in young women. Unifocal lesions are associated with invasive cancer and are more common in older women. Initially, growth is superficial but later extends into the urethra, the vagina, and the anus. In approximately 50% of late cases, superficial inguinal and femoral lymph nodes become involved (Schilder & Stehman, 2012).

Simple biopsy with histologic evaluation reveals the diagnosis. The areas of pathologic involvement are identified by staining the vulva with toluidine blue (1%), allowing an absorption time of 3 to 5 minutes, and then washing with acetic acid (2% to 3%); abnormal tissue retains the dye. Biopsy is necessary to rule out such conditions as sexually transmitted infections (e.g., chancroid, granuloma inguinale, syphilis), basal cell carcinoma, and CIS. In situ malignancies are initially small, red, white, or pigmented friable papules. In Paget disease the lesions are red, moist, and elevated. Melanomas appear as bluish black, pigmented, or papillary lesions. Melanomas metastasize through the bloodstream and lymphatics (Schilder & Stehman, 2012).

Medical and Surgical Management

Treatment varies, depending on the extent of the disease. Laser surgery, cryosurgery, or electrosurgical excision may be used to treat VIN. A disadvantage to these treatments is that healing is slow, and the treated area is painful. A local wide excision may be performed for localized lesions. Recurrence can occur after these treatments, so follow-up is important (Frumovitz & Bodurka, 2012).

Several types of vulvectomy procedures are used for CIS and invasive cancer. A *skinning vulvectomy* involves removal of the superficial vulvar skin; it is rarely performed.

A *simple vulvectomy* involves removal of all of the vulva (external genital organs including the mons pubis, labia majora and minora, and possibly the clitoris). The clitoris usually can be saved if cancer is not present.

For invasive disease, a *partial* or *complete radical vulvectomy* is performed. A partial vulvectomy is the removal of part of the vulva and deep tissues; a complete vulvectomy includes the removal of the whole vulva, deep tissues, and the clitoris (Fig. 11-18). These procedures are not used often.

Skin grafts may be done if a large area of skin is removed during the vulvectomy; however, most surgeries can be closed without grafts. If grafts are needed, a surgeon who performs reconstruction surgery may be consulted (ACS, 2014b).

The inguinal nodes may be removed through an inguinal (groin) node dissection. Usually only lymph nodes on the same side as the cancer are removed; however, nodes on both sides may be removed if the cancer is in the middle (see Fig. 11-18). Swelling of the leg often is a problem after this surgery.

A *sentinel node biopsy* may be done instead of the inguinal node dissection. This procedure involves injecting blue dye or radioactive material into the tumor site. A scan is performed to identify the sentinel (first) node to pick up the dye or radioactive material. The node is removed for microscopic study. If cancer cells are found, the rest of the lymph nodes are removed, but if cancer is not found, further lymph node removal is not done. This procedure continues to be studied for use with vulvar cancers (ACS, 2014b).

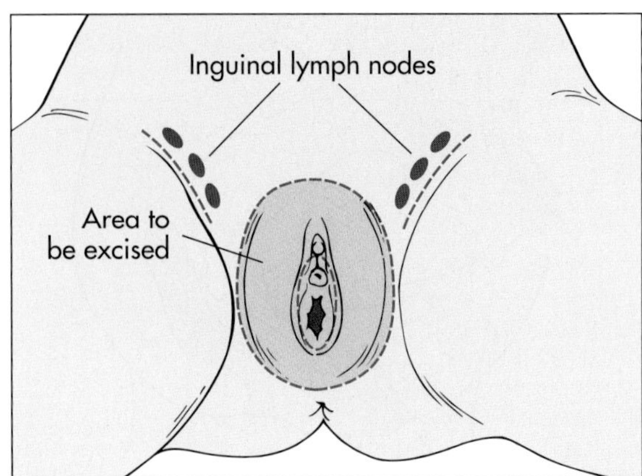

FIG 11-18 Radical vulvectomy. Note dotted lines denoting vulvectomy incision and inguinal groin incisions.

External radiation therapy can be used to shrink tumors before surgery, but it is not the primary treatment. Postoperative external radiation therapy can be used for women who are at risk for recurrence. Radiation treatment causes dermatitis and ulceration that are uncomfortable for the woman.

Chemotherapy has not been very effective as a treatment except for the topical application of 5-fluorouracil for VIN or CIS. This treatment is painful and not used often. Chemotherapy continues to be investigated in combination with radiation as an adjunct to surgery in advanced cancer of the vulva (ACS, 2014b).

Nursing Interventions

Nursing care for the woman with vulvar cancer is similar to that for other gynecologic malignancies. A history of symptoms and a physical examination as well as an assessment of the woman's understanding of the surgical procedure and her emotional state should be done.

Nursing diagnoses for women with vulvar cancer are similar to those for other gynecologic cancers.

Interventions for the woman treated with laser therapy include applying topical steroids to the area, administering sitz baths and drying the area with a hair dryer, applying local anesthetics, or giving oral pain medication as needed. Women need to be informed that pain may get worse 3 to 4 days after the treatment.

Because there can be recurrences, information about vulvar self-examination and the need for follow-up with a health care provider is reinforced. Information about community support groups may be helpful, although a study by Likes, Russell, & Tillmanns (2008) found that women reported increased anxiety after having contact with Internet support groups.

A woman undergoing radical vulvectomy requires some special nursing actions in addition to routine postoperative care (see Teaching for Self-Management). She will need instructions about wound care and infection prevention as well as about possible complications, such as a change in her urine stream (may go to one side) related to tissue removal around the urethral opening, and lymphedema (Schilder & Stehman, 2012).

TEACHING FOR SELF-MANAGEMENT

Care After Vulvectomy

- Avoid sexual activity for 4 to 6 weeks or as your health care provider directs.
- Rest frequently.
- Avoid crossing your legs, sitting, or standing for long periods.
- Avoid tight, constricting clothing, and wear cotton underwear.
- Keep wound area clean and dry. Rinse area with warm water and pat dry after voiding.
- Continue wound care as prescribed (e.g., irrigate with solution of warm water; pack with gauze; dry using hair dryer on coolest setting). Report to your health care provider any swelling, redness, unusual tenderness, drainage, or foul odor of incision site.
- Report any temperature greater than 39° C (102.2° F).
- Eat a well-balanced diet to promote healing.
- Take all medications as prescribed.
- Elevate your legs periodically to prevent pelvic congestion.
- Call your health care provider or clinic if there are concerns or problems.

The woman is at high risk for sexual dysfunction related to the effects of the surgery. For example, she may have concerns that her partner will be repulsed by the scarring and loss of the vulva. She also may have concerns about reaching orgasm and vaginal numbness or painful vaginal penetration. Nursing actions that focus on minimizing these risks include the following:

- Encouraging verbalization of feelings
- Providing privacy for discussion
- Encouraging open communication between the woman and her partner
- Discussing when sexual activity can be safely resumed
- Discussing alternative methods to achieve sexual satisfaction
- Providing information about use of vaginal dilators and water-soluble lubricants for painful vaginal intercourse
- Providing resources for counseling if necessary

Cancer of the Vagina

Vaginal carcinomas account for 1% to 3% of gynecologic malignancies, with more than 50% of cases occurring between the ages of 70 and 90 years (Slomovitz & Coleman, 2012). Most lesions are squamous cell carcinomas and are secondary rather than primary carcinomas of the vagina. Vaginal intraepithelial neoplasia (VAIN) is uncommon. Clear-cell adenocarcinoma is even rarer. It is found primarily in young women (ages 15 to 30 years) and is related to intrauterine exposure to DES (Badurka & Frumovitiz, 2012).

The etiology is unknown, but vaginal cancer may be caused by chronic vaginal irritation, vaginal trauma, and genital viruses (e.g., HPV). Women with VAIN often have had cancer or currently have cancer of another part of the genital tract (Slomovitz & Coleman, 2012). Vaginal lesions, usually seen in the upper third of the vagina, often extend into the bladder and the rectum in late stages. Metastasis can occur early because of the rich lymphatic drainage in the vaginal area.

Some women with vaginal cancer are asymptomatic. Diagnosis often comes after an abnormal Pap test. Symptoms associated with vaginal cancer include bleeding after coitus or examination, dyspareunia, and watery discharge. Bladder involvement results in urinary frequency or urgency; rectal extension causes painful defecation. A pelvic examination may reveal a single lesion, although multiple lesions are common (Slomovitz & Coleman, 2012).

Colposcopy examination and biopsy of Schiller-stained areas disclose the diagnosis. Therapy for vaginal cancer is directed by the extent of the lesion and the age and condition of the woman. Local excision is the preferred therapy for localized lesions. Topical application of 5-fluorouracil cream has been used with varying results. Laser surgery can be used to treat VAIN. Radical hysterectomy and removal of the upper vagina with dissection of the pelvic nodes or internal and external radiation are options for invasive cancer. Radiation therapy is the usual treatment of choice (Slomovitz & Coleman, 2012). If a vaginectomy is performed, sexual function will be lost without reconstructive surgery. Chemotherapy has not been effective in treating vaginal cancer, although studies are ongoing on the effectiveness of chemotherapy in combination with radiation. In early-stage cancer, 5-year survival rates are greater than 80%, with stage II survival rates in the 50% range (Slomovitz & Coleman, 2012).

Nursing care for the woman with vaginal cancer is similar to that for other gynecologic cancers. Women who are sexually active should be encouraged to continue sexual intercourse or to use a vaginal dilator to maintain vaginal patency (Slomovitz & Coleman, 2012). Sexual counseling or referral may be needed.

Cancer of the Uterine Tubes

Primary carcinoma of the uterine (fallopian) tube (usually the distal one third) is one of the rarest cancers of the female genital tract (less than 1%), with a peak incidence between ages 50 and 60 years (Bidus, Maxwell, & Rose, 2012). The cause is unknown. Most women are asymptomatic in the early stages of tubal cancer. Vaginal bleeding is the most common symptom of tubal cancer, but clear vaginal discharge and lower abdominal pain also occur frequently. An enlarging unilateral pelvic mass or ascites may occur and is often misdiagnosed as ovarian carcinoma or endometrial carcinoma. Differential diagnosis of tubal cancer is usually made postoperatively. Because uterine tube cancer is so rare, there is no established management. Current therapy guidelines parallel those established for ovarian carcinoma; therefore, tumor-reducing surgery such as a TAH with BSO, omentectomy (removal of connective tissue covering the organs), and lymph node sampling are performed (Bidus et al.). Postoperative therapy consists of chemotherapy with cisplatin or other platinum-based drugs combined with paclitaxel, sometimes followed by second-look surgery to determine whether further treatment is needed. Radiation therapy is sometimes used if the disease is limited to the tube, ovary, and uterus, although reports of its effectiveness vary. The overall 5-year survival rate for all stages is 69%; the 5-year survival rates for stages I and II are approximately 80% (Bidus et al.).

Nursing care for the woman with uterine tube cancer is similar to that of the woman with ovarian cancer.

Cancer and Pregnancy

Cancer occurs with relative infrequency during the reproductive years. Approximately 1 of every 1000 pregnant women will have cancer (Salani, Eisenhauer, & Copeland, 2012). These malignancies may be responsible for up to one third of maternal deaths. Although all forms of neoplasms have been documented in conjunction with pregnancy, the most frequently occurring types are breast cancer, cervical cancer, melanomas, ovarian cancer, leukemia and lymphomas, and thyroid cancers. Other cancers, including other gynecologic cancers, rarely are diagnosed in pregnancy (Salani et al.). When pregnancy and cancer coincide, therapeutic issues are complex, and intense reactions occur in the woman, her family, and the health care team. Women are confronted with issues such as continuing or terminating the pregnancy. The selection and timing of therapies such as chemotherapy, radiation, and surgery are affected by the pregnancy. Add to this the conflicting feelings the woman has (i.e., the joy of pregnancy versus the fear and anxiety associated with cancer), and the task of providing comprehensive care for her and her family presents a formidable challenge to the health care team. A brief discussion of the most frequent types of cancers that occur during pregnancy and the current therapies associated with them follows.

Cancer of the Breast

Approximately 1% to 2% of women are pregnant or lactating at the time of diagnosis of cancer of the breast (Tewari, 2012). Breast cancer complicates about 1 in 3000 pregnancies. The survival rate for women who are diagnosed with breast cancer while pregnant may be as low as 15% to 20% because the disease is generally in the advanced stages when first diagnosed (Salani et al., 2012). Diagnosis is often delayed because breast engorgement may obscure the mass from palpation, and increased density of the tissue makes mammographic visualization more difficult. In addition, increased vascularity and lymphatic drainage in the breast of a pregnant woman may increase the speed of metastasis. Treatment is the same as for a nonpregnant woman, although surgery is usually the treatment of choice for breast cancer in pregnancy (Tewari). If an invasive tumor is found, it must be determined whether the tissue is positive or negative for estrogen receptors (ERs). ER-negative tumors spread more rapidly than ER-positive tumors and are more common in pregnancy (Salani et al.).

Maternal-fetal management involves consideration of the gestational age of the fetus, the extent of disease, the tumor growth potential, and the proposed treatment. Termination of the pregnancy in early stages of the disease appears to have no effect on survival. There is little evidence to suggest that pregnancy affects the malignant process. Therapeutic abortion may become an issue in the presence of advanced disease and may be deemed necessary to achieve effective palliation. In the first trimester, lumpectomy or partial mastectomy is the most commonly used surgical procedure, but radical mastectomy is tolerated well in these women. For advanced disease in the second or third trimester, alkylating agents, 5-fluorouracil, doxorubicin, and cyclophosphamide are relatively safe for the fetus. Radiation therapy is avoided if at all possible until after the birth, because even with careful shielding, the fetus may still receive sufficient radiation to produce detrimental effects (Salani et al., 2012; Tewari, 2012).

There is no agreement about whether a postpartum woman with breast cancer should breastfeed, although many surgeons recommend formula feeding. There are theoretic concerns that if one of the oncogenes for breast cancer is a virus, as many have postulated, the remaining breast may be contaminated, and the virus may be passed to the newborn, possibly acting as a latent inducer of breast carcinoma. Another reason is that lactation increases vascularity in the remaining breast, which may contain a neoplasm as well (Tewari, 2012).

Breastfeeding after lumpectomy is possible, but the site of the incision may interrupt the milk ducts or prevent the nipple from extending during feeding. Breastfeeding is contraindicated if the woman is receiving chemotherapy. Women receiving radiation have diminished ability to lactate in the irradiated breast (Salani et al., 2012; Tewari, 2012).

Pregnancy incidence after mastectomy is influenced by many factors, including prior treatment and duration of survival. In general, women with good prognoses (e.g., no positive nodes) are likely to be counseled to wait at least 2 years before attempting pregnancy (Tewari, 2012).

Cancer of the Cervix

The incidence of cervical cancer concurrent with pregnancy is reported to be about 1 in 2200 pregnancies, making it the most common reproductive tract cancer associated with pregnancy (Salani et al., 2012). The outcome for a woman with cervical cancer is roughly the same as that for a nonpregnant woman (Tewari, 2012).

Cervical abnormalities are diagnosed during pregnancy with an abnormal Pap test. If the report suggests that the pregnant woman has a squamous intraepithelial lesion, a colposcopy, possibly with directed biopsy, is done. If invasive disease is not found, treatment is delayed until after the woman gives birth. Colposcopy is often repeated every 6 to 8 weeks until the birth and again postpartum (Salani et al., 2012). Conization is not advised during pregnancy unless necessary to rule out invasive cancer because it is associated with bleeding, miscarriage, and preterm birth (Tewari, 2012).

The therapy of invasive carcinoma of the cervix during pregnancy is affected by many factors. The stage of the disease and the trimester in which the cancer is diagnosed are important. Equally important are the beliefs and desires of the woman and her family in terms of initiating therapy that can interrupt the pregnancy, as opposed to postponing the therapy until fetal viability is achieved. If the woman chooses not to continue the pregnancy, external radiation to the pelvis is done. Miscarriage usually occurs, and then internal radiation is done. If miscarriage does not occur, a modified radical hysterectomy may be performed. If the woman desires to continue the pregnancy, treatment of early-stage invasive cervical cancer can be delayed until 34 to 36 weeks, without harmful effects on the woman. Cesarean birth is usually performed after the mother has received antenatal steroids and fetal lung maturity is documented; radiation therapy is then initiated (Salani et al., 2012; Tewari, 2012).

Leukemia

The average age for pregnant women with acute leukemia is 28 years; incidence during pregnancy is about 1 in 75,000 (Tewari, 2012). Pregnancy seems to have no specific effect on the course of the disease, but vigorous therapy is detrimental to early gestation. Preterm labor and postpartum hemorrhage are associated with acute leukemia (Tewari). Acute myelocytic leukemia (60% of cases) has a more fulminant course and requires immediate therapy; in the presence of chronic myelocytic leukemia, therapy can be delayed somewhat. Some pregnant women with the chronic form of the disease who had chemotherapy and radiation therapy directed at the spleen have given birth to apparently healthy infants. The decision to terminate the pregnancy rests with the woman and her family; however, prompt, aggressive therapy is always advisable if remission is to be achieved. Decisions may be influenced by the aggressiveness of the disease.

Hodgkin Disease

Hodgkin disease is a malignant lymphoma that affects many younger people and complicates about one in 6000 pregnancies. Younger women (less than 40 years) have a better prognosis (Tewari, 2012).

Pregnancy appears to have no effect on the disease and vice versa, other than those effects resulting from therapy (Salani et al., 2012). Radiation therapy of the nodes and multiagent chemotherapy result in about a 90% cure rate. Unless gestation is well into the third trimester, delay in initiating therapy should be minimal, which brings up the dilemma of therapeutic abortion. Radiation therapy to diseased areas above the diaphragm can be initiated during the third trimester with proper shielding of the fetus (Salani et al.). Chemotherapy is strongly contraindicated during the first trimester, but certain agents (antitumor antibiotics and antimicrotubule agents) appear safe to use in the second and third trimesters. Termination of the pregnancy during the course of the disease is not definitely indicated (Tewari, 2012).

Melanoma

Malignant melanoma may be one of the rare cancers that can be affected by pregnancy. This is suggested by some reports in which pregnancy has been shown to induce or exacerbate a melanoma. These suggestions are based on changes that occur naturally during pregnancy and include hyperpigmentation, an increase in melanocyte-stimulating hormone (MSH), and increased estrogen production. ERs have been identified in about half of all melanomas. Although pregnancy has been implicated in the more rapid metastases to regional lymph nodes, stage for stage there does not seem to be a significant difference in the survival of pregnant and nonpregnant women (Salani et al., 2012; Tewari, 2012). As a result, most authorities recommend that women who have histories of malignant melanoma delay pregnancy for 2 to 3 years after surgical excision, because this is the period of highest risk for recurrence (Salani et al.; Tewari).

Diagnosis is established by biopsy. Therapy consists of radical local excision. For most other malignancies, the placenta is resistant to invasion by maternal cancer. Although melanoma accounts for few cases of malignant disease during pregnancy, it is the most common cancer to metastasize to the placenta (Tewari, 2012).

Thyroid Cancer

The incidence of thyroid cancer in pregnancy is not established. Normally the thyroid gland enlarges during pregnancy, and an asymptomatic nodular mass is a common finding. Diagnosis is usually by cytologic testing of fine-needle aspirate. Thyroid suppression is the preferred treatment during pregnancy for a benign lesion. For a papillary or follicular malignancy found in the first or second trimester, the woman is advised to have a thyroidectomy in the second trimester followed by thyroid suppression (Tewari, 2012). If a tumor is found in the third trimester, surgery can be delayed until after the birth. With other thyroid malignancies, treatment is individualized based on the wishes of the woman and her family (Tewari).

MEDICATION ALERT

Radioactive iodine is contraindicated in pregnancy and lactation.

Colon Cancer

The incidence of colon cancer in pregnancy is approximately 1 in 13,000 (Terwari, 2012). The signs and symptoms such as constipation, hemorrhoids, and backache are often attributed to pregnancy, resulting in diagnosis at a more advanced stage. Colonoscopy and biopsy are usually not done in pregnancy because these procedures can cause placental abruption and fetal injury from maternal hypoxia or hypotension.

Management of the cancer is based on the weeks of gestation and tumor stage. In a woman who is less than 20 weeks of gestation, surgery may be performed to remove the tumor. If she is at more than 20 weeks, surgery may be delayed until after the birth. Chemotherapy and radiation are usually not used in pregnancy for colon cancer but may be used after the birth (Salani et al., 2012; Terwari, 2012).

Cancer Therapy and Pregnancy

Decisions about the type and timing of therapy for cancer in the pregnant woman evoke moral and philosophic dilemmas, as well as complex medical judgments and intense emotional responses.

Ethical Considerations. When a pregnant woman has cancer and her survival is contingent on treatment that will harm the fetus, the health care team must work with the woman and her significant others to make decisions about how to proceed with her care. If a one-client model of ethical decision making is used, the risk-benefit analysis is applied to the maternal-fetal unit. The pregnant woman decides what is best for her and the fetus. The woman may accept or refuse treatment. If a two-client model is used for decision making, more weight is given to fetal well-being, but the pregnant woman cannot be forced to accept harm to herself for the sake of the fetus. Thus she could elect to accept treatment.

The fetus is at risk with either chemotherapy or radiation therapy. The effect of cancer therapy on the fetus can include death, miscarriage, teratogenesis, alteration in growth and development, alterations in function, and genetic mutation. The long-term effects on the fetus are unknown. These theoretic dangers must be weighed against the potential detrimental effects to the mother if treatment is withheld (Gilbert, 2011).

Timing of Therapy. Timing of therapy is an important issue to discuss. Because most cancer therapy (except surgery) is geared toward having a differential and noxious effect on rapidly growing tissue, the fetus is most at risk during the first trimester, when organogenesis and rapid tissue growth occur. Surgery offers the least potential risk to the fetus; however, the risk of miscarriage and preterm labor may be increased. Surgery is usually scheduled in the second trimester and has been discussed in the previous sections on gynecologic cancers in nonpregnant women.

Chemotherapy is avoided in the first trimester if at all possible. Although use of most chemotherapeutic agents has had isolated reports of fetal abnormalities, data on the agents used after the first trimester have recorded surprisingly few fetal abnormalities. The placenta may act as a barrier against the chemotherapeutic agents; therefore, although risk still exists, the judicious use of chemotherapy after the first trimester can result in live births with few congenital abnormalities. Acute drug toxicities may occur if treatment has occurred just before birth. Breastfeeding by women who are taking chemotherapeutic drugs is not recommended because most of these drugs may be excreted in breast milk (Salani et al., 2012; Terwari, 2012).

Radiation therapy presents its own set of issues. During embryonic development, tissues are extremely radiosensitive. If cells are genetically altered or killed during this time, the child either fails to survive or has specific organ damage. From a radiologic stance, there are three significant periods in embryonic development (Tewari, 2012):

1. Preimplantation: If irradiation does not destroy the fertilized egg, it probably does not affect it significantly.
2. Critical period of organogenesis: During this period, especially between days 18 and 38, the organism is most vulnerable; microcephaly, anencephaly, eye damage, growth restriction, spina bifida, and foot damage may occur.
3. After day 40: Large doses may still cause observable malformation and damage to the central nervous system.

Radiation therapy should be delayed until the postpartum period if possible (Salani et al., 2012).

Pregnancy After Cancer Treatment. If cancer therapy has not included the removal of the uterus, ovaries, or uterine (fallopian) tubes, there is a possibility that the woman may still be able to become pregnant. Although her menstrual cycle may have resumed, pregnancy may be difficult to achieve. Therapy that has affected the pituitary or thyroid gland may make conception difficult. Radiation appears to have the most deleterious effects on the endocrine system. The use of chemotherapy may result in temporary or permanent sterility, depending on the drug, the dose, and the length of time since the therapy was completed. Rates of ovarian failure are increased with pelvic irradiation (Tewari, 2012).

Of growing concern is the increase in the number of childhood and adolescent cancer survivors. Long-term effects of therapy on fertility, including incidence of congenital anomalies, are not well known. Counseling issues to be discussed with the pregnant woman after cancer treatment include the risk of recurrence and the likely sites of recurrence, how the prior cancer treatment can affect fertility or reproductive outcome, and if a future pregnancy will adversely affect a tumor that is estrogen-receptor positive (Salani et al., 2012).

For recovery from the disease and treatment to be complete, a delay of at least 2 years from the end of therapy to conception often is advised (Tewari, 2012). Before conception, a woman who has had cancer should have a complete physical examination to rule out complications that may place her or a fetus in jeopardy. Cardiac, pulmonary, hematologic, neurologic, renal, or gonadal function can be impaired. The woman and the potential father (if partnered) may be referred for reproductive and genetic counseling as well.

Gestational Trophoblastic Neoplasia

Gestational trophoblastic disease (GTD) encompasses a spectrum of disorders arising from the placental trophoblast. It includes hydatidiform mole (see Chapter 28), invasive mole, and choriocarcinoma. *Gestational trophoblastic neoplasia (GTN)* refers to persistent trophoblastic tissue that is presumed to be malignant (Ko & Soper, 2012).

Table 11-2 describes the clinical classifications of GTN. For several reasons, GTN is recognized as the most curable gynecologic malignancy. There is a sensitive marker produced by the tumor (hCG); the tumor is extremely sensitive to various chemotherapeutic agents; high risk factors in the disease process can be identified, allowing individualized therapy; and the aggressive use of multiple treatment methods is possible.

Malignant disease follows normal pregnancy in about 25% of cases and hydatidiform mole in about 50% of cases. Miscarriage or ectopic pregnancy or another gestational event precedes about 25% of cases (Ko & Soper, 2012). Metastasis occurs most often in the lungs, vagina, liver, and brain.

Continued bleeding after evacuation of a hydatidiform mole is usually the most suggestive symptom of GTN. Other clinical signs include abdominal pain and uterine and ovarian enlargement. Signs of metastasis include pulmonary symptoms (e.g., dyspnea, cough). The diagnosis is usually confirmed by increasing or plateauing hCG levels after evacuation of a molar pregnancy. Once diagnosis is confirmed, other clinical studies (e.g., CT scan of lungs and brain, chest x-ray, pelvic ultrasound, and liver scan) can determine the extent of the disease (Ko & Soper, 2012).

For women who wish to preserve their fertility and who have low risk nonmetastatic or low risk metastatic GTN, single-agent chemotherapy is chosen. Methotrexate has been the treatment of choice for years. High-dose methotrexate followed by folinic

TABLE 11-2 Clinical Classification for Women with Malignant GTN

CLASSIFICATION	CRITERIA
Nonmetastatic disease	No evidence of disease outside uterus
Metastatic disease	Any disease outside uterus
Good prognosis metastatic disease	Short duration (<4 months) Low pretreatment hCG titer <40,000 milli-International Units/ml No prior term pregnancy No metastasis to brain or liver No prior chemotherapy
Poor prognosis metastatic disease	Any one risk factor: Long duration (>4 months) High pretreatment hCG titer >40,000 milli-International Units/ml Brain or liver metastasis Prior term pregnancy Prior chemotherapy

GTN, Gestational trophoblastic neoplasia; *hCG,* human chorionic gonadotropin.
From Ko, E.M., & Soper, J.T. (2012). Gestational trophoblastic disease. In P.J. DiSaia, W.T. Creasman, R.S. Mannel, & D.S. Mutch (Eds.), *Clinical gynecologic oncology* (8th ed.). Philadelphia: Saunders.

acid rescue within 24 hours also has shown excellent results and causes fewer toxic effects (Ko & Soper, 2012). Dactinomycin has been used with equally good results and is used for women with liver or renal disease, both of which are contraindications for methotrexate. Hysterectomy with adjuvant chemotherapy is often the choice of treatment for nonmetastatic tumors in women who have completed their childbearing (Ko & Soper).

Women who have metastasis are classified as having either a good or poor prognosis, depending on the absence or presence of brain or liver metastasis, unsuccessful prior chemotherapy, symptoms lasting longer than 4 months, and serum β-hCG levels greater than 40,000 milli-International Units/ml. Treatment progresses from single-agent chemotherapy in the good-prognosis metastatic GTN to multiple-agent chemotherapy and multiple methods of treatment for the poor-prognosis group. Cure rates for the good-prognosis group are almost as positive as for those with nonmetastatic disease, both approaching 100% (Ko & Soper, 2012).

Therapy is continued until negative hCG levels are obtained. After successful chemotherapy follow-up by serum hCG levels varies. One schedule is to obtain levels every 2 weeks for 3 months, every month for up to a year after completing therapy, and every 6 to 12 months up to 3 to 5 years (Ko & Soper, 2012; McGee & Covens, 2012). Physical examinations are done at least yearly as are chest x-rays if indicated. Contraception is needed until the woman has been in remission for 6 months to 1 year. Oral contraceptives are preferred, but barrier methods are acceptable if oral contraceptives are contraindicated (Ko & Soper; McGee & Covens). During a subsequent pregnancy, pelvic ultrasonography is recommended because the woman is at higher risk (1% to 2%) to develop another molar pregnancy. Serum hCG levels should be obtained 6 weeks after the birth (McGee & Covens).

KEY POINTS

- Gynecologic disorders diminish the quality of life for affected women and their families.
- Structural disorders of the uterus and vagina related to pelvic relaxation and urinary incontinence can be a delayed result of childbearing, but they can be seen in young or childless women.
- Bladder training and pelvic muscle exercises can significantly decrease or relieve mild to moderate urinary incontinence.
- The development of neoplasms, whether benign or malignant, can have a significant physical and emotional effect on a woman and her family.
- Abnormal uterine bleeding is the most common symptom of leiomyomas or fibroid tumors.
- Various alternatives to hysterectomy exist for structural and benign disorders of the uterus; women need to be informed about the risks and benefits to make an informed decision about treatment.
- Endometrial cancer is the most common reproductive system malignancy.
- Hysterectomy is the usual treatment for early-stage endometrial cancer.
- Human papillomavirus infection is the primary cause of cervical cancer and is linked to vulvar cancer in women younger than 50 years.
- The squamocolumnar junction is an important landmark identified with neoplastic changes of the cervix.
- Preinvasive cancer of the cervix may be treated with techniques such as electrosurgical excision, cryotherapy, and laser therapy to save the structure of the cervix, particularly in women who desire to retain childbearing ability.
- External and internal radiation therapy in combination is as successful as surgery in treating early stages of cancer of the cervix.
- A Pap test can detect approximately 90% of early cervical dysplasias.
- Cancer of the ovary causes more deaths than any other female genital tract cancer.
- Nurses can control their exposure to radiation by increasing the distance from the radiation source, by limiting the time of exposure, and by using lead shielding.
- Cancer is relatively infrequent during pregnancy, occurring about once in every 1000 pregnancies.
- Radiation or chemotherapy treatment of a pregnant woman who has cancer places the fetus at risk for death, miscarriage, teratogenesis, and alterations in growth and development.
- Gestational trophoblastic neoplasms are highly curable but require close monitoring of hCG levels after treatment.

REFERENCES

American Cancer Society (ACS). (2014a). *Cancer facts and figures 2014*. Atlanta: Author.

American Cancer Society (ACS). (2014b). Vulvar cancer. Available at www.cancer.org.

Benson, S., Hahn, S., Tan, S., et al. (2010). Maladaptive coping with illness; women with polycystic ovary syndrome. *Journal of Obstetric, Gynecologic and Neonatal Nursing, 39*(1), 37–45.

Bidus, M. A., Maxwell, G. L., & Rose, G. S. (2012). Fallopian tube cancer. In P. J. DiSaia, W. T. Creasman, R. S. Mannel, & D. S. Mutch (Eds.), *Clinical gynecologic oncology* (8th ed.). Philadelphia: Saunders.

Bodurka, D. C., & Frumovitz, M. (2012). Malignant diseases of the vagina. Intraepithelial neoplasia, carcinoma, sarcoma. In V. Katz, G. Lentz, R. Lobo, & D. Gershenson (Eds.), *Comprehensive gynecology* (5th ed.). Philadelphia: Mosby.

Bugge, C., Adams, E. J., Gopinath, D., & Reid, F. (2013). Pessaries (mechanical devices) for pelvic organ prolapsed in women. *The Cochrane Database of Systematic Reviews, 2013*, 2, CD004010.

Chu, C., & Rubin, S. (2012). Basic principles of chemotherapy. In P. J. DiSaia, W. T. Creasman, R. S. Mannel, & D. S. Mutch (Eds.), *Clinical gynecologic oncology* (8th ed). Philadelphia: Saunders.

Coleman, L., & Lentz, R. (2012). Infections of the lower and upper genital tract: Vulva, vagina, cervix, toxic shock syndrome, HIV infections. In G. Lentz, R. Lobo, D. Gershenson, & V. Katz (Eds.), *Comprehensive gynecology* (6th ed.). Philadelphia: Mosby.

Coleman, R., Ramirez, P., & Gershenson, D. (2012). Neoplastic diseases of the ovary. Screening, benign and malignant epithelial cell neoplasms, sex-cord stromal tumors. In G. Lentz, R. Lobo, D. Gershenson, & V. Katz (Eds.), *Comprehensive gynecology* (6th ed.). Philadelphia: Mosby.

Creasman, W. (2012). Preinvasive disease of the cervix. In P. J. DiSaia, W. T. Creasman, R. S. Mannel, & D. S. Mutch (Eds.), *Clinical gynecologic oncology* (8th ed.). Philadelphia: Saunders.

Creasman, W. T., & Miller, D. S. (2012). Adenocarcinoma of the uterus. In P. J. DiSaia, W. T. Creasman, R. S. Mannel, & D. S. Mutch (Eds.), *Clinical gynecologic oncology* (8th ed.). Philadelphia: Saunders.

Eckert, L. O., & Lentz, G. M. (2012). Infections of the lower and upper genital tracts. Vulva, vagina, cervix, toxic shock syndrome, endometritis, and salpingitis. In G. Lentz, R. Lobo, D. Gershenson, & V. Katz (Eds.), *Comprehensive gynecology* (6th ed.). Philadelphia: Mosby.

Eisenhauer, E. L., Salani, R., & Copeland, L. J. (2012). Epithelial ovarian cancer. In P. J. DiSaia, W. T. Creasman, R. S. Mannel, & D. S. Mutch (Eds.), *Clinical gynecologic oncology* (8th ed.). Philadelphia: Saunders.

Gilbert, E. (2011). *Manual of high risk pregnancy & delivery* (5th ed.). St. Louis: Mosby.

Guo, Y., Tian, X., & Wang, L. (2013). Laparoscopically assisted vaginal hysterectomy vs vaginal hysterectomy: Meta analysis. *Journal of Minimally Invasive Gynecology, 20*(10), 15–21.

Gupta, J. K., Sinha, A., Lumsden, M. A., & Hickey, M. (2012). Uterine artery embolization for symptomatic uterine fibroids. *The Cochrane Database of Systematic Reviews, 2012*, 5, CD005073.

Hay-Smith, J., Herderschee, R., Dumoulin, C., & Herbison, P. (2012). Comparison of approaches to pelvic floor muscle training for urinary incontinence in women: An abridged Cochrane systematic review. *European Journal of Rehabilitative Medicine, 48*(4), 689–705.

Hersh, L., & Salzman, B. (2013). Clinical management of urinary incontinence in women. *American Family Physician, 87*(9), 634–640.

Huang, G., & Coviello, A. (2012). Clinical update on screening, diagnosis, and management of metabolic disorders and cardiovascular risk factors associated with polycystic ovary syndrome. *Current Opinion in Endocrinology, Diabetes, and Obesity, 19*(6), 512–519.

Katz, V. (2012). Benign gynecologic lesions: Vulva, vagina, cervix, uterus, oviduct, ovary. In G. Lentz, R. Lobo, D. Gershenson, & V. Katz (Eds.), *Comprehensive gynecology* (6th ed.). Philadelphia: Mosby.

Kives, S., Lefebvre, G., Wolfman, W., et al.,. (2010). Supracervical hysterectomy. *Journal of Obstetrics and Gynaegology Canada, 32*(1), 62–68.

Ko, E. M., & Soper, J. T. (2012). Gestational trophoblastic disease. In P. J. DiSaia, W. T. Creasman, R. S. Mannel, & D. S. Mutch (Eds.), *Clinical gynecologic oncology* (8th ed.). Philadelphia: Saunders.

Lentz, G. (2012a). Anatomic defects of the abdominal wall and pelvic floor. In G. Lentz, R. Lobo, D. Gershenson, & V. Katz (Eds.), *Comprehensive gynecology* (6th ed.). Philadelphia: Mosby.

Lentz, G. (2012b). Urogynecology. In G. Lentz, R. Lobo, D. Gershenson, & V. Katz (Eds.), *Comprehensive gynecology* (6th ed.). Philadelphia: Mosby.

Likes, W., Russell, C., & Tillmanns, T. (2008). Women's experiences with vulvar intraepithelial neoplasia. *Journal of Obstetric, Gynecologic and Neonatal Nursing, 37*(6), 640–646.

Lobo, R. (2012). Hyperandrogenism: Physiology, etiology, differential diagnosis, management. In G. Lentz, R. Lobo, D. Gershenson, & V. Katz (Eds.), *Comprehensive gynecology* (6th ed.). Philadelphia: Mosby.

McGee, J., & Covens, A. (2012). Gestational trophoblastic disease: Hydatidiform mole, nonmetastatic and metastatic gestational trophoblastic tumor: Diagnosis and management. In G. Lentz, R. Lobo, D. Gershenson, & V. Katz (Eds.), *Comprehensive gynecology* (6th ed.). Philadelphia: Mosby.

Mitchell, E. S., & Woods, N. F. (2013). Correlates of urinary incontinence during the menopausal transition and early menopause: Observations from the Seattle Midlife Women's Health Study. *Climacteric, 16*(6), 653–662.

Moyer, V. A., & U.S. Preventive Services Task Force (2012). Screening for cervical cancer: U.S. Preventive Services Task Force recommendation statement. *Annals of Internal Medicine, 156*(12), 880–891.

Nelson, A., & Gambone, J. (2010). Congenital anomalies and benign conditions of the uterine corpus and cervix. In N. Hacker, J. Gambone, & C. Hobel (Eds.), *Hacker and Moore's essentials of obstetrics and gynecology* (5th ed.). Philadelphia: Saunders.

Noller, K. (2012). Intraepithelial neoplasia of the lower genital tract (cervix, vulva): Etiology, screening, diagnostic techniques, management. In G. Lentz, R. Lobo, D. Gershenson, & V. Katz (Eds.), *Comprehensive gynecology* (6th ed.). Philadelphia: Mosby.

Pauls, R. N. (2010). Impact of gynecological surgery on female sexual function. *International Journal of Impotence Research, 22*(2), 105–114.

Pisco, J., Bilhim, T., Duarte, M., & Santos, D. (2009). Management of uterine artery embolization for fibroids as an outpatient procedure. *Journal of Vascular and Interventional Radiology, 20*(6), 730–735.

Reed, B. D., Harlow, S. D., Sen, A., et al. (2012). Prevalence and demographic characteristics of vulvodynia in a population-based sample. *American Journal of Obstetrics and Gynecology, 206*(2), 170e1–170e9.

Sabry, M., & Al-Hendy, A. (2012). Innovative oral treatments of uterine leiomyomas. *Obstetrics and Gynecology International*, 943635 published online Feb 16, 2012.

Salani, R., Eisenhauer, E. L., & Copeland, L. J. (2012). Malignant disease and pregnancy. In S. G. Gabbe, J. R. Niebyl, J. L. Simpson, et al. (Eds.), *Obstetrics: Normal and problem pregnancies* (6th ed.). Philadelphia: Saunders.

Saslow, D., Solomon, D., Lawson, H. W., et al. (2012). American Cancer Society, American Society for Colposcopy and Cervical Pathology, and American Society for Clinical Pathology screening guidelines for the prevention and early detection of cervical cancer. *CA: A Cancer Journal for Clinicians, 62*(3), 147–172.

Schilder, J. M., & Stehman, F. B. (2012). Invasive cancer of the vulva. In P. J. DiSaia, W. T. Creasman, R. S. Mannel, & D. S. Mutch (Eds.), *Clinical gynecologic oncology* (8th ed.) Philadelphia: Saunders.

Slomovitz, B., & Coleman, R. (2012). Invasive cancer of the vagina and urethra. In P. J. DiSaia, W. T. Creasman, R. S. Mannel, & D. S. Mutch (Eds.), *Clinical gynecologic oncology* (8th ed.). Philadelphia: Saunders.

Soliman, P. T., & Lu, K. H. (2012). Neoplastic diseases of the uterus. Endometrial hyperplasia, endometrial carcinoma, sarcoma: Diagnosis and management. In G. Lentz, R. Lobo, D. Gershenson, & V. Katz (Eds.), *Comprehensive gynecology* (6th ed.). Philadelphia: Mosby.

Tarnay, C., & Bhatia, N. (2010). Genitourinary dysfunction: Pelvic organ prolapse, urinary incontinence, and infection. In N. Hacker, J. Gambone, & C. Hobel (Eds.), *Hacker and Moore's essentials of obstetrics and gynecology* (5th ed.). Philadelphia: Saunders.

Tewari, K. S. (2012). Cancer in pregnancy. In P. J. DiSaia, W. T. Creasman, R. S. Mannel, & D. S. Mutch (Eds.), *Clinical gynecologic oncology* (8th ed.). Philadelphia: Saunders.

Tewari, K. S., & Monk, B. J. (2012). Invasive cervical cancer. In P. J. DiSaia, W. T. Creasman, R. S. Mannel, & D. S. Mutch (Eds.), *Clinical gynecologic oncology* (8th ed.). Philadelphia: Saunders.

van der Kooij, S. M., Ankum, W. M., & Hehenkamp, W. J. (2012). Review of non-surgical/minimally invasive treatments for uterine fibroids. *Current Opinion in Obstetrics and Gynecology, 24*(6), 368–375.

Ventolini, G. (2011). Measuring treatment outcomes in women with vulvodynia. *Journal of Clinical Medicine Research, 3*(2), 59–64.

Workman, M. L. (2013). Care of patients with cancer. In D. D. Ignatavicius, & M. L. Workman (Eds.), *Medical-surgical nursing: Patient-centered collaborative care* (7th ed.). St. Louis: Saunders.

Wu, J., Hundley, A., Fulton, R., & Myers, E. (2009). Forecasting the prevalence of pelvic floor disorders in U.S. women: 2020 to 2050. *Obstetrics & Gynecology, 114*(6), 1278–1283.

Yashar, C. (2012). Basic principles of gynecologic radiotherapy. In P. J. DiSaia, W. T. Creasman, R. S. Mannel, & D. S. Mutch (Eds.), *Clinical gynecologic oncology* (8th ed.). Philadelphia: Saunders.

Yen, J., Chen, Y., Long, C., Chang, Y., Yen, C., & Ko, C. (2008). Risk factors for major depressive disorder and the psychological impact of hysterectomy: A prospective investigation. *Psychosomatics, 49*(2), 137–142.

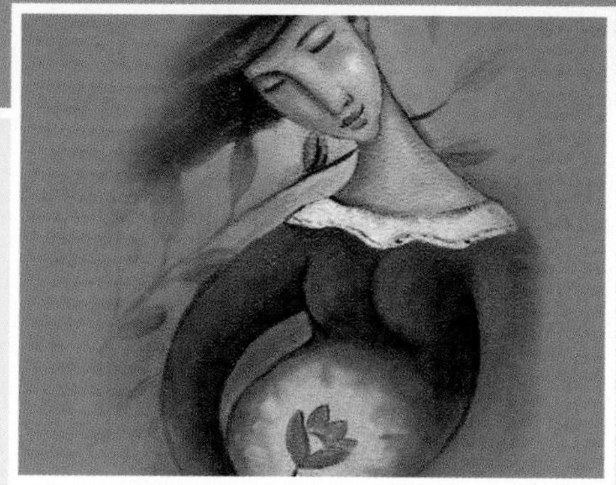

CHAPTER 12

Conception and Fetal Development

Shannon E. Perry

http://evolve.elsevier.com/Lowdermilk/MWHC/

LEARNING OBJECTIVES

- Summarize the process of fertilization.
- Describe the development, structure, and functions of the placenta.
- Describe the composition and functions of amniotic fluid.
- Identify three organs or tissues arising from each of the three primary germ layers.
- Summarize the significant changes in growth and development of the embryo and fetus.
- Analyze the potential effects of teratogens during vulnerable periods of embryonic and fetal development.
- Relate selected congenital defects to stage of fetal development.

This chapter presents an overview of the process of fertilization and the development of the normal embryo and fetus.

CONCEPTION

Conception, defined as the union of a single egg and sperm, marks the beginning of a pregnancy. Conception occurs not as an isolated event but as part of a sequential process, which includes gamete (egg and sperm) formation, ovulation (release of the egg), fertilization (union of the gametes), and implantation in the uterus. An explanation of cell division by mitosis and meiosis precedes discussion of gametogenesis.

Cell Division

Cells are reproduced by two different methods: mitosis and meiosis. In mitosis, body cells replicate to yield two cells with the same genetic makeup as the parent cell. First the cell makes a copy of its deoxyribonucleic acid (DNA), and then it divides. Each daughter cell receives one copy of the genetic material. Mitotic division facilitates growth and development or cell replacement.

Meiosis, the process by which germ cells divide and decrease their chromosomal number by half, produces gametes (eggs and sperm). Each homologous pair of chromosomes contains one chromosome received from the mother and one from the father; thus meiosis results in cells that contain one of each of the 23 pairs of chromosomes. Because these germ cells contain 23 single chromosomes, half of the genetic material of a normal somatic cell, they are called *haploid*. This halving of the genetic material is accomplished by replicating the DNA once and then dividing twice. When the female gamete (egg or ovum) and the male gamete (spermatozoon) unite to form the zygote, the diploid number of human chromosomes (46, or 23 pairs) is restored.

The process of DNA replication and cell division in meiosis allows different *alleles* (genes on corresponding loci that code for variations of the same trait) for genes to be distributed at random by each parent and then rearranged on the paired chromosomes. The chromosomes then separate and proceed to different gametes. Many combinations of genes are possible on each chromosome because parents have genotypes derived from four different grandparents. This random mixing of alleles accounts for the variation of traits seen in the offspring of the same two parents.

Gametogenesis

Oogenesis, the process of egg (ovum) formation, begins during fetal life in the female. All the cells that may undergo meiosis in a woman's lifetime are contained in her ovaries at birth. The majority of the estimated 2 million primary oocytes (the cells that undergo the first meiotic division) degenerate spontaneously. Only 400 to 500 ova will mature during the approximately 35 years of a woman's reproductive life. The primary oocytes begin the first meiotic division (i.e., they replicate their DNA) during fetal life but they remain suspended at this stage until puberty (Fig. 12-1, *A*). Then, usually monthly, one primary oocyte matures and completes the first meiotic division, yielding two unequal cells: the secondary oocyte and a small polar body. Both contain 22 autosomes and one X sex chromosome.

At ovulation the second meiotic division begins. However, the ovum does not complete the second meiotic division unless fertilization occurs. At fertilization, when the sperm is united with the mature ovum, a second polar body and the zygote (the united egg and sperm) are produced (see Fig. 12-1, *C*). The three polar bodies degenerate.

When a male reaches puberty, his testes begin the process of spermatogenesis. The cells that undergo meiosis in the male are called *spermatocytes*. The primary spermatocyte, which

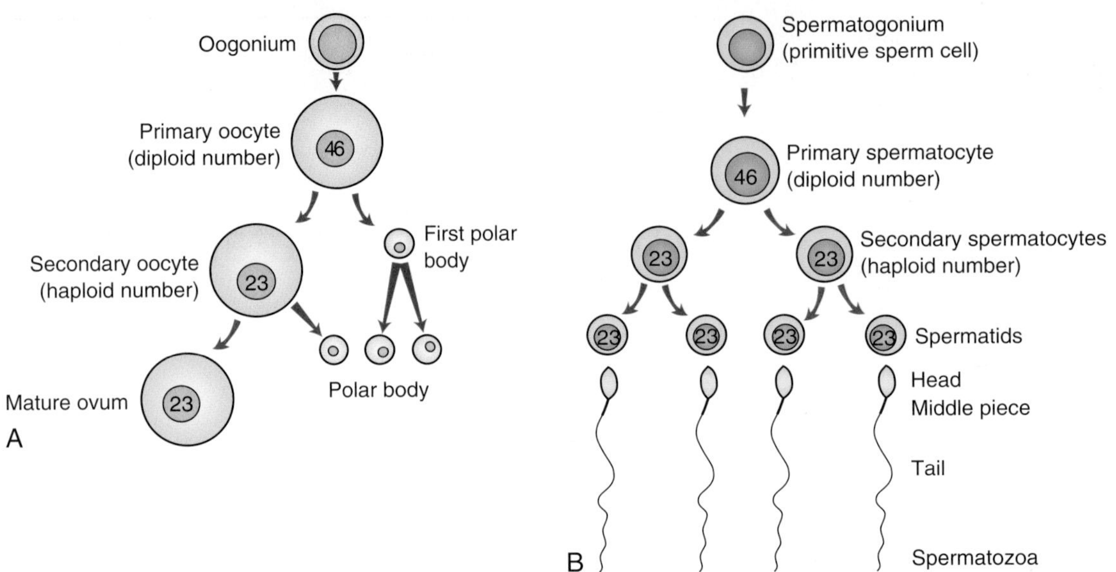

FIG 12-1 Gametogenesis. **A,** Oogenesis. Gametogenesis in the female produces one mature ovum and three polar bodies. Note the relative difference in overall size between the ovum and sperm. **B,** Spermatogenesis. Gametogenesis of the male produces four mature gametes, the sperm.

undergoes the first meiotic division, contains the diploid number of chromosomes. The cell has already copied its DNA before division, so four alleles for each gene are present. The cell is still considered diploid because the copies are bound together (i.e., one allele plus its copy on each chromosome).

During the first meiotic division two haploid secondary spermatocytes are formed. Each secondary spermatocyte contains 22 autosomes and one sex chromosome; one contains the X chromosome (plus its copy), and the other, the Y chromosome (plus its copy). During the second meiotic division the male produces two gametes with an X chromosome and two gametes with a Y chromosome, all of which will develop into viable sperm (see Fig. 12-1, *B*). When homologous chromosomes fail to separate during gametogenesis (nondisjunction), some gametes have 24 chromosomes and others have 22. If a gamete with 24 chromosomes unites with a normal gamete with 23 chromosomes, the resulting zygote has 47 chromosomes. This produces a trisomy as occurs in Down syndrome. When a gamete with 22 chromosomes unites with a normal gamete with 23 chromosomes, a zygote with 45 chromosomes results, producing a monosomy. Abnormal gametogenesis can occur in both sex chromosomes and in autosomes (Moore, Persaud, & Torchia, 2013). (See also Chapter 3.)

Ovum

Meiosis occurs in the female in the ovarian follicles and produces an egg, or ovum. Each month one ovum matures with a host of surrounding supportive cells. At ovulation the ovum is released from the ruptured ovarian follicle. High estrogen levels increase the motility of the uterine tubes so their cilia are able to capture the ovum and propel it through the tube toward the uterine cavity. An ovum cannot move by itself.

Two protective layers surround the ovum (Fig. 12-2). The inner layer is a thick, acellular layer, the *zona pellucida.* The outer layer, the *corona radiata,* is composed of elongated cells.

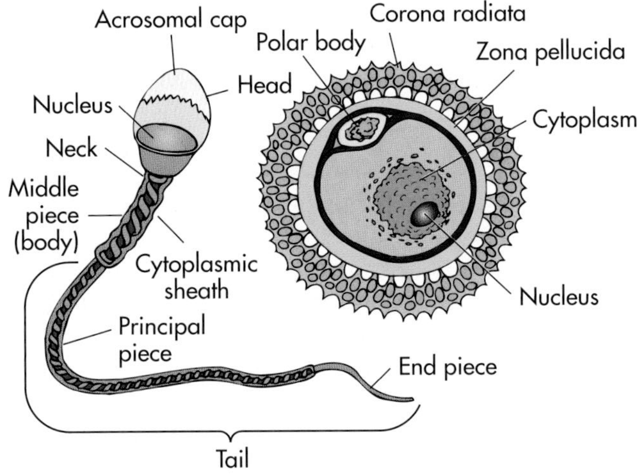

FIG 12-2 Sperm and ovum.

Ova are considered fertile for about 24 hours after ovulation. If not fertilized by a sperm, the ovum degenerates and is resorbed.

Sperm

Ejaculation during sexual intercourse normally propels about a teaspoon of semen containing as many as 200 to 500 million sperm, into the vagina. The sperm swim propelled by the flagellar movement of their tails. Some sperm can reach the site of fertilization within 5 minutes, but average transit time is 4 to 6 hours. Sperm remain viable within the woman's reproductive system for an average of 2 to 3 days. Most sperm are lost in the vagina, within the cervical mucus, or in the endometrium, or they enter the uterine tube that contains no ovum.

As the sperm travel through the female reproductive tract, enzymes are produced to aid in their capacitation. *Capacitation* is a physiologic change that removes the protective coating

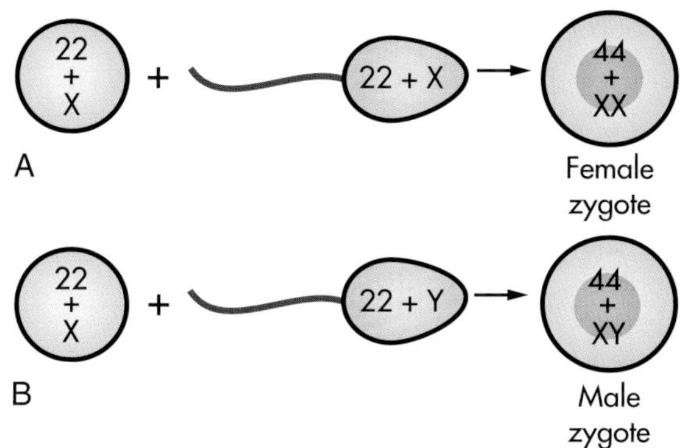

FIG 12-3 Fertilization. **A,** Ovum fertilized by X-bearing sperm to form female zygote. **B,** Ovum fertilized by Y-bearing sperm to form male zygote.

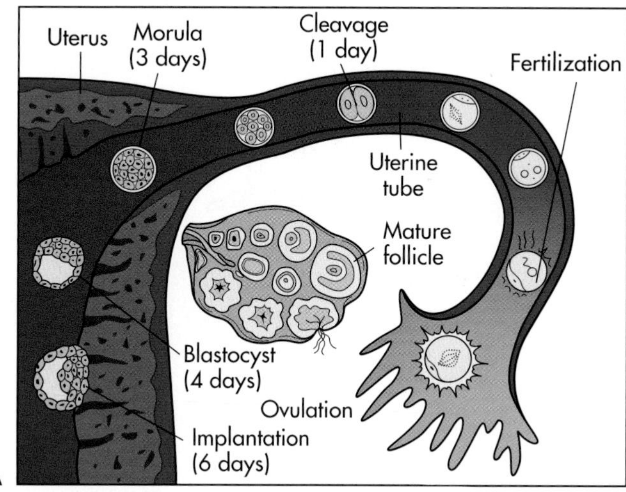

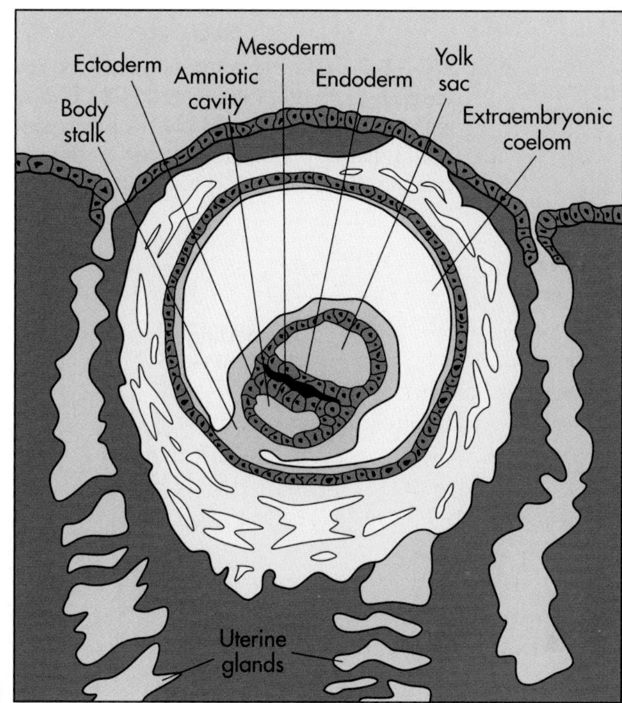

FIG 12-4 First weeks of human development. **A,** Follicular development in the ovary, ovulation, fertilization, and transport of the early embryo down the uterine tube and into the uterus, where implantation occurs. **B,** Blastocyst embedded in endometrium. Germ layers forming. (**A** from Carlson, B. [2004]. *Human embryology and developmental biology* (3rd ed.). Philadelphia: Mosby; **B** adapted from Langley, L. [1980]. *Dynamic anatomy and physiology* [5th ed.]. New York: McGraw-Hill.)

from the heads of the sperm. Small perforations then form in the acrosome (a cap on the sperm) and allow enzymes (e.g., hyaluronidase) to escape (see Fig. 12-2). These enzymes are necessary for the sperm to penetrate the protective layers of the ovum before fertilization.

Fertilization

Fertilization takes place in the ampulla (outer third) of the uterine tube. When a sperm successfully penetrates the membrane surrounding the ovum, both sperm and ovum are enclosed within the membrane, and the membrane becomes impenetrable to other sperm; this process is termed the *zona reaction.* The second meiotic division of the secondary oocyte is then completed, and the nucleus of the ovum becomes the female pronucleus. The head of the sperm enlarges to become the male pronucleus, and the tail degenerates. The nuclei fuse, and the chromosomes combine, restoring the diploid number (46) (Fig. 12-3). Conception, the formation of the zygote (the first cell of the new individual), has been achieved.

Mitotic cellular replication, called *cleavage,* begins as the zygote travels the length of the uterine tube into the uterus. This transit takes 3 to 4 days. Because the fertilized egg divides rapidly with no increase in size, successively smaller cells, blastomeres, are formed with each division. A 16-cell morula, a solid ball of cells, is produced within 3 days and is still surrounded by the protective zona pellucida (Fig. 12-4, *A*). Further development occurs as the morula floats freely within the uterus. Fluid passes through the zona pellucida into the intercellular spaces between the blastomeres, separating them into two parts, the trophoblast (which gives rise to the placenta) and the embryoblast (which gives rise to the embryo). A cavity forms within the cell mass as the spaces come together, forming a structure called the *blastocyst cavity.* When the cavity becomes recognizable, the whole structure of the developing embryo is known as the blastocyst. Stem cells are derived from the inner cell mass of the blastocyst. The outer layer of cells surrounding the blastocyst cavity is the trophoblast. The trophoblast differentiates into villous and extravillous trophoblast (Fig. 12-5).

Implantation

The zona pellucida degenerates, the trophoblast cells displace endometrial cells at the implantation site, and the blastocyst embeds in the endometrium, usually in the anterior or posterior fundal region. Between 6 and 10 days after conception, the trophoblast secretes enzymes that enable it to burrow into the endometrium until the entire blastocyst is covered. This is known as implantation. Endometrial blood vessels erode, and some women have slight implantation bleeding (slight spotting or bleeding at the time of the first missed menstrual period). Chorionic villi, finger-like projections, develop out of the trophoblast and extend into the blood-filled spaces of the endometrium. These villi are vascular processes that obtain oxygen and nutrients from the maternal bloodstream and dispose of carbon dioxide and waste products into the maternal blood.

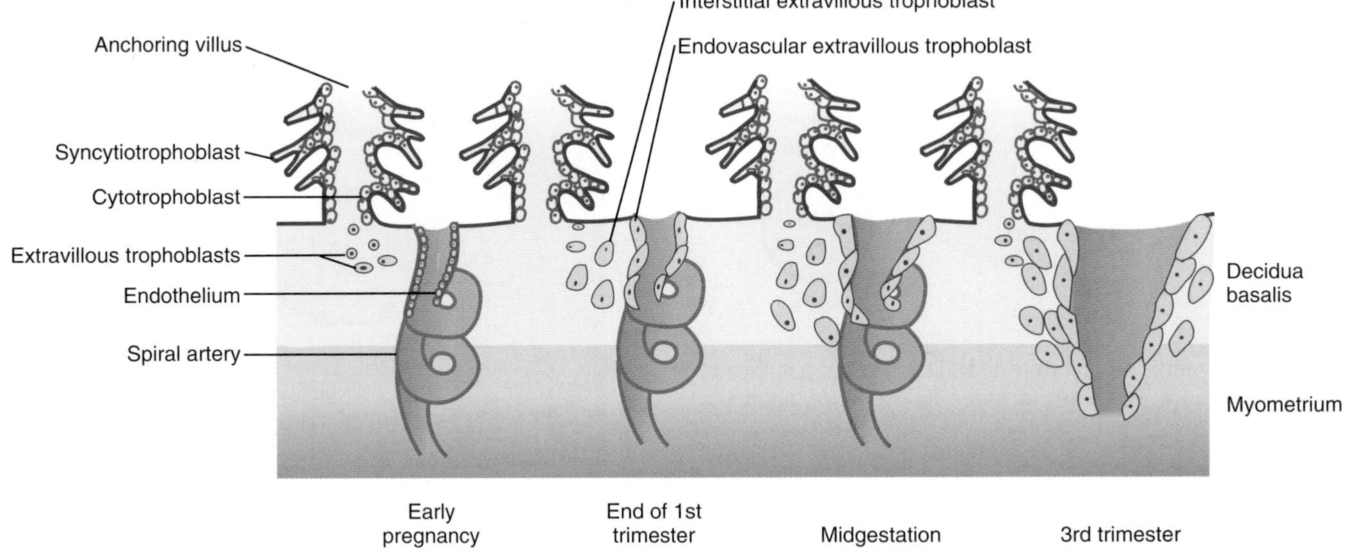

FIG 12-5 Extravillous trophoblasts are found outside the villus and can be subdivided into endovascular and interstitial categories. Endovascular trophoblasts invade and transform spiral arteries during pregnancy to create low-resistance blood flow that is characteristic of the placenta. Interstitial trophoblasts invade the decidua and surround spiral arteries. (From Cunningham, F., Leveno, K., Bloom, S., et al. [2014]. *Williams obstetrics* [24th ed.]. New York: McGraw-Hill.)

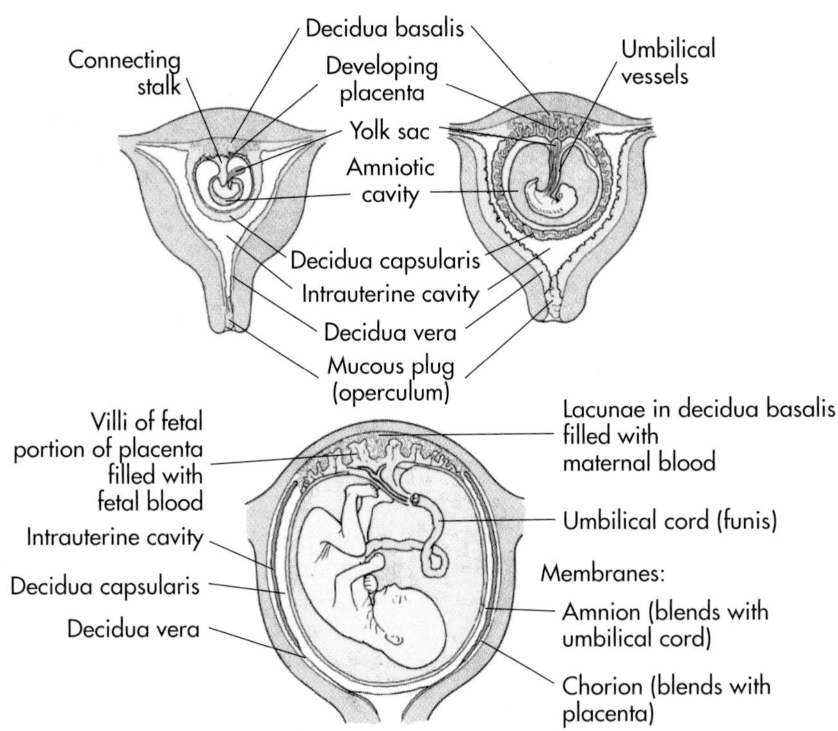

FIG 12-6 Development of the fetal membranes. Note gradual obliteration of intrauterine cavity as decidua capsularis and decidua vera meet. Also note thinning of uterine wall. Chorionic and amniotic membranes are in apposition to each other but may be peeled apart.

After implantation the endometrium is termed the *decidua.* The portion directly under the blastocyst, where the chorionic villi tap into the maternal blood vessels, is the **decidua basalis**. The portion covering the blastocyst is the *decidua capsularis,* and the portion lining the rest of the uterus is the *decidua vera* (Fig. 12-6).

EMBRYO AND FETUS

Pregnancy lasts approximately 10 lunar months, 9 calendar months, 40 weeks, or 280 days. Length of pregnancy is computed from the first day of the last menstrual period (LMP) until the day of birth. However, conception occurs approximately

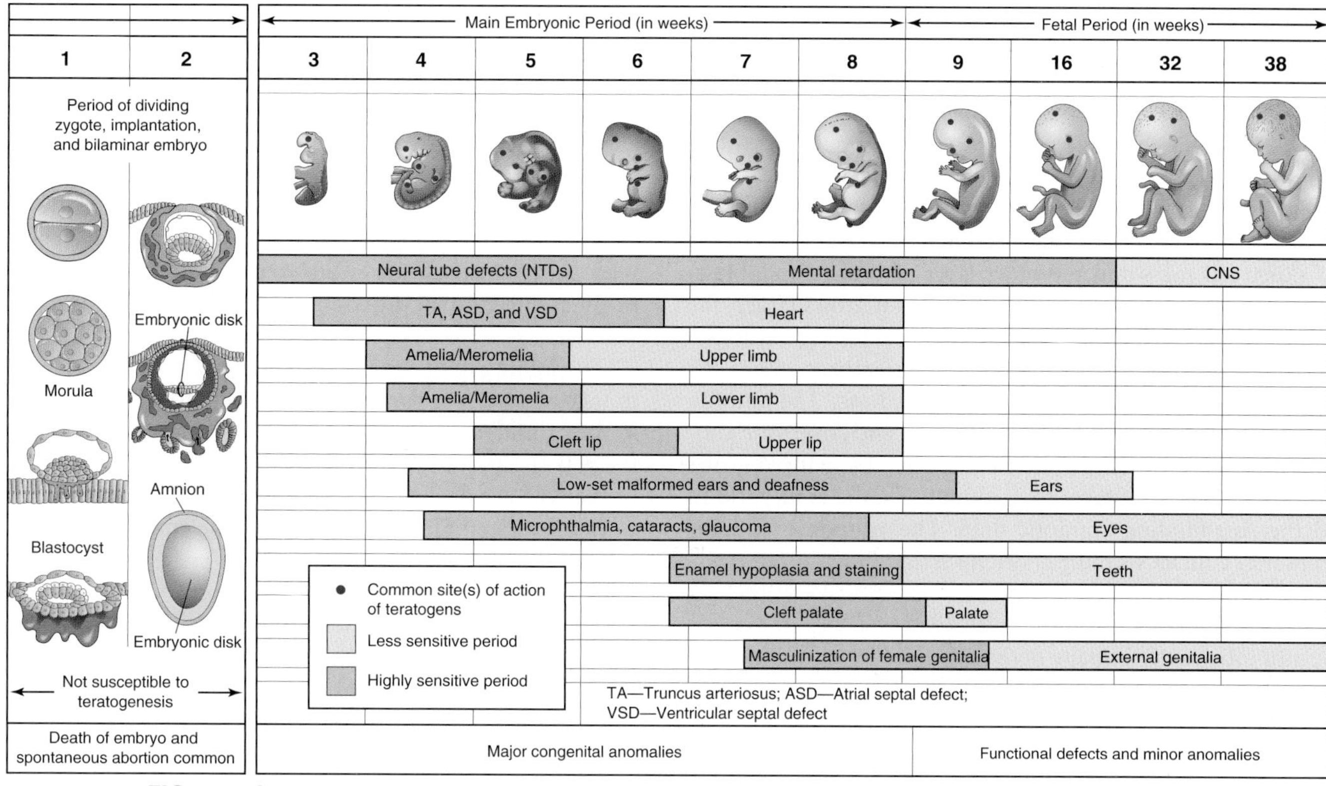

FIG 12-7 Sensitive or critical periods in human development. During the first 2 weeks of development the embryo usually is not susceptible to teratogens. After that time a teratogen damages all or most of the cells, resulting in death of the embryo, or damages only a few cells, allowing the conceptus to recover and the embryo to develop without birth defects. The dark color denotes highly sensitive periods; the light color indicates stages that are less sensitive to teratogens. (From Moore, K.L., Persaud, T.V.N., & Torchia, M.G. [2013]. *Before we are born: Essentials of embryology and birth defects* [8th ed.]. Philadelphia: Saunders.)

2 weeks after the first day of the LMP; thus the postconception age of the fetus is 2 weeks less, for a total of 266 days, or 38 weeks. Postconception age is used in the discussion of fetal development.

Intrauterine development is divided into three stages: ovum or preembryonic, embryo, and fetus (Fig. 12-7). The stage of the ovum lasts from conception until day 14. This period covers cellular replication, blastocyst formation, initial development of the embryonic membranes, and establishment of the primary germ layers.

Primary Germ Layers

During the third week after conception, the embryonic disk differentiates into three primary germ layers: the ectoderm, the mesoderm, and the endoderm (or entoderm) (see Fig. 12-4, *B*). All tissues and organs of the embryo develop from these three layers.

The upper layer of the embryonic disk, the *ectoderm,* gives rise to the epidermis, the glands (anterior pituitary, cutaneous, and mammary), the nails and hair, the central and peripheral nervous systems, the lens of the eye, the tooth enamel, and the floor of the amniotic cavity.

The middle layer, the *mesoderm,* develops into the bones and teeth, the muscles (skeletal, smooth, and cardiac), the dermis and connective tissue, the cardiovascular system and spleen, and the urogenital system.

The lower layer, the *endoderm,* gives rise to the epithelium lining the respiratory and digestive tracts, and the glandular cells of associated organs, including the oropharynx, the liver and pancreas, the urethra, the bladder, and the vagina. The endoderm forms the roof of the yolk sac.

Development of the Embryo

The stage of the embryo lasts from day 15 until approximately 8 weeks after conception, when the embryo measures 3 cm from crown to rump. This embryonic stage is the most critical time in the development of the organ systems and the main external features. Developing areas with rapid cell division are the most vulnerable to malformation caused by environmental teratogens (substances or exposure that causes abnormal development). At the end of the eighth week, all organ systems and external structures are present, and the embryo is unmistakably human (see Fig. 12-7 and Visible Embryo, www.visembryo.com/baby, for a pictorial view of normal and abnormal development).

Membranes

At the time of implantation, two fetal membranes that will surround the developing embryo begin to form. The chorion develops from the trophoblast and contains the chorionic villi on its surface. The villi burrow into the decidua basalis and increase in size and complexity as the vascular processes develop into the placenta. The chorion becomes the covering of the fetal side of the placenta. It contains the major umbilical blood vessels as they branch out over the surface of the placenta. As the embryo grows the decidua capsularis stretches. The chorionic villi on this side atrophy and degenerate, leaving a smooth chorionic membrane.

The inner cell membrane, the amnion, develops from the interior cells of the blastocyst. The cavity that develops between this inner cell mass and the outer layer of cells (trophoblast) is the amniotic cavity (see Fig. 12-4, *B*). As it grows larger, the amnion forms on the side opposite the developing blastocyst (see Figs. 12-4 and 12-6). The developing embryo draws the amnion around itself, forming a fluid-filled sac. The amnion becomes the covering of the umbilical cord and covers the chorion on the fetal surface of the placenta. As the embryo grows larger, the amnion enlarges to accommodate the embryo/fetus and the surrounding amniotic fluid. The amnion eventually comes into contact with the chorion surrounding the fetus.

Amniotic Fluid

The amniotic cavity initially derives its fluid by diffusion from the maternal blood. Fluid secreted by the respiratory and gastrointestinal tracts of the fetus also enters the amniotic cavity (Moore, Persaud, & Torchia, 2013). The amount of fluid increases weekly; 700 to 1000 ml of transparent liquid is normally present at term. The amniotic fluid volume changes constantly. The fetus swallows fluid, and fluid flows into and out of the fetal lungs. Beginning in week 11, the fetus urinates into the fluid, increasing its volume.

Amniotic fluid serves many functions. It helps maintain a constant body temperature. It serves as a source of oral fluid and a repository for waste and assists in maintenance of fluid and electrolyte homeostasis. It allows freedom of movement for musculoskeletal development. It cushions the fetus from trauma by blunting and dispersing outside forces. It acts as a barrier to infection and allows fetal lung development (Moore et al., 2013). The fluid keeps the embryo from tangling with the membranes, facilitating symmetric growth. If the embryo does become tangled with the membranes, amputations of extremities or other deformities can occur from constricting amniotic bands.

The volume of amniotic fluid is an important factor in assessing fetal well-being throughout pregnancy. Having less than 300 ml of amniotic fluid (oligohydramnios) is associated with fetal renal abnormalities. Having more than 2 L of amniotic fluid (hydramnios [polyhydramnios]) is associated with gastrointestinal and other malformations.

Amniotic fluid contains albumin, urea, uric acid, creatinine, lecithin, sphingomyelin, bilirubin, fructose, fat, leukocytes, proteins, epithelial cells, enzymes, and lanugo hair. Study of fetal cells in amniotic fluid through amniocentesis yields much information about the fetus. Genetic studies (karyotyping) provide knowledge about the sex and the number and structure of chromosomes (see Chapter 3). Other studies, such as the *lecithin/sphingomyelin* (L/S) ratio, determine the health or maturity of the fetus (see Chapters 26 and 35).

Yolk Sac

When the amniotic cavity and amnion are forming, another blastocyst cavity forms on the other side of the developing embryonic disk (see Fig. 12-4, *B*). This cavity becomes surrounded by a membrane, forming the *yolk sac*. The yolk sac aids in transferring maternal nutrients and oxygen, which have diffused through the chorion, to the embryo. Blood vessels form to aid transport. Blood cells and plasma are manufactured in the yolk sac during the second and third weeks while uteroplacental circulation is being established and is forming primitive blood cells until hematopoietic activity begins. At the end of the third week the primitive heart begins to beat and circulate the blood through the embryo, the connecting stalk, the chorion, and the yolk sac.

The folding in of the embryo during the fourth week results in incorporation of part of the yolk sac into the embryo's body as the primitive digestive system. Primordial germ cells arise in the yolk sac and move into the embryo. The shrinking remains of the yolk sac degenerate (see Fig. 12-6). By the fifth or sixth week the remnant has separated from the embryo.

Umbilical Cord

By day 14 after conception, the embryonic disk, the amniotic sac, and the yolk sac are attached to the chorionic villi by the connecting stalk. During the third week the blood vessels develop to supply the embryo with maternal nutrients and oxygen. During the fifth week the embryo has curved inward on itself from both ends, bringing the connecting stalk to the ventral side of the embryo. The connecting stalk becomes compressed from both sides by the amnion and forms the narrower umbilical cord (see Fig. 12-6). Two arteries carry blood from the embryo to the chorionic villi, and one vein returns blood to the embryo. Approximately 1% of umbilical cords contain only two vessels: one artery and one vein (Blackburn, 2012). This occurrence is sometimes associated with congenital malformations.

The cord rapidly increases in length. At term the cord is 2 cm in diameter and ranges from 30 to 90 cm long (with an average of 55 cm). It spirals on itself and loops around the embryo/fetus. A true knot is rare, but false knots occur as folds or kinks in the cord and can jeopardize circulation to the fetus. Connective tissue called *Wharton's jelly* prevents compression of the blood vessels and ensures continued nourishment of the embryo or fetus. Compression can occur if the cord lies between the fetal head and the maternal pelvis or is twisted around the fetal body. When the cord is wrapped around the fetal neck, it is called a nuchal cord.

Because the placenta develops from the chorionic villi, the umbilical cord is usually located centrally. A peripheral location is less common and is termed *battledore placenta.* The blood vessels are arrayed out from the center to all parts of the placenta.

Placenta

Structure

The placenta begins to form at implantation. During the third week after conception the trophoblast cells of the chorionic villi continue to invade the decidua basalis. As the uterine capillaries are tapped, the endometrial spiral arteries fill with maternal blood. The chorionic villi grow into the spaces with two layers of cells: the outer syncytium and the inner cytotrophoblast. A third layer develops into anchoring septa, dividing the projecting decidua into separate areas called cotyledons. In each of the 15 to 20 cotyledons, the chorionic villi branch out, and a

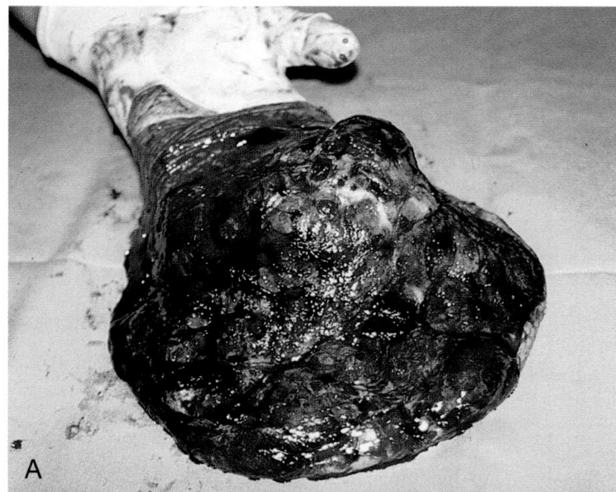

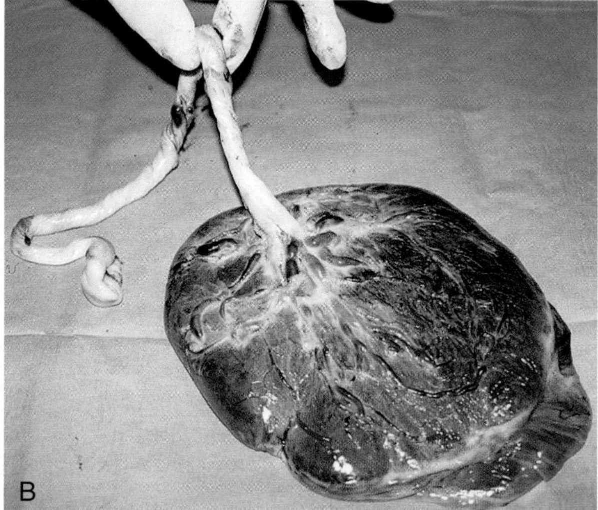

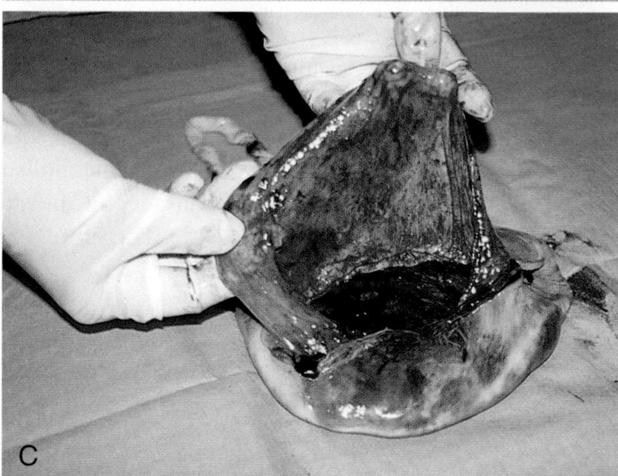

FIG 12-8 Term placenta. **A,** Maternal (or uterine) surface, showing cotyledons and grooves. **B,** Fetal (or amniotic) surface, showing blood vessels running under amnion and converging to form umbilical vessels at attachment of umbilical cord. **C,** Amnion and smooth chorion are arranged to show that they are (1) fused and (2) continuous with margins of placenta. (Courtesy Marjorie Pyle, RNC, Lifecircle, Costa Mesa, CA.)

complex system of fetal blood vessels forms. Each cotyledon is a functional unit. The whole structure is the placenta (Fig. 12-8).

The maternal-placental-embryonic circulation is in place by day 17, when the embryonic heart starts beating. By the end of the third week, embryonic blood is circulating between the embryo and the chorionic villi. In the intervillous spaces, maternal blood supplies oxygen and nutrients to the embryonic capillaries in the villi (Fig. 12-9). Waste products and carbon dioxide diffuse into the maternal blood.

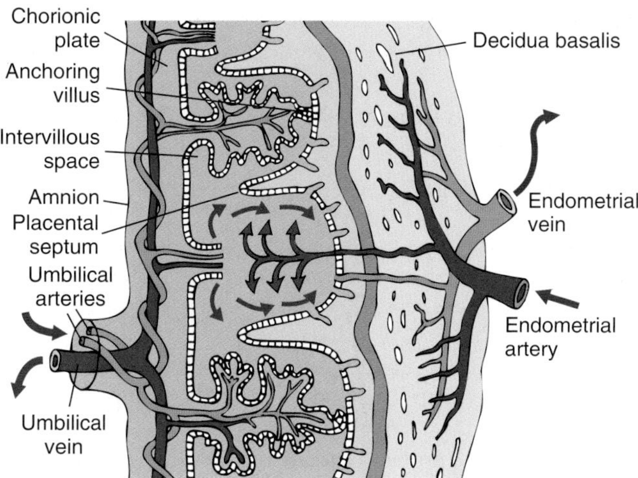

FIG 12-9 Schematic drawing of the placenta illustrating how it supplies oxygen and nutrition to the embryo and removes its waste products. Deoxygenated blood leaves the fetus through the umbilical arteries and enters the placenta, where it is oxygenated. Oxygenated blood leaves the placenta through the umbilical vein, which enters the fetus via the umbilical cord.

The placenta functions as a means of metabolic exchange. Exchange is minimal at this time because the two cell layers of the villous membrane are too thick. Permeability increases as the cytotrophoblast thins and disappears; by the fifth month, only the single layer of syncytium is left between the maternal blood and the fetal capillaries. The syncytium is the functional layer of the placenta. By the eighth week, genetic testing can be done on a sample of chorionic villi by aspiration biopsy; however, limb defects have been associated with chorionic villus sampling done before 10 weeks. The structure of the placenta is complete by the twelfth week. The placenta continues to grow wider until 20 weeks, when it covers about half of the uterine surface. It then continues to grow thicker. The branching villi continue to develop within the body of the placenta, increasing the functional surface area.

Functions

Endocrine gland function. One of the early functions of the placenta is as an endocrine gland that produces four hormones necessary to maintain the pregnancy and support the embryo and fetus. The hormones are produced in the syncytium.

The protein hormone human chorionic gonadotropin (hCG) can be detected in the maternal serum by 8 to 10 days after conception, shortly after implantation. This hormone is the basis for pregnancy tests. The hCG preserves the function of the ovarian corpus luteum, ensuring the continued supply of estrogen and progesterone needed to maintain the pregnancy. Miscarriage occurs if the corpus luteum stops functioning before the placenta is producing sufficient estrogen and progesterone. The hCG reaches its maximum level at 50 to 70 days and then begins to decrease.

The other protein hormone produced by the placenta is *human chorionic somatomammotropin* (hCS), formerly known

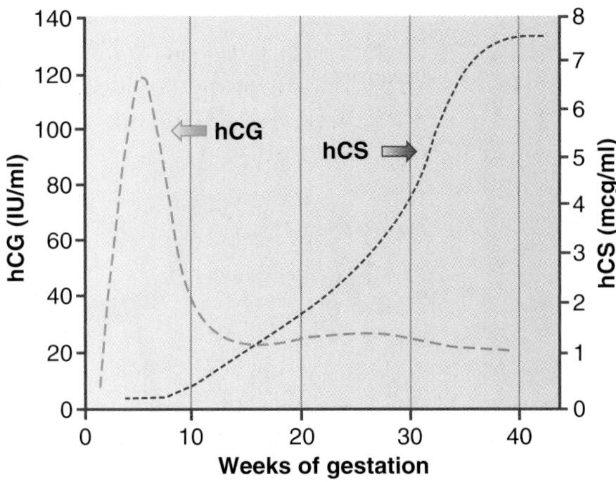

FIG 12-10 Distinct profile for the concentrations of human chorionic gonadotropin (hCG) and human chorionic somatomammotropin (hCS) in serum of women through normal pregnancy. *IU,* International Units. (Adapted from Cunningham, F., Leveno, K., Bloom, S., et al. [2014]. *Williams obstetrics* [24th ed.]. New York: McGraw-Hill.)

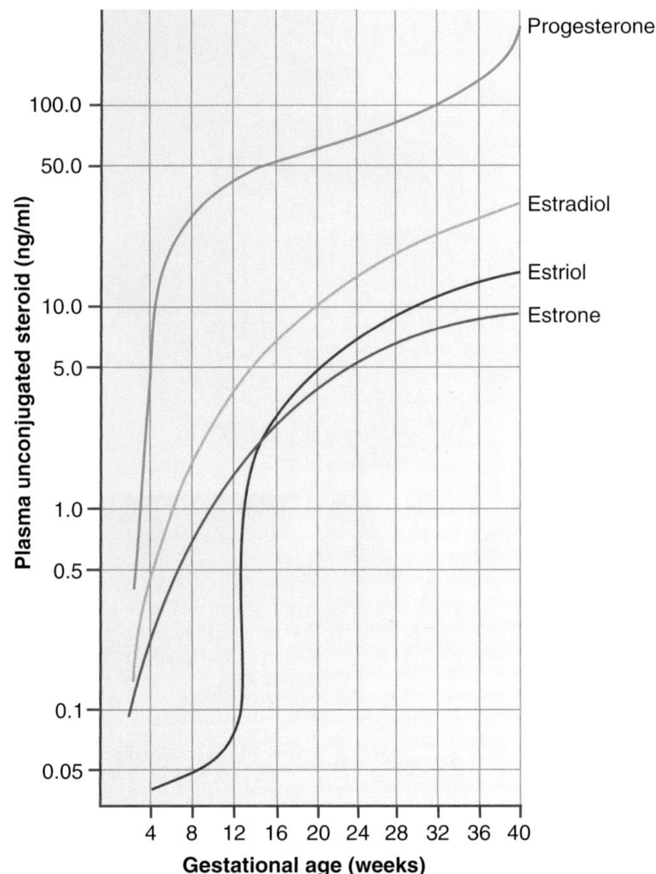

FIG 12-11 Plasma level of progesterone, estradiol, estrone, and estriol in women during the course of gestation. (From Cunningham, F., Leveno, K., Bloom, S., et al. [2014]. *Williams obstetrics* [24th ed.]. New York: McGraw-Hill.)

as human placental lactogen (hPL). This substance is similar to a growth hormone and stimulates the maternal metabolism to supply nutrients needed for fetal growth. hCS increases the resistance to insulin, facilitates glucose transport across the placental membrane, and stimulates breast development to prepare for lactation (Fig. 12-10).

The placenta eventually produces more of the steroid hormone *progesterone* than the corpus luteum does during the first few months of pregnancy. Progesterone maintains the endometrium, decreases the contractility of the uterus, and stimulates maternal metabolism and development of breast alveoli.

By 7 weeks after fertilization the placenta is producing most of the maternal estrogens, which are steroid hormones. The major estrogen secreted by the placenta is estriol, whereas the ovaries produce mostly estradiol. Estriol levels may be measured to determine placental functioning. Estrogen stimulates uterine growth and uteroplacental blood flow. It causes a proliferation of the breast glandular tissue and stimulates myometrial contractility. Placental estrogen production increases greatly toward the end of pregnancy. One theory for the cause of the onset of labor is the decline in the ratio of circulating levels of progesterone to the increased levels of estrogen (Fig. 12-11).

Metabolic functions. The metabolic functions of the placenta are respiration, nutrition, excretion, and storage. Oxygen diffuses from the maternal blood across the placental membrane into the fetal blood, and carbon dioxide diffuses in the opposite direction. In this way the placenta functions as lungs for the fetus.

Carbohydrates, proteins, calcium, and iron are stored in the placenta for ready access to meet fetal needs. Water, inorganic salts, carbohydrates, proteins, fats, and vitamins pass from the maternal blood supply across the placental membrane into the fetal blood, supplying nutrition. Water and most electrolytes with a molecular weight less than 500 readily diffuse through the membrane. Hydrostatic and osmotic pressures aid in the flow of water and some solutions. Facilitated and active transport assist in the transfer of glucose, amino acids, calcium, iron, and substances with higher molecular weights. Amino acids and calcium are transported against the concentration gradient between the maternal blood and fetal blood.

The fetal concentration of glucose is lower than the glucose level in the maternal blood because of its rapid metabolism by the fetus. This fetal requirement demands larger concentrations of glucose than simple diffusion can provide. Therefore, maternal glucose moves into the fetal circulation by active transport.

Pinocytosis is a mechanism used for transferring large molecules, such as albumin and gamma globulins, across the placental membrane. This mechanism conveys the maternal immunoglobulins that provide early passive immunity to the fetus.

Metabolic waste products of the fetus cross the placental membrane from the fetal blood into the maternal blood. The maternal kidneys then excrete them. Many viruses can cross the placental membrane and infect the fetus. Some bacteria and protozoa first infect the placenta and then the fetus. Drugs also can cross the placental membrane and may harm the fetus. Caffeine, alcohol, nicotine, carbon monoxide, and other toxic substances in cigarette smoke, as well as prescription and recreational drugs (such as cocaine and marijuana) readily cross the placenta (Box 12-1).

Although no direct link exists between the fetal blood in the vessels of the chorionic villi and the maternal blood in the intervillous spaces, only one cell layer separates the maternal and fetal blood. Breaks occasionally occur in the placental

BOX 12-1 Developmentally Toxic Exposures in Humans

- Aminopterin
- Androgens
- Angiotensin-converting enzyme inhibitors
- Carbamazepine
- Cigarette smoking
- Cocaine
- Coumarin anticoagulants
- Cytomegalovirus
- Diethylstilbestrol
- Ethanol (>1 drink/day)
- Etretinate
- Hyperthermia
- Iodides
- Ionizing radiation (>10 rad)
- Isotretinoin
- Lead
- Lithium
- Methimazole
- Methyl mercury
- Parvovirus B19
- Penicillamine
- Phenytoin
- Radioiodine
- Rubella
- Syphilis
- Tetracycline
- Thalidomide
- Toxoplasmosis
- Trimethadione
- Valproic acid
- Varicella

membrane. Fetal erythrocytes then leak into the maternal circulation, and the mother may develop antibodies to the fetal red blood cells (isoimmunized). This is often the way an Rh-negative mother becomes sensitized to the erythrocytes of her Rh-positive fetus. (See discussions of isoimmunization in Chapters 21 and 36.)

Although the placenta and the fetus are analogous to living tissue transplants, they are not destroyed by the host mother (Mor & Abrahams, 2013). Either the placental hormones suppress the immunologic response or the tissue evokes no response.

Adequate circulation necessary for placental function. Placental function depends on the maternal blood pressure supplying circulation. Maternal arterial blood, under pressure in the small uterine spiral arteries, spurts into the intervillous spaces (see Fig. 12-9). As long as rich arterial blood continues to be supplied, pressure is exerted on the blood already in the intervillous spaces, pushing it toward drainage by the low-pressure uterine veins. At term gestation, 10% of the maternal cardiac output goes to the uterus.

If there is interference with the circulation to the placenta, the placenta cannot supply the embryo or fetus. Vasoconstriction, such as that caused by hypertension and cocaine use, diminishes uterine blood flow. Decreased maternal blood pressure or cardiac output also diminishes uterine blood flow.

When a woman lies on her back with the pressure of the uterus compressing the vena cava, blood return to the right atrium is diminished (see discussion of supine hypotension in Chapter 19 and Fig. 19-5). Excessive maternal exercise that diverts blood to the muscles away from the uterus compromises placental circulation. Optimal circulation is achieved when the woman is lying at rest on her side. Decreased uterine circulation can lead to intrauterine growth restriction of the fetus and to infants who are small for gestational age.

Braxton Hicks contractions, painless contractions that occur intermittently after the first trimester, appear to enhance the movement of blood through the intervillous spaces, aiding placental circulation. Prolonged contractions or too-short intervals between contractions during labor, however, reduce blood flow to the placenta.

Fetal Maturation

The stage of the fetus lasts from 9 weeks (when the fetus becomes recognizable as a human being) until the pregnancy ends. Changes during the fetal period are not so dramatic, because refinement of structure and function is taking place. The fetus is less vulnerable to teratogens, except for those affecting functioning of the central nervous system.

Viability refers to the capability of the fetus to survive outside the uterus and is usually defined by fetal weight and pregnancy duration for statistical and legal purposes. A standard definition is 20 weeks gestation and birthweight of 350 g, 400 g, or 500 g, but this varies by state. Nurses must be aware of the laws in their states. With modern technology and advancements in maternal and neonatal care, infants who are 22 to 25 weeks of gestation are on the threshold of viability (Cunningham, Leveno, Bloom, et al., 2014). The limitations on survival outside the uterus when an infant is born at this early stage are based on central nervous system function and the oxygenation capability of the lungs.

Fetal Circulatory System

The cardiovascular system is the first organ system to function in the developing human. Blood vessel and blood cell formation begins in the third week and supplies the embryo with oxygen and nutrients from the mother. By the end of the third week the tubular heart begins to beat, and the primitive cardiovascular system links the embryo, connecting stalk, chorion, and yolk sac. During the fourth and fifth weeks the heart develops into a four-chambered organ. By the end of the embryonic stage the heart is developmentally complete.

The fetal lungs do not function for respiratory gas exchange, so a special circulatory pathway, the ductus arteriosus, bypasses the lungs. Oxygen-rich blood from the placenta flows rapidly through the umbilical vein into the fetal abdomen (Fig. 12-12). When the umbilical vein reaches the liver, it divides into two branches; one branch circulates some oxygenated blood through the liver. Most of the blood passes through the ductus venosus into the inferior vena cava. There it mixes with the deoxygenated blood from the fetal legs and abdomen on its way to the right atrium. Most of this blood passes straight through the right atrium and through the foramen ovale, an opening into the left atrium. There it mixes with the deoxygenated blood returning from the fetal lungs through the pulmonary veins.

The blood flows into the left ventricle and is squeezed out into the aorta, where the arteries supplying the heart, head, neck, and arms receive most of the oxygen-rich blood. This pattern of supplying the highest levels of oxygen and nutrients to the head, neck, and arms enhances the cephalocaudal (head-to-rump) development of the embryo/fetus. Deoxygenated blood returning from the head and arms enters the right atrium through the superior vena cava. This blood is directed downward into the right ventricle, where it is squeezed into the pulmonary artery. A small amount of blood circulates through the resistant lung tissue, but the majority follows the path with less resistance through the ductus arteriosus into the aorta, distal to the point of exit of the arteries supplying the head and arms with oxygenated blood. The oxygen-poor blood flows through the abdominal aorta into the internal iliac arteries, where the umbilical arteries direct most of it back through the umbilical cord to the placenta. There the blood gives up its wastes and carbon dioxide

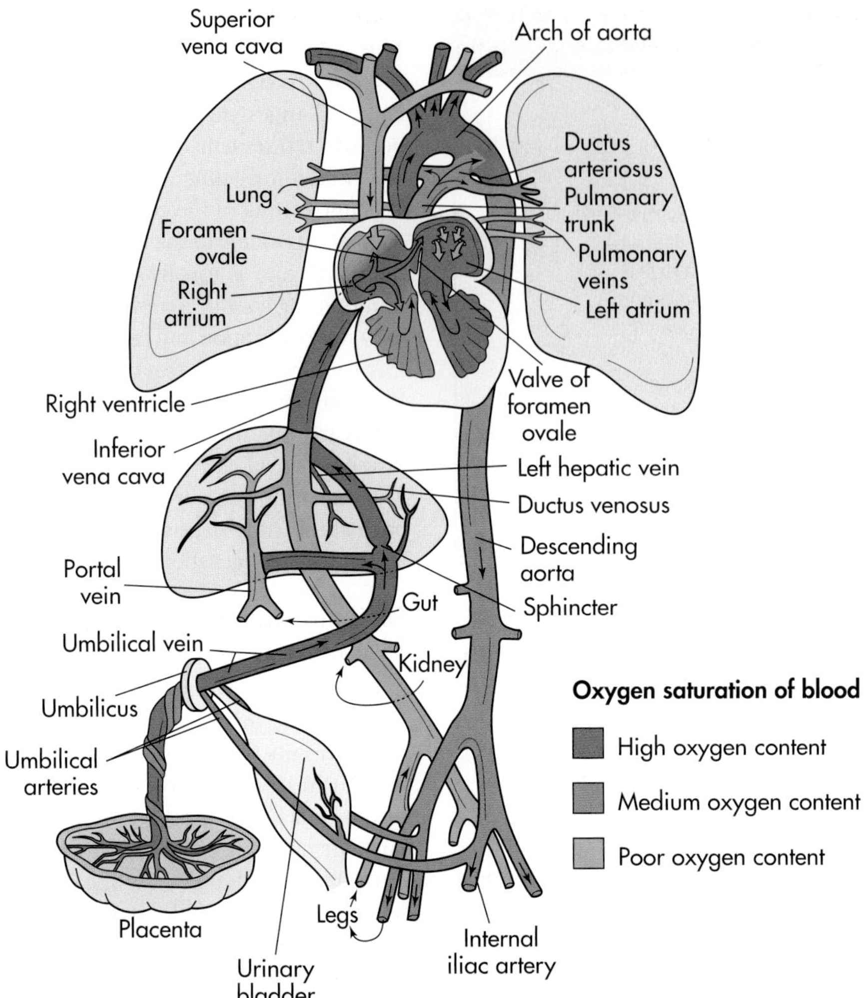

FIG 12-12 Schematic illustration of the fetal circulation. The colors indicate the oxygen saturation of the blood, and the arrows show the course of the blood from the placenta to the heart. The organs are not drawn to scale. Observe that three shunts permit most of the blood to bypass the liver and lungs: (1) ductus venosus, (2) foramen ovale, and (3) ductus arteriosus. A small amount of highly oxygenated blood from the inferior vena cava remains in the right atrium and mixes with poorly oxygenated blood from the superior vena cava. This medium oxygenated blood then passes into the right ventricle. The poorly oxygenated blood returns to the placenta for oxygen and nutrients through the umbilical arteries. (From Moore, K.L., Persaud, T.V.N., & Torchia, M.G. [2013]. *Before we are born: Essentials of embryology and birth defects* [8th ed.]. Philadelphia: Saunders).

in exchange for nutrients and oxygen. The blood remaining in the iliac arteries flows through the fetal abdomen and legs, ultimately returning through the inferior vena cava to the heart.

The following three special characteristics enable the fetus to obtain sufficient oxygen from the maternal blood:

- Fetal hemoglobin has a high affinity for oxygen and carries 20% to 30% more oxygen than maternal hemoglobin.
- The hemoglobin concentration of the fetus is about 50% greater than that of the mother.
- The fetal heart rate is 110 to 160 beats/minute, making the cardiac output per unit of body weight higher than that of an adult.

Hematopoietic System

Hematopoiesis, the formation of blood, occurs in the yolk sac (see Fig. 12-4, *B*) beginning in the third week. Hematopoietic stem cells seed the fetal liver during the fifth week, and hematopoiesis begins there during the sixth week. This accounts for the relatively large size of the liver between the seventh and ninth weeks. Stem cells seed the fetal bone marrow, spleen, thymus, and lymph nodes between weeks 8 and 11 (for more information about stem cells see http://stemcells.nih.gov).

The antigenic factors that determine blood type are present in the erythrocytes soon after the sixth week. For this reason the Rh-negative woman is at risk for isoimmunization in any pregnancy that lasts longer than 6 weeks after fertilization.

Respiratory System

The respiratory system begins development during embryonic life and continues through fetal stages and into childhood. The development of the respiratory tract begins in week 4 and continues through week 17 with formation of the larynx, trachea, bronchi, and lung buds. Between 16 and 24 weeks the bronchi and terminal bronchioles enlarge, and vascular structures and primitive alveoli are formed. Between 24 weeks and term more alveoli form. Specialized alveolar cells, type I and type II cells, secrete pulmonary surfactants to line the interior of the alveoli. After 32 weeks sufficient surfactant is present in developed alveoli to provide infants with a good chance of survival.

Pulmonary Surfactants. The detection of the presence of pulmonary surfactants, surface-active phospholipids, in amniotic fluid has been used to determine the degree of fetal lung maturity, or the ability of the lungs to function after birth. Lecithin (L) is the most critical alveolar surfactant required for postnatal lung expansion. It is detectable at approximately 21 weeks and increases in amount after week 24. Another pulmonary phospholipid, sphingomyelin (S), remains constant in amount. Thus the measure of lecithin in relation to sphingomyelin, or the L/S ratio, is used to determine fetal lung maturity. When the L/S ratio reaches 2:1, the infant's lungs are considered to be mature. This occurs approximately in the middle of the third trimester (Mercer, 2013).

Certain maternal conditions that cause decreased maternal placental blood flow, such as maternal hypertension, placental dysfunction, infection, or corticosteroid use, can accelerate fetal lung maturity. This apparently is caused by the resulting fetal hypoxia, which stresses the fetus and increases the blood levels of corticosteroids that accelerate alveolar and surfactant development.

Conditions such as gestational diabetes and chronic glomerulonephritis can inhibit fetal lung maturity. Using intrabronchial synthetic surfactant to treat respiratory distress syndrome in the newborn has greatly improved the chances of preterm infant survival.

Fetal respiratory movements have been seen on ultrasound examination as early as week 11. These fetal respiratory movements can aid in development of the chest wall muscles and regulate lung fluid volume. The fetal lungs produce fluid that expands the air spaces in the lungs. The fluid drains into the amniotic fluid or is swallowed by the fetus.

Shortly before birth, secretion of lung fluid decreases. The normal birth process squeezes out approximately one third of the fluid. Infants born by cesarean may have respiratory difficulty at birth, which is partially attributed to not having the benefit of this squeezing process (Ramachandrappa & Jain, 2008). The fluid remaining in the lungs at birth is usually reabsorbed into the infant's bloodstream within 2 hours of birth.

Gastrointestinal System

During the fourth week the shape of the embryo changes from being almost straight to a C shape, as both ends fold in toward the ventral surface. A portion of the yolk sac is incorporated into the body from head to tail as the primitive gut (digestive system).

The foregut produces the pharynx, part of the lower respiratory tract, the esophagus, the stomach, the first half of the duodenum, the liver, the pancreas, and the gallbladder. These structures evolve during the fifth and sixth weeks. The malformations that can occur in these areas are esophageal atresia, hypertrophic pyloric stenosis, duodenal stenosis or atresia, and biliary atresia (see Chapter 36).

The midgut becomes the distal half of the duodenum, the jejunum and the ileum, the cecum and the appendix, and the proximal half of the colon. The midgut loop projects into the umbilical cord between weeks 5 and 10. A malformation (omphalocele) results if the midgut fails to return to the abdominal cavity, causing the intestines to protrude from the umbilicus (see Fig. 36-8, *A*). Meckel diverticulum is the most common malformation of the midgut. It occurs when a remnant of the yolk stalk that failed to degenerate attaches to the ileum, leaving a blind sac.

The hindgut develops into the distal half of the colon, the rectum and parts of the anal canal, the urinary bladder, and the urethra. Anorectal malformations are the most common abnormalities of the digestive system.

The fetus swallows amniotic fluid beginning in the fifth month. Gastric emptying and intestinal peristalsis occur. Fetal nutrition and elimination needs are taken care of by the placenta. As the fetus nears term, fetal waste products accumulate in the intestines as dark green to black, tarry meconium. Normally this substance is passed through the rectum within 24 hours of birth. Sometimes with a breech presentation or fetal hypoxia, meconium is passed in utero into the amniotic fluid. The failure to pass meconium after birth can indicate atresia somewhere in the digestive tract, an imperforate anus (see Fig. 36-9), or meconium ileus, in which a firm meconium plug blocks passage (seen in infants with cystic fibrosis).

The metabolic rate of the fetus is relatively low, but the fetus has great growth and development needs. Beginning in week 9 the fetus synthesizes glycogen for storage in the liver. Between 26 and 30 weeks the fetus begins to lay down stores of brown fat in preparation for extrauterine cold stress. Thermoregulation in the neonate requires increased metabolism and adequate oxygenation.

The gastrointestinal system is mature by 36 weeks. Digestive enzymes (except pancreatic amylase and lipase) are present in sufficient quantity to facilitate digestion. The neonate cannot digest starches or fats efficiently. Little saliva is produced.

Hepatic System

The liver and biliary tract develop from the foregut during the fourth week of gestation. The embryonic liver is prominent, occupying most of the abdominal cavity. Bile, a constituent of meconium, begins to form in the twelfth week.

Glycogen is stored in the fetal liver beginning at week 9 or 10. At term, glycogen stores are twice those of the adult. Glycogen is the major source of energy for the fetus and neonate stressed by intrauterine hypoxia, extrauterine loss of the maternal glucose supply, the work of breathing, or cold.

Iron also is stored in the fetal liver. If the maternal intake is sufficient, the fetus can store enough iron to last for 5 months after birth.

During fetal life the liver does not have to conjugate bilirubin for excretion because the unconjugated bilirubin is cleared by the placenta. Therefore, the glucuronyl transferase enzyme needed for conjugation is present in the fetal liver in amounts less than those required after birth. This predisposes the neonate, especially the preterm infant, to hyperbilirubinemia.

Coagulation factors II, VII, IX, and X cannot be synthesized in the fetal liver because of the lack of vitamin K synthesis in the sterile fetal gut. This coagulation deficiency persists after birth for several days and is the rationale for the prophylactic administration of vitamin K to the newborn.

Renal System

The kidneys form during the fifth week and begin to function approximately 4 weeks later. Urine is excreted into the amniotic fluid and forms a major part of the amniotic fluid volume. Oligohydramnios is indicative of renal dysfunction. Because the placenta acts as the organ of excretion and maintains fetal water and electrolyte balance, the fetus does not need functioning kidneys while in utero. At birth, however, the kidneys are required immediately for excretory and acid-base regulatory functions.

A fetal renal malformation can be diagnosed in utero. Corrective or palliative fetal surgery may treat the malformation successfully, or plans can be made for treatment immediately after birth.

At term the fetus has fully developed kidneys. However, the glomerular filtration rate (GFR) is low, and the kidneys lack the ability to concentrate urine. This makes the newborn more susceptible to both overhydration and dehydration.

Most newborns void within 24 hours of birth. With the loss of the swallowed amniotic fluid and the metabolism of nutrients provided by the placenta, the amount voided for the first days of life is scanty until fluid intake increases.

Neurologic System

The nervous system originates from the ectoderm during the third week after fertilization. The open neural tube forms during the fourth week. It initially closes at what will be the junction of the brain and spinal cord, leaving both ends open. The embryo folds in on itself lengthwise at this time, forming a head fold in the neural tube at this junction. The cranial end of the neural tube closes, and then the caudal end closes. During week 5, different growth rates cause more flexures in the neural tube, delineating three brain areas: the forebrain, the midbrain, and the hindbrain.

The forebrain develops into the eyes (cranial nerve II) and the cerebral hemispheres. The development of all areas of the cerebral cortex continues throughout fetal life and into childhood. The olfactory system (cranial nerve I) and the thalamus also develop from the forebrain. Cranial nerves III and IV (oculomotor and trochlear) form from the midbrain. The hindbrain forms the medulla, the pons, the cerebellum, and the remainder of the cranial nerves. Brain waves can be recorded on an electroencephalogram by week 8.

The spinal cord develops from the long end of the neural tube. Another ectodermal structure, the neural crest, develops into the peripheral nervous system. By the eighth week nerve fibers traverse throughout the body. At term the fetal brain is approximately one fourth the size of an adult brain. Neurologic development continues. Stressors on the fetus and neonate (e.g., chronic poor nutrition or hypoxia, drugs, environmental toxins, trauma, disease) cause damage to the central nervous system long after the vulnerable embryonic time for malformations in other organ systems. Neurologic insult can result in cerebral palsy, neuromuscular impairment, intellectual disability, and learning disabilities.

Sensory Awareness. Purposeful movements of the fetus have been demonstrated in response to a firm touch transmitted through the mother's abdomen. Because the fetus can feel pressure and pain, anesthesia is required for invasive procedures.

Fetuses respond to sound by 24 weeks. Different types of music evoke different movements. The fetus can be soothed by the sound of the mother's voice. Acoustic stimulation can be used to evoke a fetal heart rate response. The fetus becomes accustomed (i.e., habituates) to noises heard repeatedly. Hearing is fully developed at birth.

The fetus is able to distinguish taste. By the fifth month, when the fetus is swallowing amniotic fluid, a sweetener added to the fluid causes the fetus to swallow faster. The fetus also reacts to temperature changes. A cold solution placed into the amniotic fluid can cause fetal hiccups.

The fetus can see. Eyes have both rods and cones in the retina by the seventh month. A bright light shone on the mother's abdomen in late pregnancy causes abrupt fetal movements. During sleep time, rapid eye movements have been observed similar to those occurring in children and adults while dreaming.

Endocrine System

The thyroid gland develops along with structures in the head and neck during the third and fourth weeks. The secretion of thyroxine begins during the eighth week. Maternal thyroxine does not readily cross the placenta; therefore, the fetus who does not produce thyroid hormones will be born with congenital hypothyroidism. If untreated, hypothyroidism can result in severe intellectual disability. Hypothyroidism is included in routine newborn screening after birth.

The adrenal cortex is formed during the sixth week and produces hormones by the eighth or ninth week. As term approaches, the fetus produces more cortisol. This is believed to aid in initiation of labor by decreasing the maternal progesterone and stimulating production of prostaglandins.

The pancreas forms from the foregut during the fifth through eighth weeks. The islets of Langerhans develop during the twelfth week. Insulin is produced by week 20. In fetuses of mothers with uncontrolled diabetes, maternal hyperglycemia produces fetal hyperglycemia, stimulating hyperinsulinemia and islet cell hyperplasia. This results in a macrosomic (large) fetus. The hyperinsulinemia also blocks lung maturation, placing the neonate at risk for respiratory distress (see Chapter 34) and hypoglycemia when the maternal glucose source is lost at birth (see Chapters 23 and 29). Control of the maternal glucose level before and during pregnancy minimizes problems for the fetus and infant.

Reproductive System

Sex differentiation begins in the embryo during the seventh week. Female and male external genitalia are indistinguishable until after the ninth week. Distinguishing characteristics of female and male genitalia appear around the ninth week and are fully differentiated by the twelfth week. When a Y chromosome is present, testes are formed. By the end of the embryonic period, testosterone is being secreted and causes formation of the male genitalia. By week 28 the testes begin descending into the scrotum. After birth low levels of testosterone continue to be secreted until the pubertal surge.

The female, with two X chromosomes, forms ovaries and female external genitalia. By the sixteenth week oogenesis has been established. At birth the ovaries contain the female's lifetime supply of ova. Most female hormone production is delayed until puberty. However, the fetal endometrium responds to maternal hormones, and withdrawal bleeding or vaginal discharge (*pseudomenstruation*) can occur at birth when these hormones are lost. The high level of maternal estrogen also stimulates mammary engorgement and secretion of fluid ("witch's milk") in newborn infants of both sexes.

CLINICAL REASONING CASE STUDY

Ultrasound Examination During Pregnancy

Veronica is 16 weeks pregnant. She has taken a folic acid supplement since 3 months before she became pregnant. On ultrasound a neural tube defect, myelomeningocele, was detected. Veronica is extremely upset and states that she took folic acid from before the time she was pregnant until now. She asks how this defect could have happened and what she should do about it. What information should the nurse provide Veronica?

1. Evidence—Is there sufficient evidence to draw conclusions about what information the nurse should provide Veronica?
2. Assumptions—What assumptions can be made about the following factors related to neural tube defects:
   a. Veronica's knowledge of folic acid and the cause of myelomeningocele
   b. Veronica's concern for her fetus
   c. Veronica's knowledge of myelomeningocele and its treatment
   d. Veronica's need for genetic counseling
3. What implications and priorities for nursing care can be made at this time?
4. Does the evidence objectively support your conclusion?

Musculoskeletal System

Bones and muscles develop from the mesoderm by the fourth week of embryonic development. At that time the cardiac muscle is already beating. The mesoderm next to the neural tube forms the vertebral column and ribs. The parts of the vertebral column grow toward each other to enclose the developing spinal cord. Ossification, or bone formation, begins. If there is a defect in the bony fusion, various forms of spina bifida can occur. A large defect affecting several vertebrae may allow the membranes and spinal cord to pouch out from the back, producing neurologic deficits and skeletal deformity.

The flat bones of the skull develop during the embryonic period, and ossification continues throughout childhood. At birth connective tissue sutures exist where the bones of the skull meet.

The areas where more than two bones meet (called *fontanels*) are especially prominent. The sutures and fontanels allow the bones of the skull to mold, or move during birth, enabling the head to pass through the birth canal (see Fig. 23-9).

The bones of the shoulders, arms, hips, and legs appear in the sixth week as a continuous skeleton with no joints. Differentiation occurs, producing separate bones and joints. Ossification continues through childhood to allow growth. Beginning in the seventh week, muscles contract spontaneously. By week 11 or 12 the fetus makes respiratory movements, moves all extremities, and changes position in utero. The fetus can suck his or her thumb and swim in the amniotic fluid pool, turn somersaults, and occasionally tie a knot in the umbilical cord. Arm and leg movements are visible on ultrasound examination, although the mother does not perceive them until sometime between 16 and 20 weeks.

Integumentary System

The epidermis begins as a single layer of cells derived from the ectoderm at 4 weeks. By the seventh week there are two layers of cells. The cells of the superficial layer are sloughed and become mixed with the sebaceous gland secretions to form the white, cheesy vernix caseosa, the material that protects the fetus's skin. The vernix is thick at 24 weeks but becomes scant by term.

The basal layer of the epidermis is the germinal layer, which replaces lost cells. Until 17 weeks the skin is thin and wrinkled, with blood vessels visible underneath. The skin thickens and all layers are present at term. After 32 weeks, as subcutaneous fat is deposited under the dermis, the skin becomes less wrinkled and red.

By 16 weeks the epidermal ridges are present on the palms of the hands, the fingers, the bottom of the feet, and the toes. Handprints and footprints are unique to each infant.

Hairs form from hair bulbs in the epidermis that project into the dermis. Cells in the hair bulb keratinize to form the hair shaft. As the cells at the base of the hair shaft proliferate, the hair grows to the surface of the epithelium. Very fine hairs, called lanugo, appear first at 12 weeks on the eyebrows and upper lip. By 20 weeks they cover the entire body. At this time the eyelashes, eyebrows, and scalp hair are beginning to grow. By 28 weeks the scalp hair is longer than the lanugo, which thins and may disappear by term gestation.

Fingernails and toenails develop from thickened epidermis at the tips of the digits beginning during the tenth week. They grow slowly. Fingernails usually reach the fingertips by 32 weeks, and toenails reach toe tips by 36 weeks.

Immunologic System

During the third trimester albumin and globulin are present in the fetus. The only immunoglobulin that crosses the placenta, immunoglobulin G (IgG), provides passive acquired immunity to specific bacterial toxins. The fetus produces IgM by the end of the first trimester. These are produced in response to blood group antigens, gram-negative enteric organisms, and some viruses. IgA is not produced by the fetus; however, colostrum, the precursor to breast milk, contains large amounts of IgA and can provide passive immunity to the neonate who is breastfed.

The normal-term neonate can fight infection but not so effectively as an older child. The preterm infant is at much greater risk for infection.

Table 12-1 summarizes embryonic and fetal development.

Multifetal Pregnancy

Twins

The incidence of twinning is 1 in 43 births. There has been a steady rise in multiple births since 1973 (Benirschke, 2013). This is partly attributed to the availability of assisted reproductive technologies and the increasing age at which women give birth as well as use of ovulation-enhancing drugs (Benirschke).

Dizygotic Twins. When two mature ova are produced in one ovarian cycle, both have the potential to be fertilized by separate sperm. This results in two zygotes, or dizygotic twins

(Fig. 12-13). There are always two amnions, two chorions, and two placentas, that may be fused (Fig. 12-14). These dizygotic, or fraternal, twins can be the same sex or different sexes and are genetically no more alike than siblings born at different times. Dizygotic twinning occurs in families, more often among African-American women than among Caucasian women and least often among Asian women. Dizygotic twinning increases in frequency with maternal age up to 35 years, with parity, and with the use of fertility drugs.

Monozygotic Twins. Identical, or monozygotic, twins develop from one fertilized ovum, which then divides (Fig. 12-15). They are the same sex and have the same genotype. If division occurs soon after fertilization, two embryos, two amnions, two chorions, and two placentas that can be fused will develop. Most often, division occurs between 4 and 8 days after fertilization, and there are two embryos, two amnions, one chorion, and one placenta. Rarely, division occurs after the eighth day after fertilization. In this case there are two embryos within a common amnion and a common chorion with one placenta. This often causes circulatory problems because the umbilical cords may tangle together, and one or both fetuses may die. Monozygotic twinning occurs approximately 3.5 to

TABLE 12-1 Milestones in Human Development Before Birth Since Last Menstrual Period

	4 WEEKS	8 WEEKS	12 WEEKS
External Appearance	Body flexed, C-shaped; arm and leg buds present; head at right angles to body 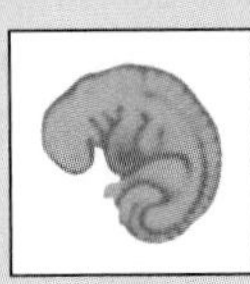	Body fairly well formed; nose flat, eyes far apart; digits well formed; head elevating; tail almost disappeared; eyes, ears, nose, and mouth recognizable 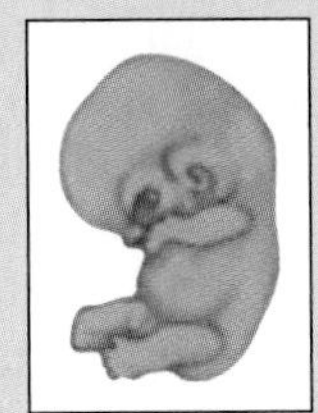 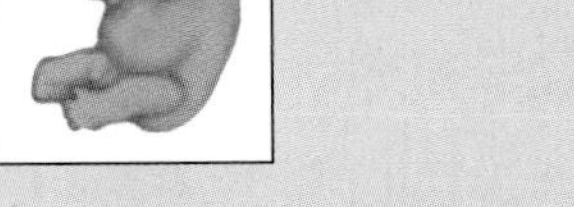	Nails appearing; resembles a human; head erect but disproportionately large; skin pink, delicate 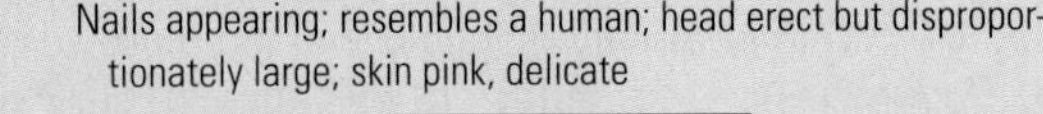 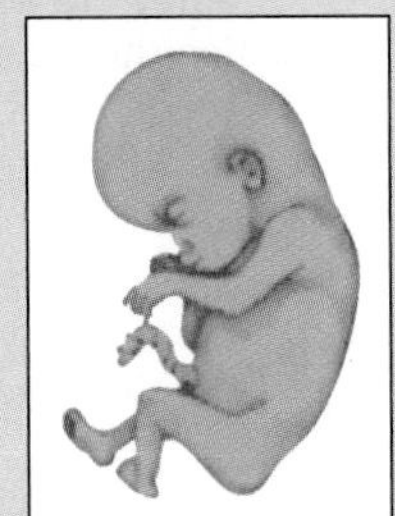
Crown-to-Rump Measurement; Weight	0.4-0.5 cm; 0.4 g	2.5-3 cm; 2 g	6-9 cm; 19 g
Gastrointestinal System	Stomach at midline and fusiform; conspicuous liver; esophagus short; intestine a short tube	Intestinal villi developing; small intestines coil within umbilical cord; palatal folds present; liver very large	Bile secreted; palatal fusion complete; intestines have withdrawn from cord and assume characteristic positions
Musculoskeletal System	All somites present	First indication of ossification—occiput, mandible, and humerus; fetus capable of some movement; definitive muscles of trunk, limbs, and head well represented	Some bones well outlined, ossification spreading; upper cervical to lower sacral arches and bodies ossify; smooth muscle layers indicated in hollow viscera
Circulatory System	Heart develops, double chambers visible, begins to beat; aortic arch and major veins completed	Main blood vessels assume final plan; enucleated red cells predominate in blood	Blood forming in marrow
Respiratory System	Primary lung buds appear	Pleural and pericardial cavities forming; branching bronchioles; nostrils closed by epithelial plugs	Lungs acquire definite shape; vocal cords appear
Renal System	Rudimentary ureteral buds appear	Earliest secretory tubules differentiating; bladder-urethra separates from rectum	Kidney able to secrete urine; bladder expands as a sac
Nervous System	Well-marked midbrain flexure; no hindbrain or cervical flexures; neural groove closed	Cerebral cortex begins to acquire typical cells; differentiation of cerebral cortex, meninges, ventricular foramina, cerebrospinal fluid circulation; spinal cord extends entire length of spine	Brain structural configuration almost complete; cord shows cervical and lumbar enlargements; fourth ventricle foramina are developed; sucking present
Sensory Organs	Eye and ear appearing as optic vessel and otocyst	Primordial choroid plexuses develop; ventricles large relative to cortex; development progressing; eyes converging rapidly; internal ear developing; eyelids fuse	Earliest taste buds indicated; characteristic organization of eye attained
Genital System	Genital ridge appears (fifth week)	Testes and ovaries distinguishable; external genitalia sexless but begin to differentiate	Sex recognizable; internal and external sex organs specific

TABLE 12-1 Milestones in Human Development Before Birth Since Last Menstrual Period—cont'd

	16 WEEKS	20 WEEKS	24 WEEKS
External Appearance	Head still dominant; face looks human; eyes, ears, and nose approach typical appearance on gross examination; arm/leg ratio proportionate; scalp hair appears 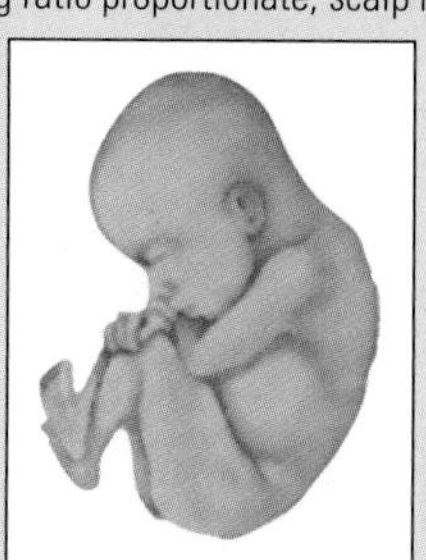	Vernix caseosa appears; lanugo appears; legs lengthen considerably; sebaceous glands appear 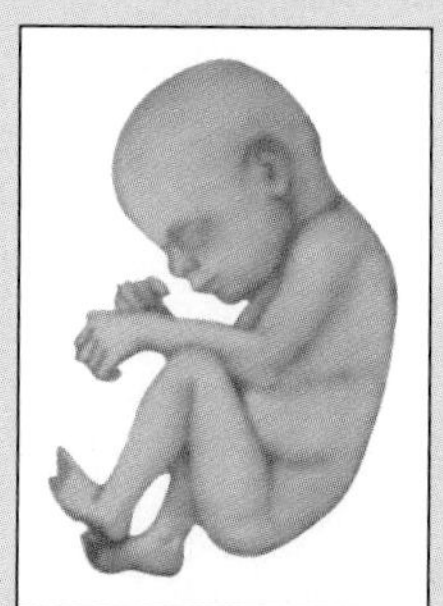	Body lean but fairly well proportioned; skin red and wrinkled; vernix caseosa present; sweat glands forming 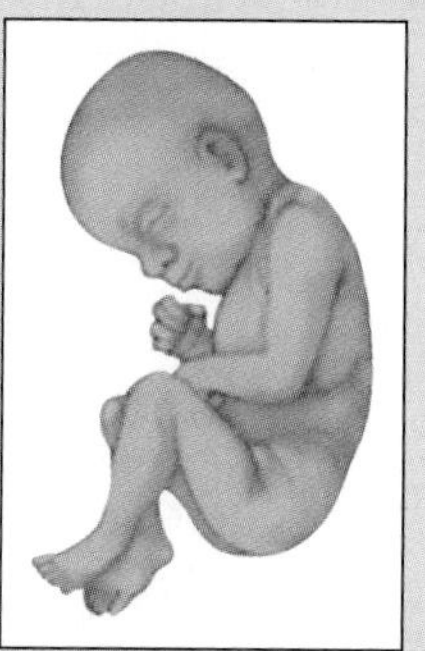
Crown-to-Rump Measurement; Weight	11.5-13.5 cm; 100 g	16-18.5 cm; 300 g	23 cm; 600 g
Gastrointestinal System	Meconium in bowel; some enzyme secretion; anus open	Enamel and dentine depositing; ascending colon recognizable	
Musculoskeletal System	Most bones distinctly indicated throughout body; joint cavities appear; muscular movements can be detected	Sternum ossifies; fetal movements strong enough for mother to feel	
Circulatory System	Heart muscle well developed; blood formation active in spleen		Blood formation increases in bone marrow and decreases in liver
Respiratory System	Elastic fibers appear in lungs; terminal and respiratory bronchioles appear	Nostrils reopen; primitive respiratory-like movements begin	Alveolar ducts and sacs present; lecithin begins to appear in amniotic fluid (weeks 26 to 27)
Renal System	Kidney in position; attains typical shape and plan		
Nervous System	Cerebral lobes delineated; cerebellum assumes some prominence	Brain grossly formed; cord myelination begins; spinal cord ends at level of first sacral vertebra (S1)	Cerebral cortex layered typically; neuronal proliferation in cerebral cortex ends
Sensory Organs	General sense organs differentiated	Nose and ears ossify	Can hear
Genital System	Testes in position for descent into scrotum: vagina open		Testes at inguinal ring in descent to scrotum

Continued

TABLE 12-1 Milestones in Human Development Before Birth Since Last Menstrual Period—cont'd

	28 WEEKS	30-31 WEEKS	36-40 WEEKS
External Appearance	Lean body, less wrinkled and red; nails appear	Subcutaneous fat beginning to collect; more rounded appearance; skin pink and smooth; has assumed birth position 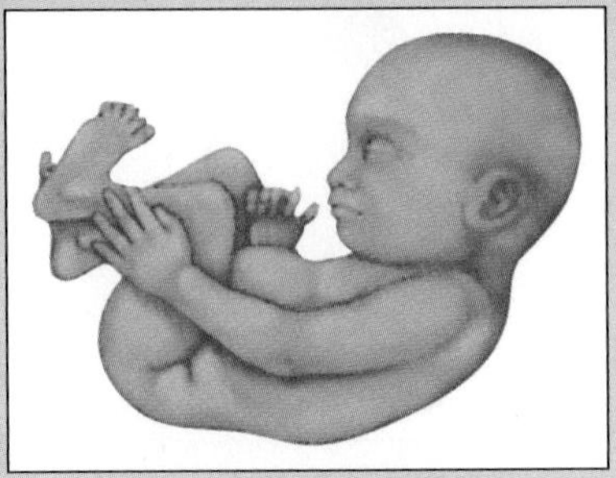	36 weeks: Skin pink, body rounded; general lanugo disappearing; body usually plump 40 weeks: Skin smooth and pink; scant vernix caseosa; moderate to profuse hair; lanugo on shoulders and upper body only; nasal and alar cartilage apparent
Crown-to-Rump Measurement; Weight	27 cm; 1100 g	31 cm; 1800-2100 g	36 weeks: 35 cm; 2200-2900 g; 40 weeks: 40 cm; 3200+ g
Musculoskeletal System	Astragalus (talus, ankle bone) ossifies; weak, fleeting movements, minimum tone	Middle fourth phalanges ossify; permanent teeth primordia seen; can turn head to side	36 weeks: Distal femoral ossification centers present; sustained, definite movements; fair tone; can turn and elevate head 40 weeks: Active, sustained movement; good tone; may lift head
Respiratory System	Lecithin forming on alveolar surfaces	L/S ratio = 1.2:1	36 weeks: L/S ratio >2:1 40 weeks: Pulmonary branching only two thirds complete
Renal System			36 weeks: Formation of new nephrons ceases
Nervous System	Appearance of cerebral fissures, convolutions rapidly appearing; indefinite sleep-wake cycle; cry weak or absent; weak suck reflex		36 weeks: End of spinal cord at level of third lumbar vertebra (L3); definite sleep-wake cycle 40 weeks: Myelination of brain begins; patterned sleep-wake cycle with alert periods; strong suck reflex
Sensory Organs	Eyelids reopen; retinal layers completed, light-receptive; pupils capable of reacting to light	Sense of taste present; aware of sounds outside mother's body	
Genital System		Testes descending to scrotum	40 weeks: Testes in scrotum; labia majora well developed

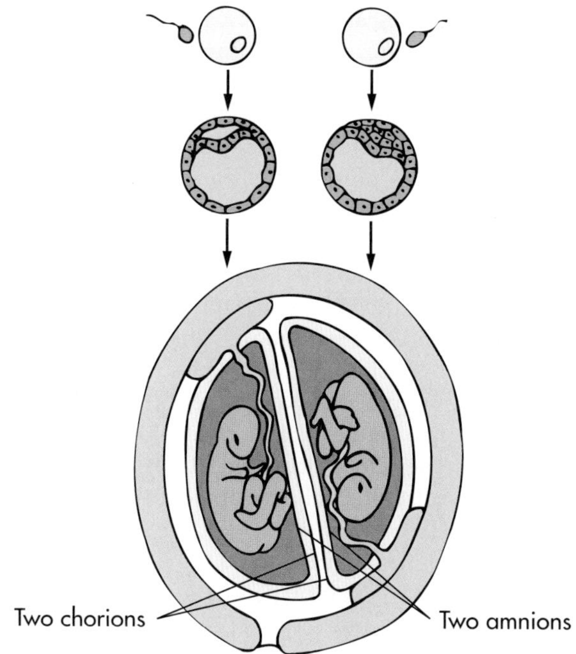

FIG 12-13 Formation of dizygotic twins, with fertilization of two ova, two implantations, two placentas, two chorions, and two amnions.

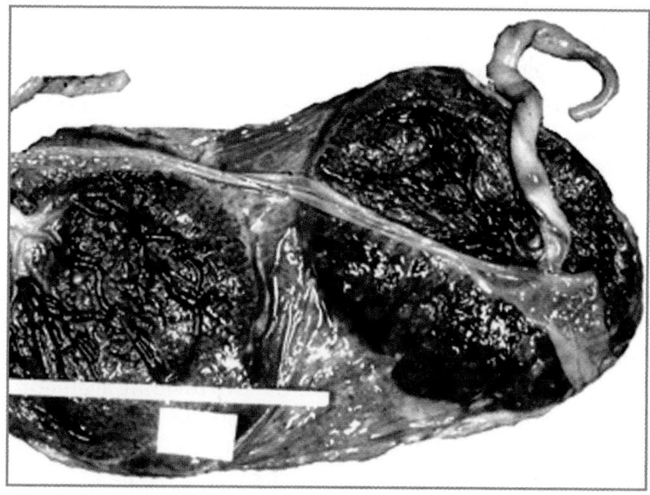

FIG 12-14 Diamniotic dichorionic (separate) twin placenta. (From Benirschke, K. [2013]. Multiple gestation. The biology of twinning. In R. Creasy, R. Resnik, J. Iams, et al. (Eds.), *Creasy and Resnik's maternal-fetal medicine: Principles and practice* (7th ed.). Philadelphia: Saunders.

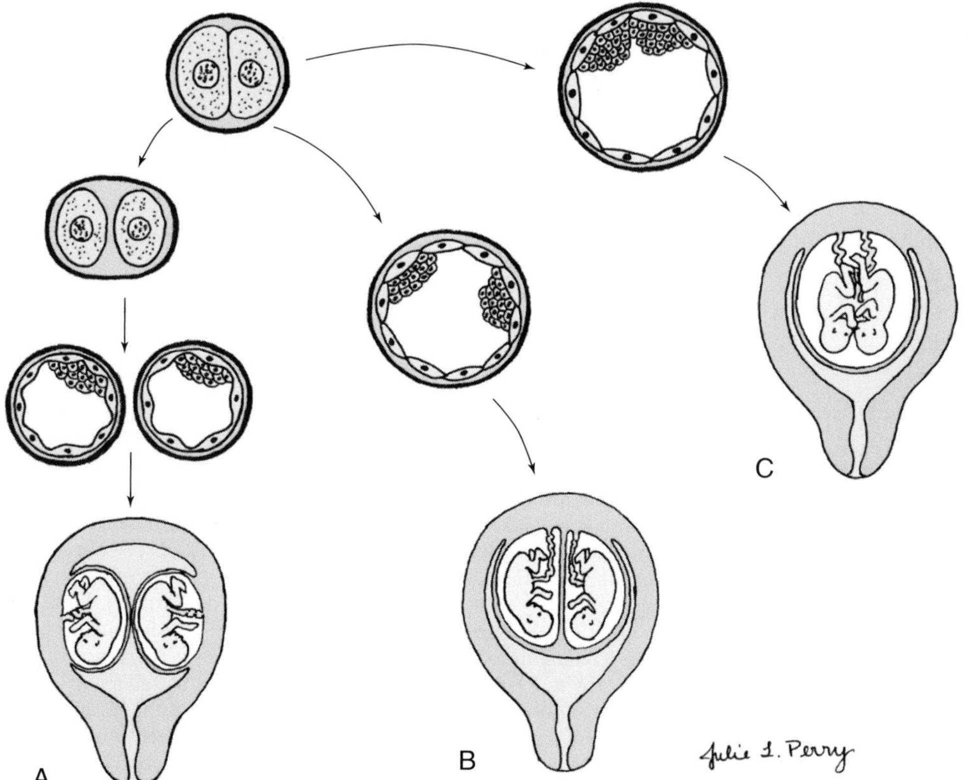

FIG 12-15 Formation of monozygotic twins. **A,** One fertilization: blastomeres separate, resulting in two implantations, two placentas, and two sets of membranes. **B,** One blastomere with two inner cell masses, one fused placenta, one chorion, and separate amnions. **C,** One blastomere with incomplete separation of cell mass, resulting in conjoined twins.

4 per 1000 births (Benirschke, 2013). There is no association with race, heredity, maternal age, or parity. Fertility drugs increase the incidence of monozygotic twinning.

Conjoined, or "Siamese," twins are a type of monozygotic twins in which cleavage is incomplete and occurs late (13 to 15 days postconception) (see Fig. 12-15). The estimated frequency is 1.5 in 100,000 births (Malone & D'Alton, 2013). Prenatal diagnosis is possible with three-dimensional ultrasonography. Cesarean birth minimizes trauma to mother and fetuses.

Other Multifetal Pregnancies

The occurrence of **multifetal pregnancies** with three or more fetuses has increased with the use of fertility drugs and in vitro fertilization. Triplets occur in approximately 1 of 1341 pregnancies (Benirschke, 2013). They can occur from the division of one zygote into two, with one of the two dividing again, producing identical triplets. Triplets also can be produced from two zygotes, one dividing into a set of identical twins, and the second zygote developing as a single fraternal sibling, or from three zygotes. Quadruplets, quintuplets, sextuplets, and so on, likewise have similar possible derivations.

NONGENETIC FACTORS INFLUENCING DEVELOPMENT

Congenital disorders may be inherited, may be caused by environmental factors, or may be a result of inadequate maternal nutrition. *Congenital* means that the condition was present at birth. Some congenital malformations may be caused by teratogens, that is, environmental substances or exposures that result in functional or structural disability. In contrast to other forms of developmental disabilities, disabilities caused by teratogens are theoretically totally preventable. Known human teratogens are certain drugs and chemicals, infections, exposure to radiation, and certain maternal conditions such as diabetes and phenylketonuria (PKU) (see Box 12-1). A teratogen has the greatest effect on the organs and parts of an embryo during its periods of rapid growth and differentiation. This occurs during the embryonic period, specifically from days 15 to 60. During the first 2 weeks of development, teratogens either have no effect or have effects so severe that they cause miscarriage. Brain growth and development continue during the fetal period, and teratogens can severely affect mental development throughout gestation (see Fig. 12-7).

In addition to genetic makeup and the influence of teratogens, the adequacy of maternal nutrition influences development. The embryo and fetus must obtain the nutrients needed from the mother's diet; they cannot tap the maternal reserves. Malnutrition during pregnancy produces low-birth-weight newborns who are susceptible to infection. Malnutrition also affects brain development during the latter half of gestation and can result in intellectual disabilities in the child. Inadequate folic acid is associated with neural tube defects.

KEY POINTS

- Human gestation lasts approximately 280 days after the last menstrual period or 266 days after conception.
- Fertilization occurs in the uterine tube within 24 hours of ovulation. The zygote undergoes mitotic divisions, creating a 16-cell morula.
- Implantation begins 6 days after fertilization.
- The organ systems and external features develop during the embryonic period, that is, the third to the eighth week after fertilization.
- Refinement of structure and function occurs during the fetal period, and the fetus becomes capable of extrauterine survival.
- During critical periods in human development, the embryo and fetus are vulnerable to environmental teratogens.
- There has been a steady rise in the incidence of multifetal pregnancies, which is partly due to the use of fertility drugs and in vitro fertilization, the increasing age at which women give birth, and ovulation-enhancing drugs.

REFERENCES

Benirschke, K. (2013). Multiple gestation: The biology of twinning. In R. Creasy, R. Resnik, J. Iams, et al. (Eds.), *Creasy and Resnik's maternal-fetal medicine: Principles and practice* (7th ed.). Philadelphia: Saunders.

Blackburn, S. T. (2012). *Maternal, fetal, & neonatal physiology. A clinical perspective* (4th ed.). St. Louis, MO: Saunders Elsevier.

Cunningham, F., Leveno, K., Bloom, S., et al. (2014). *Williams obstetrics* (24th ed.). New York: McGraw-Hill.

Malone, F., & D'Alton, M. (2013). Multiple gestation: Clinical characteristics and management. In R. Creasy, R. Resnik, J. Iams, et al. (Eds.), *Creasy and Resnik's maternal-fetal medicine: Principles and practice* (7th ed.). Philadelphia: Saunders.

Mercer, B. (2013). Assessment and induction of fetal pulmonary maturity. In R. Creasy, R. Resnik, J. Iams, et al. (Eds.), *Creasy and Resnik's maternal-fetal medicine: Principles and practice* (7th ed.). Philadelphia: Saunders.

Moore, K. L., Persaud, T. V. N., & Torchia, M. G. (2013). *Before we are born. Essentials of embryology and birth defects* (8th ed.). Philadelphia: Saunders.

Mor, G., & Abrahams, V. (2013). The immunology of pregnancy. In R. Creasy, R. Resnik, J. Iams, et al. (Eds.), *Creasy and Resnik's maternal-fetal medicine: Principles and practice* (6th ed.). Philadelphia: Saunders.

Ramachandrappa, A., & Jain, L. (2008). Elective cesarean section: Its impact on neonatal respiratory outcome. *Clinics in Perinatology*, *35*(2), 373–393.

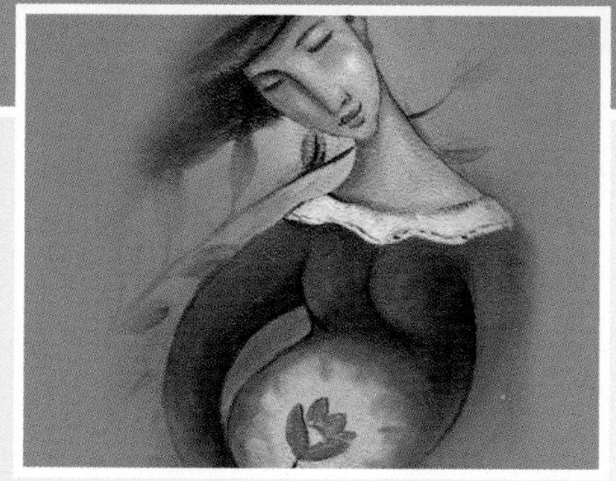

CHAPTER 13

Anatomy and Physiology of Pregnancy

Kathryn R. Alden

http://evolve.elsevier.com/Lowdermilk/MWHC/

LEARNING OBJECTIVES

- Determine gravidity and parity using the two- and five-digit systems.
- Describe the various types of pregnancy tests, including the timing of tests and interpretation of results.
- Explain the expected maternal anatomic and physiologic adaptations to pregnancy.
- Differentiate among presumptive, probable, and positive signs of pregnancy.
- Identify maternal hormones produced during pregnancy, their target organs, and their major effects on pregnancy.

The goal of maternity care is a healthy pregnancy with a physically safe and emotionally satisfying outcome for mother, infant, and family. Consistent health supervision and surveillance are of utmost importance. However, many maternal adaptations are unfamiliar to pregnant women and their families. Helping the pregnant woman recognize the relationship between her physical status and the plan for her care assists her in making decisions and encourages her to participate in her own care.

GRAVIDITY AND PARITY

An understanding of the following terms used to describe pregnancy and the pregnant woman is essential to the study of maternity care:

Gravida: A woman who is pregnant

Gravidity: Pregnancy

Nulligravida: A woman who has never been pregnant and is not currently pregnant

Primigravida: A woman who is pregnant for the first time

Multigravida: A woman who has had two or more pregnancies

Parity: The number of pregnancies in which the fetus or fetuses have reached 20 weeks of gestation, not the number of fetuses (e.g., twins) born. Parity is not affected by whether the fetus is born alive or is stillborn (i.e., showing no signs of life at birth).

Nullipara: A woman who has not completed a pregnancy with a fetus or fetuses beyond 20 weeks of gestation

Primipara: A woman who has completed one pregnancy with a fetus or fetuses who have reached 20 weeks of gestation

Multipara: A woman who has completed two or more pregnancies to 20 weeks of gestation or more

Preterm: A pregnancy that has reached 20 weeks of gestation but ends before completion of 37 weeks of gestation

Late preterm: A pregnancy that has reached between 34 weeks 0 days and 36 weeks 6 days of gestation

Early term: A pregnancy that has reached between 37 weeks 0 days and 38 weeks 6 days of gestation (American College of Obstetricians and Gynecologists [ACOG] Committee on Obstetric Practice & Society for Maternal-Fetal Medicine [SMFM], 2013)

Full term: A pregnancy that has reached between 39 weeks 0 days and 40 weeks 6 days of gestation (ACOG Committee on Obstetric Practice & SMFM, 2013)

Late term: A pregnancy that has reached between 41 weeks 0 days and 41 weeks 6 days of gestation (ACOG Committee on Obstetric Practice & SMFM, 2013)

Post term: A pregnancy that has reached between 42 weeks 0 days and beyond of gestation (ACOG Committee on Obstetric Practice & SMFM, 2013)

Viability: The capacity to live outside the uterus; there are no clear limits of gestational age or weight. Infants born at 22 to 25 weeks of gestation are considered to be on the threshold of viability and are especially vulnerable to brain injury if they survive.

Gravidity and parity information is obtained during history-taking interviews. Obtaining and documenting this information accurately is important in planning care for a pregnant woman.

Information may be recorded in client records in a variety of ways because no one standardized system exists. It is important that the nurse understand the documentation system used by the health care facility.

TABLE 13-1 Obstetric History Using Five-Digit and Two-Digit System

	FIVE-DIGIT SYSTEM					TWO-DIGIT SYSTEM
	G	T	P	A	L	G/P
CONDITION	GRAVIDITY	TERM BIRTH	PRETERM BIRTHS	ABORTIONS AND MISCARRIAGES	LIVING CHILDREN	GRAVIDITY/ PARITY
Olivia is pregnant for the first time.	1	0	0	0	0	1/0
She carries the pregnancy to term, and the neonate survives.	1	1	0	0	1	1/1
She is pregnant again.	2	1	0	0	1	2/1
Her second pregnancy ends in miscarriage at 10 weeks.	2	1	0	1	1	2/1
During her third pregnancy, she gives birth at 36 weeks to twins.	3	1	1	1	3	3/2

Two commonly used systems of summarizing the obstetric history are discussed here. Gravidity and parity can be described with only two digits: the first digit indicates the number of pregnancies the woman has had, including the present one, and parity the number of pregnancies that have reached 20 weeks of gestation. For example, the abbreviation gravida 1, para 0 (1/0) means that a woman is pregnant for the first time (primigravida) and has not carried a pregnancy to 20 weeks (nullipara). If a woman had twins at 36 weeks with her first pregnancy, she would be gravida 1, para 1.

Another system consisting of five digits is commonly used. This system provides more information about the woman's obstetric history, although it may not provide accurate information about parity because it provides information about births and not pregnancies reaching 20 weeks of gestation. The first digit represents gravidity, the second digit represents the total number of term births, the third indicates the number of preterm births, the fourth identifies the number of abortions (miscarriage [spontaneous abortion] or elective termination of pregnancy before 20 weeks), and the fifth is the number of children currently living. The acronym GTPAL (gravidity, term, preterm, abortions, living children) can be helpful in remembering this system of notation. For example, if a woman pregnant only once gives birth at week 35 and the infant survives, the abbreviation that represents this information is "1-0-1-0-1." During her next pregnancy the abbreviation is "2-0-1-0-1." Additional examples are in Table 13-1.

While the GTPAL notation for obstetric history is commonly used, the current recommendation is that term pregnancy (beyond 37 weeks) is classified as early term, full term, late term, or post term. Use of this uniform classification by clinicians, researchers, and public health officials will facilitate the provision of quality health care, clinical research, and data reporting (ACOG Committee on Obstetric Practice & SMFM, 2013).

PREGNANCY TESTS

Early detection of pregnancy allows for early initiation of prenatal care. Human chorionic gonadotropin (hCG) is the earliest biologic marker for pregnancy. Pregnancy tests are based on the recognition of hCG or a beta (β) subunit of hCG. Production of β-hCG begins as early as the day of implantation and can be detected in maternal serum or urine as soon as 7 to 8 days before the expected menses. hCG levels usually double approximately every 2 days for the first 4 weeks of pregnancy. The level of hCG rises until it peaks at 60 to 70 days and then declines to lowest levels at about 100 to 130 days as the placenta becomes the primary source of estrogen and progesterone. Plasma levels of hCG remain at this lower level for the remainder of the pregnancy. Higher than normal levels of hCG are associated with abnormal gestation (e.g., fetus with Down syndrome, gestational trophoblastic disease) or multiple gestation. Abnormally slow increase in hCG or lower levels can indicate impending miscarriage or ectopic pregnancy (Liu, 2014).

Serum and urine pregnancy tests are performed in clinics, offices, women's health centers, and laboratory settings. Urine tests can also be done at home. Both serum and urine tests can provide accurate results.

Quantitative serum testing—the β-hCG test—has a high level of accuracy because it measures the exact amount of hCG in the blood and can detect even small amounts. hCG levels greater than 25 International Units/L are diagnostic for pregnancy. For serum testing, a 7- to 10-ml sample of venous blood is collected (Pagana & Pagana, 2013).

Sandwich-type immunoassay testing is the most popular method of testing for pregnancy and is the basis for most home pregnancy tests. It uses a specific monoclonal antibody (anti-hCG) with enzymes that bond with hCG in urine. Many different pregnancy tests are available (Fig. 13-1). With these one-step tests the woman usually applies urine to a strip or absorbent-tipped applicator and reads the results. The test kits come with directions for collection of the specimen, the testing procedure, and reading of results.

The accuracy of the results is related to following the instructions correctly. However, instructions for some home pregnancy tests do not comply with the recommended guidelines for use of plain language, and many instructions are written at a seventh-grade reading level or above, which limits understanding by some users. A positive test result is indicated by a simple color change reaction or a digital reading. Most manufacturers of the kits provide a toll-free telephone number to call if users have concerns or questions about test procedures or results. A common error in performing home pregnancy tests is doing the test too early in pregnancy before a significant rise in hCG level; this can cause a false-negative result (Pagana & Pagana, 2013) (see Clinical Reasoning Case Study).

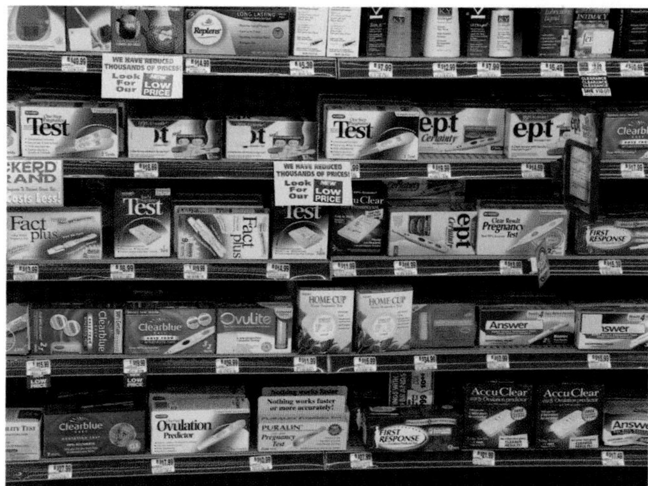

FIG 13-1 Many pregnancy test products are available over the counter. (Courtesy Dee Lowdermilk, Chapel Hill, NC.)

COMMUNITY ACTIVITY

- Review web-based information about home pregnancy tests. Explore websites such as www.babycenter.com and www.parents.com. Assess the accuracy of information.
- Visit a pharmacy in your neighborhood. How many different types of home pregnancy test kits are available in the pharmacy? Read the labels on three different types of home pregnancy test kits. Do the kits include material for more than one test? Are the directions printed in more than one language? After reading the directions, do you have questions about how to perform the test or how to interpret the results? If so, what does that say about the likelihood that the tests will be used correctly?

CLINICAL REASONING CASE STUDY

Pregnancy Testing

When her menstrual period was 10 days late, Regine purchased a home pregnancy test on her way home from work and performed the test that evening. The result was negative. Regine and her partner have been trying to get pregnant so that the baby will be born when she is on summer break from her teaching job at the elementary school. She is disappointed that the test was negative and she calls the clinic to ask the nurse if she should come in for a blood test to see if she is pregnant.

1. Evidence—Is there sufficient evidence to draw conclusions about the advice the nurse should provide to Regine?
2. Assumptions—What assumptions can be made about the following issues?
   a. Proper use of home pregnancy tests
   b. Factors that can affect results of home pregnancy tests
   c. Human chorionic gonadotropin (hCG) levels in pregnancy
3. What are the implications and priorities for providing information to Regine?
4. Does the evidence objectively support your conclusion?

Interpreting the results of pregnancy tests requires some judgment. The type of pregnancy test and its degree of sensitivity (the ability to detect low levels of a substance) and specificity (the ability to discern the absence of a substance) must be considered in conjunction with the woman's history. This includes the date of her last normal menstrual period, her usual cycle length, and results of previous pregnancy tests. It is important to know about any medications or other substances she is taking. Medications such as anticonvulsants and tranquilizers can cause false-positive results, whereas diuretics and promethazine can cause false-negative results (Pagana & Pagana, 2013). Improper collection of the specimen, hormone-producing tumors, and laboratory errors can also cause inaccurate results.

Women who use a home pregnancy test should be advised about the variations in accuracy and to use caution when interpreting results. Whenever there is any question, further evaluation or retesting may be appropriate (see Teaching for Self-Management).

TEACHING FOR SELF-MANAGEMENT

Home Pregnancy Testing

1. Follow the manufacturer's instructions carefully. Do not omit steps.
2. Review the manufacturer's list of foods, medications, and other substances that can affect the test results.
3. Use a first-voided morning urine specimen.
4. If the test done at the time of your missed period is negative, repeat the test in 1 week if you still have not had a period.
5. If you have questions about the test, contact the manufacturer.
6. Contact your health care provider for follow-up if the test result is positive or if the test result is negative and you still have not had a period.

ADAPTATIONS TO PREGNANCY

Maternal physiologic adaptations are attributed to the hormones of pregnancy and to mechanical pressures arising from the enlarging uterus and other tissues. These adaptations protect the woman's normal physiologic functioning, meet the metabolic demands that pregnancy imposes on her body, and provide a nurturing environment for fetal development and growth. Although pregnancy is a normal phenomenon, problems can occur.

Signs of Pregnancy

Some physiologic adaptations are recognized as the signs and symptoms of pregnancy. Three commonly used categories of these signs and symptoms are:

- Presumptive—those changes felt by the woman (e.g., amenorrhea, fatigue, breast changes)
- Probable—those changes observed by an examiner (e.g., Hegar sign, ballottement, pregnancy tests)
- Positive—those signs attributed only to the presence of the fetus (e.g., hearing fetal heart tones, visualizing the fetus, palpating fetal movements)

Table 13-2 summarizes these signs of pregnancy in relation to when they might occur and gives other possible causes for their occurrence.

Reproductive System and Breasts

Uterus

Changes in Size, Shape, and Position. High levels of estrogen and progesterone stimulate phenomenal uterine growth in the first trimester. Early uterine enlargement results from increased vascularity and dilation of blood vessels, hyperplasia (production of new muscle fibers and fibroelastic tissue) and

TABLE 13-2 Signs of Pregnancy

TIME OF OCCURRENCE (GESTATIONAL AGE)	SIGN	OTHER POSSIBLE CAUSE
Presumptive		
3-4 wk	Breast changes	Premenstrual changes, oral contraceptives
4 wk	Amenorrhea	Stress, vigorous exercise, early menopause, endocrine problems, malnutrition
4-14 wk	Nausea, vomiting	Gastrointestinal virus, food poisoning
6-12 wk	Urinary frequency	Infection, pelvic tumors
12 wk	Fatigue	Stress, illness
16-20 wk	Quickening	Gas, peristalsis
Probable		
5 wk	Goodell sign	Pelvic congestion
6-8 wk	Chadwick sign	Pelvic congestion
6-12 wk	Hegar sign	Pelvic congestion
4-12 wk	Positive pregnancy test (serum)	Hydatidiform mole, choriocarcinoma
6-12 wk	Positive pregnancy test (urine)	False-positive result may be caused by pelvic infection, tumors
16 wk	Braxton Hicks contractions	Myomas, other tumors
16-28 wk	Ballottement	Tumors, cervical polyps
Positive		
5-6 wk	Visualization of fetus by real-time ultrasound examination	No other causes
6 wk	Fetal heart tones detected by ultrasound	No other causes
16 wk	Visualization of fetus by radiographic study	No other causes
8-17 wk	Fetal heart tones detected by Doppler ultrasound stethoscope	No other causes
17-19 wk	Fetal heart tones detected by fetal stethoscope	No other causes
19-22 wk	Fetal movements palpated by examiner	No other causes
Late pregnancy	Fetal movements visible to examiner	No other causes

hypertrophy (enlargement of preexisting muscle fibers and fibroelastic tissue), and development of the decidua. By 7 weeks of gestation, the uterus is the size of a large hen's egg; by 10 weeks, it is the size of an orange (twice its nonpregnant size); and by 12 weeks, it is the size of a grapefruit. After the third month, uterine enlargement is primarily the result of mechanical pressure of the growing fetus.

As the uterus enlarges it also changes in shape and position. At conception the uterus is shaped like an upside-down pear. During the second trimester, as the muscular walls strengthen and become more elastic, the uterus becomes spherical or globular. Later, as the fetus lengthens, the uterus becomes larger and more ovoid and rises out of the pelvis into the abdominal cavity.

The pregnancy may "show" after the fourteenth week, although this depends to some degree on the woman's height and weight. Abdominal enlargement may be less apparent in the nullipara with good abdominal muscle tone (Fig. 13-2). Posture also influences the type and degree of abdominal enlargement that occurs. In normal pregnancies the uterus enlarges at a predictable rate.

As the uterus grows it can be palpated above the symphysis pubis sometime between the twelfth and fourteenth weeks of pregnancy (Fig. 13-3). The uterus rises gradually to the level of the umbilicus at 22 to 24 weeks of gestation and nearly reaches the xiphoid process at term. Between weeks 38 and 40, fundal height decreases as the fetus begins to descend into the pelvis (**lightening**) in preparation for birth (see Fig. 13-3, *dashed line*). Generally lightening occurs in the nullipara about 2 weeks before the onset of labor and in the multipara at the start of labor.

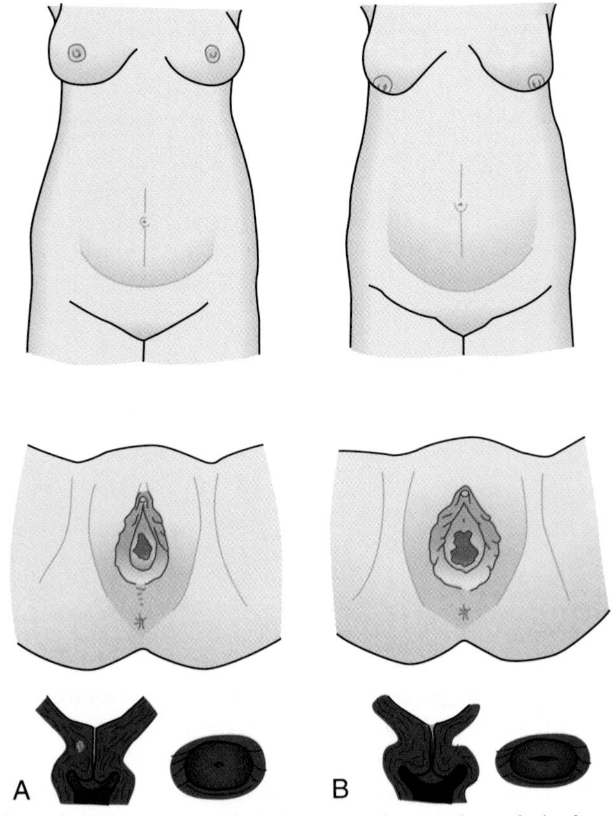

FIG 13-2 Comparison of abdomen, vulva, and cervix in **A,** nullipara, and **B,** multipara, at the same stage of pregnancy.

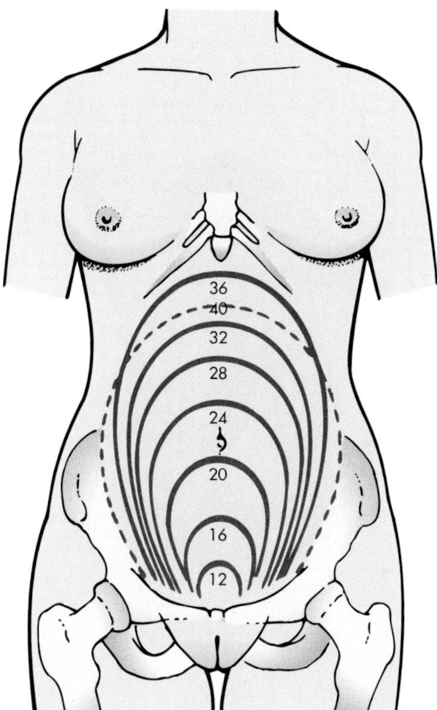

FIG 13-3 Height of fundus by weeks of normal gestation with a single fetus. *Dashed line,* Height after lightening. (From Seidel, H.M., Ball, J.W., Dains, J.E., et al. [2011]. *Mosby's guide to physical examination* [7th ed.]. St. Louis: Mosby.)

Uterine enlargement is determined by measuring fundal height (see Fig. 14-8). This measurement is commonly used to estimate the weeks of gestation. However, variations in the position of the fundus or the fetus, variations in the amount of amniotic fluid present, the presence of more than one fetus, maternal obesity, and differences in examiner technique can reduce the accuracy of this estimation.

Generally the uterus rotates to the right as it enlarges and rises in the abdomen, probably because of the presence of the rectosigmoid colon on the left side. However, the extensive hypertrophy (enlargement) of the round ligaments keeps the uterus in the midline. Eventually the growing uterus touches the anterior abdominal wall and displaces the intestines to either side of the abdomen (Fig. 13-4). When a pregnant woman is standing, most of her uterus rests against the anterior abdominal wall and contributes to altering her center of gravity.

At approximately 6 weeks of gestation, softening and compressibility of the lower uterine segment (uterine isthmus) occurs (Hegar sign) (Fig. 13-5). This results in exaggerated uterine anteflexion during the first 3 months of pregnancy. In this position the uterine fundus presses on the urinary bladder, causing the woman to have urinary frequency.

Changes in Contractility. Soon after the fourth month of pregnancy, uterine contractions can be felt through the abdominal wall. These are referred to as Braxton Hicks contractions. Braxton Hicks contractions are irregular and painless contractions that occur intermittently throughout pregnancy. Although Braxton Hicks contractions are not painful, some women complain that they are annoying. After the twenty-eighth week, these contractions become more definite, but they usually cease with walking or exercise. Braxton Hicks contractions can be mistaken for true labor; however, they do not increase in intensity or duration or cause cervical dilation. Conversely, premature labor contractions can be mistaken for Braxton Hicks contractions, which can lead to a delay in seeking treatment.

Uteroplacental Blood Flow. Placental perfusion depends on the maternal blood flow to the uterus. Blood flow increases rapidly as the uterus increases in size. Although uterine blood flow increases 10-fold, the fetoplacental unit grows even more rapidly (Norwitz, Mahendroo, & Lye, 2014). Consequently, more oxygen is extracted from the uterine blood during the latter part of pregnancy. In a normal-term pregnancy, one sixth of the total maternal blood volume is within the uterine vascular system. The rate of blood flow through the uterus averages 450 to 650 ml/minute at term, and oxygen consumption of the gravid uterus increases to meet fetal needs. Three factors known to decrease uterine blood flow are low maternal arterial pressure, contractions of the uterus, and maternal supine position. Estrogen stimulation can increase uterine blood flow. Doppler ultrasound examination may be used to measure uterine blood flow velocity, especially in pregnancies at risk because of conditions associated with decreased placental perfusion (e.g., hypertension, intrauterine growth restriction, diabetes mellitus, multiple gestation) (Blackburn, 2013).

By using an ultrasound device or a fetal stethoscope to auscultate fetal heart tones, the examiner may also hear the uterine souffle or bruit, a rushing or blowing sound of maternal blood flowing through uterine arteries to the placenta that is synchronous with the maternal pulse. The funic souffle, which is synchronous with the fetal heart rate and is caused by fetal blood coursing through the umbilical cord, may also be heard, as well as the fetus's actual heartbeat (see Fig. 14-7).

Cervical Changes. In a normal, unscarred cervix, softening of the cervical tip can be observed about the beginning of the sixth week. This probable sign of pregnancy, Goodell sign, is brought about by increased vascularity, slight hypertrophy, and hyperplasia (increase in number of cells). The muscle and its collagen-rich connective tissue become loose, edematous, highly elastic, and increased in volume. The glands near the external os proliferate beneath the stratified squamous epithelium, giving the cervix the velvety appearance characteristic of pregnancy. Friability (tissue is easily damaged) is increased and can result in slight bleeding after vaginal examination or after coitus with deep penetration.

Pregnancy can also cause the squamocolumnar junction, the site for obtaining cells for cervical cancer screening, to be located away from the cervix. Because of these changes, evaluation of abnormal Papanicolaou (Pap) tests during pregnancy can be complicated. However, careful assessment of all pregnant women is important because approximately 3% of all invasive cervical cancers occur during pregnancy (Salani, Eisenhauer, & Copeland, 2012).

The cervix of the nullipara is rounded. Lacerations of the cervix can occur during the birth process. After birth, with or without lacerations, the cervix becomes more oval in the horizontal plane and the external os appears as a transverse slit (see Fig. 13-2).

Changes Related to the Presence of the Fetus. Passive movement of the unengaged fetus is called ballottement

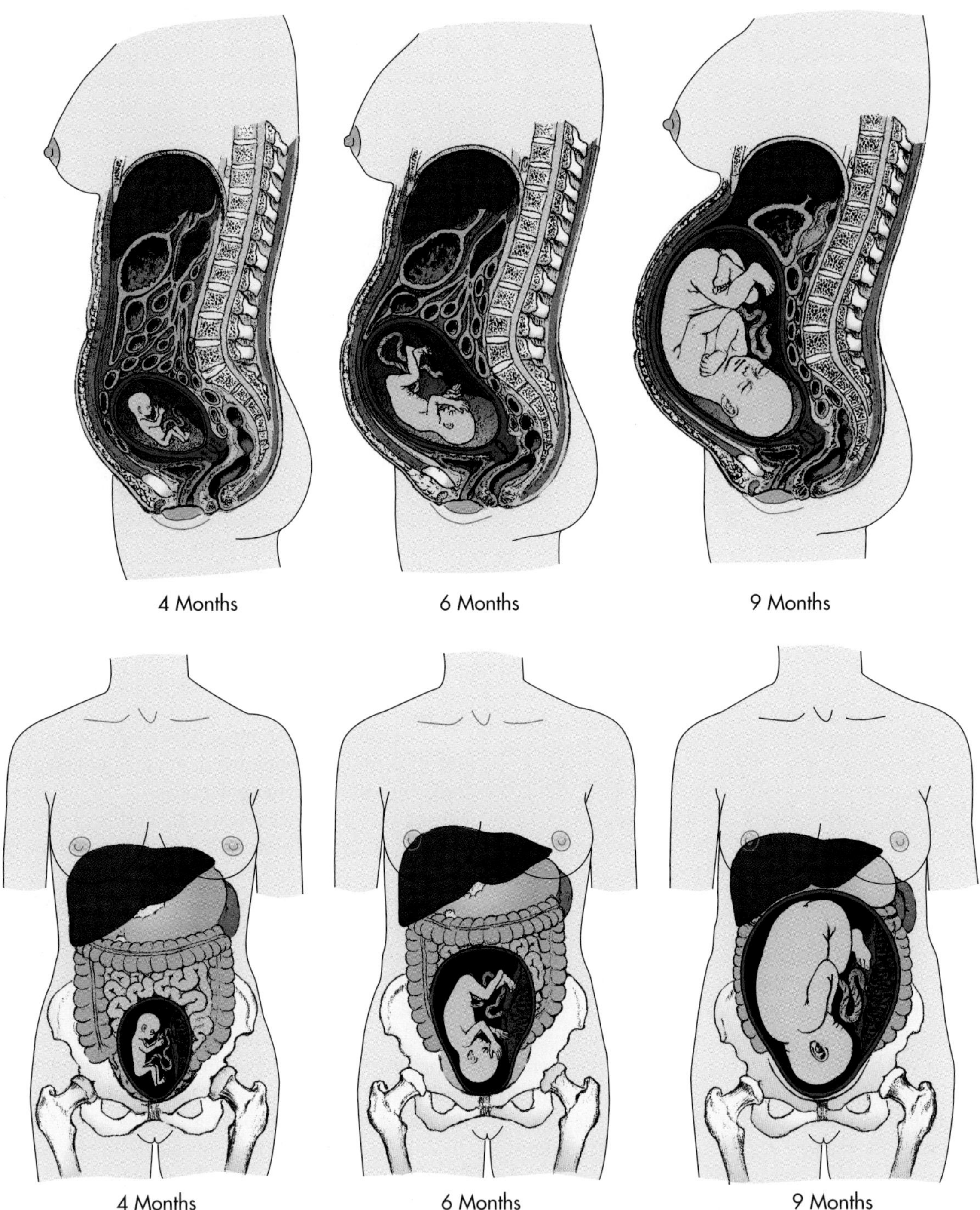

FIG 13-4 Displacement of internal abdominal structures and diaphragm by the enlarging uterus at 4, 6, and 9 months of gestation.

and can be identified by the examiner generally between the sixteenth and eighteenth weeks. Ballottement is a technique of palpating a floating structure by bouncing it gently and feeling it rebound. To palpate the fetus, the examiner places a finger within the vagina and taps gently upward on the cervix, causing the fetus to rise. The fetus then sinks, and a gentle tap is felt on the finger (Fig. 13-6).

Quickening is the first recognition of fetal movements, or "feeling life." It can be detected by the multiparous woman as early as 14 to 16 weeks. The nulliparous woman may not notice these sensations until the eighteenth week or later. Quickening is commonly described as a flutter and is difficult to distinguish from peristalsis. Fetal movements gradually increase in intensity and frequency as pregnancy progresses. The week in which quickening occurs provides a tentative clue in dating the duration of gestation.

Vagina and Vulva

Pregnancy hormones prepare the vagina for stretching during labor and birth by causing the vaginal mucosa to thicken, the connective tissue to loosen, the smooth muscle to hypertrophy, and the vaginal vault to lengthen. Increased vascularity results

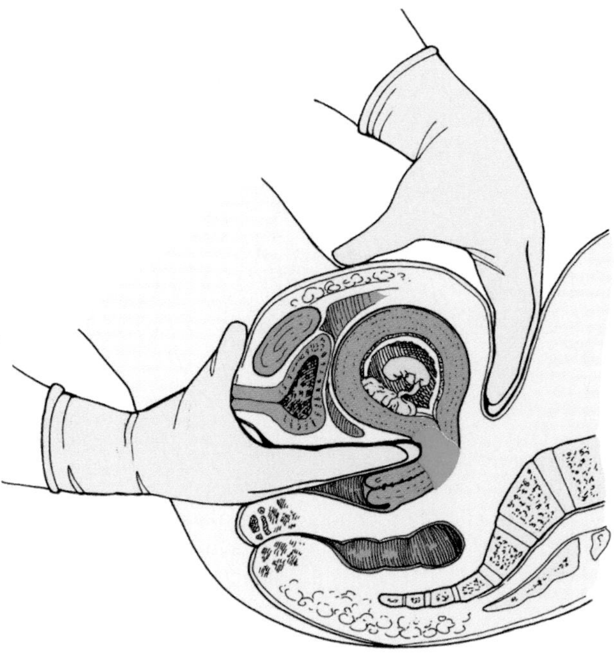

FIG 13-5 Hegar sign. Bimanual examination for assessing compressibility and softening of isthmus (lower uterine segment) while the cervix is still firm.

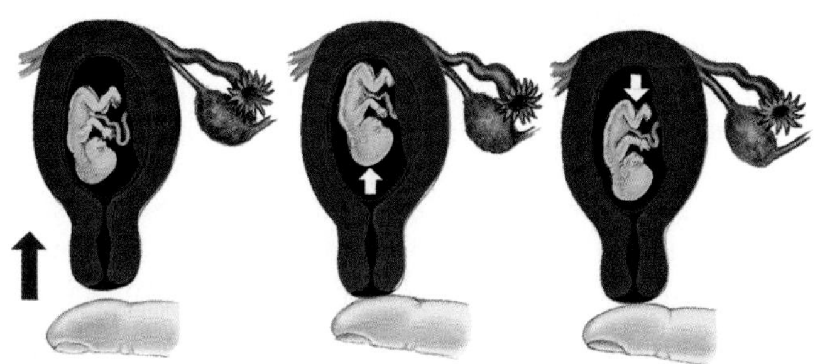

FIG 13-6 Internal ballottement (18 weeks).

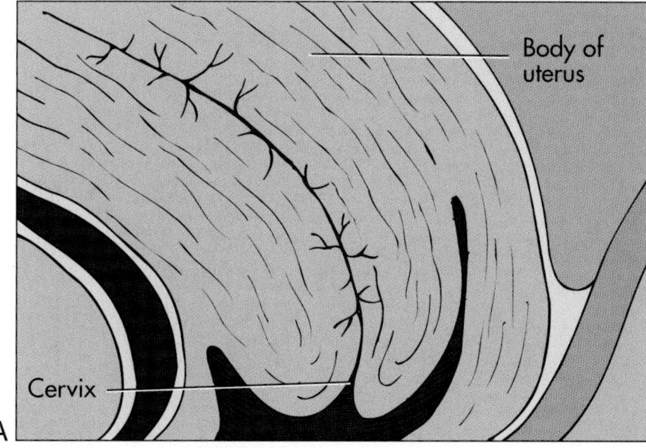

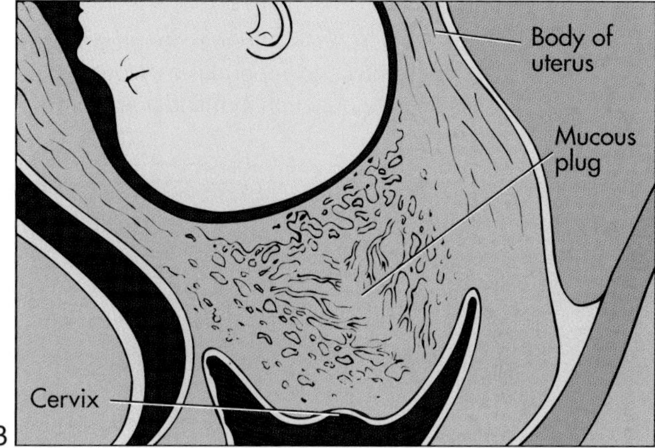

FIG 13-7 **A**, Cervix in nonpregnant woman. **B**, Cervix during pregnancy.

in a violet-blue vaginal mucosa and cervix. This is known as the Chadwick sign and can be evident as early as the sixth week but is easily noted by the eighth week of pregnancy (Blackburn, 2013).

Leukorrhea is a white or slightly gray mucoid discharge with a faint musty odor. This copious mucoid fluid occurs in response to cervical stimulation by estrogen and progesterone. The fluid is whitish because of the presence of many exfoliated vaginal epithelial cells caused by the hyperplasia of normal pregnancy. This normal vaginal discharge is never pruritic or blood stained. The mucus fills the endocervical canal, resulting in the formation of the mucus plug (operculum) (Fig. 13-7). The operculum acts as a barrier against bacterial invasion during pregnancy.

During pregnancy the pH of vaginal secretions is more acidic, ranging from about 3.5 to about 6.0 (nonpregnant, 4.0 to 5.0), because of increased production of lactic acid. Although this acidic environment provides more protection from some organisms, the pregnant woman is more vulnerable to other infections, especially yeast infections because the glycogen-rich environment of the vagina is more susceptible to *Candida albicans.*

The increased vascularity of the vagina and other pelvic viscera results in a marked increase in sensitivity. The increased sensitivity can lead to a high degree of sexual interest and arousal, especially during the second trimester of pregnancy. The increased congestion, plus the relaxed walls of the blood vessels and the heavy uterus, can result in edema and varicosities of the vulva. The edema and varicosities usually resolve during the postpartum period.

External structures of the perineum are enlarged during pregnancy because of an increase in vasculature, hypertrophy of the perineal body, and deposition of fat (Fig. 13-8). The labia majora of nulliparous women approximate (come together) and obscure the vaginal introitus; those of the parous woman separate and gape after childbirth and perineal or vaginal injury. See Figure 13-2 for a comparison of the nullipara and the multipara in relation to the pregnant abdomen, vulva, and cervix.

Breasts

Fullness, heightened sensitivity, tingling, and heaviness of the breasts begin in the early weeks of gestation in response to increased levels of estrogen and progesterone. Breast sensitivity varies from mild tingling to sharp pain. Nipples and areolae become more pigmented; secondary pinkish areolae develop, extending beyond the primary areolae; and nipples become more erectile. Hypertrophy of the sebaceous (oil) glands embedded in the primary areolae, called Montgomery tubercles, may be seen around the nipples. Within the tubercles are sebaceous and sweat glands that secrete lubricating and antiinfective substances to help protect the nipples and areolae during breastfeeding.

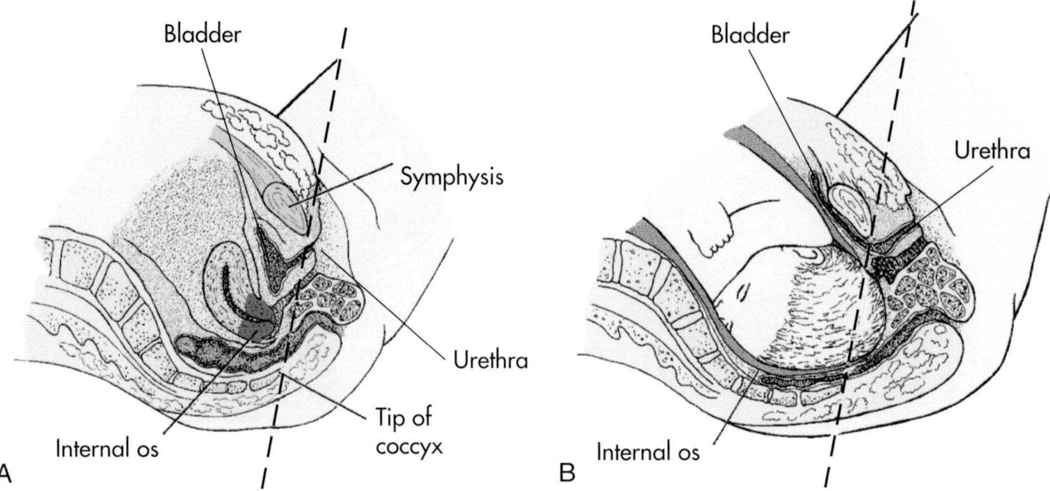

FIG 13-8 A, Pelvic floor in nonpregnant woman. B, Pelvic floor at end of pregnancy. Note marked hypertrophy and hyperplasia below *dotted line* joining tip of coccyx and inferior margin of symphysis. Note elongation of bladder and urethra as a result of compression. Fat deposits are increased.

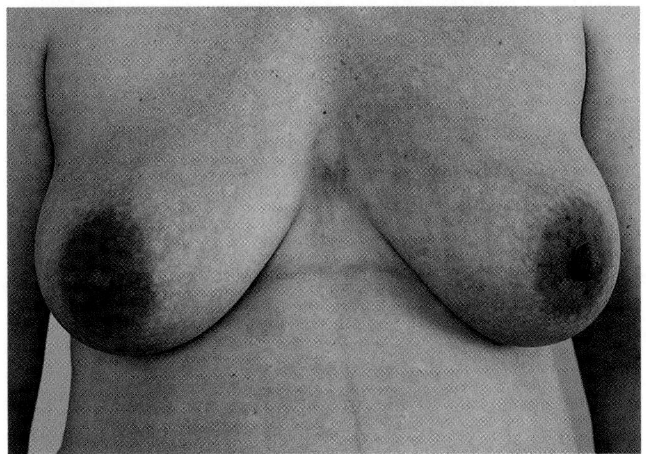

FIG 13-9 Enlarged breasts in pregnancy with venous network and darkened areolae and nipples. (From Seidel, H.M., Ball, J.W., Dains, J.E., et al. [2011]. *Mosby's guide to physical examination* [7th ed.]. St. Louis: Mosby.)

The richer blood supply causes the vessels beneath the skin to dilate. Once barely noticeable, the blood vessels become visible, often appearing in an intertwining bluish network beneath the surface of the skin. Venous congestion in the breasts is more obvious in primigravidas. Striae gravidarum, or stretch marks, can appear at the outer aspects of the breasts.

During the second and third trimesters, growth of the mammary glands accounts for the progressive breast enlargement (Fig. 13-9). The high levels of luteal and placental hormones in pregnancy promote proliferation of the lactiferous ducts and lobule-alveolar tissue so that palpation of the breasts reveals a generalized coarse nodularity. Glandular tissue displaces connective tissue, resulting in the tissue becoming softer and looser.

Although development of the mammary glands is functionally complete by midpregnancy, lactation is inhibited until the progesterone level decreases after birth. A thin, clear, viscous secretory material (precolostrum) can be found in the acinar cells by the third month of gestation. Colostrum, the yellow to yellowish-orange premilk fluid secreted during the second trimester may be expressed from the nipples as early as 16 weeks of gestation (Lawrence & Lawrence, 2011). See Chapter 25 for a discussion of lactation.

General Body Systems

Cardiovascular System

Maternal adjustments to pregnancy involve extensive anatomic and physiologic changes in the cardiovascular system. Cardiovascular adaptations protect the woman's normal physiologic functioning, meet the metabolic demands pregnancy imposes on her body, and provide for fetal developmental and growth needs.

Slight cardiac hypertrophy (enlargement) is probably secondary to increased blood volume and cardiac output that occur in pregnancy. The heart returns to its normal size after birth. As the diaphragm is displaced upward by the enlarging uterus, the heart is elevated upward and rotated forward to the left (Fig. 13-10). The apical impulse, or point of maximal intensity (PMI), is shifted upward and laterally about 1 to 1.5 cm. The degree of shift depends on the duration of pregnancy and the size and position of the uterus.

The changes in heart size and position and the increases in blood volume and cardiac output contribute to auscultatory changes common in pregnancy. There is more audible splitting of S_1 and S_2, and S_3 can be readily heard after 20 weeks of gestation. More than 95% of women develop systolic murmurs; they are most audible over the left sternal border. These changes are transient and disappear in most women shortly after they give birth.

Maternal heart rate begins to increase at about 5 weeks of gestation, reaching a peak of 10 to 15 beats/minute over the prepregnancy baseline by 32 weeks and persisting until term. In the late third trimester, this increased heart rate helps to maintain cardiac output (Monga & Mastrobattista, 2014).

The pregnant woman may experience palpitations and the cardiac rhythm can be disturbed. She can experience sinus dysrhythmia, premature atrial contractions, and premature ventricular systole. In the healthy woman with no underlying heart disease, no therapy is needed. Women with preexisting heart disease need close medical and obstetric supervision during pregnancy (see Chapter 30).

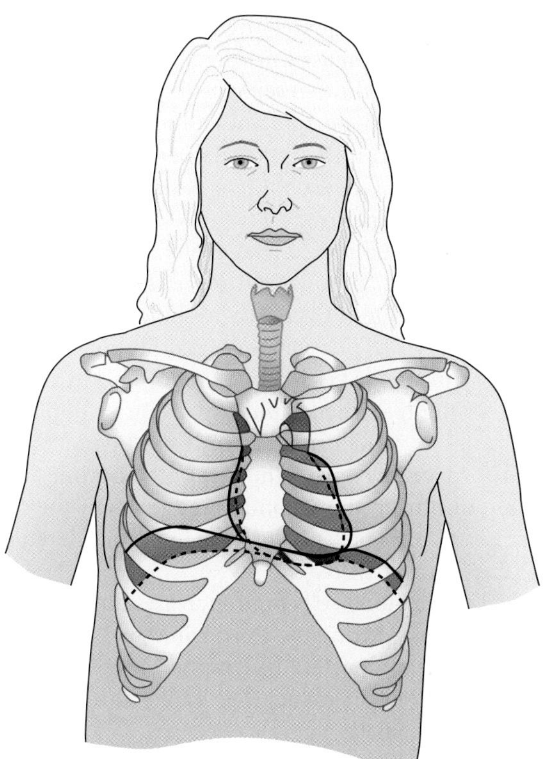

FIG 13-10 Changes in position of heart and in pregnancy. *Broken line,* Nonpregnant state; *solid line,* change that occurs in pregnancy.

Blood Pressure. Arterial blood pressure (brachial artery) varies with age, activity level, presence of health problems, circadian rhythm, use of alcohol, smoking, and pain. Additional factors to consider during pregnancy include maternal position and type of blood pressure apparatus. Maternal anxiety can elevate readings. If an elevated reading is found, the woman is given time to rest and the reading is repeated.

Maternal position affects readings. Brachial blood pressure is highest when the woman is sitting; lowest when she is lying in the lateral recumbent position; and intermediate when she is supine, except for some women who experience hypotensive syndrome (see later discussion). Therefore, at each prenatal visit the reading should be obtained in the same arm and with the woman in a seated position with her back and arm supported and her upper arm at the level of the right atrium. The position and arm used should be recorded along with the reading.

The proper-size cuff is essential for accurate readings. A cuff that is too small yields a falsely high reading; a cuff that is too large yields a falsely low reading (Box 13-1).

Caution should be used when comparing auscultatory and oscillatory blood pressure readings because discrepancies can occur. Automated monitors can give inaccurate readings in women with hypertensive conditions.

During pregnancy maternal blood pressure remains the same or decreases slightly. This is due to reduced systemic vascular resistance caused primarily by the vasodilatory effects of progesterone, prostaglandins, and relaxin. The uteroplacental vascular system holds a large percentage of the maternal blood volume, which also contributes to decreased systemic vascular resistance (Monga & Mastrobattista, 2014). Systemic vascular resistance is lowest at 16 to 34 weeks and increases gradually, approximating nonpregnant values by term. During the first trimester, systolic blood pressure usually remains the same as the prepregnancy level but can decrease slightly as pregnancy advances. Diastolic blood pressure begins to decrease in the first trimester, continues to drop until 24 to 32 weeks, and gradually increases, returning to prepregnancy levels by term (Blackburn, 2013).

BOX 13-1 Procedure for Blood Pressure Measurement

1. Use correct cuff size; cuff should cover approximately 80% of the upper arm or be 1.5 times the length of the upper arm.
2. Measure blood pressure (BP) after the woman sits for 5 minutes.
3. Instruct the woman to refrain from tobacco or caffeine use 30 minutes before BP measurement.
4. Measure BP with the woman sitting or semi-reclining with her feet flat, not dangling.
5. The arm should be supported on a desk at the level of the heart.
6. Measurements with an automated device should be checked with a manual device.
7. Diastolic pressure should be recorded at Korotkoff phase V (disappearance of sound).
8. If the BP is elevated, have the woman rest for 5 to 10 minutes and then retake it.
9. BP may vary by more than 10 mm Hg from one arm to the other; record the higher reading.
10. Take the average of two readings at least 1 minute apart.

Data from Peters, R. (2008). High blood pressure in pregnancy. *Nursing for Women's Health,* 12(5), 412-421.

BOX 13-2 Calculation of Mean Arterial Pressure

- Blood pressure: 106/70
- Formula:

Systolic + 2 (diastolic) /3
106 + 2 (70) /3
106 + 140/3
246/3 = 82 mm Hg

Calculating the *mean arterial pressure* (MAP) (mean of the blood pressure in the arterial circulation) can increase the diagnostic value of the findings. MAP is useful in predicting gestational hypertensive disorders in the second and third trimesters (Gaillard, Bakker, Willemsen, et al., 2011). Normal MAP readings in the nonpregnant woman are 86 ± 7.5 mm Hg. MAP readings during pregnancy range from 84 to 87 ± 7 (Galan & Goetzl, 2012). Box 13-2 illustrates one way to calculate MAP.

Some degree of compression of the vena cava occurs in any woman who lies on her back during the second half of pregnancy. Cardiac output is reduced by as much as 25% to 30% when a pregnant woman is turned from left lateral recumbent to supine position. Some women experience a fall of more than 30 mm Hg in their systolic pressure. After 4 to 5 minutes, a reflex bradycardia is noted, cardiac output is reduced by half, and the woman feels faint. This condition is called *supine hypotensive syndrome* or *vena caval syndrome* (Monga & Mastrobattista, 2014) (see Fig. 19-5).

Compression of the iliac veins and inferior vena cava by the uterus causes increased venous pressure and reduced blood flow in the legs, except when the woman is in the lateral position. These alterations contribute to the dependent edema, varicose veins in the legs and vulva, and hemorrhoids that develop in the latter part of term pregnancy.

Blood Volume and Composition. Total blood volume (TBV), consisting of plasma and red blood cell volume, increases significantly during pregnancy by approximately 30% to 45%. During the first half of pregnancy TBV increases rapidly, peaks around 28 to 34 weeks, and then stabilizes or decreases slightly by term (Blackburn, 2013). In a singleton pregnancy, plasma volume increases by approximately 1200 to 1500 ml, or 45% above prepregnancy levels by 32 weeks of gestation, decreasing slightly by term. By term, there is an increase in red blood cell mass of 250 to 450 ml, or approximately 20% to 30% over prepregnancy values (Monga & Mastrobattista, 2014). The percentage of increase depends on the amount of iron available (Blackburn). Increased blood volume is a protective mechanism. It is essential for meeting the blood volume needs of the hypertrophied vascular system of the enlarged uterus, for adequately hydrating fetal and maternal tissues when the woman assumes an erect or supine position, and for providing a fluid reserve to compensate for blood loss during birth and postpartum. Blood volume increases are greater with multiple gestation. Peripheral vasodilation allows for a normal blood pressure despite the increased blood volume in pregnancy.

Because the plasma increase is greater than the increase in red blood cell (RBC) production, there is a decrease in normal hemoglobin values (12 to 16 g/dl blood) and hematocrit values (37% to 47%). This state of hemodilution is referred to as *physiologic anemia.* The decrease is more noticeable during the second trimester, when rapid expansion of blood volume occurs faster than RBC production. If the hemoglobin value drops to 11 g/dl or less during the first or third trimester or less than 10.5 g/dl during the second trimester or if the hematocrit decreases to 32% or less, the woman is considered anemic (Hark & Catalano, 2012).

The total white blood cell count increases during the second trimester and peaks during the third trimester. This increase is primarily in the granulocytes; the lymphocyte count stays about the same throughout pregnancy. See Table 13-3 for laboratory values during pregnancy.

TABLE 13-3 Laboratory Values for Pregnant and Nonpregnant Women

VALUES	NONPREGNANT	PREGNANT
Hematologic		
Complete Blood Count		
Hemoglobin, g/dl	12-16*	>11*
Hematocrit, packed cell volume, %	37-47	>33*
RBC volume, per ml	1400	1650
Plasma volume, per ml	2400	40%-45% increase
RBC count, million/mm^3	4.2-5.4	5-6.25; 20%-30% increase
White blood cells, total per mm^3	5000-10,000	5000-15,000
Neutrophils, %	55-70	60-85
Lymphocytes, %	20-40	15-40
Erythrocyte sedimentation rate, mm/hr	20	Elevated in second and third trimesters
Mean corpuscular hemoglobin concentration (MCHC) (g/dl packed RBCs) g/dl packed RBCs	32-36	No change
Mean corpuscular hemoglobin (MCH) (pg), pg	27-31	No change
Mean corpuscular volume (MCV), per mm^3	80-95	No change
Blood Coagulation and Fibrinolytic Activity†		
Factor VII	65-140	Increases in pregnancy, returns to normal in early puerperium
Factor VIII	55-145	Increases during pregnancy and immediately after birth
Factor IX	60-140	Same as factor VII
Factor X	45-155	Same as factor VII
Factor XI	65-135	Decreases in pregnancy
Factor XII	50-150	Same as factor VII
Prothrombin time (PT), sec	11-12.5	Decreases slightly in pregnancy
Partial thromboplastin time (PTT), sec	60-70	Decreases slightly in pregnancy and decreases during second and third stages of labor (indicates clotting at placental site)
Bleeding time, min	1-9 (Ivy method)	No appreciable change
Coagulation time, min	6-10 (Lee-White method)	No appreciable change
Platelets, per mm^3	150,000-400,000	No significant change until 3-5 days after birth and then increases rapidly (may predispose woman to thrombosis) and gradually returns to normal
Fibrinolytic activity		Decreases in pregnancy and then abruptly returns to normal (protection against thromboembolism)
Fibrinogen, mg/dl	200-400	Levels increase late in pregnancy
Mineral/Vitamin Concentrations		
Vitamin B_{12}, folic acid, ascorbic acid	Normal	Moderate decrease

TABLE 13-3 Laboratory Values for Pregnant and Nonpregnant Women—cont'd

VALUES	NONPREGNANT	PREGNANT
Blood Glucose		
Fasting, mg/dl	70-105	60-90 before breakfast; 60-105 before lunch, supper, bedtime snack
2-hr postprandial, mg/dl	<140	<120
Acid-Base Values in Arterial Blood		
Po_2, mm Hg	80-100	104-108 (increased)
Pco_2, mm Hg	35-45	27-32 (decreased)
Sodium bicarbonate (HCO_3), mEq/L	21-28	18-31 (decreased)
Blood pH	7.35-7.45	7.40-7.45 (slightly increased, more alkaline)
Hepatic		
Bilirubin, total, mg/dl	≤1	Unchanged
Serum cholesterol, mg/dl	120-200	Increases from 16-32 wk of pregnancy; remains at this level until after birth
Serum alkaline phosphatase, units/L	30-120	Increases from wk 12 of pregnancy to 6 wk after birth
Serum albumin, g/dl	3.5-5	Increases 25% by term
Renal		
Bladder capacity, ml	1300	1500
Renal plasma flow, ml/min	490-700	Increases by 25%-30%
Glomerular filtration rate, ml/min	88-128	Increases by 30%-50%
Nonprotein nitrogen, mg/dl	25-40	Decreases
Blood urea nitrogen, mg/dl	10-20	Decreases
Serum creatinine, mg/dl	0.5-1.1	Decreases
Serum uric acid, mg/dl	2.7-7.3	Decreases but returns to prepregnancy level by end of pregnancy
Urine glucose	Negative	Present in 20% of pregnant women
Intravenous pyelogram	Normal	Slight to moderate hydroureter and hydronephrosis; right kidney larger than left kidney

pg, picogram; *RBC,* Red blood cell.

*At sea level. Permanent residents of higher levels (e.g., Denver) require higher levels of hemoglobin.

†Pregnancy represents a hypercoagulable state.

Data from Blackburn, S. (2013). *Maternal, fetal, & neonatal physiology: A clinical perspective* (4th ed.). St. Louis: Saunders; Gordon, M.C. (2012). Maternal physiology. In S.G. Gabbe, J.R. Niebyl, J.L. Simpson, et al. (Eds.), *Obstetrics: Normal and problem pregnancies* (6th ed.). Philadelphia: Saunders; Landon, M.B., Catalano, P.J., & Gabbe, S.G. (2012). Diabetes mellitus complicating pregnancy. In S.G. Gabbe, J.R. Niebyl, J.L. Simpson, et al. (Eds.), *Obstetrics: Normal and problem pregnancies* (6th ed.). Philadelphia: Saunders; Pagana, K.D., & Pagana, T.J. (2013). *Mosby's diagnostic and laboratory test reference* (11th ed.). St. Louis: Mosby; Samuels, P. (2012). Hematology complications of pregnancy. In S.G. Gabbe, J.R. Niebyl, J.L. Simpson, et al. (Eds.), *Obstetrics: Normal and problem pregnancies* (6th ed.). Philadelphia: Saunders.

Cardiac Output. Cardiac output increases 30% to 50% over the nonpregnant rate by week 32 of pregnancy; it declines to about a 20% increase at 40 weeks of gestation. This elevated cardiac output is largely a result of increased stroke volume and heart rate and occurs in response to increased tissue demands for oxygen (Monga & Mastrobattista, 2014). Cardiac output increases with any exertion such as labor and birth. Table 13-4 summarizes cardiovascular changes in pregnancy.

Circulation and Coagulation Times. Pregnancy is considered a hypercoagulable state in which women are at a five- to sixfold increased risk for thromboembolic disease (Gordon, 2012). The circulation time decreases slightly by week 32 and returns to near normal by term. There is a greater tendency for blood to coagulate (clot) during pregnancy because of increases in various clotting factors (i.e., factors VII, VIII, IX, X, and fibrinogen) and decreases in factors that inhibit coagulation (e.g., protein S). This tendency, combined with the fact that fibrinolytic activity (the splitting up or dissolving of a clot) is depressed during pregnancy and the postpartum period, provides a protective function to decrease the chance of bleeding but also makes the woman more vulnerable to thrombosis, especially after cesarean birth.

TABLE 13-4 Cardiovascular Changes in Pregnancy

PARAMETER	CHANGE
Heart rate	Increases 10 to 15 beats/min
Blood pressure	
Systolic	Slight or no decrease from prepregnancy levels
Diastolic	Slight decrease to midpregnancy (24-32 wk) and gradual return to prepregnancy levels by end of pregnancy
Blood volume	Increases by 1200 to 1500 ml or 40% to 45% above prepregnancy level
Cardiac output	Increases 30% to 50%

Data from Gordon, M.C. (2012). Maternal physiology. In S.G. Gabbe, J.R. Niebyl, J.L. Simpson, et al. (Eds.), *Obstetrics: Normal and problem pregnancies* (6th ed.). Philadelphia: Saunders

Respiratory System

Structural and ventilatory adaptations occur during pregnancy to provide for maternal and fetal needs. Maternal oxygen requirements increase in response to the acceleration in metabolic rate and the need to add to the tissue mass in the uterus and breasts. In addition, the fetus requires oxygen and a way to eliminate carbon dioxide.

TABLE 13-5 Respiratory Changes in Pregnancy

PARAMETER	CHANGE
Respiratory rate	Unchanged or slightly increased
Tidal volume	Increased 33%
Vital capacity	Unchanged
Inspiratory capacity	Increased 6%
Expiratory reserve volume	Decreased 20%
Total lung capacity	Unchanged to slightly decreased
Minute ventilation	Increased 30% to 50%
Oxygen consumption	Increased 20% to 40%

Data from Monga, M., & Mastrobattista, J.M. (2014). Maternal cardiovascular, respiratory, and renal adaptation to pregnancy. In R.K. Creasy, R. Resnik, J.D. Iams, et al. (Eds.), *Creasy & Resnik's maternal-fetal medicine: Principles and practice* (7th ed.). Philadelphia: Saunders.

Elevated levels of estrogen cause the ligaments of the rib cage to relax, permitting increased chest expansion. The transverse diameter of the thoracic cage increases by about 2 cm and the circumference by 6 cm. The costal angle increases, and the lower rib cage appears to flare out. The chest may not return to its prepregnant state after birth (Seidel, Ball, Dains, et al., 2011).

The diaphragm is displaced by as much as 4 cm during pregnancy. With advancing pregnancy, chest breathing replaces abdominal breathing and it becomes less possible for the diaphragm to descend with inspiration. Thoracic breathing is accomplished primarily by the diaphragm rather than by the costal muscles (Blackburn, 2013).

The upper respiratory tract becomes more vascular in response to elevated levels of estrogen. As the capillaries become engorged, edema and hyperemia develop within the nose, pharynx, larynx, trachea, and bronchi. This congestion within the tissues of the respiratory tract gives rise to several conditions commonly seen during pregnancy, including nasal and sinus stuffiness, epistaxis (nosebleed), changes in the voice, and marked inflammatory response to even a mild upper respiratory infection (Gordon, 2012).

Increased vascularity of the upper respiratory tract also can cause the tympanic membranes and eustachian tubes to swell, giving rise to symptoms of impaired hearing, earaches, or a sense of fullness in the ears.

Pulmonary Function. Respiratory changes in pregnancy are related to the elevation of the diaphragm and changes in the chest wall. Changes in the respiratory center result in a lowered threshold for carbon dioxide. The actions of progesterone and estrogen are presumed to be responsible for the increased sensitivity of the respiratory center to carbon dioxide. See Table 13-5 for respiratory changes in pregnancy. Although pulmonary function is not impaired by pregnancy, diseases of the respiratory tract can be more serious during this time. One important factor responsible for this can be the increase in oxygen requirements.

Basal Metabolic Rate. The basal metabolic rate (BMR) increases during pregnancy. The elevation in BMR reflects increased oxygen demands of the uterine-placental-fetal unit and greater oxygen consumption because of increased maternal cardiac work. This increase varies considerably, depending on the prepregnancy nutritional status of the woman and fetal growth. By the third trimester the BMR is increased by 10% to 20% over the nonpregnant state. The BMR returns to nonpregnant levels by 5 to 6 days after birth. Peripheral vasodilation and acceleration of sweat gland activity help dissipate the excess heat resulting from the increased BMR during pregnancy. Pregnant women can experience heat intolerance. Lassitude and fatigability after only slight exertion are experienced by many women in early pregnancy. These feelings, along with a greater need for sleep, can persist and be caused in part by the increased metabolic activity.

Acid-Base Balance. By about the tenth week of pregnancy, there is a decrease of about 5 mm Hg in the partial pressure of carbon dioxide (Pco_2). Progesterone may be responsible for increasing the sensitivity of the respiratory center receptors so that tidal volume increases and Pco_2 decreases, the base excess (HCO_3, or bicarbonate) decreases, and pH increases slightly. These alterations in acid-base balance indicate that pregnancy is a state of respiratory alkalosis (Gordon, 2012) (see Table 13-3). These changes also facilitate the transport of CO_2 from the fetus and O_2 release from the mother to the fetus.

Renal System

The kidneys are responsible for maintaining electrolyte and acid-base balance, regulating extracellular fluid volume, excreting waste products, and conserving essential nutrients.

Anatomic Changes. Changes in renal structure result from hormonal activity (estrogen and progesterone), pressure from an enlarging uterus, and an increase in blood volume. As early as the tenth week of pregnancy, the renal pelves and the ureters dilate. Dilation of the ureters is more pronounced above the pelvic brim, in part because they are compressed between the uterus and the pelvic brim. In most women the ureters below the pelvic brim are normal size. The smooth-muscle walls of the ureters undergo hyperplasia and hypertrophy and muscle tone relaxation. The ureters elongate, become tortuous, and form single or double curves. In the latter part of pregnancy the renal pelvis and ureter dilate more on the right side than on the left because the heavy uterus is displaced to the right by the sigmoid colon (Monga & Mastrobattista, 2014).

Because of these changes, a larger volume of urine is held in the pelves and ureters and urine flow rate is slowed. Urinary stasis or stagnation has several consequences:

- A lag occurs between the time urine is formed and when it reaches the bladder. Therefore, clearance test results may reflect substances contained in glomerular filtrate several hours before.
- Stagnated urine is an excellent medium for the growth of microorganisms. In addition, the urine of pregnant women contains more nutrients, including glucose, that increase the pH (making the urine more alkaline). This makes pregnant women more susceptible to urinary tract infection (Cheung & Lafayette, 2013).

Bladder irritability, nocturia, and urinary frequency and urgency (without dysuria) are commonly reported in early pregnancy. These bladder symptoms may return near term, especially after lightening occurs.

Urinary frequency results initially from increased bladder sensitivity and later from compression of the bladder (see Fig. 13-8). In the second trimester the bladder is pulled up out of the true pelvis into the abdomen. The urethra lengthens to

7.5 cm as the bladder is displaced upward. The pelvic congestion that occurs in pregnancy is reflected in hyperemia of the bladder and urethra. This increased vascularity causes the bladder mucosa to be easily traumatized. Bladder tone may decrease, which increases the bladder capacity to 1500 ml. At the same time, the bladder is compressed by the enlarging uterus, resulting in the urge to void even if the bladder contains only a small amount of urine.

Functional Changes. In normal pregnancy renal function is altered considerably. Renal plasma flow (RPF) rises significantly from early in pregnancy, peaking by the end of the first trimester. RPF remains elevated above nonpregnant levels throughout pregnancy, although it begins to decrease somewhat as term approaches (Colombo, 2012). By the end of the first trimester, glomerular filtration rate (GFR) has increased by 50% and remains elevated throughout pregnancy. These changes are caused by pregnancy hormones; an increase in blood volume; and the woman's posture, physical activity, and nutritional intake. The woman's kidneys must manage the increased metabolic and circulatory demands of the maternal body as well as the excretion of fetal waste products. The increase in GFR results in increased creatinine clearance and a reduction in serum creatinine, blood urea nitrogen (BUN), and uric acid levels (Gordon, 2012).

Renal function is most efficient when the woman lies in the lateral recumbent position and least efficient when the woman assumes a supine position. A side-lying position increases renal perfusion, which increases urine output and decreases edema. When the pregnant woman is lying supine, the heavy uterus compresses the vena cava and the aorta, and cardiac output decreases. As a result, blood flow to the brain and heart is continued at the expense of other organs, including the kidneys and uterus.

Fluid and Electrolyte Balance. Selective renal tubular reabsorption maintains sodium and water balance, regardless of changes in dietary intake and losses through sweat, vomitus, or diarrhea. About 950 mg of sodium is cumulatively retained during pregnancy to meet fetal needs, although maternal serum levels of sodium decrease by 3 to 4 mmol/L (Gordon, 2012). To prevent excessive sodium depletion, the maternal kidneys undergo a significant adaptation by increasing tubular reabsorption. Because of the need for increased maternal intravascular and extracellular fluid volume, additional sodium is needed to expand fluid volume and maintain an isotonic state.

MEDICATION ALERT

As efficient as the renal system is, it can be overstressed by excessive dietary sodium intake or restriction or by use of diuretics. Severe hypovolemia and reduced placental perfusion are two consequences of using diuretics during pregnancy.

The capacity of the kidneys to excrete water is more efficient during the early weeks than later in pregnancy. As a result, some women feel thirsty in early pregnancy because of the greater amount of water loss. The pooling of fluid in the legs in the latter part of pregnancy decreases renal blood flow and GFR. This pooling is sometimes referred to as *physiologic or dependent edema* and requires no treatment. The normal diuretic response to the water load is triggered when the woman lies down, preferably on her side, and the pooled fluid reenters general circulation.

Normally the kidney reabsorbs almost all the glucose and other nutrients from the plasma filtrate. However, in pregnant women tubular reabsorption of glucose is impaired, causing glucosuria to occur at varying times and to varying degrees (Cheung & Lafayette, 2013). Nonpregnant women excrete less than 100 mg/day, whereas pregnant women with normal blood glucose levels excrete 1 to 10 g of glucose each day (Gordon, 2012). The mechanism by which this occurs is unclear, although it may be related to the increased GFR and tubular flow rate that exceeds the capacity for tubular reabsorption of glucose (Blackburn, 2013). Although glucosuria can be found in normal pregnancies (2+ levels can be seen with increased anxiety states), the possibility of diabetes mellitus and gestational diabetes must be considered.

During normal pregnancy there is an increase in urinary excretion of protein and albumin, most notable after 20 weeks of gestation (Cheung & Lafayette, 2013). This is due to increased GFR and impaired proximal tubular function. It is considered abnormal when proteinuria exceeds 300 mg/24 hours or albuminuria is greater than 30 mg/24 hours. The amount of protein excreted is not an indication of the severity of renal disease, nor does an increase in protein excretion in a pregnant woman with known renal disease necessarily indicate a progression in her disease. However, a pregnant woman with hypertension and proteinuria must be evaluated carefully because she may be at greater risk for adverse pregnancy outcomes (Gordon, 2012).

Integumentary System

Alterations in hormone balance and mechanical stretching are responsible for several changes in the integumentary system during pregnancy. Hyperpigmentation is stimulated by the anterior pituitary hormone *melanotropin,* which is increased during pregnancy. Darkening of the nipples, areolae, axillae, and vulva occurs at about the sixteenth week of gestation. Melasma (also called chloasma or mask of pregnancy) is a blotchy, brownish hyperpigmentation of the skin over the cheeks, nose, and forehead, especially in pregnant women with dark complexions. Melasma appears in 50% to 70% of pregnant women, beginning after the sixteenth week and increasing gradually until term. The sun intensifies this pigmentation in susceptible women. Melasma caused by normal pregnancy usually fades after birth but often recurs with oral contraceptive use or subsequent pregnancies (Kroumpouzos, 2012).

The linea nigra (Fig. 13-11) is a pigmented line extending from the symphysis pubis to the top of the fundus in the midline. This line is known as the linea alba before hormone-induced pigmentation. In primigravidas, the extension of the linea nigra, beginning in the third month, keeps pace with the rising height of the fundus; in multigravidas, the entire line often appears earlier than the third month. Not all pregnant women develop linea nigra, and some women notice hair growth along the line with or without the change in pigmentation.

Striae gravidarum (see Fig. 13-11) appear in 50% to 80% of pregnant women during the second half of pregnancy. Striae reflect separation within the underlying connective (collagen) tissue of the skin. These slightly depressed streaks tend to

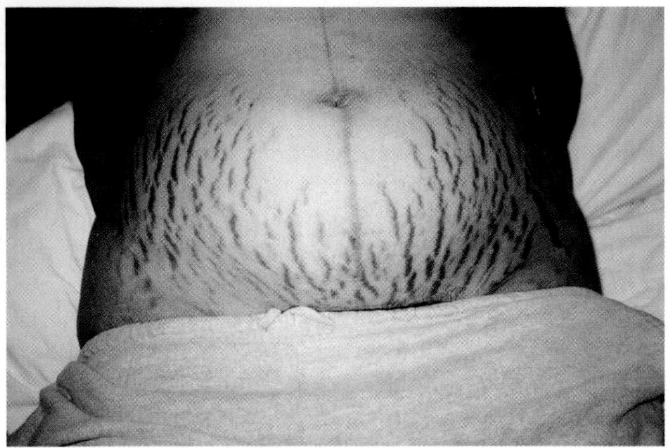

FIG 13-11 Striae gravidarum and linea nigra in a dark-skinned person. (Courtesy Shannon Perry, Phoenix, AZ.)

occur over areas of maximum stretch (the abdomen, thighs, and breasts). The stretching sometimes causes a sensation that resembles itching. The tendency to develop striae may be familial (Rapini, 2014). After birth they usually fade, although they never disappear completely. No topical therapy has been shown to affect the course of striae, although pulsed laser therapy can reduce redness of early lesions (Rapini).

Angiomas are commonly referred to as vascular spiders. These tiny star-shaped or branched, slightly raised, and pulsating end-arterioles are usually found on the neck, thorax, face, and arms. They occur as a result of elevated levels of circulating estrogens. The spiders are bluish and do not blanch with pressure. Vascular spiders appear during the second to fifth months of pregnancy in about 65% of Caucasian women and 10% of African-American women. The spiders usually disappear after birth (Blackburn, 2013).

Pinkish red, diffusely mottled, or well-defined blotches are seen over the palmar surfaces of the hands in about 70% of Caucasian women and 30% of African-American women during pregnancy (Krompouzos, 2012). These color changes, called **palmar erythema,** are related primarily to increased estrogen levels.

Some dermatologic conditions have been identified as unique to pregnancy or as having an increased incidence during pregnancy. The most common dermatologic symptom during pregnancy is itching (pruritis). Mild pruritus, also known as **pruritus gravidarum,** usually occurs over the abdomen. Less than 2% of women have significant pruritus that requires further evaluation (Krompouzos, 2012). The problem usually resolves during the postpartum period.

The most common specific dermatosis is **pruritic urticarial papules and plaques of pregnancy (PUPPP),** affecting 1 in 130 to 1 in 300 pregnancies. PUPPP is more common in multiple gestations. Although it can cause significant maternal discomfort, it does not cause adverse outcomes for the mother or fetus. Mild PUPPP is usually treated with oral antihistamines and topical antipruritic and corticosteroid creams. Oral steroids may be needed in more severe cases (Krompouzos, 2012) (see Chapter 30 and Fig. 30-1).

The effect of pregnancy on acne is variable. In some women the skin clears and looks radiant. Acne can worsen or occur for the first time during pregnancy or postpartum. Commonly used topical treatments for acne (e.g., benzyl peroxide, topical antibiotics) are considered safe during pregnancy; topical retinoids should be avoided in the first trimester (Tyler & Zirwas, 2013).

MEDICATION ALERT

Women with severe acne taking isotretinoin (e.g., Accutane) should avoid pregnancy while receiving the treatment because it is teratogenic and is associated with fetal loss and major fetal malformations (Tyler & Zirwas, 2013).

Nail and hair growth may be accelerated. Some women notice thinning and softening of the nails. Hirsutism, the excessive growth of hair or growth of hair in unusual places, is commonly reported. An increase in fine hair growth can occur but tends to disappear after pregnancy. However, growth of coarse or bristly hair does not usually disappear after pregnancy. The rate of scalp hair loss slows during pregnancy; increased hair loss may be noted in the postpartum period (Rapini, 2014).

Increased blood supply to the skin leads to increased perspiration. Women feel hotter during pregnancy, possibly related to a progesterone-induced increase in body temperature and the increased BMR.

Musculoskeletal System

The gradually changing body and increasing weight of pregnancy usually cause noticeable changes in a woman's posture (Fig. 13-12). The great abdominal distention that causes the pelvis to tilt forward, decreased abdominal muscle tone, and increased weight bearing require a realignment of the spinal curvatures. The woman's center of gravity shifts forward. An increase in the normal lumbosacral curve (lordosis) develops, and a compensatory curvature in the cervicodorsal region (exaggerated anterior flexion of the head) develops to help her maintain balance. Aching, numbness, and weakness of the upper extremities can result. Large breasts and a stoop-shouldered stance further accentuate the lumbar and dorsal curves. The ligamentous and muscular structures of the middle and lower spine can be severely stressed. These and related changes often cause musculoskeletal discomfort such as back pain, especially in older women or those with a back disorder or a faulty sense of balance.

The hormones relaxin and progesterone cause loosening of ligaments of the pubic symphysis and sacroiliac joints to facilitate labor and birth. By 28 to 32 weeks of gestation, the symphysis widens from approximately 3 to 4 mm to 7.7 to 7.9 mm. Separation of the symphysis pubis and the instability of the sacroiliac joints can cause pain and difficulty in walking. A waddling gait is common. Obesity or multifetal pregnancy tends to increase the pelvic instability (Gordon, 2012).

SAFETY ALERT

Pregnant women are at increased risk of falling due to the shifting center of gravity, impaired balance, and joint laxity.

The muscles of the abdominal wall stretch and ultimately lose some tone. During the third trimester the rectus abdominis muscles can separate **(diastasis recti abdominis)** (Fig. 13-13),

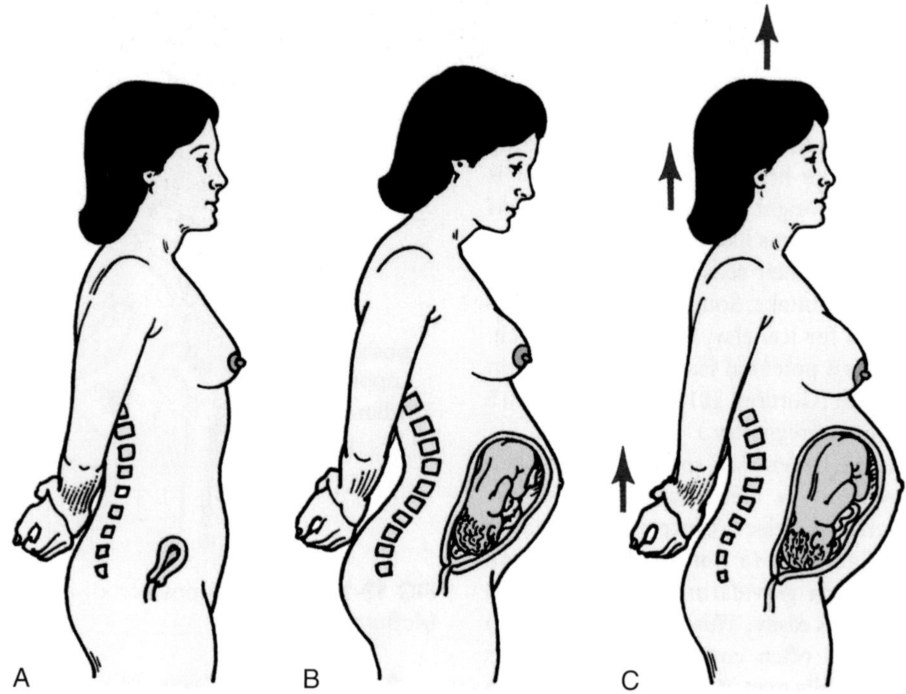

FIG 13-12 Postural changes during pregnancy. **A,** Nonpregnant. **B,** Incorrect posture during pregnancy. **C,** Correct posture during pregnancy.

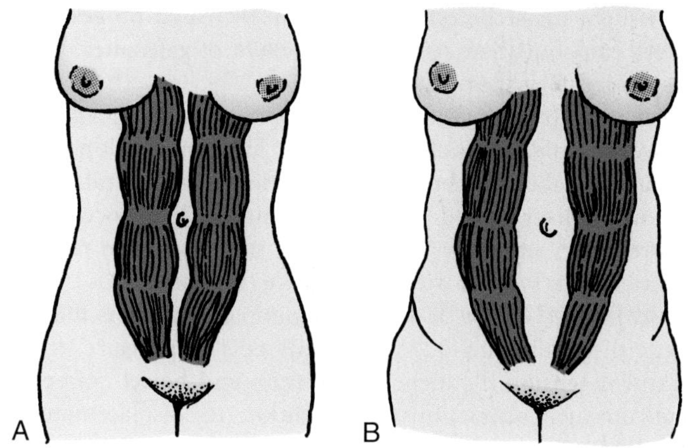

FIG 13-13 Possible change in rectus abdominis muscles during pregnancy. **A,** Normal position in nonpregnant woman. **B,** Diastasis recti abdominis in pregnant woman.

allowing abdominal contents to protrude at the midline. The umbilicus flattens or protrudes. After birth, the muscles gradually regain tone. However, separation of the muscles can persist.

Neurologic System

Little is known about specific alterations in function of the neurologic system during pregnancy aside from hypothalamic-pituitary neurohormonal changes. Specific physiologic alterations resulting from pregnancy can cause the following neurologic or neuromuscular symptoms:

- Compression of pelvic nerves or vascular stasis caused by enlargement of the uterus can result in sensory changes in the legs.
- Dorsolumbar lordosis can cause pain because of traction on nerves or compression of nerve roots.
- Edema involving the peripheral nerves can result in carpal tunnel syndrome during the last trimester. The syndrome is characterized by paresthesia (abnormal sensation such as burning or tingling) and pain in the hand, radiating to the elbow. The sensations are caused by edema that compresses the median nerve beneath the carpal ligament of the wrist. Smoking and alcohol consumption can impair the microcirculation and worsen the symptoms. The dominant hand is usually affected most, although many women report symptoms in both hands. Symptoms usually regress after pregnancy. In some cases, surgical treatment is necessary.
- Acroesthesia (numbness and tingling of the hands) is caused by the stoop-shouldered stance (see Fig. 13-11, *B*) assumed by some women during pregnancy. The condition is associated with traction on segments of the brachial plexus.
- Tension headache is common when anxiety or uncertainty complicates pregnancy. However, vision problems such as refractive errors, sinusitis, or migraine may also be responsible for headaches.
- Lightheadedness, faintness, and even syncope (fainting) are common during early pregnancy. Vasomotor instability, postural hypotension, or hypoglycemia may be responsible.
- Hypocalcemia can cause neuromuscular problems such as muscle cramps or tetany.

Gastrointestinal System

Appetite. During pregnancy a woman's appetite and food intake fluctuate. Early in pregnancy some women have nausea with or without vomiting ("morning sickness"), possibly in response to increasing levels of hCG and altered carbohydrate metabolism (Gordon, 2012). Nausea and vomiting of pregnancy (NVP) appears at about 4 to 6 weeks of gestation and usually subsides by the end of the third month (first trimester) of pregnancy (see Chapter 15). Severity varies from mild distaste for certain foods to more severe vomiting. The condition can be triggered by the sight or odor of various foods. By the end of the second trimester the appetite increases in response to increasing metabolic needs. Rarely does NVP have harmful effects on the embryo, the fetus, or the woman. Whenever the vomiting is severe or persists beyond the first trimester or when it is accompanied by fever, pain, or weight loss, further evaluation is necessary and medical intervention is likely.

Women can have changes in their sense of taste, leading to cravings and changes in dietary intake. Some women have nonfood cravings (pica) such as for ice, clay, and laundry starch. Pica should be considered as a potential factor in cases of iron deficiency or poor weight gain (Gordon, 2012). (See Chapter 15 for a discussion of nutrition in pregnancy.)

Mouth. The gums become hyperemic, spongy, and swollen during pregnancy. They tend to bleed easily because the increasing levels of estrogen cause selective increased vascularity and connective tissue proliferation (a nonspecific gingivitis). An epulis (gingival granuloma gravidarum) is a red, raised nodule on the gums that bleeds easily. This lesion may develop around the third month and often continues to enlarge as pregnancy progresses. It is usually managed by avoiding trauma to the gums (e.g., using a soft toothbrush). An epulis commonly regresses spontaneously after birth.

Some pregnant women complain of ptyalism (excessive salivation), which can be caused by the unconscious decrease in swallowing by the woman when nauseated or caused by stimulation of salivary glands by eating starch.

Esophagus, Stomach, and Intestines. Increased progesterone causes decreased tone and motility of smooth muscles, resulting in esophageal regurgitation (reflux), slower emptying time of the stomach, and reverse peristalsis. As a result, the woman can experience acid indigestion, or heartburn (pyrosis), beginning as early as the first trimester and intensifying through the third trimester.

The incidence of hiatal hernia is increased during pregnancy as a result of the upward displacement of the stomach by the enlarging uterus, which causes a widening of the hiatus of the diaphragm. Hiatal hernia occurs more often in multiparas and older or obese women.

In response to increased needs during pregnancy, iron is absorbed more readily in the small intestine. Even when the woman is deficient in iron, it continues to be absorbed in sufficient amounts for the fetus to have a normal hemoglobin level.

Smooth muscle relaxation and reduced peristalsis caused by increased progesterone and estrogen result in an increase in water absorption from the colon and can cause constipation (Gordon, 2012). Constipation can also result from food choices, lack of fluids, iron supplementation, decreased activity level, abdominal distention by the pregnant uterus, and displacement and compression of the intestines. If the pregnant woman has hemorrhoids and is constipated, the hemorrhoids can evert or bleed during straining at stool.

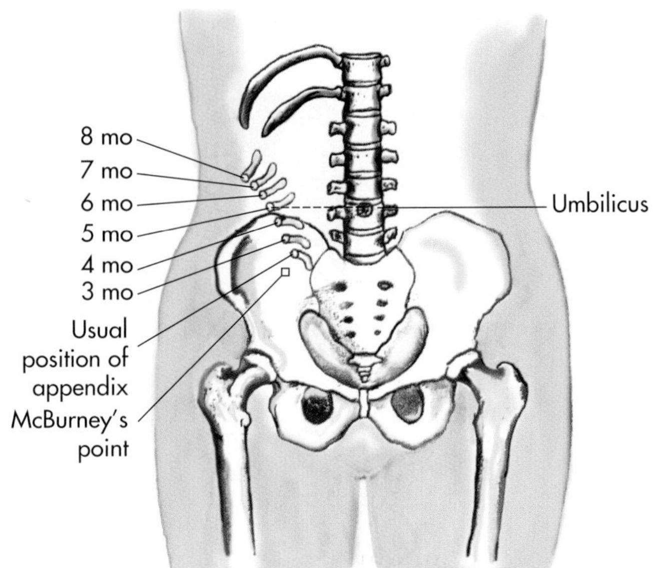

FIG 13-14 Change in position of appendix in pregnancy. Note McBurney's point.

Gallbladder and Liver. The gallbladder is often distended because of its decreased muscle tone during pregnancy. Increased emptying time and thickening of bile caused by prolonged retention are typical changes. These features, together with slight hypercholesterolemia from increased progesterone levels, can contribute to the development of gallstones during pregnancy (Blackburn, 2013).

Hepatic function is difficult to appraise during pregnancy. However, only minor changes in liver function develop. Occasionally intrahepatic cholestasis (retention and accumulation of bile in the liver caused by factors within the liver) occurs late in pregnancy in response to placental steroids. It can result in severe itching with or without jaundice (Rapini, 2014).

Abdominal Discomfort. Intraabdominal alterations that can cause discomfort include pelvic heaviness or pressure, round ligament tension, flatulence, distention and bowel cramping, and uterine contractions. In addition to displacement of intestines, pressure from the expanding uterus causes an increase in venous pressure in the pelvic organs. Although most abdominal discomfort is a consequence of normal maternal alterations, the health care provider must be constantly alert to the possibility of disorders such as bowel obstruction or an inflammatory process.

Appendicitis can be difficult to diagnose in pregnancy because the appendix is displaced upward and laterally, high and to the right, away from McBurney's point (Fig. 13-14).

Endocrine System

Profound endocrine changes are essential for pregnancy maintenance, normal fetal growth, and postpartum recovery. Hormones, their sources, and their effects on the pregnancy are presented in Table 13-6.

TABLE 13-6 Hormones and Effects of Changes During Pregnancy

HORMONE	SOURCE	EFFECTS OF CHANGES DURING PREGNANCY
Human chorionic gonadotropin (hCG)	Fertilized ovum and chorionic villi	Maintains corpus luteum production of estrogen and progesterone until placenta takes over the function
Progesterone	Corpus luteum until 14 wk of gestation, then the placenta	Suppresses secretion of FSH and LH by the anterior pituitary; maintains pregnancy by relaxing smooth muscles, decreasing uterine contractility; causes fat to deposit in subcutaneous tissues over the maternal abdomen, back, and upper thighs; decreases mother's ability to use insulin
Estrogen	Corpus luteum until 14 wk of gestation, then the placenta	Suppresses secretion of FSH and LH by the anterior pituitary; causes fat to deposit in subcutaneous tissues over the maternal abdomen, back, and upper thighs; promotes enlargement of genitals, uterus, and breasts; increases vascularity; relaxes pelvic ligaments and joints; interferes with folic acid metabolism; increases the level of total body proteins; promotes retention of sodium and water; decreases secretion of hydrochloric acid and pepsin; decreases mother's ability to use insulin
Serum prolactin	Anterior pituitary	Prepares breasts for lactation
Oxytocin	Posterior pituitary	Stimulates uterine contractions; stimulates milk ejection from breasts
Human chorionic somatomammotropin (previously called *human placental lactogen)*	Placenta	Acts as a growth hormone; contributes to breast development; decreases maternal metabolism of glucose; increases the amount of fatty acids for metabolic needs
Thyroxine-binding globulin, thyroxine, triiodothyronine	Thyroid	With adequate iodine intake, little or no enlargement of thyroid gland. Total T_3 and T_4 levels are slightly increased, peak by midpregnancy; by term are 10% to 15% lower than nonpregnant.
Parathyroid	Parathyroid	Controls calcium and magnesium metabolism
Insulin	Pancreas	Increases production of insulin to compensate for insulin antagonism caused by placental hormones; effect of insulin antagonists is to decrease tissue sensitivity to insulin or ability to use insulin
Cortisol	Adrenal glands	Stimulates production of insulin; increases peripheral resistance to insulin
Aldosterone	Adrenal glands	Stimulates reabsorption of excess sodium from the renal tubules

FSH, Follicle-stimulating hormone; LH, luteinizing hormone.

KEY POINTS

- The biochemical, physiologic, and anatomic adaptations that occur during pregnancy are profound and revert to the nonpregnant state after birth and lactation.
- Maternal adaptations are attributed to the hormones of pregnancy and to mechanical pressures arising from the enlarging uterus and other tissues.
- Adaptations to pregnancy protect the woman's normal physiologic functioning, meet the metabolic demands that pregnancy imposes, and provide for fetal developmental and growth needs.
- Accuracy of results of home pregnancy tests is dependent on following instructions correctly.
- Presumptive, probable, and positive signs of pregnancy aid in the diagnosis of pregnancy; only positive signs (identification of a fetal heart tone, verification of fetal movements, and visualization of the fetus) can establish the diagnosis of pregnancy.
- Physiologic anemia of pregnancy results from increase in plasma volume greater than the increase in red blood cells.
- During pregnancy maternal blood pressure remains the same or decreases slightly.
- Heart rate increases 10 to 15 beats/minute by 32 weeks of gestation and persists until term.
- Respiratory rate is unchanged during pregnancy, although tidal volume and minute ventilation increase by 30% to 50%.
- Pregnancy is a hypercoagulable state with increased risk for thrombotic disease.
- Dilation of renal pelves and ureters during pregnancy increases the risk of urinary tract infection.
- Balance and coordination are affected by changes in joints and in the woman's center of gravity as pregnancy progresses.
- Decreased muscle tone during pregnancy contributes to heartburn, reflux, and constipation.
- Endocrine changes are essential to maintaining pregnancy and promoting fetal growth.

REFERENCES

American College of Obstetricians and Gynecologists (ACOG) Committee on Obstetric Practice & Society for Maternal-Fetal Medicine (SMFM). (2013). Committee opinion no. 579: Definition of term pregnancy. *Obstetrics and Gynecology, 122*(5), 1139–1140.

Blackburn, S. (2013). *Maternal, fetal, & neonatal physiology: A clinical perspective* (4th ed.). St. Louis: Saunders.

Cheung, K. L., & Lafayette, R. A. (2013). Renal physiology of pregnancy. *Advances in Chronic Kidney Disease, 20*(3), 209–214.

Columbo, D. F. (2012). Renal disease. In S. G. Gabbe, J. R. Niebyl, J. L. Simpson, et al. (Eds.), *Obstetrics: Normal and problem pregnancies* (6th ed.). Philadelphia: Saunders.

Gaillard, R., Bakker, R., Willemsen, S. P., et al. (2011). Blood pressure tracking during pregnancy and the risk of gestational hypertensive disorders: The Generation R study. *European Heart Journal, 32*(24), 3088–3097.

Galan, H. L., & Goetzl, L. (2012). Normal values in pregnancy. In S. G. Gabbe, J. R. Niebyl, J. L. Simpson, et al. (Eds.), *Obstetrics: Normal and problem pregnancies* (6th ed.). Philadelphia: Saunders.

Gordon, M. C. (2012). Maternal physiology. In S. G. Gabbe, J. R. Niebyl, J. L. Simpson, et al. (Eds.), *Obstetrics: Normal and problem pregnancies* (6th ed.). Philadelphia: Saunders.

Hark, L., & Catalano, P. M. (2012). Nutritional management during pregnancy. In S. G. Gabbe, J. R. Niebyl, J. L. Simpson, et al. (Eds.), *Obstetrics: Normal and problem pregnancies* (6th ed.). Philadelphia: Saunders.

Kroumpouzos, G. (2012). Skin disease in pregnancy and puerperium. In S. G. Gabbe, J. R. Niebyl, J. L. Simpson, et al. (Eds.), *Obstetrics: Normal and problem pregnancies* (6th ed.). Philadelphia: Saunders.

Lawrence, R. A., & Lawrence, R. M. (2011). *Breastfeeding: A guide for the medical profession* (7th ed.). St. Louis: Mosby.

Liu, J. H. (2014). Endocrinology of pregnancy. In R. K. Creasy, R. Resnik, J. D. Iams, et al. (Eds.), *Creasy & Resnik's maternal-fetal medicine: Principles and practice* (7th ed.). Philadelphia: Saunders.

Monga, M., & Mastrobattista, J. M. (2014). Maternal cardiovascular, respiratory, and renal adaptation to pregnancy. In R. K. Creasy, R. Resnik, J. D. Iams, et al. (Eds.), *Creasy & Resnik's maternal-fetal medicine: Principles and practice* (7th ed.). Philadelphia: Saunders.

Norwitz, E. R., Mahendroo, M., & Lye, S. J. (2014). Biology of parturition. In R. K. Creasy, R. Resnik, J. D. Iams, et al. (Eds.), *Creasy & Resnik's maternal-fetal medicine: Principles and practice* (7th ed.). Philadelphia: Saunders.

Pagana, K. D., & Pagana, T. J. (2013). *Mosby's diagnostic and laboratory test reference* (11th ed.). St. Louis: Mosby.

Rapini, R. P. (2014). The skin and pregnancy. In R. K. Creasy, R. Resnik, J. D. Iams, et al. (Eds.), *Creasy & Resnik's maternal-fetal medicine: Principles and practice* (7th ed.). Philadelphia: Saunders.

Salani, R., Eisenhauer, E. L., & Copeland, L. J. (2012). Malignant diseases and pregnancy. In S. G. Gabbe, J. R. Niebyl, J. L. Simpson, et al. (Eds.), *Obstetrics: Normal and problem pregnancies* (6th ed.). Philadelphia: Saunders.

Seidel, H. M., Ball, J. W., Dains, J. E., et al. (2011). *Mosby's guide to physical examination* (7th ed.). St. Louis: Mosby.

Tyler, K. H., & Zirwas, M. J. (2013). Pregnancy and dermatologic therapy. *Journal of the American Academy of Dermatology, 68*(4), 663–671.

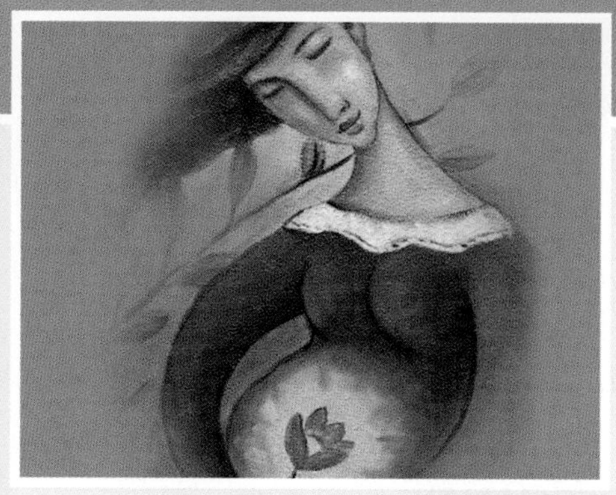

CHAPTER 14

Nursing Care of the Family During Pregnancy

Denise G. Link

http://evolve.elsevier.com/Lowdermilk/MWHC/

LEARNING OBJECTIVES

- Describe strategies for confirming pregnancy and estimating the date of birth.
- Summarize the physical, psychosocial, and behavioral changes that usually occur as the expectant mother and other family members adapt to pregnancy.
- Evaluate the benefits of prenatal care and problems of accessibility for some women.
- Outline the patterns of health care used to assess maternal and fetal health status at initial and follow-up visits during pregnancy.
- Select the typical nursing assessments, diagnoses, interventions, and methods of evaluation in providing care for the pregnant woman.
- Plan education needed by pregnant women to understand and manage physical discomforts related to pregnancy and to recognize signs and symptoms of potential complications.
- Evaluate the effect of age, parity, and number of fetuses on the response of the family to the pregnancy and on the prenatal care provided.
- Analyze the effects of cultural beliefs and practices on care of women during pregnancy.
- Compare the options for health care providers and birth setting choices that are available.

The prenatal period is a time of physical and psychologic preparation for birth and parenthood. Becoming a parent is considered one of the maturational milestones of adult life. It is a time of intense learning for parents and those close to them. The prenatal period provides a unique opportunity for nurses and other members of the health care team to influence family health. During this period essentially healthy women seek regular care and guidance. The nurse's health promotion interventions can affect the well-being of the woman, her unborn child, and the rest of her family for many years.

Regular prenatal visits, ideally beginning soon after the first missed menstrual period, offer opportunities to safeguard the health of the expectant mother and her infant. Prenatal health care enables discovery, diagnosis, and treatment of preexisting maternal disorders and any disorders that develop during the pregnancy. Prenatal care is designed to monitor the growth and development of the fetus and to identify abnormalities that will interfere with the course of normal labor. Prenatal care also provides education and support for self-management and parenting.

Pregnancy spans 9 months, but health care providers do not use the familiar monthly calendar to determine fetal age or to discuss the pregnancy. Instead, they use lunar months, which last 28 days, or 4 weeks. Normal pregnancy lasts about 10 lunar months, which is the same as 40 weeks or 280 days. Health care providers also refer to early, middle, and late pregnancy as trimesters. The first trimester lasts from weeks 1 through 13; the second, from weeks 14 through 26; and the third, from weeks 27 through 40. A pregnancy is considered to be at term if it advances to the completion of 37 weeks. The focus of this chapter is on meeting the health needs of the expectant family over the course of pregnancy, which is known as the *prenatal period*.

DIAGNOSIS OF PREGNANCY

Women suspect pregnancy when they miss a menstrual period. Many women come to the first prenatal visit after a positive home pregnancy test; however, the clinical diagnosis of pregnancy before the second missed period is difficult in some women. Physical variations, obesity, or tumors, for example, confound even the experienced examiner. Accuracy is important, however, because emotional, social, health, or legal consequences of an inaccurate diagnosis, either positive or negative, can be extremely serious.

Signs and Symptoms

The physical cues of pregnancy vary greatly; therefore, the diagnosis of pregnancy is uncertain for a time. Many of the indicators of pregnancy are clinically useful in the diagnosis of pregnancy and are classified as presumptive, probable, or positive (see Table 13-2).

Presumptive indicators of pregnancy include subjective symptoms and objective signs. Subjective symptoms are reported by the woman and include amenorrhea, nausea and vomiting (morning sickness), breast tenderness, urinary frequency, and fatigue. *Quickening*, the mother's first perception of fetal movement, is noted between weeks 16 and 20. Objective signs that are validated by the examiner include elevation of basal body temperature (BBT), breast and abdominal enlargement, and changes in the uterus and vagina. Other visible changes occur in the skin, such as striae gravidarum, deeper pigmentation of the areola, melasma (mask of pregnancy), and linea nigra (pigmented line on the abdomen). The presumptive indicators of pregnancy can be caused by conditions other than gestation; therefore, these signs alone are not reliable for diagnosis of pregnancy.

Probable indicators of pregnancy are detected by an examiner and are related mainly to physical changes in the uterus. Objective signs include uterine enlargement, Braxton Hicks contractions, placental souffle (sound of blood passing through the placenta), ballottement (examiner is able to feel the fetus float during a vaginal examination), and a positive pregnancy test. When combined with presumptive signs and symptoms, they strongly suggest pregnancy, but they are not conclusive.

The *positive* indicators of pregnancy are directly attributed to the fetus and include the presence of a fetal heartbeat distinct from that of the mother, fetal movement felt by someone other than the mother, and visualization of the fetus with a technique such as ultrasound examination.

Estimating Date of Birth

After the diagnosis of pregnancy the woman's first question usually concerns when she will give birth. This date has traditionally been termed the *estimated date of confinement* (EDC), although *estimated date of delivery* (EDD) also has been used. To promote a more positive perception of both pregnancy and birth, however, the term estimated date of birth (EDB) is suggested. Accurate dating of pregnancy and calculation of the EDB have implications for timing of specific prenatal screening tests, assessing fetal growth, and making critical decisions for managing pregnancy complications.

Ultrasound has become a standard procedure for determining the gestational age of the fetus. The American Institute of Ultrasound in Medicine (AIUM), in collaboration with the American College of Radiology (ACR), the American College of Obstetricians and Gynecologists (ACOG), and the Society of Radiologists in Ultrasound (SRU), published guidelines for the safe and effective use of ultrasound in prenatal care (AIUM, 2013).

Naegele's rule is a common method for calculating the EDB. It is based on the woman's accurate recall of her last menstrual period (LMP). It assumes that the woman has a 28-day cycle and that fertilization occurred on the 14th day. According to Naegele's rule, after determining the first day of the LMP, subtract 3 calendar months and add 7 days (Box 14-1). Only about 5% of women give birth spontaneously on the EDB as determined by Naegele's rule. Most women give birth during the period extending from 7 days before to 7 days after the EDB.

BOX 14-1 Use of Naegele's Rule

December 10, 2015, is the first day of the last menstrual period (LMP).

	MONTH	DAY	YEAR
LMP	12	10	2015
	−3	+7	
Estimated day of birth:	9	17	2016

The estimated date of birth (EDB) is September 17, 2016.

ADAPTATION TO PREGNANCY

Pregnancy affects all family members, and each family member must adapt to the pregnancy and interpret its meaning in light of his or her own needs. This process of family adaptation to pregnancy takes place within a cultural environment influenced by societal trends. Dramatic changes have occurred in Western society in recent years, and the nurse must be prepared to support not only traditional families in the childbearing experience but also single-parent families, reconstituted families, dual-career families, and alternative families.

Much of the research on family dynamics in pregnancy in the United States and Canada has been done with Caucasian middle-class nuclear families. Therefore, the findings may not apply to families who do not fit the traditional North American model. Adaptation of terms is appropriate to avoid embarrassment to the nurse and offense to the family. Additional research is needed on a variety of families to determine if study findings generated in traditional families are applicable to others.

Maternal Adaptation

Women of all ages use the months of pregnancy to adapt to the maternal role, a complex process of social and cognitive learning. Early in pregnancy nothing seems to be happening, and a woman may spend much time sleeping secondary to the increased fatigue of this stage. With the perception of fetal movement in the second trimester, the woman turns her attention inward to her pregnancy and to relationships with her mother and other women who have been or who are pregnant.

Pregnancy is a maturational milestone that can be stressful but also rewarding as the woman prepares for a new level of caring and responsibility. Her self-concept changes in readiness for parenthood as she prepares for her new role. She moves gradually from being self-contained and independent to being committed to a lifelong concern for another human being. This growth requires mastery of certain developmental tasks: accepting the pregnancy, identifying with the role of mother, reordering the relationships between herself and her mother and between herself and her partner, establishing a relationship with the unborn child, and preparing for the birth experience. The partner's emotional support is an important factor in successfully accomplishing these developmental tasks. Single women with limited support can have difficulty making this adaptation.

Accepting the Pregnancy

The first step in adapting to the maternal role is accepting the idea of pregnancy and assimilating the pregnant state into the woman's way of life. Mercer (1995) described this process as *cognitive restructuring* and credited Reva Rubin (1975, 1984) as the nurse theorist who pioneered our understanding of maternal role attainment. The degree of acceptance is reflected in the woman's emotional responses. Many women are upset initially when they discover they are pregnant, especially if the pregnancy is unintended. Eventual acceptance of pregnancy parallels the growing acceptance of the reality of a child. However, nonacceptance of the pregnancy does not equate with rejection of the child, because a woman can dislike being pregnant but feel love for the child to be born.

Women who are happy and pleased about their pregnancy often view it as biologic fulfillment and part of their life plan. They have high self-esteem and tend to be confident about outcomes for themselves, their babies, and other family members. Despite a general feeling of well-being, many women are surprised to experience *emotional lability,* that is, rapid and unpredictable changes in mood. These swings in emotions and increased sensitivity to others are disconcerting to the expectant mother and those around her. Increased irritability and explosions of tears and anger can alternate with feelings of great joy and cheerfulness apparently with little or no provocation.

Profound hormonal changes that are part of the maternal response to pregnancy can be responsible for mood changes. Other reasons such as concerns about finances and changes in lifestyle contribute to this seemingly erratic behavior.

Most women have ambivalent feelings during pregnancy whether the pregnancy was intended or not. Ambivalence—having conflicting feelings simultaneously—is considered a normal response for people preparing for a new role. For example, during pregnancy some women feel great pleasure that they are fulfilling a lifelong dream, but they also feel great regret that life as they know it is ending.

Even women who are pleased to be pregnant can experience feelings of hostility toward the pregnancy or unborn child from time to time. Such incidents as a partner's chance remark about the attractiveness of a slim, nonpregnant woman or news of a colleague's promotion can give rise to ambivalent feelings. Body sensations, feelings of dependence, or the realization of the responsibilities of child care also can generate such feelings.

Intense feelings of ambivalence that persist through the third trimester can indicate an unresolved conflict with the motherhood role (Mercer, 1995). After the birth of a healthy child, memories of these ambivalent feelings usually are dismissed. If the child is born with a defect, however, a woman may look back at the times when she did not want the pregnancy and feel intense guilt. She may believe that her ambivalence caused the birth defect. She then will need assurance that her feelings were not responsible for the problem.

Identifying with the Mother Role

The process of identifying with the mother role begins early in each woman's life when she is being mothered as a child. Her social group's perception of what constitutes the feminine role can subsequently influence her choosing between motherhood or a career, being married or single, being independent rather than interdependent, or being able to manage multiple roles. Practice roles, such as playing with dolls, babysitting, and taking care of siblings can increase her understanding of what being a mother involves.

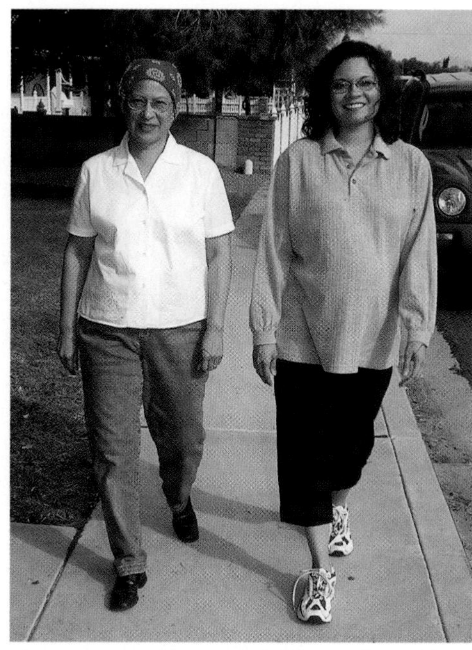

FIG 14-1 A pregnant woman and her mother enjoying a walk together. (Courtesy Michael S. Clement, MD, Mesa, AZ.)

Many women have always wanted a baby, liked children, and looked forward to motherhood. Their high motivation to become a parent promotes acceptance of pregnancy and eventual prenatal and parental adaptation. Other women have not considered in any detail what motherhood means to them. During pregnancy these women must resolve conflicts such as not wanting the pregnancy and child-related or career-related decisions.

Reordering Personal Relationships

Close relationships of a pregnant woman undergo change during pregnancy as she prepares emotionally for the new role of mother. As family members learn their new roles, periods of tension and conflict can occur. An understanding of the typical patterns of adjustment can help the nurse reassure the pregnant woman and explore issues related to social support. Promoting effective communication patterns between the expectant mother and her own mother and between the expectant mother and her partner are common nursing interventions provided during the prenatal visits.

The woman's relationship with her mother is significant in adaptation to pregnancy and motherhood. Important components in the pregnant woman's relationship with her mother are the mother's availability (past and present), her reactions to the daughter's pregnancy, respect for her daughter's autonomy, and the willingness to reminisce (Mercer, 1995).

The mother's reaction to the daughter's pregnancy signifies her acceptance of the grandchild and of her daughter. If the mother is supportive, the daughter has an opportunity to discuss pregnancy and labor with a knowledgeable and accepting woman (Fig. 14-1). Reminiscing about the pregnant woman's early childhood and sharing the prospective grandmother's account of her childbirth experience help the daughter anticipate and prepare for labor and birth.

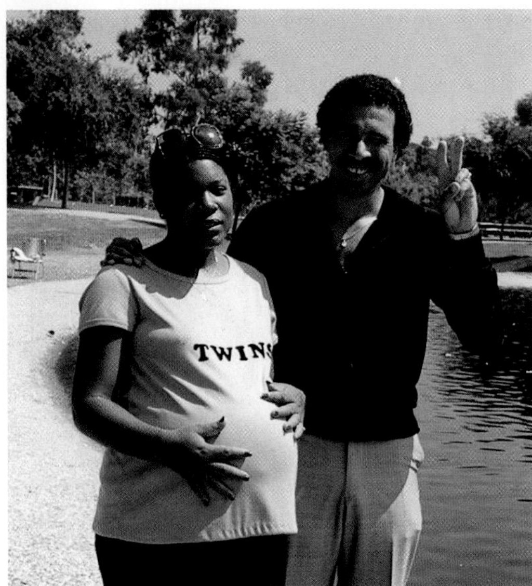

FIG 14-2 A prospective mother and father walk together. Women respond positively to their partner's interest and concern. (Courtesy Marjorie Pyle, RNC, Lifecircle, Costa Mesa, CA.)

Although the woman's relationship with her mother is significant in considering her adaptation to pregnancy, the most important person to the pregnant woman is usually the father of her child (Fig. 14-2). With same sex couples, the most important person is the partner. Women express two major needs within this relationship during pregnancy: feeling loved and valued and having the child accepted by the partner.

The marital or committed partner relationship is not static but evolves over time. The addition of a child changes forever the nature of the bond between partners. This can be a time when couples grow closer, and the pregnancy has a maturing effect on the partners' relationship as they assume new roles and discover new aspects of each other. Partners who trust and support each other are able to share mutual-dependency needs (Mercer, 1995).

Sexual expression during pregnancy is highly individual. The sexual relationship is affected by physical, emotional, and interactional factors, including misinformation about sex during pregnancy, sexual dysfunction, and physical changes in the woman. An individual may also inaccurately attribute anomalies, intellectual disability, and other injuries to the fetus and mother to sexual relations during pregnancy. Some couples fear that the birth process will dramatically change the woman's genitals. Some couples do not express their concerns to the health care provider because they are embarrassed or do not want to appear foolish.

As pregnancy progresses, changes in body shape, body image, and levels of discomfort influence both partners' desire for sexual expression. During the first trimester the woman's sexual desire usually decreases, especially if she has breast tenderness, nausea, or fatigue. As she progresses into the second trimester, however, her sense of well-being combined with the increased pelvic congestion that occurs at this time often increases her desire for sexual release. In the third trimester somatic complaints and physical bulkiness can increase her physical discomfort and again diminish her interest in sex.

Partners need to feel free to discuss their sexual responses during pregnancy with each other, their health care provider, and nurses involved in their care (see later discussion).

Establishing a Relationship with the Fetus

Emotional attachment—feelings of being tied by affection or love—begins during the prenatal period as women use fantasizing and daydreaming to prepare themselves for motherhood (Rubin, 1975, 1984). They think of themselves as mothers and imagine maternal qualities they would like to possess. Expectant parents desire to be warm, loving, and close to their child. They try to anticipate changes that the child will bring into their lives and wonder how they will react to noise, disorder, reduced freedom, and caregiving activities. The mother-child relationship progresses through pregnancy as a developmental process that unfolds in three phases.

In phase 1 the woman accepts the biologic fact of pregnancy. She needs to be able to state, "I am pregnant," and incorporate the idea of a child into her body and self-image. The woman's thoughts center on herself and the reality of her pregnancy. The child is viewed as part of herself, not a separate and unique person.

In phase 2 the woman accepts the growing fetus as distinct from herself. This is usually accomplished by the fifth month. She can now say, "I am going to have a baby." This differentiation of the child from the woman's self permits the beginning of the mother-child relationship that involves not only caring but also responsibility. Attachment of a mother to her child is enhanced by experiencing a planned or desired pregnancy, and it increases when ultrasound examination and quickening confirm the reality of the fetus. With acceptance of the reality of the child (hearing the heartbeat and feeling the fetus move) and an overall feeling of well-being, the woman enters a quiet period and becomes more introspective. A fantasy child becomes precious to her. As she seems to withdraw and concentrate her interest on the unborn child, her partner sometimes feels left out. If there are children in the family, they can become more demanding in their efforts to redirect the mother's attention to themselves.

During phase 3 of the attachment process, the woman prepares realistically for the birth and parenting of the child. She expresses the thought, "I am going to be a mother," and defines the nature and characteristics of the child. She may, for example, speculate about the child's sex (if unknown) and personality traits based on patterns of fetal activity.

Although the mother alone experiences the child within, both parents and siblings believe the unborn child responds in a very individualized, personal manner. Family members may interact a great deal with the unborn child by talking to the fetus and stroking the mother's abdomen, especially when the fetus shifts position (Fig. 14-3). The fetus may have a nickname used by family members.

Preparing for Birth

Many women actively prepare for birth by reading books and information on various websites, watching videos, attending parenting classes, and talking to other women. They seek the best caregiver possible for advice, monitoring, and caring. The multiparous woman has her own history of labor and birth that influences her approach to preparation for this birth experience.

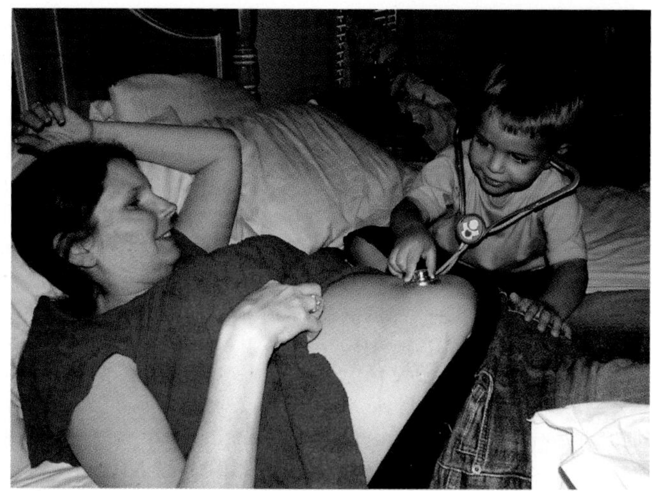

FIG 14-3 A 4-year-old likes to examine his pregnant mother's abdomen. (Courtesy Kara George, Phoenix, AZ.)

Anxiety can arise from concern about a safe passage for herself and her child during the birth process (Mercer, 1995; Rubin, 1975, 1984). Some women do not express this concern overtly, but they give cues to the nurse by making plans for care of the new baby and other children in case "anything should happen." Many women fear the pain of labor and birth because they do not understand anatomy and the birth process. Education by the nurse can alleviate many of these fears.

Toward the end of the third trimester, breathing is difficult, and fetal movements become vigorous enough to disturb the woman's sleep. Backaches, frequency and urgency of urination, constipation, and varicose veins can become troublesome. The bulkiness and awkwardness of her body interfere with the woman's ability to care for other children, perform routine work-related duties, and assume a comfortable position for sleep and rest. By this time most women become impatient for labor to begin, whether the birth is anticipated with joy, dread, or a mixture of both. A strong desire to see the end of pregnancy, to be over and done with it, makes women at this stage ready to move on to birth.

Paternal Adaptation

The father's beliefs and feelings about the ideal mother and father and his cultural expectations of appropriate behavior during pregnancy affect his response to his partner's need for him. One man may engage in nurturing behavior. Another may feel lonely and alienated as the woman becomes physically and emotionally engrossed in the unborn child. He may seek friends and relationships outside the home or become interested in a new hobby or involved with his work. Some men view pregnancy as proof of their masculinity and their dominant role. To others, pregnancy has no meaning in terms of responsibility to either mother or child. However, for most men, pregnancy is a time of preparation for the parental role with intense learning.

Accepting the Pregnancy

The ways fathers adjust to the parental role has been the subject of considerable research. In older societies the man enacted the ritual couvade; that is, he behaved in specific ways and respected taboos associated with pregnancy and giving birth so his new status was recognized and endorsed. Some men experience pregnancy-like symptoms, such as nausea, weight gain, and other physical symptoms. This phenomenon is known as the couvade syndrome. Changing cultural and professional attitudes have encouraged fathers' participation in the birth experience.

The man's emotional response to becoming a father, his concerns, and his informational needs change during the course of pregnancy. Phases of the developmental pattern become apparent. May (1982) described three phases characterizing the developmental tasks experienced by the expectant father:

- The *announcement phase* lasts from a few hours to a few weeks. The developmental task is to accept the biologic fact of pregnancy. Men react to the confirmation of pregnancy with joy or dismay, depending on whether the pregnancy is desired, unplanned, or unwanted. Ambivalence in the early stages of pregnancy is common. If pregnancy is unplanned or unwanted, some men find the alterations in life plans and lifestyles difficult to accept. Some men engage in extramarital affairs for the first time during their partner's pregnancy. Others batter their wives for the first time or escalate the frequency of battering episodes (Forsyth, Skouteris, Wertheim, et al., 2011). Chapter 5 provides information about violence against women and offers guidance on assessment and interventions.
- The second phase, the *moratorium phase,* is the period when he adjusts to the reality of pregnancy. The developmental task is to accept the pregnancy. Men appear to put conscious thought of the pregnancy aside for a time. They become more introspective and engage in many discussions about their philosophy of life, religion, childbearing, and childrearing practices and their relationships with family members, particularly with their father. Depending on the man's readiness for the pregnancy, this phase can be relatively short or persist until the last trimester.
- The third phase, the *focusing phase,* begins in the last trimester and is characterized by the father's active involvement in both the pregnancy and his relationship with his child. The developmental task is to negotiate with his partner the role he is to play in labor and to prepare for parenthood. In this phase the man concentrates on his experience of the pregnancy and begins to think of himself as a father.

Identifying with the Father Role

Each man brings to pregnancy attitudes that affect the way in which he adjusts to the pregnancy and the parental role. His memories of the fathering he received from his own father, the experiences he has had with child care, and the perceptions of the male and father roles within his social group will guide his selection of the tasks and responsibilities he will assume. Some men are highly motivated to nurture and love a child. They are excited and pleased about the anticipated role of father. Others are more detached or even hostile to the idea of fatherhood.

Reordering Personal Relationships

The partner's main role in pregnancy is to nurture and respond to the pregnant woman's feelings of vulnerability. The partner also must deal with the reality of the pregnancy. The partner's support indicates involvement in the pregnancy and preparation for attachment to the child.

Some aspects of a partner's behavior can indicate rivalry, and it can be especially evident during sexual activity. For example, some men protest that fetal movements prevent sexual gratification or feel that they are being watched by the fetus during sexual activity. However, feelings of rivalry are often unconscious and not verbalized, but expressed in subtle behaviors.

The woman's increased introspection can cause her partner to feel uneasy as she becomes preoccupied with thoughts of the child and of her motherhood, with her growing dependence on her health care provider, and with her reevaluation of the couple's relationship.

Establishing a Relationship with the Fetus

The father-child attachment can be as strong as the mother-child relationship, and fathers can be as competent as mothers in nurturing their infants. The father-child attachment also begins during pregnancy. A father may rub or kiss the maternal abdomen; try to listen, talk, or sing to the fetus; or play with the fetus as he notes movement. Calling the unborn child by name or nickname helps confirm the reality of pregnancy and promote attachment.

Men prepare for fatherhood in many of the same ways as women do for motherhood—by reading and fantasizing about the baby. Daydreaming about their role as father is common in the last weeks before the birth; however, men rarely describe their thoughts unless they are reassured that such daydreams are normal.

Nurses can help fathers identify concerns and prepare for the reality of a baby by asking questions such as:

- How do you expect the baby to look and act?
- How do you envision life as a father?
- How will you be involved in helping to care for the baby?
- How will having a baby affect your relationship with your partner?

Some fathers do not wish to answer such questions when they are asked but need time to think them through or discuss them with their partners.

As the birth date approaches, men have more questions about fetal and newborn behaviors. Some men are shocked or amazed at the smallness of clothes and furniture for the baby. If an expectant father can imagine only an older child and has difficulty visualizing or talking about an infant, this situation must be explored. The nurse can tell the father about the unborn child's ability to respond to light, sound, and touch and encourage him to feel and talk to the fetus. Discussions with new fathers, as in childbirth classes, may be welcomed.

Some men become involved by choosing the child's name and anticipating the child's sex, if it is not already known. Some couples select the name of the child as early as the first month of pregnancy. Family tradition, religious customs, and the continuation of the parent's name or names of relatives or friends are important in the selection process.

Preparing for Birth

The days and weeks immediately before the expected day of birth are characterized by anticipation and anxiety. Boredom and restlessness are common as the couple focuses on the birth process; however, during the last 2 months of pregnancy, many expectant fathers experience a surge of creative energy at home and on the job. They become dissatisfied with their present living space. If possible, they tend to act on the need to alter the environment (remodeling, painting, etc.). This activity is their way of sharing in the childbearing experience. They are able to channel the anxiety and other feelings experienced during the final weeks before birth into productive activities. This behavior earns recognition and compliments from friends, relatives, and their partners.

Major concerns for the man are getting the woman to a health care facility in time for the birth and not appearing ignorant. Many men want to be able to recognize labor and determine when it is appropriate to leave for the hospital or call the obstetric care provider. They fantasize different situations and plan what they will do in response to them or rehearse taking various routes to the hospital, timing each route at different times of the day.

Some prospective fathers have questions about the labor suite's furniture and equipment, nursing staff, and location, as well as the availability of the obstetric and anesthesia care providers. Others want to know what is expected of them when their partners are in labor. The man also may have fears concerning safe passage of his child and partner and the possible death or complications of his partner and child. It is important he verbalize these fears; otherwise he cannot help his mate deal with her spoken or unspoken apprehension.

With the exception of childbirth preparation classes, a man has few opportunities to learn ways to be an involved and active partner in this rite of passage into parenthood. Mothers often sense the tensions and apprehensions of the unprepared, unsupportive father and it can increase their fears.

Adaptation to Parenthood for the Nonpregnant Partner

The same fears, questions, and concerns may affect birth partners who are not the biologic fathers or who are the nonpregnant partner in a same sex couple. Much attention is paid to the needs of the pregnant partner, but the nonpregnant partner's needs receive less attention. Nonpregnant partners, also referred to as co-mothers, can feel excluded by heterocentric maternity care service structures, but are likely to feel included by nursing staff (Cherguit, Burns, Pettle, & Tasker, 2012). Nonpregnant partners will be better prepared for the changes that come with pregnancy and parenting if they are included and considered in the process. In addition to dealing with their own feelings and the care of their partner, nonpregnant partners in a same sex couple are often not acknowledged or accepted as a parent-to-be from within their own families and in society in general. Partners need to be kept informed, supported, and included in all activities in which the mother desires their participation. Nurses can do much to promote pregnancy and birth as a family experience by providing information about resources for same sex parents such as community and on-line support groups.

Sibling Adaptation

Sharing the spotlight with a new brother or sister can be the first major crisis for a child. The older child often experiences a sense of loss or feels jealous at being "replaced" by the new sibling. Some of the factors that influence the child's response are age, the parents' attitudes, the role of the father, the length of separation from the mother, the facility visitation policy, and the way the child has been prepared for the change.

A mother with other children must devote time and effort to reorganizing her relationships with them. She needs to prepare siblings for the baby's birth (Fig. 14-4 and Box 14-2) and begin the process of role transition in the family by including the children in the pregnancy and being sympathetic to older children's concerns about losing their places in the family hierarchy. No child willingly gives up a familiar position.

Siblings' responses to pregnancy vary with their age and dependency needs. The 1-year-old infant seems largely unaware of the process, but the 2-year-old child notices the change in his or her mother's appearance and may comment that "Mommy's fat." Toddlers' need for sameness in the environment makes children aware of any change. They can exhibit more clinging behavior and sometimes regress in toilet training or eating.

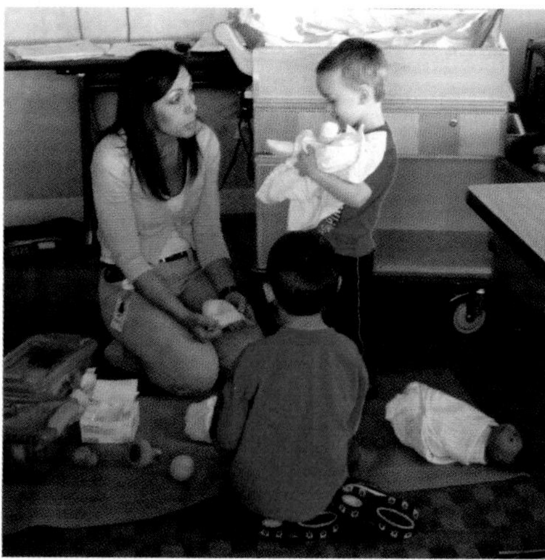

FIG 14-4 A preschooler in a sibling class learns about childbirth and infant care using dolls and a bunny. (Courtesy Julie and Darren Nelson, Loveland, CO.)

By age 3 or 4 years, children like to be told the story of their own beginning and accept a comparison of their own development with that of the present pregnancy. They like to listen to the fetal heartbeat and feel the baby moving in utero (see Fig. 14-3). Sometimes they worry about how the baby is being fed and clothed.

School-age children take a more clinical interest in their mother's pregnancy. They may want to know in more detail, "How did the baby get in there?" and "How will it get out?" Children in this age-group notice pregnant women in stores, churches, and schools and sometimes seem shy if they need to approach a pregnant woman directly. On the whole, they look forward to the new baby, see themselves as "mothers" or "fathers," and enjoy buying baby supplies and readying a place for the baby. Because they still think in concrete terms and base judgments on the here and now, they respond positively to their mother's current good health.

Early and middle adolescents preoccupied with the establishment of their own sexual identity can have difficulty accepting the overwhelming evidence of the sexual activity of their parents. They reason that if they are too young for such activity, certainly their parents are too old. They seem to take on a critical parental role and may ask, "What will people think?" or "How can you let yourself get so fat?" or "How can you let yourself get pregnant?" Many pregnant women with teenage children will confess that the attitudes of their teenagers are the most difficult aspect of their current pregnancy.

Late adolescents do not appear to be unduly disturbed. They are busy making plans for their own lives and realize that they

BOX 14-2 Sibling Adaptation: Tips for Sibling Preparation

Prenatal

- Take your child on a prenatal visit. Let the child listen to the fetal heartbeat and feel the baby move.
- Involve the child in preparations for the baby, such as helping decorate the baby's room.
- Move the child to a bed (if still sleeping in a crib) at least 2 months before the baby is due.
- Read books, show videos or DVDs, and/or take your child to sibling preparation classes, including a hospital tour.
- Answer your child's questions about the coming birth, what babies are like, and any other questions.
- Take your child to the homes of friends who have babies so that the child has realistic expectations of what babies are like.

During the Hospital Stay

- Have someone bring the child to the hospital to visit you and the baby (unless you plan to have the child attend the birth).
- When the child arrives, make sure your arms are open to embrace the child.
- Do not force interactions between the child and the baby. Often the child will be more interested in seeing you and being reassured of your love.
- Help the child explore the infant by showing how and where to touch the baby.
- Give the child a gift (from you or from you, the father or your partner, and baby).

Going Home

- Leave the child at home with a relative or babysitter or have someone such as the grandmother available to focus on the child during hospital discharge and on the trip home.
- Have someone else carry the baby from the car so that you can hug the child first.

Adjustment After the Baby Is Home

- Arrange for a special time for the child to be alone with each parent.
- Do not exclude the child during infant feeding times. The child can sit with you and the baby and feed a doll or drink juice or milk or sit quietly with a game. You can read aloud to the child while you are feeding the infant.
- Prepare small gifts for the child so that when the baby gets gifts, the sibling will not feel left out. The child can also help open the baby gifts.
- Praise the child for acting age appropriately (so that being a baby does not seem better than being older).

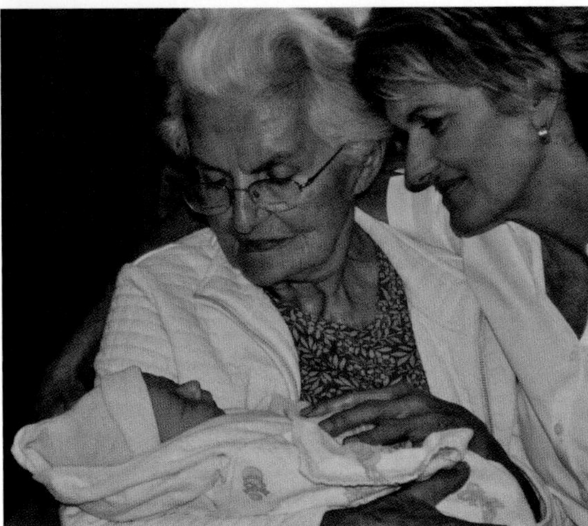

FIG 14-5 A great-grandmother and grandmother admiring the new baby. (Courtesy Barbara Wilson, West Jordan, UT.)

soon will be gone from home. Parents usually report they are comforting and act more as other adults than as children.

Grandparent Adaptation

Most grandparents are delighted at the prospect of a new baby in the family. It reawakens the feelings of their own youth, the excitement of giving birth, and their delight in the behavior of the parents-to-be when they were infants. They set up a memory store of the child's first smiles, first words, and first steps that they can use later for "claiming" the newborn as a member of the family. These behaviors provide a link between the past and present for the parents and grandparents-to-be.

In addition, the grandparent is the historian who transmits the family history, a resource person who shares knowledge based on experience; a role model; and a support person. The grandparent's presence and support can strengthen family systems by widening the circle of support and nurturance (Fig. 14-5). Other sources of information cannot replace the unique contribution that grandparents make (www.grandparents.com; www.grandparenting.org).

For some expectant grandparents a first pregnancy in a child is undeniable evidence that they are growing older. Many think of a grandparent as old, white-haired, and becoming feeble of mind and body; however, some people face grandparenthood while still in their 30s or 40s. Some individuals react negatively to the news that they will be grandparents, indicating that they are not ready for the new role.

In some family units expectant grandparents are nonsupportive and can inadvertently decrease the self-esteem of the parents-to-be. Mothers may talk about their terrible pregnancies; fathers may discuss the endless cost of rearing children; and mothers-in-law may complain that their sons are neglecting them because their concern is now directed toward the pregnant daughters-in-law.

CARE MANAGEMENT

The goal of prenatal care is to promote the health and well-being of the pregnant woman, her fetus, the newborn, and the family (Gregory, Niebyl, & Johnson, 2012). It includes education about healthy lifestyle behaviors such as nutrition and physical activity, self-care for the common pregnancy discomforts, and information about changes in the mother and growth of the developing fetus. Routine screening is offered during pregnancy to help identify existing risk factors and potential problems so that efforts to reduce risk of harm to mother or baby and management of identified conditions can be initiated at the earliest opportunity. Major emphasis is placed on preventive aspects of care, primarily to support the pregnant woman in self-management between visits with health care professionals and to help her to recognize and report changes that can signal problems early so that adverse effects for her or her unborn child can be prevented or minimized. If health behaviors must be modified in early pregnancy, nurses need to understand psychosocial factors that can influence the woman. In holistic care, nurses provide information and guidance about the physical changes and the psychosocial impact of pregnancy on the woman and members of her family. The goals of prenatal nursing care, therefore, are to foster a safe birth for the mother and infant and to promote satisfaction of the mother and family with the pregnancy and birth experience.

According to the National Center for Health Statistics (NCHS), more than 75% of women in the United States receive pregnancy care in the first trimester. Women who are least likely to begin early prenatal care are non-Hispanic African-American, non-Hispanic Native Hawaiian/Other Pacific Islander, and non-Hispanic American Indian/Alaska Native mothers (Martin, Hamilton, Sutton, et al., 2012). Although women of middle or high socioeconomic status routinely seek prenatal care, women's reasons for delaying prenatal care include cost, lack of insurance, child care, transportation barriers, or inability to take time off from work. Lack of culturally sensitive care providers, discrimination based on sexual orientation, and barriers to communication resulting from differences in language also interfere with access to care. Likewise, immigrant women who come from cultures in which prenatal care is not emphasized may not know to seek routine prenatal care. Birth outcomes in these populations are less positive, with higher rates of maternal and fetal or newborn complications. In particular, problems with low birth weight (LBW; less than 2500 g) and infant mortality are associated with lack of adequate prenatal care (Gregory et al., 2012).

The availability of advanced practice nurses (nurse practitioners and certified nurse-midwives [CNM]) as independent providers of care or in collaborative practice with physicians improves the availability and accessibility of prenatal care (American College of Nurse-Midwives [ACNM], 2012). A regular schedule of home visits by nurses aids in reducing barriers to care and contributes to improved maternal and infant outcomes (Agency for Healthcare Research and Quality [AHRQ], 2012). Under the Patient Protection and Affordable Care Act of 2010 (ACA), payment for innovative models for delivery of prenatal care, including home visits by unlicensed professionals, can reduce barriers to early prenatal care (Salinsky, 2013).

The traditional model for provision of prenatal care has been used for more than a century. The initial visit usually occurs in the first trimester, with monthly visits through week 28 of pregnancy. Thereafter, visits are scheduled every 2 weeks until week 36 and then every week until birth. Today the trend is toward individualizing the schedule of care. Women with low

BOX 14-3 Prenatal Visit Schedule

Traditional*	CenteringPregnancy†
• First visit within the first trimester (12 weeks) • Monthly visits weeks 16 through 28 • Every 2 weeks from weeks 29 to 36 • Weekly visits week 36 to birth	• First visit within the first trimester (12 weeks) • Every 4 weeks—weeks 16 to 28 • Every 2 weeks—weeks 29 to 40

Data from Centering Healthcare Institute. (2012). *CenteringPregnancy*. Available at www.centeringhealthcare.org/pages/centering-model/model-overview.php.

*Frequency of visits may be decreased in low risk women and increased in women with high risk pregnancies.

†Additional individual visits may be added as needed.

risk pregnancies may have fewer routine prenatal visits, whereas those at risk for complications may be seen more frequently than the traditional schedule (American Academy of Pediatrics [AAP] and American College of Obstetricians and Gynecologists [ACOG], 2012).

Group prenatal care is an alternative model to traditional care during pregnancy. In group prenatal care authority is shifted from the provider to the woman and other women who have similar due dates. The model creates an atmosphere that facilitates learning, encourages discussion, and develops mutual support. CenteringPregnancy (www.centeringhealthcare.org) is a well-known model of group prenatal care that involves three components: health care assessment, education, and peer support. Most care takes place in the group setting after the initial visit and continues for 10-hour sessions that begin at about 16 weeks. At each meeting, the first 30 to 40 minutes consist of assessments (by the woman herself and by the health care provider) and the remaining 60 to 75 minutes are spent in group discussion of specific issues such as discomforts of pregnancy and preparation for labor and birth (Box 14-3). Families and partners are encouraged to participate (Centering Healthcare Institute, 2012). Benefits associated with group prenatal care include improved birth outcomes such as lower rates of preterm birth, increased knowledge, improved satisfaction, and higher breastfeeding initiation rates (Herrman, Rogers, & Ehrenthal, 2012; Picklesimer, Billings, Hale, et al., 2012; Rotundo, 2011).

Prenatal care is ideally a multidisciplinary activity in which nurses work with certified nurse-midwives, nutritionists, physicians, social workers, and others. Collaboration among these individuals is necessary to provide holistic care. The case management model, which makes use of care maps and critical pathways, is one system that promotes comprehensive care with limited overlap in services. To emphasize the nursing role, care management for the initial visit and follow-up visits is organized around the central elements of the nursing process: assessment, nursing diagnoses, expected outcomes, plan of care and interventions, and evaluation.

In recent years the concept of preconception care has been recognized as an important contributor to good pregnancy outcomes (see Chapter 4). If women can be taught healthy lifestyle behaviors and then practice them before conception—specifically good nutrition, entering pregnancy with as healthy a weight as possible, adequate intake of folic acid, avoidance of alcohol and tobacco use, and prevention of sexually transmitted infections (STIs) and other health hazards—a healthier pregnancy will result. Likewise, women who have health problems related to chronic diseases such as diabetes mellitus can be counseled regarding their special needs with the intent to minimize maternal and fetal complications.

Initial Visit

Once the presence of pregnancy has been confirmed and the woman's desire to continue the pregnancy has been validated, prenatal care is begun. The assessment process begins at the initial prenatal visit and is continued throughout the pregnancy. Assessment techniques include the interview, physical examination, and laboratory tests. Because the initial visit and follow-up visits are distinctly different in content and process, they are described separately.

Prenatal Interview

The therapeutic relationship between the nurse and the woman is established during the initial assessment interview. During this interview the nurse has the opportunity to gain the woman's trust.

The pregnant woman and family members who are present should be told that the first prenatal visit is longer and more detailed than future visits. The initial evaluation includes a comprehensive health history emphasizing the current pregnancy, previous pregnancies, the family, a psychosocial profile, a physical assessment, diagnostic testing, and an overall risk assessment. A prenatal history form (paper or electronic) is used to document information obtained.

One or more family members often accompany the pregnant woman. With the woman's permission, the nurse includes those accompanying the woman in the initial prenatal interview. Observations and information about the woman's family are then included in the database. For example, if the woman has small children with her, the nurse can ask about her plans for child care during the time of labor and birth. The nurse notes any special needs that are identified during this first interview (e.g., wheelchair access, assistance in getting on and off the examining table, difficulty speaking and/or understanding English, and cognitive deficits).

Reason for Seeking Care. Although pregnant women are scheduled for routine prenatal visits, they often come to the health care provider seeking information or reassurance about a particular concern. When the woman is asked a broad, open-ended question such as, "How have you been feeling?," she may reveal problems that could otherwise be overlooked. The woman's chief concerns should be recorded in her own words to alert other personnel to the priority of needs as identified by her. At the initial visit the desire for information about what is normal in the course of pregnancy is typical.

Current Pregnancy. The presumptive signs of pregnancy, such as nausea and vomiting, can be of great concern to the woman. A review of symptoms she is experiencing and how she is coping with them helps establish a database to develop a plan of care. Some early teaching may be provided at this time.

Childbearing and Female Reproductive System History. Data are gathered on the woman's age at menarche, menstrual history, and contraceptive history; any infertility or reproductive system conditions; history of STIs; sexual history; and detailed history of all her pregnancies, including the present pregnancy, and their outcomes. The date of the last Papanicolaou (Pap) test and the result are noted. The date of her LMP is obtained to calculate the EDB.

Health History. The health history includes physical conditions or surgical procedures that can affect the pregnancy or that can be affected by the pregnancy. For example, a pregnant woman who has diabetes, hypertension, or epilepsy requires special care. A careful history of any allergies and the type of reaction, medication use, and immunizations must be included. Because most women are anxious during the initial interview, the nurse's attention to cues, such as a MedicAlert bracelet, can prompt the woman to recall allergies, chronic diseases, or medications being taken such as cortisone, insulin, or anticonvulsants.

The woman should also describe any previous surgical procedures. If a woman has undergone uterine surgery or extensive repair of the pelvic floor, a cesarean birth may be necessary; appendectomy rules out appendicitis as a cause of right lower quadrant pain in pregnancy; and spinal surgery may contraindicate the use of spinal or epidural anesthesia. The nurse notes any injury involving the pelvis as from a motor vehicle accident or childhood nutritional deficit.

Women who have chronic or handicapping conditions often forget to mention them during the initial assessment because they have become so adapted to them. Special shoes or a limp can indicate the existence of a pelvic structural defect, which is an important consideration in pregnant women. The nurse who observes these special characteristics and inquires about them with sensitivity can obtain individualized data that will provide the basis for a comprehensive nursing care plan (Signore, Spong, Krotoski, et al., 2011). Observations are vital components of the interview process because they prompt the nurse and woman to focus on the specific needs of the woman and her family.

Nutritional History. The woman's nutritional history is an important component of the prenatal history because her nutritional status has a direct effect on the growth and development of the fetus. A dietary assessment can reveal special dietary practices, food allergies, eating behaviors, the practice of *pica* (the consumption of nonfood substances), and other factors related to her nutritional status (see Box 15-7). Obese women should receive counseling about weight gain, physical activity, and healthy food choices. They should also be advised about the risk for maternal or fetal complications (ACOG Committee on Obstetric Practice, 2013a). Pregnant women are usually motivated to learn about healthy lifestyle behaviors and respond well to advice generated by this assessment. However, there is not enough rigorous research evidence to recommend any specific intervention for preventing excess weight gain during pregnancy (Muktabhant, Lumbiganon, Ngamjarus, & Dowswell, 2012). Women with a history of bariatric surgery are nutritionally at risk and should be followed closely throughout pregnancy to promote maternal and fetal well-being (Magdaleno, Pereira, Chaim, & Turato, 2012) (see Chapter 15).

History of Drug and Herbal Preparation Use. The prenatal history includes past and present use of drugs (legal over-the-counter [OTC] and prescription medications; vitamin supplements such as A, C, D, and E; herbal preparations; caffeine; alcohol; nicotine) and street drugs (e.g., marijuana, cocaine, heroin). This is because many substances cross the placenta and can therefore pose a risk to the developing fetus. See Chapter 31 for discussion of substance abuse during pregnancy. Increasing numbers of individuals are using herbal preparations, and this includes pregnant women. Therefore, it is important for health care providers to question prenatal women regarding the use of herbal preparations and document their responses. Information about allergies to medications and the type of reaction should also be obtained and recorded in the health record.

The immunization record should be reviewed for vaccinations against diseases such as rubella (German measles), varicella (chickenpox), seasonal influenza, hepatitis B, and pertussis (whooping cough) that can pose a particular risk to pregnant women or their infants during pregnancy and immediately following birth. Recommendations for vaccinations during the perinatal period are discussed later in the chapter.

Family History. The family history provides information about the woman's immediate family, including parents, siblings, and children. These data help identify familial or genetic disorders or conditions that could affect the health status of the woman or her fetus.

Social, Experiential, and Occupational History. Situational factors such as the family's ethnic and cultural background and socioeconomic status are assessed while the history is obtained. The following information may be obtained in several encounters. The woman's perception of this pregnancy is explored by asking questions that focus on the following issues:

- Is this pregnancy planned or wanted?
- Is the woman pleased, displeased, accepting, or nonaccepting?
- Will any changes related to finances, career, or living accommodations occur as a result of the pregnancy?

The family support system is assessed by questioning the mother about these areas:

- What primary support is available to her?
- Are changes needed to promote adequate support?
- What are the existing relationships among the mother, father or partner, siblings, and expectant grandparents?
- What preparations are being made for her care and that of dependent family members during labor and for the care of the infant after birth?
- Is financial, educational, or other support needed from the community?
- What are the woman's ideas about childbearing, her expectations of the infant's behavior, and her outlook on life and the maternal role?

Other questions can provide perspective on the woman's perceptions about becoming a mother. Examples of issues to explore include:

- What does the woman think it will be like to have a baby in the home?
- How is her life going to change by having a baby?
- How prepared does she feel for becoming a mother?

During interviews throughout the pregnancy nurses should remain alert to the appearance of potential parenting problems, such as depression, lack of family support, and inadequate living conditions. Nurses assess the woman's attitude toward health care, particularly during childbearing, her expectations of health care providers, and her view of the relationship between herself and the nurse.

Coping mechanisms and patterns of interacting are identified through observation and conversation with the mother. Early in the pregnancy the nurse should determine the woman's knowledge in various areas: pregnancy, maternal changes, fetal growth, self-care, and care of the newborn, including feeding. Asking about attitudes toward unmedicated or medicated labor and birth and about her knowledge of the availability of parenting skills classes is important. Before planning for nursing care, the nurse obtains information about the woman's decision-making abilities and living habits (i.e., exercise, sleep, diet, recreational interests, personal hygiene, clothing). Common concerns that can be sources of stress during childbearing include the baby's welfare, labor and birth process, behaviors of the newborn, the woman's relationship with her partner and her family, changes in body image, and physical symptoms.

The nurse explores attitudes concerning the range of acceptable sexual behavior during pregnancy by asking questions such as the following: What has your family (partner, friends) told you about sex during pregnancy? To gain insight into the woman's sexual self-concept, the nurse can ask questions such as the following: How do you feel about the changes in your appearance? How does your partner feel about your body now? How do you feel about wearing maternity clothes?

Women are questioned regarding their occupation—past and present—because this can adversely affect maternal and fetal health. For some women heavy lifting and exposure to chemicals and radiation are part of their daily work, and these activities can negatively affect the pregnancy. Standing for long periods at a retail checkout line or in front of a classroom is associated with orthostatic hypotension. For others long hours of sitting at a desk working on a computer can contribute to carpal tunnel syndrome or circulatory stasis in the legs.

History or Risk of Intimate Partner Violence. All women should be assessed for a history or risk of abuse in all forms—physical, sexual, or psychologic—particularly because the likelihood of intimate partner violence (IPV) increases during pregnancy (see Chapter 5). This screening should be done at the first prenatal visit, at least once each trimester, and at the postpartum visit (ACOG Committee on Health Care for Underserved Women, 2012). It is essential that the screening is done in a safe, private setting with the woman alone. Nurses can ask the woman screening questions with routine assessments during pregnancy. Examples of questions that might be asked include:

- Are you with a spouse or partner who threatens or physically hurts you? If yes, who?
- Within the past year or in this pregnancy, has anyone hit, slapped, kicked, or otherwise hurt you? If yes, who? Are you currently with that person?
- Has anyone forced you to have sexual activities that made you uncomfortable? If yes, who? Are you currently with that person?

Although cues from the woman's appearance, behavior or how she responds to questions can suggest the possibility, no one profile of the abused woman exists. During pregnancy the target body parts can change during abusive episodes. Women may report physical blows directed to the head, breasts, abdomen, and genitalia; verbal abuse; and sexual assault. The nurse should be prepared to offer support and community resources to women who are victims of intimate partner violence.

Abuse and pregnancy in teenagers constitute a particularly difficult situation. Adolescents can be trapped in the abusive relationship because of their inexperience, dependence on the abuser, and separation from family and friend support systems. Routine screening for abuse and sexual assault is recommended for pregnant adolescents (Centers for Disease Control and Prevention [CDC], 2013c). Because pregnancy in minor adolescent girls can be the result of sexual abuse, possibly from a relative, the nurse should know the state reporting laws and be prepared to contact protective services authorities if abuse or sexual assault is suspected (see Chapter 5 for further discussion).

Nurses should be aware that victims of human trafficking can be seen in prenatal settings because of unintended pregnancy. Similar to victims of IPV, these women are likely to exhibit signs of physical abuse or neglect such as scars, bruises, burns, unusual bald patches, or tattoos that can be a sign of branding. They are likely to be accompanied by someone who never leaves them alone and speaks for them. They may not speak English and may lack identification documents. If the woman is alone, she may have her cell phone on and in speaker mode so that the person on the other end can hear everything that is said during the visit. Nurses and other health care providers must be creative in getting the woman alone for questioning. Strategies might include sending the other person to the front desk to fill out paperwork, interviewing the woman in the restroom, or telling her she needs to go for testing and cannot take her cell phone. With the consent of suspected or confirmed victims of human trafficking, intervention plans can be developed. An excellent resource is the National Human Trafficking Resource Center (www.polarisproject.org/what-we-do/national-human-trafficking-hotline/the-nhtrc/overview) (1-888-373-7888) (Tracy & Konstantopoulos, 2012).

Review of Systems. During this portion of the interview the woman is asked to identify and describe preexisting or concurrent problems in any of the body systems, and her mental status is assessed. The nurse questions the woman about physical symptoms she has experienced, such as shortness of breath or pain. Pregnancy affects and is affected by all body systems; therefore, information on the current status of the body systems is important in planning care. For each sign or symptom described, the following additional data should be obtained: location, quality, quantity, chronology, aggravating or alleviating factors, and associated manifestations (signs or symptoms that occur with the primary symptom) (Seidel, Ball, Dains, et al., 2011).

Physical Examination

The initial physical examination provides the baseline for assessing subsequent changes. The nurse should determine the woman's needs for basic information regarding reproductive anatomy and provide this information, along with a demonstration of the equipment that may be used and an explanation of the procedure itself. The interaction requires an unhurried, sensitive, and gentle approach with a matter-of-fact attitude.

The physical examination begins with assessment of vital signs and height and weight (for calculation of body mass index [BMI]) (see Chapter 15). The bladder should be empty before pelvic examination; the woman may be asked to provide a urine specimen at this time if not already provided.

TABLE 14-1 Laboratory Tests in Prenatal Period

LABORATORY TEST	PURPOSE
Hemoglobin, hematocrit, WBC, differential	Detects anemia; detects infection
Hemoglobin electrophoresis	Identifies women with hemoglobinopathies (e.g., sickle cell anemia, thalassemia)
Blood type, Rh, and irregular antibody	Identifies women whose fetuses are at risk for developing erythroblastosis fetalis or hyperbilirubinemia in neonatal period
Rubella titer	Determines immunity to rubella
Tuberculin skin testing; chest film after 20 weeks of gestation in women with reactive tuberculin tests	Screens for exposure to tuberculosis
Urinalysis, including microscopic examination of urinary sediment; pH, specific gravity, color, glucose, albumin, protein, RBCs, WBCs, casts, acetone; hCG	Identifies women with glycosuria, renal disease, hypertensive disease of pregnancy; infection; occult hematuria; hCG for confirmation of pregnancy
Urine culture	Identifies women with asymptomatic bacteriuria
Renal function tests: BUN, creatinine, electrolytes, creatinine clearance, total protein excretion	Evaluates level of possible renal compromise in women with a history of diabetes, hypertension, or renal disease
Pap test	Screens for cervical intraepithelial neoplasia; if a liquid-based test is used, may also screen for HPV
Cervical cultures for *Neisseria gonorrhoeae, Chlamydia*	Screens for asymptomatic infection at first visit
Vaginal/anal culture	GBS test done at 35-37 weeks for infection
RPR, VDRL, or FTA-ABS	Identifies women with untreated syphilis, done at first visit
HIV antibody, hepatitis B surface antigen, toxoplasmosis	Screens for the specific infections
1-hour glucose tolerance	Screens for gestational diabetes; done at initial visit for women with risk factors; done at 24-28 weeks for pregnant women at risk whose initial screen was negative and for others who were not previously tested
3-hour glucose tolerance	Tests for gestational diabetes in women with elevated glucose level after 1-hour test; must have two elevated readings for diagnosis
Cardiac evaluation: ECG, chest x-ray, and echocardiogram	Evaluates cardiac function in women with a history of hypertension or cardiac disease

BUN, Blood urea nitrogen; *ECG,* electrocardiogram; *FTA-ABS,* fluorescent treponemal antibody absorption; *GBS,* group B streptococcus; *hCG,* human chorionic gonadotropin; *HIV,* human immunodeficiency virus; *HPV,* human papillomavirus; *RBCs,* red blood cells; *RPR,* rapid plasma reagin; *WBCs,* white blood cells; *VDRL,* Venereal Disease Research Laboratory.

Each examiner develops a routine for proceeding with the physical examination; most choose the head-to-toe progression. Heart and lung sounds are evaluated, and extremities are examined. Distribution, amount, and quality of body hair are of particular importance because the findings reflect nutritional status, endocrine function, and attention to hygiene. The thyroid gland is assessed carefully. The height of the fundus is noted if the first examination is done after the first trimester of pregnancy. During the examination the nurse must remain alert to the woman's cues that give direction to the remainder of the assessment and that indicate a potential threatening condition such as supine hypotension—low blood pressure (BP) that occurs while the woman is lying on her back, causing feelings of faintness (see Emergency Box). See Chapter 4 for a detailed description of the physical examination.

Whenever a pelvic examination is performed, the tone of the pelvic musculature and the woman's knowledge of Kegel exercises are assessed. Particular attention is paid to the size of the uterus because this is an indication of the duration of gestation. During the examination the nurse can coach the woman in breathing and relaxation techniques, as needed. One vaginal examination during early pregnancy is recommended; another is usually not performed until late in the third trimester unless indicated by the woman's health status.

Laboratory Tests

The laboratory data yielded by the analysis of the specimens obtained during the examination provide important information concerning the symptoms of pregnancy and the woman's health status.

Urine, cervical, and blood samples are requested during the initial visit for a variety of recommended screening and diagnostic tests for infectious diseases and metabolic conditions that can affect the mother and/or developing fetus. (A list of the various tests is found in Table 14-1.) Women should receive information about the various tests and the purpose for each test and be provided an opportunity to opt-out of testing. All pregnant women should receive human immunodeficiency virus (HIV) risk-reduction counseling and be notified that they will be tested for antibody to HIV as part of the routine prenatal testing unless the test is declined (AAP & ACOG, 2012) (Box 14-4). If the woman refuses testing for HIV, this should be documented. The Centers for Disease Control and Prevention (CDC) also recommend testing during the first prenatal visit for syphilis, chlamydia, and hepatitis B. Screening for *Neisseria gonorrhoeae* is done for women who are at risk (CDC, 2013d). Screening for HIV, syphilis, chlamydia, and gonorrhea is repeated in the third trimester for women who are at high risk for contracting these infections. A purified protein derivative (PPD) tuberculin test may be administered to assess exposure to tuberculosis in women who are high risk. The urine is tested for protein, glucose, and leukocytes; urine culture may also be done. During the pelvic examination Papanicolaou test and culture for chlamydia and gonorrhea are done. In addition, pregnant women and fathers with certain ancestry or a family history of various genetically linked disorders may choose to undergo genetic testing (see Chapter 3). Antenatal testing for risk factors in pregnancy is discussed in Chapter 26.

Follow-up Visits

In traditional prenatal care, visits can occur more or less frequently, often depending on individual needs, complications, and risks of the pregnant woman. The pattern of interviewing the woman first and then assessing physical changes and performing laboratory tests continues.

BOX 14-4 Human Immunodeficiency Virus Screening

- Pregnant women are ethically obligated to seek reasonable care during pregnancy and to avoid causing harm to the fetus. Women's health nurses should be advocates for the fetus while accepting of the pregnant woman's decision regarding testing and/or treatment for HIV.
- Without treatment, the incidence of perinatal transmission from an HIV-positive mother to her fetus is approximately 25%. Triple drug antiviral or highly active antiretroviral therapy (HAART) during pregnancy decreases perinatal transmission to less than 1% (CDC, 2014).
- The Centers for Disease Control and Prevention (CDC, 2014) recommend testing for HIV infections for all pregnant women as early as possible in pregnancy and a second test in the third trimester for women in certain geographic areas and those who are at high risk for HIV infection.
- Testing has the potential to identify HIV-positive women who can then be treated. Health care providers have an obligation to ensure that pregnant women are well informed about HIV symptoms, testing, and methods of decreasing maternal-fetal transmission. The CDC and the American College of Obstetricians and Gynecologists (ACOG) recommend universal opt-out screening, which means that all pregnant women are offered HIV screening but have the opportunity to opt-out if desired (ACOG Committee on Obstetric Practice, 2011a; CDC, 2014). The Association of Women's Health, Obstetric and Neonatal Nurses (AWHONN, 2008) supports this system of HIV screening that allows all pregnant women to be offered screening.

Sources: American College of Obstetricians and Gynecologists (ACOG) Committee on Obstetric Practice (2011). Committee opinion no. 418. Prenatal and perinatal human immunodeficiency virus testing—Expanded recommendations. *Obstetrics & Gynecology, 104*(5 Part 1), 1119-1124; AWHONN. (2008). *HIV screening procedures for pregnant women and newborns—Policy position statement.* Washington, DC: Author; Centers for Disease Control and Prevention. (2014). Reducing HIV transmission from mother-to-child: An opt-out approach to HIV screening. Available at www.cdc.gov/hiv/risk/gender/pregnantwomen/opt-out.html.

In prenatal care models that use a reduced-frequency screening schedule or in group prenatal care (e.g., CenteringPregnancy), the timing of follow-up visits varies, but assessments and care are similar (see Box 14-3).

Interview

Follow-up visits are briefer and less intensive than the initial prenatal visit. At each of these follow-up visits, the woman is asked to summarize relevant events that have occurred since the previous visit. She is asked about her general emotional and physiologic well-being, complaints, problems, and questions she may have. Family needs also are identified and explored (Fig. 14-6).

Emotional changes are common during pregnancy, and therefore asking whether the woman has experienced any mood swings, reactions to changes in her body image, bad dreams, or worries is reasonable. The nurse documents the reactions of the partner and other family members to the pregnancy and the woman's emotional changes.

During the third trimester it is important to assess current family situations and their effect on the woman as well as siblings' and grandparents' responses to the pregnancy and the coming child. This is a time to assess the woman and her family's knowledge of warning signs of emergencies, signs of preterm and term labor, the labor process and concerns about labor, and fetal development and methods to assess fetal well-being. The nurse should ask if the woman is planning to attend childbirth preparation classes and what she knows about management of discomfort during labor.

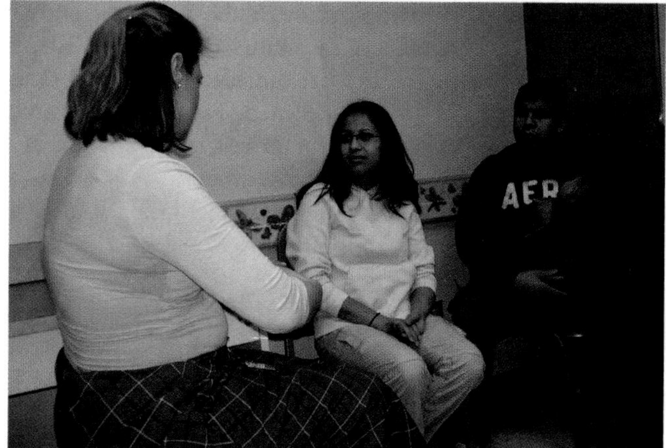

FIG 14-6 A prenatal interview. (Courtesy Dee Lowdermilk, Chapel Hill, NC.)

A review of the woman's physical systems is appropriate at each prenatal visit, and any suspicious signs or symptoms are assessed in depth. This review of systems includes identifying any discomforts reflecting adaptations to pregnancy. The nurse inquires about success with self-care measures as well as outcomes of prescribed therapy.

Physical Examination

Reevaluation is a constant aspect of a pregnant woman's care. Physiologic changes are documented as the pregnancy progresses and reviewed for possible deviations from normal progress.

At each visit physical parameters are measured. BP is measured using the same arm at every visit. The woman's weight is assessed, and the appropriateness of the gestational weight gain is evaluated in relationship to her BMI. Urine may be checked by dipstick, and the presence and degree of edema are noted. For examination of the abdomen, the woman lies on her back with her arms by her side and head supported by a pillow. A small wedge is placed under her right hip to tilt her slightly to the left. The bladder should be empty. Abdominal inspection is followed by measurement of the height of the fundus (see Fig. 14-8). While the woman lies on her back, the nurse should be alert for the occurrence of supine hypotension (see the Emergency box).

EMERGENCY

Supine Hypotension

Signs and Symptoms
- Pallor
- Dizziness, faintness, breathlessness
- Tachycardia
- Nausea
- Clammy (damp, cool) skin; sweating

Interventions
- Position woman on her side until her signs and symptoms subside and vital signs stabilize within normal limits.

The information provided through the interview and the physical examination reflects the status of maternal adaptations. When any of the findings are outside the expected range, an in-depth examination is performed. For example, careful interpretation of BP is important in the risk factor analysis of all pregnant women. Signs and symptoms other than hypertension also can be present that indicate potential complications (see Signs of Potential Complications).

SIGNS OF POTENTIAL COMPLICATIONS

First, Second, and Third Trimesters

SIGNS AND SYMPTOMS	POSSIBLE CAUSES
First Trimester	
Severe vomiting	Hyperemesis gravidarum
Chills, fever	Infection
Burning on urination	Infection
Diarrhea	Infection
Abdominal cramping; vaginal bleeding	Miscarriage, ectopic pregnancy
Second and Third Trimesters	
Persistent, severe vomiting	Hyperemesis gravidarum, hypertension, preeclampsia
Sudden discharge of fluid from vagina before 37 weeks	Preterm premature rupture of membranes (PPROM)
Vaginal bleeding, severe abdominal pain	Miscarriage, placenta previa, abruptio placentae
Chills, fever, burning on urination, diarrhea	Infection
Severe backache or flank pain	Kidney infection or stones; preterm labor
Change in fetal movements: absence of fetal movements after quickening, any unusual change in pattern or amount	Fetal jeopardy or intrauterine fetal death
Uterine contractions; pressure; cramping before 37 weeks	Preterm labor
Visual disturbances: blurring, double vision, or spots	Hypertensive conditions, preeclampsia
Swelling of face or fingers and over sacrum	Hypertensive conditions, preeclampsia
Headaches: severe, frequent, or continuous	Hypertensive conditions, preeclampsia
Muscular irritability or convulsions	Hypertensive conditions, preeclampsia
Epigastric or abdominal pain (perceived as heartburn or severe stomachache)	Hypertensive conditions, preeclampsia, abruptio placentae
Glycosuria, positive glucose tolerance test reaction	Gestational diabetes mellitus

Fetal Assessment

Gestational Age. In an uncomplicated pregnancy fetal gestational age is estimated after the duration of pregnancy and the EDB are determined. Fetal gestational age is determined from the menstrual history, contraceptive history, pregnancy test result, and the following findings obtained during the clinical evaluation:

- First uterine evaluation: date, size
- Fetal heart first heard: date, method (Doppler stethoscope, fetoscope)
- Date of quickening
- Current fundal height, estimated fetal weight (EFW)
- Current week of gestation by history of LMP and/or ultrasound examination
- Ultrasound examination: date, week of gestation, biparietal diameter (BPD)
- Reliability of dates

Quickening usually occurs between 16 and 20 weeks of gestation and is initially experienced as a fluttering sensation. The mother's report should be recorded. Multiparous women often perceive fetal movement earlier than primigravidas.

The use of ultrasound examination (also called a *sonogram*) in early pregnancy has become routine, and many health care providers have this equipment available in the office or clinic. This procedure may be used to establish the duration of pregnancy if the woman cannot give a precise date for her LMP or if the size of the uterus does not conform to the EDB as calculated by Naegele's rule. Ultrasound can detect a multiple gestation pregnancy and provide information about the well-being of the fetus or fetuses (see Chapter 26 for further discussion).

Fetal Heart Tones. The fetal heart tones (FHT) are checked on routine visits. Early in pregnancy the fetal heartbeat can be detected during ultrasound examination. Late in the first trimester the heartbeat can be heard with a Doppler device that transmits fetal heart tones through a speaker or attached ear pieces (Fig. 14-7, *B*). As the uterus grows and becomes an abdominal organ, the fetal heartbeat can also be auscultated with a fetoscope (see Fig. 14-7, *A*). Many practitioners use the Doppler device because it allows the mother and others who are present to easily hear the fetal heartbeat. Another tool for assessing fetal heart tones is the Pinard horn, which is a fetoscope commonly used by midwives and in much of Europe (see Fig. 14-7, *C*).

To detect the heartbeat before the fetal position can be palpated by Leopold maneuvers (see Chapter 19), the Doppler or fetoscope is moved around the abdomen until the heartbeat is heard. Each nurse develops a set pattern for searching the abdomen for the heartbeat—for example, starting first in the midline about 2 to 3 cm above the symphysis pubis, then moving to the left lower quadrant, and so on. The heartbeat is counted for 1 minute, and the quality and rhythm noted. A normal rate and rhythm are other good indicators of fetal health. Once the heartbeat is noted, its absence is cause for immediate investigation.

Health Status. The assessment of fetal health status often includes consideration of fetal movement. Absence of fetal movement is correlated with fetal death; women who report decreased fetal movement have an increased risk for adverse outcomes (AAP & ACOG, 2012). The mother is instructed to note the extent and timing of fetal movements and to report immediately if the pattern changes or if movement ceases. The woman may be instructed to count movements daily over a 1- or 2-hour period. Her perception of four or more movements in an hour is considered reassuring. There is no standard recommendation for the ideal number of movements or kicks or for the duration of daily fetal movement assessment. The most important consideration is the mother's perception that fetal movements have decreased relative to previous levels (AAP & ACOG).

Fetal health status is investigated intensively if any maternal or fetal complications arise (e.g., gestational hypertension, intrauterine growth restriction (IUGR), premature rupture of

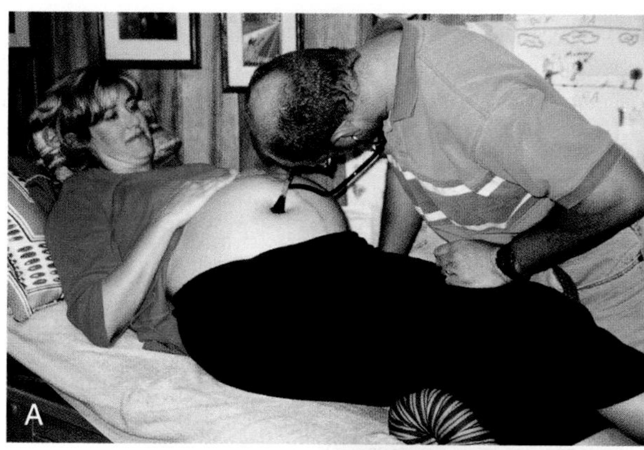

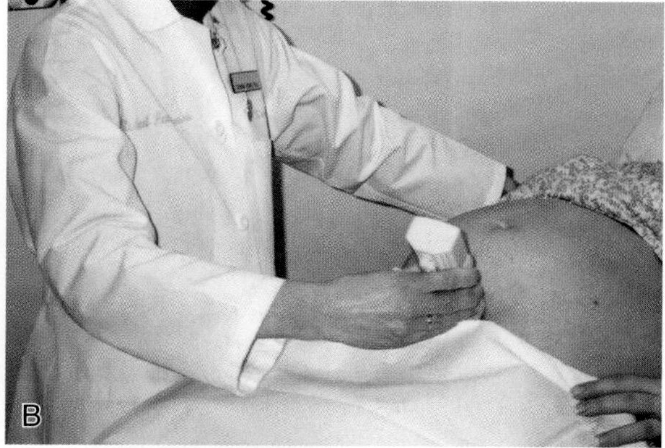

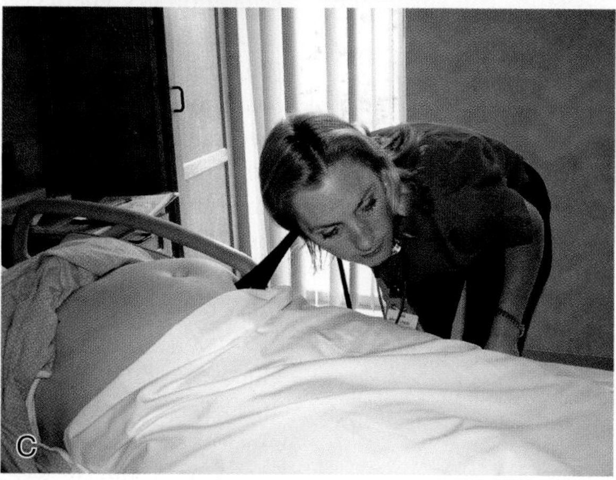

FIG 14-7 Detecting fetal heartbeat. **A,** Father can listen to the fetal heart with a fetoscope (first detectable at 18 to 20 weeks with a fetoscope). **B,** Doppler ultrasound stethoscope (fetal heartbeat detectable at 12 weeks). **C,** Pinard fetoscope. Note: Hands should not touch fetoscope while listening. (**A,** Courtesy Shannon Perry, Phoenix, AZ. **B,** Courtesy Dee Lowdermilk, Chapel Hill, NC. **C,** Courtesy Julie Perry Nelson, Loveland, CO.)

membranes [PROM], irregular or absent FHR, or decreased or absent fetal movements after quickening). Careful, precise, and concise recording of the woman's responses and laboratory results contributes to the continuous supervision vital to promoting the well-being of the mother and fetus.

Fundal Height. During the second trimester the uterus becomes an abdominal organ. The fundal height (measurement of the height of the uterus above the symphysis pubis) is one indicator of fetal growth. The measurement also provides a gross estimate of the duration of pregnancy. From gestational weeks (GW) 18 to 30, the height of the fundus in centimeters is approximately the same as the number of weeks of gestation (±2 GW), if the woman's bladder is empty at the time of measurement. As much as a 3-cm variation is possible if the bladder is full. For example, a woman of 28 weeks of gestation, with an empty bladder, would measure from 26 to 30 cm. The fundal height measurement can aid in identifying risk factors. A stable or decreased fundal height can indicate intrauterine growth restriction (IUGR); an excessive increase can indicate the presence of multifetal gestation (more than one fetus) or polyhydramnios.

A disposable paper metric tape measure is preferred for measuring fundal height; plastic retractable tape measures should be cleaned after use and prior to retraction. To increase the reliability of the measurement, the same person examines the pregnant woman at each of her prenatal visits, but often this is not possible. All clinicians who examine a particular pregnant woman should be consistent in their measurement technique. Ideally a protocol should be established for the health care setting in which the measurement technique is explicitly set forth, and the woman's position on the examining table, the measuring device, and method of measurement used are specified. Conditions under which the measurements are taken also can be described in the woman's records, including whether the bladder was empty and whether the uterus was relaxed or contracted at the time of measurement.

Various positions for measuring fundal height have been described. The woman can be supine with her head elevated and/or knees flexed. Measurements obtained with the woman in the various positions differ, making it even more important to standardize the fundal height measurement technique.

Placement of the tape measure also can vary. The tape can be placed in the middle of the woman's abdomen and the measurement made from the upper border of the symphysis pubis to the upper border of the fundus, with the tape measure held in contact with the skin for the entire length of the uterus (Fig. 14-8, *A*). In another measurement technique, the upper curve of the fundus is not included in the measurement. Instead, one end of the tape measure is held at the upper border of the symphysis pubis with one hand, and the other hand is placed at the upper border of the fundus. The tape is placed between the middle and index fingers of the other hand, and the point where these fingers intercept the tape measure is taken as the measurement (see Fig. 14-8, *B*).

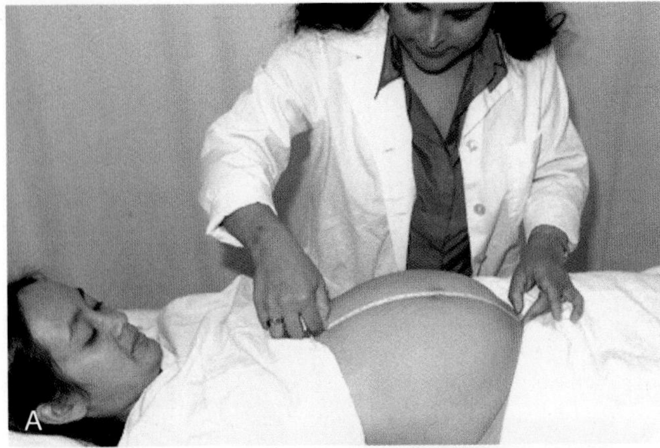

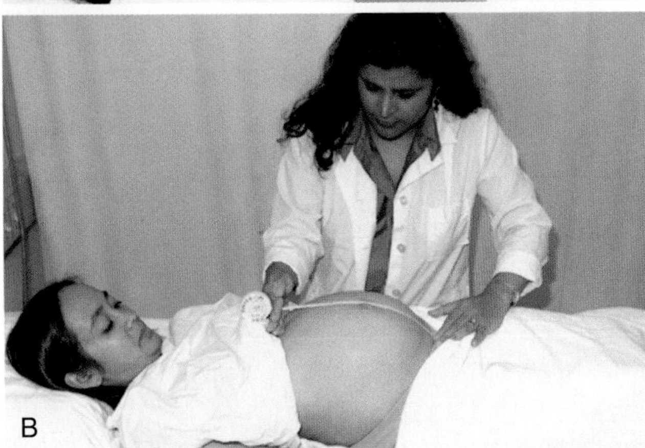

FIG 14-8 Measurement of fundal height from symphysis pubis that **A**, includes the upper curve of the fundus and **B**, does not include the upper curve of the fundus. Note position of hands and measuring tape. (Courtesy Chris Rozales, San Francisco, CA.)

Laboratory Tests

The number of routine laboratory tests done during follow-up visits in pregnancy is limited. A clean-catch urine specimen is obtained to test for glucose, protein, nitrites, and leukocytes at each visit. Urine specimens for culture and sensitivity are obtained, and cervical and vaginal smears and blood tests are repeated as necessary.

Sequential integrated screening (SIS) is an option for women who begin prenatal care before 14 weeks of gestation; it involves two blood tests and one ultrasound. This multiple marker screen can identify the following conditions: Down syndrome (trisomy 21), trisomy 18, neural tube defects (anencephaly and spina bifida), abdominal wall defects (gastroschisis and omphalocele), and Smith-Lemli-Opitz syndrome. The first blood test is performed between 10 and 13 weeks of gestation to measure two biochemical markers—pregnancy-associated placental protein (PAPP-A) and free beta-human chorionic gonadotropin (β-hCG). The second step for SIS is an ultrasound between 11 and 14 weeks of gestation to assess for nuchal translucency. The final step in SIS is performed between 15 and 20 weeks of pregnancy and measures the levels of four substances normally found in a pregnant woman's blood: alpha-fetoprotein (AFP), human chorionic gonadotropin (hCG), unconjugated estriol, and inhibin-A. This second group of four tests is also known as quad marker screening. Maternal serum marker levels that are higher or lower than normal are associated with increased risk of chromosomal abnormalities (see Chapter 26). Women who begin their prenatal care between the fourteenth and twentieth weeks of pregnancy are too advanced in their pregnancy to be offered the first two steps in SIS, but can be offered the quad marker screening alone (Wapner, 2014). Noninvasive prenatal testing (NIPT) is a new genetic test used to identify fetuses at risk for trisomies 21, 18, and 13 and sex chromosome abnormalities. NIPT detects fetal deoxyribonucleic acid (DNA) circulating in the maternal blood (cell-free DNA) as a result of the breakdown of fetal cells. Positive NIPT results should be followed by a confirmatory test such as chorionic villus sampling or amniocentesis (National Coalition for Health Professional Education in Genetics, 2012).

The American College of Obstetricians and Gynecologists (2013) recommends glucose screening for all pregnant women. Assessment for risk factors can be done through review of the medical history, screening for clinical risk factors, or measurement of blood glucose levels. Risk factors that warrant early screening include obesity, history of gestational diabetes mellitus (GDM), or known impairment of glucose metabolism. If GDM is not diagnosed with early screening, blood glucose testing is repeated at 24 to 28 weeks. The standard screening test for GDM is a 1-hour, 50-g oral glucose tolerance test (GTT). If the glucose level is elevated, further testing is done using a 3-hour, 100-g GTT (see Chapter 29).

Group B streptococcus (GBS) testing is recommended between 35 and 37 weeks of gestation; cultures collected earlier will not accurately predict GBS status at time of birth. All pregnant women should have GBS testing, even those who are scheduled for a cesarean birth, because labor can begin or membranes can rupture prior to the routine administration of prophylactic antibiotics. Women with a history of GBS in a previous pregnancy should be retested with each pregnancy (ACOG Committee on Obstetric Practice, 2013d).

See Chapter 26 for other diagnostic tests available to assess the health status of the pregnant woman and fetus.

Nursing Interventions

After obtaining information through the assessment process, the data are analyzed to identify deviations from the norm and unique needs of the pregnant woman and her family. Care is optimized with a collaborative approach involving the physician or CNM, nurse, other relevant health care professionals, the woman, her partner, and her family.

The nurse-client relationship is critical in setting the tone for further interaction. The techniques of active listening with an attentive expression, using touch and eye contact (if culturally appropriate), have their place, as does recognizing the woman's feelings and her right to express these feelings. The interaction may occur in various formal or informal settings. A clinical setting, home visits, or telephone conversations all provide opportunities for contact and can be used effectively.

Education for Self-Management

The expectant mother needs information on many topics. The nurse who is observant, listens, and is familiar with typical concerns of expectant parents can anticipate the questions that will be asked and can encourage mothers and their partners to discuss what is on their minds. Printed literature can be given to supplement the individualized teaching the nurse provides. To be most effective, educational materials should be appropriate for the pregnant woman's or couple's ethnicity, culture, and literacy level and the agency's resources. Women often avidly read books, pamphlets, and web information related to their own pregnancy experience. Nurses should be familiar with the educational materials that are distributed to expectant parents as well as popular web-based resources related to pregnancy. Nurses can direct pregnant women and their families to reliable websites that contain accurate information.

Because family members are common sources for health information, it is also important to include them in health education endeavors during pregnancy (U.S. Department of Health and Human Services Office of Disease Prevention and Promotion, 2013). This can enhance their ability to be supportive of the pregnant woman as she progresses through pregnancy.

Pregnant women who receive conflicting advice or instruction are likely to grow increasingly frustrated with members of the health care team and the care provided. Several topics that can cause concerns in pregnant women are discussed in the following sections.

Expected Maternal and Fetal Changes. Most expectant parents are curious about the growth and development of the fetus and the changes that occur in the mother's body during pregnancy. Mothers are often more tolerant of the discomforts related to the continuing pregnancy if they understand the underlying causes. Educational literature (printed, electronic, or web-based materials) that describes fetal and maternal changes can be used to explain changes as they occur. Couples can track the development of their growing fetus through websites such as www.babycenter.com/fetal-development or www.parents.com/pregnancy/stages/fetal-development.

Nutrition. Good nutrition is important for the maintenance of maternal health during pregnancy and the provision of adequate nutrients for embryonic and fetal development. Assessing a woman's nutritional status and weight gain and providing ongoing education about nutrition are part of the nurse's responsibilities in providing prenatal care. Education for pregnant women includes recommendations about daily intake of nutrients, calories, vitamins, and minerals. Based on the woman's BMI, the recommended weight gain during pregnancy is discussed. Additional information regarding nutrition during pregnancy may include foods high in iron, the importance of taking prenatal vitamins, and recommendations to avoid alcohol and to limit caffeine intake. Pregnant women are instructed about how to avoid food-borne illnesses such as listeriosis. At each visit the nurse assesses for practice of pica. In some settings a nutritionist counsels women individually or conducts classes for pregnant women about nutrition during pregnancy. Nurses can refer women to a nutritionist if a need is identified during the nursing assessment. (For detailed information concerning maternal and fetal nutritional needs and related nursing care, see Chapter 15.)

Personal Hygiene. During pregnancy the sebaceous (sweat) glands are highly active because of hormonal influences, and women often perspire freely. They can be informed that the increase is normal and that their previous patterns of perspiration will return after the postpartum period. Baths and warm showers can be therapeutic because they relax tense, tired muscles; help counter insomnia; and make the pregnant woman feel fresh. Tub bathing is not restricted even in late pregnancy because little water enters the vagina unless under pressure. However, late in pregnancy, when the woman's center of gravity lowers, she is at risk for falling. Tub bathing is contraindicated after rupture of the membranes.

Prevention of Urinary Tract Infections. Because of physiologic changes that occur in the renal system during pregnancy (see Chapter 13), infections of the lower urinary tract (acute urethritis, acute cystitis) are common. *Escherichia coli (E. coli)* is the most common causative organism for urinary tract infection (UTI) in pregnant women (Duff, 2012). Although UTIs can be asymptomatic, typical symptoms include frequency, urgency, dysuria, dribbling, and hesitancy; gross hematuria can occur. Women should be instructed to inform their health care provider promptly if they experience these symptoms. Urinary tract infections pose a risk to the mother and fetus, and thus their prevention or early treatment is essential. Oral antibiotics are commonly prescribed.

The nurse can assess the woman's understanding and use of appropriate hand hygiene techniques before and after urinating and the importance of wiping the perineum from front to back. Soft, absorbent toilet tissue, preferably white and unscented, should be used; harsh, scented, or printed toilet paper can cause irritation. Bubble bath or other bath oils should be avoided because these can irritate the urethra. Women should wear all-cotton undergarments and cotton-lined pantyhose and avoid tight-fitting slacks or jeans for long periods; anything that allows a buildup of heat and moisture in the genital area can foster the growth of bacteria.

Some women do not consume enough fluid. The nurse should advise her to drink at least 2 L (eight glasses) of liquid a day, preferably water, to maintain an adequate fluid intake that ensures frequent urination. Pregnant women should not limit fluids in an effort to reduce the frequency of urination. Women need to know that if urine appears dark (concentrated), they must increase their fluid intake.

The nurse should review healthy urination practices with the woman. Women are told not to ignore the urge to urinate because holding urine lengthens the time bacteria are in the bladder and allows them to multiply. Women should plan ahead when they are faced with situations that can require them to delay urination (e.g., a long car ride). They always should urinate before going to bed at night. Bacteria can be introduced during intercourse; therefore, women are advised to urinate before and after intercourse, and then drink a large glass of water to promote additional urination. Consumption of cranberry juice has been offered as an intervention to prevent UTI. The effectiveness of cranberry juice in the prevention of UTIs is dependent on long-term adherence to daily consumption of about 10 ounces of juice (Jepson, Williams, & Craig, 2012). The value of recommending cranberry juice to prevent UTI must include consideration of cost, sugar content, and additional calories. Low-sugar or pure cranberry juices may be recommended. Some women take cranberry pills as an alternative to drinking juice.

Kegel Exercises. Kegel exercises (deliberate contraction and relaxation of the pubococcygeus muscle) strengthen the muscles around the reproductive organs and improve muscle tone. Many women are not aware of the muscles of the pelvic floor until it is pointed out that these are the muscles used during urination and sexual intercourse that can be consciously controlled. The muscles of the pelvic floor encircle the vaginal outlet, and they need to be exercised because an exercised muscle can then stretch and contract readily at the time of birth. Practice of pelvic muscle exercises during pregnancy also results in fewer complaints of urinary incontinence in late pregnancy and postpartum (Kocaöz, Erogul, & Sivaslioglu, 2013).

Several ways of performing Kegel exercises have been described. The method described in the Teaching for Self-Management box: Kegel Exercises in Chapter 4 demonstrates evidence-based nursing care. This method was developed by nurses involved in a research utilization project for continence in women. Teaching has been effective if the woman reports an increased ability to control urine flow and greater muscular control during sexual intercourse.

Preparation for Breastfeeding. During the first prenatal visit, the nurse asks if the woman is planning to breastfeed. A woman's decision about the method of infant feeding is usually made before pregnancy; thus it is essential to educate women of childbearing age about the benefits of breastfeeding. The woman and her partner are encouraged to decide which method of feeding is suitable for them; however, the benefits of breastfeeding should be emphasized. Once the couple has been given information about the advantages and disadvantages of breastfeeding and formula-feeding, they can make an informed choice. Most women who choose to breastfeed do so because they are aware of the numerous benefits (see Chapter 25). Lack of knowledge about the benefits of breastfeeding and perceived personal and social disadvantages to breastfeeding can influence a woman not to breastfeed. Modesty issues, lack of support by the partner and family, incompatibility with lifestyle, and lack of confidence are among the reasons cited by women who decide to formula-feed their infants (Lawrence & Lawrence, 2011; Nelson, 2012).

Assessment of breasts during the prenatal period can reveal potential concerns related to breastfeeding. Scars on the breast can indicate previous breast reduction surgery, which can affect milk production. The woman may have breast implants; this may affect successful breastfeeding. Asymmetry of the breasts or tubular-shaped breasts suggest a lack of glandular tissue and potential problems with adequate milk production. Examination of the breasts can reveal flat or inverted nipples, which can affect the baby's ability to successfully latch on to the breast. To determine if nipples are inverted, a woman can perform a test on her nipples to determine freedom of protrusion (Fig. 14-9). The woman places her thumb and forefinger on her areola and presses inward gently. A normal nipple will evert or stand erect while an inverted nipple will appear to withdraw (Lawrence & Lawrence, 2011).

Exercises to break the adhesions that cause the nipple to invert do not work and can cause uterine contractions. Some clinicians recommend the prenatal use of breast shells (Fig. 14-10) during the last trimester for women with flat or inverted nipples, although evidence to support their effectiveness is lacking. They can be uncomfortable and cause irritation to the nipple or areola. Breast stimulation is contraindicated in women at risk for preterm labor; therefore, the decision to suggest the use of breast shells to women with flat or inverted nipples must be made judiciously (Lawrence & Lawrence, 2011).

There is no special preparation of the nipples or breasts for breastfeeding. The woman is taught to cleanse the nipples with warm water to keep the ducts from being blocked with dried colostrum. Soap, ointments, alcohol, and tinctures should not be applied because they remove protective oils that keep the nipples supple. Breast pads with plastic liners should be avoided (Lawrence & Lawrence, 2011).

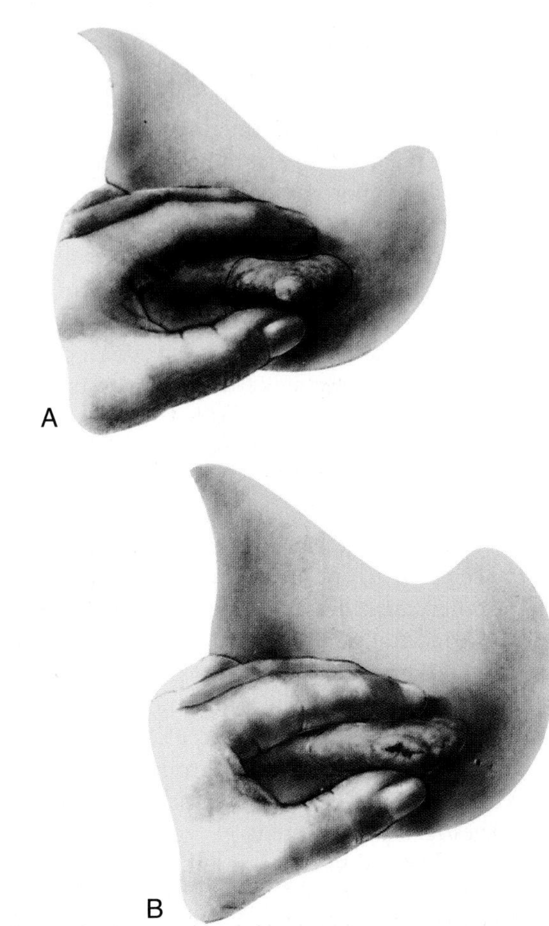

FIG 14-9 Test for inverted nipples **A,** Normal nipple everts with gentle pressure. **B,** Inverted nipple inverts with gentle pressure. (Adapted from Lawrence, R.A., & Lawrence, R.M. [2011]. *Breastfeeding: A guide for the medical profession* [7th ed.]. St. Louis: Mosby.)

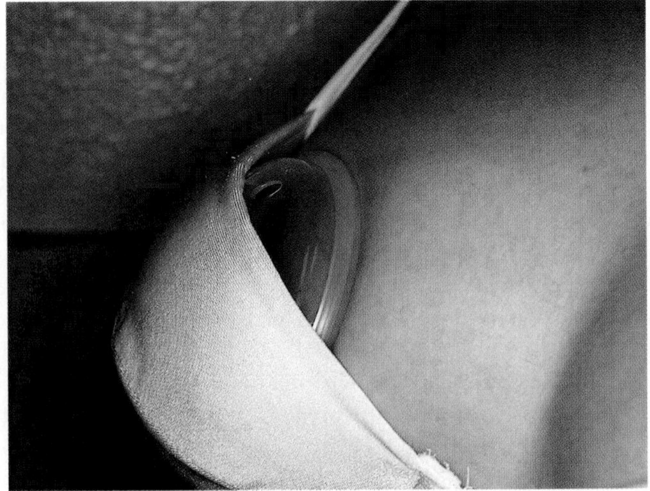

FIG 14-10 Breast shell in place inside bra; sometimes recommended for flat or inverted nipples. (Courtesy Michael S. Clement, MD, Mesa, AZ.)

TEACHING FOR SELF-MANAGEMENT BOX

Exercise Tips for Pregnant Women

- *Consult your health care provider* when you know or suspect you are pregnant. Discuss your health and pregnancy history, your current exercise regimen, and the exercises you would like to continue throughout pregnancy.
- *Seek help* in determining an exercise routine that is well within your limit of tolerance, especially if you have not been exercising regularly.
- *Consider decreasing weight-bearing exercises* (jogging, running) and concentrating on non–weight-bearing activities such as swimming, cycling, or stretching. If you are a runner, starting in your seventh month, you may wish to walk instead.
- *Avoid risky activities* such as surfing, mountain climbing, skydiving, and racquetball because such activities, which require precise balance and coordination, can be dangerous. Avoid activities that require holding your breath and bearing down (Valsalva maneuver). Jerky, bouncy motions also should be avoided.
- *Exercise regularly* every day if possible, as long as you are healthy, to improve muscle tone and increase or maintain your stamina. Exercising sporadically can place undue strain on your muscles. Thirty minutes of moderate physical exercise is recommended. This activity can be broken up into shorter segments with rest in between. For example, exercise for 10 to 15 minutes, rest for 2 to 3 minutes, and then exercise for another 10 to 15 minutes.
- *Consider decreasing your exercise level* as your pregnancy progresses. The normal alterations of advancing pregnancy, such as decreased cardiac reserve and increased respiratory effort, can produce physiologic stress if you exercise strenuously for a long time.
- *Take your pulse* every 10 to 15 minutes while you are exercising. If it is more than 140 beats/min, slow down until it returns to a maximum of 90 beats/min. You should be able to converse easily while exercising. If you cannot, you need to slow down.
- *Avoid becoming overheated* for extended periods. It is best not to exercise for more than 35 minutes, especially in hot, humid weather. As your body temperature rises, the heat is transmitted to your fetus. Prolonged or repeated elevation of fetal temperature can result in birth defects, especially during the first 3 months of pregnancy. Your temperature should not exceed 38° C.
- *Do not use hot tubs and saunas.*
- *Perform warm-up and stretching exercises* to prepare your joints for more strenuous exercise and lessen the likelihood of strain or injury to your joints. After the fourth month of pregnancy you should not perform exercises flat on your back.
- *Include a cool-down period* of mild activity involving your legs after an exercise period to help bring your respiration, heart, and metabolic rates back to normal and prevent blood from pooling in the exercised muscles.
- *Rest for 10 minutes after exercising,* lying on your side. As the uterus grows it puts pressure on a major vein in your abdomen that carries blood to your heart. Lying on your side removes the pressure and promotes return circulation from your extremities and muscles to your heart, thereby increasing blood flow to your placenta and fetus. You should rise gradually from the floor to prevent dizziness or fainting (orthostatic hypotension).
- *Stay hydrated.* Drink two or three 8-ounce glasses of water after you exercise to replace the body fluids lost through perspiration. While exercising, drink water whenever you feel the need.
- *Increase your caloric intake* to replace the calories burned during exercise and provide the extra energy needs of pregnancy. Choose high-protein foods such as fish, milk, cheese, eggs, and meat.
- *Take your time.* This is not the time to be competitive or train for activities requiring speed or long endurance.
- *Wear a supportive bra.* Your increased breast weight can cause changes in posture and put pressure on the ulnar nerve.
- *Wear supportive shoes.* As your uterus grows your center of gravity shifts and you compensate for this by arching your back. These natural changes can make you feel off balance and more likely to fall.
- *Stop exercising immediately* if you experience shortness of breath, dizziness, numbness, tingling, pain of any kind, more than four uterine contractions per hour, decreased fetal activity, or vaginal bleeding, and consult your health care provider.
- *Recognize signs of danger,* including vaginal bleeding*; blurred vision*; nausea; dizziness; fainting*; breathlessness; heart palpitations; increased swelling in your hands, feet, and ankles; sharp pain in the abdomen and chest*; and sudden change in body temperature.
- *Avoid the following exercises* during pregnancy: downhill snow skiing because the center of gravity changes and there is a risk for falls; contact sports such as ice hockey, soccer, and basketball; and scuba diving because the pressure from the water could put the fetus at risk for decompression sickness.

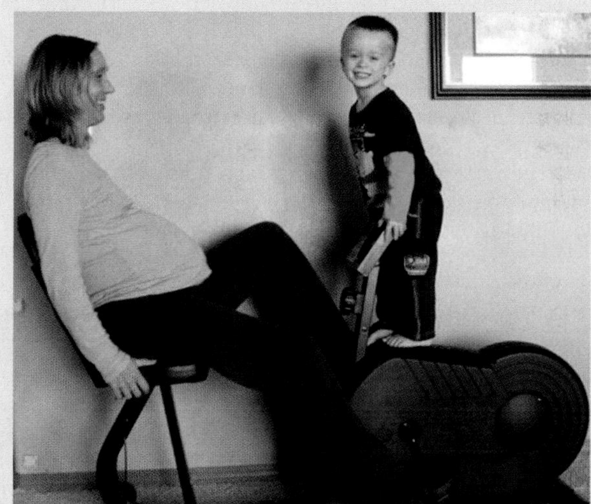

Riding recumbent bicycle provides exercise while supplying back support. Big brother becomes involved. (Courtesy Julie Perry Nelson, Loveland, CO.)

Sources: American College of Obstetricians and Gynecologists (ACOG) Committee on Obstetric Practice. (2009). Committee opinion no. 267: Exercise during pregnancy and the postpartum period. Available at www.acog.org/Resources_And_Publications/Committee_Opinions/Committee_on_Obstetric_Practice/Exercise_During_Pregnancy_and_the_Postpartum_Period; American College of Obstetricians and Gynecologists. (2011). Exercise during pregnancy (FAQ 0119). Available at https://www.acog.org/~/media/For%20Patients/faq119.pdf?dmc=1&ts=20140602T2215146111.

*If you experience any of these signs, contact your physician or midwife immediately.

A bra that fits well and provides support promotes comfort as breasts increase in size during pregnancy. The woman who plans to breastfeed may want to purchase a nursing bra that will accommodate her increased breast size during the last few months of pregnancy and during lactation.

Dental Health. Dental care during pregnancy is especially important because nausea during pregnancy can lead to poor oral hygiene, allowing dental caries to develop. Fluoride toothpaste should be used daily. Inflammation and infection of the gingival and periodontal tissues can occur. Research links periodontal disease with preterm births and LBW and an increased risk for preeclampsia (Jared & Boggess, 2012).

Early in prenatal care, the nurse should ask the woman about her last dental visit. If it was more than 6 months earlier, she should schedule a dental examination soon (Oral Health Care During Pregnancy Expert Workgroup, 2012).

Because calcium and phosphorus in the teeth are fixed in enamel, the old adage "for every child a tooth" is not true. There is no scientific evidence to support the belief that filling teeth or even dental extraction involving the administration of local or nitrous oxide-oxygen anesthesia precipitates miscarriage or preterm labor. Antibacterial therapy should be considered for prevention of sepsis, especially in pregnant women who have had rheumatic heart disease or nephritis.

Diagnosis and treatment of oral health problems, including necessary dental x-rays and the use of local anesthetics or nitrous oxide-oxygen anesthesia, are considered safe during pregnancy. Dental care and nonemergent procedures are best scheduled during the second trimester when the woman is past the stage of feeling nauseated and can sit comfortably in the chair. To avoid supine hypotension during dental procedures, the pregnant woman in her second or third trimester is positioned in the dental chair with a small pillow under her right hip (Oral Health Care During Pregnancy Expert Workgroup, 2012).

Physical Activity. Physical activity promotes a feeling of well-being in the pregnant woman. It improves circulation, promotes relaxation and rest, and counteracts boredom, as it does in the nonpregnant woman (Price, Amini, & Kappeler, 2012). Detailed exercise tips for pregnancy are presented in the Teaching for Self-Management box: Exercise Tips for Pregnant Women. Exercises that help relieve the low back pain that often arises during the second trimester because of the increased weight of the fetus are demonstrated in Figure 14-11 (see Clinical Reasoning Case Study).

CLINICAL REASONING CASE STUDY

Exercise in Pregnancy

Lourdes is 16 weeks pregnant with her second child. She wants to avoid gaining extra weight during this pregnancy and would like to continue her exercise habits: walking and Zumba classes. What guidance can you give to Lourdes?

1. Evidence—Is the evidence sufficient to make a recommendation for or against exercising during pregnancy?
2. Assumptions—Describe the underlying assumptions for each of the following issues:
   a. Physiologic changes in pregnancy that affect balance, movement, respiration, and cardiac function
   b. Maternal physiologic response during exercise
   c. Benefits of exercise
3. What implications and priorities for nursing care can be drawn at this time?
4. Does the evidence objectively support your conclusion?

Posture and Body Mechanics. Skeletal and musculature changes and hormonal changes in pregnancy can predispose the woman to backache and possible injury. As pregnancy progresses, the woman's center of gravity changes, pelvic joints soften and relax, and stress is placed on abdominal musculature. Poor posture and body mechanics contribute to the discomfort and potential for injury. To minimize these problems, women can learn good body posture and body mechanics (Fig. 14-12). Strategies to prevent or relieve backache are presented in the Teaching for Self-Management box: Posture and Body Mechanics.

Rest and Relaxation. Nurses encourage women to plan regular rest periods, particularly as pregnancy advances. The side-lying position is recommended because it promotes uterine perfusion and fetoplacental oxygenation by eliminating pressure on the ascending vena cava and descending aorta, which can lead to supine hypotension (Fig. 14-13). The woman

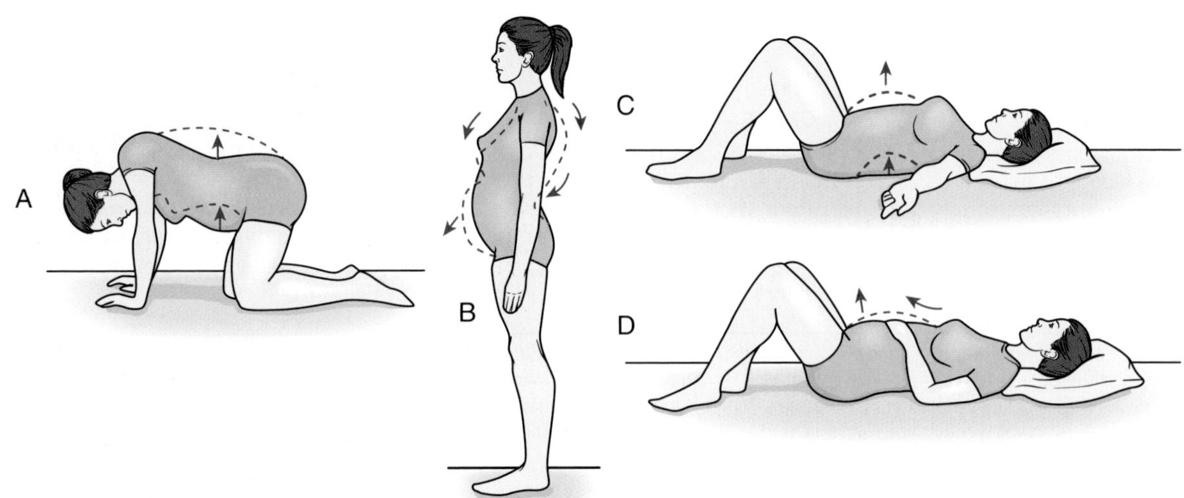

FIG 14-11 Exercises. **A, B,** and **C,** Pelvic rocking relieves low backache (excellent for relief of menstrual cramps as well). **D,** Abdominal breathing aids relaxation and lifts abdominal wall off uterus.

TEACHING FOR SELF-MANAGEMENT

Posture and Body Mechanics

To Prevent or Relieve Backache

Do pelvic tilt:

- Pelvic tilt (rock) on hands and knees (see Fig. 14-11, *A*) and while sitting in straight-back chair
- Pelvic tilt (rock) in standing position against a wall, or lying on floor (see Fig. 14-11, *B* and *C*)
- Perform abdominal muscle contractions during pelvic tilt while standing, lying, or sitting to help strengthen rectus abdominis muscle (see Fig. 14-11, *D*).

Use good body mechanics.

- Use leg muscles to reach objects on or near floor. Bend at the knees, not from the back. Knees are bent to lower body to squatting position. Feet are kept 12 to 18 inches apart to provide a solid base to maintain balance (see Fig. 14-12, *A*).
- Lift with the legs. To lift a heavy object (e.g., young child) one foot is placed slightly in front of the other and kept flat as woman lowers herself onto one knee. She lifts the weight, holding it close to her body and never higher than her chest. To stand up or sit down she places one leg slightly behind the other as she raises or lowers herself (see Fig. 14-12, *B*).

To Restrict the Lumbar Curve

- For prolonged standing (e.g., ironing, employment), place one foot on low footstool or box; change positions often.
- Move car seat forward so that knees are bent and higher than hips. If needed, use a small pillow to support the low back area.
- Sit in chairs low enough to allow both feet to be placed on floor, preferably with knees higher than hips.

To Prevent Round Ligament Pain and Strain on Abdominal Muscles

- Implement suggestions given in Table 14-2.

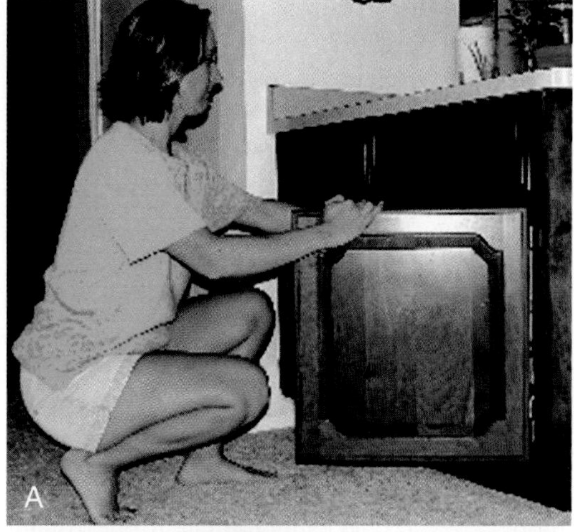

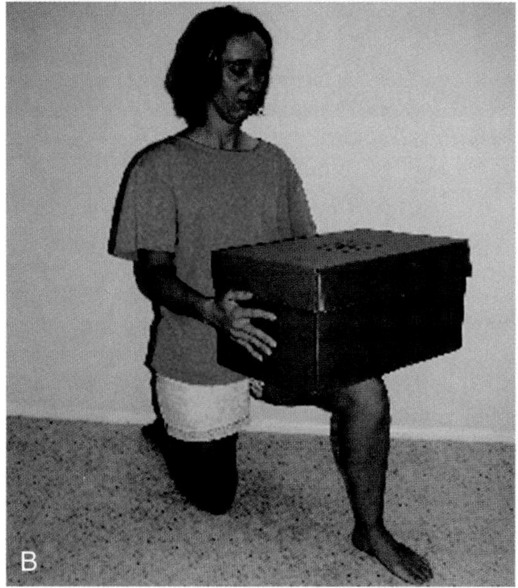

FIG 14-12 Correct body mechanics. **A,** Squatting. **B,** Lifting. (Courtesy Julie Perry Nelson, Loveland, CO.)

should be shown how to rise slowly from a side-lying position to prevent placing strain on the back and to minimize the orthostatic hypotension caused by changes in position common in the later part of pregnancy. To stretch and rest back muscles at home or work, the nurse can show the woman the way to do the following exercises:

- Stand behind a chair. Support and balance self by using the back of the chair (Fig. 14-14). Squat for 30 seconds; stand for 15 seconds. Repeat 6 times, several times per day, as needed.
- While sitting in a chair, lower head to knees for 30 seconds. Raise head. Repeat 6 times, several times per day, as needed.

Conscious relaxation is the process of releasing tension from the mind and body through deliberate effort and practice. The techniques for conscious relaxation are numerous and varied. Box 14-5 gives some guidelines. The ability to relax consciously and intentionally is beneficial for the following reasons:

- To relieve the normal discomforts related to pregnancy
- To reduce stress and therefore diminish pain perception during the childbearing cycle
- To heighten self-awareness and trust in one's own ability to control responses and functions
- To help cope with stress in everyday life situations.

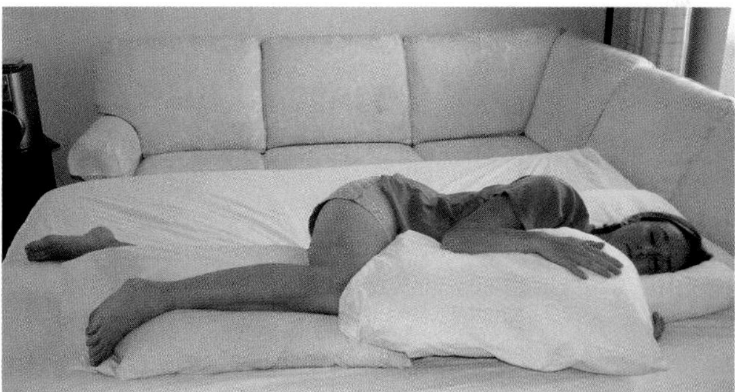

FIG 14-13 Side-lying position for rest and relaxation. (Courtesy Julie Perry Nelson, Loveland, CO.)

Employment. Employment of pregnant women usually has no adverse effects on pregnancy outcomes. Job discrimination that is based strictly on pregnancy is illegal. However, some job environments pose potential risk to the fetus (e.g., dry-cleaning plants, chemistry laboratories, parking garages). Excessive fatigue is usually the deciding factor in the termination of employment. Strategies to improve safety during pregnancy are described in the Teaching for Self-Management box: Safety During Pregnancy.

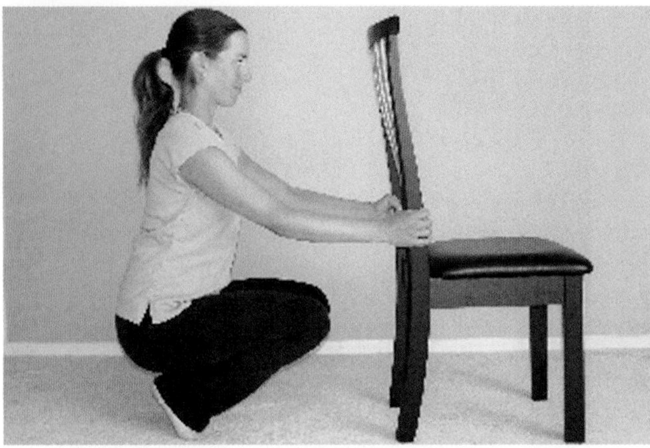

FIG 14-14 Squatting for muscle relaxation and strengthening and for keeping leg and hip joints flexible. (Courtesy Julie Perry Nelson, Loveland, CO.)

TEACHING FOR SELF-MANAGEMENT

Safety During Pregnancy

Changes in the body resulting from pregnancy include relaxation of the joints, alteration to the center of gravity, faintness, and discomforts. Problems with coordination and balance are common. Therefore, the woman should follow these guidelines:

- Use correct body mechanics.
- Use safety features on tools and vehicles (e.g., safety seat belts, shoulder harnesses, headrests, goggles, helmets) as specified.
- Avoid activities requiring coordination, balance, and concentration.
- Take rest periods; reschedule daily activities to meet rest and relaxation needs.

The developing fetus is vulnerable to environmental teratogens. Many potentially dangerous chemicals—cleaning agents, paints, sprays, herbicides, and pesticides—are present in the home, yard, and workplace. The soil and water supply may be unsafe. Therefore, the woman should follow these guidelines:

- Read all labels for ingredients and proper use of a product.
- Ensure adequate ventilation with clean air.
- Dispose of wastes appropriately.
- Wear gloves when handling chemicals.
- Change job assignments or workplace as necessary.
- Avoid travel to high-altitude regions above 12,000 feet.

Women with sedentary jobs need to walk around at intervals to counter the usual sluggish circulation in the legs. They also should neither sit nor stand in one position for long periods, and they should avoid crossing their legs at the knees, because all of these activities can increase the risk of varices and thrombophlebitis. Standing for long periods also increases the risk of preterm labor. The pregnant woman's chair should provide adequate back support. Use of a footstool can prevent pressure on veins, relieve strain on varicosities, minimize edema of the feet, and prevent backache.

Clothing. Some women continue to wear their usual clothes during pregnancy as long as they fit and feel comfortable. If maternity clothing is needed, outfits can be purchased new or found at thrift shops or garage sales in good condition. Comfortable, loose clothing is recommended. Tight bras and belts, stretch pants, garters, tight-top knee socks, panty girdles, and other constrictive clothing should be avoided because tight clothing over the perineum increases the risk of vaginitis and miliaria (heat rash), and impaired circulation in the legs can cause varicosities.

BOX 14-5 Conscious Relaxation Tips

Preparation—Loosen clothing, assume a comfortable sitting or side-lying position with all parts of your body well supported with pillows. The use of soothing music is optional.

Beginning—Allow yourself to feel warm and comfortable. Inhale and exhale slowly and imagine peaceful relaxation coming over each part of your body, starting with the neck and working down to the toes. People who learn conscious relaxation often speak of feeling relaxed even if some discomfort is present.

Maintenance—Use imagery (fantasy or daydream) to maintain the state of relaxation. Using *active imagery,* imagine yourself moving or doing some activity and experiencing its sensations. Using *passive imagery,* imagine yourself watching a scene such as a lovely sunset.

Awakening—Return to the wakeful state gradually. Slowly begin to take in stimuli from the surrounding environment.

Further retention and development of the skill—Practice regularly for some periods each day (e.g., at the same hour for 10 to 15 minutes each day to feel refreshed, revitalized, and invigorated).

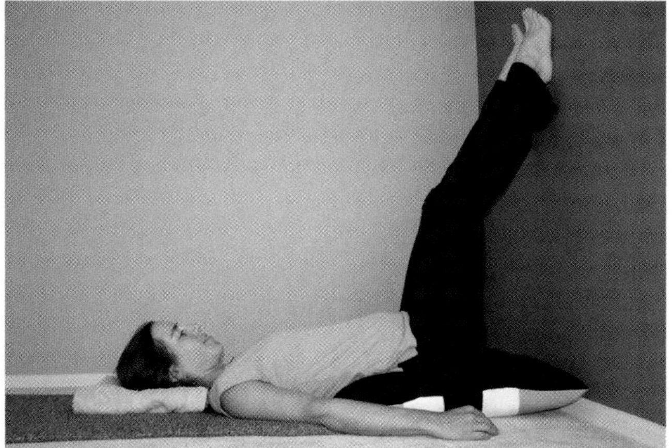

FIG 14-15 Position for resting legs and reducing edema and varicosities. Encourage the woman with vulvar varicosities to include a pillow under her hips. (Courtesy Julie Perry Nelson, Loveland, CO.)

Maternity bras are constructed to accommodate the increased breast weight, chest circumference, and size of breast tail tissue (under the arm). A well-fitting support bra can help prevent neckache and backache.

Maternal support hose give considerable comfort and promote greater venous emptying in women with large varicose veins. Ideally, support stockings should be put on before the woman gets out of bed in the morning. Figure 14-15 demonstrates a position for resting the legs and reducing swelling and varicosities.

Comfortable shoes that provide firm support and promote good posture and balance are advisable. Very high heels and platform shoes are not recommended because of the changes in the pregnant woman's center of gravity and softening of the pelvic joints in later pregnancy which can cause her to lose her balance. In addition, in the third trimester, the woman's pelvis

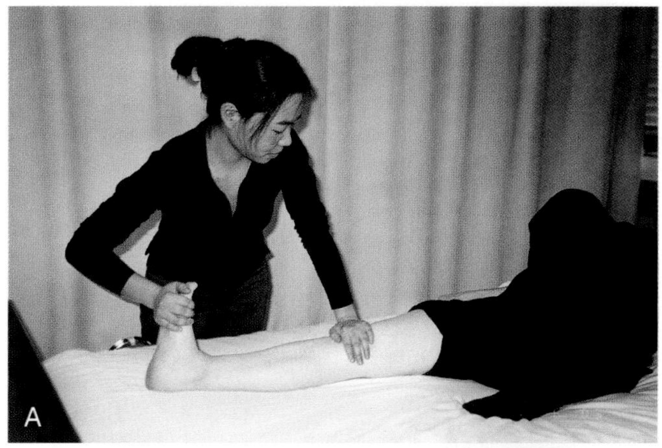

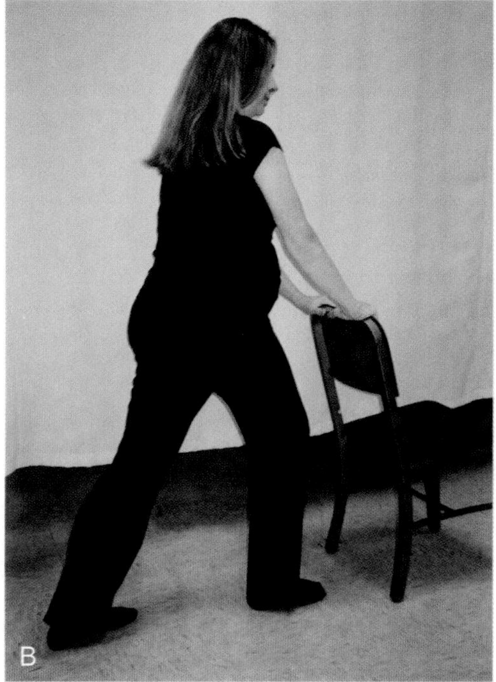

FIG 14-16 Relief of muscle spasm (leg cramps). **A,** Another person dorsiflexes foot with knee extended. **B,** Woman stands and leans forward, thereby dorsiflexing foot of the affected leg. (Courtesy Shannon Perry, Phoenix, AZ.)

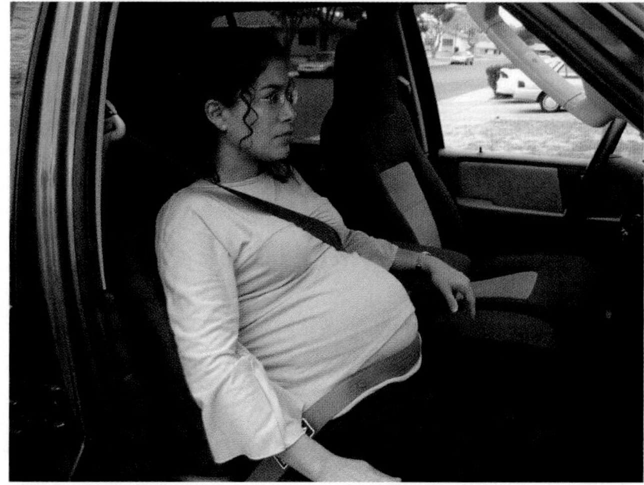

FIG 14-17 Proper use of seatbelt and headrest. (Courtesy Brian and Mayannyn Sallee, Anchorage, AK.)

tilts forward, and her lumbar curve increases. The resulting leg aches and cramps are aggravated by nonsupportive shoes. Exercises to relieve leg cramps are shown in Figure 14-16.

Travel. Travel is not contraindicated in low risk pregnant women; women with high risk pregnancies are advised to avoid long-distance travel after fetal viability has been reached to avert possible economic and psychologic consequences of giving birth to a preterm infant far from home. Travel to areas in which medical care is poor, water is untreated, or malaria is prevalent should be avoided. Women who contemplate foreign travel should be aware that many health insurance carriers do not cover a birth in a foreign setting or even hospitalization for preterm labor. In addition, some vaccinations for foreign travel are contraindicated during pregnancy (e.g., BCG vaccine for tuberculosis). Pregnant women who are accustomed to living and working abroad need to seek advice from their health care provider.

Pregnant women who travel for long distances should schedule periods of activity and rest. While sitting, the woman can practice deep breathing, foot circling, and alternately contracting and relaxing different muscle groups. She should avoid becoming fatigued. Although travel in itself is not a cause of adverse outcomes such as miscarriage or preterm labor, certain precautions are recommended while traveling in a car. For example, women riding in a car should wear automobile restraints and stop to walk every hour.

Motor vehicle accidents are a major cause of maternal morbidity and mortality, second only to violence (Schwaitzberg, Mahoney, & Newton, 2013). Lack of seatbelt use during pregnancy is associated with a greater risk of fetal death (Luley, Fitzpatrick, Grotegut, et al., 2013). A combination lap belt and shoulder harness is the most effective automobile restraint, and both should be used whether the mother is a driver or passenger seated in the front or back seats. The lap belt should be worn low across the pelvic bones as snugly as is comfortable. The shoulder harness should be worn above the gravid uterus and below the neck to prevent chafing (Fig. 14-17). The pregnant woman should sit upright. The headrest should be used to prevent whiplash injury. Airbags if present should remain engaged, but the steering wheel should be tilted upward, away from the abdomen and the seat moved back away from the steering wheel as much as possible.

Airline travel in large commercial jets poses little risk to a healthy pregnant woman. She is advised to inquire about restrictions or recommendations from her carrier. Most health care providers allow air travel up to 36 weeks of gestation for domestic travel and 32 to 35 weeks for international destinations in women without health- or pregnancy-related complications. Metal detectors used at airport security checkpoints emit low levels of radiation and should not pose an increased risk of harm to the fetus (CDC, 2014). Exposure to cosmic radiation while in flight is below the dose that can cause harm at any stage of gestation (Health Physics Society, 2012). The 8% humidity at which the cabins of commercial airlines are maintained can result in some water loss; hydration (with water) should therefore be maintained. Sitting in the cramped seat of an airliner for prolonged periods can increase the risk of superficial and deep vein thrombosis therefore, the woman is encouraged to take a walk around the aircraft during each hour of travel and to wear graduated compression stockings to minimize this risk (CDC).

TABLE 14-2 Discomforts Related to Pregnancy

DISCOMFORT	PHYSIOLOGY	EDUCATION FOR SELF-MANAGEMENT
First Trimester		
Breast changes: pain, tingling, tenderness, enlargement	Hypertrophy of mammary glandular tissue and increased vascularization, pigmentation, and size and prominence of nipples and areolae caused by hormonal stimulation	Wear supportive maternity bras with pads to absorb discharge, may be worn at night; wash with warm water and keep dry; breast tenderness may interfere with sexual expression or foreplay but is temporary
Urgency and frequency of urination	Vascular engorgement and altered bladder function caused by hormones; bladder capacity reduced by enlarging uterus and fetal presenting part	Empty bladder regularly; perform Kegel exercises; limit fluid intake before bedtime; wear perineal pad; report pain or burning sensation to primary health care provider
Languor and malaise; fatigue (early pregnancy, most common)	Unexplained; may be caused by increasing levels of estrogen, progesterone, and hCG or by elevated basal body temperature; psychologic response to pregnancy and its required physical and psychologic adaptations	Rest as needed; eat well-balanced diet to prevent anemia
Nausea and vomiting, also known as morning sickness, occurs in 50%-75% of pregnant women; starts between first and second missed periods and lasts until about fourth missed period; can occur any time during day; fathers also may have symptoms	Cause unknown; may result from hormonal changes, possibly hCG; may be partly emotional, reflecting pride in, ambivalence about, or rejection of pregnant state	Avoid empty or overloaded stomach; maintain good posture—give stomach ample room; stop smoking; eat dry carbohydrate on awakening; remain in bed until feeling subsides, or alternate dry carbohydrate every other hour with fluids such as hot herbal decaffeinated tea, milk, or clear coffee until feeling subsides; eat five or six small meals per day; avoid fried, odorous, spicy, greasy, or gas-forming foods; wear acupressure bands used to treat motion sickness; ginger or acupuncture may be helpful; vitamin B6 + doxylamine (Diclegis®) may be ordered if weight loss occurs; consult primary health care provider if intractable vomiting occurs
Ptyalism (excessive salivation) can occur starting 2 to 3 weeks after first missed period	Possibly caused by elevated estrogen levels; may be related to reluctance to swallow because of nausea	Use astringent mouthwash, chew gum, eat hard candy as comfort measures
Gingivitis and epulis (hyperemia, hypertrophy, bleeding, tenderness of the gums); condition disappears spontaneously 1 to 2 months after birth	Increased vascularity and proliferation of connective tissue from estrogen stimulation	Eat well-balanced diet with adequate protein and fresh fruits and vegetables; brush teeth gently with soft toothbrush and observe good dental hygiene; avoid infection; see dentist
Nasal stuffiness; epistaxis (nosebleed)	Hyperemia of mucous membranes related to increased estrogen levels	Use humidifier; avoid trauma; normal saline nose drops or spray may be used
Leukorrhea: often noted throughout pregnancy	Hormonally stimulated cervix becomes hypertrophic and hyperactive, producing abundant amount of mucus	Not preventable; do not douche; wear perineal pads; perform hygienic practices such as wiping front to back; report to primary health care provider if accompanied by pruritus, foul odor, or change in character or color
Psychosocial dynamics, mood swings, mixed feelings	Hormonal and metabolic adaptations; feelings about female role, sexuality, timing of pregnancy, and resultant changes in life and lifestyle	Participate in pregnancy support group; communicate concerns to partner, family, and health care provider; request referral for supportive services if needed (financial assistance)
Second Trimester		
Pigmentation deepens: darkening of areola and vulva; linea negra; melasma (mask of pregnancy), acne, oily skin	Melanocyte-stimulating hormone (from anterior pituitary)	Not preventable; usually resolves during puerperium
Spider nevi (angiomas) appear over neck, thorax, face, and arms during second or third trimester	Focal networks of dilated arterioles (end arteries) from increased concentration of estrogens	Not preventable; they fade slowly during late puerperium; rarely disappear completely
Pruritus (noninflammatory)	Unknown cause; various types: nonpapular; closely aggregated pruritic papules	Keep fingernails short and clean; contact primary health care provider for diagnosis of cause
	Increased excretory function of skin and stretching of skin possible factors	Not preventable; use comfort measures for symptoms; distraction; tepid baths with sodium bicarbonate or oatmeal added to water; lotions and oils; change of soaps or reduction in use of soap; loose clothing; oral or topical antihistamines or topical steroid cream if recommended by health care provider
Palpitations	Unknown; should not be accompanied by persistent cardiac irregularity	Not preventable; contact primary health care provider if accompanied by symptoms of cardiac decompensation
Supine hypotension (vena cava syndrome) and bradycardia	Caused by pressure of gravid uterus on ascending vena cava when woman is supine; reduces uteroplacental and renal perfusion	Side-lying position or semi-sitting posture, with knees slightly flexed (see Emergency box: Supine Hypotension)
Faintness and, rarely, syncope (orthostatic hypotension) may persist throughout pregnancy	Vasomotor lability or postural hypotension from hormones; in late pregnancy may be caused by venous stasis in lower extremities	Moderate exercise, deep breathing, vigorous leg movement; avoid sudden changes in position and warm crowded areas; move slowly and deliberately; keep environment cool; avoid hypoglycemia by eating five or six small meals per day; wear elastic hose; sit as necessary; if symptoms are serious, contact primary health care provider
Food cravings	Cause unknown; craving influenced by culture or geographic area	Not preventable; satisfy craving unless it interferes with well-balanced diet; report unusual cravings to primary health care provider

TABLE 14-2 **Discomforts Related to Pregnancy—cont'd**

DISCOMFORT	PHYSIOLOGY	EDUCATION FOR SELF-MANAGEMENT
Heartburn (pyrosis or acid indigestion): burning sensation, occasionally with burping and regurgitation of a little sour-tasting fluid	Progesterone slows gastrointestinal (GI) tract motility and digestion, reverses peristalsis, relaxes cardiac sphincter, and delays emptying time of stomach; stomach displaced upward and compressed by enlarging uterus	Limit or avoid gas-producing or fatty foods and large meals; maintain good posture; sip milk for temporary relief; drink hot herbal tea; primary health care provider may prescribe antacid between meals; contact primary health care provider for persistent symptoms
Constipation	GI tract motility slowed because of progesterone, resulting in increased resorption of water and drying of stool; intestines compressed by enlarging uterus; predisposition to constipation because of oral iron supplementation	Drink 2 L (8 to 10 glasses) of water per day; include roughage in diet; engage in moderate exercise; maintain regular schedule for bowel movements; use relaxation techniques and deep breathing; do not take stool softener, laxatives, mineral oil, other drugs, or enemas without first consulting primary health care provider
Flatulence with bloating and belching	Reduced GI motility because of progesterone, allowing time for bacterial action that produces gas; swallowing air	Chew foods slowly and thoroughly; avoid gas-producing foods, fatty foods, large meals; exercise; maintain regular bowel habits
Varicose veins (varicosities): can be associated with aching legs and tenderness; can be present in legs and vulva; hemorrhoids are varicosities in perianal area	Hereditary predisposition; relaxation of smooth muscle walls of veins because of hormones causing tortuous dilated veins in legs and pelvic vasocongestion; condition aggravated by enlarging uterus, gravity, and bearing down for bowel movements; thrombi from leg varices rare but can occur in hemorrhoids	Avoid lengthy standing or sitting, constrictive clothing, and constipation and bearing down with bowel movements; moderate exercise; rest with legs and hips elevated (see Fig. 14-15); wear support stockings; thrombosed hemorrhoid may be evacuated; relieve swelling and pain with warm sitz baths, local application of astringent compresses
Headaches (through week 26)	Emotional tension (more common than vascular migraine headache); eye strain (refractory errors); vascular engorgement and congestion of sinuses resulting from hormone stimulation	Conscious relaxation; contact primary health care provider for constant "splitting" headache to assess for preeclampsia; OTC analgesics may be used if recommended by health care provider (e.g., acetaminophen)
Carpal tunnel syndrome (involves thumb, second, and third fingers, lateral side of little finger)	Compression of median nerve resulting from changes in surrounding tissues; pain, numbness, tingling, burning; loss of skilled movements (typing); dropping of objects	Not preventable; elevate affected arms; splinting of affected hand may help; regressive after pregnancy; surgery is curative
Periodic numbness, tingling of fingers (acrodysesthesia)	Brachial plexus traction syndrome resulting from drooping of shoulders during pregnancy (occurs especially at night and early morning)	Maintain good posture; wear supportive maternity bra; condition will disappear after birth if lifting and carrying baby do not aggravate it
Round ligament pain (tenderness)	Stretching of ligament caused by enlarging uterus	Not preventable; rest, maintain good body mechanics to avoid overstretching ligament; relieve cramping by squatting or bringing knees to chest; sometimes heat helps
Joint pain, backache, and pelvic pressure; hypermobility of joints	Relaxation of symphyseal and sacroiliac joints because of hormones, resulting in unstable pelvis; exaggerated lumbar and cervicothoracic curves caused by change in center of gravity resulting from enlarging abdomen	Maintain good posture and body mechanics; avoid fatigue; wear low-heeled shoes; abdominal support may be useful; conscious relaxation; sleep on firm mattress; apply local heat or ice; get back rubs; do pelvic tilt exercises; rest; condition will disappear 6 to 8 weeks after the birth
Third Trimester		
Shortness of breath and dyspnea occur in 60% of pregnant women	Expansion of diaphragm limited by enlarging uterus; diaphragm is elevated about 4 cm; some relief after lightening	Good posture; sleep with extra pillows; avoid overloading stomach; stop smoking; contact health care provider if symptoms worsen to rule out anemia, emphysema, and asthma
Insomnia (later weeks of pregnancy)	Fetal movements, muscle cramping, urinary frequency, shortness of breath, or other discomforts	Reassurance; conscious relaxation; back massage or effleurage; support of body parts with pillows; warm milk or warm shower or bath before bedtime
Psychosocial responses: mood swings, mixed feelings, increased anxiety	Hormonal and metabolic adaptations; feelings about impending labor, birth, and parenthood	Reassurance and support from significant other and health care providers; improved communication with partner, family, and others
Urinary frequency and urgency return	Vascular engorgement and altered bladder function caused by hormones; bladder capacity reduced by enlarging uterus and fetal presenting part	Empty bladder regularly; Kegel exercises; limit fluid intake before bedtime; reassurance; wear perineal pad; contact health care provider for pain or burning sensation
Perineal discomfort and pressure	Pressure from enlarging uterus, especially when standing or walking; worse with multifetal gestation	Rest, conscious relaxation, and good posture; contact health care provider for assessment and treatment if pain is present
Braxton Hicks contractions	Intensification of uterine contractions in preparation for work of labor	Reassurance; rest; change of position; practice breathing techniques when contractions are bothersome; effleurage; differentiate from preterm labor
Leg cramps (gastrocnemius spasm), especially when reclining	Compression of nerves supplying lower extremities because of enlarging uterus; reduced level of diffusible serum calcium or elevation of serum phosphorus; aggravating factors: fatigue, poor peripheral circulation, pointing toes when stretching legs or when walking, drinking more than 1 L (1 qt) of milk per day	Check for Homans sign; if negative, use massage and heat over affected muscle; dorsiflex foot until spasm relaxes (see Fig. 14-16); stand on cold surface; oral supplementation with calcium carbonate or calcium lactate tablets; aluminum hydroxide gel, 30 ml, with each meal removes phosphorus by absorbing it (consult primary health care provider before taking these remedies)
Ankle edema (nonpitting) to lower extremities	Edema aggravated by prolonged standing, sitting, poor posture, lack of exercise, constrictive clothing, or hot weather	Ample fluid intake for natural diuretic effect; put on support stockings before arising; rest periodically with legs and hips elevated (see Fig. 14-15); exercise moderately; contact health care provider if generalized edema develops; diuretics are contraindicated

Medications and Herbal Preparations. Although much has been learned in recent years about fetal drug toxicity, the possible teratogenicity of many medications, both prescription and OTC, is still unknown. This is especially true for new medications and combinations of drugs. Moreover, certain subclinical errors or deficiencies in intermediate metabolism in the fetus may cause an otherwise harmless drug to be converted into a hazardous one. The greatest danger of drug-caused developmental defects in the fetus extends from the time of fertilization through the first trimester, a time when the woman may not realize she is pregnant. Self-treatment must be discouraged. The use of all drugs, including OTC medications, herbs, and vitamins, should be limited and a careful record kept of all therapeutic and nontherapeutic agents used.

The use of complementary and alternative medicine by pregnant women is widespread (Frawley, Adams, Sibbritt, et al., 2013). There is limited research evidence about the safety of herbal preparations, especially during pregnancy. Although the use of complementary and alternative therapies is consistent with the holistic, woman-centered approach to care, caution is warranted in their use because of the lack of evidence related to their safety and efficacy.

MEDICATION ALERT

Although complementary and alternative medicine (CAM) may benefit the woman during pregnancy, some practices should be avoided because they can increase the risk for complications. It is important to ask the woman about OTC products (including herbals and vitamins) she is using.

Immunizations. Immunization with live or attenuated live viruses is contraindicated during pregnancy because of potential teratogenicity; recommended vaccination with these agents should be part of postpartum care. Live-virus vaccines include those for measles (rubeola and rubella), varicella (chickenpox), and mumps, as well as the Sabin (oral) poliomyelitis vaccine (no longer used in the United States). Vaccines that can be administered during pregnancy include combined tetanus-diphtheria-acellular pertussis (Tdap), recombinant hepatitis B, and influenza (inactivated) vaccines (CDC, 2013a).

Reported cases of pertussis (whooping cough) have increased significantly in the United States and Canada in recent years. Pertussis can cause serious and life-threatening complications in mothers and infants. To provide maximal maternal antibody response and transfer passive immunity to the infant, Tdap should be administered between 27 and 36 weeks of pregnancy. Maternal antipertussis antibodies are short lived and antibody levels drop significantly during the first year after vaccination. As a result, it is unlikely that a Tdap vaccination in one pregnancy will transfer passive immunity from mother to infant in a subsequent pregnancy. Therefore, the recommendation is to administer Tdap to a pregnant woman during each pregnancy regardless of her prior vaccination history. If Tdap is not administered during pregnancy, it should be given immediately postpartum. Adolescents and adults (parents, grandparents, siblings, child care workers, and health care personnel) who will have close contact with an infant less than 12 months of age should receive a single dose of Tdap if not vaccinated previously (CDC, 2013e).

All women who are pregnant during the influenza season (November through March) should be offered an influenza vaccination. The injectable inactivated influenza vaccine is safe throughout pregnancy. The intranasal influenza vaccine is contraindicated during pregnancy because it contains a live virus (AAP & ACOG, 2012; CDC, 2011).

Alcohol, Cigarette Smoke, Caffeine, and Drugs. A safe level of alcohol consumption during pregnancy has not been established. Complete abstinence is strongly advised in order to avoid any risk of pregnancy complications. Maternal alcoholism is associated with high rates of miscarriage and fetal alcohol spectrum disorders (FASDs); the risk for miscarriage in the first trimester is dose related (three or more drinks per day) (CDC, 2013b).

Cigarette smoking or continued exposure to secondhand smoke (even if the mother does not smoke) is associated with IUGR and an increase in perinatal and infant morbidity and mortality. Smoking is associated with an increased frequency of preterm labor, PROM, abruptio placentae, placenta previa, and fetal death, possibly resulting from decreased placental perfusion. Smoking cessation activities should be incorporated into routine prenatal care (ACOG Committee on Obstetric Practice, 2013c). All women who smoke should be strongly encouraged to quit or at least reduce the number of cigarettes they smoke.

Caffeine crosses the placenta easily and the fetus does not produce the enzymes that inactivate caffeine. Conflicting results have been obtained in studies investigating caffeine intake and the occurrence of spontaneous abortion, preterm birth, fetal death, congenital malformations, and fetal growth restriction (Sengpiel, Elind, Bacelis, et al., 2013). Because other effects are unknown, pregnant women are advised to limit their caffeine intake, particularly coffee, because it has high caffeine content per unit of measure (see Table 15-5). The ACOG Committee on Obstetric Practice (2013b) recommends 200 mg as the recommended maximum daily intake of caffeine during pregnancy.

Any drug or environmental agent that enters the pregnant woman's bloodstream has the potential to cross the placenta and harm the fetus. Marijuana, heroin, and cocaine are common examples. Although the problem of substance abuse in pregnancy is considered a major public health concern and comprehensive care of drug-addicted women improves maternal and neonatal outcomes, few facilities are available for treatment of these women (see Chapters 32 and 35).

Normal Discomforts. Pregnant women have physical symptoms that would be considered abnormal in the nonpregnant state. They have an increased need for explanations of the causes of the discomforts and for advice on ways to relieve them. The discomforts of the first trimester are fairly specific. Information about the physiology, prevention, and self-management of discomforts experienced during the three trimesters is given in Table 14-2. Box 14-6 lists alternative and complementary therapies that may be safely used during pregnancy. Nurses can do much to allay a first-time mother's anxiety about such symptoms by telling her about them in advance and using terminology that the woman (or couple) can understand. Understanding the rationale for treatment

BOX 14-6 Alternative Therapies Used in Pregnancy

Touch and Energetic Therapies
Massage
Acupressure
Therapeutic touch
Healing touch
Mind-body healing
Imagery
Meditation, prayer, reflection
Biofeedback
Aromatherapy
Other modalities that may fall outside of nurse practice guidelines unless the nurse has completed additional training or certification:
- Herbs
- Homeopathy
- Traditional Chinese medicine

promotes their participation in their care. Interventions should be individualized, with attention given to the woman's lifestyle and culture (see Nursing Care Plan).

Recognizing Potential Complications. One of the most important responsibilities of care providers is to alert the pregnant woman to signs and symptoms that indicate a potential complication of pregnancy. The woman needs to know how and to whom to report such warning signs. She and her family should receive a printed list of warning signs, written at the appropriate literacy level and in their language, that warrant a call to the health care provider (HCP) or clinic; phone numbers for the HCP or clinic should be listed.

The nurse answers questions as they arise during pregnancy. Pregnant women often have difficulty deciding when to report signs and symptoms. The mother is encouraged to refer to the printed list of potential complications and to listen to her body. If she senses that something is wrong, she should call her care provider. Several signs and symptoms must be discussed more

NURSING CARE PLAN

Discomforts of Pregnancy and Warning Signs

NURSING DIAGNOSIS	EXPECTED OUTCOME	NURSING INTERVENTIONS	RATIONALES
First Trimester			
Anxiety related to deficient knowledge about schedule of prenatal visits throughout pregnancy as evidenced by woman's questions and concerns	Woman will verbalize correct appointment schedule for duration of pregnancy and feelings of being "in control."	Provide information regarding schedule of visits, tests, and other assessments and interventions that will be occurring throughout pregnancy.	To empower woman to function in collaboration with caregiver and diminish anxiety
		Allow woman time to describe level of anxiety.	To establish basis for care
		Provide information to woman regarding prenatal classes and labor area tours.	To decrease feelings of anxiety about unknown
Imbalanced Nutrition: Less Than Body Requirements related to nausea and vomiting as evidenced by woman's report and weight loss	Woman will gain 1 to 2.5 kg (2.2 to 5.5 lb) during first trimester.	Verify prepregnant weight.	To plan realistic diet according to individual woman's nutritional needs
		Obtain diet history.	To identify current meal patterns and foods that may be implicated in nausea
		Advise woman to consume small, frequent meals and avoid having empty stomach.	To avoid further nausea episodes
		Suggest that woman eat a simple carbohydrate such as dry crackers before arising in morning.	To avoid empty stomach and decrease incidence of nausea and vomiting
		Advise woman to call health care provider if vomiting is persistent and severe.	To identify possible incidence of hyperemesis gravidarum
Fatigue related to hormonal changes in first trimester as evidenced by woman's complaints	Woman will report decreased number of episodes of fatigue.	Advise woman to rest as needed.	To avoid increasing feeling of fatigue
		Advise woman to eat well-balanced diet.	To meet increased metabolic demands and avoid anemia
		Discuss use of support systems to help with household responsibilities.	To decrease workload at home and decrease fatigue
		Reinforce to woman the transitory nature of first-trimester fatigue.	To provide emotional support
		Explore with woman a variety of techniques to prioritize roles.	To decrease family expectations

Continued

NURSING CARE PLAN—cont'd

Discomforts of Pregnancy and Warning Signs

NURSING DIAGNOSIS	EXPECTED OUTCOME	NURSING INTERVENTIONS	RATIONALES
Second Trimester			
Constipation related to progesterone influence on gastrointestinal (GI) tract as evidenced by woman's report of altered patterns of elimination	Woman will report return to normal bowel elimination pattern after implementation of interventions.	Provide information to woman regarding pregnancy-related causes: progesterone slowing GI motility, growing uterus compressing intestines, and influence of iron supplementation.	To provide basic information for self-management during pregnancy
		Assist woman to plan diet that will promote regular bowel movements, such as increasing amount of oral fluid intake to at least 8 to 10 glasses (2 L) of water a day, increasing the amount of fiber in daily diet, and maintaining moderate exercise program.	To promote self-management care
		Reinforce for woman that she should not take any laxatives, stool softeners, or enemas without first consulting the health care provider.	To prevent any injuries to woman or fetus
Readiness for Enhanced Knowledge about course of first pregnancy as evidenced by woman's questions regarding possible complications of second and third trimesters	Woman will correctly list signs of potential complications that can occur during second and third trimesters and exhibit no overt signs of stress.	Provide information concerning potential complications or warning signs that can occur during second and third trimesters, including possible causes of signs and importance of calling health care provider immediately.	To ensure identification and treatment of problems in timely manner
		Provide a written list of complications.	To have a reference list for emergencies
Third Trimester			
Fear related to inexperience regarding onset and processes of labor as evidenced by woman's questions and statement of concerns	Woman will verbalize basic understanding of signs of labor onset and when to call health care provider, identify resources for childbirth education, and express increasing confidence in readiness to cope with labor.	Provide information regarding signs of labor onset and when to call health care provider; give written information regarding local childbirth education classes.	To empower and promote self-management
		Promote ongoing effective communication with health care provider.	To promote trust and decrease fear of unknown
		Provide woman with decision-making opportunities.	To promote effective coping
		Provide opportunity for woman to verbalize fears regarding childbirth.	To assist in decreasing fear through discussion
Disturbed Sleep Pattern related to discomforts or insomnia of third trimester as evidenced by woman's report of inadequate rest	Woman will report improvement of quality and quantity of rest and sleep.	Assess current sleep pattern, and review need for increased requirement during pregnancy.	To identify need for change in sleep patterns
		Suggest change of position to side-lying with pillows between legs or to semi-Fowler position.	To increase support and decrease any problems with dyspnea or heartburn
		Reinforce possibility of use of various sleep aids such as relaxation techniques, reading, and decreased activity before bedtime.	To decrease possibility of anxiety or physical discomforts before bedtime
Ineffective Sexuality Pattern related to changes in comfort level and fatigue	Woman will verbalize feelings regarding changes in sexual desire, and woman and her partner will express satisfaction with sexual activities.	Assess couple's usual sexuality patterns.	To determine how patterns have been altered by pregnancy
		Provide information regarding expected changes in sexuality patterns during pregnancy.	To correct any misconceptions
		Allow couple to express feelings in nonjudgmental atmosphere.	To promote trust
		Refer couple for counseling as appropriate.	To assist couple to cope with sexuality pattern changes
		Suggest alternative sexual positions.	To decrease pressure on enlarging abdomen of woman and increase sexual comfort and satisfaction of couple

extensively. These include vaginal bleeding, alteration in fetal movements, symptoms of gestational hypertension, rupture of membranes, and preterm labor (see Signs of Potential Complications box: First, Second, and Third Trimesters).

Recognizing Preterm Labor. Teaching each expectant mother to recognize preterm labor is necessary for early diagnosis and treatment. Preterm labor is the occurrence of uterine contractions after the twentieth week but before the thirty-seventh week of pregnancy that, if untreated, cause the cervix to open earlier than normal and result in preterm birth. Warning signs and symptoms of preterm labor are discussed in Chapter 32.

Sexual Counseling

Sexual counseling of expectant couples includes countering misinformation, providing reassurance of normality, and suggesting alternative behaviors. The uniqueness of each couple is considered within a biopsychosocial framework (see Teaching for Self-Management box: Sexuality in Pregnancy). Nurses can initiate discussion about sexual adaptations during pregnancy, based on sound knowledge about the physical, social, and emotional responses to sex during pregnancy. Not all maternity nurses are comfortable dealing with the sexual concerns of their clients. Nurses should be aware of their personal strengths and limitations in dealing with sexual content and be prepared to make referrals if necessary.

TEACHING FOR SELF-MANAGEMENT

Sexuality in Pregnancy

- Be aware that maternal physiologic changes, such as breast enlargement and tenderness, nausea, fatigue, abdominal changes, perineal enlargement, leukorrhea, pelvic vasocongestion, and orgasmic responses can affect sexuality and sexual expression.
- Discuss concerns about sexuality during pregnancy with your partner.
- Keep in mind that cultural prescriptions ("do's") and proscriptions ("don'ts") can affect your attitudes and responses.
- Although your libido can be depressed during the first trimester, it often increases during the second trimester.
- Discuss and explore with your partner:
  - Alternative behaviors (e.g., mutual masturbation, foot massage, cuddling)
  - Alternative positions (e.g., female superior, side-lying) for sexual intercourse
- Intercourse is safe as long as it is not uncomfortable. There is no correlation between intercourse and miscarriage, but observe the following precautions:
  - Abstain from intercourse if you experience uterine cramping or vaginal bleeding; report these symptoms to your physician or midwife as soon as possible.
  - Abstain from intercourse (or any activity that results in orgasm) if you have a history of premature dilation of the cervix, until otherwise advised by your health care provider.
- Continue to use risk-reducing sexual behaviors. Women at risk for acquiring or conveying sexually transmitted infections should use condoms during sexual intercourse throughout pregnancy.

Many women merely need permission to be sexually active during pregnancy. Many others, however, need to be given information about the physiologic changes that occur during pregnancy, have the myths that are associated with sex during pregnancy dispelled, and participate in open discussions of positions for intercourse that decrease pressure on the gravid abdomen (Fig. 14-18). Such tasks are within the purview of the nurse and should be an integral component of the health care rendered.

Some couples need to be referred for sex therapy or family therapy. Couples with long-standing problems with sexual dysfunction that are intensified by pregnancy are candidates for sex therapy. Whenever a sexual problem is a symptom of a more serious relationship problem, family therapy can be beneficial.

Using the History. The couple's sexual history provides a basis for counseling, but history taking also is an ongoing process. The couple's receptivity to changes in attitudes, body image, partner relationships, and physical status are relevant topics throughout pregnancy. The history reveals the woman's knowledge of female anatomy and physiology and her attitudes about sex during pregnancy, as well as her perceptions of the pregnancy, the health status of the couple, and the quality of their relationship.

Countering Misinformation. Many myths and much of the misinformation related to sex and pregnancy are masked by seemingly unrelated issues. For example, a discussion about the baby's ability to hear and see in utero can be prompted by questions about the baby being an "unseen observer" of the couple's sexual activities. The counselor must be extremely sensitive to the concerns behind such questions when counseling in this highly charged emotional area.

Safety and Comfort During Sexual Activity. For most women, there are no restrictions on sexual intercourse during pregnancy. However, pregnant women should be aware that they are likely to experience alternations in sexual desire and comfort during sexual activity. Uterine activity can increase with sexual intercourse; this can be related to breast stimulation, orgasm, or prostaglandins in male ejaculate. For the majority of women, this is not a problem. However, a history of more than one miscarriage, a threatened miscarriage in the first trimester, impending miscarriage in the second trimester, and PROM, bleeding, or abdominal pain during the third trimester may warrant caution regarding coitus and orgasm (Gregory et al., 2012).

Solitary and mutual masturbation and oral-genital intercourse may be used by couples as alternatives to penile-vaginal intercourse. Partners who enjoy cunnilingus (oral stimulation of the clitoris or vagina) can feel "turned off" by the normal increase in the amount and odor of vaginal discharge during pregnancy. Couples who practice cunnilingus should be cautioned against the blowing of air into the vagina, particularly during the last few weeks of pregnancy when the cervix can be slightly open. An air embolism can occur if air is forced between the uterine wall and the fetal membranes and enters the maternal vascular system through the placenta.

Showing the woman or couple pictures of possible variations of coital position often is helpful (Fig. 14-18). The female-superior, side-by-side, rear-entry, and side-lying are possible alternatives to the traditional male-superior position. The woman astride (superior position) allows her to control the angle and depth of penetration, as well as to protect her breasts and abdomen. During the third trimester, the side-by-side position or any position that places less pressure on the pregnant abdomen and requires less energy will likely be preferred.

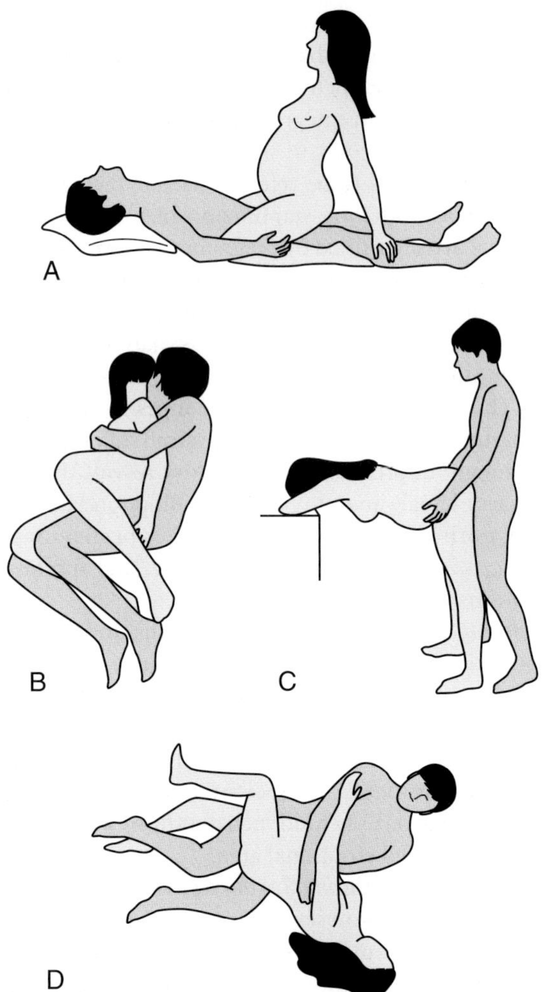

FIG 14-18 Positions for sexual intercourse during pregnancy. **A,** Female superior. **B,** Side by side. **C,** Rear entry. **D,** Facing each other.

Some women, especially multiparas, have significant breast tenderness in the first trimester. The nurse can recommend a coital position that avoids direct pressure on the breasts and decreased breast fondling during sexual activity. The woman also should be reassured that this condition is normal and temporary.

During the first and third trimesters, some women complain of lower abdominal cramping and backache after orgasm. A back rub can often relieve some of the discomfort and provide a pleasant experience. A tonic uterine contraction, often lasting up to a minute, replaces the rhythmic contractions of orgasm during the third trimester. Changes in the FHR without fetal distress also have been reported.

Risk-reduction measures against the acquisition and transmission of STIs (e.g., syphilis, gonorrhea, chlamydia, herpes simplex virus [HSV], HIV) are advised during sexual activity at all times, including during pregnancy. Because these diseases can be transmitted to the woman and her fetus, using condoms is recommended throughout pregnancy if the woman is at risk for acquiring an STI (e.g., adolescents) (AAP & ACOG, 2012).

Psychosocial Support

Esteem, affection, trust, concern, consideration of cultural and religious responses, and listening are all components of the emotional support given to the pregnant woman and her family. The woman's satisfaction with her relationships—partner and family—and their support, her feeling of competence, and her sense of being in control are important issues to be addressed in the third trimester. A discussion of fetal responses to stimuli, such as sound and light, as well as patterns of sleeping and waking, can be helpful. Other common concerns for the pregnant woman and her partner include fear of pain, loss of control, and possible birth of the infant before reaching the hospital; anxieties about parenthood; parental concerns about the safety of the mother and unborn child; siblings and their acceptance of the new baby; social and economic responsibilities; and issues arising from conflicts in cultural, religious, or personal value systems. In addition, the woman may have concerns about the father's or partner's commitment to the pregnancy and to the couple's relationship. Providing the prospective parents with an opportunity to discuss their concerns and validating the normality of their responses can meet their needs to varying degrees. Anticipatory guidance and health promotion strategies can help partners cope with their concerns. Nurses can facilitate and encourage open dialogue between the expectant mother and her partner.

VARIATIONS IN PRENATAL CARE

The course of prenatal care described thus far may seem to suggest that the experiences of childbearing women are similar and that nursing interventions are uniformly consistent across all populations. Although typical patterns of response to pregnancy are easily recognized and many aspects of prenatal care indeed are consistent, pregnant women and their families enter the health care system with unique concerns and needs. The nurse's ability to assess unique needs and to tailor interventions to the woman and her family is the hallmark of expertise in providing care. Variations that influence prenatal care include culture, maternal age, medical and obstetric history, and number of fetuses.

Cultural Influences

All health care professionals are responsible for providing safe, evidence-based care that helps people to attain and maintain their optimal state of health. Services that are offered in a way that respects people's cultural and linguistic preferences have been demonstrated to improve the quality of health care and to reduce health disparities. The U.S. Department of Health and Human Services Office of Minority Health (2013) has developed standards for the delivery of culturally and linguistically appropriate health care; the standards can be accessed at http://minorityhealth.hhs.gov.

Prenatal care as we know it is a phenomenon of Western health practices. In the U.S. model of health care, women are encouraged to seek prenatal care as early as possible in pregnancy by visiting a physician or certified nurse-midwife. This recommendation not only is unfamiliar but also seems strange to women of other cultures.

Many cultural variations are found in prenatal care. Even if the prenatal care described is familiar to a woman, some practices can conflict with the beliefs and practices of a subculture group to which she belongs. Because of these and other factors, such as lack of money, lack of transportation, and language barriers, women from diverse cultures may not seek prenatal care until late in pregnancy or they may not participate in the prenatal care system at all. A concern for modesty can be a deterrent to seeking prenatal care. For some women, exposing body parts, especially to a male, is considered a serious violation of their modesty. For many women, an invasive procedure such as a vaginal examination is so threatening that they cannot discuss it, even with their own husbands. Many women prefer a female health care provider. Too often, health care providers assume women lose this modesty during pregnancy and labor, but actually most women value and appreciate efforts to maintain their modesty.

Because pregnancy is considered a normal process and the woman is in a state of health, many cultural groups regard care from a health care professional to be necessary only in times of illness. Therefore, the services of a clinician are considered inappropriate during pregnancy. Western medicine's view of problems in pregnancy can differ from that of members of other cultural groups.

Although pregnancy is considered normal by many, certain practices are expected of women of all cultures to promote a good outcome. **Cultural prescriptions** tell women what to do, and **cultural proscriptions** establish taboos. The purposes of these practices are to prevent maternal illness resulting from a pregnancy-induced imbalanced state and to protect the vulnerable fetus. Prescriptions and proscriptions regulate the woman's emotional response, clothing, activity, rest, sexual activity, and dietary practices. Exploring her beliefs, perceptions of the meaning of childbearing, and health care practices can help health care professionals foster the woman's self-actualization, promote attainment of the maternal role, and positively influence her relationship with her partner.

To provide culturally responsive care, nurses must be knowledgeable about practices and customs, although it is not possible to know all there is to know about every culture and subculture or the many lifestyles that exist. It is important to learn about the varied cultures in the setting where each nurse practices. When exploring cultural beliefs and practices related to childbearing, the nurse can support and nurture those beliefs that promote physical or emotional adaptation. However, if potentially harmful beliefs or activities are identified, the nurse should sensitively provide education and propose modifications (see Community Activity).

COMMUNITY ACTIVITY

Select an immigrant or other minority group in your community and identify childbearing-related beliefs and practices that are unique to that group. Are there stores in the area that sell items that meet that group's needs? Does the community center have activities or classes that are directed toward the group? Are perinatal education programs available that provide essential information while incorporating cultural patterns? Are classes available in languages other than English? What could you, as a nurse, contribute to the community that would help meet the needs of that group?

Emotional Response

Virtually all cultures emphasize the importance of maintaining a socially harmonious and agreeable environment for a pregnant woman. A lifestyle with minimal stress is important in promoting positive outcomes for the mother and baby. Harmony with other people must be fostered, and visits from extended family members may be required to demonstrate pleasant and noncontroversial relationships. If discord exists in a relationship, it is usually dealt with in culturally prescribed ways.

Some cultural proscriptions involve forms of magic. For example, some Mexicans believe pregnant women should not be allowed to witness an eclipse of the moon because it can cause a cleft palate in the infant. They also believe that exposure to an earthquake can precipitate preterm birth, miscarriage, or a breech presentation. In some cultures a pregnant woman must not ridicule someone with an affliction for fear her child might be born with the same handicap. A mother should not hate a person lest her child resemble that person. Dental work should not be done during pregnancy because it may cause a baby to have a cleft lip. A folk belief widely held in many cultures is that the pregnant woman should refrain from raising her arms above her head and from tying knots because such movements tie knots in the umbilical cord and can cause it to wrap around the baby's neck. Another belief is that placing a knife under the bed of a laboring woman will "cut" her pain.

Physical Activity and Rest

Norms that regulate the physical activity of mothers during pregnancy vary tremendously. Some cultural groups encourage women to be active, to walk, and to engage in normal, although not strenuous, activities to ensure that the baby is healthy and not too large. Conversely, some groups believe that any activity is dangerous, and family members willingly take over the work of the pregnant woman, believing that this inactivity protects the mother and child. The mother is encouraged simply to produce the succeeding generation. If health care professionals are unaware of this belief, they can misinterpret their behavior as laziness or nonadherence with the desired prenatal health care regimen. It is important for the nurse to find out how each pregnant woman views activity and rest.

Clothing

Although most cultural groups do not prescribe specific clothing to be worn during pregnancy, modesty is an expectation of many. Amulets, medals, and beads are worn by women from some cultures to promote health or protect the woman and fetus from danger. For example, some Mexican women of the U.S. Southwest and women of Central America wear a cord beneath the breasts and knotted over the umbilicus. This cord, called a *muñeco,* is thought to prevent morning sickness and ensure a safe birth (Fig. 14-19).

Sexual Activity

In most cultures sexual activity is not prohibited until the end of pregnancy. Some groups view sexual activity as necessary to keep the birth canal lubricated. Others may have definite

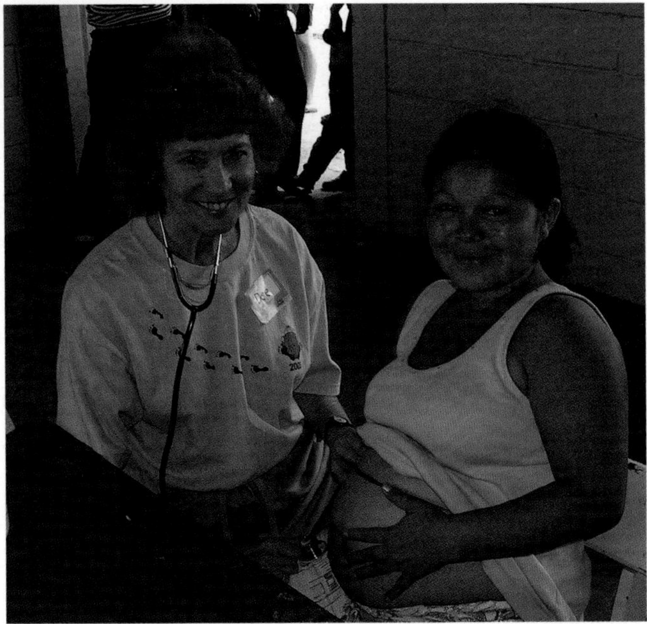

FIG 14-19 A young woman from Honduras wearing a red muñeco given to her by her mother to ensure a safe birth. (Courtesy Dee Lowdermilk, Chapel Hill, NC.)

proscriptions against sexual intercourse, requiring abstinence throughout the pregnancy because it is thought that sexual intercourse can harm the mother and fetus.

Diet

Nutritional information given by Western health care providers can be a source of conflict for some cultural groups. Such a conflict commonly is not known by health care providers unless they understand the dietary beliefs and practices of the people for whom they are caring. For example, some religious groups have strict regulations regarding preparation of food, and if meat cannot be prepared as prescribed, they omit meats from their diets. Many cultures permit pregnant women to eat only warm foods.

Age Differences

The age of the childbearing couple can have a significant influence on their physical and psychosocial adaptation to pregnancy. Normal developmental processes that occur in both very young and older mothers are interrupted by pregnancy and require a different type of adaptation to pregnancy than that of the woman of typical childbearing age. Although the individuality of each pregnant woman is recognized, special needs of

NURSING CARE PLAN

Adolescent Pregnancy

NURSING DIAGNOSIS	EXPECTED OUTCOME	INTERVENTIONS	RATIONALES
Imbalanced Nutrition: Less Than Body Requirements related to intake insufficient to meet metabolic needs of fetus and adolescent client	Adolescent will gain weight as prescribed by age, take prenatal vitamins/iron as prescribed, and maintain normal hematocrit and hemoglobin.	Assess current diet history/intake.	To determine prescriptions for additions or changes in present dietary pattern
		Compare prepregnancy weight with current weight.	To determine if pattern of weight gain is consistent with appropriate fetal growth and development
		Provide information concerning food prescriptions for appropriate weight gain, considering preferences for "fast food" and peer influences.	To correct any misconceptions and increase chances for compliance with diet
		Include adolescent's immediate family or support system during instruction.	To ensure that person preparing family meals receives information
Risk for Injury, maternal or fetal, related to inadequate prenatal care and screening	Adolescent will experience uncomplicated pregnancy and give birth to healthy fetus at term.	Provide information, using therapeutic communication and confidentiality.	To establish relationship and build trust
		Discuss importance of ongoing prenatal care and possible risks to adolescent client and fetus.	To reinforce that ongoing assessment is crucial to health and well-being of client and fetus, even if client feels well. The adolescent client is more at risk for certain complications that may be avoided or managed early if prenatal visits are maintained.
		Discuss risks of alcohol, tobacco, and recreational drug use during pregnancy.	To minimize risks to client and fetus because adolescent clients have higher abuse rate than rest of pregnant population
		Assess for evidence of sexually transmitted infection (STI), and provide information regarding sexual practices.	To minimize risk to client and fetus because adolescent is more at risk for STIs
		Screen for preeclampsia on an ongoing basis.	To minimize risk because adolescent population is more at risk for preeclampsia

Continued

NURSING CARE PLAN—cont'd

Adolescent Pregnancy

NURSING DIAGNOSIS	EXPECTED OUTCOME	INTERVENTIONS	RATIONALES
Social Isolation related to body image changes of pregnant adolescent as evidenced by client statements and concerns	Adolescent will identify support systems and report decreased feelings of social isolation.	Establish a therapeutic relationship.	To listen objectively and establish trust
		Discuss with client changes in relationships that have occurred as result of pregnancy.	To determine extent of isolation from family, peers, and baby's father
		Provide referrals and resources appropriate for developmental stage of client.	To give information for client support
		Provide information regarding parenting classes, breastfeeding classes, and childbirth preparation classes.	To give further information and group support, which lessens social isolation
Interrupted Family Processes related to adolescent pregnancy	Adolescent will reestablish relationship with her mother and baby's father.	Encourage communication with mother.	To clarify roles and relationships related to birth of infant
		Encourage communication with father of baby (if she desires continued contact).	To ascertain level of support to be expected of baby's father
		Refer to support group.	To learn more effective problem-solving methods and reduce conflict within the family
Disturbed Body Image related to situational crisis of pregnancy	Adolescent will verbalize positive comments regarding her body image during pregnancy.	Assess pregnant adolescent's perception of self related to pregnancy.	To provide basis for further interventions
		Give information regarding expected body changes occurring during pregnancy.	To provide a realistic view of these temporary changes
		Provide opportunity to discuss personal feelings and concerns.	To promote trust and support
Risk for Impaired Parenting related to immaturity and lack of experience in new role of adolescent mother	Parents will demonstrate parenting roles with confidence.	Provide information on growth and development.	To enhance knowledge so that adolescent mother can have basis for caring for her infant
		Initiate discussion of child care.	To assist adolescent in problem solving for future needs
		Assess parenting abilities of adolescent mother and father.	To provide baseline for education
		Provide information on parenting classes that are appropriate for parents' developmental stage.	To enhance knowledge, obtain support, and share common feelings and concerns
		Assist parents to identify pertinent support systems.	To give assistance with parenting as needed

expectant mothers 15 years of age or younger or those 35 years of age or older are summarized.

Adolescents

Teenage pregnancy is a worldwide problem. The United States has one of the highest teen birth rates among industrialized nations. However, the rate of teen births has declined in the United States since the 1950s. From 2011 to 2012, the teen birth rate decreased 6% to the historic low of 29.4%. Hispanic adolescents have the highest birth rate, although the rate for African-American adolescents also is high (Martin, Hamilton, Osterman et al., 2013). Most of these young women are unmarried, and many are not ready for the emotional, psychosocial, and financial responsibilities of parenthood.

Numerous adolescent pregnancy-prevention programs have had varying degrees of success. Characteristics of programs that make a difference are those that have sustained commitment to adolescents over a long time, involve the parents and other adults in the community, promote abstinence and personal responsibility, and assist adolescents to develop a clear strategy for reaching goals such as a college education or a career.

When adolescents become pregnant and decide to give birth, they are much less likely than older women to receive adequate prenatal care, often receiving no health care at all. These young women also are more likely to smoke and less likely to gain adequate weight during pregnancy. As a result, babies born to adolescents are at greatly increased risk of LBW, of serious and long-term disability, and of dying during the first year of life (Elfenbein & Felice, 2011).

Delayed entry into prenatal care can be the result of late recognition of pregnancy, denial of pregnancy, or confusion about the available services. Such a delay in care can leave an

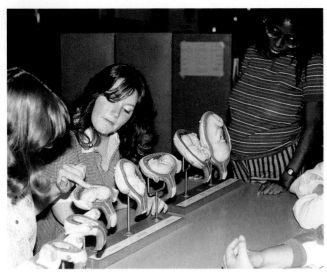

FIG 14-20 Pregnant adolescents review fetal development. (Courtesy Marjorie Pyle, RNC, Lifecircle, Costa Mesa, CA).

inadequate time before birth to attend to correctable problems. The very young pregnant adolescent is at higher risk for each of the variables associated with poor pregnancy outcomes (e.g., socioeconomic factors) and for those conditions associated with a first pregnancy, regardless of age (e.g., gestational hypertension).

The role of the nurse in reducing the risks and consequences of adolescent pregnancy is to encourage early and continued prenatal care; to provide early and ongoing education about pregnancy, birth, and parenting (Fig. 14-20); and to refer the adolescent, if necessary, for appropriate social support services, which can help decrease the effects of a negative socioeconomic environment (see Nursing Care Plan). Adolescents often see the nurse as trustworthy and someone who will maintain confidentiality, as well as provide them with accurate information. Therefore, effective communication is essential in providing care to the pregnant adolescent (U.S. Department of Health and Human Services Office of Adolescent Health, 2013) (see Nursing Care Plan).

Women Older Than 35 Years

Two groups of older parents have emerged in the population of women having a child late in their childbearing years. One group consists of multiparous women who intentionally or unintentionally become pregnant in the peri-menopausal period. The other group consists of primigravidas: women who have deliberately delayed childbearing until their late 30s or early 40s and those who previously were unable to conceive due to fertility problems and became pregnant through assisted reproductive technology.

In contemporary times, women living in high-income countries who become pregnant after the age of 35 are more likely to be healthy, well educated, and of higher socioeconomic status than in previous decades. As a result, there is a greater likelihood of vaginal birth to a term infant of normal weight (Carolan & Frankowska, 2011). There is evidence that women whose first birth occurs at an older age may have some psychologic advantages such as fewer symptoms of anxiety and depression, and they may be more resilient (McMahon, Boivin, Gibson, et al., 2011).

However, in general, pregnancy for women older than age 35 is associated with increased risk of miscarriage, stillbirth, diabetes, hypertension, placenta previa, placental abruption, and cesarean birth (Carolan & Frankowska, 2011). These women are more likely than younger primiparas to have infants with chromosomal abnormalities, LBW infants, preterm birth, and multiple gestation (Johnson & Tough, 2012).

Multiparous Women. For some multiparous women over the age of 35, pregnancy is desired, such as with a new marriage or partner. For others, it may be unplanned. Some multiparous women have never used contraceptives because of personal choice or lack of knowledge concerning contraceptives. Others may have used contraceptives successfully during the childbearing years, but as menopause approaches they cease menstruating regularly or stop using contraceptives and consequently become pregnant.

Pregnancy can bring feelings of joy as women consider continuing the maternal role and expanding the family. For some older multiparas, pregnancy can evoke feelings of isolation. She may feel that pregnancy separates her from her peer group and that her age is a hindrance to close associations with young mothers.

Primiparous Women. First-time birth rates for U.S. women over age 35 have steadily increased across all ethnicities. From 2000 to 2012, there was a 24% rise in first births among women ages 35 to 39 and a 35% increase for women ages 40 to 44 (Mathews & Hamilton, 2014).

Seeing women in their late 30s or 40s during their first pregnancy is no longer unusual for health care providers. Reasons for delaying pregnancy include a desire to obtain advanced education, career priorities, and use of better contraceptive measures. Women who are infertile do not delay pregnancy deliberately but can become pregnant at a later age as a result of fertility studies and therapies.

Many primigravidas over the age of 35 deliberately choose parenthood. They often are successfully established in a career and a lifestyle with a partner that includes time for self-attention, the establishment of a home with accumulated possessions, and freedom to travel. When asked the reason they chose pregnancy later in life, many reply, "Because time is running out."

The dilemma of choice includes the recognition that being a parent will have positive and negative consequences. Couples should discuss the joys, responsibilities, and challenges of childbearing and childrearing before committing themselves to this lifelong venture. Partners in this group seem to share the preparation for parenthood, planning for a family-centered birth, and desire to be loving and competent parents; however, the reality of child care can prove difficult for such parents.

First-time mothers older than 35 years select the "right time" for pregnancy; this time is influenced by their awareness of the increasing possibility of infertility or of genetic defects in infants of older women. Such women seek information about pregnancy from books, friends, and electronic resources. They actively try to prevent fetal disorders and are careful in searching for the best possible maternity care. They identify sources of stress in their lives. They have concerns about having enough energy and stamina to meet the demands of parenting and their new roles and relationships.

If older women with a history of infertility become pregnant through assisted reproductive technology, they can suddenly have negative or ambivalent feelings about the pregnancy. They can experience a multifetal pregnancy that can create emotional and physical problems. Adjusting to parenting two or more infants requires adaptability and additional resources.

During pregnancy parents explore the possibilities and responsibilities of changing identities and new roles. They must prepare a safe and nurturing environment during pregnancy and after birth. They must integrate the child into an established family system and negotiate new roles (parent roles, sibling roles, grandparent roles) for family members.

Adverse perinatal outcomes are more common in older primiparas than in younger women, even when they receive good prenatal care. The occurrence of these complications is quite stressful for the new parents, and nursing interventions that provide information and psychosocial support are needed, as well as care for physical needs.

Multifetal Pregnancy

With the increased use of assistive reproductive technology and ovulation induction agents, the incidence of multifetal pregnancy has risen (AAP & ACOG, 2012). In the United States, the twin birth rate has stabilized at 33.1 per 1000 live births. The birth rate for triplets and higher order multiples is 124.4 per 1000 live births; this is a drop from 153.5 per 1000 live births in 2009 (Martin, Hamilton, Osterman, et al., 2013).

A multifetal pregnancy, or pregnancy with more than one fetus, places the mother and fetuses at increased risk for adverse outcomes. The maternal blood volume is increased, resulting in an increased strain on the maternal cardiovascular system. Anemia often develops because of a greater demand for iron by the fetuses. Marked uterine distention, increased pressure on the adjacent viscera and pelvic vasculature, and diastasis of the rectus abdominis muscles can occur (see Fig. 13-13). Women are at increased risk for gestational diabetes, hypertension, and preeclampsia (AAP & ACOG). Placenta previa develops more commonly in multifetal pregnancies because of the large size or placement of the placentas. Premature separation of the placenta can occur before the second and any subsequent fetuses are born (Gilbert, 2011).

Multifetal pregnancies often end prematurely. The risk of preterm labor and birth increases with the number of fetuses. Spontaneous rupture of membranes is common. Fetuses are likely to experience growth restriction or discordant growth. There can be local shunting of blood between placentas (twin-to-twin transfusion); this causes the recipient twin to be larger and the donor twin to be small, pallid, dehydrated, malnourished, and hypovolemic. However, the larger twin can develop congenital heart failure during the first 24 hours after birth. The risk of death of one or more fetuses increases significantly with higher order multiples (Newman & Unal, 2012).

If the presence of more than three fetuses is diagnosed, parents may receive counseling regarding selective reduction to reduce the incidence of premature birth and improve the opportunities for the remaining fetuses to grow to term gestation (ACOG Committee on Ethics, 2013). This situation poses an ethical dilemma for many couples, especially those who have worked hard to overcome problems with infertility and have strong values regarding right to life. Nurses can initiate discussions with couples to help them identify resources (e.g., a minister, priest, rabbi, or mental health counselor) to aid in the decision-making process (see Chapter 37).

The likelihood of a multifetal pregnancy is increased if any one or a combination of the following factors is noted during a careful assessment:

- History of dizygotic twins in the female lineage
- Use of fertility drugs
- More rapid uterine growth for the number of weeks of gestation
- Polyhydramnios
- Palpation of more than the expected number of small or large fetal parts
- Asynchronous fetal heartbeats or more than one fetal electrocardiographic tracing
- Ultrasound evidence of more than one fetus

The diagnosis of multifetal pregnancy comes as a shock to many expectant parents. They need additional support and education to help them cope with the changes they face.

The prenatal care for women with multifetal pregnancies includes changes in the pattern of care and modifications in other aspects. Prenatal visits are scheduled more frequently. Frequent ultrasound examinations, nonstress tests, and FHR monitoring will be performed. The mother needs information related to self-management of a multifetal pregnancy because guidelines differ in comparison with a singleton pregnancy. Specific instruction should be provided regarding nutrition so that she consumes a well-balanced diet with adequate caloric intake and gains weight appropriately. Other pertinent information includes maternal adaptations during pregnancy, management of discomforts, and the risk of preterm labor and birth, including warning signs and when to call the provider. The uterine distention associated with multifetal pregnancy can cause the backache commonly experienced by pregnant women to be even worse. Maternal support hose may be worn to control leg varicosities. If risk factors such as premature dilation of the cervix or bleeding are present, abstinence from orgasm and nipple stimulation during the last trimester is recommended to help avert preterm labor. Some practitioners recommend bed rest beginning at 20 weeks in women carrying multiple fetuses to prevent preterm labor. Other practitioners question the value of prolonged bed rest. If bed rest is recommended, the mother assumes a lateral position to promote increased placental perfusion. If birth is delayed until after the thirty-sixth week, the risk of morbidity and mortality decreases for the neonates.

Multiple newborns can place a strain on finances, space, workload, and the woman's and family's coping capabilities. Lifestyle changes can be necessary. Parents need assistance in making realistic plans for the care of the infants (e.g., whether to breastfeed and whether to raise them as "alike" or as separate people). Parents should be referred to national organizations such as Parents of Twins and Triplets (www.nashvilleparent.com/directories/parents-of-twins-and-triplets-organization-potato), Mothers of Twins (www.nomotc.org), and the La Leche League (www.llli.org) for further support.

PERINATAL EDUCATION

The goal of perinatal education is to assist women and their family members to make informed, safe decisions about pregnancy, labor and birth, infant care, and early parenthood. It also is to assist them to comprehend the long-lasting potential that empowering birth experiences have in the lives of women and that early experiences have on the development of children and the family.

Classes for Expectant Parents

The perinatal education program is an expansion of the earlier childbirth education movement that originally offered a set of classes in the third trimester of pregnancy to prepare parents for birth. Today perinatal education programs consist of a menu of class series and activities from preconception through the early months of parenting.

Expectant parents and their families have different interests and information needs as the pregnancy progresses. Parents may select a variety of classes such as:

- Early pregnancy ("early bird") classes provide fundamental information including (1) early fetal development, (2) physiologic and emotional changes of pregnancy, (3) human sexuality, and (4) the nutritional needs of the mother and fetus. The classes often address environmental and workplace hazards. Exercises, nutrition, warning signs, drugs, and self-medication also are topics of interest and concern.
- Midpregnancy classes emphasize the woman's participation in self-management. Classes provide information on preparation for breastfeeding and formula feeding, infant care, basic hygiene, common discomforts and simple safe remedies, infant health, parenting, and planning for labor and birth.
- Late pregnancy classes emphasize different methods of coping with labor and birth, and these are often the basis for various prenatal classes. These include Lamaze, Bradley, and Dick-Read. These classes usually include a tour of the birthing facility. Because fear of pain in labor is a key issue for many women, childbirth preparation classes provide information on management of discomfort during labor and birth. Topics include nonpharmacologic methods to reduce discomfort such as relaxation and breathing techniques, imagery and visualization, and biofeedback. Pharmacologic interventions such as intravenous medications and epidural analgesia are also discussed. An emphasis on nonpharmacologic pain management strategies helps couples manage the labor and birth with dignity and increased comfort. Most instructors teach a flexible approach, which helps couples learn and master many techniques to use during labor (see Chapter 17 for further discussion).
- Perinatal education programs offer classes to meet specific learning needs. These include classes for adolescents, first-time mothers older than age 35, single women, adoptive parents, parents of multiples, or women with special needs such as those with visual or hearing impairments. In some agencies, classes are also offered in languages other than English. Refresher classes for parents with children not only review coping techniques for labor and birth but also help couples prepare for sibling reactions and adjustments to a new baby. Cesarean birth classes are available for couples who have this kind of birth scheduled because of breech presentation or other risk factors. Other classes focus on vaginal birth after cesarean (VBAC) because many women can successfully give birth vaginally after previous cesarean birth.

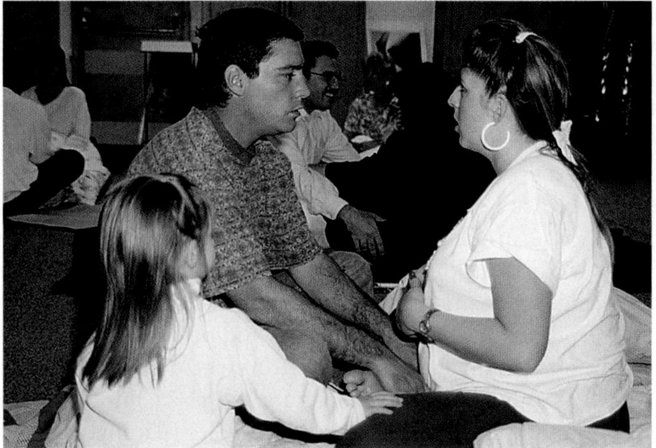

FIG 14-21 Learning relaxation exercises in a family-centered childbirth education class. (Courtesy Marjorie Pyle, RNC, Lifecircle, Costa Mesa, CA).

For the most part, the pregnant woman and her partner attend perinatal education classes, although sometimes a friend or parent is the designated support person (Fig. 14-21). There are also classes for grandparents and siblings to prepare them for their attendance at birth or the arrival of the baby. Siblings often see a film about birth and learn ways they can help welcome the baby. They also learn to cope with changes that include a reduction in parental time and attention. Grandparents learn about current child care practices and how to help their adult children adapt to parenting in a supportive way.

Perinatal classes include discussion of support systems that people can use during pregnancy, labor and birth, and in the postpartum period. Such support systems help parents function independently and effectively. During all the classes the open expression of feelings and concerns about any aspect of pregnancy, birth, and parenting is welcomed. Perinatal education is focused on health promotion and emphasizes how a healthy body is best able to adapt to the changes that accompany pregnancy. Without this context of health, routine care and testing for risks can contribute to a mindset of families that pregnancy is a state of illness as opposed to a healthy mind-body-spirit event.

Some of the decisions the childbearing family must consider are the decision to have a baby, followed by choices of a health care provider and type of care (a midwifery model [natural oriented] versus a medical [intervention oriented] model); the place for birth (hospital, birthing center, home); the type of infant feeding (breast or formula); and infant care. If a woman has had a cesarean birth, she may consider having a vaginal birth. Perinatal education can provide information to help childbearing families make informed decisions about these issues.

Previous pregnancy and childbirth experiences are important influences on current learning needs. The woman's (and support person's) age, cultural background, personal philosophy with regard to labor and birth, socioeconomic status, spiritual beliefs, and learning styles are assessed to develop the best plan to help the woman meet her needs.

PERINATAL CARE CHOICES

Often the first decision the woman makes is to select her primary health care provider for the pregnancy and birth. This decision usually affects where the birth will take place. The nurse can provide information about the different types of obstetric health care providers and the kind of care to expect from each one. Women are encouraged to ask potential care providers a series of pertinent questions (Box 14-7).

Physicians

According to the National Center for Health Statistics (NCHS), physicians (obstetricians, family medicine physicians, osteopathic physicians) attended 92% of hospital births and 5% of home births in the United States (MacDorman, Mathews, & Declercq, 2014). Family practice physicians and osteopathic physicians provide care for primarily low risk pregnant women and refer high risk women to obstetricians. Obstetricians see low risk and high risk pregnant women. Care often includes pharmacologic and medical management of problems as well as use of technologic procedures.

Midwives

Increasing numbers of pregnant women are choosing certified nurse-midwives (CNM) and certified midwives (CM) as their obstetric care providers. From 2005 to 2012, there was a 6% increase in CNM/CM attended births, accounting for 7.6% of all hospital births and 30.4% of out-of-hospital births. Out-of-hospital births attended by CNMs and CMs occurred in freestanding birth centers (2.55%) and homes (2.47%) (Martin, Hamilton, Osterman, et al., 2013).

The midwifery model of care emphasizes the natural ability of women to experience pregnancy, labor, and birth with minimal intervention. Compared with the medical model of care, midwifery care throughout pregnancy, labor, and birth is associated with benefits for mothers and babies. These include reduced use of epidurals and fewer episiotomies and instrument-assisted births. Midwifery care is associated with an increased likelihood of spontaneous vaginal birth (Sandall, Soltani, Gates, et al., 2013).

The services provided by midwives are dependent on their licensing and certification as well as the practice regulations in each state. Women who are interested in midwifery care should be knowledgeable about the various types of midwives, the care that is available, where they are allowed to practice and attend births, and reimbursement by insurance companies.

In the United States there are three types of credentialed professional midwives: certified nurse midwives (CNM), certified midwives (CM), and certified professional midwives (CPM). CMs and CPMs are known as direct-entry midwives. CNMs are legally approved to practice in all 50 states and the District of Columbia. Fewer states allow CMs and CPMs to practice.

Certified Nurse-Midwives

Certified nurse-midwives (CNM) are registered nurses with education in the two disciplines of nursing and midwifery. They are certified by the American College of Nurse Midwives (ACNM). Nurse midwifery programs are graduate level; since 2010, ACNM has mandated that entry into practice requires at least a master's degree. CNMs are trained to provide women's health care throughout the lifespan, not just during pregnancy and birth. Nurse-midwives practice collaboratively with physicians or independently with an arrangement for physician backup. They usually see low risk women. Care is often noninterventionist, and the woman and her family are encouraged to be active participants in the care. Certified nurse-midwives co-manage and/or refer pregnant women with complications to physicians.

BOX 14-7 Questions to Ask When Seeking a Maternity Care Provider

The Coalition for Improving Maternity Services (CIMS, 2013), a group of more than 50 nursing and maternity care–oriented organizations, produced a document to assist women in selecting their perinatal care. After some explanation of choices, the nurse can encourage women to ask potential care providers the following questions:

- Who can be with me during labor and birth?
- What happens during a normal labor and birth in your setting?
- How do you allow for differences in culture and beliefs?
- May I walk and move around during labor? What position do you suggest for birth?
- How do you make sure everything goes smoothly when my nurse, doctor, nurse-midwife, or agency works with one another?
- What things do you normally do to a woman in labor?
- How do you help mothers stay as comfortable as they can be? Besides drugs, how do you help mothers relieve the pain of labor?
- What if my baby is born early or has special problems?
- Do you circumcise babies?
- How do you help mothers who want to breastfeed?

Modified from Coalition for Improving Maternity Services (CIMS). (2000). *Having a baby? 10 questions to ask.* Available at www.motherfriendly.org/Resources/Documents/Having_a_Baby-English.pdf.

Direct-Entry Midwives

Certified midwives (CM) are trained in midwifery schools, colleges, or universities. A nursing degree is not required, although a bachelor's degree and specific health and science courses are required prior to entering a CM training program. Certified midwives are credentialed by the ACNM based on a certification examination; a graduate degree is required for entry into practice.

Certified professional midwives (CPM) meet the standards of certification set by the North American Registry of Midwives (NARM) in collaboration with Midwives Alliance of North America (MANA). They are educated in midwifery programs in colleges, universities, or midwifery schools, or through self-study and apprenticeship.

Traditional or Lay Midwives

Independent or *lay midwives* are also known as traditional or community-based midwives. These midwives are not certified. They are usually trained through self-study and apprenticeship. It is up to the woman seeking care from a lay midwife to assess the level of experience and expertise of a lay midwife. Lay midwives can legally practice and are licensed in some states, although there are specific requirements and guidelines that must be followed. Care by lay midwives is usually not covered by third-party payers.

Doulas

A doula is trained to provide physical, emotional, and informational support to women and their partners during labor and birth. The doula does not become involved with clinical tasks. Today many couples, no matter which type of childbirth classes they take, also use a doula for labor support.

Continuous labor support provided by a doula has been shown to decrease the use of pain medication, increase satisfaction, and increase the likelihood of a spontaneous vaginal birth. There are no known risks associated with labor support by a doula (Hodnett, Gates, Hofmeyr, & Sakala, 2012).

A doula typically meets with the woman and her husband or partner before labor. At this meeting she ascertains the woman's expectations and desires for the birth experience. With this information as her guide during labor and birth, the doula focuses her efforts on assisting the woman to achieve her goals. Doulas work collaboratively with other health care providers and the husband or other supportive individuals, but their primary goal is to assist the woman. Doulas who are also trained medical interpreters can enhance the care of women with limited English proficiency (Maher, Crawford-Carr, & Neidigh, 2012).

Doulas can be found through community contacts, health care providers, or childbirth educators; a number of organizations offer information or referral services. It is important that the expectant mother is comfortable with the doula who will be attending her. (See Box 14-8 for a list of questions to ask when arranging for a doula.) Doula International (DONA) is an organization that certifies doulas (www.dona.org). Although the doula role originally developed as an assistant during labor, some women benefit from assistance during the postpartum period. There are small but growing numbers of postnatal doulas who provide assistance to the new mother as she develops competence with infant care, feeding, and other maternal tasks.

BOX 14-8 Questions to Ask When Choosing a Doula

To discover the specific training, experience, and services offered by anyone who provides labor support, potential clients, nursing supervisors, physicians, midwives, and others should ask the following questions of that person:

- What training have you had?
- Tell me about your experience with birth, both personally and as a doula.
- What is your philosophy about childbirth and supporting women and their partners through labor?
- May we meet to discuss our birth plans and the role you will play in supporting me through childbirth?
- May we call you with questions or concerns before and after the birth?
- When do you try to join women in labor? Do you come to our home or meet us at the hospital?
- Do you meet with us after the birth to review the labor and answer questions?
- Do you work with one or more backup doulas for times when you are not available? May we meet them?
- What is your fee?

Adapted from Doula International. (2012). *Position paper: The birth doula's contribution to modern maternity care.* Available at www.dona.org/pdfs/position_papers/BIRTH%20Paper--%204%20page.pdf.

Birth Plans

The birth plan is a natural evolution of a contemporary wellness-oriented lifestyle in which women assume a level of responsibility for their own health. The birth plan is a tool with which parents can explore their childbirth options and choose those that are most important to them. The plan must be viewed as tentative because the realities of what is feasible may change as the actual labor and birth unfold. It is understood to be a preference list based on a best-case scenario.

It is useful for the nurse in a prenatal practice setting to initiate a discussion of choices and birth planning during the first and second prenatal visits. Some maternity practices provide printed material describing available options and giving answers to commonly asked questions, and tours of the birth setting are offered by almost all birthing facilities. The nurse can provide couples with pertinent information and make them aware of the various options for care and the advantages and consequences of each so they can begin making informed decisions. Early plans can be modified as the couple learns more details in their childbirth classes. Topics for the expectant parents to consider when creating a birth plan are listed in Box 14-9.

The birth plan can serve as a means of open communication between the pregnant woman and her partner and between the couple and health care providers. An early introduction to the idea of a birth plan allows the couple time to think about events or situations that could make their childbearing experience more meaningful and those they would prefer to avoid (Anderson & Kilpatrick, 2012).

BOX 14-9 Creating a Birth Plan

Topics for birth plan discussion and decision making may include any or all of the following:

Partner's participation: Attend prenatal visits? Childbirth and parent education classes? Present during labor? During birth? During cesarean birth?

Birth setting: Hospital delivery room or birthing room (if available)? A birthing center? Home?

Labor management: Walk around during labor? Use a rocking chair? Use a shower? Use a Jacuzzi, if available? Intermittent versus continuous use of an electronic fetal monitor? Have music or dimmed lighting? Have older children or other people present? Is telemetry monitoring available? Consider stimulation of labor? Consider medication—what kind?

Birth: Positions—Side-lying? On hands and knees, kneeling, or squatting? Use a birthing bed or delivery table? Will you be photographing, videotaping, or recording any of the labor or birth? Who would you like to be present—partner, older siblings, other family members, or friends? What do you know about the use of forceps? Episiotomy? Will your partner want to cut the umbilical cord? Emergency considerations/contingencies (e.g., cesarean)?

Immediately after birth: Do you want to hold the baby skin-to-skin right away? Breastfeed immediately?

Postpartum care: What kind of care do you anticipate—labor, delivery, recovery, postpartum room; mother-baby couplet care? How long does your insurance company provide coverage for you to stay? Would you like to attend self-management classes, or do you prefer to get such information from media sources? On which subjects?

Traditionally, birth plans are created prenatally and implemented on admission to the labor and birth unit. However, when women without predesigned birth plans are admitted, nurses can use a template with simple questions about preferences for care to help them develop a simple birth plan (Anderson & Kilpatrick, 2012). This is in accordance with the Association of Women's Health, Obstetric and Neonatal Nurses (AWHONN) position statement on nursing support of laboring women, specifically creating individualized care plans for laboring women based on their needs, desires, and expectations (AWHONN, 2011).

Birth Setting Choices

With careful thought the concept of natural or family- or woman-centered maternity care can be implemented in any setting. The three primary options for birth settings are the hospital, free-standing birth center, and home. Women consider several factors in choosing a setting for birth, including the preference of their health care provider, characteristics of the birthing unit, and reimbursement by third party payors.

While the majority of births occurs in hospital settings, there has been an increase in out-of-hospital births from 0.87% in 2004 to 1.36% in 2012. Of those births, 66% were at home, 29% occurred in free-standing birth centers, and the remaining 5% took place in a physician's office, clinic, or other location (MacDorman, Mathews, & Declercq, 2014).

Hospital

The types of labor and birth services in hospital settings vary greatly, from the traditional labor and delivery rooms with separate postpartum and newborn units to in-hospital birthing centers where all or almost all care takes place in a single unit.

Labor, delivery, and recovery (LDR) and labor, delivery, recovery, and postpartum (LDRP) rooms offer families a comfortable, private space for labor and birth (Fig. 14-22). Women are admitted to LDR units, labor and give birth, and spend the first 1 to 2 hours postpartum there for immediate recovery and to have time with their families to bond with their newborns. After this period, the mothers and newborns move to a postpartum unit and nursery or mother-baby unit for the duration of their stay.

In LDRP units, the same nursing staff usually provides total care from admission through postpartum discharge. The woman and her family may stay in this unit for 6 to 48 hours after giving birth. The units are furnished to provide a homelike atmosphere, as LDR units are, but have accommodations for family members to stay overnight (see Fig. 14-22, *A*).

Both units have fetal monitors, emergency resuscitation equipment for mother and newborn, and heated cribs or warming units for the newborn. Often this equipment is out of sight in cabinets or closets when it is not being used (see Fig. 14-22, *B*).

Birth Centers

Free-standing birth centers are usually built in locations separate from the hospital but are often located nearby so that quick transfer of the woman or newborn can occur when needed. These birth centers offer families a safe and cost-effective alternative to hospital or home birth. The centers are usually staffed by CNMs or physicians who also have privileges at the local hospital. Only women at low risk for complications are included for care.

Birth centers typically have homelike accommodations, including a double bed for the couple and a crib for the newborn (Fig. 14-23, *A*). Emergency equipment and drugs are usually in cabinets, out of view but easily accessible. Private bathroom facilities are incorporated into each birth unit. There may be an early labor lounge or a living room and small kitchen (see Fig. 14-23, *B*). The family is admitted to the birth center for labor and birth and will remain there until discharge, which often takes place within 6 hours of the birth.

Services provided by the free-standing birth centers include those necessary for safe management of low risk pregnant women during the childbearing cycle. Attendance at birthing and parenting classes is required of all clients. Expectant families develop birth plans. They must understand that some situations require transfer to a hospital, and they must agree to abide by those guidelines.

Birth centers and hospitals with comprehensive birthing programs usually provide resources for parents such as a lending library that includes books and DVDs, reference files on related topics, and supplies and reference materials for childbirth educators. The centers may also have referral files for community resources that offer services relating to birth and early parenting, including support groups (e.g., for single parents, for

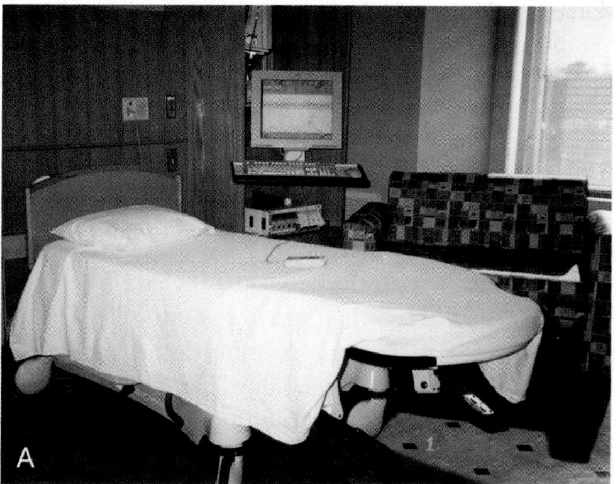

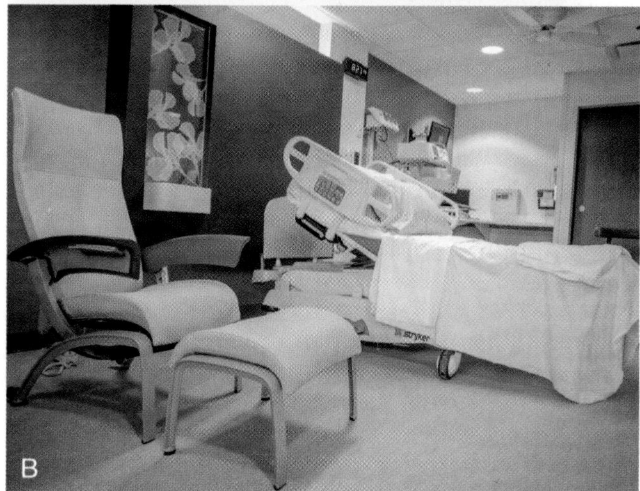

FIG 14-22 Labor, delivery, recovery, and postpartum (LDRP) units. (**A**, Courtesy Dee Lowdermilk, Chapel Hill, NC. **B**, Courtesy Mercy Hospital, St. Louis, MO.)

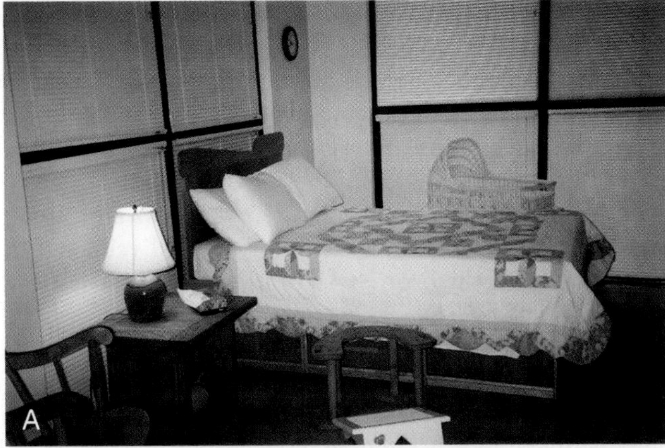

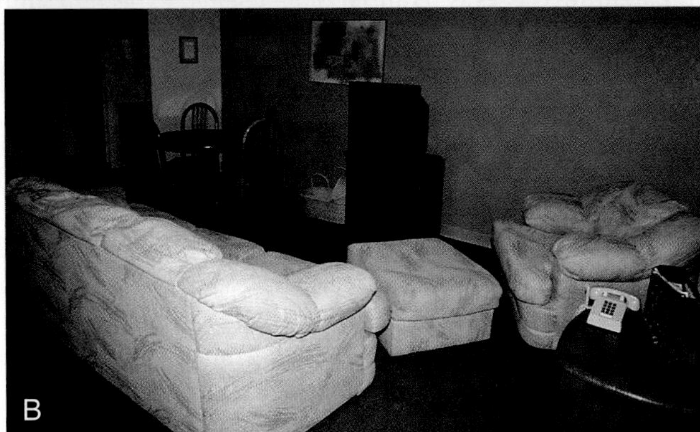

FIG 14-23 Birth center. **A,** Note double bed, baby crib, and birthing stool. **B,** Lounge and kitchen. (**A,** Courtesy Dee Lowdermilk, Chapel Hill, NC. **B,** Courtesy Michael S. Clement, MD, Mesa, AZ. Photo location: Bethany Birth Center, Phoenix, AZ.)

postbirth support, and for parents of twins), genetic counseling, women's issues, and consumer action.

Ambulance service and emergency procedures must be readily available. Fees vary with the services provided by birthing centers but typically are less than or equal to those charged by local hospitals. Some base fees on the ability of the family to pay (a reduced-fee sliding scale). Several third-party payers, as well as Medicaid and the Civilian Health and Medical Programs of the Uniformed Services (TRICARE/CHAMPVA, recognize and reimburse these centers.

Home Birth

Home birth has always been popular in certain countries, such as the Netherlands. In developing countries, hospitals or adequate lying-in facilities often are unavailable to most pregnant women, and home birth is a necessity. Although the number of home births in the United States has increased in recent years, still less than 1% of all births takes place in the home (MacDorman et al., 2014).

Home birth remains a controversial topic in American health care. Organizations such as the ACOG and the American Medical Association (AMA) agree that the safest setting for birth is a hospital or birthing center that meets standards set forth by AAP and ACOG or a free-standing birth center that meets standards of the Accreditation Association for Ambulatory Health Care (ACOG Committee on Obstetric Practice, 2011; AMA, 2008). ACOG emphasizes the need to inform women considering planned home birth about risks and benefits; although they note that absolute risk may be low, they cite a two- to threefold increased risk for neonatal death with home birth compared with planned hospital birth (ACOG Committee on Obstetric Practice). Research findings based on cohort and observational studies do not support this stance. Large-scale studies have documented the safety of planned home birth for healthy, low risk women who are attended by CNMs and when there is a system in place for transfer to a hospital facility (Cheyney, Bovbjerg, Everson, et al., 2014; Cox, Schlegel, Payne, et al., 2013; McIntyre, 2012). The National Perinatal Association (2008) and the American College of Nurse-Midwives (ACNM, 2011) support planned home birth for carefully selected low risk women within a system that provides hospitalization as needed.

In response to the increase in home births, opponents are disseminating documentation about the risks of home births for mother and infant and actively discouraging families from choosing a home birth when there are safe and compassionate hospitals and birth centers available (Chervenak, McCullough, Brent, et al., 2013). National groups supporting home birth are the Home Oriented Maternity Experience (HOME) and the National Association of Parents for Safe Alternatives in Childbirth (NAPSAC). These groups work to foster more humane childbearing practices at all levels, integrating the alternatives for childbirth to meet the needs of the total population.

There are advantages of planned home birth. The family is in control of the experience. The birth may be more physiologically normal in familiar surroundings. The mother may be more relaxed than she would be in the hospital environment. Care providers who participate in home births tend to be more support oriented and less intervention oriented. The family can assist in and be a part of the happy event, and contact with the newborn is immediate and sustained. In addition, home birth may be less expensive than a hospital or birth center. Serious infection may be less likely, assuming strict aseptic principles are followed, because people generally are relatively immune to their own home bacteria.

KEY POINTS

- The prenatal period is a preparatory one both physically, in terms of fetal growth and parental adaptations, and psychologically, in terms of anticipation of parenthood.
- Pregnancy affects parent-child, sibling-child, and grandparent-child relationships.
- Discomforts and changes of pregnancy can cause anxiety for the woman and her family and require sensitive attention and a plan for teaching self-management measures.
- Education about safety during activity and exercise is essential given maternal anatomic and physiologic responses to pregnancy.
- Important components of the initial prenatal visit include detailed and carefully documented findings from the interview, a comprehensive physical examination, and selected laboratory tests.

KEY POINTS—cont'd

- Follow-up visits are shorter than the initial visit and are important for monitoring the health of the mother and fetus and providing anticipatory guidance as needed.
- Even in normal pregnancy the nurse must remain alert to hazards such as supine hypotension, signs and symptoms of potential complications, and signs of family maladaptations.
- Blood pressure is evaluated based on absolute values and length of gestation and interpreted in light of modifying factors.
- Each pregnant woman needs to know how to recognize and report signs of potential complications such as preterm labor.
- There is an increased incidence of physical, mental, and verbal abuse during pregnancy.
- Culture, age, parity, and multifetal pregnancy can have a significant effect on the course and outcome of the pregnancy.
- Nurses must ask pregnant women and their families about preferences, practices, and customs related to childbearing to provide culturally sensitive care.
- Childbirth education teaches tuning in to the body's inner wisdom and strategies that enhance women's ability to cope effectively with labor and birth.
- Perinatal education strives to promote healthier pregnancies and family lifestyles.
- Nurses can assist pregnant women and their families to make informed decisions about care providers, birth settings, and labor support.

REFERENCES

Agency for Healthcare Research and Quality (AHRQ). (2012). Healthcare Innovations Exchange: *Nurse home visits improve outcomes for low-income, first-time mothers and their children*. Available at www.innovations.ahrq.gov/content.aspx?id=2229.

American Academy of Pediatrics (AAP) Committee on Fetus and Newborn and American College of Obstetricians and Gynecologists (ACOG) Committee on Obstetric Practice. (2012). *Guidelines for perinatal care* (7th ed.). Washington, DC: Author.

American College of Nurse-Midwives. (2011). *Legal recognition*. Available at midwife.org/Legal-Recognition.

American College of Nurse-Midwives (ACNM). (2011). *Position statement: Home birth*. Available at www.midwife.org/ACNM/files/ACNMLibraryData/UPLOADFILENAME/000000000251/Home%20Birth%20Aug%202011.pdf.

American College of Nurse-Midwives (ACMN). (2012). *Midwifery: Evidence-based practice*. Silver Spring, MD: Author. Available at www.midwife.org/ACNM/files/ccLibraryFiles/Filename/000000002128/Midwifery%20Evidence-based%20Practice%20Issue%20Brief%20FINALMAY%202012.pdf.

American College of Obstetricians and Gynecologists (ACOG). (2013). Practice bulletin no. 137: Gestational diabetes mellitus. *Obstetrics and Gynecology, 122*(2 Pt 1), 406–416.

American College of Obstetricians and Gynecologists (ACOG) Committee on Ethics. (2013). Committee opinion no. 553: Multifetal pregnancy reduction. *Obstetrics and Gynecology, 121*(2), 405–410.

American College of Obstetricians and Gynecologists (ACOG) Committee on Health Care for Underserved Women. (2012). Committee opinion no. 518: Intimate partner violence. *Obstetrics and Gynecology, 119*(2), 412–417.

American College of Obstetricians and Gynecologists (ACOG) Committee on Obstetric Practice. (2011). Committee opinion no. 476: Planned home birth. *Obstetrics and Gynecology, 117*(2 Part 1), 425–428.

American College of Obstetricians and Gynecologists (ACOG) Committee on Obstetric Practice. (2013a). Committee opinion no. 54: *Obesity in pregnancy*. Available at www.acog.org/Resources%20And%20Publications/Committee%20Opinions/Committee%20on%20Obstetric%20Practice/Obesity%20in%20Pregnancy.aspx.

American College of Obstetricians and Gynecologists (ACOG) Committee on Obstetric Practice. (2013b). Committee opinion no. 462: *Moderate caffeine consumption during pregnancy*. Available at www.acog.org/Resources%20And%20Publications/Committee%20Opinions/Committee%20on%20Obstetric%20Practice/Moderate%20Caffeine%20Consumption%20During%20Pregnancy.aspx.

American College of Obstetricians and Gynecologists (ACOG) Committee on Obstetric Practice. (2013c). Committee opinion no. 471: *Smoking cessation during pregnancy*. Available at www.acog.org/Resources%20And%20Publications/Committee%20Opinions/Committee%20on%20Health%20Care%20for%20Underserved%20Women/Smoking%20Cessation%20During%20Pregnancy.aspx.

American College of Obstetricians and Gynecologists (ACOG) Committee on Obstetric Practice. (2013d). Committee opinion no. 485: *Prevention of early-onset group B streptococcal disease in newborns*. Available at www.acog.org/~/media/Committee%20Opinions/Committee%20on%20Obstetric%20Practice/co485.pdf?dmc.

American Institute of Ultrasound in Medicine (AUIM). (2013). AIUM practice guideline for the performance of obstetric ultrasound examinations. *Journal of Ultrasound in Medicine, 32*(6), 1083–1101.

American Medical Association (AMA). (2008). *Home deliveries, resolution no. 205*. Available at http://elephantcircle.net/wp-content/uploads/2011/01/AMA-Resolution-205.pdf.

Anderson, C. J., & Kilpatrick, C. (2012). Patients' birth plans: Theories, strategies, and implications for nurses. *Nursing for Women's Health, 16*(3), 211–218.

Association of Women's Health, Obstetric and Neonatal Nurses (AWHONN). (2011). Nursing support for laboring women. *Journal of Obstetric, Gynecologic, and Neonatal Nursing, 40*(5), 665–666.

Carolan, M., & Frankowska, D. (2011). Advanced maternal age and adverse perinatal outcome: A review of the evidence. *Midwifery, 27*(6), 793–801.

Centering Healthcare Institute. (2012). *CenteringPregnancy*. Available at www.centeringhealthcare.org/pages/centering-model/model-overview.php.

Centers for Disease Control and Prevention (CDC). (2011). *Pregnant women and influenza*. Available at www.cdc.gov/flu/protect/vaccine/pregnant.htm.

Centers for Disease Control and Prevention (CDC). (2013a). Advisory Committee on Immunization Practices recommended immunization schedules for persons aged 0 through 18 years and adults aged 19 years and older—United States, 2013. *MMWR Morbidity and Mortality Weekly Report, 62*(Suppl 1), 1–19.

Centers for Disease Control and Prevention (CDC). (2013b). *Fetal alcohol spectrum disorders*. Available at www.cdc.gov/ncbddd/fasd.

Centers for Disease Control and Prevention (CDC). (2013c). *Intimate partner violence*. Available at www.cdc.gov/violence prevention/intimatepartnerviolence.

Centers for Disease Control and Prevention (CDC). (2013d). *STDs and pregnancy—CDC fact sheet*. Available at www.cdc.gov/std/pregnancy/stdfact-pregnancy.htm.

Centers for Disease Control and Prevention. (2013e). Updated recommendations for use of tetanus toxoid, reduced diphtheria toxoid, and acellular pertussis vaccine (Tdap) in pregnant women—Advisory Committee on Immunization Practices (ACIP), 2012. *MMWR Morbidity and Mortality Weekly Report, 62*(07), 131–135.

Centers for Disease Control and Prevention (CDC). (2014). *Advising travelers with specific needs. In CDC health information for international travel 2014*. Available at www.nc.cdc.gov/travel/yellowbook/2014/chapter-8-advising-travelers-with-specific-needs/pregnant-travelers.

Cherguit, J., Burns, J., Pettle, S., & Tasker, F. (2012). Lesbian co-mothers' experiences of maternity healthcare services. *Journal of Advanced Nursing, 69*(6), 1269–1278.

Chervenak, F., McCullough, L., Brent, R., et al. (2013). Planned home birth: The professional responsibility response. *American Journal of Obstetrics & Gynecology, 208*(1), 31–38.

Cheyney, M., Bovbjerg, M., Everson, C., et al. (2014). Outcomes of care for 16,924 planned home births in the United States: The Midwives Alliance of North America Statistics Project, 2004-2009. *Journal of Midwifery and Women's Health, 59*(1), 17–27.

Cox, K. J., Schlegel, R., Payne, P., et al. (2013). Outcomes of planned home births attended by certified nurse-midwives in southeastern Pennsylvania, 1983-2008. *Journal of Midwifery & Women's Health, 58*(2), 145–149.

Duff, P. (2012). Maternal and perinatal infection-bacterial. In S. G. Gabbe, J. R. Niebyl, J. L. Simpson, et al. (Eds.), *Obstetrics: Normal and problem pregnancies* (6th ed.). Philadelphia: Saunders.

Elfenbein, D., & Felice, M. (2011). Adolescent pregnancy. In M. Kliegman, B. Stanton, J. St. Geme, et al. (Eds.), *Nelson textbook of pediatrics* (19th ed.). Philadelphia: Elsevier.

Forsyth, C., Skouteris, H., Wertheim, E., et al. (2011). Men's emotional responses to their partner's pregnancy and their views on support and information received. *Australian & New Zealand Journal of Obstetrics & Gynaecology, 51*(1), 53–56.

Frawley, J., Adams, J., Sibbritt, D., et al. (2013). Prevalence and determinants of complementary and alternative medicine use during pregnancy: Results from a nationally representative sample of Australian pregnant women. *Australian & New Zealand Journal of Obstetrics & Gynaecology, 53*(4), 347–352.

Gilbert, E. (2011). *Manual of high risk pregnancy & delivery* (5th ed.). St. Louis: Mosby.

Gregory, K. D., Niebyl, J. R., & Johnson, T. R. (2012). Preconception and prenatal care: Part of the continuum. In S. G. Gabbe, J. R. Niebyl, J. L. Simpson, et al. (Eds.), *Obstetrics: Normal and problem pregnancies* (6th ed.). Philadelphia: Saunders.

Health Physics Society. (2012). *Pregnancy and flying*. Available at www.hps.org/publicinformation/ate/faqs/pregnancyandflying.html.

Herrman, J. W., Rogers, S., & Ehrenthal, D. B. (2012). Women's perceptions of CenteringPregnancy: A focus group study. *MCN: The American Journal of Maternal/Child Nursing, 37*(1), 19–26.

Hodnett, E., Gates, S., Hofmeyr, G., & Sakala, C. (2012). Continuous support for women during childbirth. *The Cochrane Database of Systematic Reviews 2012, 10*, CD003766.

Jared, H., & Boggess, K. (2012). Periodontal diseases and adverse pregnancy outcomes: A review of the evidence and implications for practice. *American Dental Hygienists' Association*. Available at www.cdeworld.com/courses/20006.

Jepson, R., Williams, G., & Craig, J. (2012). Cranberries for preventing urinary tract infections (Cochrane Review). *The Cochrane Database of Systematic Reviews 2013, 10*, CD001321.

Johnson, J. A., & Tough, S. (2012). Delayed child-bearing. *Journal of Obstetrics and Gynaecology of Canada, 34*(1), 80–93.

Kocaöz, S., Erogul, K., & Sivaslioglu, A. (2013). Role of pelvic floor muscle exercises in the prevention of stress urinary incontinence during pregnancy and the postpartum period. *Gynecologic and Obstetric Investigation, 75*(1), 34–40.

Lawrence, R. A., & Lawrence, R. M. (2011). *Breastfeeding: A guide for the medical profession* (7th ed.). St. Louis: Mosby.

Luley, T., Fitzpatrick, C., Grotegut, C., et al. (2013). Perinatal implications of motor vehicle accident trauma during pregnancy: Identifying populations at risk. *American Journal of Obstetrics and Gynecology, 208*(6), 466 e1-466.e5.

MacDorman, M. F., Mathews, T. J., & Declercq, E. (2014). *Trends in out-of-hospital births in the United States, 1990-2012. NCHS data brief no. 144*. Hyattsville, MD: National Center for Health Statistics. Available at www.cdc.gov/nchs/data/databriefs/db144.htm.

Magdaleno, R., Pereira, B. G., Chaim, E. A., & Turato, E. R. (2012). Pregnancy after bariatric surgery: A current view of maternal, obstetrical, and perinatal challenges. *Archives of Gynecology and Obstetrics, 285*(3), 559–566.

Maher, S., Crawford-Carr, A., & Neidigh, K. (2012). The role of the interpreter/doula in the maternity setting. *Nursing for Women's Health, 16*(6), 472–481.

Martin, J. A., Hamilton, B. E., Osterman, M. J., et al. (2013). Births: Final data for 2012. *National Vital Statistics Reports, 62*(9). Hyattsville, MD: National Center for Health Statistics. Available at www.cdc.gov/nchs/data/nvsr/nvsr62/nvsr62_09.pdf.

Martin, J. A., Hamilton, B. E., Sutton, P. D., et al. (2012). Births: Final data for 2010. *National Vital Statistics Reports, 61*(1). Hyattsville, MD: National Center for Health Statistics. Available at www.cdc.gov/nchs/data/nvsr/nvsr61/nvsr61_01.pdf.

Mathews, T. J., & Hamilton, B. E. (2014). *First births to older women continue to rise. NCHS data brief no. 152*. Hyattsville, MD: National Center for Health Statistics. Available at http://www.cdc.gov/nchs/data/databriefs/db152.pdf.

May, K. (1982). Three phases of father involvement in pregnancy. *Nursing Research, 31*(6), 337–342.

McIntyre, M. (2012). Safety of non-medically led primary maternity care models: A critical review of the international literature. *Australian Health Review, 36*(2), 140–147.

McMahon, C. A., Boivin, J., Gibson, F. L., et al. (2011). Age at first birth, mode of conception and psychological well-being in pregnancy: Findings from the parental age and transition to parenthood Australia (PATPA) study. *Human Reproduction, 26*(6), 1389–1398.

Mercer, R. (1995). *Becoming a mother*. New York: Springer.

Muktabhant, B., Lumbiganon, P., Ngamjarus, C., & Dowswell, T. (2012). Interventions for preventing excessive weight gain during pregnancy. *The Cochrane Database of Systematic Reviews 2012, 4*, CD007145.

National Coalition for Health Professional Education in Genetics. (2012). *Non-invasive prenatal testing (NIPT) factsheet*. Available at www.nchpeg.org/index.php?option=com_content&;view=article&id=384&Itemid=255.

National Perinatal Association. (2008). *Position paper: Choice of birth setting*. Available at www.nationalperinatal.org/advocacy/pdf/Choice-of-Birth-Setting.pdf.

Nelson, A. M. (2012). A meta-synthesis related to infant feeding decision making. *MCN: The American Journal of Maternal/Child Nursing, 37*(4), 247–252.

Newman, R., & Unal, E. R. (2012). Multiple gestations. In S. G. Gabbe, J. R. Niebyl, J. L. Simpson, et al. (Eds.), *Obstetrics: Normal and problem pregnancies* (6th ed.). Philadelphia: Elsevier.

Oral Health Care During Pregnancy Expert Workgroup. (2012). *Oral health care during pregnancy: A national consensus statement – summary of an expert workgroup meeting*. Washington, DC: National Maternal and Child Oral Health Resource Center. Available at http://www.mchoralhealth.org/PDFs/Oralhealthpregnancyconsensusmeetingsummary.pdf.

Picklesimer, A. H., Billings, D., Hale, N., et al. (2012). The effect of CenteringPregnancy group prenatal care on preterm birth in a low-income population. *American Journal of Obstetrics and Gynecology, 206*(5), 415.e1-415.e7.

Price, B., Amini, S., & Kappeler, K. (2012). Exercise in pregnancy: Effect on fitness and obstetric outcomes—a randomized trial. *Medicine and Science in Sports and Exercise, 44*(12), 2263–2269.

Rotundo, G. (2011). CenteringPregnancy: The benefits of group prenatal care. *Nursing for Women's Health, 15*(6), 508–518.

Rubin, R. (1975). Maternal tasks in pregnancy. *The Maternal and Child Nursing Journal, 4*(3), 143–153.

Rubin, R. (1984). *Maternal identity and the maternal experience.* New York: Springer.

Salinsky, E. (2013). *Effect of provider payment reforms on maternal and child health services.* NGA paper: National Governor's Association, May, 2013.

Sandall, J., Soltani, H., Gates, S., et al. (2013). Midwife-led continuity models versus other models of care for childbearing women. *The Cochrane Database of Systematic Reviews, 2013, 8,* CD004667.

Schwaitzberg, S., Mahoney, B., & Newton, E. (2013). *Trauma and pregnancy. Medscape Reference.* Available at http://emedicine.medscape.com/article/435224-overview#showall.

Seidel, H., Ball, J., Dains, J., et al. (2011). *Mosby's guide to physical examination* (7th ed.). St. Louis: Mosby.

Sengpiel, V., Elind, E., Bacelis, J., et al. (2013). Maternal caffeine intake during pregnancy is associated with birth weight but not with gestational length: Results from a large prospective observational cohort study. *BMC Medicine, 11*(42), 1–18.

Signore, C., Spong, C., Krotoski, D., et al. (2011). Pregnancy in women with physical disabilities. *Obstetrics and Gynecology, 117*(4), 935–947.

Tracy, E. E., & Konstantopoulos, W. M. (2012). Human trafficking: A call for heightened awareness and advocacy by obstetrician-gynecologists. *Obstetrics and Gynecology, 119*(5), 1045–1047.

U.S. Department of Health and Human Services Office of Adolescent Health. (2013). *Teen pregnancy and childbearing.* Available at www.hhs.gov/ash/oah/adolescent-health-topics/reproductive-health/teen-pregnancy.

U.S. Department of Health and Human Services Office of Disease Prevention and Health Promotion. (2013). *Maternal, infant, and child health. Healthy People 2020.* Available at http://healthypeople.gov/2020.

U.S. Department of Health and Human Services Office of Minority Health. (2013). *National standards for culturally and linguistically appropriate services (CLAS) in health and health care.* Available at www.thinkculturalhealth.hhs.gov.

Wapner, R. J. (2014). Prenatal diagnosis of congenital disorders. In R. K. Creasy, R. Resnik, J. D. Iams, et al. (Eds), *Creasy and Resnik's maternal-fetal medicine* (7th ed). Philadelphia: Elsevier.

15 CHAPTER

Maternal and Fetal Nutrition

Mary Courtney Moore

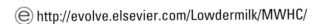

http://evolve.elsevier.com/Lowdermilk/MWHC/

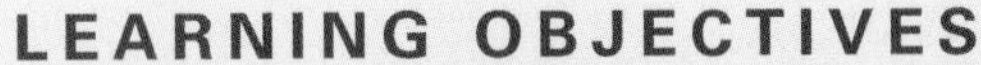

LEARNING OBJECTIVES

- Discuss recommendations for maternal weight gain during pregnancy.
- Compare the recommended level of intake of energy sources, protein, and key vitamins and minerals during pregnancy and lactation.
- Give examples of the food sources that provide the nutrients required for optimal maternal nutrition during pregnancy and lactation.
- Examine the role of nutritional supplements during pregnancy.
- List nutritional risk factors during pregnancy.
- Analyze examples of eating patterns of women from two different ethnic or cultural backgrounds, and identify potential dietary concerns. Assess nutritional status during pregnancy.
- Discuss nutritional considerations for pregnant women who are obese and those who have had bariatric surgery.
- Describe food safety precautions for pregnant women.

Nutrition is one of the many factors that influence the outcome of pregnancy (Fig. 15-1). However, maternal nutritional status is an especially significant factor because it is potentially alterable and because good nutrition before and during pregnancy is an important preventive measure for a variety of problems. These problems include birth of low birth weight (LBW) (birth weight of 2500 g or less) and preterm infants. Evidence is growing that a mother's nutrition and lifestyle affect the long-term health of her children. Thus the importance of good nutrition must be emphasized to all women of childbearing potential. Key components of nutritional care during the preconception period and pregnancy include (Harnisch, Harnisch, & Harnisch, 2012):

- Nutrition assessment that includes appropriate weight for height, adequacy and quality of dietary intake and habits, and preexisting issues that can affect nutritional status and planning, such as maternal phenylketonuria (PKU) or smoking
- Diagnosis of nutrition-related problems or risk factors such as diabetes and obesity
- Interventions based on an individual's dietary goals and plan to promote appropriate weight gain, ingestion of a variety of foods, appropriate use of dietary supplements, and physical activity
- Evaluation as an integral part of the nursing care provided to women during the preconception period and pregnancy, with referral to a nutritionist or dietitian as necessary.

NUTRIENT NEEDS BEFORE CONCEPTION

The first trimester of pregnancy is crucial in terms of embryonic and fetal organ development. A healthful diet before conception is the best way to ensure that adequate nutrients are available for the developing fetus. Folate or folic acid intake is of particular concern in the periconception period. Folate is the form in which this vitamin is found naturally in foods, and folic acid is the form used to fortify grain products and other foods and vitamin supplements. Neural tube defects (NTDs), or failures in closure of the neural tube, are more common in infants of women with poor folic acid intake. Proper closure of the neural tube is required for normal formation of the spinal cord, and the neural tube begins to close within the first month of gestation, often before the woman realizes that she is pregnant. Therefore, all adolescents and women who are capable of becoming pregnant should take 0.4 mg of folic acid every day, in addition to consuming dietary sources of folate (Box 15-1). During pregnancy the supplement is increased to 0.6 mg daily. A woman who has had a pregnancy involving a child with NTD should take a 4.0-mg folic acid supplement daily even if not planning another pregnancy. If she decides to become pregnant, she should consult with her health care provider before conception to determine whether a larger supplement is advisable (Centers for Disease Control and Prevention [CDC], 2012).

Maternal and fetal risks in pregnancy are increased when the mother is significantly underweight or overweight when pregnancy begins. Moreover, the child born to a woman who is obese during pregnancy is more likely to be obese and diabetic as an adult. Overweight and obese women who lose weight before pregnancy are likely to have healthier pregnancies (Box 15-2). Counseling in regard to healthy diet and lifestyle

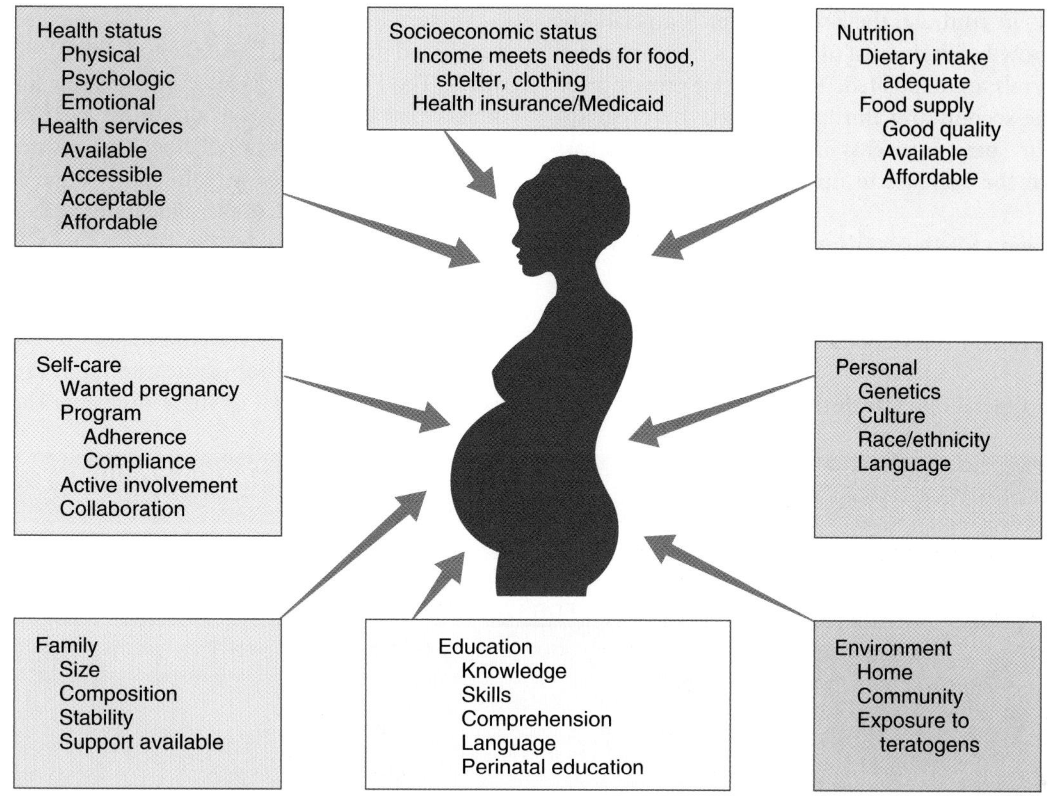

FIG 15-1 Factors that influence the outcome of pregnancy.

BOX 15-1 Food Sources of Folate*

Foods Providing 500 mcg or More per Serving
- Liver: chicken, turkey, goose (100 g [3.5 oz])

Foods Providing 200 mcg or More per Serving
- Liver: lamb, beef, veal (100 g [3.5 oz])
- Rice, enriched, cooked (1 cup)
- Breakfast cereals, ready-to-eat, fortified (1 cup)

Foods Providing 100 mcg or More per Serving
- Legumes, cooked (½ cup)
  - Peas: black-eyed, chickpea (garbanzo)
  - Beans: black, kidney, pinto, red, navy
  - Lentils
- Vegetables (½ cup)
  - Asparagus
  - Spinach, cooked
- Papaya (1 medium)
- Wheat germ (¼ cup)

Foods Providing 50 mcg or More per Serving
- Vegetables (½ cup)
  - Broccoli
  - Beans: lima beans, baked beans, or pork and beans
  - Greens: collards or mustard, cooked
  - Okra, cooked
  - Spinach, raw
- Fruits (½ cup)
  - Avocado
  - Orange or orange juice
- Pasta, cooked (1 cup)

Foods Providing 20 mcg or More per Serving
- Bread (1 slice)
- Egg (1 large)
- Corn (½ cup)

*See www.nutrition.gov/whats-food for additional food sources of folate.

BOX 15-2 Bariatric Obstetric Care

Obstetricians are seeing more morbidly obese pregnant women, including women who weigh over 250 kg (550 lb). Obesity creates many risks for pregnant women, including hypertension, thromboembolic complications, diabetes, and preterm birth. To manage their conditions and to meet their logistical needs, a new medical subspecialty—bariatric obstetrics—has arisen. Extra-wide blood pressure cuffs, scales that can accommodate up to 400 kg (880 pounds), and extra-wide surgical tables designed to hold the weight of these women are used. Special techniques for ultrasound examination and longer surgical instruments for cesarean birth are required.

practices, as well as behavioral modification techniques, should be available to women before they become pregnant (American College of Obstetricians and Gynecologists [ACOG] Committee on Obstetric Practice, 2013).

NUTRIENT NEEDS DURING PREGNANCY

Nutrient needs are determined, at least in part, by the stage of gestation. During the first trimester the synthesis of fetal tissues places relatively few demands on maternal nutrition. Therefore, during the first trimester, when the embryo or fetus is very small, the needs are only slightly increased over those before pregnancy. In contrast, the last trimester is a period of noticeable fetal growth, when most of the fetal stores of energy sources and minerals are deposited. Thus as fetal growth progresses during the second and third trimesters, the pregnant woman's need for some nutrients increases greatly. Factors that contribute to the increase in nutrient needs include the following:

- Development and growth of the uterine-placental-fetal unit
- Increase in maternal blood volume and red blood cell production
- Maternal mammary development in preparation for lactation
- 20% increase in metabolic rate during pregnancy

Dietary Reference Intakes (DRIs) (www.iom.edu) have been established in the United States and Canada and are updated regularly. The DRIs include recommendations for daily nutritional intakes that meet the needs of almost all (97% to 98%) of the healthy members of the population. They are divided into age, sex, and life-stage categories (e.g., infancy, pregnancy, and lactation) and can be used as goals in planning individuals' diets (Table 15-1).

Energy Needs

Energy (kilocalories [kcal]) needs are met by carbohydrate, fat, and protein in the diet. No specific recommendations exist for the amount of carbohydrate and fat in the diet of pregnant women, but the intake of these nutrients should be adequate

TABLE 15-1 Recommendations for Daily Intakes of Selected Nutrients During Pregnancy and Lactation

NUTRIENT (UNITS)	RECOMMENDATION FOR NONPREGNANT WOMAN*	RECOMMENDATION FOR PREGNANCY*	RECOMMENDATION FOR LACTATION*	ROLE IN RELATION TO PREGNANCY AND LACTATION	FOOD SOURCES
Energy (kilocalories [kcal] or kilojoules [kJ] †)	Variable	First trimester, same as nonpregnant; second trimester, nonpregnant needs + 340 kcal (1424 kJ); third trimester, nonpregnant needs + 452 kcal (1892 kJ)	First 6 months, nonpregnant needs + 330 kcal (1382 kJ); second 6 months, nonpregnant needs + 400 kcal (1675 kJ)	Growth of fetal and maternal tissues; milk production	Carbohydrate, fat, and protein
Protein (g)	46	First trimester, same as nonpregnant; second and third trimesters, 71 g‡	Nonpregnant needs + 25 g	Synthesis of the products of conception; growth of maternal tissue and expansion of blood volume; secretion of milk protein during lactation	Meats, eggs, cheese, yogurt, legumes (dry beans and peas, peanuts), nuts, grains
Water (L) in food and beverages	2.7	3	3.8	Expansion of blood volume, excretion of wastes; milk secretion	Water and beverages made with water, milk, juices; all foods, especially frozen desserts, fruits, lettuce and other fresh vegetables
Fiber (g)	25	28	29	Promotes regular bowel elimination; reduces long-term risk for heart disease, diverticulosis, and diabetes	Whole grains, bran, vegetables, fruits, nuts and seeds
Minerals					
Calcium (mg)	1300/1000	1300/1000	1300/1000	Fetal skeleton and tooth formation; maintenance of maternal bone and tooth mineralization	Milk, cheese, yogurt, sardines or other fish eaten with bones left in, dark green leafy vegetables except spinach or Swiss chard, calcium-set tofu, baked beans, tortillas
Iron (mg)	15/18	27	10/9	Maternal hemoglobin formation, fetal liver iron storage	Liver, meats, whole grain or enriched breads and cereals, dark green leafy vegetables, legumes, dried fruits
Zinc (mg)	9/8	12/11	13/12	Component of numerous enzyme systems, possibly important in preventing congenital malformations	Liver, shellfish, meats, whole grains, milk
Iodine (mcg)	150	220	290	Increased maternal metabolic rate	Iodized salt, seafood, milk and milk products, commercial yeast breads, rolls, and donuts
Magnesium (mg)	360/310-320	400/350-360	360/310-320	Involved in energy and protein metabolism, tissue growth, muscle action	Nuts, legumes, cocoa, meats, whole grains

TABLE 15-1 **Recommendations for Daily Intakes of Selected Nutrients During Pregnancy and Lactation—cont'd**

NUTRIENT (UNITS)	RECOMMENDATION FOR NONPREGNANT WOMAN*	RECOMMENDATION FOR PREGNANCY*	RECOMMENDATION FOR LACTATION*	ROLE IN RELATION TO PREGNANCY AND LACTATION	FOOD SOURCES
Fat-Soluble Vitamins					
A (mcg)	700	750/770	1200/1300	Essential for cell development, tooth bud formation, bone growth	Dark green leafy vegetables, dark yellow vegetables and fruits, liver, fortified margarine and butter
D (IU)	600	600	600	Involved in absorption of calcium and phosphorus, improves mineralization	Fortified milk and breakfast cereals; salmon, tuna, and other oily fish; butter, liver
E (mg)	15	15	19	Antioxidant (protects cell membranes from damage), especially important for preventing breakdown of red blood cells (RBCs)	Vegetable oils, green leafy vegetables, whole grains, liver, nuts and seeds, cheese, fish
Water-Soluble Vitamins					
C (mg)	65/75	80/85	115/120	Tissue formation and integrity, especially connective tissue; enhancement of iron absorption	Citrus fruits, strawberries, melons, broccoli, tomatoes, peppers, raw dark green leafy vegetables
Folate (mg)	0.4	0.6	0.5	Prevention of neural tube defects, increased maternal RBC formation	Fortified ready-to-eat cereals and other grain products, green leafy vegetables, oranges, broccoli, asparagus, artichokes, liver
B_6 or pyridoxine (mg)	1.2/1.3	1.9	2	Involved in protein metabolism	Meats, liver, dark green vegetables, whole grains
B_{12} (mcg)	2.4	2.6	2.8	Production of nucleic acids and proteins, especially important in formation of RBCs and neural functioning	Milk and milk products, eggs, meats, liver, fortified soy milk

*When two values appear, separated by a diagonal slash, the first is for females younger than 19 years and the second is for those 19 to 50 years of age.
†The international metric unit of energy measurement is the joule (J). 1 kcal = 4.184 kJ.
‡Add an additional 25 g in twin pregnancies.
Data from Otten, J.J., Helwig, J.P., & Meyers, L.D. (Eds). (2006). *Dietary reference intakes: The essential guide to nutrient requirements.* Washington, DC: National Academies Press; Ross, A.C., Taylor, C.L., Yaktine, A.L., & Del Valle, H.B. (Eds.). (2011). *Dietary reference intakes for calcium and vitamin D.* Washington, DC: National Academies Press.

to support the recommended weight gain. Longitudinal assessment of weight gain during pregnancy is the best way to determine whether the kcal intake is adequate; very underweight or active women may require more than the recommended increase in kcal to sustain the desired rate of weight gain. Although protein can provide energy, it is unique in its ability to provide amino acids for the synthesis of new tissues (see discussion later in this chapter).

The recommended energy (kcal) intake corresponds to the recommended pattern of gain (see Table 15-1). There is no increment for the first trimester; an additional 340 kcal per day and 462 kcal per day over the prepregnant intake is recommended during the second and third trimesters, respectively (Panel on Dietary Reference Intakes for Macronutrients, Institute of Medicine [IOM], 2005). These recommendations are most appropriate for singleton pregnancy and may need to be adjusted in multiple gestation. The amount of food providing the needed increase in energy is not large. The 340 additional kcal needed during the second trimester can be provided by two additional servings from any one of the following groups: dairy (all low fat or fat free), fruits, vegetables, and grains. In the third trimester an additional half a serving will provide the needed kcal.

Weight Gain

The desirable weight gain during pregnancy varies among women. The primary factor to consider in making a weight gain recommendation is the appropriateness of the prepregnancy weight for the woman's height—that is, whether the woman's weight was normal before pregnancy or whether she was underweight or overweight. Whenever possible, the woman should achieve a weight in the normal range for her height before pregnancy. Maternal and fetal risks in pregnancy are increased when the mother is significantly underweight or overweight before pregnancy and when weight gain during pregnancy is either too low or too high. Severely underweight women are more likely to have preterm labor and to give birth to LBW infants. Both normal-weight and underweight women with inadequate weight gain during pregnancy have an increased risk of giving birth to an infant with intrauterine growth restriction (IUGR). Greater than expected weight gain during pregnancy can occur for many reasons, including multiple gestation, edema, gestational hypertension, and overeating.

At the first health care visit the pregnant woman should be helped to establish a weight gain goal for pregnancy that is based on her prepregnancy weight (ACOG Committee on Obstetric Practice, 2013). Progress toward this goal should be monitored at each visit. A commonly used method of evaluating the appropriateness of weight for height is the body mass index (BMI), which is calculated by the following formula:

$$BMI = \frac{Weight}{Height^2}$$

in which the weight is in kilograms and height is in meters. Thus for a woman who weighed 51 kg before pregnancy and is 1.57 m tall:

$$BMI = \frac{51\ kg}{(1.57\ m)^2},\ \text{or } 20.7$$

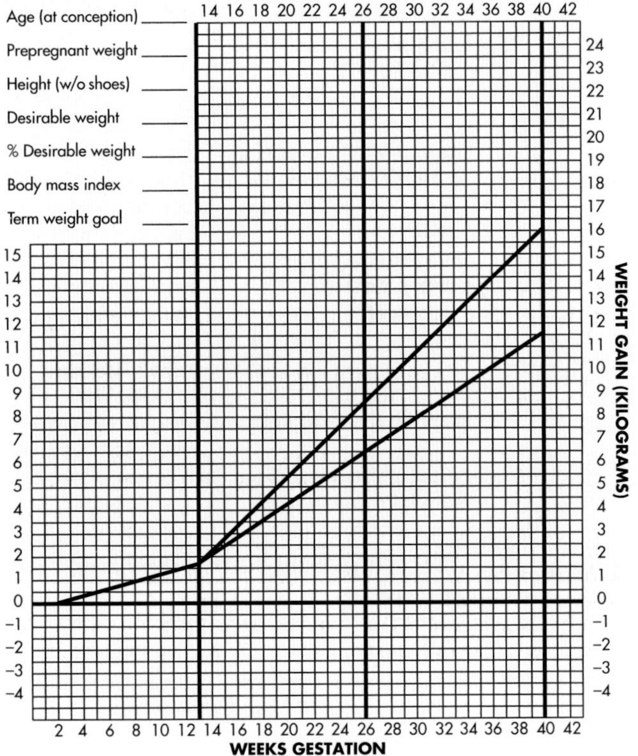

FIG 15-2 Chart for plotting prenatal weight gain for normal-weight women.

Prepregnant BMI can be classified into the following categories: less than 18.5, underweight or low; 18.5 to 24.9, normal; 25 to 29.9, overweight or high; and greater than 30, obese. The BMI can be calculated on this website: www.nhlbi.nih.gov/guidelines/obesity/BMI/bmicalc.htm.

The Institute of Medicine (IOM) (2009) issued guidelines for weight gain during pregnancy based on the prepregnancy BMI. For women with single fetuses, recommendations are that women with normal BMI should gain 11.3 to 15.9 kg (25 to 35 lb) during pregnancy (Fig. 15-2). Table 15-2 lists recommended weight gain for pregnancies with single fetuses and twin gestations for women who are normal weight, underweight, and overweight. Women's views of appropriate weight gain during pregnancy are likely to be affected by their racial or cultural backgrounds.

Pattern of Weight Gain. The optimal rate of weight gain depends on the stage of pregnancy. During the first and second trimesters, growth takes place primarily in maternal tissues; during the third trimester growth occurs primarily in fetal tissues. During the first trimester of singleton pregnancy, the average total weight gain is only 1 to 2 kg (2.2 to 4.4 lb). Thereafter, the recommended weight gain increases to approximately 0.5 kg (1.1 lb) per week for an underweight woman and 0.4 kg (0.9 lb) per week for a woman of normal weight. The recommended weekly weight gain for overweight women during the second and third trimesters is 0.3 kg (0.7 lb), and for obese women, 0.2 kg (0.4 lb) (Table 15-2).

The reasons for an inadequate weight gain (less than 1 kg [2.2lb] per month for normal-weight women or less than 0.5 kg [1.1 lb] per month for obese women during the last two trimesters) or

TABLE 15-2 Weight Gain During Pregnancy

PREPREGNANCY WEIGHT CATEGORY	BODY MASS INDEX	RECOMMENDED RANGE OF TOTAL WEIGHT	RECOMMENDED RATES OF WEIGHT GAIN IN THE SECOND AND THIRD TRIMESTERS (MEAN RANGE/WK)*
• Underweight	• Less than 18.5	• 12.7-18.1 kg (28-40 lb)	• 0.45-0.6 kg (1-1.3 lb)
• Normal weight	• 18.5-24.9	• 11.3-15.9 kg (25-35 lb)	• 0.36-0.45 kg (0.8-1 lb)
• Overweight	• 25-29.9	• 6.8-11.3 kg (15-25 lb)	• 0.23-0.32 kg (0.5-0.7 lb)
• Obese (includes all classes)	• 30 and greater	• 5-9.1 kg (11-20 lb)	• 0.18-0.27 kg (0.4-0.6 lb)

For twin gestations the recommended total weight gain is 21 to 28 kg (46 to 62 lb) for women who are underweight before conception; 17 to 25 kg (37 to 54 lb) for normal-weight women; 14 to 23 kg (31 to 50 lb) for overweight women; and 11 to 19 kg (25 to 42 lb) for obese women. The provisional recommendations for women with more than two fetuses suggest that women who were normal weight before pregnancy should gain 17 to 25 kg (37 to 54 lb), overweight women should gain 14 to 23 kg (31 to 50 lb), and obese women should gain 11 to 19 kg (25 to 42 lb). There is no recommendation for women who were underweight before pregnancy (Institute of Medicine, 2009).

*Based on weight gain of 0.5-2.2 kg (1.1 to 4.4 lb) during first trimester.

From Institute of Medicine. (2009). *Weight gain during pregnancy: Reexamining the guidelines.* Washington, DC: National Academies Press.

excessive weight gain (more than 3 kg [6.6 lb] per month) should be evaluated thoroughly. Possible reasons for deviations from the expected rate of weight gain, besides inadequate or excessive dietary intake, include measurement or recording errors or differences in weight of clothing or time of day. An exceptionally high gain is likely to be caused by an accumulation of fluids, and a gain of more than 3 kg (6.6 lb) in a month, especially after the twentieth week of gestation, often is associated with the development of preeclampsia.

Hazards of Restricting Adequate Weight Gain. An obsession with thinness and dieting pervades the North American culture. Figure-conscious women may find it difficult to make the transition from guarding against weight gain before pregnancy to valuing weight gain during pregnancy. In counseling these women the nurse emphasizes the positive effects of good nutrition as well as the adverse effects of maternal malnutrition (manifested by poor weight gain) on infant growth and development.

This counseling includes information on the components of weight gain during pregnancy (Table 15-3) and the amount of this weight that will be lost at birth. Because lactation can help reduce maternal energy stores gradually (Lawrence & Lawrence, 2011), this also provides an opportunity to promote breastfeeding.

Pregnancy is not a time for a weight reduction diet. Even overweight or obese pregnant women need to gain at least enough weight to equal the weight of the products of conception (fetus, placenta, and amniotic fluid). If they limit their energy intake to prevent weight gain, they can also excessively limit their intake of important nutrients. Moreover, dietary restriction results in catabolism of fat stores, which in turn augments the production of ketones. The long-term effects of mild ketonemia during pregnancy are not known, but ketonuria is associated with preterm labor. It should be stressed to obese women (and to all pregnant women) that the quality of the weight gain is important, with emphasis placed on consuming nutrient-dense foods and avoiding empty-calorie foods.

Excessive Weight Gain. In the United States, 60% of women who give birth are overweight or obese; only 30% follow the weight gain recommendations for pregnancy, with most women gaining excessive amounts (CDC, 2014). Obesity during pregnancy is associated with increased use of health care services and longer hospital stays. During pregnancy an emphasis on regular physical activity and a healthy dietary intake can help avert excessive weight gain (see Clinical Reasoning Case Study). Excessive weight gained during pregnancy can be difficult to lose after pregnancy, thus contributing to chronic overweight or obesity—an etiologic factor in a host of chronic diseases, including hypertension, diabetes mellitus, and arteriosclerotic heart disease. The woman who gains 18 kg or more is especially at risk (Box 15-3). Food energy intake and particularly intake of fat is likely to be high among pregnant women, especially low-income women (see Evidence-Based Practice box).

TABLE 15-3 Tissues Contributing to Maternal Weight Gain at 40 Weeks of Gestation

TISSUE	KILOGRAMS	POUNDS
Fetus	3.2-3.9	7-8.5
Placenta	0.9-1.1	2-2.5
Amniotic fluid	0.9	2
Increase in uterine tissue	0.9	2
Breast tissue	0.5-1.8	1-4
Increased blood volume	1.8-2.3	4-5
Increased tissue fluid	1.4-2.3	3-5
Increased stores (fat)	1.8-2.7	4-6

CLINICAL REASONING CASE STUDY

Nutrition and the Pregnant Woman with Excessive Weight Gain

Claudia, a 29-year-old Hispanic woman, has been followed at the clinic since her twelfth week of pregnancy. At her first visit she was overweight (5′2″ tall, 70.9 kg [156 lb]). She received counseling about healthy diet choices for pregnancy. At today's clinic appointment (24 weeks of gestation), you record that she has gained a total of 10 kg (22 lb) since her first visit. You are asked to develop with Claudia a nutrition and lifestyle plan that provides for optimal fetal growth while helping to curb excessive weight gain. You know that it is important to include consideration of personal preferences and cultural factors in your plan. With Claudia, identify barriers to implementing the plan.

1. Evidence—Is there sufficient evidence to draw conclusions about an appropriate nutrition plan, considering personal preferences and cultural factors?
2. Assumptions—Describe underlying assumptions about each of the following issues:
   a. Dietary Reference Intakes for pregnancy and lactation
   b. Indicators of nutritional risk in pregnancy
   c. Daily food guide for pregnancy and lactation
   d. Lifestyle factors contributing to overweight; physical activities that may be acceptable to the client, whose cultural background does not encourage physical activity among girls and women
   e. Effects of weight gain during pregnancy on future health of the woman and her infant
3. What implications and priorities for nursing care can be drawn at this time? What interventions and teaching are likely to be indicated?
4. Does the evidence objectively support your conclusion?

BOX 15-3 Indicators of Nutritional Risk in Pregnancy

- Adolescence or less than 2 years post menarche
- Frequent pregnancies: three within 2 years
- Poor fetal outcome in a previous pregnancy
- Poverty/food insecurity
- Poor diet habits with resistance to change
- Use of tobacco, alcohol, or drugs
- Weight at conception under or over normal weight
- Problems with weight gain
  - Any weight loss
  - Weight gain of less than 1 kg (2.2 lb)/month after the first trimester
  - Weight gain of more than 3 kg (6.6 lb)/month after the first trimester
- Multifetal pregnancy
- Low hemoglobin and/or hematocrit values
- Diabetes
- Chronic illness, including an eating disorder, that affects intake, absorption, or metabolism of nutrients

EVIDENCE-BASED PRACTICE

Weight Management in Pregnancy

Ask the Question

For obese and overweight pregnant women, are weight management interventions safe and beneficial to the mother and baby?

Search for the Evidence

Search Strategies

- English language research-based publications on pregnancy, obesity, weight gain, diet, and exercise were included.
- Exclusions included trials in developing countries with food shortages.

Databases Used

- Cochrane Collaborative Database, National Guideline Clearinghouse (Agency for Healthcare Research and Quality [AHRQ]), CINAHL, PubMed, UpToDate, and the professional website for the Association of Women's Health, Obstetric and Neonatal Nurses (AWHONN)

Critical Appraisal of the Evidence

- Obesity in pregnancy is associated with offspring with attention deficit hyperactivity disorder (ADHD) in childhood, eating disorders in adolescence, and psychotic disorders in adulthood (Van Lieshout, Taylor, & Boyle, 2011).
- Weight management interventions for obese pregnant women result in significantly decreased weight gain and significantly less preeclampsia and shoulder dystocia (Thangaratinam, Rogozinska, Jolly, et al., 2012).
- The most effective interventions are dietary, resulting in decreased risk for preeclampsia, gestational hypertension, and preterm birth, with no harm to the fetus (Thangaratinam et al.).
- In a systematic review, researchers found that goal setting is a useful technique for achieving optimal weight gain. Obese women may require further counseling (Brown, Sinclair, Liddle, et al., 2012).
- Regular activity improves maternal glycemic control and fetal outcomes. Caregivers should recommend physical activity to most pregnant women as safe and beneficial (Ferraro, Gaudet, & Adamo, 2012).

Apply the Evidence: Nursing Implications

- Preconception counseling should include prevention of obesity, ideally from childhood. Obese women are at risk for cardiac and pulmonary diseases, gestational hypertension and diabetes, and obstructive sleep apnea. Obesity in pregnancy can result in higher risk for congenital abnormalities, operative birth, and surgical complications (ACOG, 2013).
- Nurses are frequently the primary educators for pregnant women. Counseling obese pregnant women about nutrition and food choices and using collaborative goal setting for weight gain can prevent pregnancy risks and avoid weight gain that may persist beyond pregnancy.
- Activity needs to be frequent, fun, and affordable. An excellent idea is encouraging the woman to walk with other women, which provides social support and increased safety. In addition, the nurse can advocate for low-cost indoor facilities in the community.

Quality and Safety Competencies: Evidence-Based Practice*

Knowledge

- Explain the role of evidence in determining best clinical practice.
- Both nutrition counseling and motivation work best for weight management in pregnancy.

Skills

- Locate evidence reports related to clinical practice topics and guidelines.
- Dietary and activity interventions are safe and beneficial in pregnancy for obese women.

Attitudes

- Appreciate the importance of regularly reading relevant professional journals.
- Systematic reviews and professional guidelines highlight interventions that have evidence of success, such as motivational goal setting for weight management.

References

American College of Obstetricians and Gynecologists (ACOG). (2013). Committee opinion no. 549: Obesity in pregnancy. *Obstetrics and Gynecology, 121*(1), 213–217.

Brown, M. J., Sinclair, M., Liddle, D., et al. (2012). A systematic review investigating healthy lifestyle interventions incorporating goal setting strategies for preventing excess gestational weight gain. *PLoS One, 7*(7), e39503.

Ferraro, Z. M., Gaudet, L., & Adamo, K. B. (2012). The potential impact of physical activity during pregnancy on maternal and neonatal outcome. *Obstetrical and Gynecological Survey, 67*(2), 99–110.

Thangaratinam, S., Rogozinska, E., Jolly, K., et al. (2012). Interventions to reduce or prevent obesity in pregnant women: A systematic review. *Health Technology Assessment, 16*(31), 1–192.

Van Lieshout, R. J., Taylor, V. H., & Boyle, M. H. (2011). Pre-pregnancy and pregnancy obesity and neurodevelopmental outcomes in offspring: A systematic review. *Obesity Reviews, 12*(5), e548–e559.

Pat Mahaffee Gingrich

*Adapted from Quality and Safety Education for Nurses (QSEN) at www.qsen.org.

When obesity is present (either preexisting obesity or obesity that develops during pregnancy), there is an increased likelihood of preeclampsia; gestational diabetes; macrosomia and cephalopelvic disproportion; operative vaginal birth; emergency cesarean birth; postpartum hemorrhage; wound, genital tract, or urinary tract infection; birth trauma; and late fetal death (American Academy of Pediatrics [AAP] & ACOG, 2012; Langford, Joshu, Chang, et al., 2011). Maternal obesity is also associated with increased risk of miscarriage, congenital anomalies, growth abnormalities, and stillbirth (AAP & ACOG, 2012). In addition, the infant of a woman who is obese during pregnancy is more likely to be obese and to develop diabetes as an adult.

Protein

Adequate protein is needed for tissue growth during pregnancy that results from:

- The rapid growth of the fetus
- The enlargement of the uterus and its supporting structures, the mammary glands, and the placenta

- The increase in the maternal circulating blood volume and the subsequent demand for increased amounts of plasma protein to maintain colloidal osmotic pressure
- The formation of amniotic fluid

The recommendation for daily protein intake during pregnancy is approximately 71 g/day, which is an increase of 25 g/day over the nonpregnant level (Otten, Helwig, & Meyers, 2006). Milk, meat, eggs, yogurt, and cheese are complete protein foods with a high biologic value. Legumes (dried beans and peas), whole grains, and nuts are also valuable sources of protein. In addition, these protein-rich foods are a source of other nutrients such as calcium, iron, and B vitamins. Plant sources of protein often provide needed dietary fiber. The recommended daily food plan (Table 15-4) is a guide to the amounts of these foods that supply the quantities of protein needed.

Protein intake in many people in the United States is relatively high; thus, many women may not need to increase their intake at all during pregnancy. Three servings of milk, yogurt, or cheese (four for adolescents) and two servings (5 to 6 ounces [140 to 168 g]) of meat, poultry, or fish supplies most of the recommended protein for a pregnant woman. Additional protein is provided by vegetables and breads, cereals, rice, or pasta. Pregnant adolescents, women from impoverished backgrounds, and women adhering to unusual diets such as a macrobiotic (highly restricted vegetarian) diet are those whose protein intake is most likely to be inadequate. High-protein supplements are not recommended during pregnancy because of potentially harmful effects on the fetus.

Omega-3 Fatty Acids

The long-chain polyunsaturated fatty acids (LC-PUFAs) docosahexaenoic acid (DHA) and arachidonic acid (AA) are considered essential to brain development and neurologic function. Supplementation of omega-3 (n-3) LC-PUFA during pregnancy has been associated with reduced risk of preterm birth and improved neurologic and visual development in the offspring. However, there is a lack of conclusive evidence on the specific beneficial effects of DHA supplementation (Gould, Smithers, & Makrides, 2013; Lo, Sienna, Mamak, et al., 2012). Many providers recommend at least 300 mg/day of DHA for pregnant women. Some prenatal vitamins contain DHA; fish oil supplements are another source of DHA. Women can get adequate amounts of DHA by eating 8 to 12 ounces of seafood per week. Because of the risk of fetal neurotoxicity of methylmercury, pregnant women are cautioned to select fish species known to have lower levels of methylmercury.

TABLE 15-4 Daily Food Guide for Pregnancy and Lactation

FOOD GROUP	DAILY AMOUNT OF FOOD RECOMMENDED FOR WOMEN*	SERVING SIZE
Grains	6- to 8-ounce equivalents At least half of grain servings should be whole grains. *Whole grains* are those that contain the entire grain kernel (bran, germ, endosperm) (e.g., whole wheat or whole cornmeal, oatmeal, quinoa, bulgur, and brown rice). *Refined grains* have been milled to remove the bran and germ (e.g., white flour, white bread, degermed cornmeal, white rice, and masa harina and corn or flour tortillas, unless they are labeled as whole grain).	1-ounce equivalent = 1 slice bread; ¾ to 1 cup ready-to-eat cereal, ½ cup cooked rice, pasta, or cooked cereal; 1 small muffin; or 1 small (6″) tortilla
Vegetables Vary the vegetables consumed to take advantage of the different nutrients they offer. Remember that half the plate should be fruits and vegetables.	2½ to 3 cups Dark green (e.g., kale, collards, spinach, broccoli) and red/orange (e.g., winter squash, pumpkin, and sweet potato) vegetables should be included often.	1 cup = 2 cups raw leafy greens; 1 cup of other vegetables, raw or cooked; or 1 cup of vegetable juice
Fruits	2 cups	1 cup = 1 cup raw, frozen, or canned fruit; 1 cup 100% juice; or ½ cup dried fruit
Dairy	3 cups Most dairy choices should be fat free or low fat.	1 cup = 1 cup (8 ounces) milk or yogurt; 1½ ounces natural cheese; 2 ounces processed cheese (e.g., American); 2 cups cottage cheese; 1 cup frozen yogurt or 1½ cups ice cream (choose fat free or low fat most often); 1 cup calcium-fortified soy milk
Protein foods	5½- to 6½-ounce equivalents Most meat and poultry choices should be lean or low fat. Fish, nuts, and seeds contain healthy oils, so choose these foods frequently.	1-ounce equivalent = 1 ounce (30 g) cooked meat, poultry, or fish; ¼ cup cooked dried beans or peas†; 1 egg; 1 tablespoon (15 ml) peanut butter; ½ ounce nuts or seeds
Oils It is not essential to consume 5-6 teaspoons/day, but limiting intake to that amount helps to avoid excessive weight gain.	5-6 teaspoons (25-30 ml) Choose oils rather than solid fats. Solid fats are fats that are solid at room temperature, such as butter, shortening, stick margarine, and pork, chicken, or beef fat. Read the label: choose products with no *trans* fats, limit intake of saturated fats, and choose oils high in monounsaturated and polyunsaturated fats.	1 teaspoon = 1 teaspoon liquid oil (e.g., olive, canola, sunflower, safflower, peanut, soybean, cottonseed) or soft margarine (tub or squeeze bottle); 1 tablespoon mayonnaise-type or Italian salad dressing; ¾ tablespoon Thousand Island salad dressing; 8 large olives‡; ⅙ medium avocado‡; ⅓ ounce dry-roasted nuts or peanuts‡

*These are approximate amounts and should be individualized. Intake may have to be increased for women with a more active lifestyle or multiple gestation, those who are underweight before pregnancy, or those exhibiting poor gestational weight gain. Needs during lactation may be greater than these recommendations.

†Beans are also part of the vegetable group.

‡Avocados and olives are part of the vegetable group; nuts and seeds are part of the protein foods group. These foods are also high in oils.

SAFETY ALERT

High levels of mercury can harm the developing nervous system of the fetus or young child, and certain fish are especially high in mercury. Women who may become pregnant, women who are pregnant or nursing, and young children need to follow some precautions: (1) avoid eating shark, swordfish, king mackerel, and tilefish; (2) check local advisories about the safety of fish caught by family and friends in local bodies of water, but if no advisory is available, limit intake of these fish to 6 ounces and eat no other fish that week; and (3) eat as much as 12 ounces a week of a variety of commercially caught fish and shellfish low in mercury, such as shrimp, salmon, pollock, catfish, and canned light tuna (but limit intake of albacore or "white" tuna and tuna steaks, which contain more mercury, to 6 ounces per week) (U.S. Food and Drug Administration [FDA], 2013b).

Fluids

Water is the main substance of cells, blood, lymph, amniotic fluid, and other vital body fluids. It is essential during the exchange of nutrients and waste products across cell membranes. It also aids in maintaining body temperature. A good fluid intake promotes regular bowel function, which is sometimes a problem during pregnancy. The recommended daily intake is about 8 to 10 glasses (2.3 L) of fluid. Water, milk, and decaffeinated or herbal tea are good sources. Foods in the diet should supply an additional 700 ml or more of fluid. Dehydration can increase the risk of cramping, contractions, and preterm labor.

Minerals and Vitamins

In general, the nutrient needs of pregnant women, with perhaps the exception of folate and iron, can be met through dietary sources. Counseling about the need for a varied diet rich in vitamins and minerals should be a part of early prenatal care of every pregnant woman and should be reinforced throughout pregnancy (see Community Activity box). It has been suggested that taking a micronutrient supplement (including vitamins and trace minerals) before and during pregnancy reduces the risk for congenital defects, LBW, and preterm birth, as well as preeclampsia. There is no conclusive evidence to support this suggestion; further research is needed on maternal and fetal benefits of micronutrient supplementation. Supplements are especially advisable for women with known nutritional risk factors (Box 15-4). It is important that the pregnant woman understand that the use of a vitamin-mineral supplement does not lessen the need to consume a nutritious, well-balanced diet.

COMMUNITY ACTIVITY

Visit a prenatal clinic. Identify sources of nutrition education that are evident in the waiting room. Does the clinic employ a nutritionist or dietitian? Who provides nutrition counseling in the clinic? Do all clinic clients receive nutrition counseling, in either individual or group settings? What ethnic and language groups are served by the clinic? Are print materials available in multiple languages? Are interpreters available? Are there sources for free materials on nutrition that could be placed in the clinic? Identify strengths and weaknesses of nutrition education in that setting. Develop a feasible plan for improving nutrition education in the clinic.

Iron

Women are at increased risk for iron deficiency during pregnancy related to the associated increased iron requirements. Iron is needed to allow transfer of adequate iron to the fetus and to permit expansion of the maternal red blood cell (RBC) mass. Beginning in the latter part of the first trimester, the blood volume of the mother increases steadily, peaking at about 1500 ml more than that in the nonpregnant state. In twin gestations the increase is at least 500 ml greater than that in singleton pregnancies. Plasma volume increases more than RBC mass, with the difference between plasma and RBCs being greatest during the second trimester. The relative excess of plasma causes a modest decrease in the hemoglobin concentration and hematocrit, known as **physiologic anemia of pregnancy**. This is a normal adaptation during pregnancy.

Poor iron status, which can result in iron deficiency anemia, is relatively common among women in the childbearing years. Anemic women are poorly prepared to tolerate hemorrhage at the time of birth. In addition, women who have iron deficiency anemia during early pregnancy are at increased risk for preterm birth. Iron deficiency during the third trimester apparently does not carry the same risk. In the United States, anemia is most common among adolescents, African-American women, and women of lower socioeconomic status.

The recommended iron intake for pregnant women is 27 mg/day, compared with 18 mg/day in nonpregnant females (Otten et al., 2006). A supplement of 30 mg of ferrous iron daily starting by 12 weeks of gestation helps ensure an adequate iron intake. Prenatal vitamins typically contain 30 mg

BOX 15-4 Calcium Sources for Women Who Do Not Drink Milk

Each of the following provides approximately the same amount of calcium as 1 cup of milk:

Fish
- 3-oz can of sardines
- 4½ -oz can of salmon (if bones are eaten)

Beans and Legumes
- 3 cups cooked dried beans
- 2½ cups refried beans
- 2 cups baked beans with molasses
- 1 cup tofu (calcium added)

Greens
- 1 cup collards
- 1½ cups kale or turnip greens

Baked Products
- 3 pieces cornbread
- 4 slices French toast
- 2 (7-inch diameter) waffles

Fruits
- 11 dried figs
- 1⅛ cups orange juice with calcium added

Sauces
- 3 oz creamy pesto sauce
- 5 oz cheese sauce

of iron. Iron supplements can be poorly tolerated during the nausea prevalent in the first trimester, and starting the supplement after this point may improve tolerance. If maternal iron deficiency anemia is present (preferably diagnosed by measurement of serum ferritin, a storage form of iron), increased dosages (60 to 120 mg daily) may be required; iron supplements are often recommended for women who are pregnant with multiple fetuses (Hark & Catalano, 2012). Certain foods taken with an iron supplement can promote or inhibit absorption of iron from the supplement. See the Teaching for Self-Management box: Iron Supplementation later in the chapter. Even when a woman is taking an iron supplement, she should also include good food sources of iron in her daily diet (see Table 15-1).

Calcium

There is no increase in the DRI of calcium during pregnancy and lactation (see Table 15-1). The DRI (1000 mg daily for women 19 years and older and 1300 mg for those younger than 19 years [Ross, Taylor, Yaktine, & Del Valle, 2011]) appears to provide sufficient calcium for fetal bone and tooth development while maintaining maternal bone mass. Milk and yogurt are especially rich sources of calcium, providing approximately 300 mg per cup (240 ml). Nevertheless, many women do not consume these foods or do not consume adequate amounts to provide the recommended intakes of calcium. One problem that can interfere with milk consumption is lactose intolerance, the inability to digest milk sugar (lactose) caused by the lack of the lactase enzyme in the small intestine. It is relatively common in adults, particularly African-Americans, Asians, Native Americans, and Inuits (Alaska Natives). Milk consumption can cause abdominal cramping, bloating, and diarrhea in these populations, although many lactose-intolerant individuals can tolerate small amounts of milk without symptoms. Yogurt, sweet acidophilus milk, buttermilk, cheese, chocolate milk, and cocoa may be tolerated even when fresh fluid milk is not. Commercial lactase supplements (e.g., Lactaid®) are widely available to consume with milk, and many supermarkets stock lactase-treated milk, making it possible for lactose-intolerant people to drink milk. An alternative to cow's milk is calcium-fortified almond milk; natural almond milk does not contain adequate calcium. However, almond milk is lower in protein than cow's milk.

In some cultures it is uncommon for adults to drink milk. For example, Puerto Ricans and other Hispanic people may use milk only as an additive in coffee. Pregnant women from these cultures may need to consume nondairy sources of calcium (see Box 15-4). If calcium intake appears low and the woman does not change her dietary habits despite counseling, a daily supplement containing 600 mg of elemental calcium may be needed. Calcium supplements may also be recommended when a pregnant woman experiences leg cramps caused by an imbalance in the calcium-to-phosphorus ratio.

Other Minerals and Electrolytes

Magnesium. Diets of women in the childbearing years are likely to be low in magnesium, and as many as half of pregnant and lactating women may have inadequate intakes. Adolescents and low-income women are especially at risk. The recommended daily intake during pregnancy is 400 mg (Otten et al., 2006). Dairy products, nuts, whole grains, and green leafy vegetables are good sources of magnesium.

Sodium. During pregnancy the need for sodium increases slightly, primarily because the body water is expanding (e.g., the expanding blood volume). Sodium is essential for maintaining body water balance. In the past, dietary sodium was routinely restricted in an effort to control the peripheral edema that commonly occurs during pregnancy. It is now recognized that moderate peripheral edema is normal, occurring as a response to the fluid-retaining effects of elevated levels of estrogen. Sodium is not routinely restricted in pregnancy, and restriction has not proved effective in reducing the rates of preeclampsia. Severe sodium restriction can make it difficult for pregnant women to achieve an adequate diet. Grain, milk, and meat products, which are good sources of nutrients needed during pregnancy, are significant sources of sodium. In addition, sodium restriction can stress the adrenal glands and the kidneys as they attempt to retain adequate sodium. In general, sodium restriction is necessary only if the woman has a medical condition such as renal or liver failure or hypertension that warrants it.

Excessive intake of sodium is discouraged during pregnancy because it can contribute to development of hypertension in salt-sensitive individuals. An adequate sodium intake for pregnant and lactating women, as well as for nonpregnant women in the childbearing years, is estimated to be 1.5 g/day, with a recommended upper limit of intake of 2.3 g/day (Otten et al., 2006). Table salt (sodium chloride) is the richest source of sodium, with approximately 2.3 g of sodium in 1 teaspoon (5 g) of salt. Most canned foods contain added salt unless the label states otherwise. Large amounts of sodium are also found in many processed foods, including smoked or cured meats, cold cuts, and corned beef; frozen entrees and meals; baked goods; mixes for casseroles or bread products; soups; and condiments. Products low in nutritive value and excessively high in sodium include pretzels, potato and other chips (except salt free), pickles, catsup, prepared mustard, steak and Worcestershire sauces, some soft drinks, and bouillon. A moderate sodium intake can usually be achieved by salting food lightly during cooking, adding no additional salt at the table, and avoiding low-nutrient, high-sodium foods.

Potassium. Diets including adequate intakes of potassium are associated with reduced risk for hypertension. Potassium has been identified as one of the nutrients most likely to be lacking in the diets of women of childbearing years. A diet including 8 to 10 servings of unprocessed fruits and vegetables daily, along with moderate amounts of low-fat meats and dairy products, reduces sodium intake while providing adequate amounts of potassium (Frisoli, Schmieder, Grodzicki, & Messerli, 2011).

Zinc. Zinc is a constituent of numerous enzymes involved in major metabolic pathways. Zinc deficiency is associated with malformations of the central nervous system in infants. When large amounts of iron and folic acid are consumed, the absorption of zinc is inhibited and the serum zinc levels are reduced as a result. Because iron and folic acid supplements are commonly prescribed during pregnancy, pregnant women should be encouraged to consume good sources of zinc daily (see Table 15-1). The recommended intake for pregnant women is 11 mg/day (Otten et al., 2006). Women with anemia who receive high-dose iron supplements also need supplements of zinc and copper.

Fat-Soluble Vitamins

The fat-soluble vitamins include vitamins A, D, E, and K. Fat-soluble vitamins are stored in the body tissues; in the event of prolonged overdoses, these vitamins can reach toxic levels. Because of the high potential for toxicity, pregnant women are advised to take fat-soluble vitamin supplements only as prescribed. Toxicity from dietary sources is very unlikely.

Adequate intake of vitamin A is needed so that sufficient amounts of the vitamin can be stored in the fetus. A well-chosen diet, including adequate amounts of deep yellow and dark green vegetables—leafy greens, broccoli, and carrots—and fruits such as cantaloupe and apricots, provides sufficient amounts of carotenes that can be converted in the body to vitamin A. Congenital malformations such as spina bifida and cleft palate have occurred in infants of mothers who took excessive amounts of preformed vitamin A (from supplements) during pregnancy; thus extra supplements, in addition to the commonly prescribed prenatal vitamins, are not recommended routinely for pregnant women (Hark & Catalano, 2012).

Vitamin D plays an important role in the absorption and metabolism of calcium. The main food sources of this vitamin are enriched or fortified foods such as milk and ready-to-eat cereals. Vitamin D is also produced in the skin by the action of ultraviolet light (in sunlight). A severe deficiency can lead to neonatal hypocalcemia and tetany, as well as to poor development of tooth enamel. Women with lactose intolerance, those on vegan diets, and others who do not include milk in their diet for any reason are at risk for vitamin D deficiency. Other risk factors are dark skin (African-American women are at high risk for deficiency), habitual use of clothing that covers most of the skin, and living in northern latitudes where sunlight exposure is limited, especially during the winter. Use of recommended amounts of sunscreen with a sun protection factor (SPF) rating of 15 or greater reduces skin vitamin D production by as much as 99%, thus bringing about a need for regular intake of fortified foods or a supplement. Health care providers may prescribe vitamin D supplements of 1000 to 2000 IU/day for women with low serum vitamin D levels (AAP & ACOG, 2012).

Vitamin E is needed to protect against the increased oxidative stress associated with pregnancy. Oxidative stress above that usually associated with pregnancy has been proposed as an explanation for the etiology of preeclampsia, although supplementation with vitamin E has not been shown to prevent preeclampsia (Conde-Aqudelo, Romero, Kusanovic, & Hassan, 2011). Vegetable oils and nuts are especially good sources of vitamin E, and whole grains and green leafy vegetables are moderate sources.

Water-Soluble Vitamins

Body stores of water-soluble vitamins are much smaller than those of fat-soluble vitamins, and the water-soluble vitamins, in contrast to fat-soluble vitamins, are readily excreted in the urine. Therefore, good sources of these vitamins must be consumed frequently. Toxicity with overdose is less likely than it is when taking fat-soluble vitamins.

Folate and Folic Acid. Because of the increase in RBC production during pregnancy, as well as the nutritional requirements of the rapidly growing cells in the fetus and placenta, pregnant women should consume about 50% more folic acid than nonpregnant women, or about 0.6 mg (600 mcg) daily. In the United States, all enriched grain products (which include most white breads, flour, and pasta) must contain folic acid at a level of 1.4 mg/kg of flour. All women of childbearing potential need careful counseling about including good sources of folate in their diets (see Box 15-1).

Vitamin C. Vitamin C, or ascorbic acid, plays an important role in tissue formation and enhances iron absorption (Hark & Catalano, 2012). The recommended intake of vitamin C during pregnancy is 85 mg/day. The vitamin C needs of most women are readily met by a diet that includes at least one or two daily servings of citrus fruit or juice or another good source of the vitamin (see Table 15-1), but women who smoke need more.

Vitamin B_6. Pyridoxine, or vitamin B_6, is essential for carbohydrate, protein, and fat metabolism and is involved in the synthesis of red blood cells, antibodies, and neurotransmitters. Although the recommended intake during pregnancy is 1.9 mg/day, there is evidence that larger doses (10 to 25 mg) are effective for some women in reducing nausea and vomiting (Hark & Catalano, 2012).

Vitamin B_{12}. Vitamin B_{12} is involved in production of nucleic acids and proteins; it is especially important in formation of RBCs and in neural functioning. It is found naturally only in animal products (milk and dairy products, eggs, meats, liver, fish, and poultry). Commercial dried cereals, as well as some plant milks (almond, rice, or soy), and other vegan products are fortified with vitamin B_{12}. For women who do not include these sources of the vitamin in their diets, a daily or weekly supplement is essential. The recommended daily intake during pregnancy is 2.6 mcg/day (Otten et al., 2006).

Other Nutritional Issues During Pregnancy

Alcohol

Alcohol use is contraindicated throughout pregnancy. There is no safe amount or type of alcohol during pregnancy and there is no time during pregnancy when alcohol consumption is without risk. Because alcohol is a teratogen, it can cause birth defects, impaired cognitive and psychomotor development, and emotional and behavioral problems. Fetal alcohol syndrome can result from maternal alcohol consumption; this severe disorder involves growth restriction, central nervous system abnormalities, and facial dysmorphia (ACOG Committee on Health Care for Underserved Women, 2013) (see Chapter 31).

Women who have been consuming alcohol during pregnancy should be advised to stop immediately to prevent further risk to the fetus. On discovering they are pregnant, many women who have been consuming low levels of alcohol will be very concerned about potential effects on the fetus. Health care providers should inform them that having consumed low levels of alcohol during pregnancy is not an indication for terminating pregnancy (ACOG Committee on Health Care of Underserved Women, 2013).

Caffeine

The safety of caffeine use in pregnancy is not yet clear. Data suggest that excess caffeine intake can contribute to intrauterine growth restriction (IUGR) (Sengpiel, Elind, Bacelis, et al.,

TABLE 15-5 Caffeine* Content of Common Beverages and Foods

BEVERAGE OR FOOD	CAFFEINE (mg)
Coffee (8 oz [240 ml])	95
Espresso (1 oz [30 ml])	64
Tea, black, brewed (8 oz [240 ml])	47
Tea, ready-to-drink, with lemon (12 oz [360 ml])	7
Tea, green, brewed (8 oz [240 ml])	50
Tea, white, brewed (8 oz [240 ml])	35
Energy drink, 5-hour energy (2 oz [60 ml])	207
Energy drink, Rockstar (8 oz [240 ml])	79
Energy drink, Red Bull (8.4 oz [250 ml])	77
Energy drink, Vault (8 oz [250 ml])	47
Energy drink, AMP (8 oz [240 ml])	74
Cola beverage, regular (12 oz [360 ml])	29
Hot chocolate, homemade or from mix (8 oz [240 ml])	5
Dark chocolate bar (1 oz [30 g])	23
Candy bar, milk chocolate with almonds (1.5 oz [45 g])	7

*Maximum caffeine intake during pregnancy: 200 mg/day (ACOG Committee on Obstetric Practice, 2013).

Data from American College of Obstetricians and Gynecologists (ACOG) Committee on Obstetric Practice. (2013b). Committee opinion no. 462: *Moderate caffeine consumption during pregnancy.* Available at www.acog.org/Resources%20And%20Publications/Committee%20Opinions/Committee%20on%20Obstetric%20Practice/Moderate%20Caffeine%20Consumption%20During%20Pregnancy.aspx; Chin, J., Merves, M., Goldberger, B., et al. (2008). Caffeine content of brewed teas. *Journal of Analytical Toxicology 32*(8), 702-704; Reissig, C., Strain, E., & Griffiths, R. (2009). Caffeinated energy drink—A growing problem. *Drug and Alcohol Dependence, 99*(1-3), 1-10; U.S. Department of Agriculture, Agricultural Research Service: *USDA national nutrient database for standard reference, release 25,* 2012, Nutrient Data Laboratory home page. Available at www.ars.usda.gov/ba/bhnrc/ndl.

2013). In their review, Jahanfar and Jaafara (2013) found that there is insufficient evidence to determine whether caffeine has any effect on pregnancy outcome. Although the evidence about caffeine is far from conclusive, ACOG and the March of Dimes recommend a daily intake of no more than 200 mg of caffeine (ACOG Committee on Obstetric Practice, 2013; March of Dimes, 2012). Caffeine is found not only in coffee but also in tea, some soft drinks, and chocolate (Table 15-5).

Artificial Sweeteners

Aspartame (NutraSweet, Equal), acesulfame potassium (Sunett), and sucralose (Splenda)—artificial sweeteners commonly used in low- or no-calorie beverages and low-calorie food products—have not been found to have adverse effects on the normal mother or fetus and therefore are approved by the U.S. Food and Drug Administration (FDA) for use during pregnancy. Aspartame, which contains phenylalanine, should be avoided by pregnant women with PKU. Stevia (stevioside) is a sweetener sold as a dietary supplement; no acceptable daily intake has been established for stevia. Agave is another dietary supplement sweetener, but little is known about its safety or effects in pregnancy.

Pica and Food Cravings

Pica, which is the practice of consuming nonfood substances (e.g., clay, soil, and laundry starch) or excessive amounts of foodstuffs low in nutritional value (e.g., cornstarch, ice or freezer frost, baking powder, or baking soda), is often influenced by the woman's cultural background (Fig. 15-3). One

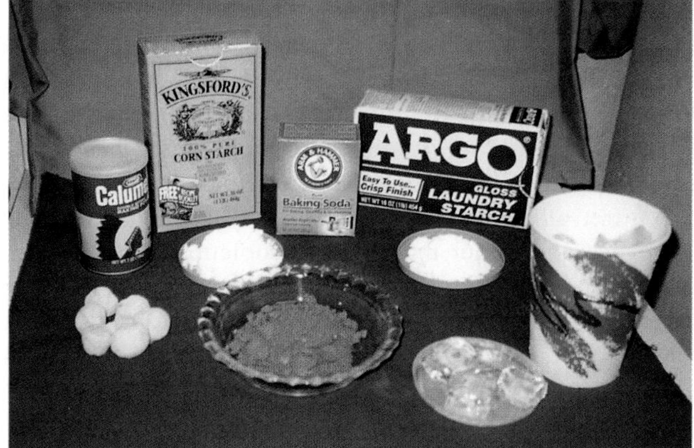

FIG 15-3 Nonfood substances consumed in pica: red clay from Georgia, Nzu from East Nigeria, baking powder, cornstarch, baking soda, laundry starch, and ice. Some individuals practice poly-pica, consuming more than one of these or other nonfood substances. (Courtesy Shannon Perry, Phoenix, AZ.)

problem with pica is that regular and heavy consumption of low-nutrient products can cause more nutritious foods to be displaced from the diet. As an example, cornstarch ingestion is popular among African-American women. It is a source of "empty" calories; half a cup (64 g) provides 240 kcal but almost no vitamins, minerals, or protein. Overuse of cornstarch can contribute to development of gestational diabetes. In addition, the pica items consumed can interfere with the absorption of nutrients, especially minerals. Women with pica have been found to have lower hemoglobin levels than those without pica.

Moreover, there is a risk that nonfood items are contaminated with heavy metals or other toxic substances. Among Mexican-American women, consumption of *tierra* includes both soil and pulverized Mexican pottery. Lead contamination of soils and soil-based products has caused high levels of lead in pregnant women and their newborns. Regular household use of Mexican pottery in cooking or serving food or ingestion of ground pottery must be included in interviews or questionnaires regarding nutrition intake of pregnant women. The possibility of pica must be considered when pregnant women are found to be anemic, and the nurse should provide counseling about the health risks associated with pica.

The practice of pica, as well as details of the types and amounts of products ingested, is likely to be discovered only by the sensitive interviewer who has developed a relationship of trust with the woman. It has been proposed that pica and food cravings (e.g., the urge to have ice cream, pickles, or pizza) during pregnancy are caused by an innate drive to consume nutrients missing from the diet. However, research has not supported this hypothesis.

Many women experience food cravings during pregnancy. In general, consuming foods to satisfy the cravings is not harmful. However, there is some concern that it can lead to dietary imbalances, especially if the cravings involve pica. The nurse can suggest choosing healthy alternatives for cravings, eating small amounts of the craved foods (buying single servings), eating regularly and including healthy snacks to avoid drops in blood glucose levels, and using distraction to curb the craving (take a walk or make a call to a friend).

Adolescent Pregnancy Needs

Many adolescent females have diets that provide less than the recommended intakes of key nutrients, including calcium and iron. Pregnant adolescents and their infants are at increased risk for complications during pregnancy and birth. Growth of the pelvis is delayed in comparison with growth in stature, and this helps explain why cephalopelvic disproportion and other mechanical problems associated with labor are common among young adolescents. Competition for nutrients between the growing adolescent and the fetus can also contribute to some of the poor outcomes apparent in teen pregnancies. Recommended weight gain goals do not differ from those of adult women. Pregnant adolescents are encouraged to choose a weight gain goal at the upper end of the range for their BMI. BMI is calculated as for adult women (IOM, 2009) rather than by using the adolescent BMI growth charts available from the Centers for Disease Control and Prevention (CDC).

Adolescent females who have given birth are more likely to be obese than those who have not (Chang, Choi, Richardson, & Davis, 2013); thus, the adolescent mother needs careful teaching regarding nutritional intake and physical activity to control body weight in the postpartum period.

Efforts to improve the nutritional health of pregnant adolescents focus on:

- Improving the nutrition knowledge, meal planning, and selection and food preparation skills of young women
- Promoting access to prenatal care
- Developing nutrition interventions and educational programs that are effective with adolescents
- Striving to understand the factors that create barriers to change in the adolescent population

Physical Activity During Pregnancy

Moderate exercise during pregnancy yields numerous benefits, including improving muscle tone, potentially shortening the course of labor, and promoting a sense of well-being. Almost all pregnant women, except the few with medical or obstetric problems that contraindicate physical activity, should engage in a minimum of 30 minutes of moderate physical exercise on most, if not all, days of the week (see Chapter 14). A liberal amount of fluid should be consumed before, during, and after exercise because dehydration can trigger preterm labor. Caloric intake may need to be adjusted according to physical activity.

CARE MANAGEMENT

During pregnancy, nutrition plays a key role in achieving an optimal outcome for the mother and her unborn baby. The motivation to learn about nutrition is usually greater during pregnancy because parents strive to "do what's right for the baby." Optimal nutrition cannot eliminate all problems that can arise during pregnancy, but it does establish a good foundation for supporting the needs of the mother and her developing fetus.

Assessment

Ideally a nutritional assessment is performed before conception so that any recommended changes in diet, lifestyle, and weight can be undertaken before the woman becomes pregnant. At the initial prenatal visit, information on nutrition and diet is obtained from an interview and review of the woman's health records, physical examination, and laboratory results.

Obstetric and Gynecologic Effects on Nutrition

Nutrition reserves can be depleted in the multiparous woman or one who has had frequent pregnancies (especially three pregnancies within 2 years). A history of preterm birth or the birth of an LBW or small for gestational age (SGA) infant can indicate inadequate dietary intake. Maternal diabetes mellitus can be associated with the birth of a large for gestational age (LGA) infant.

Contraceptive methods also can affect reproductive health. Increased menstrual blood loss often occurs during the first 3 to 6 months after placement of an intrauterine contraceptive device; consequently, the user can have low iron stores or even iron deficiency anemia. Oral contraceptive agents are associated with decreased menstrual losses and increased iron stores.

Health History

Chronic maternal illnesses such as diabetes mellitus, renal disease, liver disease, cystic fibrosis or other malabsorptive disorders, seizure disorders and the use of anticonvulsant agents, hypertension, and PKU can affect a woman's nutritional status and dietary needs. In women with illnesses that have resulted in nutrition deficits or that require dietary treatment (e.g., diabetes mellitus, PKU), it is extremely important for nutritional care to be started and for the condition to be optimally controlled before conception. A registered dietitian can provide in-depth counseling for the woman who requires medical nutrition therapy during pregnancy and lactation.

Usual Maternal Diet

The nurse interviews the pregnant woman to determine her usual food and beverage intake, any dietary modifications, food allergies and intolerances, medications and nutrition supplements being taken, cultural practices related to nutrition such as pica, and the adequacy of her income and other resources to meet her nutrition needs. In addition, the nurse inquires about the presence and severity of nutrition-related discomforts of pregnancy such as nausea and vomiting, constipation, and pyrosis (heartburn). The nurse should be alert to any evidence of eating disorders such as anorexia nervosa, bulimia, or frequent and rigorous dieting before or during pregnancy. Box 15-5 provides a simple tool for obtaining diet history information. When potential problems are identified, further assessment is needed. The health care provider is notified and a nutritional consultation may be needed.

The effect of food allergies and intolerances on nutritional status varies. Lactose intolerance is of special concern in pregnant and lactating women because no other food group equals milk and milk products in terms of calcium content. If a woman has lactose intolerance, the interviewer should explore her intake of other calcium sources (see Box 15-4).

The assessment must include an evaluation of the woman's financial status and her knowledge of sound dietary practices. The quality of the diet improves with increasing

BOX 15-5 Food Intake Questionnaire

Which of the following did you eat or drink yesterday? If the way you ate yesterday wasn't the way you usually eat, choose a recent day that was typical for you.

FOOD OR DRINK	NUMBER OF SERVINGS
Beer, wine, other alcoholic drinks	______
Tea	______
Coffee	______
Caffeinated	______
Decaffeinated	______
Fruit drink (not 100% juice)	______
Water	______
Soft drinks	______
Milk	______
Cheese	______
Macaroni and cheese	______
Other foods with cheese (e.g., lasagna, enchiladas, cheeseburgers)	______
Pizza	______
Yogurt	______
Orange or grapefruit	______
Bananas	______
Peaches or apricots	______
Orange or grapefruit juice	______
Fruit juice other than orange or grapefruit	______
Melon (e.g., watermelon, cantaloupe, honeydew)	______
Berries (type)	______
Apples	______
Other fruit	______
Broccoli	______
Kale or other leafy greens	______
Lettuce or salad	______
Corn	______
Potatoes (other than fried)	______
Other vegetables	______
Chicken, turkey, beef, or pork	______
Egg	______
Nuts	______
Hot dog	______
Cold cuts (e.g., bologna)	______
Roll/bagel	______
Noodles	______
Chips	______
Cake	______
Donut or pastry	______
Cookie	______
Pie	______

Are you often bothered by any of the following? (Circle all that apply)

Nausea Vomiting Heartburn Constipation

Are you on a special diet? No ______ Yes ______ If yes, what kind?__________

Do you try to limit the amount or kind of food you eat to control your weight? No_____ Yes________

Do you avoid any foods for health or religious reasons? No ______ Yes ______ If yes, which foods?______________

Do you take any prescribed drugs or medications? No ______ Yes ______ If yes, what are they?______________

Do you take any over-the-counter medications (e.g., aspirin, cold medicines, acetaminophen [Tylenol])? No ______ Yes ______
If yes, what are they? ____________________

Do you take any herbal supplements? No ______ Yes ______ If yes, what are they? ______________

Do you ever have trouble affording the food you need? No ______ Yes ______

Do you have any help getting the food you need? No ______ Yes ______ If yes, what kind? Food Stamps/SNAP ____ WIC ____
School Lunch or Breakfast ____ Food from a Food Pantry, Soup Kitchen, or Food Bank ____ Other ____________

socioeconomic status and educational level. Poor women may not have access to adequate refrigeration and cooking facilities and may find it difficult to obtain adequate nutritious food.

Physical Examination

Anthropometric (body) measurements provide short- and long-term information on a woman's nutritional status and are thus essential to the assessment. At a minimum, the woman's height and weight are determined at her initial prenatal visit, and her weight is measured at each subsequent visit (see earlier discussion of BMI).

A careful physical examination can reveal objective signs of malnutrition (Table 15-6). It is important to note, however, that some of these signs are nonspecific and that the physiologic changes of pregnancy can complicate the interpretation of physical findings. For example, lower extremity edema often occurs when calorie and protein deficiencies are present but it can also be a normal finding in the third trimester of pregnancy. The interpretation of physical findings is made easier by a thorough health history and by laboratory testing when indicated.

TABLE 15-6 Physical Assessment of Nutritional Status

SIGNS OF GOOD NUTRITION	SIGNS OF POOR NUTRITION
General Appearance	
Alert, responsive, energetic, good endurance	Listless, apathetic, cachectic, easily fatigued, looks tired
Muscles	
Well developed, firm, good tone, some fat under skin	Flaccid, poor tone, tender, "wasted" appearance
Gastrointestinal Function	
Good appetite and digestion, normal regular elimination, no palpable organs or masses	Anorexia, indigestion, constipation or diarrhea, liver or spleen enlargement
Cardiovascular Function	
Normal heart rate and rhythm, no murmurs, normal blood pressure for age	Rapid heart rate, enlarged heart, abnormal rhythm, elevated blood pressure
Hair	
Shiny, lustrous, firm, not easily plucked, healthy scalp	Stringy, dull, brittle, dry, thin and sparse, depigmented, can be easily plucked
Skin (General)	
Smooth, slightly moist, good color	Rough, dry, scaly, pale, pigmented, irritated, easily bruised, petechiae
Face and Neck	
Skin color uniform, smooth, pink, healthy appearance; no enlargement of thyroid gland; lips not chapped or swollen	Scaly, swollen, skin dark over cheeks and under eyes, lumpiness or flakiness of skin around nose and mouth; thyroid enlarged; lips swollen, angular lesions or fissures at corners of mouth
Oral Cavity	
Reddish pink mucous membranes and gums; no swelling or bleeding of gums; tongue healthy pink or deep red in appearance, not swollen or smooth, surface papillae present; teeth bright and clean, no cavities, no pain, no discoloration	Gums spongy, bleed easily, inflamed or receding; tongue swollen, scarlet and raw, magenta color, beefy, hyperemic and hypertrophic papillae, atrophic papillae; teeth with unfilled caries, absent teeth, worn surfaces, mottled
Eyes	
Bright, clear, shiny, no sores at corners of eyelids, membranes moist and healthy pink color, no prominent blood vessels or mound of tissue (Bitot spots) on sclera, no fatigue circles beneath	Eye membranes pale, redness of membrane, dryness, signs of infection, redness and fissuring of eyelid corners, dryness of eye membrane, dull appearance of cornea, blue sclerae
Extremities	
No tenderness, weakness, or swelling; nails firm and pink	Edema, tender calves, tingling, weakness; nails spoon-shaped, brittle
Skeleton	
No malformations	Bowlegs, knock-knees, chest deformity at diaphragm, beaded ribs, prominent scapulae

Laboratory Testing

The only nutrition-related laboratory testing needed by most pregnant women is a hematocrit or hemoglobin measurement to screen for anemia. Because of the physiologic anemia of pregnancy, the reference values for hemoglobin and hematocrit must be adjusted during pregnancy. The lower limit of the normal range for hemoglobin during pregnancy is 11 g/dl in the first and third trimesters and 10.5 g/dl in the second trimester (compared with 12 g/dl in the nonpregnant state). The lower limit of the normal range for hematocrit is 33% during the first and third trimesters and 32% in the second trimester (compared with 36% in the nonpregnant state) (CDC, 2011). Diagnostic values for anemia are higher in women who smoke or live at high altitudes because the decreased oxygen carrying capacity of their RBCs causes them to produce more RBCs than other women produce.

A woman's history or physical findings can indicate the need for additional testing. These tests might include a complete blood cell count with a differential to identify megaloblastic or macrocytic anemia and measurement of levels of specific vitamins or minerals believed to be lacking in the diet.

Nutritional Care and Teaching

For many women with uncomplicated pregnancies, the nurse serves as the primary source of nutrition education. The registered dietitian, who has specialized training in diet evaluation and planning, nutritional needs during illness, ethnic and cultural food patterns, as well as translating nutrient needs into food patterns, frequently serves as a consultant. Pregnant women with serious nutritional problems, those with intervening illnesses such as diabetes (either preexisting or gestational), and any others requiring in-depth dietary counseling should be referred to the dietitian. The nurse, dietitian, physician, and certified nurse-midwife collaborate in helping the woman achieve nutrition-related expected outcomes. Nutritional care and teaching generally involve:

- Educating the woman about nutritional needs during pregnancy and the components of an adequate diet, if necessary
- Helping her individualize her diet so that she achieves an adequate intake while conforming to her personal, cultural, financial, and health circumstances

- Discussing with her strategies for coping with the nutrition-related discomforts of pregnancy
- Helping her use nutrition supplements appropriately
- Consulting with and making referrals to other professionals or services as indicated

For women with limited financial resources, two programs in the United States provide nutrition services: the Supplemental Nutrition Assistance Program (SNAP or food stamps) and the Special Supplemental Nutrition Program for Women, Infants and Children (WIC), which provides vouchers for selected foods for pregnant and lactating women as well as for infants and children at nutritional risk. WIC foods include items such as eggs, milk (or cheese, soy milk, or tofu), juice, fortified cereals, legumes, and peanut butter. WIC participants receive nutrition counseling, and the program encourages breastfeeding.

Nutrition counseling can take place in a one-on-one interview or in a group setting. In either case, teaching should emphasize the importance of choosing a varied diet composed of readily available foods (rather than specialized diet supplements) (see the Nursing Care Plan). Good nutrition practices (and avoidance of poor practices such as smoking and alcohol or drug use) are essential content for prenatal classes designed for women in early pregnancy.

Daily Food Guide and Menu Planning. MyPlate (www.choosemyplate.gov) can be used as a guide to making daily food choices during pregnancy and lactation, just as it is during other stages of the life cycle. A woman can create a profile, and the MyPlate program will generate an individualized daily food plan. Additional individualized information and resources for professionals are available from the website. The importance of consuming adequate amounts from the milk, yogurt, and cheese group should be emphasized, especially for adolescents

NURSING CARE PLAN

Nutrition During Pregnancy

NURSING DIAGNOSIS	EXPECTED OUTCOME	NURSING INTERVENTIONS	RATIONALES
Deficient Knowledge related to nutritional requirements during pregnancy	Woman will describe nutritional requirements and exhibit evidence of incorporating requirements into her diet.	Review basic nutritional requirements for healthy diet by using recommended dietary guidelines and MyPlate.	To provide knowledge baseline for discussion
		Discuss increased nutrient needs (calories, protein, minerals, vitamins) that occur as the result of being pregnant.	To increase knowledge needed for altered dietary requirements
		Discuss relation between weight gain and fetal growth.	To reinforce interdependence of fetus and mother
		Calculate appropriate total weight gain range during pregnancy using woman's body mass index as a guide, and discuss recommended rates of weight gain during various trimesters of pregnancy.	To provide concrete measures of dietary success
		Review food preferences, cultural eating patterns or beliefs, and prepregnancy eating patterns.	To enhance integration of new dietary needs
		Discuss how to fit nutritional needs into usual dietary patterns and how to alter any identified nutritional deficits or excesses.	To increase chances of success with dietary alterations
		Discuss food aversions or cravings that can occur during pregnancy and strategies to deal with these if they are detrimental to the fetus (e.g., pica).	To ensure well-being of fetus
		Have woman keep a food diary delineating eating habits, dietary alterations, aversions, and cravings.	To track eating habits and potential problem areas

Continued

NURSING CARE PLAN—cont'd

Nutrition During Pregnancy

NURSING DIAGNOSIS	EXPECTED OUTCOME	NURSING INTERVENTIONS	RATIONALES
Imbalanced Nutrition: Less Than Body Requirements related to inadequate intake of needed nutrients	Woman's weekly weight gain will be increased to appropriate rate using her body mass index (BMI) and recommended weight gain ranges as guidelines.	Review recent diet history (including food aversions) using food diary, 24-hour recall, or food frequency approach.	To ascertain dietary inadequacies contributing to insufficient weight gain
		Review normal activity and exercise routines and discuss eating patterns and reasons that lead to decreased food intake (e.g., morning sickness, pica, fear of becoming fat, stress, boredom).	To determine level of energy expenditure and to identify habits that contribute to inadequate weight gain
		Review optimal weight gain guidelines and their rationale.	To ensure that woman is knowledgeable about healthful weight gain rates
		Set target weight gains for remaining weeks of pregnancy.	To establish set goals
		Review increased nutrient needs (calories, protein, minerals, vitamins) that occur as the result of being pregnant.	To ensure woman is knowledgeable about altered dietary requirements
		Review relation between weight gain and fetal growth.	To reinforce that adequate weight gain is needed to promote fetal well-being
		Discuss with woman what changes can be made in diet, activity, and lifestyle.	To enhance chances of meeting set weight gain goals and nutrient needs of mother and fetus
		If woman has fear of being fat, if symptoms of eating disorder are evident, or if problems in adjusting to changing body image surface, refer her to appropriate mental health professional for evaluation.	Because intensive treatment and follow-up may be required to ensure fetal health
Nausea related to physiologic alterations of first trimester of pregnancy	Nausea will not be so severe that it interferes with adequate nutrient intake or substantially reduces quality of life.	Assess state of hydration and assess pattern of weight gain during pregnancy.	To ensure that woman does not have deficient fluid volume; to ensure that nausea is not preventing adequate energy intake
		Review nausea history (i.e., frequency of episodes of nausea, likelihood of nausea progressing to vomiting, factors precipitating or associated with nausea, and any relief measures that woman has tried).	To determine severity of problem and to begin to identify effective and ineffective measures for coping with nausea
		Review measures for prevention or relief of nausea and vomiting (morning sickness).	To ensure that woman is knowledgeable about measures that are often effective in alleviating morning sickness
		Discuss with woman what relief measures she will try.	To determine whether she understands how to implement measures

and women younger than 25 years, who are still actively adding calcium to their skeletons; adolescents need at least three or four servings from the milk group daily.

The daily food plan in Table 15-4 is consistent with MyPlate and can be used for educating women about nutritional needs during pregnancy and lactation. This food plan is general enough to be used by women from a wide variety of cultures, including those who follow a vegetarian diet. The nurse or dietician can help the woman plan daily menus that follow the food plan and are affordable, have realistic preparation times, and are compatible with personal preferences and cultural practices. Women who follow a healthy eating pattern before and during pregnancy reduce their risk of developing complications such as gestational diabetes (Asemi, Tabassi, Samimi, et al., 2013; Tobias, Zhang, Chavarro, et al., 2012). A healthy pattern emphasizes intake of whole grains; fruits and vegetables; low-fat dairy products; nuts, seeds, and legumes; and lean meats, poultry, and fish while limiting intake of solid fats, fatty or processed meats, and sweets.

Food Safety. Food-borne illnesses can cause adverse maternal and fetal effects. The woman's understanding of safe food-handling practices should be assessed. The nurse can provide simple instructions that are essential to preventing food-borne illnesses. According to the FDA (2013d), there are four simple steps:

- Clean: Cleanse hands, food preparation surfaces, and utensils frequently.
- Separate: Avoid contact between raw meat, fish, or poultry and other foods that will not be cooked before consumption.
- Cook: Cook foods to a proper temperature.
- Chill: Store foods properly and refrigerate promptly.

Pregnant women have altered immune function that places them at increased risk for developing food-borne illnesses such as listeriosis and toxoplasmosis that can cause maternal illness, miscarriage, and severe fetal effects such as cognitive impairment, hearing loss, blindness, or death. To prevent listeriosis, foods that should be avoided altogether during pregnancy include soft cheeses made from unpasteurized milk, including Brie, feta, Camembert, Roquefort, queso blanco, and queso fresco; raw cookie dough and cake batter; sushi, raw oysters, and other raw or undercooked fish and seafood; unpasteurized juice and cider, including fresh squeezed; unpasteurized milk; raw or undercooked sprouts; and ham, chicken, or seafood salads and similar products that are made in a store. Even if they are labeled as ready to serve, these foods should be thoroughly cooked if they are to be consumed during pregnancy: hot dogs, luncheon meats, cold cuts, fermented or dry sausage, and other deli-style meat and poultry; eggs; fresh meat, poultry, and fish; poultry stuffing (preferably bake in a separate dish, rather than inside the bird); and refrigerated smoked seafood, meat paste, or pâté (canned versions can be consumed). To prevent infection from *Salmonella* and *Campylobacter*, pregnant women should not consume raw eggs, raw milk, and raw or undercooked meats; commercial products with pasteurized eggs and milk may be used. Women can develop toxoplasmosis from eating raw or undercooked meat or from using utensils or cutting boards that were in contact with raw meat; toxoplasmosis can result from contact with contaminated cat feces or garden soil (FDA, 2013a, b, and c; Hark & Catalano, 2012).

Medical Nutrition Therapy. During pregnancy and lactation the food plan for women with special medical nutrition therapy may have to be modified. The registered dietitian can instruct these women about their diets and assist them in meal planning. However, the nurse should understand the basic principles of the diet and be able to reinforce the teaching.

The nurse should be especially aware of the dietary modifications necessary for women with diabetes mellitus (either gestational or preexisting). This disease is relatively common, and fetal morbidity and mortality occur more often in pregnancies complicated by hyperglycemia or hypoglycemia (see discussion of diabetes in Chapter 29). Every effort should be made to maintain blood glucose levels in the normal range throughout pregnancy. The food plan of the woman with diabetes usually includes four to six meals and snacks daily, with the daily carbohydrate intake distributed fairly evenly among the meals and snacks. The complex carbohydrates—fibers and starches—should be well represented in the diet. To maintain strict control of the blood glucose level, the pregnant woman with diabetes usually must monitor her own blood glucose daily.

Nutrition-Related Concerns During Pregnancy. It is important for the pregnant woman to understand the need for adequate weight gain during pregnancy and to be able to evaluate her own gain in terms of the desirable pattern. Many women, particularly those who have worked hard to control their weight before pregnancy, find it difficult to understand why the weight gain goal is so high when a newborn infant is so small. The nurse can explain that maternal weight gain consists of increases in the weight of many tissues, not just the growing fetus (see Table 15-3).

Dietary overindulgence, which can result in excessive fat stores that persist after giving birth, should be discouraged. Nevertheless, it is best not to focus solely on weight gain

TEACHING FOR SELF-MANAGEMENT

Iron Supplementation

- A diet rich in vitamin C (in citrus fruits, tomatoes, melons, and strawberries) and heme iron (in meats) increases the absorption of iron supplements; therefore, include these in the diet often.
- Bran, tea, coffee, milk, oxalates (in spinach and Swiss chard), and egg yolk decrease iron absorption. Avoid consuming them at the same time as the iron supplement.
- Iron is absorbed best if it is taken when the stomach is empty, so it is best to take it between meals with a beverage other than tea, coffee, or milk.
- Iron may be taken at bedtime if abdominal discomfort occurs when it is taken between meals.
- If an iron dose is missed, take it as soon as it is remembered if that is within 12 hours of the scheduled dose. Do not double up on the dose.
- Keep the supplement in a childproof container and out of the reach of any children in the household.
- The iron can cause stools to be black or dark green. This is normal.
- Constipation is common with iron supplementation. A diet high in fiber with adequate fluid intake (about 8 to 10 glasses [2 L] of fluids daily) will help to avoid constipation.

because this can result in feelings of stress and guilt in the woman who does not follow the preferred pattern of gain; instead, the nurse emphasizes a healthy diet plan. Teaching regarding weight gain during pregnancy is summarized in Table 15-2.

Iron Supplementation. The nutrition supplement most commonly needed during pregnancy is iron. However, a variety of dietary factors can affect the completeness of absorption of an iron supplement, and some women experience discomfort when taking the supplement. The Teaching for Self-Management box: Iron Supplementation summarizes important points regarding iron supplementation.

Nutrition-Related Discomforts of Pregnancy

Nausea and Vomiting. Nausea and vomiting of pregnancy (NVP) is most common during the first trimester. Usually NVP causes only mild to moderate problems nutritionally, although it can be a source of substantial discomfort. The pregnant woman may find the suggestions in Box 15-6 helpful in alleviating NVP. Antiemetic medications, vitamin B_6, ginger, and P6 acupressure may be effective in reducing the severity of nausea.

SAFETY ALERT

Ginger has anticoagulant properties and should be avoided by women receiving anticoagulant therapy or other drugs or herbal agents that can prolong clotting time (Tiran, 2012).

Hyperemesis gravidarum, or severe and persistent vomiting causing weight loss, dehydration, and electrolyte abnormalities, occurs in up to 1% of pregnant women (see Chapter 29). Intravenous fluid and electrolyte replacement, enteral tube feeding, and in some instances total parenteral nutrition have been used to nourish women with hyperemesis gravidarum. There is very limited evidence that acupressure and ginger might provide some relief.

Constipation. Improved bowel function generally results from increasing the intake of fiber (e.g., whole grains, fresh fruit, and raw or lightly steamed vegetables). Fiber helps create a bulky stool that stimulates intestinal peristalsis. The recommendation for pregnant women for fiber is 28 g daily. An adequate fluid intake (at least 50 ml/kg/day) helps hydrate the fiber and increase the bulk of the stool. Making a habit of regular physical activity that uses large muscle groups (walking, swimming, water aerobics) also helps stimulate bowel motility. Pregnant women may take psyllium fiber supplements (Hark & Catalano, 2012).

Heartburn. Heartburn, or *pyrosis*, is usually caused by reflux of gastric contents into the esophagus. This condition can be minimized by eating small, frequent meals rather than two or three larger meals daily. Fluids increase the distention of the stomach, so it can help if they are not consumed with foods. The woman needs to drink adequate amounts between meals. Avoiding spicy foods can possibly help alleviate the problem. Reflux can be exacerbated by lying down immediately after eating and wearing clothing that is tight across the abdomen. Walking after eating can aid in reducing heartburn. Use of antacids may be recommended by the health care provider.

Vegetarian Diets. Foods basic to almost all vegetarian diets are vegetables, fruits, legumes, nuts, seeds, and grains, but with many variations. *Lacto-vegetarians* include milk products. Lacto-ovovegetarians consume eggs and dairy products in addition to plant products. Strict vegetarians, or *vegans,* consume only plant products. All of these types of vegetarian diets, if well planned, can be nutritionally adequate for pregnant and lactating women Pregnant women who adhere to vegan diets need to be attentive to their intake of protein, iron, calcium, and vitamin B_{12}.

Plant proteins tend to be "incomplete," in that they lack one or more amino acids required for growth and the maintenance of body tissues. However, consuming a variety of different plant proteins—grains, dried beans and peas, nuts, and seeds—on a daily basis can provide all of the essential amino acids. Because vitamin B_{12} is found naturally only in foods of animal origin, the vegan diet is deficient in vitamin B_{12}. As a result, strict vegetarians should take a supplement or regularly consume vitamin B_{12}–fortified foods such as fortified plant milks two or three times a day. Vitamin B_{12} deficiency can result in megaloblastic anemia, glossitis (inflamed red tongue), and neurologic deficits in the mother. Infants born to affected mothers are likely to have megaloblastic anemia and exhibit neurodevelopmental delays. The diet should be carefully planned to include adequate

BOX 15-6 Suggestions for Managing Nausea and Vomiting During Pregnancy

- Eat dry, starchy foods such as dry toast, melba toast, or crackers on awakening in the morning and at other times when nausea occurs.
- Avoid consuming excessive amounts of fluids early in the day or when nauseated (but compensate by drinking fluids at other times).
- Eat small amounts frequently (every 2 to 3 hours), and avoid large meals that distend the stomach.
- Avoid skipping meals and thus becoming extremely hungry, which can worsen nausea. Have a snack such as cereal with milk, a small sandwich, or yogurt before bedtime.
- Avoid sudden movements. Get out of bed slowly.
- Decrease intake of fried and other fatty foods. Try high-carbohydrate foods such as toast, rice, or potatoes. Some women find high-protein meals or snacks helpful.
- Breathe fresh air to help relieve nausea. Keep the environment well ventilated (e.g., open a window), go for a walk outside, or decrease cooking odors by using an exhaust fan.
- Eat foods served at cool temperatures and foods that give off little aroma. Avoid spicy foods.
- Avoid brushing your teeth immediately after eating.
- Try salty and tart foods (e.g., potato chips or lemonade) during periods of nausea. Sucking a lemon slice may help.
- Try herbal teas such as those made with raspberry leaf or peppermint to decrease nausea.
- Try ginger (ginger-ale soda, ginger tea, ginger snaps, ginger jam on toast).
- Try sucking on flavored lollipops (e.g., Preggie Pops®).
- Wear acupressure bands (seabands) used for motion sickness around the wrist.
- If nausea and vomiting are severe and/or if weight loss occurs, notify your health care provider. Some providers recommend a combination of vitamin B_6 and doxylamine. For more severe problems, other medications may be prescribed. Do not take any medication without consulting your health care provider.

minerals. Iron and zinc may not be as well absorbed from plant foods as they are from meats, and calcium intake can be low if milk products are avoided.

Cultural Influences. Consideration of a woman's cultural food preferences enhances communication and provides a greater opportunity for following the agreed-on pattern of intake. The nurse needs to be aware of what constitutes a typical diet for each cultural or ethnic group present in his or her client population, although variations can occur within a group. Thus a careful exploration of individual preferences is needed. Although ethnic and cultural food beliefs can seem at first glance to conflict with the dietary instruction provided by physicians, nurses, and dietitians, it is often possible for the empathic health care provider to identify cultural beliefs that are congruent with the modern understanding of pregnancy and fetal development. Many cultural food practices have some merit or the culture would not have survived. Food cravings during pregnancy are considered normal by many cultures, but the kinds of cravings often are culturally specific. Cultural influences on food intake usually lessen if the woman and her family become more integrated into the dominant culture. Nutritional beliefs and the practices of selected cultural groups are summarized in Table 15-7.

Postpartum Nutrition. A nutritionally sound, balanced diet is important in the postpartum period as the woman's body is recovering from birth and going through the normal physiologic changes of the postpartum period (see Chapter 20).

An important goal of postpartum nutrition is for the woman to lose the weight gained during pregnancy and attain a healthy weight. Retaining the weight gained during pregnancy can contribute to overweight and obesity and the development of later health problems including metabolic syndrome, cardiovascular disease, and diabetes. Obese women and normal-weight women who gain more than the recommended amount of weight during pregnancy are less likely to breastfeed than normal-weight women with appropriate weight gain. Obesity is associated with lower breastfeeding initiation rates, decreased duration of breastfeeding, lower milk supply, and delayed onset of lactogenesis II ("milk coming in") (Turcksin, Bel, Galjaard, & Devlieger, 2012).

The woman who does not breastfeed can lose weight gradually if she consumes a balanced diet that provides slightly less

TABLE 15-7 Popular Foods of Various Cultural and Ethnic Groups and Their Place in MyPlate

CULTURAL OR ETHNIC GROUP OR EATING PATTERN	FOOD GROUPS				
	GRAIN	VEGETABLE	FRUIT	DAIRY	PROTEIN
Mexican	Tortilla Taco shell Posole (corn soup) Rice Postres (pastries)*	Red: Tomato Starchy: Corn Other: Avocado Chayote (Mexican squash) Jicama (root vegetable) Nopales (cactus leaves)	Mango Papaya Plantano (cooking banana) Zapote (sweet, yellowish fruit)	Queso blanco (white Mexican cheese) Custard (1 cup = 1 cup milk serving) Leche (milk)	Chorizo (sausage)* Chicken, beef, goat, or pork Beans, dried, cooked
African-American soul food (Southern-style cooking)	Biscuit Cornbread Grits, rice, macaroni, or noodles Hominy Crackers Hushpuppies	Dark green: Collard, kale, mustard, or turnip greens Orange: Sweet potatoes Other: Okra Snap, pole (green), lima, and butter beans Turnips Summer squash (yellow or zucchini) Coleslaw	Blackberries Melons Muscadines (grapes) Peaches	Buttermilk	Pork (cured ham and uncured cuts), chicken, beef, fish Peas or beans (black-eyed, crowder, purple-hull, or cream)
Vegetarian	Whole-grain bread Cereal, cooked or ready-to-eat Brown rice Whole-grain pasta Bagel	All	All	Milk and cheese (lacto-vegetarians) Soy or almond milk, calcium fortified Soy cheese	Cooked dried beans or peas Tofu (soybean curd) or tempeh (fermented soy) Nuts or seeds Peanut butter Egg (ovovegetarians)
Italian	Breadsticks, breads Gnocchi (dumplings) Polenta (cornmeal mush) Risotto (creamy rice dish) Pastas	Dark green: Spinach Other: Artichoke Eggplant Mushrooms Marinara sauce	Berries Figs Pomegranates	Cheeses (e.g., mozzarella, Parmesan, Romano, ricotta) Gelato (Italian ice cream)	Veal or beef Fish Sausage* Luncheon meats* Lentils Squid Almonds, pistachios

Continued

TABLE 15-7 Popular Foods of Various Cultural and Ethnic Groups and Their Place in MyPlate—cont'd

CULTURAL OR ETHNIC GROUP OR EATING PATTERN	FOOD GROUPS				
	GRAIN	VEGETABLE	FRUIT	DAIRY	PROTEIN
Chinese	Rice or millet Rice vermicelli (thin rice pasta) Cellophane noodles (bean thread) Steamed rolls Rice congee (soup) Rice sticks	Other: Pea pods Yard-long beans Baby corn Bamboo shoots Straw mushrooms Eggplant Bitter melon	Guava Lychee Persimmon Pummelo Kumquat Star fruit	Soy milk	Pork, fish, chicken Shrimp, crab, lobster Tofu or tempeh
Indian (south Asia)	Breads: roti (chapati), naan, paratha, batura, puris, dosa, idli Rice or rice pilau Pooha, upma, sabudana	Dark green: Saag (mixed greens and potatoes) Spinach Other: Green peppers Cabbage Eggplant Green beans Methi (fenugreek leaves) Cucumbers Chutney or vegetable pickles	Mangos Dates Raisins Melons Figs Fruit juices and nectars	Yogurt	Dal (lentils, mung beans, other dried beans) Beef, chicken (many Indians are vegetarian)
Native American†	Bread Fry bread (Navajo) Wild rice or oats Popcorn Tortilla Mush (cooked cereal)	Orange: Winter squash (hard outer shell) Starchy: Potato Corn Other: Rhubarb	Berries Cherries Plums Apples Peaches		Wild game (deer, rabbit, elk, beaver) Lamb Salmon and other fish Clams, mussels Crab Duck or quail
Middle Eastern	Rice or bulgur (cracked wheat) Couscous Bread Pita	Orange and red: Pumpkin or winter squash (butternut) Tomatoes Other: Peppers Grape leaves Cucumbers Fava beans Eggplant	Apricots Grapes Melons Dried fruits: dates, raisins, apricots	Yogurt	Lamb, goat, fish Almonds Pistachio nuts Dried beans and peas, lentils Eggs

*High fat, use sparingly.
†Varies widely depending on tribal grouping and locale.

than her daily energy expenditure, although overweight and obese women with excessive weight gain during pregnancy have an increased likelihood of failing to return to their prepregnancy weights (ACOG Committee on Obstetric Practice, 2013). Women should have realistic expectations for weight loss after pregnancy. For some it can take months or years to return to their prepregnancy weight. Postpartum complications such as thyroiditis can interfere with weight loss. A reasonable weight loss goal for nonlactating women is 0.5 to 0.9 kg (1.1 to 2 lb) per week; a loss of 1 kg (2.2 lb) per month is recommended for most lactating women. Those at risk for obesity and overweight need follow-up to ensure that they know how to make wise food choices, primarily from fruits, vegetables, whole grains, lean meats, and low-fat dairy products. An hour of moderately vigorous physical activity (e.g., walking, jogging, swimming, cycling, aerobic dance) most days of the week will improve the woman's ability to lose weight gradually and maintain the weight loss.

Nutrient Needs During Lactation. Nutritional needs during lactation are similar in many ways to those during pregnancy. Needs for energy (calories), protein, calcium, iodine, zinc, the B vitamins (thiamine, riboflavin, niacin, pyridoxine, and vitamin B_{12}), and vitamin C remain greater than nonpregnant needs. The recommendations for some of these (e.g., vitamin C, zinc, and protein) are slightly to moderately higher than during pregnancy (see Table 15-1). This allowance covers the amount of the nutrients released in the milk, as well as the needs of the mother for tissue maintenance. In the case of iron and folic acid, the recommendation during lactation is lower than that during pregnancy. Both of these nutrients are essential for RBC formation and thus for maintaining the increase in the blood volume that occurs during pregnancy. With the decrease in maternal blood volume to nonpregnant levels after birth, maternal iron and folic acid needs also decrease. Many lactating women have a delay in the return of menses, which also conserves blood cells and reduces iron and folic acid needs. It is especially important that the calcium intake is adequate; if it is not, a supplement of 600 mg of calcium per day may be needed.

According to the IOM, the recommended energy intake for the first 6 months is an increase of 330 kcal more than the woman's nonpregnant intake; this means an average daily intake of approximately 2700 calories (Panel on Dietary Reference Intakes for Macronutrients, IOM, 2005). The AAP recommends that breastfeeding women who are well nourished should add 450 to 500 kcal/day to a balanced diet (AAP Section on Breastfeeding, 2012). Because of the deposition of energy stores, the woman who has gained the optimal amount of weight during pregnancy is heavier after birth than at the beginning of pregnancy. As a result of the caloric demands of lactation, the lactating mother usually experiences a gradual but steady weight loss. Most women rapidly lose several kilograms during the first month after birth, whether or not they breastfeed. After the first month, the average loss during lactation is 0.5 to 1 kg (1.1 to 2.2 lb) a month, and a woman who is overweight may be able to lose up to 2 kg without decreasing her milk supply.

Fluid intake must be adequate to maintain milk production, but the mother's level of thirst is the best guide to the right amount. There is no need to consume more fluids than those needed to satisfy thirst (Scott, 2013).

Smoking, alcohol intake, and excessive caffeine intake should be avoided during lactation. Smoking not only can impair milk production but also exposes the infant to the risk of passive smoking. It is speculated that the infant's psychomotor development may be affected by maternal alcohol use, and alcohol use may impair the milk-ejection reflex. Caffeine intake can lead to a reduced iron concentration in milk and consequently contribute to the development of anemia in the infant. The caffeine concentration in milk is only approximately 1% of the mother's plasma level, but caffeine levels build up in the infant. Breastfed infants of mothers who drink large amounts of coffee or caffeine-containing soft drinks can be unusually active and wakeful (Scott, 2013).

KEY POINTS

- A woman's nutritional status before, during, and after pregnancy contributes, to a significant degree, to her well-being and that of her developing fetus and newborn.
- Many physiologic changes occurring during pregnancy influence the need for additional nutrients and the efficiency with which the body uses them.
- Both the total maternal weight gain and the pattern of weight gain are important determinants of the outcome of pregnancy.
- The appropriateness of the woman's prepregnancy weight for height (BMI) is a major determinant of her recommended weight gain during pregnancy.
- Nutritional risk factors include adolescent pregnancy; abuse of nicotine, alcohol, or drugs; bizarre or faddish food habits; a low or high weight for height; and frequent pregnancies.
- Iron supplementation is usually routinely recommended during pregnancy. Other supplements may be warranted when nutritional risk factors are present.
- Food safety is important for pregnant women to prevent adverse maternal and fetal effects.
- Women who are pregnant should consume seafood that is low in methylmercury.
- The nurse and the woman are influenced by cultural and personal values and beliefs during nutrition counseling.
- Pregnancy complications that can be nutrition-related include anemia, gestational hypertension, gestational diabetes, and IUGR.
- Dietary modifications can be effective interventions for some of the common discomforts of pregnancy, including nausea and vomiting, constipation, and heartburn.

REFERENCES

American Academy of Section on Breastfeeding. (2012). Breastfeeding and the use of human milk. *Pediatrics, 129*(3), e827–e841.

American Academy of Pediatrics (AAP), & American College of Obstetricians and Gynecologists (ACOG). (2012). *Guidelines for perinatal care* (7th ed.). Elk Grove Village, IL & Washington, DC. Author.

American College of Obstetricians and Gynecologists. (2013). (ACOG) Committee on Health Care for Underserved Women. (2011, reaffirmed). In Committee opinion no. 496: At-risk drinking and alcohol dependence: Obstetric and gynecologic implications. Available at www.acog.org/~/media/Committee%20Opinions/Committee%20on%20Health%20Care%20for%20Underserved%20Women/co496.pdf.

American College of Obstetricians and Gynecologists (ACOG) Committee on Obstetric Practice. (2011, reaffirmed 2013). Committee opinion no. 462: Moderate caffeine consumption during pregnancy. Available at www.acog.org/Resources%20And%20Publications/Committee%20Opinions/Committee%20on%20Obstetric%20Practice/Moderate%20Caffeine%20Consumption%20During%20Pregnancy.aspx.

American College of Obstetricians & Gynecologists Committee on Obstetric Practice. (2013). Committee opinion no. 549: Obesity in pregnancy. *Obstetrics and Gynecology, 121*(1), 213–217.

Asemi, Z., Tabassi, Z., Samimi, M., et al. (2013). Favourable effects of the Dietary Approaches to Stop Hypertension diet on glucose tolerance and lipid profiles in gestational diabetes: A randomised clinical trial. *British Journal of Nutrition, 109*(11), 2024–2030.

Centers for Disease Control and Prevention. (2011). Pediatric and pregnancy nutrition surveillance system: PNSS health indicators. Available at http://www.cdc.gov/pednss/what_is/pnss_health_indicators.htm.

Centers for Disease Control and Prevention. (2014). *Pregnancy complications.* Available at www.cdc.gov/reproductivehealth/MaternalInfantHealth/PregComplications.htm.

Centers for Disease Control and Prevention. (2014). *Pregnancy complications.* Available at www.cdc.gov/reproductive-health/MaternalInfantHealth/PregComplications.htm.

Chang, T., Choi, H., Richardson, C. R., & Davis, M. M. (2013). Implications of teen birth for overweight and obesity in adulthood. *American Journal of Obstetrics and Gynecology, 209*(2), 110.e1–110.e7.

Conde-Aqudelo, A., Romero, R., Kusanovic, J. P., & Hassan, S. S. (2011). Supplementation with vitamins C and E during pregnancy for the prevention of preeclampsia and other adverse maternal and perinatal outcomes: A systematic review and metaanalysis. *American Journal of Obstetrics and Gynecology, 204*(6), 503.e1–503.e12.

Frisoli, T. M., Schmieder, R. E., Grodzicki, T., & Messerli, F. H. (2011). Beyond salt: Lifestyle modifications and blood pressure. *European Heart Journal, 32*(24), 3081–3087.

Gould, J. F., Smithers, L. G., & Makrides, M. (2013). The effect of maternal omega-3 (n-3) LCPUFA supplementation on early childhood cognitive and visual development: A systematic review and meta-analysis of randomized controlled trials. *American Journal of Clinical Nutrition, 97*(3), 532–544.

Harnisch, J. M., Harnisch, P. H., & Harnisch, D. R. (2012). Family medicine obstetrics: Pregnancy and nutrition. *Primary Care, 39*(1), 39–54.

Hark, L., & Catalano, P. M. (2012). Nutritional management during pregnancy. In S. G. Gabbe, J. R. Niebyl, J. L. Simpson, et al. (Eds.), *Obstetrics: Normal and problem pregnancies* (6th ed.). Philadelphia: Elsevier.

Institute of Medicine. (2009). *Weight gain during pregnancy: Reexamining the guidelines.* Washington, DC: National Academies Press.

Jahanfar, S., & Jaafara, S. H. (2013). Effects of restricted caffeine intake by mother on fetal, neonatal and pregnancy outcome. *The Cochrane Database of Systematic Reviews, 2013,* 2 CD006965.

Langford, A., Joshu, C., Chang, J. J., et al. (2011). Does gestational weight gain affect the risk of adverse maternal and infant outcomes in overweight women? *Maternal and Child Health Journal, 15*(7), 860–865.

Lawrence, R. M., & Lawrence, R. A. (2011). *Breastfeeding: A guide for the medical profession* (7th ed.). St. Louis: Mosby.

Lo, A., Sienna, J., Mamak, E., et al. (2012). The effects of maternal supplementation of polyunsaturated fatty acids on visual, neurobehavioural, and developmental outcomes of the child: A systematic review of the randomized trials. *Obstetrics and Gynecology International, article ID 591531, 2012,* 1–9.

March of Dimes. (2012). *Eating and nutrition.* Available at www.marchofdimes.com/pregnancy/caffeine-in-pregnancy.aspx.

Otten, J. J., Helwig, J. P., & Meyers, L. D. (2006). *Dietary reference intakes: The essential guide to nutrient requirements.* Washington, DC: National Academies Press.

Panel on Dietary Reference Intakes for Macronutrients, & Institute of Medicine. (2005). *Dietary reference intakes for energy, carbohydrate, fiber, fat, fatty acids, cholesterol, protein, and amino acids.* Washington, DC: National Academies Press.

Ross, A. C., Taylor, C. L., Yaktine, A. L., et al: (2011). *Dietary reference intakes for calcium and vitamin D.* Washington, DC: National Academies Press.

Scott, M. (2013). Nutrition for lactating women. In R. Mannel, P. J. Martens, & M. Walker (Eds.), *Core curriculum for lactation consultant practice.* Burlington, MA: Jones and Bartlett.

Sengpiel, V., Elind, E., Bacelis, J., et al. (2013). Maternal caffeine intake during pregnancy is associated with birth weight but not with gestational length: Results from a large prospective observational cohort study. *BMC Medicine,* (11), 42.

Tiran, D. (2012). Ginger to reduce nausea and vomiting during pregnancy: Evidence of effectiveness is not the same as proof of safety. *Complementary Therapies in Clinical Practice, 18*(1), 22–25.

Tobias, D. K., Zhang, C., Chavarro, J., et al. (2012). Prepregnancy adherence to dietary patterns and lower risk of gestational diabetes mellitus. *American Journal of Clinical Nutrition, 96*(2), 289–295.

Turcksin, R., Bel, S., Galjaard, S., & Devlieger, R. (2012). Maternal obesity and breastfeeding intention, initiation, intensity, and duration: A systematic review. *Maternal and Child Nutrition, 10*(2), 166–183.

U.S. Food & Drug Administration (FDA). (2013a). Food safety for moms-to-be: While you're pregnant—listeria. Available at www.fda.gov/Food/FoodborneIllnessContaminants/PeopleAtRisk/ucm083320.htm.

U.S. Food & Drug Administration (FDA). (2013b). Food safety for moms-to-be: While you're pregnant—methylmercury. Available at www.fda.gov/Food/FoodborneIllnessContaminants/PeopleAtRisk/ucm083324.htm.

U.S. Food & Drug Administration (FDA). (2013c). Food safety for moms-to-be: While you're pregnant—toxoplasma. Available at www.fda.gov/food/foodborneillnesscontaminants/peopleatrisk/ucm083327.htm.

U.S. Food & Drug Administration (FDA). (2013d). *While you're pregnant—What is foodborne illness?* Available at www.fda.gov/Food/FoodborneIllness-Contaminants/PeopleAtRisk/ucm083316.htm.

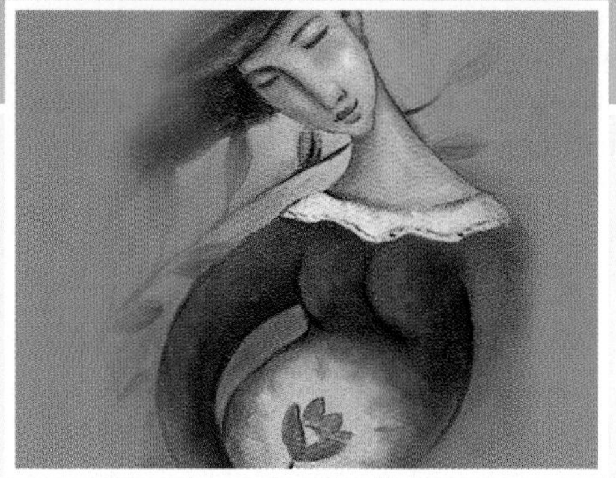

CHAPTER 16

Labor and Birth Processes

Kitty Cashion

http://evolve.elsevier.com/Lowdermilk/MWHC/

LEARNING OBJECTIVES

- Explain the five major factors that affect the labor process.
- Describe the anatomic structure of the bony pelvis.
- Recognize the normal measurements of the diameters of the pelvic inlet, cavity, and outlet.
- Explain the significance of the size and position of the fetal head during labor and birth.
- Summarize the cardinal movements of the mechanism of labor for a vertex presentation.
- Examine the maternal anatomic and physiologic adaptations to labor.
- Describe factors thought to contribute to the onset of labor.
- Describe fetal adaptations to labor.

During late pregnancy a woman and fetus prepare for the labor process. The fetus has grown and developed in preparation for extrauterine life. The woman has undergone various physiologic adaptations during pregnancy that prepare her for giving birth and for motherhood. Labor and birth represent the end of pregnancy, the beginning of extrauterine life for the newborn, and a change in the lives of the family. This chapter discusses the factors affecting labor, the process involved, the normal progression of events, and the adaptations made by both the woman and fetus.

FACTORS AFFECTING LABOR

At least five factors affect the process of labor and birth. These are easily remembered as the five P's: *p*assenger (fetus and placenta), *p*assageway (birth canal), *p*owers (contractions), *p*osition of the mother, and *p*sychologic response. The first four factors are presented here as the basis for understanding the physiologic process of labor. The fifth factor is discussed in Chapter 19. The following factors may also affect the process of labor and birth. VandeVusse (1999) identified external forces including place of birth, preparation, type of provider (especially nurses), and procedures. Physiology (sensations) was identified as an internal force. These factors are discussed generally in Chapter 19 as they relate to nursing care during labor. Further research investigating essential forces of labor is recommended.

Passenger

The way the passenger, or fetus, moves through the birth canal is determined by the following interacting factors: the size of the fetal head, fetal presentation, fetal lie, fetal attitude, and fetal position. Because the placenta also must pass through the birth canal, it can also be considered a passenger; however, the placenta rarely interferes with the process of labor in a normal vaginal birth. An exception is the case of placenta previa (see Chapter 28).

Size of the Fetal Head

Because of its size and relative rigidity, the fetal head has a major effect on the birth process. The fetal skull is composed of two parietal bones, two temporal bones, the frontal bone, and the occipital bone (Fig. 16-1, *A*). These bones are united by membranous sutures: sagittal, lambdoidal, coronal, and frontal (see Fig. 16-1, *B*). Membrane-filled spaces called fontanels are located where the sutures intersect. During labor, after rupture of membranes, palpation of fontanels and sutures during vaginal examination reveals fetal presentation, position, and attitude.

The two most important fontanels are the anterior and posterior (see Fig. 16-1, *B*). The larger of these, the anterior fontanel, is diamond shaped, is about 3 cm by 2 cm, and lies at the junction of the sagittal, coronal, and frontal sutures. It closes by 18 months after birth. The posterior fontanel lies at the junction of the sutures of the two parietal bones and the occipital bone, is triangular, and is about 1 cm by 2 cm. It closes 6 to 8 weeks after birth.

Sutures and fontanels make the skull flexible to accommodate the infant brain, which continues to grow for some time after birth. However, because the bones are not firmly united, slight overlapping of the bones, or molding of the shape of the head, occurs during labor. This capacity of the bones to slide over one another also permits adaptation to the various diameters of the maternal pelvis. Molding can be extensive, but the heads of most newborns assume their normal shape within 3 days after birth.

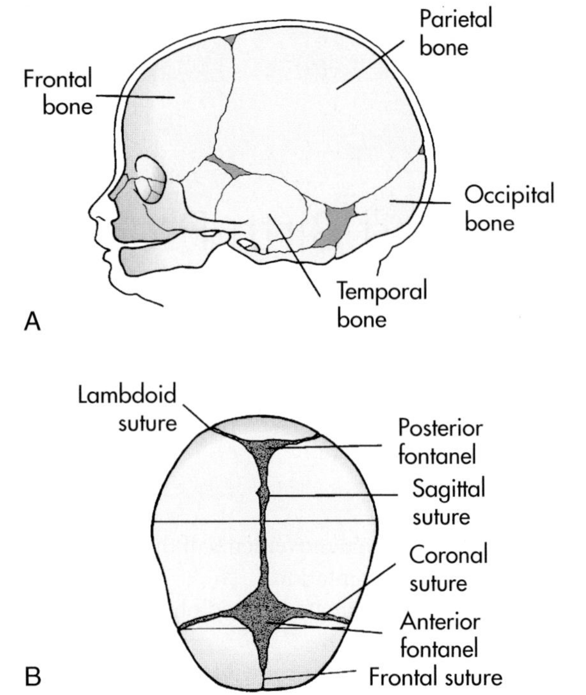

FIG 16-1 Fetal head at term. **A,** Bones. **B,** Sutures and fontanels.

Although the size of the fetal shoulders may affect passage, their position can be altered relatively easily during labor, so one shoulder may occupy a lower level than the other. This creates a shoulder diameter that is smaller than the skull, facilitating passage through the birth canal. After the birth of the head and shoulders, the rest of the body usually emerges quickly (Cunningham, Leveno, Bloom, et al., 2014).

Fetal Presentation

Presentation refers to the part of the fetus that enters the pelvic inlet first and leads through the birth canal during labor. The three main presentations are *cephalic presentation* (head first), occurring in 96% of births (Fig. 16-2); *breech presentation* (buttocks, feet, or both first), occurring in 3% of births (Fig. 16-3, *A-C*); and *shoulder presentation,* seen in 1% of births (see Fig. 16-3, *D*). The **presenting part** is that part of the fetus that lies closest to the internal os of the cervix. It is the part of the fetal body first felt by the examining finger during a vaginal examination. In a cephalic presentation the presenting part is usually the occiput; in a breech presentation it is the sacrum; in the shoulder presentation it is the scapula. When the presenting part is the occiput, the presentation is noted as vertex (see Fig. 16-2). Factors that determine the presenting

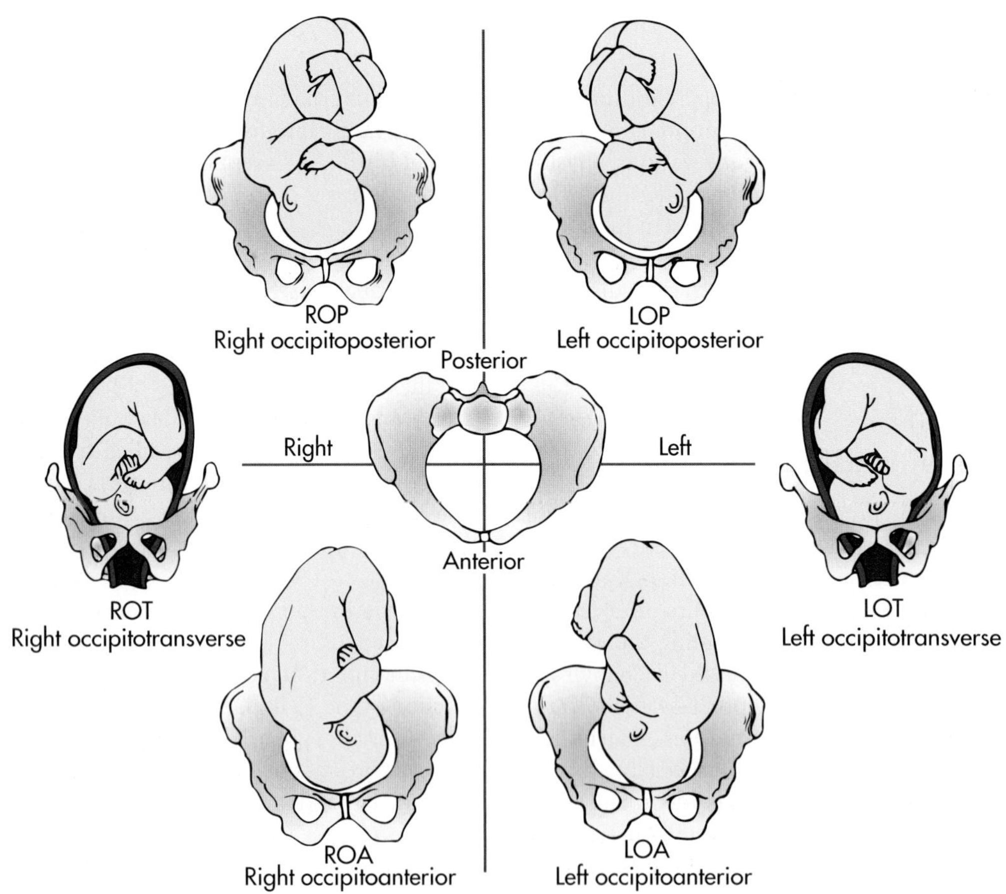

FIG 16-2 Examples of fetal vertex (occiput) presentations in relation to front, back, or side of maternal pelvis.

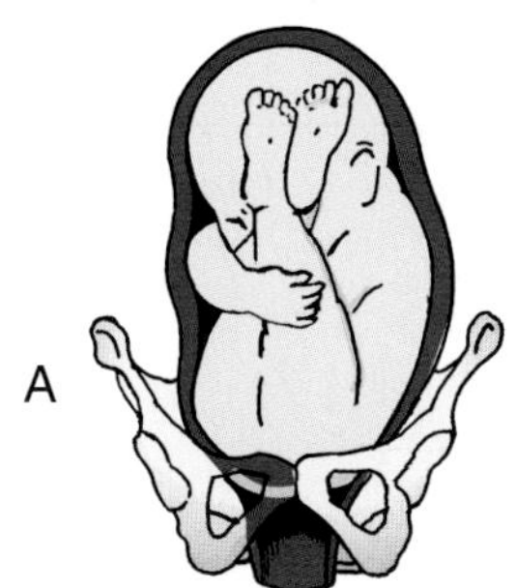

Frank breech
Lie: Longitudinal or vertical
Presentation: Breech (incomplete)
Presenting part: Sacrum
Attitude: Flexion, except for legs at knees

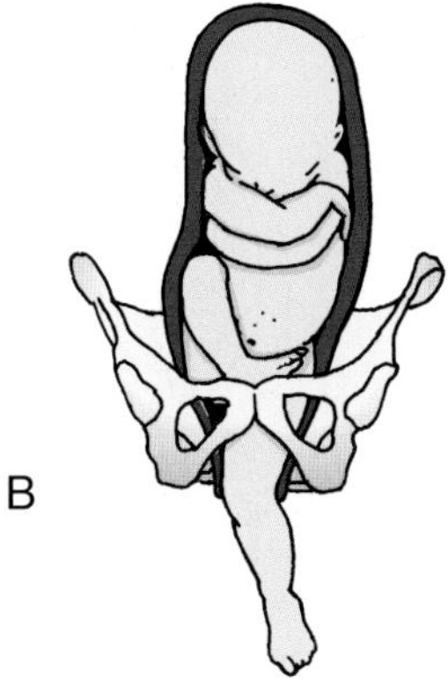

Single footling breech
Lie: Longitudinal or vertical
Presentation: Breech (incomplete)
Presenting part: Sacrum
Attitude: Flexion, except for one leg extended at hip and knee

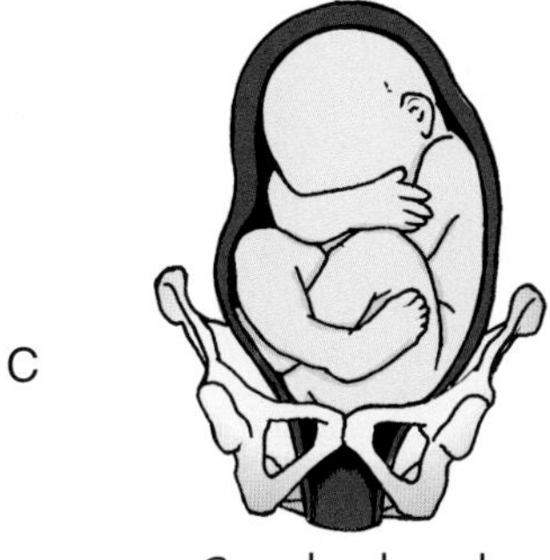

Complete breech
Lie: Longitudinal or vertical
Presentation: Breech (sacrum and feet presenting)
Presenting part: Sacrum (with feet)
Attitude: General flexion

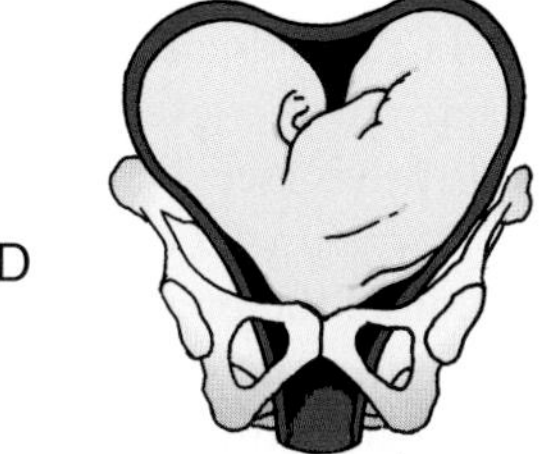

Shoulder presentation
Lie: Transverse or horizontal
Presentation: Shoulder
Presenting part: Scapula
Attitude: Flexion

FIG 16-3 Fetal presentations. **A** through **C**, Breech (sacral) presentations. **D**, Shoulder presentation.

part include fetal lie, fetal attitude, and extension or flexion of the fetal head.

Fetal Lie

Lie is the relation of the long axis (spine) of the fetus to the long axis (spine) of the mother. The two primary lies are longitudinal, or vertical, in which the long axis of the fetus is parallel with the long axis of the mother (see Fig. 16-2); and transverse, horizontal, or oblique, in which the long axis of the fetus is at a right angle diagonal to the long axis of the mother (see Fig. 16-3, *D*). Longitudinal lies, which are present in more than 99% of term labors, are either cephalic or breech presentations, depending on the fetal structure that first enters the mother's pelvis. Vaginal birth cannot occur when the fetus stays in a transverse lie. An oblique lie, one in which the long axis of the fetus is lying at an angle to the long axis of the mother, is less common and usually converts to a longitudinal or transverse lie during labor (Cunningham et al., 2014).

Fetal Attitude

Attitude is the relation of the fetal body parts to one another. The fetus assumes a characteristic posture (attitude) in utero partly because of the mode of fetal growth and partly because of the way the fetus conforms to the shape of the uterine cavity. Normally the back of the fetus is rounded so that the chin is flexed on the chest, the thighs are flexed on the abdomen, and the legs are flexed at the knees. The arms are crossed over the thorax, and the umbilical cord lies between the arms and the legs. This attitude is termed *general flexion* (see Fig. 16-2).

Deviations from the normal attitude may cause difficulties in childbirth. For example, in a cephalic presentation the fetal head may be extended or flexed in a manner that presents a head diameter that exceeds the limits of the maternal pelvis, leading to prolonged labor, forceps- or vacuum-assisted birth, or cesarean birth.

Certain critical diameters of the fetal head are usually measured. The biparietal diameter, which is about 9.25 cm at term, is the largest transverse diameter and an important indicator of fetal head size (Fig. 16-4, *B*). In a well-flexed cephalic presentation, the biparietal diameter is the widest part of the head entering the pelvic inlet. Of the several anteroposterior diameters, the smallest and the most critical one is the suboccipitobregmatic diameter (about 9.5 cm at term). When the head is in complete flexion, this diameter allows the fetal head to pass through the

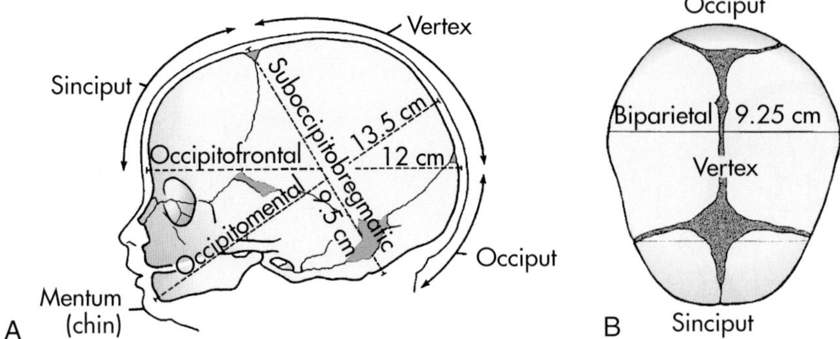

FIG 16-4 Diameters of the fetal head at term. **A,** Cephalic presentations: occiput, vertex, and sinciput; and cephalic diameters: suboccipitobregmatic, occipitofrontal, and occipitomental. **B,** Biparietal diameter.

true pelvis easily (see Fig. 16-4, *A*; Fig. 16-5, *A*). As the head is more extended, the anteroposterior diameter widens, and the head may not be able to enter the true pelvis (see Fig. 16-5).

Fetal Position

The presentation, or presenting part, indicates that portion of the fetus that overlies the pelvic inlet. Position is the relationship of a reference point on the presenting part (occiput, sacrum, mentum [chin], or sinciput [deflexed vertex]) to the four quadrants of the mother's pelvis (see Fig. 16-2). Position is denoted by a three-part abbreviation. The first letter of the abbreviation denotes the location of the presenting part in the right (R) or left (L) side of the mother's pelvis. The middle letter stands for the specific presenting part of the fetus (O for occiput, S for sacrum, M for mentum [chin], and Sc for scapula [shoulder]). The final letter stands for the location of the presenting part in relation to the anterior (A), posterior (P), or transverse (T) portion of the maternal pelvis. For example, ROA means that the occiput is the presenting part and is located in the right anterior quadrant of the maternal pelvis (see Fig. 16-2). LSP means that the sacrum is the presenting part and is located in the left posterior quadrant of the maternal pelvis (see Fig. 16-3).

Station is the relationship of the presenting fetal part to an imaginary line drawn between the maternal ischial spines and is a measure of the degree of descent of the presenting part of the fetus through the birth canal. The placement of the presenting part is measured in centimeters above or below the ischial spines (Fig. 16-6). For example, when the lowermost portion of the presenting part is 1 cm above the spines, it is noted as being minus (−) 1. At the level of the spines the station is said to be 0 (zero). When the presenting part is 1 cm below the spines, the station is said to be plus (+) 1. Birth is imminent when the presenting part is at +4 to +5 cm. The station of the presenting part should be determined when labor begins so that the rate of descent of the fetus during labor can be determined accurately.

Engagement is the term used to indicate that the largest transverse diameter of the presenting part (usually the biparietal diameter) has passed through the maternal pelvic brim or inlet into the true pelvis and usually corresponds to station 0. It often occurs in the weeks just before labor begins in nulliparas and may occur before labor or during labor in multiparas. Engagement can be determined by abdominal or vaginal examination.

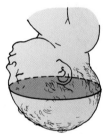

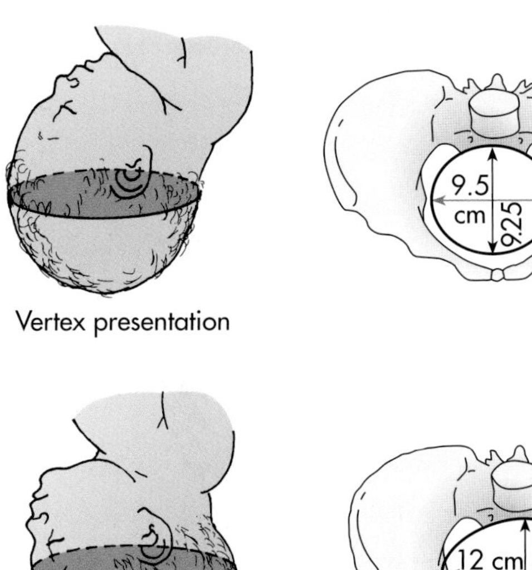

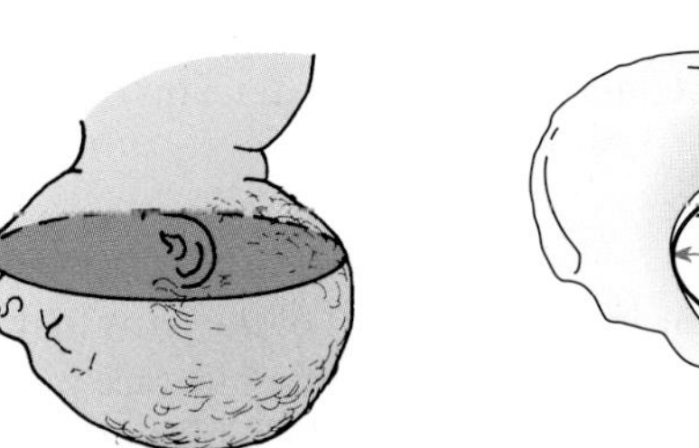

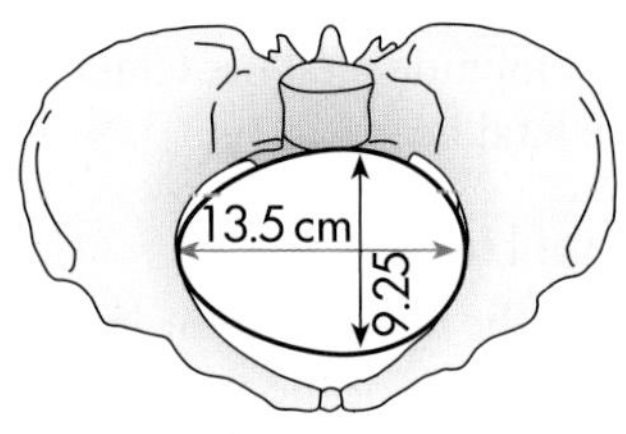

FIG 16-5 Head entering pelvis. Biparietal diameter is indicated with shading (9.25 cm). **A,** Suboccipitobregmatic diameter: complete flexion of head on chest so that smallest diameter enters. **B,** Occipitofrontal diameter: moderate extension (military attitude) so that large diameter enters. **C,** Occipitomental diameter: marked extension (deflection), so that the largest diameter, which is too large to permit head to enter pelvis, is presenting.

Passageway

The passageway, or birth canal, is composed of the mother's rigid bony pelvis and the soft tissues of the cervix, the pelvic floor, the vagina, and the introitus (the external opening to the vagina). Although the soft tissues, particularly the muscular layers of the pelvic floor, contribute to vaginal birth of the fetus, the maternal

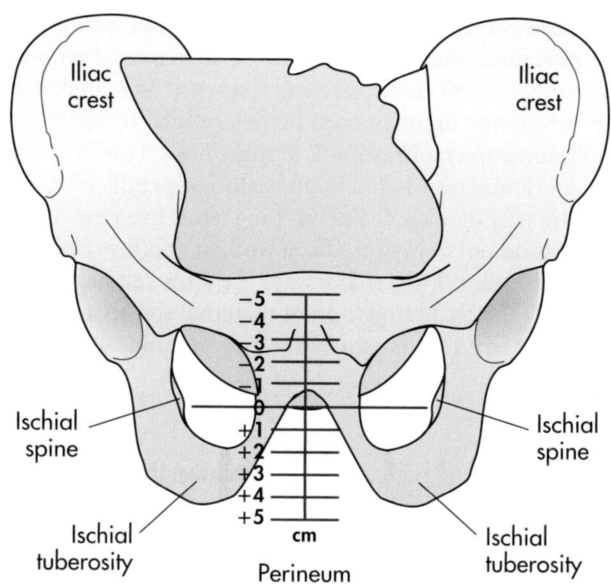

FIG 16-6 Stations of presenting part, or degree of descent. The lowermost portion of the presenting part is at the level of the ischial spines, station 0.

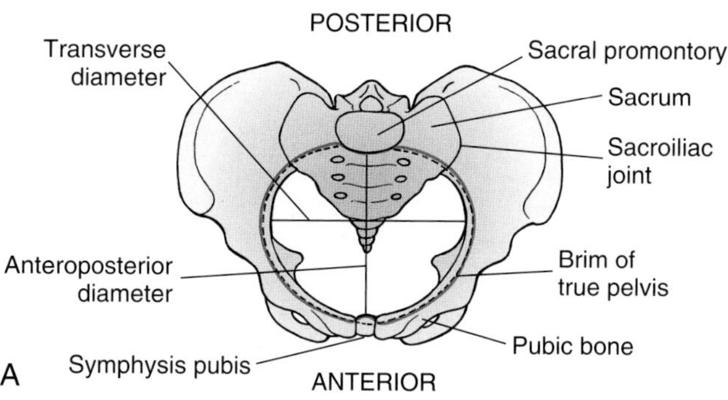

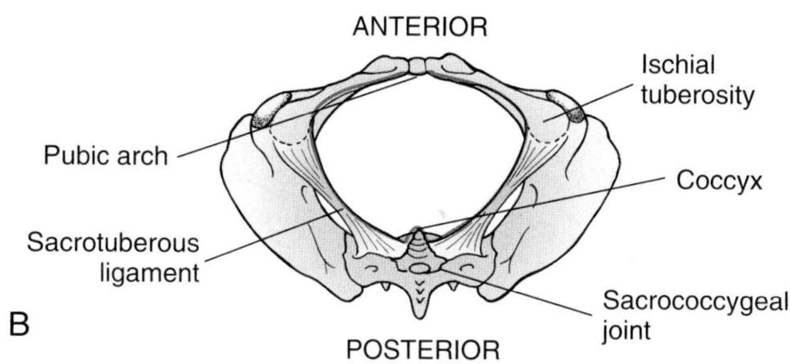

FIG 16-7 Female pelvis. **A,** Pelvic brim from above. **B,** Pelvic outlet from below, as seen by health care provider when the woman is lying supine.

pelvis plays a far greater role in the labor process because the fetus must successfully accommodate itself to this relatively rigid passageway. The determination of the size and shape of the pelvis can be done at the initial prenatal visit or on admission in labor. This information can then be used in the assessment of labor progress (Thorp & Laughon, 2014).

Bony Pelvis

The anatomy of the bony pelvis is described in Chapter 4. The following discussion focuses on the importance of pelvic configurations as they relate to the labor process. (It may be helpful to refer to Fig. 4-4.)

The bony pelvis is formed by the fusion of the ilium, the ischium, the pubis, and the sacral bones. The four pelvic joints are the symphysis pubis, the right and left sacroiliac joints (Fig. 16-7, *A*), and the sacrococcygeal joint (see Fig. 16-7, *B*). The bony pelvis is separated by the brim, or inlet, into two parts: the false pelvis and the true pelvis. The false pelvis is the part above the brim and plays no part in childbearing. The true pelvis, the part involved in birth, is divided into three planes: the inlet, or brim; the midpelvis, or cavity; and the outlet.

The pelvic inlet, which is the upper border of the true pelvis, is formed anteriorly by the upper margins of the pubic bone, laterally by the iliopectineal lines along the innominate bones, and posteriorly by the anterior, upper margin of the sacrum and the sacral promontory.

The pelvic cavity, or midpelvis, is a curved passage with a short anterior wall and a much longer concave posterior wall. It is bounded by the posterior aspect of the symphysis pubis, the ischium, a portion of the ilium, the sacrum, and the coccyx.

The pelvic outlet is the lower border of the true pelvis. Viewed from below it is ovoid, somewhat diamond shaped, and bounded by the pubic arch anteriorly, the ischial tuberosities laterally, and the tip of the coccyx posteriorly (see Fig. 16-7, *B*). In the latter part of pregnancy the coccyx is movable (unless it has been broken in a fall during skiing or skating, for example, and has fused to the sacrum during healing).

The pelvic canal varies in size and shape at various levels. The diameters at the plane of the pelvic inlet, midpelvis, and outlet, plus the axis of the birth canal (Fig. 16-8), determine whether vaginal birth is possible and the manner by which the fetus may pass down the birth canal.

The subpubic angle, which determines the type of pubic arch, together with the length of the pubic rami and the intertuberous diameter, is of great importance. Because the fetus must first pass beneath the pubic arch, a narrow subpubic angle will be less accommodating than a rounded, wide arch. The method of measurement of the subpubic arch is shown in Fig. 16-9. A summary of obstetric measurements is given in Table 16-1.

The four basic types of pelves are classified as follows:

1. *Gynecoid* (the classic female type)
2. *Android* (resembling the male pelvis)
3. *Anthropoid* (oval shaped, with a wider anteroposterior diameter)
4. *Platypelloid* (the flat pelvis)

The gynecoid pelvis is the most common, with major gynecoid pelvic features present in 50% of all women. Anthropoid and android features are less common, and platypelloid pelvic features are the least common. Mixed types of pelves are more common than are pure types (Cunningham et al., 2014). Examples of pelvic variations and their effects on mode of birth are given in Table 16-2.

Assessment of the bony pelvis can be performed during the first prenatal evaluation and need not be repeated if the pelvis is of adequate size and suitable shape. In the third trimester of pregnancy the examination of the bony pelvis may be more thorough and the results more accurate because there is relaxation and increased mobility of the pelvic joints and ligaments owing to hormonal influences. Widening of the joint of the symphysis pubis and the resulting instability may cause pain in any or all of the pelvic joints.

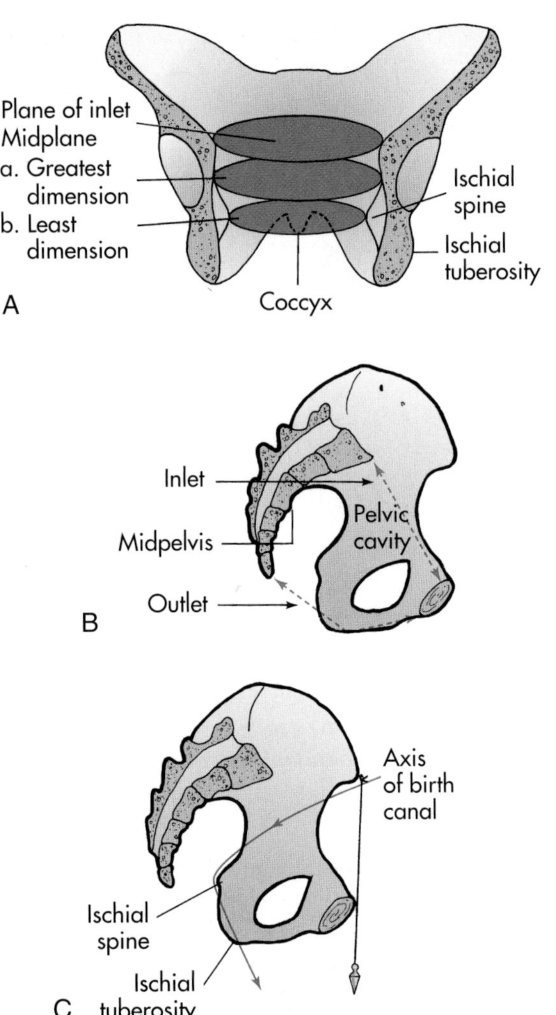

FIG 16-8 Pelvic cavity. **A,** Inlet and midplane. Outlet not shown. **B,** Cavity of true pelvis. **C,** Note curve of sacrum and axis of birth canal.

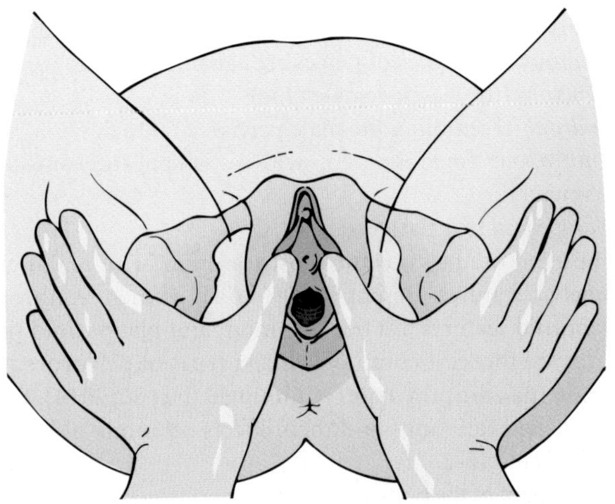

FIG 16-9 Estimation of angle of subpubic arch. With both thumbs, examiner externally traces descending rami down to tuberosities. (From Barkauskas, V., Baumann, L., & Darling-Fisher, C. [2002]. *Health and physical assessment* [3rd ed.]. St. Louis: Mosby.)

Because the examiner does not have direct access to the bony structures and because the bones are covered with varying amounts of soft tissue, size and shape are estimated. Precise bony pelvis measurements can be determined by use of computed tomography, ultrasound, or x-ray films. However, radiographic examination is rarely done during pregnancy because the x-rays may damage the developing fetus. Even precise measurements do not always predict a woman's ability to give birth vaginally because of the many ways the fetus can negotiate the pelvis and the accommodation of maternal soft tissues. Therefore, pelvimetry results would rarely contraindicate a trial of labor.

Soft Tissues

The soft tissues of the passageway include the stretchy lower uterine segment, the cervix, the pelvic floor muscles, the vagina, and the introitus. Before labor begins, the uterus is composed of the uterine body (corpus) and the cervix (neck). After labor has begun, uterine contractions cause the uterine body to have a thick and muscular upper segment and a thin-walled, passive, muscular lower segment. A *physiologic retraction ring* separates the two segments (Fig. 16-10). The lower uterine segment gradually stretches to accommodate the intrauterine contents as the wall of the upper segment thickens and its accommodating capacity is reduced. The contractions of the uterine body thus exert downward pressure on the fetus, pushing it against the cervix.

The cervix effaces (thins) and dilates (opens) sufficiently to allow the first fetal portion to descend into the vagina. As the fetus descends, the cervix is actually drawn upward and over this first portion.

The pelvic floor is a muscular layer that separates the pelvic cavity above from the perineal space below. This structure helps the fetus rotate anteriorly as it passes through the birth canal. As noted, the soft tissues of the vagina develop throughout pregnancy until at term the vagina can dilate to accommodate the fetus and permit its passage to the external world.

Powers

Involuntary and voluntary powers combine to expel the fetus and the placenta from the uterus. Involuntary uterine contractions, called the *primary powers,* signal the beginning of labor. Once the cervix has dilated, voluntary bearing-down efforts by the woman, called the *secondary powers,* augment the force of the involuntary contractions.

Primary Powers

The involuntary contractions originate at certain pacemaker points in the thickened muscle layers of the upper uterine segment. From the pacemaker points, contractions move downward over the uterus in waves, separated by short rest periods. Terms used to describe these involuntary contractions include *frequency* (the time from the beginning of one contraction to the beginning of the next), *duration* (length of contraction), and *intensity* (strength of contraction at its peak).

The primary powers are responsible for the effacement and dilation of the cervix and descent of the fetus. Effacement of the cervix means the shortening and thinning of the cervix during the first stage of labor. The cervix, normally 2 to 3 cm long and about 1 cm thick, is obliterated, or "taken up," by a shortening of the uterine muscle bundles during the thinning of the lower uterine segment that occurs in advancing labor. Only a thin edge of the cervix can be palpated when effacement is complete. Effacement generally progresses significantly in first-time term pregnancy before more than slight dilation occurs. In subsequent pregnancies effacement and dilation of the cervix tend to progress together. Degree of effacement is expressed in percentages from 0% to 100% (e.g., a cervix is 50% effaced) (Fig. 16-11, *A-C*).

Dilation of the cervix is the enlargement or widening of the cervical opening and the cervical canal that occurs once

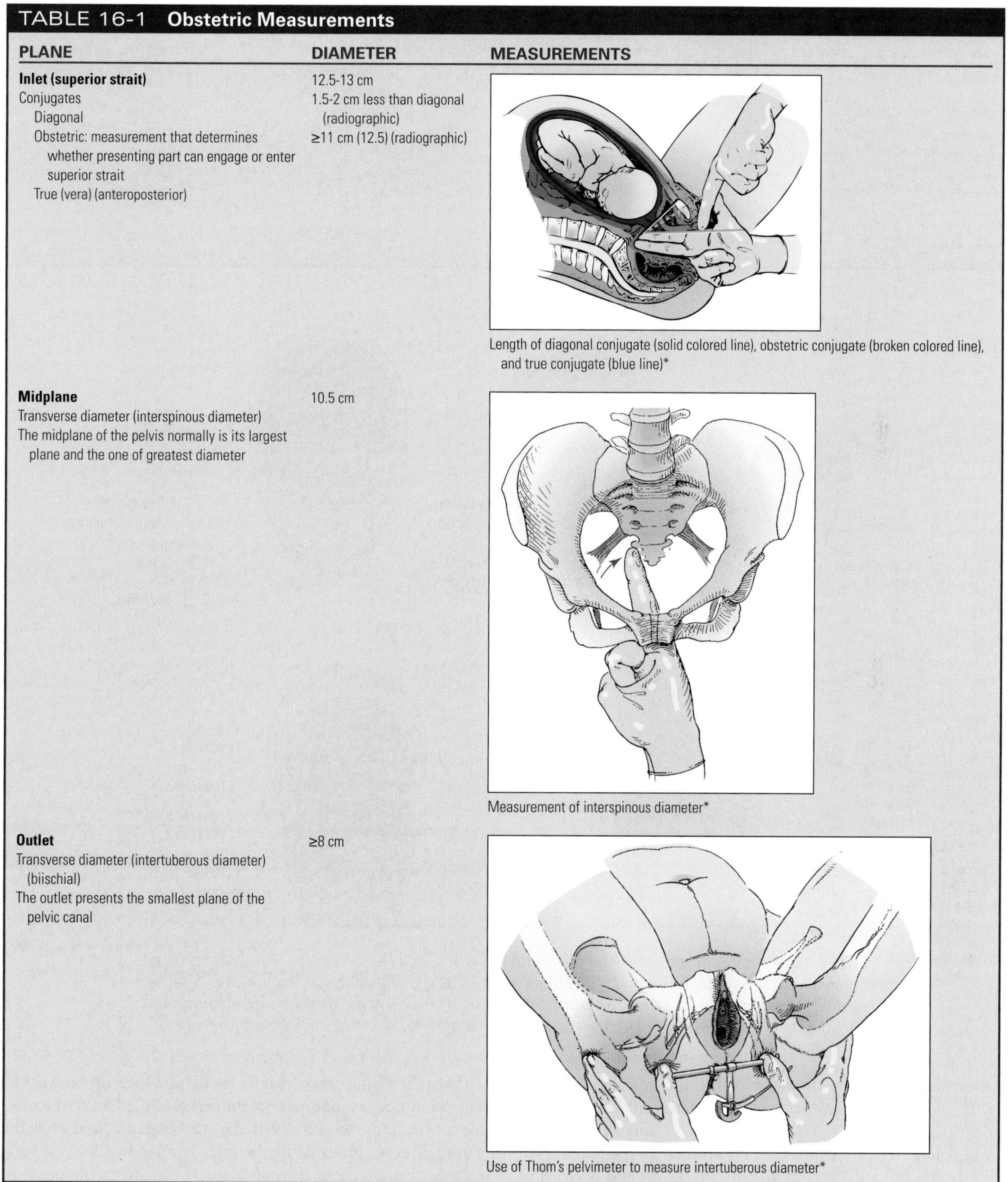

TABLE 16-1 Obstetric Measurements

PLANE	DIAMETER	MEASUREMENTS
Inlet (superior strait) Conjugates Diagonal Obstetric: measurement that determines whether presenting part can engage or enter superior strait True (vera) (anteroposterior)	12.5-13 cm 1.5-2 cm less than diagonal (radiographic) ≥11 cm (12.5) (radiographic)	Length of diagonal conjugate (solid colored line), obstetric conjugate (broken colored line), and true conjugate (blue line)*
Midplane Transverse diameter (interspinous diameter) The midplane of the pelvis normally is its largest plane and the one of greatest diameter	10.5 cm	Measurement of interspinous diameter*
Outlet Transverse diameter (intertuberous diameter) (biischial) The outlet presents the smallest plane of the pelvic canal	≥8 cm	Use of Thom's pelvimeter to measure intertuberous diameter*

*From Seidel, H., Ball, J., Dains, J., et al. (2011). *Mosby's guide to physical examination* (7th ed.). St. Louis: Mosby.

TABLE 16-2 Comparison of Pelvic Types

	GYNECOID	ANDROID	ANTHROPOID	PLATYPELLOID
	(50% of Women)	**(23% of Women)**	**(24% of Women)**	**(3% of Women)**
Brim	Slightly ovoid or transversely rounded	Heart shaped, angulated	Oval, wider anteroposteriorly	Flattened anteroposteriorly, wide transversely
Shape	Round	Heart	Oval	Flat
Depth	Moderate	Deep	Deep	Shallow
Side walls	Straight	Convergent	Straight	Straight
Ischial spines	Blunt, somewhat widely separated	Prominent, narrow interspinous diameter	Prominent, often with narrow interspinous diameter	Blunted, widely separated
Sacrum	Deep, curved	Slightly curved, terminal portion often beaked	Slightly curved	Slightly curved
Subpubic arch	Wide	Narrow	Narrow	Wide
Usual mode of birth	Vaginal Spontaneous Occipitoanterior position	Cesarean Vaginal Difficult, with forceps	Vaginal Forceps Spontaneous Occipitoposterior or occipitoanterior position	Vaginal Spontaneous

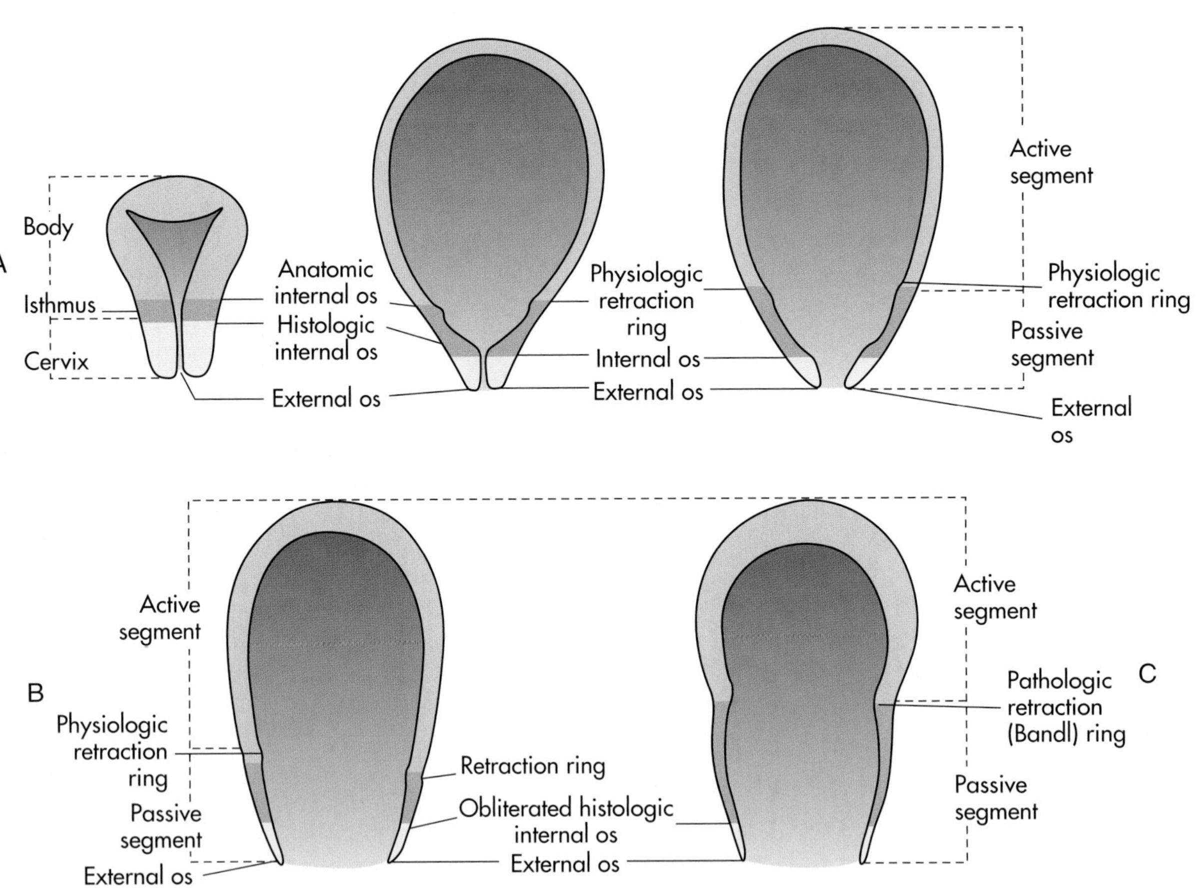

FIG 16-10 **A,** Uterus in normal labor in early first stage and, **B,** in second stage. Passive segment is derived from lower uterine segment (isthmus) and cervix, and physiologic retraction ring is derived from anatomic internal os. **C,** Uterus in abnormal labor in second-stage dystocia. Pathologic retraction (Bandl) ring that forms under abnormal conditions develops from the physiologic ring.

labor has begun. The diameter of the cervix increases from being closed to full dilation (approximately 10 cm) to allow birth of a term fetus. When the cervix is fully dilated (and completely retracted), it can no longer be palpated (see Fig. 16-11, *D*). Full cervical dilation marks the end of the first stage of labor.

Dilation of the cervix occurs by the drawing upward of the musculofibrous components of the cervix, caused by strong uterine contractions. Pressure exerted by the amniotic fluid while the membranes are intact or by the force applied by the presenting part also can promote cervical dilation. Scarring of the cervix as a result of prior infection or surgery may slow cervical dilation.

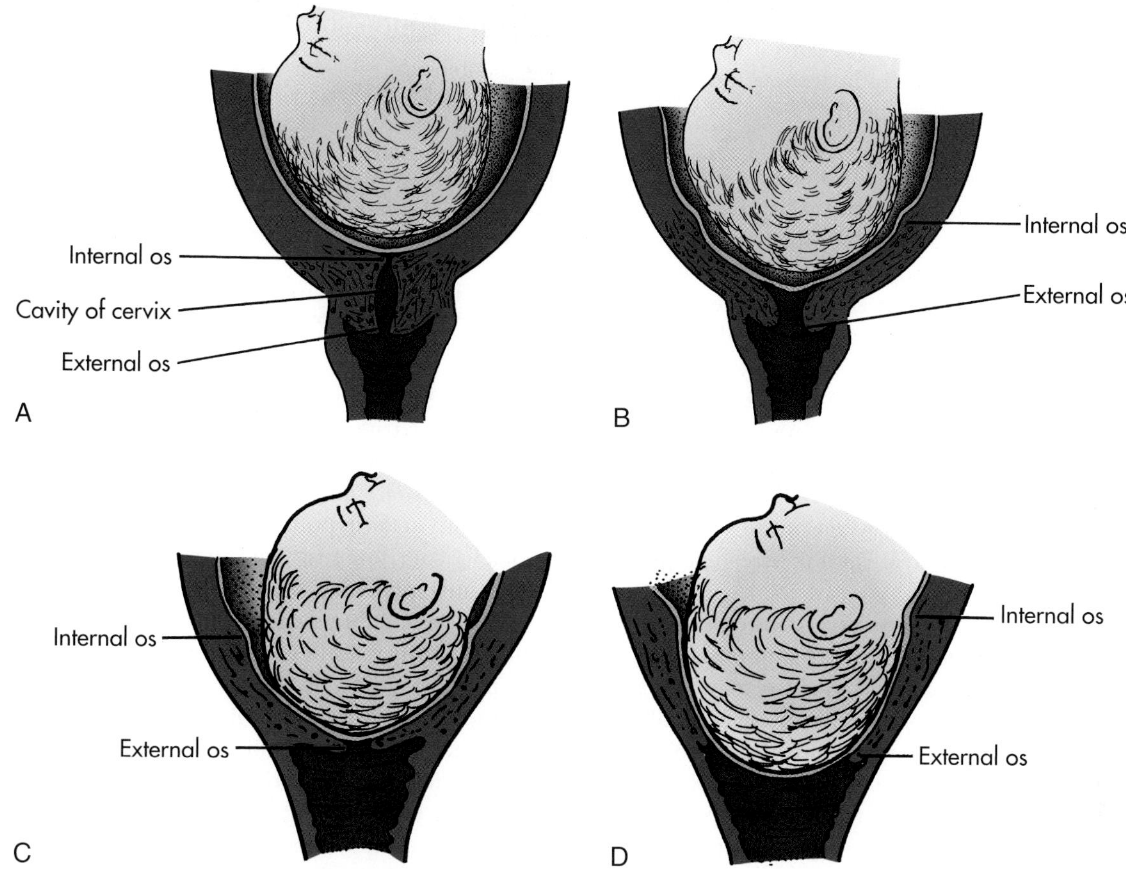

FIG 16-11 Cervical effacement and dilation. Note how cervix is drawn up around presenting part (internal os). Membranes are intact, and head is not well applied to cervix. **A,** Before labor. **B,** Early effacement. **C,** Complete effacement (100%). Head is well applied to cervix. **D,** Complete dilation (10 cm). Cranial bones overlap somewhat, and membranes are still intact.

In the first and second stages of labor, increased intrauterine pressure caused by contractions exerts pressure on the descending fetus and the cervix. When the presenting part of the fetus reaches the perineal floor, mechanical stretching of the cervix occurs. Stretch receptors in the posterior vagina cause release of endogenous oxytocin that triggers the maternal urge to bear down, or the *Ferguson reflex.*

Uterine contractions are usually independent of external forces. For example, laboring women who are paralyzed because of spinal cord lesions above the twelfth thoracic vertebra have normal but painless uterine contractions. In addition, use of epidural analgesia during labor does not decrease the frequency or intensity of contractions (Cunningham et al., 2014).

Secondary Powers

As soon as the presenting part reaches the pelvic floor, the contractions change in character and become expulsive. The laboring woman experiences an involuntary urge to push. She uses secondary powers (bearing-down efforts) to aid in expulsion of the fetus as she contracts her diaphragm and abdominal muscles and pushes. These bearing-down efforts result in increased intraabdominal pressure that compresses the uterus on all sides and adds to the power of the expulsive forces.

The secondary powers have no effect on cervical dilation, but they are of considerable importance in the expulsion of the infant from the uterus and vagina after the cervix is fully dilated. When and how a woman pushes in the second stage of labor are much-debated topics. Continued study is needed to determine the effectiveness and appropriateness of strategies used by nurses to teach pushing techniques, the suitability and effectiveness of various pushing techniques related to abnormal fetal heart patterns, and the standards for length of pushing in terms of maternal and fetal outcomes. See Chapter 19 for further discussion regarding pushing during the second stage of labor.

Position of the Laboring Woman

Position affects the woman's anatomic and physiologic adaptations to labor. Frequent changes in position relieve fatigue, increase comfort, and improve circulation. Therefore, a laboring woman should be encouraged to find positions that are most comfortable to her.

Positioning for second-stage labor may be determined by the woman's preference, but choices are limited by her condition or that of the fetus, the environment, and the health care provider's confidence in assisting in a birth in a specific position. See Chapter 19 for further discussion of positioning during labor and birth.

PROCESS OF LABOR

The term *labor* refers to the process of moving the fetus, placenta, and membranes out of the uterus and through the birth canal. Various changes take place in the woman's reproductive system in the days and weeks before labor begins. Labor itself can be discussed in terms of the mechanisms involved in the process and the stages through which the woman moves.

Signs Preceding Labor

In first-time pregnancies the uterus sinks downward and forward about 2 weeks before term, when the fetus's presenting part (usually the fetal head) descends into the true pelvis. This settling is called *lightening*, or dropping, and usually happens gradually. After lightening, women feel less pressure below the ribcage and breathe more easily, but usually more bladder pressure results from this shift. Consequently, a return of urinary frequency occurs. In a multiparous woman, lightening may not take place until after uterine contractions are established and true labor is in progress.

The woman may complain of persistent low backache and sacroiliac distress as a result of relaxation of the pelvic joints. She may identify strong and frequent but irregular uterine (Braxton Hicks) contractions.

The vaginal mucus becomes more profuse in response to the extreme congestion of the vaginal mucous membranes. Brownish or blood-tinged cervical mucus *(bloody show)* may be passed. The cervix becomes soft (ripens) and partially effaced and may begin to dilate. The membranes may rupture spontaneously.

Other phenomena are common in the days preceding labor: (1) loss of 0.5 to 1.5 kg (approximately 1 to 3½ pounds) in weight, caused by water loss resulting from electrolyte shifts that in turn are produced by changes in estrogen and progesterone levels; and (2) a surge of energy. Women speak of having a burst of energy that they often use to clean the house and put everything in order. Less commonly, some women have diarrhea, nausea, vomiting, and indigestion. Box 16-1 lists signs that may precede labor (see Clinical Reasoning Case Study).

CLINICAL REASONING CASE STUDY

"I Think I'm in Labor"

Erica is a 15-year-old G 1 P 0 at 39 weeks of gestation. She presents by ambulance to the triage area in your labor and birth unit and announces, "I'm here to have my baby. I think I'm in labor." Erica reports that she saw a thick brownish red vaginal discharge several days ago and noticed bright red vaginal spotting when wiping after peeing earlier today. She states that she has lower abdominal cramping ("It feels like the cramps I have with my periods") but denies leakage of vaginal fluid. Erica also reports active fetal movement. In answer to your question she replies that her current pain level is 8 on a scale of 1 to 10, while alternating between texting on her phone and chatting with her mother, who accompanied her to the hospital.

1. Evidence—Is there sufficient evidence at this time to draw a conclusion about whether Erica is in labor?
2. Assumptions—Describe an underlying assumption about each of the following issues:
   a. Characteristics of false labor
   b. Indications of true labor
   c. Basic teaching for Erica and her mother at this time
   d. Criteria necessary for discharging Erica from the labor and birth unit
3. What implications and priorities for nursing care can be drawn at this time?
4. Does the evidence objectively support your conclusion?

BOX 16-1 Signs Preceding Labor

- Lightening
- Return of urinary frequency
- Backache
- Stronger Braxton Hicks contractions
- Weight loss of 0.5 to 1.5 kg (approximately 1 to 3½ pounds)
- Surge of energy
- Increased vaginal discharge; bloody show
- Cervical ripening
- Possible rupture of membranes

Onset of Labor

The onset of true labor cannot be ascribed to a single cause. Many factors, including changes in the maternal uterus, cervix, and pituitary gland, are involved. Hormones produced by the normal fetal hypothalamus, pituitary, and adrenal cortex probably contribute to the onset of labor. Progressive uterine distention, increasing intrauterine pressure, and aging of the placenta seem to be associated with increasing myometrial irritability. This is a result of increased concentrations of estrogen and prostaglandins, as well as decreasing progesterone levels. The mutually coordinated effects of these factors result in the occurrence of strong, regular, rhythmic uterine contractions (Blackburn, 2013; Kilpatrick & Garrison, 2012). The outcome of these factors working together is normally the birth of the fetus and the expulsion of the placenta; however, how certain alterations trigger others and how proper checks and balances are maintained are not known.

Stages of Labor

The course of labor at or near term gestation in a woman without complications and a fetus in vertex presentation consists of (1) regular progression of uterine contractions, (2) effacement and progressive dilation of the cervix, and (3) progress in descent of the presenting part. Four stages of labor are recognized; an overview is discussed here. These stages are discussed in greater detail, along with nursing care for the laboring woman and family, in Chapter 19.

The *first stage of labor* is considered to last from the onset of regular uterine contractions to full effacement and dilation of the cervix. Commonly the onset of labor is difficult to establish because the woman may be admitted to the labor unit just before birth, and the beginning of labor may be only an estimate. The first stage is much longer than the second and third stages combined. Great variability is the rule, however, depending on the factors discussed previously in this chapter. The first stage of labor has traditionally been divided into three phases: a latent phase, an active phase, and a transition phase. In women who labor with epidural anesthesia, however, a separate transition phase may not always be identified based on maternal physical sensations and behavior (Simpson & O'Brien-Abel, 2014). During the latent phase there is more progress in effacement of the cervix and little increase in descent. During the active and transition phases there is more rapid dilation of the cervix and increased rate of descent of the presenting part.

The *second stage of labor* lasts from the time the cervix is fully dilated to the birth of the fetus. It is composed of two phases: the latent (passive fetal descent) phase and the active pushing

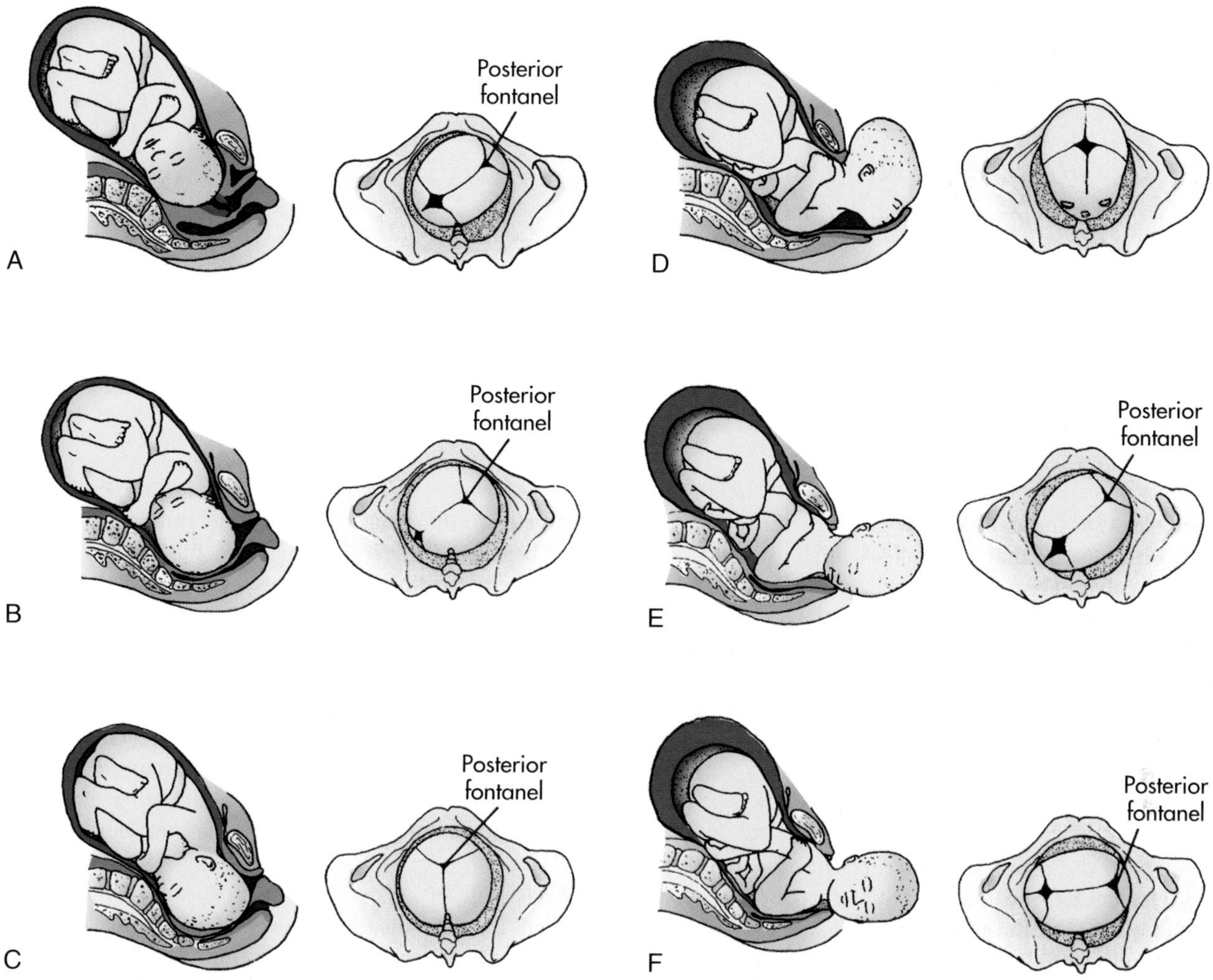

FIG 16-12 Cardinal movements of the mechanism of labor. Left occipitoanterior (LOA) position. Pelvic figures show the position of the fetal head as seen by the birth attendant. **A,** Engagement and descent. **B,** Flexion. **C,** Internal rotation to occipitoanterior position (OA). **D,** Extension. **E,** External rotation beginning (restitution). **F,** External rotation.

phase. During the latent phase the fetus continues to descend passively through the birth canal and rotate to an anterior position as a result of ongoing uterine contractions. The urge to bear down during this phase is not strong, and some women do not experience it at all. During the active pushing phase the woman has strong urges to bear down as the presenting part of the fetus descends and presses on the stretch receptors of the pelvic floor.

The *third stage of labor* lasts from the birth of the fetus until the placenta is delivered. The placenta normally separates with the third or fourth strong uterine contraction after the infant has been born. After it has separated, the placenta can be delivered with the next uterine contraction.

The *fourth stage of labor* begins with the delivery of the placenta and includes at least the first 2 hours after birth. During this stage the woman begins to recover physically from birth, so it is an important time to observe for complications, such as abnormal bleeding (see Chapter 33).

Mechanism of Labor

As already discussed, the female pelvis has varied contours and diameters at different levels, and the presenting part of the passenger is large in proportion to the passage. Therefore, for vaginal birth to occur, the fetus must adapt to the birth canal during the descent. The turns and other adjustments necessary in the human birth process are termed the *mechanism of labor* (Fig. 16-12). The seven cardinal movements of the mechanism of labor that occur in a vertex presentation are engagement, descent, flexion, internal rotation, extension, external rotation (restitution), and finally birth by expulsion. Although these movements are discussed separately, in actuality a combination of movements occurs simultaneously. For example, engagement involves both descent and flexion.

Engagement

When the biparietal diameter of the head passes the pelvic inlet, the head is said to be engaged in the pelvic inlet (see Fig. 16-12, *A*). In most nulliparous women, this occurs before the onset of active labor because the firmer abdominal muscles direct the presenting part into the pelvis. In multiparous women, because the abdominal musculature is more relaxed, the head often remains freely movable above the pelvic brim until labor is established.

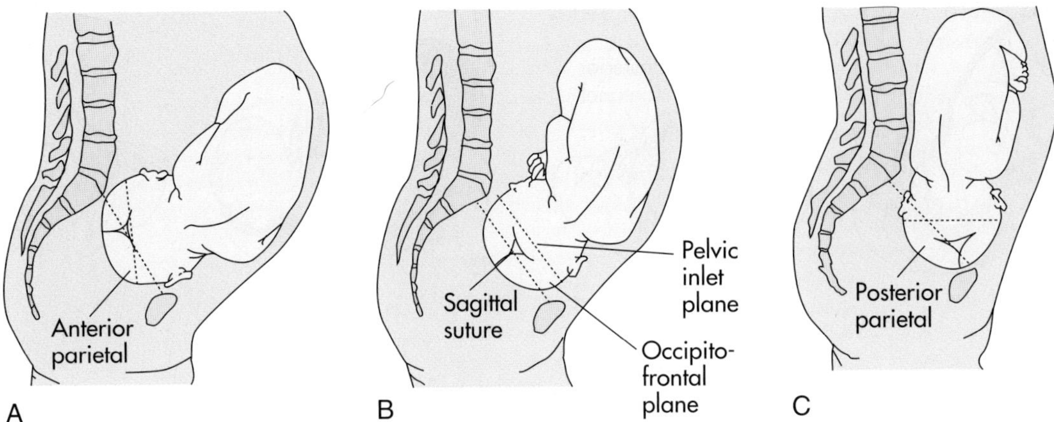

FIG 16-13 Synclitism and asynclitism. **A,** Anterior asynclitism. **B,** Normal synclitism. **C,** Posterior asynclitism.

Asynclitism. The head usually engages in the pelvis in a synclitic position—one that is parallel to the anteroposterior plane of the pelvis. Frequently asynclitism occurs (the head is deflected anteriorly or posteriorly in the pelvis), which can facilitate descent because the head is being positioned to accommodate to the pelvic cavity (Fig. 16-13). Extreme asynclitism can cause cephalopelvic disproportion, even in a normal-size pelvis, because the head is positioned so that it cannot descend.

Descent

Descent refers to the progress of the presenting part through the pelvis. Descent depends on at least four forces: (1) pressure exerted by the amniotic fluid, (2) direct pressure exerted by the contracting fundus on the fetus, (3) force of the contraction of the maternal diaphragm and abdominal muscles in the second stage of labor, and (4) extension and straightening of the fetal body. The effects of these forces are modified by the size and shape of the maternal pelvic planes and the size of the fetal head and its capacity to mold.

The degree of descent is measured by the station of the presenting part (see Fig. 16-6). As mentioned, little descent occurs during the latent phase of the first stage of labor. Descent accelerates in the active phase when the cervix has dilated to 5 to 6 cm. It is especially apparent when the membranes have ruptured.

In a first-time pregnancy descent is usually slow but steady; in subsequent pregnancies it may be rapid. Progress in descent of the presenting part is assessed by abdominal palpation and vaginal examination until the presenting part can be seen at the introitus (see Chapter 19).

Flexion

As soon as the descending head meets resistance from the cervix, pelvic wall, or pelvic floor, it normally flexes so that the chin is brought into closer contact with the fetal chest (see Fig. 16-12, *B*). Flexion permits the smaller suboccipitobregmatic diameter (9.5 cm) rather than the larger diameters to present to the outlet.

Internal Rotation

The maternal pelvic inlet is widest in the transverse diameter; therefore, the fetal head passes the inlet into the true pelvis in the occipitotransverse position. The outlet is widest in the anteroposterior diameter; for the fetus to exit, the head must rotate. Internal rotation begins at the level of the ischial spines but is not completed until the presenting part reaches the lower pelvis. As the occiput rotates anteriorly, the face rotates posteriorly. With each contraction the fetal head is guided by the bony pelvis and the muscles of the pelvic floor. Eventually the occiput will be in the midline beneath the pubic arch. The head is almost always rotated by the time it reaches the pelvic floor (see Fig. 16-12, *C*). Both the levator ani muscles and the bony pelvis are important for achieving anterior rotation. A previous childbirth injury or regional anesthesia may compromise the function of the levator sling.

Extension

When the fetal head reaches the perineum for birth, it is deflected anteriorly by the perineum. The occiput passes under the lower border of the symphysis pubis first, and then the head emerges by extension: first the occiput, then the face, and finally the chin (see Fig. 16-12, *D*).

Restitution and External Rotation

After the head is born it rotates briefly to the position it occupied when it was engaged in the inlet. This movement is referred to as restitution (see Fig. 16-12, *E*). The 45-degree turn realigns the infant's head with the back and shoulders. The head can then be seen to rotate further. This external rotation occurs as the shoulders engage and descend in maneuvers similar to those of the head (see Fig. 16-12, *F*). As noted, the anterior shoulder descends first. When it reaches the outlet, it rotates to the midline and is delivered from under the pubic arch. The posterior shoulder is guided over the perineum until it is free of the vaginal introitus.

Expulsion

After birth of the shoulders, the head and shoulders are lifted up toward the mother's pubic bone and the trunk of the baby is born by flexing it laterally in the direction of the symphysis pubis. When the baby has completely emerged, birth is complete, and the second stage of labor ends.

PHYSIOLOGIC ADAPTATION TO LABOR

In addition to the maternal and fetal anatomic adaptations that occur during birth, physiologic adaptations must occur.

Accurate assessment of the laboring woman and fetus requires knowledge of these expected adaptations.

Fetal Adaptation

Several important physiologic adaptations occur in the fetus. These changes occur in fetal heart rate, fetal circulation, respiratory movements, and other behaviors.

Fetal Heart Rate

Fetal heart rate (FHR) monitoring provides reliable and predictive information about the condition of the fetus related to oxygenation. The average FHR at term is 140 beats/minute; the normal range is 110 to 160 beats/minute. Earlier in gestation the FHR is higher, with an average of approximately 160 beats/minute at 20 weeks of gestation. The rate decreases progressively as the maturing fetus reaches term. However, temporary accelerations and slight early decelerations of the FHR can be expected in response to spontaneous fetal movement, vaginal examination, fundal pressure, uterine contractions, abdominal palpation, and fetal head compression. Stresses to the uterofetoplacental unit result in characteristic FHR patterns (see Chapter 18 for further discussion).

Fetal Circulation

Fetal circulation can be affected by many factors, including maternal position, uterine contractions, blood pressure, and umbilical cord blood flow. Uterine contractions during labor tend to decrease circulation through the spiral arterioles and subsequent perfusion through the intervillous space. Most healthy fetuses are well able to compensate for this stress and exposure to increased pressure while moving passively through the birth canal during labor. Usually the umbilical cord moves freely in the amniotic fluid. However, it can be compressed during uterine contractions (Blackburn, 2013; Miller, Miller, & Tucker, 2013).

Fetal Respiration

Certain changes stimulate chemoreceptors in the aorta and carotid bodies to prepare the fetus for initiating respirations immediately after birth (Blackburn, 2013; Rozance & Rosenberg, 2012). These changes include the following:

- Fetal lung fluid is cleared from the air passages as the infant passes through the birth canal during labor and (vaginal) birth.
- Fetal oxygen pressure (Po_2) decreases.
- Arterial carbon dioxide pressure (Pco_2) increases.
- Arterial pH decreases.
- Bicarbonate level decreases.
- Fetal respiratory movements decrease during labor.

Maternal Adaptation

As the woman progresses through the stages of labor, various body system adaptations cause her to exhibit both objective signs and subjective symptoms (Box 16-2).

Cardiovascular Changes

During each contraction an average of 400 ml of blood is emptied from the uterus into the maternal vascular system. By the end of the first stage of labor cardiac output during contractions is increased by 51% above baseline pregnancy values at term. Cardiac output peaks about 10 to 30 minutes after both vaginal and cesarean birth and returns to its prelabor baseline within the first postpartum hour. A drop in maternal heart rate accompanies this increase in cardiac output (Gordon, 2012).

Changes in blood pressure also occur. In general, both systolic and diastolic pressures increase during contractions and return to baseline levels between contractions. Systolic values increase more than diastolic values (Blackburn, 2013).

Supine hypotension (see Fig. 19-5) occurs when the ascending vena cava and descending aorta are compressed. The laboring woman is at greater risk for supine hypotension when the uterus is particularly large because of multifetal pregnancy, hydramnios, or obesity or when the woman is dehydrated or hypovolemic. In addition, anxiety and pain, as well as some medications, can cause hypotension.

The woman should be discouraged from using the Valsalva maneuver (holding one's breath and tightening abdominal muscles) for pushing during the second stage. This activity increases intrathoracic pressure, reduces venous return, and increases venous pressure. The cardiac output and blood pressure increase and the pulse slows temporarily. During the Valsalva maneuver fetal hypoxia may occur. The process is reversed when the woman takes a breath.

The white blood cell (WBC) count can increase (Blackburn, 2013). Although the mechanism leading to this increase in WBCs is unknown, it may be secondary to physical or emotional stress or to tissue trauma. Labor is strenuous, and physical exercise alone can increase the WBC count.

Some peripheral vascular changes occur, perhaps in response to cervical dilation or to compression of maternal vessels by the fetus passing through the birth canal. Flushed cheeks, hot or cold feet, and eversion of hemorrhoids may result.

Respiratory Changes

Increased physical activity with greater oxygen consumption is reflected in an increase in the respiratory rate. Hyperventilation may cause respiratory alkalosis (an increase in pH), hypoxia, and hypocapnia (decrease in carbon dioxide). In the unmedicated woman in the second stage of labor, oxygen consumption almost doubles. Anxiety also increases oxygen consumption.

BOX 16-2 Maternal Physiologic Changes During Labor

- Cardiac output increases 10% to 15% in first stage, 30% to 50% in second stage.
- Heart rate increases slightly in first and second stages.
- Blood pressure (both systolic and diastolic) increases during contractions and returns to baseline levels between contractions. Systolic values increase more than diastolic values.
- White blood cell (WBC) count increases.
- Respiratory rate increases.
- Temperature may be slightly elevated.
- Proteinuria may occur.
- Gastric motility and absorption of solid food are decreased; nausea and vomiting may occur during transition to secondstage labor.
- Blood glucose level decreases.

Renal Changes

During labor, spontaneous voiding may be difficult for various reasons: tissue edema caused by pressure from the presenting part, discomfort, analgesia, and embarrassment. Proteinuria of 1+ is a normal finding because it can occur in response to the breakdown of muscle tissue from the physical work of labor.

Integumentary Changes

The integumentary system changes are evident, especially in the great stretching of tissue that occurs in the area of the vaginal introitus. The degree of distensibility varies with the individual. Despite this ability to stretch, even in the absence of episiotomy or lacerations minute tears in the skin around the vaginal introitus do occur.

Musculoskeletal Changes

The musculoskeletal system is stressed during labor. Diaphoresis, fatigue, proteinuria (1+), and possibly an increased temperature accompany the marked increase in muscle activity. Backache and joint aches (unrelated to fetal position) occur as a result of increased joint laxity at term. The labor process itself and the woman's pointing her toes can cause leg cramps.

Neurologic Changes

Sensorial changes occur as the woman moves through the phases of the first stage of labor and as she moves from one stage to the next. Initially she may be euphoric. Euphoria gives way to increased seriousness, then to amnesia between contractions during the second stage, and finally to elation or fatigue after giving birth. Endogenous endorphins (morphine-like chemicals produced naturally by the body) raise the pain threshold and produce sedation. In addition, physiologic anesthesia of perineal tissues, caused by pressure of the presenting part, decreases perception of pain.

Gastrointestinal Changes

During labor gastrointestinal motility and absorption of solid foods are decreased, and stomach-emptying time is slowed. Nausea and vomiting of undigested food eaten after the onset of labor are common. Nausea and belching also occur as a reflex response to full cervical dilation. The woman may state that diarrhea accompanied the onset of labor, or the nurse may palpate the presence of hard or impacted stool in the rectum.

Endocrine Changes

The onset of labor may be triggered by decreasing levels of progesterone and increasing levels of estrogen, prostaglandins, and oxytocin (Simpson & O'Brien-Abel, 2014). Metabolism increases, and blood glucose levels may decrease with the work of labor.

KEY POINTS

- Labor and birth are affected by the five P's: *p*assenger, *p*assageway, *p*owers, *p*osition of the woman, and *p*sychologic response.
- Because of its size and relative rigidity, the fetal head is a major factor in determining the course of birth.
- The diameters at the plane of the pelvic inlet, the midpelvis, and the outlet plus the axis of the birth canal determine whether vaginal birth is possible and the manner in which the fetus passes down the birth canal.
- Involuntary uterine contractions act to expel the fetus and placenta during the first stage of labor; these are augmented by voluntary bearing-down efforts during the second stage.
- The first stage of labor lasts from the time dilation begins to the time when the cervix is fully dilated.
- The second stage of labor lasts from the time of full cervical dilation to the birth of the infant.
- The third stage of labor lasts from the infant's birth to the expulsion of the placenta.
- The fourth stage of labor begins with the delivery of the placenta and includes at least the first 2 hours after birth.
- The cardinal movements of the mechanism of labor are engagement, descent, flexion, internal rotation, extension, restitution and external rotation, and expulsion of the infant.
- Although the events precipitating the onset of labor are unknown, many factors, including changes in the maternal uterus, cervix, and pituitary gland, are thought to be involved.
- A healthy fetus with an adequate uterofetoplacental circulation is able to compensate for the stress of uterine contractions.
- As the woman progresses through labor, various body systems adapt to the birth process.

REFERENCES

Blackburn, S. (2013). *Maternal, fetal, and neonatal physiology: A clinical perspective* (4th ed.). St. Louis: Saunders.

Cunningham, F., Leveno, K., Bloom, S., et al. (2014). *Williams obstetrics* (24th ed.). New York: McGraw-Hill Education.

Gordon, M. (2012). Maternal physiology. In S. Gabbe, J. Niebyl, & J. Simpson (Eds.), *Obstetrics: Normal and problem pregnancies* (6th ed.). Philadelphia: Saunders.

Kilpatrick, S., & Garrison, E. (2012). Normal labor and delivery. In S. Gabbe, J. Niebyl, & J. Simpson (Eds.), *Obstetrics: Normal and problem pregnancies* (6th ed.). Philadelphia: Saunders.

Miller, L., Miller, D., & Tucker, S. (2013). *Mosby's pocket guide to fetal monitoring: A multidisciplinary approach* (7th ed.). St. Louis: Mosby.

Rozance, P., & Rosenberg, L. (2012). The neonate. In S. Gabbe, J. Niebyl, & J. Simpson (Eds.), *Obstetrics: Normal and problem pregnancies* (6th ed.). Philadelphia: Saunders.

Simpson, K., & O'Brien-Abel, N. (2014). Labor and birth. In K. Rice Simpson & P. Creehan (Eds.), *AWHONN's perinatal nursing* (4th ed.). Philadelphia: Lippincott Williams & Wilkins.

Thorp, J. M., & Laughon, S. K. (2014). Clinical aspects of normal and abnormal labor. In R. K. Creasy, R. Resnik, J. D. Iams, et al. (Eds.), *Creasy and Resnik's maternal-fetal medicine: Principles and practice* (7th ed.). Philadelphia: Saunders.

VandeVusse, L. (1999). The essential forces of labor revisited: 13 Ps reported in women's birth stories. *MCN: The American Journal of Maternal/Child Nursing, 24*(4), 176–184.

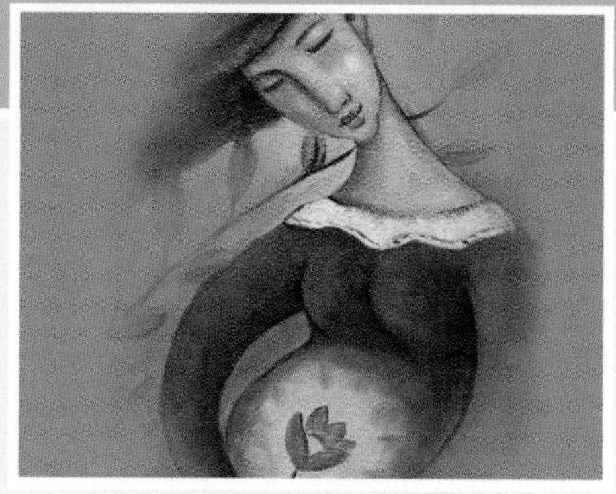

CHAPTER 17

Maximizing Comfort for the Laboring Woman

Cheryl R. Zauderer

http://evolve.elsevier.com/Lowdermilk/MWHC/

LEARNING OBJECTIVES

- Identify nonpharmacologic strategies, including breathing and relaxation techniques, used to enhance relaxation and promote comfort during labor and birth.
- Compare pharmacologic methods used to relieve discomfort in different stages of labor and for vaginal or cesarean birth.
- Discuss the effects of medication management for the mother and its effect on the newborn both during and after birth.
- Construct an evidence-based plan to manage the discomfort that a woman experiences during childbirth.
- Explain the nurse's role and responsibilities while providing care for a woman receiving analgesia or anesthesia during labor.
- Describe the nurse's role in promoting comfort and safety throughout the labor and birth process.

Although labor and birth are considered to be natural processes, laboring women experience a significant amount of discomfort and pain, as well as a variety of other challenging sensations. Pain is a highly individualized phenomenon with sensory and emotional components. Even though most women experience discomfort or pain during labor and birth it is the intensity of discomfort that is unique to the individual. Pregnant women are generally concerned about the discomfort and pain that they will experience during labor and birth and about how they will respond to and cope with it. A large variety of nonpharmacologic and pharmacologic methods are available to help the woman or the couple maximize her comfort during the labor process. The methods that are selected depend on the situation, availability, and preferences of the woman, her partner, and her health care provider.

PAIN DURING LABOR AND BIRTH

Neurologic Origins

The pain and discomfort of labor have two origins: visceral and somatic. During the first stage of labor, uterine contractions cause cervical dilation and effacement. Uterine ischemia (decreased blood flow and therefore local oxygen deficit) results from compression of the arteries supplying the myometrium during uterine contractions. Pain impulses during the first stage of labor are transmitted via the T1 to T12 spinal nerve segment and accessory lower thoracic and upper lumbar sympathetic nerves. These nerves originate in the uterine body and cervix (Blackburn, 2013).

The pain from distention of the lower uterine segment, stretching of cervical tissue as it effaces and dilates, pressure and traction on adjacent structures (e.g., uterine tubes, ovaries, ligaments) and nerves, and uterine ischemia during the first stage of labor is visceral pain. It is located over the lower portion of the abdomen. Referred pain occurs when pain that originates in the uterus radiates to the abdominal wall, lumbosacral area of the back, iliac crests, gluteal area, thighs, and lower back (Blackburn, 2013).

During most of the first stage of labor the woman usually has discomfort only during contractions, and is free of pain between contractions. Some women, especially those whose fetus is in a posterior position, experience continuous contraction-related low back pain, even in the interval between contractions. As labor progresses and pain becomes more intense and persistent, women become fatigued and discouraged, often experiencing difficulty coping with contractions (Blackburn, 2013; Burke, 2014).

During the second stage of labor the woman has somatic pain, which is often described as intense, sharp, burning, and well localized. This pain results from:

- Distention and traction on the peritoneum and uterocervical supports during contractions
- Pressure against the bladder and rectum
- Stretching and distention of perineal tissues and the pelvic floor to allow passage of the fetus
- Lacerations of soft tissue (e.g., cervix, vagina, and perineum)

As women concentrate on the work of bearing down to give birth, they may report a decrease in pain intensity (Blackburn, 2013; Burke, 2014). Pain impulses during the second stage of labor are transmitted via the pudendal nerve through S2 to S4 spinal nerve segments and the parasympathetic system (Blackburn).

Pain experienced during the third stage of labor, and the afterpains of the early postpartum period are uterine, similar to the pain experienced early in the first stage of labor. Areas of discomfort during labor are shown in Figure 17-1.

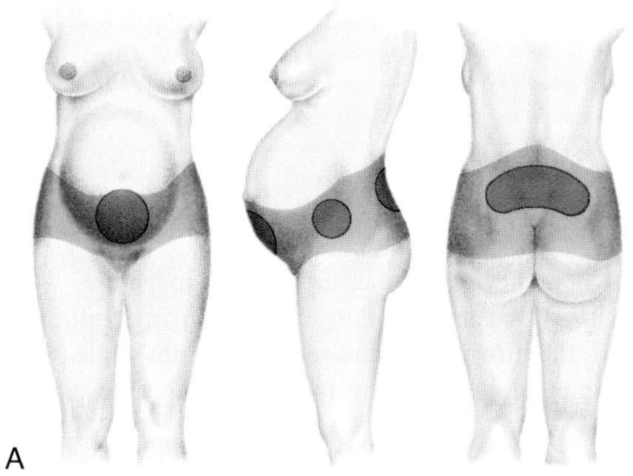

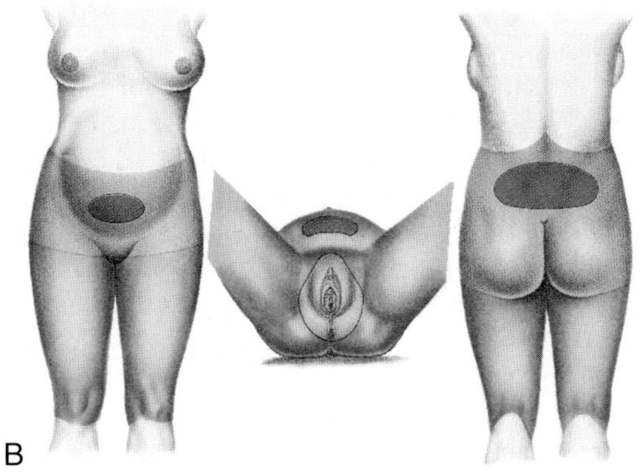

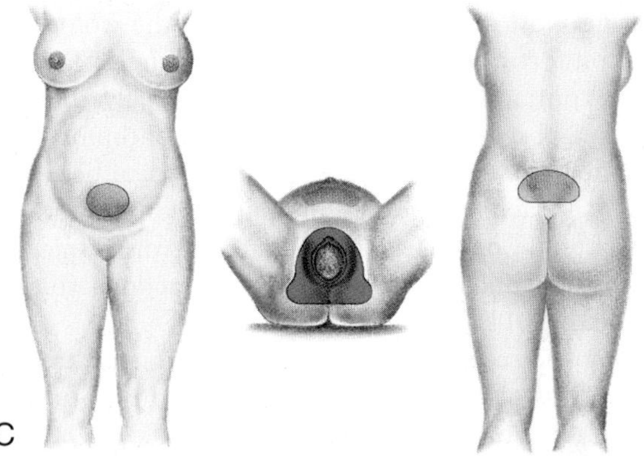

FIG 17-1 Discomfort during labor. **A,** Distribution of labor pain during first stage. **B,** Distribution of labor pain during transition and early phase of second stage. **C,** Distribution of pain during late second stage and actual birth. (*Gray* areas indicate mild discomfort; *light pink* areas indicate moderate discomfort; *dark red* areas indicate intense discomfort.)

Perception of Pain

Although the pain threshold is remarkably similar in everyone regardless of gender and social, ethnic, or cultural differences, these differences play a definite role in the person's perception of and behavioral responses to pain. Fear and lack of information can certainly increase the amount of pain and discomfort a laboring woman experiences. On the other hand, knowledge, a positive attitude, and support result in decreased pain perception and less use of medication during labor (Weatherspoon, 2011).

Pain tolerance refers to the level of pain a laboring woman is willing to endure. When this level is exceeded, she will seek measures to relieve the pain. Factors that influence her pain tolerance level and her request for pharmacologic pain relief measures include her desire for a natural, vaginal birth; her preparation for childbirth; her level of anxiety; the nature of her support during labor; and her willingness and ability to participate in nonpharmacologic measures for comfort (Weatherspoon, 2011).

Expression of Pain

Pain results in physiologic effects and sensory and emotional (affective) responses. During childbirth the pain or discomfort experienced gives rise to identifiable physiologic effects. Sympathetic nervous system activity is stimulated in response to intensifying pain, resulting in increased catecholamine levels. Blood pressure and heart rate increase. Maternal respiratory patterns change in response to an increase in oxygen consumption. Hyperventilation, sometimes accompanied by respiratory alkalosis, can occur as pain intensifies and more rapid, shallow breathing techniques are used during contractions. Pallor and diaphoresis may be seen. Gastric acidity increases, and nausea and vomiting are common in the active and transition phases of the first stage of labor. Placental perfusion may decrease, and uterine activity may diminish, potentially prolonging labor and affecting fetal well-being.

Certain emotional (affective) expressions of pain often are seen. Such changes include increasing anxiety with lessened perceptual field, writhing, crying, groaning, gesturing (hand clenching and wringing), and excessive muscular excitability throughout the body

FACTORS INFLUENCING PAIN RESPONSE

Pain during childbirth is unique to each woman. How she perceives or interprets that pain is influenced by a variety of physiologic, psychologic, emotional, social, cultural, and environmental factors.

Physiologic Factors

A variety of physiologic factors can affect the intensity of the childbirth experience. Uterine contractions, cervical dilation, and effacement are important aspects of labors, and can be the cause of discomfort and pain (Nur Rachmawati, 2012). Fatigue, anxiety, the interval and duration of contractions, fetal size and position, rapidity of fetal descent, maternal position, and maternal mobility during labor also affect a woman's perception of the intensity of childbirth contractions.

Beta-endorphins are endogenous opioids secreted by the pituitary gland that act on the central and peripheral nervous systems to reduce pain. The level of beta-endorphins increases during pregnancy and birth in humans. Beta-endorphins are associated with feelings of euphoria and analgesia. The pain threshold may rise as beta-endorphin levels increase, enabling women in labor to tolerate acute pain (Blackburn, 2013).

Culture

The population of pregnant women reflects the increasingly multicultural nature of society in the United States. As nurses care for women and families from a variety of cultural backgrounds, they must have knowledge and understanding of how culture mediates pain. Although all women expect to experience at least some pain and discomfort during childbirth, it is their culture and religious belief system that determine how they will perceive, interpret, respond to, and manage the pain. Cultural influences may impose certain behavioral expectations regarding acceptable and unacceptable behavior when experiencing pain (Burke, 2014). Women with strong religious beliefs, for example, often accept pain as a necessary and inevitable part of bringing a new life into the world, whereas others tend to vocalize their pain by moaning, breathing rhythmically, or shouting (Andrews & Boyle, 2012).

An understanding of the beliefs, values, expectations, and practices of various cultures narrows the cultural gap and helps the nurse assess the laboring woman's pain experience more accurately. The nurse can then provide appropriate, culturally sensitive care by using pain relief measures that preserve the woman's sense of control and self-confidence (see Cultural Considerations box). Recognize that although a woman's behavior in response to pain may vary according to her cultural background, it may not accurately reflect the intensity of the pain she is experiencing. Assess the woman for the physiologic effects of pain, and listen to the words she uses to describe the sensory and affective qualities of her pain.

CULTURAL CONSIDERATIONS

Some Cultural Beliefs About Childbirth and Pain

The following examples demonstrate how women of different cultural backgrounds may react to pain. Because they are generalizations, the nurse must assess each woman experiencing pain related to childbirth.

- Chinese women may not exhibit reactions to pain, although exhibiting pain during childbirth is acceptable. They consider accepting something when it is first offered as impolite; therefore, pain interventions must be offered more than once. Acupuncture may be used for pain relief.
- Arab or Middle Eastern women may be vocal in response to labor pain. They may prefer medication for pain relief.
- Japanese women may be stoic in response to labor pain, but they may request medication when pain becomes severe.
- Southeast Asian women may endure severe pain before requesting relief.
- Hispanic women may be stoic until late in labor, when they may become vocal and request pain relief.
- Native-American women may use medications or remedies made from indigenous plants. They are often stoic in response to labor pain.
- African-American women may express pain openly. Use of medication for pain relief varies.

Anxiety

Anxiety is commonly associated with increased pain during labor. Mild anxiety is considered normal for a woman during labor and birth. However, excessive anxiety and fear cause more catecholamine secretion, which increases the stimuli to the brain from the pelvis because of decreased blood flow and increased muscle tension. This action, in turn, magnifies pain perception. Therefore, as anxiety and fear heighten, muscle tension increases, the effectiveness of uterine contractions decreases, the experience of discomfort increases, and a cycle of increased fear and anxiety begins (Blackburn, 2013). Ultimately this cycle will slow the progress of labor. The woman's confidence in her ability to cope with pain will be diminished, potentially resulting in reduced effectiveness of the pain relief measures being used.

Previous Experience

Previous experience with pain and childbirth may affect a woman's description of her pain and her ability to cope with the pain. Childbirth for a healthy young woman may be her first experience with significant pain, and as a result, she may not have developed effective pain coping strategies. She may describe the intensity of even early labor pain as pain "as bad as it can be." The nature of previous childbirth experiences also may affect a woman's responses to pain. For women who have had a difficult and painful previous birth experience, anxiety and fear from this past experience may lead to increased pain perception.

Sensory labor pain for nulliparous women is often greater than for multiparous women during early labor (dilation less than 5 cm) because their reproductive tract structures are less flexible. However, during the transition phase of the first stage of labor and during the second stage of labor, multiparous women may experience greater sensory pain than nulliparous women because their flexible tissue increases the speed of fetal descent and thereby intensifies discomfort. The firmer tissue of nulliparous women results in a slower, more gradual descent (Archie & Roman, 2013).

Parity may affect the perception of labor pain because nulliparous women often have longer labors and therefore greater fatigue. Fatigue magnifies pain, thus causing many women to have an increased perception of the intensity of pain during labor.

Gate-Control Theory of Pain

Intense pain stimuli can at times be ignored. This is possible because certain nerve cell groupings within the spinal cord, brainstem, and cerebral cortex have the ability to modulate the pain impulse through a blocking mechanism. This **gate-control theory of pain** helps explain the way hypnosis and the pain relief techniques taught in childbirth preparation classes work to relieve the pain of labor. According to this theory pain sensations travel along sensory nerve pathways to the brain, but only a limited number of sensations, or messages, can travel through these nerve pathways at one time. Using distraction techniques such as massage or effleurage, stroking, music, focal points, and imagery reduces or completely blocks the capacity of nerve pathways to transmit pain. These distractions are thought to work by closing down a hypothetic gate in the spinal cord, thus preventing pain signals from reaching the brain. The perception of pain is thereby diminished (Dean, Gwilym, & Carr, 2013).

In addition, when the laboring woman engages in neuromuscular and motor activity, activity within the spinal cord itself further modifies the transmission of pain. Cognitive work involving concentration on breathing and relaxation requires selective and directed cortical activity that activates and closes the gating mechanism as well. As labor intensifies, more complex cognitive techniques are required to maintain effectiveness. The main impetus behind the gate-control theory as it relates to pain is to introduce the brain to a positive stimulus by using all of the five senses. The brain then begins to accept the more positive stimulus, while paying less attention to negative stimuli such as discomfort or pain. Stimulating the senses will not create a pain-free environment, but it can help decrease the discomforts of labor.

Comfort

Although the predominant medical approach to labor is that it is painful, and the pain must be removed, an alternative view is that labor is a natural process in which women can experience comfort and transcend the discomfort or pain to reach the joyful outcome of birth. Having needs and desires met promotes a feeling of comfort. The most helpful interventions in enhancing comfort are a caring nursing approach and a supportive presence.

Support

Evidence indicates that a woman's satisfaction with her labor and birth experience is determined by how well her personal expectations of childbirth were met and the quality of support and interaction she received from her caregivers and partners (Box 17-1). In addition, satisfaction is influenced by the degree to which she was able to stay in control of her labor and to participate in decision making regarding her labor, including the nonpharmacologic and pharmacologic pain relief measures to be used (Devereaux & Sullivan, 2013).

The value of the continuous supportive presence of a person (e.g., doula, childbirth educator, family member, friend, nurse, or partner) during labor who provides physical comforting, facilitates communication, and offers information and guidance to the woman in labor has long been known. Emotional support is demonstrated by giving praise and reassurance and conveying a positive, calm, and confident demeanor when caring for the woman in labor (Borders, Wendland, Haozous, et al., 2013). Women who have continuous support beginning early in labor are less likely to use pain medications or epidural analgesia or anesthesia and are more likely to experience a spontaneous vaginal birth and express satisfaction with their childbirth experience. Interestingly, research findings concluded that a more positive effect was achieved when continuous support was provided by people other than hospital staff members (Hodnett, Gates, Hofmeyr, & Sakala, 2013).

BOX 17-1 Suggested Measures for Supporting a Woman in Labor

- Provide companionship and reassurance.
- Offer positive reinforcement and praise for her efforts.
- Encourage participation in distracting activities and nonpharmacologic measures for comfort.
- Give nourishment (if allowed by primary health care provider).
- Assist with personal hygiene.
- Offer information and advice.
- Involve the woman in decision making regarding her care.
- Interpret the woman's wishes to other health care providers and to her support group.
- Create a relaxing environment.
- Use a calm and confident approach.
- Support and encourage the woman's support people by role-modeling labor support measures and providing time for breaks.

Environment

When the childbearing woman experiences discomfort in labor, the quality of her environment can contribute to her having a more positive experience. The woman's environment includes the individuals present (e.g., how they communicate; their philosophy of care, including a belief in the value of nonpharmacologic pain relief measures; practice policies; and quality of support) and the physical space in which the labor occurs. Women who are in a supportive environment feel more in control and therefore are more likely to have a better labor and birth experience. Studies have shown a correlation between control in childbirth and increased satisfaction with the entire childbirth experience (Meyer, 2013).

Women usually prefer to be cared for by familiar caregivers in a comfortable, homelike setting. The environment should be safe and private, allowing a woman to feel free to be herself as she tries out different comfort measures. Stimuli such as light, noise, and temperature should be adjusted according to her preferences. The environment should have space for movement, position changes, ambulation, and equipment such as birthing balls. Comfortable chairs, tubs, and showers should be readily available to facilitate participation in a variety of nonpharmacologic pain relief measures. Bringing items from home such as pillows, objects for a focal point, music, iPad, or DVDs can enhance the familiarity of the environment.

NONPHARMACOLOGIC PAIN MANAGEMENT

Relieving or reducing pain is important. Commonly it is not the amount of pain the woman experiences but whether she meets the goals she set for herself to cope with the pain that influences her perception of the birth experience as good or bad. The observant nurse looks for clues to the woman's desired level of control in the management of pain and its relief.

The labor and birth nurse can use a variety of nonpharmacologic methods for pain relief while providing support and encouragement to the laboring woman and her partner. Nonpharmacologic measures are often simple and safe, have few if any major adverse reactions, are relatively inexpensive, and can be used throughout labor. Additionally, they provide the woman with a sense of control over her childbirth as she makes choices about the measures that are best for her. During the prenatal period she should explore a variety of nonpharmacologic measures. Techniques she usually finds helpful in relieving stress and enhancing relaxation (e.g., music, meditation, massage, warm baths) may be very effective as components of a plan for managing labor pain. The woman should be encouraged to communicate to her health care providers her preferences for relaxation and pain relief measures and to actively participate in their implementation (see Clinical Reasoning Case Study).

CLINICAL REASONING CASE STUDY

Making Decisions Regarding Pain Management for Labor

Diana is a 33-year-old G 2 P 1, who has just been admitted to the labor and birth unit in active labor at 39 weeks of gestation. Her cervix is dilated to 7 cm on admission. Diana attended childbirth classes and is considered to have a low risk pregnancy. According to her birth plan, she wants to have a natural childbirth, without pharmacologic interventions. Diana was not satisfied with her experience during the labor and birth of her first child. For that birth she had an epidural, which required an IV and an indwelling urinary catheter. Because Diana was unable to push effectively during second stage labor she had a vacuum-assisted birth and a third-degree episiotomy. Diana does not want to repeat her prior birth experience this time. She is also very concerned about receiving medications that could harm her baby. Soon after admission Diana expresses discomfort and states, "I don't know if I can do this. I think I need an epidural!"

1. Evidence—Is there sufficient evidence regarding nonpharmacologic and pharmacologic pain relief measures in labor to make recommendations to Diana?
2. Assumptions—Describe the underlying assumptions about each of the following issues:
   a. Timing of transitional phase of first stage labor and possible epidural
   b. Effectiveness of physical and emotional support on the labor process
   c. Approaches that are proven to reduce the use of pharmacologic measures
3. What implications and priorities for nursing care can be drawn at this time?
4. Does the evidence objectively support your conclusion?

Many of the nonpharmacologic methods for relief of discomfort are taught in different types of prenatal preparation classes, or the woman or couple may have read various books and magazine articles on the subject in advance. Many of these methods require practice for best results (e.g., hypnosis, patterned breathing and controlled relaxation techniques, biofeedback, focal point, distraction), although the nurse may use some of them successfully without the woman or couple having prior knowledge (e.g., slow-paced breathing, massage and touch, effleurage, counterpressure, relaxation, music, hot or cold packs, movement or positioning). Women should be encouraged to try a variety of methods and to seek alternatives, including pharmacologic methods, when the measure being used is no longer effective (Burke, 2014).

Because of the increased use of epidural analgesia or anesthesia, nurses may be less likely to encourage women to use nonpharmacologic pain relief measures, in part because these methods may be viewed as more complex and time consuming than monitoring a woman receiving an epidural. In addition, new nurses may not have had the opportunity to develop skill in the implementation of these methods. It is imperative that perinatal nurses develop a commitment to and expertise in using a variety of nonpharmacologic pain relief strategies in order for women in labor to be comfortable using them. Although research data to support the effectiveness of many of these nonpharmacologic measures are limited, there are sufficient reports of their benefits from women and health care providers to recommend that nurses encourage their use. These methods are less invasive and safer for mother and baby. Nonpharmacologic methods of pain relief also allow the normal course of labor to progress more efficiently, as opposed to pharmacologic methods, which tend to interrupt or even slow the labor process. Pharmacologic methods may also influence subsequent neonatal behavior and its effect on breastfeeding. The analgesic effect of many nonpharmacologic measures is comparable to or even superior to opioids that are administered parenterally (Jones, Othman, Dowswell, et al., 2012) (Box 17-2).

Childbirth Preparation Methods

The childbirth education movement began in the 1950s. Today most health care providers recommend or offer childbirth preparation classes for expectant parents. Historically, popular childbirth methods taught in the United States were the Dick-Read method, the Lamaze (psychoprophylaxis) method, and the Bradley (husband-coached childbirth) method. Although these three organizations continue to exist, they are now less focused on a "method" approach. Rather, women are assisted to develop their birth philosophy and inner knowledge and then choose from a variety of skills to use to cope with the labor process. Many childbirth educators teach a variety of techniques that originated in several different organizations or publications. Women are encouraged to choose the techniques that work best for them.

Gaining popularity are methods developed and promoted by Birthing From Within (www.birthingfromwithin.com), Birthworks (www.birthworks.org), Association of Labor Assistants and Childbirth Educators (ALACE) (www.alace.org), Childbirth and Postpartum Professional Association (CAPPA) (www.cappa.net), and HypnoBirthing (www.hypnobirthing.com), to name a few. These methods offer classes and other services that focus on fostering a woman's confidence in her innate ability

BOX 17-2 Nonpharmacologic Strategies to Encourage Relaxation and Relieve Pain

Cutaneous Stimulation Strategies

- Counterpressure
- Effleurage (light massage)
- Therapeutic touch and massage
- Walking
- Rocking
- Changing positions
- Application of heat or cold
- Transcutaneous electrical nerve stimulation (TENS)
- Acupressure
- Water therapy (showers, whirlpool baths)
- Intradermal water block

Sensory Stimulation Strategies

- Aromatherapy
- Breathing techniques
- Music
- Imagery
- Use of focal points

Cognitive Strategies

- Childbirth education
- Hypnosis
- Biofeedback

to give birth. The woman or couple is helped to recognize the uniqueness of their pregnancy and childbirth experience.

Relaxation and Breathing Techniques

Focusing and Relaxation Techniques

By reducing tension and stress, focusing and relaxation techniques allow a woman in labor to rest and conserve energy for the task of giving birth. *Attention-focusing* and *distraction* techniques are forms of care that are effective to some degree in relieving labor pain (Jones et al., 2012). Some women bring a favorite object such as a photograph or stuffed animal to the labor room and focus their attention on this object during contractions. Others choose to fix their attention on some object in the labor room. As the contraction begins, they focus on their chosen object and perform a breathing technique to reduce their perception of pain.

With *imagery* the woman focuses her attention on a pleasant scene, a place where she feels relaxed, or an activity she enjoys. She can imagine walking through a restful garden or breathing in light, energy, and a healing color and breathing out worries and tension. Choosing the subject for the imagery and practicing the technique during pregnancy enhance effectiveness during labor.

During childbirth preparation classes the coach can learn how to palpate a woman's body to detect tense and contracted muscles. The woman then learns how to relax the tense muscle in response to the gentle stroking of the muscle by the coach (Fig. 17-2). In a common feedback mechanism, the woman and her coach say the word "relax" at the onset of each contraction and throughout it as needed. With practice the coach can effectively use support, feedback, and touch to facilitate the woman's relaxation and thereby reduce tension and stress and enhance the progress of labor (Burke, 2014).

Women may find that drinking herbal tea during labor can help them to relax (e.g., chamomile), to reduce nausea (e.g., lemon balm, peppermint), and to enhance energy and reduce fatigue (e.g., ginger, ginseng). Drinking tea can have the additional benefit of maintaining fluid balance (Walls, 2009).

The nurse can assist the woman by providing a quiet and relaxed environment, offering cues as needed, and recognizing signs of tension (e.g., frowning, change in tone of voice, clenching of fists). A relaxed environment for labor is created by controlling sensory stimuli (e.g., light, noise, temperature), and reducing interruptions. Nurses should remain calm and unhurried in their approach and sit rather than stand at the bedside whenever possible (Burke, 2014).

Breathing Techniques

Different approaches to childbirth preparation stress varying breathing techniques to provide distraction, thereby reducing the perception of pain and helping the woman maintain control throughout contractions. In the first stage of labor such breathing techniques can promote relaxation of the abdominal muscles and thereby increase the size of the abdominal cavity. This lessens discomfort generated by friction between the uterus and abdominal wall during contractions. Because the muscles of the genital area also become more relaxed, they do not interfere with fetal descent. In the second stage, breathing is used to increase abdominal pressure and thereby assist in expelling the fetus. Breathing also can be used to relax the pudendal muscles to prevent precipitate expulsion of the fetal head (Fig. 17-3).

For couples who have prepared for labor by practicing relaxing and breathing techniques, a simple review with occasional reminders may be all that is necessary to help them along. For those who have had no preparation, instruction and practice in simple breathing and relaxation techniques can be given early in labor and often are surprisingly successful. Nurses can also model breathing techniques and breathe in synchrony with the woman and her partner. Motivation is high, and readiness to learn is enhanced by the reality of labor.

Various breathing techniques can be used for controlling pain during contractions (Box 17-3). The nurse needs to determine what, if any, techniques the laboring couple know before giving them instruction. Simple patterns are more easily learned. **Paced breathing** is most associated with prepared childbirth and includes slow-paced, modified-paced, and patterned-paced (pant-blow) breathing techniques. Each labor is different, and nursing support includes assisting

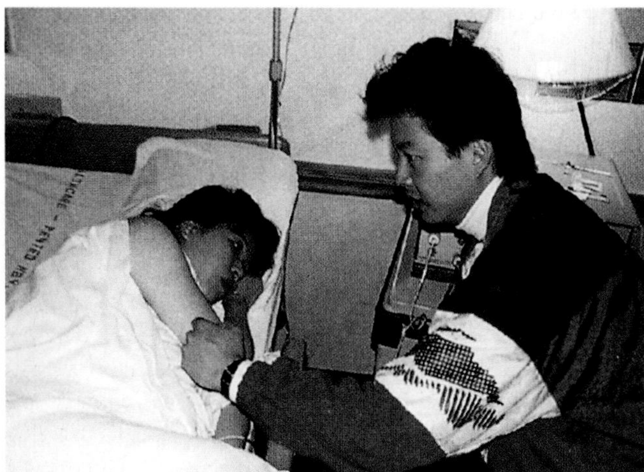

FIG 17-2 A laboring woman using focusing and breathing techniques during a uterine contraction with coaching from her partner. (Courtesy Marjorie Pyle, RNC, Lifecircle, Costa Mesa, CA.)

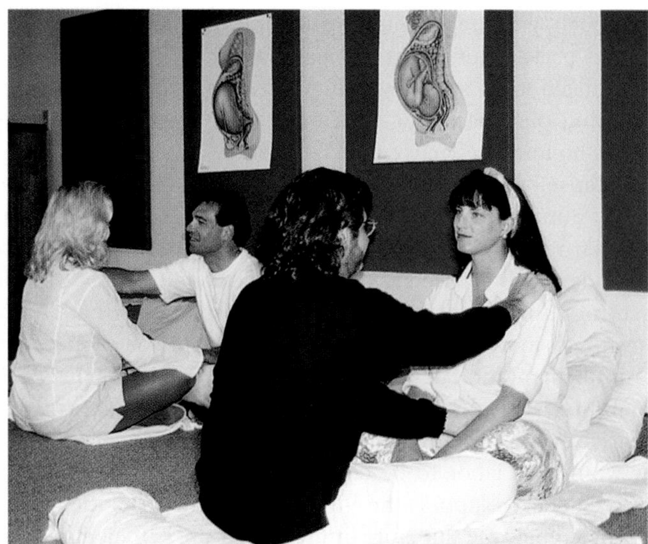

FIG 17-3 Expectant parents learning relaxation techniques. (Courtesy Marjorie Pyle, RNC, Lifecircle, Costa Mesa, CA.)

couples to adapt breathing techniques to their individual labor experience.

All patterns begin with a deep, relaxing, cleansing breath to "greet the contraction" and end with another deep breath exhaled to "gently blow the contraction away." These deep breaths ensure adequate oxygen for mother and baby and signal that a contraction is beginning or has ended. As the breath is exhaled, respiratory and voluntary muscles relax (Burke, 2014). In general, *slow-paced breathing* is performed at approximately half the woman's normal breathing rate and is initiated when she can no longer walk or talk through contractions. The woman should take approximately six to eight breaths per minute. Slow-paced breathing aids in relaxation and provides optimum oxygenation. The woman should continue to use this technique for as long as it is effective in reducing the perception of pain and maintaining control. As contractions increase in frequency and intensity, the woman often needs to change to a more complex breathing technique, which is shallower and faster than her normal rate of breathing, but should not exceed twice her resting respiratory rate. This *modified-paced breathing* pattern requires that she remain alert and concentrate more fully on breathing, thus blocking more painful stimuli than the simpler slow-paced breathing pattern does (Perinatal Education Associates, 2014).

The most difficult time to maintain control during contractions comes during the transition phase of the first stage of labor, when the cervix dilates from 8 cm to 10 cm. Even for the woman who has prepared for labor, concentration on breathing techniques is difficult to maintain. *Patterned-paced (pant-blow) breathing* is suggested during this phase. It is performed at the same rate as modified-paced breathing and consists of panting breaths combined with soft blowing breaths at regular intervals. The patterns may vary (i.e., *pant, pant, pant, pant, blow* [4:1 pattern] or *pant, pant, pant, blow* [3:1 pattern]) (Perinatal Education Associates, 2014). An undesirable reaction to this type of breathing is hyperventilation. The woman and her support person must be aware of and watch for symptoms of the resultant respiratory alkalosis: lightheadedness, dizziness, tingling of the fingers, or circumoral numbness. Having the woman breathe into a paper bag held tightly around her mouth and nose may eliminate respiratory alkalosis. This enables her to rebreathe carbon dioxide and replace the bicarbonate ions. The woman also can breathe into her cupped hands if no bag is available. Maintaining a breathing rate that is no more than twice the normal rate will lessen chances of hyperventilation. The partner can help the woman maintain her breathing rate with visual, tactile, or auditory cues.

As the fetal head reaches the pelvic floor, the woman may feel the urge to push and may automatically begin to exert downward pressure by contracting her abdominal muscles. During second-stage pushing, the woman should find a breathing pattern that is relaxing and feels good to her and is safe for her baby. Any regular or rhythmic breathing that avoids prolonged breath holding during pushing should maintain a good oxygen flow to the fetus (Perinatal Education Associates, 2014).

The woman can control the urge to push by taking panting breaths or by slowly exhaling through pursed lips (as though blowing out a candle). This type of breathing can be used to overcome the urge to push when the cervix is not fully prepared (e.g., less than 8 cm dilated, not retracting) and to facilitate a slow birth of the fetal head.

BOX 17-3 Paced Breathing Techniques

Cleansing Breath

- Relaxed breath in through nose and out through mouth. Used at the beginning and end of each contraction.

Slow-Paced Breathing (Approximately 6 to 8 Breaths per Minute)

- Performed at approximately half the normal breathing rate (number of breaths per minute divided by 2)
- IN-2-3-4/OUT-2-3-4/IN-2-3-4/OUT-2-3-4 ...

Modified-Paced Breathing (Approximately 32 to 40 Breaths per Minute)

- Performed at about twice the normal breathing rate (number of breaths per minute multiplied by 2)
- IN-OUT/IN-OUT/IN-OUT/IN-OUT ...
- For more flexibility and variety, the woman may combine the slow and modified breathing by using the slow breathing for beginnings and ends of contractions and modified breathing for more intense peaks. This technique conserves energy, lessens fatigue, and reduces risk for hyperventilation.

Patterned-Paced or Pant-Blow Breathing (Same Rate as Modified)

- Enhances concentration
- 3:1 Patterned breathing IN-OUT/IN-OUT/IN-OUT/IN-BLOW (repeat through contraction)
- 4:1 Patterned breathing IN-OUT/IN-OUT/IN-OUT/IN-OUT/IN-BLOW (repeat through contraction)

Adapted from Nichols, F. (2000). Paced breathing techniques. In F.H. Nichols & S.S. Humenick (Eds.), *Childbirth education: Practice, research, and theory* (2nd ed.). Philadelphia: Saunders; Perinatal Education Associates. (2014). *Breathing.* Available at www.birthsource.com/scripts/article.asp?articleid=211.

Effleurage and Counterpressure

Effleurage (light massage) and counterpressure have brought relief to many women during the first stage of labor. The gate-control theory may supply the reason for the effectiveness of these measures. **Effleurage** is light stroking, usually of the abdomen, in rhythm with breathing during contractions. It is used to distract the woman from contraction pain. Often the presence of monitor belts makes it difficult to perform effleurage on the abdomen; therefore, a thigh or the chest may be used. As labor progresses, hyperesthesia (hypersensitivity to touch) may make effleurage uncomfortable and thus less effective.

Counterpressure is steady pressure applied by a support person to the sacral area with a firm object (e.g., tennis ball) or the fist or heel of the hand. Pressure can also be applied to both hips (double hip squeeze) or to the knees (Burke, 2014). Application of counterpressure helps the woman cope with the sensations of internal pressure and pain in the lower back. It is especially helpful for back pain caused by pressure of the occiput against spinal nerves when the fetal head is in a posterior position. Counterpressure lifts the occiput off these nerves, thereby providing pain relief. The support person will need to be relieved occasionally because application of counterpressure is hard work.

Touch and Massage

Touch and massage have been an integral part of the traditional care process for women in labor. A variety of massage techniques have been shown to be safe and effective during labor (Jones et al., 2012).

Touch can be as simple as holding the woman's hand, stroking her body, and embracing her. When using touch to communicate caring, reassurance, and concern, it is important that the woman's preferences for touch (e.g., who can touch her, where they can touch her, and how they can touch her) and responses to touch be determined. A woman with a history of sexual abuse or certain cultural beliefs may be uncomfortable with touch. Women who perceive touch during labor as positive have less pain, anxiety, and need for pain medication (Weatherspoon, 2011). Touch also can involve very specialized techniques that require manipulation of the human energy field.

Therapeutic touch (TT) uses the concept of energy fields within the body called *prana*. Prana are thought to be deficient in some people who are in pain. TT uses laying-on of hands by a specially trained person to redirect energy fields associated with pain. Research has demonstrated the effectiveness of TT to enhance relaxation, reduce anxiety, and relieve pain (Jones et al., 2012); however, little is known about the use or effectiveness of TT for relieving labor pain.

Head, hand, back, and foot massage may be very effective in reducing tension and enhancing comfort. Some evidence suggests that massage may improve management of labor pain (Jones et al., 2012). Hand and foot massage may be especially relaxing in advanced labor when hyperesthesia limits a woman's tolerance for touch on other parts of her body. Combining massage with aromatherapy oil or lotion enhances relaxation both during and between contractions. The woman and her partner should be encouraged to experiment with different types of massage during pregnancy to determine which might feel best and be most relaxing during labor.

Application of Heat and Cold

Warmed blankets, warm compresses, heated rice bags, a warm bath or shower, or a moist heating pad can enhance relaxation and reduce pain during labor. Heat relieves muscle ischemia and increases blood flow to the area of discomfort. Heat application is effective for back pain caused by a posterior position or general backache from fatigue.

Cold application such as cold cloths, frozen gel packs, or ice packs applied to the back, the chest, or the face during labor may be effective in increasing comfort when the woman feels warm. They also may be applied to areas of musculoskeletal pain. Cooling relieves pain by reducing the muscle temperature and relieving muscle spasms (Burke, 2014). However, a woman's culture may make the use of cold during labor unacceptable.

Heat and cold may be used alternately for a greater effect. Neither heat nor cold should be applied over ischemic or anesthetized areas because tissues can be damaged. One or two layers of cloth should be placed between the skin and a hot or cold pack to prevent damage to the underlying integument.

Acupressure and Acupuncture

Acupressure and acupuncture can be used in pregnancy, in labor, and postpartum to relieve pain and other discomforts. Pressure, heat, or cold is applied to acupuncture points called *tsubos*. These points have an increased density of neuroreceptors and increased electrical conductivity. Acupressure is said to promote circulation of blood, the harmony of yin and yang, and the secretion of neurotransmitters, thus maintaining normal body functions and enhancing well-being (Gisin, Poat, Fierz, & Frei, 2013; Melchart, Jack, & Kashanian, 2011). Acupressure is best applied over the skin without using lubricants. Pressure is usually applied with the heel of the hand, fist, or pads of the thumbs and fingers (Fig. 17-4). Tennis balls or other devices also may be used. Pressure is applied with contractions initially and then continuously as labor progresses to the transition phase at the end of the first stage of labor (Gisin et al.; Hawkins & Bucklin, 2012; Melchart et al.). Synchronized breathing by the caregiver and the woman is suggested for greater effectiveness. Acupressure points are found on the neck, the shoulders, the wrists, the lower back including sacral points, the hips, the area below the kneecaps, the ankles, the nails on the small toes, and the soles of the feet. Acupressure may help to reduce pain and decrease the use of pharmacologic pain relief measures during labor. More research on its use is suggested (Arendt & Tessmer-Tuck, 2013).

Acupuncture is the insertion of fine needles into specific areas of the body to restore the flow of *qi* (energy) and to decrease pain, which is thought to obstruct the flow of energy. Effectiveness may be attributed to the alteration of chemical neurotransmitter levels in the body or to the release of endorphins as a result of hypothalamic activation. A trained certified therapist should do acupuncture. Arranging to have a qualified and credentialed acupuncture provider available during labor and birth may be challenging (Hawkins & Bucklin, 2012). Evidence indicates that acupuncture may be beneficial for relief of labor pain; however, further study is indicated (Gisin et al., 2013; Hawkins & Bucklin).

Transcutaneous Electrical Nerve Stimulation

Transcutaneous electrical nerve stimulation (TENS) involves the placing of two pairs of flat electrodes on either side of the woman's thoracic and sacral spine (Fig. 17-5). These electrodes

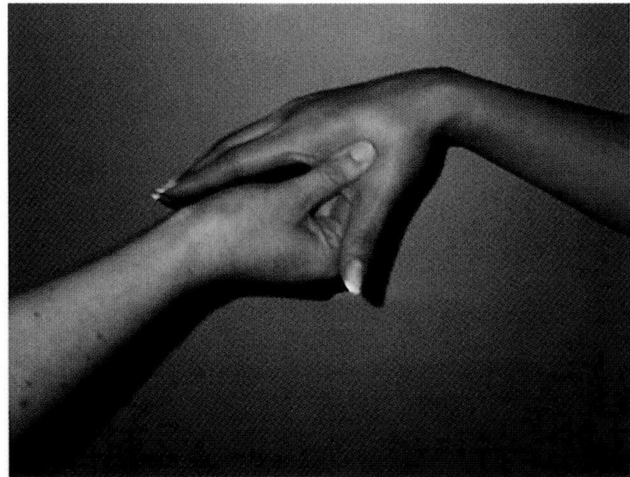

FIG 17-4 Ho-Ku acupressure point (back of hand where thumb and index finger come together) used to enhance uterine contractions without increasing pain. (Courtesy Julie Perry Nelson, Loveland, CO.)

provide continuous low-intensity electrical impulses or stimuli from a battery-operated device. During a contraction the woman increases the stimulation from low to high intensity by turning control knobs on the device. High intensity should be maintained for at least 1 minute to facilitate release of endorphins. Women describe the resulting sensation as a tingling or buzzing. TENS is most useful for lower back pain during the early first stage of labor. Women tend to rate the device as helpful although its use does not decrease pain. It appears that the electrical impulses or stimuli somehow make the pain less disturbing. There are no serious safety concerns associated with the use of TENS (Francis, 2012; Hawkins & Bucklin, 2012).

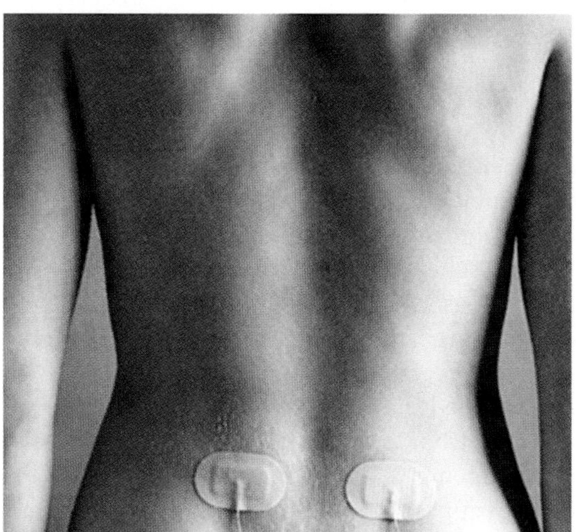

FIG 17-5 Placement of transcutaneous electrical nerve stimulation (TENS) electrodes on back for relief of labor pain.

Water Therapy (Hydrotherapy)

Bathing, showering, and jet hydrotherapy (whirlpool baths) with warm water (e.g., at or below body temperature) are nonpharmacologic measures that can promote comfort and relaxation during labor (Fig. 17-6). The warm water stimulates the release of endorphins, relaxes fibers to close the gate on pain, promotes better circulation and oxygenation, and helps soften the perineal tissues. Most women find immersion in water to be soothing, relaxing, and comforting. While immersed, they may find it easier to let go and allow labor to take its course (Gilbert, 2011). Some evidence suggests that immersion in water may improve management of labor pain (Arendt & Tessmer-Tuck, 2013; Jones et al., 2012).

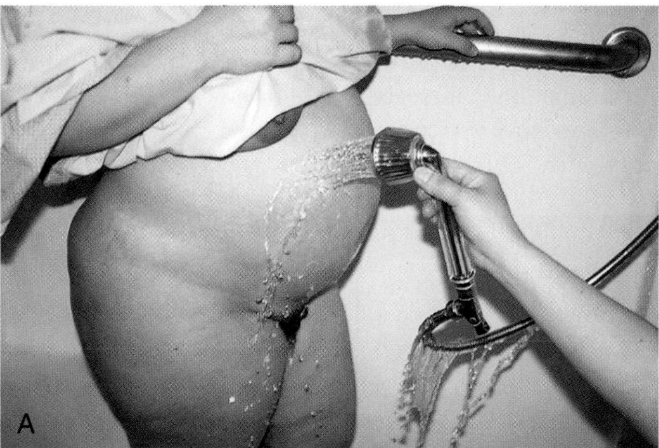

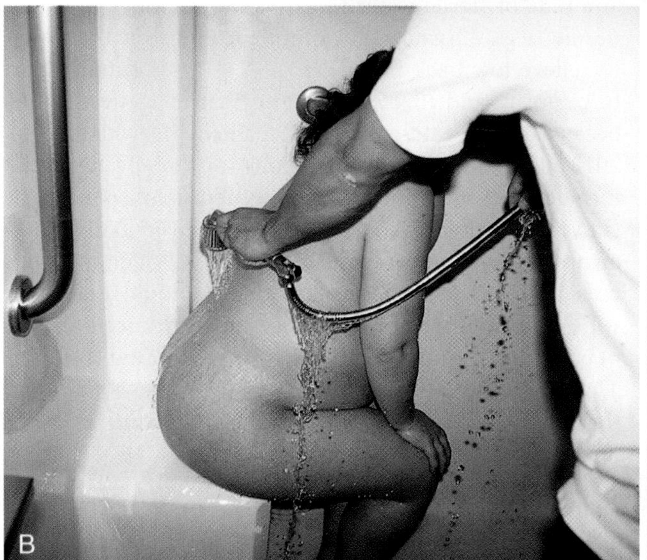

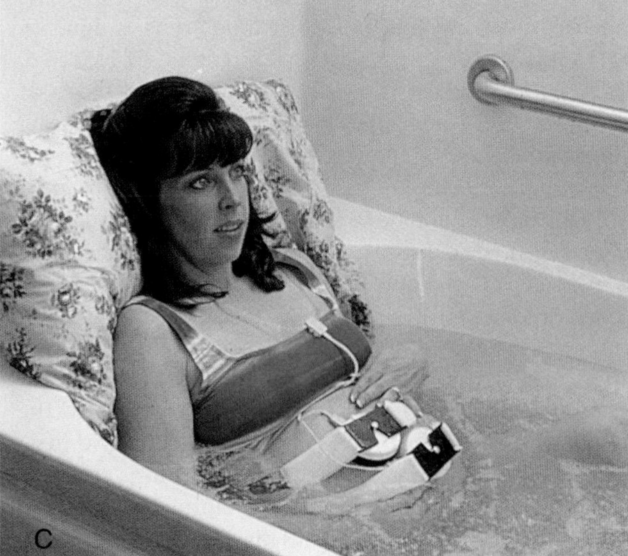

FIG 17-6 Water therapy during labor. **A**, Use of shower during labor. **B**, Woman experiencing back labor relaxes as partner sprays warm water on her back. **C**, Laboring woman relaxes in Jacuzzi. Note that fetal monitoring can continue during time in the Jacuzzi. (**A** and **B**, Courtesy Marjorie Pyle, RNC, Lifecircle, Costa Mesa, CA; **C**, courtesy Spacelabs Medical, Redmond, WA.)

Prior to initiating hydrotherapy measures, agency policy should be consulted to determine if the approval of the laboring woman's primary health care provider is required and if criteria need to be met in terms of the status of the maternal and fetal unit (e.g., stable vital signs and fetal heart rate [FHR] and pattern, stage of labor, etc.). In order to reduce the risk of a prolonged labor, hydrotherapy is usually initiated when the woman is in active labor, at approximately 5 cm. It is at this time that she may be getting discouraged and will welcome the change that hydrotherapy offers. Remember to preserve her modesty because she may be shy about the exposure of her body when getting into a tub or shower (Creehan, 2008).

In addition to pain relief and relaxation, hydrotherapy offers other benefits. If a woman is having "back labor" as the result of an occiput posterior or transverse position, assuming a hands-and-knees or a side-lying position in the tub enhances spontaneous fetal rotation to the occiput anterior position as a result of increased buoyancy. Because less effort is needed to change positions while in the water, women are encouraged to assume upright positions and to alter positions more frequently, facilitating the progress of their labors and helping them cope with labor-associated stressors (see Community Activity box) (Smith, Levett, Collins, & Jones, 2012). Additionally, hydrotherapy results in less use of pharmacologic pain relief measures, decreased use of epidural anesthesia, fewer forceps- or vacuum-assisted births, fewer episiotomies, less perineal trauma, and increased maternal satisfaction with the birth experience (Arendt & Tessmer-Tuck, 2013; Burke, 2014).

COMMUNITY ACTIVITY

Interview several women who have given birth, and explore the positions they used while in labor. Which positions were most helpful, and why? Which did they find least helpful? Did any of the women use hydrotherapy? Share your findings with your fellow students.

When hydrotherapy is in use, FHR monitoring is done by Doppler, fetoscope, or wireless external monitor (see Fig. 17-6, *C*). Placement of internal electrodes is contraindicated for jet hydrotherapy. Several studies have investigated the risks of using hydrotherapy with ruptured membranes. Findings have shown no increases in chorioamnionitis, postpartum endometritis, neonatal infections, or antibiotic use (Burke, 2014). However, care must be taken to use tubs that can be cleansed easily and thoroughly. A unit protocol should be developed for cleaning the tubs.

There is no limit to the time women can stay in the bath, and often they are encouraged to stay in it as long as desired. However, most women use jet hydrotherapy for 30 to 60 minutes at a time. During the bath, if the woman's temperature and the FHR increase, if the labor process becomes less effective (e.g., slows or becomes too intense), or if relief of pain is reduced, the woman can come out of the bath and return at a later time. Repeated baths with occasional breaks may be more effective in relieving pain in long labors than extended amounts of time in the water. The water temperature should be maintained at 36° to 37° C (96.8° to 98.6° F), with the water covering the woman's abdomen to gain maximum effect from the hydrostatic pressure and buoyancy of the water. Her shoulders should remain out of the water to facilitate the dissipation of heat (Burke, 2014; Creehan, 2008).

The American Academy of Pediatrics Committee on Fetus and Newborn has expressed concerns about actual birthing in water because of the lack of research demonstrating its safety. There are rare but reported instances of asphyxia or infection that have occurred during or as a result of underwater birth (Arendt & Tessmer-Tuck, 2013; Hawkins & Bucklin, 2012). This group believes that underwater birth should be considered an experimental procedure, performed only after informed parental consent has been obtained (Hawkins & Bucklin).

In a joint statement, the Royal College of Obstetricians & Gynaecologists (RCOG) and the Royal College of Nurse Midwives support laboring in water for healthy women with uncomplicated pregnancies at term (RCOG, 2006). While these groups acknowledge safety concerns related to respiratory problems in newborns, cord avulsion, and waterborne infection when women give birth under water, they state that these complications appear to occur rarely if good practice guidelines related to infection control, management of cord rupture, and strict adherence to eligibility criteria are followed (RCOG).

Using a shower provides comfort through the application of heat as the handheld showerhead is directed to areas of discomfort (see Fig. 17-6, *A* and *B*). The coach or partner can participate in this comfort measure by holding and directing the showerhead.

SAFETY ALERT

Because warm water can cause dizziness, a shower stool should be available, and the woman should be assisted when getting in and out of the tub.

Intradermal Water Block

An intradermal water block involves the injection of small amounts of sterile water (e.g., 0.05 to 0.1 ml) by using a fine needle (e.g., 25 gauge) into four locations on the lower back to relieve low back pain (Fig. 17-7). It is a simple procedure to perform, and there is evidence that it is effective, perhaps because of the gate-control mechanism (Hawkins & Bucklin, 2012). Other possible explanations for the effectiveness of the intradermal water block are the mechanism of counterirritation (i.e., reducing localized pain in one area by irritating the skin in an area nearby) or an increase in the level of endogenous opioids (endorphins) produced by the injections. Intense stinging will occur for about 20 to 30 seconds after injection, but relief of back pain for up to 2 hours has been reported (Burke, 2014). The procedure can be repeated, although the woman may find that the stinging that occurs with administration creates too much discomfort.

Aromatherapy

Aromatherapy uses oils distilled from plants, flowers, herbs, and trees to promote health and to treat and balance the mind, body, and spirit. These essential oils are highly concentrated, complex essences, and are mixed with lotions or creams before they are applied to the skin (e.g., for a back massage). Certain essential

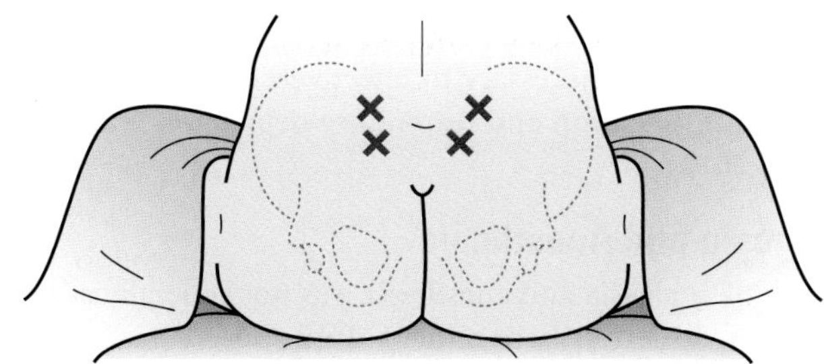

FIG 17-7 Intradermal injections of 0.1 ml of sterile water in the treatment of women with back pain during labor. Sterile water is injected into four locations on the lower back, two sites lateral to the lumbosacral spine and two sites 2 to 3 cm below and 1 to 2 cm medial to the original two injection sites; 0.1 ml of sterile water is injected between the dermal layers to raise a small bleb on the skin surface at each of the four sites. Simultaneous injections administered by two clinicians will decrease the pain of the injections. During labor the injections are administered consecutively during a contraction, with the total number of injections being completed within 20 to 30 seconds (From Leeman, L., Fontaine, P., King, V., Klein, M., & Ratcliffe, S. [2003]. The nature and management of labor pain: Part I. Nonpharmacologic pain relief. *American Family Physician 68*[6], 1109-1112. Copyright 2003 Michael Norviel.)

oils can tone the uterus, encourage contractions, reduce pain, relieve tension, diminish fear and anxiety, and enhance the feeling of well-being. Lavender, rose, and jasmine oils can promote relaxation and reduce pain. Rose oil also acts as an antidepressant and uterine tonic, and jasmine oil strengthens contractions and decreases feelings of panic in addition to reducing pain. Essential oils of bergamot or rosemary can be diffused or used in a massage oil to relieve exhaustion (Gilbert, 2011). Oils may be used by adding a few drops to a warm bath or to warm water used for soaking compresses that can be applied to the body. Drops of essential oils can be put on a pillow or on a woman's brow or palms or used as an ingredient in creating massage oil. They may also be inhaled as a steam or a smoke (Arendt & Tessmer-Tuck, 2013; Gilbert). Certain odors or scents can evoke pleasant memories and feelings of love and security. As a result, it's helpful for a woman to choose the scents that she will use. Aromatherapy has not been shown to improve labor outcomes. However, there is likely little harm associated with its use, other than the possibility of an allergic reaction (Arendt & Tessmer-Tuck).

Music

Music, recorded or live, can provide a distraction, enhance relaxation, and lift spirits during labor, thereby reducing the woman's level of stress, anxiety, and perception of pain. It can be used to promote relaxation in early labor and to stimulate movement as labor progresses. Music can help to create a more relaxed atmosphere in the birth room, leading to a more relaxed approach by health care providers (Burke, 2014). Women should be encouraged to prepare their musical preferences in advance and to bring an electronic music device to the hospital or birthing center. They should choose familiar music that is associated with pleasant memories, which can also facilitate the process of guided imagery. Use of a headset or earphones may increase the effectiveness of the music because other sounds will be shut out. Live music provided at the bedside by a support person may be very helpful in transmitting energy that decreases tension and elevates mood. Changing the tempo of the music to coincide with the rate and rhythm of each breathing technique may facilitate proper pacing. Although promising, there is insufficient evidence at the present time to support the effectiveness of music as a method of pain relief during labor. Further research is recommended (Smith et al., 2012).

Hypnosis

Hypnosis is a form of deep relaxation, similar to daydreaming or meditation (see www.hypnobirthing.com). While under hypnosis women are in a state of focused concentration and the subconscious mind can be more easily accessed. Women who attend certain childbirth preparation classes may be taught to perform self-hypnosis. Hypnosis techniques used for labor and birth place an emphasis on enhancing relaxation and diminishing fear, anxiety, and perception of pain. A few negative effects of hypnosis have been reported, including mild dizziness, nausea, and headache. These negative effects seem to be associated with failure to dehypnotize the woman properly. Although some initial small studies found hypnosis to be beneficial, a Cochrane systematic review showed no difference between women who were hypnotized and those who were not in regard to their use of pain medication during labor or their satisfaction with pain relief or the overall birth experience (Arendt & Tessmer-Tuck, 2013).

Biofeedback

Biofeedback may provide another relaxation technique that can be used for labor. Biofeedback is based on the theory that if a person can recognize physical signals, certain internal physiologic events can be changed (i.e., whatever signs the woman has that are associated with her pain). For biofeedback to be effective, the woman must be educated during the prenatal period to become aware of her body and its responses and how to relax. The woman must learn how to use thinking and mental processes (e.g., focusing) to control body responses and functions. Informational biofeedback helps couples develop awareness of their bodies and use strategies to change their responses to stress. If the woman responds to pain during a contraction with tightening of muscles, frowning, moaning, and breath holding, her partner uses verbal and touch feedback to help her relax. Formal biofeedback, which uses machines to detect skin temperature, blood flow, or muscle tension, also can prepare women to intensify their relaxation responses. Biofeedback-assisted relaxation techniques are not always successful in reducing labor pain. They may initially reduce pain or discomfort in labor, but as labor progresses women often need pain medication as well. There is insufficient evidence at this time to show that biofeedback is effective for managing labor pain (Barragán Loayza, Solà, & Juandó Prats, 2011).

PHARMACOLOGIC PAIN MANAGEMENT

Pharmacologic measures for pain management should be implemented before pain becomes so severe that catecholamines increase and labor is prolonged. Pharmacologic and nonpharmacologic measures, when used together, increase the level of pain relief and create a more positive labor experience for the woman and her family. Nonpharmacologic measures can be used for relaxation and pain relief, especially in early labor. Pharmacologic measures can be implemented as labor becomes more active and discomfort and pain intensify. Less pharmacologic intervention often is required because nonpharmacologic measures enhance relaxation and potentiate the analgesic effect. However, women in the United States are increasingly using pharmacologic measures, especially epidural analgesia, to relieve their pain during labor and birth. In one survey, nearly two-thirds of women received regional anesthesia to relieve pain during labor or during vaginal or cesarean birth (Cunningham, Leveno, Bloom, et al., 2014). Pharmacologic measures for pain management are generally used in hospital settings rather than in birthing centers or for home births.

SAFETY ALERT

Whenever medications are administered, nurses must remain alert for adverse reactions (e.g., difficulty breathing) and be prepared to administer antidotes or summon assistance if necessary. Remember that adverse reactions can occur even if the woman has received the same medication in the past without problems.

Sedatives

Sedatives relieve anxiety and induce sleep. They can be given to a woman experiencing a prolonged latent phase of labor when there is a need to lessen the intensity of the contractions, decrease anxiety, or promote sleep. They can also be given to augment analgesics and reduce nausea when an opioid is used.

Barbiturates such as secobarbital sodium (Seconal) can cause undesirable side effects including respiratory and vasomotor depression, affecting the woman and newborn. Because of the potential for neonatal central nervous system (CNS) depression, barbiturates should be avoided if birth is anticipated within 12 to 24 hours. The depressant effects are increased if a barbiturate is administered with another CNS depressant such as an opioid analgesic. However, pain will be magnified if a barbiturate is given without an analgesic to women experiencing pain because normal coping mechanisms may be blunted. As a result of these disadvantages, barbiturates are seldom used during labor (Burke, 2014; Hawkins & Bucklin, 2012).

Phenothiazines (e.g., promethazine [Phenergan]) do not relieve pain. In the past, promethazine was often given with opioids to enhance the analgesic effects of opioids, as well as to decrease anxiety and apprehension, increase sedation, and reduce nausea and vomiting. However, research has shown that promethazine actually impairs the analgesic efficacy of opioids. Metoclopramide (Reglan), an antiemetic, has been found to effectively potentiate the effects of analgesics. Therefore, its use is recommended, rather than promethazine (Hawkins & Bucklin, 2012).

Benzodiazepines (e.g., diazepam [Valium], lorazepam [Ativan]), when given with an opioid analgesic, seem to enhance pain relief and reduce nausea and vomiting. Because benzodiazepines cause significant maternal amnesia, however, their use should be avoided during labor. A major disadvantage of diazepam is that it disrupts thermoregulation in newborns, making them less able to maintain body temperature. Flumazenil (Romazicon) is a specific benzodiazepine antagonist that can be administered if necessary to effectively reverse benzodiazepine-induced sedation and respiratory depression (Hawkins & Bucklin, 2012).

Analgesia and Anesthesia

The use of analgesia and anesthesia was not generally accepted as part of obstetric management until Queen Victoria used chloroform during the birth of her son in 1853. Since then much study has gone into the development of pharmacologic measures for controlling discomfort during the birth period. The goal of researchers is to develop methods that will provide adequate pain relief to women without increasing maternal or fetal risk or affecting the progress of labor.

Nursing management of obstetric analgesia and anesthesia combines the nurse's expertise in maternity care with a knowledge and understanding of anatomy and physiology and of medications and their therapeutic effects, adverse reactions, and methods of administration.

Anesthesia encompasses analgesia, amnesia, relaxation, and reflex activity. Anesthesia abolishes pain perception by interrupting the nerve impulses to the brain. The loss of sensation may be partial or complete, sometimes with the loss of consciousness.

The term **analgesia** refers to the alleviation of the sensation of pain or the raising of the threshold for pain perception without loss of consciousness.

The type of analgesic or anesthetic chosen is determined in part by the stage of labor of the woman and by the method of birth planned (Box 17-4).

BOX 17-4 Pharmacologic Control of Discomfort by Stage of Labor and Method of Birth

First Stage
- Opioid agonist analgesics
- Opioid agonist-antagonist analgesics
- Epidural (block) analgesia
- Combined spinal-epidural (CSE) analgesia
- Nitrous oxide

Second Stage
- Nerve block analgesia and anesthesia
    - Local infiltration anesthesia
    - Pudendal block
    - Spinal (block) anesthesia
    - Epidural (block) analgesia
    - CSE analgesia
- Nitrous oxide

Vaginal Birth
- Local infiltration anesthesia
- Pudendal block
- Epidural (block) analgesia and anesthesia
- Spinal (block) anesthesia
- CSE analgesia and anesthesia
- Nitrous oxide

Cesarean Birth
- Spinal (block) anesthesia
- Epidural (block) anesthesia
- General anesthesia

Systemic Analgesia

Systemic analgesics (opioids) can be administered as intermittent intravenous (IV) or intramuscular (IM) doses by health care providers or by the woman herself using patient-controlled analgesia (PCA). With PCA, the woman self-administers small doses of an opioid analgesic by using a pump programmed for dose and frequency. Overall, a lower total amount of analgesic is used. Women appreciate the sense of autonomy provided by this method of pain relief, as well as the elimination of treatment delays while the nurse obtains and administers the medication (Hawkins & Bucklin, 2012).

Opioids provide sedation and euphoria, but their analgesic effect in labor is limited. The pain relief they provide is incomplete, temporary, and more effective in the early part of active labor (Anderson, 2011). All opioids cause side effects, the most serious of which is respiratory depression. Other undesirable opioid side effects include sedation, nausea and vomiting, dizziness, altered mental status, euphoria, decreased gastric motility, delayed gastric emptying, and urinary retention (Anderson). Prolonged gastric emptying time increases the risk for aspiration if general anesthesia becomes necessary in a woman who has received opioids (Hawkins & Bucklin, 2012). Bladder and bowel elimination can be inhibited. Because heart rate (e.g., bradycardia, tachycardia), blood pressure (e.g., hypotension), and respiratory effort (e.g., depression) can be adversely affected, opioid analgesics should be used cautiously in women with respiratory and cardiovascular disorders. Safety precautions should be taken after opioid administration, because several opioid side effects increase the risk for injury.

Opioids readily cross the placenta. Effects on the fetus and newborn can be profound, including absent or minimal FHR variability during labor and significant neonatal respiratory depression requiring treatment after birth (Hawkins & Bucklin, 2012).

SAFETY ALERT

Opioids decrease maternal heart and respiratory rate and blood pressure, which affects fetal oxygenation. Therefore, maternal vital signs and FHR and pattern must be assessed and documented before and after administration of opioids for pain relief.

Classifications of **analgesic** drugs used to relieve the pain of childbirth include **opioid (narcotic) agonists** and **opioid (narcotic) agonist-antagonists.** Choice of which medication to use often depends on the primary health care provider's preferences and the characteristics of the laboring woman. The type of systemic analgesic used therefore often varies among obstetric units.

Opioid Agonist Analgesics. Opioid (narcotic) agonist analgesics commonly used in obstetrics are meperidine (Demerol) and fentanyl (Sublimaze) (Hawkins & Bucklin, 2012). As pure opioid agonists they stimulate major opioid receptors, mu and kappa. They have no amnesic effect but create a feeling of well-being or euphoria and enhance a woman's ability to rest between contractions. Because opioids can inhibit uterine contractions, prolonging labor, they should not be administered until labor is well established unless they are being used to enhance therapeutic rest during a prolonged latent phase of labor (Burke, 2014).

Meperidine hydrochloride is a synthetic opioid that is the most widely used systemic medication for labor pain (Cunningham et al., 2014). Its widespread use is probably related to its low cost, the fact that care providers are quite familiar with the drug, and studies that were done many years ago that found that it caused less respiratory depression than morphine (see Medication Guide: Meperidine Hydrochloride [Demerol]). However, its use during labor is becoming more controversial because of undesirable side effects, particularly in the neonate (Anderson, 2011). Both meperidine and normeperidine, an active metabolite of meperidine, cross the placenta and cause prolonged neonatal sedation and neurobehavioral changes. These metabolite-related effects cannot be reversed with naloxone (Anderson). Because meperidine and normeperidine have long half-lives, the neonatal effects can persist for the first 2 to 3 days of life (Hawkins & Bucklin, 2012).

MEDICATION GUIDE

Meperidine Hydrochloride (Demerol)

Classification
Opioid agonist analgesic

Action
Synthetic opioid agonist analgesic that stimulates both mu and kappa opioid receptors to decrease the transmission of pain impulses. Meperidine 100 mg is roughly equivalent in analgesic effect to morphine 10 mg, but it is reported to cause less maternal respiratory depression. Intravenously, the onset of action begins in 5 minutes and the duration of action is 2 to 4 hours.

Indication
Moderate to severe labor pain and postoperative pain after cesarean birth

Dosage and Route
IV: 25 to 50 mg every 1 to 2 hours
PCA Pump: 15 mg every 10 minutes as needed until birth

Adverse Effects
Tachycardia, sedation, nausea and vomiting, dizziness, altered mental status, euphoria, decreased gastric motility, delayed gastric emptying, and urinary retention

Nursing Considerations
Implement safety measures as appropriate, including use of side rails and assistance with ambulation; continue use of nonpharmacologic pain relief measures. Do not give if birth is expected to occur within 1 to 4 hours after administration because infants born to women who received meperidine during labor may have respiratory depression, peaking at 2 to 3 hours after administration of the drug. Respiratory depression caused by normeperidine, an active metabolite of meperidine, cannot be reversed by naloxone. Both meperidine and normeperidine have long half-lives. Therefore, neonates whose mothers received meperidine during labor can exhibit sedation and neurobehavioral changes for the first 2 to 3 days of life.

Data from Anderson, D. (2011). A review of systemic opioids commonly used for labor pain relief. *Journal of Midwifery & Women's Health, 56*(3), 222-239; Hawkins, J., Bucklin, B. (2012). Obstetrical anesthesia. In S. Gabbe, J. Niebyl, J. Simpson, et al. (Eds.), *Obstetrics: Normal and problem pregnancies* (6th ed.). Philadelphia: Saunders.

Fentanyl citrate (Sublimaze) is a potent short-acting opioid agonist analgesic (see Medication Guide: Fentanyl Citrate [Sublimaze]). It rapidly crosses the placenta, so it is present in fetal blood within 1 minute after IV maternal administration (Anderson, 2011). As compared with meperidine, fentanyl provides equivalent analgesia with fewer neonatal effects and less maternal sedation and nausea. Fentanyl is used as a labor analgesic because of its rapid onset of action, short half-life, and lack of a metabolite (Anderson). A disadvantage of fentanyl is that more frequent dosing is required because of its relatively short duration of action (Hawkins & Bucklin, 2012). As a result, this medication is most commonly administered by PCA pump, intrathecally, or epidurally, alone or in combination with a local anesthetic agent.

Opioid (Narcotic) Agonist-Antagonist Analgesics. An agonist is an agent that activates or stimulates a receptor to act; an antagonist is an agent that blocks a receptor or a medication designed to activate a receptor. Butorphanol (Stadol) and nalbuphine (Nubain) are commonly used opioid (narcotic) agonist-antagonist analgesics (Hawkins & Bucklin, 2012). These medications are agonists at kappa opioid receptors and either antagonists or weak agonists at mu opioid receptors. In the doses used during labor, these mixed opioids provide adequate analgesia without causing significant respiratory depression in the mother or neonate. Their major advantage is their ceiling effect for respiratory depression; higher doses do not produce additional respiratory depression. They are less likely to cause nausea and vomiting, but sedation may be as great or greater when compared with pure opioid agonists (Anderson, 2011; Hawkins & Bucklin). As a result of these effects, parenteral opioid agonist-antagonist analgesics are used more commonly during labor than the opioid agonist analgesics. IM, subcutaneous, and IV routes of administration can be used, but the IV route is preferred. This classification of opioid analgesics, especially nalbuphine, is not suitable for women with an opioid dependence because the antagonist activity could precipitate withdrawal symptoms (abstinence syndrome) in both the mother and her newborn (Hawkins & Bucklin) (see the Medication Guide: Butorphanol Tartrate [Stadol], Medication Guide: Nalbuphine Hydrochloride [Nubain], and the Signs of Potential Complications box).

MEDICATION GUIDE

Fentanyl Citrate (Sublimaze)

Classification
Opioid agonist analgesic

Action
Opioid agonist analgesic that stimulates both mu and kappa opioid receptors to decrease the transmission of pain impulses. Has a rapid onset of action with a short duration (0.5 to 1 hour IV; 1 to 2 hours IM).

Indication
Moderate to severe labor pain and postoperative pain after cesarean birth

Dosage and Route
IV: 50 to 100 mcg every hour
IM: 50 to 100 mcg every hour

Adverse Effects
Sedation, respiratory depression, nausea, and vomiting

Nursing Considerations
Assess for respiratory depression; naloxone should be available as an antidote. Implement safety measures as appropriate, including use of side rails and assistance with ambulation; continue use of nonpharmacologic pain relief measures. Because of its short duration of action, frequent dosing will be necessary when given intravenously. Maximum total dose for labor is usually 500 to 600 mcg.

Data from Anderson, D. (2011). A review of systemic opioids commonly used for labor pain relief. *Journal of Midwifery & Women's Health, 56*(3), 222-239.

MEDICATION GUIDE

Butorphanol Tartrate (Stadol)

Classification
Opioid agonist-antagonist analgesic

Action
Mixed agonist-antagonist analgesic that stimulates kappa opioid receptors and blocks or weakly stimulates mu opioid receptors, resulting in good analgesia but with less respiratory depression and nausea and vomiting when compared with opioid agonist analgesics. Butorphanol produces a maternal ceiling effect on pain relief and respiratory depression. IV administration of 2 mg of butorphanol produces respiratory depression similar to that of 10 mg of morphine IV or 70 mg of meperidine IV, but 4 mg of butorphanol will produce less respiratory depression than 20 mg of morphine or 140 mg of meperidine. Whether given intravenously or intramuscularly, the drug's duration of action is 4 to 6 hours.

Indication
Moderate to severe labor pain and postoperative pain after cesarean birth

Usual Dosage and Route
IV: 1 to 2 mg every 3 to 4 hours as needed
IM: 1 to 2 mg every 3 to 4 hours as needed

Adverse Effects
Confusion, sedation, hallucinations, "floating" feeling, drowsiness, transient nonpathologic sinusoidal-like fetal heart rate pattern, respiratory depression, nausea and vomiting

Nursing Considerations
May precipitate withdrawal symptoms in opioid-dependent women and their newborns. Assess maternal vital signs, degree of pain, fetal heart rate (FHR), and uterine activity before and after administration. Observe for maternal respiratory depression, notifying primary health care provider if maternal respirations are ≤12 breaths/minute. Encourage voiding every 2 hours, and palpate for bladder distention. If birth occurs within 1 to 4 hours of dose administration, observe newborn for respiratory depression. Implement safety measures as appropriate, including use of side rails and assistance with ambulation. Continue use of nonpharmacologic pain relief measures.

Data from Anderson, D. (2011). A review of systemic opioids commonly used for labor pain relief. *Journal of Midwifery & Women's Health, 56*(3), 222-239.

MEDICATION GUIDE

Nalbuphine Hydrochloride (Nubain)

Classification
Opioid agonist-antagonist analgesic

Action
Mixed agonist-antagonist analgesic that stimulates kappa opioid receptors and blocks or weakly stimulates mu opioid receptors, resulting in good analgesia but with less respiratory depression and nausea and vomiting when compared with opioid agonist analgesics. Nalbuphine's analgesic effect is equivalent to morphine, on a milligram-to-milligram basis. Produces a maternal ceiling effect on pain relief and respiratory depression after 30 mg of the drug has been administered. Duration of action is 2 to 4 hours when given intravenously and 4 to 6 hours when given intramuscularly.

Indication
Moderate to severe labor pain and postoperative pain after cesarean birth

Dosage and Route
IV: 10 mg every 3 hours as needed
IM: 10 mg every 3 hours as needed

Adverse Effects
Sedation, drowsiness, nausea, vomiting, dizziness, respiratory depression, temporary absent or minimal fetal heart rate (FHR) variability

Nursing Considerations
May precipitate withdrawal symptoms in opioid-dependent women and their newborns. Assess maternal vital signs, degree of pain, FHR, and uterine activity before and after administration. Observe for maternal respiratory depression, notifying primary health care provider if maternal respirations are ≤12 breaths/minute. Encourage voiding every 2 hours, and palpate for bladder distention. If birth occurs within 1 to 4 hours of dose administration, observe newborn for respiratory depression. Implement safety measures as appropriate, including use of side rails and assistance with ambulation. Continue use of nonpharmacologic pain relief measures.

Data from Anderson, D. (2011). A review of systemic opioids commonly used for labor pain relief. *Journal of Midwifery & Women's Health, 56*(3), 222-239.

SIGNS OF POTENTIAL COMPLICATIONS

Maternal Opioid Abstinence Syndrome (Opioid/Narcotic Withdrawal)

- Yawning, rhinorrhea (runny nose), sweating, lacrimation (tearing), mydriasis (dilation of pupils)
- Anorexia
- Irritability, restlessness, generalized anxiety
- Tremors
- Chills and hot flashes
- Piloerection ("gooseflesh" or "chill bumps")
- Violent sneezing
- Weakness, fatigue, and drowsiness
- Nausea and vomiting
- Diarrhea, abdominal cramps
- Bone and muscle pain, muscle spasms, kicking movements

Opioid (Narcotic) Antagonists. Opioids such as meperidine and fentanyl can cause excessive CNS depression in the mother, the newborn, or both, although the current practice of giving lower doses of opioids intravenously has reduced the incidence and severity of opioid-induced CNS depression. Opioid (narcotic) antagonists such as naloxone (Narcan) can promptly reverse the CNS depressant effects, especially respiratory depression, in most situations. As stated earlier, however, naloxone cannot reverse the effects of normeperidine, an active metabolite of meperidine. In addition, the antagonist counters the effect of the stress-induced levels of endorphins. An opioid antagonist is especially valuable if labor is more rapid than expected and birth is anticipated when the opioid is at its peak effect. The antagonist may be given intravenously, or it can be administered intramuscularly (see the Medication Guide: Naloxone Hydrochloride [Narcan]). The woman should be told that the pain that was relieved with the use of the opioid analgesic will return with the administration of the opioid antagonist.

MEDICATION GUIDE

Naloxone Hydrochloride (Narcan)

Classification
Opioid antagonist

Action
Blocks both mu and kappa opioid receptors from the effects of opioid agonists

Indication
Reverses opioid-induced respiratory depression in woman or newborn; may be used to reverse pruritus from epidural opioids

Dosage and Route
Adult
Opioid overdose: 0.4 to 2 mg IV, may repeat IV at 2- to 3-min intervals until a maximum of 10 mg has been given; if IV route unavailable, IM or subcutaneous administration may be used

Newborn
Opioid-induced depression: 0.1 mg/kg (concentration is 1.0 mg/ml solution). IV is the preferred route of administration. May also be given IM, but the onset of action will be delayed compared to IV administration.

Adverse Effects
Maternal hypotension or hypertension, tachycardia, hyperventilation, nausea and vomiting, sweating, and tremulousness

Nursing Considerations
The woman should delay breastfeeding until medication is out of her system (approximately 2 hours after the last dose is given). Do not give to the woman or the newborn if the woman is opioid dependent—may cause abrupt withdrawal in the woman and newborn. If given to the woman for reversal of respiratory depression caused by opioid analgesic, pain will return suddenly. The duration of action of naloxone is shorter than that of most opioids. Therefore, the woman must be monitored closely for the return of opioid depression when the effects of naloxone are gone. Additional doses of naloxone may be necessary to maintain reversal.

Data on newborn administration from American Academy of Pediatrics (AAP) & American Heart Association (AHA). (2011). *Textbook of neonatal resuscitation* (6th ed.). Dallas, TX: AHA.

> **MEDICATION ALERT**
>
> An opioid antagonist (e.g., naloxone [Narcan]) is contraindicated for opioid-dependent women because it may precipitate abstinence syndrome (withdrawal symptoms). For the same reason, opioid agonist-antagonist analgesics such as butorphanol (Stadol) and nalbuphine (Nubain) should not be given to opioid-dependent women (see the Signs of Potential Complications box).

Nerve Block Analgesia and Anesthesia

A variety of local anesthetic agents are used in obstetrics to produce regional analgesia (some pain relief and motor block) and regional anesthesia (complete pain relief and motor block). Most of these agents are related chemically to cocaine and end with the suffix *-caine*. This helps to identify a local anesthetic.

The principal pharmacologic effect of local anesthetics is the temporary interruption of the conduction of nerve impulses, notably pain. Examples of common agents given are bupivacaine (Marcaine), chloroprocaine (Nesacaine), lidocaine (Xylocaine), ropivacaine (Naropin), and mepivacaine (Carbocaine). Rarely, people are sensitive (allergic) to one or more local anesthetics. Such a reaction may include respiratory depression, hypotension, and other serious adverse effects. Epinephrine, antihistamines, oxygen, and supportive measures should reverse these effects. Administering tiny amounts of the drug to test for an allergic reaction may identify sensitivity.

Local Perineal Infiltration Anesthesia. Local perineal infiltration anesthesia may be used when an episiotomy is to be performed or when lacerations must be sutured after birth in a woman who does not have regional anesthesia. Rapid anesthesia is produced by injecting approximately 10 to 20 ml of 1% lidocaine or 2% chloroprocaine into the skin and then subcutaneously into the region to be anesthetized. Epinephrine often is added to the solution to localize and intensify the effect of the anesthesia in a region and to prevent excessive bleeding and systemic absorption by constricting local blood vessels. Injections can be repeated to keep the woman comfortable while post-birth repairs are completed.

Pudendal Nerve Block. Pudendal nerve block, administered late in the second stage of labor, is useful if an episiotomy is to be performed or if forceps or a vacuum extractor is to be used to facilitate birth. It can also be administered during the third stage of labor if an episiotomy or lacerations must be repaired (American Academy of Pediatrics [AAP] & American College of Obstetricians and Gynecologists [ACOG], 2012). A pudendal nerve block is considered to be a reasonably safe and simple procedure to provide pain relief for vaginal birth (Cunningham et al., 2014; Hawkins & Bucklin, 2012). Although a pudendal nerve block does not relieve the pain from uterine contractions, it does relieve pain in the lower vagina, the vulva, and the perineum (Fig. 17-8, *A*). A pudendal nerve block should be administered 10 to 20 minutes before perineal anesthesia is needed.

The pudendal nerve traverses the sacrosciatic notch just medial to the tip of the ischial spine on each side. Injection of an anesthetic solution at or near these points anesthetizes the pudendal nerves peripherally (Fig. 17-9). The transvaginal approach is generally used because it is less painful for the woman, has a higher rate of success in blocking pain, and tends to cause fewer fetal complications (Hawkins & Bucklin, 2012). Pudendal block does not change maternal hemodynamic or respiratory functions, vital signs, or the FHR. However, the bearing-down reflex is lessened or lost completely.

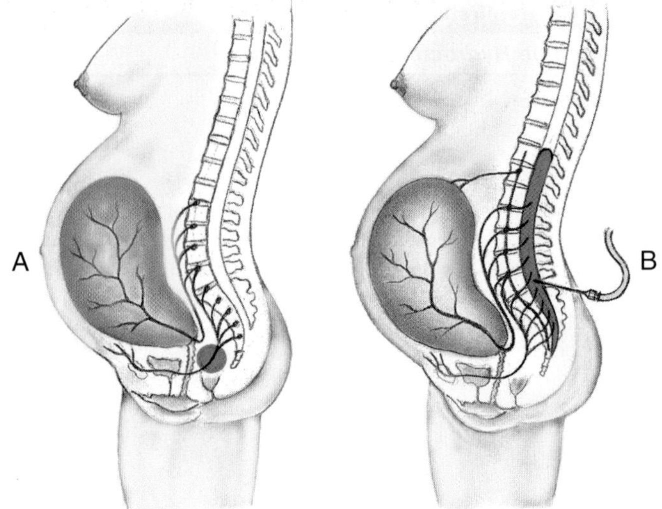

FIG 17-8 Pain pathways and sites of pharmacologic nerve blocks. **A,** Pudendal nerve block: suitable during second and third stages of labor and for repair of episiotomy or lacerations. **B,** Epidural block: suitable for all stages of labor and types of birth, and for repair of episiotomy and lacerations.

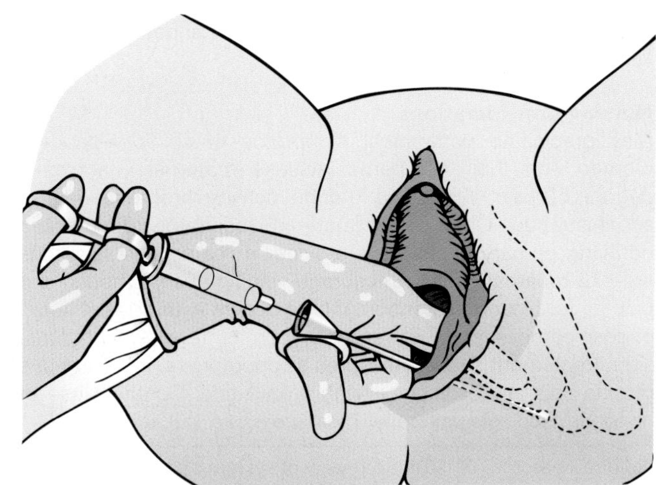

FIG 17-9 Pudendal nerve block. Use of introducer (needle guide) and Luer-Lok syringe to inject medication.

Spinal Anesthesia. In spinal anesthesia (block), a solution containing a local anesthetic alone or in combination with an opioid agonist analgesic is injected through the third, fourth, or fifth lumbar interspace into the subarachnoid space (Fig. 17-10, *A* and *B*), where the anesthetic solution mixes with cerebrospinal fluid (CSF). Low spinal anesthesia (block) may be used for vaginal birth, but it is not suitable for labor. Spinal anesthesia (block) used for cesarean birth provides anesthesia from the nipple (T6) to the feet. If it is used for vaginal birth, the anesthesia level is from the hips (T10) to the feet (see Fig. 17-10, *C*).

For spinal anesthesia (block), the woman sits or lies on her side (e.g., modified Sims position) with back curved to widen the intervertebral space to facilitate insertion of a small-gauge spinal needle and injection of the anesthetic solution into the spinal canal. The nurse supports the woman and encourages

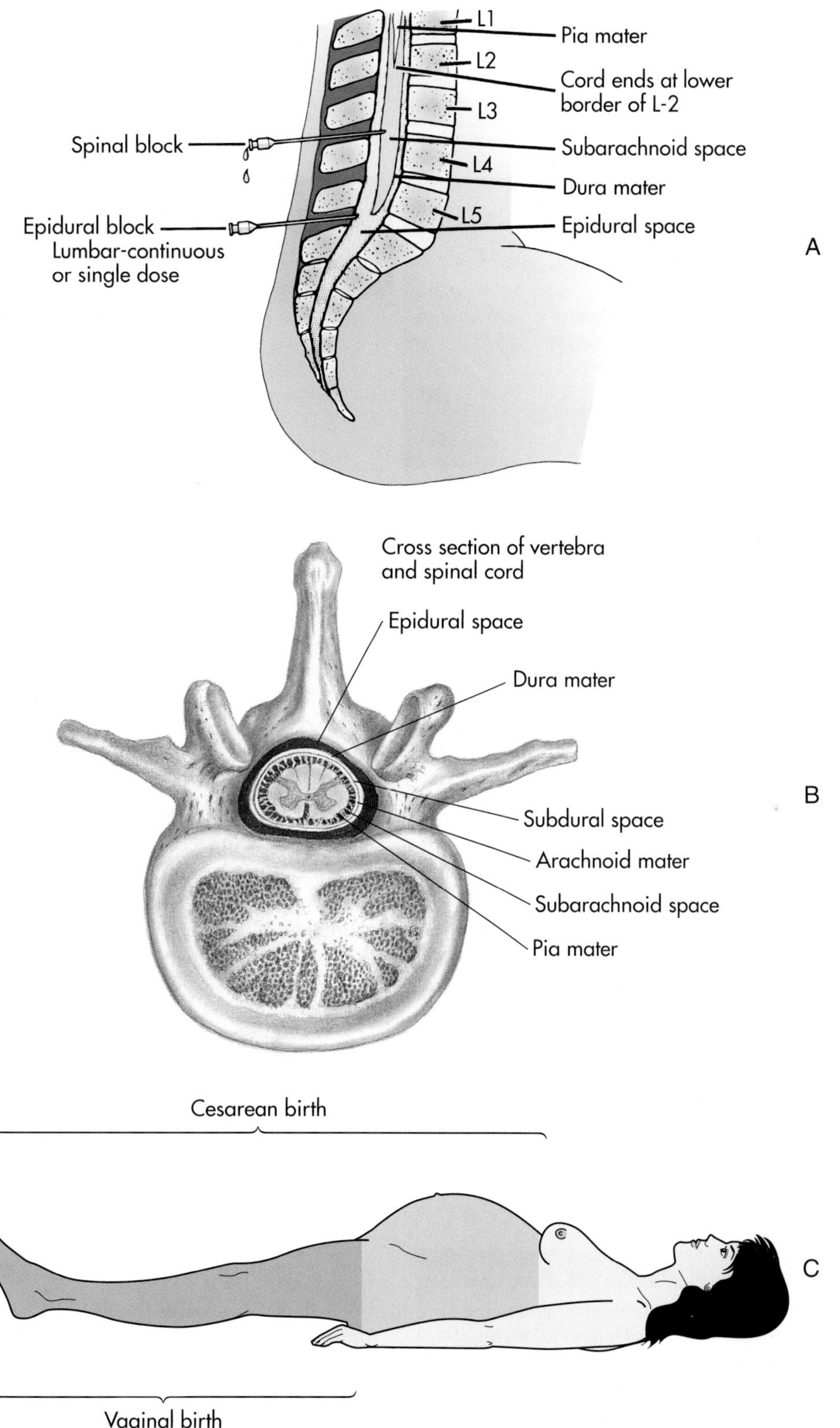

FIG 17-10 **A,** Membranes and spaces of spinal cord and levels of sacral, lumbar, and thoracic nerves. **B,** Cross section of vertebra and spinal cord. **C,** Level of anesthesia necessary for cesarean birth and for vaginal births.

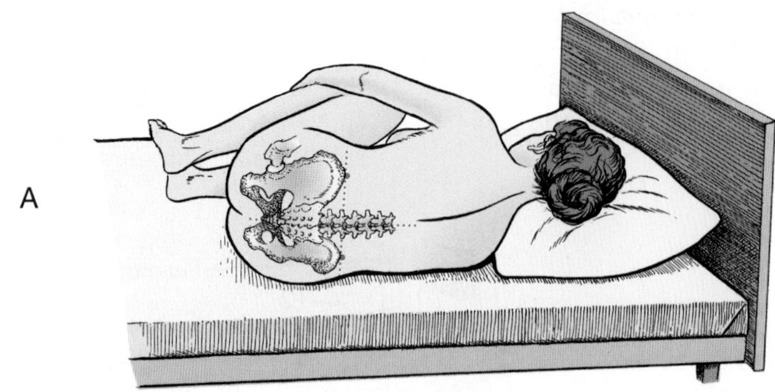

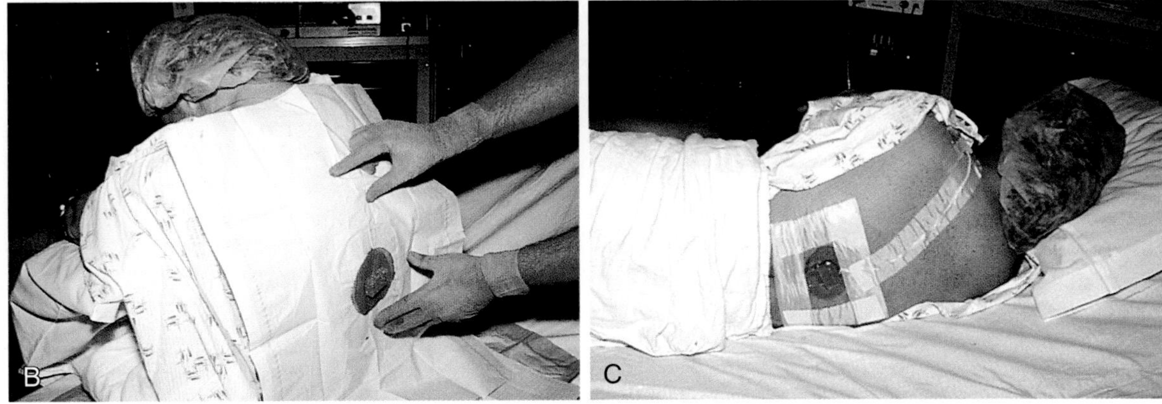

FIG 17-11 Positioning for spinal and epidural blocks. **A,** Lateral position. **B,** Upright position. **C,** Catheter for epidural is taped to the woman's back with the port segment located near her shoulder. (**B** and **C,** Courtesy Michael S. Clement, MD, Mesa, AZ.)

her to use breathing and relaxation techniques because she must remain still during the placement of the spinal needle. The needle is inserted and the anesthetic injected between contractions. After the anesthetic solution has been injected, the woman may be positioned upright to allow the heavier (hyperbaric) anesthetic solution to flow downward to obtain the lower level of anesthesia suitable for a vaginal birth. To obtain the higher level of anesthesia desired for cesarean birth she will be positioned supine with head and shoulders slightly elevated. In order to prevent supine hypotensive syndrome, the uterus is displaced laterally by tilting the operating table or placing a wedge under one of her hips. Usually the level of the block will be complete and fixed within 5 to 10 minutes after the anesthetic solution is injected but it can continue to creep upward for 20 minutes or longer (Hawkins & Bucklin, 2012). The anesthetic effect will last 1 to 3 hours, depending on the type of agent used (Fig. 17-11).

SAFETY ALERT

To reduce the risk for transmission of pathogens, (1) the woman's back is cleansed before the procedure, and (2) during the induction of spinal and epidural anesthesia or analgesia, the anesthesia care provider wears sterile gloves and a face mask. Also, spinal or epidural anesthesia or analgesia should not be initiated if the woman has a tattoo at the site where the needle would be inserted.

Marked hypotension, impaired placental perfusion, and an ineffective breathing pattern may occur during spinal anesthesia. Before induction of the spinal anesthetic, maternal vital signs are assessed and a 20- to 30-minute electronic fetal monitoring (EFM) strip is obtained and evaluated. In addition, the woman's fluid balance is assessed. A bolus of IV fluid (usually 500 to 1000 ml of lactated Ringer's or normal saline solution) may be administered 15 to 30 minutes before induction of the anesthetic to decrease the potential for hypotension caused by sympathetic blockade (vasodilation with pooling of blood in the lower extremities decreases cardiac output). Although the practice guidelines for obstetric anesthesia published by the American Society of Anesthesiologists (2007) state that this preanesthetic fluid bolus is not required, it is still usually administered in most clinical settings. Fluid that is used for the bolus should not contain dextrose, which could contribute to neonatal hypoglycemia (Hawkins & Bucklin, 2012).

After induction of the anesthetic, maternal blood pressure, pulse, and respirations and fetal heart rate and pattern must be assessed and documented every 5 to 10 minutes. If signs of serious maternal hypotension (e.g., a drop in systolic blood pressure to 100 mm Hg or less or below 20% of the baseline blood pressure) or fetal distress (e.g., bradycardia, minimal or absent variability, late decelerations) develop, emergency care must be given (Burke, 2014) (see the Emergency box).

EMERGENCY

Maternal Hypotension with Decreased Placental Perfusion

Signs and Symptoms

- Maternal hypotension (20% decrease from preblock baseline level or ≤100 mm Hg systolic)
- Fetal bradycardia
- Absent or minimal FHR variability

Interventions

- Turn woman to lateral position or place pillow or wedge under hip to displace uterus
- Maintain IV infusion at rate specified, or increase administration per hospital protocol
- Administer oxygen by nonrebreather face mask at 10 to 12 L/minute or per protocol.
- Elevate the woman's legs.
- Notify the primary health care provider, anesthesiologist, or nurse anesthetist.
- Administer IV vasopressor (e.g., ephedrine 5 to 10 mg or phenylephrine 50 to 100 mcg) per protocol if previous measures are ineffective.
- Remain with woman; continue to monitor maternal blood pressure and fetal heart rate (FHR) every 5 minutes until her condition is stable or per primary health care provider's order.

Because the woman is unable to sense her contractions, she must be instructed when to bear down during a vaginal birth. Use of a combination of local anesthetic agent and an opioid reduces the degree of motor function loss, enhancing a woman's ability to push effectively. If the birth occurs in a delivery room (rather than a labor-delivery-recovery room), the woman will need assistance in the transfer to a recovery bed after expulsion of the placenta and perineal repair if required.

Advantages of spinal anesthesia include ease of administration and absence of fetal hypoxia with maintenance of maternal blood pressure within a normal range. Maternal consciousness is maintained, excellent muscular relaxation is achieved, and blood loss is not excessive.

Disadvantages of spinal anesthesia include possible medication reactions (e.g., allergy), hypotension, and an ineffective breathing pattern; cardiopulmonary resuscitation may be needed. When a spinal anesthetic is given, the need for operative birth (e.g., episiotomy, forceps-assisted birth, or vacuum-assisted birth) tends to increase because voluntary expulsive efforts are reduced or eliminated. After birth the incidence of bladder and uterine atony, as well as postdural puncture headache, is higher.

Leakage of CSF from the site of puncture of the dura mater (membranous covering of the spinal cord) is thought to be the major causative factor in *postdural puncture headache* (PDPH), commonly referred to as a spinal headache. Spinal headache is much more likely to occur when the dura is accidentally punctured during the process of administering an epidural block. The needle used for an epidural block has a much larger gauge than the one used for spinal anesthesia and thus creates a bigger opening in the dura, resulting in a greater loss of CSF (i.e., "wet tap"). Presumably, postural changes cause the diminished volume of CSF to exert traction on pain-sensitive CNS structures.

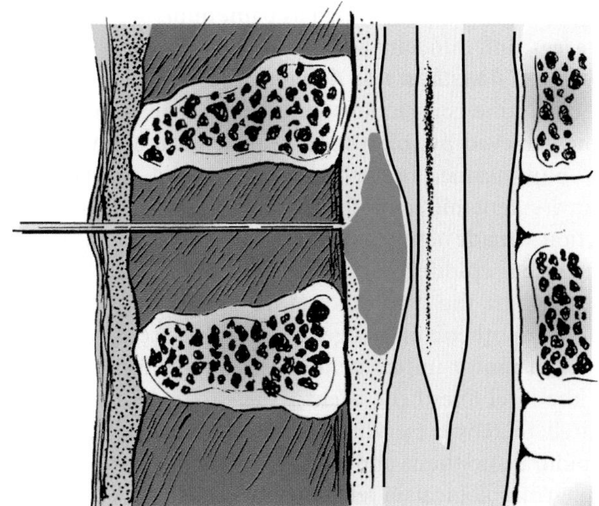

FIG 17-12 Blood-patch therapy for spinal headache.

Characteristically, assuming an upright position triggers or intensifies the headache, whereas assuming a supine position achieves relief (Hawkins & Bucklin, 2012). The resulting headache, auditory problems (e.g., tinnitus), and visual problems (e.g., blurred vision, photophobia) begin within 2 days of the puncture and may persist for days or weeks.

The likelihood of headache after dural puncture can be reduced, however, if the anesthesia care provider uses a small-gauge spinal needle and avoids making multiple punctures of the meninges. Passing an epidural catheter through the dural opening at the time of puncture to provide continuous spinal anesthesia, with removal of the catheter 24 hours later, may help prevent spinal headache. Injecting preservative-free saline through the spinal catheter before removing it also may decrease the incidence of headache. Hydration and bed rest in the prone position have been recommended as preventive measures, but have not been proven to be of much value (Hawkins & Bucklin, 2012).

Conservative management for a PDPH includes administration of oral analgesics and methylxanthines (e.g., caffeine or theophylline). Methylxanthines cause constriction of cerebral blood vessels and may provide symptomatic relief. An autologous epidural blood patch is the most rapid, reliable, and beneficial relief measure for PDPH. The woman's blood (i.e., 20 ml) is injected slowly into the lumbar epidural space, creating a clot that patches the tear or hole in the dura mater. Treatment with a blood patch is considered if the headache is severe or debilitating or does not resolve after conservative management. The blood patch is remarkably effective and is nearly complication free (Hawkins & Bucklin, 2012) (Fig. 17-12).

The woman should be observed for alteration in vital signs, pallor, clammy skin, and leakage of CSF for 1 to 2 hours after the blood patch is performed. If no complications occur she may then resume normal activity. She should, however, be instructed to avoid coughing or straining for the first day after the blood patch (Hawkins & Bucklin, 2012). She is also taught to avoid analgesics that affect platelet aggregation (e.g., nonsteroidal antiinflammatory drugs [NSAIDs]) for 2 days, drink plenty of fluids, and observe for signs of infection at the site and for neurologic symptoms such as pain, numbness and tingling in the legs, and difficulty with walking or elimination.

Epidural Anesthesia or Analgesia (Block). Relief from the pain of uterine contractions and birth (vaginal and cesarean) can be achieved by injecting a suitable local anesthetic agent (e.g., bupivacaine, ropivacaine), an opioid analgesic (e.g., fentanyl, sufentanil), or both into the epidural (peridural) space. Injection is made between the fourth and fifth lumbar vertebrae for a lumbar epidural block (see Figs. 17-8, *B*, and 17-10, *A*). Depending on the type, amount, and number of medications used, an anesthetic or analgesic effect will occur with varying degrees of motor impairment. The combination of an opioid with the local anesthetic agent reduces the dose of anesthetic required, thereby preserving a greater degree of motor function.

Epidural anesthesia and analgesia is currently the most effective pharmacologic pain relief method for labor. As a result, it is used by most women in the United States (Hawkins & Bucklin, 2012). For relieving the discomfort of labor and vaginal birth, a block from T10 to S5 is required. For cesarean birth, a block from at least T8 to S1 is essential. The diffusion of epidural anesthesia depends on the location of the catheter tip, the dose and volume of the anesthetic agent used, and the woman's position (e.g., horizontal or head-up). The woman must cooperate and maintain her position without moving during the insertion of the epidural catheter in order to prevent misplacement, neurologic injury, or hematoma formation.

MEDICATION ALERT

Epidural anesthesia effectively relieves the pain caused by uterine contractions. For most women, however, it does not completely remove the pressure sensations that occur as the fetus descends in the pelvis.

For the induction of an epidural block, the woman is positioned as for a spinal block. She may sit with her back curved or assume a modified Sims position with her shoulders parallel, legs slightly flexed, and back arched. It is important to avoid severe spinal flexion because it could compress the epidural space, increasing the risk for dural puncture (Burke, 2014) (see Fig. 17-11). A large-bore needle is inserted into the epidural space. A catheter is then threaded through the needle until its tip rests in the epidural space. The needle is then removed and the catheter is taped in place. After the epidural catheter is inserted and secured, a small amount of medication, called a test dose, is injected to be sure that the catheter has not been accidentally placed in the subarachnoid (spinal) space or in a blood vessel (Hawkins & Bucklin, 2012).

Initiating epidural anesthesia may be difficult when the woman is obese. She may find it harder to assume a position necessary for catheter placement. In addition, excess adipose tissue can obscure the anatomic landmarks used to identify the location of the appropriate insertion site. Morbidly obese women are also more likely to have accidental dural puncture (Jevitt, 2009). Although epidural catheter placement can present technical challenges, use of regional anesthesia can provide adequate pain management for the obese woman during labor and birth. Placing the catheter in early labor when the woman is more comfortable and is able to fully cooperate is a recommended solution (Burke, 2014; Hawkins & Bucklin, 2012). Early placement of a functioning epidural may reduce the potential complications associated with intubation during an emergent delivery. Note that epidural anesthesia presents less risk for the obese woman than does general anesthesia (AAP & ACOG, 2012).

After the epidural has been initiated, the woman is positioned preferably on her side so that the uterus does not compress the ascending vena cava and descending aorta, which can impair venous return, reduce cardiac output and blood pressure, and decrease placental perfusion. Her position should be alternated from side to side every hour. Upright positions and ambulation may be possible, depending on the degree of motor impairment. Oxygen should be available if hypotension occurs despite maintenance of hydration with IV fluid and displacement of the uterus to the side. Ephedrine or phenylephrine (vasopressors used to increase maternal blood pressure) and increased IV fluid infusion may be needed (see the Emergency box: Maternal Hypotension with Decreased Placental Perfusion). The fetal heart rate and pattern, contraction pattern, and progress in labor must be monitored carefully because the woman may not be aware of changes in the strength of the uterine contractions or the descent of the presenting part.

Several methods can be used for an epidural block. An intermittent block is achieved by using repeated injections of anesthetic solution; it is the least common method. The most common method is the continuous block, achieved by using a pump to infuse the anesthetic solution through an indwelling plastic catheter. Patient-controlled epidural analgesia (PCEA) is the newest method; it uses an indwelling catheter and a programmed pump that allows the woman to control the dosing. This method has been found to provide optimal analgesia with higher maternal satisfaction and enhanced sense of control during labor while decreasing the total amount of medication, including local anesthetic, used (Capogna & Stirparo, 2013). The advantages of an epidural block are numerous:

- The woman remains alert and is more comfortable and able to participate.
- Good relaxation is achieved.
- Airway reflexes remain intact.
- Only partial motor paralysis develops.
- Gastric emptying is not delayed.
- Blood loss is not excessive.

Fetal complications are rare but may occur in the event of rapid absorption of the medication or marked maternal hypotension. The dose, volume, type, and number of medications used can be modified (1) to allow the woman to push, to assume upright positions, and even to walk; (2) to produce perineal anesthesia; and (3) to permit forceps-assisted, vacuum-assisted, or cesarean birth if required.

The disadvantages of epidural block also are numerous. The woman's ability to move freely and to maintain control of her labor is limited, related to the use of numerous medical interventions (e.g., an intravenous infusion and electronic monitoring) and the occurrence of orthostatic hypotension and dizziness, sedation, and weakness of the legs. CNS effects (Box 17-5) can occur if a solution containing a local anesthetic agent is accidentally injected into a blood vessel or if excessive amounts of local anesthetic are given. High spinal or "total spinal" anesthesia,

BOX 17-5 Side Effects of Epidural and Spinal Anesthesia

- Hypotension
- Local anesthetic toxicity
  - Lightheadedness
  - Dizziness
  - Tinnitus (ringing in the ears)
  - Metallic taste
  - Numbness of the tongue and mouth
  - Bizarre behavior
  - Slurred speech
  - Convulsions
  - Loss of consciousness
- Fever
- Urinary retention
- Pruritus (itching)
- Limited movement
- Longer second stage labor
- Increased use of oxytocin
- Increased likelihood of forceps- or vacuum-assisted birth
- High or total spinal anesthesia

resulting in respiratory arrest, can occur if the relatively high dosage used with an epidural block is accidentally injected into the subarachnoid space. Women who receive an epidural have a higher rate of fever (i.e., intrapartum temperature of 38° C [100.4° F] or higher), especially when labor lasts longer than 12 hours; the temperature elevation most likely is related to thermoregulatory changes, although infection cannot be ruled out. The elevation in temperature can result in fetal tachycardia and neonatal workup for sepsis, whether or not signs of infection are present (see Box 17-5).

Hypotension as a result of sympathetic blockade can occur in about 10% to 30% of women who receive regional (spinal or epidural) analgesia during labor (Witcher & McLendon, 2013) (see Emergency box: Maternal Hypotension with Decreased Placental Perfusion). Hypotension can result in a significant decrease in uteroplacental perfusion and oxygen delivery to the fetus. Urinary retention and stress incontinence can occur in the immediate postpartum period. This temporary difficulty in urinary elimination could be related not only to the effects of the epidural block and the need for catheterization but also the increased duration of labor and need for forceps- or vacuum-assisted birth associated with the block. Pruritus (itching) is a side effect that often occurs with the use of an opioid, especially fentanyl. A relationship between epidural analgesia and longer second-stage labor, use of oxytocin, and forceps- or vacuum-assisted birth has been documented (Cunningham et al., 2014). Research findings have been unable to demonstrate a significant increase in cesarean birth associated with epidural analgesia (Hawkins & Bucklin, 2012). For some women the epidural block is not effective, and a second form of analgesia is required to establish effective pain relief. When women progress rapidly in labor, pain relief may not be obtained before birth occurs.

Combined Spinal-Epidural Analgesia. In the combined spinal-epidural (CSE) analgesia technique, sometimes referred to as a *walking epidural,* an epidural needle is inserted into the epidural space. Before the epidural catheter is placed, a smaller-gauge spinal needle is inserted through the bore of the epidural needle into the subarachnoid space. A small amount of opioid or combination of opioid and local anesthetic is then injected intrathecally to rapidly provide analgesia. Afterward the epidural catheter is inserted as usual. The CSE technique is an increasingly popular approach that can be used to block pain transmission without compromising motor ability. The concentration of opioid receptors is high along the pain pathway in the spinal cord, in the brainstem, and in the thalamus. Because these receptors are highly sensitive to opioids, a small quantity of an opioid-agonist analgesic produces marked pain relief lasting for several hours. If additional pain relief is needed, medication can be injected through the epidural catheter (see Fig. 17-10, *A*). The most common side effects of CSE are pruritus, urinary retention, immediate or delayed respiratory depression, and nausea. Naloxone can be given intravenously to manage these side effects without decreasing the degree of analgesia achieved (Hawkins & Bucklin, 2012). CSE analgesia is also associated with a greater incidence of FHR abnormalities than is epidural analgesia alone, necessitating close assessment of fetal heart rate and pattern (Cunningham et al., 2014).

Although women can walk (hence the term walking epidural), they often choose not to do so because of sedation and fatigue, abnormal sensations in and weakness of the legs, and a feeling of insecurity. Often health care providers are reluctant to encourage or assist women to ambulate for fear of injury. However, women can be assisted to change positions and use upright positions during labor and birth.

Epidural and Intrathecal (Spinal) Opioids. Opioids also can be used alone, eliminating the effect of a local anesthetic altogether. The use of epidural or intrathecal opioids without the addition of a local anesthetic agent during labor has several advantages. Opioids administered in this manner produce a rapid onset of pain relief but do not cause maternal hypotension or affect vital signs. The woman feels contractions but not pain. Her ability to bear down during the second stage of labor is preserved because the pushing reflex is not lost, and her motor power remains intact.

Fentanyl, sufentanil, or preservative-free morphine can be used. Fentanyl and sufentanil produce short-acting analgesia (1.5 to 3.5 hours), and morphine can provide pain relief for 4 to 7 hours. Morphine can be combined with fentanyl or sufentanil. Using short-acting opioids with multiparous women and morphine with nulliparous women or women with a history of long labors is appropriate. Because opioids alone usually do not provide adequate analgesia, however, they are most often given in combination with a local anesthetic (Cunningham et al., 2014).

A more common indication for the administration of epidural or intrathecal analgesics is the relief of postoperative pain. For example, a woman who gives birth by cesarean can receive fentanyl or morphine through a catheter. The catheter can then be removed, and the woman is usually free of pain for 24 hours. Occasionally the catheter is left in place in the epidural space in case another dose is needed.

Women receiving epidurally administered morphine after a cesarean birth can ambulate sooner than women who do not. The early ambulation and freedom from pain also facilitate bladder emptying, enhance peristalsis, and prevent clot formation (e.g., thrombophlebitis) in the lower extremities. Women may require additional medication for breakthrough pain during the first 24 hours after surgery. If so, they will usually be given an NSAID such as ketorolac (Toradol), indomethacin (Indocin), or ibuprofen (Motrin) rather than a narcotic.

Side effects of opioids administered by the epidural and intrathecal routes include nausea, vomiting, diminished peristalsis, pruritus, urinary retention, and delayed respiratory depression. These effects are more common when morphine is administered. Antiemetics, antipruritics, and opioid antagonists are used to relieve these symptoms. For example, naloxone or metoclopramide may be administered. Hospital protocols or detailed physician orders should provide specific instructions for the treatment of these side effects. Use of epidural opioids is not without risk. Respiratory depression is a serious concern; for this reason the woman's respiratory status should be assessed and documented every hour for 24 hours or as designated by hospital protocol. Naloxone should be readily available for use if the respiratory rate decreases to less than 10 breaths per minute or if the oxygen saturation rate decreases to less than 89%. Administration of oxygen by nonrebreather face mask also can be initiated, and the anesthesia care provider should be notified.

Contraindications to Subarachnoid and Epidural Blocks. Contraindications to epidural analgesia (Burke, 2014; Cunningham et al., 2014; Hawkins & Bucklin, 2012) include the following:

- Active or anticipated serious maternal hemorrhage. Acute hypovolemia leads to increased sympathetic tone to maintain the blood pressure. Any anesthetic technique that blocks the sympathetic fibers can produce significant hypotension that can endanger the mother and fetus.
- Maternal hypotension
- Coagulopathy: If a woman is receiving anticoagulant therapy (e.g., last dose of low-molecular-weight heparin within 12 hours) or has a bleeding disorder, injury to a blood vessel may cause the formation of a hematoma that may compress the cauda equina or the spinal cord and lead to serious CNS complications.
- Infection at the injection site. Infection can be spread through the peridural or subarachnoid spaces if the needle traverses an infected area.
- Increased intracranial pressure caused by a mass lesion
- Allergy to the anesthetic drug
- Maternal refusal or inability to cooperate
- Some types of maternal cardiac conditions

Epidural Block Effects on Newborn. Analgesia or anesthesia during labor and birth has little or no lasting effect on the physiologic status of the newborn. There is no evidence that the administration of maternal analgesia or anesthesia during labor and birth has a significant effect on the child's later mental and neurologic development (AAP & ACOG, 2012).

Nitrous Oxide for Analgesia

Nitrous oxide was used more widely for labor analgesia in the United States in the past but never as extensively as in other countries. However, interest in using nitrous oxide during labor has increased in the United States (Rooks, 2011). Nitrous oxide mixed with oxygen can be inhaled in a low concentration (50% or less) to provide analgesia during the first and second stages of labor. At the lower doses used for analgesia, it helps women relax, gives them a sense of control, and reduces their perception of pain even though they may still be aware that pain is present (Rooks, 2011).

A face mask is used to self-administer the gas. The woman places the mask over her mouth and nose as soon as a contraction begins. When she inhales, a valve opens and the gas is released. When inhalation stops, the valve closes, which prevents accidental overdosing. Scavenging equipment collects the woman's exhalations to protect health care workers from repetitive occupational exposure to nitrous oxide (Rooks, 2012).

The nurse should observe the woman for nausea, vomiting, dizziness, and drowsiness, the most common side effects of nitrous oxide (Klomp, van Poppel, Jones, et al., 2012). The use of nitrous oxide does not appear to depress uterine contractions or cause adverse reactions in the fetus and newborn. Its ease of use and rapid onset of action make it a good option for labor analgesia (Rooks, 2011; Rooks, 2012).

General Anesthesia

General anesthesia rarely is used for uncomplicated vaginal birth. It is used for only about 10% of cesarean births in the United States (Hawkins & Bucklin, 2012). General anesthesia may be necessary if a spinal or epidural block is contraindicated or if circumstances necessitate rapid birth (vaginal or emergent cesarean) without sufficient time or available personnel in the birth setting to perform a block (Witcher & McLendon, 2013). In addition, being awake and aware during major surgery may be unacceptable for some women having a cesarean birth. The major risks associated with general anesthesia are difficulty with or inability to intubate and aspiration of gastric contents (Cunningham et al., 2014; Hawkins and Bucklin). Anesthesia care providers are more likely to encounter difficulty with intubating morbidly obese women, especially in an emergency situation, than women of normal weight (Witcher & McLendon).

If general anesthesia is being considered, give the woman nothing by mouth and ensure that an IV infusion is in place. If time allows, premedicate the woman with a nonparticulate (clear) oral antacid (e.g., sodium citrate/citric acid [Bicitra]) to neutralize the acidic contents of the stomach. Aspiration of highly acidic gastric contents will damage lung tissue. Some anesthesia care providers also order the administration of a histamine (H_2)-receptor blocker such as famotidine (Pepcid) or ranitidine (Zantac) to decrease gastric acid production and metoclopramide (Reglan) to accelerate gastric emptying (Cunningham et al., 2014; Hawkins & Bucklin, 2012). Before the anesthesia is given, a wedge should be placed under one of the woman's hips to displace the uterus. Uterine displacement prevents compression of the aorta and vena cava, which maintains cardiac output and placental perfusion (Cunningham et al.; Hawkins & Bucklin).

Prior to anesthesia induction, the woman will be preoxygenated with 100% oxygen by nonrebreather face mask for 2 to 3 minutes. This is especially important in pregnant women,

EVIDENCE-BASED PRACTICE

Nitrous Oxide: Laughing Gas for Labor

Ask the Question

Is nitrous oxide a safe and effective form of pain relief that can be recommended for laboring women?

Search for the Evidence

Search Strategies English language research-based publications since 2011 on nitrous oxide, laughing gas, labor pain relief were included.

Databases Used Cochrane Collaborative Database, National Guideline Clearinghouse (AHRQ), CINAHL, PubMed, UpToDate, and the professional websites for ACOG and AWHONN.

Critical Appraisal of the Evidence

Nitrous oxide is a patient-controlled analgesia/anesthesia used for pain relief since the 1880s. It has been commonly used for labor analgesia in Canada and the United Kingdom for decades. It is delivered via mask, which the laboring woman holds to her face during contractions. Its recent introduction into practice in the United States is limited by the supply of equipment to blend the mixture of 50/50 nitrous oxide and oxygen (Likis, Andrews, Collins, et al., 2014).

- Nitrous oxide increases endorphin and dopamine levels, diminishing pain and anxiety.
- Systematic analyses comparing epidural to nitrous oxide have not shown a difference between the Apgar scores or special care admission rates between the two groups (Likis et al., 2014). Further research is needed for long-term effects.
- When compared with nitrous oxide, epidurals were associated with more hypotension, fever, motor blockade, urinary retention, and instrumental and cesarean births for fetal distress, although there was no difference in cesarean rates overall (Jones, Othman, Doswell, et al., 2012).
- Although nitrous oxide does not relieve pain as well as an epidural, it does provide other benefits: it is inexpensive, less invasive than epidural, requires less intensive monitoring, and does not limit mobility (Likis et al., 2014).
- The most common side effects of nitrous oxide are nausea, vomiting, dizziness, and drowsiness (Klomp, van Poppel, Jones, et al., 2012).

Apply the Evidence: Nursing Implications

- Some women will want the maximum pain relief of epidurals, while others may be willing to trade that for the benefits of sense of control, mobility, and limited monitoring of nitrous oxide (Rooks, 2012).
- Because nitrous has a rapid onset and clearance, it can be an excellent choice for women who want to wait for an epidural, whose epidural is not effective, or who come in too late for an epidural (Likis et al., 2014).
- Nitrous oxide is effective within a minute (Klomp et al., 2012). Women can start with nitrous oxide and easily move to another pain relief method, as needed.
- Health care providers are exposed to ambient gas vapors in close settings. The effects of this are unknown. Appropriate ventilation greatly diminishes this exposure (Likis et al., 2014).
- Because nitrous oxide produces euphoria and dissociation with pain, future research on women's satisfaction with the method may be a better measure than "pain relief" (Likis et al., 2014).

Quality and Safety Competencies: Evidence-Based Practice*

Knowledge

Describe how the strength and relevance of available evidence influence the choice of interventions in provision of client-centered care.

Nurses use high-level evidence to offer pain relief options to women in labor, based on the client's preferences.

Skills

Participate in structuring the work environment to facilitate integration of new evidence into standards of practice.

Nurses and health care providers learn safe and effective nitrous oxide administration, and educate clients.

Attitudes

Value the need for continuous improvement in clinical practice based on new knowledge.

Nurses advocate for appropriate pain relief, and collaborate in research on outcomes, including client satisfaction.

References

Jones, L., Othman, M., Doswell, T., et al. (2012). Pain management for women in labour: An overview of systematic reviews. In *The Cochrane Database of Systematic Reviews 2012* (3). Chichester, UK: John Wiley & Sons.

Klomp, T., van Poppel, M., Jones, L., et al. (2012). Inhaled analgesia for pain management in labour. In *The Cochrane Database of Systematic Reviews 2012* (9). Chichester, UK: John Wiley & Sons.

Likis, F. E., Andrews, J. C., Collins, M. R., et al. (2014). Nitrous oxide for the management of labor pain: A systematic review. *Anesthesia & Analgesia, 118*(1), 153–168.

Rooks, J. P. (2012). Labor pain management other than neuraxial: What do we know and where do we go next? *Birth, 39*(4), 318–322.

Pat Mahaffee Gingrich

*Adapted from QSEN at www.qsen.org.

who are more likely than other adults to rapidly become hypoxemic if there is a delay in successful intubation. For many years, thiopental, a short-acting barbiturate, was widely used to induce anesthesia. However, the drug is no longer available in the United States. Its manufacturer stopped production because the drug was also used for capital punishment. Propofol (Diprivan), etomidate, or ketamine are now used instead. They are administered intravenously to render the woman unconscious (Cunningham et al., 2014). Next, succinylcholine, a muscle relaxer, is administered to facilitate passage of an endotracheal tube (Cunningham et al.; Hawkins & Bucklin, 2012). Sometimes the nurse is asked to assist with applying cricoid pressure before intubation as the woman begins to lose consciousness. This maneuver blocks the esophagus and prevents aspiration should the woman vomit or regurgitate (Fig. 17-13). Pressure is released once the endotracheal tube is securely in place.

After the woman is intubated, nitrous oxide and oxygen in a 50:50 mixture are administered. A low concentration of a volatile halogenated agent (e.g., isoflurane) also may be administered to increase pain relief and to reduce maternal awareness and recall (Cunningham et al., 2014; Hawkins & Bucklin, 2012).

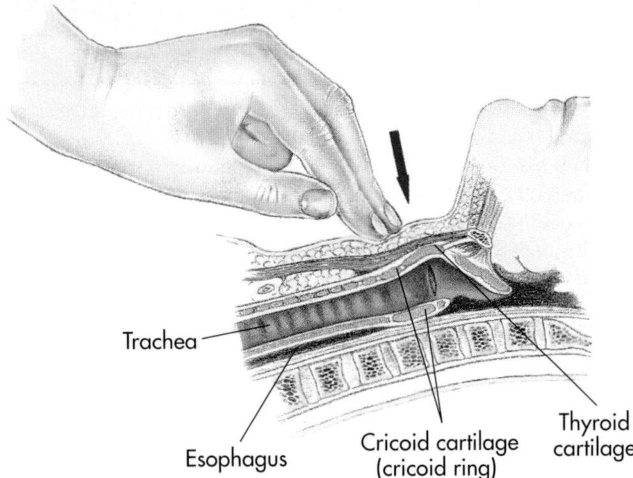

FIG 17-13 Technique of applying pressure on cricoid cartilage to occlude esophagus to prevent pulmonary aspiration of gastric contents during induction of general anesthesia.

In higher concentrations, isoflurane or methoxyflurane relaxes the uterus quickly and facilitates intrauterine manipulation, version, and extraction. However, at higher concentrations these agents cross the placenta readily and can produce narcosis in the fetus and could reduce uterine tone after birth, increasing the risk for hemorrhage. Because of this risk for neonatal narcosis, it is critical that the baby be delivered as soon as possible after inducing anesthesia to reduce the degree of fetal exposure to the anesthetic agents and the CNS depressants administered.

Priorities for recovery room care are to maintain an open airway and cardiopulmonary function and to prevent postpartum hemorrhage. Women who had surgery under general anesthesia will require pain medication soon after regaining consciousness. Routine postpartum care is organized to facilitate parent-infant attachment as soon as possible and to answer the mother's questions. When appropriate, the nurse assesses the mother's readiness to see her baby, as well as her response to the anesthesia and to the event that necessitated general anesthesia (e.g., emergency cesarean birth when vaginal birth was anticipated).

CARE MANAGEMENT

The choice of pain relief interventions depends on a combination of factors, including the woman's special needs and wishes, the availability of the desired method or methods, the knowledge and expertise in nonpharmacologic and pharmacologic methods of the health care providers involved in the woman's care, and the phase and stage of labor. (See the Nursing Care Plan for possible nursing diagnoses and interventions.)

Nonpharmacologic Interventions

The nurse supports and assists the woman as she uses nonpharmacologic interventions for pain relief and relaxation. During labor the nurse should ask the woman how she feels to evaluate the effectiveness of the specific pain management techniques used. Appropriate interventions can then be planned or continued for effective care, such as trying other nonpharmacologic methods or combining nonpharmacologic methods with medications. A pain scale, in which 0 represents no pain and 10 represents pain as bad as it could possibly be, is often used to evaluate a woman's pain before and after pain relief interventions are implemented. Comparing the woman's answers provides a way to objectively evaluate the effectiveness of pain relief interventions. Sometimes a coping scale, rather than a pain scale, is used to evaluate how well the woman is dealing with the discomfort of labor.

Pharmacologic Interventions

Informed Consent

Pregnant women have the right to be active participants in determining the best pain care approach to use during labor and birth. The primary health care provider and anesthesia care provider are responsible for fully informing women of the alternative methods of pharmacologic pain relief available in the birth setting. A description of the various anesthetic techniques and what they entail is essential to informed consent, even if the woman received information about analgesia and anesthesia earlier in her pregnancy. The initial discussion of pain management options ideally should take place in the third trimester so the woman has time to consider alternatives. Nurses play a part in the informed consent by clarifying and describing procedures or by acting as the woman's advocate and asking the primary health care provider for further explanations. The three essential components of an informed consent are:

- First, the procedure and its advantages and disadvantages must be thoroughly explained.
- Second, the woman must agree with the plan of labor pain care as explained to her.
- Third, her consent must be given freely without coercion or manipulation from her health care provider.

LEGAL TIP: Informed Consent for Anesthesia

The woman receives (in an understandable manner) the following:

- Explanation of alternative methods of anesthesia and analgesia available
- Description of the anesthetic, including its effects and the procedure for its administration
- Description of the benefits, discomforts, risks, and consequences for the mother, the fetus, and the newborn
- Explanation of how complications can be treated
- Information that the anesthetic is not always effective
- Indication that the woman may withdraw consent at any time
- Opportunity to have any question answered
- Opportunity to have components of the consent explained in the woman's own words

The consent form will:

- Be written or explained in the woman's primary language
- Have the woman's signature
- Have the date of consent
- Carry the signature of the anesthetic care provider, certifying that the woman has received and expresses understanding of the explanation

! NURSING ALERT

In some cultures a husband is expected to consent to procedures performed on his wife. Although in the United States the woman gives consent and signs any necessary forms, she may not be willing to do so unless her husband also approves.

NURSING CARE PLAN

Nonpharmacologic Pain Management

NURSING DIAGNOSIS	EXPECTED OUTCOME	INTERVENTIONS	RATIONALES
Anxiety related to lack of confidence in ability to cope effectively with pain during labor	Woman will express decrease in anxiety and experience satisfaction with her labor and birth performance.	Assess whether woman and significant other have attended childbirth classes, their knowledge of labor process, and their current level of anxiety.	To plan supportive strategies that address couple's specific needs
		Encourage support person to remain with woman in labor.	To provide support and increase probability of positive response to comfort measures
		Teach or review nonpharmacologic techniques available to decrease anxiety and pain during labor (e.g., focusing, relaxation and breathing techniques, effleurage, and sacral pressure).	To enhance chances of success in using techniques
		Explore other techniques that woman or significant other may have learned in childbirth classes (e.g., hypnosis, hydrotherapy, acupressure, biofeedback, therapeutic touch, aromatherapy, imaging, music).	To provide more options for coping strategies
		Explore use of transcutaneous electrical nerve stimulation if ordered by primary health care provider.	To provide increased perception of control over pain and increase in release of endogenous opiates (endorphins)
		Assist woman to change positions and to use pillows.	To reduce stiffness, aid circulation, and promote comfort
		Assess bladder for distention, and encourage voiding often.	To avoid bladder distention, subsequent discomfort, and potential for suppression of uterine contractions
		Encourage rest between contractions.	To minimize fatigue
		Keep woman and significant other informed about progress.	To allay anxiety
		Guide couple through labor stages and phases, helping them use and modify comfort techniques that are appropriate to each phase.	To ensure greatest effectiveness of techniques used
		Support couple if pharmacologic measures are required to increase pain relief, explaining safety and effectiveness.	To reduce anxiety and maintain self-esteem and sense of control over labor process
Readiness for Enhanced Childbearing Process related to desire for healthy outcome of labor and birth	Woman will participate in planning care for labor.	Discuss woman's birth plan and knowledge about birth process.	To collect data for nursing plan of care
		Provide information about labor process.	To correct any misconceptions
		Inform woman about her labor status and the fetus's well-being.	To promote comfort and confidence
		Discuss rationales for all interventions.	To incorporate woman into plan of care
		Incorporate nonpharmacologic interventions into plan of care.	To increase woman's sense of control during labor
		Provide emotional support and ongoing positive feedback.	To enhance positive coping mechanisms

Timing of Administration

Nonpharmacologic measures can be used to relieve pain and stress and enhance progress at any time in labor.

It is often the nurse who notifies the primary health care provider that the woman is in need of pharmacologic measures to relieve her discomfort. Orders are often written for the administration of pain medication as needed by the woman and based on the nurse's clinical judgment. In the past, pharmacologic measures for pain relief were usually not implemented until labor had advanced to the active phase of the first stage of labor and the cervix had dilated approximately 4 to 5 cm, to avoid suppressing the progress of labor. However, it is now known that epidural anesthesia in early labor does not increase the rate of cesarean birth. Whereas it may shorten the duration of first-stage labor in some women, epidural anesthesia lengthens it in others (Hawkins & Bucklin, 2012). It is no longer recommended that women in labor reach a certain level of cervical dilation or fetal station before receiving epidural anesthesia (AAP & ACOG, 2012; Cunningham et al., 2014). It is, however, still recommended that the administration of systemic opioid analgesics be delayed until labor is well established (Burke, 2014).

Preparation for Procedures

The methods of pain relief available to the woman are reviewed and information is clarified as necessary. The procedure and what will be asked of the woman (e.g., to maintain flexed position during insertion of epidural needle) must be explained.

The woman also can benefit from knowing the way that the medication is to be given, the interval before the medication takes effect, and the expected pain relief from the medication. Skin-preparation measures are described, and an explanation is given for the need to empty the bladder before the analgesic or anesthetic is administered and the reason for keeping the bladder empty. When an indwelling catheter is to be threaded into the epidural space, the woman should be told that she may have a momentary twinge down her leg, hip, or back and that this feeling is not a sign of injury (Box 17-6).

Administration of Medication

Accurate monitoring of the progress of labor forms the basis for the nurse's judgment that a woman needs pharmacologic control of discomfort. Knowledge of the medications used during childbirth is essential. The most effective route of administration is selected for each woman; then the medication is prepared and administered correctly.

Any medication can cause a minor or severe allergic reaction. As part of the assessment for such allergic reactions, the nurse should monitor the woman's vital signs, respiratory effort, cardiovascular status, integument, and platelet and white blood cell count. The woman is observed for side effects of drug therapy, especially drowsiness and dyspnea. Minor reactions can consist of rash, rhinitis, fever, shortness of breath, or pruritus. Management of the less acute allergic response is not an emergency.

Severe allergic reactions (anaphylaxis) may occur suddenly and lead to shock or death. The most dramatic form of anaphylaxis is sudden, severe bronchospasm, upper airway obstruction, and hypotension (Norred, 2012). Signs of anaphylaxis are largely caused by contraction of smooth muscles and may begin with irritability, extreme weakness, nausea, and vomiting. This may lead to dyspnea, cyanosis, convulsions, and cardiac arrest. Anaphylaxis must be diagnosed and treated immediately. Initial treatment usually consists of placing the woman in a supine position, injecting epinephrine intramuscularly, administering fluid intravenously, supporting the airway with ventilation if necessary, and giving oxygen. If the response to these measures is inadequate, IV epinephrine should be given (Norred). Cardiopulmonary resuscitation may be necessary (see Chapter 30).

Intravenous Route. The preferred route of administration of medications such as meperidine, fentanyl, butorphanol, or nalbuphine is through IV tubing, administered into the port nearest the point of insertion of the infusion (proximal port). The medication is given slowly, in small doses, during a contraction. It may be given over a period of three to five consecutive contractions if needed to complete the dose. It is given during contractions to decrease fetal exposure to the medication because uterine blood vessels are constricted during contractions and the medication stays within the maternal vascular system for several seconds before the uterine blood vessels reopen. The IV infusion is then restarted slowly to prevent a bolus of medication from being administered. With this method of injection, the amount of medication crossing the placenta to the fetus is minimized. The IV route has the following advantages:

- Onset of pain relief is rapid and more predictable.
- Pain relief is obtained with small doses of the drug.
- Duration of effect is more predictable.

Intramuscular Route. Although analgesics are still sometimes given intramuscularly (IM), it is not the preferred route of administration for the woman in labor. The advantages of using the IM route are quick administration and no need to start an IV line.

Disadvantages of the IM route include:

- Onset of pain relief is delayed.
- Higher doses of medication are required.
- Medication is released at an unpredictable rate from the muscle tissue and is available for transfer across the placenta to the fetus.

The maternal medication levels (after IM injections) are unequal because of uneven distribution (maternal uptake) and metabolism. IM injections given in the upper arm (deltoid muscle) seem to result in more rapid absorption and higher blood levels of the medication than when administered in other sites (Bricker & Lavender, 2002). If regional anesthesia is planned later in labor, the deltoid muscle is the preferred site. The autonomic blockade from the regional (e.g., epidural) anesthesia increases blood flow to the gluteal region and accelerates absorption of medication that may be sequestered there. Administration of opioids subcutaneously in the upper arm avoids this risk and, as a result, is often used as an alternative to an IM injection.

Regional (Epidural or Spinal) Anesthesia. According to professional standards (Association of Women's Health, Obstetric and Neonatal Nurses [AWHONN], 2012), the nonanesthetist registered nurse is permitted to monitor the status of the woman receiving regional anesthesia, the fetus, and the progress of labor; replace empty infusion syringes or

BOX 17-6 Nursing Interventions for the Woman Receiving Epidural or Spinal Anesthesia

Prior to the Block

- Assist primary health care provider or anesthesia care provider with explaining the procedure and obtaining the woman's informed consent.
- Assess maternal vital signs, level of hydration, labor progress, and fetal heart rate (FHR) and pattern.
- Start an IV line and infuse a bolus of fluid (Ringer's lactate or normal saline) if ordered (e.g., 500 to 1000 ml 15 to 30 minutes prior to induction of the anesthesia).
- Obtain laboratory results (hematocrit or hemoglobin level, other tests as ordered).
- Assess the woman's level of pain using a pain scale (from 0 [no pain] to 10 [pain as bad as it could possibly be]).
- Assist the woman to void.

During Initiation of the Block

- Assist the woman with assuming and maintaining the proper position.
- Verbally guide the woman through the procedure, explaining sounds and sensations as she experiences them.
- Assist the anesthesia care provider with documentation of vital signs, time and amount of medications given, etc.
- Monitor maternal vital signs (especially blood pressure) and FHR as ordered.
- Have oxygen and suction readily available.
- Monitor for signs of local anesthetic toxicity (see Box 17-5) as the test dose of medication is administered.

While the Block Is in Effect

- Continue to monitor maternal vital signs and FHR as ordered (continuous monitoring of maternal heart rate [electrocardiogram (ECG)] and blood pressure may be ordered to monitor for accidental intravenous injection of medication).
- Continue to assess the woman's level of pain with every check of vital signs using a pain scale (from 0 [no pain] to 10 [pain as bad as it could possibly be]).
- Monitor for bladder distention.
  - Assist with spontaneous voiding on a bedpan or toilet.
  - Insert a urinary catheter if necessary.
- Encourage or assist the woman to change positions from side to side every hour.
- Promote safety.
  - Keep the side rails up on the bed.
  - Place the telephone and call light within easy reach.
  - Instruct the woman not to get out of bed without help.
  - Make sure there is no prolonged pressure on anesthetized body parts.
- Keep the epidural catheter insertion site clean and dry.
- Continue to monitor for anesthetic side effects (see Box 17-5).

While the Block Is Wearing Off After Birth

- Assess regularly for the return of sensory and motor function.
- Continue to monitor maternal vital signs as ordered.
- Monitor for bladder distention.
  - Assist with spontaneous voiding on the bedpan or toilet.
  - Insert a urinary catheter if necessary.
- Promote safety.
  - Keep the side rails up on the bed.
  - Place the telephone and call light within easy reach.
  - Instruct the woman not to get out of bed without help.
  - Make sure there is no prolonged pressure on anesthetized body parts.
- Keep the epidural catheter insertion site clean and dry.
- Continue to monitor for anesthetic side effects (see Box 17-5).

bags with the same medication and concentration; stop the infusion and initiate emergency measures if the need arises; and remove the catheter if properly educated to do so. Only qualified, licensed anesthesia care providers are permitted to insert a catheter and initiate epidural anesthesia, verify catheter placement, inject medication through the catheter, or alter the medication or medications, including the type, the amount, or the rate of infusion.

SAFETY ALERT

Safe regional anesthesia administration requires specialized education, experience, and competence. There is potential for significant maternal and fetal morbidity and mortality associated with some obstetric anesthesia complications. Therefore, a licensed, credentialed anesthesia care provider should manage regional anesthesia and analgesia during labor and birth and be readily available to manage obstetric anesthesia-related emergencies (AWHONN, 2012).

Because spinal nerve blocks can reduce bladder sensation, resulting in difficulty voiding, the woman should empty her bladder before the induction of the block and should be encouraged to void at least every 2 hours thereafter. The nurse should palpate for bladder distention and measure urinary output to ensure that the bladder is being completely emptied. A distended bladder can inhibit uterine contractions and fetal descent, resulting in a slowing of the progress of labor. For this reason, an indwelling urinary catheter (Foley) is often routinely inserted immediately after epidural or spinal anesthesia is initiated and left in place for the remainder of the first stage of labor.

The status of the maternal-fetal unit and the progress of labor must be established before the block is performed. The nurse must assist the woman to assume and maintain the correct position for induction of epidural and spinal anesthesia (see Fig. 17-11, *A* and *B*).

Depending on the level of motor blockade, the woman should be assisted to remain as mobile as possible. When in bed, her position should be alternated from side to side every hour to ensure adequate distribution of the anesthetic solution and to maintain circulation to the uterus and placenta.

SAFETY ALERT

After receiving an epidural block or opioid intravenously for pain, the woman should not be allowed to ambulate alone. She must either remain in bed or request assistance before attempting to get out of bed. The nurse assesses the woman for signs of orthostatic hypotension and return of sensation and motor function of the lower extremities prior to ambulation.

Health care providers should be aware that effective epidural anesthesia prolongs the second stage of labor by 15 to 30 minutes. A longer second stage of labor does not negatively affect maternal or fetal outcome, however, as long as the FHR tracing is normal, maternal hydration and analgesia are adequate, and there is ongoing progress in the descent of the fetal head. Therefore, operative interventions (e.g., the use of forceps or vacuum) to hasten the birth solely because the second stage is prolonged are unnecessary. Reducing the density of the epidural block during the second stage of labor, delaying pushing until the woman feels the urge to do so, and avoiding arbitrary definitions for the "normal" duration of second-stage labor are suggested as interventions to decrease the risk of operative vaginal birth (Hawkins & Bucklin, 2012). (See Chapter 19 for a full discussion of second-stage labor management.) Box 17-6 summarizes the nursing interventions for women receiving epidural or spinal anesthesia.

Safety and General Care

The nurse monitors and records the woman's response to nonpharmacologic pain relief methods and to medication(s). This includes the degree of pain relief, the level of apprehension, the return of sensations and perception of pain, and allergic or adverse reactions (e.g., hypotension, respiratory depression, fever, pruritus, and nausea and vomiting). The nurse continues to monitor maternal vital signs and fetal heart rate and pattern at frequent intervals, the strength and frequency of uterine contractions, changes in the cervix and station of the presenting part, the presence and quality of the bearing-down reflex, bladder filling, and state of hydration. Determining the fetal response after administration of analgesia or anesthesia is vital. The woman is asked if she (or the family) has any questions. The nurse also assesses the woman's and her family's understanding of the need for ensuring her safety (e.g., keeping side rails up, calling for assistance as needed).

The time that elapses between the administration of an opioid and the baby's birth is documented. Medications given to the newborn to reverse opioid effects are recorded. After birth, the woman who has had spinal, epidural, or general anesthesia is assessed for return of sensory and motor function in addition to the usual postpartum assessments. Both the nurse and the anesthesia provider are responsible for documenting assessments and care in relation to the epidural.

KEY POINTS

- Nonpharmacologic pain and stress management strategies are valuable for managing labor discomfort alone or in combination with pharmacologic methods.
- The gate-control theory of pain and the stress response are the bases for many of the nonpharmacologic methods of pain relief.
- The type of analgesic or anesthetic to be used is determined by maternal and health care provider preference, the stage of labor, and the method of birth.
- Sedatives may be appropriate for women in prolonged early labor when there is a need to decrease anxiety or promote sleep or therapeutic rest.
- Naloxone (Narcan) is an opioid (narcotic) antagonist that can reverse narcotic effects, especially respiratory depression.
- Pharmacologic control of pain during labor requires collaboration among the health care providers and the laboring woman.
- The nurse must understand medications, their expected effects, potential side effects, and methods of administration.
- Maintenance of maternal fluid balance is essential during spinal and epidural nerve blocks.
- Maternal analgesia or anesthesia potentially affects neonatal neurobehavioral response.
- The use of opioid agonist-antagonist analgesics in women with preexisting opioid dependence may cause symptoms of abstinence syndrome (opioid withdrawal).
- Epidural anesthesia and analgesia is the most effective available pharmacologic pain relief method for labor. It is used by the majority of women in the United States.
- General anesthesia is rarely used for vaginal birth but may be used for cesarean birth or whenever rapid anesthesia is needed in an emergency childbirth situation.

REFERENCES

American Academy of Pediatrics (AAP) & American College of Obstetricians and Gynecologists (ACOG). (2012). *Guidelines for perinatal care* (7th ed.). Washington, DC: ACOG.

American Society of Anesthesiologists Task Force on Obstetric Anesthesia. (2007). Practice guidelines for obstetric anesthesia. *Anesthesiology, 106*(4), 843–863.

Anderson, D. (2011). A review of systemic opioids commonly used for labor pain relief. *Journal of Midwifery & Women's Health, 56*(3), 222–239.

Andrews, M. M., & Boyle, J. S. (2012). *Transcultural concepts in nursing care* (5th ed.). Philadelphia: Lippincott Williams & Wilkins.

Archie, C. L., & Roman, A. S. (2013). Normal & abnormal labor & delivery. In A. H. DeCherney, L. Nathan, N. Laufer, & A. S. Roman (Eds.), *Current diagnosis & treatment: Obstetrics & gynecology* (11th ed.). New York: The McGraw-Hill Companies, Inc.

Arendt, K. W., & Tessmer-Tuck, J. A. (2013). Nonpharmacologic labor analgesia. *Clinics in Perinatology, 40*(3), 351–371.

Association of Women's Health, Obstetric and Neonatal Nurses (AWHONN). (2012). Role of the registered nurse in the care of the pregnant woman receiving analgesia and anesthesia by catheter techniques: Clinical position statement. *Journal of Obstetric, Gynecologic, & Neonatal Nursing, 41*(3), 455–457.

Barragán Loayza, I., Solà, I., & Juandó Prats, C. (2011). Biofeedback for pain management during labour. *The Cochrane Database of Systematic Reviews*, 6, CD006168.

Blackburn, S. (2013). *Maternal, fetal, and neonatal physiology: A clinical perspective* (3rd ed.). St. Louis: Mosby.

Borders, N., Wendland, C., Haozous, E., et al. (2013). Midwives' verbal support of nulliparous women in second-stage labor. *Journal of Obstetric, Gynecologic, & Neonatal Nursing, 42*(3), 311–320.

Bricker, L., & Lavender, T. (2002). Parenteral opioids for labor pain relief: A systematic review. *American Journal of Obstetrics and Gynecology, 186*(Suppl 5), S94–S109.

Burke, C. (2014). Pain in labor: Nonpharmacologic and pharmacologic management. In K. Rice Simpson, & P. Creehan (Eds.), *AWHONN's perinatal nursing* (4th ed.). Philadelphia: Lippincott Williams & Wilkins.

Capogna, G., & Stirparo, S. (2013). Techniques for the maintenance of epidural labor analgesia. *Current Opinion in Anaesthesiology, 26*(3), 261–267.

Creehan, P. (2008). Pain relief and comfort measures in labor. In K. Rice Simpson, & P. Creehan (Eds.), *AWHONN's perinatal nursing* (3rd ed.). Philadelphia: Lippincott Williams & Wilkins.

Cunningham, F., Leveno, K., Bloom, et al. (2014). *Williams obstetrics* (24th ed.). New York: McGraw-Hill Education.

Dean, B. J. F., Gwilym, S. E., & Carr, A. J. (2013). Why does my shoulder hurt? A review of the neuroanatomical and biochemical basis of shoulder pain. *British Journal of Sports Medicine, 47*(17), 1095–1104.

Devereaux, Y., & Sullivan, H. (2013). Doula support while laboring: Does it help achieve a more natural birth? *International Journal of Childbirth Education, 28*(2), 54–61.

Francis, R. (2012). TENS (transcutaneous electrical nerve stimulation) for labour pain. *Practising Midwife, 15*(5), 20–23.

Gilbert, E. (2011). *Manual of high risk pregnancy & delivery* (5th ed.). St. Louis: Mosby.

Gisin, M., Poat, A., Fierz, K., & Frei, I. (2013). Women's experiences of acupuncture during labour. *British Journal of Midwifery, 21*(4), 254–262.

Hawkins, J., & Bucklin, B. (2012). Obstetrical anesthesia. In S. Gabbe, J. Niebyl, & J. Simpson (Eds.), *Obstetrics: Normal and problem pregnancies* (6th ed.). Philadelphia: Saunders.

Hodnett, E. D., Gates, S., Hofmeyr, G., & Sakala, C. (2013). Continuous support for women during childbirth. *The Cochrane Database of Systematic Reviews, 7*, CD003766.

Jevitt, C. (2009). Pregnancy complicated by obesity: Midwifery management. *Journal of Midwifery & Women's Health, 54*(6), 445–451.

Jones, L., Othman, M., Dowswell, T., et al. (2012). Pain management for women in labor: An overview of systematic reviews. *The Cochrane Database of Systematic Reviews, 3*, CD009234.

Klomp, T., van Poppel, M., Jones, L., et al. (2012). Inhaled analgesia for pain management in labour. In *The Cochrane Database of Systematic Reviews 2012, 9*, CD009351.

Melchart, D., Jack, M., & Kashanian, M. (2011). Acupressure may relieve pain, delivery time and oxytocin use during labour. *Focus on Alternative & Complementary Therapies, 16*(1), 40–41.

Meyer, S. (2013). Control in childbirth: A concept analysis and synthesis. *Journal of Advanced Nursing, 69*(1), 218–228.

Norred, C. L. (2012). Anesthetic-induced anaphylaxis. *American Association of Nurse Anesthetists Journal, 80*(2), 129–150.

Nur Rachmawati, I. (2012). Maternal reflection on labour pain management and influencing factors. *British Journal of Midwifery, 20*(4), 263–270.

Perinatal Education Associates. (2014). *Breathing*. Available at www.birthsource.com.

Rooks, J. P. (2012). Labor pain management other than neuraxial: What do we know and where do we go next? *Birth, 39*(4), 318–322.

Rooks, J. (2011). Safety and risks of nitrous oxide labor analgesia: A review. *Journal of Midwifery & Women's Health, 56*(6), 557–565.

Royal College of Obstetricians & Gynaecologists (RCOG). (2006). *Immersion in Water During Labour and Birth (RCOG / Royal College of Midwives Joint Statement No. 1)*. London, UK: RCOG.

Smith, C. A., Levett, K. M., Collins, C. T., & Jones, L. (2012). Massage, reflexology and other manual methods for pain management in labour. *The Cochrane Database of Systematic Reviews, 2*, CD009290.

Walls, D. (2009). Herbs and natural therapies for pregnancy, birth, and breastfeeding. *International Journal of Childbirth Education, 24*(2), 29–37.

Weatherspoon, D. (2011). Current practices in easing discomfort from labor and delivery: Alternative and medical practices. *International Journal of Childbirth Education, 25*(4), 44–48.

Witcher, P., & McLendon, K. (2013). Anesthesia emergencies in the obstetric setting. In N. Troiano, C. Harvey, & B. Chez (Eds.), *AWHONN's high risk and critical care obstetrics* (3rd ed.). Philadelphia: Lippincott Williams & Wilkins.

18 CHAPTER

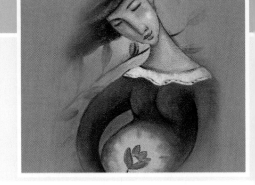

Fetal Assessment During Labor

Kitty Cashion

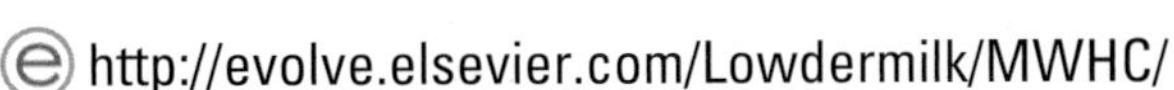
http://evolve.elsevier.com/Lowdermilk/MWHC/

LEARNING OBJECTIVES

- Identify typical signs of normal and abnormal fetal heart rate (FHR) patterns.
- Compare FHR monitoring performed by intermittent auscultation with external and internal electronic methods.
- Explain the baseline FHR and evaluate periodic changes.
- Describe nursing measures that can be used to maintain FHR patterns within normal limits.
- Differentiate among the nursing interventions used for managing specific FHR patterns, including tachycardia and bradycardia, absent or minimal variability, and late and variable decelerations.
- Review the documentation of the monitoring process necessary during labor.

The ability to assess the fetus by auscultation of the fetal heart was initially described more than 300 years ago. With the advent of the fetoscope and stethoscope after the turn of the 20th century, the listener could hear clearly enough to count the FHR. When electronic FHR monitoring made its debut for clinical use in the early 1970s, the anticipation was that its use would result in less intrapartum asphyxia and thus fewer cases of cerebral palsy. Consequently the use of electronic fetal monitoring (EFM) rapidly expanded (Garite, 2012). However, the rate of cerebral palsy has not declined since that time and is not likely to decrease, because more preterm infants are surviving (Gilbert, 2011). Prematurity is the leading cause of cerebral palsy. Intrapartum asphyxia accounts for 25% of cases or less of this disorder (Garite).

Still, EFM is a useful tool for visualizing FHR patterns on a monitor screen or printed tracing. It continues to be the primary mode of intrapartum fetal assessment in the United States and is the most commonly performed obstetric procedure in that country (American College of Obstetricians and Gynecologists [ACOG], 2009; Miller, Miller, & Tucker, 2013). Pregnant women should be informed about the equipment and procedures used and the risks, benefits, and limitations of intermittent auscultation (IA) and EFM. This chapter discusses the basis for intrapartum fetal monitoring, the types of monitoring, and nursing assessment and management of abnormal fetal status.

BASIS FOR MONITORING

Fetal Response

Because labor is a period of physiologic stress for the fetus, frequent monitoring of fetal status is part of the nursing care during labor. The fetal oxygen supply must be maintained during labor to prevent fetal compromise and to promote newborn health after birth. The fetal oxygen supply can decrease in a number of ways:

- Reduction of blood flow through the maternal vessels as a result of maternal hypertension (chronic hypertension, preeclampsia, or gestational hypertension), hypotension (caused by supine maternal position, hemorrhage, or epidural analgesia or anesthesia), or hypovolemia (caused by hemorrhage)
- Reduction of the oxygen content in the maternal blood as a result of hemorrhage or severe anemia
- Alterations in fetal circulation, occurring with compression of the umbilical cord (transient, during uterine contractions [UCs], or prolonged, resulting from cord prolapse), placental separation or complete abruption, or head compression (head compression causes increased intracranial pressure and vagal nerve stimulation with an accompanying decrease in the FHR)
- Reduction in blood flow to the intervillous space in the placenta secondary to uterine hypertonus (generally caused by excessive exogenous oxytocin) or secondary to deterioration of the placental vasculature associated with post-term gestation or maternal disorders such as hypertension or diabetes mellitus

Fetal well-being during labor can be measured by the response of the FHR to UCs. A group of fetal monitoring experts recommended that FHR tracings demonstrating certain reassuring characteristics be described as *normal* (category I) (Box 18-1).

Uterine Activity

Table 18-1 describes normal uterine activity (UA) during labor.

BOX 18-1 Three-Tier Fetal Heart Rate Classification System

Category I

Category I fetal heart rate (FHR) tracings include all of the following:

- Baseline rate 110 to 160 beats/minute (bpm)
- Baseline FHR variability: moderate
- Late or variable decelerations: absent
- Early decelerations: either present or absent
- Accelerations: either present or absent

Category II

Category II FHR tracings include all FHR tracings not categorized as category I or category III. Examples of category II tracings include any of the following:

- Baseline rate
  - Bradycardia not accompanied by absent baseline variability
  - Tachycardia
- Baseline FHR variability
  - Minimal baseline variability
  - Absent baseline variability not accompanied by recurrent decelerations
  - Marked baseline variability
- Accelerations
  - No acceleration produced in response to fetal stimulation
- Periodic or episodic decelerations
  - Recurrent variable decelerations accompanied by minimal or moderate baseline variability
  - Prolonged decelerations (≥2 minutes but <10 minutes)
  - Recurrent late decelerations with moderate baseline variability
  - Variable decelerations with other characteristics, such as slow return to baseline, "overshoots" or "shoulders"

Category III

Category III FHR tracings include:

- Absent baseline variability and any of the following:
  - Recurrent late decelerations
  - Recurrent variable decelerations
  - Bradycardia
- Sinusoidal pattern

From Macones, G. A., Hankins, G. D., Spong, C. Y., et al. (2008). The 2008 National Institute of Child Health and Human Development Workshop Report on Electronic Fetal Monitoring: Update on definitions, interpretation, and research guidelines. *Journal of Obstetric, Gynecologic, & Neonatal Nursing,* 37(5):510-515

Fetal Compromise

The goals of intrapartum FHR monitoring are to identify and differentiate the normal (reassuring) patterns from the abnormal (nonreassuring) patterns, which can be indicative of fetal compromise. Although the 2008 National Institute of Child Health and Human Development (NICHD) workshop (Macones, Hankins, Spong, et al., 2008) and the ACOG (2009) recommend use of the terms *normal* and *abnormal* to describe FHR tracings, the terms *reassuring* and *nonreassuring* are still frequently used clinically.

Abnormal FHR patterns are those associated with fetal hypoxemia, which is a deficiency of oxygen in the arterial blood. If uncorrected, hypoxemia can deteriorate to severe fetal hypoxia, an inadequate supply of oxygen at the cellular level that can cause metabolic acidosis. The term asphyxia is used when fetal hypoxia results in metabolic acidosis (Garite, 2012) (see Box 18-1 for examples of abnormal [category III] FHR tracings).

TABLE 18-1 Normal Uterine Activity During Labor

CHARACTERISTIC	DESCRIPTION
Frequency	Contraction frequency overall generally ranges from two to five per 10 minutes during labor, with lower frequencies seen in first stage of labor and higher frequencies (up to five contractions in 10 minutes) seen during second stage of labor
Duration	Contraction duration remains fairly stable throughout first and second stages, ranging from 45-80 seconds, not generally exceeding 90 seconds
Strength	Uterine contractions generally range from peaking at 40-70 mm Hg in first stage of labor to more than 80 mm Hg in second stage. Contractions palpated as "mild" will likely peak at less than 50 mm Hg if measured internally, whereas contractions palpated as "moderate" or greater will likely peak at 50 mm Hg or greater if measured internally.
Resting tone	Average resting tone during labor is 10 mm Hg; if using palpation, should palpate as "soft" (i.e., easily indented, no palpable resistance)
Relaxation time	Relaxation time is commonly 60 seconds or more in first stage and 45 seconds or more in second stage
Montevideo units (MVUs)	MVUs usually range from 100-250 in first stage; may rise to 300-400 in the second stage. Contraction intensities of 40 mm Hg or more and MVUs of 80-120 are generally sufficient to initiate spontaneous labor. MVUs are used only with internal monitoring of contractions.

Data from Macones, G.A., Hankins, G.D., Spong, C.Y., et al. (2008). The 2008 National Institute of Child Health and Human Development Workshop Report on Electronic Fetal Monitoring: Update on definitions, interpretation, and research guidelines. *Journal of Obstetric, Gynecologic, & Neonatal Nursing, 37*(5):510-515; Miller, L., Miller, D., & Tucker, S. [2013]. *Mosby's pocket guide to fetal monitoring: A multidisciplinary approach* [7th ed.]. St. Louis: Mosby.

MONITORING TECHNIQUES

The ideal method of fetal assessment during labor, IA or EFM, continues to be debated. Although IA is a high-touch, low-technology method of assessing fetal status during labor that places fewer restrictions on maternal activity, more than 85% of laboring women in the United States are monitored electronically for at least part of their labor (ACOG, 2009; Miller et al., 2013). The continued use of EFM in place of IA is thought to be because of concerns about liability and the increased nurse-client ratio required with IA. Because all surveillance methods, including EFM, have limitations, some health care providers believe that the evidence supports a return to the use of IA for low risk laboring women (ACOG, 2009; Miller et al.).

Intermittent Auscultation

Intermittent auscultation (IA) involves listening to fetal heart sounds at periodic intervals to assess the FHR. IA of the fetal heart can be performed with a Pinard fetoscope (see Fig. 14-7, *C*), Doppler ultrasound (see Fig. 18-1, *A*), an ultrasound stethoscope (see Fig. 18-1, *B*), or a DeLee-Hillis fetoscope (see Fig. 18-1, *C*). Doppler ultrasound and ultrasound stethoscopes transmit ultra-high-frequency sound waves, reflecting movement of the fetal heart, and convert these sounds into an electronic signal that can be counted. The fetoscope is applied to the listener's forehead because bone conduction amplifies the fetal heart sounds for counting. Box 18-2 describes how to perform IA.

EVIDENCE-BASED PRACTICE

Fetal Cardiac Assessment During Labor: How Are You Doing in There?

Ask the Question

For low risk women, which assessments of fetal cardiac function during labor provide better outcomes?

Search for the Evidence

Search Strategies English language research-based publications on fetal assessment, monitoring, labor, labour, cardiotocography, auscultation, pulse oximetry, electrocardiogram, scalp pH, scalp lactate were included.

Exclusions included preterm, postterm, high risk

Databases Used Cochrane Collaborative Database, Joanna Briggs Institute, National Guideline Clearinghouse (AHRQ), CINAHL, PubMed, UpToDate, and the professional websites for AWHONN and SOGC

Critical Appraisal of the Evidence

Intermittent auscultation of fetal heart rate can be accomplished with a fetal stethoscope, a Pinard fetoscope, or a hand-held Doppler ultrasound device. Admission electronic fetal monitoring for 20 to 30 minutes is intended to identify risk for fetal distress.

- Routine admission 20-minute electronic fetal monitoring (EFM) assessment is associated with higher rates of continuous fetal monitoring, fetal scalp blood sampling, and a 20% higher risk for cesarean birth than intermittent auscultation. There are no significant differences in instrumental vaginal births, artificial rupture of membranes, labor augmentation, or perinatal death. These findings do not support routine admission EFM strips for low-risk term laboring women, due to the risk for overtreatment (Devane, Lalor, Daly, et al., 2012).

Inadequate fetal oxygenation leads to abnormal fetal heart rate and electrocardiogram (ECG) patterns, including elevation or suppression of the ST segment. Monitoring the fetal ECG requires cervical dilation of at least 3 cm, and ruptured membranes, in order to directly access the fetal presenting part.

- EFM plus ECG results in fewer fetal scalp blood samples, fewer instrumental deliveries, and fewer admissions to special care nursery units than EFM alone. However, there are no differences in cesarean births, and no differences in these neonatal outcomes: severe acidosis, encephalopathy, low Apgar scores at 5 minutes, or need for intubation. The reviewers suggest that fetal ECG may be useful in decision making when contemplating continuous EFM (Neilson, 2013).

A poorly oxygenated fetus will develop acidosis, lower pH, and increased blood lactate. Fetal blood sampling requires cervical dilation and ruptured membranes. Fetal lactate sampling requires much less blood volume than pH, making it more successful.

- Fetal lactate sampling (also called fetal scalp blood sampling) can be done using a point-of-care machine, like a glucometer, and reliably correlates with cord artery pH, Apgar scores <7 at 5 minutes, and metabolic acidemia, regardless of large or growth-restricted status of the fetus (Holzmann, Cnattingius, & Nordstrom, 2012).

Apply the Evidence: Nursing Implications

- Evidence that a routine admission EFM strip is not recommended for low risk term labor may meet with resistance in institutions that have made this their practice for decades. Evaluating and communicating the evidence becomes paramount for changing long-term institutional habits.
- Overtreatment, such as unnecessary cesarean births, may be a result of fear of litigation, and create additional risks and costs. New evidence of client safety of intermittent auscultation should reassure caregivers and low risk laboring women.
- A limited assessment of ECG plus EFM is probably not any better than EFM alone, except when continuous EFM is being contemplated. The decision to initiate continuous EFM usually greatly decreases the mobility of laboring women, and may prolong labor and increase the cascade of interventions.
- Both ECG and scalp blood sampling require rupture of membranes. If this does not occur spontaneously, there is debate about the benefits versus risks of artificially rupturing membranes (increased maternal contraction pain, fetal infection, fetal distress). It falls to nurses to maintain perineal hygiene, including minimizing cervical examinations and documenting invasive procedures (Hastings-Toma, Bernard, Brody, et al., 2013).
- Fetal lactate sampling uses a very narrow capillary tube of blood, which is collected after a small incision in the fetal scalp or presenting part. Parents will probably find this distressing, and need to understand the reasons for it, the small risk for infection, and the puncture site they may notice on their newborn.

Quality and Safety Competencies: Quality Improvement*

Knowledge

Recognize that nursing and other health profession students are parts of systems of care and care processes that affect outcomes for clients and families.

Nurses can use evidence to advocate for change in institutional habits, such as overtesting that leads to overtreatment.

Skills

Seek information about outcomes of care for populations served in care setting.

Seek out the highest level evidence and demonstrate its relevance to this setting.

Attitudes

Appreciate the value of what individuals and teams can to do to improve care.

Education of the whole health care team is necessary to improve buy-in for institutional change.

References

Devane, D., Lalor, J. G., Daly, S., et al. (2012). *Cardiotocography versus intermittent auscultation of fetal heart on admission to labour ward for assessment of fetal wellbeing. The Cochrane Database of Systematic Reviews 2012.* Chichester, UK: John Wiley & Sons. 2.

Hastings-Toma, M., Bernard, R., Brody, M. G., et al. (2013). Chorioamnionitis: Prevention and management. *MCN: The American Journal of Maternal/Child Nursing, 38*(4), 206–212.

Holzmann, M., Cnattingius, S., & Nordstrom, L. (2012). Lactate production as a response to intrapartum hypoxia in the growth-restricted fetus. *British Journal of Obstetrics and Gynaecology, 119*(10), 1265–1269.

Neilson, J. P. (2013). *Fetal electrocardiogram (ECG) for fetal monitoring during labour. The Cochrane Database of Systematic Reviews 2012.* Chichester, UK: John Wiley & Sons. 4.

Pat Mahaffee Gingrich

*Adapted from QSEN at www.qsen.org.

IA is easy to use, inexpensive, and less invasive than EFM. It is often more comfortable for the woman and gives her more freedom of movement. Other care measures, such as ambulation and the use of baths or showers, are easier to carry out when IA is used. However, IA may be difficult to perform in obese women. A transvaginal fetal Doppler probe is available. It provides closer proximity to the uterus, making it easier to auscultate the FHR when the woman is obese or early in gestation (Miller et al., 2013). Because IA is intermittent, significant events may occur during a time when the FHR is not being auscultated. Also IA does not provide a permanent documented visual record of the FHR and cannot be used to assess visual patterns of the FHR variability or periodic changes (Miller et al.). When using IA the nurse can assess the baseline FHR, rhythm, and increases and decreases from baseline.

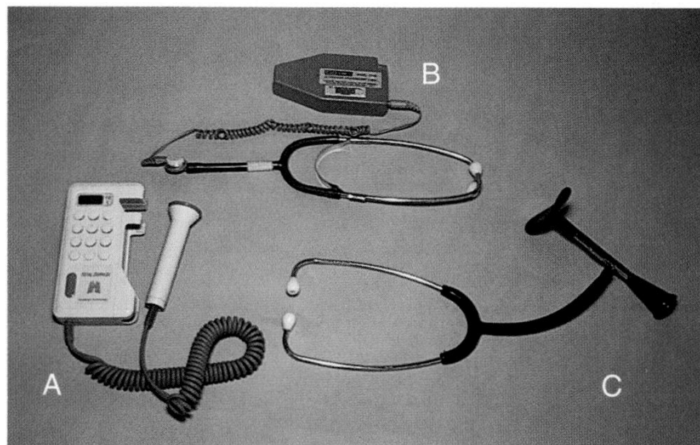

FIG 18-1 **A,** Ultrasound Doppler. **B,** Ultrasound stethoscope. **C,** DeLee-Hillis fetoscope. (Courtesy Michael S. Clement, MD, Mesa, AZ.)

BOX 18-2 Procedure for Intermittent Auscultation of the Fetal Heart Rate

1. Palpate maternal abdomen to identify fetal presentation and position.
2. Apply ultrasonic gel to device if using Doppler ultrasound. Place listening device (see Fig. 18-1, *A*) over area of maximal intensity and clarity of fetal heart sounds to obtain clearest and loudest sound, which is easiest to count. This location is usually over the fetal back. If using fetoscope, firm pressure may be needed.
3. Count maternal radial pulse while listening to FHR to differentiate it from fetal rate.
4. Palpate abdomen for presence or absence of UA to count FHR between contractions.
5. Count FHR for 30 to 60 seconds after a uterine contraction to identify auscultated baseline rate and changes (increases or decreases) in it.
6. Auscultate FHR before, during, and after contraction to identify FHR during the contraction or as a response to the contraction and to assess for absence or presence of increases or decreases in FHR.
7. When distinct discrepancies in FHR are noted during listening periods, auscultate for longer period during, after, and between contractions to identify significant changes that may indicate need for another mode of FHR monitoring.

FHR, Fetal heart rate; *UA,* uterine activity.
From Miller, L., Miller, D., & Tucker S. (2013). *Mosby's pocket guide to fetal monitoring: A multidisciplinary approach* (7th ed.). St. Louis: Mosby.

Nursing Interventions

The American College of Nurse-Midwives (ACNM) reviewed references from the United States, Great Britain, and Canada regarding the recommended frequency of IA in low risk women and found consistent recommendations for every 15 minutes in the active phase of the first stage of labor and every 5 minutes in the second stage of labor (Miller et al., 2013). The seventh edition of *Guidelines for Perinatal Care* (American Academy of Pediatrics [AAP] & ACOG, 2012) suggests performing IA every 30 minutes in the active phase of the first stage of labor and every 15 minutes in the second stage. The Association of Women's Health, Obstetric and Neonatal Nurses (AWHONN) recommends auscultation of the FHR every 15 to 30 minutes in the active phase of the first stage labor, and every 5 to 15 minutes in the active phase of the second stage of labor (Lyndon, O'Brien-Abel, & Simpson, 2014). However, the optimal frequency for IA in low risk women during labor has not been determined (Nageotte, 2014).

! NURSING ALERT

When the FHR is auscultated and documented the descriptive terms associated with EFM (e.g., moderate variability, variable deceleration) cannot be used because most of the terms are visual descriptions of the patterns produced on the monitor tracing. However, terms that are numerically defined such as bradycardia and tachycardia can be used. When the FHR is auscultated, it should be described as a baseline number or range and as having a regular or irregular rhythm. The presence or absence of accelerations or decelerations both during and after contractions should also be noted (Lyndon et al., 2014; Miller et al., 2013).

Every effort should be made to use the method of fetal assessment the woman desires, if possible. However, auscultation of the FHR in accordance with the frequency guidelines suggested earlier may be difficult in today's busy labor and birth units. When used as the primary method of fetal assessment, auscultation requires a one-to-one nurse-to-client staffing ratio. If acuity and census change so that auscultation standards are no longer met, the nurse must inform the physician or nurse-midwife that continuous EFM will be used until staffing can be arranged to meet the standards.

The woman can become anxious if the examiner cannot readily count the fetal heartbeats. It often takes time for the inexperienced listener to locate the heartbeat and find the area of maximal intensity. To allay the mother's concerns, she can be told that the nurse is "finding the spot where the sounds are loudest." If it takes considerable time to locate the fetal heartbeat, the examiner can reassure the mother by offering her an opportunity to listen, too. If the examiner cannot locate the fetal heartbeat, assistance should be requested. In some cases ultrasound can be used to help locate the fetal heartbeat. Seeing the FHR on the ultrasound screen will be reassuring to the mother if there was initial difficulty in locating the best area for auscultation.

When using IA, uterine activity is assessed by palpation. The examiner should keep his or her fingertips placed over the fundus before, during, and after contractions. The contraction intensity is usually described as mild, moderate, or strong. Duration is measured in seconds, from the beginning to the end of the contraction. The frequency of contractions is measured in minutes, from the beginning of one contraction to the beginning of the next. The examiner should keep his or her hand on the fundus after the contraction is over to evaluate uterine resting tone or relaxation between contractions. Resting tone between contractions is usually described as soft or hard (Lyndon et al., 2014).

Accurate and complete documentation of fetal status and uterine activity is especially important when IA and palpation are being used because no paper tracing record or computer storage of these assessments is provided as is the case with continuous EFM. Labor flow records or computer charting systems that prompt notations of all assessments are useful for ensuring such comprehensive documentation.

TABLE 18-2 External and Internal Modes of Monitoring

EXTERNAL MODE	INTERNAL MODE
Fetal Heart Rate	
Ultrasound transducer: High-frequency sound waves reflect mechanical action of the fetal heart. Noninvasive. Does not require rupture of membranes or cervical dilation. Used during both the antepartum and intrapartum periods.	*Spiral electrode:* Converts the fetal ECG as obtained from the presenting part to the FHR via a cardiotachometer. Can be used only when membranes are ruptured and the cervix is sufficiently dilated during the intrapartum period. Electrode penetrates the fetal presenting part by 1.5 mm and must be attached securely to ensure a good signal.
Uterine Activity	
Tocotransducer: Monitors frequency and duration of contractions by means of a pressure-sensing device applied to the maternal abdomen. Used during both the antepartum and intrapartum periods.	*Intrauterine pressure catheter (IUPC):* Monitors the frequency, duration, and intensity of contractions. The two types of IUPCs are a fluid-filled system and a solid catheter. Both measure intrauterine pressure at the catheter tip and convert the pressure into millimeters of mercury on the uterine activity panel of the strip chart. Both can be used only when membranes are ruptured and the cervix is sufficiently dilated during the intrapartum period.

ECG, Electrocardiogram; *FHR*, fetal heart rate.

Electronic Fetal Monitoring

The purpose of electronic FHR monitoring is the ongoing assessment of fetal oxygenation. FHR tracings are analyzed for characteristic patterns that suggest fetal hypoxic events and metabolic acidosis during labor. When hypoxia or metabolic acidosis is suspected in labor, interventions to resolve the problem can be implemented in a timely manner before permanent damage or death occurs (Garite, 2012). The two modes of EFM are the external mode, which uses external transducers placed on the maternal abdomen to assess FHR and UA, and the internal mode, which uses a spiral electrode applied to the fetal presenting part to assess the FHR and an intrauterine pressure catheter (IUPC) to assess UA and uterine resting tone. The differences between the external and internal modes of EFM are summarized in Table 18-2.

External Monitoring

Separate transducers are used to monitor the FHR and UCs (Fig. 18-2). The ultrasound transducer works by reflecting high-frequency sound waves off a moving interface: in this case, the fetal heart and valves. It is sometimes difficult to reproduce a continuous and precise record of the FHR because of artifact introduced by fetal and maternal movement. Maternal obesity, occiput posterior position of the fetus, and anterior attachment of the placenta can cause weak or absent signals (AWHONN, 2009). The FHR is printed on specially formatted paper and simultaneously displayed on a screen if the fetal monitor is connected to a computer. Once the area of maximal intensity of the FHR has been located, conductive gel is applied to the surface of the ultrasound transducer, and the transducer is then positioned over this area and held securely in place using an elastic belt.

The tocotransducer (tocodynamometer) measures UA transabdominally. The device is placed over the fundus above the umbilicus and held securely in place using an elastic belt (see Fig. 18-2, *B*). UCs or fetal movements depress a

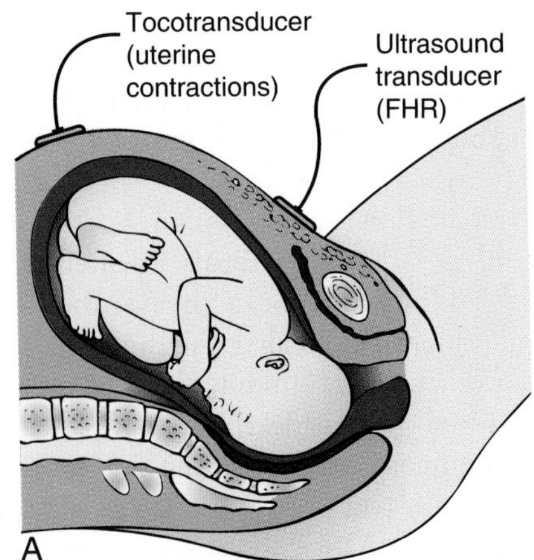

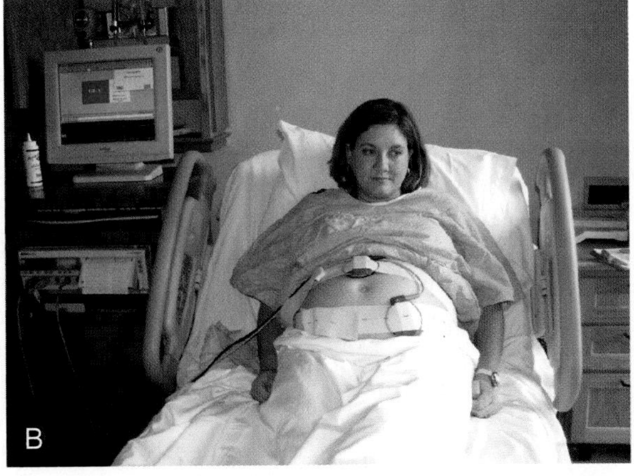

FIG 18-2 **A,** External noninvasive fetal monitoring with tocotransducer and ultrasound transducer. **B,** Ultrasound transducer is placed over the area where fetal heart rate is best heard, usually below the umbilicus and tocotransducer is placed on the uterine fundus. *FHR,* Fetal heart rate. (**B,** Courtesy Julie Perry Nelson, Loveland, CO.)

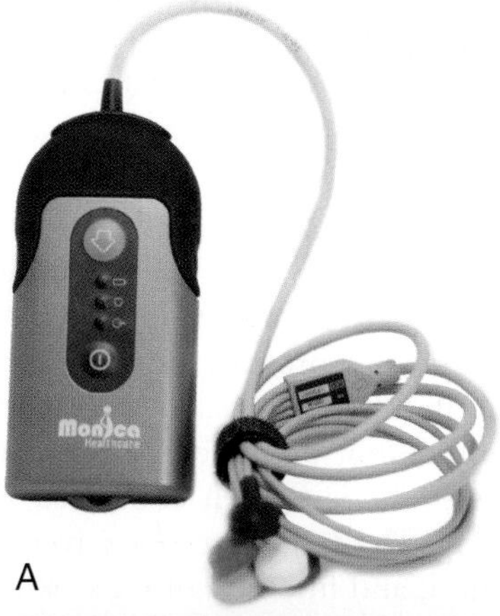

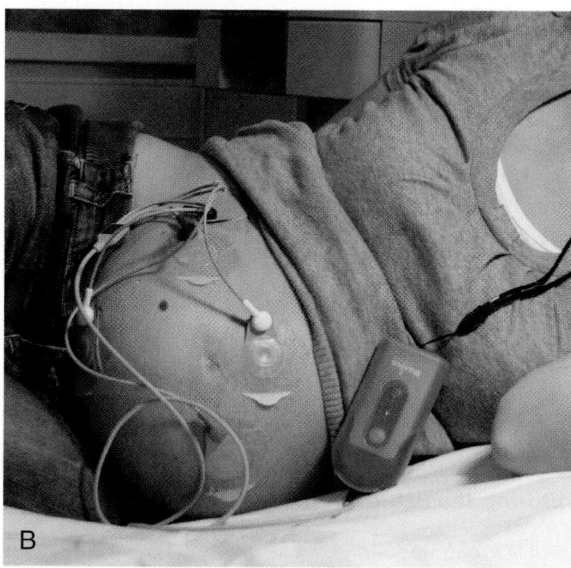

FIG 18-3 The Monica AN24 is a wireless and beltless device that can be used with existing monitors to obtain fetal heart rate via abdominal electrocardiogram (ECG). **B,** Electrodes placed on maternal abdomen monitor ECG from fetal and maternal heart and electromyogram (EMG) from uterine muscle. (Courtesy Monica Healthcare Ltd., Nottingham, UK.)

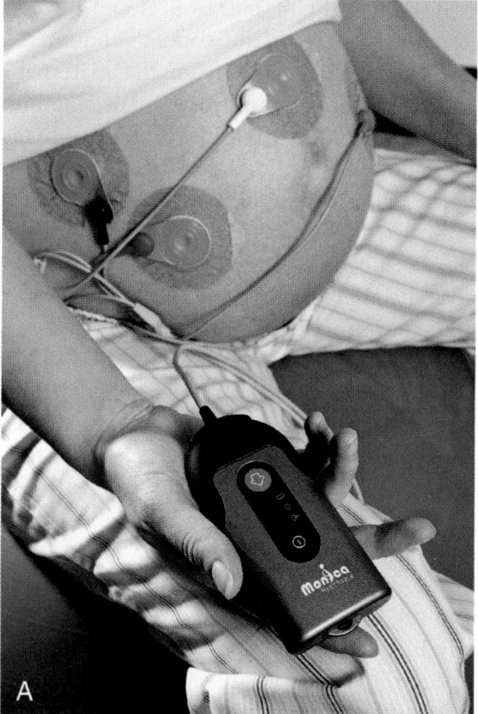

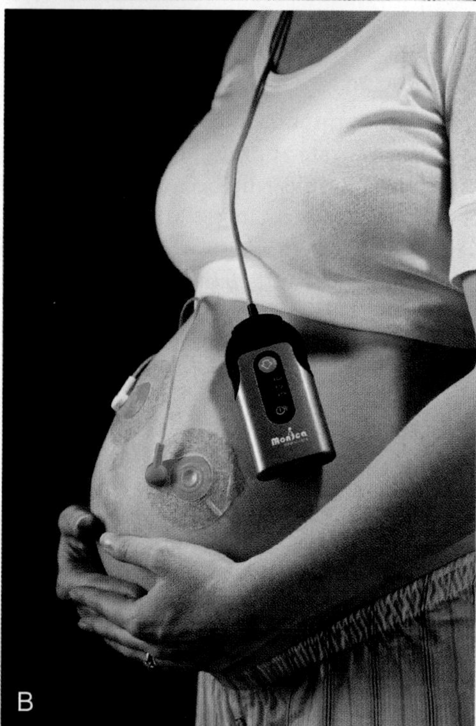

FIG 18-4 **A,** Woman sitting on birthing ball, and **B,** woman ambulating, both wearing Monica AN24. (Courtesy Monica Healthcare Ltd., Nottingham, UK.)

pressure-sensitive surface on the side next to the abdomen. The tocotransducer can measure and record the frequency and approximate duration of UCs but not their intensity. This method is especially valuable for measuring UA during the first stage of labor in women with intact membranes or for antepartum testing. If the woman is obese, the tocotransducer may be unable to detect the exact frequency and duration of UCs.

Because the tocotransducer of most electronic fetal monitors is designed for assessing UA in a term pregnancy, it may not be sensitive enough to detect preterm UA. When monitoring the woman in preterm labor, remember that the fundus may be located below the level of the umbilicus. The nurse may need to rely on the woman to indicate when UCs are occurring and to use palpation as an additional way of assessing contraction frequency and validating the monitor tracing.

The external transducers are easily applied by the nurse but often must be repositioned as the woman or fetus changes position. The woman is asked to assume a semi-Fowler or lateral position. Use of external transducers confines the woman to bed or chair.

Portable telemetry monitors allow observation of the FHR and UC patterns by means of centrally located electronic display stations. These portable units permit the woman to walk around during electronic monitoring.

In 2011 another type of external monitor became available for use in the United States. It was used in several European countries before its debut in the United States. The Monica AN24 uses abdominally obtained electronic impulses to monitor both FHR and UA (Fig. 18-3, *A* and *B*). The monitor uses five electrodes placed on the woman's abdomen to directly monitor the electrocardiogram from the maternal and fetal hearts and the electromyogram from the uterine muscle. This information is transmitted wirelessly, via Bluetooth technology, to an interface device that allows the FHR and UA data to print or display on a standard fetal monitor (Miller et al., 2013).

The Monica AN24 eliminates much of the problem caused by signal loss resulting from maternal or fetal movement or maternal obesity that often occurs with traditional external monitors. The monitor also more accurately measures the frequency, peak, and duration of UCs than does the traditional tocotransducer, although it does not provide actual intensity measurement in millimeters of mercury (mm Hg) as an IUPC does. Other advantages of the Monica AN24 are that it eliminates the need for abdominal belts and frequent readjustment of the tocotransducer and ultrasound transducer and provides some client mobility. The woman may move up to 50 feet away from the interface device without signal loss (Fig. 18-4, *A* and *B*). In the United States the Monica AN24 is approved for use only in pregnancies that have reached 36 completed weeks or more of gestation (Miller et al., 2013). The Monica AN24 monitor may not be readily available for use in all labor and birth settings.

Internal Monitoring

The technique of continuous internal FHR or UA monitoring provides a more accurate appraisal of fetal well-being during labor than external monitoring because it is not interrupted by fetal or maternal movement or affected by maternal size (Fig. 18-5). For this type of monitoring the membranes must be ruptured, the cervix sufficiently dilated (at least 2 to 3 cm), and the presenting part low enough to allow placement of the spiral electrode or IUPC or both. Internal and external modes of monitoring (i.e., internal FHR with external UA or external FHR with internal UA) may be combined without difficulty.

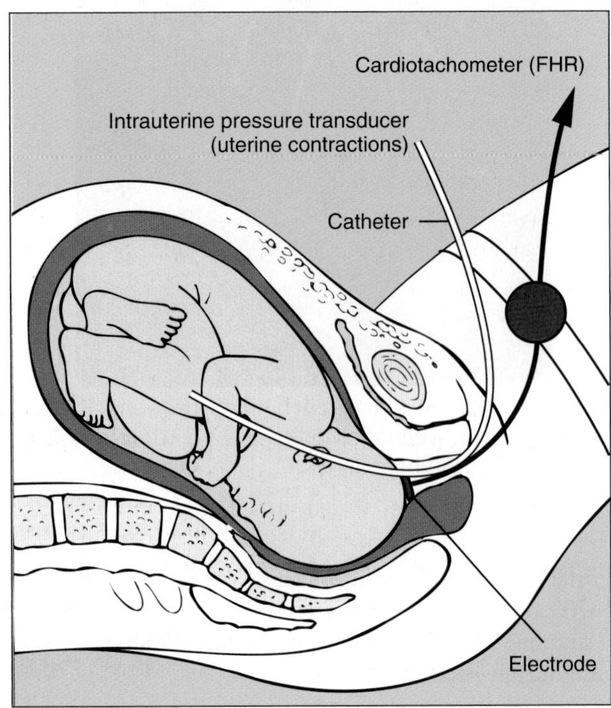

FIG 18-5 Diagrammatic representation of internal invasive fetal monitoring with intrauterine pressure catheter and spiral electrode in place (membranes ruptured and cervix dilated).

Internal monitoring of the FHR is accomplished by attaching a small spiral electrode to the presenting part. For UA to be monitored internally an IUPC is introduced into the uterine cavity. The catheter has a pressure-sensitive tip that measures changes in intrauterine pressure. As the catheter is compressed during a contraction, pressure is placed on the pressure transducer. This pressure is then converted into a pressure reading in mm Hg. The IUPC can objectively measure the frequency, duration, and intensity of UCs, as well as uterine resting tone.

Because it can precisely measure the intensity of individual UCs, the IUPC can be used to evaluate the adequacy of UA for achieving progress in labor. Montevideo units (MVUs) are calculated by subtracting the baseline uterine pressure from the peak contraction pressure for each contraction that occurs in a 10-minute window, and then adding together the pressures generated by each contraction that occurs during that period of time. Spontaneous labor usually begins when MVUs are between 80 and 120. Uterine activity during normal labor rarely exceeds 250 MVUs (see Table 18-1) (Cunningham, Leveno, Bloom, et al., 2014; Miller et al., 2013).

CLINICAL REASONING CASE STUDY

Monitoring the Fetus of an Obese Woman

Tameka is a 23-year-old G 4 P 2 0 1 2 at 35 weeks of gestation. She has had chronic hypertension since age 16 and is morbidly obese. Today she weighs 305 pounds. Tameka was sent from the antepartum testing area to the labor and birth unit for prolonged monitoring because she had a nonreactive nonstress test (NST) and her blood pressure was elevated at her appointment today. You are Tameka's nurse. After spending half an hour admitting her to the unit you walk out to the nurses' station and announce to your colleagues, "I am *so* frustrated! No matter what I do, I just can't keep that baby on the monitor!"

1. Evidence—Is there sufficient evidence at this time to draw a conclusion about the best way to monitor Tameka's fetus?
2. Assumptions—Describe an underlying assumption regarding use of the following modes of monitoring for Tameka's fetus:
   a. Intermittent auscultation
   b. External (ultrasound transducer)
   c. Internal (spiral electrode)
   d. Monica AN24
3. What implications and priorities for nursing care can be drawn at this time?
4. Does the evidence objectively support your conclusion?

Display

The FHR and UA are displayed on the monitor paper or computer screen, with the FHR in the upper section and UA in the lower section. Figure 18-6 contrasts the internal and external modes of electronic monitoring. Note that each small square on the monitor paper or screen represents 10 seconds; each larger box of six squares equals 1 minute

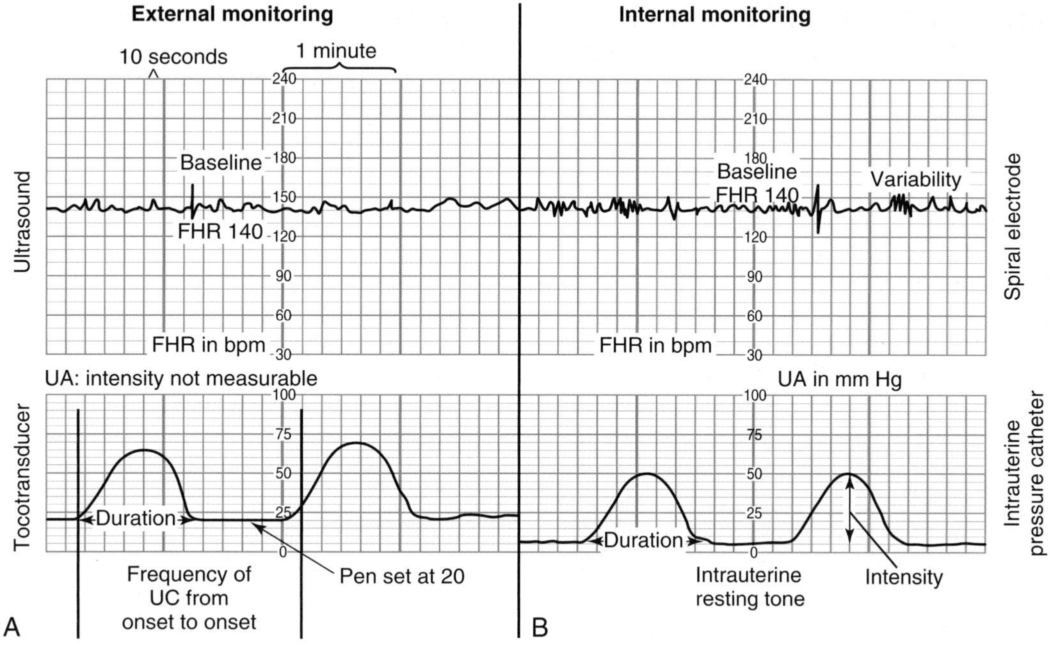

FIG 18-6 Display of fetal heart rate (FHR) and uterine contractions (UC) as seen using the external mode of monitoring (**A**) as compared to the internal mode of monitoring (**B**). (From Miller, L., Miller, D., & Tucker, S. [2013]. *Mosby's pocket guide to fetal monitoring: A multidisciplinary approach* [7th ed.]. St. Louis: Mosby.)

(when paper is moving through the monitor at the rate of 3 cm/minute).

FETAL HEART RATE PATTERNS

Characteristic FHR patterns are associated with fetal and maternal physiologic processes and have been identified for many years. Because EFM was introduced into clinical practice before consensus was reached in regard to standardized terminology, however, variations in the description and interpretation of common fetal heart rate patterns were often great. In 1997 the NICHD published a proposed nomenclature system for EFM interpretation with standardized definitions for FHR monitoring. The NICHD recommendations were not widely incorporated into clinical practice, however, until they were endorsed by the ACOG in 2005. AWHONN and ACNM also endorsed use of the NICHD standard terminology. All three organizations cited concerns regarding client safety and the need for improved communication among caregivers as reasons for using standard EFM definitions in clinical practice (Miller et al., 2013).

In April 2008 the NICHD, the ACOG, and the Society for Maternal-Fetal Medicine partnered to sponsor another workshop to revisit the FHR definitions recommended by the NICHD in 1997. The 1997 FHR definitions were reaffirmed at this workshop. In addition, new definitions related to UA were recommended, as well as a three-tier system of FHR pattern interpretation and categorization (see Box 18-1) (Macones et al., 2008).

Baseline Fetal Heart Rate

The intrinsic rhythmicity of the fetal heart, the central nervous system (CNS), and the fetal autonomic nervous system control the FHR. An increase in sympathetic response results in acceleration of the FHR, whereas an increase in parasympathetic response produces a slowing of the FHR. Usually a balanced increase of sympathetic and parasympathetic response occurs during contractions, with no observable change in the baseline FHR.

The **baseline fetal heart rate** is the average rate during a 10-minute segment that excludes periodic or episodic changes, periods of marked variability, and segments of the baseline that differ by more than 25 beats/minute. There must be at least 2 minutes of interpretable baseline data in a 10-minute segment of tracing in order to determine the baseline FHR (Macones et al., 2008). After 10 minutes of tracing is observed the approximate mean rate is rounded to the closest 5 beats/minute interval (AWHONN, 2009). For example, if the FHR rate varies between 130 and 140 beats/minute over a 10-minute period, the baseline is recorded as 135 beats/minute. The normal range at term is 110 to 160 beats/minute. In the preterm fetus the baseline rate is slightly higher.

Variability

Variability of the FHR can be described as irregular waves or fluctuations in the baseline FHR of two cycles per minute or greater (Macones et al., 2008). It is a characteristic of the baseline FHR and does not include accelerations or decelerations of the FHR. Variability is quantified in beats per minute and is measured from the peak to the trough of a single cycle. Four possible categories of variability have been identified: absent, minimal, moderate, and marked (Fig. 18-7). In the past, variability was described as either long term or short term (beat to beat). The NICHD definitions do not distinguish between long- and short-term variability, however, because in actual practice they are visually determined as a unit (NICHD, 1997).

Depending on other characteristics of the FHR tracing, absent or minimal variability is classified as either abnormal

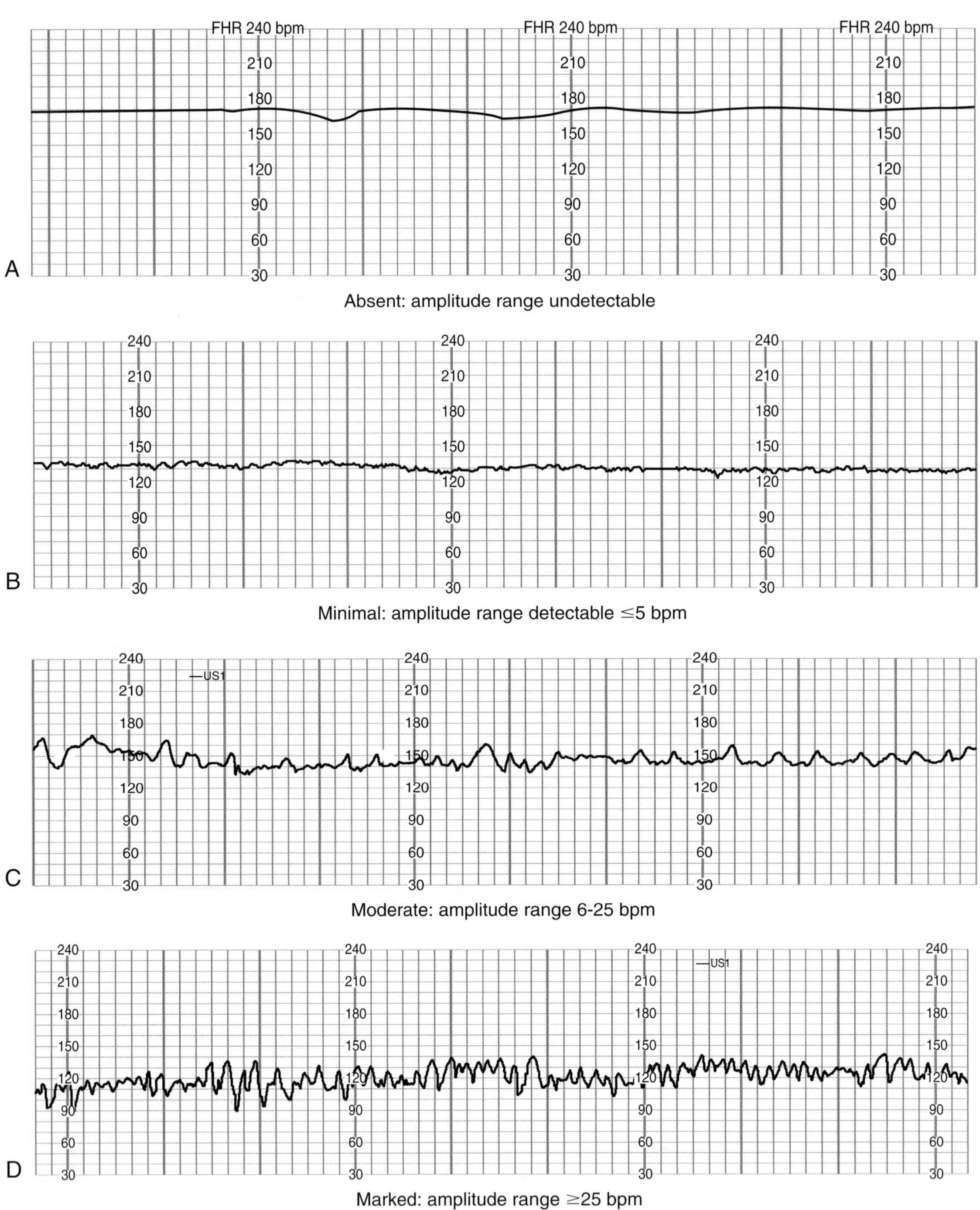

FIG 18-7 Fetal heart rate variability. **A,** Absent: amplitude range undetectable. **B,** Minimal: amplitude range detectable ≤5 beats/minute. **C,** Moderate: amplitude range 6-25 beats/minute. **D,** Marked: amplitude range ≥25 beats/minute. *FHR,* Fetal heart rate. (From Miller, L., Miller, D., & Tucker, S. [2013]. *Mosby's pocket guide to fetal monitoring: A multidisciplinary approach* [7th ed.]. St. Louis: Mosby.)

or indeterminate (Macones et al., 2008) (see Fig. 18-7, *A* and *B*). It can result from fetal hypoxemia and metabolic acidemia. Other possible causes of absent or minimal variability include congenital anomalies and preexisting neurologic injury. CNS depressant medications, including analgesics, narcotics (meperidine [Demerol]), barbiturates (secobarbital [Seconal], and pentobarbital [Nembutal]), tranquilizers (diazepam [Valium]), phenothiazines (promethazine [Phenergan]), and general anesthetics are other possible causes of minimal variability. In addition, minimal variability can occur with tachycardia, prematurity, or when the fetus is temporarily in a sleep state (Miller et al., 2013). These sleep states do not usually last longer than 30 minutes.

Moderate variability is considered normal (see Fig. 18-7, *C*). Its presence is highly predictive of a normal fetal acid-base balance (absence of fetal metabolic acidemia). Moderate variability indicates that FHR regulation is not significantly affected by fetal sleep cycles, tachycardia, prematurity, congenital anomalies, preexisting neurologic injury, or CNS depressant medications (Macones et al., 2008; Miller et al., 2013).

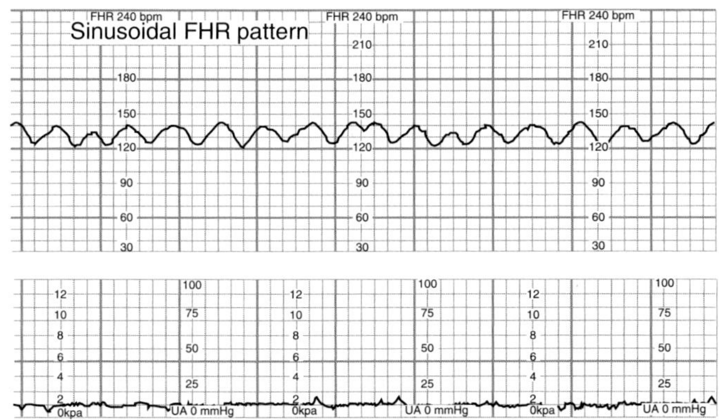

FIG 18-8 Sinusoidal pattern. *FHR*, Fetal heart rate. (From Miller, L., Miller, D., & Tucker, S. [2013]. *Mosby's pocket guide to fetal monitoring: A multidisciplinary approach* [7th ed.]. St. Louis: Mosby.)

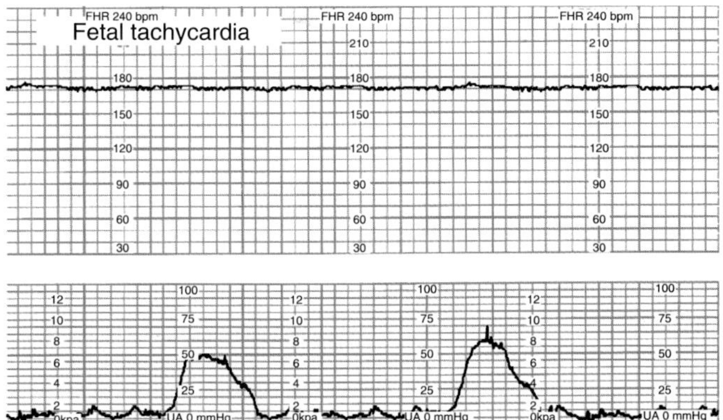

FIG 18-9 Fetal tachycardia. (From Miller, L., Miller, D., & Tucker, S. [2013]. *Mosby's pocket guide to fetal monitoring: A multidisciplinary approach* [7th ed.]. St. Louis: Mosby.)

The significance of marked variability (see Fig. 18-7, *D*) is unknown due to limited scientific evidence (Macones et al., 2008).

A sinusoidal pattern—a regular smooth, undulating wavelike pattern—is not included in the definition of FHR variability. This uncommon pattern classically occurs with severe fetal anemia (Fig. 18-8). Variations of the sinusoidal pattern have been described in association with chorioamnionitis, fetal sepsis, and administration of narcotic analgesics (Miller et al., 2013).

Tachycardia

Tachycardia is a baseline FHR greater than 160 beats/minute for 10 minutes or longer (Fig. 18-9). It can be considered an early sign of fetal hypoxemia, especially when associated with late decelerations and minimal or absent variability. Fetal tachycardia can result from maternal or fetal infection, such as prolonged rupture of membranes with amnionitis; from maternal hyperthyroidism or fetal anemia; or in response to medications such as atropine, hydroxyzine (Vistaril), terbutaline (Brethine), or illicit drugs such as cocaine or methamphetamines. Table 18-3 lists causes, clinical significance, and nursing interventions for tachycardia.

TABLE 18-3 Tachycardia and Bradycardia

TACHYCARDIA	BRADYCARDIA
Definition	
FHR >160 beats/minute lasting >10 minutes	FHR <110 beats/minute lasting >10 minutes
Possible Causes	
Early fetal hypoxemia Fetal cardiac arrhythmias Maternal fever Infection (including chorioamnionitis) Parasympatholytic drugs (atropine, hydroxyzine) Beta-sympathomimetic drugs (terbutaline) Maternal hyperthyroidism Fetal anemia Drugs (caffeine, cocaine, methamphetamines)	Atrioventricular dissociation (heart block) Structural defects Viral infections (e.g., cytomegalovirus) Medications Fetal heart failure Maternal hypoglycemia Maternal hypothermia
Clinical Significance	
Persistent tachycardia in absence of periodic changes does not appear serious in terms of neonatal outcome (especially true if tachycardia is associated with maternal fever); tachycardia is abnormal when associated with late decelerations, severe variable decelerations, or absent variability.	Baseline bradycardia alone is not specifically related to fetal oxygenation. The clinical significance of bradycardia depends on the underlying cause and the accompanying FHR patterns, including variability, accelerations, or decelerations.
Nursing Interventions	
Dependent on cause; reduce maternal fever with antipyretics as ordered and cooling measures; oxygen at 10 L/minute by nonrebreather face mask may be of some value; carry out health care provider's orders based on alleviating cause	Dependent on cause

FHR, Fetal heart rate.

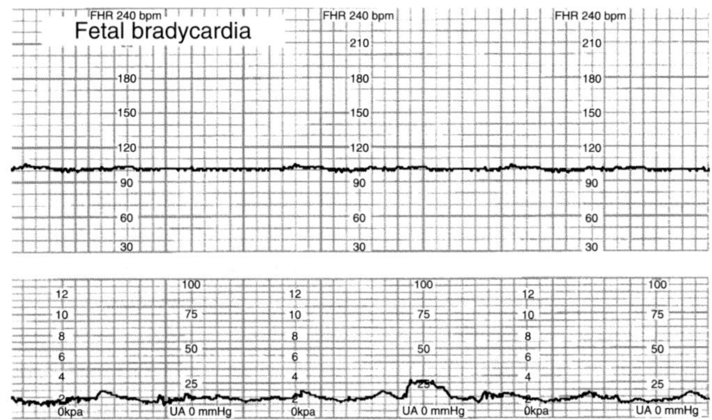

FIG 18-10 Fetal bradycardia. (From Miller, L., Miller, D., & Tucker, S. [2013]. *Mosby's pocket guide to fetal monitoring: A multidisciplinary approach* [7th ed.]. St. Louis: Mosby.)

Bradycardia

Bradycardia is a baseline FHR of fewer than 110 beats/minute for 10 minutes or longer (Fig. 18-10). True bradycardia occurs rarely and is not specifically related to fetal oxygenation. It must be distinguished from a prolonged deceleration because the causes and management of these two conditions are very different. Bradycardia is often caused by some type of fetal cardiac problem such as structural defects involving the pacemakers or conduction system or fetal heart failure. Other causes of

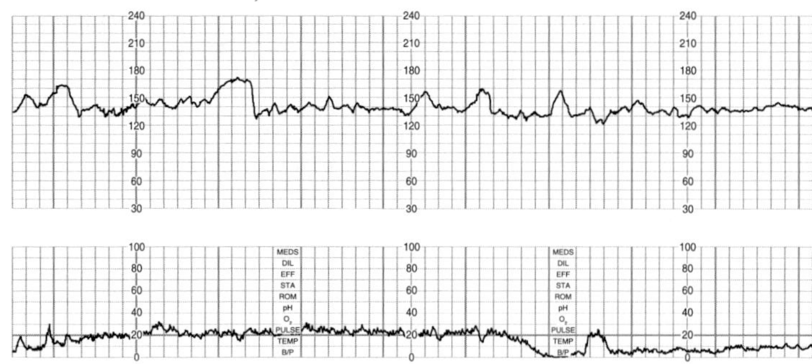

FIG 18-11 Accelerations of fetal heart rate in a term pregnancy. (From Miller, L., Miller, D., & Tucker, S. [2013]. *Mosby's pocket guide to fetal monitoring: A multidisciplinary approach* [7th ed.]. St. Louis: Mosby.)

bradycardia include viral infections (e.g., cytomegalovirus), maternal hypoglycemia, and maternal hypothermia. The clinical significance of the bradycardia depends on the underlying cause and accompanying FHR patterns, including variability and the presence of accelerations or decelerations (Miller et al., 2013). (See Table 18-3 for a list of causes, clinical significance, and nursing interventions for bradycardia.)

Periodic and Episodic Changes in Fetal Heart Rate

Changes in FHR from the baseline are categorized as periodic or episodic. Periodic changes are those that occur with UCs. Episodic changes are those that are not associated with UCs. These patterns include both accelerations and decelerations (Macones et al., 2008).

Accelerations

Acceleration of the FHR is defined as a visually apparent abrupt (onset to peak less than 30 seconds) increase in FHR above the baseline rate (Fig. 18-11). The peak is at least 15 beats/minute above the baseline, and the acceleration lasts 15 seconds or more, with a return to baseline less than 2 minutes from the beginning of the acceleration. Before 32 weeks of gestation the definition of an acceleration is a peak of 10 beats/minute or more above the baseline and a duration of at least 10 seconds. Acceleration of the FHR for more than 10 minutes is considered a change in baseline rate (Miller et al., 2013).

Accelerations can be either periodic or episodic. They may occur in association with fetal movement or spontaneously. If accelerations do not occur spontaneously, they can be elicited by fetal scalp stimulation or vibroacoustic stimulation. Similar to moderate variability, accelerations are considered an indication of fetal well-being. Their presence is highly predictive of a normal fetal acid-base balance (absence of fetal metabolic acidemia) (Miller et al., 2013). Box 18-3 lists causes, clinical significance, and nursing interventions for accelerations.

BOX 18-3 Accelerations

Causes
- Spontaneous fetal movement
- Vaginal examination
- Electrode application
- Fetal scalp stimulation
- Fetal reaction to external sounds
- Breech presentation
- Occiput posterior position
- Uterine contractions
- Fundal pressure
- Abdominal palpation

Clinical Significance
Normal pattern. Acceleration with fetal movement signifies fetal well-being representing fetal alertness or arousal states.

Nursing Interventions
None required

Decelerations

A *deceleration* (caused by dominance of a parasympathetic response) may be benign or abnormal. FHR decelerations are categorized as early, late, variable, or prolonged. They are described by their visual relation to the onset and end of a contraction and by their shape.

Early Decelerations. Early deceleration of the FHR is a visually apparent gradual (onset to lowest point ≥30 seconds) decrease in and return to baseline FHR associated with UCs. It is thought to be caused by transient fetal head compression and is considered a normal and benign finding (Macones et al., 2008; Miller et al., 2013). Generally the onset, *nadir* (lowest point), and recovery of the deceleration correspond to the beginning, peak, and end of the contraction (Figs. 18-12 and 18-13). For this reason, an early deceleration is sometimes called the "mirror image" of a contraction.

Early decelerations may occur during UCs, during vaginal examinations, as a result of fundal pressure, and during placement of the internal mode of fetal monitoring. When present, they usually occur during the first stage of labor when the cervix is dilated 4 to 7 cm. Early decelerations are also sometimes seen during the second stage when the woman is pushing.

Because early decelerations are considered to be benign, interventions are not necessary. The value of identifying early decelerations is so they can be distinguished from late or variable decelerations, which can be abnormal and for which interventions are appropriate. Box 18-4 lists causes, clinical significance, and nursing interventions for early decelerations.

Late Decelerations. Late deceleration of the FHR is a visually apparent gradual decrease in and return to baseline FHR associated with UCs (Macones et al., 2008). The deceleration begins after the contraction has started, and the nadir of the deceleration occurs after the peak of the contraction. The deceleration usually does not return to baseline until after the contraction is over (Figs. 18-14 and 18-15).

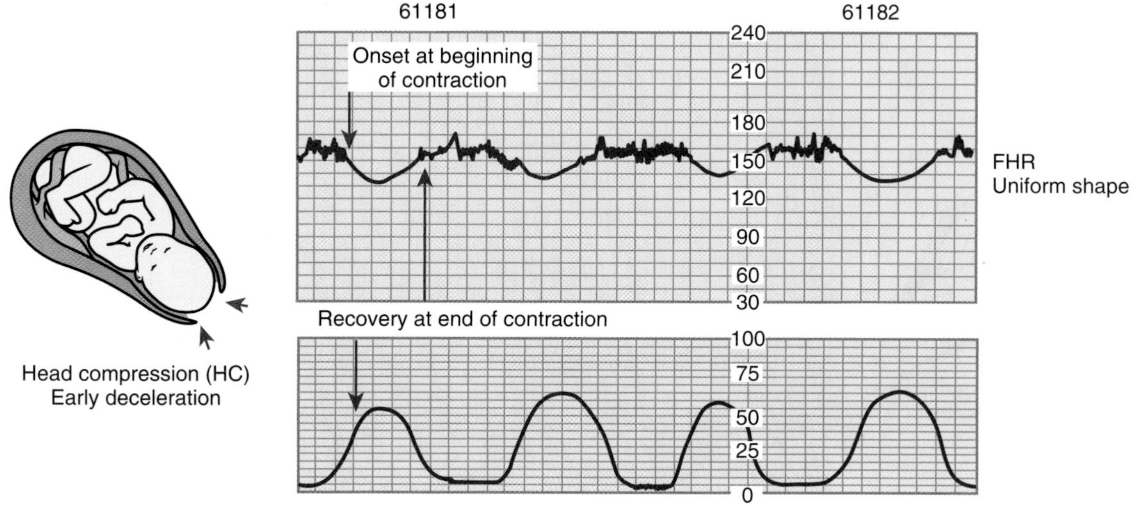

FIG 18-12 Line drawing illustrating early decelerations. *FHR,* Fetal heart rate. (From Tucker, S. [2004]. *Pocket guide to fetal monitoring and assessment* [5th ed.]. St. Louis: Mosby.)

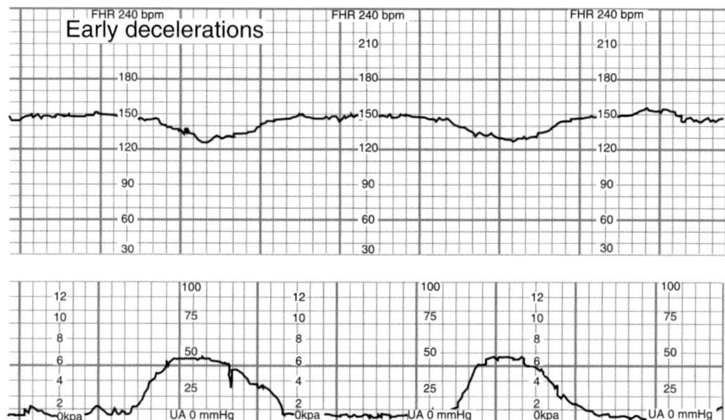

FIG 18-13 Electronic fetal monitor tracing showing early decelerations. *FHR,* Fetal heart rate; *UA,* uterine activity. (From Miller, L., Miller, D., & Tucker, S. [2013]. *Mosby's pocket guide to fetal monitoring: A multidisciplinary approach* [7th ed.]. St. Louis: Mosby.)

BOX 18-4 Early Decelerations

Cause

Head compression resulting from the following:

- Uterine contractions
- Vaginal examination
- Fundal pressure
- Placement of internal mode of monitoring

Clinical Significance

Normal pattern; not associated with fetal hypoxemia, acidemia, or low Apgar scores

Nursing Interventions

None required

Traditionally late decelerations have been attributed to uteroplacental insufficiency. However, in reality a number of factors can disrupt oxygen transfer to the fetus, even with mild UCs and a normally functioning placenta (Miller et al., 2013). These factors include maternal hypotension, *uterine tachysystole* (e.g., more than five contractions in 10 minutes averaged over a 30-minute window), preeclampsia, late term or postterm pregnancy, amnionitis, small for gestational age fetuses, maternal diabetes, placenta previa, placental abruption, conduction anesthetics, maternal cardiac disease, and maternal anemia. Rarely fetal oxygenation can be interrupted sufficiently to result in metabolic acidemia. For that reason late decelerations should be considered an ominous sign when they are associated with absent or minimal variability (Miller et al.). The most common cause of late decelerations is uterine tachysystole, usually caused by oxytocin (Pitocin) administration (Garite, 2012). The clinical significance and nursing interventions for late decelerations are described in Box 18-5.

Variable Decelerations. Variable deceleration of the FHR is defined as a visually abrupt (onset to nadir less than 30 seconds) decrease in FHR below the baseline. The decrease is at least 15 beats/minute or more below the baseline, lasts at least 15 seconds, and returns to baseline in less than 2 minutes from the time of onset (Macones et al., 2008). Variable decelerations occur any time during the UC phase and are caused by compression of the umbilical cord (Figs. 18-16 and 18-17).

The appearance of variable decelerations differs from those of early and late decelerations, which closely approximate the shape of the corresponding UC. Instead, variable decelerations have a U, V, or W shape, characterized by a rapid descent and ascent to and from the nadir of the deceleration (see Figs. 18-16 and 18-17). Some variable decelerations are preceded and followed by brief accelerations of the FHR known as *shoulders,* which is an appropriate compensatory response to compression of the umbilical vein.

Occasional variables have little clinical significance. Recurrent variable decelerations, however, indicate repetitive disruption in the fetus's oxygen supply. This can result in hypoxemia and metabolic acidemia. Variable decelerations are most commonly found during the transition phase of first stage labor or the second stage of labor as a result of umbilical cord compression and stretching during fetal descent (Garite, 2012). Box 18-6 lists causes, clinical significance, and nursing interventions for variable decelerations.

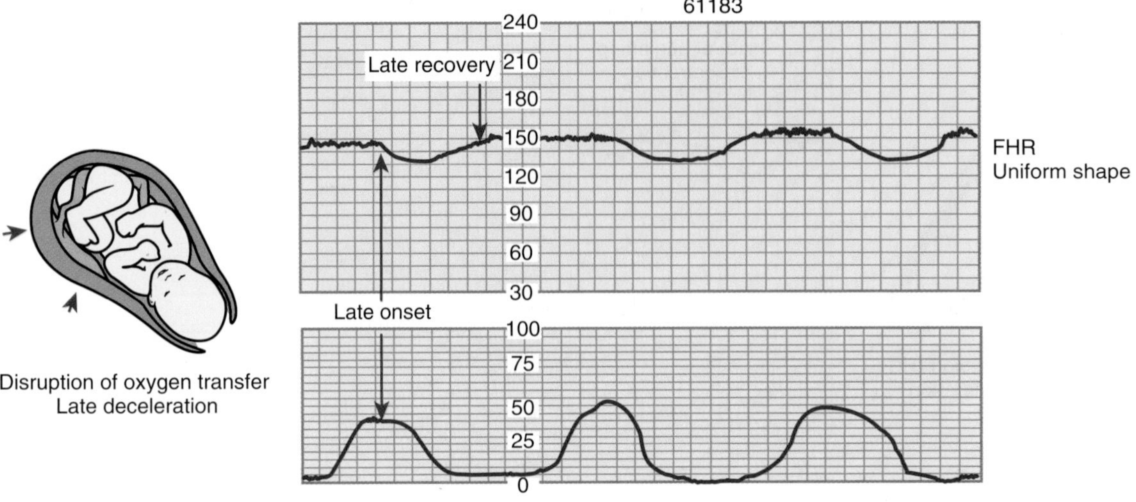

FIG 18-14 Line drawing illustrating late decelerations. *FHR,* Fetal heart rate. (Modified from Tucker, S. [2004]. *Pocket guide to fetal monitoring and assessment* [5th ed.]. St. Louis: Mosby.)

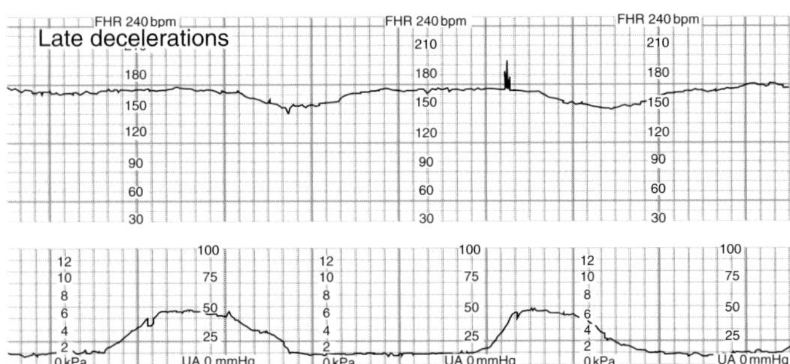

FIG 18-15 Electronic fetal monitor tracing showing late decelerations. *FHR,* Fetal heart rate; *UA,* uterine activity. (From Miller, L., Miller, D., & Tucker, S. [2013]. *Mosby's pocket guide to fetal monitoring: A multidisciplinary approach* [7th ed.]. St. Louis: Mosby.)

Prolonged Decelerations. A prolonged deceleration is a visually apparent decrease (may be either gradual or abrupt) in FHR of at least 15 beats/minute below the baseline and lasting more than 2 minutes but less than 10 minutes. A deceleration lasting more than 10 minutes is considered a baseline change (Macones et al., 2008) (Fig. 18-18).

Prolonged decelerations are caused when the mechanisms responsible for late or variable decelerations last for an extended period (more than 2 minutes). Examples of conditions that can cause an interruption in the fetal oxygen supply long enough to produce a prolonged deceleration include maternal hypotension, uterine tachysystole or rupture, extreme placental insufficiency, and prolonged cord compression or prolapse (Garite, 2012; Miller et al., 2013). The presence and degree of hypoxia are thought to correlate with the depth and duration of the deceleration, how abruptly it returns to the baseline, how much variability is lost during the deceleration, and whether rebound tachycardia and loss of variability occur after the deceleration (Garite).

! NURSING ALERT

Nurses should notify the physician or nurse-midwife immediately and initiate appropriate treatment of abnormal patterns when they see a prolonged deceleration.

BOX 18-5 Late Decelerations

Cause

Disruption of oxygen transfer from environment to fetus caused by the following:

- Uterine tachysystole
- Maternal supine hypotension
- Epidural or spinal anesthesia
- Placenta previa
- Placental abruption
- Hypertensive disorders
- Postmaturity
- Intrauterine growth restriction
- Diabetes mellitus
- Intraamniotic infection

Clinical Significance

Abnormal pattern associated with fetal hypoxemia, acidemia, and low Apgar scores; considered ominous if persistent and uncorrected, especially when associated with absent or minimal baseline variability

Nursing Interventions

The usual priority is as follows:

1. Change maternal position (lateral).
2. Correct maternal hypotension by elevating legs.
3. Increase rate of maintenance IV solution.
4. Palpate uterus to assess for tachysystole.
5. Discontinue oxytocin if infusing.
6. Administer oxygen at 8 to 10 L/minute by nonrebreather face mask.
7. Notify physician or nurse-midwife.
8. Consider internal monitoring for a more accurate fetal and uterine assessment.
9. Assist with birth (cesarean or vaginal assisted) if the pattern cannot be corrected.

IV, Intravenous.

CARE MANAGEMENT

Care of the woman receiving EFM in labor begins with evaluation of the EFM equipment. The nurse must ensure that the monitor is recording FHR and UA accurately and that the

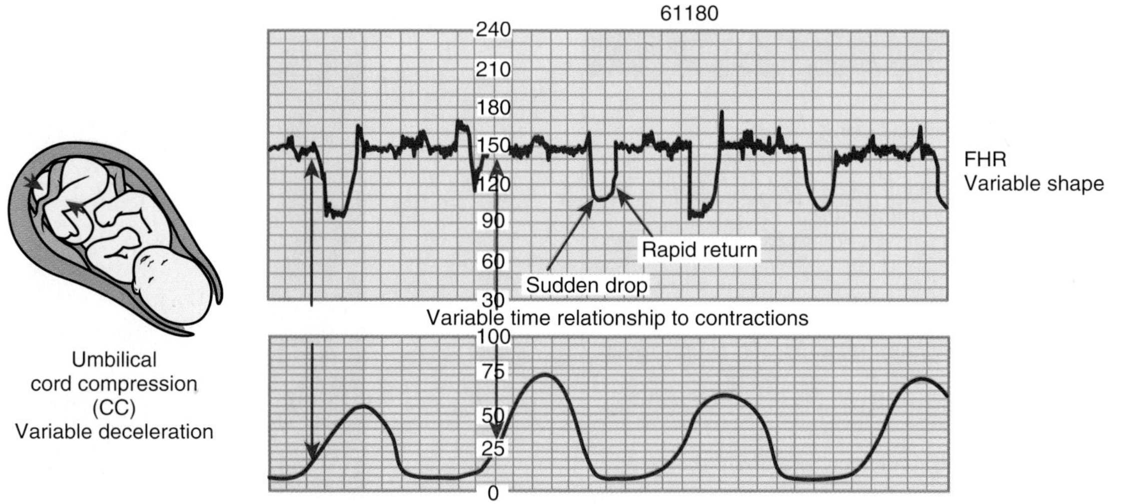

FIG 18-16 Line drawing illustrating variable decelerations. *FHR*, Fetal heart rate. (From Tucker, S. [2004]. *Pocket guide to fetal monitoring and assessment* [5th ed.]. St. Louis: Mosby.)

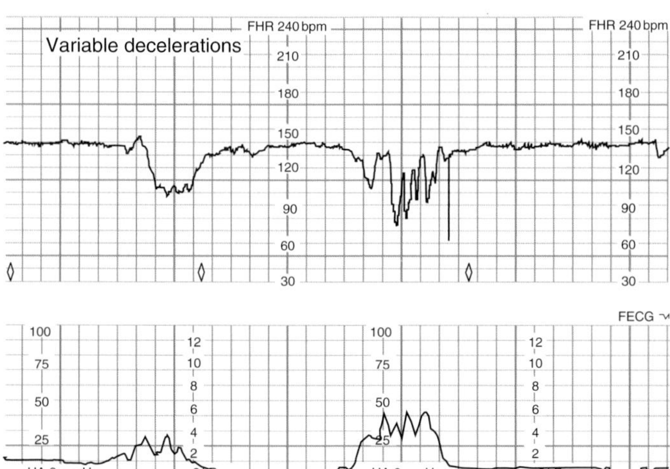

FIG 18-17 Electronic fetal monitor tracing showing variable decelerations. *FHR*, Fetal heart rate; *FECG*, fetal electrocardiogram. (From Miller, L., Miller, D., & Tucker, S. [2013]. *Mosby's pocket guide to fetal monitoring: A multidisciplinary approach* [7th ed.]. St. Louis: Mosby.)

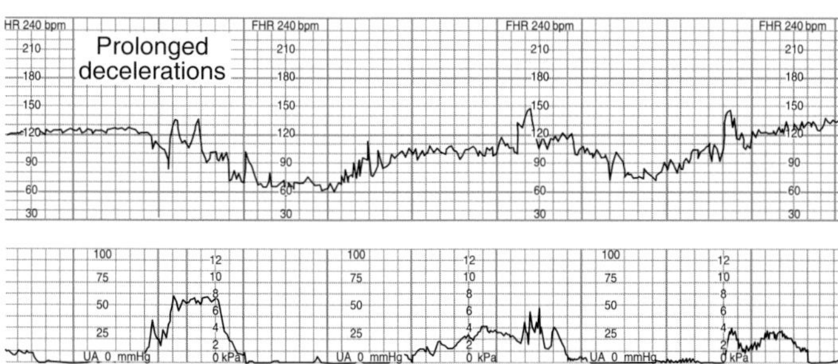

FIG 18-18 Prolonged decelerations. *FHR*, Fetal heart rate; *UA*, uterine activity. (From Miller, L., Miller, D., & Tucker, S. [2013]. *Mosby's pocket guide to fetal monitoring: A multidisciplinary approach* [7th ed.]. St. Louis: Mosby.)

BOX 18-6 Variable Decelerations

Cause

Umbilical cord compression caused by the following:

- Maternal position with cord between fetus and maternal pelvis
- Cord around fetal neck, arm, leg, or other body part
- Short cord
- Knot in cord
- Prolapsed cord

Clinical Significance

Variable decelerations occur in approximately 50% of all labors and usually are transient and correctable

Nursing Interventions

The usual priority is as follows:

1. Change maternal position (side to side, knee-chest).
2. Discontinue oxytocin if infusing.
3. Administer oxygen at 8 to 10 L/minute by nonrebreather face mask.
4. Notify physician or nurse-midwife.
5. Assist with vaginal or speculum examination to assess for cord prolapse.
6. Assist with amnioinfusion if ordered.
7. Assist with birth (vaginal assisted or cesarean) if the pattern cannot be corrected.

tracing is interpretable. If external monitoring is not adequate, changing to a fetal spiral electrode or IUPC may be necessary. A checklist for fetal monitoring equipment can be used to evaluate the equipment functions (Box 18-7).

After ensuring that the monitor is recording properly, the FHR and UA tracings are evaluated regularly throughout labor. *Guidelines for Perinatal Care*, published jointly by the American Academy of Pediatrics (AAP) and ACOG (2012), recommends that the FHR tracing be evaluated at least every 30 minutes during the first stage of labor and every 15 minutes during the second stage of labor in low risk women. If risk factors are present, the FHR tracing should be evaluated more frequently: every 15 minutes in the first stage of labor and every 5 minutes in the second stage of labor.

BOX 18-7 Checklist for Fetal Monitoring Equipment

Preparation of Monitor
1. Is the paper inserted correctly (if using paper)?
2. Are transducer cables plugged securely into the appropriate port on the monitor?
3. Is the paper speed set to 3 cm/minute?
4. Was the monitor date and time verified (when using electronic documentation)?

Ultrasound Transducer
1. Has ultrasound transmission gel been applied to the transducer?
2. Was the fetal heart rate (FHR) tested and noted on the monitor strip?
3. Was the FHR compared with the maternal pulse and noted?
4. Does a signal light flash or an audible beep occur with each heartbeat?
5. Is the belt secure and snug but comfortable for the laboring woman?

Tocotransducer
1. Is the tocotransducer firmly positioned at the site of the least maternal tissue?
2. Has it been applied without gel or paste?
3. Was the uterine activity (UA) baseline adjusted between contractions to print at the 20-mm Hg line?
4. Is the belt secure and snug but comfortable for the laboring woman?

Spiral Electrode
1. Is the connector attached firmly to the electrode pad (on the leg plate or abdomen)?
2. Is the spiral electrode attached to the presenting part of the fetus?
3. Is the inner surface of the electrode pad pre-gelled or covered with electrode gel?
4. Is the electrode pad properly secured to the woman's thigh or abdomen?

Internal Catheter or Strain Gauge
1. Is the length line on the catheter visible at the introitus?
2. Is it noted on the monitor paper that a UA test or calibration was performed?
3. Has the monitor been set to zero according to the manufacturer's directions?
4. Is the intrauterine pressure catheter properly secured to the woman?
5. Is the baseline resting tone of the uterus documented?

From Miller, L., Miller, D., & Tucker, S. (2013). *Mosby's pocket guide to fetal monitoring: A multidisciplinary approach* (7th ed.). St. Louis: Mosby.

Assessing FHR and UA patterns, implementing independent nursing interventions, documenting observations and actions according to the established standard of care, and reporting abnormal patterns to the primary care provider (e.g., physician, nurse-midwife) are the responsibilities of the nurse providing care to women in labor.

Technology has made access to and communication regarding electronic FHR tracings much more convenient for health care providers. Many hospitals use central monitor displays, which provide the opportunity to view the tracings of several

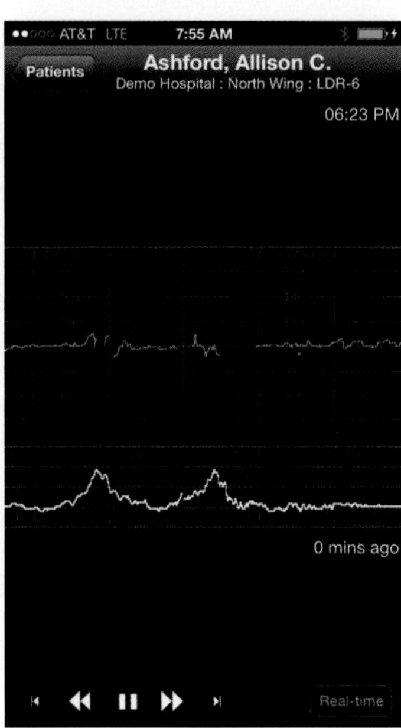

FIG 18-19 Providers can access near real-time fetal heart rate tracings and review client data using their mobile phones. (© 2014 AirStrip Technologies. All rights reserved. Trademarks not belonging to AirStrip Technologies are the property of their respective companies.)

women at the same time at the nurses' station. Health care providers can also access the FHR tracings of one woman or several clients from remote locations, including office and home. It is also possible to access FHR tracings and other client data using mobile phones (Fig. 18-19) (Miller et al., 2013).

Electronic Fetal Monitoring Pattern Recognition and Interpretation

Nurses must evaluate many factors to determine whether an FHR pattern is normal or abnormal. They evaluate these factors based on the presence of other obstetric complications, progress in labor, and use of analgesia or anesthesia. They also must consider the estimated time interval until birth. Therefore, interventions are based on clinical judgment of a complex, integrated process. Several different organizations offer EFM courses for nurses and other health care professionals. It is also possible to earn certification in EFM.

Categorizing Fetal Heart Rate Tracings

As mentioned, a three-tier system of categorizing FHR tracings is recommended (see Box 18-1). Category I FHR

LEGAL TIP: Fetal Monitoring Standards

Nurses who care for women during childbirth are legally responsible for correctly interpreting FHR patterns, initiating appropriate nursing interventions based on those patterns, and documenting the outcomes of those interventions. Perinatal nurses are responsible for the timely notification of the physician or nurse-midwife in the event of abnormal FHR patterns. They also are responsible for initiating the institutional chain of command should differences in opinion arise among health care providers concerning the interpretation of the FHR pattern and the intervention required.

tracings are normal and strongly predictive of normal fetal acid-base status at the time of observation. These tracings may be followed in a routine manner and do not require any specific action. Category II FHR tracings are indeterminate. This category includes all tracings that do not meet category I or category III criteria. Category II tracings require continued observation and evaluation. Category III FHR tracings are abnormal. Immediate evaluation and prompt intervention are required when these patterns are identified (Macones et al., 2008).

Nursing Management of Abnormal Patterns

The five essential components of the FHR tracing that must be evaluated regularly are baseline rate, baseline variability, accelerations, decelerations, and changes or trends over time. Whenever one of these five essential components is assessed as abnormal, corrective measures must be taken immediately. The purpose of these actions is to improve fetal oxygenation (Miller et al., 2013). The term *intrauterine resuscitation* is sometimes used to refer to specific interventions initiated when an abnormal FHR pattern is noted. Basic corrective measures include providing supplemental oxygen, instituting maternal position changes, and increasing intravenous fluid administration. These interventions are implemented to improve uterine and intervillous space blood flow and increase maternal oxygenation and cardiac output (Miller et al.). Box 18-8 lists basic interventions to improve maternal and fetal oxygenation status.

Depending on the underlying cause of the abnormal FHR pattern, other interventions, such as correcting maternal hypotension, reducing UA, and altering second-stage pushing techniques also may be instituted (Miller et al., 2013). Box 18-8 lists interventions for these specific problems. Some of the items listed are not independent nursing interventions. Any medications administered, for example, must be authorized either through inclusion in a specific unit protocol or by a written or verbal order. Some interventions are specific to the FHR pattern. (See Table 18-3 and Boxes 18-5 and 18-6 for nursing interventions for tachycardia, late decelerations, and variable decelerations.) Based on the FHR response to these interventions the primary health care provider decides whether additional interventions should be instituted or whether immediate assisted vaginal or cesarean birth should be performed.

BOX 18-8 Management of Abnormal Fetal Heart Rate Patterns

Basic Interventions

- Administer oxygen by nonrebreather face mask at a rate of 10 L/minute for approximately 15 to 30 minutes.
- Assist the woman to a side-lying (lateral) position.
- Increase maternal blood volume by increasing the rate of the primary IV infusion.

Interventions for Specific Problems

- Maternal hypotension
  - Increase the rate of the primary IV infusion.
  - Change to lateral or Trendelenburg positioning.
  - Administer ephedrine or phenylephrine per unit protocol or standing order if other measures are unsuccessful in increasing blood pressure.
- Uterine tachysystole
  - Reduce or discontinue the dose of any uterine stimulants in use (e.g., oxytocin [Pitocin]).
  - Administer a uterine relaxant (tocolytic) (e.g., terbutaline [Brethine]).
- Abnormal fetal heart rate pattern during the second stage of labor
  - Use open-glottis pushing.
  - Use fewer pushing efforts during each contraction.
  - Make individual pushing efforts shorter.
  - Push only with every other or every third contraction.
  - Push only with a perceived urge to push (in women with regional anesthesia).

IV, Intravenous.

OTHER METHODS OF ASSESSMENT AND INTERVENTION

A major shortcoming of EFM is its high rate of false-positive results. Even the most abnormal patterns are poorly predictive of neonatal morbidity. Therefore, other methods of assessment have been developed to evaluate fetal status. Fetal scalp stimulation and vibroacoustic stimulation and umbilical cord acid-base determination are frequently performed. Fetal scalp blood sampling is another available assessment technique. Amnioinfusion and tocolytic therapy are interventions often used in an attempt to improve abnormal FHR patterns.

Assessment Techniques

Fetal Scalp Stimulation and Vibroacoustic Stimulation

Several research studies undertaken in the 1980s found that an FHR acceleration in response to digital or vibroacoustic stimulation was highly predictive of a normal scalp blood pH. The two methods of fetal stimulation used most often in clinical practice are scalp stimulation (using digital pressure during a vaginal examination) and vibroacoustic stimulation (using an artificial larynx or fetal acoustic stimulation device on the maternal abdomen over the fetal head for 1 to 5 seconds). Another stimulation method is placing a specialized halogen light source on the maternal abdomen. The desired result of these stimulation methods is an acceleration in the FHR of at least 15 beats/minute for at least 15 seconds (Miller et al., 2013). An FHR acceleration indicates the absence of metabolic acidemia. If the fetus does not respond to stimulation with an acceleration, fetal compromise is not necessarily indicated; however, further evaluation of fetal well-being is needed. Fetal stimulation should be performed at times when the FHR is at baseline. Neither fetal scalp stimulation nor vibroacoustic stimulation should be instituted if FHR decelerations or bradycardia is present (Miller et al.).

Umbilical Cord Blood Acid-Base Determination

In assessing the immediate condition of the newborn after birth, a sample of cord blood is a useful adjunct to the Apgar score, especially if there has been an abnormal or confusing FHR tracing during labor or neonatal depression at birth.

TABLE 18-4 Approximate Normal Values for Cord Blood

VESSEL	pH	P_{CO_2} (mm Hg)	P_{O_2} (mm Hg)	BASE DEFICIT (mmol/L)
Artery	7.2-7.3	45-55	15-25	<12
Vein	7.3-7.4	35-45	25-35	<12

From Miller, L., Miller, D., & Tucker, S. (2013). *Mosby's pocket guide to fetal monitoring: A multidisciplinary approach* (7th ed.). St. Louis: Mosby.

TABLE 18-5 Types of Acidemia

VALUE	RESPIRATORY	METABOLIC	MIXED
pH	<7.20	<7.20	<7.20
P_{CO_2}	Elevated	Normal	Elevated
Base deficit	<12 mmol/L	≥12 mmol/L	≥12 mmol/L

From Miller, L., Miller, D., & Tucker, S. (2013). *Mosby's pocket guide to fetal monitoring: A multidisciplinary approach* (7th ed.). St. Louis: Mosby.

Generally the procedure is performed by withdrawing blood from both the umbilical artery and the umbilical vein. Both samples are then tested for pH, carbon dioxide pressure (P_{CO_2}), oxygen pressure (P_{O_2}), and base deficit or base excess (Garite, 2012; Miller et al., 2013). Umbilical arterial values reflect fetal condition, whereas umbilical vein values indicate placental function (Miller et al.).

The ACOG (2012) suggests obtaining cord blood values in the following clinical situations: cesarean birth for fetal compromise, low 5-minute Apgar score, severe intrauterine growth restriction, abnormal FHR tracing, maternal thyroid disease, intrapartum fever, and multifetal gestation. Normal umbilical artery and vein cord blood values are listed in Table 18-4. Normal findings preclude the presence of acidemia at or immediately before birth. If acidemia is present (e.g., pH less than 7.20), the type of acidemia is determined (respiratory, metabolic, or mixed) by analyzing the blood gas values (Table 18-5) (Miller et al., 2013).

Fetal Scalp Blood Sampling

Sampling of the fetal scalp blood for pH determination was first described in the 1960s and performed extensively in the 1970s. The procedure is performed by obtaining a sample of fetal scalp blood through the dilated cervix after the membranes have ruptured. Its use is limited by many factors, including the requirement for cervical dilation and membrane rupture, technical difficulty of the procedure, need for repetitive pH determinations, and uncertainty regarding interpretation and application of results. This procedure is now seldom used in the United States but remains a common practice in many other countries (Miller et al., 2013).

Interventions

Amnioinfusion

Amnioinfusion is infusion of room-temperature isotonic fluid (usually normal saline or lactated Ringer's solution) into the uterine cavity if the volume of amniotic fluid is low. Without the buffer of amniotic fluid the umbilical cord can easily become compressed during contractions or fetal movement, diminishing the flow of blood between the fetus and placenta. The purpose of amnioinfusion is to relieve intermittent umbilical cord compression that results in variable decelerations and transient fetal hypoxemia by restoring the amniotic fluid volume to a normal or near-normal level (Miller et al., 2013). Women with an abnormally small amount of amniotic fluid (oligohydramnios) or no amniotic fluid (anhydramnios) are candidates for this procedure. Conditions that can result in oligohydramnios or anhydramnios include uteroplacental insufficiency, premature rupture of membranes, and anomalies that prevent or reduce fetal urine production.

Risks of amnioinfusion are overdistention of the uterine cavity and increased uterine tone. Fluid is administered through an IUPC either by gravity flow or by an infusion pump. Usually a bolus of fluid is administered over 20 to 30 minutes, and then the infusion is slowed to a maintenance rate. Likely no more than 1000 ml of fluid will need to be administered. The fluid can be warmed for the preterm fetus by infusing it through a blood warmer (Miller et al., 2013).

Intensity and frequency of UCs should be continually assessed during the procedure. The recorded uterine resting tone during amnioinfusion appears higher than normal because of resistance to outflow and turbulence at the end of the catheter. Uterine resting tone should not exceed 40 mm Hg during the procedure. The amount of fluid return must be estimated and documented during amnioinfusion to prevent overdistention of the uterus. The volume of fluid returned should be approximately the same as the amount infused (Miller et al., 2013).

Tocolytic Therapy

Tocolysis (relaxation of the uterus) can be achieved by administering drugs that inhibit UCs. This therapy can be used as an adjunct to other interventions in managing fetal stress when the fetus is exhibiting abnormal patterns associated with increased UA. Tocolysis improves blood flow through the placenta by inhibiting UCs. It may be implemented by the primary health care provider when other interventions to reduce UA such as maternal position change and discontinuance of an oxytocin infusion have not diminished the UCs effectively. Tocolytics can be administered when women are having excessive spontaneous UCs. They are also frequently administered after a decision for cesarean birth has been made while preparations for surgery are under way. The most commonly used tocolytic in these situations is terbutaline (Brethine) given subcutaneously. Terbutaline works quickly and has been demonstrated to improve Apgar scores and cord pH values without apparent complications such as postpartum hemorrhage (Garite, 2012). If the FHR and UC patterns improve, the woman may be allowed to continue labor; if no improvement is seen, immediate cesarean birth may be needed.

CLIENT AND FAMILY TEACHING

Although the use of EFM can be reassuring to many parents, it can be a source of anxiety to some. Therefore, the nurse must be particularly sensitive and respond appropriately to the

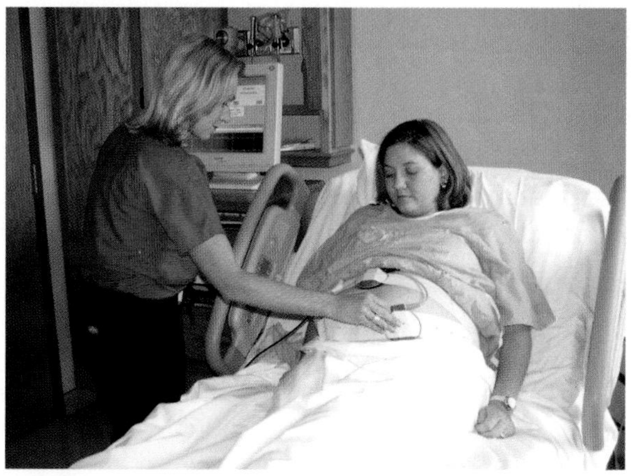

FIG 18-20 Nurse explains electronic fetal monitoring as ultrasound transducer monitors the fetal heart rate. (Courtesy Julie Perry Nelson, Loveland, CO.)

BOX 18-9 Client and Family Teaching When Electronic Fetal Monitor Is Used

The following guidelines relate to client teaching and the functioning of the monitor.

- Explain the purpose of monitoring.
- Explain each procedure.
- Provide rationale for maternal position other than supine.
- Explain that fetal status can be continuously assessed by electronic fetal monitoring (EFM), even during contractions.
- Explain that the lower tracing on the monitor strip paper shows uterine activity (UA); the upper tracing shows the fetal heart rate (FHR).
- Reassure woman and partner that prepared childbirth techniques can be implemented without difficulty.
- Explain that during external monitoring effleurage can be performed on sides of abdomen or upper portion of thighs.
- Explain that breathing patterns based on the time and intensity of contractions can be enhanced by the observation of uterine activity on the monitor strip, which shows the onset of contractions.
- Note peak of contraction; knowing that the contraction will not get stronger and is halfway over is usually helpful.
- Note diminishing intensity.
- Coordinate with appropriate breathing and relaxation techniques.
- Reassure woman and partner that the use of internal monitoring does not restrict movement, although she is confined to bed.*
- Explain that use of external monitoring usually requires the woman's cooperation during positioning and movement.
- Reassure woman and partner that use of monitoring does not imply fetal jeopardy.

*Portable telemetry monitors allow the FHR and uterine contraction patterns to be observed on centrally located display stations. These portable units permit ambulation during electronic monitoring.

emotional, informational, and comfort needs of the woman in labor and those of her family (Fig. 18-20 and Box 18-9).

Part of the nurse's role includes acting as a partner with the woman to achieve a high-quality birthing experience. In addition to teaching and supporting the woman and her family with understanding of the labor and birth process, breathing techniques, use of equipment, and pain management techniques, the nurse can assist with two factors that have an effect on fetal status: positioning and pushing. The nurse should ask for the woman's cooperation in avoiding the supine position. Instead, the woman should be encouraged to maintain a side-lying position or semi-Fowler position with a lateral tilt to the uterus. In addition, the nurse should instruct the woman to keep her mouth and glottis open and to let air escape from her lungs during the pushing process. Both of these interventions help to improve fetal oxygenation. See Chapter 19 for further discussion of maternal positioning and pushing techniques.

DOCUMENTATION

Clear and complete documentation in the woman's medical record is essential. Each FHR and UA assessment must be completely documented in the woman's medical record. More and more hospitals are moving to use of the electronic medical record and computerized charting. With computerized charting, each required component usually appears on the screen so it will be addressed routinely. Computerized charting often includes forced choices that greatly increase the use of standardized FHR terminology by all members of the health care team. In the past, nurses were often encouraged to chart both on the monitor strip and in the medical record. However, charting directly on the monitor strip is unnecessary when an electronic medical record is used (Fig. 18-21). Any information that is handwritten on the monitor strip will not be recorded in the computer record. Furthermore, given that the EFM tracing is stored on a computer, the paper strips are destroyed after the woman is discharged. No permanent record of the handwritten charting exists.

In institutions that still use a paper chart, documentation on the woman's monitor strip is started before initiating monitoring and consists of identifying information plus other relevant data. This documentation is continued and updated according to institutional protocol as monitoring continues and labor progresses.

In some institutions observations noted and interventions implemented are recorded on the monitor strip to produce a comprehensive document that chronicles the course of labor and the care rendered. In other institutions this documentation is confined to the labor flow record. Advocates of documenting on both the medical record and the EFM strip cite as advantages of this approach the ease of writing directly on the strip while at the bedside and the improved accuracy in documenting critical events and the interventions implemented. Others believe that charting on the EFM strip constitutes duplicate documentation of the information noted in the medical record, and thus it is unnecessary additional paperwork for the nurse.

A disadvantage of documenting on both the EFM strip and the medical record is that the times noted for events and interventions on the EFM strip frequently do not correlate with what is later documented in the medical record. These inaccuracies can lead people involved in the retrospective review process carried out during litigation to infer that documentation errors have occurred. Therefore, if institutional policy mandates documentation both on the monitor strip and in the medical record, the nurse must make sure the times and notations of events and interventions recorded in each place agree.

Fetal Monitor Integration

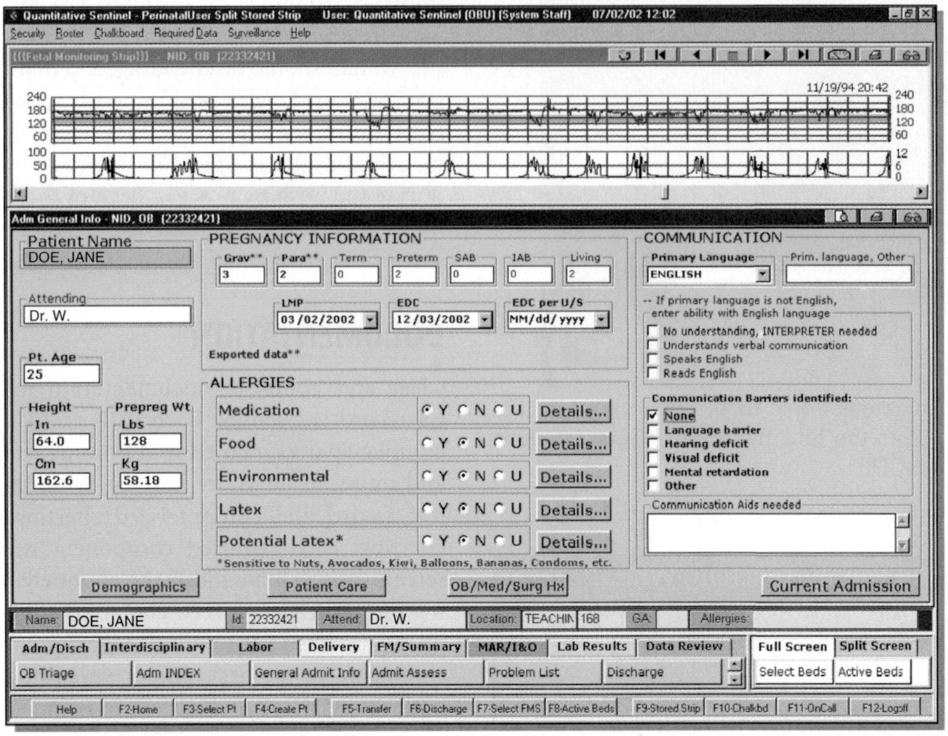

FIG 18-21 With integration of the fetal monitor tracing into the electronic medical record, the nurse can view the fetal tracing while charting. (Courtesy General Electric Healthcare Technologies, Barrington, IL.)

KEY POINTS

- Fetal well-being during labor is gauged by the response of the FHR to UCs.
- Standardized definitions for many common FHR patterns have been adopted for use in clinical practice by the ACNM, ACOG, and AWHONN.
- The five essential components of the FHR tracing are baseline rate, baseline variability, accelerations, decelerations, and changes or trends over time.
- The monitoring of fetal well-being includes FHR and UA assessment and assessment of maternal vital signs.
- The FHR can be monitored by either IA or EFM. The FHR and UA can be assessed by EFM using either the external or internal monitoring mode.
- Assessing FHR and UA patterns, implementing independent nursing interventions, and reporting abnormal patterns to the physician or nurse-midwife are the nurse's responsibilities.
- The AWHONN and ACOG have established and published health care provider standards and guidelines for FHR monitoring.
- The emotional, informational, and comfort needs of the woman and her family must be addressed when the mother and her fetus are being monitored.
- Documentation of fetal assessment is initiated and updated according to institutional protocol.

REFERENCES

American Academy of Pediatrics (AAP) and American College of Obstetricians and Gynecologists (ACOG). (2012). *Guidelines for perinatal care* (7th ed.). Washington, DC: ACOG.

American College of Obstetricians and Gynecologists (ACOG). (2009). *Intrapartum fetal heart rate monitoring: Nomenclature, interpretation, and general management principles. ACOG practice bulletin no. 106.* Washington, DC: ACOG.

American College of Obstetricians and Gynecologists (ACOG). (2012). *Umbilical cord blood gas and acid-base analysis. ACOG committee opinion no. 348.* Washington, DC: ACOG.

Association of Women's Health, Obstetric and Neonatal Nurses. (2009). *Fetal heart monitoring principles and practices* (4th ed.). Dubuque, IA: Kendall/Hunt.

Cunningham, F., Leveno, K., Bloom, S., et al. (2014). *Williams obstetrics* (24th ed.). New York: McGraw-Hill Education.

Garite, T. (2012). Intrapartum fetal evaluation. In S. Gabbe, J. Niebyl, & J. Simpson (Eds.), *Obstetrics: Normal and problem pregnancies* (6th ed.). Philadelphia: Saunders.

Gilbert, E. (2011). *Manual of high risk pregnancy & delivery* (5th ed.). St. Louis: Mosby.

Lyndon, A., O'Brien-Abel, N., & Simpson, K. (2014). Fetal assessment during labor. In K. Rice Simpson, & P. Creehan (Eds.), *AWHONN's perinatal nursing* (4th ed.). Philadelphia: Lippincott Williams & Wilkins.

Macones, G., Hankins, G., Spong, C., et al. (2008). The 2008 National Institute of Child Health and Human Development Workshop Report on Electronic Fetal Monitoring: Update on definitions, interpretation, and research guidelines. *Journal of Obstetric, Gynecologic, and Neonatal Nursing, 37*(5), 510–515.

Miller, L., Miller, D., & Tucker, S. (2013). *Mosby's pocket guide to fetal monitoring: A multidisciplinary approach* (7th ed.). St. Louis: Mosby.

Nageotte, M. (2014). Intrapartum fetal surveillance. In R. K. Creasy, R. Resnik, J. D. Iams, et al. (Eds.), *Creasy and Resnik's maternal-fetal medicine: Principles and practice* (7th ed.). Philadelphia: Saunders.

National Institute of Child Health and Human Development (NICHD) Research Planning Workshop. (1997). Electronic fetal heart rate monitoring: Research guidelines for interpretation. *American Journal of Obstetrics and Gynecology, 177*(6), 1385–1390.

19 CHAPTER

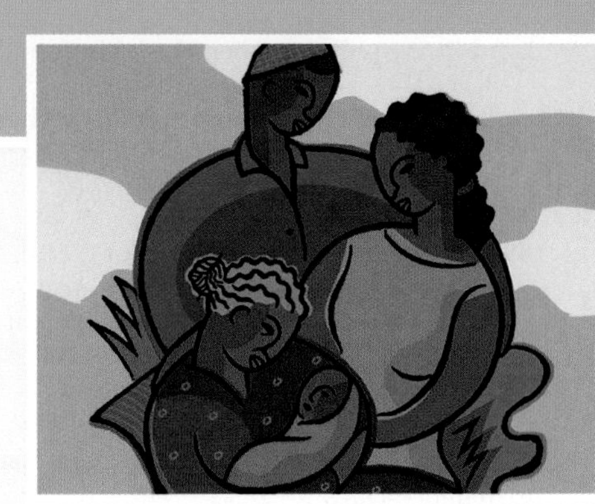

Nursing Care of the Family During Labor and Birth

Deborah S. Walker

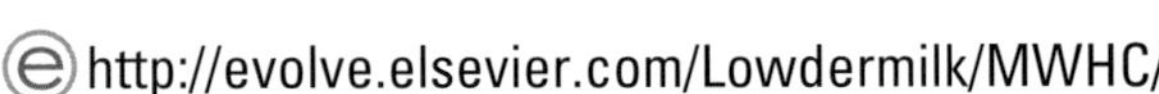

http://evolve.elsevier.com/Lowdermilk/MWHC/

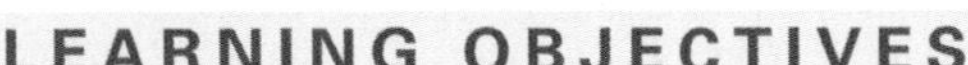

LEARNING OBJECTIVES

- Review the data included in the initial assessment of the woman in labor.
- Describe the ongoing assessment of maternal progress during the first, second, third, and fourth stages of labor.
- Recognize the physical and psychosocial findings indicative of maternal progress during labor.
- Describe fetal assessment during labor.
- Identify signs of developing complications during labor and birth.
- Incorporate evidence-based nursing interventions into a comprehensive plan of care relevant to each stage of labor.
- Recognize the importance of support (family, partner, doula, nurse) in fostering maternal confidence and facilitating the progress of labor and birth.
- Analyze the influence of cultural and religious beliefs and practices on the process of labor and birth.
- Describe the role and responsibilities of the nurse during emergency childbirth.
- Evaluate the effect of perineal trauma on the woman's reproductive and sexual health.

The labor and childbirth processes are natural phenomena during which most women benefit from a philosophy of minimal intervention. The minimal intervention philosophy acknowledges that most pregnancies, labors, and births are normal and that intervention creates the potential for iatrogenic maternal-fetal injuries (Simpson & O'Brien-Abel, 2014). This is an exciting and potentially anxious time for the woman and her significant others (support persons, family members). In a relatively short period of time, they experience one of the most profound changes in their lives. Birth may take place in the hospital, birth center, or home setting or unexpectedly at any number of locations. The woman and her significant others may be cared for by a team of caregivers including nurses, doulas, nurse-midwives, and physicians. During labor and birth, nurses provide comprehensive care for women and families by using evidence-based knowledge of physiologic and psychosocial processes and selected pharmacologic and nonpharmacologic measures.

For most women labor begins with regular uterine contractions, continues with hours of hard work during cervical dilation and birth, and ends as the woman begins to recover physically from birth and she and her significant others begin the attachment process with the newborn. Nursing care management focuses on assessment and support of the woman and her significant others throughout labor and birth, with the goal of ensuring the best possible outcome for all involved. The focus of this chapter is on nursing care that facilitates normal birth processes.

COMMUNITY ACTIVITY

- Compare and contrast childbirth education classes offered by a hospital with those offered by a community group.
- Visit the website of a hospital that offers childbirth education classes in your community. Review the client information about the childbirth classes. If you are not able to find this information on their website, contact one of the instructors. What is the philosophy of the class? Is a specific type of childbirth method taught? Are the classes offered by nurses, nurse-midwives, physicians, or someone else? How long are the classes; one class versus a series of classes? What information is covered in the class(es)? Are significant others welcome to attend? Is breastfeeding information given? Is skin-to-skin contact immediately following birth discussed? How much of the information relates to hospital policies and practices rather than to childbirth coping strategies and newborn care? Are women encouraged to develop a birth plan?
- Visit the website of a community group offering childbirth education classes in your city or state that teaches a specific method such as Lamaze or Bradley. If you cannot find the information on the website, contact one of the instructors. What is the philosophy of the method? What are the credentials and education of the instructor? Are the classes offered as a series or one time only? Are significant others and children welcome? Where do women/families attending these classes plan to give birth? Are women encouraged to develop a birth plan?

FIRST STAGE OF LABOR

The first stage of labor begins with the onset of regular uterine contractions and ends with full cervical effacement and dilation. The first stage of labor consists of three phases: the latent (early) phase (through 3 cm of dilation), the active phase (4 to 7 cm of dilation), and the transition phase (8 to 10 cm of dilation).

CARE MANAGEMENT

Most nulliparous women planning a hospital or birth center birth seek admission in the latent (early) phase because they have not experienced labor before and are unsure of the "right" time to come in. Multiparous women usually do not come to the birth center or hospital until they are in the active phase of the first stage of labor. Even though no two labors are identical, women who have given birth before often are less anxious about the process, unless their previous experience was negative.

Assessment

Assessment begins at the first contact with the woman, whether by telephone or in person. Many women call the hospital or birthing center first for validation that it is all right for them to come in for evaluation or admission or that they can remain at home. Many hospitals, however, discourage the nurse from giving advice regarding what to do because of legal liability. Nurses are often instructed to tell women who call with questions to call their nurse-midwife or physician or to come to the hospital if they feel the need to be checked. The nature of the telephone conversation, including any advice or instructions given, should be documented in the woman's record (Gilbert, 2011).

A pregnant woman may first call her nurse-midwife or physician or go to the hospital or birth center while in false labor or early in the latent phase of the first stage of labor. She may feel discouraged, angry, or confused on learning that the contractions that feel so strong and regular to her are not true contractions because they are not causing cervical dilation or that they are still not strong or frequent enough for admission. During the third trimester of pregnancy, women should be instructed about the stages of labor and the signs indicating its onset. They should be informed that they will usually not be admitted if the cervix is dilated 3 cm or less (see Teaching for Self-Management).

If the woman lives near the hospital or birth center and has adequate support and transportation, she may be encouraged to stay at home or return home to allow labor to progress (e.g., until the uterine contractions are more frequent and intense). The ideal setting at this time for the woman at low risk for obstetric complications is usually the familiar environment of her home, where she can move around freely and eat and drink at will. The woman who lives at a considerable distance from the hospital or birth center, who lacks adequate support and transportation, or who has a history of rapid labors in the past, however, may be admitted in latent labor. The same measures used by the woman at home should be offered to the woman admitted in early labor.

A warm shower is often relaxing during early labor. However, warm baths before labor is well established could inhibit uterine contractions and prolong the labor process (Waterbirth International, 2013). Soothing back, foot, and hand massage or a warm drink of preferred liquids such as tea or milk can help the woman rest and even sleep, especially if false or early labor is occurring at night. Diversional activities such as walking outdoors or in the house, reading, watching television, "playing" on a computer or smart phone, or talking with friends can reduce the perception of early discomfort, help the time pass, and decrease anxiety.

When the woman arrives at the birth center or hospital perinatal unit, assessment is the top priority (Fig. 19-1). The nurse first performs a screening assessment by using the techniques of interview and physical assessment and reviews the laboratory and diagnostic test findings to determine the health status of the woman and her fetus and the progress of her labor. The nurse also notifies the nurse midwife or physician. If the woman is admitted, a detailed systems assessment is done.

When the woman is admitted to a hospital, she is usually moved from an observation area to the labor room; the labor, delivery, and recovery (LDR) room; or the labor, delivery, recovery, and postpartum (LDRP) room. If the woman wishes, include her partner in the assessment and admission process. The nurse can direct significant other(s) not participating in this process to the appropriate waiting area. In the hospital setting the woman undresses and puts on her own gown

TEACHING FOR SELF-MANAGEMENT

How to Distinguish True Labor from False Labor

True Labor

Contractions

- Occur regularly, becoming stronger, lasting longer, and occurring closer together
- Become more intense with walking
- Are usually felt in the lower back, radiating to the lower portion of the abdomen
- Continue despite use of comfort measures

Cervix (by Vaginal Examination)

- Shows progressive change (softening, effacement, and dilation signaled by the appearance of bloody show)
- Moves to an increasingly anterior position

Fetus

- Presenting part usually becomes engaged in the pelvis, which results in increased ease of breathing; at the same time, the presenting part presses downward and compresses the bladder, resulting in urinary frequency

False Labor

Contractions

- Occur irregularly or become regular only temporarily
- Often stop with walking or position change
- Can be felt in the back or the abdomen above the umbilicus
- Can often be stopped through the use of comfort measures

Cervix (by Vaginal Examination)

- May be soft but with no significant change in effacement or dilation or evidence of bloody show
- Is often in a posterior position

Fetus

- Presenting part is usually not engaged in the pelvis

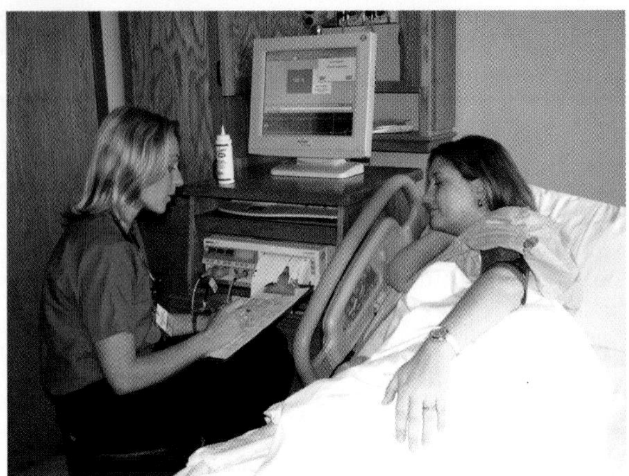

FIG 19-1 Woman being assessed for admission to the labor and birth unit. (Courtesy Julie Perry Nelson, Loveland, CO.)

LEGAL TIP: Obstetric Triage and EMTALA

The Emergency Medical Treatment and Active Labor Act (EMTALA) is a federal regulation enacted to protect pregnant women during an emergency regardless of their insurance status or ability to pay for care. According to the EMTALA, pregnant women who present with contractions or who may be in labor are considered unstable and must be assessed, stabilized, and treated at the hospital where they present regardless of their insurance status or ability to pay (Wilson-Griffin, 2014). Nurses working in labor and birth units must be familiar with their responsibilities according to the EMTALA regulations, which include providing services to pregnant women when they experience an urgent pregnancy problem (e.g., labor, decreased fetal movement, rupture of membranes, or recent trauma) and fully documenting all relevant information (e.g., assessment findings, interventions implemented, and client responses to care measures provided). A pregnant woman presenting in an obstetric triage area is considered to be in "true" labor until a qualified health care provider certifies that she is not. Agencies need to have specific policies and procedures in place so that compliance with the EMTALA regulations is achieved while safe and efficient care is provided (Miller, Miller, & Tucker, 2013).

or a hospital gown. The nurse places an identification band on the woman's wrist. Her personal belongings are put away safely or given to family members, according to agency policy. Women who participate in expectant parents classes often bring a birth bag or Lamaze bag with them. The nurse then shows the woman and her partner the layout and operation of the unit and room, how to use the call light and telephone system, and how to adjust lighting in the room and the different bed positions.

The nurse assures the woman that she is in competent, caring hands and that she and those to whom she gives permission can ask questions related to her care and status and that of her fetus at any time during labor. The nurse can minimize the woman's anxiety by explaining terms commonly used during labor. The woman's interest, response, and prior experience guide the depth and breadth of these explanations.

Most hospitals have specific forms, whether paper or electronic, that are used to obtain important assessment information when a woman in labor is being evaluated or admitted (Fig. 19-2, *A* and *B*). More and more hospitals now use an electronic health record (EHR); almost all documentation is done on a computer. Sources of data include the prenatal record, the initial interview, physical examination to determine baseline physiologic parameters (e.g., vital signs), laboratory and diagnostic test results, select psychosocial and cultural factors, and the clinical evaluation of labor status.

Prenatal Data

The nurse reviews the prenatal record to identify the woman's individual needs and risks. Copies of prenatal records are generally filed in the hospital's perinatal unit at some time during the woman's pregnancy (usually in the third trimester) or accessed by computer so that they are readily available on admission. If the woman has had no prenatal care or her prenatal records are unavailable, the nurse must obtain certain baseline information. If the woman is having discomfort, the nurse should ask questions between contractions when the woman can concentrate more fully on her answers. At times, the partner or support person(s) may need to be secondary sources of essential information. According to the Health Insurance Portability and Accountability Act (HIPAA), the woman must give permission for other individuals to be involved in the exchange of information regarding her care. Ideally, this permission should be obtained during pregnancy and a signed form included in her health records.

Knowing the woman's age is important so that the nurse can individualize care to the needs of her age group. For example, a 14-year-old girl and a 40-year-old woman have different but specific needs, and their ages place them at risk for different problems. Accurate height and weight measurements are important. A pregnancy weight gain greater than recommended may place the woman at a higher risk for cephalopelvic disproportion and cesarean birth. This is especially true for women who are petite and have gained 16 kg (35 lb) or more. A prepregnancy body mass index (BMI) greater than 30 is also a cause for concern. Other factors to consider are the woman's general health status, current medical conditions or allergies, respiratory status, and previous surgical procedures.

The nurse should carefully review the woman's prenatal records, taking note of her obstetric and pregnancy history including gravidity; parity; and problems such as history of vaginal bleeding, gestational hypertension, anemia, pregestational or gestational diabetes, infections (e.g., bacterial, viral, sexually transmitted), and immunodeficiency status. In addition, the expected date of birth (EDB) should be confirmed. Other important data found in the prenatal record include patterns of maternal weight gain, physiologic measurements such as maternal vital signs (blood pressure, temperature, pulse, respirations), fundal height, baseline fetal heart rate (FHR), and laboratory and diagnostic test results. See Table 14-1 for a list of common prenatal laboratory tests. Common diagnostic and fetal assessment tests performed prenatally include amniocentesis, nonstress test (NST), biophysical profile (BPP), and ultrasound examination. See Chapter 26 for more information.

If this labor and birth experience is not the woman's first, the nurse needs to note the characteristics of her previous

Centricity Perinatal - Perinatal User View User: Susan Smith, RN 10/5/13 09:57

HOME Security Patient Roster Surveillance Admission Patient Progress Graphs Labs Discharge Print System MD View Eval View PP View WBN View NICU View Atlas

Jones, Mary ID# 0102030405 Unit/Bed: Train Train2 Age: G/P EGA: GBS: Allergies:

Admission | Labor FS | Shift Assess | Delivery/OR | RR/Chg/BC | I&O/MAR | SBAR | Stored Strip | Split Screen

Adm General Info - Jones, Mary (0102030405)

Patient Name: Jones, Mary Pt. Age Demographics Send Outbound Now M / d /yyyy H :mm

PREGNANCY INFORMATION
EDC M / d /yyyy EDC per U/S M / d /yyyy LMP M / d /yyyy
Grav** Para** Term Preterm SAB IAB Living
Cesareans VBAC's Ectopic Multiple Births

Source of PNC
Month of 1st Prenatal Visit
Date last PNV M / d /yyyy Total # of Visits
Fetal Center Patient Yes
Prepreg Wt Lbs Kg
Height In Cm

ALLERGIES
Medication Latex
Medication Allergies
Food Allergies Environmental Allergies

COMMUNICATION
Primary Language
-- If primary language is not English, enter ability with English language
No understanding, INTERPRETER needed
Understands verbal communication
Speaks English
Reads English
Prim. language, Other
Communication Barriers identified: None, Language barrier, Hearing deficit, Visual deficit, Mental retardation, Other
Communication Aids needed

DRUG AND ALCOHOL USE
Alcohol Y N Details...
Cigarettes Y N Details...
Marijuana Y N Details

A General Admit | Prenatal Labs | History | Current Admit | Med Reconcile | DC Meds List | Admit Assess | CarePlans

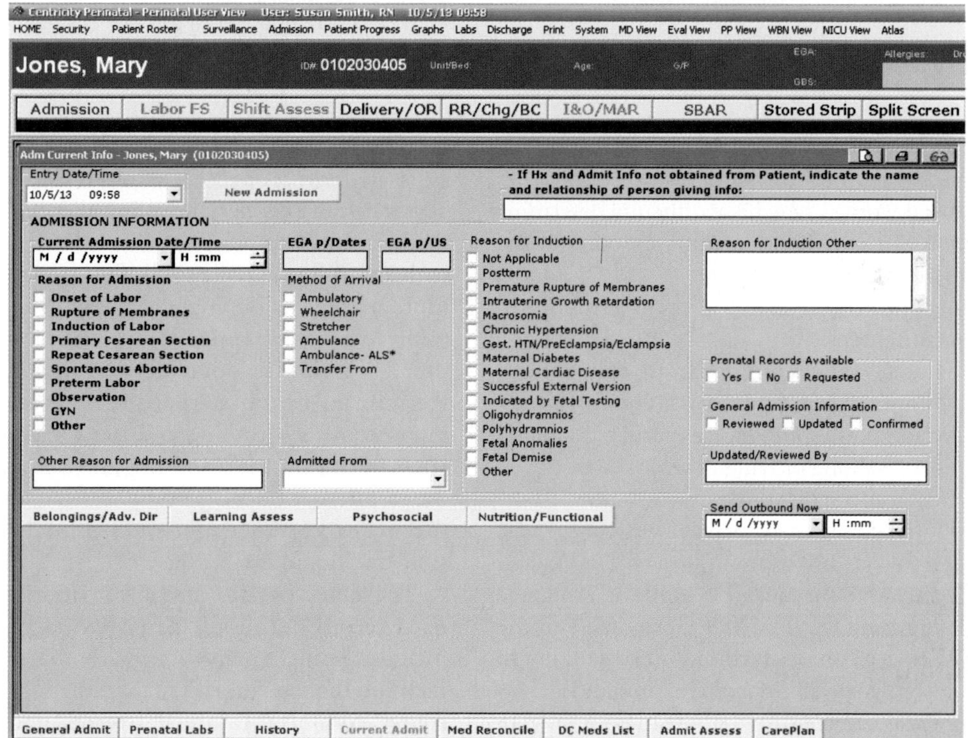

Centricity Perinatal - Perinatal User View User: Susan Smith, RN 10/5/13 09:58

HOME Security Patient Roster Surveillance Admission Patient Progress Graphs Labs Discharge Print System MD View Eval View PP View WBN View NICU View Atlas

Jones, Mary ID# 0102030405 Unit/Bed: Age: G/P EGA: GBS: Allergies:

Admission | Labor FS | Shift Assess | Delivery/OR | RR/Chg/BC | I&O/MAR | SBAR | Stored Strip | Split Screen

Adm Current Info - Jones, Mary (0102030405)

Entry Date/Time 10/5/13 09:58 New Admission

- If Hx and Admit Info not obtained from Patient, indicate the name and relationship of person giving info:

ADMISSION INFORMATION
Current Admission Date/Time M / d /yyyy H :mm
EGA p/Dates EGA p/US
Reason for Admission: Onset of Labor, Rupture of Membranes, Induction of Labor, Primary Cesarean Section, Repeat Cesarean Section, Spontaneous Abortion, Preterm Labor, Observation, GYN, Other
Method of Arrival: Ambulatory, Wheelchair, Stretcher, Ambulance, Ambulance- ALS*, Transfer From
Reason for Induction: Not Applicable, Postterm, Premature Rupture of Membranes, Intrauterine Growth Retardation, Macrosomia, Chronic Hypertension, Gest. HTN/PreEclampsia/Eclampsia, Maternal Diabetes, Maternal Cardiac Disease, Successful External Version, Indicated by Fetal Testing, Oligohydramnios, Polyhydramnios, Fetal Anomalies, Fetal Demise, Other
Reason for Induction Other
Prenatal Records Available: Yes No Requested
General Admission Information: Reviewed Updated Confirmed
Updated/Reviewed By
Other Reason for Admission Admitted From
Send Outbound Now M / d /yyyy H :mm

Belongings/Adv. Dir | Learning Assess | Psychosocial | Nutrition/Functional

B General Admit | Prenatal Labs | History | Current Admit | Med Reconcile | DC Meds List | Admit Assess | CarePlan

FIG 19-2 Admission screens in an electronic health record. **A**, General admission screen. **B**, Current admission screen. (Courtesy Kitty Cashion, Memphis, TN).

experiences. This information includes the duration of previous labors, the types of pain relief measures, including anesthesia used, the type of birth (e.g., spontaneous vaginal, forceps-assisted, vacuum-assisted, or cesarean birth), and the condition of the newborn. Explore the woman's perception of her previous labor and birth experiences because this perception may influence her attitude toward her current experience.

Interview

The woman's primary reason for coming to the hospital is determined in the interview. Her primary reason may be, for example, that her bag of waters (BOW, amniotic membranes) ruptured, with or without contractions. The woman may also have come in for a period of observation reserved for women who are unsure about the onset of their labor. This allows time for the diagnosis of labor without official hospital admission

BOX 19-1 Procedure: Tests for Rupture of Membranes

Nitrazine Test for pH
- Explain procedure to the woman or couple.

Procedure
- Wash hands and put on sterile gloves.
- Use a cotton-tipped applicator impregnated with Nitrazine dye for determining pH (differentiates amniotic fluid, which is slightly alkaline, from urine and purulent material [pus], which are acidic).
- Dip the cotton-tipped applicator deep into the vagina to pick up fluid (procedure may be performed during speculum examination).

Read Results
- Membranes probably intact: identifies vaginal and most body fluids that are acidic:

Yellow	pH 5
Olive-yellow	pH 5.5
Olive-green	pH 6

- Membranes probably ruptured: identifies amniotic fluid that is alkaline:

Blue-green	pH 6.5
Blue-gray	pH 7
Deep blue	pH 7.5

- Realize that false test results are possible because of presence of bloody show, insufficient amniotic fluid, or semen.
- Provide pericare as needed.
- Remove gloves and wash hands.

Document Results
- Results are reported as positive or negative.

Test for Ferning or Fern Pattern
- Explain procedure to woman or couple.

Procedure
- Wash hands, put on sterile gloves, obtain specimen of fluid (usually during sterile speculum examination).
- Spread a drop of fluid from vagina on clean glass slide with sterile cotton-tipped applicator.
- Allow fluid to dry.
- Examine the slide under microscope; observe for appearance of ferning (a frondlike crystalline pattern) (do not confuse with cervical mucus test, when high levels of estrogen cause ferning).
- Observe for absence of ferning (alerts staff to possibility that amount of specimen was inadequate or that specimen was urine, vaginal discharge, or blood).
- Provide pericare as needed.
- Remove gloves and wash hands.

Document Results
- Results are reported as positive or negative.

and minimizes or avoids cost to the woman when used by the hospital and approved by her health insurance plan.

Even the experienced woman may have difficulty determining the onset of labor. She is asked to recall the events of the previous days and to describe the following:

- Time and onset of contractions and progress in terms of frequency, duration, and intensity
- Location and character of discomfort from contractions (e.g., back pain, abdominal or suprapubic discomfort)
- Persistence of contractions despite changes in maternal position and activity (e.g., walking or lying down)
- Presence and character of vaginal discharge or "show"
- The status of amniotic membranes, such as a gush or seepage of fluid (spontaneous rupture of membranes [SROM]). If there has been a discharge that may be amniotic fluid, she is asked the date and time the fluid was first noted and the fluid's characteristics (e.g., amount, color, unusual odor). In many instances, a sterile speculum examination and Nitrazine (pH) and *fern tests* can confirm that the membranes are ruptured (Box 19-1).

These descriptions help the nurse assess the degree of progress in the process of labor. Bloody show is distinguished from bleeding by the fact that it is pink and feels sticky because of its mucoid nature. There is very little bloody show in the beginning, but the amount increases with effacement and dilation of the cervix. A woman may report a small amount of brownish to bloody discharge that may be attributed to cervical trauma resulting from vaginal examination or coitus (intercourse) within the past 48 hours.

Assessing the woman's respiratory status is important in case general anesthesia is needed in an emergency. The nurse determines this status by asking the woman if she has a "cold" or related symptoms (e.g., stuffy nose, sore throat, or cough). The status of allergies, including allergies to latex and tape, and medications routinely used in obstetrics, such as opioids (e.g., hydromorphone [Dilaudid], butorphanol [Stadol], fentanyl [Sublimaze], nalbuphine [Nubain]), anesthetic agents (e.g., bupivacaine, lidocaine, ropivacaine), and antiseptics (Betadine) is reviewed. Some allergic responses cause swelling of the mucous membranes of the respiratory tract, which could interfere with breathing and the administration of inhalation anesthesia. Because vomiting and subsequent aspiration into the respiratory tract can complicate an otherwise normal labor, the nurse records the time and type of the woman's most recent solid and liquid intake.

The nurse obtains any information not found in the prenatal record during the admission assessment. Pertinent data include the birth plan (Box 19-2), the choice of infant feeding method, the type of pain management (including nonpharmacologic comfort measures) preferred, and the name of the pediatric health care provider. She or he obtains a client profile that identifies the woman's preparation for childbirth, the support person or family members desired during childbirth and their availability, and ethnic or cultural expectations and needs. The nurse also determines the woman's use of alcohol, drugs, and tobacco during pregnancy.

The nurse reviews the birth plan. If no written plan has been prepared, the nurse helps the woman formulate a birth plan by describing options available and determining the woman's wishes and preferences. As caregiver and advocate, the nurse integrates the woman's desires into the nursing care plan while explaining what may or may not be possible given the hospital's

BOX 19-2 The Birth Plan

The birth plan should include the woman's or couple's preferences related to:

- Presence of birth companions such as the partner, older children, parents, friends, and doula, and the role each will play
- Presence of other persons such as students, male attendants, and interpreters
- Clothing to be worn
- Environmental modifications such as lighting, music, privacy, focal point, items from home such as pillows
- Labor activities such as preferred positions for labor and for birth, ambulation, birth balls, showers and whirlpool baths, oral food and fluid intake
- List of comfort and relaxation measures
- Labor and birth medical interventions such as pharmacologic pain relief measures, intravenous therapy, electronic monitoring, induction or augmentation measures, and episiotomy
- Care and handling of the newborn immediately after birth such as immediate skin-to-skin contact, cutting of the cord, eye care, breastfeeding
- Cultural and religious requirements related to the care of the mother, newborn, and placenta

The childbirth website—www.childbirth.org—provides couples with an interactive birth plan along with examples of birth plans and descriptions of the options that can be included.

policies. She or he also prepares the woman for the possibility that her plan may change as labor progresses and assures her that the staff will provide information so that she can make informed decisions. The woman must also understand that the longer her "wish list", the less is the likelihood that all of her expectations will be met.

The nurse should discuss with the woman and her partner their plans for preserving childbirth memories through the use of photography and videotaping. Information should be provided about the agency's policies regarding these practices and under what circumstances they are allowed. Protection of privacy and safety and infection control are major concerns for the expectant parents and the agency. To avoid future embarrassment and distress, the nurse should clarify with the woman exactly what parts of her childbirth she wishes to have photographed and the degree of detail. Remind women and their families that pictures should not be posted on social media sites without the knowledge and consent of every person who appears in the picture.

LEGAL TIP: Recording of Childbirth

The woman's record should reflect that the childbirth was recorded. Some hospitals and health care providers do not allow videotaping of the birth because of concerns related to legal liability.

Psychosocial Factors

The woman's general appearance and behavior (and that of her partner) provide valuable clues to the type of supportive care she will need. However, keep in mind that general appearance and behavior may vary, depending on the stage and phase of labor (Table 19-1 and Box 19-3).

Women with a History of Sexual Abuse. Labor can trigger memories of sexual abuse, especially during intrusive procedures such as vaginal examinations. Monitors, intravenous (IV) lines, and epidurals can make the woman feel a loss of control or feel as if she is being confined to bed and "restrained." Being observed by students and having intense sensations in the uterus and genital area, especially at the time when she must push the baby out, can also trigger negative memories.

The nurse can help the abuse survivor associate the sensations she is experiencing with the process of childbirth and not with her past abuse. Help maintain her sense of control by explaining all procedures and why they are needed, validating her needs, and paying close attention to her requests. Wait for the woman to give permission before touching her, and accept her often extreme reactions to labor (Simpson & O'Brien-Abel, 2014). Avoid words and phrases that can cause the woman to recall the words of her abuser (e.g., "open your legs," "relax and it won't hurt so much"). Limit the number of procedures that invade her body (e.g., vaginal examinations, urinary catheter, internal monitor, forceps or vacuum extractor) as much as possible. Encourage her to choose a person (e.g., doula, friend, family member) to be with her during labor to provide continuous support and comfort and to act as her advocate. Nurses are advised to care for all laboring women in this manner because it is not unusual for a woman to choose not to reveal a history of sexual abuse. Careful attention to these care measures can help a woman perceive her childbirth experience in positive terms.

Stress in Labor

The way in which women and their support persons or family members approach labor is related to how they have been socialized to the childbearing process as well as how they deal with other stressors in their lives. Their reactions reflect their life experiences regarding childbirth—physical, social, cultural, and religious. Society communicates its expectations regarding acceptable and unacceptable maternal behaviors during labor and birth. These expectations may be used by some women as the basis for evaluating their own actions during childbirth. An idealized perception of labor and birth may be a source of guilt and cause a sense of failure if the woman finds the process less than joyous, especially when the pregnancy is unplanned or is the product of a dysfunctional or terminated relationship. Often women have heard horror stories or have seen friends or relatives going through labors that appear anything but easy. Multiparous women often base their expectations of the present labor on their previous childbirth experiences.

Discuss the feelings a woman has about her pregnancy and fears regarding childbirth. This discussion is especially important if the woman is a primigravida who has not attended childbirth classes but has obtained information on childbirth from reality birth television shows or is a multiparous woman who has had a previous negative childbirth experience. Women in labor usually have a variety of concerns that they will voice if asked but may not volunteer. Major fears and concerns relate to the process and effects of childbirth, maternal and fetal well-being, and the attitude and actions of the health care staff. Every effort should be made to provide support and to encourage those with her to be supportive. Women who have continuous labor support are more likely to have a spontaneous vaginal birth and are less

TABLE 19-1 Expected Maternal Progress During First Stage of Labor

CRITERION	0-3 cm (LATENT)	4-7 cm (ACTIVE)	8-10 cm (TRANSITION)
	PHASES MARKED BY CERVICAL DILATION*		
Duration†	About 6-8 hours	About 3-6 hours	About 20-40 minutes
Contractions			
Strength	Mild to moderate	Moderate to strong	Strong to very strong
Rhythm	Irregular	More regular	Regular
Frequency	5-30 minutes apart	3-5 minutes apart	2-3 minutes apart
Duration	30-45 seconds	40-70 seconds	45-90 seconds
Descent			
Station of presenting part	Nulliparous: 0 Multiparous: −2 cm to 0	Varies: +1 to +2 cm Varies: +1 to +2 cm	Varies: +2 to +3 cm Varies: +2 to +3 cm
Show			
Color	Brownish discharge, mucus plug, or pale pink mucus	Pink to bloody mucus	Bloody mucus
Amount	Scant	Scant to moderate	Copious
Behavior and appearance‡	Excited; thoughts center on self, labor, and baby; may be talkative or silent, calm or tense; some apprehension; pain controlled fairly well; alert, follows directions readily; open to instructions	Becomes more serious, doubtful of pain control, more apprehensive; desires companionship and encouragement; attention more inwardly directed; fatigue evidenced; malar (cheeks) flush; has some difficulty following directions	Pain described as severe; backache common; frustration, fear of loss of control, and irritability may be voiced; expresses doubt about ability to continue; vague in communications; amnesia between contractions; writhing with contractions; nausea and vomiting, especially if hyperventilating; hyperesthesia; circumoral pallor, perspiration of forehead and upper lip; shaking tremor of thighs; feeling of need to defecate, pressure on anus

*In the nullipara, effacement is often complete before dilation begins; in the multipara it occurs simultaneously with dilation.

†Duration of each phase is influenced by such factors as parity, maternal emotions, position, level of activity, and fetal size, presentation, and position. For example, the labor of a nullipara tends to last longer, on average, than the labor of a multipara. Women who ambulate and assume upright positions or change positions frequently during labor tend to experience a shorter first stage. Descent is often prolonged in breech presentations and occiput posterior positions.

‡Women who have epidural analgesia for pain relief may not demonstrate some of these behaviors.

BOX 19-3 Psychosocial Assessment of the Laboring Woman

Verbal Interactions
- Does the woman ask questions?
- Can she ask for what she needs?
- Does she talk to her support person(s)?
- Does she talk freely with the nurse or respond only to questions?

Body Language
- Does she change positions or lie rigidly still?
- What is her anxiety level?
- How does she react to being touched by the nurse or support person?
- Does she avoid eye contact?
- Does she look tired? If she appears tired, ask her how much rest she has had in the past 24 hours.

Perceptual Ability
- Is there a language barrier?
- Are repeated explanations necessary because her anxiety level interferes with her ability to comprehend?
- Can she repeat what she has been told or otherwise demonstrate her understanding?

Discomfort Level
- To what degree does the woman describe what she is experiencing including her pain experience?
- How does she react to a contraction?
- How does she react to assessment and care measures?
- Are any nonverbal pain messages noted?
- Can she ask for comfort measures?

likely to have intrapartum analgesia or anesthesia, a cesarean or an operative vaginal birth, and a baby with a low 5-minute Apgar score; or to report dissatisfaction with their childbirth experiences (Hodnett, Gates, Hofmeyr, & Sakala, 2013).

The father, coach, or significant other also experiences stress during labor. The nurse can assist and support these individuals by identifying their needs and expectations, helping to make sure these are met, and interpreting events that are occurring. The nurse can determine what role the support person intends to fulfill and whether he or she is prepared for that role by making observations and asking herself or himself such questions as, "Has the couple attended childbirth classes?" "What role does this person expect to play?" "Does he or she do all the talking?" "Is he or she nervous, anxious, aggressive, or hostile?" "Does he or she look hungry, tired, worried, or confused?" "Does he or she watch television, sleep, or stay out of the room instead of paying attention to the woman?" "Where does he or she sit?" "Does he or she touch the woman; what is the character of the touch?" Be sensitive to the needs of support persons and provide teaching and support as appropriate. In many instances the support these people provide to the laboring woman may be in direct proportion to the support they receive from the nurses and other health care providers.

Cultural Factors

Nearly 1 million immigrants come to the United States each year, half of whom are women of childbearing age. More than 30% of the U.S. population belongs to a cultural group other than non-Hispanic white. It is expected that by the year

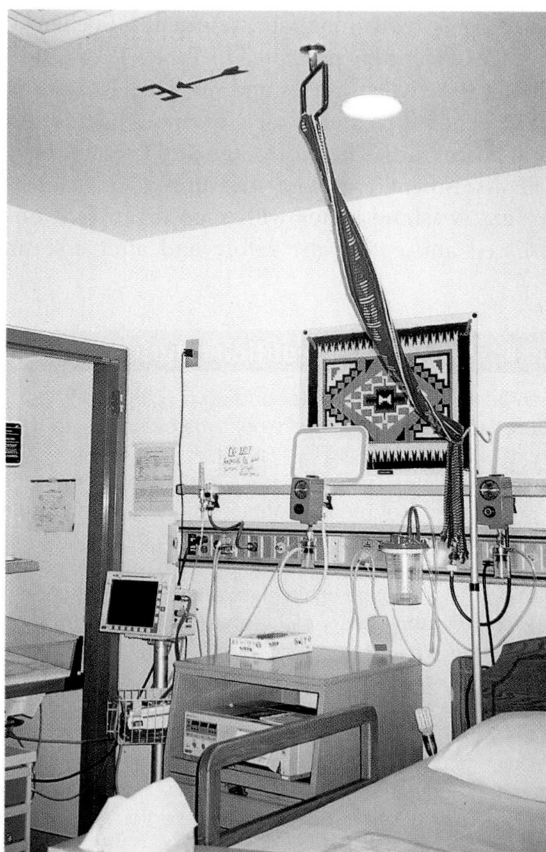

FIG 19-3 Birthing room specific to a Native-American population. Note the arrow pointing east, the rug on the wall, and the rope or sash belt hanging from the ceiling. (Courtesy Patricia Hess, San Francisco, CA; Chinle Comprehensive Health Care Center, Chinle, AZ.)

2050 members of cultural groups other than non-Hispanic white will make up more than half of the U.S. population (Callister, 2014). As the population becomes more diverse, it is increasingly important to note the woman's ethnic or cultural and religious values, beliefs, and practices in order to anticipate nursing interventions to add or eliminate from an individualized, mutually acceptable plan of care that provides a feeling of safety and control (Fig. 19-3). Nurses should be committed to providing culturally sensitive care and to developing an appreciation and respect for cultural diversity (Callister). Encourage the woman to request specific caregiving behaviors and practices that are important to her. In some cases if a special request contradicts usual practices in that setting, the woman or the nurse can ask the woman's nurse-midwife or physician to write an order to accommodate the special request. For example, in many cultures, it is unacceptable to have a male caregiver examine a pregnant woman. In some cultures it is traditional to take the placenta home; in others, the woman has only certain nourishments during labor. Some women believe that cutting the body, as with an episiotomy, allows her spirit to leave her body and that rupturing the membranes prolongs, not shortens, labor. It is always important to listen respectfully and carefully explain the rationale for recommended care measures (see the Cultural Considerations box).

CULTURAL CONSIDERATIONS BOX

Birth Practices in Different Cultures

Somalia: Because Somalis in general do not like to show any sign of weakness, women are extremely stoic during childbirth

Japan: Natural childbirth methods practiced; may labor silently; may eat during labor; father may be present

China: Stoic response to pain; father not usually present; side-lying position preferred for labor and birth because this position is thought to reduce infant trauma

India: Natural childbirth methods preferred; father not usually present; female relatives usually present

Iran: Father not present; female support and female caregivers preferred

Mexico: May be stoic about discomfort until second stage, and then may request pain relief; father and female relatives may be present

Laos: May use squatting position for birth; father may or may not be present; female attendants preferred

Data from D'Avanzo, C. (2008). *Mosby's pocket guide to cultural health assessment* (4th ed.). St. Louis: Mosby.

Within cultures, women may have an idea of the "right" way to behave in labor and may react to the pain experienced in that way. These behaviors can range from total silence to moaning or screaming, but they do not necessarily indicate the degree of pain being experienced. A woman who moans with contractions may not be in as much physical pain as a woman who is silent but winces during contractions. Some women believe that screaming or crying out in pain is shameful if a man is present. If the woman's support person is her mother, she may perceive the need to "behave" more strongly than if her support person is the father of the baby. She will perceive herself as failing or succeeding based on her ability to follow these "standards" of behavior. Conversely, a woman's behavior in response to pain may influence the support received from significant others. In some cultures, women who lose control and cry out in pain may be scolded, whereas in other cultures, support persons will become more helpful.

Culture and Father Participation. A companion is an important source of support, encouragement, and comfort for women during childbirth. The woman's cultural and religious background influences her choice of birth companion as do trends in the society in which she lives. For example, in Western societies the father is often viewed as the ideal birth companion. For many years European-American couples traditionally attended childbirth classes together as an expected activity, although this is not as common today. Laotian (Hmong) husbands also traditionally participate actively in the labor process. In some other cultures the father may be available, but his presence in the labor room with the mother may not be considered appropriate, or he may be present but resist active involvement in her care. Such behavior could be perceived by the nursing staff to indicate a lack of concern, caring, or interest. Women from many cultures prefer female caregivers and want to have at least one female companion present during labor and birth. They are also usually very concerned about modesty. If couples from these cultures immigrate to the United States or Canada, their roles may change. The nurse needs to talk to the woman and her support persons to determine the roles they will assume.

The Non–English-Speaking Woman in Labor. A woman's level of anxiety in labor increases when she does not understand what is happening to her or what is being said. Non–English-speaking women often feel a complete loss of control over their situation if no health care provider is present who speaks their language. They can panic and withdraw or become physically abusive when someone tries to do something they perceive might harm them or their babies. A support person is sometimes able to serve as an interpreter. However, caution is warranted because the interpreter may not be able to convey exactly what the nurse or others are saying or what the woman is saying, which can increase the woman's stress level even more.

Ideally, a bilingual or bicultural nurse will care for the woman. Alternatively a hospital employee or volunteer interpreter may be contacted for assistance (see Box 2-2). Ideally, the interpreter is from the woman's culture. For some women, a female is more acceptable than a male interpreter. If no one in the hospital is able to interpret, call a service so that interpretation can take place over the telephone. Even when the nurse has limited ability to communicate verbally with the woman, in most instances the woman appreciates his or her efforts to do so. Speaking slowly, avoiding complex words and medical terms, and using gestures can help a woman and her partner understand. Often the woman understands English much better than she speaks it.

Physical Examination

The initial physical examination includes a general systems assessment and an assessment of fetal status. During the examination uterine contractions are assessed and a vaginal examination is performed. The findings of the admission physical examination serve as a baseline for assessing the woman's progress from that point. The information obtained from a complete and accurate assessment during the initial examination serves as the basis for determining whether the woman should be admitted and what her ongoing care should be. Expected maternal progress and minimal assessment guidelines during the first stage of labor are presented in Tables 19-1 and 19-2.

Birth is a time when nurses and other health care providers may be exposed to a great deal of maternal and newborn blood and body fluids. Therefore, Standard Precautions should guide all assessment and care measures (Box 19-4). Hand hygiene (e.g., washing hands with soap or application of an alcohol-based antiseptic rub) before and after assessing the

BOX 19-4 Standard Precautions During Childbirth

- Wash hands before and after putting on gloves and performing procedures; cleansing alcohol rubs can be used if hands are not visibly soiled.
- Wear gloves (clean or sterile, as appropriate) when performing procedures that require contact with the woman's genitalia and body fluids, including bloody show (e.g., during vaginal examination, amniotomy, hygienic care of the perineum, insertion of an internal scalp electrode and intrauterine pressure monitor, and urinary catheterization).
- Wear a mask that has a shield or protective eyewear, and cover gown when assisting with the birth. Cap and shoe covers are worn for cesarean birth but are optional for vaginal birth in a birthing room. Gowns worn by the nurse-midwife or physician who is attending the birth should have a waterproof front and sleeves and should be sterile. Mask also should be worn during spinal puncture or insertion of an epidural catheter.
- Drape the woman with sterile towels and sheets as appropriate. Explain to the woman what can and cannot be touched.
- Help the woman's partner put on appropriate coverings for the type of birth, such as cap, mask, gown, and shoe covers. Show the partner where to stand and what can and cannot be touched.
- Wear gloves and gown when handling the newborn immediately after birth.
- Use an appropriate method to suction the newborn's airway, such as a bulb syringe or mechanical wall suction.

TABLE 19-2 Nursing Assessments in First-Stage Labor

LABOR PHASE	TIME FRAME	SPECIFIC ASSESSMENTS
Latent	Every 30-60 minutes	Maternal blood pressure, pulse, and respirations Fetal heart rate (FHR) and pattern Uterine activity Presence of vaginal show
	Every 30 minutes	Changes in maternal appearance, mood, affect, energy level, and condition of partner or coach
	Every 2-4 hours	Temperature (every 4 hours until membranes rupture, then every 2 hours)
	As needed	Vaginal examination to identify progress in labor
Active	Every 30 minutes	Maternal blood pressure, pulse, and respirations
	Every 15-30 minutes	FHR and pattern Uterine activity Presence of vaginal show
	Every 15 minutes	Changes in maternal appearance, mood, affect, energy level, and condition of partner or coach
	Every 2-4 hours	Temperature (every 4 hours until membranes rupture, then every 2 hours)
	As needed	Vaginal examination to identify progress in labor
Transition	Every 15-30 minutes	Maternal blood pressure, pulse, and respirations
	Every 15-30 minutes	FHR and pattern
	Every 10-15 minutes	Uterine activity Presence of vaginal show
	Every 5 minutes	Changes in maternal appearance, mood, affect, energy level, and condition of partner or coach
	Every 2-4 hours	Temperature (every 4 hours until membranes rupture, then every 2 hours)
	As needed	Vaginal examination to identify progress in labor

woman and providing care is critical in preventing infection transmission. The nurse should explain assessment findings to the woman and her partner whenever possible. Throughout labor, accurate documentation, following agency policy, is done as soon as possible after a procedure has been performed (Fig. 19-4). If in-room computer stations are used, make sure to turn the computer so that your back is not to the woman while you are documenting.

General Systems Assessment. On admission, the nurse should perform a brief systems assessment. This includes an assessment of the heart, lungs, and skin and an examination to determine the presence and extent of edema of the face, hands, sacrum, and legs. It also includes testing of deep tendon reflexes and for clonus, if indicated. Also note the woman's weight. Increasing numbers of women are overweight or obese. Excessive size can make nursing care during labor and birth more difficult and places the woman at risk for complications such as operative birth, infection, and blood clots. See Chapter 32 for further information.

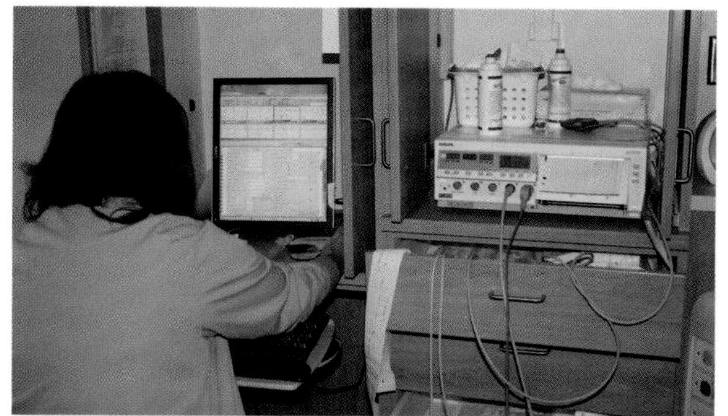

FIG 19-4 Nurse documenting assessment findings on computer in a labor, delivery, recovery, postpartum room. (Courtesy Shannon Perry, Phoenix, AZ.)

Vital Signs. Assess vital signs (temperature, pulse, respirations, and blood pressure using a correct size cuff) on admission. The initial values are used as the baseline for comparison for all future measurements. If the blood pressure is elevated, reassess it 30 minutes later, between contractions, to obtain a reading after the woman has relaxed. Encourage the woman to lie on her side to prevent supine hypotension and the resulting fetal hypoxemia (Fig. 19-5). Monitor her temperature so you can identify signs of infection or a fluid deficit (e.g., dehydration associated with inadequate intake of fluids).

Leopold Maneuvers (Abdominal Palpation). Leopold maneuvers are performed with the woman briefly lying on her back (Box 19-5). These maneuvers help to answer three important questions: (1) What fetal part is in the uterine fundus? (2) Where is the fetal back located? (3) What is the presenting fetal part?

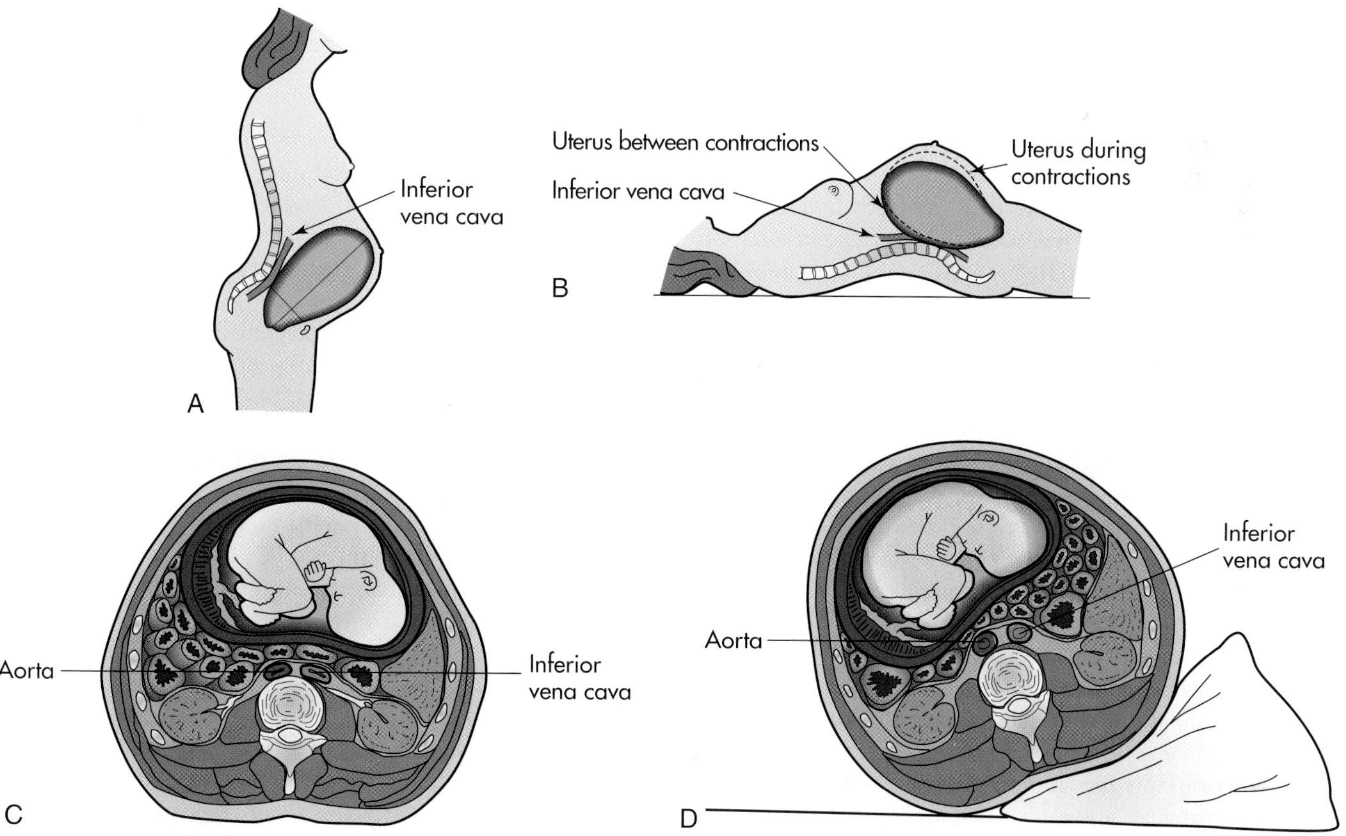

FIG 19-5 Supine hypotension. Note relation of pregnant uterus to ascending vena cava in standing position (**A**), and in the supine position (**B**). **C**, Compression of aorta and inferior vena cava with woman in supine position. **D**, Compression of these vessels is relieved by placement of a wedge pillow under the woman's right side.

BOX 19-5 Procedure: Leopold Maneuvers

- Wash hands.
- Ask woman to empty bladder.
- Position woman supine with one pillow under her head and with her knees slightly flexed.
- Place small rolled towel under woman's right or left hip to displace uterus off major blood vessels (prevents supine hypotensive syndrome; see Fig. 19-5, *D*).
- If right-handed, stand on woman's right, facing her (if left-handed, stand on woman's left):
  - Identify fetal part that occupies the fundus. The head feels round, firm, freely movable, and palpable by ballottement; the breech feels less regular and softer. This maneuver identifies fetal lie (longitudinal or transverse) and presentation (cephalic or breech) (Fig. A).
  - Using palmar surface of one hand, locate and palpate the smooth convex contour of the fetal back and the irregularities that identify the small parts (feet, hands, elbows). This maneuver helps identify fetal presentation (Fig. B).
  - With right hand, determine which fetal part is presenting over the inlet to the true pelvis. Gently grasp the lower pole of the uterus between the thumb and fingers, pressing in slightly (Fig. C). If the head is presenting and not engaged, determine the attitude of the head (flexed or extended).
  - Turn to face the woman's feet. Using both hands, outline the fetal head (Fig. D) with the palmar surface of the fingertips. When the presenting part has descended deeply, only a small portion of it may be outlined. Palpation of the cephalic prominence helps identify the attitude of the head. If the cephalic prominence is found on the same side as the small parts, this means that the head must be flexed and the vertex is presenting (see Fig. D). If the cephalic prominence is on the same side as the back, this indicates that the presenting head is extended and the face is presenting.
- Document fetal presentation, position, and lie and whether presenting part is flexed or extended, engaged, or free floating. Use agency's protocol for documentation (e.g., "Vtx, LOA, floating").

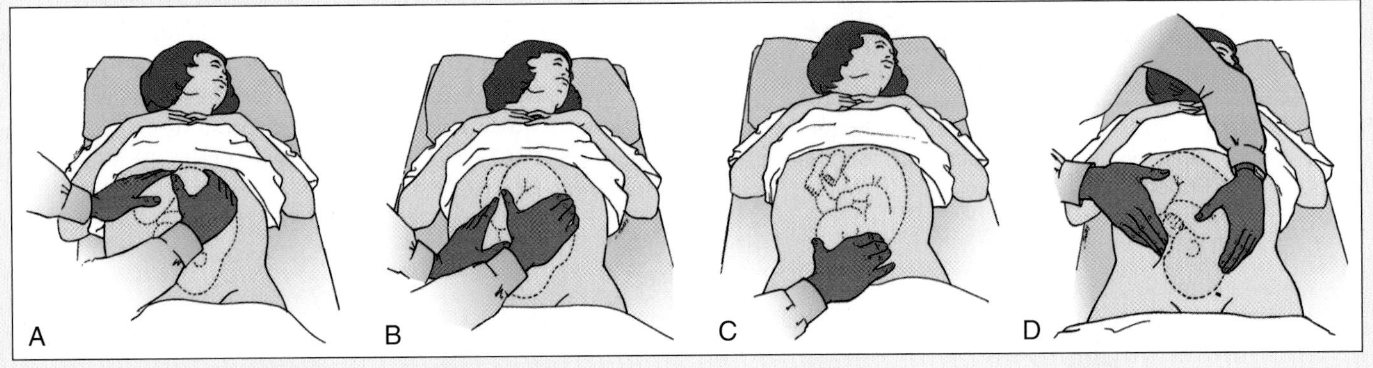

Assessment of Fetal Heart Rate and Pattern. The point of maximal intensity (PMI) of the FHR is the location on the maternal abdomen at which the FHR is heard the loudest. It is usually directly over the fetal back. In a vertex presentation you can usually hear the FHR below the mother's umbilicus in either the right or the left lower quadrant of the abdomen. In a breech presentation you usually hear the FHR above the mother's umbilicus. Table 19-2 summarizes the assessments recommended for determining fetal status. In addition, you must assess the FHR after ROM because this is the most common time for the umbilical cord to prolapse, after any change in the contraction pattern or maternal status, and before and after the woman receives medication or a procedure is performed.

Assessment of Uterine Contractions. A general characteristic of effective labor is regular uterine activity (i.e., contractions becoming more frequent with increased duration), but uterine activity is not directly related to labor progress. Uterine contractions are the primary powers that act involuntarily to expel the fetus and the placenta from the uterus. Several methods are used to evaluate uterine contractions, including the woman's subjective description, palpation and timing of contractions by a health care provider, and electronic monitoring.

Each contraction exhibits a wavelike pattern. It begins with a slow increment (the "building up" of a contraction from its onset), gradually reaches a peak, and then diminishes rapidly (decrement, the "letting down" of the contraction). An interval of rest ends when the next contraction begins. The outward appearance of the woman's abdomen during and between contractions and the pattern of a typical uterine contraction are shown in Figure 19-6.

A uterine contraction is described in terms of the following characteristics:

- *Frequency:* How often uterine contractions occur; the time that passes from the beginning of one contraction to the beginning of the next contraction
- *Intensity:* The strength of a contraction at its peak
- *Duration:* The time that passes between the onset and the end of a contraction
- *Resting tone:* The tension in the uterine muscle between contractions; relaxation of the uterus

Uterine contractions are assessed by palpation or by using external or internal electronic monitors (see Chapter 18 for further discussion). Frequency and duration can be measured by all three methods of uterine activity monitoring. The accuracy of determining intensity and resting tone varies by the method used. The woman's description and examiner's palpation are more subjective and less precise ways of determining the intensity of uterine contractions and resting tone than are the external or internal electronic monitors. The following terms describe what is felt on palpation:

- *Mild:* Slightly tense fundus that is easy to indent with fingertips (feels like pressing finger to tip of nose)

EVIDENCE-BASED PRACTICE

Correcting Fetal Malpresentations: Version and Moxibustion

Ask the Question

For women near term with noncephalic fetal presentation, what are the options to maximize the chance of a vaginal birth?

Search for the Evidence

Search Strategies English language research-based publications since 2011 on external cephalic version, moxibustion, postural, obesity, and tocolytics were included.

Databases Used Cochrane Collaborative Database, National Guideline Clearinghouse (AHRQ), CINAHL, PubMed, UpToDate, and the professional websites for ACOG and AWHONN

Critical Appraisal of the Evidence

Noncephalic presentation (breech or transverse) makes vaginal birth risky or impossible and is a common reason for scheduled cesarean birth. Malpresentations can sometimes be corrected. Ideally correction occurs before engagement of the presenting part in the pelvis ("dropping"), yet close enough to term to maintain the position until birth and minimize the risk of preterm birth.

External cephalic version (ECV) is an ultrasound-guided, hands-on procedure to externally manipulate the fetus into a cephalic lie. It is done at 36 to 37 weeks, in the hospital setting.

- Beta stimulants to relax the uterus, such as terbutaline, have the best evidence for premedication (Cluver, Hofmeyr, Gyte, & Sinclair, 2012).
- Successful outcome of a vaginal birth is most likely for multiparous women with adequate amniotic fluid (Mowat & Gardener, 2013).
- Even with successful ECV, women are still at a greater risk for cesarean birth, especially if they are nulliparous and labor is induced (Kuppens, Hutton, Hasaart, et al., 2013).

Postural management, the practice of positioning women with their pelvis elevated, does not have sufficient evidence to support it as an effective corrective technique (Hofmeyr & Kulier, 2012).

Moxibustion, the Chinese practice of burning lungwort close to acupuncture point 67, the tip of the fifth toe, has promising evidence. Meta-analysis of eight trials found that moxibustion was associated with less need for oxytocin. When combined with acupuncture or postural management, moxibustion may result in fewer cesarean births (Coyle, Smith, & Peat, 2012).

Apply the Evidence: Nursing Implications

Promoting cephalic vaginal birth is protective against the complications of cesarean birth, which includes a high risk for future cesarean births.

- Even with uterine relaxers, ECV is very uncomfortable or painful, and carries its own risks for placental abruption, cord accident, and emergent cesarean birth. Women benefit from having a support person present.
- Moxibustion is a welcome noninvasive technique that shows promise and does no harm. Proper training is required to avoid burns and respiratory reaction. Of practical concern to consider is the venting of smoke, to avoid triggering smoke alarms. Lack of familiarity probably impedes its uptake.

Women with malposition need to understand the mechanics of vaginal birth, and the risk factors for all options. Some women may prefer a cesarean birth, even with its increased risks.

Quality and Safety Competencies: Evidence-Based Practice*

Knowledge

Discriminate between valid and invalid reasons for modifying evidence-based clinical practice based on clinical expertise or patient or family preferences.

ECV is well accepted, but painful and risky. Postural management has insufficient evidence, but moxibustion may be a noninvasive and safe way to correct malposition.

Skills

Consult with clinical experts before deciding to deviate from evidence-based protocols.

The skill and preparation of the practitioner and team are paramount for client safety and efficacy.

Attitudes

Acknowledge your own limitations in knowledge and clinical expertise before determining when to deviate from evidence-based best practices.

Keeping knowledge and skills up-to-date is essential for all members of the health team.

References

Cluver, C., Hofmeyr, G. J., Gyte, G. M., & Sinclair, M. (2012). Interventions for helping to turn breech babies to head first presentation when using cephalic version. In *The Cochrane Database of Systematic Reviews 2012*, 1. Chichester, UK: John Wiley & Sons.

Coyle, M. E., Smith, C. A., & Peat, B. (2012). Cephalic version by moxibustion for breech presentation. In *The Cochrane Database of Systematic Reviews 2012*, 5. Chichester, UK: John Wiley & Sons.

Hofmeyr, G. J., & Kulier, R. (2012). Cephalic version by postural management for breech presentation. In *The Cochrane Database of Systematic Reviews 2012*, 10. Chichester, UK: John Wiley & Sons.

Kuppens, S. M., Hutton, E. K., Hasaart, T. H., et al. (2013). Mode of delivery following successful external cephalic version: Comparison with spontaneous cephalic presentations at birth. *Journal of Obstetrics and Gynaecology of Canada, 35*(10), 883–888.

Mowat, A., & Gardener, G. (2013). Predictors of successful external cephalic version in an Australian maternity hospital. *The Australian & New Zealand Journal of Obstetrics & Gynaecology* (Epub ahead of print, Dec 23, 2013).

Pat Mahaffee Gingrich

*Adapted from QSEN at www.qsen.org.

- *Moderate:* Firm fundus that is difficult to indent with fingertips (feels like pressing finger to chin)
- *Strong:* Rigid boardlike fundus that is almost impossible to indent with fingertips (feels like pressing finger to forehead)

Women in labor tend to describe the pain of contractions in terms of the sensations they are experiencing in the lower abdomen or back, which are sometimes unrelated to the firmness of the uterine fundus. Therefore, their assessment of the strength of their contractions can be less accurate than that of the health care provider, although the amount of discomfort reported is valid.

External electronic monitoring provides some information about the strength of uterine contractions when the appearance

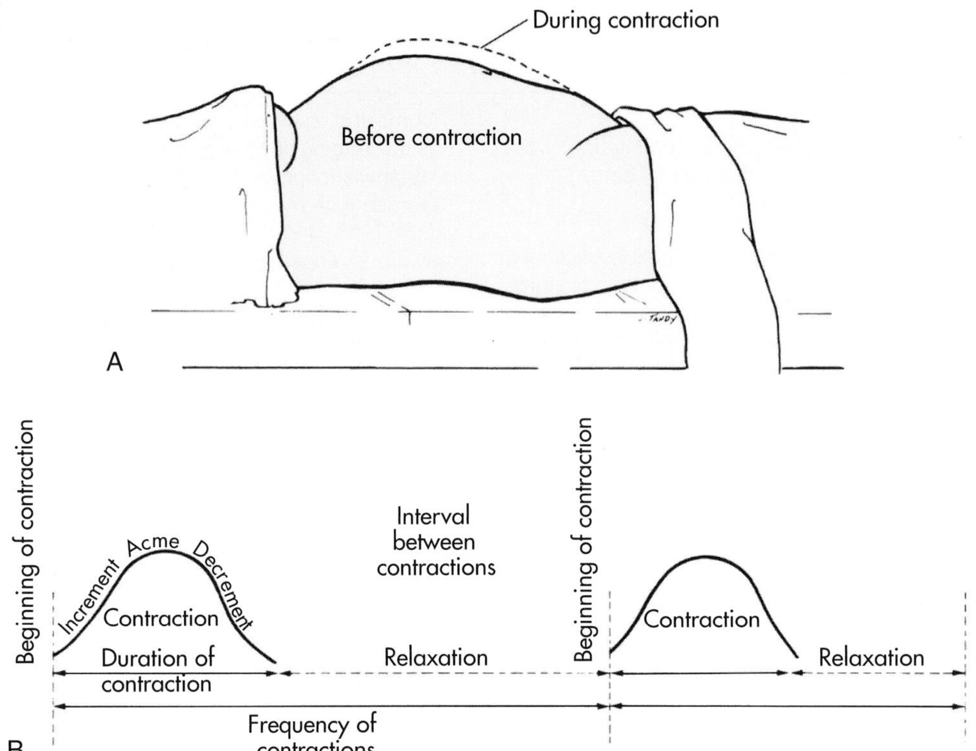

FIG 19-6 Assessment of uterine contractions. **A,** Abdominal contour before and during uterine contraction. **B,** Wavelike pattern of contractile activity.

of contractions on admission is compared with those that occur later in labor. Internal electronic monitoring with an intrauterine pressure catheter, however, is the most accurate way of assessing the intensity of uterine contractions and uterine resting tone.

On admission to a hospital, uterine contractions and FHR and pattern are usually monitored electronically for at least a 20- to 30-minute period as a baseline. The minimal times for assessing uterine activity during the various phases of stage one labor are listed in Table 19-2. The findings expected as the first stage of labor progresses are summarized in Table 19-1.

SAFETY ALERT

If you find the characteristics of contractions to be abnormal, either exceeding or falling below what is considered acceptable in terms of the standard characteristics, report this finding to the nurse-midwife or physician.

You must consider uterine activity in the context of its effect on cervical effacement and dilation and on the degree of descent of the presenting part (see Chapter 16). You must also consider the effect on the fetus. You can verify the progress of labor effectively through the use of graphic charts (partograms) on which you plot cervical dilation and station (descent). This type of graphic charting assists in early identification of deviations from expected labor patterns. Figure 19-7 provides examples of partograms. Hospitals and birthing centers may develop their own assessment graphs that may include data not only on dilation and descent but also maternal vital signs, FHR, and uterine activity.

SAFETY ALERT

The nurse should recognize that active labor can actually last longer than the expected labor patterns because all women are different. This finding is not a cause for concern unless the maternal-fetal unit exhibits signs of stress (e.g., abnormal FHR patterns, maternal fever).

Vaginal Examination. The vaginal examination reveals whether the woman is in true labor and enables the examiner to determine whether the membranes have ruptured (Fig. 19-8). Because this examination is often stressful and uncomfortable for the woman and may introduce microorganisms into the vagina if the membranes are ruptured, perform it only when indicated by the status of the woman and her fetus. For example, perform a vaginal examination on admission, prior to administering medications (e.g., analgesics, increasing oxytocin infusion), when significant change has occurred in uterine activity, on maternal request or perception of perineal pressure or the urge to bear down, when membranes rupture, or when you note variable decelerations of the FHR. A full explanation of the examination and support of the woman are important in reducing the stress and discomfort associated with the examination (Simpson & O'Brien-Abel, 2014) (Box 19-6).

Laboratory and Diagnostic Tests

Analysis of Urine Specimen. A clean-catch urine specimen may be obtained to gather further data about the pregnant woman's health. Analysis of the specimen is a convenient and simple procedure that can provide information about her hydration status (e.g., specific gravity, color, amount), nutritional status (e.g.,

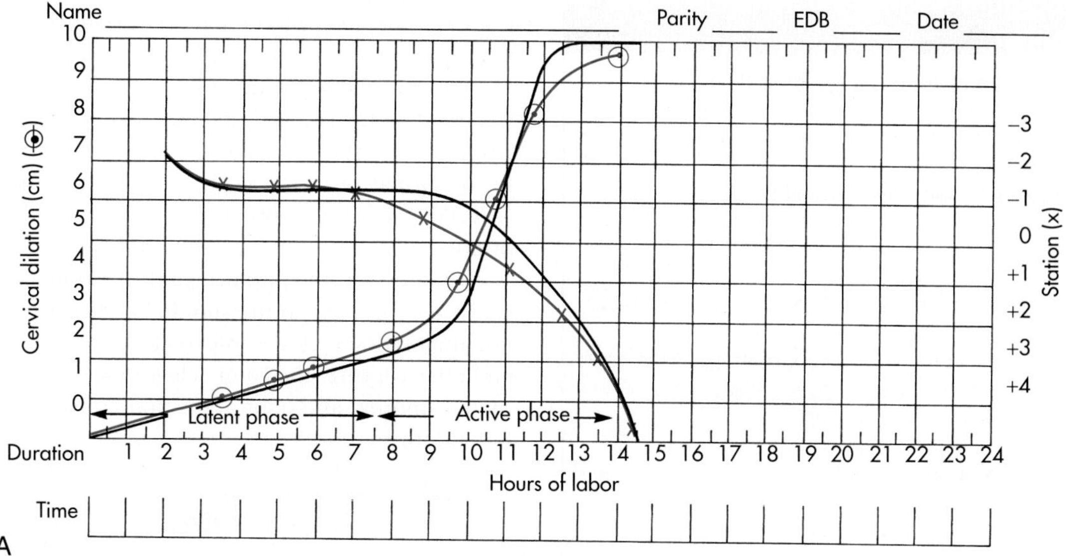

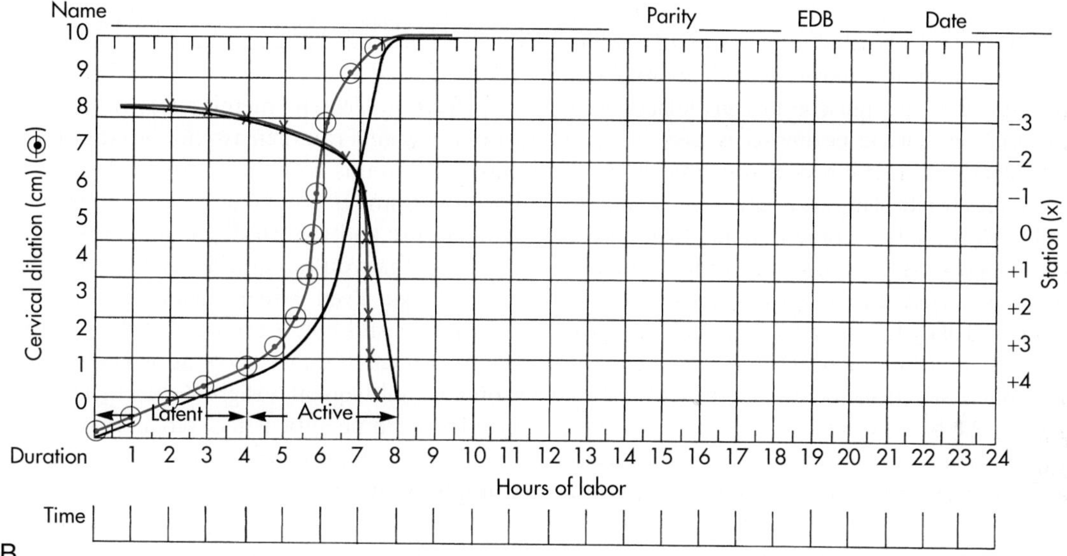

FIG 19-7 Partograms for assessment of patterns of cervical dilation and descent. Individual woman's labor patterns *(colored)* are superimposed on prepared labor graph *(black)* for comparison. **A,** Labor of a nulliparous woman. **B,** Labor of a multiparous woman. The rate of cervical dilation is plotted with the circled plot points. A line drawn through these symbols depicts the slope of the curve. Station is plotted with X's. A line drawn through the X's reveals the pattern of descent.

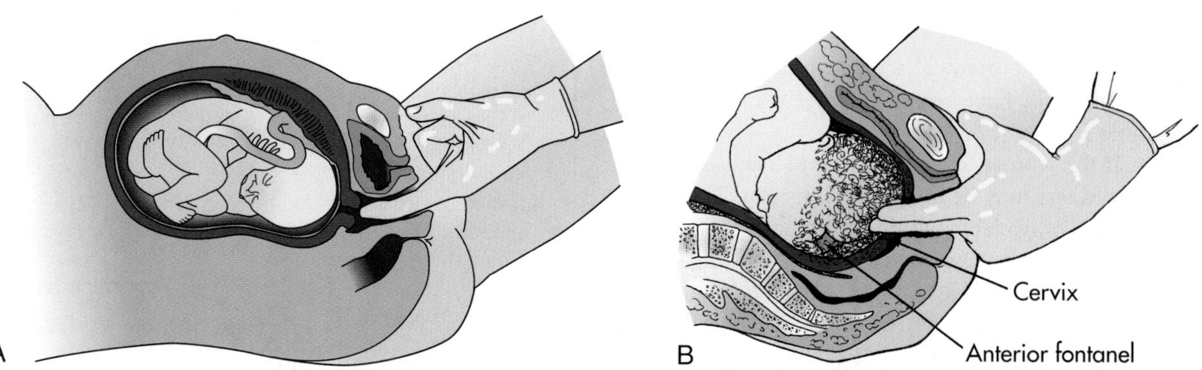

FIG 19-8 Vaginal examination. **A,** Undilated, uneffaced cervix; membranes intact. **B,** Palpation of sagittal suture line. Cervix effaced and partially dilated.

BOX 19-6 Procedure: Vaginal Examination of the Laboring Woman

- Use a sterile glove and antiseptic solution or soluble gel for lubrication.
- Position the woman to prevent supine hypotension. Drape to ensure privacy.
- Cleanse the perineum and vulva, if needed.
- After obtaining the woman's permission to touch her, gently insert the index and middle fingers into the woman's vagina.
- Determine:
  - Cervical dilation, effacement, and position (e.g., posterior, mid, anterior)
  - Presenting part, position, and station; molding of the head with development of caput succedaneum (may affect accuracy of determination of station)
  - Status of membranes (intact, bulging, or ruptured)
  - Characteristics of amniotic fluid (e.g., color, clarity, and odor), if membranes are ruptured
- Explain the findings of the examination to the woman.
- Document your findings and report them to the nurse-midwife or physician.

ketones), infection status (e.g., leukocytes), or the status of possible complications such as preeclampsia, shown by finding protein in the urine. In many hospitals this test must be done in the laboratory rather than at the bedside, even if a urine dipstick is used.

Blood Tests. The blood tests performed vary with the hospital protocol and the woman's health status. Currently, all blood tests must be performed in the hospital laboratory rather than on the perinatal unit. Often blood samples are obtained from the hub of the catheter when an IV is started or a heplock or saline lock is inserted. A hematocrit will likely be ordered. More comprehensive blood assessments such as white blood cell count, red blood cell count, hemoglobin level, hematocrit, and platelet values are included in a complete blood count (CBC). A CBC may be ordered for women with a history of infection, anemia, gestational hypertension, or other disorders. Many hospitals require that a CBC be done before epidural anesthesia is initiated. Any woman whose human immunodeficiency virus (HIV) status is undocumented at the time of labor should be screened with a rapid HIV test unless she declines (opts-out) testing (Centers for Disease Control and Prevention [CDC], Branson, Handsfield, et al., 2006).

Most hospitals require that a "type and screen," to determine the woman's blood type and Rh status, be performed on admission. Even if these tests have already been performed during pregnancy, the hospital's laboratory or blood bank must verify the results in-house. If the woman had no prenatal care or if her prenatal records are not available, a prenatal screen will likely be drawn on admission. The prenatal screen includes laboratory tests that would normally have been drawn at the initial prenatal visit (see Table 14-1).

Other Tests. If the woman's group B streptococcus status is not known, a rapid test may be done on admission. The rapid test results are usually available within an hour or so and will determine if the woman must be given antibiotics during labor.

Assessment of Amniotic Membranes and Fluid. Labor is initiated at term by SROM in approximately 25% of pregnant women. A lag period, rarely exceeding 24 hours, may precede the onset of labor. Membranes (the BOW) also can rupture spontaneously any time during labor, but most commonly in the transition phase of the first stage of labor. Box 19-1 explains how to determine if membranes are ruptured. If the membranes do not rupture spontaneously, the BOW may be ruptured artificially at some time during labor. However, this practice is discouraged if there is no medical reason because it can increase the laboring woman's sensation of pressure and pain and is not necessary for a normal birth to occur. Artificial rupture of membranes (AROM), called an amniotomy, is performed by the physician or nurse-midwife using a plastic AmniHook or a surgical clamp.

Whether the membranes rupture spontaneously or artificially, the time of rupture should be recorded. Other necessary documentation includes information regarding the FHR before and after rupture, the color (clear or meconium stained), estimated amount, and odor of the fluid. (See Chapter 32 for additional information.)

SAFETY ALERT

The umbilical cord may prolapse when the membranes rupture. The FHR and pattern should be monitored closely for several minutes immediately after ROM to determine fetal well-being, and the findings should be documented.

Infection. When membranes rupture, microorganisms from the vagina can then ascend into the amniotic sac, causing chorioamnionitis and placentitis to develop. For this reason, limit the number of vaginal examinations and assess maternal temperature and vaginal discharge frequently (at least every 2 hours) so that you can quickly identify an infection developing after ROM. Even when membranes are intact, however, microorganisms may ascend and cause infection.

Assessment findings serve as a baseline for evaluating the woman's subsequent progress during labor. Although some problems can be anticipated, others may appear unexpectedly during the clinical course of labor (see the Signs of Potential Complications box).

SIGNS OF POTENTIAL COMPLICATIONS

Labor

- Intrauterine pressure of ≥80 mm Hg or resting tone of ≥20 mm Hg (both determined by internal monitoring with intrauterine pressure catheter [IUPC])
- Contractions lasting ≥90 seconds
- More than five contractions in a 10-minute period (contractions occur more frequently than every 2 minutes)
- Relaxation between contractions lasting <30 seconds
- Fetal bradycardia or tachycardia; absent or minimal variability not associated with fetal sleep cycle or temporary effects of central nervous system (CNS) depressant drugs given to the woman; late, variable, or prolonged fetal heart rate (FHR) decelerations
- Irregular FHR; suspected fetal arrhythmias
- Appearance of meconium-stained or bloody fluid from the vagina
- Arrest in progress of cervical dilation or effacement, descent of the fetus, or both
- Maternal temperature of ≥38° C (100.4° F)
- Foul-smelling vaginal discharge
- Persistent bright or dark red vaginal bleeding

BOX 19-7 Evidence-Based Care Practices Designed to Promote, Protect, and Support Normal Labor and Birth

- Allow labor to begin on its own: encourage spontaneous labor rather than fostering elective labor inductions.
- Encourage freedom of movement throughout labor to facilitate the progress of labor and enhance maternal comfort and control of the labor process.
- Provide labor support beginning early in labor and continuing throughout the process of childbirth to relieve maternal anxiety and stress and decrease the risk for epidural anesthesia and cesarean birth; support should be provided by someone not employed by the hospital (e.g., doula).
- Avoid routine implementation of interventions (e.g., intravenous fluids, oral intake restrictions, continuous electronic fetal monitoring, labor augmentation measures [amniotomy, oxytocin administration], and epidural anesthesia).
- Support the practice of spontaneous, nondirected pushing in nonsupine positions (e.g., lateral, squatting, standing, kneeling, and semisitting) to facilitate the progress of fetal descent and shorten the second stage of labor.
- Avoid separation of the mother from her healthy baby after birth by encouraging skin-to-skin contact of mother and baby to keep newborn warm, prevent neonatal infection, enhance the newborn's physiologic adjustment to extrauterine life, and foster early breastfeeding.

Adapted from Romano, A.M. & Lothian, J.A. (2008). Promoting, protecting, and supporting normal birth: A look at the evidence. *Journal of Obstetric, Gynecologic, and Neonatal Nursing, 37*(1), 94-105.

Nursing Interventions

The nursing process provides the framework for the nursing care management of women in labor. The physical nursing care given to a woman in labor is an essential component of her care. The current emphasis on evidence-based practice supports the management of care by using this approach to enhance the safety, effectiveness, and acceptability of the physical care measures chosen to support the woman during labor and birth (Box 19-7). The various physical needs, the necessary nursing actions, and the rationale for care are presented in Table 19-3 and the Nursing Care Plan.

General Hygiene

Offer women in labor the use of showers or warm-water baths, if they are available, to enhance the feeling of well-being and to minimize the discomfort of contractions. Water immersion during active labor is associated with a decrease in the use of analgesia and reports of less maternal pain (Arendt & Tessmer-Tuck, 2013; Berghella, Baxter, & Chauhan, 2008). Also encourage women to wash their hands or use cleansing foam after voiding and performing self-hygiene measures. Change the linen if it becomes wet or stained with blood and use linen savers (Chux), changing them as needed.

Nutrient and Fluid Intake

Oral Intake. Before the 1940s women were allowed to eat and drink during labor to maintain the energy required to sustain labor and the stamina required to give birth. This practice changed, allowing the laboring woman only clear liquids or ice chips or nothing by mouth during the active phase of labor when concern arose regarding the risk of anesthesia complications and their secondary effects, if general anesthesia were required in an emergency. These secondary effects include the aspiration of gastric contents and resultant compromise in oxygen perfusion, which could endanger the lives of the mother and fetus (Sharts-Hopko, 2010; Simpson & O'Brien-Abel, 2014). There have been no randomized trials evaluating the ingestion of solid foods in labor, so current management is based mostly on expert opinion. The American College of Obstetricians and Gynecologists (ACOG), the American Society of Anesthesiologists, and the Canadian Anesthesiologists' Society recommend avoiding solid food during labor (Simpson & O'Brien-Abel). This practice is being challenged by many health care providers, however, because regional anesthesia is used more often than general anesthesia, even for emergency cesarean births. Women are awake during regional anesthesia and are able to participate in their own care and protect their airway.

An adequate intake of fluids and calories is required to meet the energy demands and fluid losses associated with childbirth. The progress of labor slows, with a more rapid development of hypoglycemia and ketosis if these demands are not met and fat is metabolized. Reduced energy for bearing-down efforts (pushing) increases the risk for a forceps- or vacuum-assisted birth. This is most likely to occur in women who begin to labor early in the morning after a night without caloric intake. When women are permitted to consume fluid and food freely, they typically regulate their own oral intake, eating light foods (e.g., eggs, yogurt, ice cream, dry toast and jelly, fruit) and drinking fluids during early labor and tapering off to the intake of clear fluids and sips of water or ice chips as labor intensifies and the second stage approaches (Sharts-Hopko, 2010).

Common hospital practice is to allow clear liquids (e.g., water, tea, fruit juices without pulp, clear sodas, coffee, sports drinks, fruit ice, Popsicles, gelatin, broth) during early labor, tapering off to ice chips and sips of water as labor progresses and becomes more active. Herbal teas can provide not only hydration but also other beneficial effects. Chamomile tea can enhance relaxation, lemon balm or peppermint tea can reduce nausea, and teas of ginger or ginseng root are energizing (Walls, 2009). A woman's culture may influence what she will eat and drink during labor. In addition, women who use nonpharmacologic pain relief measures and labor at home or in birthing centers are more likely to eat and drink during labor. The amount of solid and liquid carbohydrates to offer a woman in labor is still unclear. Although it is known that energy needs increase as labor becomes prolonged, there is limited evidence regarding the effect of oral carbohydrate intake in enhancing the progress of labor and reducing the risk for dystocia (Sharts-Hopko, 2010).

A Cochrane database review of this topic concluded that there is no justification for restricting food or fluid intake during labor in women at low risk for complications (Singata, Tranmer, & Gyte, 2013). Nurses should follow the orders of the woman's primary health care provider when offering the woman food or fluid during labor. However, as advocates, nurses can facilitate change by informing others of the current research findings that support the safety and effectiveness of the oral intake of food and fluid during labor and initiating such research themselves.

NURSING CARE PLAN

Care of the Woman in Labor

NURSING DIAGNOSIS	EXPECTED OUTCOME	INTERVENTIONS	RATIONALES
Anxiety related to labor and the birthing process	Woman reports decreased anxiety level using an anxiety scale (from 0 [no anxiety] to 10 [anxiety as bad as it could possibly be]).	Orient woman and significant others to labor and birth unit and explain admission protocol.	To allay initial feelings of anxiety
		Assess woman's knowledge, experience, and expectations of labor; note any signs or expressions of anxiety, nervousness, or fear.	To establish baseline for intervention
		Discuss expected progression of labor and describe what to expect during process.	To decrease anxiety associated with the unknown
		Identify specific source(s) of anxiety.	To better target interventions
		Actively involve woman in care decisions during labor, interpret sights and sounds of environment (monitor sights and sounds, unit activities), and share information on progression of labor (vital signs, fetal heart rate [FHR], dilation, effacement).	To increase her sense of control and lessen fears
Acute Pain related to increasing frequency and intensity of contractions	Woman reports decreased pain level using a pain scale (from 0 [no pain] to 10 [pain as bad as it could possibly be]).	Assess woman's level of pain and strategies that she has used to cope with it.	To establish baseline for intervention
		Encourage significant other to remain as support person during labor process.	To assist with support and comfort measures because measures are often more effective when delivered by a familiar person
		Assist the woman and support person(s) in use of specific nonpharmacologic pain methods such as conscious relaxation, breathing techniques, hypnosis, music, distraction, imagery, massage, and touch.	To increase relaxation, help woman cope with the intensity of contractions, and promote use of controlled thought and direction of energy
		Provide comfort measures such as frequent mouth care to prevent dry mouth, application of damp cloth to forehead, and changing of damp gown or bed covers.	To relieve discomfort associated with diaphoresis
		Help the woman to move around and change position such as squatting or using a birthing ball or birthing stool.	To reduce stiffness, promote comfort, and facilitate progress of birth
		Explain which analgesics and anesthesia are available for use during labor and birth.	To provide knowledge to help woman make decisions about pain control
		Administer analgesics or assist with regional anesthesia (e.g., epidural) as ordered or desired.	To provide effective pain relief during labor and birth
Impaired Urinary Elimination related to sensory impairment secondary to labor	Woman's bladder is emptied at least every 2 hours, either by spontaneous voiding or urinary catheter.	Palpate bladder superior to symphysis frequently (at least every 2 hours).	To detect full bladder that occurs from increased fluid intake and inability to feel urge to void
		Encourage frequent voiding (at least every 2 hours) and catheterize if necessary.	To avoid bladder distention because it impedes progress of fetus down birth canal and may result in trauma to bladder
		Help woman to bathroom or commode to void, if appropriate; provide privacy, and use techniques to stimulate voiding such as running water.	To facilitate bladder emptying with an upright position (natural) and relaxation

NURSING CARE PLAN—cont'd

Care of the Woman in Labor

NURSING DIAGNOSIS	EXPECTED OUTCOME	INTERVENTIONS	RATIONALES
Ineffective Coping related to the birthing process	Woman actively participates in birth process with no evidence of injury to her or her fetus.	Constantly monitor events of labor and birth, including physiologic responses of woman and fetus and emotional responses of woman and partner.	To ensure maternal, partner, and fetal well-being
		Provide ongoing feedback to woman and partner.	To decrease anxiety and enhance participation
		Continue to provide comfort measures and minimize distractions (e.g., dim the room lights and speak quietly).	To decrease discomfort and aid in focus on birth process
		Encourage woman to experiment with various positions.	To assist downward movement of fetus
		Ensure that woman takes deep cleansing breaths before and after each contraction.	To enhance gas exchange and oxygen transport to fetus
		Encourage woman to push spontaneously when urge to bear down is perceived during contraction.	To aid descent and rotation of fetus
		Encourage woman to exhale, holding breath for short periods while bearing down.	To avoid holding breath and triggering Valsalva maneuver, thereby increasing intrathoracic and cardiovascular pressure and decreasing the amount of oxygen that reaches uterus and placenta, placing fetus at risk
		Have woman take deep breaths and relax between contractions.	To reduce fatigue and increase effectiveness of pushing efforts
		Have mother pant as fetal head crowns.	To control birth of head and reduce risk for perineal trauma or fetal head injury
		Explain to woman and labor partner what is expected in the third stage of labor.	To enlist cooperation
		Have woman maintain her position.	To facilitate delivery of placenta
Fatigue related to energy expenditure required during labor and birth	Woman's energy levels are restored.	Educate woman and partner about need for rest and help them plan strategies (e.g., restricting visitors, increasing role of support systems performing functions associated with daily routines) that allow specific times for rest and sleep.	To ensure that woman can restore depleted energy levels in preparation for caring for new infant
		Monitor woman's fatigue level and amount of rest received.	To ensure restoration of energy
		Group care activities as much as possible.	To allow for periods of uninterrupted rest

Intravenous Intake. Fluids commonly are administered intravenously to the laboring woman to maintain hydration, especially if labor is long and the woman is unable to ingest a sufficient amount of fluid orally or if she is receiving epidural or intrathecal anesthesia. In most cases an electrolyte solution without glucose (e.g., Ringer's lactate or normal saline) is adequate and does not introduce excess glucose into the bloodstream. The latter is important because an excessive maternal glucose level results in fetal hyperglycemia and fetal hyperinsulinism. After birth the neonate's high level of insulin reduces his or her glucose stores, and hypoglycemia results. Infusions containing glucose can also reduce sodium levels in the woman and the fetus, leading to transient neonatal tachypnea. If maternal ketosis occurs, the nurse-midwife or physician can order an IV solution containing a small amount of dextrose to provide the glucose needed to assist in fatty acid metabolism.

SAFETY ALERT

Nurses should carefully monitor the intake and output of laboring women receiving IV fluids because they face an increased danger of hypervolemia as a result of the fluid retention that occurs during pregnancy.

TABLE 19-3 Physical Nursing Care During Labor

NEED	NURSING ACTIONS	RATIONALE
General Hygiene		
Showers or bed baths, Jacuzzi bath	Assess for progress in labor	Determines appropriateness of the activity
	Supervise showers closely if woman is in true labor	Prevents injury from fall; labor may be accelerated
	Suggest allowing warm water to flow over back	Aids relaxation; increases comfort
Perineum	Cleanse frequently, especially after rupture of membranes and when show increases	Enhances comfort and reduces risk of infection
Oral hygiene	Offer toothbrush or mouthwash, or wash the teeth with an ice-cold wet washcloth as needed	Refreshes mouth; helps counteract dry, thirsty feeling
Hair	Brush, braid per woman's wishes	Improves morale; increases comfort
Handwashing	Offer washcloths or cleansing foam before and after voiding and as needed	Maintains cleanliness; prevents infection
Face	Offer cool washcloth	Provides relief from diaphoresis; cools and refreshes
Gowns and linens	Change as needed	Improves comfort; enhances relaxation
Nutrient and Fluid Intake		
Oral	Offer fluids and solid foods as ordered by nurse-midwife or physician and desired by laboring woman	Provides hydration and calories; enhances positive emotional experience and maternal control
Intravenous (IV)	Establish and maintain IV line as ordered	Maintains hydration; provides venous access for medications
Elimination		
Voiding	Encourage voiding at least every 2 hours	A full bladder may impede descent of presenting part; overdistention may cause bladder atony and injury, as well as postpartum voiding difficulty
Ambulatory woman	Allow ambulation to bathroom according to orders of nurse-midwife or physician, if:	
	The presenting part is engaged	Reinforces normal process of urination
	The membranes are not ruptured	Precautionary measure to protect against prolapse of umbilical cord
	The woman is not medicated	Precautionary measure to protect against injury
Woman on bed rest	Offer bedpan	Prevents complications of bladder distention and ambulation
	Encourage upright position on bedpan, allow tap water to run; place woman's hands in warm water; pour warm water over the vulva; give positive suggestion	Encourages voiding
	Provide privacy	Shows respect for woman
	Put up side rails on bed	Prevents injury from fall
	Place call bell and telephone within reach	Reinforces safe care
	Offer washcloth or cleansing foam for hands	Maintains cleanliness; prevents infection
	Wash vulvar area	Maintains cleanliness; enhances comfort; prevents infection
Catheterization	Catheterize according to orders of nurse-midwife or physician or hospital protocol if measures to facilitate voiding are ineffective	Prevents complications of bladder distention
	Insert catheter between contractions	Minimizes discomfort
	Avoid force if obstacle to insertion is noted	"Obstacle" may be caused by compression of urethra by presenting part
Bowel elimination—sensation of rectal pressure	Perform vaginal examination	Prevents misinterpretation of rectal pressure from the presenting part as the need to defecate
		Determines degree of descent of presenting part
	Help the woman ambulate to bathroom, or offer bedpan if rectal pressure is not from presenting part	Reinforces normal process of bowel elimination and safe care
	Cleanse perineum immediately after passage of stool	Reduces risk of infection and sense of embarrassment

Elimination

Voiding. Encourage voiding every 2 hours. A distended bladder may impede descent of the presenting part, slow or stop uterine contractions, and lead to decreased bladder tone or uterine atony after birth. Women who receive epidural analgesia or anesthesia are especially at risk for the retention of urine. Therefore, the need to void should be assessed more frequently with them.

Assist the woman to the bathroom to void or use a bedside commode, unless any of the following apply: the nurse-midwife or physician has ordered bed rest; the woman is receiving epidural analgesia or anesthesia; internal monitoring is being used; or ambulation will compromise the status of the laboring woman or her fetus. External monitoring can usually be interrupted long enough for the woman to go to the bathroom.

If using a bedpan is necessary, encourage spontaneous voiding by providing privacy and having the woman sit upright (as she would on a toilet). Other interventions to encourage urination, either in the bathroom or on the bedpan, are having the woman listen to the sound of water slowly running from a faucet, placing her hands in warm water, having her blow bubbles into a glass of water using a straw, or pouring warm water over the vulva and perineum using a peri bottle.

Catheterization. If the woman is unable to void and her bladder is distended, she may need to be catheterized. Many hospitals have protocols or standing orders that rely on the nurse's judgment concerning the need for catheterization. Before performing the catheterization, clean the vulva and perineum because vaginal show and amniotic fluid may be present. If an obstacle that prevents advancement of the catheter is present, this obstacle is most likely the presenting part. If you cannot advance the catheter, stop the procedure and notify the nurse-midwife or physician of the difficulty.

Bowel Elimination. Most women do not have bowel movements during labor because of decreased intestinal motility. Stool that has formed in the large intestine often moves downward toward the anorectal area as a result of pressure exerted by the fetal presenting part as it descends. This stool is often expelled during second-stage pushing and birth. However, the passage of stool with bearing-down efforts increases the risk of infection and may embarrass the woman, thereby reducing the effectiveness of her pushing efforts. To prevent these problems, the nurse should immediately cleanse the perineal area to remove any stool, while reassuring the woman that the passage of stool at this time is a normal and expected event, because the same muscles used to expel the baby also expel stool.

Routine use of enemas on hospital admission for women at term has shown only modest benefits. There is a trend toward lower infection rates and the newborns have fewer lower respiratory tract infections and less need for antibiotics. However, because enemas cause discomfort for women and increase the costs of giving birth, the small benefits do not outweigh the disadvantages of this practice (Berghella et al., 2008). In addition, a Cochrane review of this topic found that the evidence does not support the routine use of enemas during labor (Reveiz, Gaitan, & Cuervo, 2013).

When the presenting part is deep in the pelvis, even in the absence of stool in the anorectal area, the woman may feel rectal pressure and think she needs to defecate. If the woman expresses the urge to defecate, the nurse should perform a vaginal examination to assess cervical dilation and station. When a multiparous woman experiences the urge to defecate, this often means birth will follow quickly.

Ambulation and Positioning

Upright positions and mobility during labor may be more pleasant for laboring women. These practices have also been associated with improved uterine contraction intensity and shorter labors, less need for pain medications, reduced rate of operative birth (e.g., cesarean birth, forceps- and vacuum-assisted birth), increased maternal autonomy and control, distraction from the discomforts of labor, and an opportunity for close interaction with the woman's partner and care provider as they help her assume upright positions and remain mobile (Lawrence, Lewis, Hofmeyr, & Styles, 2013; Simpson & O'Brien-Abel, 2014; Zwelling, 2010). No harmful effects have been observed from maternal activity and position changes. However, confinement to bed is the norm for laboring women in U.S. hospitals. The increased use of epidurals during childbirth accompanied by multiple medical interventions (e.g., electronic fetal monitors, IV infusions) and reduced motor control contribute to this practice, thereby interfering with a woman's freedom of movement and often slowing labor progress.

It is important to encourage ambulation if membranes are intact, after ROM if the fetal presenting part is engaged, and if the woman has not received medication for pain (Fig. 19-9). The woman also may find it comfortable to stand and lean forward on her partner, doula, or nurse for support at times during

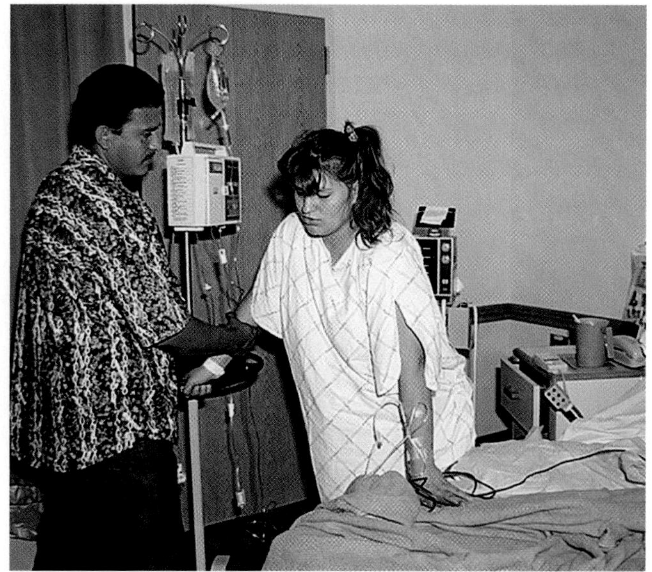

FIG 19-9 Woman preparing to walk with partner. (Courtesy Marjorie Pyle, RNC, Lifecircle, Costa Mesa, CA.)

labor (Fig. 19-10, *A*). In some circumstances, ambulation may be contraindicated because of maternal or fetal status.

When the woman lies in bed, she usually changes her position spontaneously as labor progresses. If she does not change position every 30 to 60 minutes, assist her to do so. The side-lying (lateral) position is preferred because it promotes optimal uteroplacental and renal blood flow and increases fetal oxygen saturation (Fig. 19-11, *B*). If the woman wants to lie supine, the nurse should place a pillow under one hip as a wedge to prevent the uterus from compressing the aorta and vena cava (see Fig. 19-5). Sitting is not contraindicated unless it adversely affects fetal status, which you can determine by checking the FHR and pattern. If the fetus is in the occiput posterior position, it may be helpful to encourage the woman to squat during contractions because this position increases the pelvic diameter, allowing the head to rotate to a more anterior position (see Fig. 19-11, *A*). A hands-and-knees position during contractions (see Fig. 19-10, *B*) or a lateral position on the same side as the fetal spine also are recommended to facilitate the rotation of the fetal occiput from a posterior to an anterior position, as gravity pulls the fetal back forward. These positions also provide access to the back for application of counterpressure by the partner, doula, or nurse (Hanson, 2009; Simpson & O'Brien-Abel, 2014; Simpson, Cesario, Morin, et al., 2008; Zwelling, 2010) (see Fig. 19-11, *B*). Women with epidural anesthesia may not be able to squat or assume a hands-and-knees position depending on the degree of motor involvement resulting from the epidural.

Much research continues to focus on acquiring a better understanding of the physiologic and psychologic effects of maternal position in labor. Box 19-8 describes a variety of positions that are commonly used and recommended.

The woman can use a birth ball (gymnastic ball, physical therapy ball) to support her body as she assumes a variety of labor and birth positions (Fig. 19-12). She can sit on the ball while leaning over the bed or lean over the ball to support her upper body and reduce stress on her arms and hands when she assumes a hands-and-knees position. The birth ball can encourage pelvic mobility and pelvic and perineal relaxation when the

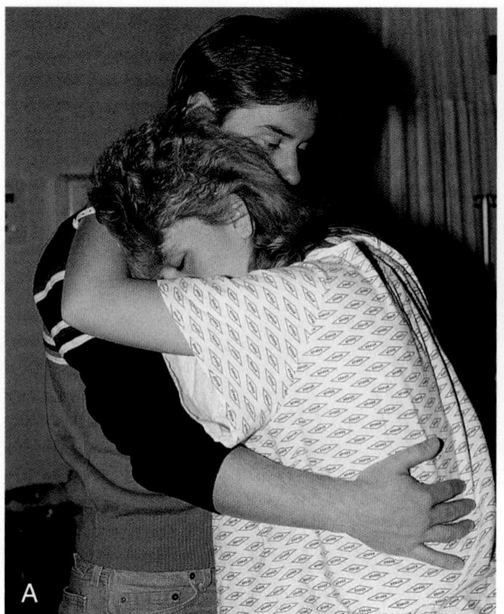

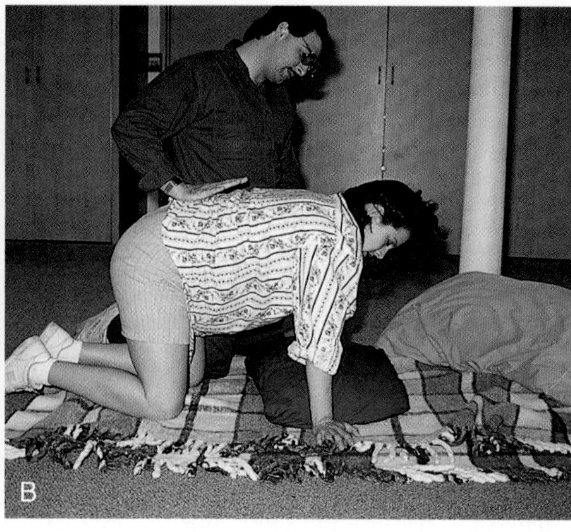

FIG 19-10 A, Woman standing and leaning forward with support. B, Woman in hands-and-knees position. (Courtesy Marjorie Pyle, RNC, Lifecircle, Costa Mesa, CA.)

woman sits on the firm yet pliable ball and rocks in rhythmic movements. Warm compresses applied to the perineum and lower back can maximize this relaxation and comfort effect. The birth ball should be large enough that, when the woman sits, her knees are bent at a 90-degree angle and her feet are flat on the floor and approximately 2 feet apart.

SAFETY ALERT

A woman may experience dizziness as she changes upright positions during labor. It is essential that the nurse or support person be present to provide assistance should dizziness occur.

Supportive Care During Labor and Birth

Support during labor and birth involves emotional support, physical care and comfort measures, and advice and information. The value of the continuous supportive presence of a person (e.g., doula, childbirth educator, family member, friend, nurse, partner) during labor has long been known. Women who have continuous support beginning in early labor are less likely to use pain medication or epidurals, more likely to have a spontaneous vaginal birth, and less likely to report dissatisfaction with their birth experience. No harmful effects from continuous labor support have been identified. To the contrary, there is good evidence that labor support improves important health outcomes (Association of Women's Health, Obstetric and Neonatal Nurses [AWHONN], 2011; Berghella et al., 2008; Hodnett et al., 2013).

Labor rooms should be airy, clean, and homelike. The laboring woman should feel safe in this environment and free to be herself and to use the comfort and relaxation measures she prefers. To enhance relaxation, turn off bright overhead lights when not needed, and keep noise and intrusions to a minimum. Control the temperature to ensure the laboring woman's comfort. The room

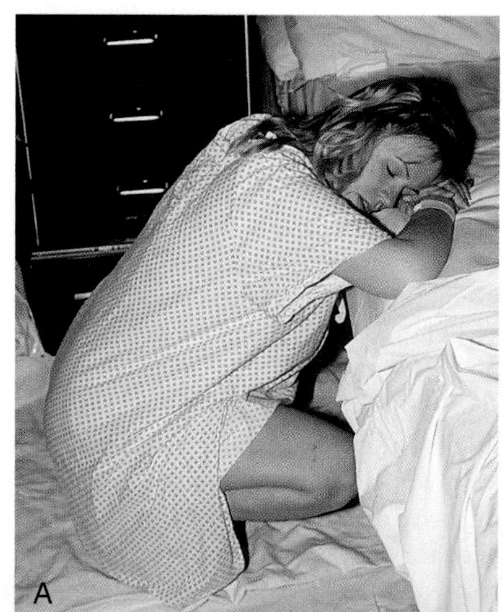

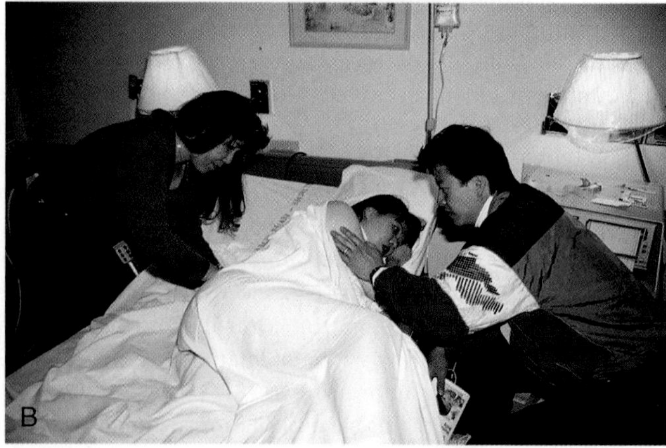

FIG 19-11 Maternal positions for labor. A, Squatting. B, Lateral position. Support person is applying sacral pressure while partner provides encouragement. (Courtesy Marjorie Pyle, RNC, Lifecircle, Costa Mesa, CA.)

BOX 19-8 Common Maternal Positions* During Labor and Birth

Semirecumbent Position (See Figs. 19-14, *B*, and 19-15, *B*)

With the woman sitting with her upper body elevated to at least a 30-degree angle, place a wedge or small pillow under her hip to prevent vena cava compression and reduce the likelihood of supine hypotension (see Fig. 19-5).

- The greater the angle of elevation, the more gravity or pressure is exerted that promotes fetal descent, the progress of contractions, and the widening of pelvic dimensions.
- This position is convenient for providing care measures and for external fetal monitoring.

Lateral Position (See Figs. 19-11, *B*, and 19-14, *A*)

Have the woman alternate between a left and right side-lying position, and provide abdominal and back support as needed for comfort.

- Removes pressure from the vena cava and back, enhances uteroplacental perfusion, and relieves backache
- Facilitates internal rotation of fetus in a posterior position to an anterior position (woman should lie on same side as fetal spine)
- Makes it easier to perform back massage or counterpressure
- Associated with less frequent, but more intense, contractions
- May be more difficult to obtain good external fetal monitor tracings
- May be used as a birthing position
- Takes pressure off perineum, allowing it to stretch gradually
- Reduces risk for perineal trauma

Upright Position

The gravity effect enhances the contraction cycle and fetal descent: the weight of the fetus places increasing pressure on the cervix; the cervix is pulled upward, facilitating effacement and dilation; impulses from the cervix to the pituitary gland increase, causing more oxytocin to be secreted; and contractions are intensified, thereby applying more forceful downward pressure on the fetus, but they are less painful.

- Fetus is aligned with pelvis, and pelvic diameters are widened slightly
- Effective upright positions include:
  - Ambulation (see Fig. 19-9)
  - Standing and leaning forward with support provided by coach (see Fig. 19-10, *A*), end of bed, back of chair, or birth ball; relieves backache and facilitates application of counterpressure or back massage
  - Sitting up in bed, in chair, in birthing chair, on toilet, or on bedside commode (see Fig. 19-14, *B*)
  - Squatting (see Figs. 19-11, *A*, and 19-15, *E*)

Hands-and-Knees Position—Position for Posterior Positions of the Presenting Part (See Figs. 19-10, *B*, and 19-12)

Assume an "all fours" position or lean over an object (e.g., birth ball) while on the knees in bed or on a covered floor; this allows for pelvic rocking.

- Relieves backache characteristic of "back labor"
- Facilitates internal rotation of the fetus by increasing mobility of the coccyx, increasing the pelvic diameters, and using gravity to turn the fetal back and rotate the head (NOTE: A side-lying position, double hip squeeze, or knee squeeze also can facilitate internal rotation.)

*Assess the effect of each position on the laboring woman's comfort and anxiety level, progress of labor, and fetal heart rate and pattern. Alternate positions every 30 to 60 minutes, allowing the woman to take control of her position changes.

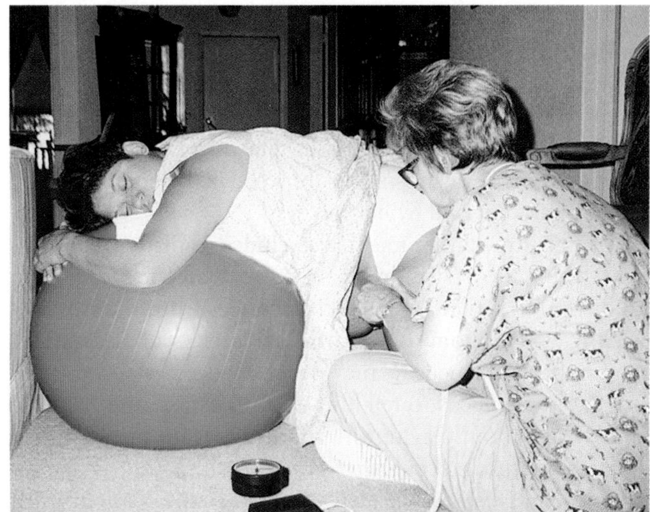

FIG 19-12 Woman laboring using birth ball. (Courtesy Polly Perez, Cutting Edge Press, Johnson, VT.)

should be large enough to accommodate a comfortable chair for the woman's support person, the monitoring equipment, and hospital personnel. Encourage women to bring their own pillows to make the hospital surroundings more homelike and to facilitate position changes. Environmental modifications should reflect the preferences of the woman, including the number of visitors and availability of a telephone, television, and music.

Labor Support by the Nurse. Supportive nursing care for a woman in labor includes:

- Helping her maintain control and participate to the extent she wishes in the birth of her infant
- Providing continuity of care that is nonjudgmental and respectful of her cultural and religious values and beliefs
- Meeting her expected outcomes for her labor
- Listening to her concerns and encouraging her to express her feelings
- Acting as her advocate, supporting her decisions and respecting her choices as appropriate, and relating her wishes as needed to other health care providers
- Helping her conserve her energy and cope effectively with her pain and discomfort by using a variety of comfort measures that are acceptable to her
- Helping control her discomfort
- Acknowledging her efforts during labor including her strength and courage, as well as those of her partner, and providing positive reinforcement
- Protecting her privacy, modesty, and dignity

Women who have attended childbirth education programs that teach the psychoprophylactic (Lamaze) approach will know something about the labor process, coaching techniques, and comfort measures. The nurse plays a supportive role and keeps the woman and her partner informed of the labor progress. If necessary, review the methods learned in class and practiced at home because it may be difficult for the woman to effectively

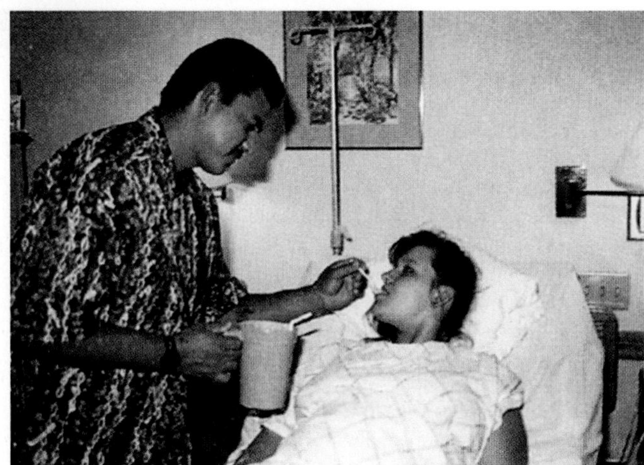

FIG 19-13 Partner providing comfort measures. (Courtesy Marjorie Pyle, RNC, Lifecircle, Costa Mesa, CA.)

use these methods and techniques now that she is in labor and in an unfamiliar setting.

Even when a laboring woman has not attended childbirth classes, the nurse can teach her simple breathing and relaxation techniques during the early phase of labor. In this case the nurse provides more of the coaching and supportive care until the support person feels ready to take on a more active coaching role (see Chapter 17). The nurse can demonstrate comfort measures while encouraging the support person to assist and the laboring woman to express her needs and feelings. Observing the comforting approaches of the nurse can help the partner learn effective comfort measures.

Comfort measures vary with the situation (Fig. 19-13). The nurse can draw on the woman's list of comfort measures and relaxation techniques learned during the pregnancy and through life experiences. Such measures include maintaining a comfortable, calm, supportive atmosphere in the labor and birth area; using touch therapeutically (e.g., heat or cold applied to the lower back in the event of back labor, a cool cloth applied to the forehead, massage); providing nonpharmacologic measures to relieve discomfort (e.g., hydrotherapy); and most important, just being there (see Tables 19-1 and 19-4). See Chapter 17 for a full discussion of pharmacologic and nonpharmacologic comfort measures.

Most women in labor respond positively to touch, but you should obtain permission before using any touching measures. Women appreciate gentle assistance by staff members. Back rubs and counterpressure may be offered, especially if the woman is experiencing back labor. Teach the support person to exert counterpressure against the woman's sacrum over the occiput of the head of a fetus in a posterior position (see Fig. 19-11, *B*). Double hip or knee squeezes can also be helpful in reducing back pain. The back pain is caused by the occiput pressing on spinal nerves, and counterpressure lifts the occiput off these nerves, providing some relief from pain. The partner will need to be relieved after a while, however, because exerting counterpressure is hard work. Hand and foot massage also can be soothing and relaxing.

The woman's perception of the soothing qualities of touch may change as labor progresses. Many women become more sensitive to touch (hyperesthesia) as labor progresses. This is a typical response during the transition phase (see Table 19-1). They may tell their coach to leave them alone or not to touch them. The partner who is unprepared for this normal response may feel rejected and may react by withdrawing active support. The nurse can reassure him or her that this response is a positive indication that the first stage is ending and the second stage is approaching. Women with increased sensitivity to touch may tolerate it better on surfaces of the body where hair does not grow, such as the forehead, the palms of the hands, and the soles of the feet.

Labor Support by the Father or Partner. Although a woman or a man other than the father may be the woman's partner, the father of the baby is usually the support person during labor. He is often able to provide the comfort measures and touch that the laboring woman needs. When the woman becomes focused on her pain, sometimes the partner can persuade her to try nonpharmacologic variations of comfort measures. In addition, he usually is able to interpret the woman's needs and desires for staff members.

The feelings of a first-time father change as labor progresses. Although he is often calm at the onset of labor, feelings of fear and helplessness begin to dominate as labor becomes more active and the father realizes that it is more stressful than he anticipated. A study of Swedish fathers' birth experiences found that although about three quarters of the men reported positive or very positive experiences, less positive experiences were associated with emergency cesarean birth, assisted vaginal birth, and dissatisfaction with their partners' medical care. The interactions of health care providers with the fathers and the fathers' perception of the health care providers' competence were also related to the fathers' birth experiences (Johansson, Rubertsson, Radestad, & Hildingsson, 2012). Staff members should tell the father that his presence is helpful and encourage him to be involved in the care of the woman to the extent to which he and his partner are comfortable. He should be reassured that he is not assuming the responsibility for observation and management of his partner's labor, but that his responsibility is to support her as the labor progresses. The nurse can suggest alternative comfort measures when those he is using are no longer helpful or are rejected by his partner.

The first-time father may feel excluded as birth preparations begin during the transition phase. Once the second stage begins and birth nears, the father's focus changes from the woman to the baby who is about to be born. The father will be exposed to many sights and smells he may never have experienced. Therefore, the nurse needs to tell him what to expect and make him comfortable about leaving the room to regain his composure should something occur that surprises him, but make sure that someone else is available to support the woman during his absence.

Nursing actions that support the father convey several important concepts: first, he is a person of value; second, he can be a partner in the woman's care; and third, childbearing is a team effort. Box 19-9 details ways in which the nurse can support the father-partner. A well-informed father can make an important contribution to the health and well-being of the mother and child, their family interrelationship, and his self-esteem.

Labor Support by Doulas. Continuity of care has been cited by women as a critical component of a satisfying childbirth

BOX 19-9 Guidelines for Supporting the Father*

- Orient him to the labor room and the unit; explain location of the cafeteria, toilet, waiting room, and nursery; give information about visiting hours; introduce personnel by name and describe their functions.
- Inform him of sights and smells he can expect; encourage him to leave the room if necessary.
- Respect his or the couple's decision about the degree of his involvement. Offer them freedom to make decisions.
- Tell him when his presence has been helpful, and continue to reinforce this throughout labor.
- Offer to teach him comfort measures; demonstrate or role-play these measures.
- Inform him frequently of the progress of the labor and the woman's needs. Keep him informed about procedures to be performed.
- Prepare him for changes in the woman's behavior and physical appearance.
- Remind him to eat; offer him snacks and fluids if possible.
- Relieve him of the job of support person as necessary. Offer him blankets if he is to sleep in a chair by the bedside.
- Acknowledge the stress experienced by each partner during labor and birth, and identify normal responses.
- Attempt to modify or eliminate unsettling stimuli, such as extra noise and extra light; create a relaxing and calm environment.

*These guidelines are appropriate for any support person or partner.

experience. A specially trained, experienced female labor attendant called a doula can meet this need. The doula is a professional or lay labor-support person who is present during labor in addition to the labor and birth nurse (Burke, 2014). The primary role of the doula is to focus on the laboring woman and to provide physical and emotional support by using soft, reassuring words of praise and encouragement; touching; stroking; and hugging. The doula also administers comfort measures to reduce pain and enhance relaxation and coping, walks with the woman, helps her to change positions, and coaches her bearing-down efforts. Doulas provide information about labor progress and explain procedures and events. They advocate for the woman's right to participate actively in managing her labor.

The doula also supports the woman's partner, who often feels unqualified to be the sole labor support and may find it difficult to watch the woman when she is experiencing pain. The doula can encourage and praise the partner's efforts, create a partnership as caregivers, and provide respite care. Doulas also facilitate communication between the laboring woman and her partner, as well as between the couple and the health care team (Simkin, 2012).

Doula support during labor is associated with decreased use of analgesia, decreased incidence of operative birth, increased incidence of spontaneous vaginal birth, and increased maternal satisfaction with the childbirth experience (Berghella et al., 2008).

The roles of the nurse and the doula are complementary. They should work together as a team, recognizing and respecting the role each plays in supporting and caring for the woman and her partner during the childbirth process. Both the nurse and the doula provide supportive care measures. The nurse also focuses on monitoring the status of the maternal-fetal unit, implementing clinical care protocols (including pharmacologic interventions), and documenting assessment findings, actions, and responses (Simkin, 2012).

Labor Support by Grandparents. When grandparents act as labor coaches, it is especially important to support and treat them with respect. They may have ways to deal with pain based on their experience. Grandparents should be encouraged to help as long as their actions do not compromise the status of the mother or the fetus. The nurse treats grandparents with dignity and respect by acknowledging the value of their contributions to parental support and recognizing the difficulty parents have in witnessing the woman's discomfort or crisis. If they have never witnessed a birth, the nurse may need to provide explanations of what is happening. Many of the activities used to support fathers also are appropriate for grandparents (see Box 19-9).

Siblings During Labor and Birth

Preparing siblings for acceptance of the new child helps promote the attachment process and may help older children accept this change. The older child or children who know they are important to the family become active participants. Rehearsal for the event before labor is essential.

The age and developmental level of children influence their responses; therefore, preparation for the children to be present during labor is adjusted to meet each child's needs (see Box 14-2). The child younger than 2 years shows little interest in pregnancy and labor. However, for the older child, such preparation may reduce fears and misconceptions. Parents need to be prepared for labor and birth themselves and feel comfortable about the process and the presence of their children. Most parents have a "feel" for their children's maturational level and their physical and emotional ability to observe and cope with the events of the labor and birth process. Preparation can include a description of the anticipated sights, events (e.g., ROM, monitors, IV infusions), smells, and sounds; a labor and birth demonstration; a tour of the birthing unit; and an opportunity to be around a real newborn. Storybooks about the birth process can be read to or by children to prepare them for the event. Films are available for preparing preschool and school-age children to participate in the labor and birth experience. Children must learn that their mother will be working hard during labor and birth. She will not be able to talk to them during contractions. She may groan, scream, grunt, and pant at times as well as say things she would not say otherwise (e.g., "I can't take this anymore," "Take this baby out of me," or "This pain is killing me"). You can tell them that labor is uncomfortable, but that their mother's body is made for the job.

Most agencies require that a specific person be designated to watch over the children who are participating in their mother's childbirth experience, to provide them with support, explanations, diversions, and comfort as needed. Health care providers involved in attending women during birth must be comfortable with the presence of children and the unpredictability of their questions, comments, and behaviors.

Emergency Interventions

Although rare, emergency conditions that require immediate nursing intervention can arise with startling speed. See Chapter 18 for information on management of abnormal

FHR. Management of other emergency situations, including meconium-stained amniotic fluid, shoulder dystocia, prolapsed umbilical cord, ruptured uterus, and amniotic fluid embolus, is discussed in Chapter 32.

SECOND STAGE OF LABOR

The second stage of labor is the stage in which the infant is born. This stage begins with full cervical dilation (10 cm) and complete effacement (100%) and ends with the baby's birth. The force exerted by uterine contractions, gravity, and maternal bearing-down efforts facilitates achievement of the expected outcome of a spontaneous, uncomplicated vaginal birth. The median duration of second-stage labor is 50 to 60 minutes in nulliparous women and 20 to 30 minutes in multiparous women. In addition to parity, maternal size and fetal weight, position, and descent influence the length of this stage. The use of epidural anesthesia often increases the length of the second stage of labor because the epidural blocks or reduces the woman's urge to bear down and limits her ability to attain an upright position to push. The upper limits for the duration of normal second-stage labor are (Wing & Farinelli, 2012):

- Nulliparous women: 2 hours with no regional anesthesia use
  3 hours with use of regional anesthesia
- Multiparous women: 1 hour with no regional anesthesia use
  2 hours with regional anesthesia

A prolonged second stage is diagnosed after these time limits are reached. A thorough assessment of the status of the maternal-fetal unit should be made as well as a determination regarding the likely effectiveness and safety of further bearing-down efforts (Simpson et al., 2008).

The second stage of labor is composed of two phases: the latent phase and the active pushing phase. Maternal verbal and nonverbal behaviors, uterine activity, the urge to bear down, and fetal descent characterize these phases (Hanson, 2009; Simpson et al., 2008).

The latent ("laboring down") phase is a period of rest and relative calm. During this phase the fetus continues to descend passively through the birth canal and rotate to an anterior position as a result of ongoing uterine contractions. The woman is quiet and often relaxes with her eyes closed between contractions. The urge to bear down is not strong, and some women do not experience it at all or only during the acme (peak) of a contraction. Delayed pushing has been shown to result in significant decreases in pushing time, significant increases in the duration of second-stage labor, and a reduction in the number of operative vaginal births. On the other hand, no differences in the number of cesarean births, perineal lacerations or episiotomies, or fetal complications have been linked to delayed pushing (Kelly, Johnson, Lee, et al., 2010). In a randomized clinical trial, allowing a woman to rest during this phase and waiting until the urge intensified to begin pushing significantly reduced the amount of time spent pushing but did not significantly increase the total length of second-stage labor. In this study maternal fatigue scores, perineal injuries, and FHR decelerations were similar in the immediate- and delayed-pushing groups (Gillesby, Burns, Dempsey, et al., 2010). Another study also found a significant decrease in pushing time in nulliparous women with epidural anesthesia who practiced delayed pushing during second-stage labor (Gillesby et al.).

Careful monitoring with assurance of normal fetal status should be used during delayed pushing. If descent is slow and the woman becomes anxious, she should be encouraged to change positions frequently or to stand by the bedside to use the advantage of gravity and movement to facilitate descent and progress to the active pushing phase signaled by a perception of the need to bear down (Hanson, 2009).

During the active pushing (descent) phase the woman has strong urges to bear down as the Ferguson reflex is activated when the presenting part presses on the stretch receptors of the pelvic floor. At this point the fetal station is usually +1 and the position is anterior. This stimulation causes the release of oxytocin from the posterior pituitary gland, which provokes stronger expulsive uterine contractions. The woman becomes more focused on bearing-down efforts, which become rhythmic. She changes positions frequently to find a more comfortable pushing position. The woman often announces the onset of contractions and becomes more vocal as she bears down. The urge to bear down intensifies as descent progresses and the presenting part reaches the perineum. The woman may be more verbal about the pain she is experiencing; she may scream or swear and may act out of control.

The nurse encourages the woman to "listen" to her body as she progresses through the phases of the second stage of labor. When a woman listens to her body to tell her when to bear down, she is using an internal locus of control and often feels more satisfied with her efforts to give birth to her baby. This enhances her sense of self-esteem and accomplishment and her efforts become more effective. Always encourage the woman's trust in her own body and her ability to give birth to her baby. Validate the woman's experience of pressure, stretching, and straining as normal and a signal that the descent of the fetus is progressing and that her body is capable of withstanding birth. Honestly explain what is happening and describe the progress being made.

CARE MANAGEMENT

Box 19-10 describes nursing care during the second stage of labor. The only certain objective sign that the second stage of labor has begun is the inability to feel the cervix during vaginal examination, indicating that the cervix is fully dilated and effaced. The precise moment that this occurs is not easily determined because it depends on when a vaginal examination is performed to validate full dilation and effacement. This makes timing of the actual duration of the second stage difficult. Other signs that suggest the onset of the second stage include the urge to push or feeling the need to have a bowel movement. These signs commonly appear at the time the cervix reaches full dilation. However, they can appear earlier in labor. Women with an epidural block may not exhibit such signs.

Women who are laboring without regional anesthesia can experience an irresistible urge to bear down before full dilation. For some, this occurs as early as 5 cm dilation. This is most often related to the station of the presenting part below the level of the ischial spines of the maternal pelvis. This occurrence creates a conflict between the woman, whose body is telling her to

BOX 19-10 Nursing Care in Second-Stage Labor

Assessment

Signs That Suggest the Onset of the Second Stage

Urge to push or feeling need to have a bowel movement
Sudden appearance of sweat on upper lip
An episode of vomiting
Increased bloody show
Shaking of extremities
Increased restlessness; verbalization (e.g., "I can't go on.")
Involuntary bearing-down efforts

Physical Assessment

Assess every 5 to 30 minutes: maternal blood pressure, pulse, and respirations.
Assess every 5 to 15 minutes, depending on risk status: fetal heart rate and pattern.
Assess every 10 to 15 minutes: vaginal show, signs of fetal descent, and changes in maternal appearance, mood, affect, energy level, and condition of partner/coach.
Assess every contraction and bearing-down effort.

Interventions

Latent ("Laboring Down") Phase

Help to rest in a position of comfort; encourage relaxation to conserve energy.
Promote progress of fetal descent and onset of urge to bear down by encouraging position changes, pelvic rock, ambulation, showering.

Active Pushing (Descent) Phase

Help to change position and encourage spontaneous bearing-down efforts.
Help to relax and conserve energy between contractions.
Provide comfort and pain-relief measures as needed.
Cleanse perineum promptly if fecal material is expelled.
Coach to pant during contractions and to gently push between contractions when head is emerging.
Provide emotional support, encouragement, and positive reinforcement of efforts.
Keep woman informed regarding progress.
Create a calm and quiet environment.
Offer mirror to watch birth.

push, and her health care providers, who may believe that pushing the fetal presenting part against an incompletely dilated cervix will result in cervical edema and lacerations, as well as slow the labor progress. Evaluate the premature urge to bear down as a sign of labor progress, possibly indicating the onset of the second stage of labor. Base the timing of when a woman pushes in relation to whether her cervix is fully dilated on research evidence rather than on tradition or routine practice. Pushing with the urge to bear down at the acme of a contraction may be safe and effective for a woman if her cervix is soft, retracting, and 8 cm or more dilated and if the fetus is at +1 station and rotating to an anterior position (Roberts, 2002).

Assessment continues during the second stage of labor. Professional standards and agency policy determine the specific type and timing of assessments, as well as the way in which findings are documented (see Box 19-10). Signs and symptoms of impending birth (Table 19-4) may appear unexpectedly, requiring immediate action by the nurse (Box 19-11).

The nurse continues to monitor maternal-fetal status and events of the second stage and provide comfort measures for the mother. This includes helping her change position; providing mouth care; maintaining clean, dry bedding; and keeping extraneous noise, conversation, and other distractions (e.g., laughing, talking of attending personnel in or outside the labor area) to a minimum. The woman is encouraged to indicate other support measures she would like (see Table 19-3; Nursing Care Plan).

In the hospital, birth may occur in an LDR, LDRP, or delivery room. If the mother is to be transferred to the delivery room for birth, perform the transfer early enough to avoid rushing her. The birth area also is readied (see later discussion).

Preparing for Birth

Maternal Position

No single position for childbirth exists. Labor is a dynamic, interactive process involving the woman's uterus, pelvis, and voluntary muscles. In addition, angles between the baby and the woman's pelvis constantly change as the infant turns and flexes down the birth canal. The woman may want to assume various positions for childbirth. She should be encouraged to change positions frequently and assisted in attaining and maintaining her position(s) of choice (Figs. 19-14 and 19-15). Supine, semirecumbent, or lithotomy positions are still widely used in Western societies despite evidence that an upright position shortens labor (Chang, Chou, Lin, et al., 2011).

Birth attendants play a major role in influencing a woman's choice of positions for birth, with nurse-midwives tending to advocate nonlithotomy positions (e.g., upright, lateral) for the second stage of labor. An upright position (walking, sitting, kneeling, or squatting) offers a number of advantages. Gravity can promote the descent of the fetus. Uterine contractions are generally stronger and more efficient in effacing and dilating the cervix, resulting in shorter labor (Blackburn, 2013; Lawrence et al., 2013; Zwelling, 2010). An upright position also is beneficial to the mother's cardiac output, thereby increasing perfusion of the uterus. The use of upright and lateral positions is also associated with less pain and perineal damage, fewer episiotomies and abnormal FHR patterns, and fewer operative vaginal births (Berghella et al., 2008; Chang et al., 2011; Simpson et al., 2008; Zwelling, 2010). The benefits of upright positions may be related to:

- Straightening of the longitudinal axis of the birth canal and improving the alignment of the fetus for passage through the pelvis
- Application of gravity to direct the fetal head toward the pelvic inlet, thereby facilitating descent
- Enlargement of pelvic dimensions and restriction of the encroachment of the sacrum and coccyx into the pelvic outlet
- Increased uteroplacental circulation, resulting in more intense, efficient uterine contractions
- Enhancement of the woman's ability to bear down effectively, thereby minimizing maternal exhaustion

Squatting is highly effective in facilitating the descent and birth of the fetus. It is one of the best and most natural positions for second stage labor and has been associated with the same benefits as other upright and lateral positions (Simpson et al., 2008). Women should assume a modified, supported squat until the fetal head is engaged, at which time a deep squat can be

TABLE 19-4 Expected Maternal Progress in the Second Stage of Labor

CRITERION	LATENT ("LABORING DOWN") PHASE (AVERAGE DURATION, 10-30 MINUTES)	ACTIVE PUSHING (DESCENT) PHASE (AVERAGE DURATION VARIES)*
Contractions		
Intensity	Period of physiologic lull for all criteria; period of peace and rest	Significant increase becoming overwhelmingly strong and expulsive
Frequency		Every 2 to 2.5 minutes progressing to every 1 to 2 minutes
Duration		90 seconds
Descent, station	0 to +2	+2 to +4; rate of descent increases and Ferguson reflex† is activated; fetal head becomes visible at introitus, and birth occurs
Show: color and amount		Significant increase in dark red bloody show; bloody show accompanies emergence of head
Spontaneous bearing-down efforts	Slight to absent, except at peak of strongest contractions	Increased urge to bear down; becomes stronger as fetus descends to vaginal introitus and reaches perineum
Vocalization	Quiet; concern over progress	Grunting sounds or expiratory vocalizations; announces contractions; may scream or swear
Maternal behavior	Experiences sense of relief that transition to second stage is finished Feels fatigued and sleepy Feels a sense of accomplishment and optimism because the "worst is over" Feels in control	Senses increased urge to push and describes increasing pain; describes *ring of fire* (burning sensation of acute pain as vagina stretches and fetal head crowns) Expresses feeling of powerlessness Shows decreased ability to listen to or concentrate on anything but giving birth Alters respiratory pattern: has short 4- to 5-second breath holds with regular breaths in between, 5 to 7 times per contraction Frequent repositioning Often shows excitement immediately after birth of head

*Duration of descent phase can vary, depending on maternal parity, effectiveness of bearing-down efforts, and presence of spinal anesthesia or epidural analgesia.
†Pressure of presenting part on stretch receptors of pelvic floor stimulates release of oxytocin from posterior pituitary, resulting in more intense uterine contractions.
Data from Hanson, L. (2009). Second-stage labor care, *Journal of Perinatal & Neonatal Nursing, 23*(1), 31-39; AWHONN. (2008). *Nursing care and management of the second stage of labor: Evidence-based clinical practice guideline* (2nd ed.). Washington, DC: Author; Roberts, J.E. (2002). The "push" for evidence: Management of the second stage. *Journal of Midwifery & Women's Health, 1*, 2-15; Simkin, P., & Ancheta, R. (2000). *The labor progress*. Malden, MA: Blackwell Science.

used. A firm surface is required for this position, and the woman will need side support (see Fig. 19-11, *A*). In a birthing bed, a squat bar is available that she can use to help support herself (Fig. 19-15, *E*). A birth ball can also help a woman maintain the squatting position. The fetus will be aligned with the birth canal, and pelvic and perineal relaxation is facilitated as she sits on the ball or holds it in front of her for support as she squats (see Box 19-8).

When a woman uses the supported standing position for bearing down, her weight is borne on both femoral heads, allowing the pressure in the acetabulum to cause the transverse diameter of the pelvic outlet to increase by up to 1 cm. This can be helpful if descent of the head is delayed because the occiput has not rotated from the lateral (transverse diameter of pelvis) to the anterior position. Birthing chairs or rocking chairs may be used to provide women with a good physiologic position to enhance bearing-down efforts during childbirth (see Box 19-8), although some women may feel restricted by a chair. The upright position also provides a potential psychologic advantage in that it allows the mother to see the birth as it occurs and to maintain eye contact with the attendant.

Oversized beanbag chairs and large floor pillows can be used for both labor and birth. They can mold around and support the mother in whatever position she selects. These chairs are of particular value for mothers who wish to be actively involved in the birth process. Birthing stools can be used to support the woman in an upright position similar to squatting. Some women may feel more comfortable sitting on the toilet or commode during pushing because they are concerned about stool incontinence during this stage. Encourage them to empty their bladder to avoid the effects of a distended bladder. You must closely monitor these women, however, and ask them to move from the toilet before birth becomes imminent. Because sitting on chairs, stools, toilets, or commodes can increase perineal edema and blood loss, assist the woman to change her position frequently (e.g., every 10 to 15 minutes).

The side-lying, or lateral, position, with the upper part of the woman's leg held by the nurse or coach or placed on a pillow, is an effective position for the second stage of labor (see Fig. 19-14, *A*, and Box 19-8). Some women prefer a semisitting (semirecumbent) position instead (see Fig. 19-15, *B*, and Box 19-8). If the semirecumbent position is used, do not force the woman's legs against her abdomen as she bears down. This position will increase perineal stretching and the risk for perineal trauma as well as spinal and lower extremity neurologic injuries (Simpson & O'Brien-Abel, 2014; Simpson et al., 2008). The hands-and-knees position is yet another effective position for birth (see Fig. 19-10, *B*, and Box 19-8).

The birthing bed can be set for different positions according to the woman's needs (see Fig. 19-15; Fig. 19-16). The woman can squat, kneel, sit, recline, or lie on her side, choosing the position most comfortable for her without having to climb into bed for the birth. At the same time, the birthing bed provides excellent access and visualization for the attendant to perform examinations, place electrodes, and assist the woman giving birth. You can position the bed for the administration of anesthesia and it is ideal to help women receiving an epidural to assume different positions to facilitate birth. You can also use the bed to transport the woman to the operating room if a cesarean birth is necessary. The woman can use squat bars, over-the-bed tables, birth balls, and pillows for support.

BOX 19-11 Guidelines for Assistance at the Emergency Birth of a Fetus in the Vertex Presentation

1. The woman usually assumes the position most comfortable for her. A lateral position is often recommended to facilitate a controlled birth of the head, thereby minimizing the risk for perineal trauma and neonatal head injury.
2. Reassure the woman that birth is usually uncomplicated in these situations. Use eye-to-eye contact and a calm, relaxed manner. If there is someone else available, such as the partner, that person could help support the woman in the position, assist with coaching, and provide positive reinforcement and praise of her efforts.
3. Wash your hands and put on gloves, if available.
4. Place under the woman's buttocks whatever clean material is available.
5. Avoid touching the vaginal area to decrease the possibility of infection.
6. As the head begins to crown, you should perform the following tasks:
   a. Tear the amniotic membranes if they are still intact.
   b. Instruct the woman to pant or pant-blow, thus minimizing the urge to push.
   c. Place the flat side of your hand on the exposed fetal head and apply *gentle* pressure toward the vagina to prevent the head from "popping out." The mother may participate by placing her hand under yours on the emerging head. NOTE: Rapid birth of the fetal head must be prevented because a rapid change of pressure within the molded fetal skull follows, which may result in dural or subdural tears. Rapid birth also may cause vaginal or perineal lacerations.
7. After the birth of the head, check to see if the umbilical cord is around the baby's neck. If it is, *gently* try to slip it over the baby's head or pull it *gently* to get some slack so that you can slip it over the shoulders.
8. Support the baby's head as external rotation occurs. Then with one hand on each side of the baby's head, exert *gentle* pressure downward so that the anterior shoulder emerges under the symphysis pubis and acts as a fulcrum; then, as *gentle* pressure is exerted upward, the posterior shoulder, which has passed over the sacrum and coccyx, emerges.
9. Be alert! Hold the baby securely because the rest of the body may emerge quickly. The baby will be slippery!
10. Cradle the baby's head and back in one hand and the buttocks in the other. Keep the baby's head down to drain away the mucus. Use a bulb syringe, if needed, to remove mucus from the baby's mouth and then from the nose.
11. Dry the baby quickly to prevent rapid heat loss and immediately place the baby on the mother's abdomen. Keep the baby at the same level as the mother's uterus until the cord stops pulsating. NOTE: The baby should be kept at the same level as the mother's uterus to prevent the baby's blood from flowing to or from the placenta and resulting in hypovolemia or hypervolemia. Also, do not "milk" the cord.
12. With the baby on the mother's abdomen, cover the baby (remember to keep the head warm, too) with a warmed blanket or the mother's clothing, and have her cuddle the baby. Compliment her (them) on a job well done, and on the baby, if appropriate.
13. Wait for the placenta to separate. *Do not* tug on the cord. NOTE: Inappropriate traction may tear the cord, separate the placenta, or invert the uterus. Signs of placental separation include a slight gush of dark blood from the introitus, lengthening of the cord, and change in the uterine contour from a discoid to globular shape.
14. Instruct the mother to push to deliver the separated placenta. Gently ease out the placental membranes using an up-and-down motion until the membranes are removed. If birth occurs outside a hospital setting, to minimize complications, do not cut the cord without proper clamps and a sterile cutting tool. Inspect the placenta for intactness. Place the baby on the placenta and wrap the two together for additional warmth.
15. Check the firmness of the uterus. Gently massage the fundus and demonstrate to the mother how she can massage her own fundus properly.
16. If supplies are available, clean the mother's perineal area and apply a peripad.
17. In addition to gentle massage of the fundus, the following measures can be taken to prevent or minimize hemorrhage:
   a. Put the baby to the mother's breast as soon as possible. Sucking or nuzzling and licking the nipple stimulates the release of oxytocin from the posterior pituitary. NOTE: If the baby does not or cannot nurse, manually stimulate the mother's nipples.
   b. Do not allow the mother's bladder to become distended. Assess the bladder for fullness and encourage her to void if fullness is found.
   c. Expel any clots from the mother's uterus after ensuring that the fundus is firm.
18. Comfort or reassure the mother and her family or friends. Keep the mother and the baby warm. Give her fluids if available and tolerated.
19. If there is more than one baby, identify the infants in order of birth (using letters *A*, *B*, etc.).
20. Make notations regarding the following aspects of the birth:
   a. Fetal presentation and position
   b. Presence of cord around neck (nuchal cord) or other parts and number of times cord encircled part
   c. Color, character, and estimated amount of amniotic fluid, if rupture of membranes occurred immediately before birth
   d. Time of birth
   e. Estimated time of determination of Apgar score (e.g., 1 and 5 minutes after birth), resuscitation efforts implemented, and ultimate condition of baby
   f. Gender of baby
   g. Time of placental expulsion, as well as the appearance and completeness of the placenta
   h. Maternal condition: affect, behavior, and demeanor, amount of bleeding, and status of uterine tonicity
   i. Any unusual occurrences during the birth (e.g., maternal or paternal response, verbalizations, or gestures in response to birth of baby)

Bearing-Down Efforts

As the fetal head reaches the pelvic floor, most women experience the urge to bear down. Reflexively the woman will begin to exert downward pressure by contracting her abdominal muscles while relaxing her pelvic floor. This bearing down is an involuntary response to the Ferguson reflex. A strong expiratory grunt or groan (vocalization) often accompanies pushing when the woman exhales as she pushes. This natural vocalization by women during open-glottis bearing-down efforts should not be discouraged.

When coaching women to push, encourage them to push as they feel like pushing (instinctive, spontaneous pushing)

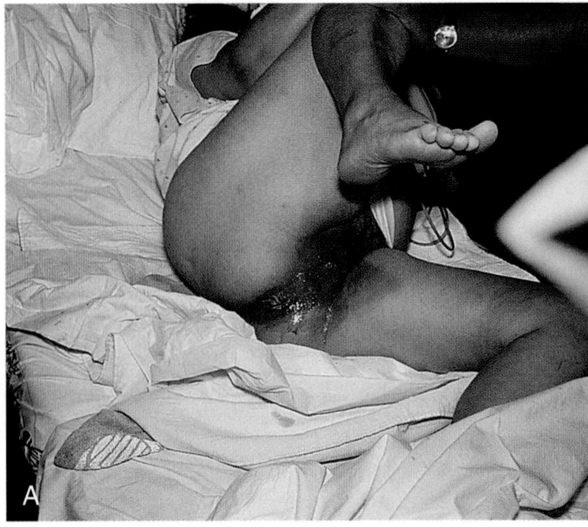

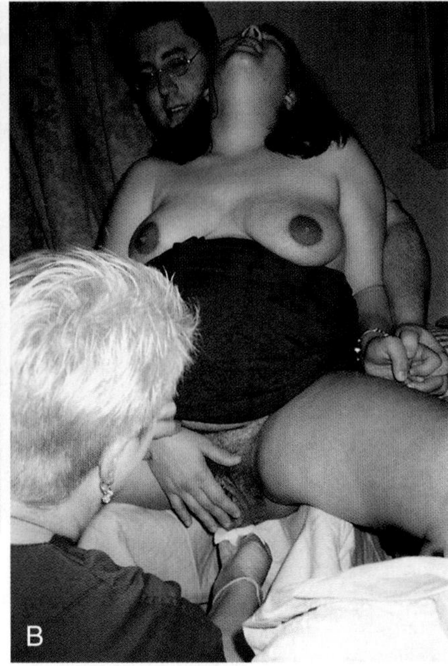

FIG 19-14 **A,** Pushing, side-lying position. Perineal bulging can be seen. **B,** Pushing, semisitting position. Nurse-midwife assists mother to feel top of fetal head. (**A,** Courtesy Michael S. Clement, MD, Mesa, AZ. **B,** Courtesy Roni Wernik, Palo Alto, CA.)

rather than to give a prolonged push on command (directed, closed-glottis pushing). Prolonged breath-holding, or sustained, directed bearing down is still a common practice, often beginning at 10-cm dilation and before the urge to bear down is perceived. The woman is coached to hold her breath, closing her glottis, and to push while the nurse or partner counts to 10. This method of bearing down is strongly discouraged because it may trigger the Valsalva maneuver, which occurs when the woman closes her glottis (closed-glottis pushing), which increases intrathoracic and cardiovascular pressure. This reduces cardiac output and decreases perfusion of the uterus and the placenta. Adverse effects associated with prolonged breath-holding and forceful pushing efforts include fetal hypoxia and subsequent acidosis, increased risk for pelvic floor damage (structural and neurogenic), and perineal trauma (Blackburn, 2013; Hanson, 2009; Simpson & O'Brien-Abel, 2014; Simpson et al., 2008). The benefits of spontaneous pushing efforts rather than sustained Valsalva pushes include less fatigue and enhanced comfort. In addition, these more effective bearing-down efforts result in less time spent actively pushing (Hanson, 2009; James, 2011; Simpson & O'Brien-Abel, 2014). Based on this evidence, it is essential that labor and birth nurses advocate for the practice of delayed and spontaneous bearing-down efforts with the woman in an upright or lateral position (Hanson, 2009).

A woman can become confused and anxious when she is being told to do something in conflict with what her body is telling her. Using phrases such as "You are doing so well; do it again," "You are moving the baby down," and "Follow what your body is telling you," rather than "Push, push, push," encourages a woman to feel confident in her body and what she is feeling (Hanson, 2009).

Monitor the woman's breathing so that she does not hold her breath for more than 6 to 8 seconds at a time followed by a slight exhale (a combination of open-glottis and voluntary closed-glottis pushing). Remind her to ventilate her lungs fully by taking deep cleansing breaths before and after each contraction. Bearing down while exhaling (open-glottis pushing) and taking breaths between bearing-down efforts help to maintain adequate oxygen levels for the mother and fetus, thus enhancing fetal well-being. The active pushing phase of the second stage of labor is considered to be the most physiologically stressful part of labor. Therefore, every effort should be made to ensure that women use nondirected spontaneous pushing to conserve energy and maximize the effect of each bearing-down effort. A woman's bearing-down efforts naturally will become more forceful and frequent as the second stage progresses to birth (Simpson et al., 2008).

A woman may reach the second stage of labor and then experience a lack of readiness to complete the process and give birth to her baby. She may have doubts about her readiness to be a mother or may desire to wait for her support person or nurse-midwife or physician to arrive. Fear, anxiety, or embarrassment regarding unfamiliar or painful sensations and behaviors during pushing (e.g., sounds made, passage of stool) may be other inhibiting factors. Fear that the baby will be in danger once it emerges from the protective intrauterine environment also may be present. By recognizing that a woman may experience a need to hold back the birth of her baby, you can address the woman's concerns and effectively coach her during this stage of labor.

To ensure the slow birth of the fetal head, encourage the woman to control the urge to bear down by coaching her to take panting breaths or exhale slowly through pursed lips as the baby's head crowns. At this point the woman needs simple, clear directions from one person. Amnesia between contractions often occurs in the second stage of labor; therefore, you may have to rouse the woman to get her to cooperate in the bearing-down process. Parents who have attended childbirth

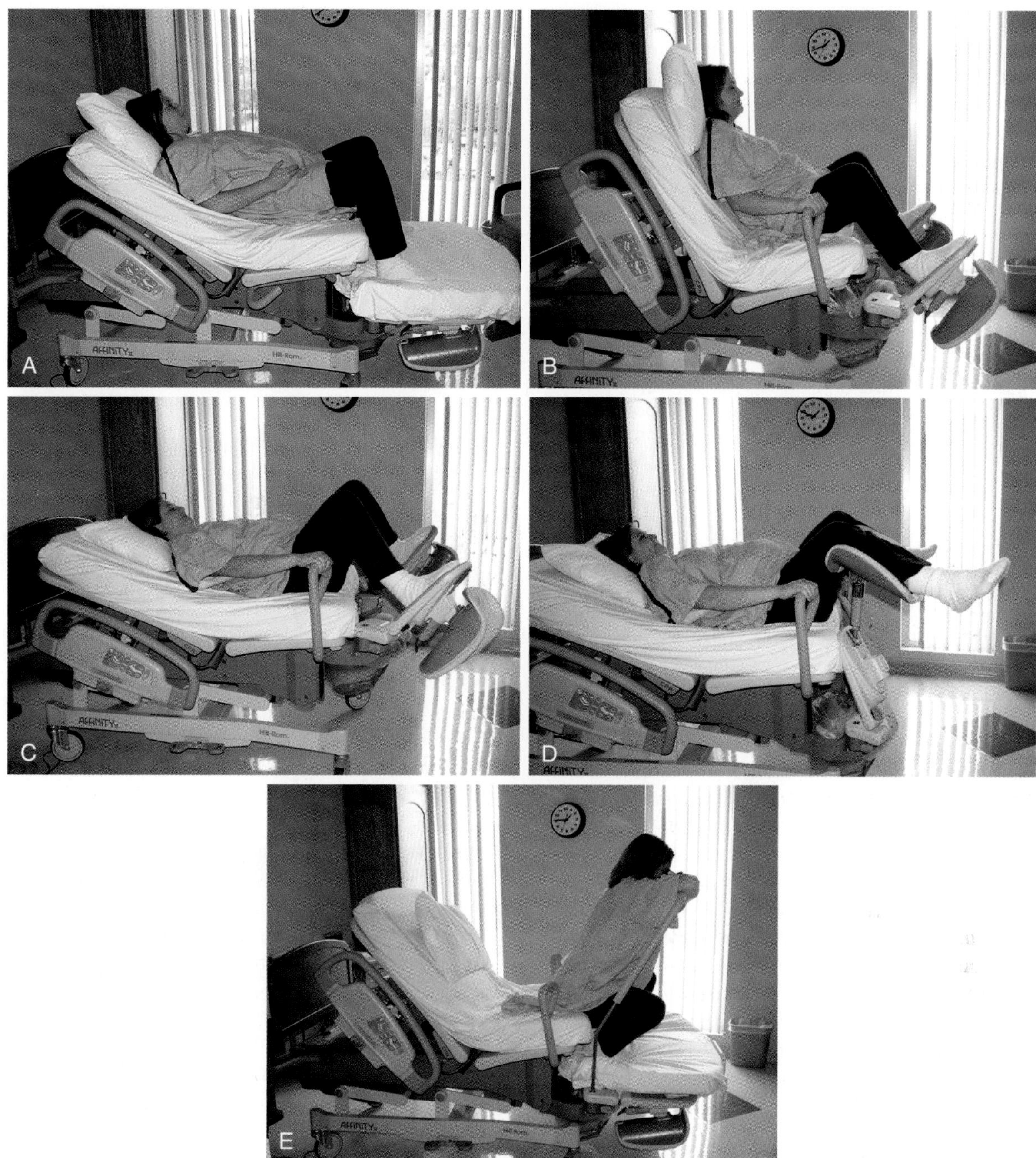

FIG 19-15 The versatility of today's birthing bed makes it practical in a variety of settings. Note: Obstetric (OB) table used for lithotomy position. **A,** Labor bed. **B,** Birth chair. **C,** Birth bed. **D,** OB table. **E,** Squatting or birth bar. (Courtesy Julie Perry Nelson, Loveland, CO.)

education classes may have devised a set of verbal cues for the laboring woman to follow.

Fetal Heart Rate and Pattern

As noted, you must check the fetal heart rate regularly (see Chapter 18 for further discussion). If the baseline rate begins to slow, if absent or minimal variability occurs, or if deceleration patterns (e.g., late, variable, or prolonged decelerations) develop, initiate interventions promptly. Turn the woman onto her side to reduce the pressure of the uterus against the ascending vena cava and descending aorta (see Fig. 19-5). Oxygen can be administered by nonrebreather mask at 10 L/min (Miller et al., 2013). These interventions are often all that is necessary to restore a normal pattern. If the FHR and pattern do not become normal immediately, notify the nurse-midwife or physician because the woman may need medical intervention to give birth. See Chapter 18 for more interventions related to abnormal FHR.

Support of the Father or Partner

During the second stage the woman needs continuous support and coaching (see Table 19-4 and Box 19-10). Because the coaching process is often physically and emotionally tiring for support persons, the nurse offers them nourishment and fluids and encourages them to take short breaks as needed (see Box 19-9). If birth occurs in an LDR or LDRP room, the support person usually wears street clothes. Instruct the support person who attends the birth in a delivery or operating room to put on a cover gown or scrub clothes, mask, hat, and shoe covers, if required by agency policy. The nurse also specifies support measures that can be used for the laboring woman and points out areas of the room in which the partner can move freely.

Encourage partners to be present at the birth of their infants if doing so is in keeping with their cultural and personal expectations and beliefs. The presence of partners maintains the psychologic closeness of the family unit, and the partner can continue to provide the supportive care given during labor. The woman and her partner need to have an equal opportunity to initiate the attachment process with the baby.

LEGAL TIP: Documentation

Documentation of all observations (e.g., maternal vital signs, FHR and pattern, progress of labor) and nursing interventions, including the woman's response, should be done concurrent with care. The course of labor and the maternal-fetal response may change without warning. All documentation must be accurate, complete, timely, and according to agency policy.

Supplies, Instruments, and Equipment

To prepare for birth in any setting, the birthing table is usually set up during the transition phase of first stage labor for nulliparous women and during the active phase for multiparous women.

Prepare the birthing bed or table, and arrange instruments on the instrument table or delivery cart (Fig. 19-17). Follow standard procedures for gloving, identifying and opening sterile packages, adding sterile supplies to the instrument table, unwrapping sterile instruments, and handing them to the nurse-midwife or physician. Ready the crib or radiant warmer and equipment for the support and stabilization of the infant (Fig. 19-18).

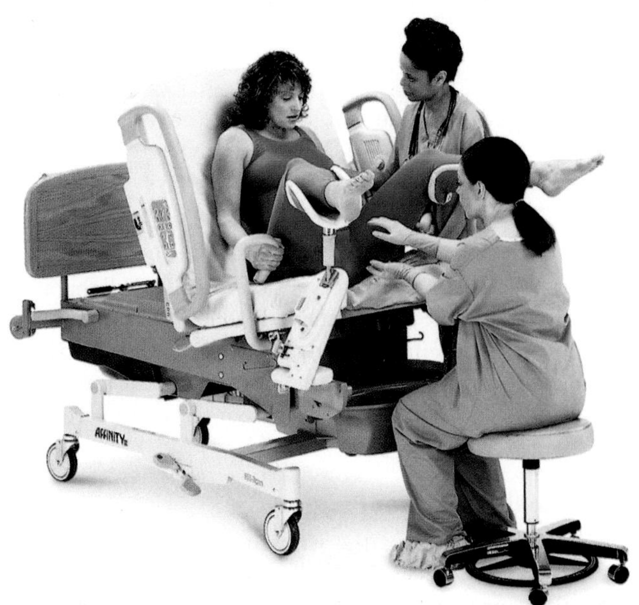

FIG 19-16 Birth bed. (Courtesy Hill-Rom, Batesville, IN.)

The items used for birth may vary among different facilities; therefore, consult each facility's procedure manual to determine the protocols specific to that facility.

The nurse estimates the time until the birth will occur and notifies the nurse-midwife or physician if he or she is not in the woman's room. Even the most experienced nurse can miscalculate the time left before birth occurs; therefore, every nurse who attends a woman in labor must be prepared to assist with an emergency birth if the physician or nurse-midwife is not present (see Box 19-11).

Birth in a Delivery Room or Birthing Room

The woman will need assistance if she must move from the labor bed to the delivery table (Fig. 19-19). The various positions assumed for birth in a delivery room are the Sims or lateral

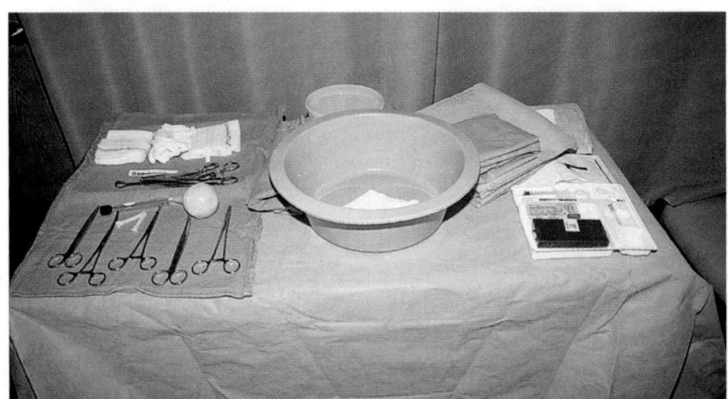

FIG 19-17 Instrument table. (Courtesy Marjorie Pyle, RNC, Lifecircle, Costa Mesa, CA.)

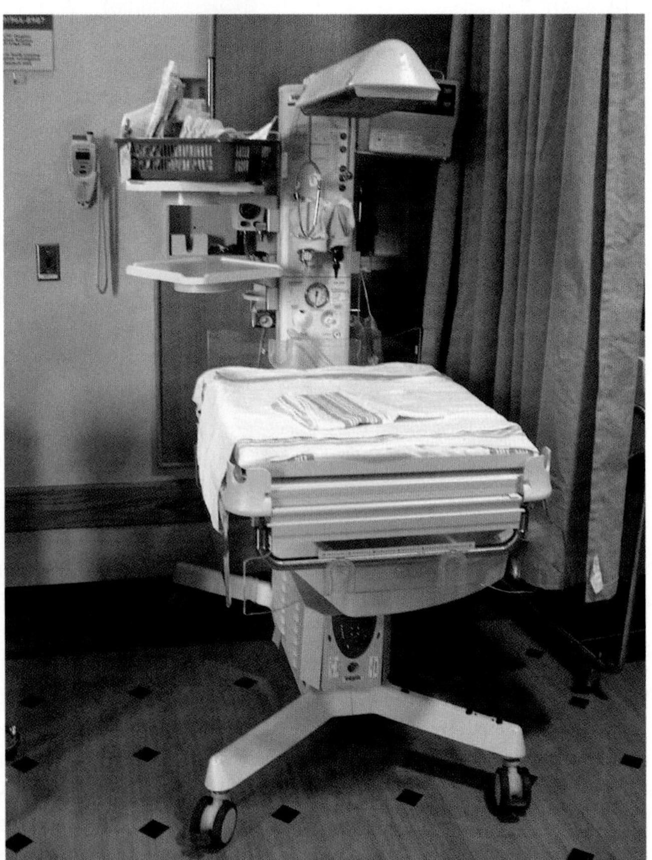

FIG 19-18 Radiant warmer for newborn. (Courtesy Dee Lowdermilk, Chapel Hill, NC.)

position in which the attendant supports the upper part of the woman's leg, the dorsal position (supine position with one hip elevated), and the lithotomy position.

The lithotomy position makes dealing with some complications that arise more convenient for the nurse-midwife or physician (see Fig. 19-15, *D*). To place the woman in this position, bring her buttocks to the edge of the bed or table and place her legs in stirrups. Take care to pad the stirrups, to raise and place both legs simultaneously, and to adjust the shanks of the stirrups so that the calves of the legs are supported. No pressure should be placed on the popliteal space. Stirrups that are not the same height will strain ligaments in the woman's back as she bears down, leading to considerable discomfort in the postpartum period. The lower portion of the table may be dropped down and rolled back under the table.

The maternal position for birth in a birthing room varies from a lithotomy position with the woman's feet in stirrups or resting on footrests or with her legs held and supported by the nurse or support person, to one in which her feet rest on footrests while she holds on to a squat bar, to a side-lying position with the woman's upper leg supported by the coach, nurse, or squat bar. Once the woman is positioned, the foot of the bed is removed so that the nurse-midwife or physician attending the birth can gain better perineal access for performing an episiotomy, delivering a large baby, using forceps or vacuum extractor, or getting access to the emerging head to facilitate suctioning. Alternately, the foot of the bed can be left in place and lowered slightly to form a ledge that allows access for birth and serves as a place to lay the newborn (see Fig. 19-15, *A*).

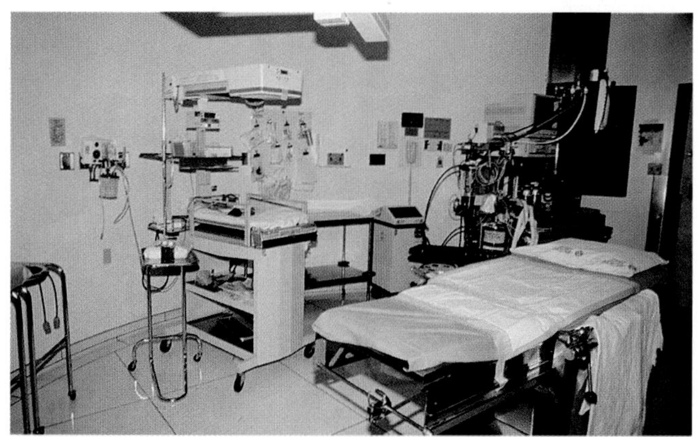

FIG 19-19 Delivery room. (Courtesy Michael S. Clement, MD, Mesa, AZ.)

Once the woman is positioned for birth either in a delivery room or birthing room, the vulva and perineum are cleansed. Hospital or birthing center protocols and the preferences of nurse-midwives or physicians for cleansing may vary.

The nurse continues to coach and encourage the woman and monitor the fetal status. Keep the nurse-midwife or physician informed of the FHR and pattern. Prepare or obtain an oxytocic medication such as oxytocin (Pitocin) so that it is ready to be administered immediately after expulsion of the placenta. Always follow Standard Precautions as care is administered during the process of labor and birth (see Box 19-4).

In the hospital delivery room, the nurse-midwife or physician may put on a cap, a mask that has a shield or protective eyewear, and shoe covers. After washing hands, the provider puts on a sterile gown (with waterproof front and sleeves) and sterile gloves. Nurses attending the birth also may need to wear caps, protective eyewear, masks, gowns, and gloves. The woman may then be draped with sterile drapes. In the birthing room, Standard Precautions are observed, but the amount and types of protective coverings worn by those in attendance may vary.

Maintain contact with the parents by touching, verbal comforting, describing progress, explaining the reasons for care, and sharing in the parents' joy at the birth of their baby.

Mechanism of Birth: Vertex Presentation. The three phases of the spontaneous birth of a fetus in a vertex presentation are (1) birth of the head, (2) birth of the shoulders, and (3) birth of the body and extremities (see Chapter 16).

With voluntary bearing-down efforts, the head appears at the introitus (Fig. 19-20, *A* to *D*). Crowning occurs when the widest part of the head (the biparietal diameter) distends the vulva just before birth. Immediately before birth, the perineal musculature becomes greatly distended. If an episiotomy (incision into the perineum to enlarge the vaginal outlet) is necessary, it is done at this time to minimize soft-tissue damage. A local anesthetic may be administered if necessary before performing an episiotomy. Box 19-12 shows the process of normal vaginal childbirth using a series of photographs.

The physician or nurse-midwife may use a hands-on approach to control the birth of the head, believing that guarding the perineum results in a gradual birth that will prevent fetal intracranial injury, protect maternal tissues, and reduce

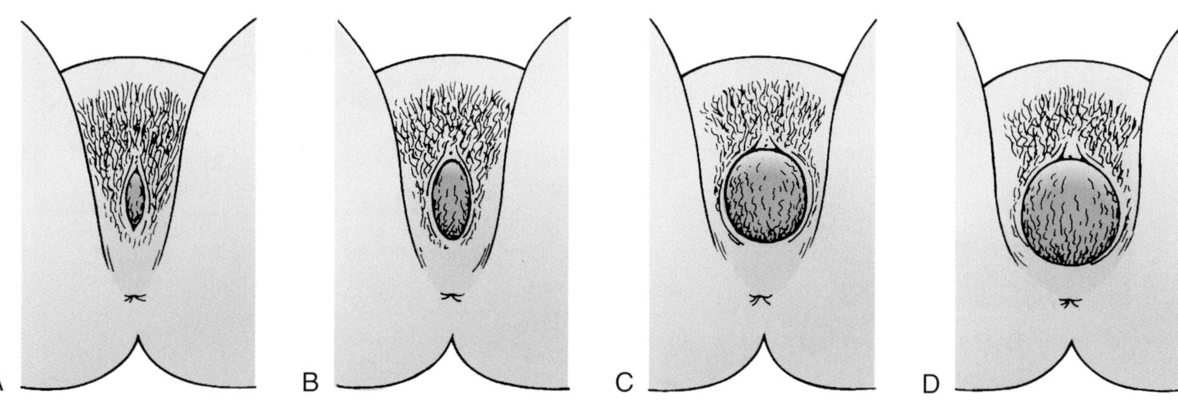

FIG 19-20 Beginning birth with vertex presenting. **A,** Anteroposterior slit. **B,** Oval opening. **C,** Circular shape. **D,** Crowning.

BOX 19-12 Normal Vaginal Childbirth

First Stage

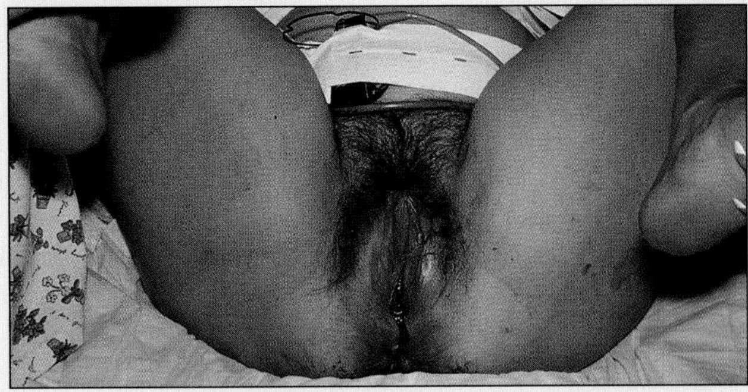

Anteroposterior slit. Vertex visible during contraction.

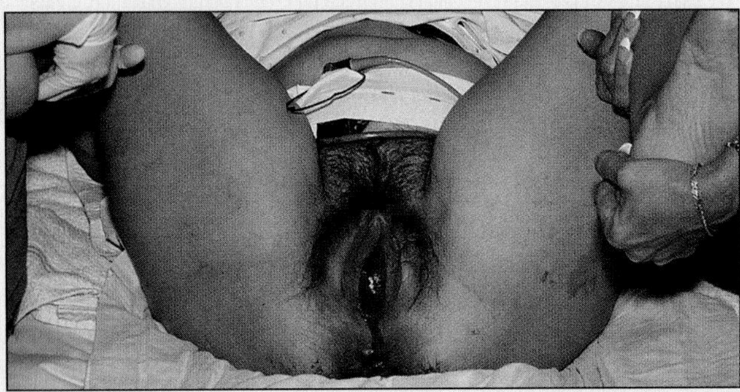

Oval opening. Vertex presenting. NOTE: Nurse *(on left)* is wearing gloves, but support person *(on right)* is not.

Second Stage

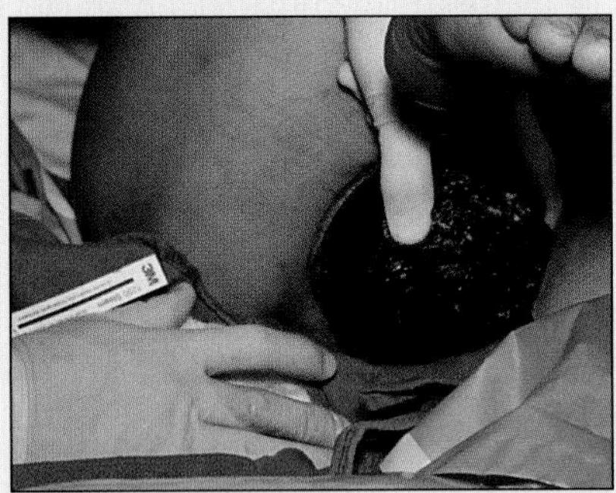

Crowning.

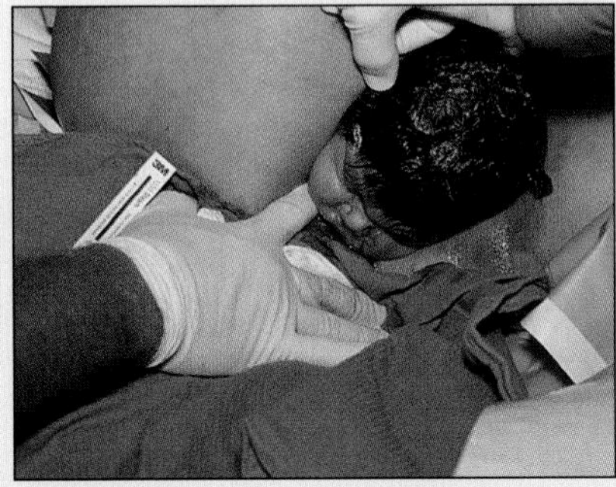

Nurse-midwife using Ritgen maneuver as head is born by extension.

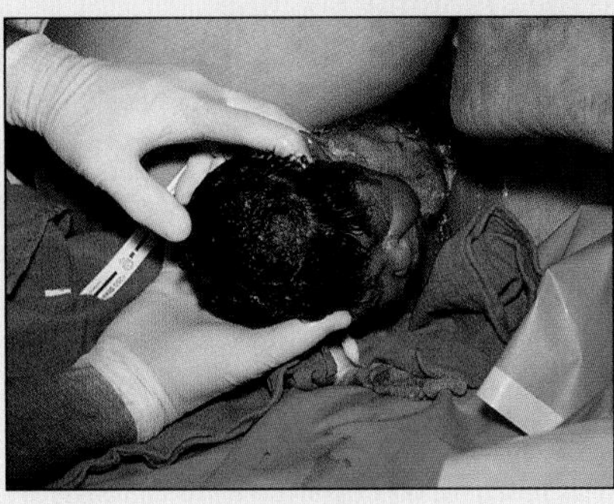

After nurse-midwife checks for nuchal cord, she supports head during external rotation and restitution.

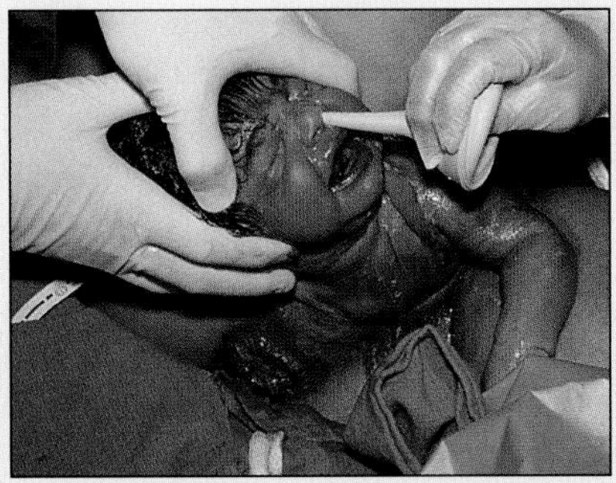

Use of bulb syringe to suction mucus.

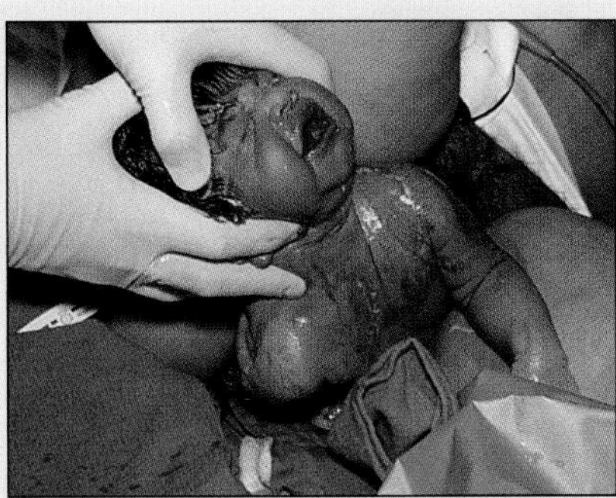

Birth of posterior shoulder.

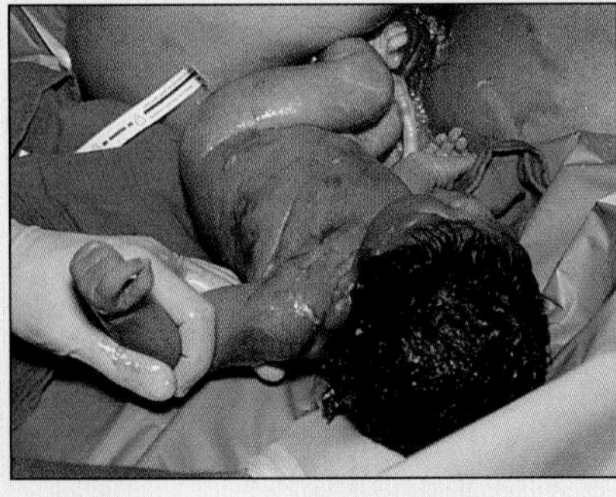

Birth of newborn by slow expulsion.

BOX 19-12 **Normal Vaginal Childbirth—cont'd**

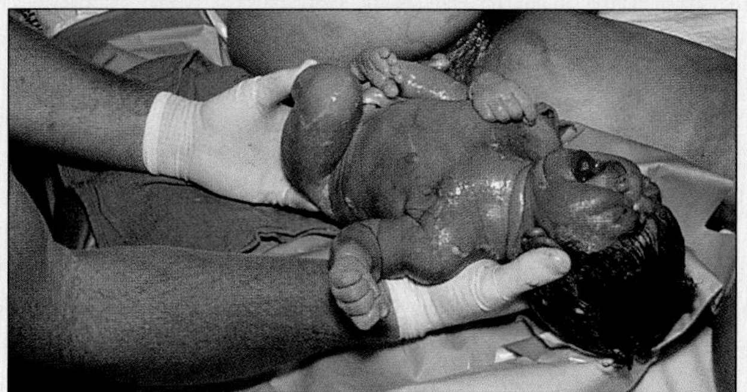

Second stage complete. Note that newborn is not completely pink yet.

Third Stage

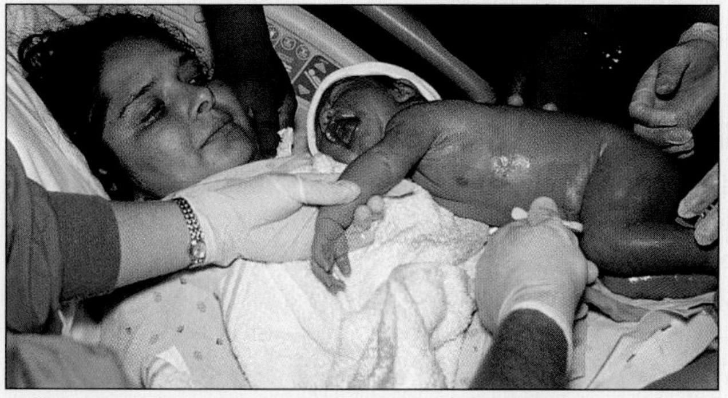

Newborn placed on mother's abdomen while cord is clamped and cut.

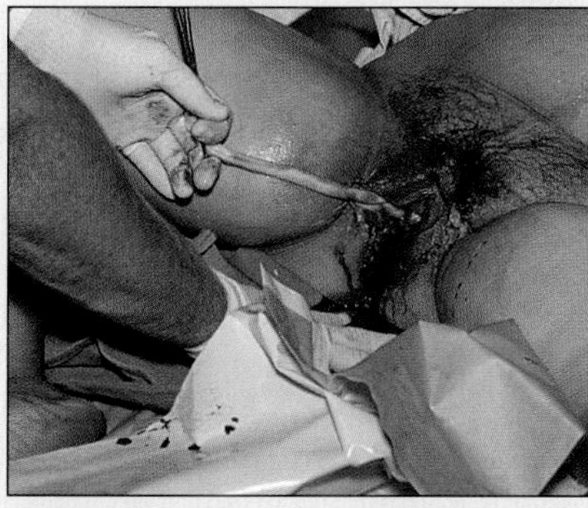

Note increased bleeding as placenta separates.

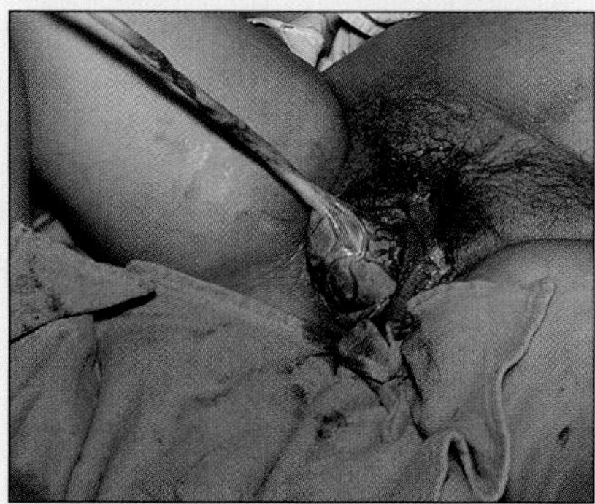

Expulsion of placenta.

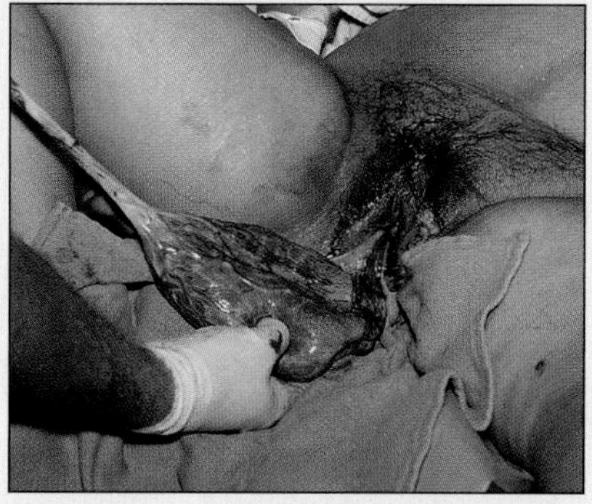

Expulsion is complete, marking the end of the third stage.

The Newborn

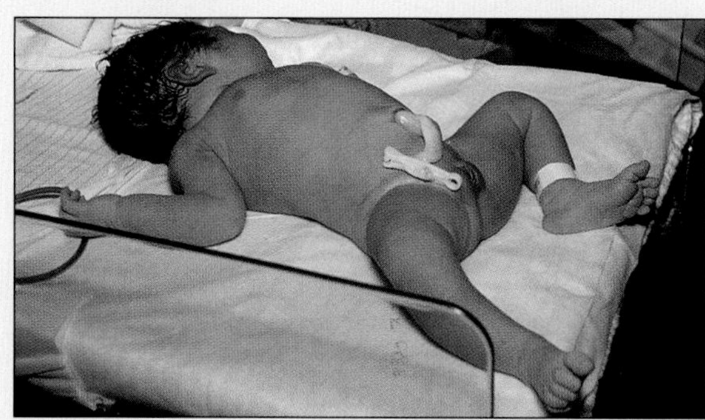

Newborn awaiting assessment. Note that color is almost completely pink.

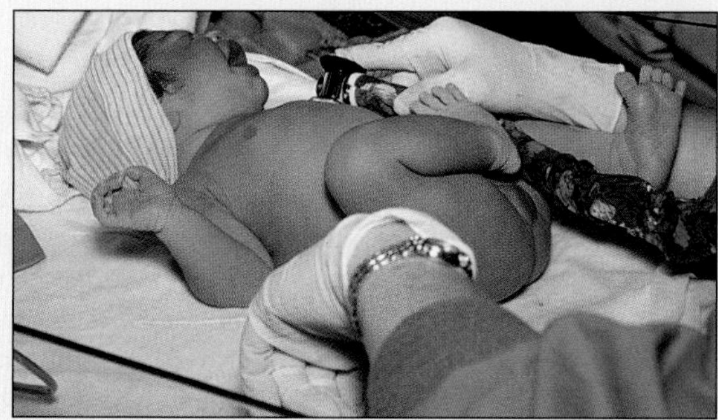

Newborn assessment under radiant warmer.

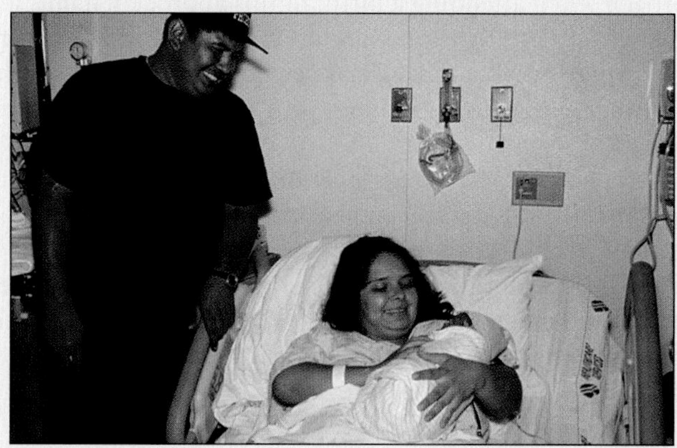

Parents admiring their newborn.

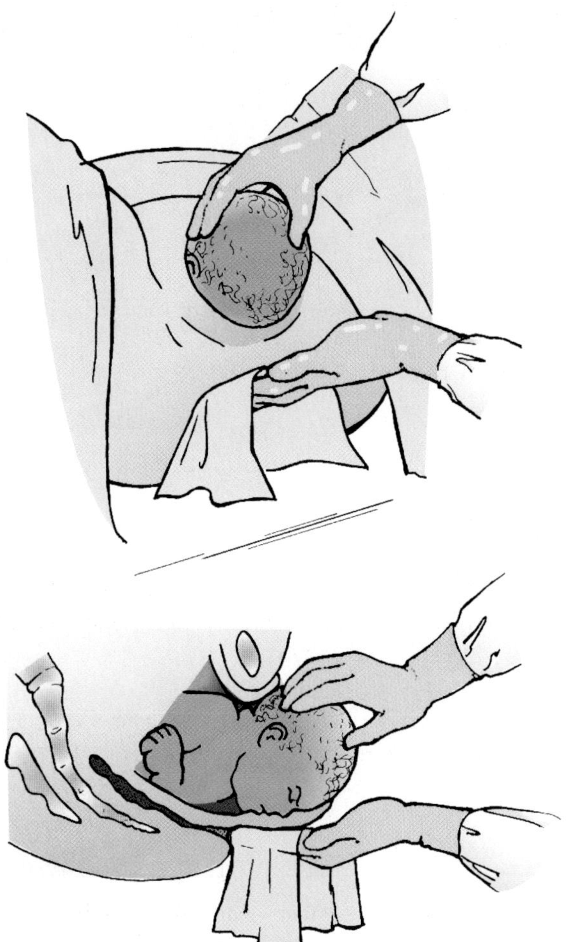

FIG 19-21 Birth of head with modified Ritgen maneuver. Note control to prevent too-rapid birth of head.

postpartum perineal pain. This approach involves (1) applying pressure against the rectum, drawing it downward to aid in flexing the head as the back of the neck catches under the symphysis pubis; (2) applying upward pressure from the coccygeal region (modified *Ritgen maneuver*) (Fig. 19-21) to extend the head during the actual birth, thereby protecting the musculature of the perineum; and (3) assisting the mother with voluntary control of the bearing-down efforts by coaching her to pant while letting uterine forces expel the fetus.

Some health care providers use a hands-poised (hands-off) approach when attending a birth. In this approach, hands are prepared to place light pressure on the fetal head to prevent rapid expulsion. The provider does not place hands on the perineum or use them to assist with birth of the shoulders and body.

The hands-on and hands-poised approaches have similar results in terms of perineal and vaginal tears, but the hands-on technique is associated with a higher incidence of third-degree tears and episiotomies. In one study the hands-poised approach resulted in fewer third-degree tears (Berghella et al., 2008). However, the hands-on approach may result in less perineal pain.

The umbilical cord often encircles the neck (nuchal cord) but rarely so tightly as to cause hypoxia. After the head is born, gentle palpation is used to feel for the cord. If present, the health care provider slips the cord gently over the head if possible. If the loop is tight or if there is a second loop, he or she will probably clamp the cord twice, cut between the clamps, and unwind the cord from around the neck before the birth is allowed to continue. Mucus, blood, or meconium in the nasal or oral passages may prevent the newborn from breathing. To eliminate this problem, moist gauze sponges are used to wipe the nose and mouth. A bulb syringe may be inserted first into the mouth and oropharynx and then into both nares to aspirate contents.

Fundal Pressure. Fundal pressure is the application of gentle, steady pressure against the fundus of the uterus to facilitate the vaginal birth. Use of fundal pressure by nurses is *not* advised because there is no standard technique available for this maneuver. Historically it has been used when the administration of analgesia and anesthesia decreased the woman's ability to push during the birth, in cases of shoulder dystocia, and when second-stage fetal bradycardia or other abnormal FHR patterns were present. However, no legal, professional, or regulatory standards exist for its use and no evidence related to its effectiveness in facilitating a safe vaginal birth is available (Simpson et al., 2008).

Immediate Assessments and Care of the Newborn

The time of birth is the precise time when the entire body is out of the mother and must be recorded. In the case of multiple births, each birth is noted in the same way. If the newborn's condition is not compromised, he or she should be dried and placed on the mother's abdomen immediately after birth and covered with a warm, dry blanket. The cord may be clamped at this time, and the nurse-midwife or physician may ask if the woman's partner would like to cut the cord. If so, the partner is given a sterile pair of scissors and instructed to cut the cord 1 inch (2.5 cm) above the clamp.

The care given immediately after the birth focuses on assessing and stabilizing the newborn. AWHONN (2010) recommends that at least two nurses be present for each birth. One nurse is responsible for care of the newborn while the other nurse assists the nurse-midwife or physician with delivery of the placenta and care of the mother. The "baby nurse" must watch the infant for any signs of distress and initiate appropriate interventions. AWHONN also recommends that, in cases of multiple births, each baby has his own nurse (AWHONN).

Perform a brief assessment of the newborn immediately while the mother is holding the infant. This assessment includes assigning Apgar scores at 1 and 5 minutes after birth (see Table 24-1). Maintaining a patent airway, supporting respiratory effort, and preventing cold stress by drying and, preferably, covering the newborn with a warmed blanket while on his mother's abdomen skin-to-skin or, less optimally, placing him or her under a radiant warmer are the major priorities in terms of the newborn's immediate care. You can postpone further examination, identification procedures, and care until later in the third stage of labor or early in the fourth stage.

Perineal Trauma Related to Childbirth

Most acute injuries and lacerations of the perineum, vagina, uterus, and their support tissues occur during childbirth. Alternative measures for perineal management, such as application of warm compresses and gentle perineal massage and stretching have been suggested to lessen the degree of perineal lacerations and trauma. Perineal massage during the last month of pregnancy has clear benefits of reducing perineal trauma during birth and pain afterward for women who had not given birth vaginally before. A Cochrane review found that warm compresses during the second stage of labor may be beneficial in reducing the incidence of third- and fourth-degree lacerations (Aasheim, Nilsen, Lukasse, & Reinar, 2011).

Some degree of trauma to the soft tissues of the birth canal and adjacent structures occurs during every birth. The tendency to sustain lacerations varies with each woman; that is, the soft tissue in some women may be less distensible. Damage usually is more pronounced in nulliparous women because the tissues are firmer and more resistant than are those in multiparous women. Heredity is also a factor. For example, the tissue of light-skinned women, especially those with reddish hair, is not as readily distensible as that of darker-skinned women, and healing may be less efficient. Other risk factors associated with perineal trauma include maternal nutritional status, birth position, pelvic anatomy (e.g., narrow subpubic arch with a constricted outlet), fetal malpresentation and position (e.g., breech, occiput posterior position), large (macrosomic) infants, use of forceps or vacuum to facilitate birth, prolonged second-stage labor, and rapid labor in which there is insufficient time for the perineum to stretch.

Some injuries to the supporting tissues, whether they are acute or nonacute and whether they were repaired or not, may lead to genitourinary and sexual problems later in life (e.g., pelvic relaxation, uterine prolapse, cystocele, rectocele, dyspareunia, urinary and bowel dysfunction) (see Chapter 11). Performing Kegel exercises in the prenatal and postpartum periods improves and restores the tone and strength of the perineal muscles (see Chapter 4, Teaching for Self-Management box: Kegel Exercises). Health practices, including good nutrition and appropriate hygienic measures, help maintain the integrity and suppleness of the perineal tissues, enhance healing, and prevent infection.

Perineal Lacerations. Perineal lacerations usually occur as the fetal head is being born. The extent of the laceration is defined in terms of its depth (Cunningham, Leveno, Bloom, et al., 2014):

First degree: Laceration that extends through the skin and vaginal mucous membrane but not the underlying fascia and muscle

Second degree: Laceration that extends through the fascia and muscles of the perineal body, but not the anal sphincter

Third degree: Laceration that involves the external anal sphincter

Fourth degree: Laceration that extends completely through the rectal mucosa, disrupting both the external and internal anal sphincters

Perineal injury often is accompanied by small lacerations on the medial surfaces of the labia minora below the pubic rami and to the sides of the urethra (periurethral) and clitoris. Lacerations in this highly vascular area often result in profuse bleeding. Third- and fourth-degree lacerations must be carefully repaired so that the woman retains fecal continence. Simple perineal injuries usually heal without permanent disability, regardless of whether they were repaired. However, repairing a new perineal injury to prevent future complications is easier than correcting long-term damage.

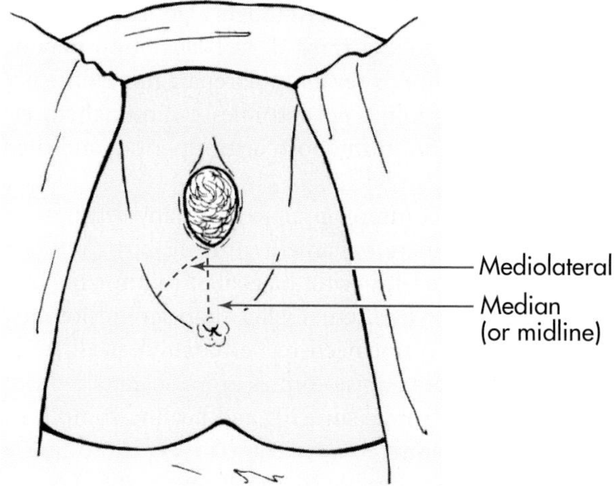

FIG 19-22 Types of episiotomies.

Vaginal and Urethral Lacerations. Vaginal lacerations often occur in conjunction with perineal lacerations. Vaginal lacerations tend to extend up the lateral walls (sulci) and, if deep enough, involve the levator ani muscle. Additional injury may occur high in the vaginal vault near the level of the ischial spines. Vaginal vault lacerations are often circular and may result from use of forceps to rotate the fetal head, rapid fetal descent, or precipitous birth.

Cervical Injuries. Cervical injuries occur when the cervix retracts over the advancing fetal head. These cervical lacerations occur at the lateral angles of the external os. Most lacerations are shallow and bleeding is minimal. Larger lacerations may extend to the vaginal vault or beyond it into the lower uterine segment; serious bleeding may occur. Extensive lacerations may follow hasty attempts to enlarge the cervical opening artificially or to deliver the fetus before full cervical dilation is achieved. Injuries to the cervix can have adverse effects on future pregnancies and childbirths.

Episiotomy. An episiotomy is an incision in the perineum used to enlarge the vaginal outlet (Fig. 19-22). Its use has steadily declined in recent years due to a lack of sound, rigorous research to support its benefits. Episiotomies are performed in approximately 10% of births in the United States (Martin, Hamilton, Ventura, et al., 2011). This practice is even less common in Europe and Canada, probably because of the more routine use in those countries of the side-lying position for birth. This position places less tension on the perineum, making possible a gradual stretching of the perineum with fewer indications for episiotomy. Whenever possible, giving birth over an intact perineum provides the best outcomes (e.g., less blood loss, less risk of infection, and less postpartum pain).

Different types of episiotomies may be performed, classified by the site and direction of the incision (see Fig. 19-22); the type that provides the best outcome is unknown (Berghella et al., 2008). Midline (median) episiotomy is most commonly used in the United States. It is effective, easily repaired, and generally the least painful. However, midline episiotomies also are associated with a higher incidence of third- and fourth-degree lacerations (Cunningham et al., 2014). Sphincter tone is usually restored after primary healing and a good repair. Mediolateral episiotomy is used in operative births when the need for posterior extension is likely. Although a fourth-degree laceration may be prevented, a third-degree laceration may occur. The blood loss is also greater and the repair more difficult and painful than with midline episiotomies (Cunningham et al.). It is also more painful in the postpartum period, and the pain lasts longer.

An increasingly common practice in many settings now is to support the perineum manually during birth rather than performing an episiotomy with the goal of minimizing trauma. If tears occur, they are often smaller than an episiotomy, are repaired easily or do not need to be repaired at all, and heal quickly with less pain. Episiotomies are associated with more posterior perineal trauma, suturing and healing complications, and later pain with intercourse. Therefore, episiotomy should be avoided whenever possible (Berghella et al., 2008).

THIRD STAGE OF LABOR

The third stage of labor lasts from the birth of the baby until the placenta is expelled.

CARE MANAGEMENT

The goal in the management of the third stage of labor is the prompt separation and expulsion of the placenta, achieved in the easiest, safest manner. The third stage is generally by far the shortest stage of labor. The placenta is usually expelled within 10 to 15 minutes after the birth of the baby. If the third stage has not been completed within 30 minutes, the placenta is considered to be retained and interventions to hasten its separation and expulsion are usually instituted (Wing & Farinelli, 2012).

Under normal circumstances the placenta is attached to the decidual layer of the basal plate's thin endometrium by numerous fibrous anchor villi—much in the same way a postage stamp is attached to a sheet of postage stamps. After the birth of the fetus, strong uterine contractions and the sudden decrease in uterine size cause the placental site to shrink. This causes the anchor villi to break and the placenta to separate from its attachments. Normally the first few strong contractions that occur after the baby's birth cause the placenta to shear away from the basal plate. A placenta cannot detach itself from a flaccid (relaxed) uterus because the placental site is not reduced in size.

Placental Separation and Expulsion

Depending on preference, the nurse-midwife or physician may use either a passive or an active approach to manage the third stage of labor. Passive management involves patiently watching for signs that the placenta has separated from the uterine wall spontaneously and monitoring for spontaneous expulsion. This approach is commonly practiced in the United States (Burke, 2010). Active management of third-stage labor is practiced in many countries around the world. Components of active management include administering an oxytocic medication (e.g., oxytocin [Pitocin]) when the anterior shoulder is birthed or immediately following the birth of the fetus, clamping and cutting the umbilical cord within 3 minutes after birth, and gently controlling cord traction following uterine contraction and separation of the placenta. Evidence-based literature and the World Health Organization now recommend active management of the third stage of labor because its use decreases the rate of postpartum hemorrhage caused by uterine atony (Burke, 2010; Cunningham et al., 2014).

To assist in the delivery of the placenta, the woman is instructed to push when signs of separation have occurred (Fig. 19-23). If possible, the woman should expel the placenta during a uterine contraction. Alternate compression and elevation of the fundus along with minimal, controlled traction on the umbilical cord may also be used to facilitate delivery of the placenta and amniotic membranes. Oxytocics are usually administered after the placenta is removed when active management of third stage labor is not implemented because they stimulate the uterus to contract, thereby helping to prevent hemorrhage (Box 19-13).

Whether the placenta first appears by its shiny fetal surface (Schultze mechanism) or turns to show its dark roughened maternal surface first (Duncan mechanism) is of no clinical importance.

After the placenta and the amniotic membranes emerge, the nurse-midwife or physician examines them for intactness to ensure that no portion remains in the uterine cavity (i.e., no fragments of the placenta or membranes are retained) (Fig. 19-24). At this time the nurse will obtain a sample of blood from the umbilical cord to be used for determining the baby's blood type and Rh status. Some parents will also have made arrangements to have blood from the cord collected for storage and possible future use.

When the third stage of labor has been completed the nurse-midwife or physician examines the woman for any perineal, vaginal, or cervical lacerations requiring repair. The nurse may need to assist by providing adequate lighting or exposure of the woman's perineum and vagina so that a thorough examination can be performed. If an episiotomy was performed, it will be sutured. Immediate repair promotes healing, limits residual damage, and decreases the possibility of infection. The woman usually feels some discomfort while the nurse-midwife or physician carries out the postbirth vaginal examination. Help the woman to use breathing and relaxation or distraction techniques to assist her in dealing with the discomfort. During this time the "baby nurse" performs a quick assessment of the newborn's physical condition and places matching identification bands on baby and mother. Weighing the baby, eye prophylaxis, and a vitamin K injection can be delayed until after the initial bonding time with the parents.

After any necessary repairs have been completed, cleanse the vulvar area gently with warm water or normal saline, and apply a perineal pad or an ice pack to the perineum. Reposition the birthing bed or table, and lower the woman's legs simultaneously from the stirrups if she gave birth in a lithotomy position. Remove any drapes, and place dry linen under the woman's buttocks. Provide her with a clean gown and a blanket, which is warmed, if needed.

Some women and their families may have culturally based beliefs regarding the care of the placenta and the manner of its disposal after birth, viewing the care and disposal of the placenta as a way of protecting the newborn from bad luck and illness. In Spanish the placenta is referred to as *el compañero* or "the companion" of the child (Callister, 2014). A request by the woman to take the placenta home and dispose of it according to her

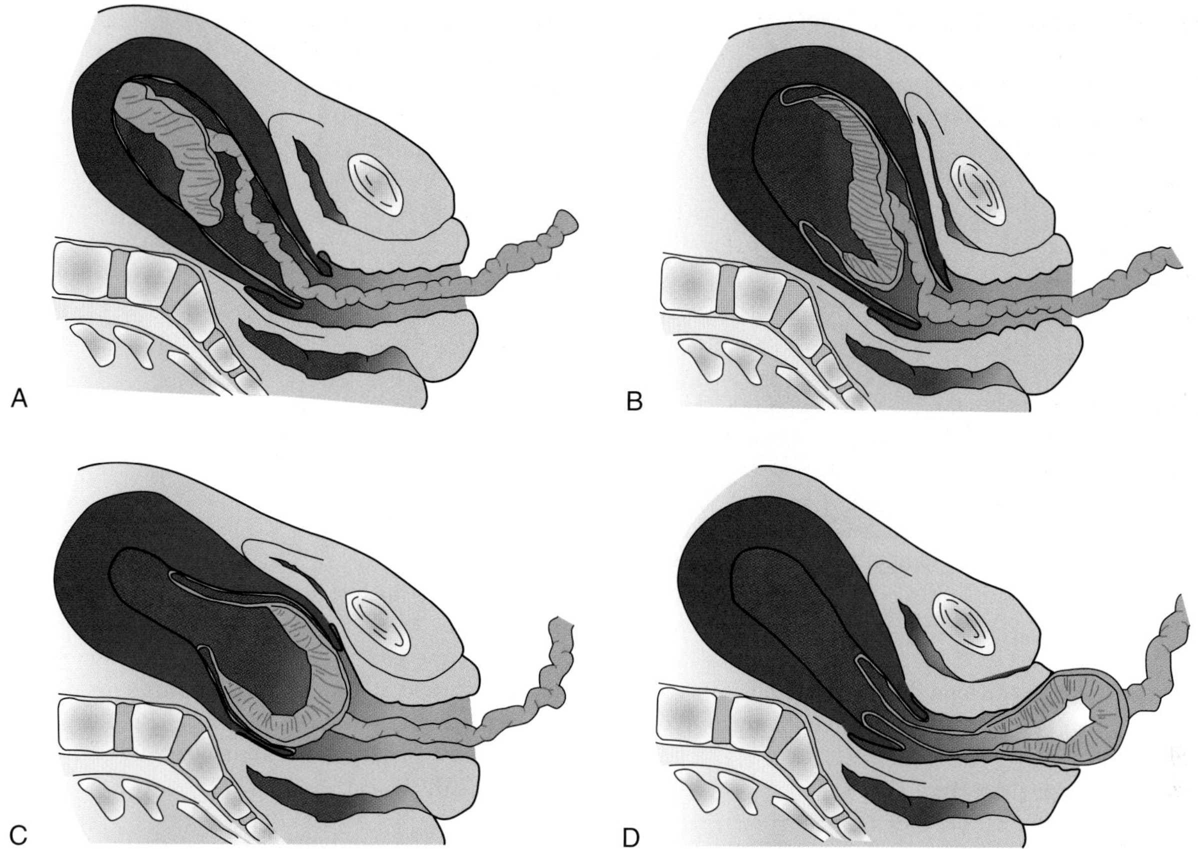

FIG 19-23 Third stage of labor. **A,** Placenta begins to separate in central portion, accompanied by retroplacental bleeding. Uterus changes from discoid to globular shape. **B,** Placenta completes separation and enters lower uterine segment. Uterus has globular shape. **C,** Placenta enters vagina, cord is seen to lengthen, and there may be an increase in bleeding. **D,** Expulsion (delivery) of placenta and completion of third stage.

BOX 19-13 Nursing Care in Third-Stage Labor

Assessment

Signs That Suggest the Onset of the Third Stage

A firmly contracting fundus

A change in the uterus from a discoid to a globular ovoid shape as the placenta moves into the lower uterine segment

A sudden gush of dark blood from the introitus

Apparent lengthening of the umbilical cord as the placenta descends to the introitus

The finding of vaginal fullness (the placenta) on vaginal or rectal examination or of fetal membranes at the introitus

Physical Assessment

Assess every 15 minutes: maternal blood pressure, pulse, and respirations.

Assess for signs of placental separation and amount of bleeding.

Assist with determination of Apgar score at 1 and 5 minutes after birth (see Table 24-1).

Assess maternal and paternal response to completion of childbirth process and their reaction to the newborn.

Interventions

Assist to bear down to facilitate expulsion of the separated placenta.

Administer an oxytocic medication as ordered to ensure adequate contraction of the uterus, thereby preventing hemorrhage.

Provide nonpharmacologic and pharmacologic comfort and pain relief measures.

Perform hygienic cleansing measures.

Keep mother/partner informed of progress of placental separation and expulsion and perineal repair if appropriate.

Explain purpose of medications administered.

Introduce parents to their baby and facilitate the attachment process by delaying eye prophylaxis; wrap mother and baby together for skin-to-skin contact.

Provide private time for parents to bond with new baby; help them create memories.

Encourage breastfeeding if desired.

customs sometimes conflicts with health care agency policies, especially those related to infection control and the disposal of biologic wastes. Many cultures follow specific rules regarding the disposal of the placenta in terms of method (burning, drying, burying, eating), site for disposal (in or near the home), and timing of disposal (immediately after birth, time of day, astrologic signs). Disposal rituals may vary according to the gender of the child and the length of time before another child is desired. Some cultures believe that eating the placenta is a means of restoring a woman's well-being after birth or ensuring high-quality breast milk. Health care providers can provide culturally sensitive health care by encouraging women and their families to express

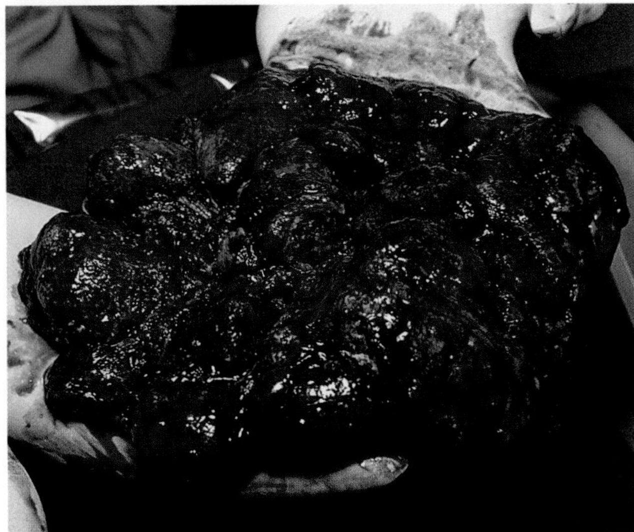

FIG 19-24 Examination of the placenta. (Courtesy Michael S. Clement, MD, Mesa, AZ.)

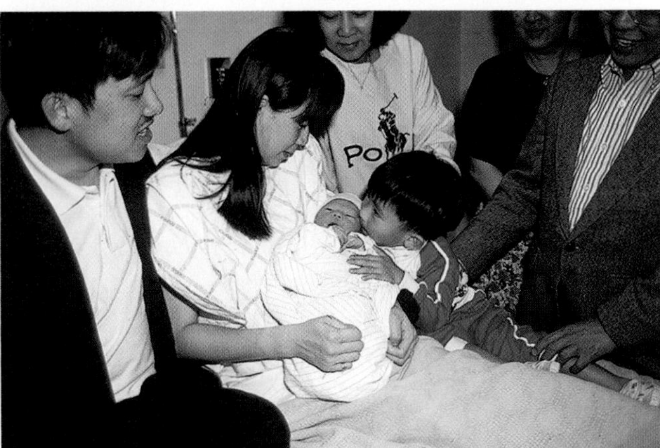

FIG 19-25 Big brother becomes acquainted with new baby sister. (Courtesy Marjorie Pyle, RNC, Lifecircle, Costa Mesa, CA.)

their wishes regarding the care and disposal of the placenta and by establishing a policy to fulfill these requests (D'Avanzo, 2008).

FOURTH STAGE OF LABOR

The first 1 to 2 hours after birth, sometimes called the fourth stage of labor, is a crucial time for mother and newborn. Both are not only recovering from the physical process of birth but also becoming acquainted with each other and additional family members. During this time maternal organs undergo their initial readjustment to the nonpregnant state, and the functions of body systems begin to stabilize.

CARE MANAGEMENT

In most hospitals the mother remains in the labor and birth area during this recovery time. In an institution where LDR rooms are used, the woman stays in the same room where she gave birth. In traditional settings women are taken from the delivery room to a separate recovery area for observation. Arrangements for care of the newborn vary during the fourth stage of labor. In many settings the baby remains with the mother, and the labor or birth nurse cares for both of them. In other institutions the baby is taken to the nursery for several hours of observation after an initial bonding period with the parents, siblings, and perhaps other family members (Fig. 19-25).

Assessment

If the recovery nurse has not previously cared for the new mother, he or she begins with an oral report from the nurse who attended the woman during labor and birth and a review of the prenatal, labor, and birth records. Of primary importance are conditions that could predispose the mother to hemorrhage, such as precipitous labor, a large baby, grand multiparity (i.e., having given birth to five or more viable infants), or induced labor. For healthy women, hemorrhage is the most dangerous potential complication during the fourth stage of labor.

During the fourth stage of labor the mother is assessed frequently (Box 19-14). The American Academy of Pediatrics (AAP) and the ACOG recommend that blood pressure and pulse be assessed at least every 15 minutes for the first 2 hours after birth. Temperature should be assessed every 4 hours for the first 8 hours after birth and then at least every 8 hours (AAP & ACOG, 2012).

Postanesthesia Recovery

The woman who has given birth by cesarean or has received regional anesthesia for a vaginal birth requires special attention during the recovery period. Obstetric recovery areas are held to the same standard of care that would be expected of any other postanesthesia recovery (PAR) unit (AAP & ACOG, 2012). A PAR score is determined for each woman on arrival and is updated as part of every 15-minute assessment. Components of the PAR score include activity, respirations, blood pressure, level of consciousness, and color.

If the woman received general anesthesia, she should be awake and alert and oriented to time, place, and person. Her respiratory rate should be within normal limits, and her oxygen saturation level at least 95%, as measured by a pulse oximeter. If the woman received epidural or spinal anesthesia, she should be able to raise her legs, extended at the knees, off the bed, or flex her knees, place her feet flat on the bed, and raise her buttocks well off the bed. The numb or tingling, prickly sensation should be entirely gone from her legs. The length of time required to recover from regional anesthesia varies greatly. Often it takes several hours for these anesthetic effects to disappear completely.

> **SAFETY ALERT**
>
> Regardless of her obstetric status, no woman should be discharged from the recovery area until she has completely recovered from the effects of anesthesia.

Nursing Interventions

Care of the New Mother

If food and fluids were restricted, especially if excessive fluid loss occurred during labor and birth (blood, perspiration, or

BOX 19-14 Assessment During the Fourth Stage of Labor

Blood Pressure
- Measure blood pressure every 15 minutes for the first 2 hours.

Pulse
- Assess rate and regularity. Measure every 15 minutes for the first 2 hours.

Temperature
- Determine temperature at the beginning of the recovery period. Temperature should then be assessed every 4 hours for the first 8 hours after birth and then at least every 8 hours.

Fundus
- Position woman with knees flexed and head flat.
- Just below umbilicus, cup hand and press firmly into abdomen. At the same time, stabilize the uterus at the symphysis with the opposite hand (see Fig. 20-1).
- If fundus is firm (and bladder is empty), with uterus in midline, measure its position relative to woman's umbilicus. Lay fingers flat on abdomen under umbilicus; measure how many fingerbreadths (fb) or centimeters (cm) fit between umbilicus and top of fundus. Fundal height is documented according to agency guidelines. For example, if the fundus is 1 fb or 1 cm above the umbilicus, fundal height may be recorded as either +1, u+1, or 1/u. If the fundus is 1 fb or 1 cm below the umbilicus, fundal height may be recorded as either −1, u−1, or u/1.
- If fundus is not firm, massage it gently to contract and expel any clots before measuring distance from umbilicus.
- Place hands appropriately; massage gently only until firm.
- Expel clots while keeping hands placed as in Figure 20-1. With upper hand, firmly apply pressure downward toward vagina; observe perineum for amount and size of expelled clots.

Bladder
- Assess distention by noting location and firmness of uterine fundus and by observing and palpating bladder. A distended bladder is seen as a suprapubic rounded bulge that is dull to percussion and fluctuates like a water-filled balloon. When the bladder is distended, the uterus is usually boggy in consistency, well above the umbilicus, and to the woman's right side.
- Assist woman to void spontaneously. Measure amount of urine voided.
- Catheterize as necessary.
- Reassess after voiding or catheterization to make sure the bladder is not palpable and the fundus is firm and in the midline.

Lochia
- Observe lochia on perineal pads and on linen under the mother's buttocks. Determine amount and color; note size and number of clots; note odor.
- Observe perineum for source of bleeding (e.g., episiotomy, lacerations).

Perineum
- Ask or assist woman to turn onto her side and flex upper leg on hip.
- Lift upper buttock.
- Observe perineum in good lighting.
- Assess episiotomy or laceration repair for redness (erythema), edema, ecchymosis (bruising), drainage, and approximation (REEDA).
- Assess for presence of hemorrhoids.

emesis), the woman will be very hungry and thirsty soon after birth. In the absence of complications, a woman who has given birth vaginally may have fluids and a regular diet as soon as she desires (AAP & ACOG, 2012). In the immediate postpartum period, women who give birth by cesarean are usually restricted to clear liquids and ice chips.

As soon as they have had a chance to bond with the baby and eat, most new mothers are ready for a nap or at least a quiet period of rest. Following this rest period, the woman may want to shower and change clothes. Most new mothers are capable of self-management or are assisted in these activities by family members or support persons.

Care of the Family

Most parents enjoy being able to hold, explore, and examine the baby immediately after birth. Both parents can assist with thoroughly drying the infant. Usually the infant is wrapped in a receiving blanket and given to the mother or father/partner to hold. Skin-to-skin contact is encouraged. The nurse places the unwrapped infant on the woman's chest or abdomen and then covers the baby and mother with a warm blanket. Holding the newborn next to her skin helps the mother maintain the baby's body heat and provides skin-to-skin contact. Stockinette caps are often used to keep the newborn's head warm and prevent heat loss.

Many women wish to begin breastfeeding their newborns at this time to take advantage of the infant's alert state *(first period of reactivity)* and to stimulate the production of oxytocin that promotes contraction of the uterus and prevents hemorrhage. In Baby Friendly hospitals, breastfeeding is initiated within the first hour after birth, and any unnecessary separation of mother and baby is strongly discouraged. However, some women prefer to wait to breastfeed until they have had time to rest. Be aware that in some cultures breastfeeding is not acceptable to some women until the milk comes in. In the Hispanic culture, for example, the colostrum is thought to be bad or old milk (Callister, 2014). Therefore, women may wait several days after giving birth before initiating breastfeeding.

Family-Newborn Relationships. The woman's reaction to the sight of her newborn may range from excited outbursts of laughing, talking, and even crying, to apparent apathy. A polite smile and nod may be her only acknowledgment of the comments of nurses and the nurse-midwife or physician. Occasionally the reaction is one of anger or indifference; the woman turns away from the baby, concentrates on her own pain, and sometimes makes hostile comments. These varied reactions can arise from pleasure, exhaustion, or deep disappointment. When evaluating parent-newborn interactions after birth, the nurse should consider the cultural characteristics of the woman and her family and the expected behaviors of that culture. In some cultures the birth of a male child is preferred, and women may grieve when a female child is born (Callister, 2014).

CLINICAL REASONING CASE STUDY

Encouraging Skin-to-Skin Contact Immediately After Birth

A nurse returning from international travel during which she was able to observe childbirth in different cultures noted that generally babies were cradled naked on the mother's abdomen or chest immediately after birth. She noted that the babies were calm, breastfed readily, and had stable vital signs. She also noted that the nurses respected the time that mothers and babies spent together and delayed any unnecessary interventions until at least an hour after birth.

The nurse approached her unit manager to discuss what she learned regarding how skin-to-skin contact immediately following birth promotes, protects, and supports well-being, attachment, and breastfeeding. The manager expressed great interest, and asked the nurse to present an in-service program for the medical and nursing staff regarding this issue as a first step in implementing skin-to-skin contact. What should this nurse include in her in-service program to convince the medical and nursing staff that there is evidence to support skin-to-skin contact immediately following birth and that delaying unnecessary interventions can be safe and effective for women and their newborns?

1. Evidence—Is there sufficient evidence to support the safety and effectiveness of immediate skin-to-skin contact?
2. Assumptions—What assumptions can be made about the following issues related to skin-to-skin contact?
   a. Benefits of an approach that promotes, protects, and supports skin-to-skin contact
   b. Management approaches that should be emphasized during the labor and birth
   c. Necessity of gaining the support of both the medical and nursing staff to effectively implement this change in practice on the unit.
3. What implications and priorities for nursing care can be drawn at this time?
4. Does the evidence objectively support your conclusion?

Whatever the reaction and its cause, the woman needs continuing acceptance and support from all staff. Make a notation regarding the parents' reaction to the newborn in the recovery record. Assess this reaction by asking yourself such questions as, "How do the parents look?" "What do they say?" "What do they do?" Conduct further assessment of the parent-newborn relationship as you give care during the period of recovery. This assessment is especially important if you notice warning signs (e.g., passive or hostile reactions to the newborn, disappointment with gender or appearance of the newborn, absence of eye contact, or limited interaction of parents with each other) immediately after birth. Nurses should discuss any warning signs with the woman's nurse-midwife or physician.

Siblings, who may have appeared only remotely interested in the final phases of the second stage, tend to experience renewed interest and excitement when the newborn appears. They can be encouraged to hold the baby (see Fig. 19-25).

Parents usually respond to praise of their newborn. Many need to be reassured that the dusky appearance of their baby's hands and feet immediately after birth is normal until circulation is well established. If appropriate, explain the reason for the molding of the newborn's head. Communicate information about hospital routine. Recognize, however, that the cultural background of the parents may influence their expectations regarding the care and handling of their newborn immediately after birth. For example, Korean mothers may believe that the head should not be touched because it is the most sacred part of a person's body. Hispanic mothers may believe that the "evil eye" or too much praise of the baby will cause illness, restlessness, or excessive crying (Callister, 2014). Hospital staff members, by their interest and concern, can provide the environment for making this a satisfying experience for parents, family, and significant others.

KEY POINTS

- The onset of labor may be difficult to determine for both nulliparous and multiparous women.
- The familiar environment of her home is most often the ideal place for a woman during the latent phase of the first stage of labor.
- The nurse assumes much of the responsibility for assessing the progress of labor and for keeping the nurse-midwife or physician informed about that progress and deviations from expected findings.
- The fetal heart rate and pattern reveal the fetal response to the stress of the labor process.
- Assessing the laboring woman's urinary output and bladder is critical to ensure her progress and to prevent bladder injury.
- Regardless of the actual labor and birth experience, the woman's or couple's perception of the birth experience is most likely to be positive when events and performances are consistent with expectations, especially in terms of maintaining control and adequacy of pain relief.
- The woman's level of anxiety may increase when she does not understand what is being said to her about her labor because of the medical terminology used or because of a language barrier.
- Coaching, emotional support, and comfort measures assist the woman to use her energy constructively in relaxing and working with the contractions.
- The progress of labor is enhanced when a woman changes her position frequently during the first stage of labor.
- Doulas provide a continuous, supportive presence during labor that can have a positive effect on the process of childbirth and its outcome.
- The cultural beliefs and practices of a woman and her significant others, including her partner, can have a profound influence on their approach to labor and birth.
- Siblings present for labor and birth need preparation and support for the event.
- Women with a history of sexual abuse often experience profound stress and anxiety during childbirth.
- Inability to palpate the cervix during vaginal examination indicates that complete effacement and full dilation have occurred and is the only certain, objective sign that the second stage has begun.
- Women may have an urge to bear down at various times during labor; for some it may be before the cervix is fully dilated and for others it may not occur until the active phase of the second stage of labor.

KEY POINTS—cont'd

- When encouraged to respond to the rhythmic nature of the second stage of labor, the woman normally changes body positions, bears down spontaneously, and vocalizes (open-glottis pushing) when she perceives the urge to push (Ferguson reflex).
- Women should bear down several times during a contraction using the open-glottis pushing method. They should avoid sustained closed-glottis pushing because this will inhibit oxygen transport to the fetus.
- Nurses can use the role of advocate to prevent routine use of episiotomy and reduce the incidence of lacerations by empowering women to take an active role in their birth and by educating health care providers about approaches to managing childbirth that reduce the incidence of perineal trauma.
- Objective signs indicate that the placenta has separated and is ready to be expelled; excessive traction (pulling) on the umbilical cord before the placenta has separated can result in maternal injury.
- During the fourth stage of labor, the woman's fundal tone, lochial flow, and vital signs should be assessed frequently to ensure that she is physically recovering well after giving birth.
- Most parents and families enjoy being able to hold, explore, and examine the baby immediately after the birth.

REFERENCES

Aasheim, V., Nilsen, A. B., Lukasse, M., & Reinar, L. M. (2011). Perineal techniques during the second stage of labour for reducing perineal trauma. *The Cochrane Database of Systematic Reviews*, 2011, 12, CD006672.

American Academy of Pediatrics (AAP) & American College of Obstetricians and Gynecologists (ACOG). (2012). *Guidelines for perinatal care* (7th ed.). Washington, DC: ACOG.

Arendt, K. W., & Tessmer-Tuck, J. A. (2013). Nonpharmacologic labor analgesia. *Clinics in Perinatology*, *40*(3), 351–371.

Association of Women's Health, Obstetric and Neonatal Nurses (AWHONN). (2011). AWHONN position statement: Nursing support of laboring women. *Journal of Obstetric, Gynecologic, and Neonatal Nursing*, *40*(5), 665–666.

Association of Women's Health, Obstetric and Neonatal Nurses (AWHONN). (2010). *Guidelines for professional registered nurse staffing for perinatal units.* Washington, DC: AWHONN.

Berghella, V., Baxter, J., & Chauhan, S. (2008). Evidence-based labor and delivery management. *American Journal of Obstetrics and Gynecology*, *199*(5), 445–454.

Blackburn, S. T. (2013). *Maternal, fetal, and neonatal physiology: A clinical perspective* (4th ed.). St. Louis: Saunders.

Burke, C. (2010). Active versus expectant management of the third stage of labor and implementation of a protocol. *Journal of Perinatal and Neonatal Nursing*, *24*(3), 215–228.

Burke, C. (2014). Pain in labor: Nonpharmacologic and pharmacologic management. In K. Rice Simpson, & P. Creehan (Eds.), *AWHONN's perinatal nursing* (4th ed.). Philadelphia: Lippincott Williams & Wilkins.

Callister, L. C. (2014). Integrating cultural beliefs and practices when caring for childbearing women and families. In K. Rice Simpson, & P. Creehan (Eds.), *AWHONN's perinatal nursing* (4th ed.). Philadelphia: Lippincott Williams & Wilkins.

Centers for Disease Control and Prevention, Branson, B., Handsfield, H., et al. (2006). Revised recommendations for HIV testing of adults, adolescents, and pregnant women in health-care settings. *MMWR Morbidity and Mortality Weekly Report*, *55*(RR-14), 1–17.

Chang, S. C., Chou, M. M., Lin, K. C., et al. (2011). Effects of a pushing intervention on pain, fatigue and birthing experiences among Taiwanese women during the second stage of labour. *Midwifery*, *27*(6), 825–831.

Cunningham, F., Leveno, K., Bloom, S., et al. (2014). *Williams obstetrics* (24th ed.). New York: McGraw-Hill Education.

D'Avanzo, C. (2008). *Mosby's pocket guide to cultural health assessment* (4th ed.). St. Louis: Mosby.

Gilbert, E. (2011). *Manual of high risk pregnancy & delivery* (5th ed.). St. Louis: Mosby.

Gillesby, E., Burns, S., Dempsey, A., et al. (2010). Comparison of delayed versus immediate pushing during second stage of labor for nulliparous women with epidural anesthesia. *Journal of Obstetric, Gynecologic, and Neonatal Nursing*, *39*(6), 635–644.

Hanson, L. (2009). Second-stage labor care: Challenges in spontaneous bearing down. *Journal of Perinatal and Neonatal Nursing*, *23*(1), 31–39.

Hodnett, E. D., Gates, S., Hofmeyr, G., & Sakala, C. (2013). Continuous support for women during childbirth. *The Cochrane Database of Systematic Reviews*, 2013, 7, CD003766.

James, D. (2011). Routine obstetrical interventions: Research agenda for the next decade. *Journal of Perinatal and Neonatal Nursing*, *25*(2), 148–152.

Johansson, M., Rubertsson, C., Radestad, I., & Hildingsson, I. (2012). Childbirth—An emotionally demanding experience for fathers. *Sexual and Reproductive Healthcare*, *3*(1), 11–20.

Kelly, M., Johnson, E., Lee, V., et al. (2010). Delayed versus immediate pushing in second stage of labor. *MCN: The American Journal of Maternal/Child Nursing*, *35*(2), 81–88.

Lawrence, A., Lewis, L., Hofmeyr, G., & Styles, C. (2013). Mothers' position during the first stage of labour. *The Cochrane Database of Systematic Reviews*, 2013, 2, CD003934.

Martin, J. A., Hamilton, B. E., Ventura, S. J., et al. (2011). Births: Final data for 2009. *National Vital Statistics Reports*, *60*(1), 1–72.

Miller, L. A., Miller, D. A., & Tucker, S. M. (2013). *Mosby's pocket guide to fetal monitoring: A multidisciplinary approach* (7th ed.). St. Louis: Mosby.

Reveiz, L., Gaitan, H., & Cuervo, L. (2013). Enemas during labour. *The Cochrane Database of Systematic Reviews*, 2013, 4, CD000330.

Roberts, J. (2002). The "push" for evidence: Management of the second stage. *Journal of Midwifery & Women's Health*, *47*(1), 2–15.

Sharts-Hopko, N. (2010). Oral intake during labor: A review of the evidence. *MCN: The American Journal of Maternal/Child Nursing*, *35*(4), 197–203.

Simkin, P. (2012). Doulas of North America (DONA) international position paper: The birth doula's contribution to modern maternity care. Available at www.DONA.org.

Simpson, K., & O'Brien-Abel, N. (2014). Labor and birth. In K. Rice Simpson, & P. Creehan (Eds.), *AWHONN's perinatal nursing* (4th ed.). Philadelphia: Lippincott Williams & Wilkins.

Simpson, K., Cesario, S., Morin, K., et al. (2008). *Nursing care and management of the second stage of labor: Evidence-based clinical practice guideline* (2nd ed.). Washington, DC: Association of Women's Health, Obstetric and Neonatal Nurses.

Singata, M., Tranmer, J., & Gyte, G. (2013). Restricting oral fluid and food intake during labour. *The Cochrane Database of Systematic Reviews*, 2013, 1, CD003930.

Walls, D. (2009). Herbs and natural therapies for pregnancy, birth, and breastfeeding. *International Journal of Childbirth Education*, *24*(2), 29–37.

Waterbirth International. (2013). *Waterbirth-FAQs*. Available at http://waterbirth.org.

Wilson-Griffin, J. (2014). Maternal-fetal transport. In K. Rice Simpson, & P. Creehan (Eds.), *AWHONN's perinatal nursing* (4th ed.). Philadelphia: Lippincott Williams & Wilkins.

Wing, D., & Farinelli, C. (2012). Abnormal labor and induction of labor. In S. Gabbe, J. Niebyl, J. Simpson, et al. (Eds.), *Obstetrics: Normal and problem pregnancies* (6th ed.). Philadelphia: Saunders.

Zwelling, E. (2010). Overcoming the challenges: Maternal movement and positioning to facilitate labor progress. *MCN: The American Journal of Maternal/Child Nursing, 35*(2), 72–78.

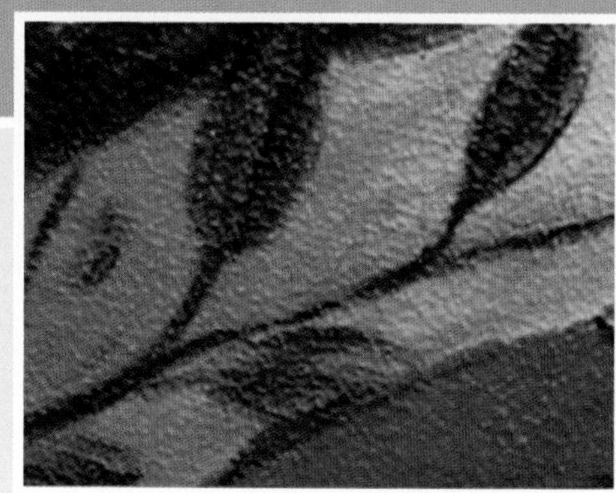

CHAPTER 20

Postpartum Physiologic Changes

Kathryn R. Alden

http://evolve.elsevier.com/Lowdermilk/MWHC/

LEARNING OBJECTIVES

- Describe the anatomic and physiologic changes that occur during the postpartum period.
- Discuss characteristics of uterine involution and lochial flow and describe ways to measure them.
- List expected values for vital signs and blood pressure, deviations from normal findings, and probable causes of the deviations.

The postpartum period is the interval between birth and the return of the reproductive organs to their normal nonpregnant state. This period is sometimes referred to as the puerperium, or *fourth trimester of pregnancy*. Although the puerperium has traditionally been considered to last 6 weeks, this time frame varies among women. The physiologic changes that occur during the reversal of the processes of pregnancy are distinctive, but they are normal. To provide care during the recovery period that is beneficial to the mother, her infant, and her family, the nurse must synthesize knowledge of maternal anatomy and physiology of the recovery period, the newborn's physical and behavioral characteristics, infant care activities, and the family's response to the birth. This chapter focuses on anatomic and physiologic changes that occur in the mother during the postpartum period.

REPRODUCTIVE SYSTEM AND ASSOCIATED STRUCTURES

Uterus

Involution Process

The return of the uterus to a nonpregnant state after birth is called involution. This process begins immediately after expulsion of the placenta with contraction of the uterine smooth muscle.

At the end of the third stage of labor, the uterus is in the midline, approximately 2 cm below the level of the umbilicus, with the fundus resting on the sacral promontory. At this time the uterus weighs approximately 1000 g.

Within 12 hours the fundus can rise to approximately 1 cm above the umbilicus (Fig. 20-1). By 24 hours after birth the uterus is about the same size as it was at 20 weeks of gestation. Involution progresses rapidly during the next few days. The fundus descends 1 to 2 cm every 24 hours. By the sixth postpartum day the fundus is normally located halfway between the umbilicus and the symphysis pubis. The uterus should not be palpable abdominally after 2 weeks and should have returned to its nonpregnant location by 6 weeks after birth (Blackburn, 2013).

The uterus, which at full term weighs approximately 11 times its prepregnancy weight, involutes to approximately 500 g by 1 week after birth and to 350 g by 2 weeks after birth. At 6 weeks postpartum, it weighs 60 to 80 g.

Increased estrogen and progesterone levels are responsible for stimulating the massive growth of the uterus during pregnancy. Prenatal uterine growth results from both hyperplasia (an increase in the number of muscle cells) and hypertrophy (an enlargement of the existing cells). After birth the decrease in these hormones causes autolysis—the self-destruction of excess hypertrophied tissue. The additional cells laid down during pregnancy remain and account for the slight increase in uterine size after each pregnancy.

Subinvolution is the failure of the uterus to return to a nonpregnant state. The most common causes of subinvolution are retained placental fragments and infection (see Chapter 33).

Contractions

Postpartum hemostasis is achieved primarily by compression of intramyometrial blood vessels as the uterine muscle contracts rather than by platelet aggregation and clot formation. The hormone *oxytocin,* released from the pituitary gland, strengthens and coordinates these uterine contractions, which compress blood vessels and promote hemostasis. During the first 1 to 2 postpartum hours, uterine contractions can decrease in intensity and become uncoordinated. Because it is vital that the uterus remains firm and well contracted, exogenous oxytocin

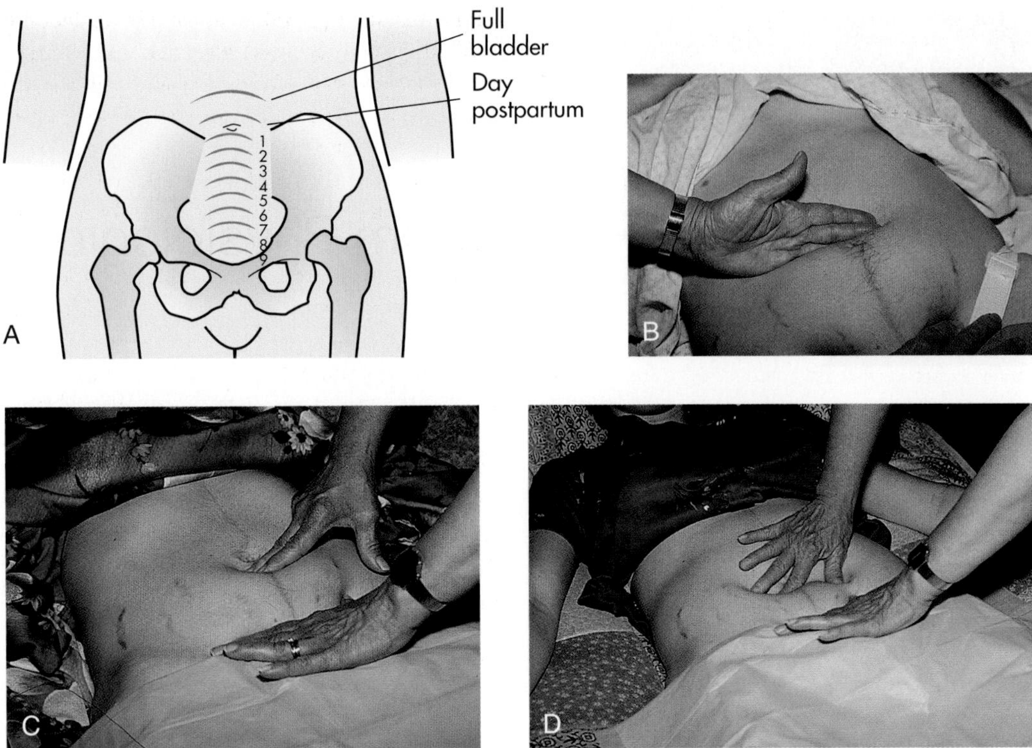

FIG 20-1 Assessment of involution of uterus after birth. **A,** Normal progress, days 1 through 9. **B,** Size and position of uterus 2 hours after birth. **C,** Two days after birth. **D,** Four days after birth. (**B** through **D,** Courtesy Marjorie Pyle, RNC, Lifecircle, Costa Mesa, CA.)

(Pitocin) is usually administered intravenously or intramuscularly immediately after expulsion of the placenta. The uterus is very sensitive to oxytocin during the first week or so after birth. Breastfeeding immediately after birth and in the early days postpartum increases the release of oxytocin, which decreases blood loss and reduces the risk for postpartum hemorrhage (Lawrence & Lawrence, 2011).

In first-time mothers uterine tone is good, the fundus generally remains firm, and the woman usually perceives only mild uterine cramping. Periodic relaxation and vigorous contractions are more common in subsequent pregnancies and can cause uncomfortable cramping called afterpains (afterbirth pains), which typically resolve in 3 to 7 days. Afterpains are more noticeable after births in which the uterus was overdistended (e.g., macrosomic infant, multifetal gestation, polyhydramnios). Breastfeeding and exogenous oxytocic medication usually intensify these afterpains because both stimulate uterine contractions.

Placental Site

Immediately after the placenta and membranes are expelled, vascular constriction and thromboses reduce the placental site to an irregular nodular and elevated area. Upward growth of the endometrium causes sloughing of necrotic tissue and prevents the scar formation characteristic of normal wound healing. This unique healing process enables the endometrium to resume its usual cycle of changes and permit implantation and placentation in future pregnancies. Endometrial regeneration is completed by postpartum day 16, except at the placental site. Regeneration at the placental site usually is not complete until 6 weeks after birth (Blackburn, 2013).

Lochia

Postbirth uterine discharge, commonly called lochia, initially is bright red (lochia rubra) and may contain small clots. For the first 2 hours after birth the amount of uterine discharge should be about that of a heavy menstrual period. After that time the lochial flow should steadily decrease.

Lochia rubra is dark red and consists mainly of blood and decidual and trophoblastic debris. The flow pales, becoming pink or brown (lochia serosa) after 3 to 4 days. Lochia serosa consists of old blood, serum, leukocytes, and tissue debris. In most women, about 10 to 14 days after birth the drainage becomes yellow to white (lochia alba). Lochia alba consists of leukocytes, decidua, epithelial cells, mucus, serum, and bacteria. Lochia can persist up to 4 to 8 weeks after birth. If the woman receives an oxytocic medication, regardless of the route of administration, the flow of lochia is often scant until the effects of the medication wear off. The amount of lochia is usually less after a cesarean birth because the surgeon suctions the blood and fluids from the uterus or wipes the uterine lining before closing the incision. Flow of lochia usually increases with ambulation and breastfeeding. Lochia tends to pool in the vagina when the woman is lying in bed; the woman then can experience a gush of blood when she stands. This gush should not be confused with hemorrhage.

Persistence of lochia rubra in the postpartum period suggests continued bleeding as a result of retained fragments of the placenta or membranes. It is not uncommon for women to experience a sudden, but brief, increase in bleeding 7 to 14 days after birth when sloughing of eschar over the placental site occurs. If this increase in bleeding does not subside within 1 to 2 hours, the woman needs to be evaluated for possible retained placental fragments (Katz, 2012).

BOX 20-1 Lochial and Nonlochial Bleeding

Lochial Bleeding

Lochia usually trickles from the vaginal opening. The steady flow is greater as the uterus contracts.

A gush of lochia can appear as the uterus is massaged. If it is dark in color, it has been pooled in the relaxed vagina, and the amount soon lessens to a trickle of bright red lochia (in the early puerperium).

Nonlochial Bleeding

If the bloody discharge spurts from the vagina, and the uterus is firmly contracted, there can be cervical or vaginal tears in addition to the normal lochia.

If the amount of bleeding continues to be excessive and bright red, a tear can be the source.

About 10% to 15% of women still have normal lochia serosa discharge at their 6-week postpartum examination (Katz, 2012). However, the continued flow of lochia serosa or lochia alba by 3 to 4 weeks after birth can indicate endometritis, particularly if the woman has fever, pain, or abdominal tenderness. Lochia should smell like normal menstrual flow; an offensive odor usually indicates infection.

Not all postpartal vaginal bleeding is lochia; vaginal bleeding after birth can be caused by unrepaired vaginal or cervical lacerations. Box 20-1 distinguishes between lochial and nonlochial bleeding.

Cervix

The cervix is soft immediately after birth. The ectocervix (portion of the cervix that protrudes into the vagina) appears bruised and has some small lacerations, creating optimal conditions for the development of infection. Over the next 12 to 18 hours it shortens and becomes firmer. The cervical os, which dilated to 10 cm during labor, closes gradually. Within 2 to 3 days postpartum, it has shortened, become firm, and regained its form. The cervix up to the lower uterine segment remains edematous, thin, and fragile for several days after birth. By the second or third postpartum day, the cervical dilation has decreased to 2 to 3 cm, and by 1 week after birth, it is approximately 1 cm dilated (Blackburn, 2013). The external cervical os never regains its prepregnancy appearance; it no longer has a circular shape but, instead, appears as a jagged slit often described as a "fish mouth" (see Fig. 13-2). Lactation delays the production of cervical and other estrogen-influenced mucus and affects mucosal characteristics.

Vagina and Perineum

Postpartum estrogen deprivation is responsible for the thinness of the vaginal mucosa and the absence of rugae. The smooth-walled vagina that was greatly distended during birth gradually decreases in size and regains tone, although it never completely returns to its prepregnancy state. Rugae reappear within 3 weeks, but they are never as prominent as in the nulliparous woman. Most rugae are permanently flattened. The mucosa remains atrophic in the lactating woman, at least until menstruation resumes. Thickening of the vaginal mucosa occurs with the return of ovarian function. Estrogen deficiency is responsible for a decreased amount of vaginal lubrication; vaginal dryness is more prevalent among breastfeeding mothers. Localized dryness and coital discomfort (dyspareunia) can persist until ovarian function returns and menstruation resumes. The use of a water-soluble lubricant during sexual intercourse is usually recommended.

Immediately after birth the introitus is erythematous and edematous, especially in the area of an episiotomy or laceration repair. It is barely distinguishable from that of a nulliparous woman if lacerations or an episiotomy have been carefully repaired, hematomas are prevented or treated early, and the woman practices good hygiene during the first 2 weeks after birth.

Most episiotomies and laceration repairs are visible only if the woman is lying on her side with her upper buttock raised or if she is placed in the lithotomy position. A good light source is essential for visualization of some repairs. Healing of an episiotomy or laceration is the same as any surgical incision. Signs of infection (pain, redness, warmth, swelling, or discharge) or lack of approximation (separation of the edges of the incision) can occur. Initial healing occurs within 2 to 3 weeks, but 4 to 6 months can be required for the repair to heal completely (Blackburn, 2013). If forceps were used for the birth, the woman may have experienced vaginal or cervical lacerations; hematomas of the pelvic soft tissues can also occur with forceps-assisted birth (see Chapter 32).

Hemorrhoids (anal varicosities) are commonly seen. Internal hemorrhoids can evert while the woman is pushing during birth. Women often experience associated symptoms such as itching, discomfort, and bright red bleeding with defecation. Hemorrhoids usually decrease in size within 6 weeks of childbirth.

Pelvic Muscular Support

The supporting structure of the uterus and vagina can be injured during birth; this can contribute to later gynecologic problems. Supportive tissues of the pelvic floor that are torn or stretched during birth can require up to 6 months to regain tone. Kegel exercises, which help strengthen perineal muscles and encourage healing, are recommended after birth (see Teaching for Self-Management: Kegel Exercises, Chapter 4). Later in life, women can experience pelvic relaxation—the lengthening and weakening of the fascial supports of pelvic structures. These structures include the uterus, upper posterior vaginal wall, urethra, bladder, and rectum. Although relaxation can occur in any woman, it is commonly a direct but delayed complication of birth (see Chapter 11).

ENDOCRINE SYSTEM

Placental Hormones

Significant hormonal changes occur during the postpartum period. Expulsion of the placenta results in dramatic decreases in the hormones produced by that organ.

Estrogen and progesterone levels drop markedly after expulsion of the placenta and reach their lowest levels 1 week after birth. Decreased estrogen levels are associated with the diuresis of excess extracellular fluid accumulated during pregnancy. In nonlactating women, estrogen levels begin to increase by 2 weeks after birth and by postpartum day 17 are higher than in women who breastfeed (Katz, 2012).

Human chorionic gonadotropin (hCG) disappears fairly quickly from maternal circulation. However, because removing hCG from the extravascular and intracellular spaces takes additional time, the hormone can be detected in the maternal system for 3 to 4 weeks after birth (Blackburn, 2013).

Metabolic Changes

Decreases in human chorionic somatomammotropin (formerly called *human placental lactogen*), estrogens, cortisol, and the placental enzyme *insulinase* reverse the diabetogenic effects of pregnancy, resulting in significantly lower blood glucose levels in the immediate puerperium. Mothers with type 1 diabetes will likely require much less insulin for several days after birth. Because these normal hormonal changes make the puerperium a transitional period for carbohydrate metabolism, it is more difficult to interpret results of glucose tolerance tests at this time.

Thyroid volume gradually returns to normal by 3 months after birth. Levels of thyroxine and triiodothyronine decrease to prepregnant levels within 4 weeks. There is an increased risk of a transient autoimmune thyroiditis in the postpartum period (Katz, 2012).

The basal metabolic rate remains elevated for the first 1 to 2 weeks after birth (James, 2014). It gradually returns to prepregnancy levels.

Pituitary Hormones and Ovarian Function

Prolactin levels in blood rise progressively throughout pregnancy. After birth, as levels of progesterone decrease, prolactin levels increase. In a woman who breastfeeds, prolactin levels are highest during the first month after birth and remain elevated above nonpregnant levels as long as she is breastfeeding. Serum prolactin levels are influenced by the frequency of breastfeeding, the duration of each feeding, and the degree to which supplementary feedings are used. Individual differences in the strength of an infant's sucking stimulus also affect prolactin levels. In nonlactating women, prolactin levels decline after birth and reach the prepregnant range by the third postpartum week (Katz, 2012).

Lactating and nonlactating women differ considerably in the timing of their first ovulation and when menstruation resumes. Ovulation occurs as early as 27 days after birth in nonlactating women, with a mean time of about 7 to 9 weeks. About 70% of nonbreastfeeding women resume menstruating by 12 weeks after birth. The mean time to ovulation in women who breastfeed is about 6 months (Katz, 2012). The persistence of elevated serum prolactin levels in breastfeeding women appears to be responsible for suppressing ovulation. In lactating women both the resumption of ovulation and the return of menses are determined in large part by breastfeeding patterns. For example, ovulation is delayed longer in women who breastfeed exclusively compared with women who breastfeed and offer supplemental infant formula to their infants. Because of the uncertainty about the return of ovulation and menstruation, discussion of contraceptive options early in the puerperium is necessary. The first menstrual flow after birth is usually heavier than normal. Within three or four cycles, the amount of menstrual flow returns to the prepregnancy volume.

URINARY SYSTEM

The hormonal changes of pregnancy (i.e., high steroid levels) contribute to an increase in renal function; diminishing steroid levels after birth may partly explain the reduced renal function that occurs during the puerperium. Kidney function returns to normal within 1 month after birth. About 6 to 8 weeks are required for the pregnancy-induced hypotonia and dilation of the ureters and renal pelves to return to the nonpregnant state In a small percentage of women dilation of the urinary tract can persist for 3 months or longer, increasing the risk of developing a urinary tract infection.

Urine Components

The renal glycosuria induced by pregnancy disappears by 1 week postpartum, but lactosuria can occur in lactating women. The blood urea nitrogen increases during the puerperium as autolysis of the involuting uterus occurs. Plasma creatinine levels return to normal by 6 weeks postpartum. Pregnancy-associated proteinuria resolves by 6 weeks after birth (Blackburn, 2013). Ketonuria can occur in women with an uncomplicated birth or after a prolonged labor with dehydration.

Fluid Loss

Within 12 hours of birth women begin to lose excess tissue fluid accumulated during pregnancy. Postpartal diuresis, caused by decreased estrogen levels, removal of increased venous pressure in the lower extremities, and loss of the remaining pregnancy-induced increase in blood volume, aids the body in ridding itself of excess fluid. Urine output of 3000 ml or more each day during the first 2 to 3 days is common. Profuse diaphoresis often occurs, especially at night, for the first 2 to 3 days after birth. Fluid loss through perspiration and increased urinary output accounts for a weight loss of approximately 2.25 kg (5 lb) during the early puerperium.

Urethra and Bladder

Birth-induced trauma, increased bladder capacity after birth, and the effects of conduction anesthesia can result in a decreased urge to void. In addition, pelvic soreness caused by the forces of labor, vaginal or perineal lacerations, or episiotomy can reduce or alter the voiding reflex. Decreased voiding combined with postpartal diuresis can result in bladder distention.

Immediately after birth, excessive bleeding can occur if the bladder becomes distended because it pushes the uterus up and to the side and prevents it from contracting firmly. Later in the puerperium, overdistention can make the bladder more susceptible to infection and impede the resumption of normal voiding. With adequate bladder emptying, bladder tone is usually restored by 5 to 7 days after birth.

Some women experience *stress incontinence* during the postpartum period. This is more likely to occur after vaginal than cesarean birth. Stress incontinence can be related to tissue trauma to the pelvic floor occurring with maternal expulsive efforts and increased size of the neonate. Coached pushing versus uncoached (non-Valsalva) pushing can increase the risk of damage to the pelvic floor and subsequent stress incontinence (James, 2014) (see Chapter 11).

GASTROINTESTINAL SYSTEM

Most new mothers are very hungry after full recovery from analgesia, anesthesia, and fatigue. Requests for extra portions of food and frequent snacks are common.

A spontaneous bowel evacuation may not occur for 2 to 3 days after birth. This delay can be explained by slowed peristalsis related to decreased muscle tone in the intestines during labor and the immediate puerperium, prelabor diarrhea, lack of food, or dehydration. The mother often anticipates discomfort during the bowel movement because of perineal tenderness as a result of an episiotomy, lacerations, or hemorrhoids and resists the urge to defecate. Regular bowel habits should be reestablished when bowel tone returns.

Third- and fourth-degree perineal lacerations that involve the anal sphincter are associated with an increased risk for postpartum anal incontinence. Women with this problem are more often incontinent of flatus than of stool. If anal incontinence lasts more than 6 months, studies should be conducted to determine the specific cause and appropriate treatment (Katz, 2012).

BREASTS

Promptly after birth, a decrease occurs in the concentrations of hormones (i.e., estrogen, progesterone, hCG, prolactin, cortisol, and insulin) that stimulated breast development during pregnancy. The time required for these hormones to return to prepregnancy levels is determined in part by whether or not the mother breastfeeds her infant.

Breastfeeding Mothers

During the first 24 hours after birth, there is little if any change in the breast tissue. Colostrum, or early milk, a clear yellow fluid, can be expressed from the breasts. The breasts gradually become fuller and heavier as the colostrum transitions to mature milk by about 72 to 96 hours after birth; this is often referred to as the "milk coming in," or lactogenesis II. The breasts can feel warm, firm, and somewhat tender. Bluish white milk with a skim-milk appearance (true milk) can be expressed from the nipples. As milk glands and milk ducts fill with milk, breast tissue can feel somewhat nodular or lumpy. Unlike the lumps associated with fibrocystic breast changes or cancer (which can be palpated consistently in the same location), the nodularity associated with milk production tends to shift in position. Some women experience engorgement at this time due to an increase in blood and lymphatic fluid as milk production increases. Engorged breasts are hard and uncomfortable; the fullness of the nipple tissue can make it difficult for the infant to latch on and feed. With frequent breastfeeding and proper care, engorgement is a temporary condition that typically lasts only 24 to 48 hours (see Chapter 25).

Nonbreastfeeding Mothers

The breasts generally feel nodular in contrast to the granular feel of breasts in nonpregnant women. The nodularity is bilateral and diffuse. Prolactin levels drop rapidly. Colostrum is present for the first few days after birth. Palpation of the breasts on the second or third day as milk production begins can reveal tissue tenderness in some women. On the third or fourth postpartum day, engorgement can occur. The breasts are distended (swollen), firm, tender, and warm to the touch. Breast distention is caused primarily by the temporary congestion of veins and lymphatics rather than by an accumulation of milk. Milk is present but should not be expressed. Axillary breast tissue (the tail of Spence) and any accessory breast or nipple tissue along the milk line can be involved. Engorgement resolves spontaneously, and discomfort decreases usually within 24 to 36 hours. A breast binder or well-fitted supportive bra, ice packs, fresh cabbage leaves, and/or mild analgesics may be used to relieve discomfort. Nipple stimulation is avoided. If suckling or milk expression is never begun (or is discontinued), lactation ceases within a few days to a week.

CARDIOVASCULAR SYSTEM

Blood Volume

Changes in blood volume after birth depend on several factors, such as blood loss during birth and the amount of extravascular water (physiologic edema) mobilized and excreted. Pregnancy-induced hypervolemia (an increase in blood volume to 40% to 45% above nonpregnancy levels) allows most women to tolerate considerable blood loss during birth. The average blood loss for a vaginal birth of a single fetus ranges from 300 to 500 ml (10% of blood volume). The typical blood loss for women who give birth by cesarean is 500 to 1000 ml (15% to 30% of blood volume). During the first few days after birth the plasma volume decreases further as a result of diuresis (Blackburn, 2013).

Maternal physiologic changes in the puerperium enable the woman to cope with the blood loss that normally occurs during birth by increasing her circulation blood volume. These changes are: (1) elimination of uteroplacental circulation that reduces the size of the maternal vascular bed by 10% to 15%; (2) loss of placental endocrine function that removes the stimulus for vasodilation; and (3) mobilization of extravascular water stored during pregnancy. By the third postpartum day, the plasma volume has been replenished as extravascular fluid returns to the intravascular space (Katz, 2012) (see Clinical Reasoning Case Study).

CLINICAL REASONING CASE STUDY

Maternal Postpartum Blood Loss and Fatigue

You are caring for four women on the postpartum unit: two had vaginal births and two had cesarean births. Each of the women has complained about feeling tired and has expressed concern about the amount of blood she lost during birth. Before providing client education related to fatigue after birth and blood loss, you review the clients' records with attention to estimated blood loss, hemoglobin and hematocrit values, intake and output, and nursing notes.

1. Evidence—Is there sufficient evidence to draw conclusions about the relation between tiredness (fatigue) after birth and blood loss?
2. Assumptions—What assumptions can be made about the following factors?
   a. Comparison of amount of blood loss between women who give birth vaginally and by cesarean
   b. Postpartum norms for hematocrit and hemoglobin for women who give birth vaginally and by cesarean
   c. Causes of fatigue after birth
   d. Interventions to alleviate fatigue and replace blood lost at birth
3. What implications and priorities for nursing care can be drawn at this time?
4. Does the evidence objectively support your conclusion?

Cardiac Output

Pulse rate, stroke volume, and cardiac output increase throughout pregnancy. Dramatic changes in maternal hemodynamic status occur with birth of the newborn and delivery of the placenta. The immediate blood loss reduces plasma volume without reducing cardiac output. This is due to the compensatory influx of nearly 500 ml of blood into the maternal system from the uteroplacental bed, a rapid decrease in uterine blood flow, and mobilization of extracellular fluid. Typically cardiac output is increased immediately after birth by 60% to 80% over prelabor values; it returns to prelabor values within 1 hour. By 2 weeks after birth, cardiac output decreases by 30% and gradually decreases to prepregnant levels by 6 to 8 weeks postpartum in the majority of women (Blackburn, 2013).

Vital Signs

Few alterations in vital signs are seen under normal circumstances (Table 20-1). Heart rate is increased immediately after birth and can remain elevated for the first hour. Puerperal bradycardia is common, with heart rate decreasing to 40 to 50 beats/minute (James, 2014).

There is a transient increase in blood pressure of approximately 5% during the first few days after birth (Katz, 2012). It can take weeks or months for pulse and blood pressure to return to prepregnancy levels. Increase in blood pressure greater than 140/90 when measured on two or more occasions at least 6 hours apart can indicate preeclampsia.

Respiratory function rapidly returns to nonpregnant levels after birth. After the uterus is emptied, the diaphragm descends, the normal cardiac axis is restored, and the point of maximal impulse and the electrocardiogram are normalized.

TABLE 20-1 Vital Signs After Childbirth

NORMAL FINDINGS	DEVIATIONS FROM NORMAL FINDINGS AND PROBABLE CAUSES
Temperature	
During first 24 hours, temperature can increase to 38° C (100.4° F) as a result of dehydrating effects of labor. After 24 hours, the woman should be afebrile.	A diagnosis of puerperal sepsis is suggested if an increase in maternal temperature to 38° C (100.4° F) is noted after the first 24 hours after birth and recurs or persists for 2 days. Other possible causes are mastitis, endometritis, urinary tract infections, and other systemic infections.
Pulse	
Pulse, along with stroke volume and cardiac output, remains elevated for the first hour or so after birth. It gradually decreases over the first 48 hours postpartum. Puerperal bradycardia (40-50 beats/min) is common.	A rapid pulse rate or one that is increasing can indicate hypovolemia as a result of hemorrhage.
Respirations	
The respiratory rate, which was unchanged or slightly increased during pregnancy, should be within the woman's normal prepregnancy range soon after birth.	Hypoventilation (respiratory depression) can occur after an unusually high subarachnoid (spinal) block or epidural opioid medication after a cesarean birth.
Blood Pressure	
Blood pressure shows a transient increase of approximately 5% over the first few days after birth, returning to prepregnancy levels over weeks or months. Orthostatic hypotension, as indicated by feelings of faintness or dizziness immediately after standing up, can develop in the first 48 hours as a result of the splanchnic engorgement that can occur after birth.	A low or decreasing blood pressure can indicate hypovolemia secondary to hemorrhage; however, it is a late sign, and other symptoms of hemorrhage usually are present. An increased reading can result from excessive use of vasopressor or oxytocic medications. Because gestational hypertension can persist into or occur first in the postpartum period, routine evaluation of blood pressure is needed. If a woman complains of headache, hypertension must be ruled out as a cause before analgesics are administered.

Blood Components

Hematocrit and Hemoglobin

In women with an average blood loss during birth, the hematocrit level drops moderately for 3 to 4 days, then begins to increase, and reaches nonpregnant levels by 8 weeks postpartum (Katz, 2012). A postpartum hematocrit can be lower than normal if the blood loss was increased or if the hypervolemia of pregnancy was less than normal.

White Blood Cell Count

Normal leukocytosis of pregnancy averages approximately 12,000/mm^3. During the first 4 to 7 days after birth, values between 20,000 and 25,000/mm^3 are common. Leukocytosis, coupled with the increase in erythrocyte sedimentation rate that normally occurs, can obscure the diagnosis of acute infection.

Coagulation Factors

Clotting factors and fibrinogen are normally increased during pregnancy and remain elevated in the immediate puerperium. When combined with vessel damage and immobility, this hypercoagulable state causes an increased risk for venous thromboembolism, especially after a cesarean birth. Fibrinolytic activity also increases during the first few days after birth (Katz, 2012). Factors I, II, VIII, IX, and X decrease to nonpregnant levels within a few days. Fibrin split products, probably released from the placental site, can be found in maternal blood.

Varicosities

Varicosities (varices) of the legs (Fig. 20-2) and around the anus (hemorrhoids) are common during pregnancy. All varices, even the less common vulvar varices, regress (empty) rapidly immediately after birth. Total or nearly total regression of varicosities is expected in the postpartum period.

RESPIRATORY SYSTEM

When birth occurs there is an immediate decrease in intraabdominal pressure, which allows for greater excursion of the diaphragm. With decreased pressure on the diaphragm and reduced pulmonary blood flow, chest wall compliance increases. Rib cage elasticity can take months to return to a prepregnancy state. The costal angle that was increased during pregnancy may

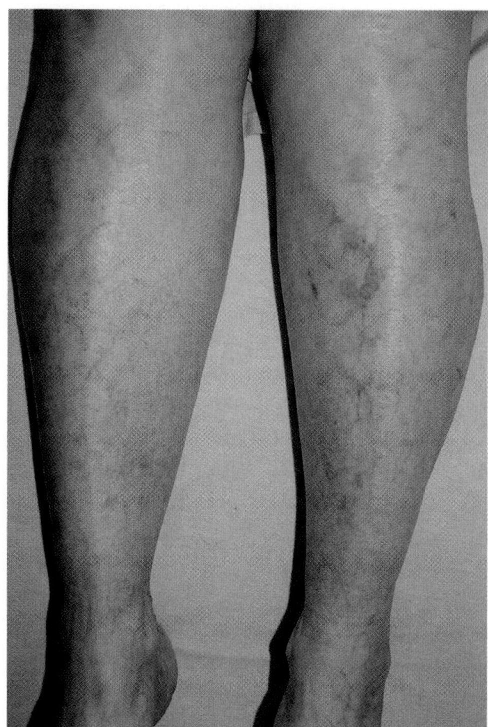

FIG 20-2 Varicosities in legs. (Courtesy Cheryl Briggs, RNC, Annapolis, MD.)

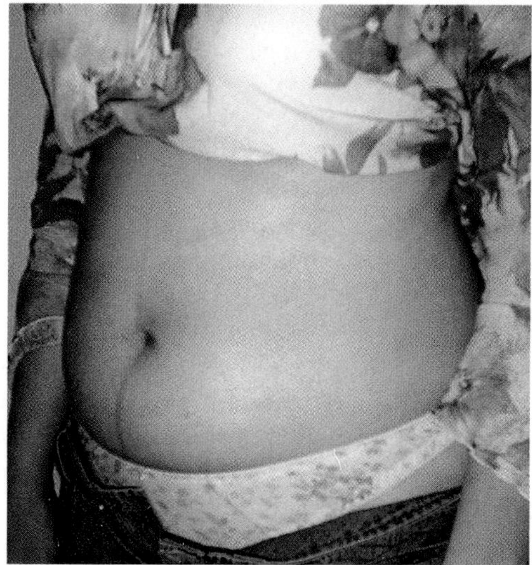

FIG 20-3 Abdominal wall 6 weeks after vaginal birth is almost back to prepregnancy appearance. Note that the linea nigra is still visible. (Courtesy Jodi Brackett, Phoenix, AZ.)

not completely return to the prepregnancy level. The decline in progesterone that occurs with loss of the placenta causes $Paco_2$ levels to rise (Blackburn, 2013).

NEUROLOGIC SYSTEM

Neurologic changes during the puerperium result from a reversal of maternal adaptations to pregnancy and from trauma during labor and birth.

Pregnancy-induced neurologic discomforts disappear after birth. Elimination of physiologic edema through the diuresis that follows birth relieves carpal tunnel syndrome by easing compression of the median nerve. The periodic numbness and tingling of fingers usually disappear after the birth unless lifting and carrying the baby aggravate the condition. Nasal stuffiness, tinnitus, and laryngeal changes resolve within a few days postpartum.

Headaches are common in the first postpartum week; they are usually bilateral and frontal (Blackburn, 2013). However, headache requires careful assessment. Postpartum headaches can be caused by various conditions, including postpartum-onset preeclampsia, stress, and leakage of cerebrospinal fluid into the extradural space during placement of the needle for administration of epidural or spinal anesthesia.

MUSCULOSKELETAL SYSTEM

Abdomen

When the woman stands during the first days after birth, her abdomen protrudes and gives her a still-pregnant appearance. During the first 2 weeks after birth, the abdominal wall is relaxed. It takes about 6 weeks for the abdominal wall to return almost to its prepregnancy state (Fig. 20-3). The return of muscle tone depends on previous tone, proper exercise, and the amount of adipose tissue. Occasionally, with or without overdistention because of a large fetus or multiple fetuses, the abdominal wall muscles separate, a condition termed *diastasis recti abdominis* (see Fig. 13-13, *B*). Persistence of this separation can be disturbing to the woman, but surgical correction rarely is necessary. With time the separation becomes less apparent.

Other adaptations of the mother's musculoskeletal system that occur during pregnancy are reversed in the puerperium. These adaptations include the relaxation and subsequent hypermobility of the joints and the change in the mother's center of gravity in response to the enlarging uterus. The joints are completely stabilized by 6 to 8 weeks after birth. Although all other joints return to their normal prepregnancy state, those in the parous woman's feet do not. The new mother may notice a permanent increase in her shoe size. Back pain usually resolves in a few weeks or months following birth.

INTEGUMENTARY SYSTEM

Melasma (chloasma or "mask of pregnancy") usually disappears in the postpartum period but persists in about 30% of women (Kroumpouzos, 2012). Hyperpigmentation of the areolae and linea nigra may not regress completely after birth. Some women will have permanent darker pigmentation of those areas. Striae gravidarum (stretch marks) on the breasts, abdomen, and thighs may fade but usually do not disappear completely.

Vascular abnormalities such as spider angiomas (nevi) and palmar erythema generally regress in response to the rapid decline in estrogens after birth. For some women, spider nevi persist indefinitely.

For the first 3 months after birth, women often report hair loss when they brush or comb their hair. The abundance of fine hair seen during pregnancy usually disappears after giving birth; however, any coarse or bristly hair that appears during pregnancy usually remains. Fingernails return to their prepregnancy consistency and strength.

IMMUNE SYSTEM

In the postpartum period the woman's immune (lymphoreticular) system, which was mildly suppressed during pregnancy, gradually returns to its prepregnant state, although the exact timeline is unclear (Blackburn, 2013). This rebound of the immune system can trigger "flare-ups" of autoimmune conditions such as multiple sclerosis or lupus erythematosus (Katz, 2012).

KEY POINTS

- The rapid decrease in estrogen and progesterone levels after expulsion of the placenta is responsible for triggering many of the anatomic and physiologic changes in the puerperium.
- Within 6 weeks after birth, the physiologic changes induced by pregnancy have reverted to their normal state.
- Assessing lochia and fundal height is essential to monitor the progress of normal involution and to identify potential problems.
- The uterus involutes rapidly after birth and returns to the true pelvis within 2 weeks.
- The return of ovulation and menses is determined in part by whether the woman breastfeeds her infant.
- Few alterations in vital signs are seen after birth under normal circumstances.
- Hypercoagulability, vessel damage, and immobility predispose the woman to venous thromboembolism.
- Marked diuresis, decreased bladder sensitivity, and overdistention of the bladder can lead to problems with urinary elimination.
- Pregnancy-induced hypervolemia, combined with several postpartum physiologic changes, allows the woman to tolerate considerable blood loss at birth.

REFERENCES

Blackburn, S. T. (2013). *Maternal, fetal, and neonatal physiology* (4th ed.). St. Louis: Saunders.

James, D. C. (2014). Postpartum care. In K. R. Simpson, & P. A. Creehan (Eds.), *Perinatal nursing* (4th ed.). Philadelphia: Lippincott Williams & Wilkins.

Katz, V. L. (2012). Postpartum care. In S. G. Gabbe, J. R. Niebyl, J. L. Simpson, et al. (Eds.), *Obstetrics: Normal and problem pregnancies* (6th ed.). Philadelphia: Saunders.

Kroumpouzos, G. (2012). Skin disease in pregnancy and puerperium. In S. G. Gabbe, J. R. Niebyl, J. L. Simpson, et al. (Eds.), *Obstetrics: Normal and problem pregnancies* (6th ed.). Philadelphia: Saunders.

Lawrence, R. M., & Lawrence, R. A. (2011). *Breastfeeding: A guide for the medical profession* (7th ed.). St. Louis: Mosby.

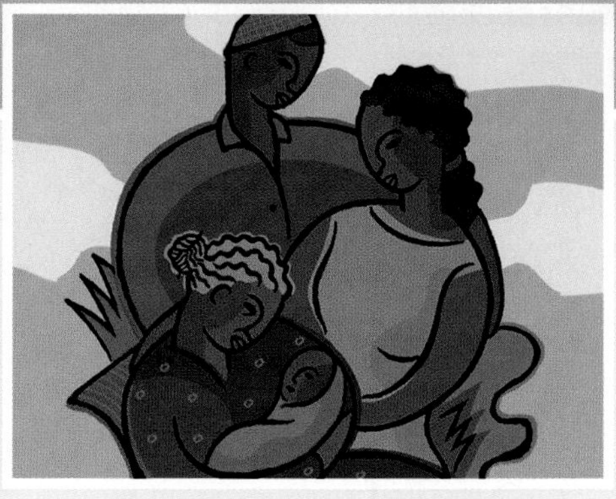

CHAPTER 21

Nursing Care of the Family During the Postpartum Period

Jennifer T. Alderman

http://evolve.elsevier.com/Lowdermilk/MWHC/

LEARNING OBJECTIVES

- Describe components of a systematic postpartum assessment.
- Recognize signs of potential complications in the postpartum woman.
- Formulate a nursing care plan for a woman and her family in the postpartum period.
- Explain the influence of cultural beliefs and practices on postpartum care.
- Identify psychosocial needs of the woman and family in the early postpartum period.
- Prepare a plan for postpartum teaching for self-management.
- Describe the nurse's role in these postpartum follow-up strategies: home visits, telephone follow-up, warm lines and help lines, support groups, and referrals to community resources.

At no other time is family-centered maternity care more important than in the postpartum period. Nursing care is provided in the context of the family unit and focuses on assessment and support of the woman's physiologic and emotional adaptation after birth. During the early postpartum period, components of nursing care include assisting the mother with rest and recovery from labor and birth, assessing physiologic and psychologic adaptation after birth, preventing complications, educating regarding self-management and infant care, and supporting the mother and her partner during the initial transition to parenthood. In addition, the nurse considers the needs of other family members and includes strategies in the nursing care plan to assist the family in adjusting to the new baby.

The approach to the care of women after birth is wellness oriented. In the United States most women remain hospitalized no more than 1 or 2 days after vaginal birth, and some as few as 6 hours. Because so much important information needs to be shared with these women in a very short time, their care must be thoughtfully planned and provided. This chapter discusses nursing care of the woman and her family in the postpartum period extending into the fourth trimester—the first 3 months after birth.

TRANSFER FROM THE RECOVERY AREA

After the initial recovery period has been completed, and provided that her condition is stable, the woman may be transferred to a postpartum room in the same or another nursing unit. In facilities with labor, delivery, recovery, postpartum (LDRP) rooms, the woman is not moved and the nurse who provides care during the recovery period usually continues caring for the woman. In many settings, women who have received general or regional anesthesia must be cleared for transfer from the recovery area by a member of the anesthesia care team. In other settings, a nurse makes the determination.

In preparing the transfer report, the recovery nurse uses information from the records of admission, birth, and recovery (Fig. 21-1). Information that must be communicated to the postpartum nurse includes the woman's name, age, identity of the health care provider; gravidity and parity; anesthetic used; any medications given; duration of labor and time of rupture of membranes; whether labor was induced or augmented; type of birth and perineal repair; blood type and Rh status; group B streptococcus (GBS) status; status of rubella immunity; human immunodeficiency virus (HIV), hepatitis B, and syphilis serology test results; other infections identified during pregnancy (e.g., gonorrhea, chlamydia), and whether these were treated; type and amount of intravenous fluids; physiologic status since birth; description of fundus, lochia, bladder, and perineum; sex and weight of infant; time of birth; name of pediatric care provider; chosen method of feeding; any abnormalities noted; and assessment of initial parent-infant interaction.

Most of this information is also documented for the nursing staff in the newborn nursery if the infant is transferred to that unit (in some settings, the newborn never leaves the mother's room). In addition, specific information should be provided regarding the newborn's Apgar scores (see Chapter 24), weight, voiding, stooling, and whether fed since birth. Nursing

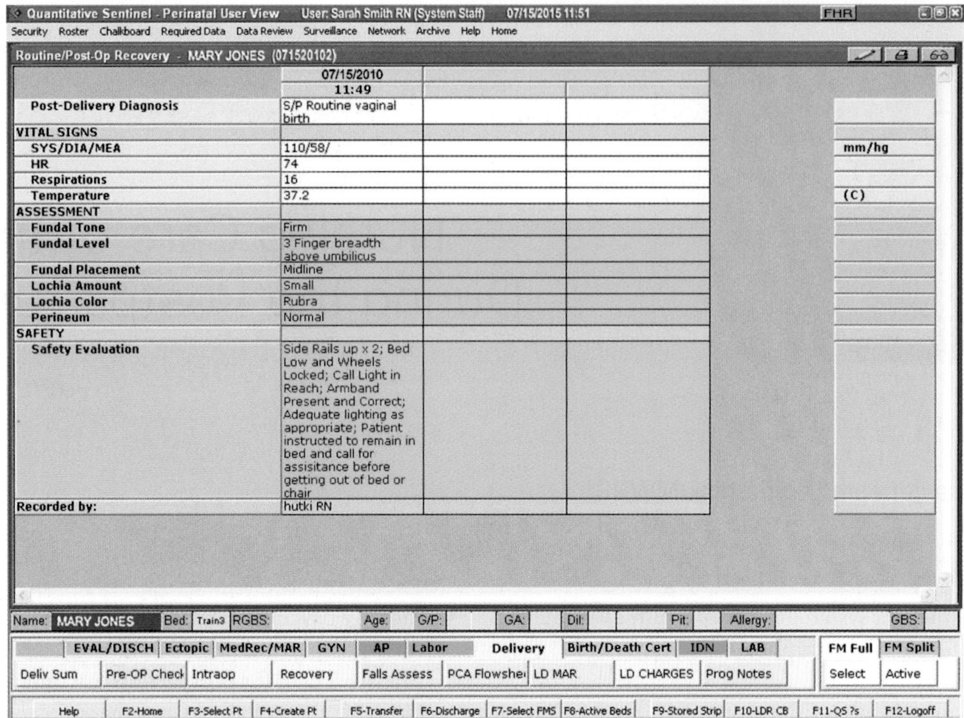

Quantitative Sentinel - Perinatal User View User: Sarah Smith RN (System Staff) 07/15/2015 11:51 FHR

Security Roster Chalkboard Required Data Data Review Surveillance Network Archive Help Home

Routine/Post-Op Recovery - MARY JONES (071520102)

	07/15/2010 11:49			
Post-Delivery Diagnosis	S/P Routine vaginal birth			
VITAL SIGNS				
SYS/DIA/MEA	110/58/			mm/hg
HR	74			
Respirations	16			
Temperature	37.2			(C)
ASSESSMENT				
Fundal Tone	Firm			
Fundal Level	3 Finger breadth above umbilicus			
Fundal Placement	Midline			
Lochia Amount	Small			
Lochia Color	Rubra			
Perineum	Normal			
SAFETY				
Safety Evaluation	Side Rails up x 2; Bed Low and Wheels Locked; Call Light in Reach; Armband Present and Correct; Adequate lighting as appropriate; Patient instructed to remain in bed and call for assisitance before getting out of bed or chair			
Recorded by:	hutki RN			

Name: MARY JONES Bed: Train3 RGBS: Age: G/P: GA: Dil: Pit: Allergy: GBS:

EVAL/DISCH | Ectopic | MedRec/MAR | GYN | AP | Labor | Delivery | Birth/Death Cert | IDN | LAB | FM Full | FM Split

Deliv Sum | Pre-OP Check | Intraop | Recovery | Falls Assess | PCA Flowsheet | LD MAR | LD CHARGES | Prog Notes | Select | Active

Help | F2-Home | F3-Select Pt | F4-Create Pt | F5-Transfer | F6-Discharge | F7-Select FMS | F8-Active Beds | F9-Stored Strip | F10-LDR CB | F11-QS ?s | F12-Logoff

FIG 21-1 Portion of a vaginal birth recovery screen in an electronic record. (Courtesy Kitty Cashion, Memphis, TN.)

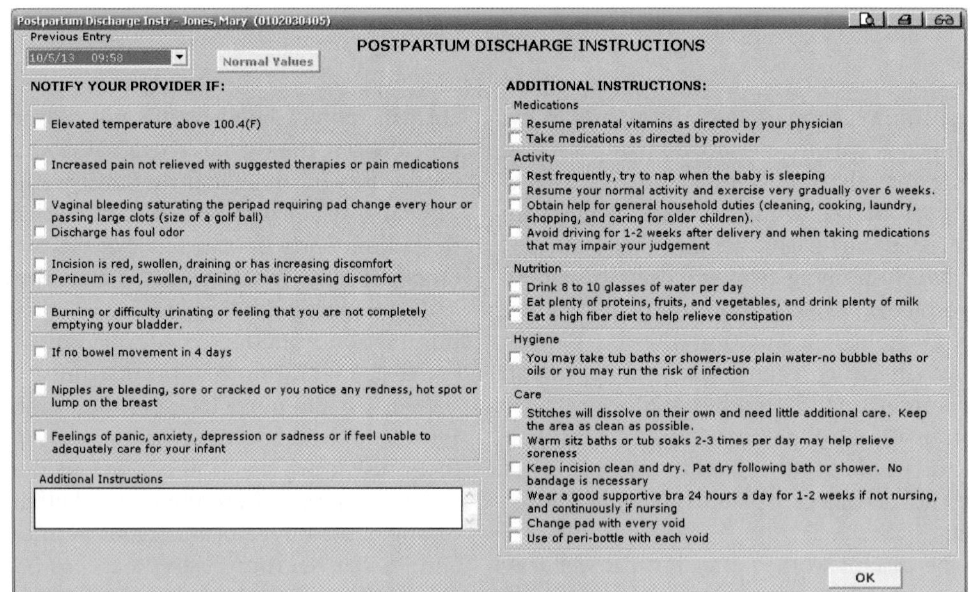

Postpartum Discharge Instr - Jones, Mary (0102030405)

Previous Entry 10/5/13 09:58 Normal Values

POSTPARTUM DISCHARGE INSTRUCTIONS

NOTIFY YOUR PROVIDER IF:

- Elevated temperature above 100.4(F)
- Increased pain not relieved with suggested therapies or pain medications
- Vaginal bleeding saturating the peripad requiring pad change every hour or passing large clots (size of a golf ball)
- Discharge has foul odor
- Incision is red, swollen, draining or has increasing discomfort
- Perineum is red, swollen, draining or has increasing discomfort
- Burning or difficulty urinating or feeling that you are not completely emptying your bladder.
- If no bowel movement in 4 days
- Nipples are bleeding, sore or cracked or you notice any redness, hot spot or lump on the breast
- Feelings of panic, anxiety, depression or sadness or if feel unable to adequately care for your infant

Additional Instructions

ADDITIONAL INSTRUCTIONS:

Medications
- Resume prenatal vitamins as directed by your physician
- Take medications as directed by provider

Activity
- Rest frequently, try to nap when the baby is sleeping
- Resume your normal activity and exercise very gradually over 6 weeks.
- Obtain help for general household duties (cleaning, cooking, laundry, shopping, and caring for older children).
- Avoid driving for 1-2 weeks after delivery and when taking medications that may impair your judgement

Nutrition
- Drink 8 to 10 glasses of water per day
- Eat plenty of proteins, fruits, and vegetables, and drink plenty of milk
- Eat a high fiber diet to help relieve constipation

Hygiene
- You may take tub baths or showers-use plain water-no bubble baths or oils or you may run the risk of infection

Care
- Stitches will dissolve on their own and need little additional care. Keep the area as clean as possible.
- Warm sitz baths or tub soaks 2-3 times per day may help relieve soreness
- Keep incision clean and dry. Pat dry following bath or shower. No bandage is necessary
- Wear a good supportive bra 24 hours a day for 1-2 weeks if not nursing, and continuously if nursing
- Change pad with every void
- Use of peri-bottle with each void

OK

FIG 21-2 Part of a postpartum discharge teaching screen in an electronic medical record. (Courtesy Kitty Cashion, Memphis, TN.)

interventions that have been completed (e.g., eye prophylaxis, vitamin K injection) as well as identification procedures done (e.g., footprints, armbands) must be recorded.

In recent years many inpatient nursing units, including perinatal care areas, have changed the way the nurse-to-nurse handoff report is given. Bedside reporting is increasingly being used instead of the traditional report given at the nurses' station. Bedside reporting has been shown to improve client safety and client satisfaction. Clients feel more involved in their plan of care, which increases their satisfaction. Additionally, holding report at the bedside has enabled many nurses to both visualize and communicate with the client at the time of report, which improves client safety (Novak & Fairchild, 2012).

PLANNING FOR DISCHARGE

From their initial contact with the postpartum woman, nurses prepare the new mother for her return to home. Planning for discharge begins with the first interaction between the nurse, the woman, and her family and continues until they leave the hospital or birthing facility (Fig. 21-2).

The length of hospital stay after giving birth depends on many factors, including the physical condition of the mother and the newborn, mental and emotional status of the mother, social support at home, client education needs for self-management and infant care, and financial constraints.

Women who give birth in birthing centers may be discharged within a few hours, after the woman's and infant's conditions are stable. Mothers and newborns who are at low risk for complications may be discharged from the hospital within 24 to 36 hours after vaginal birth. This short time frame is often called early postpartum discharge, shortened hospital stay, and 1-day maternity stay. Early discharge was popular in the late 1980s and early 1990s, but concerns related to the health and safety of mothers and newborns led to legislation promoting longer hospital stays. The passage of the Newborns' and Mothers' Health Protection Act of 1996 provided minimum federal standards for health plan coverage for mothers and their newborns (American Academy of Pediatrics [AAP] Committee on Fetus and Newborn, 2010). Under this act all health plans are required to allow the new mother and newborn to remain in the hospital for a minimum of 48 hours after an uncomplicated vaginal birth and for 96 hours after a cesarean birth, unless the attending provider in consultation with the mother decides on early discharge.

Criteria for Discharge

The American Academy of Pediatrics (AAP) recommends that the hospital stay for a mother with a healthy term newborn should be of sufficient length to identify early problems and determine that the mother and family are prepared and able to care for the neonate at home. The health of the mother and her newborn should be stable, the mother should be able and confident to provide care for her infant, and there should be adequate support systems in place and access to follow-up care (AAP Committee on Fetus and Newborn, 2010).

It is essential that nurses consider the individual needs of the woman and her newborn and provide care that is intentionally planned to meet these needs. Hospital-based maternity nurses continue to play key roles as caregivers, teachers, and advocates for mothers, newborns, and families in developing and implementing effective home-care strategies. Postpartum order sets and maternal-newborn teaching checklists that address the mother's learning needs can be used to accomplish client care tasks and educational outcomes.

CARE MANAGEMENT: PHYSICAL NEEDS

The nursing plan of care includes both the postpartum woman and her infant. It is also family centered, considering the needs and concerns of the family and focusing on family unity (Waller-Wise, 2012). Although in some hospitals the nursery nurse retains primary responsibility for the infant, most perinatal settings use the couplet or mother/baby model of care (Association of Women's Health, Obstetric and Neonatal Nurses [AWHONN], 2010). Nurses in these settings have been educated in both mother and infant care and function as primary nurses for both mother and infant, even if the infant is kept in the nursery. This approach is a variation of rooming-in, in which the mother and infant room together and mother and nurse share the infant's care. The organization of the mother's care must take the newborn's feeding and care needs into consideration.

Ongoing Physical Assessment

Ongoing assessments are performed throughout hospitalization. In addition to vital signs, physical assessment of the postpartum woman focuses on evaluation of the breasts, uterine fundus, lochia, perineum, bladder and bowel function, vital signs, and legs (Table 21-1).

Routine Laboratory Tests

Several laboratory tests may be performed in the immediate postpartum period. Hemoglobin and hematocrit values are often evaluated on the first postpartum day to assess blood loss during birth, especially after cesarean birth. In some hospitals a clean-catch or catheterized urine specimen is obtained and sent for routine urinalysis or culture and sensitivity, especially if an indwelling urinary catheter was inserted during the intrapartum period. In addition, if the woman's rubella immunity and Rh status are unknown, tests to determine her status and need for possible treatment should be performed at this time.

Nursing Interventions

Based on the available data (e.g., medical record) and assessment findings, the nurse plans with the woman which nursing measures are appropriate and which are to be given priority. The nursing care plan includes periodic assessments to detect deviations from normal physical changes, measures to relieve discomfort or pain, safety measures to prevent injury and infection, and education and counseling measures designed to promote the woman's feelings of competence in self-management and infant care. The nurse evaluates continually and is ready to change the plan if indicated. Almost all hospitals use standardized care plans as a base. Nurses individualize care of the postpartum woman and neonate according to their specific needs (see the Nursing Care Plan). Signs of potential problems that may be identified during the assessment process are listed in Table 21-1.

Nurses assume many roles while implementing the nursing care plan. They provide direct physical care, educate new mothers and their families, and provide anticipatory guidance and counseling. Perhaps most important, they nurture the woman by providing encouragement and support as she begins to assume the many tasks of motherhood. Nurses who take the time to "mother the mother" do much to increase feelings of self-confidence in new mothers. Nurses are careful to include the woman's spouse or partner and other primary support persons in education and counseling.

The first step in providing individualized care is to confirm the woman's identity by checking her wristband. At the same time the infant's identification number is matched with the corresponding band on the mother's wrist and in some instances the father's or partner's wrist. The nurse determines how the mother wishes to be addressed and notes her preference in her medical record and her nursing care plan.

NURSING CARE PLAN

Postpartum Care—Vaginal Birth

NURSING DIAGNOSIS	EXPECTED OUTCOME	NURSING INTERVENTIONS	RATIONALES
Risk for Fluid Volume Deficit related to uterine atony/ hemorrhage	Fundus is firm, lochia is moderate, and there is no evidence of hemorrhage.	Monitor lochia (color, amount, consistency) and count sanitary pads if lochia is heavy.	To evaluate amount of bleeding
		Monitor and palpate fundus for location and tone to determine status of uterus and direct further interventions.	To assess for uterine atony, the most common cause of postpartum hemorrhage
		Monitor intake and output, assess for bladder fullness, and encourage voiding.	To prevent bladder distention because a full bladder interferes with involution of uterus
		Monitor vital signs (increased pulse and respirations, decreased blood pressure) and skin temperature and color.	To detect signs of hemorrhage/shock
		Monitor postpartum hematology studies.	To assess effects of blood loss
		If the fundus is boggy, apply gentle massage and assess tone response.	To promote uterine contractions and increase uterine tone (do not overstimulate because doing so can cause fundal relaxation)
		Express uterine clots.	To promote uterine contraction
		Explain to woman process of involution and teach her to assess and massage fundus and report any persistent bogginess.	To involve her in self-management and increase sense of self-control
		Administer uterotonic agents per health care provider's order and evaluate effectiveness.	To promote continuing uterine contraction
		Administer fluids, blood, blood products, or plasma expanders as ordered.	To replace lost fluid and lost blood volume
Acute Pain related to postpartum physiologic changes (hemorrhoids, episiotomy, breast engorgement, sore/damaged nipples)	Woman exhibits signs of decreased discomfort.	Assess location, type, and quality of pain.	To direct intervention
		Explain to woman source and reasons for pain, its expected duration, and treatments.	To decrease anxiety and increase sense of control
		Administer prescribed pain medications and monitor effectiveness.	To provide pain relief
		If pain is perineal (lacerations, episiotomy, hemorrhoids), apply ice packs in first 24 hours.	To reduce edema and vulvar irritation and reduce discomfort
		Encourage sitz baths using cool water the first 24 hours.	To reduce edema and discomfort
		Use warm water for sitz baths after 24 hours.	To promote circulation and reduce discomfort
		Apply witch hazel compresses.	To reduce edema
		Teach woman to use prescribed perineal creams, sprays, or ointments.	To depress response of peripheral nerves
		Teach woman to tighten buttocks before sitting and to sit on flat, hard surfaces.	To compress buttocks and reduce pressure on perineum (avoid donuts and soft pillows because they separate buttocks and decrease venous blood flow, increasing pain)
		If nipples are sore or damaged, assess infant positioning and latch; assist mother to correct problems.	To prevent further nipple soreness and damage
		If nipples are sore, have woman rub expressed milk into them after feeding and leave nipples open to air.	To promote healing
		Apply hydrogel pads between feedings.	To promote comfort
		Wear breast shells over sore nipples.	To prevent irritation
		If breasts are engorged, have breastfeeding woman feed frequently, hand express or pump as needed, and apply ice packs and/ or cabbage leaves intermittently between feedings.	To reduce tissue swelling and promote milk flow

NURSING CARE PLAN—cont'd

Postpartum Care—Vaginal Birth

NURSING DIAGNOSIS	EXPECTED OUTCOME	NURSING INTERVENTIONS	RATIONALES
		Suggest that woman take a warm shower before breastfeeding.	To stimulate milk flow and relieve stasis
		If pain is from breast and woman is not breastfeeding, encourage use of well-fitting supportive bra or breast binder and application of ice packs or cold cabbage leaves.	To suppress milk production and reduce tissue swelling from engorgement
Sleep Pattern Disturbance related to excitement, discomfort, and environmental interruptions	Woman sleeps for uninterrupted periods of time and feels rested after waking.	Establish woman's routine sleep patterns and compare with current sleep pattern, exploring things that interfere with sleep.	To determine scope of problem and direct interventions
		Individualize nursing routines to fit woman's natural body rhythms (i.e., sleep-wake cycles); provide a sleep-promoting environment (i.e., darkness, quiet, adequate ventilation, appropriate room temperature); prepare for sleep using woman's usual routines (i.e., back rub, soothing music, warm milk); teach use of guided imagery and relaxation techniques.	To promote optimal conditions for sleep
		Avoid things or routines that can interfere with sleep (i.e., caffeine, foods that induce heartburn, fluids, strenuous mental/physical activity).	To enhance quality of sleep
		Administer sedative or pain medication as prescribed.	To enhance quality of sleep
		Advise woman/partner to limit visitors and activities.	To avoid further taxation and fatigue
		Teach woman to use infant nap time as a nap time to rest.	To nap and replenish energy and decrease fatigue
Risk for Altered Patterns of Urinary Elimination related to perineal trauma and effects of anesthesia	Woman will void within 3 to 4 hours after birth and empty bladder completely.	Assess position and character of uterine fundus and bladder.	To ascertain if any further interventions are indicated because of displacement of fundus or distention of bladder
		Measure intake and output.	To assess adequacy of fluid intake and urine output; a full or distended bladder increases the risk for uterine atony
		Encourage voiding by assisting woman to bathroom, running water over perineum, running water in sink, and providing privacy.	To encourage voiding
		Encourage oral fluid intake.	To replace any fluids lost during birth and prevent dehydration
		Catheterize as necessary with indwelling or straight method.	To ensure bladder emptying and prevent uterine atony

The woman and her family are oriented to their surroundings. Familiarity with the unit, routines, resources, and personnel reduces one potential source of anxiety—the unknown. The mother is reassured through knowing whom and how she can call for assistance and what she can expect in the way of supplies and services. If the woman's usual daily routine before admission differs from the routine of the facility, the nurse works with the woman to develop a mutually acceptable routine.

Nurses discuss infant security precautions with the mother and her family because infant abductions are an ongoing concern. Between 1983 and 2013, 132 infants were abducted from health care facilities in the United States; 58% of the babies were taken from the mother's room and 13% were taken from the nursery (National Center for Missing and Exploited Children, 2014). The Joint Commission (1999) calls for hospitals to have a management plan to prevent infant abductions. As a result, many units have special limited-entry systems.

TABLE 21-1 **Postpartum Assessment and Signs of Potential Complications**

ASSESSMENT	NORMAL FINDINGS	SIGNS OF POTENTIAL COMPLICATIONS
Blood pressure (BP)	Consistent with BP baseline during pregnancy; can have orthostatic hypotension for 48 hours	Hypertension: anxiety, preeclampsia, essential hypertension Hypotension: hemorrhage
Temperature	36.2°-38° C (97.2°-100.4° F)	>38° C (100.4° F) after 24 hours: infection
Pulse	50-90 beats/min	Tachycardia: pain, fever, dehydration, hemorrhage
Respirations	16-24 breaths/min	Bradypnea: effects of opioid medications Tachypnea: anxiety; may be sign of respiratory disease
Breath sounds	Clear to auscultation	Crackles: possible fluid overload
Breasts	Days 1-2: soft Days 2-3: filling Days 3-5: full, soften with breastfeeding (milk is "in")	Firmness, heat, pain: engorgement
Nipples	Skin intact; no soreness reported	Redness, bruising, cracks, fissures, abrasions, blisters: usually associated with latching problems
Uterus (fundus)	Firm, midline; first 24 hours at level of umbilicus; involutes ≈1 cm/day	Soft, boggy, higher than expected level: uterine atony Lateral deviation: distended bladder
Lochia	Days 1-3: rubra (dark red) Days 3-10: serosa (brownish red or pink) After 10 days: alba (yellowish white) Amount: scant to moderate Few clots Fleshy odor	Large amount of lochia, large clots: uterine atony, vaginal or cervical laceration Foul odor: infection
Perineum	Minimal edema Laceration or episiotomy: edges approximated Pain minimal to moderate: controlled by analgesics, nonpharmacologic techniques, or both	Pronounced edema, bruising, hematoma Redness, warmth, drainage: infection Excessive discomfort first 1-2 days: hematoma; after day 3: infection
Rectal area	No hemorrhoids; if hemorrhoids are present, soft and pink	Discolored hemorrhoidal tissue, severe pain: thrombosed hemorrhoid
Bladder	Able to void spontaneously; no distention; able to empty completely; no dysuria Diuresis begins ≈12 hours after birth; can void 3000 ml/day	Overdistended bladder possibly causing uterine atony, excessive lochia Dysuria, frequency, urgency: infection
Abdomen and bowels	Abdomen soft, active bowel sounds in all quadrants Bowel movement by day 2 or 3 after birth Cesarean: incision dressing clean and dry; suture line intact	No bowel movement by day 3 or 4: constipation; diarrhea Abdominal incision—redness, edema, warmth, drainage: infection
Legs	Deep tendon reflexes (DTRs) 1+ to 2+ Peripheral edema possibly present Homan sign* negative	DTRs ≥3+: preeclampsia Redness, tenderness, pain, thrombophlebitis*
Energy level	Able to care for self and infant; able to sleep	Lethargy, extreme fatigue, difficulty sleeping: postpartum depression
Emotional status	Excited, happy, interested or involved in infant care	Sad, tearful, disinterested in infant care: postpartum blues or depression

*Homan sign was traditionally included in routine postpartum assessments; however, it is no longer common practice due to concern about its limited sensitivity and specificity in diagnosing venous thromboembolism and the potential risk of dislodging a clot when the test is performed.

Nurses teach mothers and their families to check the identity of any person who comes to remove the baby from their room. Hospital personnel usually wear picture identification badges. On some units all staff members wear matching scrubs or special badges. Other units use closed-circuit television, computer monitoring systems, or fingerprint identification pads. As a rule, the infant is never carried in a staff member's arms outside the mother's room, but is always wheeled in a bassinet.

SAFETY ALERT

Nurses play a critical role in educating parents about measures to prevent infant abduction. Parents should be instructed how to identify legitimate hospital personnel, to never leave the newborn in the hospital room without direct supervision, and to request a second staff member to verify the identity of any questionable person who wants to take the baby from the mother's room. Parents should be instructed to use caution when posting photos of the new baby on the Internet and publishing public notices about the birth (AAP and American College of Obstetricians and Gynecologists [ACOG], 2012).

Nurses and new parents must work together to ensure the safety of newborns in the hospital environment (Hiner, Pyka, Burks, et al., 2012).

Preventing Excessive Bleeding

All women who have given birth are at risk for excessive bleeding that can progress to postpartum hemorrhage (see Chapter 33). The most frequent cause of excessive bleeding after birth is uterine atony (i.e., failure of the uterine muscle to contract firmly). The two most important interventions for preventing excessive bleeding are maintaining good uterine tone and preventing bladder distention. If uterine atony occurs, the relaxed uterus distends with blood and clots, blood vessels in the placental site are not clamped off, and excessive bleeding results. Although the cause of uterine atony is not always clear, it often results from retained placental fragments.

Excessive blood loss after birth can also be caused by vaginal or vulvar hematomas or unrepaired lacerations of the vagina or cervix. These potential sources might be suspected if excessive vaginal bleeding occurs in the presence of a firmly contracted uterus.

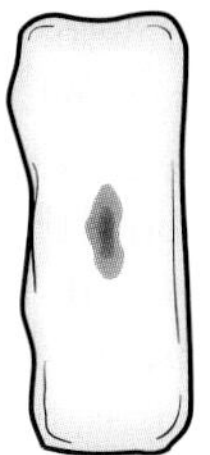
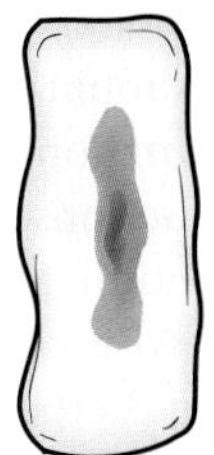
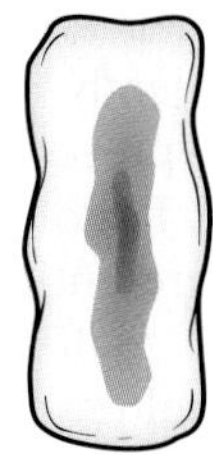
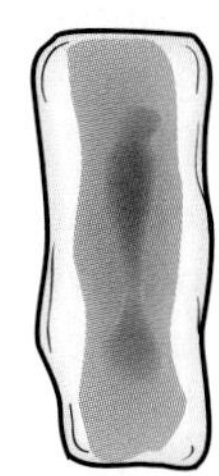

FIG 21-3 Blood loss after birth is assessed by the extent of perineal pad saturation as *(from left to right)* scant (<2.5 cm), light (<10 cm), moderate (>10 cm), or heavy (one pad saturated within 2 hours).

SAFETY ALERT

A perineal pad saturated in 15 minutes or less and pooling of blood under the buttocks are indications of excessive blood loss, requiring immediate assessment, intervention, and notification of the primary health care provider.

Accurate visual estimation of blood loss is an important nursing responsibility. Blood loss is usually described subjectively as scant, light, moderate, or heavy (profuse). Figure 21-3 shows examples of perineal pad saturation corresponding to each of these descriptions.

Although postpartal blood loss can be estimated by observing the amount of drainage on a perineal pad, judging the amount of lochial flow is difficult if based only on observation of perineal pads. More objective estimates of blood loss include measuring serial hemoglobin or hematocrit values, weighing blood clots and items saturated with blood (1 ml equals 1 g), and establishing how many milliliters are required to saturate the perineal pads being used.

Any estimation of lochial flow is inaccurate and incomplete without considering the time factor. The woman who saturates a perineal pad in 1 hour or less is bleeding much more heavily than the woman who saturates one perineal pad in 8 hours.

Nurses in general tend to overestimate rather than underestimate blood loss. Different brands of perineal pads vary in their saturation volume and soaking appearance. For example, blood placed on some brands tends to soak down into the pad, whereas on other brands it tends to spreads outward. Nurses should determine saturation volume and soaking appearance for the brands used in their institution so that they can improve accuracy of blood loss estimation.

SAFETY ALERT

The nurse always checks for blood under the mother's buttocks as well as on the perineal pad. Although the amount on the perineal pad can appear to be small, blood can flow between the buttocks onto the linens under the mother. When this happens, excessive bleeding can go undetected.

When excessive bleeding occurs, vital signs are monitored closely. Blood pressure is not a reliable indicator of impending shock from early postpartum hemorrhage because compensatory mechanisms prevent a significant drop in blood pressure until the woman has lost 30% to 40% of her blood volume (see Chapter 33). Respirations, pulse, skin condition, urinary output, and level of consciousness are more sensitive means of identifying hypovolemic shock (see the Emergency box). The frequent physical assessments performed during the fourth stage of labor are designed to provide prompt identification of excessive bleeding. Nurses maintain vigilance for excessive bleeding throughout the hospital stay as they perform periodic assessment of the uterine fundus and lochia.

EMERGENCY

Hypovolemic Shock

Signs and Symptoms

- Persistent significant bleeding occurs—perineal pad is soaked within 15 minutes; may not be accompanied by a change in vital signs or maternal color or behavior.
- The woman states she feels weak, lightheaded, "funny," or nauseated or that she "sees stars."
- The woman begins to act anxious or exhibits air hunger.
- The woman's skin color turns ashen or grayish.
- Skin feels cool and clammy.
- Pulse rate increases.
- Blood pressure decreases.

Interventions

- Notify the primary health care provider.
- If the uterus is atonic, massage gently and expel clots to cause it to contract; compress uterus manually, as needed, using two hands. Add oxytocic agent to intravenous drip, as ordered.
- Give oxygen by nonrebreather face mask at 10 L/min.
- Tilt the woman onto her side or elevate the right hip; elevate her legs to at least a 30-degree angle.
- Provide additional or maintain existing intravenous (IV) infusion of lactated Ringer's solution or normal saline solution to restore circulatory volume (woman should have two patent IV lines; insert second IV using 16- to 18-gauge IV catheter).
- Administer blood or blood products, as ordered.
- Monitor vital signs.
- Insert an indwelling urinary catheter to monitor kidney perfusion.
- Administer emergency drugs, as ordered.
- Prepare for possible surgery or other emergency treatments or procedures.
- Document the incident, medical and nursing interventions instituted, and the woman's response to interventions.

Maintaining Uterine Tone

A major intervention to alleviate uterine atony and restore uterine muscle tone is stimulation by gently massaging the fundus until firm (Fig. 21-4). Fundal massage can cause a temporary increase in the amount of vaginal bleeding seen as pooled blood leaves the uterus. Clots can also be expelled. The uterus can remain boggy even after massage and clot expulsion.

Fundal massage can be a very uncomfortable procedure. If the nurse explains the purpose of fundal massage as well as the causes and dangers of uterine atony, the woman will likely be more cooperative. Teaching the woman to massage her own fundus enables her to maintain some control and decreases her anxiety.

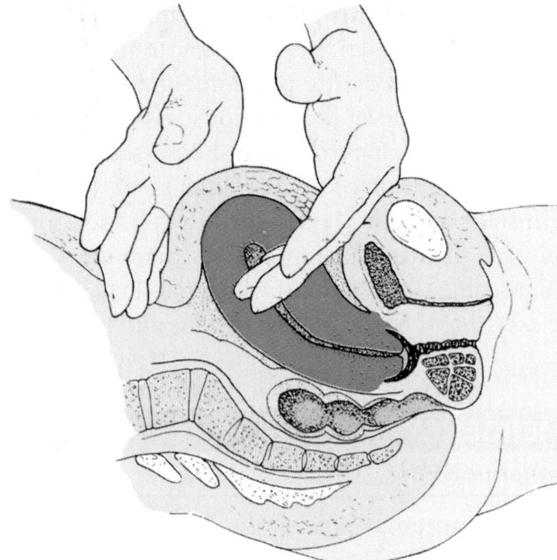

FIG 21-4 Palpating fundus of uterus during the postpartum period. Note that upper hand is cupped over fundus; lower hand dips in above symphysis pubis and supports uterus while it is massaged gently.

When uterine atony and excessive bleeding occur, additional interventions likely to be used are administration of intravenous fluids and oxytocic medications (drugs that stimulate contraction of the uterine smooth muscle). (See Medication Guide in Chapter 33 for information about common oxytocic medications.)

Preventing Bladder Distention

Uterine atony and excessive bleeding after birth can be the result of bladder distention. A full bladder causes the uterus to be displaced above the umbilicus and well to one side of midline in the abdomen. It also prevents the uterus from contracting normally.

Women can be at risk of bladder distention resulting from urinary retention based on intrapartum factors including epidural anesthesia, episiotomy, extensive vaginal or perineal lacerations, instrument-assisted birth, or prolonged labor. Women who have had indwelling catheters, such as with cesarean birth, can experience some difficulty as they initially attempt to void after the catheter is removed. Nurses who are aware of these risk factors can be proactive in preventing complications.

Nursing interventions for a postpartum woman focus on helping the woman empty her bladder spontaneously as soon as possible. The first priority is to assist the woman to the bathroom or onto a bedpan if she is unable to ambulate. Having the woman listen to running water, placing her hands in warm water, or pouring water from a squeeze bottle over her perineum may stimulate voiding. Other techniques include assisting the woman into the shower or sitz bath and encouraging her to void; relaxation techniques can also be helpful. Administering analgesics, if ordered, may be indicated because some women fear voiding because of anticipated pain. If these measures are unsuccessful, a sterile catheter may be inserted to drain the urine.

Preventing Infection

Nurses in the postpartum setting are acutely aware of the importance of preventing infection. One important means of preventing infection is by maintaining a clean environment. Bed linens should be changed as needed. Disposable pads and drawsheets are changed frequently. Women should wear slippers when walking about to prevent contamination of the linens when they return to bed. Personnel must be conscientious about their hand hygiene to prevent cross-infection. Standard Precautions must be practiced. Staff members with colds, coughs, or skin infections (e.g., a cold sore on the lip [herpes simplex virus, type 1]) must follow hospital protocol when in contact with postpartum women. In many hospitals, staff members with open herpetic lesions, strep throat, conjunctivitis, upper respiratory infections, or diarrhea are encouraged to avoid contact with mothers and infants by staying home until the condition is no longer contagious. Visitors with signs of illness are not permitted to enter the postpartum unit.

Perineal lacerations and episiotomies can increase the risk of infection as a result of interruption in skin integrity. Proper perineal care helps prevent infection in the genitourinary area and aids the healing process. Educating the woman to wipe from front to back (urethra to anus) after voiding or defecating is a simple first step. In many hospitals a squeeze bottle filled with warm water or an antiseptic solution is used after each voiding to cleanse the perineal area. The woman should change her perineal pad from front to back each time she voids or defecates and wash her hands thoroughly before and after doing so (Box 21-1).

Promoting Comfort

Most women experience some degree of discomfort during the postpartum period. Common causes of discomfort include pain from uterine contractions (afterpains), perineal lacerations or episiotomy, hemorrhoids, sore nipples, and breast engorgement. The woman's description of the location, type, and severity of her pain is the best guide in choosing appropriate interventions. To confirm the location and extent of discomfort, the nurse inspects and palpates areas of pain as appropriate for redness, swelling, discharge, and heat, and observes for body tension, guarded movements, and facial tension. Blood pressure, pulse, and respirations can be elevated in response to acute pain. Diaphoresis can accompany severe pain. A lack of objective signs does not necessarily mean there is no pain because there can be a cultural component to the expression of pain. Nursing interventions are intended to eliminate the pain sensation entirely or reduce it to a tolerable level that allows the woman to care for herself and her newborn. Nurses may use nonpharmacologic and pharmacologic interventions to promote comfort. Pain relief is enhanced by using more than one method or route.

Nonpharmacologic Interventions. Various nonpharmacologic measures are used to reduce postpartum discomfort. These include distraction, imagery, therapeutic touch, relaxation, acupressure, aromatherapy, hydrotherapy, massage therapy, music therapy, and transcutaneous electrical nerve stimulation (TENS).

For women who are experiencing discomfort associated with uterine contractions, application of warmth (e.g., heating pad) or lying prone can be helpful. Interaction with the infant can also provide distraction and decrease this discomfort. Because afterpains are more severe during and after breastfeeding, interventions are planned to provide the most timely and effective relief. Simple interventions that can decrease the discomfort associated with an episiotomy or perineal

BOX 21-1 Interventions for Episiotomy, Lacerations, and Hemorrhoids

Explain procedure and rationale before implementation.

Cleansing
- Wash hands before and after cleansing perineum and changing pads.
- Wash perineum with mild soap and warm water at least once daily.
- Cleanse from symphysis pubis to anal area.
- Apply peripad from front to back, protecting inner surface of pad from contamination.
- Wrap soiled pad and place in covered waste container.
- Change pad with each void or defecation or at least four times per day.
- Assess amount and character of lochia with each pad change.

Ice Pack
- Apply a covered ice pack to perineum from front to back:
  - During first 24 hours to decrease edema formation and increase comfort
  - After first 24 hours following birth as needed to provide anesthetic effect

Squeeze Bottle
- Demonstrate use and assist woman; explain rationale.
- Fill bottle with tap water warmed to approximately 38° C (100.4° F) (comfortably warm on wrist).
- Instruct woman to position nozzle between her legs so squirts of water reach perineum as she sits on toilet seat. Explain that it will take whole bottle of water to cleanse the perineum.
- Remind her to blot dry with toilet paper or clean wipes.
- Remind her to avoid contamination from anal area by wiping "front to back."
- Apply clean pad.

Sitz Bath

Built-in Type
- Prepare bath by thoroughly scrubbing with cleaning agent and rinsing.
- Pad with towel before filling.
- Fill one third to one half full with water of correct temperature 38° to 40.6° C (100.4° to 105.1° F). Some women prefer cool sitz baths. Ice is added to water to lower temperature to a comfortable level.
- Encourage woman to use at least twice a day for 20 minutes.
- Place call bell within easy reach.
- Teach woman to enter bath by tightening gluteal muscles and keeping them tightened and then relaxing them after she is in bath.
- Place dry towels within reach.
- Ensure privacy.
- Check woman in 15 minutes.

Disposable Type
- Clamp tubing and fill bag with warm water.
- Raise toilet seat; place bath in bowl with overflow opening directed toward back of toilet.
- Place container above toilet bowl.
- Attach tube into groove at front of bath.
- Loosen tube clamp to regulate rate of flow; fill bath to about one half full; continue as for built-in sitz bath.

Topical Applications
- Apply anesthetic cream or spray after cleansing perineal area: use sparingly three or four times per day.
- Apply witch hazel pads (Tucks) after voiding or defecating; woman pats perineum dry from front to back and applies witch hazel pads.
- Apply hemorrhoidal cream as ordered to anal area after cleansing.

lacerations include encouraging the woman to lie on her side whenever possible. Other interventions include application of an ice pack; topical application (if ordered) of anesthetic spray or cream; cleansing with water from a squeeze bottle; and a cleansing shower, tub bath, or sitz bath. Many of these interventions are also effective for hemorrhoids, especially ice packs, sitz baths, and topical applications (such as witch hazel pads). (Box 21-1 gives additional specific information about these interventions.)

Sore nipples in breastfeeding mothers are most likely related to ineffective latch technique. Assessment and assistance with feeding can help alleviate the cause. To ease discomfort associated with sore nipples, the mother may apply topical preparations such as purified lanolin or hydrogel pads (see Chapter 25).

Breast engorgement can occur whether the woman is breastfeeding or formula feeding. The discomfort associated with engorged breasts may be reduced by applying ice packs or cabbage leaves (or both) to the breasts, and wearing a well-fitted support bra. Antiinflammatory medications such as ibuprofen can also be helpful in relieving some of the discomfort. Decisions about specific interventions for engorgement are based on whether the woman chooses breastfeeding or bottle feeding (see Chapter 25).

Pharmacologic Interventions. Pharmacologic interventions are commonly used to relieve or reduce postpartum discomfort. Most health care providers routinely order a variety of analgesics to be administered as needed, including both opioid and nonopioid (e.g., nonsteroidal antiinflammatory drugs [NSAIDs]). In some hospitals NSAIDs are administered on a scheduled basis, especially if the woman had perineal repair. Topical application of antiseptic or anesthetic ointment or spray can be used for perineal pain. Patient-controlled analgesia (PCA) pumps and epidural analgesia are commonly used to provide pain relief after cesarean birth.

MEDICATION ALERT

The nurse should carefully monitor all women receiving opioids because respiratory depression and decreased intestinal motility are side effects.

Many women want to participate in decisions about analgesia. Severe pain, however, can interfere with active participation in choosing pain relief measures. If an analgesic is to be given, the nurse must make a clinical judgment of the type, appropriate dosage, and frequency from the medications ordered. The woman is informed of the prescribed analgesic and its common side effects; this teaching is documented.

Breastfeeding mothers often have concerns about the effects of an analgesic on the infant. Although nearly all drugs present in maternal circulation are also found in breast milk, many analgesics commonly used during the postpartum period are considered relatively safe for breastfeeding mothers and infants. Often the timing of medications can be adjusted to minimize infant exposure. A mother may be given pain medication immediately after breastfeeding so that the interval between medication administration and the next breastfeeding session is as long as possible. The decision to administer medications of any kind to a breastfeeding mother must always be made by carefully weighing the woman's need against actual or potential risks to the infant. Resources are readily accessible for nurses and health care providers to examine the safety of medications for breastfeeding mothers (e.g., LactMed [http://toxnet.nlm.nih.gov/cgi-bin/sis/htmlgen?LACT]).

If acceptable pain relief has not been obtained in 1 hour and there is no change in the initial assessment, the nurse may need to contact the primary care provider for additional pain relief orders or further directions. Unrelieved pain results in fatigue, anxiety, and a worsening perception of the pain. It might also indicate the presence of a previously unidentified or untreated problem.

Promoting Rest. *Postpartum fatigue* (PPF) is more than just feeling tired; it is a common complex physiologic and psychologic phenomenon. Physical fatigue or exhaustion can be associated with long labor or cesarean birth; hospital routines and infant care demands such as breastfeeding also contribute to maternal fatigue. Fatigue can also be associated with anemia, infection, or thyroid dysfunction. The excitement and exhilaration experienced after the birth of the infant makes resting difficult. Physical discomfort can interfere with sleep. Well-intentioned visitors can interrupt periods of rest in the hospital and at home.

Symptoms of PPF and depressive symptoms are interrelated. Depressive symptoms can affect fatigue, whereas fatigue can lead to or worsen depressive symptoms. Depression-related PPF can be differentiated from nondepression-related fatigue based on whether depressive symptoms are reduced when fatigue is decreased (Doering & Durfor, 2011).

Fatigue is likely to worsen over the first 6 weeks after birth, often because of situational factors. After discharge from the hospital, fatigue increases as the woman provides care and feeding for the newborn in combination with other family and household responsibilities such as caring for other children, preparing meals, and doing laundry. Many women have partners, family members, or friends to provide much-needed assistance, whereas others can be without any help at all. The nurse needs to inquire about resources available to the woman after discharge and help her plan accordingly.

Interventions are planned to meet the woman's individual needs for sleep and rest while she is in the hospital. Comfort measures and medications to promote sleep may be necessary. The side-lying position for breastfeeding minimizes fatigue in nursing mothers. Support and encouragement of mothering behaviors help reduce anxiety. Hospital and nursing routines can be adjusted to meet needs of individual mothers. In addition, the nurse can help the family limit visitors and provide a comfortable chair or bed for the partner or other family member who is staying with the new mother.

Because PPF can be very debilitating, follow-up after hospital discharge is important. Screening for PPF can be accomplished with a nurse-initiated telephone call at 2 weeks, as well as at the routine 6-week postpartum visit with the health care provider. Nurses in the pediatric care provider's office or clinic should also be alert for signs of PPF. The infant will be seen within the first few days after birth—before the woman sees her obstetric care provider.

Some physiologic factors contributing to PPF are amenable to intervention and can be identified even before birth. These include sleeping problems during pregnancy, anemia, infection or inflammation, and thyroid dysfunction. The medical records of women with known risk factors can be flagged to alert hospital staff to their special needs (Doering & Durfor, 2011).

Promoting Ambulation. Early ambulation is associated with a reduced incidence of venous thromboembolism (VTE); it also promotes the return of strength. Free movement is encouraged once anesthesia wears off unless an opioid analgesic has been administered. After the initial recovery period the mother is encouraged to ambulate frequently.

In the early postpartum period women can feel lightheaded or dizzy when standing. The rapid decrease in intraabdominal pressure after birth results in a dilation of blood vessels supplying the intestines (splanchnic engorgement) and causes blood to pool in the viscera. This condition contributes to the development of orthostatic hypotension when the woman who has recently given birth sits or stands up, first ambulates, or takes a warm shower or sitz bath. When assisting a woman to ambulate, the nurse needs to consider the baseline blood pressure, amount of blood loss, and type, amount, and timing of analgesic or anesthetic medications administered.

Women who have had regional (epidural or spinal) anesthesia can experience slow return of sensory and motor function in their lower extremities, increasing the risk of falls with early ambulation. Careful assessment by the postpartum nurse can prevent falls. Factors that the nurse should consider are the time lapse since epidural or spinal medication was given; the woman's ability to bend both knees, place both feet flat on the bed, and lift buttocks off the bed without assistance; medications since birth; vital signs; and estimated blood loss with birth. Before allowing the woman to ambulate the nurse assesses the ability of the woman to stand unassisted beside her bed, simultaneously bending both knees slightly, and then standing with knees locked. If the woman is unable to balance herself, she can be safely eased back into bed without injury (Lockwood & Anderson, 2013).

SAFETY ALERT

To promote safety and prevent injury it is important to have hospital personnel present the first time the woman gets out of bed after birth because she can feel weak, dizzy, faint, or lightheaded. The woman is instructed to call for assistance before getting out of bed the first time and any time thereafter if she feels dizzy or weak. The partner or family members who are present are instructed as well.

Preventing VTE is important. Women who must remain in bed after giving birth are at increased risk for this complication. Antiembolic stockings (TED hose) or a sequential compression device (SCD boots) may be ordered prophylactically. If a woman remains in bed longer than 8 hours (e.g., for postpartum magnesium sulfate therapy for preeclampsia), exercise to promote circulation in the legs is indicated, using the following routine:

- Alternate flexion and extension of the feet.
- Rotate the ankles in a circular motion.
- Alternate flexion and extension of the legs.
- Press the back of the knees to the bed surface; relax.

If the woman is susceptible to VTE, she is encouraged to walk about actively for true ambulation and is discouraged from sitting immobile in a chair. Women with varicosities are encouraged to wear support hose. If a thrombus is suspected, as evidenced by warmth, redness, or tenderness in the suspected leg, the primary health care provider should be notified. Meanwhile the woman should be confined to bed, with the affected limb elevated on pillows.

Promoting Exercise. Postpartum exercise can begin soon after birth, although the woman should be encouraged to start with simple exercises and gradually progress to more strenuous ones. Figure 21-5 illustrates a number of exercises appropriate for the new mother. Abdominal exercises are postponed until approximately 4 to 6 weeks after cesarean birth.

Kegel exercises to strengthen muscle tone are extremely important, particularly after vaginal birth. Kegel exercises help women regain the muscle tone that is often lost as pelvic tissues are stretched and torn during pregnancy and birth. Women who maintain muscle strength benefit years later by retaining urinary continence.

Women must learn to perform Kegel exercises correctly (see Teaching for Self-Management box: Kegel Exercises, Chapter 4). Some women perform the exercises incorrectly and can increase the risk of incontinence, which can occur when inadvertently bearing down on the pelvic floor muscles, thrusting the perineum outward. The health care provider can assess the woman's technique during the pelvic examination at her follow-up visit by inserting two fingers intravaginally and noting whether the pelvic floor muscles correctly contract and relax.

Promoting Nutrition

During the hospital stay most women have a good appetite and eat well. They may request that family members bring favorite or culturally appropriate foods. Cultural dietary preferences must be respected. This interest in food presents an ideal opportunity for nutritional counseling on dietary needs after pregnancy, with specific information related to breastfeeding, preventing constipation and anemia, promoting weight loss, and promoting healing and well-being (see Chapter 15).

A well-balanced diet helps promote healing and health in the postpartum period. The recommended caloric intake for the moderately active, nonlactating postpartum woman is 1800 to 2200 kcal/day. Lactating women need an additional 450 to 500 kcal/day, which can usually be met with simple adjustments in a normally balanced diet. Women who are underweight, exercise excessively, or are breastfeeding more than one infant need additional calories. Dietary intake for lactating women should include 200 to 300 mg of the omega-3 long-chain polyunsaturated fatty acids (docosahexaenoic acid [DHA]) so that there is adequate DHA in the breast milk. The addition of one or two portions of fish with low mercury content provides the additional DHA. Women on selected vegan diets and those who are poorly nourished may need to take DHA and multivitamin supplements (AAP Section on Breastfeeding, 2012).

Prenatal vitamins may be continued until 6 weeks after birth or until the supply has been used. Iron supplements may be prescribed for women with low hemoglobin and hematocrit levels.

Promoting Normal Bladder and Bowel Patterns

Bladder Function. The mother should void spontaneously within 6 to 8 hours after giving birth. The first several voidings should be measured to document adequate emptying of the bladder. A volume of at least 150 ml is expected for each voiding. Some women experience difficulty in emptying the bladder, possibly as a result of diminished bladder tone, edema from trauma, or fear of discomfort. Nursing interventions for inability to void and bladder distention are discussed in the section "Preventing Bladder Distention."

Bowel Function. After birth, women can be at risk for constipation related to side effects of medications (opioid analgesics, iron supplements, magnesium sulfate), dehydration, immobility, or the presence of episiotomy, perineal lacerations, or hemorrhoids. The woman can be fearful of pain with the first bowel movement.

Nursing interventions to promote normal bowel elimination include educating the woman about measures to prevent constipation, such as ambulation and increasing the intake of fluids and fiber. Alerting the woman to side effects of medications such as opioid analgesics (e.g., decreased gastrointestinal tract motility) can encourage her to implement measures to reduce the risk of constipation. Stool softeners or laxatives may be necessary during the early postpartum period. These are used only at the direction of the health care provider.

> **SAFETY ALERT**
>
> Rectal suppositories and enemas should not be administered to women with third- or fourth-degree perineal lacerations. These measures to treat constipation can be very uncomfortable and can cause hemorrhage or damage to the suture line. They can also predispose the woman to infection.

Some mothers experience gas pains; this is more common following cesarean birth. Ambulation or rocking in a rocking chair can stimulate passage of flatus and provide relief. Antiflatulent medications may be ordered. The mother can avoid foods (e.g., legumes, beans, broccoli) that tend to produce gas.

Promoting Breastfeeding

The ideal time to initiate breastfeeding is within the first 1 to 2 hours after birth. Newborns should be placed in skin-to-skin contact with their mothers as soon as possible after birth and remain there for at least an hour. Nurses can encourage mothers to observe their babies for signs that they are ready to breastfeed and then assist the mothers as needed to initiate breastfeeding (Baby-Friendly USA, 2011). During this first hour most infants

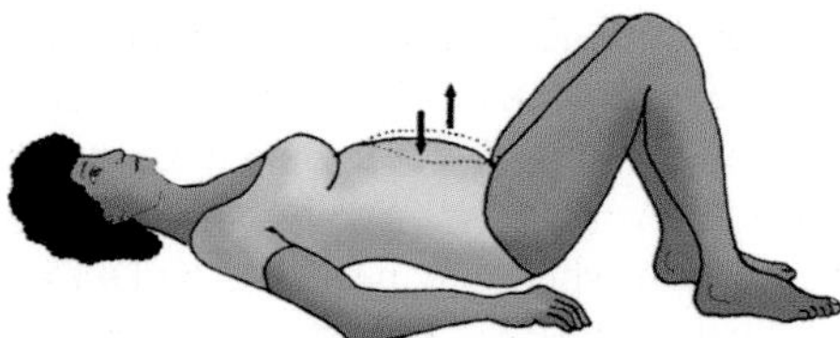

Abdominal Breathing. Lie on back with knees bent. Inhale deeply through nose. Keep ribs stationary and allow abdomen to expand upward. Exhale slowly but forcefully while contracting the abdominal muscles; hold for 3 to 5 seconds while exhaling. Relax.

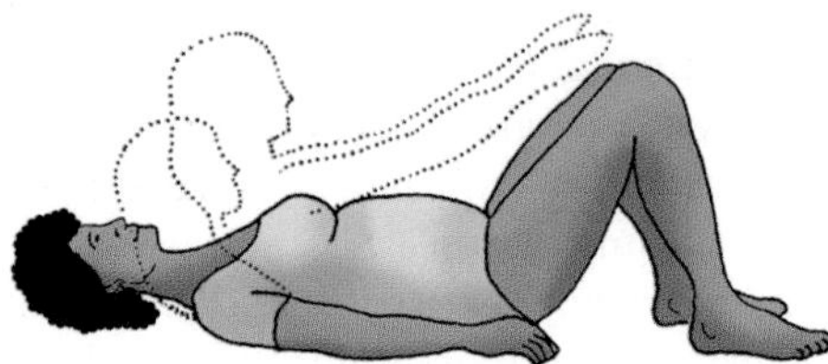

Reach for the Knees. Lie on back with knees bent. While inhaling deeply, lower chin onto chest. While exhaling, raise head and shoulders slowly and smoothly and reach for knees with arms outstretched. The body should rise only as far as the back will naturally bend while waist remains on floor or bed (about 6 to 8 inches). Slowly and smoothly lower head and shoulders back to starting position. Relax.

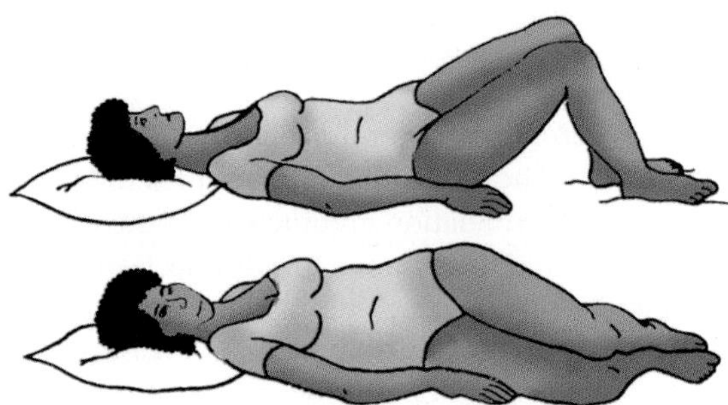

Double Knee Roll. Lie on back with knees bent. Keeping shoulders flat and feet stationary, slowly and smoothly roll knees over to the right to touch floor or bed. Maintaining a smooth motion, roll knees back over to the left until they touch floor or bed. Return to starting position and relax.

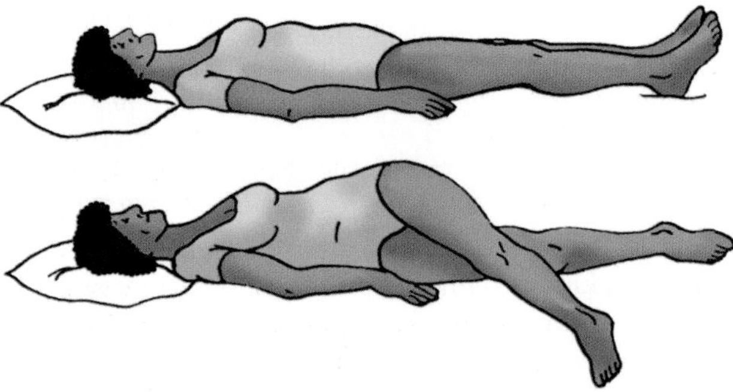

Leg Roll. Lie on back with legs straight. Keeping shoulders flat and legs straight, slowly and smoothly lift left leg and roll it over to touch the right side of floor or bed and return to starting position. Repeat, rolling right leg over to touch left side of floor or bed. Relax.

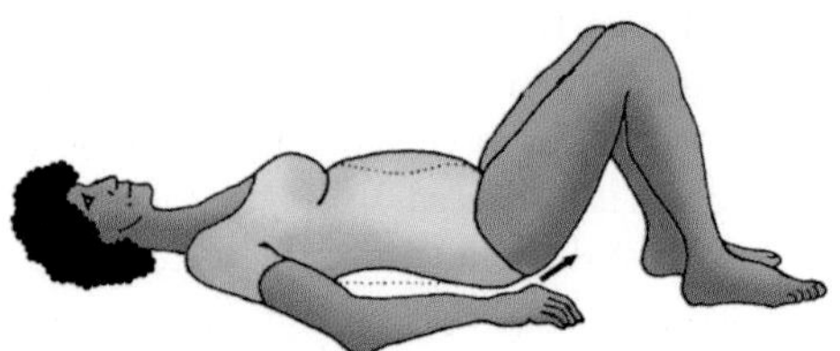

Combined Abdominal Breathing and Supine Pelvic Tilt (Pelvic Rock). Lie on back with knees bent. While inhaling deeply, roll pelvis back by flattening lower back on floor or bed. Exhale slowly but forcefully while contracting abdominal muscles and tightening buttocks. Hold for 3 to 5 seconds while exhaling. Relax.

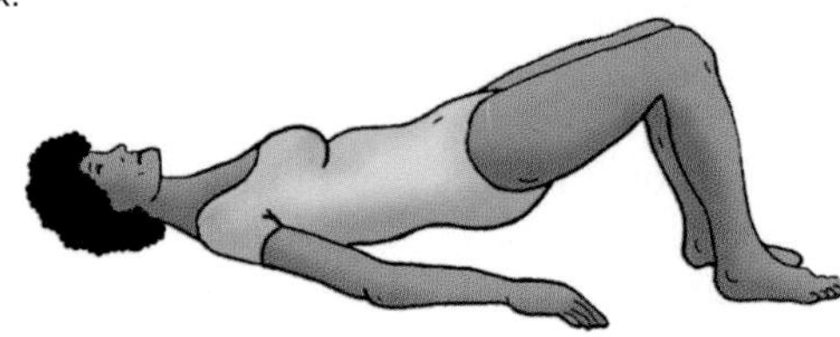

Buttocks Lift. Lie on back with arms at sides, knees bent, and feet flat. Slowly raise buttocks and arch back. Return slowly to starting position.

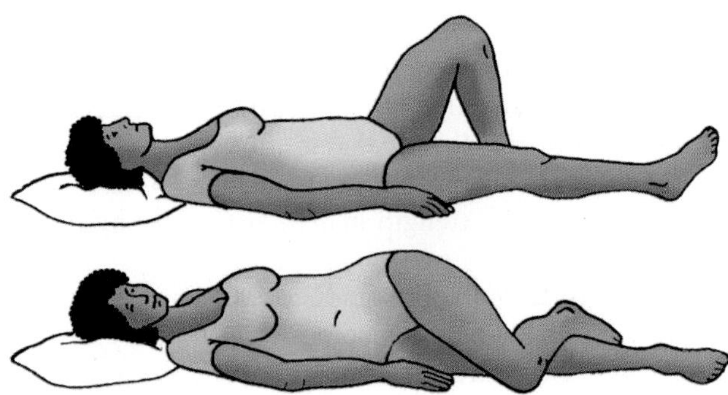

Single Knee Roll. Lie on back with right leg straight and left leg bent at the knee. Keeping shoulders flat, slowly and smoothly roll left knee over to the right to touch floor or bed and then back to starting position. Reverse position of legs. Roll right knee over to the left to touch floor or bed and return to starting position. Relax.

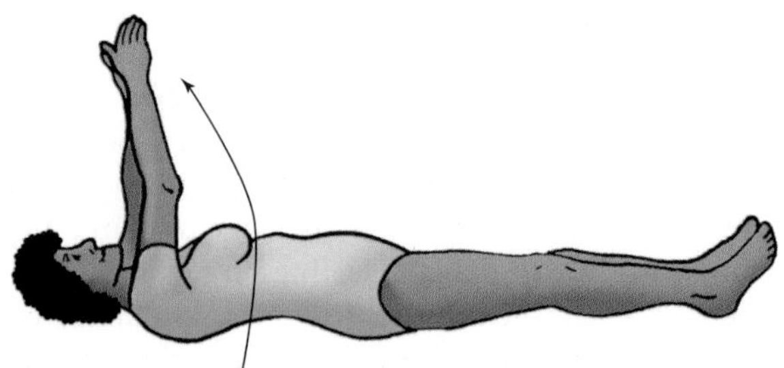

Arm Raises. Lie on back with arms extended at 90-degree angle from body. Raise arms so they are perpendicular and hands touch. Lower slowly.

FIG 21-5 Postpartum exercise should begin as soon as possible. The woman should start with simple exercises and gradually progress to more strenuous ones.

are alert and ready to nurse. Breastfeeding aids in contracting the uterus and preventing maternal hemorrhage. This initial breastfeeding session allows the nurse to assess the mother's basic knowledge of breastfeeding and the physical appearance of the breasts and nipples. Throughout the hospital stay, nurses provide education and assistance for the breastfeeding mother, making appropriate referrals to lactation consultants as needed. Nurses also provide information about community breastfeeding support groups (see Chapter 25 for further information on assisting the breastfeeding woman.)

COMMUNITY ACTIVITY

Women breastfeed longer if they feel supported in their breastfeeding efforts. Nurses and lactation consultants provide support during inpatient stays after birth. Women can find support in the community in various groups. Social support interventions that include peer support are successful in increasing the duration of exclusive breastfeeding and satisfaction with breastfeeding. In their discharge planning nurses can refer breastfeeding mothers to community groups such as La Leche League for support. Community and home health care nurses can facilitate breastfeeding efforts through organizing or facilitating support groups. Mothers experienced in breastfeeding can facilitate these efforts.

Identify sources of breastfeeding support in your community. Are these resources free and available in various parts of the community? What form does the support take? Are there group classes? Individual consultation? Who provides the consultation? Make a list of the resources you identified and share the list with your clinical group.

Lactation Suppression. Lactation suppression is necessary when a woman has decided not to breastfeed or in the case of neonatal death. The woman wears a well-fitted support bra continuously for at least the first 72 hours after giving birth. She should avoid breast stimulation, including running warm water over the breasts, newborn suckling, or expressing milk. Some nonbreastfeeding mothers experience severe breast engorgement (swelling of breast tissue caused by increased blood and lymph supply to the breasts as the body produces milk, occurring about 72 to 96 hours after birth). Breast engorgement can usually be managed satisfactorily with nonpharmacologic interventions.

Periodic application of ice packs to the breasts can help decrease the discomfort associated with engorgement. Although there is lack of scientific evidence to support effectiveness, cabbage leaves are often recommended to help relieve engorgement; formula-feeding mothers may be told to place fresh green cabbage leaves over their breasts and to replace the leaves when they are wilted. A mild analgesic or antiinflammatory medication can reduce discomfort associated with engorgement. Medications that were once prescribed for lactation suppression (e.g., estrogen, estrogen and testosterone, and bromocriptine) are no longer used.

Health Promotion for Planning Future Pregnancies and Children

Rubella Vaccination. For women who have not had rubella or who are serologically non-immune (titer of 1:8 or enzyme immunoassay level less than 0.8), a subcutaneous injection of rubella vaccine is recommended in the postpartum period prior to hospital discharge to prevent the possibility of contracting rubella in future pregnancies; this is given as the measles, mumps, rubella (MMR) vaccine. Women are cautioned to avoid becoming pregnant for 28 days after receiving the rubella vaccine because of the potential teratogenic risk to the fetus (CDC, 2014). The live attenuated rubella virus is not communicable in breast milk; therefore, breastfeeding mothers can be vaccinated. However, because the virus is shed in urine and other body fluids, the vaccine should not be given if the mother or other household members are immunocompromised. Fever, transient arthralgia, rash, and lymphadenopathy are common side effects of the rubella vaccine (McLean, Fiebelkorn, Temte, & Wallace, 2013).

Varicella Vaccination. The Centers for Disease Control and Prevention (CDC) recommend that varicella vaccine be administered before discharge in postpartum women who have no immunity. A second dose is given at the postpartum follow-up visit (4 to 8 weeks after the first dose) (CDC, 2014).

LEGAL TIP: Rubella and Varicella Vaccination

Informed consent for rubella and varicella vaccination in the postpartum period includes information about possible side effects and the risk of teratogenic effects on the fetus. Women must understand that they must not become pregnant for 28 days after being vaccinated (CDC, 2014).

Tetanus-Diphtheria-Acellular Pertussis Vaccine. Tetanus-diphtheria-acellular pertussis (Tdap) vaccine is recommended for postpartum women who have not previously received the vaccine; it is given before discharge from the hospital or as early as possible in the postpartum period to protect women from pertussis and to decrease the risk of infant exposure to pertussis. Women should be advised that other adults and children who will be around the newborn should be vaccinated with Tdap if they have not previously received the vaccine. Women who receive the vaccine can continue to breastfeed (CDC, 2013).

Preventing Rh Isoimmunization. Injection of Rh immune globulin (a solution of gamma globulin that contains Rh antibodies) within 72 hours after birth prevents sensitization in the Rh-negative woman who has had a fetomaternal transfusion of Rh-positive fetal red blood cells (RBCs) (see the Medication Guide). Rh immune globulin promotes lysis of fetal Rh-positive blood cells before the mother forms her own antibodies against them.

The administration of 300 mcg (1 vial) of Rh immune globulin is usually sufficient to prevent maternal sensitization. If a large fetomaternal transfusion is suspected, however, the dosage needed should be determined by performing a Kleihauer-Betke test, which detects the amount of fetal blood in the maternal circulation. If more than 30 ml of fetal blood is present in maternal circulation, the dosage of Rh immune globulin must be increased (AAP & ACOG, 2012).

MEDICATION GUIDE

Rh Immune Globulin, RhoGAM, Gamulin Rh, HypRho-D, Rhophylac

Action

Suppression of immune response in nonsensitized women with Rh-negative blood who receive Rh-positive blood cells because of fetomaternal hemorrhage, transfusion, or accident

Indications

Routine antepartum prevention at 28 weeks of gestation in women with Rh-negative blood; suppress antibody formation after birth, miscarriage, pregnancy termination, abdominal trauma, ectopic pregnancy, amniocentesis, version, or chorionic villus sampling

Dosage and Route

Standard dose: 1 vial (300 mcg) IM in deltoid or gluteal muscle; microdose: 1 vial (50 mcg) IM in deltoid muscle; Rh_0(D) immune globulin (Rhophylac) can be given IM or IV (available in prefilled syringes).

Adverse Effects

Myalgia, lethargy, localized tenderness and stiffness at injection site, mild and transient fever, malaise, headache; rarely nausea, vomiting, hypotension, tachycardia, possible allergic response

Nursing Considerations

- Give standard dose to mother at 28 weeks of gestation as prophylaxis or after an incident or exposure risk that occurs after 28 weeks of gestation (e.g., amniocentesis, second-trimester miscarriage or abortion, and after version).
- Give standard dose within 72 hours after birth if neonate is Rh+.
- Give microdose for first trimester miscarriage or abortion, ectopic pregnancy, chorionic villus sampling.
- Verify that the woman is Rh negative and has not been sensitized, if postpartum that Coombs' test is negative, and that baby is Rh positive. Provide explanation to the woman about the procedure, including the purpose, possible side effects, and effect on future pregnancies. Have the woman sign a consent form if required by agency. Verify correct dosage and confirm lot number and woman's identity before giving injection (verify with another registered nurse or by other procedure per agency policy); document administration per agency policy. Observe client for at least 20 minutes after administration for allergic response.
- Document lot number and expiration date in the client record.
- The medication is made from human plasma (a consideration if woman is a Jehovah's Witness). The risk of transmitting infectious agents, including viruses, cannot be eliminated completely.

IM, Intramuscular; *IV*, intravenous.

MEDICATION ALERT

Rh immune globulin suppresses the immune response. Therefore, the woman who receives both Rh immune globulin and a live virus immunization such as rubella must be tested in 3 months to see if she has developed rubella immunity. If not, she will need another dose of the vaccine (McLean et al., 2013).

There is some disagreement about whether Rh immune globulin should be considered a blood product. Health care providers need to discuss the most current information about this issue with women whose religious beliefs conflict with having blood products administered to them (e.g., Jehovah's Witnesses).

CARE MANAGEMENT: PSYCHOSOCIAL NEEDS

Meeting the psychosocial needs of new parents involves assessing their reactions to the birth experience, feelings about themselves, and interactions with the new baby (Fig. 21-6) and other family members. Specific interventions are planned to increase the parents' knowledge and self-confidence as they assume the care and responsibility of the new baby and integrate this new member into their existing family structure in a way that meets their cultural expectations (see Chapters 22 and 24).

Taking time to assess maternal emotional needs and to address concerns before discharge can promote better psychologic health and adjustment to parenting. Ongoing support for postpartum women is also needed. Even though issues such as fatigue are often evident during the hospital stay, this type of support will likely be an ongoing concern after discharge when the woman is providing care for the newborn, herself, and other family members. Postpartum support is especially beneficial to at-risk populations such as low-income primiparas, those at risk for family dysfunction and child abuse, and those at risk for postpartum depression (PPD).

Sometimes the psychosocial assessment indicates serious actual or potential problems that must be addressed. The Signs of Potential Complications box identifies psychosocial characteristics and behaviors that warrant ongoing evaluation after hospital discharge. Women exhibiting these needs should be referred to appropriate community resources for assessment and management.

Effect of the Birth Experience

Many women need to review and reflect on labor and birth and to look retrospectively at their own intrapartal behavior. Their

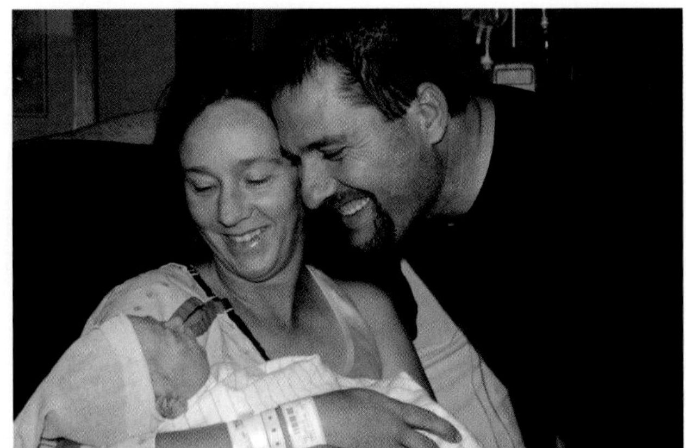

FIG 21-6 Parents getting acquainted with their new son. (Courtesy Julie and Darren Nelson, Loveland, CO.)

SIGNS OF POTENTIAL COMPLICATIONS

Postpartum Psychosocial Concerns

The following signs suggest potentially serious complications and should be reported to the health care provider or clinic (these may be noticed by the partner or other family members):

- Unable or unwilling to discuss labor and birth experience
- Refers to self as ugly and useless
- Excessively preoccupied with self (body image)
- Markedly depressed
- Lacks a support system
- Partner or other family members react negatively to the baby
- Refuses to interact with or care for baby; for example, does not name baby, does not want to hold or feed baby, is upset by vomiting and wet or soiled diapers (cultural appropriateness of actions must be considered)
- Expresses disappointment over baby's sex
- Sees baby as messy or unattractive
- Baby reminds mother of family member or friend she does not like
- Has difficulty sleeping
- Experiences loss of appetite

partners can have similar needs. If their birth experience was different from their birth plan (e.g., induction, epidural anesthesia, cesarean birth), both partners may need to mourn the loss of their expectations before they can adjust to the reality of their actual birth experience. Inviting them to review the events and describe how they feel helps the nurse assess how well they understand what happened and how well they have been able to put their birth experience into perspective.

Maternal Self-Image

An important assessment concerns the woman's self-concept, body image, and sexuality. How the new mother feels about herself and her body during the postpartum period can affect her behavior and adaptation to parenting. The woman's self-concept and body image can also affect her sexuality.

Feelings related to sexual adjustment after birth are often a cause of concern for new parents. Women who have recently given birth can be reluctant to resume sexual intercourse for fear of pain or may worry that coitus will damage healing perineal tissue. Because many new parents are anxious for information but reluctant to bring up the subject, postpartum nurses can matter-of-factly include the topic of postpartum sexuality during their routine physical assessment and teaching. Partners often have questions and concerns as well; it is helpful to include them in teaching sessions or discussions regarding sexuality in the postpartum period.

Adaptation to Parenthood and Parent-Infant Interactions

The psychosocial assessment includes evaluating adaptation to parenthood as evidenced by the mother's and father's (partner's) reactions to and interactions with the new baby. Clues indicating successful adaptation begin to appear early in the postbirth period as parents react positively to the newborn infant and continue the process of establishing a relationship with their child.

Parents are adapting well to their new roles when they exhibit a realistic perception and acceptance of their newborn's needs and limited abilities, immature social responses, and helplessness. Examples of positive parent-infant interactions include taking pleasure in the infant and in providing care, responding appropriately to infant cues, and providing comfort (see Chapter 24). If these indicators are missing, the nurse needs to investigate further in an attempt to identify what is hindering the normal adaptation process. The nurse can ask questions to determine if the woman is experiencing the normal "baby blues" or if there is a more serious underlying condition. Screening for PPD through use of a simple tool such as the Edinburgh Postnatal Depression Scale (EPDS) can be done before hospital discharge. Screening for PPD should also be done after discharge (see Chapter 31). The AAP recommends that pediatric care providers routinely perform maternal screening for PPD during infant follow-up visits at 1, 2, and 4 months (AAP Committee on Psychosocial Aspects of Child and Family Health, 2010) (see Clinical Reasoning Case Study).

? CLINICAL REASONING CASE STUDY

Risk for Postpartum Depression

Elisabeth, a 38-year old multipara, has just given birth to her fourth baby. The ages of her other children are 8, 4, and 2. During the morning nursing assessment, Elisabeth was noted to be tearful and stated that she was feeling "overwhelmed" and "very unsure" of herself and how to take care of the new baby, although she has three previous children. She shared that her mother was diagnosed with cancer 2 months ago and is undergoing treatment. Her husband will be starting a much-needed new job next week and will not be able to get any time off for a while. Other family members do not live close by except for her sister, who is out of town often due to her job responsibilities. Elisabeth is concerned about how she will manage taking care of a newborn and three other children with a seemingly depleted support system.

1. Evidence—Is there sufficient evidence to support counseling women with psychosocial concerns in the immediate postpartum period?
2. Assumptions—What assumptions can be made about the following issues?
   a. Elisabeth is at risk for postpartum depression
   b. Elisabeth's lack of a support system
   c. Elisabeth's ability to connect with community resources after discharge
3. What implications and priorities for nursing care can be drawn at this time?
4. Does the evidence objectively support your conclusion?

Family Structure and Functioning

A woman's adjustment to her role as mother is affected greatly by her relationships with her partner, her mother and other relatives, and any other children (Fig. 21-7). Nurses can help ease the new mother's return home by identifying possible conflicts among family members and by helping the woman plan strategies for dealing with these problems before discharge. Such a conflict can arise when couples have very different ideas about parenting. Dealing with the stresses of sibling rivalry and unsolicited grandparent advice also can affect the woman's transition to motherhood. Only by asking about other nuclear and extended family members can the nurse discover potential problems in such relationships and help plan workable solutions for them.

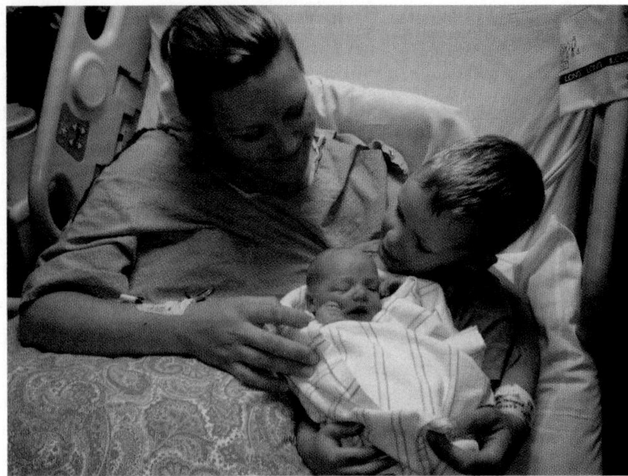

FIG 21-7 Older sibling cuddles with mother and new baby. (Courtesy Jennifer Hobgood, Creedmoor, NC.)

Effect of Cultural Diversity

The final component of a complete psychosocial assessment is the woman's cultural beliefs, values, and practices. Cultural beliefs and traditions strongly influence the behaviors of the woman and her family during the postpartum period. Nurses are likely to come into contact with women from many different countries and cultures. All cultures have developed safe and satisfying methods of caring for new mothers and babies. The nurse can identify some cultural beliefs and practices through observation and interaction with the mother and her family. Only by understanding and respecting the values and beliefs of each woman can the nurse design a plan of care to meet the individual's needs.

To identify cultural beliefs and practices when planning and implementing care, the nurse conducts a cultural assessment. It can be accomplished most easily through conversation with the mother and her partner. Some hospitals have assessment tools designed to identify cultural beliefs and practices that can influence care. Components of the cultural assessment include the ability to read and write English, primary language spoken, family involvement and support, dietary preferences, infant care, attachment, religious or cultural beliefs, folk medicine practices, nonverbal communication, and personal space preferences.

Postpartum care occurs within a sociocultural context. Rest, seclusion, dietary restraints, and ceremonies honoring the mother are common traditional practices that are followed for the promotion of the health and well-being of the mother and baby. In some cultures the postpartum period is considered a time of increased vulnerability for the mother. To protect her there are restrictions on activity, diet, bathing, and infant caretaking.

The postpartum period is seen by some cultures as a time of impurity for the mother. For as many days or weeks as she has lochial flow, she is considered "impure" and has limited contact with others. Sexual activity is prohibited during this time (Mattson, 2011).

In many Asian cultures the balance between yin and yang (cold and hot) is necessary for balance and harmony with the environment. Postpartum practices focus on helping the mother achieve this balance. Pregnancy is considered a "hot" condition. It is believed that birth depletes the mother's body of heat through loss of blood and inner energy; this places her in a "cold" state for about 40 days until her womb is healed. The woman consumes only "hot" foods and beverages. Examples of foods that are considered "hot" include rice, eggs, beef, and chicken soup. Seaweed soup is consumed by postpartum women for the purpose of increasing milk production and helping to rid the body of lochia. Family members often bring in foods from home (Callister, 2014). To help prevent the loss of heat from the body, the mother may be discouraged from showering or bathing for several days or weeks; however, there is attention to perineal care and hygiene. The temperature of the hospital room is warmer than usual. The mother likely spends most of the time in bed to prevent cold air from entering the body and she has minimal contact with the infant. Family members provide care for the mother and the newborn. For example, in the Korean culture, the mother-in-law is charged with caring for her daughter-in-law and newly born grandchild during the postpartum period (Callister).

> **! NURSING ALERT**
>
> Women whose cultural beliefs involve achieving balance between hot and cold prefer warm or hot beverages. They will not drink cold beverages or ice water. They are likely to refuse routine application of cold packs or pads to the perineum because this conflicts with beliefs about preventing loss of heat.

Hispanic and Latino women who have immigrated to the United States or other Western nations often observe the period of 40 days (6 weeks) after birth as *la cuarentena*. During this time the woman's body is perceived to be "open" and vulnerable to drafts; la cuarentena is about "closing the body." Traditional practices associated with la cuarentena include a liquid diet of nutritious drinks, soups, and broths in the early postpartum period; binding the abdomen; avoiding cool air; and maintaining sexual abstinence. Activity is restricted and the mother stays at home (Waugh, 2011). A common concern of Hispanic and Latino women is the "evil eye" or *mal de ojo*. They believe that if someone admires or covets the infant but does not touch him or her, it can cause bad luck, illness, or even death. In an attempt to ward off the evil eye, some mothers place a bracelet with a black onyx hand, *la manita de azabache*, on or near the newborn (Callister, 2014).

The nurse should not assume that a mother desires to use traditional health practices that represent a particular cultural group merely because she is a member of that culture. Many young women who are first- or second-generation Americans follow their cultural traditions only when older family members are present or not at all.

It is important that nurses consider all cultural aspects when planning care and not use their own cultural beliefs as the framework for that care. Although the beliefs and behaviors of other cultures can seem different or strange, they should be encouraged as long as the mother wants to conform to them and she and the baby have no ill effects.

MEDICATION ALERT

The nurse needs to determine whether a woman is using any complementary or alternative therapies (i.e., "folk medicine") during the postpartum period because active ingredients in some herbal preparations can have adverse physiologic effects when used in combination with prescribed medicines.

The Cultural Considerations box lists some common cultural beliefs about the postpartum period and family planning.

DISCHARGE TEACHING

Self-Management and Signs of Complications

Discharge planning begins at the time of admission to the unit and should be reflected in the nursing care plan developed for each woman. For example, a great deal of time during the hospital stay is usually spent in teaching about maternal self-management and care of the newborn because the goal is for all women to be capable of providing basic care for themselves and their infants at the time of discharge. In addition, every woman must be taught to recognize physical and psychologic signs and symptoms that might indicate problems and how to obtain advice and assistance quickly if these signs appear. Table 21-1 and the Signs of Potential Complications box: Postpartum Psychosocial Concerns earlier in this chapter list several common indications of maternal physical and psychosocial problems in the postpartum period. (See Chapter 31 and Chapter 33 for more information on postpartum complications.) Before discharge, women need basic instruction regarding a variety of self-management topics such as nutrition, exercise, family planning, the resumption of sexual intercourse, prescribed medications, and routine mother-baby follow-up care.

Because of the limited time available for teaching, nurses must target their teaching on expressed needs of the woman. Giving the woman a list of topics and asking her to indicate her learning needs help the nurse maximize teaching efforts and can increase retention of information. Providing written materials on postpartum self-management, breastfeeding, and infant care that the woman can consult after discharge is helpful.

Just before the time of discharge the nurse reviews the woman's records to see that laboratory reports, medications, signatures, and other items are in order. Some hospitals have a checklist to use before the woman's discharge. The nurse verifies that medications, if ordered, have arrived on the unit; that any valuables kept secured during the woman's stay have been returned to her and that she has signed a receipt for them; and that the infant is ready to be discharged. The woman's and the baby's identification bands are checked carefully.

SAFETY ALERT

No medication that can cause drowsiness should be administered to the mother before discharge if she is the one who will be holding the baby when they leave the hospital. In most instances the woman is seated in a wheelchair and given the baby to hold. Some families leave unescorted and ambulatory, depending on hospital protocol. The newborn must be secured in a car seat for the drive home.

In many hospitals new mothers (breastfeeding and formula feeding) are routinely presented with gift bags that contain samples of infant formula. This practice is not consistent with

CULTURAL CONSIDERATIONS

Examples of Cultural Beliefs and Practices in the Postpartum Period

Postpartum Care

- *Chinese, Mexican, Korean, and Southeast Asian women* may wish to consume only warm foods and hot drinks to replace blood loss and restore the balance of hot and cold in their bodies. These women desire to stay warm and avoid bathing, exercises, and hair washing for 7 to 30 days after childbirth. Self-management is usually not a priority; care by family members is preferred. The woman has respect for elders and authority. Some women wear abdominal binders. They may prefer not to give their babies colostrum.
- *Chinese women* follow specific restrictions on diet and activity for the first month; this is referred to as "doing the month."
- *Arabic women* eat special meals designed to restore their energy. They are expected to stay at home for 40 days after birth to avoid illness resulting from exposure to the outside air.
- *Haitian women* often wear a belt or piece of linen pulled tightly around the waist to prevent gas from entering the body; they may request to take the placenta home to bury or burn. For 6 to 11 weeks after birth, they typically follow a strict regimen of baths, vapor baths, teas, and dressing warmly.
- *Muslim women* follow strict religious laws on modesty and diet. A Muslim woman must keep her hair, body, arms to the wrist, and legs to the ankles covered at all times. She cannot be alone in the presence of a man other than her husband or a male relative. Observant Muslims will not eat pork or pork products and are obligated to eat meat slaughtered according to Islamic laws (halal meat). If halal meat is not available, kosher meat, seafood, or a vegetarian diet is usually accepted.
- *Ethiopian women* stay secluded for a minimum of 40 days after birth. They consume special foods such as a gruel of oats and honey to increase breast milk production.

Family Planning

- Birth control is government mandated in mainland *China*. Most *Chinese women* have an intrauterine device (IUD) inserted after the birth of their first child. Women do not want hormonal methods of contraception because they fear putting these medications into their bodies.
- *Hispanic women* may choose the rhythm method or natural family planning because most are Catholic.
- *(East) Indian men* are encouraged to have voluntary sterilization by vasectomy.
- *Muslim couples* may practice contraception by mutual consent as long as its use is not harmful to the woman. Acceptable contraceptive methods include foam and condoms, the diaphragm, and natural family planning.
- *Hmong women* highly value and desire large families, which limits birth control practices.
- *Arabic women* value large families, and sons are especially prized.

the Baby-Friendly Hospital USA Initiative (2011). Prepackaged formula should not be given to mothers who are breastfeeding. Such "gifts" are associated with earlier cessation of breastfeeding.

Sexual Activity and Contraception

Discussing sexual activity with women and their partners is important before they leave the hospital because many couples resume sexual activity before the traditional postpartum follow-up visit with the health care provider 6 weeks after birth. For most women the risk of hemorrhage or infection is minimal by approximately 2 weeks postpartum. Couples may be anxious about the topic but uncomfortable and unwilling to bring it up. The nurse needs to discuss the physical and psychologic effects that giving birth can have on sexual activity (see Teaching for Self-Management).

Many factors can influence the timing and quality of sexual activity after birth. Postpartum perineal pain and dyspareunia (painful intercourse) are common among women with perineal lacerations or episiotomy. Some women who had an episiotomy report discomfort with intercourse for months after birth.

TEACHING FOR SELF-MANAGEMENT

Resuming Sexual Activity After Birth

- Unless your health care provider indicates otherwise, you can safely resume sexual activity (intercourse) by the second to fourth week after birth, when bleeding has stopped and the perineum is healed. Most women resume sexual activity by 5 to 6 weeks after birth, although this varies and is often related to perineal discomfort. Perineal lacerations or episiotomy increases the chances of discomfort with intercourse. For the first 6 weeks to 6 months, vaginal lubrication might be decreased, especially among breastfeeding women. Your physiologic reactions to sexual stimulation for the first 3 months after birth may be slower and less intense. The strength of the orgasm may be reduced.
- A water-soluble gel or contraceptive cream or jelly might be recommended for lubrication. If some vaginal tenderness is present, your partner can be instructed to insert one or more clean, lubricated fingers into the vagina and rotate them to help the vagina relax and identify possible areas of discomfort. A position in which you have control of the depth of the insertion of the penis also is useful. The side-by-side or female-on-top position may be most comfortable.
- The presence of the baby influences sexual activity and enjoyment. Parents hear every sound made by the baby; conversely you may be concerned that the baby hears every sound you make. In either case any phase of the sexual response cycle can be interrupted by hearing the baby cry or move, leaving both of you frustrated and unsatisfied. In addition, the amount of psychologic energy expended by you in child-care activities can lead to fatigue. Newborns require a great deal of attention and time.
- Some women have reported feeling sexual stimulation and orgasms when breastfeeding their babies. This is not abnormal. Breastfeeding mothers often are interested in returning to sexual activity before nonbreastfeeding mothers.
- You should be instructed to perform the Kegel exercises correctly to strengthen your pubococcygeal muscle. This muscle is associated with bowel and bladder function and vaginal feeling during intercourse.

Discomfort is more severe and lasts longer with third- and fourth-degree lacerations (see Evidence-Based Practice box). Breastfeeding mothers often experience vaginal dryness related to high levels of prolactin and low estrogen levels. Changes in family structure and altered sleep patterns can make it difficult for a couple to find time for privacy and intimacy. Postpartum depression is associated with decreased sexual desire; medication used to treat PPD can reduce sexual desire and inhibit orgasm (Leeman & Rogers, 2012).

Contraceptive options should also be discussed with heterosexual women (and their partners, if present) before discharge so that they can make informed decisions about fertility management before resuming sexual activity. Waiting to discuss contraception at the 6-week checkup can be too late. Ovulation can occur as soon as 1 month after birth, particularly in women who formula-feed their infants. Breastfeeding mothers should be informed that breastfeeding is not a reliable means of contraception and that other methods should be used; nonhormonal methods are best because oral contraceptives can interfere with milk production. Women who are undecided about contraception at the time of discharge need information about using condoms with spermicidal foam or creams until the first postpartum checkup. Contraceptive options are discussed in detail in Chapter 8.

Medications

Women routinely continue to take their prenatal vitamins during the postpartum period. Breastfeeding mothers may continue prenatal vitamins for the duration of breastfeeding. Supplemental iron may be prescribed for mothers with lower than normal hemoglobin levels. Women with extensive episiotomies or perineal lacerations (third or fourth degree) are usually prescribed stool softeners to take at home. Pain medications (opioid and nonopioid) may be prescribed, especially for women who had cesarean births. The nurse should make certain that the woman knows the route, dosage, frequency, and common side effects of all medications that she will be taking at home. Written information about the medications is usually included in the discharge instructions.

Follow-Up After Discharge

Routine Schedule of Care

Women who have experienced uncomplicated vaginal births are commonly scheduled for the traditional 6-week postpartum examination. Women who have had a cesarean birth are often seen in the health care provider's office or clinic within 2 weeks after hospital discharge. The date and time for the follow-up appointment should be included in the discharge instructions. If an appointment has not been made before the woman leaves the hospital, she should be encouraged to call the health care provider's office or clinic to schedule one.

Parents who have not already done so need to make plans for newborn follow-up at the time of discharge. Breastfeeding infants are routinely seen by the pediatric health care provider or clinic within 3 to 5 days after birth or 48 to 72 hours after hospital discharge and again at approximately 2 weeks of age (AAP Section on Breastfeeding, 2012). Formula-feeding infants may be seen for the first time at 2 weeks of age. If an appointment for a specific date and time

EVIDENCE-BASED PRACTICE

Perineal Trauma and Postpartum Sexual Function

Ask the Question

Which perinatal interventions for perineal trauma minimize pain and prevent sexual dysfunction?

Search for the Evidence

Search Strategies English language research-based publications on perineal trauma, birth, postpartum, sexual were included.

Databases Used Cochrane Collaborative Database, National Guideline Clearinghouse (AHRQ), CINAHL, PubMed, and UpToDate

Critical Appraisal of the Evidence

- Sexual dysfunction can affect more than half of all women at 2 to 3 months after birth. One major cause is dyspareunia (painful intercourse) after perineal trauma, especially third- and fourth-degree lacerations requiring repair. Other causes may include decreased libido and lower estrogen resulting from breastfeeding, postpartum depression, and fatigue.
- Both episiotomy and second-degree lacerations with repair are associated with lower libido, orgasm, sexual satisfaction, and greater dyspareunia than in women with intact perineums (Rathfisch, Dikencik, Kazilkaya, et al., 2010). Routine episiotomy during birth is not recommended.
- Warm compresses and perineal massage during first- and second-stage birth significantly decrease third- and fourth-degree tears (Aasheim, Nilsen, Lukasse, et al., 2011).
- Evidence is still mixed for whether to suture or not suture first- and second-degree lacerations. Although small studies find little difference between groups for pain and wound complications, despite slower wound healing the unsutured group still experiences greater satisfaction than the sutured group (Elharmeel, Chaudhary, Tan, et al., 2011).

Apply the Evidence: Nursing Implications

Women can be embarrassed to discuss sexual function with their partners and/or with their health care team. Nurses are ideally placed to initiate and keep the dialog going throughout childbearing. Leeman and Rogers (2012) recommend the following clinical approach for assessing and preventing postpartum sexual dysfunction:

- Discussion of anatomy, physiology, and sexual function should begin in early pregnancy and continue throughout the postpartum period, including a brief valid and reliable sexual function survey.
- Antenatal perineal massage should be taught to minimize perineal damage.
- Perineal management at birth should include limited use of instrumental delivery, especially forceps, and avoiding episiotomy, along with careful assessment and repair of anal sphincter lacerations with synthetic, absorbable sutures.
- Before hospital discharge initiate discussions with woman and partner regarding pain, dyspareunia, resumption of intercourse, and contraception. Women should know the hypoestrogenic and sensitivity changes that they can experience as a result of breastfeeding and the need for additional vaginal lubrication.
- At postpartum visits assess urine, bowel, and sexual function; inspect perineum; and assess and discuss mood and intimacy challenges such as fatigue and timing issues. Suggesting alternate positions may help increase comfort during intercourse. Evaluate satisfaction with contraceptive method.

Quality and Safety Competencies: Evidence-Based Practice*

Knowledge

Describe evidence-based practice to include the components of research evidence, clinical expertise, and patient/family values.

Sexuality is affected by birth. Nurses can sensitively initiate discussion of sexual intimacy.

Skills

Base individualized care plan on client values, clinical expertise, and evidence.

The nurse models a view of human sexuality as a healthy and normal part of one's quality of life.

Attitudes

Value the concept of evidence-based practice as integral to determining best clinical practice.

The nurse can educate the woman and partner and dispel myths about sexuality.

References

Aasheim, V., Nilsen, A. B., Lukasse, M., et al. (2011). Perineal techniques during the second stage of labour for reducing perineal trauma. *The Cochrane Database of Systematic Reviews*, 2011, *12*, CD006672.

Elharmeel, S. M., Chaudhary, Y., Tan, S., et al. (2011). Surgical repair of spontaneous perineal tears that occur during childbirth versus no intervention. *The Cochrane Database of Systematic Reviews*, 2011, *8*, CD008534.

Leeman, L. M., & Rogers, R. G. (2012). Sex after childbirth. *Obstetrics and Gynecology, 119*(3), 647–655.

Rathfisch, G., Dikencik, B. K., Kazilkaya, B. N., et al. (2010). Effects of perineal trauma on postpartum sexual function. *Journal of Advanced Nursing, 66*(12), 2640–2649.

Pat Mahaffee Gingrich

*Adapted from QSEN at www.qsen.org/.

was not made for the infant before leaving the hospital, the parents should be encouraged to call the office or clinic soon after their arrival home.

Home Visits

Home visits to mothers and babies within a few days of discharge can help bridge the gap between hospital care and routine visits to health care providers. Nurses can assess the mother, the infant, and the home environment; answer questions and provide education and emotional support; and make referrals to community resources if necessary. Some families hire postpartum doulas to help during the early postpartum period. The support provided by nurses and other trained community health workers can enhance parent-infant interaction and parenting skills; home visits also help to promote mutual support between the mother and her partner. Breastfeeding outcomes can be enhanced through home visitation programs (Paul, Beiler, Schaefer, et al., 2012; Yonemoto, Dowswell, Nagai, & Mori, 2013).

Home nursing care may not be available, even if needed, because no agencies are available to provide the service or no coverage is in place for payment by third-party payers. If care is available, a referral form containing information about the mother and baby should be completed at hospital discharge and sent immediately to the home care agency.

The home visit is most commonly scheduled on the woman's second day home from the hospital, but it can be scheduled on any of the first 4 days at home, depending on the individual family's situation and needs. Additional visits are planned throughout the first week, as needed. The home visits may be extended beyond that time if the family's needs warrant it and if a home visit is the most appropriate option for carrying out the follow-up care required to meet the specific needs identified.

During the home visit the nurse conducts a systematic assessment of mother and newborn to determine physiologic adjustment and identify any existing complications. The assessment also focuses on the mother's emotional adjustment and her knowledge of self-management and infant care. Conducting the assessment in a private area of the home provides an opportunity for the mother to ask questions on potentially sensitive topics such as breast care, constipation, sexual activity, or family planning. The nurse assesses family adjustment to the newborn and addresses any concerns during the home visit.

During the newborn assessment the nurse can demonstrate and explain normal newborn behavior and capabilities and encourage the mother and family to ask questions or express concerns they have. The home care nurse verifies if the blood sample for newborn screening has been drawn (see Chapter 24). If the baby was discharged from the hospital before 24 hours of age, a blood sample for the newborn screen may be drawn by the home care nurse, or the family will need to take the infant to the health care provider's office or clinic.

Telephone Follow-Up

In addition to or instead of a home visit, many providers are implementing one or more postpartum telephone follow-up calls to their clients for assessment, health teaching, and identification of complications to effect timely intervention and referrals. Telephone follow-up may be offered by hospitals, private physicians, clinics, or private agencies. It may be either a separate service or combined with other strategies for extending postpartum care. Telephone nursing assessments are frequently used as follow-up to postpartum home visits to reassess a woman's knowledge about the signs and symptoms of adequate intake by the breastfeeding infant or, after initiating home phototherapy, to assess the caregiver's knowledge regarding equipment complications.

Warm Lines. The warm line is another type of telephone link between the new family and concerned caregivers or experienced parent volunteers. A warm line is a help line or consultation service, not a crisis intervention line. The warm line is appropriately used for dealing with less extreme concerns that seem urgent at the time the call is placed but are not actual emergencies. Calls to warm lines commonly relate to infant feeding, prolonged crying, or sibling rivalry. Families are encouraged to call when concerns arise. Telephone numbers for warm lines should be given to parents before hospital discharge.

Support Groups

The woman adjusting to motherhood may desire interaction and conversation with other women who are having similar experiences. Postpartum women who have met earlier in prenatal clinics or on the hospital unit can begin to associate for mutual support. Members of childbirth classes who attend a postpartum reunion may decide to extend their relationship during the fourth trimester. Fathers or partners also benefit from participation in support groups.

A postpartum support group enables mothers and partners/fathers to share with and support each other as they adjust to parenting. Many new parents find it reassuring to discover that they are not alone in their feelings of confusion and uncertainty. An experienced parent can often impart concrete information that is valuable to other group members. Inexperienced parents can imitate the behavior of others in the group whom they perceive as particularly capable.

Referral to Community Resources

To develop an effective referral system the nurse should have an understanding of the needs of the woman and family and of the organization and community resources available for meeting those needs. Locating and compiling information about available community services contributes to the development of a referral system. The nurse also needs to develop his or her own resource file of local and national services that are frequently useful to postpartum families.

KEY POINTS

- Postpartum care is family centered and modeled on the concept of health.
- Cultural beliefs and practices affect the maternal and family response to the postpartum period.
- The nursing care plan includes assessments to detect deviations from normal, comfort measures to relieve discomfort or pain, and safety measures to prevent injury or infection.
- Common nursing interventions in the postpartum period focus on preventing excessive bleeding, bladder distention, infection; providing nonpharmacologic and pharmacologic relief of discomfort associated with the episiotomy, lacerations, or breastfeeding; and instituting measures to promote or suppress lactation.
- Teaching and counseling measures are designed to promote the woman's feelings of competence in self-management and infant care.
- Meeting the psychosocial needs of new mothers involves taking into consideration the composition and functioning of the entire family.
- Early discharge classes, telephone follow-up, home visits, warm lines, and support groups are effective means of facilitating physiologic and psychologic adjustments in the postpartum period.

REFERENCES

American Academy of Pediatrics (AAP), & Committee on Psychosocial Aspects of Child and Family Health. (2010). Incorporating recognition and management of perinatal and postpartum depression into pediatric practice. *Pediatrics, 126*(5), 1032–1039.

American Academy of Pediatrics (AAP) Section on Breastfeeding. (2012). Breastfeeding and the use of human milk. *Pediatrics, 129*(3), e827–e841.

American Academy of Pediatrics (AAP), & Committee on Fetus and Newborn. (2010). Hospital stay for healthy term infants. *Pediatrics, 125*(2), 405–409.

American Academy of Pediatrics (AAP) Committee on Fetus and Newborn and American College of Obstetricians and Gynecologists (ACOG) Committee on Obstetric Practice. (2012). *Guidelines for perinatal care* (7th ed.). Washington, DC: Author.

Association of Women's Health, Obstetric, & Neonatal Nurses (AWHONN). (2010). *Guidelines for professional registered nurse staffing for perinatal units.* Washington, DC: Author.

Baby-Friendly, USA (2011). *Guidelines and evaluation criteria for facilities seeking Baby-Friendly designation.* Sandwich, MA: Baby-Friendly USA. Available at www.babyfriendlyusa.org/get-started/the-guidelines-evaluation-criteria.

Callister, L. C. (2014). Integrating cultural beliefs and practices when caring for childbearing women and families. In K. R. Simpson, & P. A. Creehan (Eds.), *Perinatal nursing* (4th ed.). Philadelphia: Wolters Kluwer/Lippincott Williams & Wilkins.

Centers for Disease Control and Prevention. (2013). Updated recommendations for use of tetanus toxoid, reduced diphtheria toxoid, and acellular pertussis vaccine (Tdap) in pregnant women—Advisory Committee on Immunization Practices (ACIP), 2012. *MMWR Morbidity and Mortality Weekly Report, 62*(07), 131–135.

Centers for Disease Control and Prevention (CDC). (2014). *Guidelines for vaccinating pregnant women.* Available at www.cdc.gov/vaccines/pubs/preg-guide.htm#mmr.

Doering, J., & Durfor, S. L. (2011). The process of "preserving toward normalcy" after childbirth. *MCN: The American Journal of Maternal/Child Nursing, 36*(4), 258–265.

Hiner, J., Pyka, J., Burks, C., et al. (2012). Preventing infant abductions: An infant security program transitioned into an interdisciplinary model. *Journal of Perinatal and Neonatal Nursing, 26*(1), 47–56.

Leeman, L. M., & Rogers, R. G. (2012). Sex after childbirth. *Obstetrics and Gynecology, 119*(3), 647–655.

Lockwood, S., & Anderson, K. (2013). Postpartum safety: A patient-centered approach to fall prevention. *MCN: The American Journal of Maternal/Child Nursing, 38*(1), 15–18.

Mattson, S. (2011). Ethnocultural considerations in the childbearing period. In S. Mattson, & J. E. Smith (Eds.), *Core curriculum for maternal-newborn nursing* (4th ed.). St. Louis: Saunders.

McLean, H. Q., Fiebelkorn, A. P., Temte, J. L., & Wallace, G. S. (2013). Prevention of measles, rubella, congenital rubella syndrome, and mumps, 2013: Summary recommendations of the Advisory Committee on Immunization Practices (ACIP). *MMWR Morbidity and Mortality Weekly Report, 62*(RR04), 1–34.

National Center for Missing and Exploited Children (NCMEC). (2014). *Newborn/infant abductions.* Alexandria, VA: NCMEC. Available at http://www.missingkids.com/en_US/documents/InfantAbductionStats.pdf.

Novak, K., & Fairchild, R. (2012). Bedside reporting and SBAR: Improving patient communication and satisfaction. *Journal of Pediatric Nursing, 27*(6), 760–762.

Paul, I. M., Beiler, J. S., Schaefer, E. W., et al. (2012). A randomized trial of single home nursing visits vs office-based care after nursery/maternity discharge: The Nurses for Infants Through Teaching and Assessment After the Nursery (NITTANY) Study. *Archives of Pediatric and Adolescent Medicine, 166*(3), 263–270.

The Joint Commission (TJC). (1999). *Sentinel event alert: Infant abductions, preventing future occurrences.* Available at www.jointcommission.org/assets/1/18/SEA_9.pdf.

Waller-Wise, R. (2012). Mother-baby care: The best for patients, nurses, and hospitals. *Nursing for Women's Health, 16*(4), 273–278.

Waugh, L. J. (2011). Beliefs associated with Mexican immigrant families' practice of la cuarentena during postpartum recovery. *Journal of Obstetric, Gynecologic and Neonatal Nursing, 40*(6), 732–741.

Yonemoto, N., Dowswell, T., Nagai, S., & Mori, R. (2013). Schedules for home visits in the early postpartum period. *The Cochrane Database of Systematic Reviews, 2013,* 7, CD009326.

22 CHAPTER

Transition to Parenthood

Diana McCarty

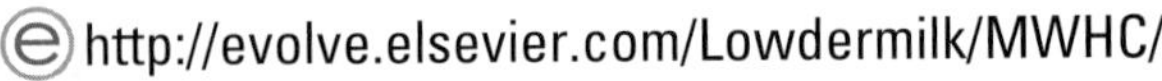

LEARNING OBJECTIVES

- Identify parental and infant behaviors that facilitate and those that inhibit parental attachment.
- Describe sensual responses that strengthen attachment.
- Examine the process of becoming a mother and becoming a father.
- Compare maternal adjustment and paternal adjustment to parenthood.
- Describe nursing interventions that facilitate parent-infant adjustment.
- Examine the effects of the following on parenting responses and behavior: parental age (i.e., adolescence and older than 35 years), social support, culture, same sex parenting, socioeconomic conditions, personal aspirations, and sensory impairment.
- Describe sibling adjustment.
- Discuss grandparent adaptation.

Becoming a parent brings great joy and amazement to most people. The **transition to parenthood** involves change and adaptation as the family adjusts to life with a new baby. It is the first months of having a child when parents define their parental roles and adjust to parenthood. It can create a period of instability, whether parenthood is biologic or adoptive and whether the parents are married husband-wife couples, cohabiting couples, single mothers, single fathers, or same sex couples. Parenting is a process of role attainment and role transition. The transition is an ongoing process as the parents and infant develop and change.

PARENTAL ATTACHMENT, BONDING, AND ACQUAINTANCE

The process by which a parent comes to love and accept a child and a child comes to love and accept a parent is known as **attachment.** Attachment occurs through the process of *bonding*. In their bonding theory, Klaus and Kennell (1976) proposed that there is a sensitive period during the first few minutes or hours after birth when mothers and fathers must have close contact with their infants to optimize the child's later development. Klaus and Kennell (1982) later revised their theory of parent-infant bonding, modifying their claim of the critical nature of immediate contact with the infant after birth. They acknowledged the adaptability of human parents, stating that more than minutes or hours are needed for parents to form an emotional relationship with their infants. The terms *attachment* and *bonding* continue to be used interchangeably.

Attachment is developed and maintained by proximity and interaction with the infant, through which the parent becomes acquainted with the infant, identifies the infant as an individual, and claims the infant as a member of the family. Positive feedback between the parent and the infant through social, verbal, and nonverbal responses (whether real or perceived) facilitates the attachment process. Attachment occurs through a mutually satisfying experience. A mother commented on her son's grasp reflex, "I put my finger in his hand, and he grabbed right on. It is just a reflex, I know, but it felt good anyway" (Fig. 22-1).

The concept of attachment includes **mutuality;** that is, the infant's behaviors and characteristics elicit a corresponding set of parental behaviors and characteristics. The infant displays signaling behaviors such as crying, smiling, and cooing that initiate the contact and bring the caregiver to the child. These behaviors are followed by executive behaviors such as rooting, grasping, and postural adjustments that maintain the contact. Most caregivers are attracted to an alert, responsive, cuddly infant but find it less desirable to interact with an irritable, apparently disinterested infant. Attachment occurs more readily with the infant whose temperament, social capabilities, appearance, and sex fit the parent's expectations. If the infant does not meet these expectations, the parent's disappointment can delay the attachment process. Table 22-1 presents a comprehensive list of classic infant behaviors affecting parental attachment. Table 22-2 presents a corresponding list of parental behaviors that affect infant attachment.

An important part of attachment is **acquaintance.** Parents use eye contact (Fig. 22-2), touching, talking, and exploring to become acquainted with their infant during the immediate postpartum period. Adoptive parents undergo the same process when they first meet their new child. During this period families engage in the **claiming process,** which is the identification of the new baby

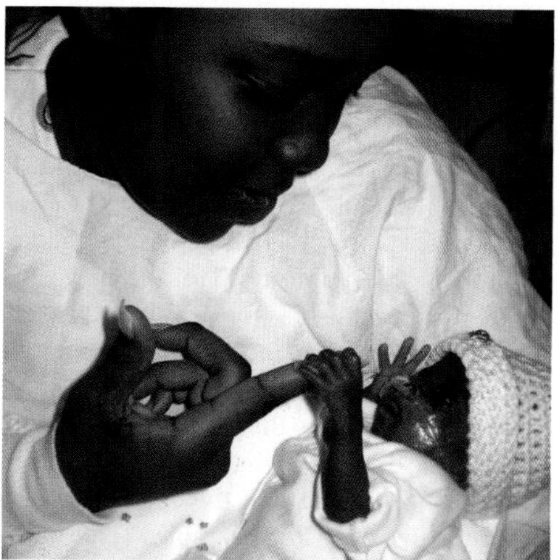

FIG 22-1 Hands. (Courtesy Cheryl Briggs, RNC, Annapolis, MD.)

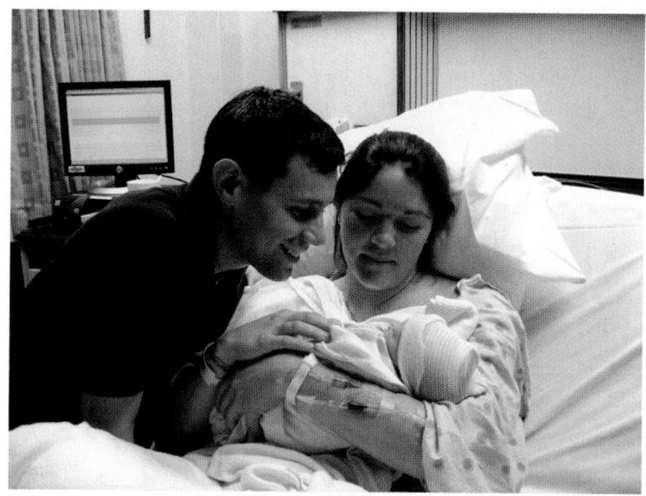

FIG 22-2 Early acquaintance between parents and newborn as mother holds infant in en face position. (Courtesy Kathryn Alden, Chapel Hill, NC.)

TABLE 22-1 Infant Behaviors Affecting Parental Attachment

FACILITATING BEHAVIORS	INHIBITING BEHAVIORS
Visually alert; eye-to-eye contact; tracking or following parent's face	Sleepy; eyes closed most of the time; gaze aversion
Appealing facial appearance; randomness of body movements reflecting helplessness	Resemblance to person parent dislikes; hyperirritability or jerky body movements when touched
Smiles	Bland facial expression; infrequent smiles
Vocalization; crying only when hungry or wet	Crying for hours on end; colicky
Grasp reflex	Exaggerated motor reflex
Anticipatory approach behaviors for feedings; sucks well; feeds easily	Feeds poorly; regurgitates; vomits often
Enjoys being cuddled and held	Resists holding and cuddling by crying, stiffening body
Easily consolable	Inconsolable; unresponsive to parenting, caretaking tasks
Activity and regularity somewhat predictable	Unpredictable feeding and sleeping schedule
Attention span sufficient to focus on parents	Inability to attend to parent's face or offered stimulation
Differential crying, smiling, and vocalizing; recognizes and prefers parents	Shows no preference for parents over others
Approaches through locomotion	Unresponsive to parent's approaches
Clings to parent; puts arms around parent's neck	Seeks attention from any adult in room
Lifts arms to parents in greeting	Ignores parents

Adapted from Gerson, E. (1973). *Infant behavior in the first year of life.* New York: Raven Press.

TABLE 22-2 Parental Behaviors Affecting Infant Attachment

FACILITATING BEHAVIORS	INHIBITING BEHAVIORS
Looks; gazes; takes in physical characteristics of infant; assumes en face position; eye contact	Turns away from infant; ignores infant's presence
Hovers; maintains proximity; directs attention to, points to infant	Avoids infant; does not seek proximity; refuses to hold infant when given opportunity
Identifies infant as unique individual	Identifies infant with someone parent dislikes; fails to recognize any of infant's unique features
Claims infant as family member; names infant	Fails to place infant in family context or identify infant with family member; has difficulty naming
Touches; progresses from fingertip to fingers to palms to encompassing contact	Fails to move from fingertip touch to palmar contact and holding
Smiles at infant	Maintains bland countenance or frowns at infant
Talks to, coos, or sings to infant	Wakes infant when infant is sleeping; handles roughly; hurries feeding by moving nipple continually
Expresses pride in infant	Expresses disappointment, displeasure in infant
Relates infant's behavior to familiar events	Does not incorporate infant into life
Assigns meaning to infant's actions and sensitively interprets infant's needs	Makes no effort to interpret infant's actions or needs
Views infant's behaviors and appearance in positive light	Views infant's behavior as exploiting, deliberately uncooperative; views appearance as distasteful, ugly

Adapted from Mercer, R. (1983). Parent-infant attachment. In L. Sonstegard, K. Kowalski, & B. Jennings (Eds.), *Women's health* (vol. 2). New York: Grune & Stratton.

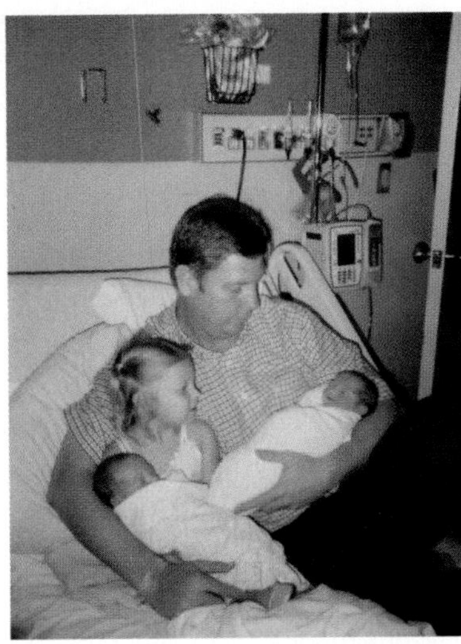

FIG 22-3 Father looks for resemblance between newborns and older daughter. (Courtesy Cheryl Briggs, RNC, Annapolis, MD.)

(Fig. 22-3). The child is first identified in terms of "likeness" to other family members, then in terms of "differences," and finally in terms of "uniqueness." The unique newcomer is thus incorporated into the family. Mothers and fathers examine their infant carefully and point out characteristics that the child shares with other family members and that are indicative of a relationship between them. Maternal comments such as the following reveal the claiming process: "Everyone says, 'He's the image of his father,' but I found one part like me—his toes are shaped like mine."

On the other hand, some mothers react negatively. They "claim" the infant in terms of the discomfort or pain the baby causes. The mother interprets the infant's normal responses as being negative toward her and reacts to her child with dislike or indifference. She does not hold the child close or touch the child in a comforting way. For example, "The nurse put the baby into Lydia's arms. She promptly laid him across her knees and glanced up at the television. 'Stay still until I finish watching; you've been enough trouble already.'"

Nursing interventions related to the promotion of parent-infant attachment are numerous and varied (Table 22-3).

TABLE 22-3 Examples of Parent-Infant Attachment Interventions

INTERVENTION LABEL AND DEFINITION	ACTIVITIES
Attachment Promotion Facilitation of development of parent-infant relationship	Provide opportunity for parent or parents to see, hold, and examine newborn immediately after birth. Encourage parent or parents to hold infant close to body. Assist parent or parents to participate in infant care. Provide rooming-in while in hospital.
Environmental Management: Attachment Process Manipulation of individuals' surroundings to facilitate development of parent-infant relationship	Create environment that fosters privacy. Individualize daily routine to meet parents' needs. Permit father or significant other to sleep in room with mother. Develop policies that permit presence of significant others as much as desired.
Family Integrity Promotion: Childbearing Family Facilitation of growth of individuals or families who are adding infant to family unit	Prepare parent or parents for expected role changes involved in becoming a parent. Prepare parent or parents for responsibilities of parenthood. Monitor effects of newborn on family structure. Reinforce positive parenting behaviors.
Lactation Counseling Use of interactive helping process to assist in achieving and maintaining successful breastfeeding	Correct misconceptions, misinformation, and inaccuracies about breastfeeding. Assess feeding techniques and assist as needed. Evaluate parents' understanding of infant's feeding cues (e.g., rooting, sucking, alertness). Determine frequency of feedings in relation to infant's needs. Demonstrate breast massage and discuss its advantages to increasing milk supply. Provide education, encouragement, and support.
Parent Education: Infant Instruction on nurturing and physical care needed during first year of life	Determine parents' knowledge, readiness, and ability to learn about infant care. Provide anticipatory guidance about developmental changes during first year of life. Teach parent or parents skills to care for newborn. Demonstrate ways in which parent or parents can stimulate infant's development. Discuss infant's capabilities for interaction. Demonstrate quieting techniques.
Risk Identification: Childbearing Family Identification of individual or family likely to experience difficulties in parenting and assigning priorities to strategies to prevent parenting problems	Determine developmental stage of parent or parents. Review prenatal history for factors that predispose individuals or family to complications. Ascertain understanding of English or other language used in community. Monitor behavior that may indicate problem with attachment. Plan for risk-reduction activities in collaboration with individual or family.

Modified from Bulechek, G., Butcher, H., Dochterman, J., & Vagner, C. (2013). *Nursing interventions classification (NIC)* (6th ed.). St. Louis: Mosby.

They can enhance positive parent-infant contacts by heightening parental awareness of an infant's responses and ability to communicate. As the parent attempts to become competent and loving in that role, nurses can bolster the parent's self-confidence and ego. Nurses can identify actual and potential problems and collaborate with other health care professionals who will provide care for the parents after discharge. Nursing considerations for fostering maternal-infant bonding among special populations can vary (see the Cultural Considerations box).

CULTURAL CONSIDERATIONS

Fostering Bonding in Women of Varying Ethnic and Cultural Groups

Childbearing practices and rituals of other cultures are not always congruent with standard practices associated with bonding in the Anglo-American culture. For example, Chinese families traditionally use extended family members to care for the newborn so that the mother can rest and recover, especially after a cesarean birth. Some Native-American, Asian, and Hispanic women do not initiate breastfeeding until their breast milk comes in. Haitian families do not name their babies until after the confinement month. The amount of eye contact varies among cultures as well. Yup'ik Eskimo mothers almost always position their babies so that they can make eye contact.

Nurses should become knowledgeable about the childbearing beliefs and practices of diverse cultural and ethnic groups. Because individual cultural variations exist within groups, nurses need to clarify with the client and family members or friends what cultural norms they follow. Incorrect judgments can be made about parent-infant bonding if nurses do not practice culturally sensitive care.

Modified from D'Avanzo, C. (2008). *Mosby's pocket guide to cultural health assessment* (4th ed.). St. Louis: Mosby.

Assessment of Attachment Behaviors

One of the most important areas of assessment is careful observation of specific behaviors thought to indicate the formation of emotional bonds between the newborn and the family, especially the mother. Unlike physical assessment of the neonate, which has concrete guidelines to follow, assessment of parent-infant attachment relies more on skillful observation and interviewing. Rooming-in of mother and infant and liberal visiting privileges for father or partner, siblings, and grandparents provide nurses with excellent opportunities to observe interactions and identify behaviors that demonstrate positive or negative attachment. Attachment behaviors can be easily observed during infant feeding sessions. Box 22-1 presents guidelines for assessment of attachment behaviors.

During pregnancy, and often even before conception occurs, parents develop an image of the "ideal" or "fantasy" infant. At birth the fantasy infant becomes the real infant. How closely the dream child resembles the real child influences the bonding process. Assessing such expectations during pregnancy and at the time of the infant's birth allows identification of discrepancies in the parents' view of the fantasy child versus the real child.

The labor process significantly affects the immediate attachment of mothers to their newborn infants. Factors such as a long labor, feeling tired or "drugged" after birth, and problems with breastfeeding, preterm birth, and being separated from the infant at birth can delay the development of initial positive feelings toward the newborn (Flacking, Lehtonen, Thomson, et al., 2012; Hoffenkamp, Tooten, Hall, et al., 2012). Referral to groups such as La Leche League International (www.lli.org) or Postpartum Support International (www. Postpartum.net) can be helpful.

BOX 22-1 Assessing Attachment Behavior

- When the infant is brought to the parents, do they reach out for the infant and call the infant by name? (Recognize that in some cultures parents may not name the infant in the early newborn period.)
- Do the parents speak about the infant in terms of identification—who the infant resembles, and what appears special about their infant over other infants?
- When parents are holding the infant, what kind of body contact is seen—do parents feel at ease in changing the infant's position, are fingertips or whole hands used, and does the infant have parts of the body they avoid touching or parts of the body they investigate and scrutinize?
- When the infant is awake, what kinds of stimulation do the parents provide—do they talk to the infant, to each other, or to no one, and how do they look at the infant—direct visual contact, avoiding eye contact, or looking at other people or objects?
- How comfortable do the parents appear in terms of caring for the infant? Do they express any concern regarding their ability or disgust for certain activities, such as changing diapers?
- What type of affection do they demonstrate to the newborn, such as smiling, stroking, kissing, or rocking?
- If the infant is fussy, what kinds of comforting techniques do the parents use, such as rocking, swaddling, talking, or stroking?

PARENT-INFANT CONTACT

Early Contact

Early close contact can facilitate the attachment process between parent and child. Although a delay in contact does not necessarily mean that attachment will be inhibited, additional psychologic energy can be necessary to achieve the same effect. To date, no scientific evidence has demonstrated that immediate contact after birth is essential for the human parent-child relationship.

Early skin-to-skin contact between the mother and newborn immediately after birth and during the first hour facilitates maternal affectionate and attachment behaviors (Hung & Berg, 2011; Thukral, Sankar, Agarwal, et al., 2012). The newborn is placed in the prone position on the mother's bare chest; the baby and mother are covered with a warm blanket and a cap is placed on the infant's head to prevent heat loss. This practice promotes early and effective breastfeeding and increases breastfeeding duration. It is also associated with less infant crying, improved thermoregulation (especially in low birth weight infants), and improved cardiorespiratory stability in late preterm infants (Moore, Anderson, Bergman, & Dowswell, 2012).

Parents who are unable to have early contact with their newborn (e.g., the infant was transferred to the intensive care nursery) can be reassured that such contact is not essential for parent-infant attachment. Otherwise, adopted infants would not form affectionate ties with their parents. Nurses need to stress that the parent-infant relationship is a process that occurs over time.

Extended Contact

Rooming-in is common in family-centered care. With this practice the infant stays in the room with the mother. In some facilities the newborn never leaves the mother's presence; nurses perform the initial assessment and care in the room with the parents. In other hospitals the infant is transferred to the postpartum or mother-baby unit from the transitional nursery (if the facility uses one) after showing satisfactory extrauterine adjustment. Nurses encourage the father or partner to actively participate in caring for the infant. They can also encourage siblings and grandparents to visit and become acquainted with the infant. Whether the method of family-centered care is rooming-in, mother-baby or couplet care, or a family birth unit, mothers, their partners, and family members are equal and integral parts of the developing family.

Extended contact with the infant should be available for all parents but especially for those at risk for parenting inadequacies, such as adolescents and low-income women. Postpartum nurses need to consider and encourage activities that optimize family-centered care (Welch, Hofer, Brunelli, et al., 2012).

COMMUNICATION BETWEEN PARENT AND INFANT

The parent-infant relationship is strengthened through the use of sensual responses and abilities by both partners in the interaction. The nurse should keep in mind that cultural variations are often seen in these interactive behaviors.

The Senses

Touch

Touch, or the tactile sense, is used extensively by parents as a means of becoming acquainted with the newborn. Many mothers reach out for their infants as soon as they are born. Mothers lift their infants to their breasts, enfold them in their arms, and cradle them. Once the infant is close, the mother begins the exploration process with her fingertips, one of the most touch-sensitive areas of the body. Within a short time she uses her palm to caress the baby's trunk and eventually enfolds the infant. Similar progression of touching is demonstrated by fathers, partners, and other caregivers. Gentle stroking motions are used to soothe and quiet the infant; patting or gently rubbing the infant's back is a comfort after feedings. Infants also pat the mother's breast as they nurse. Both seem to enjoy sharing each other's body warmth. Parents seem to have an innate desire to touch, pick up, and hold the infant (Fig. 22-4). They comment on the softness of the baby's skin and note details of the baby's appearance. As parents become increasingly sensitive to the infant's like or dislike for different types of touch, they draw closer to the baby.

Touching behaviors by mothers vary in different cultural groups. For example, minimal touching and cuddling is a traditional Southeast Asian practice thought to protect the infant from evil spirits. Because of tradition and spiritual beliefs, women in India and Bali have practiced infant massage since ancient times.

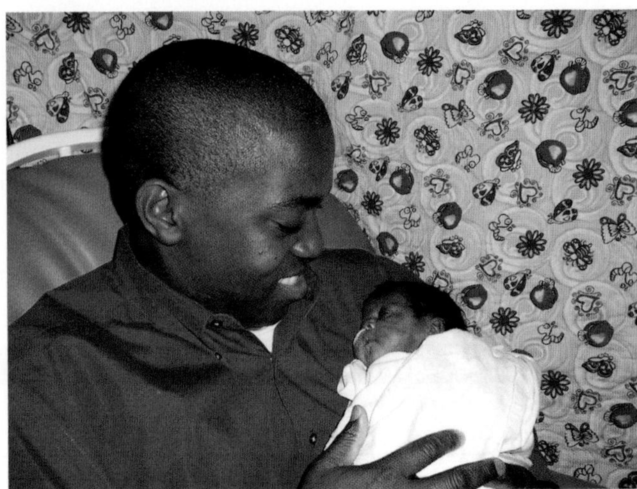

FIG 22-4 Father interacts with his newborn son. (Courtesy Cheryl Briggs, RNC, Annapolis, MD.)

Eye Contact

Parents repeatedly demonstrate interest in having eye contact with the baby. Some mothers remark that once their babies have looked at them, they feel much closer to them. Parents are intent on getting their babies to open their eyes and look at them. In North American culture, eye contact appears to reinforce the development of a trusting relationship and is an important factor in human relationships at all ages. In other cultures, eye contact is perceived differently. For example, in Mexican culture, sustained direct eye contact is considered to be rude, immodest, and dangerous for some. This danger can arise from the *mal de ojo* (evil eye), resulting from excessive admiration. Women and children are thought to be more susceptible to mal de ojo.

As newborns become functionally able to sustain eye contact with their parents, they spend time in mutual gazing, often in the en face position, in which the parent's and infant's faces are approximately 30 cm (12 inches) apart and on the same plane (see Fig. 22-2). Nurses, physicians, or nurse midwives can facilitate eye contact immediately after birth by positioning the infant on the mother's abdomen or chest with the mother's and the infant's faces on the same plane. Dimming the lights encourages the infant's eyes to open. To promote eye contact, instillation of prophylactic antibiotic ointment in the infant's eyes can be delayed until the infant and parents have had some time together in the first hour after birth.

Voice

The shared response of parents and infants to each other's voices is remarkable. Parents wait tensely for the first cry. Once that cry has reassured them of the baby's health, they begin comforting behaviors. As the parents speak, the infant is alerted and turns toward them. Infants respond to higher-pitched voices and can distinguish their mother's voice from others soon after birth.

Odor

Another behavior shared by parents and infants is a response to each other's odor. Mothers comment on the smell of their

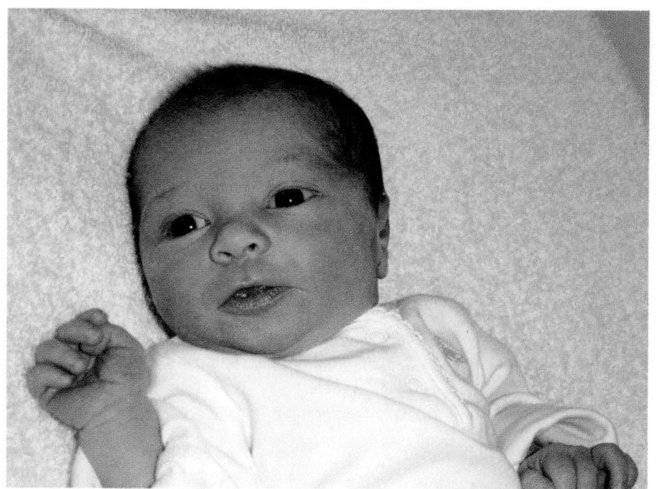

FIG 22-5 Infant in alert state. (Courtesy Kathryn Alden, Chapel Hill, NC.)

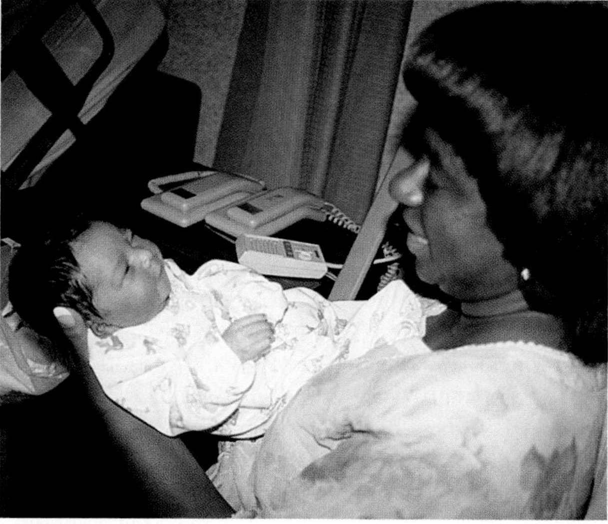

FIG 22-6 Sharing a smile: an example of synchrony. (Courtesy Marjorie Pyle, RNC, Lifecircle, Costa Mesa, CA.)

babies when first born and have noted that each infant has a unique odor. Infants learn rapidly to distinguish the odor of their mother's breast milk.

Entrainment

Newborns move in time with the structure of adult speech, which is termed entrainment. They wave their arms, lift their heads, and kick their legs, seemingly "dancing in tune" to a parent's voice. Culturally determined rhythms of speech are ingrained in the infant long before he or she uses spoken language to communicate. This shared rhythm also gives the parent positive feedback and establishes a positive setting for effective communication.

Biorhythmicity

Biorhythmicity refers to the infant being in tune with the mother's natural rhythms. The mother's heartbeat or a recording of a heartbeat can soothe a crying infant. One of the newborn's tasks is to establish a personal biorhythm. Parents can help in this process by giving consistent loving care and using their infant's alert state to develop responsive behavior and increase social interactions and opportunities for learning (Fig. 22-5).

Reciprocity and Synchrony

Reciprocity is a type of body movement or behavior that provides the observer with cues. The observer or receiver interprets those cues and responds to them. Reciprocity often takes several weeks to develop with a new baby. For example, when the newborn fusses and cries, the mother responds by picking up and cradling the infant, the baby becomes quiet and alert and establishes eye contact, and the mother verbalizes, sings, and coos while the baby maintains eye contact. The baby then averts the eyes and yawns; the mother decreases her active response. If the parent continues to stimulate the infant, the baby can become fussy.

The term synchrony refers to the "fit" between the infant's cues and the parent's response. When parent and infant experience a synchronous interaction, it is mutually rewarding (Fig. 22-6). Parents need time to interpret the infant's cues correctly. For example, the infant develops a specific cry in response to different situations such as boredom, loneliness, hunger, and discomfort. The parent may need assistance in interpreting these cries, along with trial and error interventions, before synchrony develops.

PARENTAL ROLE AFTER BIRTH

Adaptation involves stabilizing tasks, a coming to terms with commitments. Parents demonstrate growing competence in child care activities and become increasingly more attuned to their infant's behavior.

Transition to Parenthood

Historically the transition to parenthood was viewed as a crisis. The current perspective is that parenthood is a developmental transition rather than a major life crisis. The transition to parenthood is a time of disorder and disequilibrium, as well as satisfaction and joy, for mothers and their partners. Usual methods of coping often seem ineffective during this time. Some parents are so distressed that they are unable to be supportive of each other. Because men typically identify their spouses or partners as their primary or only source of support, the transition can be comparatively harder for the fathers. They often feel deprived when the mothers, who are also experiencing stress, cannot provide their usual level of support. Many parents are unprepared for the strong emotions such as helplessness, inadequacy, and anger that arise when dealing with a crying infant. However, the parenthood role allows adults to develop and display a selfless, warm, and caring side of themselves that may not otherwise be expressed.

For the majority of mothers and their partners the transition to parenthood is an opportunity rather than a time of crisis. Parents try new coping strategies as they work to master their new roles and reach new developmental levels. As they work through the transition, they often find personal strength and resourcefulness.

Parental Tasks and Responsibilities

Parents need to reconcile the actual child with the fantasy and dream child. This process means coming to terms with the infant's physical appearance, sex, innate temperament, and physical status. If the real child differs greatly from the fantasy child, some parents delay acceptance of the child. In some instances, they never accept the child.

Many parents know the sex of the infant before birth because of the use of ultrasound assessments. For those who do not have this information, disappointment over the baby's sex can take time to resolve. The parents may provide adequate physical care but have difficulty in being sincerely involved with the infant until this internal conflict has been resolved. As one mother remarked, "I really wanted a boy. I know it is silly and irrational, but when they said, 'She's a lovely little girl,' I was so disappointed and angry—yes, angry—I could hardly look at her. Oh, I looked after her okay, her feedings and baths and things, but I couldn't feel excited. To tell the truth, I felt like a monster not liking my child. Then one day, she was lying there and she turned her head and looked right at me. I felt a flooding of love for her come over me, and we looked at each other a long time. It's okay now. I wouldn't change her for all the boys in the world."

The normal appearance of the neonate—size, color, molding of the head, or bowed appearance of the legs—is startling for some parents. Nurses can encourage parents to examine their babies and to ask questions about newborn characteristics.

Parents need to become adept in the care of the infant, including caregiving activities, noting the communication cues given by the infant to indicate needs, and responding appropriately to the infant's needs. The more quickly parents become competent in child care activities, the more quickly they can direct their psychologic energy toward observing and responding to these communication cues. Self-esteem grows with competence. Breastfeeding helps mothers believe that they are contributing in a unique way to the welfare of the infant. The parent may interpret the infant's response to the parental care and attention as a comment on the quality of that care. Infant behaviors that parents interpret as positive responses to their care include being consoled easily, enjoying being cuddled, and making eye contact. Spitting up frequently after feedings, crying, and being unpredictable are often perceived as negative responses to parental care. Continuation of these infant responses that parents view as negative can result in alienation of parent and infant.

Some people view assistance, including advice by husbands, partners, wives, mothers, mothers-in-law, and health care professionals, as supportive. Others view advice as criticism or an indication of how inept these people judge the new parents to be. Criticism, real or imagined, of the new parents' ability to provide adequate physical care, nutrition, or social stimulation for the infant can be devastating. By providing encouragement and praise for parenting efforts, nurses can enhance the new parents' confidence.

Parents must establish a place for the newborn within the family group. Whether the infant is the firstborn or the last born, all family members must adjust their roles to accommodate the newcomer.

TABLE 22-4 Phases of Maternal Postpartum Adjustment

PHASE	CHARACTERISTICS
Dependent: **taking-in phase**	First 24 hours (range, 1 to 2 days) Focus: self and meeting of basic needs: Reliance on others to meet needs for comfort, rest, closeness, and nourishment Excited and talkative Desire to review birth experience
Dependent-independent: **taking-hold phase**	Starts second or third day; lasts 10 days to several weeks Focus: care of baby and competent mothering: Desire to take charge Still has need for nurturing and acceptance by others Eagerness to learn and practice—optimal period for teaching by nurses Handling of physical discomforts and emotional changes Possible experience with "blues"
Interdependent: **letting-go phase**	Focus: forward movement of family as unit with interacting members: Reassertion of relationship with partner Resumption of sexual intimacy Resolution of individual roles

Data from Rubin, R. (1961). Basic maternal behavior. *Nursing Outlook*, 9(11), 683-686.

Becoming a Mother

Rubin (1961) identified three phases of maternal role attainment in which the mother adjusts to her parental role. These phases extend over the first several weeks and are characterized by dependent behavior, dependent-independent behavior, and interdependent behavior (Table 22-4). Rubin's research was conducted when the length of stay in the hospital was longer (3 to 5 or more days). With today's early discharge, women seem to move through the phases faster.

Mercer (2004) suggested that the concept of *maternal role attainment* be replaced with *becoming a mother* to signify the transformation and growth of the mother's identity. Becoming a mother implies more than attaining a role. It includes learning new skills and increasing her confidence in herself as she meets new challenges in caring for her child or children.

Mercer and Walker (2006) identified four stages in the process of becoming a mother: "(a) commitment, attachment to the unborn baby, and preparation for delivery and motherhood during pregnancy; (b) acquaintance/attachment to the infant, learning to care for the infant, and physical restoration during the first 2 to 6 weeks following birth; (c) moving toward a new normal; and (d) achievement of a maternal identity through redefining self to incorporate motherhood (around 4 months)" (Mercer & Walker, pp. 568-569). The time of achievement of the stages is variable and the stages can overlap. Achievement is influenced by maternal and infant variables and the social environment.

Maternal sensitivity or maternal responsiveness is an important determinant of the maternal-infant relationship. It can be defined as the quality of a mother's sensitive behaviors that are based on her awareness, perception, and responsiveness to infant cues and behaviors. Maternal sensitivity significantly influences the infant's physical, psychologic, and cognitive development. Maternal qualities inherent to this sensitivity include awareness and responsiveness to infant cues, affect, timing, flexibility, acceptance, and conflict negotiation. Maternal sensitivity develops over time in a reciprocal give-and-take relationship with the infant (Tharner, Luijk, Raat, et al., 2012).

The transition to motherhood requires adjustment for the mother and her family. Not all mothers experience the transition to motherhood in the same way. Circumstances such as problems in postpartum recovery or giving birth to a high risk infant add to the disruption. For some women becoming a mother entails multiple losses. For example, for a single woman a loss of the family of origin can occur when the family does not accept her decision to have the child. There can be loss of a relationship with the father of the baby, with friends, and with her own sense of self. Some women describe a loss of dreams that includes loss of job, financial security, and a future profession. Accompanying these losses is a loss of support.

Reality-based perinatal education programs help to prepare mothers and decrease their anxiety. Live classes allow time for questions to be answered and for mothers to lend support to one another. Mothers need to know that during the first months of parenthood it is common to feel overwhelmed and insecure and to experience physical and mental fatigue. They need to be assured that this situation is temporary and that 3 to 6 months can be needed to become comfortable in caregiving and in being a mother. Maternal support by professionals should not end with hospital discharge but, instead, extend over the next 4 to 6 months. Nurses can advocate for the extension of support services well into the postpartum period (Mercer & Walker, 2006; Shapiro, Nahm, Gottman, & Content, 2011).

During pregnancy and after birth nurses can discuss the usual postpartum concerns that mothers experience. They can provide anticipatory guidance on coping strategies, such as resting when the infant sleeps and planning with an extended family member or friend to do the housework for the first week or two after the baby is born. Once a mother is home, periodic telephone calls from a nurse who cared for her in the birth setting can provide the mother with an opportunity to vent her concerns and get support and advice from "her" nurse. Nurses should plan additional supportive counseling for first-time mothers inexperienced in child care, women whose careers had provided outside stimulation, women who lack friends or family members with whom to share delights and concerns, and adolescent mothers. When, possible, postpartum home visits should be included in the postpartum care.

In summary, nurses have the unique opportunity to experience the miracle of a birth and provide valuable client and family education and emotional support that will help during and after this exciting and overwhelming time of transition to parenthood (Husmillo, 2013).

Postpartum "Blues"

The "pink" period surrounding the first day or two after birth, characterized by heightened joy and feelings of well-being, is often followed by a "blue" period. Approximately 50% to 80% of women of all ethnic and racial groups experience the postpartum blues, or "baby blues." During the blues, women are emotionally labile and often cry easily for no apparent reason. This lability seems to peak around the fifth day and subsides by the tenth day. Other symptoms of postpartum blues include depression, a let-down feeling, restlessness, fatigue, insomnia, headache, anxiety, sadness, and anger. Biochemical, psychologic, social, and cultural factors have been explored as possible causes of postpartum blues; however, the cause remains unknown.

Whatever the cause, the early postpartum period appears to be one of emotional and physical vulnerability for new mothers, who are often psychologically overwhelmed by the reality of parental responsibilities. Mothers feel deprived of the supportive care they received from family members and friends during pregnancy. Some mothers regret the loss of the mother–unborn child relationship and mourn its passing. Still others experience a let-down feeling when labor and birth are complete. The majority of women experience fatigue after birth, which is compounded by the around-the-clock demands of the new baby. Postpartum fatigue increases the risk of postpartum depressive symptoms and can have a negative effect on maternal role attainment (Kurth, Spichiger, Stutz, et al., 2010). A few questions on a discharge checklist can help mothers assess their level of blues and decide when to seek advice from their nurse, nurse-midwife, or physician. Home visits and telephone follow-up calls by a nurse are important to assess the mother's pattern of blue feelings and behavior over time. To help mothers cope with postpartum blues, nurses can suggest various strategies (see Teaching for Self-Management box).

TEACHING FOR SELF-MANAGEMENT

Coping with Postpartum Blues

- Remember that the "blues" are normal and that both the mother and the father or partner can experience them.
- Get plenty of rest; nap when the baby does if possible. Go to bed early and let friends and family know when to visit and how they can help. (Remember, you are not Supermom.)
- Use relaxation techniques learned in birthing classes (or ask the nurse to teach you and your partner some techniques).
- Do something for yourself. Take advantage of the time your partner or family members care for the baby—soak in the tub (a 20-minute soak can be the equivalent of a 2-hour nap), or go for a walk.
- Plan a day out of the house—go to the mall with the baby, being sure to take a stroller or carriage, or go out to eat with friends without the baby. Many communities have churches or other agencies that provide child care programs such as Mothers' Morning Out.
- Talk to your partner about the way you feel—for example, about feeling tied down, how the birth met your expectations, and things that will help you (do not be afraid to ask for specifics).
- If you are breastfeeding, give yourself and your baby time to learn.
- Seek out and use community resources such as La Leche League or community mental health centers. One nationally recognized resource is:
  Postpartum Support International
  927 North Kellogg Ave.
  Santa Barbara, CA 93111
  (805) 967-7636
  www.postpartum.net

Although the postpartum blues are usually mild and short-lived, approximately 10% to 15% of women experience a more severe syndrome termed *postpartum depression* (PPD). Symptoms of PPD can range from mild to severe, with women having good days and bad days. Fathers can also experience PPD. Screening for PPD should be performed with both mothers and fathers. PPD can go undetected because new parents generally do not voluntarily admit to this kind of emotional distress out of embarrassment, guilt, or fear. Nurses need to include teaching about how to differentiate symptoms of the blues and PPD and urge parents to report depressive symptoms promptly if they occur (see Chapter 31).

Becoming a Father

The realities of the first few weeks at home with a newborn cause fathers to change their expectations, set new priorities, and redefine their role. They develop strategies for balancing work, their own needs, and the needs of their partner and infant. Men become increasingly more comfortable with infant care. During this time they may struggle for recognition and positive feedback from their partner, the infant, and others. They can feel excluded from support and attention by health care providers. Infant smiles enhance involvement and the father-infant relationship (Table 22-5).

First-time fathers often perceive the first 4 to 10 weeks of parenthood in much the same way that mothers do. It is a period characterized by uncertainty, increased responsibility, disruption of sleep, and inability to control time needed to care for the infant while reestablishing the relationship with their partner (Yu, Hung, Chan, et al., 2012). The realities of these first few weeks at home with a newborn often cause fathers to change their expectations, set new priorities, and redefine their roles. They begin to develop strategies for balancing work with their own needs and the needs of their partner and infant (de Montigny, Lacharité, & Devault, 2012)

Research on paternal adjustment to parenthood suggests that men go through predictable phases during their transition to parenthood as they seek to become involved fathers (Goodman, 2005). In the first phase men enter parenthood with intentions of being an emotionally involved father with deep connections to the infant. They consider how they were parented by their own father. Many desire to parent differently from their own father, whereas others plan to adopt the parenting style of their father (Chin, Hall, & Daiches, 2011).

The second phase is a time of confronting reality, when men realize that their expectations were inconsistent with the realities of life with a newborn during the first few weeks. During this period fathers experience intense emotions. Many acknowledge that their expectations were of limited value once they were immersed in the reality of parenthood. Feelings that often accompany this reality are sadness, ambivalence, jealousy, frustration, and an overwhelming desire to be more involved. Some men are surprised that establishing a relationship with the infant is more gradual than expected. Fathers often feel alone, having no one with whom to discuss their feelings during this time because mothers are often preoccupied with infant care and their own transition to parenting.

The third phase is working to create the role of involved father. Men strive to become increasingly more comfortable with infant care. Uncertainty about child care skills can lead to feelings of anxiety (Goodman, 2005). Communicating with other new fathers about their experiences can help alleviate some of this anxiety (Chin et al., 2011). During this time they may struggle for recognition and positive feedback from their partner, the infant, and others and may feel excluded from support and attention by health care providers. Leaving their partner and the newborn to return to work after the birth can be difficult for fathers; many find it challenging to balance their time between work and spending time with their families. Some men reprioritize their activities or negotiate work hours to allow them to be at home more often (Chin et al.).

The final phase of becoming an involved father is one of reaping rewards, the most significant being reciprocity from the infant, such as a smile. This phase typically occurs around 6 weeks to 2 months. Increased sociability of the infant enhances this father-infant relationship (Goodman, 2005).

In North American culture, neonates have a powerful effect on their fathers who become intensely involved with their babies. The term used for the father's absorption, preoccupation, and interest in the infant is **engrossment.** Characteristics of engrossment include some of the sensual responses relating to touch and eye-to-eye contact that were discussed earlier and the father's keen awareness of features both unique and similar to himself that validate his claim to the infant. The father feels strong attraction to the newborn. Fathers spend considerable time "communicating" with the infant and taking delight in the infant's response to them (Fig. 22-7). Fathers experience increased self-esteem and a sense of being proud, bigger, more mature, and older after seeing their baby for the first time.

TABLE 22-5 Early Development of the Involved Father Role

PHASES	CHARACTERISTICS
Expectations and intentions	Desire for emotional involvement and deep connection with infant
Confronting reality	Dealing with unrealistic expectations, frustration, disappointment, feelings of guilt, helplessness, and inadequacy
Creating the role of involved father	Altering expectations, establishing new priorities, redefining role, negotiating changes with partner, learning to care for infant, increasing interaction with infant, struggling for recognition
Reaping rewards	Infant smile, sense of meaning, completeness and immortality

From Goodman, J. (2005). Becoming an involved father of an infant. *Journal of Obstetric, Gynecologic and Neonatal Nursing, 34*(2), 190-200.

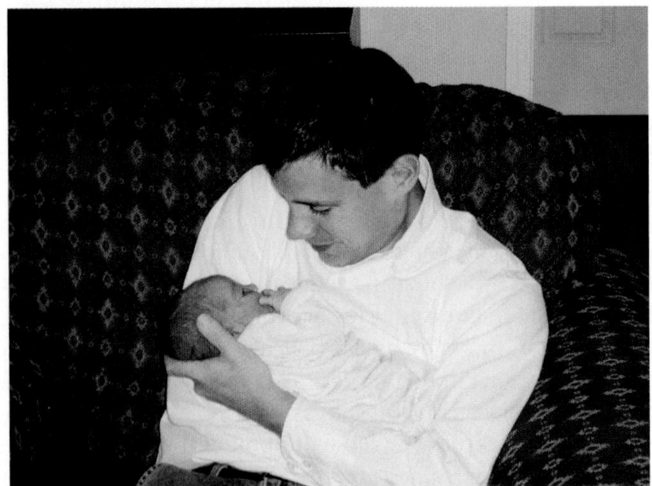

FIG 22-7 Engrossment. Father is absorbed in looking at his newborn. (Courtesy Kathryn Alden, Chapel Hill, NC.)

Fathers spend less time than mothers with infants, and their interactions with infants tend to be characterized by stimulating social play rather than caretaking. The variations in infant stimulation from both parents provide a wider social experience for the infant.

Fathers receive less interpersonal and professional support compared with mothers and can feel excluded from prenatal appointments and perinatal classes (Chin et al., 2011; Steen, Downe, Bamford, & Edozien, 2012). They need information and encouragement during pregnancy and in the postpartum period related to infant care, parenting, and relationship changes. During the postpartum hospital stay, nurses can arrange to teach infant care when the father is present and provide anticipatory guidance for fathers about the transition to parenthood. Separate prenatal and parenting classes and parenting support groups for fathers can provide them with an opportunity to discuss their concerns and have some of their needs met. To prepare fathers for the transition to parenthood, perinatal education should include information on role changes associated with parenting, the importance of parenting "teamwork," the increased risk of mental distress and depression, the mother's experience and how to provide support, how to interpret and respond to infant behaviors, and how to deal with infant crying (May & Fletcher, 2013). Postpartum telephone calls and home visits by the nurse should include time for assessment of the father's adjustment and needs (Chin et al.).

Adjustment for the Couple

The transition to parenthood brings about changes in the relationship between the mother and her partner. A strong, healthy marriage or couple relationship is the best foundation for parenthood, although even the best relationships are often shaken with the addition of a new baby. During the first few weeks after birth, parents experience many emotions. Even though they may feel an overwhelming love and a sense of amazement toward their newborn, they can also feel a great responsibility. Even if the mother and her partner have been to prenatal classes, read books or Internet sources, or sought advice from family or friends, they are usually surprised by the realities of life with a new baby and the changes in their relationship. Because men and women experience pregnancy and birth differently, the expectation is that they will also vary in their transition to parenthood.

Common issues that couples face as they become parents include changes in their relationship with one another, division of household and infant care responsibilities, financial concerns, balancing work and parental responsibilities, and social activities (Menéndez, Hidalgo, Jiménez, & Moreno, 2011). To assist new parents in their transition, nurses can encourage them during pregnancy and in the postpartum period to share personal expectations with each other and to assess their relationship periodically. Couples need to schedule time into their busy lives for one-on-one conversation and try to have regular "dates" or time apart from the infant. The mother and her partner need to express appreciation for one another and for their baby. Support from family, friends, and community health professionals should be identified early and used as needed during pregnancy and in the postpartum period and beyond. The couple who is willing to experiment with new approaches to their lifestyle and habits can find the transition to parenthood less difficult.

Resuming Sexual Intimacy

Nurses can provide opportunities for parents to discuss concerns and ask questions about resuming sexual intimacy. The couple may begin to engage in sexual intercourse during the second to fourth week after the baby is born. Some couples begin earlier, as soon as it can be accomplished without discomfort, depending on factors such as timing and vaginal dryness. Sexual intimacy enhances the adult aspect of the family, and the adult pair shares a closeness denied to other family members. Changes in a woman's sexual desire after birth are related to hormonal shifts, increased breast size, uneasiness with a body that has yet to return to a prepregnant size, chronic fatigue related to sleep deprivation, and physical exhaustion. Partners can feel alienated when they observe the intimate mother-infant relationship, and some are frank in expressing feelings of jealousy toward the infant. The resumption of sexual intimacy seems to bring the parents' relationship back into focus. Before and after birth, nurses should review with new parents their plans for other pregnancies and their preferences for contraception. (See Teaching for Self-Management box: Resuming Sexual Intimacy in Chapter 21.)

Infant-Parent Adjustment

It has long been recognized that newborns participate actively in shaping their parents' reaction to them. Behavioral characteristics of the infant influence parenting behaviors. The infant and the parent each have unique rhythms, behaviors, and response styles that are brought to every interaction. Infant-parent interactions can be facilitated in any of the following three ways: (1) modulation of rhythm, (2) modification of behavioral repertoires, and (3) mutual responsivity. Nurses can teach parents about these three aspects of infant-parent interaction through discussions, written materials, and media resources describing infant capabilities. A creative approach is to make a video recording of the parent-infant pair during an interaction and then use that recording to discuss the pair's rhythm, behavioral repertoire, and responsivity.

Rhythm. To modulate rhythm, both parent and infant must be able to interact. Therefore, the infant must be in the alert state, one of the most difficult of the sleep-wake states to maintain. The alert state (Fig. 22-8) occurs most often during a feeding or in face-to-face play. The parent must work hard to help the infant maintain the alert state long enough and often enough for interactions to take place. The en face position is usually assumed (see Fig. 22-8, *D*). Multiparous mothers in particular are very sensitive and responsive to the infant's feeding rhythms.

Mothers learn to reserve stimulation for pauses in sucking activity and not to talk or smile excessively while the infant is sucking because the infant will stop feeding to interact with her. With maturity the infant can sustain longer interactions by modulating activity rhythms, that is, limb movement, sucking, gaze alternation, and habituation. Meanwhile, the parent becomes more attuned to the infant's rhythms and learns to modulate the rhythms, facilitating a rhythmic turn-taking interaction.

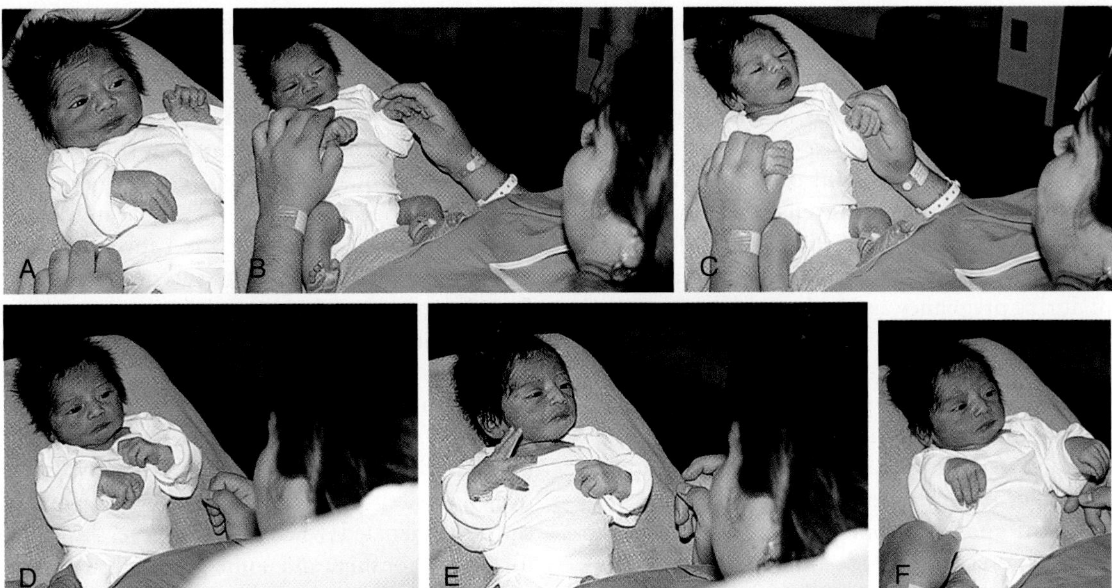

FIG 22-8 Holding newborn in en face position, mother interacts with her daughter, 6 hours old. **A,** Infant is quiet and alert. **B,** Mother begins talking to daughter. **C,** Infant responds, opens mouth like her mother. **D,** Infant gazes at her mother. **E,** Infant waves hand. **F,** Infant glances away, resting; hands relax. (Courtesy Marjorie Pyle, RNC, Lifecircle, Costa Mesa, CA.)

Behavioral Repertoires. Both the infant and the parent have a repertoire of behaviors they can use to facilitate interactions. Fathers and mothers engage in these behaviors depending on the extent of contact and caregiving of the infant. Nurses can teach parents to recognize, interpret, and respond to infant behaviors. An innovative program called HUG Your Baby (Help, Understanding and Guidance for Young Families: www.hugyourbaby.org) is designed to prepare health care professionals to teach parents how to understand their newborns and prevent problems related to crying, sleeping, eating, attachment, and bonding.

The infant's behavioral repertoire includes gazing, vocalizing, and facial expressions. From birth the infant is able to focus, follow the human face, and alternate the gaze voluntarily, looking away from the parent's face when understimulated or overstimulated (see Fig. 22-8, *F*). One of the key responses for the parents to learn is to be sensitive to the infant's capacity for attention and inattention. Developing this sensitivity is especially important when interacting with preterm infants.

Body gestures form a part of the infant's "early language." Babies greet parents with waving hands (see Fig. 22-8, *E*) or by reaching out. They can raise an eyebrow or soften their expression to elicit loving attention. Game-playing can stimulate them to smile or laugh. Pouting or crying, arching of the back, and general squirming usually signal the end of an interaction.

The parents' repertoire includes various types of interactive behaviors such as constantly looking at the infant and noting the infant's response. New parents often remark that they are exhausted from looking at the baby and smiling. Adults also "infantilize" their speech to help the infant "listen." They do this by slowing the tempo, speaking loudly and rhythmically, and emphasizing key words. Phrases are repeated frequently. Infantilizing does not mean using "baby talk," which involves distortion of sounds.

To communicate emotions to the infant, parents often use facial expressions such as slow and exaggerated looks of surprise, happiness, and confusion. Games such as peek-a-boo and imitation of the infant's behaviors are other means of interaction. For example, if the baby smiles, so does the parent; if the baby frowns, the parent responds in kind.

Responsivity. Contingent responses (responsivity) are those that occur within a specific time and are similar in form to a stimulus behavior. The adult has the feeling of having an influence on the interaction. Infant behaviors such as smiling, cooing, and sustained eye contact, usually in the en face position, are viewed as contingent responses. The infant's responses act as rewards to the initiator and encourage the adult to continue with the game when the infant responds positively. When the adult imitates the infant, the infant appears to enjoy it. A progression occurs in the types of behaviors that parents present for the baby to imitate; for example, in early interactions, the parent will grimace rather than laugh, which is in keeping with the infant's developmental level. Such "turnabout" behaviors sustain interactions and promote harmony in the relationship.

DIVERSITY IN TRANSITIONS TO PARENTHOOD

Various factors, including age, social networks, socioeconomic conditions, and personal aspirations for the future, influence how parents respond to the birth of a child. Cultural beliefs and practices also affect parenting behaviors. Factors that are recognized to increase the risk of parenting problems include age (adolescent or older than 35 years), same sex parenting, social support, culture, socioeconomic conditions, and personal aspirations.

Age

Maternal age has a definite effect on the transition to parenting. The mother, fetus, and newborn are at highest risk when the mother is an adolescent or older than 35 years.

The Adolescent Mother

Although becoming a parent is biologically possible for the adolescent female, her egocentricity and concrete thinking often interfere with the ability to parent effectively. Adolescent mothers are more likely to give birth to preterm and/or low-birth-weight infants (Martin, Hamilton, Osterman, et al., 2013). Mortality rates are higher among infants of adolescent mothers. This can be related to inherent problems associated with preterm birth or other conditions, but it is also influenced by the mother's inexperience, lack of knowledge, and immaturity. In the United States, adolescent mothers are often poorer, less educated, and receive less prenatal care than older mothers (Geoghegan, 2013). Nevertheless, in most instances, with adequate support and developmentally appropriate teaching, adolescents can learn effective parenting skills. Strong social and functional support promotes positive outcomes for adolescent mothers.

Contrary to popular beliefs related to the detrimental effects of adolescent pregnancy, research evidence suggests that the life course for adolescent mothers is similar to that of their socioeconomic peers. In some families or communities, adolescent parenthood is considered a normal or positive life event. Even so, adolescent pregnancy and parenting are important public health concerns.

The transition to parenthood can be difficult for adolescents. Because many adolescents have their own unmet developmental needs, coping with the developmental tasks of parenthood is often difficult. Some young parents experience difficulty accepting a changing self-image and adjusting to new roles related to the responsibilities of infant care. Adolescent mothers are at increased risk for postpartum depression; this is often associated with a lack of social support and poor relations with their partner (Mollborn & Jacobs, 2011). There is an increased risk of child abuse and neglect by adolescent mothers; the risk increases when the mother experienced abuse as a child (Bartlett & Easterbrooks, 2012).

As adolescent parents move through the transition to parenthood, they can feel "different" from their peers, excluded from "fun" activities, and prematurely forced to enter an adult social role. The conflict between their own desires and the infant's demands, in addition to the low tolerance for frustration that is typical of adolescence, further contribute to the normal psychosocial stress of birth and parenting. Maintaining a relationship with the baby's father is often beneficial for the teen mother and her infant, although in adolescent pregnancy it is often found that the young father departs from the relationship.

Adolescent mothers provide warm and attentive physical care; however, they use less verbal interaction than older parents, tend to be less responsive, and interact less positively with their infants than older mothers. Interventions emphasizing verbal and nonverbal communication skills between mother and infant are important. Such intervention strategies must be concrete and specific because of the cognitive and developmental level of adolescents. In comparison with older mothers, teenage mothers have a limited knowledge of child development. They tend to expect too much of their infants too soon and often characterize their infants as being fussy. This limited knowledge can cause teenagers to respond to their infants inappropriately.

Many young mothers pattern their maternal role on what they experienced with their own mothers. Therefore, nurses need to determine the type of support that people close to the young mother are able and prepared to give, as well as the kinds of community assistance available to supplement this support. Many teen mothers can identify a source of social support, with the predominant source being their own mothers.

The need for continued assessment of the new mother's parenting abilities during this postpartum period is essential. Continued support is facilitated by involving the grandparents and other family members, as well as through home visits and group sessions for discussion of infant care and parenting concerns (Schaffer, Goodhue, Stennes, & Lanigan, 2012). Community-based programs for pregnant adolescents and adolescent parents improve access to health care, education, and other support services. Many school-based programs include a parenting and life skills curriculum as well as pregnancy prevention strategies. Serious problems can be prevented through outreach programs concerned with self-management, parent-child interactions, infant development, and child safety. As the adolescent performs her mothering role within the framework of her family, she may need to address dependence versus independence issues. The adolescent's family members also need help adapting to their new roles. Some mothers and fathers of adolescents feel they are too young and unprepared to be grandparents (see Clinical Reasoning Case Study).

The Adolescent Father

The adolescent father and mother face immediate developmental tasks that include completing the developmental tasks of

CLINICAL REASONING CASE STUDY

Transition to Parenthood for the Adolescent Couple

You are the mother/baby nurse caring for Sherika, a 16-year-old who gave birth to a baby girl 24 hours ago. John, the baby's father, is Sherika's 17-year-old "on again, off again" boyfriend who has visited once since the baby was born, but only for a couple of hours. John has held the baby briefly twice but seems to stand in the background most of the time. Sherika's mother has been at the hospital with her since admission and has been very involved in her care. Her mother has raised six children and has very strong opinions about how to take care of the baby and Sherika as she recovers from the birth. Sherika would like to breastfeed the baby, but her mother states that when she was raising her children she did not have enough milk to feed them, and insists that Sherika start with formula feeding.

1. Evidence—Is evidence sufficient to draw conclusions about the education and care needed for this family?
2. Assumptions—What assumptions can be made about the following factors?
   a. The relationship of maternal age and transition to parenthood
   b. The relationship of paternal age and transition to parenthood
   c. The need for postpartum and discharge teaching
   d. The role of family dynamics and postpartum adaptation
   e. Short- and long-term goals that would promote positive outcomes
3. What nursing care priorities can be determined at this time?
4. Does the evidence objectively support your conclusion?

adolescence, making a transition to parenthood, and sometimes adapting to marriage. These transitions are often stressful. In addition, relationships between adolescent mothers and fathers tend to be less stable than among adults and often deteriorate or dissolve soon after birth. The involvement of the father with the infant is dependent on his relationship with the mother, who also controls his access to the infant (Farrie, Lee, & Fagan, 2011).

The nurse can initiate interaction with the adolescent father during prenatal visits, labor and birth, and the postpartum hospitalization. The nurse can assess the relationship between the two adolescents and encourage them to discuss their plans for the father's involvement with the mother and infant after birth (Fagan, 2013). During the hospital stay the nurse can include the adolescent father in teaching sessions about infant care and parenting. The nurse can ask him to be present during postpartum home visits and to accompany the mother and the baby to well-baby follow-up visits at the clinic or pediatrician's office. With the adolescent mother's approval, the nurse may contact the father directly.

Adolescent fathers need support to discuss their emotional responses to the pregnancy, birth, and fatherhood. The nurse needs to be aware of the father's feelings of guilt, powerlessness, or bravado because these feelings can have negative consequences for both the parents and the child. Counseling of adolescent fathers needs to be reality oriented and should include topics such as finances, child care, parenting skills, and the father's role in the parenting experience. Teenage fathers also need to know about reproductive physiology and birth control options, as well as sexual practices that lower the risk of pregnancy and sexually transmitted infections.

The adolescent father may continue to be involved in an ongoing relationship with the young mother and his baby. In those instances he plays an important role in the decisions about child care and raising the child. He may need help to develop realistic perceptions of his role as "father to a child" and is encouraged to use coping mechanisms that are not harmful to his own, his partner's, or his child's well-being. The nurse may enlist support systems, parents, and professional agencies on his behalf.

Maternal Age Older Than 35 Years

Women older than 35 years have always continued their childbearing either by choice or because of a lack of or a failure of contraception during the perimenopausal years. Added to this group are women who have postponed pregnancy because of careers or other reasons, as well as women of infertile couples who finally become pregnant with the aid of assisted reproductive techology.

Support from partners aids in the adjustment of older mothers to changes involved in becoming a parent and seeing themselves as competent. Support from other family members and friends is also important for positive self-evaluation of parenting, a sense of well-being and satisfaction, and help in dealing with stress. Women of advanced maternal age can experience social isolation. Older mothers may have less family and social support than younger mothers. They are less likely to live near family, and their own parents may be unable to provide assistance or support because of age or health issues. Mothers of advanced maternal age are often caught in the "sandwich generation," taking on responsibility for care of aging parents while parenting young children. Social support can be lacking because their peers are probably busy with their careers and have limited time to help. Their friends are likely to have older children and have less in common with the new mother (Morgan, Merrell, Rentschler, & Chadderton, 2012).

Changes in the sexual aspect of a relationship can create stress for new midlife parents. Mothers report that it is difficult to find time and energy for a romantic rendezvous. They attribute much of this difficulty to the reality of caring for an infant, but the decreasing libido that normally accompanies getting older also contributes.

Work and career issues are sources of conflict for older mothers. Conflicts emerge over being disinterested in work, worrying about giving enough attention to work with the distractions of a new baby, and anticipating what returning to work will entail. Child care is a major factor in causing stress about work.

Another major issue for older mothers with careers is the perception of loss of control. Mothers older than 35 years, when compared with younger mothers, are at a different stage in their careers, having attained high levels of education, career, and income. The loss of control experienced when going from the consistency of a work role to the inconsistency of the parent role comes as a surprise to many older women. Helping the older mother have realistic expectations of herself and of parenthood is essential.

New mothers who are also perimenopausal can experience difficulty distinguishing fatigue, loss of sleep, decreased libido, or other physiologic symptoms as the causes of the change in their sex lives. Although many women view menopause as a natural stage of life, for midlife mothers, this cessation of menstruation coincides with the state of parenthood. The changes of midlife and menopause can add more emotional and physical stress to older mothers' lives because of the time- and energy-consuming aspects of raising a young child.

Paternal Age Older Than 35 Years

Although many older fathers describe their experience of midlife parenting as wonderful, they also recognize drawbacks. Positive aspects of fatherhood in older years include increased love and commitment between the two parents, a reinforcement of why one married in the first place, a feeling of being complete, experiencing "the child" again in oneself, more financial stability than in younger years, and more freedom to focus on parenting rather than on career. A common drawback of midlife parenting is the change that it brings about in the relationships with their partners.

Parenting in Same Sex Couples

The transition to parenting for same sex couples can present unique challenges. Whether the couple consists of two women or two men, issues such as a lack of family acceptance and support, public ignorance, and social and legal invisibility influence their ability to adapt as new parents. Attitudes of health care professionals can either positively or negatively affect the care provided to same-sex couples.

Lesbian Couple

The transition to parenting for many lesbian couples is unique in that there are two women with maternal status, one who gave birth and the other who may be referred to as "the other mother," "nonbiologic mother," "co-parent," or other term preferred by the couple. It is important for health care providers to determine the couple's preference about how they wish to be identified.

Among lesbian couples the decision to become parents is intentional. There are several methods to achieve a pregnancy. One woman can be artificially inseminated and conceive a child who is genetically related to her. The fertilized egg of one partner can be implanted into the uterus of the other who carries the pregnancy. Alternatively, one woman can be implanted with the fertilized egg from a donor so that the child is not biologically related to either partner. Evidence suggests that the birth mother has chosen to be the one to carry the baby because of a greater desire to experience the pregnancy and birth and to be genetically related to the child. Other factors that influence the decision are age, health, infertility, and career considerations. Some lesbian couples who wish to become parents use a surrogate to carry the pregnancy or they may adopt. If the couple adopts a newborn, the nurse may be involved in educating them about infant care.

Health care providers demonstrate a variety of reactions to lesbian couples ranging from rejection and exclusion to complete acceptance and inclusion. Judgmental attitudes, confusion, or lack of understanding can affect the quality of care provided to these families (Dahl, Fylkesnes, Sorlie, & Malterud, 2013). Although the traditional roles of the mother and father in heterosexual relationships are well recognized, the role of the lesbian co-parent can be questioned, misunderstood, and ignored by society and by health care providers. Intentionally or accidentally, health care providers can exclude partners or fail to acknowledge their roles in pregnancy, birth, and parenting (O'Neill, Hamer, & Dixon, 2012).

Integration of the nonchildbearing partner into care includes offering opportunities afforded male partners of heterosexual women such as "cutting the cord" and rooming in with the mother and baby during hospitalization. An option not available to male partners is to actually breastfeed the infant. The nonchildbearing female partner can stimulate milk production through induced lactation using medications and regular pumping. A supplemental feeding device containing expressed breast milk or formula can be used to provide additional milk to the breastfeeding infant (see Fig. 25-8). Women who choose not to induce lactation yet desire to have the breastfeeding experience can put the baby to breast using a supplemental feeding device.

Similar to heterosexual parents, lesbian couples face challenges in adjusting to life with a new baby. The birth mother tends to be the one most responsible for child care because she is likely to be working fewer hours than her partner. Tensions can arise between the partners in relation to their roles. This can be compounded by the lack of a formal, recognized relationship between the co-parent and the infant and the issues surrounding her legal rights in relation to her partner and the infant (Mortensen, Torsheim, Melkevik, & Thuen, 2012).

Lesbian couples face strong social sanctions regarding pregnancy and parenting. Their families may not have resolved the initial dismay and guilt over learning of their daughters' homosexuality, or they may disagree with the lesbian couple's decision to conceive and be parents. Lesbian parents deal with public ignorance, social and legal invisibility, and the lack of biologic connection to the child by using various techniques. These techniques include carefully planning and accomplishing their transition to parenthood, displaying public acts of equal mothering, sharing parenting at home, establishing a distinct parenting role within the family, and supporting each partner's sense of identity as a mother. In situations in which family support is limited or absent, the nurse can help lesbian couples locate supportive social groups, lesbian or heterosexual.

Gay Couples

Some men in same-sex relationships, or gay couples, choose to become parents by adoption or through assisted reproduction in which a gestational carrier is impregnated by artificial insemination or in vitro fertilization (Greenfield & Seli, 2011). Female-to-male transgender individuals in gay relationships have been known to become pregnant. Same-sex male couples face the same social sanctions regarding pregnancy and parenting that lesbian couples encounter.

Nurses are likely to encounter gay couples in the hospital setting if they are present for birth by a surrogate or if they are adopting a newborn and visit the hospital to spend time with the neonate and learn about infant care. Nurses can help these men locate support groups that will address their needs. They need to ensure that these families receive effective health care. Data on gay parenting are limited and focus more on developmental outcomes of the children than on parenting styles or parental caregiving. Research is needed to identify the needs of gay parents and ways to support them in their parenting endeavors.

Social Support

Social support is strongly related to positive adaptation by new parents during the transition to parenthood. Social support is multidimensional and includes the number of members in a person's social network, types of support, perceived general support, actual support received, and satisfaction with support available and received. Partner support in pregnancy has a positive influence on adaptation in the postpartum period (Goldberg & Smith, 2011; Westling, Glynn, Sandman, et al., 2012).

Across cultural groups, families and friends of new parents form an important dimension of the parent's social network. Through seeking help within the social network, new mothers learn culturally valued practices and develop role competency.

Social networks provide a support system on which parents can rely for assistance, but they also can be a source of conflict. Sometimes a large network can cause problems because it results in conflicting advice that comes from numerous people. Grandparents or in-laws are most appreciated when they assist with household responsibilities and do not intrude into the parents' privacy or judge them critically.

Because of the extent of restructuring and reorganization that occurs in a family with the birth of another child, the mothers' moods and fatigue in the postpartum period can be helped more by situation-specific support from family and friends than by general support. Situation-specific support relates to practice concerns such as physical needs and child care. For example, the practical support of a grandparent bathing the infant can help lessen a second-time mother's feelings of loss by providing her time to be with her first-born child. General support addresses the feelings of being loved, supported, and valued.

Culture

Cultural beliefs and practices are important determinants of parenting behaviors. Culture influences the interactions with the baby, as well as the parents' or the family's caregiving style.

All cultures place importance on desiring and valuing children. In Asian families, children are a source of family strength and stability, are perceived as wealth, and are objects of parental love and affection. Infants are almost always given an affectionate "cradle" name that is used during the first years of life. Differing cultural values can influence parents' interactions with health care professionals. For example, Asians are taught to be humble and obedient, to refrain from questioning authority figures (e.g., a nurse), to avoid confrontation, and to respect the yin/yang balance in nature. Because of these learned values, an Asian mother might not confront the nurse about the length of time taken to receive the medication requested for her episiotomy pain. A mother may nod and say, "Yes," in response to the nurse's directions for using an iced sitz bath but then will not use the sitz bath. The "yes," in this case, is a gesture of courtesy, meaning, "I'm listening"; it is not an indication of agreement to comply. The mother does not use the iced sitz bath because of her traditional avoidance of bathing and cold after birth. Because not all members of a cultural group adhere to traditional practices, it is necessary to validate which cultural practices are important to individual parents. This can be easily accomplished by asking the parents specific questions about their cultural beliefs and practices.

Knowledge of cultural beliefs can help the nurse make more accurate assessments and analyses of observed parenting behaviors. For example, nurses can become concerned when they observe cultural practices that appear to reflect poor maternal-infant bonding. Algerian mothers may not unwrap and explore their infants as part of the acquaintance process because in Algeria, babies are wrapped tightly in swaddling clothes to protect them physically and psychologically. The nurse may observe a Vietnamese woman who gives minimal care to her infant but refuses to cuddle or further interact with her baby. This apparent lack of interest in the newborn is this cultural group's attempt to ward off "evil spirits" and actually reflects an intense love and concern for the infant. An Asian mother might be criticized for almost immediately relinquishing the care of the infant to the grandmother and not even attempting to hold her baby when it is brought to her room. However, in Asian extended families, members show their support for a new mother's rest and recuperation by assisting with the care of the baby. Contrary to the guidance that is sometimes given to mothers in the United States about exclusive breastfeeding, a mix of breastfeeding and bottle feeding is standard practice for Japanese mothers. This tradition is related to concern for the mother's rest during the first 2 to 3 months and does not usually lead to problems with lactation; breastfeeding is widespread and successful among Japanese women.

Cultural beliefs and values give perspective to the meaning of childbirth for a new mother. Nurses can provide an opportunity for a new mother to talk about her perception of the meaning of childbearing. In helping new families adjust to parenthood, nurses must provide culturally sensitive care by following principles that facilitate nursing practice within transcultural situations (Chalmers, 2012).

Socioeconomic Conditions

Socioeconomic conditions often determine access to available resources. Parents whose economic condition is made worse with the birth of each child and who are unable to use an effective method of fertility management can find birth complicated by concern for their own health and a sense of helplessness. Mothers who are single, separated, or divorced from their husbands or without a partner, family, and friends can view the birth of a child with dread. Serious financial problems can negatively affect mothering behaviors. Similarly, fathers who are overwhelmed with financial stresses may lack effective parenting skills and behaviors.

Personal Aspirations

For some women parenthood interferes with or blocks plans for personal freedom or career advancement. Unresolved resentment affects caregiving activities and adjustment to parenting. This situation can result in indifference and neglect of the infant or in excessive concerns; the mother may set impossibly high standards for her own behavior or the child's performance.

Nursing interventions include providing opportunities for mothers to express their feelings freely to an objective listener, to discuss measures to permit personal growth, and to learn about the care of their infant. Referring the woman to a support group of other mothers "in the same situation" may also be helpful.

Nurses can be proactive in influencing changes in work policies related to maternity and paternity leaves, varying models of work sharing and family-friendly work environments. Some corporations already structure their worksites to support new mothers (e.g., by providing on-site day care facilities and lactation rooms).

PARENTAL SENSORY IMPAIRMENT

In early interactions between the parent and child, each one uses all senses—sight, hearing, touch, taste, and smell—to initiate and sustain the attachment process. A parent who has an impairment of one or more of the senses needs to maximize use of the remaining senses. Mothers with disabilities tend to value the importance of performing parenting tasks in the perceived culturally usual way.

Visually Impaired Parent

Visual impairment alone does not seem to have a negative effect on early parenting experiences. These parents, just as sighted parents, express the wonders of parenthood and encourage other visually impaired people to become parents.

Although visually impaired parents can initially feel pressure to conform to traditional, sighted ways of parenting, they soon adapt and develop methods better suited to themselves. Examples of activities that visually impaired parents perform differently include preparation of the infant's nursery, clothes, and supplies. Some parents put an entire clothing outfit together and hang it in the closet rather than keeping items separate in drawers. Some develop a labeling system for the infant's clothing and place diapering, bathing, and other care supplies where they will be easy to locate. A strength that visually impaired parents have is a heightened sensitivity to other sensory outputs. Visually impaired parents can tell when their infant is facing them because they notice the baby's breath on their faces.

One of the major difficulties that visually impaired parents experience is the skepticism, open or hidden, of health care professionals. Visually impaired people may sense reluctance on the part of others to acknowledge that they have a right to be parents. All too often nurses and physicians lack the experience to deal with the childbearing and childrearing needs of visually impaired parents, as well as parents with other disabilities, such as the hearing impaired, physically impaired, and mentally challenged. The nurse's best approach is to assess the parents' capabilities and to use that information as a basis for making plans to assist them, often in much the same way as for parents without impairments. Visually impaired mothers have made suggestions about providing care for women such as themselves during childbearing (Box 22-2). Such approaches can help avoid a sense of increased vulnerability on the parent's part. Materials for perinatal education are available in Braille.

Eye contact is important in U.S. culture. With a parent who is visually impaired, this critical factor in the parent-child attachment process is obviously missing. However, the blind parent, who may never have experienced this method of strengthening relationships, does not miss it. The infant will need other sensory input from that parent. An infant looking into the eyes of a parent who is blind can be unaware that the eyes are unseeing. Other people in the newborn's environment can also participate in active eye-to-eye contact to supply this need. A problem may arise, however, if the visually impaired parent has little facial expression. The infant, after making repeated unsuccessful attempts to engage in face play with the mother, will abandon the behavior with her and intensify it with the father or other people in the household. Nurses can provide anticipatory guidance regarding this situation and help the mother learn to nod and smile while talking and cooing to the infant.

Hearing-Impaired Parent

A parent who has a hearing impairment faces challenges in caregiving and parenting, particularly if the deafness dates from birth or early childhood. Whether one or both parents are hearing impaired, they are likely to have established an independent household. Devices that transform sound into light flashes can be placed in the infant's room to permit immediate detection of crying. Even if the parent is not speech trained, vocalizing can serve as both a stimulus and a response to the infant's early vocalizing. Deaf parents can provide additional vocal training by use of recordings and television so that from birth the child is aware of the full range of the human voice. Young children acquire sign language readily, and the first sign used is as varied as the first word.

Section 504 of the Rehabilitation Act of 1973 requires that hospitals and other institutions receiving funds from the U.S. Department of Health and Human Services use various communication techniques and resources with the deaf, including having staff members or certified interpreters who are proficient in sign language. For example, provision of written materials with demonstrations and having nurses stand where the parent can read their lips (if the parent practices lip reading) are two techniques that can be used. A creative approach is for the nursing unit to develop videos in which information on postpartum care, infant care, and parenting issues is signed by an interpreter and spoken by a nurse. A video recording in which a nurse signs while speaking is ideal. With the advent of the Internet, many resources are available to deaf parents. Box 22-3 lists suggestions for working with hearing-impaired parents.

BOX 22-2 Nursing Approaches for Working with Visually Impaired Parents

- A visually impaired parent needs an orientation to the hospital room that allows the parent to move about the room independently. For example, "Go to the left of the bed and trail the wall until you feel the first door. That is the bathroom."
- Parents who are visually impaired need explanations of routines.
- Parents who are visually impaired need to feel devices (e.g., portable sitz bath equipment, breast pump) and to hear descriptions of the devices.
- Visually impaired parents need a chance to ask questions.
- Visually impaired parents need the opportunity to hold and touch the newborn after birth.
- Nurses need to demonstrate infant care by touch and to follow with, "Now show me how you would do it."
- Nurses need to give instructions such as, "I'm going to give you the baby. The head is to your left side."

SIBLING ADAPTATION

Because the family is an interactive, open unit, the addition of a new family member affects everyone in the family. Siblings have to assume new positions within the family hierarchy. Parents often face the task of caring for the neonate while also attending to the needs of other children, and attempting to distribute their attention equitably. When the newborn is preterm or has special needs, this task can be difficult.

Reactions of siblings result from temporary separation from the mother, changes in the mother's or father's behavior, or the infant coming home. Positive behavioral changes of siblings include interest in and concern for the baby (Fig. 22-9) and increased independence. Regression in toileting and sleep habits, aggression toward the baby, and increased seeking of attention and whining are examples of negative behaviors.

The parents' attitudes toward the arrival of the baby can set the stage for the other children's reactions. Because the baby absorbs the time and attention of the important people in the other children's lives, jealousy (sibling rivalry) is common once the initial excitement of having a new baby in the home is over.

Parents, especially mothers, spend much time and energy promoting sibling acceptance of a new baby. Sibling preparation classes can help children adjust. Older children may be actively involved in preparing for the infant, and this involvement can intensify after the birth. Parents have to manage the

BOX 22-3 Nursing Approaches for Working with Hearing-Impaired Parents

- Before initiating communication, the nurse needs to be aware of the parents' preferences and capabilities: Do they wear a hearing aid? Do they read lips? Do they wish to have an interpreter?
- The nurse should make certain that the parent(s) sees the nurse approaching to avoid startling the parent.
- Before speaking, the nurse needs to be directly in front of the parent and should have that person's full attention.
- When speaking, the nurse should face the parent directly and should be at the same level.
- It is best to avoid standing in front of a light or a window while speaking to the parent.
- Keep hands away from the face while speaking to minimize distractions.
- If the parent relies on lip reading, the nurse should sit close enough so that the parent can easily see lip movements.
- The nurse should speak clearly with a regular voice volume and lip movements, while maintaining eye contact.
- Speak in short, simple sentences to facilitate understanding.
- If the parent does not understand something, it is better to find a different way to say what needs to be communicated rather than repeating the same words over and over.
- Written messages aid in communication. A small white or black erasable board can be useful.
- Educational materials should be given to hearing-impaired parents and they should be asked to read the materials prior to a teaching session. They can refer to the materials after discharge.
- Visual aids such as pictures, diagrams, or other devices should be used when doing client teaching.
- When doing parent teaching, it is helpful for a hearing person (partner or family member) to be present.
- The nurse should allow ample time to communicate with the hearing-impaired parent; being in a rush can evoke stress and create barriers to effective communication.

feeling of guilt that the older children are being deprived of parental time and attention and monitor the behavior of older children toward the more vulnerable infant and divert aggressive behavior. Box 22-4 presents strategies that parents have used to facilitate sibling acceptance of a new baby.

Siblings demonstrate acquaintance behaviors with the newborn. The acquaintance process depends on the information given to the child before the baby is born and on the child's cognitive and developmental levels. The initial behaviors of siblings with the newborn include looking at the infant and touching the head (see Fig. 22-9). The initial adjustment of older children to a newborn takes time, and parents should allow children to interact at their own pace rather than forcing them to interact. To expect a young child to accept and love a rival for the parents' affection assumes an unrealistic level of maturity. Sibling love grows as does other love, that is, by being with another person and sharing experiences. The bond between siblings involves a secure base in which one child provides support for the other, is missed when absent, and is looked to for comfort and security.

GRANDPARENT ADAPTATION

Becoming a grandparent is most often associated with great joy and happiness. Yet it is a time of transition as roles and relationships change and new opportunities arise. Emotions are varied and can change from day to day; feelings of joy, anticipation, and excitement are often intermingled with some degree of anxiety and uncertainty. Circumstances surrounding the pregnancy and birth influence the feelings, reactions, and responses of grandparents.

Pregnancy and birth necessitate redefining of intergenerational roles and relationships within the family. A primary role of the grandparents is to support, nurture, and empower their children in the parenting role. Grandparents must acknowledge that things have changed since they first became parents as they deal with changes in practices and attitudes toward pregnancy, birth, childrearing, and men's and women's roles at home and in the workplace. The degree to which grandparents understand

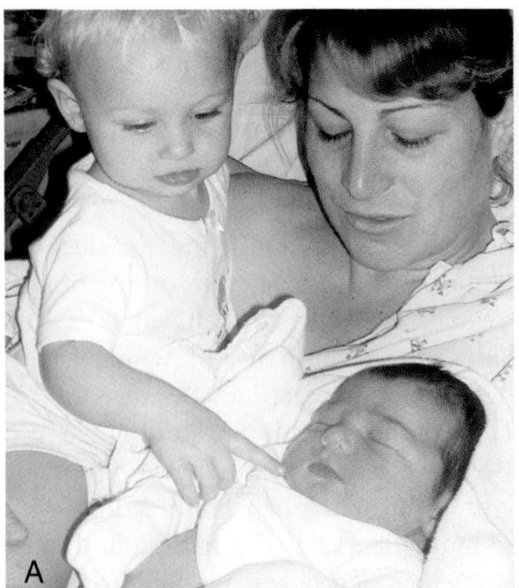

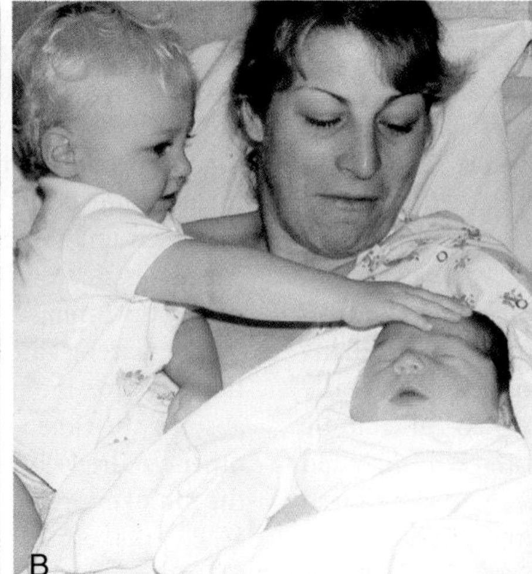

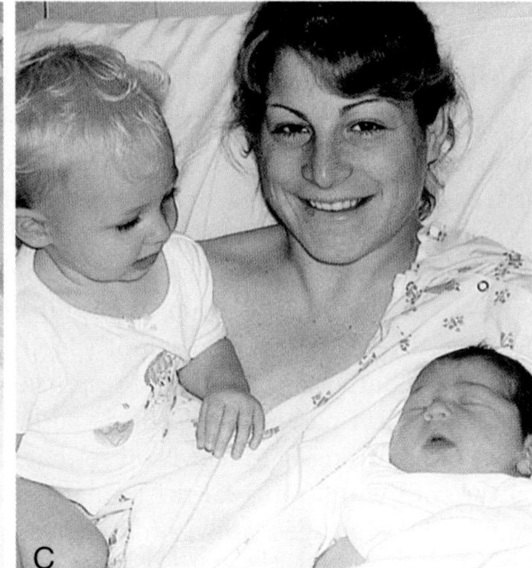

FIG 22-9 First meeting. Sister with mother during first meeting with new sibling. **A,** First tentative touch with fingertip. **B,** Relationship is more secure; touching with whole hand is now okay. **C,** Smiles indicate acceptance. (Courtesy Sara Kossuth, Los Angeles, CA.)

BOX 22-4 Strategies for Facilitating Sibling Acceptance of a New Baby

- Take your older child (or children) on a tour of your hospital room and point out similarities between this birth and his or her birth. "This is like the room I was in with you, and the baby is in the same kind of bassinet that you were in."
- Have a small gift from the baby to give to your older child each day he or she visits in the hospital.
- Give the older child a T-shirt that says "I'm a big brother" [or "sister"].
- Arrange for your children to be among the first to see the newborn. Let them hold the baby in the hospital.
- When the older child visits for the first time, make sure you are not holding the new baby. Your arms need to be open and available for the older child. Instruct the person accompanying the older child to call ahead or give a warning knock to give you time to lay the baby down or have someone else hold the baby.
- Plan individual time with each child. The father or partner can spend time with the older siblings while the mother is taking care of the baby and vice versa. Siblings like to have time and attention from both parents.
- Give preschool and early school-age siblings a newborn doll as "their baby." Give the sibling a photograph of the new baby to take to school to show off "his" or "her" baby. Older siblings may enjoy the responsibility of helping care for the newborn, such as learning how to give the baby a bottle or change a diaper. Remember to supervise interactions between the siblings and new baby.

and accept current practices can influence how supportive they are to their adult children.

At the same time that they are adjusting to grandparenthood, many grandparents are experiencing typical life transitions and events, such as retirement and a move to smaller housing, and need support from their adult children. Some may feel regret about their limited involvement because of poor health or geographic distance.

The extent of grandparent involvement in the care of the newborn depends on many factors such as the willingness to become involved, the proximity of the grandparents, and cultural expectations of the grandparents' role. For example, if the new parents live in the United States, Asian grandparents will typically come to the United States to care for the baby and the mother after birth and to care for the children once the parents return to work. In the United States, paternal grandparents, in contrast to those in other cultures, frequently consider themselves secondary to the maternal grandparents. Less seems expected of them, and they are initially less involved. Nevertheless, these grandparents are eager to help and express great pleasure in their son's fatherhood and his involvement with the baby (Fig. 22-10).

Relationships between grandparents and parents can change with the birth of a new baby. For first-time parents, pregnancy and parenthood can reawaken old issues related to dependence versus independence. Couples often do not plan on their parents' help immediately after the baby arrives. They want time "to be a family," implying a couple-baby unit, not the intergenerational family network. Contrary to their expectations, however, new parents do call on their parents for help, especially the maternal grandmother. Many grandparents are aware of their adult children's wishes for autonomy, respect these wishes, and remain available to help when asked.

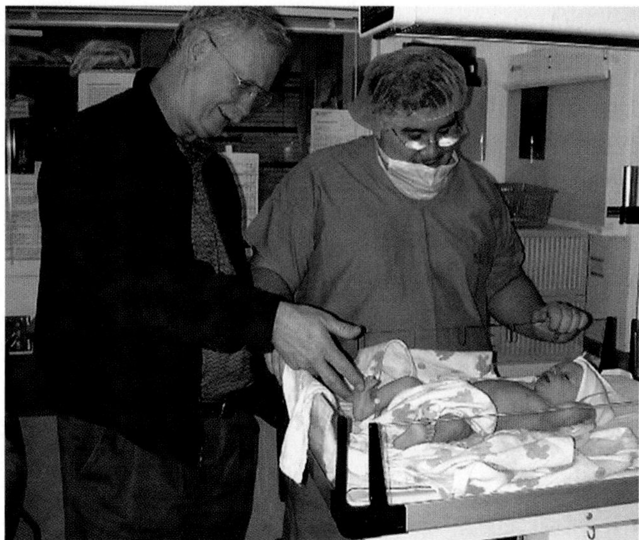

FIG 22-10 Father, grandfather, and new grandson get acquainted. (Courtesy Sharon Johnson, Petaluma, CA.)

Grandparents' classes can be used to bridge the generation gap and to help the grandparents understand their adult children's parenting concepts. The classes include information on up-to-date childbearing practices; family-centered care; infant care, feeding, and safety (car seats); and exploration of roles that grandparents play in the family unit.

Increasing numbers of grandparents are providing permanent care for their grandchildren as a result of divorce, substance abuse, child abuse or neglect, abandonment, teenage pregnancy, death, human immunodeficiency virus and acquired immunodeficiency syndrome, unemployment, incarceration, and mental health problems. This emerging trend requires the nurse to evaluate the role of the grandparent in parenting the infant. Educational and financial considerations must be addressed and available support systems identified for these families.

CARE MANAGEMENT

Numerous changes occur during the first weeks of parenthood. Nursing care management should be directed toward helping parents cope with infant care, role changes, altered lifestyle, and change in family structure resulting from the addition of a new baby. Developing skill and confidence in caring for an infant can be anxiety provoking. Anticipatory guidance can help prevent a shock of reality in the transition from hospital or birthing center to home that might negate the parents' joy or cause them undue stress.

Through education, support, and encouragement, nurses are instrumental in assisting mothers and their partners in the transition to parenthood, whether they are first-time parents or parents of several other children. Early and ongoing assessment and intervention promotes positive outcomes for parents, infants, and family members (see Nursing Care Plan).

NURSING CARE PLAN

Home Care Follow-Up: Transition to Parenthood

NURSING DIAGNOSIS	EXPECTED OUTCOME	INTERVENTIONS	RATIONALES
Deficient Knowledge of infant care related to lack of experience or lack of support	Parents provide safe and adequate care, and infant appears healthy.	Observe infant care routines (bathing, diapering, feeding, play).	To evaluate parental ease with care and adequacy of techniques
		Observe infant's appearance (height-weight ratio, head circumference, fontanels, skin tone and turgor), and assess vital signs, overall tone, reflexes, and age-appropriate developmental skills.	To evaluate for signs indicative of inadequate care
		Explore available support systems for infant care.	To determine adequacy of existing system
		Demonstrate care routines that pose difficulties, and have involved family members return demonstration.	To facilitate improvements in care
		Provide ongoing follow-up and referrals as needed.	To ensure that identified potential and actual care deficits are addressed and resolved
Disturbed Sleep Pattern related to infant demands and environmental interruptions	Woman sleeps for uninterrupted periods and states that she feels rested on waking.	Discuss woman's routine, and specify factors that interfere with sleep.	To determine scope of problem and direct interventions
		Explore ways woman and significant others can make environment more conducive to sleep (e.g., privacy, darkness, quiet, back rubs, soothing music, warm milk), and teach use of guided imagery and relaxation techniques.	To promote optimal conditions for sleep
		Eliminate factors or routines that can interfere with sleep (e.g., caffeine, foods that induce heartburn, strenuous mental or physical activity).	To prevent interference with sleep
		Advise family to limit visitors and activities.	To prevent further stress and fatigue
		Have family plan specific times to care for newborn.	To allow mother time to sleep
		Have mother learn to use infant nap time as time for her to nap as well.	To replenish energy and decrease fatigue
		Assist family to identify persons such as family members or friends who can help with household tasks, infant care, and care of other children.	To allow mother more time to rest
Impaired Home Maintenance related to addition of new family member, inadequate resources, or inadequate support systems	Home exhibits signs of safe and functional environment.	Observe home environment (e.g., available living space and sleeping arrangements; adequacy of facilities for food preparation and storage, hygiene, and toileting; overall state of repair; cleanliness; presence of safety hazards).	To determine adequacy and effective use of resources
		Observe arrangements for newborn, such as sleeping space, care equipment, and supplies (bathing, changing, feeding, transportation).	To determine adequacy of resources
		Explore who is responsible for cooking, cleaning, child care, and newborn care, and determine whether mother seems adequately rested.	To determine adequacy of support systems
		Identify and arrange referrals to needed social agencies (e.g., Temporary Assistance for Needy Families [TANF]; Special Supplemental Nutrition Program for Women, Infants and Children [WIC]; food pantries).	To address resource deficits (finances, supplies, equipment)
Interrupted Family Processes related to inclusion of new family member	Infant is successfully incorporated into family structure.	Explore with family ways that birth and neonate have changed family structure and function.	To evaluate functional and role adjustment
		Observe family's interaction with newborn, and note degree of bonding, evidence of sibling rivalry, and involvement in newborn care.	To evaluate acceptance of newest family member
		Clarify identified misinformation and misperceptions.	To promote clear communication
		Assist family in exploring options for solutions to identified problems.	To promote effective problem resolution
		Support family's efforts as they move toward adjusting and incorporating new member.	To reinforce new functions and roles
		If needed, make referrals to appropriate social services or community agencies.	To ensure ongoing support and care

COMMUNITY ACTIVITY

- Visit the website of a hospital that provides maternity services in your community. Does the hospital offer prepared childbirth, parenting, sibling or infant/child cardiorespiratory resuscitation (CPR) classes? Are group tours of the birthing center provided for expectant parents?
- Visit the website babycenter.com, which provides information for parents about pregnancy, parenting, and children's health. Review the information about postpartum emotional health, causes and treatments of baby blues, and baby blues versus postpartum depression.
- Visit the FamilyandHomeNetwork.com website, and research the availability of support groups for parents in your community.

In collaboration with the family, incorporating their priorities and preferences to meet their specific needs, nurses can:

- Provide opportunities for parent-infant interaction.
- Implement strategies to facilitate sibling acceptance of the infant (see Box 22-4).
- Provide practical suggestions for infant care (see Chapter 24).
- Provide anticipatory guidance on what to expect as the infant grows and develops including sleep-wake cycles, interpretation of infant behaviors, quieting techniques, infant developmental milestones, sensory enrichment/infant stimulation, recognizing signs of illness, well-baby follow-up and immunizations.
- Provide positive reinforcement for loving and nurturing behaviors with the infant.
- Closely monitor parents who interact in inappropriate or abusive ways with their infants, and notify an appropriate mental health practitioner or professional social worker.

While the nurse may be able to evaluate the effectiveness of some interventions before the mother and infant are discharged from the hospital, ongoing evaluation is needed. This is likely done by the infant's primary health care provider in follow-up visits.

KEY POINTS

- The birth of a child necessitates changes in the existing interactional structure of a family.
- Attachment is the process by which the parent and infant come to love and accept each other.
- Attachment is strengthened through the use of sensory responses or interactions by both partners in the parent-infant interaction.
- Women go through predictable stages in becoming a mother.
- Many mothers exhibit signs of postpartum blues (baby blues).
- Fathers experience emotions and adjustments during the transition to parenthood that are similar to, and also distinctly different from, those of mothers.
- Modulation of rhythm, modification of behavioral repertoires, and mutual responsivity facilitate infant-parent adjustment.
- Many factors influence adaptation to parenthood (e.g., age, culture, socioeconomic level, expectations of what the child will be like).
- A parent who has a sensory impairment needs to maximize use of the remaining senses.
- Sibling adjustment to a new baby requires creative parental interventions.
- Grandparents can have a positive influence on the postpartum family.
- Nurses play a major role in educating and supporting new parents in the transition to parenthood.

REFERENCES

Bartlett, J. D., & Easterbrooks, M. A. (2012). Links between physical abuse in childhood and child neglect among adolescent mothers. *Children and Youth Services Review, 34*(11), 2164–2169.

Chalmers, B. (2012). Childbirth across cultures: Research and practice. *Birth: Issues in Perinatal Care, 39*(4), 276–280.

Chin, R., Hall, P., & Daiches, A. (2011). Fathers' experiences of their transition to fatherhood: A metasynthesis. *Journal of Reproductive & Infant Psychology, 29*(1), 4–18.

Dahl, B., Fylkesnes, A. M., Sorlie, V., & Malterud, K. (2013). Lesbian women's experiences with healthcare providers in the birthing context: A meta-ethnography. *Midwifery, 29*(6), 674–681.

de Montigny, F., Lacharité, C., & Devault, A. (2012). Transition to fatherhood: Modeling the experience of fathers of breastfed infants. *Advances in Nursing Science, 35*(3), E11–E22.

Fagan, J. (2013). Adolescent parents' partner conflict and parenting alliance, fathers' prenatal involvement, and fathers' engagement with infants. *Journal of Family Issues, 0192513X13491411, first published on June 17, 2013.* http://dx.doi.org/10.1177/0192513X13491411.

Farrie, D., Lee, Y., & Fagan, J. (2011). The effect of cumulative risk on paternal engagement: Examining differences among adolescent and older couples. *Youth & Society, 43*(1), 90–117.

Flacking, R., Lehtonen, L., Thomson, G., et al. (2012). Closeness and separation in neonatal intensive care. *Acta Paediatrica, 101*(10), 1032–1037.

Geoghegan, T. (2013). *Surviving the first day: State of the world's mothers 2013.* London: Save the Children International. Available at www.savethechildrenweb.org/SOWM-2013/files/assets/common/downloads/State%20of%20the%20WorldOWM-2013.pdf.

Goldberg, A. E., & Smith, J. Z. (2011). Stigma, social context, and mental health: Lesbian and gay couples across the transition to adoptive parenthood. *Journal of Counseling Psychology, 58*(1), 139–150.

Goodman, J. (2005). Becoming an involved father of an infant. *Journal of Obstetric, Gynecologic and Neonatal Nursing, 34*(2), 190–200.

Greenfield, D. A., & Seli, E. (2011). Gay men choosing parenthood through assisted reproduction: Medical and psychosocial considerations. *Fertility and Sterility, 95*(1), 225–229.

Hoffenkamp, H. N., Tooten, A., Hall, R. A. S., et al. (2012). The impact of premature childbirth on parental bonding. *Evolutionary Psychology, 10*(3), 542–561. Available at http://search.ebscohost.com/login.aspx?direct=true&db=psyh&AN=2013-10495-011&site=ehost-live.

Hung, K. J., & Berg, O. (2011). Early skin-to-skin after cesarean to improve breast-feeding. *MCN: The American Journal of Maternal/Child Nursing, 36*(5), 318–324; quiz 325–326.

Husmillo, M. (2013). Maternal role attainment theory. *International Journal of Childbirth Education, 28*(2), 46–48.

Klaus, M., & Kennell, J. (1976). *Maternal-infant bonding*. St. Louis: Mosby.

Klaus, M., & Kennell, J. (1982). *Parent-infant bonding* (2nd ed.). St. Louis: Mosby.

Kurth, E., Spichiger, E., Stutz, E. Z., et al. (2010). Crying babies, tired mothers—Challenges of the postnatal hospital stay: An interpretive phenomenological study. *BMC Pregnancy & Childbirth, 10*, 21–30.

Martin, J. A., Hamilton, B. E., Osterman, M. J. K., et al. (2013). Births: Final data for 2012. *National Vital Statistics Reports, 63*(2). Hyattsville, MD: *National Center for Vital Statistics.* Available at www.cdc.gov/nchs/data/nvsr/nvsr62/nvsr62_09.pdf.

May, C., & Fletcher, R. (2013). Preparing fathers for the transition to parenthood: Recommendations for the content of antenatal education. *Midwifery, 29*(5), 474–478.

Menéndez, S., Hidalgo, M. V., Jiménez, L., & Moreno, M. C. (2011). Father involvement and marital relationship during transition to parenthood: Differences between dual and single-earner families. *The Spanish Journal of Psychology, 14*(2), 639–647.

Mercer, R. (2004). Becoming a mother versus maternal role attainment. *Journal of Nursing Scholarship, 36*(3), 226–232.

Mercer, R., & Walker, L. (2006). A review of nursing interventions to foster becoming a mother. *Journal of Obstetric, Gynecologic and Neonatal Nursing, 35*(5), 568–582.

Mollborn, S., & Jacobs, J. (2011). "We'll figure a way": Teenage mothers' experiences in shifting social and economic contexts. *Qualitative Sociology, 35*(1), 23–46.

Moore, E. R., Anderson, G. C., Bergman, N., & Dowswell, T. (2012). Early skin-to-skin contact for mothers and their healthy newborn infants. *The Cochrane Database of Systematic Reviews 2012, 16*, CD003519.pub3.

Morgan, P., Merrell, J., Rentschler, D., & Chadderton, H. (2012). Uncertainty during perimenopause: Perceptions of older first-time mothers. *Journal of Advanced Nursing, 68*(10), 2299–2308.

Mortensen, O., Torsheim, T., Melkevik, O., & Thuen, F. (2012). Adding a baby to the equation: Married and cohabiting women's relationship satisfaction in the transition to parenthood. *Family Process, 51*(1), 122–139.

O'Neill, K. R., Hamer, H. P., & Dixon, R. (2012). "A lesbian family in a straight world": The impact of the transition to parenthood on couple relationships in planned lesbian families. *Women's Studies Journal, 26*(2), 39–53. Available at http://search.ebscohost.com/login.aspx?direct=true&db=a9h&AN=84013284&site=ehost-live.

Rubin, R. (1961). Basic maternal behavior. *Nursing Outlook, 9*(11), 683–686.

Schaffer, M. A., Goodhue, A., Stennes, K., & Lanigan, C. (2012). Evaluation of a public health nurse visiting program for pregnant and parenting teens. *Public Health Nursing, 29*(3), 218–231.

Shapiro, A. F., Nahm, E. Y., Gottman, J. M., & Content, K. (2011). Bringing baby home together: Examining the impact of a couple-focused intervention on the dynamics within family play. *American Journal of Orthopsychiatry, 81*(3), 337–350.

Steen, M., Downe, S., Bamford, N., & Edozien, L. (2012). Not-patient and not-visitor: A metasynthesis fathers' encounters with pregnancy, birth and maternity care. *Midwifery, 28*(4), 362–371.

Tharner, A., Luijk, M. P., Raat, H., et al. (2012). Breastfeeding and its relation to maternal sensitivity and infant attachment. *Journal of Developmental and Behavioral Pediatrics, 33*(5), 396–404.

Thukral, A., Sankar, M. J., Agarwal, R., et al. (2012). Early skin-to-skin contact and breast-feeding behavior in term neonates: A randomized controlled trial. *Neonatology, 102*(2), 114–119.

Waugh, L. J. (2011). Beliefs associated with Mexican immigrant families' practice of la cuarentena during postpartum recovery. *Journal of Obstetric, Gynecologic and Neonatal Nursing, 40*(6), 732–741.

Welch, M. G., Hofer, M. A., Brunelli, S. A., et al. (2012). Family Nurture Intervention (FNI) Trial Group: Family nurture intervention (FNI): Methods and treatment protocol of a randomized controlled trial in the NICU. *BMC Pediatrics, 12*, 14.

Westling, E., Glynn, L. M., Sandman, C. A., et al. (2012). Perceived partner support in pregnancy predicts lower maternal and infant distress. *Journal of Family Psychology, 26*(3), 453–463.

Yu, C., Hung, C., Chan, T., et al. (2012). Prenatal predictors for father-infant attachment after childbirth. *Journal of Clinical Nursing, 21*(11), 1577–1583.

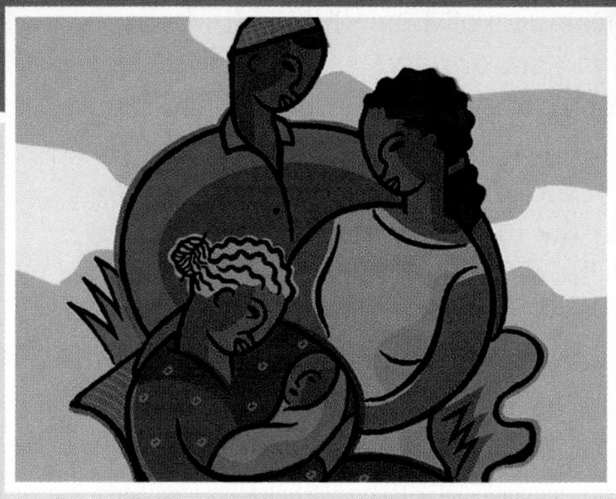

CHAPTER 23

Physiologic and Behavioral Adaptations of the Newborn

Kathryn R. Alden

http://evolve.elsevier.com/Lowdermilk/MWHC/

LEARNING OBJECTIVES

- Analyze the physiologic adaptations that the neonate must make during the transition intrauterine to extrauterine life.
- Describe the behavioral adaptations that are characteristic of the newborn during the transition period.
- Explain the mechanisms of thermoregulation in the neonate and the potential consequences of hypothermia and hyperthermia.
- Recognize newborn reflexes and differentiate characteristic responses from abnormal responses.
- Discuss the sensory and perceptual functioning of the neonate.
- Identify signs that the neonate is at risk related to problems with each body system.

The neonatal period includes the time from birth through day 28 of life. During this time the neonate must make many physiologic and behavioral adaptations to extrauterine life. Physiologic adjustment tasks are those that involve: (1) establishing and maintaining respirations; (2) adjusting to circulatory changes; (3) regulating temperature; (4) ingesting, retaining, and digesting nutrients; (5) eliminating waste; and (6) regulating weight. Behavioral tasks include: (1) establishing a regulated behavioral tempo independent of the mother, which involves self-regulating arousal, self-monitoring changes in state, and patterning sleep; (2) processing, storing, and organizing multiple stimuli; and (3) establishing a relationship with caregivers and the environment. The term infant usually makes these adjustments with little or no difficulty.

TRANSITION TO EXTRAUTERINE LIFE

The major adaptations associated with transition from intrauterine to extrauterine life occur during the first 6 to 8 hours after birth. The predictable series of events during transition are mediated by the sympathetic nervous system and result in changes that involve heart rate, respirations, temperature, and gastrointestinal function. This transition period represents a time of vulnerability for the neonate and warrants careful observation by nurses. To detect disorders in adaptation soon after birth, nurses must be aware of normal features of the transition period.

In their classic work on newborn adaptation to extrauterine life, Desmond, Rudolph, and Phitaksphraiwan (1966) proposed three stages of newborn transition. The stages are still considered valid today.

The first stage of the transition period lasts up to 30 minutes after birth and is called the *first period of reactivity*. The newborn's heart rate increases rapidly to 160 to 180 beats/minute but gradually falls after 30 minutes or so to a baseline rate of 100 to 120 beats/minute. Respirations are irregular, with a rate between 60 and 80 breaths/minute. Fine crackles can be present on auscultation. Audible grunting, nasal flaring, and retractions of the chest also can be present, but these should cease within the first hour of birth. The infant is alert and may have spontaneous startles, tremors, crying, and head movement from side to side. Bowel sounds are audible, and meconium may be passed.

After the first period of reactivity the newborn either sleeps or has a marked decrease in motor activity. This *period of decreased responsiveness* lasts from 60 to 100 minutes. During this time the infant is pink, and respirations are rapid and shallow (up to 60 breaths/minute) but unlabored. Bowel sounds are audible, and peristaltic waves may be noted over the rounded abdomen.

The *second period of reactivity* occurs roughly between 2 and 8 hours after birth and lasts from 10 minutes to several hours. Brief periods of tachycardia and tachypnea occur, associated with increased muscle tone, changes in skin color, and mucus production. Meconium is commonly passed at this time. Most healthy newborns experience this transition, regardless of gestational age or type of birth; extremely and very preterm infants do not because of physiologic immaturity.

Physiologic Adjustments

Respiratory System

As the infant emerges from the intrauterine environment and the umbilical cord is severed, profound adaptations are necessary for survival. The most critical of these is the establishment of effective respirations. Most newborns breathe spontaneously after birth and are able to maintain adequate oxygenation. Preterm infants often encounter respiratory difficulties related to their immature lungs.

Initiation of Breathing. During intrauterine life oxygenation of the fetus occurs through transplacental gas exchange. However, at birth the lungs must be established as the site of gas exchange. In utero fetal blood was shunted away from the lungs, but when birth occurs the pulmonary vasculature must be fully perfused for this purpose. Clamping the umbilical cord causes a rise in blood pressure (BP), which increases circulation and lung perfusion.

It has been recognized that there is no single trigger for newborn respiratory function. The initiation of respirations in the neonate is the result of a combination of chemical, mechanical, thermal, and sensory factors (Blackburn, 2013).

Chemical Factors. The activation of chemoreceptors in the carotid arteries and aorta results from the relative state of hypoxia associated with labor. With each labor contraction there is a temporary decrease in uterine blood flow and transplacental gas exchange, resulting in transient fetal hypoxia and hypercarbia. Although the fetus is able to recover between contractions, there appears to be a cumulative effect that results in progressive decline in Po_2, increased Pco_2, and lowered blood pH. Decreased levels of oxygen and increased levels of carbon dioxide seem to have a cumulative effect that is involved in initiating neonatal breathing by stimulating the respiratory center in the medulla. Another chemical factor may also play a role; it is thought that as a result of clamping the cord, there is a drop in levels of a prostaglandin that can inhibit respirations.

Mechanical Factors. Respirations in the newborn can be stimulated by changes in intrathoracic pressure resulting from compression of the chest during vaginal birth. As the infant passes through the birth canal, the chest is compressed. With birth this pressure on the chest is released, and the negative intrathoracic pressure helps draw air into the lungs. Crying increases the distribution of air in the lungs and promotes expansion of the alveoli. The positive pressure created by crying helps keep the alveoli open.

Thermal Factors. With birth the newborn enters the extrauterine environment, in which the temperature is significantly lower. The profound change in environmental temperature stimulates receptors in the skin, resulting in stimulation of the respiratory center in the medulla.

Sensory Factors. Sensory stimulation occurs in a variety of ways with birth. Some of these include handling the infant by the physician or nurse-midwife, suctioning the mouth and nose, and drying by the nurses. Pain associated with birth also can be a factor. The lights, sounds, and smells of the new environment also can be involved in stimulation of the respiratory center.

At term the lungs hold approximately 20 ml of fluid per kilogram. Air must be substituted for the fluid that filled the fetal respiratory tract. Traditionally it had been thought that the thoracic squeeze occurring during normal vaginal birth resulted in significant clearance of lung fluid. However, it appears that this event plays a minor role. In the days preceding labor there is reduced production of fetal lung fluid and concomitant decreased alveolar fluid volume. Shortly before the onset of labor there is a catecholamine surge that seems to promote fluid clearance from the lungs, which continues during labor (Goldsmith, 2011). The movement of lung fluid from the air spaces occurs through active transport into the interstitium, with drainage occurring through the pulmonary circulation and lymphatic system. Retention of lung fluid can interfere with the infant's ability to maintain adequate oxygenation, especially if other factors (e.g., meconium aspiration, congenital diaphragmatic hernia, esophageal atresia with fistula, choanal atresia, congenital cardiac defect, immature alveoli) that compromise respirations are present. Infants born by cesarean in which labor did not occur before birth can experience some lung fluid retention, although it typically clears without harmful effects on the infant (Hillman, Kallapur, & Jobe, 2012). These infants are also more likely to develop transient tachypnea of the newborn (TTNB) caused by the lower levels of catecholamines (Abu-Shaweesh, 2011).

The alveoli of the term infant's lungs are lined with **surfactant,** a protein manufactured in type II lung cells. Lung expansion depends largely on chest wall contraction and adequate surfactant secretion. Surfactant lowers surface tension, therefore reducing the pressure required to keep the alveoli open with inspiration, and prevents total alveolar collapse on exhalation, thereby maintaining alveolar stability. The decreased surface tension results in increased lung compliance, helping to establish the functional residual capacity of the lungs (Blackburn, 2013). With absent or decreased surfactant, more pressure must be generated for inspiration, which can soon tire or exhaust preterm or sick term infants.

Breathing movements that began in utero as intermittent become continuous after birth, although the mechanism for this is not well understood. Once respirations are established, breaths are shallow and irregular, ranging from 30 to 60 breaths/minute, with periods of breathing that include pauses in respirations lasting less than 20 seconds. These episodes of periodic breathing occur most often during the active (rapid eye movement [REM]) sleep cycle and decrease in frequency and duration with age. Apneic periods longer than 20 seconds indicate a pathologic process and should be evaluated.

Newborn infants are by preference nose breathers. The reflex response to nasal obstruction is to open the mouth to maintain an airway. This response is not present in most infants until 3 weeks after birth; therefore cyanosis or asphyxia can occur with nasal blockage.

In most newborns, auscultation of the chest reveals loud, clear breath sounds that seem very near because little chest tissue intervenes. Breath sounds should be clear and equal bilaterally, although fine rales for the first few hours are not unusual (Gardner & Hernandez, 2011). The ribs of the infant articulate with the spine at a horizontal rather than a downward slope; consequently the rib cage cannot expand with inspiration as readily as that of an adult. Because neonatal respiratory function is largely a matter of diaphragmatic contraction, abdominal breathing is characteristic of newborns. The newborn infant's chest and abdomen rise simultaneously with inspiration. Characteristics of the respiratory system of the neonate and the effects of these characteristics on respiratory function are listed in Table 23-1.

Signs of Respiratory Distress. Signs of respiratory distress can include nasal flaring, intercostal or subcostal retractions (in-drawing of tissue between the ribs or below the rib cage), or grunting with respirations. Suprasternal or subclavicular retractions with stridor or gasping most often represent an upper airway obstruction. Seesaw or paradoxical respirations (exaggerated rise in abdomen with respiration as the chest falls) instead of abdominal respirations are abnormal and should be reported. A respiratory rate of less than 30 or greater than 60 breaths/minute with the infant at rest must be evaluated. The respiratory rate of the infant can be slowed, depressed, or absent as a result of the effects of analgesics or anesthetics administered to the mother during labor and birth. Apneic episodes can be related to several events (rapid increase in body temperature, hypothermia, hypoglycemia, or sepsis) that require thorough evaluation. Tachypnea can result from inadequate clearance of lung fluid, or it can be an indication of newborn respiratory distress syndrome (RDS). Tachypnea can be the first sign of respiratory, cardiac, metabolic, or infectious illnesses (Gardner & Hernandez, 2011).

Changes in the infant's color can indicate respiratory distress. Acrocyanosis, the bluish discoloration of hands and feet, is a normal finding in the first 24 hours after birth. Transient periods of duskiness while crying are common immediately after birth; however, central cyanosis is abnormal and signifies hypoxemia. With central cyanosis the lips and mucous membranes are bluish. It can be the result of inadequate delivery of oxygen to the alveoli, poor perfusion of the lungs that inhibits gas exchange, or cardiac dysfunction. Because central cyanosis is a late sign of distress, newborns usually have significant hypoxemia when cyanosis appears.

Infants who experience mild TTNB often have signs of respiratory distress during the first 1 to 2 hours after birth as they transition to extrauterine life. Tachypnea with rates up to 100 breaths/minute can be present along with intermittent grunting, nasal flaring, and mild retractions. Supplemental oxygen may be needed. TTNB usually resolves in 24 to 48 hours (Soltau & Carlo, 2014).

In neonates with more serious respiratory problems, symptoms of distress are more pronounced and tend to last beyond the first 2 hours after birth. Respiratory rates can exceed 120 breaths/minute. Moderate to severe retractions, grunting, pallor, and central cyanosis can occur. The respiratory symptoms can be accompanied by hypotension, temperature instability, hypoglycemia, acidosis, and signs of cardiac problems. Common respiratory complications affecting neonates include RDS, meconium aspiration, pneumonia, and persistent pulmonary hypertension of the newborn (PPHN) (see Chapter 34).

TABLE 23-1 Characteristics of the Respiratory System of the Neonate

CHARACTERISTIC	EFFECT ON FUNCTION
Immature alveoli; decreased size and number of alveoli	Risk of respiratory insufficiency and pulmonary problems
Thicker alveolar wall; decreased alveolar surface area	Less efficient gas transport and exchange
Continued development of alveoli until childhood	Possible opportunity to reduce effects of discrete lung injury
Decreased lung elastic tissue and recoil	Decreased lung compliance requiring higher pressures and more work to expand; increased risk of atelectasis
Reduced diaphragm movement and maximal force potential	Less effective respiratory movement; difficulty generating negative intrathoracic pressures; risk of atelectasis
Tendency to nose breathe; altered position of larynx and epiglottis	Enhanced ability to synchronize swallowing and breathing; risk of airway obstruction; possibly more difficult to intubate
Small compliant airway passages with higher airway resistance; immature reflexes	Risk of airway obstruction and apnea
Increased pulmonary vascular resistance with sensitive pulmonary arterioles	Risk of ductal shunting and hypoxemia with events such as hypoxia, acidosis, hypothermia, hypoglycemia, and hypercarbia
Increased oxygen consumption	Increased respiratory rate and work of breathing; risk of hypoxia
Increased intrapulmonary right-left shunting	Increased risk of atelectasis with wasted ventilation; lower Pco_2
Immaturity of pulmonary surfactant system in immature infants	Increased risk of atelectasis and respiratory distress syndrome; increased work of breathing
Immature respiratory control	Irregular respirations with periodic breathing; risk of apnea; inability to rapidly alter depth of respirations

Pco_2, Partial pressure of carbon dioxide.
From Blackburn, S. (2013). *Maternal, fetal, and neonatal physiology: A clinical perspective* (4th ed.). St. Louis: Mosby.

Cardiovascular System

The cardiovascular system changes significantly after birth. The infant's first breaths, combined with increased alveolar capillary distention, inflate the lungs and reduce pulmonary vascular resistance to pulmonary blood flow from the pulmonary arteries. Pulmonary artery pressure drops, and pressure in the right atrium declines. Increased pulmonary blood flow from the left side of the heart increases pressure in the left atrium, which causes a functional closure of the foramen ovale. During the first few days of life crying can temporarily reverse the flow through the foramen ovale and lead to mild cyanosis. Soon after birth cardiac output nearly doubles and blood flow increases to the lungs, heart, kidney, and gastrointestinal (GI) tract (Hillman et al., 2012).

In utero fetal Po_2 is 20 to 30 mm Hg. After birth, when the Po_2 level in the arterial blood approximates 50 mm Hg, the ductus arteriosus constricts in response to increased oxygenation. Circulating prostaglandin E (PGE_2) levels also have an important role in closing the ductus arteriosus. In term infants it functionally closes within the first 24 hours after birth; permanent (anatomic) closure usually occurs within 3 to 4 weeks, and the ductus arteriosus becomes a ligament. The ductus arteriosus can open in response to low oxygen levels in association with hypoxia, asphyxia, or prematurity. With auscultation of the chest a patent ductus arteriosus can be detected as a heart murmur (Lott, 2014).

When the cord is clamped and severed, the umbilical arteries, the umbilical vein, and the ductus venosus are functionally closed; they are converted into ligaments within 2 to 3 months. The hypogastric arteries also occlude and become ligaments. Table 23-2 summarizes the cardiovascular changes at birth.

Heart Rate and Sounds. The heart rate for a term newborn ranges from 110 to 160 beats/minute, with brief fluctuations

TABLE 23-2 **Cardiovascular Changes at Birth**

PRENATAL STATUS	POSTBIRTH STATUS	ASSOCIATED FACTORS
Primary Changes		
Pulmonary circulation: High pulmonary vascular resistance, increased pressure in right ventricle and pulmonary arteries	Low pulmonary vascular resistance; decreased pressure in right atrium, ventricle, and pulmonary arteries	Expansion of collapsed fetal lung with air
Systemic circulation: Low pressures in left atrium, ventricle, and aorta	High systemic vascular resistance; increased pressure in left atrium, ventricle, and aorta	Loss of placental blood flow
Secondary Changes		
Umbilical arteries: Patent, carrying of blood from hypogastric arteries to placenta	Functionally closed at birth; obliteration by fibrous proliferation possibly taking 2 to 3 months, distal portions becoming lateral vesicoumbilical ligaments, proximal portions remaining open as superior vesicle arteries	Closure preceding that of umbilical vein, probably accomplished by smooth muscle contraction in response to thermal and mechanical stimuli and alteration in oxygen tension Mechanically severed with cord at birth
Umbilical vein: Patent, carrying of blood from placenta to ductus venosus and liver	Closed; becoming ligamentum teres hepatis after obliteration	Closure shortly after umbilical arteries; hence blood from placenta possibly entering neonate for short period after birth Mechanically severed with cord at birth
Ductus venosus: Patent, connection of umbilical vein to inferior vena cava	Closed; becoming ligamentum venosum after obliteration	Loss of blood flow from umbilical vein
Ductus arteriosus: Patent, shunting of blood from pulmonary artery to descending aorta	Functionally closed almost immediately after birth; anatomic obliteration of lumen by fibrous proliferation requiring 1 to 3 months, becoming ligamentum arteriosum	Increased oxygen content of blood in ductus arteriosus creating vasospasm of its muscular wall High systemic resistance increasing aortic pressure; low pulmonary resistance reducing pulmonary arterial pressure
Foramen ovale: Formation of a valve opening that allows blood to flow directly to left atrium (shunting of blood from right to left atrium)	Functionally closed at birth; constant apposition gradually leading to fusion and permanent closure within a few months or years in majority of persons	Increased pressure in left atrium and decreased pressure in right atrium, causing closure of valve over foramen

Data from Blackburn, S. (2013). *Maternal, fetal, and neonatal physiology: A clinical perspective* (4th ed.). St. Louis: Mosby.

greater and less than these values usually noted during sleeping and waking states. The range of the heart rate in the term infant is about 85 to 100 beats/minute during deep sleep and can increase to 180 beats/min or higher when the infant cries. A heart rate that is either high (more than 160 beats/minute) or low (fewer than 100 beats/minute) should be reevaluated within 30 minutes to 1 hour or when the activity of the infant changes. Immediately after birth the heart rate can be palpated by grasping the base of the umbilical cord.

The apical impulse (point of maximal impulse [PMI]) in the newborn is at the fourth intercostal space and to the left of the midclavicular line (Gardner & Hernandez, 2011). The PMI is often visible and easily palpable because of the thin chest wall; this is also called *precordial activity.*

Apical pulse rates should be determined for all infants. Auscultation should be for a full minute, preferably when the infant is asleep. An irregular heart rate in newborns is not uncommon in the first few hours of life. Sinus dysrhythmia is common. After this time an irregular heart rate not attributed to changes in activity or respiratory pattern should be evaluated. Heart sounds during the neonatal period are of higher pitch, shorter duration, and greater intensity than during adult life. The first sound (S_1) is typically louder and duller than the second sound (S_2), which is sharp. The third and fourth heart sounds are not auscultated in newborns. Most heart murmurs heard during the neonatal period have no pathologic significance, and more than half of the murmurs disappear by 6 months. However, the presence of a murmur and accompanying signs such as poor feeding, apnea, cyanosis, or pallor is considered abnormal and should be investigated. There can be significant cardiac defects without a murmur or other symptoms (Smith, 2012). This reinforces the importance of ongoing assessment.

Blood Pressure. Values for newborn BP vary with gestational age, weight, state of alertness, and cuff size. The term newborn infant's average systolic BP is 60 to 80 mm Hg, and average diastolic BP is 40 to 50 mm Hg. The mean arterial pressure (MAP) should be equivalent to the weeks of gestation. For example, an infant born at 40 weeks of gestation should have a MAP of at least 40. The BP increases by the second day of life, with minor variations noted during the first month of life. A drop in systolic BP (about 15 mm Hg) in the first hour of life is common. Crying and movement usually cause increases in the systolic BP. The measurement of BP is best accomplished with an oscillometric device while the infant is at rest. A correctly sized cuff must be used for accurate measurement of an infant's BP; the cuff should cover 75% of the distance between the axilla and elbow (Fanaroff & Fanaroff, 2012).

Policies on routine assessment of neonatal BP vary. In many agencies, unless a specific indication exists, BP is not measured in the newborn on a routine basis except as a baseline. In some institutions nurses obtain four extremity BPs in the presence of any cardiovascular symptoms such as tachycardia, murmur, abnormal pulses, poor perfusion, or abnormal precordial activity. If the systolic pressure is more than 10 mm Hg higher in the upper extremities than in the lower extremities, further diagnostic testing may be needed (Kenney, Hoover, Williams, & Iskersky, 2011).

Blood Volume. Blood volume in the term newborn averages 85 ml/kg of body weight (Luchtman-Jones & Wilson, 2011). Immediately after birth the total blood volume averages 300 ml, but this volume can increase by as much as 100 ml, depending on the length of time to cord clamping and cutting. The infant born prematurely has a relatively greater blood volume than the term newborn. This occurs because the preterm infant has a proportionately greater plasma volume, not a greater red blood cell (RBC) mass.

Early or delayed clamping of the umbilical cord changes the circulatory dynamics of the newborn. Delayed clamping expands the blood volume from the so-called placental transfusion of blood to the newborn. Delayed cord clamping (≥2 minutes after birth) has been reported to be beneficial in improving hematocrit and iron status and decreasing anemia; such benefits can last up to 6 months (Andersson, Hellström-Westas, Andersson, et al., 2011). Polycythemia that occurs with delayed clamping is usually not harmful, although there can be an increased risk of jaundice that requires phototherapy. The American College of Obstetricians and Gynecologists (ACOG, 2012) and the American Academy of Pediatrics (AAP, 2013) report that there is a lack of evidence to support or refute benefits of delayed cord clamping for term infants in rich resource settings. However, they recognize that preterm infants experience important benefits. Transitional circulation is improved, red blood cell volume is better established, and there is a reduced need for blood transfusion. The risk of intraventricular hemorrhage is significantly reduced in preterm infants when cord clamping is delayed (ACOG, 2012; AAP, 2013).

Signs of Cardiovascular Problems. Close monitoring of the infant's vital signs is important in detecting impending problems early. Persistent tachycardia (more than 160 beats/minute) can be associated with anemia, hypovolemia, hyperthermia, or sepsis. Persistent bradycardia (less than 100 beats/minute) can be a sign of a congenital heart block or hypoxemia.

The newborn's skin color can reflect cardiovascular problems. Pallor in the immediate postbirth period is often a sign of underlying problems such as anemia or marked peripheral vasoconstriction as a result of intrapartum asphyxia or sepsis. Any prolonged cyanosis other than in the hands or feet can indicate respiratory and/or cardiac problems. The presence of jaundice can indicate ABO or Rh factor incompatibility problems (see Chapter 36).

Congenital heart defects are the most common types of congenital malformations (see Chapter 36). Although the more serious defects such as tetralogy of Fallot are likely to have clinical manifestations such as cyanosis, dyspnea, and hypoxia, others such as small ventricular septal defects can be asymptomatic. The prenatal history can provide information regarding risk factors for congenital heart defects so the nurse knows to be more alert for symptoms. Maternal illness such as rubella, metabolic disease such as diabetes, and drug ingestion are associated with an increased risk of cardiac defects.

Hematopoietic System

Red Blood Cells. Because fetal circulation is less efficient at oxygen exchange than the lungs, the fetus needs additional RBCs for transport of oxygen in utero. Therefore, at birth the average levels of RBCs, hemoglobin, and hematocrit are higher than those in the adult; these levels fall slowly over the first month. At birth the RBC count ranges from 4.6 to 5.2 million/mm^3 (Blackburn, 2013). The term newborn can have a hemoglobin concentration of 14 to 24 g/dl at birth, decreasing gradually to 12 to 20 g/dl during the first 2 weeks (Pagana & Pagana, 2011). Hematocrit levels at birth range from 51% to 56%, increase slightly in the first few hours or days as fluid shifts from intravascular to interstitial spaces (Blackburn, 2013), and by 8 weeks are between 39% and 59% (Pagana & Pagana). Polycythemia (central venous hematocrit greater than 65%) can occur in term and preterm infants as a result of delayed cord clamping, maternal hypertension or diabetes, or intrauterine growth restriction.

The source of the sample is a significant factor in levels of RBCs, hemoglobin, and hematocrit because capillary blood yields higher values than venous blood. The timing of blood sampling is also significant; the slight rise in RBCs after birth is followed by a substantial drop. At birth the infant's blood contains an average of 70% fetal hemoglobin; however, because of the shorter life span of the cells containing fetal hemoglobin, the percentage falls to 55% by 5 weeks and to 5% by 20 weeks. Iron stores generally are sufficient to sustain normal RBC production for 4 to 5 months in the term infant, at which time a transient physiologic anemia can occur.

Leukocytes. Leukocytosis, with a white blood cell (WBC) count of approximately 18,000/mm^3 (range 9000 to 30,000/mm^3), is normal at birth (Pagana & Pagana, 2011). The number of WBCs increases to 23,000 to 24,000/mm^3 during the first day after birth. The initial high WBC count of the newborn decreases rapidly, and a stable level of 12,000/mm^3 is normally maintained during the neonatal period (Blackburn, 2013). Serious infection is not tolerated well by the newborn; leukocytes are slow to recognize foreign protein and localize and fight infection early in life. Sepsis can be accompanied by a concomitant rise in neutrophils; however, some infants initially have clinical signs of sepsis without a significant elevation in WBCs. In addition, events other than infection (i.e., prolonged crying, maternal hypertension, asymptomatic hypoglycemia, hemolytic disease, meconium aspiration syndrome, labor induction with oxytocin, surgery, difficult labor, high altitude, and maternal fever) can cause neutrophilia in the newborn.

Platelets. Platelet count ranges between 150,000 and 300,000/mm^3 and is essentially the same in newborns as in adults (Pagana & Pagana, 2011). The levels of factors II, VII, IX, and X found in the liver decrease during the first few days of life because the newborn cannot synthesize vitamin K. However, bleeding tendencies in the newborn are rare, and, unless the vitamin K deficiency is great, clotting is sufficient to prevent hemorrhage.

Blood Groups. The infant's blood group is determined genetically and established early in fetal life. However, during the neonatal period the strength of the agglutinogens present in the RBC membrane gradually increases. Cord blood samples may be used to identify the infant's blood type and Rh status.

Thermogenic System

Next to establishing respirations and adequate circulation, heat regulation is most critical to the newborn's survival. During the first 12 hours after birth the neonate attempts to achieve thermal balance in adjusting to the extrauterine environmental temperature. Thermoregulation is the maintenance of balance between heat loss and heat production. Newborns attempt to stabilize their core body temperatures within a narrow range. Hypothermia from excessive heat loss is a common and dangerous problem.

Anatomic and physiologic characteristics of neonates place them at risk for heat loss. Newborns have a thin layer of subcutaneous fat. The blood vessels are close to the surface of the skin. Changes in environmental temperature alter the temperature of the blood, thereby influencing temperature regulation centers in the hypothalamus. Newborns have larger body surface–to–body weight (mass) ratios than do children and adults (Blackburn, 2013).

Heat Loss. The body temperature of newborn infants depends on the heat transfer between the infant and the external environment. Factors that influence heat loss to the environment include the temperature and humidity of the air, the flow and velocity of the air, and the temperature of surfaces in contact with and around the infant. The goal of care is to provide a neutral thermal environment for the neonate in which heat balance is maintained. The neutral thermal environment is the ideal environmental temperature that allows the neonate to maintain a normal body temperature to minimize oxygen and glucose consumption (Ringer, 2013a). Heat loss in the newborn occurs by four modes:

1. *Convection* is the flow of heat from the body surface to cooler ambient air. Because of heat loss by convection, the ambient temperature in the nursery is kept at approximately 24° C (75.2° F), and newborns in open bassinets are wrapped to protect them from the cold. A cap may be worn to decrease heat loss from the infant's head.
2. *Radiation* is the loss of heat from the body surface to a cooler solid surface not in direct contact but in relative proximity. To prevent this type of loss, cribs and examining tables are placed away from outside windows, and care is taken to avoid direct air drafts.
3. *Evaporation* is the loss of heat that occurs when a liquid is converted to a vapor. In the newborn, heat loss by evaporation occurs as a result of moisture vaporization from the skin. This heat loss is intensified by failing to dry the newborn directly after birth or by drying the infant too slowly after a bath. The less mature the newborn, the more severe the evaporative heat loss. Evaporative heat loss, as a component of insensible water loss, is the most significant cause of heat loss in the first few days of life.
4. *Conduction* is the loss of heat from the body surface to cooler surfaces in direct contact. During the initial assessment, the newborn is placed on a prewarmed bed under a radiant warmer to minimize heat loss. The scales used for weighing the newborn should have a protective cover to minimize conductive heat loss.

Heat loss must be controlled to protect the infant. Control of such modes of heat loss is the basis of caregiving policies and techniques. Drying the infant quickly after birth is essential to prevent hypothermia. Skin-to-skin contact with the mother is an effective means of reducing conductive and radiant heat loss and enhancing newborn temperature control and maternal-infant interaction. The naked newborn is placed on the mother's bare chest and covered with a warm blanket; a cap may be placed on the infant's head to help conserve heat (Fig. 23-1) (Brown & Landers, 2011). An alternative is to place the neonate under a radiant warmer to reduce heat loss and promote thermoregulation.

Thermogenesis. In response to cold the neonate attempts to generate heat (thermogenesis) by increasing muscle activity. Cold infants may cry and appear restless. Because of vasoconstriction the skin can feel cool to touch, and acrocyanosis can be present. There is an increase in cellular metabolic activity, primarily in the brain, heart, and liver; this also increases oxygen and glucose consumption.

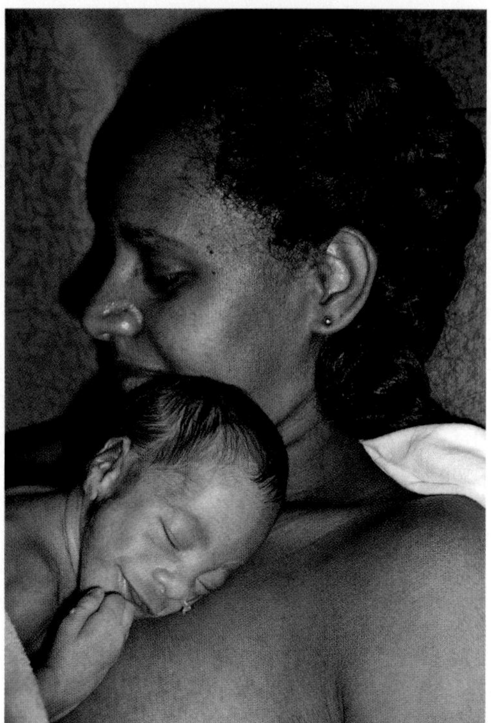

FIG 23-1 Infant in skin-to-skin contact with mother. Note infant smile. (Courtesy Cheryl Briggs, RNC, Annapolis, MD.)

In an effort to conserve heat, term newborns assume a position of flexion that helps guard against heat loss because it diminishes the amount of body surface exposed to the environment. Infants also can reduce the loss of internal heat through the body surface by constricting peripheral blood vessels.

Adults are able to produce heat through shivering; however, the shivering mechanism of heat production is rarely operable in the newborn unless there is prolonged cold exposure (Blackburn, 2013). Newborns produce heat through nonshivering thermogenesis. This is accomplished primarily by metabolism of brown fat, which is unique to the newborn; and secondarily by increased metabolic activity in the brain, heart, and liver. Brown fat is located in superficial deposits in the interscapular region and axillae and in deep deposits at the thoracic inlet, along the vertebral column, and around the kidneys. Brown fat has a richer vascular and nerve supply than ordinary fat. Heat produced by intense lipid metabolic activity in brown fat can warm the newborn by increasing heat production as much as 100%. Reserves of brown fat, usually present for several weeks after birth, are rapidly depleted with cold stress. The amount of brown fat reserve increases with the weeks of gestation. A full-term newborn has greater stores than a preterm infant (Ringer, 2013a).

Hypothermia and Cold Stress. When the neonate's temperature drops, vasoconstriction occurs as a mechanism to conserve heat. The infant can appear pale and mottled; the skin feels cool, especially on the extremities. If the hypothermia is not corrected it will progress to cold stress, which imposes metabolic

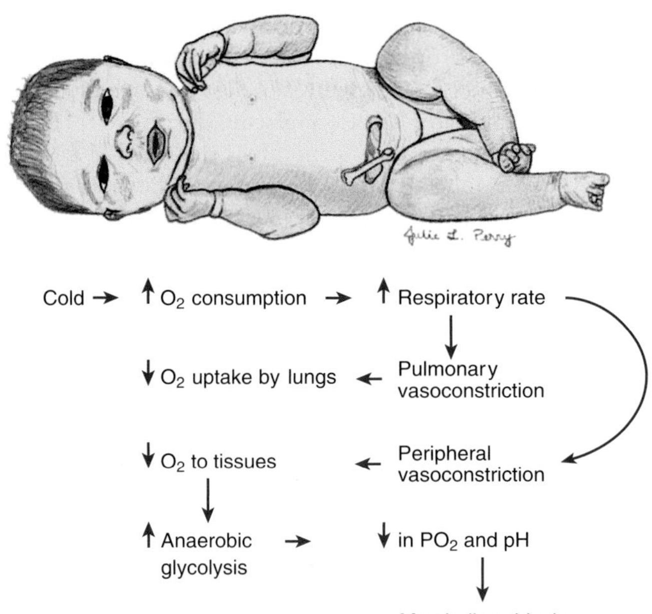

FIG 23-2 Effects of cold stress. When an infant is stressed by cold, oxygen consumption increases, and pulmonary and peripheral vasoconstriction occur, thereby decreasing oxygen uptake by the lungs and oxygen to the tissues; anaerobic glycolysis increases; and there is a decrease in Po_2 and pH, leading to metabolic acidosis.

and physiologic demands on all infants, regardless of gestational age and condition. The respiratory rate increases in response to the increased need for oxygen. In the cold-stressed infant, oxygen consumption and energy are diverted from maintaining normal brain and cardiac function and growth to thermogenesis for survival. If the infant cannot maintain an adequate oxygen tension, vasoconstriction follows and jeopardizes pulmonary perfusion. As a consequence the Po_2 is decreased, and the blood pH drops (Ringer, 2013b). Surfactant synthesis can be altered. These changes can prompt a transient respiratory distress or aggravate existing RDS. Moreover, decreased pulmonary perfusion and oxygen tension can maintain or reopen the right-to-left shunt across the ductus arteriosus.

The basal metabolic rate increases with cold stress. If cold stress is protracted, anaerobic glycolysis occurs, resulting in increased production of acids. Metabolic acidosis develops, and, if a defect in respiratory function is present, respiratory acidosis also develops (Fig. 23-2). Excessive fatty acids can displace the bilirubin from the albumin-binding sites and exacerbate hyperbilirubinemia. Hypoglycemia is another metabolic consequence of cold stress. The process of anaerobic glycolysis can deplete existing stores. If the infant is sufficiently stressed and low glucose stores are not replaced, hypoglycemia, which can be asymptomatic in the newborn, can develop (Brown & Landers, 2011; Sedin, 2011).

Hyperthermia. Although occurring less frequently than hypothermia, hyperthermia can occur and must be corrected. A body temperature greater than 37.5° C (99.5° F) is considered to be abnormally high and is typically caused by excess heat production related to sepsis or a decrease in heat loss. Hyperthermia can result from the inappropriate use of external heat sources such as radiant warmers, phototherapy, sunlight, increased environmental temperature, and the use of excessive clothing or blankets (Brown & Landers, 2011). The clinical appearance of the infant who is hyperthermic often indicates the causative mechanism. Infants who are overheated because of environmental factors such as being swaddled in too many blankets exhibit signs of heat-losing mechanisms: skin vessels dilate, skin appears flushed, hands and feet are warm to touch, and the infant assumes a posture of extension. The newborn who is hyperthermic because of sepsis appears stressed: vessels in the skin are constricted, color is pale, and hands and feet are cool. Hyperthermia develops more rapidly in a newborn than in an adult because of the relatively larger surface area of an infant. Sweat glands do not function well. Hyperthermia can cause neurologic injury and increased risk of seizures; severe cases can result in heat stroke and death (Brown & Landers, 2011; Ringer, 2013b).

Renal System

At term the kidneys occupy a large portion of the posterior abdominal wall. The bladder lies close to the anterior abdominal wall and is both an abdominal and a pelvic organ. In the newborn almost all palpable masses in the abdomen are renal in origin.

At birth a small quantity (approximately 40 ml) of urine is usually present in the bladder of a full-term infant. Many newborns void at the time of birth, although this is easily missed and may not be recorded. During the first few days term infants generally excrete 15 to 60 ml/kg/day; output gradually increases over the first month (Blackburn, 2013). The frequency of voiding varies from 2 to 6 times per day during the first and second days of life and increases during the subsequent 24 hours. After day 4, approximately 6 to 8 voidings per day of pale straw-colored urine indicate adequate fluid intake. Noting and recording the first voiding are important. An infant who has not voided by 24 hours should be assessed for adequacy of fluid intake, bladder distention, restlessness, and symptoms of pain. The health care provider should be notified.

Full-term newborns have limited capacity to concentrate urine; therefore, the specific gravity is usually low (less than 1.004) (Vogt & Dell, 2011). The ability to concentrate urine fully is attained by about 3 months of age. After the first voiding the infant's urine can appear cloudy (because of mucus content) and have a much higher specific gravity. This decreases as fluid intake increases. Normal urine during early infancy is usually straw colored and almost odorless. Sometimes pink-tinged uric acid crystal stains or "brick dust" appears on the diaper. Uric acid crystals are normal during the first week, but thereafter can be a sign of inadequate intake (Janke, 2014). Loss of fluid through urine, feces, lungs, increased metabolic rate, and limited fluid intake results in a 5% to 10% loss of the birth weight. This usually occurs over the first 3 to 5 days of life. If the mother is breastfeeding and her milk supply has not come in yet (which occurs by the third or fourth day after birth), the neonate is somewhat protected from dehydration by its increased extracellular fluid volume. The neonate should regain the birth weight within 10 to 14 days, depending on the feeding method (breast or bottle).

Fluid and Electrolyte Balance. In the term neonate approximately 75% of body weight consists of total body water (extracellular and intracellular). A reduction in extracellular fluid occurs with diuresis during the first few days after birth. The weight loss experienced by most newborns during the first few days after birth is caused primarily by extracellular water loss (Dell, 2011).

The daily fluid requirement for neonates weighing more than 1500 g is 60 to 80 ml/kg during the first 2 days of life. From 3 to 7 days the requirement is 100 to 150 ml/kg/day, and from 8 to 30 days it is 120 to 180 ml/kg/day (Dell, 2011).

At birth the glomerular filtration rate (GFR) of a newborn is approximately 30% to 50% of the adult GFR. This results in a decreased ability to remove nitrogenous and other waste products from the blood. The GFR rapidly increases during the first month of life as a result of postnatal physiologic changes, including decreased renal vascular resistance, increased renal blood flow, and increased filtration pressure.

Sodium reabsorption is decreased as a result of a lowered sodium- or potassium-activated adenosine triphosphatase activity. The decreased ability to excrete excess sodium results in hypotonic urine compared with plasma, leading to a higher concentration of sodium, phosphates, chloride, and organic acids and a lower concentration of bicarbonate ions. The infant has a higher renal threshold for glucose than adults.

Bicarbonate concentration and buffering capacity are decreased. This can lead to acidosis and electrolyte imbalance.

Signs of Renal System Problems. The renal system has a wide range of functions. Dysfunction resulting from physiologic abnormalities can range from the lack of a steady stream of urine to gross anomalies such as hypospadias and exstrophy of the bladder, which can be identified easily at birth. Enlarged or cystic kidneys can be identified as masses during abdominal palpation. Some kidney anomalies also can be detected by ultrasound examination during pregnancy (see Chapter 36).

Gastrointestinal System

The full-term newborn is capable of swallowing, digesting, metabolizing and absorbing proteins and simple carbohydrates and emulsifying fats. With the exception of pancreatic amylase, the characteristic enzymes and digestive juices are present even in low-birth-weight neonates.

In the adequately hydrated infant the mucous membrane of the mouth is moist and pink; the hard and soft palates are intact. The presence of moderate to large amounts of mucus is common in the first few hours after birth. Small whitish areas (Epstein pearls) may be found on the gum margins and at the juncture of the hard and soft palates. The cheeks are full because of well-developed sucking pads. These, like the labial tubercles (sucking calluses) on the upper lip, disappear around the age of 12 months when the sucking period is over.

Sucking is a reflex behavior that begins in utero as early as 15 to 16 weeks. Sucking behavior is influenced by neuromuscular maturity, maternal medications received during labor and birth, and the type of initial feeding. As early as 28 weeks some infants can coordinate sucking, swallowing, and breathing while breastfeeding. Bottle-feeding infants may not coordinate sucking, swallowing, and breathing until 32 to 34 weeks. A special mechanism present in healthy term newborns coordinates the sucking, swallowing, and breathing reflexes necessary for oral feeding. This is well developed in most infants by 37 weeks (Gardner & Lawrence, 2011). Sucking takes place in small bursts of 3 or 4 and up to 8 to 10 sucks at a time, with a brief pause between bursts. The infant is unable to move food from the lips to the pharynx; therefore placing the nipple (breast or bottle) well inside the baby's mouth is necessary. Peristaltic activity in the esophagus is uncoordinated in the first few days of life. It quickly becomes a coordinated pattern in healthy full-term infants, and they swallow easily.

Teeth begin developing in utero, with enamel formation continuing until about 10 years of age. Tooth development is influenced by neonatal or infant illnesses and medications and by illnesses of or medications taken by the mother during pregnancy. The fluoride level in the water supply also influences tooth development. Occasionally an infant may be born with one or more teeth. These natal teeth have poorly formed roots and as they loosen place the infant at risk of aspiration. Therefore, they are usually extracted.

The mucosal barrier in the intestines is not fully mature until 4 to 6 months of age, which allows antigens and other macromolecules such as bacteria to be transported across the intestinal wall into the systemic circulation. This increases the risk of allergies and infection (Blackburn, 2013).

The neonate's intestines are sterile at birth; bacteria are not present in the infant's GI tract. Soon after birth oral and anal orifices permit entrance of bacteria and air. Generally the highest bacterial concentration is found in the lower portion of the intestine, particularly in the large intestine. Normal colonic bacteria are established within the first week after birth; and normal intestinal flora help synthesize vitamin K, folate, and biotin. Bowel sounds can usually be heard shortly after birth.

The capacity of the newborn stomach varies widely, depending on the size of the infant, from less than 30 ml on day 1 to more than 90 ml on day 3. After birth the newborn stomach becomes increasingly more compliant and relaxed to accommodate larger volumes. Several factors such as time and volume of feedings or type and temperature of food can affect the emptying time.

Because of the immaturity of the GI system, newborns are prone to regurgitation, vomiting, and gastroesophageal reflux (GER). Regurgitation is common among newborns and is most prevalent during the first 3 months. Vomiting and regurgitation can be decreased by avoiding overfeeding, burping the infant, and positioning him or her with the head slightly elevated.

Regurgitation is not equivalent to GER, although it often accompanies GER, which is the backflow of gastric contents into the esophagus. In some infants GER is severe enough to cause dysphagia, esophagitis, and aspiration. These infants may be treated with medications to reduce gastric acidity such as antacids, histamine-blocking agents, or proton-pump inhibitors (Barksdale, Chwals, Magnuson, & Parry, 2011).

Digestion. The infant's ability to digest carbohydrates, fats, and proteins is regulated by the presence of certain enzymes. Most of these enzymes are functional at birth except for pancreatic amylase and lipase. Amylase is produced by the salivary glands after approximately 3 months and by the pancreas at approximately 6 months of age. This enzyme is necessary to convert starch into maltose and occurs in high amounts in colostrum. The other exception is lipase, also secreted by the pancreas; it is necessary for the digestion of fat. Therefore, the normal newborn is capable of digesting simple carbohydrates and proteins but has a limited ability to digest fats. Mammary lipase in human milk aids in digestion of fats by the neonate.

Lactase levels in newborns are higher than in older infants. This enzyme is necessary for digestion of lactose, the major carbohydrate in human milk and commercial infant formula.

Stools. Meconium fills the lower intestine at birth. It is formed during fetal life from the amniotic fluid and its constituents, intestinal secretions (including bilirubin), and cells (shed from the mucosa). Meconium is greenish black and viscous and contains occult blood. The first meconium stool passed is usually sterile, but within hours all meconium passed contains bacteria. Most healthy term infants pass meconium within the first 12 to 24 hours of life, and almost all do so by 48 hours. The number of stools passed varies during the first week, being most numerous between the third and sixth days. Newborns fed early pass stools sooner. Progressive changes in the stooling pattern indicate a properly functioning GI tract (Box 23-1).

Feeding Behaviors. Variations occur among infants regarding interest in food, signs of hunger, and amount ingested at one time. The amount of food that the infant takes in at any feeding depends on the infant's size, hunger level, and alertness. When put to breast some infants feed immediately, whereas others require a longer learning period. Random hand-to-mouth movement and sucking of fingers are well developed at birth and intensify when the infant is hungry. Caregivers should be alert and responsive to these hunger cues (Lawrence & Lawrence, 2011).

Signs of Gastrointestinal Problems. The time, color, and character of the infant's first stool should be noted. Failure to pass meconium can indicate bowel obstruction related to conditions such as an inborn error of metabolism (e.g., cystic fibrosis) or a congenital disorder (e.g., Hirschsprung's disease or an imperforate anus). An active rectal "wink" reflex (contraction of the anal sphincter muscle in response to touch) is a sign of good sphincter tone.

Fullness of the abdomen above the umbilicus can be caused by hepatomegaly, duodenal atresia, or distention. Abdominal distention at birth usually indicates a serious disorder such as a ruptured viscus (from abdominal wall defects) or tumors. Distention that occurs later can be the result of overfeeding or signal GI disorders. A scaphoid (sunken) abdomen, with bowel sounds heard in the chest and signs of respiratory distress, indicates a diaphragmatic hernia. Fullness below the umbilicus can indicate a distended bladder.

Some infants are intolerant of certain commercial infant formulas. If an infant is allergic or unable to digest a formula, the stools can become very soft with a high water content that is signaled by a distinct water ring around the stool on the diaper. Forceful ejection of stool and a water ring around the stool are signs of diarrhea. Care must be taken to avoid misinterpreting transitional stools for diarrhea. The loss of fluid in diarrhea can rapidly lead to fluid and electrolyte imbalance. Passage of meconium from the vagina or urinary meatus is a sign of a possible fistulous tract from the rectum.

The amount and frequency of regurgitation ("spitting up") or vomiting after feedings should be documented. Color change, gagging, and projectile (very forceful) vomiting occur in association with esophageal and tracheoesophageal anomalies. Vomiting in large amounts, especially if it is projectile, can be a sign of pyloric stenosis. Bilious emesis is suggestive intestinal obstruction or malrotation of the bowel (Barksdale et al., 2011).

BOX 23-1 Changes in Stooling Patterns of Newborns

Meconium

- The infant's first stool is composed of amniotic fluid and its constituents, intestinal secretions, shed mucosal cells, and possibly blood (ingested maternal blood or minor bleeding of alimentary tract vessels).
- Passage of meconium should occur within the first 24 to 48 hours, although it can be delayed up to 7 days in very low birth weight. The passage of meconium can occur in utero and can be a sign of fetal distress.

Transitional Stools

- Usually appear by third day after initiation of feeding
- Greenish brown to yellowish brown; thin and less sticky than meconium; can contain some milk curds

Milk Stool

- Usually appears by the fourth day
- *Breastfed infants:* Stools yellow to golden, pasty in consistency; resemble a mixture of mustard and cottage cheese, with an odor similar to sour milk
- *Formula-fed infants:* Stools pale yellow to light brown, firmer consistency, with a more offensive odor

Hepatic System

The liver and gallbladder are formed by the fourth week of gestation. In the newborn the liver can be palpated about 1 to 2 cm below the right costal margin because it is enlarged and occupies about 40% of the abdominal cavity. The infant's liver plays an important role in iron storage, carbohydrate metabolism, conjugation of bilirubin, and coagulation.

Iron Storage. The fetal liver, which serves as the site for production of hemoglobin after birth, begins storing iron in utero. The infant's iron store is proportional to total body hemoglobin content and length of gestation. At birth the term infant has an iron store sufficient to last 4 to 6 months. Iron stores of preterm and small for gestational age infants are often lower and are depleted sooner than in healthy term infants. Although both breast milk and cow's milk contain iron, the bioavailability of iron in breast milk is far superior.

The American Academy of Pediatrics (AAP) recommends that breastfed infants should receive a daily oral iron supplement (1 mg/kg) beginning at 4 months until feeding includes iron-fortified cereal or other foods fortified with iron. Formula-fed infants should receive a formula that contains supplemental iron (Baker, Greer, & the Committee on Nutrition, 2010).

Carbohydrate Metabolism. In utero the glucose concentration in the umbilical vein is approximately 80% of the maternal level. At birth the newborn is cut off from its maternal glucose supply and as a result experiences an initial decrease in serum glucose levels. Glucose levels reach a low point between 30 and 90 minutes after birth and then rise gradually. In most healthy term newborns blood glucose levels stabilize at 50 to 60 mg/dl during the first several hours after birth. Within the first week they should be approximately 60 to 80 mg/dl (Kalhan & Devaskar, 2011).

The initiation of feedings helps to stabilize the newborn's blood glucose levels. In general blood glucose levels less than 40 mg/dl are considered abnormal and warrant intervention. The hypoglycemic infant can display the classic symptoms of jitteriness, lethargy, apnea, feeding problems, or seizures; or the infant can be asymptomatic. Hypoglycemia in the initial newborn period is most often transient and easily corrected through feeding. Persistent or recurrent hypoglycemia necessitates intravenous glucose therapy and possible pharmacologic intervention.

Conjugation of Bilirubin and Newborn Jaundice. Jaundice, the visible yellowish color of the skin and sclera, is caused by elevated serum levels of unconjugated (indirect) bilirubin. The liver is responsible for the conjugation of bilirubin, which results from the breakdown of RBCs. When RBCs reach the end of their life span, their membranes rupture, and hemoglobin is released. The hemoglobin is phagocytosed by macrophages; it then splits into heme and globin. The heme is broken down by the reticuloendothelial cells, converted to bilirubin, and released in an unconjugated form. The unconjugated (indirect) bilirubin is relatively insoluble and almost entirely bound to circulating albumin, a plasma protein. Bilirubin that is not bound to albumin, or free bilirubin, can easily cross the blood-brain barrier and cause neurotoxicity (acute bilirubin encephalopathy or kernicterus).

The unconjugated bilirubin must be conjugated so it becomes soluble and excretable. In the liver the unbound bilirubin is conjugated with glucuronic acid in the presence of the enzyme glucuronyl transferase. The conjugated form of bilirubin (direct bilirubin) is soluble and excreted from liver cells as a constituent of bile. Along with other components of bile, direct bilirubin is excreted into the biliary tract system that carries the bile into the duodenum. Bilirubin is converted to urobilinogen and stercobilinogen within the duodenum through the action of the bacterial flora. Urobilinogen is excreted in urine and feces; stercobilinogen is excreted in the feces. The effectiveness of bilirubin excretion through the feces depends on the stooling pattern of the newborn and the substances in the intestine that break down conjugated bilirubin. In the newborn intestine the enzyme β-glucuronidase is able to convert conjugated bilirubin into the unconjugated form, which is subsequently reabsorbed by the intestinal mucosa and transported to the liver; this is called *enterohepatic circulation*. Feeding is important in reducing serum bilirubin levels because it stimulates peristalsis and produces more rapid passage of meconium, thus diminishing the amount of reabsorption of unconjugated bilirubin. Feeding also introduces bacteria to aid in the reduction of bilirubin to urobilinogen. Colostrum, a natural laxative, facilitates the passage of meconium (Fig. 23-3).

When levels of unconjugated bilirubin exceed the ability of the liver to conjugate it, plasma levels of bilirubin increase, and jaundice appears. Jaundice is generally noticeable first in the head, especially in the sclera and mucous membranes, and progresses gradually to the thorax, abdomen, and extremities. The degree of jaundice is determined by serum total bilirubin measurements. Jaundice is likely to appear when bilirubin levels exceed 5 to 6 mg/dl (Blackburn, 2013).

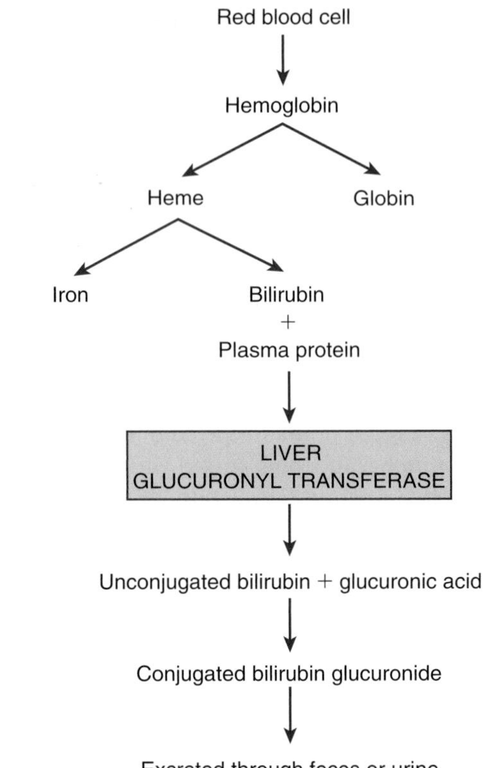

FIG 23-3 Formation and excretion of bilirubin.

The newborn is at risk for hyperbilirubinemia because of distinctive aspects of normal neonatal physiology. The higher RBC mass at birth and shorter life span of neonatal RBCs mean that there is a need for greater bilirubin synthesis. The ability of the liver to conjugate bilirubin is reduced during the first few days after birth; it can metabolize and excrete only about two thirds of the circulating bilirubin. In addition, there are fewer bilirubin binding sites because newborns have lower serum albumin levels. In the intestines conjugated bilirubin becomes unconjugated and recirculated through the enterohepatic circulation, which increases serum bilirubin levels (Blackburn, 2013).

Traditionally newborn jaundice has been categorized as either *physiologic* or *pathologic* (nonphysiologic), depending primarily on the time it appears and on serum bilirubin levels. Controversy surrounds the definitions of normal or physiologic ranges of total serum bilirubin. Total serum bilirubin levels in newborns are affected by variables such as length of gestation, age, weight, race, nutritional status, and mode of feeding (Blackburn, 2013). The time of onset of jaundice is a key factor in evaluating its cause and determining if treatment is needed. *Early-onset jaundice* is usually related to increased bilirubin production; *late-onset jaundice* is most often related to delayed elimination of bilirubin, with or without increased production (Kamath, Thilo, & Hernandez, 2011). Table 23-3 lists the varying causes of neonatal hyperbilirubinemia.

Among the factors that increase the risk of hyperbilirubinemia, prematurity is the most significant. Prematurity affects liver and brain metabolism and albumin binding sites, placing preterm and late preterm infants at greater risk for hyperbilirubinemia. Infants of Asian and Native-American

TABLE 23-3 Causes of Neonatal Unconjugated (Indirect) Hyperbilirubinemia

BASIS	CAUSES
Increased Production of Bilirubin	
Increased hemoglobin destruction	Fetomaternal blood group incompatibility (Rh, ABO) Congenital red blood cell abnormalities Congenital enzyme deficiencies (G6PD, galactosemia) Enclosed hemorrhage (cephalhematoma, bruising) Sepsis
Increased amount of hemoglobin	Polycythemia (maternal-fetal or twin-twin transfusion, SGA) Delayed cord clamping
Increased enterohepatic circulation	Delayed passage of meconium, meconium ileus, or plug Fasting or delayed initiation of feeding Intestinal atresia or stenosis
Altered Hepatic Clearance of Bilirubin	
Alteration in uridine diphosphate glucuronyl transferase production or activity	Immaturity Metabolic/endocrine disorders (e.g., Crigler-Najjar disease, hypothyroidism, disorders of amino acid metabolism)
Alteration in hepatic function and perfusion (and thus conjugating ability)	Asphyxia, hypoxia, hypothermia, hypoglycemia Sepsis (also causes inflammation) Drugs and hormones (e.g., novobiocin, pregnanediol)
Hepatic obstruction (associated with direct hyperbilirubinemia)	Congenital anomalies (biliary atresia, cystic fibrosis) Biliary stasis (hepatitis, sepsis) Excessive bilirubin load (often seen with severe hemolysis)

G6PD, Glucose-6-phosphate dehydrogenase; *SGA,* small for gestational age.
From Blackburn, S. (2013). *Maternal, fetal, and neonatal physiology: A clinical perspective* (4th ed.). St. Louis: Mosby.

ethnicity have higher bilirubin levels. Breastfeeding infants are at greater risk of hyperbilirubinemia (see later discussion).

Physiologic Jaundice. Physiologic or nonpathologic jaundice occurs in approximately 60% of newborn infants born at term and 80% of preterm infants (Kaplan, Wong, & Sibley, 2011). It appears after 24 hours of age and usually resolves without treatment.

Two phases of physiologic jaundice have been identified in full-term infants. In the first phase bilirubin levels of Caucasian and African-American infants gradually increase to approximately 5 to 6 mg/dl by 72 to 96 hours of life and decrease to a plateau of 2 to 3 mg/dl by the fifth day. In Asian and Asian-American infants bilirubin levels peak between 72 and 120 hours of age and gradually fall to 2 to 3 mg/dl by the seventh to tenth days. In the second phase of physiologic jaundice bilirubin levels gradually decrease between 5 and 10 days of life, reaching normal adult levels of 2 mg/dl or less by 14 days. This pattern varies according to racial group, method of feeding (breast versus formula), and gestational age. In preterm formula-fed infants serum bilirubin levels can peak as high as 10 to 12 mg/dl at 5 to 6 days of life and decrease slowly over a period of 2 to 4 weeks (Kaplan et al., 2011).

SAFETY ALERT

The appearance of jaundice during the first 24 hours of life or persistence beyond the ages previously delineated usually indicates a potential pathologic process that requires investigation.

Pathologic Jaundice. Although physiologic jaundice is usually considered benign, unconjugated bilirubin (indirect) can accumulate to hazardous levels and lead to a pathologic condition. Pathologic or nonphysiologic jaundice is unconjugated hyperbilirubinemia that is either pathologic in origin or severe enough to warrant further evaluation and treatment. Jaundice is usually considered pathologic or nonphysiologic if it appears within 24 hours after birth, if total serum bilirubin levels increase by more than 6 mg/dl in 24 hours, and if the serum bilirubin level exceeds 15 mg/dl at any time (Blackburn, 2013). High levels of unconjugated bilirubin are usually caused by excessive production of bilirubin through hemolysis. Hemolytic disease of the newborn caused by maternal/newborn blood group incompatibility is the most common cause of hyperbilirubinemia. It can also be caused by glucose-6-phosphate dehydrogenase (G6PD) deficiency, a genetic disorder that is more common among Asian and Native-American populations. Other causes are listed in Table 23-3.

If increased levels of unconjugated bilirubin are left untreated, neurotoxicity can result as bilirubin is transferred into the brain cells. Acute bilirubin encephalopathy refers to the acute manifestations of bilirubin toxicity that occur during the first weeks after birth. This can include a range of symptoms such as lethargy, hypotonia, irritability, seizures, coma, and death. Kernicterus refers to the irreversible, long-term consequences of bilirubin toxicity such as hypotonia, delayed motor skills, hearing loss, cerebral palsy, and gaze abnormalities (AAP Subcommittee on Hyperbilirubinemia, 2004) (see Chapter 36).

Jaundice Related to Breastfeeding. Two forms of breastfeeding-related jaundice are recognized: breastfeeding-associated jaundice and breast milk jaundice. These typically occur in otherwise healthy infants. Both types can occur in the same infant and are not easily differentiated (Blackburn, 2013).

Breastfeeding-associated jaundice (early-onset jaundice) begins at 2 to 5 days of age. Breastfeeding does not cause the jaundice; rather it is a lack of effective breastfeeding that contributes to the hyperbilirubinemia. If the infant is not feeding effectively, there is less caloric and fluid intake and possible dehydration. Hepatic clearance of bilirubin is reduced. With less intake, there are fewer stools. As a result bilirubin is reabsorbed from the intestine back into the bloodstream and must be conjugated again so it can be excreted (Blackburn, 2013; Lawrence & Lawrence, 2011).

Breast milk jaundice (late-onset jaundice) usually occurs at 5 to 10 days of age. Infants are usually feeding well and gaining weight appropriately. Rising levels of bilirubin peak during the second week and gradually diminish. Despite high levels of bilirubin that can persist for 3 to 12 weeks, these infants have no signs of hemolysis or liver dysfunction. The etiology of breast milk jaundice is uncertain. However, it seems to be related to factors in the breast milk (e.g., pregnanediol, fatty acids, and β-glucuronidase) that either inhibit the conjugation of bilirubin or decrease the excretion of bilirubin (Blackburn, 2013). (See Chapter 25 for a discussion of these conditions in relation to newborn nutrition.)

Coagulation. The liver plays an important role in blood coagulation. Coagulation factors, which are synthesized in the liver, are activated by vitamin K. The lack of intestinal bacteria needed to synthesize vitamin K results in transient blood coagulation deficiency between the second and fifth days of life. The levels of coagulation factors slowly increase to reach adult levels by the age of 9 months. The administration of intramuscular vitamin K shortly after birth helps prevent bleeding problems. Any bleeding problems noted in the newborn should be reported immediately, and tests for clotting ordered (Manco-Johnson, Rodden, & Hays, 2011).

Signs of Hepatic System Problems. Preterm infants are at risk for hepatic system problems such as hyperbilirubinemia and hypoglycemia because of their immaturity. The hematologic status of all newborns should be assessed for anemia. Because infants can develop a coagulation deficiency, a male neonate who has been circumcised must be observed closely for signs of hemorrhage. Hemorrhage also can be caused by a clotting defect, indicating a serious problem such as hemophilia.

Immune System

Beginning early in gestation the immune system of the fetus is developing the capacity to respond to foreign antigens. The development of the immune system is necessary to equip the neonate to meet the numerous environmental challenges (e.g., microorganisms) associated with life in the extrauterine world.

At birth most of the circulating antibodies in the newborn are immunoglobulin G (IgG) antibodies that were transported across the placenta from the maternal circulation. IgG is key to immunity to bacteria and viruses. This transfer of antibodies from the mother begins as early as 14 weeks of gestation and is greatest during the third trimester. By term the IgG levels in the cord blood of the infant are higher than those in maternal blood. The passive immunity afforded the infant through the placental transfer of IgG usually provides sufficient antimicrobial protection during the first 3 months of life. Production of adult concentrations of IgG is reached by 4 to 6 years of age (Kapur, Yoder, & Polin, 2011).

The fetus is capable of producing IgM by the eighth week of gestation, and low levels are present at term (less than 10% of adult levels). IgM is important for immunity to blood-borne infections and is the major immunoglobulin synthesized during the first month. By the age of 2 years IgM reaches adult levels. The production of IgA, IgD, and IgE is much more gradual, and maximal levels are not attained until early childhood (Kapur et al., 2011).

The membrane-protective IgA is missing from the respiratory and urinary tracts, and, unless the newborn is breastfed, it also is absent from the GI tract. Breast milk provides the newborn with important immunity. The secretory IgA in human milk acts locally in the intestines to neutralize bacterial and viral pathogens. It can also lessen the risk of allergy and food intolerance through modulation of exposure to foreign milk protein antigens.

The newborn is capable of producing a protective immune response to vaccines, given as early as a few hours after birth. For example, when hepatitis B vaccine is administered at birth to the infant born to a mother with hepatitis B, there is an excellent immune response. This holds true even if the infant does not receive additional hepatitis B immunoglobulin.

The WBCs of the newborn display a delayed response to invading bacteria. The influx of phagocytic cells to areas of inflammation is somewhat slowed, although the ability of these cells to attack and destroy bacteria is equivalent to that of adults (Kapur et al., 2011).

Risk for Infection. All newborns, and preterm newborns especially, are at high risk for infection during the first several months of life. During this period infection is one of the leading causes of morbidity and mortality. The newborn cannot limit the invading pathogen to the portal of entry because of the generalized hypofunctioning of the inflammatory and immune mechanisms.

Early signs of infection must be recognized so prompt diagnosis and treatment can occur. Temperature instability or hypothermia can be symptomatic of serious infection; newborns do not typically exhibit fever, although hyperthermia can occur (temperature greater than 38° C [100.4° F]). Lethargy, irritability, poor feeding, vomiting or diarrhea, decreased reflexes, and pale or mottled skin color are some of the clinical signs that suggest infection. Respiratory symptoms such as apnea, tachypnea, grunting, or retracting can be associated with infection such as pneumonia (Bodin, 2014). Any unusual discharge from the infant's eyes, nose, mouth, or other orifice must be investigated. If a rash appears, it must be evaluated closely; many normal rashes in the newborn are not associated with any infection. Infants must be protected from infections by the use of proper hand hygiene.

The greatest risk factor for neonatal infection is prematurity because of immaturity of the immune system. Other risk factors include premature rupture of membranes, chorioamnionitis, maternal fever, antenatal or intrapartal asphyxia, invasive procedures, stress, and congenital anomalies.

Integumentary System

All skin structures are present at birth. The epidermis and dermis are loosely bound and extremely thin. After 35 weeks of gestation the skin is covered by vernix caseosa (a cheeselike, whitish substance) that is fused with the epidermis and serves as a protective covering. Vernix caseosa is a complex substance that contains sebaceous gland secretions. It has emollient and antimicrobial properties and prevents fluid loss through the skin; it also has antioxidant properties. Removal of the vernix is followed by desquamation of the epidermis in most infants. There is evidence that leaving residual vernix intact after birth has positive benefits for neonatal skin such as decreasing the skin pH, decreasing skin erythema, and improving skin hydration (Association of Women's Health, Obstetric and Neonatal Nurses [AWHONN], 2013; Visscher, Utturkar, Pickens, et al., 2011).

The skin of a term infant is erythematous (red) for a few hours after birth, and then it fades to its normal color. The skin often appears blotchy or mottled, especially over the extremities. The hands and feet appear slightly cyanotic (acrocyanosis); this is caused by vasomotor instability and capillary stasis. Acrocyanosis is normal and appears intermittently over the first 7 to 10 days, especially with exposure to cold (Fig. 23-4).

The healthy term infant usually has a plump appearance because of large amounts of subcutaneous tissue and extracellular water content. Subcutaneous fat accumulated during the last trimester acts as insulation. Fine lanugo hair may be

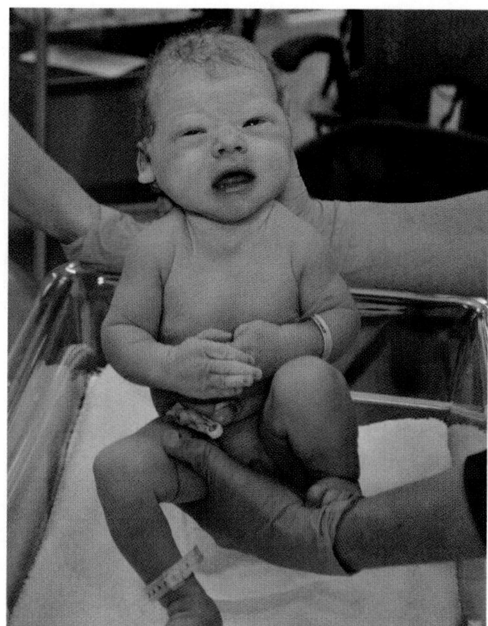

FIG 23-4 Newborn infant with acrocyanosis of upper and lower extremities. (Courtesy Barbara Wilson, West Jordan, UT.)

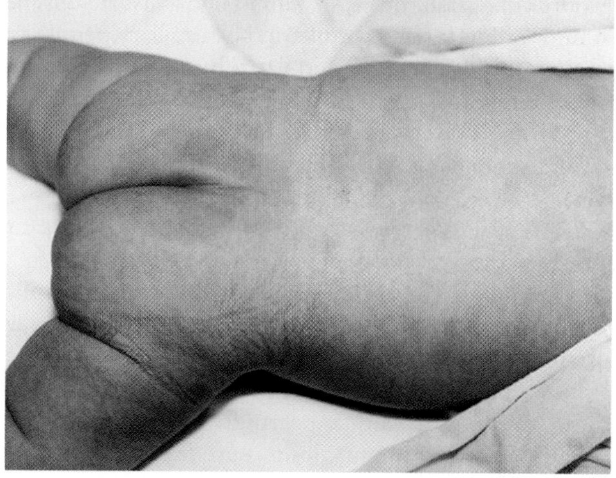

FIG 23-5 Mongolian spot.

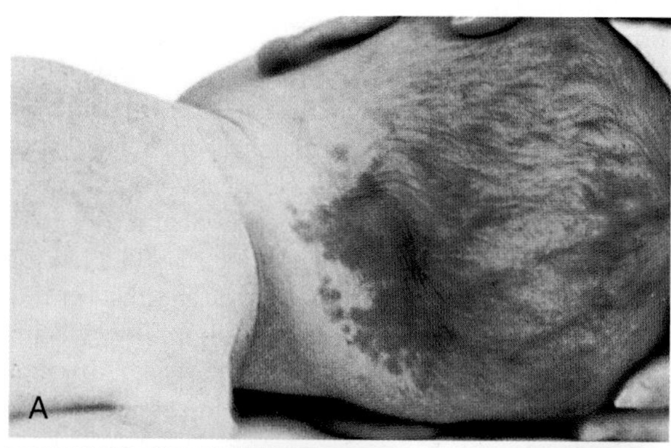

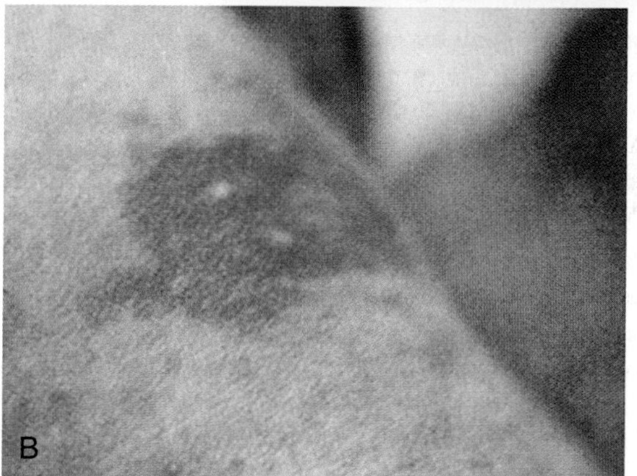

FIG 23-6 **A,** Nevus simplex or telangiectatic nevi (stork bite). **B,** Erythema toxicum. (Courtesy Mead Johnson & Co., Evansville, IN.)

noted over the face, shoulders, and back. Edema of the face and ecchymosis (bruising) or petechiae may be noted as a result of face presentation, forceps-assisted birth, or vacuum extraction.

Creases are located on the palms of the hands and the soles of the feet. The simian line, a single palmar crease, is often seen in Asian infants and infants with Down syndrome. The soles of the feet should be inspected for the number of creases during the first few hours after birth; as the skin dries, more creases appear. More creases correlate with a greater maturity rating. Preterm newborns have few, if any, creases.

Sweat Glands. Distended, small, white sebaceous glands noticeable on the newborn face are known as milia. Although sweat glands are present at birth, term infants usually do not sweat for the first 24 hours. By day 3 sweating begins on the face, then progresses to the palms. Infants can sweat as a function of body or environmental temperature; there can also be emotional sweating from crying or pain (Hoath & Narendran, 2011).

Desquamation. Desquamation (peeling) of the skin of the term infant does not occur until a few days after birth. Large generalized areas of skin desquamation present at birth can be an indication of postmaturity.

Mongolian Spots. Mongolian spots, bluish black areas of pigmentation, can appear over any part of the exterior surface of the body, including the extremities. They are noted more commonly on the back and buttocks (Fig. 23-5). These pigmented areas occur most frequently in newborns whose ethnic origins are Latin America, Asia, Africa, or the Mediterranean area. They are more common in dark-skinned individuals but can occur in 5% to 13% of Caucasians (Blackburn, 2013). Mongolian spots fade gradually over months or years.

The presence of Mongolian spots on the newborn should be documented carefully in the medical record. These normal skin pigmentations can be mistaken for bruises once the infant is discharged, which can raise suspicion of physical abuse.

Nevi. Nevus simplex, also known as salmon patches, telangiectatic nevi, "stork bites," or "angel kisses," are the result of a superficial capillary defect. They are usually small, flat, and pink and are easily blanched (Fig. 23-6, *A*). The most common sites are the upper eyelids, nose, upper lip, and nape of the neck (Blackburn, 2013). Salmon patches tend to be symmetric, with lesions occurring on both eyelids or both sides of midline. They have no clinical significance and require no treatment. Facial lesions usually fade between the first and second years of life, whereas neck lesions can be visible into adulthood (Morelli, 2011).

A port-wine stain, or nevus flammeus, is usually visible at birth and is due to an asymmetric postcapillary venule malformation. It is usually pink and flat at birth, but darkens with time, becoming red or purple and pebbly in consistency. True port-wine stains do not blanch on pressure or disappear. They are found most commonly on the face and neck (Püttgen & Cohen, 2012).

A nevus vascularis, or strawberry hemangioma, is a common type of capillary hemangioma that occurs more often in female infants. It consists of dilated newly formed capillaries occupying the entire dermal and subdermal layers with associated connective tissue hypertrophy. The typical lesion is a raised, sharply demarcated, bright or dark red rough-surfaced swelling, usually appearing on the head. In more than half of affected infants, lesions are present at birth; the remainder appear during the early weeks after birth. Most lesions reach maximum growth in 6 to 8 months, although deeper hemangiomas can continue to grow for up to 2 years. Hemangiomas usually fade or shrink with time (Hoath & Narendran, 2011).

Erythema Toxicum. Erythema toxicum, a transient rash, is also called *erythema neonatorum, newborn rash,* or *flea bite dermatitis.* It first appears in term neonates during the first 24 to 72 hours after birth and can last up to 3 weeks of age (Blackburn, 2013). It has lesions in different stages: erythematous macules, papules, and small vesicles (see Fig. 23-6, *B*). The lesions can appear suddenly anywhere on the body. The rash is thought to be an inflammatory response. Eosinophils, which help decrease inflammation, are found in the vesicles. Although the appearance is alarming, the rash has no clinical significance and requires no treatment.

Signs of Integumentary Problems. Close observation of the newborn's skin color can lead to early detection of potential problems. Any pallor, plethora (deep purplish color from increased circulating RBCs), petechiae, central cyanosis, or jaundice should be noted and described. The skin should be examined for signs of birth injuries such as forceps marks and lesions related to fetal monitoring. Bruises or petechiae can be present on the head, neck, and face of an infant born with a nuchal cord (cord around the neck) or who had a face presentation at birth. Bruising can increase the risk of hyperbilirubinemia. Petechiae can be present if increased pressure was applied to an area. Petechiae scattered over the infant's body should be reported to the health care provider because petechiae can indicate underlying problems such as low platelet count or infection.

Unilateral or bilateral periauricular papillomas (skin tags) occur fairly frequently. Their occurrence is usually a family trait and of no consequence.

Reproductive System

Female. An increase in estrogen during pregnancy followed by a drop after birth results in a mucoid vaginal discharge and even some slight bloody spotting (pseudomenstruation). External genitalia (i.e., labia majora and minora) are usually edematous with increased pigmentation. In term neonates the labia majora and minora cover the vestibule (Fig. 23-7, *A*). In preterm infants the clitoris is prominent, and the labia majora are small and widely separated. Vaginal or hymenal tags are common findings and have no clinical significance. Vernix caseosa can be present between the labia and should not be forcibly removed during bathing.

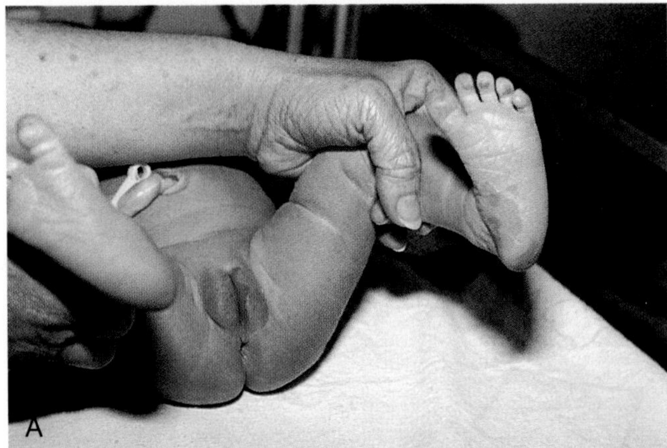

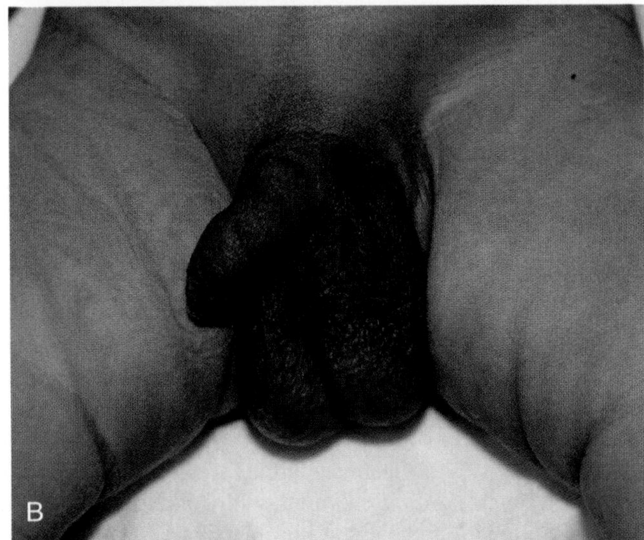

FIG 23-7 External genitalia. **A,** Genitalia in female term infant. **B,** Genitalia in uncircumcised male infant. Rugae cover scrotum, indicating term gestation. (Courtesy Marjorie Pyle, RNC, Lifecircle, Costa Mesa, CA.)

If the girl was born in the breech position, the labia can be edematous and bruised. The edema and bruising resolve in a few days; no treatment is necessary.

Male. In the uncircumcised newborn the foreskin or prepuce completely covers the glans. The foreskin adheres to the glans and is not fully retractable for 3 to 4 years. The position of the urethra should be at the tip of the penis. With hypospadias or epispadias the urethral opening is located in an abnormal position, on or adjacent to the glans, although it can appear on the penile shaft or perineum. Small, white, firm lesions called *epithelial pearls* may be seen at the tip of the prepuce.

By 28 to 36 weeks of gestation the testes can be palpated in the inguinal canal, and a few rugae appear on the scrotum. At 36 to 40 weeks of gestation the testes are palpable in the upper scrotum, and rugae appear on the anterior portion. After 40 weeks the testes can be palpated in the scrotum, and rugae cover the scrotal sac. The postterm neonate has deep rugae and a pendulous scrotum. The incidence of undescended testes is 3.7%

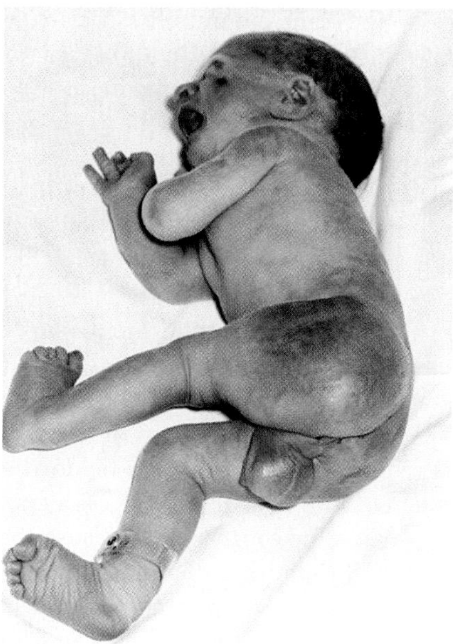

FIG 23-8 Swelling of the genitals and bruising of the buttocks after a breech birth. (From O'Doherty, N. [1986]. *Neonatology: Micro atlas of the newborn.* Nutley, NJ: Hoffman-LaRoche.)

in term males and 21% in preterm males (Shulman, Palmert, & Wherrett, 2011). Hydrocele, caused by an accumulation of fluid around the testes, can be present. Hydroceles can be easily transilluminated with a light and usually resolve without treatment.

The scrotum is usually more deeply pigmented than the rest of the skin (see Fig. 23-7, *B*), particularly in darker-skinned infants. A bluish discoloration of the scrotum suggests testicular torsion, which needs immediate attention. If the male infant is born in a breech presentation, the scrotum can be very edematous and bruised (Fig. 23-8). The swelling and discoloration subside within a few days.

Swelling of Breast Tissue. Swelling of the breast tissue in term infants of both sexes is caused by the hyperestrogenism of pregnancy. In a few infants a thin discharge (witch's milk) can be seen. This finding has no clinical significance, requires no treatment, and subsides within a few days as the maternal hormones are eliminated from the infant's body.

The nipples should be symmetric on the chest. Breast tissue and areola size increase with gestation. The areola appears slightly elevated at 34 weeks of gestation. By 36 weeks a breast bud of 1 to 2 mm is palpable; this increases to 12 mm by 42 weeks.

Signs of Reproductive System Problems. The infant must be inspected closely for ambiguous genitalia and other abnormalities. Normally in a female infant the urethral opening is located behind the clitoris. Any deviation from this can incorrectly suggest that the clitoris is a small penis, which can occur in conditions such as adrenal hyperplasia. Nearly all female infants are born with hymenal tags; absence of such tags can indicate vaginal agenesis. Fecal discharge from the vagina indicates a rectovaginal fistula. Any of these findings must be reported to the neonatal or pediatric health care provider for further evaluation.

Hypospadias (urethra is located on ventral surface of the penis) or epispadias (urethra is located on dorsal surface), undescended or maldescended testes, and other abnormalities of the male genitalia must be reported. Circumcision is contraindicated in the presence of hypospadias or epispadias because the foreskin is used in repair of these anomalies.

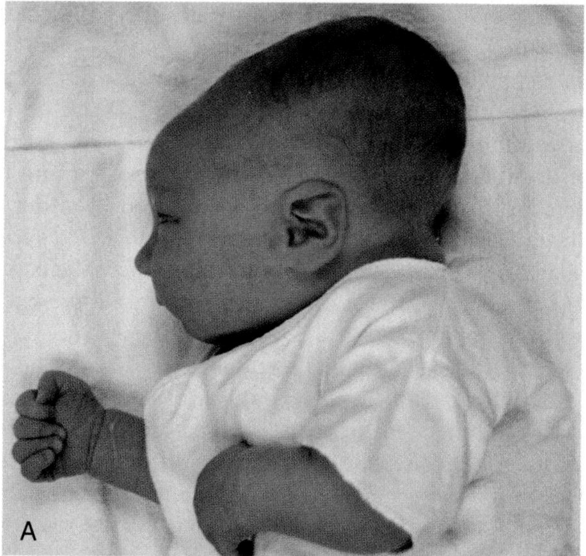

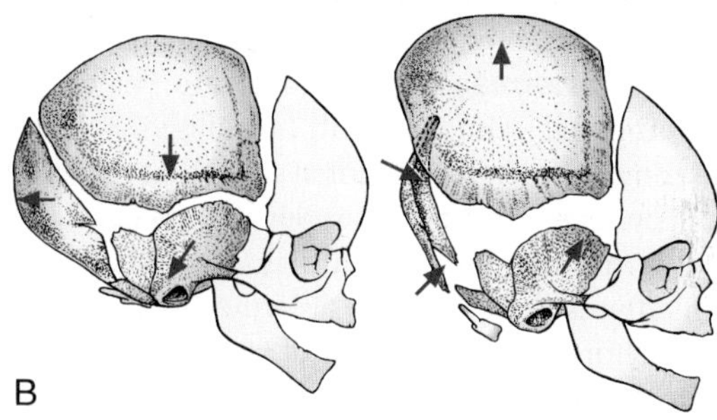

FIG 23-9 Molding. **A,** Significant molding after vaginal birth. **B,** Schematic of bones of skull when molding is present. (**A,** Courtesy Kim Molloy, Knoxville, IA.)

Inguinal hernias can be present and become more obvious when the infant cries. They are common, especially in African-American neonates, and usually require no treatment because they resolve with time.

Skeletal System

The infant's skeletal system undergoes rapid development during the first year of life. At birth more cartilage is present than ossified bone. Because of cephalocaudal (head-to-rump) development, the newborn looks somewhat out of proportion.

The head at term is approximately one fourth of the total body length. The arms are slightly longer than the legs. In the newborn the legs are about one third of the total body length. As growth proceeds the midpoint in head-to-toe measurements gradually descends from the level of the umbilicus at birth to the level of the symphysis pubis at maturity.

The face appears small in relation to the skull. The skull appears large and heavy. Cranial size and shape can be distorted by molding (the shaping of the fetal head by overlapping of the cranial bones to facilitate movement through the birth canal during labor) (Fig. 23-9).

Caput Succedaneum. Caput succedaneum is a generalized, easily identifiable edematous area of the scalp, most commonly found on the occiput (Fig. 23-10, *A*). With vertex presentation the sustained pressure of the presenting vertex against the cervix results in compression of local vessels, slowing venous return. The slower venous return causes an increase in tissue fluids within the skin of the scalp, and edema develops. This edematous area, present at birth, extends across suture lines of the skull and usually disappears spontaneously within 3 to 4 days. Infants who are born with the assistance of vacuum extraction usually have a caput in the area where the cup was applied. Bruising of the scalp is often seen in the presence of caput succedaneum.

Cephalhematoma. Cephalhematoma is a collection of blood between a skull bone and its periosteum. Therefore, a cephalhematoma does not cross a cranial suture line (see Fig. 23-10, *B*). A cephalhematoma is firmer and more well defined than a caput. Often caput succedaneum and cephalhematoma occur simultaneously. A cephalhematoma usually resolves in 2 to 8 weeks. As the hematoma resolves, hemolysis of RBCs occurs, and hyperbilirubinemia can result (Bonifacio, Gonzalez, & Ferriero, 2012).

Subgaleal Hemorrhage. Subgaleal hemorrhage is bleeding into the subgaleal compartment (see Fig. 23-10, *C*). The subgaleal compartment is a potential space that contains loosely arranged connective tissue; it is located beneath the galea aponeurosis, the tendinous sheath that connects the frontal and occipital muscles and forms the inner surface of the scalp. Subgaleal hemorrhage is the result of traction or application of shearing forces to the scalp, commonly associated with difficult operative vaginal birth, especially vacuum extraction. The scalp is pulled away from the bony calvarium; the vessels are torn, and blood collects in the subgaleal space. Blood loss can be severe, resulting in hypovolemic shock, disseminated intravascular coagulation (DIC), and death (Mangurten & Puppala, 2011).

Early detection of the hemorrhage is vital; serial head circumference measurements and inspection of the back of the neck for increasing edema and a firm mass are essential. A boggy scalp, pallor, tachycardia, and increasing head circumference can also be early signs of a subgaleal hemorrhage. Computed tomography or magnetic resonance imaging is useful in confirming the diagnosis. Replacement of lost blood and clotting factors is required in acute cases of hemorrhage. Another possible early sign of subgaleal hemorrhage is a forward and lateral positioning of the newborn's ears because the hematoma extends posteriorly. Monitoring the infant for changes in level of consciousness and decreases in hematocrit is also key to early recognition and management. An increase in serum bilirubin levels may be seen as a result of the degradation of blood cells within the hematoma (Mangurten & Puppala, 2011).

Spine. The bones in the vertebral column of the newborn form two primary curvatures—one in the thoracic region and one in the sacral region. Both are forward, concave curvatures. As the infant gains head control at approximately age 3 months, a secondary curvature appears in the cervical region. The newborn's spine appears straight and can be flexed easily. The newborn

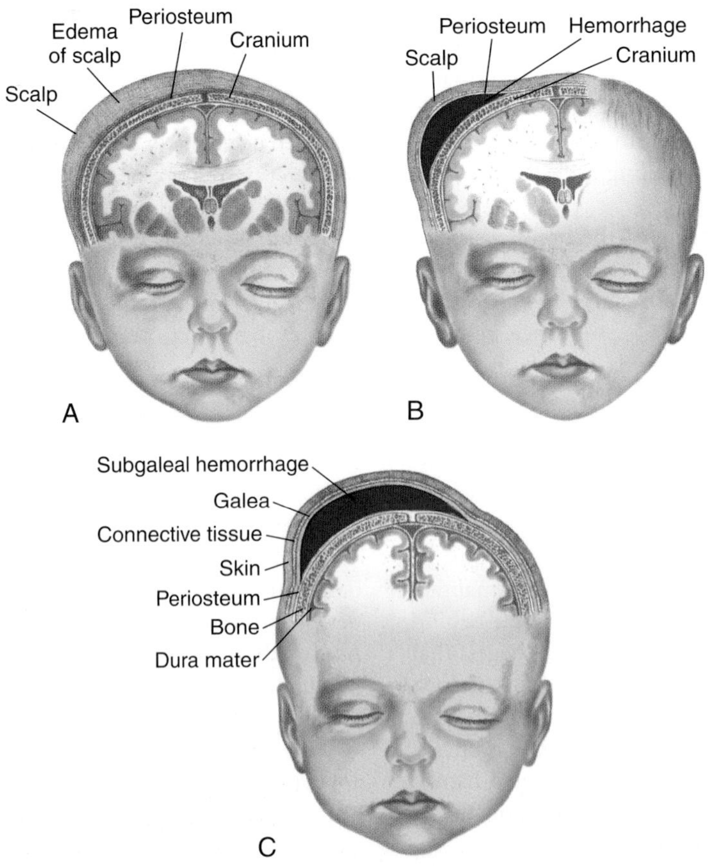

FIG 23-10 A, Caput succedaneum. B, Cephalhematoma C, Subgaleal hemorrhage. (A and C, From Seidel, H., Ball, J., Dains, J., & Benedict, G. [2006]. *Mosby's guide to physical examination* [6th ed.]. St. Louis: Mosby.)

can lift the head and turn it from side to side when prone. The vertebrae should appear straight and flat. If a pilonidal dimple is noted, further inspection is required to determine whether a sinus is present. A pilonidal dimple, especially with a sinus and nevus pilosis (hairy nevus), can be associated with spina bifida.

Extremities. The infant's extremities should be symmetric and of equal length. Fingers and toes should be equal in number (five fingers on each hand and five toes on each foot) and should have nails present. Digits may be missing *(oligodactyly)*. Extra digits *(polydactyly)* are sometimes found on hands or feet. Fingers or toes may be fused *(syndactyly)*.

The infant is examined for developmental dysplasia of the hips (DDH). In newborns with DDH the affected hip is unlikely to be dislocated at birth; instead it is easily dislocatable. Postnatal factors determine whether the hip dislocates, subluxates, or remains stable. DDH occurs more often in female infants, in breech presentations (Fig. 23-11), and in infants with family history of DDH (Cooperman & Thompson, 2011).

Signs of DDH are asymmetric gluteal and thigh skinfolds, uneven knee levels, a positive Ortolani test, and a positive Barlow test. The hips are inspected for symmetry. Gluteal and thigh skinfolds should be equal and symmetric, and legs should be of equal length (Fig. 23-12, *A*). The level of the knees in flexion should be equal (see Fig. 23-12, *C*). Hip integrity is assessed by using the Barlow test and the Ortolani maneuver. For the Barlow test the examiner places the middle finger over the greater trochanter and the thumb along the midthigh. The hip is flexed to 90 degrees and adducted, followed by gentle downward pushing of the femoral head. If the hip can be dislocated with this maneuver, the femoral head moves out of the acetabulum, and the examiner feels a "clunk." The hip is then checked to determine if the femoral head can be returned into the acetabulum using the Ortolani manuever. As the hip is abducted and upward leverage is applied, a dislocated hip returns to the acetabulum with a clunk that is felt by the examiner (White & Goldberg, 2012) (see Fig. 23-12, *B* and *D*).

SAFETY ALERT

Only expert examiners (physicians, nurse practitioners) should perform the Barlow test and Ortolani maneuver to assess for DDH. An unskilled examiner can cause injury to the newborn.

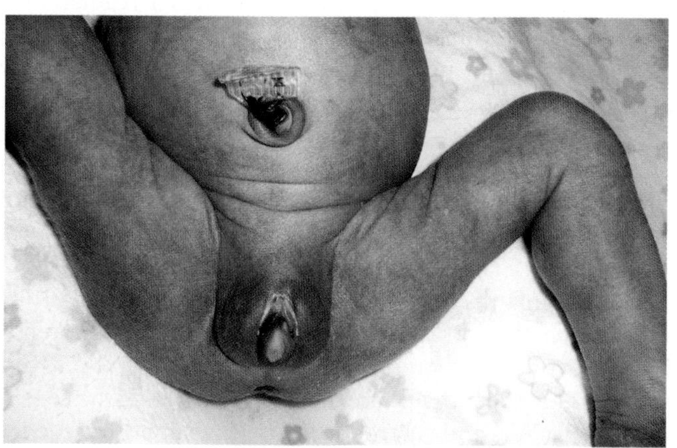

FIG 23-11 Position of infant's legs after breech birth. Note preterm genitalia. (Courtesy Cheryl Briggs, RNC, Annapolis, MD.)

Signs of Skeletal Problems. Abnormalities of the skeletal system can be congenital, developmental, drug induced, or the result of intrapartum or postnatal factors. Signs of DDH, additional digits or webbing of digits, and any other abnormality should be documented and reported to the primary health care provider.

A fractured clavicle often occurs in macrosomic infants and in those who had a difficult birth (e.g., shoulder dystocia). Unequal movement of the upper extremities or crepitus over the clavicular area can indicate fracture.

The newborn's feet can appear to be abnormally positioned. This can indicate congenital deformity or can be related to fetal positioning in utero. For example, clubfoot (talipes equinovarus), a deformity in which the foot turns inward and is fixed in a plantar-flexion position, is a congenital condition

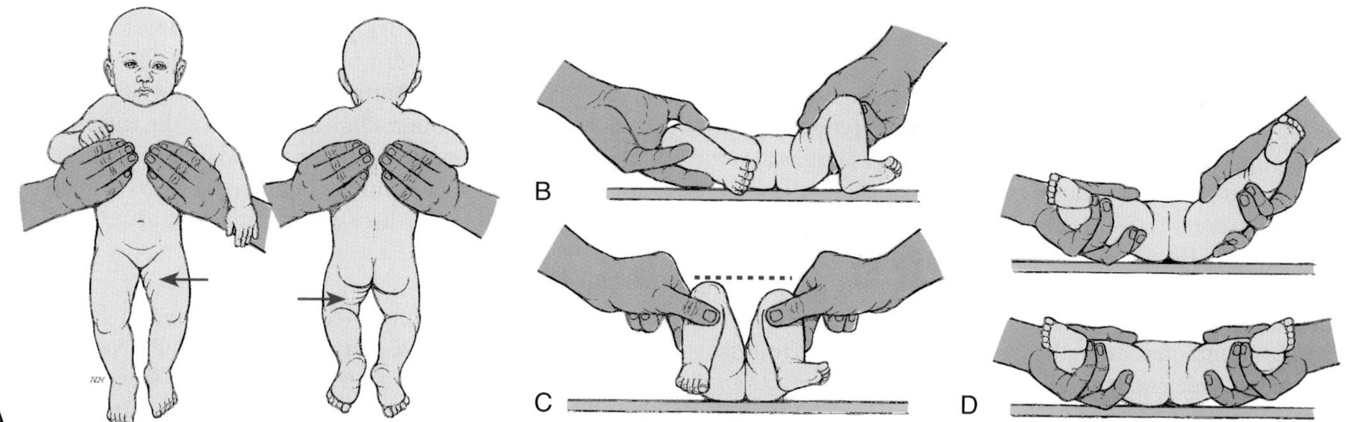

FIG 23-12 Signs of developmental dysplasia of the hip. **A,** Asymmetry of gluteal and thigh folds with shortening of the thigh (Galeazzi sign). **B,** Limited hip abduction, as seen in flexion (Ortolani test). **C,** Apparent shortening of the femur, as indicated by the level of the knees in flexion (Allis sign). **D,** Ortolani maneuver with femoral head moving in and out of acetabulum (in infants 1 to 2 months old). (From Hockenberry, M. J., & Wilson, D. (2013). *Wong's essentials of pediatric nursing* (9th ed.). St. Louis: Mosby.)

that warrants attention. If the foot is turned inward in the plantar-flexion position but can be moved into the normal position, it is likely caused by fetal positioning and should gradually resolve.

Neuromuscular System

The neuromuscular system is almost completely developed at birth. The term newborn is a responsive and reactive being with remarkable capacity for social interaction and self-organization.

Growth of the brain after birth follows a predictable pattern of rapid growth during infancy and early childhood; it becomes more gradual during the remainder of the first decade and minimal during adolescence. By the end of the first year the cerebellum ends its growth spurt, which began at approximately 30 gestational weeks.

The brain requires glucose as a source of energy and a relatively large supply of oxygen for adequate metabolism. The necessity for glucose requires careful assessment of neonates who are at risk for hypoglycemia (e.g., infants of mothers who have diabetes; infants who are macrosomic or small for gestational age; and newborns who experienced prolonged birth, hypoxia, or preterm birth).

Spontaneous motor activity can be seen as transient tremors of the mouth and chin, especially during crying episodes, and of the extremities, notably the arms and hands. Transient tremors are normal and can be observed in nearly every newborn. They most often involve the mouth and chin or the arms and hands. These tremors should not be present when the infant is quiet and should not persist beyond 1 month of age. Persistent tremors or tremors involving the total body can indicate pathologic conditions. Normal tremors, tremors (jitteriness) of hypoglycemia, and seizure activity must be differentiated so corrective care can be instituted as necessary (Verklan & Lopez, 2011).

To differentiate between tremors or jitteriness and seizure activity, the nurse can consider the following signs (Scher, 2012; Verklan & Lopez, 2011):

- Tremors or jitteriness are easily elicited by motions or voice and cease with gentle restraint of the body part, whereas seizure activity continues.
- Passive flexion and repositioning of the tremulous extremity reduces or stops the movement.
- Seizure activity is associated with ocular changes (eyes deviating or staring) and autonomic changes (apnea, tachycardia, pupil changes, increased salivation); these signs are not associated with jitteriness or tremors.

The posture of the term newborn demonstrates flexion of the arms at the elbows and the legs at the knees. Hips are abducted and partially flexed. Intermittent fisting of the hands is common.

Muscle tone and strength are directly related. The infant with normal tone and strength exhibits some resistance to passive movement such as when being pulled to sit or when the arm or leg is extended by the examiner. The hypotonic neonate shows little resistance and can feel like a "rag doll." Hypertonia is evidenced by increased resistance to passive movement.

Although neuromuscular control is very limited, it can be noted. If newborns are placed face down on a firm surface, they will turn their heads to the side. They attempt to hold their heads in line with their bodies if they are raised by their arms. Various reflexes serve to promote safety and adequate food intake.

Newborn Reflexes. The newborn has many primitive reflexes. The times at which these reflexes appear and disappear reflect the maturity and intactness of the developing nervous system. The most common reflexes found in the normal term newborn are described in Table 23-4.

Behavioral Characteristics

The healthy infant must accomplish behavioral and biologic tasks to develop normally. Behavioral characteristics form the basis of the social capabilities of the infant. Newborns progress through a hierarchy of developmental challenges as they adapt to their environment and caregivers. They must first be able to regulate their physiologic or autonomic system, including involuntary physiologic functions such as heart rate, respiration, and temperature. The next level is motor organization, in which infants regulate or control their motor behavior. This includes controlling random movements, improving muscle tone, and reducing excessive activity. The third level of behavior is *state regulation*, which refers to the ability to modulate the state of consciousness. The infant develops predictable sleep and wake states and is able to react to stress through self-regulation or communicating with the caregiver by crying and then being consoled. Finally the infant reaches the fourth level of attention and social interaction. He or she is able to attend to visual and auditory stimulation, stay alert for long periods, and engage in social interaction (Brazelton & Nugent, 2011).

This progression in behavior is the basis for the Brazelton Neonatal Behavioral Assessment Scale (NBAS) (Brazelton & Nugent, 2011). The NBAS is an interactive examination that assesses the infant's response to 28 areas organized according to the clusters in Box 23-2. It is generally used as a research or diagnostic tool and requires special training. The NBAS helps the practitioner identify where the infant falls along the continuum of behaviors and determine the type of support needed.

The Newborn Behavioral Observations (NBO) system, based on the NBAS, is a tool that is used in clinical settings to help parents identify, understand, and respond to newborn behavior (Nugent, Keefer, Minear, et al., 2007). Karl and Keefer (2011) developed a training program using the NBO system to educate clinicians about newborn behavior, self-regulation skills, and social interaction capabilities. A major benefit of this program is that nurses and other clinicians can use the information to educate and help parents interpret newborn cues and respond appropriately, which promotes attachment (Karl & Keefer). See Chapter 22 for further discussion of attachment.

Sleep-Wake States

Healthy newborns differ in their activity levels, feeding patterns, sleeping patterns, and responsiveness. Parents' reactions to their newborns are often determined by these differences. Showing parents the unique characteristics of their infant helps them develop a more positive perception of the infant and promotes increased interaction between infant and parent. Infant responses to environmental stimuli and to their caregivers depend on the infant's state or state of consciousness.

In the early newborn period infants tend to alternate periods of sleep and wakefulness that resemble their fetal inactivity

TABLE 23-4 Assessment of Newborn Reflexes

REFLEX	ELICITING THE REFLEX	CHARACTERISTIC RESPONSE	COMMENTS
Sucking and rooting	Touch infant's lip, cheek, or corner of mouth with nipple or finger.	Infant turns head toward stimulus and opens mouth.	Response is difficult if not impossible to elicit after infant has been fed; if response is weak or absent, consider preterm birth or neurologic defect. Parental guidance: Avoid trying to turn head toward breast or nipple; allow infant to root; response disappears after 3-4* mo but can persist up to 1 yr. If response is weak or absent, it can indicate prematurity or neurologic defect.
Swallowing	Feed infant; swallowing usually follows sucking and obtaining fluids.	Swallowing is usually coordinated with sucking and breathing and usually occurs without gagging, coughing, apnea, or vomiting.	If response is weak or absent, this can indicate preterm birth, effects of maternal analgesics, or illness that needs investigation. Sucking, swallowing, and breathing are often uncoordinated in preterm infant.
Grasp			
Palmar	Place finger in palm of hand.	Infant's fingers curl around examiner's fingers.	Palmar response lessens by 3-4 mo; parents enjoy this contact with infant.
Plantar	Place finger at base of toes.	Toes curl downward.	Plantar response lessens by 8 mo.

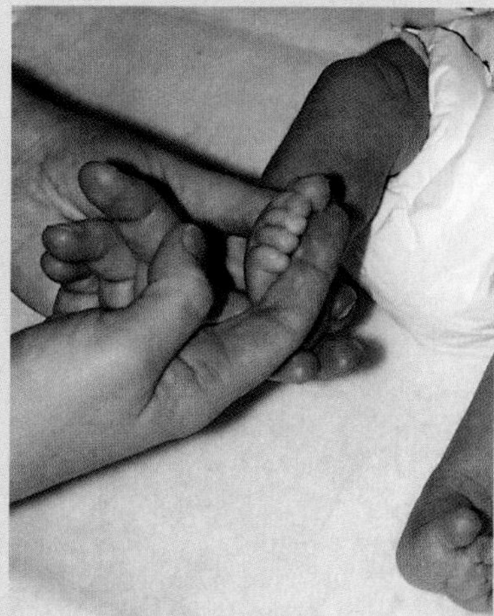

Plantar grasp reflex. (From Zitelli, B. J., & Davis, H. W. [2007]. *Atlas of pediatric physical diagnosis* [5th ed.]. St. Louis: Mosby.)

REFLEX	ELICITING THE REFLEX	CHARACTERISTIC RESPONSE	COMMENTS
Extrusion	Touch or depress tip of tongue.	Newborn forces tongue outward.	Response disappears about fourth to fifth month.
Glabellar (Myerson)	Tap over forehead, bridge of nose, or maxilla of newborn whose eyes are open.	Newborn blinks for first four or five taps.	Continued blinking with repeated taps is consistent with extrapyramidal signs.
Tonic neck or "fencing"	With infant in supine neutral position, turn head quickly to one side.	With infant facing left side, arm and leg on that side extend; opposite arm and leg flex (turn head to right, and extremities assume opposite postures).	Responses in leg are more consistent. Complete response disappears by 3-4 mo; incomplete response may be seen until third or fourth year. After 6 wk persistent response is sign of possible cerebral palsy.

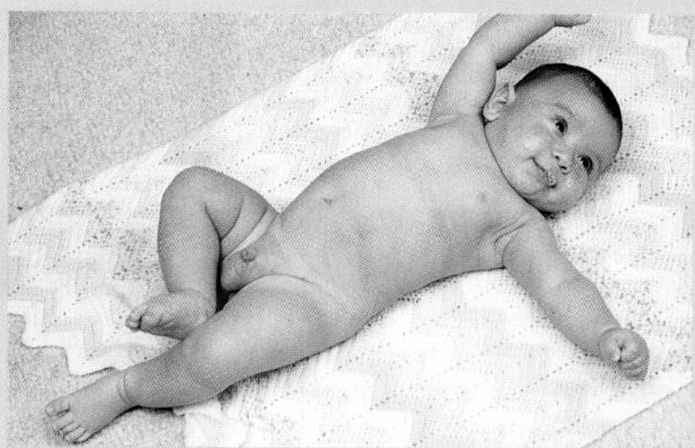

Classic pose in tonic neck reflex. (Courtesy Marjorie Pyle, RNC, Lifecircle, Costa Mesa, CA.)

*All durations for persistence of reflexes are based on time elapsed after 40 weeks of gestation (i.e., if newborn was born at 36 weeks of gestation, add 1 month to all time limits given).

Continued

TABLE 23-4 Assessment of Newborn Reflexes—cont'd

REFLEX	ELICITING THE REFLEX	CHARACTERISTIC RESPONSE	COMMENTS
Moro	Hold infant in semisitting position, allow head and trunk to fall backward to angle of at least 30 degrees (with support). Place infant supine on flat surface; perform sharp hand clap.	Symmetric abduction and extension of arms are seen; fingers fan out and form a C with thumb and forefinger; slight tremor may be noted; arms are adducted in embracing motion and return to relaxed flexion and movement. A cry may accompany or follow motor movement. Legs may follow similar pattern of response. Preterm infant does not complete "embrace"; instead arms fall backward because of weakness.	Response is present at birth; complete response may be seen until 8 wk; body jerk only is seen between 8 and 18 wk; response is absent by 6 mo if neurologic maturation is not delayed; response may be incomplete if infant is in deep sleep state; give parental guidance about normal response. Asymmetric response can connote injury to brachial plexus, clavicle, or humerus. Persistent response after 6 mo indicates possible neurologic abnormality.
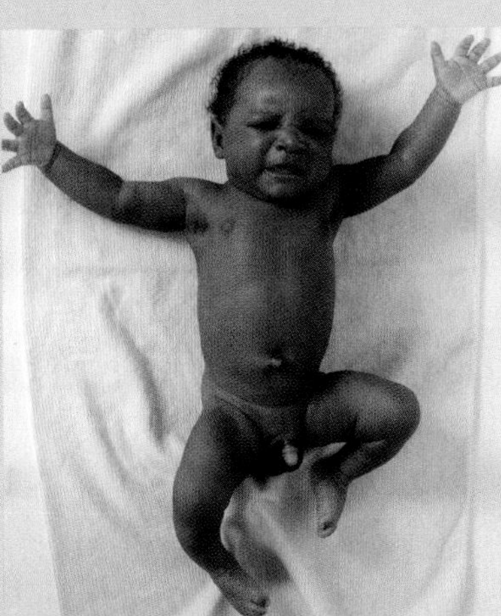 Moro reflex. (Courtesy Paul Vincent Kuntz, Texas Children's Hospital, Houston.)			
Stepping or "walking"	Hold infant vertically under arms or on trunk, allowing one foot to touch table surface.	Infant will simulate walking, alternating flexion and extension of feet; term infants walk on soles of their feet, and preterm infants walk on their toes.	Response is normally present for 3-4 wk.
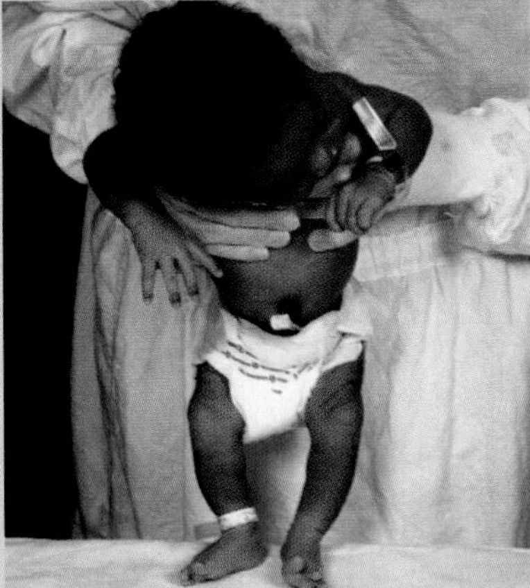 Stepping reflex. (From Dickason, E. J., Silverman, B. L., & Kaplan, J. A. [1998]. *Maternal-infant nursing care* [3rd ed.]. St. Louis: Mosby.)			
Crawling	Place newborn on abdomen.	Newborn makes crawling movements with arms and legs.	Response should disappear about 6 wk of age.
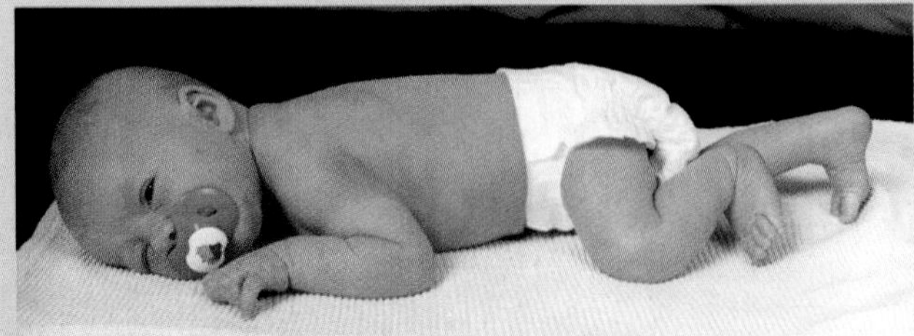 Crawling reflex. (Courtesy Paul Vincent Kuntz, Texas Children's Hospital, Houston.)			

TABLE 23-4 Assessment of Newborn Reflexes—cont'd

REFLEX	ELICITING THE REFLEX	CHARACTERISTIC RESPONSE	COMMENTS
Deep tendon	Use finger instead of percussion hammer to elicit patellar, or knee jerk, reflex; newborn must be relaxed.	Reflex jerk is present; even with newborn relaxed, nonselective overall reaction may occur.	It is usually more difficult to elicit upper extremity reflexes than lower extremity reflexes.
Crossed extension	With infant in supine position, examiner extends one leg of infant and presses down knee. Stimulation of sole of foot of fixated limb should cause free leg to flex, adduct, and extend as if attempting to push away stimulating agent.	Opposite leg flexes, adducts, and then extends.	This reflex should be present during newborn period.

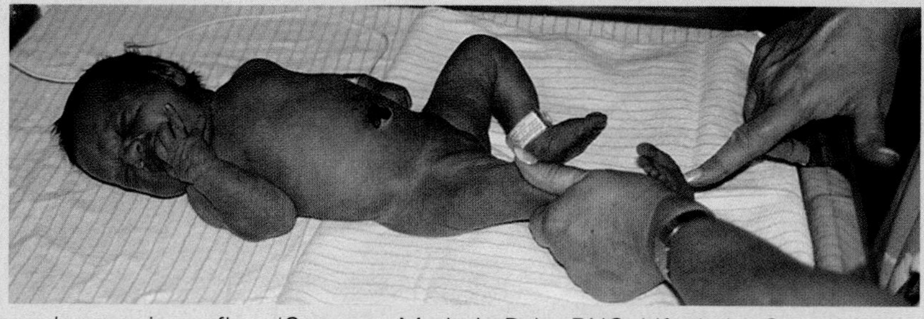

Crossed extension reflex. (Courtesy Marjorie Pyle, RNC, Lifecircle, Costa Mesa, CA.)

REFLEX	ELICITING THE REFLEX	CHARACTERISTIC RESPONSE	COMMENTS
Babinski (plantar)	On sole of foot, beginning at heel, stroke upward along lateral aspect of sole; then move finger across ball of foot.	All toes hyperextend, with dorsiflexion of big toe—recorded as a positive sign.	Absence requires neurologic evaluation; should disappear after 1 yr of age. Response depends on infant's general muscle tone, maturity, and condition.

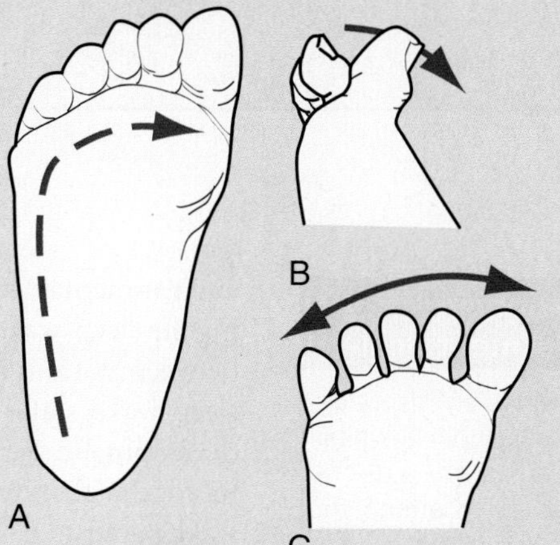

Babinski reflex. **A,** Direction of stroke. **B,** Dorsiflexion of big toe. **C,** Fanning of toes. (From Hockenberry, M. J., & Wilson, D. [2013]. *Wong's nursing care of infants and children* [9th ed.]. St. Louis: Mosby.)

REFLEX	ELICITING THE REFLEX	CHARACTERISTIC RESPONSE	COMMENTS
Pull-to-sit (traction response); postural tone	Pull infant up by wrists from supine position with head in midline.	Head lags until infant is in upright position; then head is held in same plane with chest and shoulder momentarily before falling forward; infant attempts to right head.	Response depends on general muscle tone and maturity and condition of infant.
Truncal incurvation (Galant)	Place infant prone on flat surface; run finger down back about 4-5 cm lateral to spine, first on one side and then down the other.	Trunk is flexed, and pelvis is swung toward stimulated side.	Response disappears by fourth week. Response varies but should be obtainable in all infants, including preterm. Absence suggests general depression of nervous system. With transverse lesions of cord, no response below level of lesion is present.

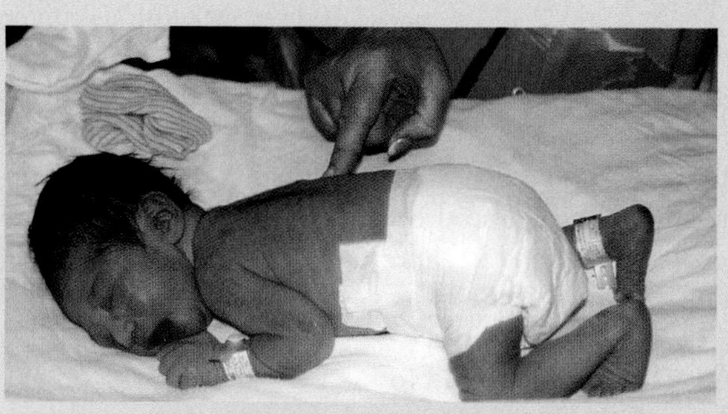

Trunk incurvation reflex. (Courtesy Marjorie Pyle, RNC, Lifecircle, Costa Mesa, CA.)

Continued

TABLE 23-4 Assessment of Newborn Reflexes—cont'd

REFLEX	ELICITING THE REFLEX	CHARACTERISTIC RESPONSE	COMMENTS
Magnet	Place infant in supine position, partially flex both lower extremities, and apply light pressure with fingers to soles of feet (Fig. A). Normally, while examiner's fingers maintain contact with soles of feet, lower limbs extend.	Both lower limbs should extend against examiner's pressure (Fig. B).	Absence suggests damage to central nervous system. Weak reflex may be seen after breech presentation *without* extended legs or may indicate sciatic nerve stretch syndrome. Breech presentation *with* extended legs may evoke exaggerated response.
Additional newborn responses: yawn, stretch, burp, hiccup, sneeze	These are spontaneous behaviors.	Responses can be slightly depressed temporarily because of maternal analgesia or anesthesia, fetal hypoxia, or infection.	Parental guidance: Most of these behaviors are pleasurable to parents. Parents need to be assured that behaviors are normal. Sneeze is usually a response to mucus in the nose and not an indicator of a cold (upper respiratory tract infection). No treatment is needed for hiccups; sucking may help. In a preterm infant these are signs of neurodevelopmental immaturity and physiologic stress.

A B

Magnet reflex. (Courtesy Michael S. Clement, MD, Mesa, AZ.)

BOX 23-2 Clusters of Neonatal Behaviors in Brazelton Neonatal Behavioral Assessment Scale

- Habituation—Ability to respond to and then inhibit responding to discrete stimulus (e.g., light, rattle, bell, pinprick) while asleep
- Orientation—Quality of alert states and ability to attend to visual and auditory stimuli while alert
- Motor performance—Quality of movement and tone
- Range of state—Measure of general arousal level or arousability of infant
- Regulation of state—How infant responds when aroused
- Autonomic stability—Signs of stress (e.g., tremors, startles, skin color) related to homeostatic (self-regulator) adjustment of the nervous system
- Reflexes—Assessment of several neonatal reflexes

From Brazelton, T., & Nugent, J. (2011). *Neonatal behavioral assessment scale* (4th ed.). London: MacKeith.

and activity patterns. Variations in the state of consciousness of infants are called sleep-wake states. The six states form a continuum from deep sleep to extreme irritability (Fig. 23-13): two sleep states (deep sleep and light sleep) and four wake states (drowsy, quiet alert, active alert, and crying) (Brazelton & Nugent, 2011). Each state has specific characteristics and state-related behaviors. The optimal state of arousal is the quiet alert state. During this state infants smile, vocalize, move in synchrony with speech, watch their parents' faces, and respond to people talking to them. They respond to internal and external environmental factors by controlling sensory input and regulating the sleep-wake states; the ability to make smooth transitions between states is called *state modulation*. The ability to regulate sleep-wake states is essential in the infant's neurobehavioral development. Term infants are better able than preterm infants to cope with external or internal factors that affect the sleep-wake patterns.

Infants use purposeful behavior to maintain the optimal arousal state as follows: (1) actively withdrawing by increasing physical distance, (2) rejecting by pushing away with hands and feet, (3) decreasing sensitivity by falling asleep or breaking eye contact by turning the head, or (4) using signaling behaviors such as fussing and crying. These behaviors permit infants to quiet themselves and reinstate readiness to interact.

The first 6 weeks of life involve a steady decrease in the proportion of active REM sleep to total sleep. A steady increase in the proportion of quiet sleep to total sleep also occurs. Periods of wakefulness increase. For the first few weeks the wakeful periods seem dictated by hunger, but soon a need for socializing appears. The newborn sleeps approximately 16 to 19 hours a day, with periods of wakefulness gradually increasing. By the fourth week of life some infants stay awake from one feeding to the next (Gardner & Goldson, 2011).

Other Factors Influencing Newborn Behavior

Gestational Age. The gestational age and level of central nervous system (CNS) maturity affect infant behavior. In the preterm neonate with an immature CNS the entire body

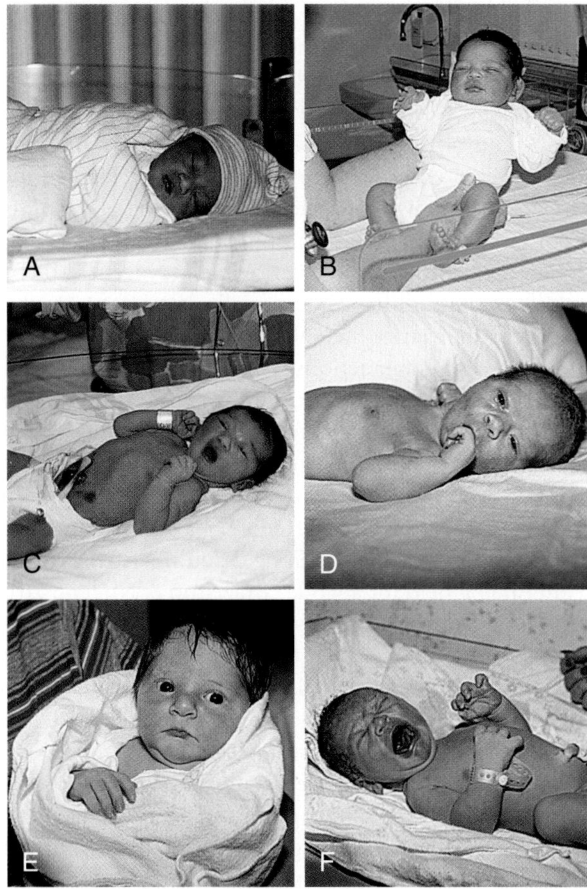

FIG 23-13 Newborn sleep-wake states. **A,** Deep sleep. **B,** Light sleep. **C,** Drowsy. **D,** Quiet alert. **E,** Active alert. **F,** Crying. (Courtesy Marjorie Pyle, RNC, Lifecircle, Costa Mesa, CA.)

responds to a pinprick of the foot, although the response may not be observed by an untrained observer. The more mature infant withdraws only the foot. CNS immaturity is reflected in reflex development, sleep-wake states, and ability (or lack thereof) to regulate or modulate a smooth transition between different states. Preterm infants have brief periods of alertness but have difficulty maintaining alertness without becoming overstimulated, which leads to autonomic instability unless intervention is implemented. Premature or sick infants show signs of fatigue or physiologic stress sooner than full-term healthy infants.

Time. The time elapsed since birth affects the behavior of infants as they attempt to become organized initially. Time elapsed since the previous feeding and time of day also can influence infants' responses.

Stimuli. Environmental events and stimuli affect the infants' behavioral responses. The newborn responds to animate and inanimate stimuli. Nurses in intensive care nurseries observe that infants respond to loud noises, bright lights, monitor alarms, and tension in the unit. If a mother is tense, nervous, or uncomfortable while feeding her infant, the infant may sense her tension and demonstrate difficulty feeding.

Medication. No conclusive evidence exists regarding the effects of maternal analgesia or anesthesia during labor on neonatal behavior. Researchers who have studied the effects of epidural medications on breastfeeding behaviors have been unable to show a cause-and-effect relationship (Hoyt, 2011).

Sensory Behaviors

From birth infants possess sensory capabilities that indicate a state of readiness for social interaction. They effectively use behavioral responses in establishing their first dialogues. These responses, coupled with the newborns' "baby appearance" (e.g., facial proportions of forehead, eyes larger than the lower portion of the face) and their small size and helplessness, rouse feelings of wanting to hold, protect, and interact with them.

Vision. At birth the eye is structurally incomplete, and the muscles are immature. The process of accommodation is not present but improves over the first 3 months of life. The pupils react to light, the blink reflex is stimulated easily, and the corneal reflex is activated by light touch. Term newborns can see objects as far away as 50 cm (2.5 feet). The clearest visual distance is 17 to 20 cm (8 to 12 inches), which is approximately the distance between the mother's and infant's faces during breastfeeding or cuddling. Newborns seem to have a preference for faces and can recognize the mother's face. This facilitates interaction and promotes bonding. They will engage the mother or caregiver with eye contact. Newborns can imitate facial expressions and motions such as protruding the tongue (Gardner & Goldson, 2011). Newborns prefer complex patterns over nonpatterned stimuli. They prefer black and white, possibly because of the greater contrast. Within 2 to 3 months they can discriminate colors (Nugent & Morell, 2011).

Hearing. Term newborns can hear and differentiate among various sounds. They will turn toward a sound and attempt to locate the source. The neonate recognizes and responds readily to the mother's voice and shows a preference for high-pitched intonation. Newborns respond to rhythmic sounds. They are accustomed to hearing the regular rhythm of the mother's heartbeat, which was a constant sound during intrauterine life. As a result they respond by relaxing and ceasing to fuss and cry if a regular heartbeat simulator is placed in their cribs; a lullaby can have the same effect (Nugent & Morell, 2011). Hearing is integral to bonding and attachment and may be more important than vision (Gardner & Goldson, 2011).

Routine hearing screening is recommended for all newborns before hospital discharge. See Chapter 24 for a discussion about screening of newborn hearing.

Smell. Newborns have a highly developed sense of smell and can detect and discriminate distinct odors. It has been shown that preterm infants as early as 28 weeks are capable of reacting to odors. They react to strong odors such as alcohol or vinegar by turning their heads away but are attracted to sweet smells. By the fifth day of life newborn infants can recognize their mother's smell. Breastfed infants are able to smell breast milk and can differentiate their mothers from other lactating women (Lawrence & Lawrence, 2011).

Taste. Young infants are particularly oriented toward the use of their mouths, both for meeting their nutritional needs for rapid growth and for releasing tension through sucking. The early development of circumoral sensation, muscle activity, and taste would seem to be preparation for survival in the extrauterine environment. The newborn can distinguish among tastes and has a preference for sweet solutions (Gardner & Goldson, 2011).

Touch. The infant is responsive to touch on all parts of the body. The face (especially the mouth), the hands, and the soles of the feet seem to be the most sensitive. Reflexes can be elicited by stroking the infant. The newborn's responses to touch suggest that this sensory system is well prepared to receive and process tactile messages (Gardner & Goldson, 2011). Touch and motion are essential to normal growth and development. However, each infant is unique, and variations can be seen in newborns' responses to touch. Birth trauma or stress and depressant drugs taken by the mother decrease the infant's sensitivity to touch or painful stimuli.

Response to Environmental Stimuli

Temperament. Each neonate has a unique repertoire of behaviors that are influenced by various factors including temperament, sensory threshold, ability to habituate, and consolability. Temperament refers to individual variations in the reaction pattern of newborns. Newborns possess individual characteristics that affect selective responses to various stimuli present in the internal and external environments. Some infants appear to be quiet by nature and can remain still for extended periods. Their movements may be smooth and relaxed most of the time, and they have little difficulty settling down for feeding, Other infants are more active and seem to be in constant motion; they seem to be excited and interested in exploring the faces and sounds around them. These infants often need help to settle; containment (swaddling), physical contact, and boundaries surrounding the neonate in the crib can facilitate a quiet alert state (Nugent & Morell, 2011).

Habituation. Habituation is a protective mechanism that allows the infant to become accustomed to environmental stimuli. It is a psychologic and physiologic phenomenon in which the response to a constant or repetitive stimulus is decreased. In the term newborn this can be demonstrated in several ways. Shining a bright light into a newborn's eyes causes a startle or squinting the first two or three times. The third or fourth flash elicits a diminished response, and by the fifth or sixth flash the infant ceases to respond (Brazelton & Nugent, 2011). The same response pattern holds true for the sounds of a rattle or stroking the bottom of the foot.

The ability to habituate allows the healthy term newborn to select stimuli that promote continued learning about the social world, thus avoiding overload. The intrauterine environment seems to have programmed the newborn to be especially responsive to human voices, soft lights, soft sounds, and sweet tastes.

The newborn quickly learns the sounds in the home environment and is able to sleep in their midst. The selective responses of the newborn indicate cerebral organization capable of memory and making choices. The ability to habituate depends on the state of consciousness, hunger, fatigue, and temperament. These factors also affect consolability, cuddliness, irritability, and crying.

Consolability. Newborns vary in the ability to console themselves or be consoled. In the crying state most newborns initiate one of several ways to reduce their distress. Hand-to-mouth movements with or without sucking and being alert to voices, noises, or visual stimuli are common. Some infants are consoled only if they are held and rocked (Brazelton & Nugent, 2011).

Cuddliness. Cuddliness is especially important to parents because they often gauge their ability to care for the child by the child's responses to their actions. The degree to which newborns relax and mold into the contours of the person holding them varies. One extreme is the infant who always resists being held with thrashing and stiffening of the body. This is in contrast to the infant who immediately relaxes when held and molds to the body of the person. Less extreme behavior is demonstrated by infants who are passive when held and those who gradually mold after being held for a while (Brazelton & Nugent, 2011).

Irritability. Some newborns cry longer and harder than others. For some the sensory threshold seems low. They are readily upset by unusual noises, hunger, wetness, or new experiences and thus respond intensely. Others with a high sensory threshold require a great deal more stimulation and variation to reach the active, alert state.

Crying. Crying is the language an infant uses most often to communicate needs. It can signal hunger, discomfort, pain, desire for attention, or fussiness. Infants may cry in response to environmental stimuli such as cold, being overstimulated, or being held by multiple persons. Responsiveness of the caregiver to the crying creates trust as the infant learns to associate the caregiver with comfort.

The amount and tone of crying vary based on gestational age, weight, and the reason for the cry (e.g., hunger, pain). A high-pitched cry can be a sign of a neurologic disorder. Some mothers state that they learn to distinguish among the cries. The breastfeeding mother's body responds physiologically to infant crying by stimulating the milk-ejection reflex ("let-down") (Gardner & Goldson, 2011).

The duration of crying also varies greatly in each infant; newborns may cry for as little as 5 minutes or as much as 2 hours or more per day. The amount of crying peaks in the second month and then decreases. There is a diurnal rhythm of crying, with more crying occurring in the evening hours.

KEY POINTS

- By full term the newborn's various anatomic and physiologic systems have reached a level of development and functioning that permits a physical existence apart from the mother.
- The neonate's most critical adaptation to extrauterine life is to establish effective respirations.
- Heat loss in the healthy term newborn can exceed the capacity to produce heat; this can lead to cold stress and metabolic and respiratory complications that threaten the newborn's well-being.
- Physiologic jaundice occurs in 60% of term infants and 80% of preterm infants.
- Jaundice is considered pathologic if it appears within the first 24 hours of life, if serum bilirubin levels increase by more than 6 mg/dl in 24 hours, or if serum bilirubin exceeds 15 mg/dl at any time.
- Some reflex behaviors are important for the newborn's survival.
- The healthy newborn has sensory abilities that indicate a state of readiness for social interaction. Sleep-wake states and other factors influence the newborn's behavior.
- Newborn behavior progresses from self-regulation of autonomic processes to social interaction.
- Each full-term newborn has a predisposed capacity to handle the multitude of stimuli in the external world.

REFERENCES

Abu-Shaweesh, J. M. (2011). Respiratory disorders in preterm and term infants. In R. J. Martin, A. A. Fanaroff, & M. C. Walsh (Eds.), *Fanaroff & Martin's neonatal-perinatal medicine* (9th ed.). St. Louis: Mosby.

American Academy of Pediatrics (AAP). (2013). Statement of endorsement: Timing of umbilical cord clamping after birth. *Pediatrics, 131*(4), e1323.

American Academy of Pediatrics (AAP) Subcommittee on Hyperbilirubinemia. (2004). Clinical practice guideline: Management of hyperbilirubinemia in the newborn infant 35 or more weeks of gestation. *Pediatrics, 114*(1), 297–316.

American College of Obstetricians and Gynecologists Committee on Obstetric Practice. (2012). Committee opinion no. 543: Timing of umbilical cord clamping after birth. *Obstetrics and Gynecology, 120*(6), 1522–1526.

Andersson, O., Hellström-Westas, L., Andersson, D., & Domellöf, M. (2011). Effect of delayed versus early umbilical cord clamping on neonatal outcomes and iron status at 4 months: A randomised controlled trial. *British Medical Journal, 343*, 1–12.

Association of Women's Health, Obstetric and Neonatal Nurses (AWHONN). (2013). *Neonatal skin care* (3rd ed.). Washington, DC: Author.

Baker, R. D., Greer, F. R., & the Committee on Nutrition. (2010). Diagnosis and prevention of iron deficiency and iron-deficiency anemia in infants and young children (0-3 years of age). *Pediatrics, 126*(5), 1040–1050.

Barksdale, E. M., Chwals, W. J., Magnuson, D. K., & Parry, R. L. (2011). Selected gastrointestinal anomalies. In R. J. Martin, A. A. Fanaroff, & M. C. Walsh (Eds.), *Fanaroff & Martin's neonatal-perinatal medicine* (9th ed.). St. Louis: Mosby.

Blackburn, S. T. (2013). *Maternal, fetal, and neonatal physiology* (4th ed.). St. Louis: Mosby.

Bodin, M. B. (2014). Immune system. In C. Kenner, & J. W. Lott (Eds.). *Comprehensive neonatal nursing care* (5th ed.). New York: Springer.

Bonifacio, S. L., Gonzalez, F., & Ferriero, D. M. (2012). Central nervous system injury and neuroprotection. In C. A. Gleason, & S. U. Devaskar (Eds.), *Avery's diseases of the newborn* (9th ed.). Philadelphia: Elsevier Saunders.

Brazelton, T., & Nugent, J. (2011). *Neonatal behavioral assessment scale* (4th ed.). London: MacKeith.

Brown, V. D., & Landers, S. (2011). Heat balance. In S. L. Gardner, B. S. Carter, M. Enzman-Hines, & J. A. Hernandez (Eds.), *Merenstein & Gardner's handbook of neonatal intensive care* (7th ed.). St. Louis: Mosby.

Cooperman, D. R., & Thompson, G. H. (2011). Musculoskeletal disorders. In R. J. Martin, A. A. Fanaroff, & M. C. Walsh (Eds.), *Fanaroff & Martin's neonatal-perinatal medicine* (9th ed.). St. Louis: Mosby.

Dell, K. M. (2011). Fluids, electrolytes, and acid-base homeostasis. In R. J. Martin, A. A. Fanaroff, & M. C. Walsh (Eds.), *Fanaroff & Martin's neonatal-perinatal medicine* (9th ed.). St. Louis: Mosby.

Desmond, M., Rudolph, A., & Phitaksphraiwan, P. (1966). The transitional care nursery: A mechanism for preventive medicine in the newborn. *Pediatric Clinics of North America, 13*(3), 651–668.

Fanaroff, A. A., & Fanaroff, J. M. (2012). Clinical examination. In S. M. Dunn, & S. K. Sinha (Eds.), *Manual of neonatal respiratory care* (3rd ed.). Philadelphia: Springer Science & Business Media.

Gardner, S. L., & Goldson, E. (2011). The neonate and the environment: Impact on development. In S. L. Gardner, B. S. Carter, M. Enzman-Hines, & J. A. Hernandez (Eds.), *Merenstein & Gardner's handbook of neonatal intensive care* (7th ed.). St Louis: Mosby.

Gardner, S. L., & Hernandez, J. A. (2011). Initial nursery care. In S. L. Gardner, B. S. Carter, M. Enzman-Hines, & J. A. Hernandez (Eds.), *Merenstein & Gardner's handbook of neonatal intensive care* (7th ed.). St Louis: Mosby.

Gardner, S. L., & Lawrence, R. A. (2011). Breast feeding the neonate with special needs. In S. L. Gardner, B. S. Carter, M. Enzman-Hines, & J. A. Hernandez (Eds.), *Merenstein & Gardner's handbook of neonatal intensive care* (7th ed.). St. Louis: Mosby.

Goldsmith, J. P. (2011). Delivery room resuscitation of the newborn. In R. J. Martin, A. A. Fanaroff, & M. C. Walsh (Eds.), *Fanaroff & Martin's neonatal-perinatal medicine* (9th ed.). St. Louis: Mosby.

Hillman, N. H., Kallapur, S. G., & Jobe, A. H. (2012). Physiology of transition from intrauterine to extrauterine life. *Clinics in Perinatology, 39*(4), 769–783.

Hoath, S. B., & Narendran, V. (2011). The skin. In R. J. Martin, A. A. Fanaroff, & M. C. Walsh (Eds.), *Fanaroff & Martin's neonatal-perinatal medicine* (9th ed.). St. Louis: Mosby.

Hoyt, M. R. (2011). Anesthetic options for labor and delivery. In R. J. Martin, A. A. Fanaroff, & M. C. Walsh (Eds.), *Fanaroff & Martin's neonatal-perinatal medicine* (9th ed.). St. Louis: Mosby.

Janke, J. (2014). Newborn nutrition. In K. R. Simpson, & P. A. Creehan (Eds.), *Perinatal nursing* (4th ed.). Philadelphia: Wolters Kluwer/Lippincott Williams & Wilkins.

Kalhan, S. C., & Devaskar, S. U. (2011). Metabolic and endocrine disorders. In R. J. Martin, A. A. Fanaroff, & M. C. Walsh (Eds.), *Fanaroff & Martin's neonatal-perinatal medicine* (9th ed.). St. Louis: Mosby.

Kamath, B. D., Thilo, E. H., & Hernandez, J. A. (2011). Jaundice. In S. L. Gardner, B. S. Carter, M. Enzman-Hines, & J. A. Hernandez (Eds.), *Merenstein & Gardner's handbook of neonatal intensive care* (7th ed.). St Louis: Mosby.

Kaplan, M., Wong, R. J., Sibley, E., & Stevenson, D. K. (2011). Neonatal jaundice and liver disease. In R. J. Martin, A. A. Fanaroff, & M. C. Walsh (Eds.), *Fanaroff & Martin's neonatal-perinatal medicine* (9th ed.). St. Louis: Mosby.

Kapur, R., Yoder, M. C., & Polin, R. A. (2011). Developmental immunology. In R. J. Martin, A. A. Fanaroff, & M. C. Walsh (Eds.), *Fanaroff & Martin's neonatal-perinatal medicine* (9th ed.). St. Louis: Mosby.

Karl, D. J., & Keefer, C. H. (2011). Use of the behavioral observation of the newborn educational trainer for teaching newborn behavior. *Journal of Obstetric, Gynecologic and Neonatal Nursing, 40*(1), 75–83.

Kenney, P. M., Hoover, D., Williams, L. C., & Iskersky, V. (2011). Cardiovascular diseases and surgical interventions. In S. L. Gardner, B. S. Carter, M. Enzman-Hines, & J. A. Hernandez (Eds.), *Merenstein & Gardner's handbook of neonatal intensive care* (7th ed.). St. Louis: Mosby.

Lawrence, R. A., & Lawrence, R. M. (2011). *Breastfeeding: A guide for the medical profession* (7th ed.). St. Louis: Mosby.

Lott, J. W. (2014). Cardiovascular system. In C. Kenner, & J. W. Lott (Eds.), *Comprehensive neonatal care* (5th ed.). New York: Springer.

Luchtman-Jones, L., & Wilson, D. B. (2011). Hematologic problems in the fetus and neonate. In R. J. Martin, A. A. Fanaroff, & M. C. Walsh (Eds.), *Fanaroff & Martin's neonatal-perinatal medicine* (9th ed.). St. Louis: Mosby.

Manco-Johnson, M., Rodden, D. J., & Hays, T. (2011). Newborn hematology. In S. L. Gardner, B. S. Carter, M. Enzman-Hines, & J. A. Hernandez (Eds.), *Merenstein & Gardner's handbook of neonatal intensive care* (7th ed.). St. Louis: Mosby.

Mangurten, H. H., & Puppala, B. L. (2011). Birth injuries. In R. J. Martin, A. A. Fanaroff, & M. C. Walsh (Eds.), *Fanaroff & Martin's neonatal-perinatal medicine* (9th ed.). St. Louis: Mosby.

Morelli, J. G. (2011). Diseases of the neonate. In R. M. Kliegman, B. F. Stanton, J. W. St. Geme, III, et al. (Eds.), *Nelson textbook of pediatrics* (19th ed.). Philadelphia: Elsevier Saunders.

Nugent, J. K., Keefer, C. H., Minear, S., et al. (2007). *Understanding newborn behavior and early relationships: The Newborn Behavioral Observations (NBO) system handbook.*. Baltimore: Brookes Publishing.

Nugent, K., & Morell, A. (2011). *Your baby is speaking to you.* Boston: Houghton Mifflin Harcourt.

Pagana, K. D., & Pagana, T. J. (2011). *Mosby's diagnostic and laboratory test reference* (9th ed.). St. Louis: Mosby.

Püttgen, K. B., & Cohen, B. A. (2012). Cutaneous congenital defects. In C. A. Gleason, & S. U. Devaskar (Eds.), *Avery's diseases of the newborn* (9th ed.). Philadelphia: Elsevier Saunders.

Ringer, S. A. (2013a). Core concepts: Thermoregulation in the newborn part I: Basic mechanisms. *Neoreviews*, *14*(4), c161–c167.

Ringer, S. A. (2013b). Core concepts: Thermoregulation in the newborn part II: Prevention of aberrant body temperature. *Neoreviews*, *14*(5), c221–c226.

Scher, M. S. (2012). Neonatal seizures. In C. A. Gleason, & S. U. Devaskar (Eds.), *Avery's diseases of the newborn* (9th ed.). Philadelphia: Elsevier Saunders.

Sedin, G. (2011). The thermal environment. In R. J. Martin, A. A. Fanaroff, & M. C. Walsh (Eds.), *Fanaroff & Martin's neonatal-perinatal medicine* (9th ed.). St. Louis: Mosby.

Shulman, R. M., Palmert, M. R., & Wherrett, D. K. (2011). Disorders of sex development. In R. J. Martin, A. A. Fanaroff, & M. C. Walsh (Eds.), *Fanaroff & Martin's neonatal-perinatal medicine* (9th ed.). St. Louis: Mosby.

Smith, J. B. (2012). Initial evaluation: History and physical examination of the newborn. In C. A. Gleason, & S. U. Devaskar (Eds.), *Avery's diseases of the newborn* (9th ed.). Philadelphia: Elsevier Saunders.

Soltau, T. D., & Carlo, W. A. (2014). Respiratory system. In C. Kenner, & J. W. Lott (Eds.), *Comprehensive neonatal care* (5th ed.). New York: Springer.

Verklan, M. T., & Lopez, S. M. (2011). Neurologic disorders. In S. L. Gardner, B. S. Carter, M. Enzman-Hines, & J. A. Hernandez (Eds.), *Merenstein & Gardner's handbook of neonatal intensive care* (7th ed.). St Louis: Mosby.

Visscher, M. O., Utturkar, R., Pickens, W. L., et al. (2011). Neonatal skin maturation—vernix caseosa and free amino acids. *Pediatric Dermatology*, *28*(2), 122–132.

Vogt, B. A., & Dell, K. M. (2011). The kidney and urinary tract. In R. J. Martin, A. A. Fanaroff, & M. C. Walsh (Eds.), *Fanaroff & Martin's neonatal-perinatal medicine* (9th ed.). St. Louis: Mosby.

White, K. K., & Goldberg, M. J. (2012). Common neonatal orthopedic ailments. In C. A. Gleason, & S. U. Devaskar (Eds.), *Avery's diseases of the newborn* (9th ed.). Philadelphia: Elsevier Saunders.

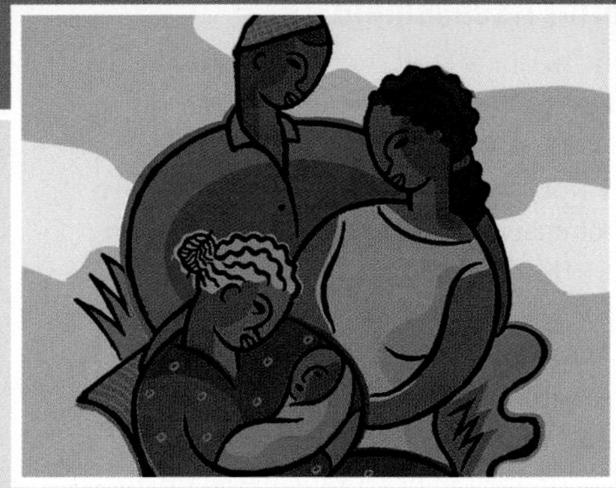

CHAPTER 24

Nursing Care of the Newborn and Family

Kathryn R. Alden

http://evolve.elsevier.com/Lowdermilk/MWHC/

LEARNING OBJECTIVES

- Explain the purpose and components of the Apgar score.
- Describe how to perform a physical assessment of a newborn.
- Describe how to perform a gestational age assessment of a newborn.
- Compare the characteristics of the preterm, late preterm, early term, full term, and postterm neonate.
- Provide nursing care to assist the newborn to transition to extrauterine life.
- Explain the elements of a safe environment.
- Discuss phototherapy and the guidelines for teaching parents about this treatment.
- Explain the purposes and methods for circumcision, the postoperative care of the circumcised infant, and parent teaching regarding circumcision.
- Describe the procedures for administering an intramuscular injection, performing a heelstick, collecting urine specimens, and venipuncture.
- Evaluate pain in the newborn based on physiologic changes and behavioral observations.
- Discuss pharmacologic and nonpharmacologic interventions to reduce neonatal pain.
- Review anticipatory guidance nurses provide to parents before discharge.

Although most infants make the necessary biopsychosocial adjustments to extrauterine existence without undue difficulty, their well-being depends on the care they receive from others. This chapter describes the assessment and care of the infant immediately after birth until discharge from the birth setting, as well as important anticipatory guidance related to ongoing infant care. A discussion of pain in the neonate and its management is included.

CARE MANAGEMENT: BIRTH THROUGH THE FIRST 2 HOURS

Care begins immediately after birth and focuses on assessing and stabilizing the newborn's condition. The nurse has the primary responsibility for the infant during this period because the physician or nurse-midwife is involved with care of the mother. The nurse must be alert for any signs of distress and initiate appropriate interventions.

The foundation for providing comprehensive, family-centered newborn care is awareness of the mother's preconception and prenatal history as well as intrapartal events. Recognition of risk factors (Box 24-1) enables the nurse to be more astute in observations and assessments and more likely to identify early signs of complications. This allows for earlier intervention and promotes positive outcomes.

SAFETY ALERT

With the possibility of transmission of viruses such as hepatitis B virus (HBV) and human immunodeficiency virus (HIV) through maternal blood and blood-stained amniotic fluid, the newborn must be considered a potential contamination source until proved otherwise. As part of Standard Precautions, nurses wear gloves when handling the newborn until blood and amniotic fluid are removed by bathing.

Immediate Care after Birth

The primary goal of care in the first moments after birth is to assist the newly born infant to transition to extrauterine life by establishing effective respirations. If the infant is at term, is crying or breathing, and has good muscle tone, routine care can begin (Kattwinkel, Perlman, Aziz, et al., 2010). The infant is placed prone skin-to-skin on the mother's abdomen or chest, and the nurse assesses the airway. Slight extension of the neck helps keep the airway patent. Drying the infant with vigorous rubbing removes moisture to prevent evaporative heat loss and provides tactile stimulation to stimulate respiratory effort. The mother and her newborn are covered with a warm blanket and a cap is placed on the infant's head (Niermeyer & Clarke, 2011).

The newborn should be breathing spontaneously. The trunk and lips should be pink; acrocyanosis is a normal finding (see Fig. 23-4) (Niermeyer & Clarke, 2011). If the neonate is apneic or has gasping respirations, positive-pressure ventilation is needed.

The heart rate is quickly assessed by grasping the base of the cord or by auscultating the left chest with a stethoscope. The nurse counts for 6 seconds and multiplies by 10 to calculate the heart rate. It should be greater than 100 beats/minute. If the newborn requires respiratory or circulatory support, the nurse and other members of the health care team (e.g., neonatologist, respiratory therapist) follow the American Heart Association guidelines for neonatal resuscitation (Kattwinkel et al., 2010). The neonatal resuscitation algorithm directs the care (Fig. 24-1).

As soon as possible after birth, the nurse places identically numbered bands on the infant's wrist and ankle, on the mother, and on the father or significant other. An electronic infant security tag or abduction system alarm should be placed on all newborns to aid in protecting against infant abduction. The infant is footprinted with ink or a scanning device within 2 hours of birth. (See later discussion of infant abduction.)

BOX 24-1 Assessment of Preconception, Prenatal, and Intrapartum Risk Factors

Preconception
- Age
- Preexisting medical conditions: diabetes, hypertension, cardiac disease, anemia, thyroid disorder, renal disease, obesity
- Genetic factors: family history
- Obstetric history: gravidity, parity, number of living children and their ages, history of stillbirth, previous infant with congenital anomalies, habitual abortion, use of assisted reproductive technology, interpregnancy spacing
- Blood type and Rh status

Prenatal
- Prenatal care: when started
- Nutrition: weight gain, diet, obesity, eating disorders
- Health-compromising behaviors: smoking, alcohol use, substance abuse
- Blood group or Rh sensitization
- Medications: prescription, over-the-counter, and complementary and alternative medications
- History of infection: sexually transmitted infections, TORCH* infections, group B streptococcus status

Intrapartum
- Length of gestation: preterm, late preterm, early term, term, or postterm
- First stage of labor: length, electronic fetal monitoring—internal or external, rupture of membranes (time, presence of meconium), signs of fetal distress (decelerations)
- Group B streptococcus status: treatment during labor
- Second stage of labor: length, vaginal or cesarean, instrument assisted—forceps or vacuum extractor, complications (shoulder dystocia, bleeding [abruptio placentae or placenta previa]), cord prolapse, maternal analgesia and/or anesthesia

*TORCH is the collective name for *t*oxoplasmosis, *o*ther infections (e.g., hepatitis), *r*ubella virus, *c*ytomegalovirus (CMV), and *h*erpes simplex virus.

Adapted from Hurst, H.M. (2015). Antepartum-intrapartum complications. In T.M. Verklan & M. Walden (Eds.), *Core curriculum for neonatal intensive care nursing* (5th ed.). St. Louis: Saunders.

Apgar Scoring and Initial Assessment

The initial assessment of the neonate is performed immediately after birth using the Apgar score (Table 24-1) and a brief physical examination (Table 24-2). A gestational age assessment is completed within the first hours of birth in a stable newborn (Fig. 24-2). A more comprehensive physical assessment is completed within 24 hours of birth (Table 24-3).

Apgar Score

The Apgar score permits a rapid assessment of the newborn's transition to extrauterine life based on five signs that indicate the physiologic state of the neonate: (1) heart rate, based on auscultation with a stethoscope or palpation of the umbilical cord; (2) respiratory effort, based on observed movement of the chest wall; (3) muscle tone, based on degree of flexion and movement of the extremities; (4) reflex irritability, based on response to suctioning of the nares or nasopharynx; and (5) generalized skin color, described as pallid, cyanotic, or pink (see Table 24-1). Evaluations are made at 1 and 5 minutes after birth and can be completed by the nurse or birth attendant. Scores of 0 to 3 indicate severe distress, scores of 4 to 6 indicate moderate difficulty, and scores of 7 to 10 indicate that the infant is having minimal or no difficulty adjusting to extrauterine life. Apgar scores do not predict future neurologic outcome but are useful for describing the newborn's transition to the extrauterine environment and the need for resuscitation (Box 24-2). If resuscitation is required, it should be initiated before the 1-minute Apgar score is determined (American College of Obstetricians and Gynecologists [ACOG] Committee on Obstetric Practice, 2010).

Initial Physical Assessment

The initial examination of the newborn (see Table 24-2) can occur while the nurse is drying and wrapping the infant, or observations can be made while the infant is lying on the mother's abdomen or in her arms immediately after birth. Efforts should be directed toward minimizing interference in the initial parent-infant acquaintance process. If the infant is breathing effectively, is pink, and has no apparent life-threatening anomalies or risk factors requiring immediate attention (e.g., infant of a mother with diabetes), further examination can be delayed until after the parents have had an opportunity to interact with the infant. Routine procedures and the admission process can be carried out in the mother's room or in a separate nursery.

Physical Assessment

Although the initial assessment after birth can reveal significant anomalies, birth injuries, and cardiopulmonary problems that have immediate implications, a more detailed, thorough physical examination should follow within 24 hours after birth (see Table 24-3). The parents' presence during this and other examinations encourages discussion of their concerns and actively involves them in the health care of their infant from birth. It also affords the nurse an opportunity to observe parental interactions with the infant. The findings provide a database for implementing the nursing process with newborns and providing anticipatory guidance for the parents. Ongoing assessments are made throughout the hospital stay; another detailed physical examination is performed before discharge.

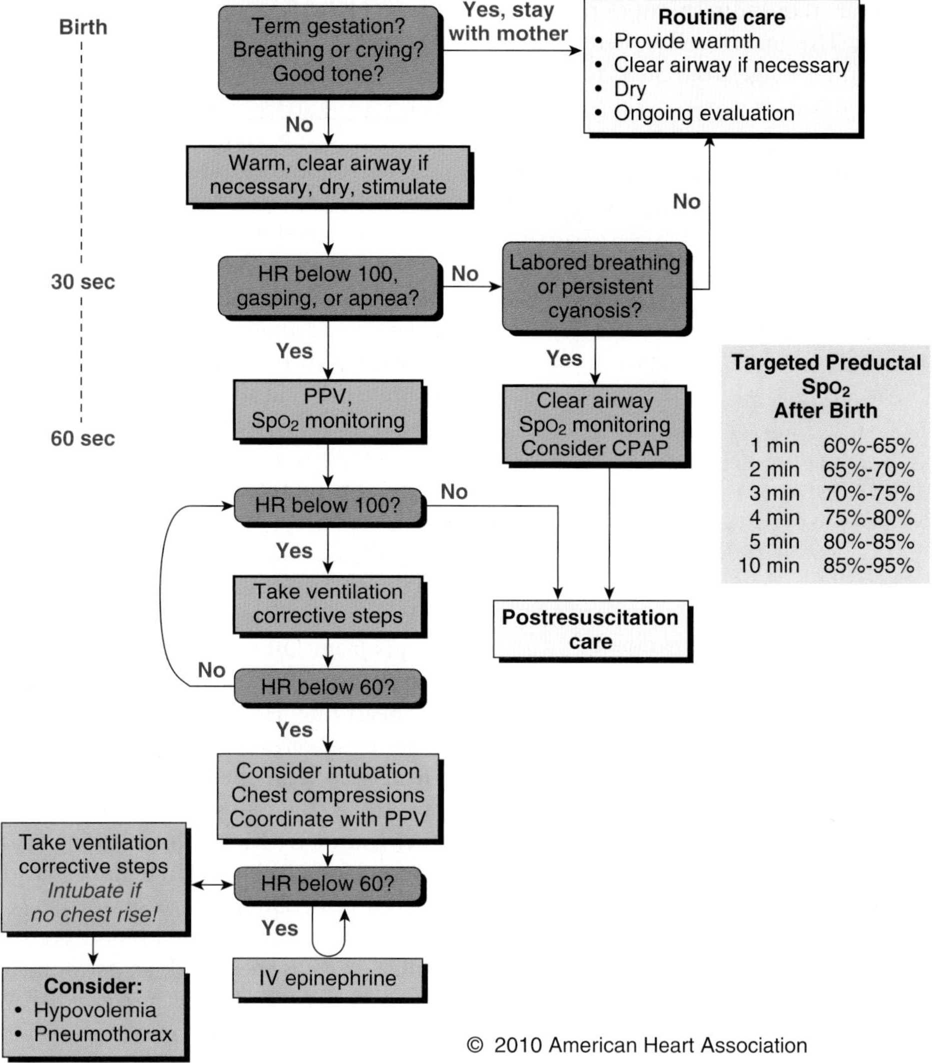

FIG 24-1 Neonatal resuscitation algorithm. *CPAP,* Continuous positive airway pressure; *HR,* heart rate; *IV,* intravenous; *PPV,* positive-pressure ventilation; *Spo₂,* blood oxygen saturation. (From Kattwinkel, J., Perlman, J.M., Aziz, K., et al. [2010]. Part 15: Neonatal resuscitation: 2010 American Heart Association guidelines for cardiopulmonary resuscitation and emergency cardiovascular care. *Circulation, 122*[Suppl 3], S909-S919. Reprinted with permission of the American Heart Association.)

TABLE 24-1 Apgar Score

SIGN	SCORE 0	1	2
Heart rate	Absent	Slow (<100/min)	>100/min
Respiratory effort	Absent	Slow, weak cry	Good cry
Muscle tone	Flaccid	Some flexion of extremities	Well flexed
Reflex irritability	No response	Grimace	Cry
Color	Blue, pale	Body pink, extremities blue	Completely pink

General Appearance

The neonate's maturity level can be gauged by assessing general appearance. Features to assess in the general survey include posture, activity, any overt signs of anomalies that can cause initial distress, presence of bruising or other birth trauma, and state of alertness. The normal resting position of the neonate is one of general flexion.

Vital Signs

The temperature, heart rate, and respiratory rate are always obtained. Blood pressure (BP) is not routinely assessed unless cardiac problems are suspected. An irregular, very slow, or very fast heart rate can indicate a need for further evaluation of circulatory status including BP measurement.

The axillary temperature is a safe, accurate measurement of temperature. Electronic thermometers have expedited this task and provide a reading within 1 minute. Temporal artery, tympanic, and oral routes for measuring temperature in the newborn are not considered accurate (Brown & Landers, 2011). Taking an infant's temperature can cause the infant to cry and struggle against the placement of the thermometer in the axilla. Before taking the temperature, the examiner can determine the apical heart rate and respiratory rate while the infant is quiet and at rest. The normal axillary temperature averages 37° C (98.6° F), with a range from 36.5° to 37.5° C (97.7° to 99.5° F).

SAFETY ALERT

Rectal temperatures should not be done on a newborn because of the risk for perforation.

TABLE 24-2 Initial Physical Assessment of the Newborn

General appearance	☐ Color pink ☐ Acrocyanosis present ☐ Flexed posture ☐ Alert ☐ Active
Respiratory system	☐ Airway patent ☐ No upper airway congestion ☐ No retractions or nasal flaring ☐ Respiratory rate, 30-60 breaths/min ☐ Lungs clear to auscultation bilaterally ☐ Chest expansion symmetric
Cardiovascular system	☐ Heart rate >100 beats/min; strong and regular ☐ No murmurs heard ☐ Pulses strong and equal bilaterally
Neurologic system	☐ Moves extremities ☐ Normotonic ☐ Symmetric features, movement Reflexes present: ☐ Sucking ☐ Rooting ☐ Moro ☐ Grasp ☐ Anterior fontanel soft and flat
Gastrointestinal system	☐ Abdomen soft, no distention ☐ Cord attached and clamped ☐ Anus appears patent
Eyes, nose, mouth	☐ Eyes clear ☐ Palate intact ☐ Nares patent
Skin	☐ No signs of birth trauma ☐ No lesions or abrasions
Genitourinary system	☐ Normal genitalia
Other	☐ No obvious anomalies
Comments:	

The respiratory rate varies with the state of alertness and activity after birth. Respirations are abdominal in nature and can be counted by observing or lightly feeling the rise and fall of the abdomen. Neonatal respirations are shallow and irregular. The respirations should be counted for a full minute to obtain an accurate count because there are periods when respirations can cease for seconds (≤20) and resume again. The examiner should also observe for symmetry of chest movement. The average respiratory rate is 40 breaths/minute but will vary between 30 and 60 breaths/minute; respiratory rate can exceed 60 breaths/minute if the newborn is very active or crying.

An apical pulse rate should be obtained on all newborns. Auscultation should be for a full minute, preferably when the infant is asleep or in a quiet alert state. The infant may need to be held and comforted during assessment. The normal heart rate ranges from 110 to 160 beats/minute when the infant is awake (Blackburn, 2013). It is common to detect brief irregularities in the heart rate. Heart rate varies with the newborn's behavioral state. Bradycardia is a heart rate less than 100 beats/minute. However, a term infant in deep sleep can have a heart rate in the 80s or 90s; the rate should increase when the infant awakens. Tachycardia is a heart rate exceeding 160 beats/minute. It is not unusual for a crying infant to have a heart rate greater than 160; the heart rate should decrease when the crying ceases.

Assessment of neonatal blood pressure is based on agency policy. If BP is measured, an oscillometric monitor calibrated for neonatal pressures is preferred. An appropriate-size cuff (width-to-arm or width-to-calf ratio of 0.45 to 0.70, or approximately ½ to ¾) is essential for accuracy. Neonatal BP usually is highest immediately after birth and falls to a minimum by 3 hours after birth. It then begins to rise steadily and reaches a plateau between 4 and 6 days after birth. This measurement is usually equal to that of the immediate postbirth BP. The BP varies with the neonate's activity; accurate measurement is best obtained while the newborn is at rest. Blood pressure varies with gestational age and chronologic age. Systolic pressure in a term neonate averages 60 to 80 mm Hg; diastolic pressure averages 40 to 50 mm Hg. The mean arterial pressure should approximate

BOX 24-2 Significance of the Apgar Score

The Apgar score was developed to provide a rapid systematic method of assessing an infant's condition at birth. When used correctly it is useful for standardized assessment and provides a mechanism to document the neonate's transition after birth. It is designed to be used for a limited time frame. Apgar scores are affected by factors such as gestational age, maternal medications, trauma, congenital anomalies, hypovolemia, and hypoxia.

Researchers have tried to correlate Apgar scores with various outcomes in the term infant such as intelligence and neurologic development. In some instances researchers have attempted to attribute causality to the Apgar score, that is, to suggest that the low Apgar score caused or predicted later problems. This use of the Apgar score is inappropriate.

There is a lack of evidence regarding the significance of the Apgar score in preterm infants. It should be used with this population of infants only for ongoing assessment in the delivery room.

The Apgar score is a useful index for monitoring neonatal response to resuscitation, especially in regard to a change in the score from 1 minute to 5 minutes after birth. However, assigning an Apgar score to a neonate during resuscitation is not equivalent to assigning a score to a newborn who is breathing spontaneously. It is important that health care professionals be consistent in assigning Apgar scores during a resuscitation.

Adapted from American College of Obstetricians and Gynecologists (ACOG) Committee on Obstetric Practice & American Academy of Pediatrics Committee on Fetus and Newborn. (2010). Committee opinion no. 333: The Apgar score. *Obstetrics and Gynecology, 107*(5), 1209–1212.

the neonate's week of gestation. According to agency protocol, four extremity blood pressures may be assessed routinely or only when a murmur is auscultated. If the upper extremity systolic pressures are more than 15 mm Hg greater than those in the lower extremities, the infant may have a cardiac defect such as coarctation of the aorta (Kenney, Hoover, Williams, & Iskersky, 2011). Peripheral pulses are also palpated as part of the assessment in any infant with a heart murmur.

Baseline Measurements of Physical Growth

Baseline measurements are taken and recorded to help assess the progress and determine the growth patterns of the neonate. These measurements may be recorded on growth charts. The following measurements are made when the neonate is assessed.

Weight. The newborn is usually weighed shortly after birth. This assessment is performed in the labor and birthing area, the mother's room, or in the nursery. Care must be taken to ensure that the scales are balanced. The totally unclothed neonate is placed in the center of the scale, which is usually covered with a disposable pad or cloth to prevent heat loss via conduction and to prevent cross-infection. The nurse should place one hand over (but not touching) the neonate to be prepared to prevent the infant from falling off the scales. Weighing the infant at the same time every day is common during the hospital stay. Birth weight of a term infant typically ranges from 2500 to 4000 g (5.5 to 8.8 lb).

Head Circumference and Body Length. The head is measured at the widest part, which is the occipitofrontal diameter. The tape measure is placed around the head just above the infant's eyebrows. The term neonate's head circumference ranges from 32 to 36.8 cm (12.6 to 14.5 in.).

The length can be difficult to obtain because of the flexed posture of the newborn. The examiner places the newborn on a flat surface and extends the leg until the knee is flat against the surface. Placing the head against a perpendicular surface and extending the leg can assist with obtaining this measurement. In the term neonate, head-to-heel length ranges from 45 to 55 cm (17.7 to 21.7 in.).

Neurologic Assessment

The physical examination includes a neurologic assessment of newborn reflexes (see Table 23-4). This assessment provides useful information about the infant's nervous system and state of neurologic maturation. Many reflex behaviors (e.g., sucking, rooting) are important for proper development. Other reflexes such as gagging and sneezing act as primitive safety mechanisms. The assessment needs to be carried out as early as possible because abnormal signs in the early neonatal period can require further investigation before the newborn is discharged home.

Gestational Age Assessment

Assessment of gestational age is important because perinatal morbidity and mortality rates are related to gestational age and birth weight. A frequently used method of determining gestational age is the New Ballard Score, which can be used to measure gestational ages of infants as young as 20 weeks of gestation (see Fig. 24-2). It assesses six external physical and six neuromuscular signs. Each sign has a numeric score, and the cumulative score correlates with a maturity rating (gestational age). The examination of infants with a gestational age of 26 weeks or less should be performed at a postnatal age of less than 12 hours. For infants with a gestational age of at least 26 weeks, the examination can be performed up to 96 hours after birth. To ensure accuracy, experts recommend that the initial examination is performed within the first 48 hours of life. Neuromuscular adjustments after birth in extremely immature neonates require a follow-up examination to further validate neuromuscular criteria (Ballard, Khoury, Wedig, et al., 1991). Box 24-3 highlights specific maneuvers used in gestational age assessment.

Classification of Newborns by Gestational Age and Birth Weight

Classification of infants at birth by both birth weight and gestational age provides a more satisfactory method for predicting mortality risks and providing guidelines for management of the neonate than estimating gestational age or birth weight alone. The infant's birth weight, length, and head circumference are plotted on standardized graphs that identify normal values for gestational age. A normal range of birth weights exists for each gestational week (see Fig. 24-2, *B*).

The infant whose weight is appropriate for gestational age (AGA) (between the 10th and 90th percentiles) can be presumed to have grown at a normal rate regardless of the length of gestation—preterm, term, or postterm. The infant who is large for gestational age (LGA) (more than the 90th percentile) can be presumed to have grown at an accelerated rate during fetal life; the small for gestational age (SGA) infant (less than the 10th percentile) can be presumed to have grown at a restricted rate during intrauterine life. When gestational age is determined according to the New Ballard Score, the newborn will fall into one of the following nine possible categories for birth weight and gestational age: AGA—term, preterm, postterm; SGA—term, preterm, postterm; or LGA—term, preterm, postterm. Birth weight influences mortality: the lower the birth weight, the higher the mortality. The same is true for gestational age: the lower the gestational age, the higher the mortality (Gardner & Hernandez, 2011).

Infants may also be classified in the following ways according to gestation (ACOG Committee on Obstetric Practice & Society for Maternal-Fetal Medicine, 2013):

- **Preterm,** *or premature*—born before completion of 37 weeks of gestation, regardless of birth weight
- **Late preterm**—34 0/7 through 36 6/7 weeks
- **Early term**—37 0/7 through 38 6/7 weeks
- **Full term**— 39 0/7 through 40 6/7 weeks
- **Late term**—41 0/7 through 41 6/7 weeks
- **Postterm**—42 0/7 weeks and beyond
- **Postmature**—born after completion of week 42 of gestation and showing the effects of progressive placental insufficiency

Early Term Infant

"Early term" (37 0/7 through 38 6/7 weeks) is a recent addition to the categories describing newborns according to gestational age. In 2011, 25.86% of births were considered early term (Martin, Hamilton, Ventura, et al., 2013). A recent increase in the number of early term infants is associated with elective inductions and elective cesarean births that are scheduled before 39 weeks. Compared with full-term infants, early term infants are at greater

ESTIMATION OF GESTATIONAL AGE BY MATURITY RATING

NEUROMUSCULAR MATURITY

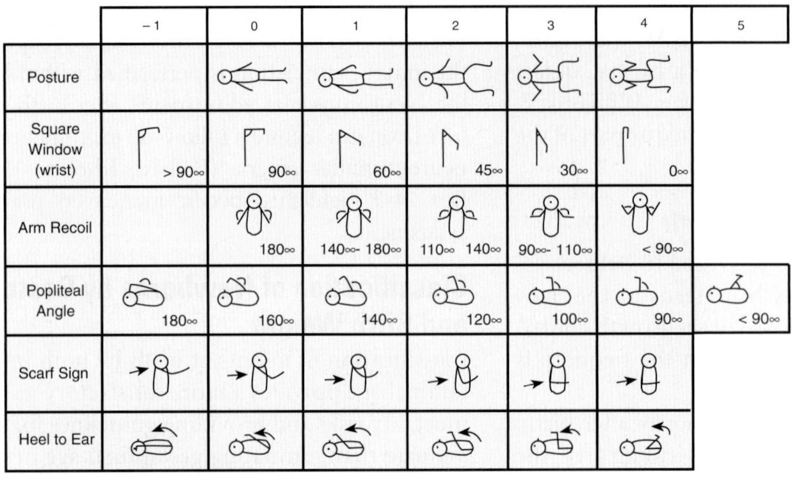

	-1	0	1	2	3	4	5
Posture							
Square Window (wrist)	> 90°	90°	60°	45°	30°	0°	
Arm Recoil		180°	140°- 180°	110° 140°	90°- 110°	< 90°	
Popliteal Angle	180°	160°	140°	120°	100°	90°	< 90°
Scarf Sign							
Heel to Ear							

PHYSICAL MATURITY

Skin	sticky, friable, transparent	gelatinous red, translucent	smooth pink, visible veins	superficial peeling &/or rash, few veins	cracking, pale areas, rare veins	parchment, deep cracking, no vessels	leathery, cracked, wrinkled
Lanugo	none	sparse	abundant	thinning	bald areas	mostly bald	
Plantar Surface	heel-toe 40-50 mm: -1 <40 mm: -2	>50 mm no crease	faint red marks	anterior transverse crease only	creases ant. 2/3	creases over entire sole	
Breast	imperceptible	barely perceptible	flat areola no bud	stippled areola 1-2 mm bud	raised areola 3-4 mm bud	full areola 5-10 mm bud	
Eye/Ear	lids fused loosely: -1 tightly: -2	lids open, pinna flat, stays folded	slightly curved pinna, soft, slow recoil	well-curved pinna, soft but ready recoil	formed & firm, instant recoil	thick cartilage, ear stiff	
Genitals (male)	scrotum flat, smooth	scrotum empty, faint rugae	testes in upper canal, rare rugae	testes descending, few rugae	testes down, good rugae	testes pendulous, deep rugae	
Genitals (female)	clitoris prominent, labia flat	prominent clitoris, small labia minora	prominent clitoris, enlarging minora	majora & minora equally prominent	majora large, minora small	majora cover clitoris & minora	

MATURITY RATING

score	weeks
-10	20
-5	22
0	24
5	26
10	28
15	30
20	32
25	34
30	36
35	38
40	40
45	42
50	44

A

FIG 24-2 Estimation of gestational age. **A,** New Ballard score for newborn maturity rating. Expanded scale includes extremely premature infants and has been refined to improve accuracy in more mature infants.

risk for short- and long-term health problems. Early term birth is associated with higher risk of hypoglycemia, respiratory problems such as respiratory distress syndrome and transient tachypnea of the newborn (TTNB), and a greater likelihood of NICU admission (Sengupta, Carrion, Shelton, et al., 2013). These infants are also at increased risk for long-term problems such as learning difficulties (e.g., attention deficit hyperactivity disorder [ADHD]) (Lindstrom, Lindblad, & Hjern, 2011). Early term infants have higher neonatal, postnatal, and infant mortality rates (Reddy, Bettegowda, Dias, et al., 2011). Nurses and other health care providers need to be aware of the vulnerability of this population of neonates and monitor them closely (Craighead, 2012).

Late Preterm Infant

The rate of preterm birth in the United States was 11.73% in 2011. The majority of preterm births are considered late preterm, occurring between $34\frac{0}{7}$ and $36\frac{6}{7}$ weeks of gestation. These late preterm infants account for 8.28% of all births (Martin et al., 2013). Elective vaginal and cesarean births before 39 weeks have contributed significantly to late preterm birth rates in the United States.

Late preterm infants have been called "the great impostors" because they are often the size and weight of term infants and are often treated as healthy newborns. Despite their appearance as term infants, late preterm infants are at increased risk for respiratory distress, temperature instability, hypoglycemia, apnea, feeding difficulties, and hyperbilirubinemia. Nurses and health care providers must be cognizant of the risk factors for late preterm infants and be continually vigilant for the development of problems related to the infant's immaturity (Phillips, Goldstein, Hougland, et al., 2013). In an effort to identify these infants, a gestational age assessment should be performed on all newborns soon after birth (Cooper, Holditch-Davis, Verklan, et al., 2012). The late preterm infant's care is further addressed in Chapter 34.

Text continued on p. 565

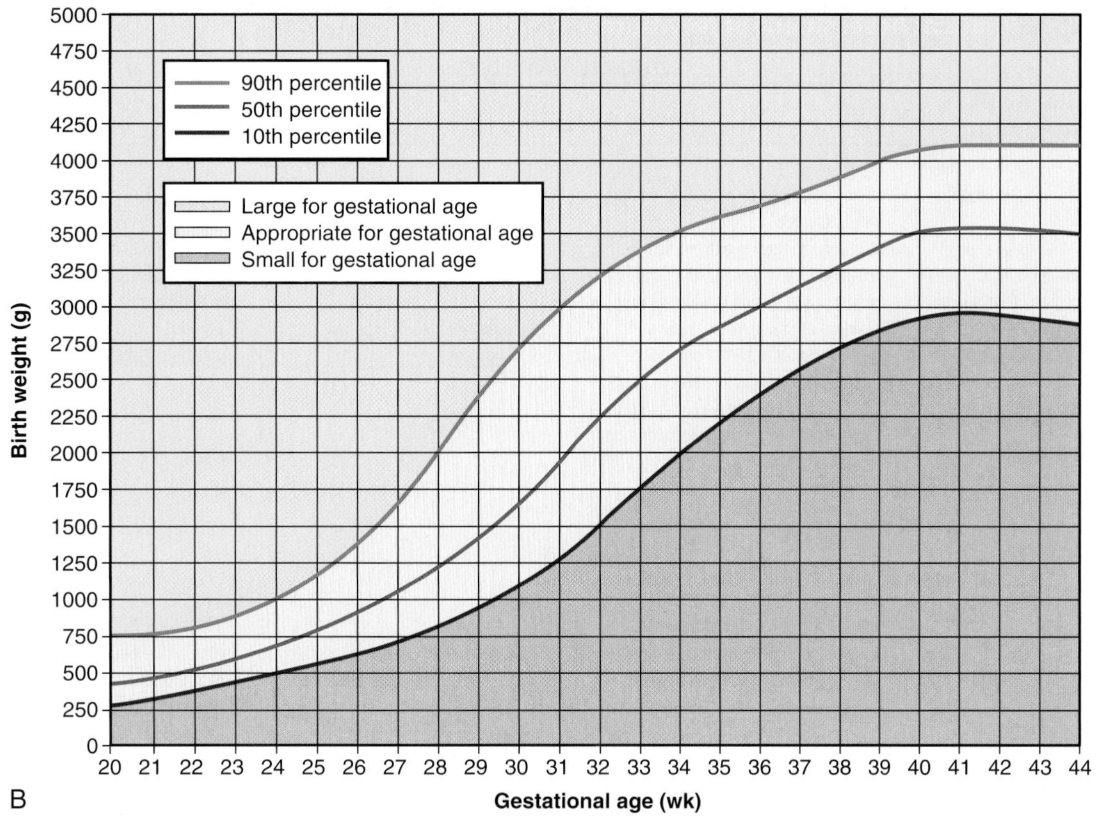

FIG 24-2, cont'd B, Intrauterine growth: birth weight percentiles based on live single births at gestational ages 20 to 44 weeks. (**A,** From Ballard, J., Khoury, J., Wedig, K., et al. [1991]. New Ballard score, expanded to include extremely premature infants. *Journal of Pediatrics, 119*[3], 417-423.)

BOX 24-3 Maneuvers Used in Assessing Gestational Age

Posture

With infant quiet and in a supine position, observe degree of flexion in arms and legs. Muscle tone and degree of flexion increase with maturity. Full flexion of the arms and legs = score 4.*

Square Window

With thumb supporting back of arm below wrist, apply gentle pressure with index and third fingers on dorsum of hand without rotating infant's wrist. Measure angle between base of thumb and forearm. Full flexion (hand lies flat on ventral surface of forearm) = score 4.*

Arm Recoil

With infant supine, fully flex both forearms on upper arms and hold for 5 seconds; pull down on hands to extend fully, and rapidly release arms. Observe rapidity and intensity of recoil to a state of flexion. A brisk return to full flexion = score 4.*

Popliteal Angle

With infant supine and pelvis flat on a firm surface, flex lower leg on thigh and then flex thigh on abdomen. While holding knee with thumb and index finger, extend lower leg with index finger of other hand. Measure degree of angle behind knee (popliteal angle). An angle of less than 90 degrees = score 5.*

Scarf Sign

With infant supine, support head in midline with one hand; use other hand to pull infant's arm across the shoulder so that infant's hand touches shoulder. Determine location of elbow in relation to midline. Elbow does not reach midline = score 4.*

Heel to Ear

With infant supine and pelvis flat on a firm surface, pull foot as far as possible (without using force) up toward ear on same side. Measure distance of foot from ear and degree of knee flexion (same as popliteal angle). Knees flexed with a popliteal angle of less than 10 degrees = score 4.*

*See Fig. 24-2 for scale and interpretation of scores.

From Hockenberry, M.J., & Wilson, D. (2015). *Wong's nursing care of infants and children* (10th ed.). St. Louis: Mosby.

TABLE 24-3 Physical Assessment of Newborn

AREA ASSESSED AND APPRAISAL PROCEDURE	NORMAL FINDINGS		DEVIATIONS FROM NORMAL RANGE: POSSIBLE PROBLEMS (ETIOLOGY)
	AVERAGE FINDINGS	NORMAL VARIATIONS	
Posture			
Inspect newborn before disturbing for assessment Refer to maternal chart for fetal presentation, position, and type of birth (vaginal, surgical), given that newborn readily assumes in utero position	Vertex: arms, legs in moderate flexion; fists clenched Resistance to having extremities extended for examination or measurement, crying possible when attempted Cessation of crying when allowed to resume curled-up fetal position (lateral) Normal spontaneous movement bilaterally asynchronous (legs moving in bicycle fashion) but equal extension in all extremities	Frank breech: legs straighter and stiff, newborn assuming intrauterine position in repose for a few days Prenatal pressure on limb or shoulder possibly causing temporary facial asymmetry or resistance to extension of extremities	Hypotonia, relaxed posture while awake (preterm or hypoxia in utero, maternal medications, neuromuscular disorder such as spinal muscular atrophy) Hypertonia (chemical dependence, central nervous system [CNS] disorder) Limitation of motion in any of extremities
Vital Signs			
Check heart rate and pulses:			
Thorax (chest)			
Inspection	Visible pulsations in left midclavicular line, fifth intercostal space		
Palpation	Apical pulse, fourth intercostal space 110-160 beats/min when awake	80-100 beats/min (sleeping) to 180 beats/min (crying); possibly irregular for brief periods, especially after crying	Tachycardia: persistent, ≥180 beats/min (respiratory distress syndrome [RDS]; pneumonia) Bradycardia: persistent, ≤80 beats/min (congenital heart block, maternal lupus)
Auscultation Apex: mitral valve Second interspace, left of sternum: pulmonic valve Second interspace, right of sternum: aortic valve Junction of xiphoid process and sternum: tricuspid valve	Quality: *first sound* (closure of mitral and tricuspid valves) and *second sound* (closure of aortic and pulmonic valves) sharp and clear	Murmur, especially over base or at left sternal border in interspace 3 or 4 (foramen ovale anatomically closing at approximately 1 yr)	Murmur (possibly functional) Dysrhythmias: irregular rate Sounds: Distant (pneumopericardium) Poor quality Extra Heart on right side of chest (dextrocardia, often accompanied by reversal of intestines)
Peripheral pulses: femoral, brachial, popliteal, posterior tibial	Peripheral pulses equal and strong		Weak or absent peripheral pulses (decreased cardiac output, thrombus, possible coarctation of aorta if weak on left and strong on right) Bounding
Assess temperature:			
Axillary: method of choice Temporal and intraauricular thermometers not effective in measuring newborn temperature	Axillary: 37° C (98.6° F) Temperature stabilized by 8-10 hr of age	36.5°-37.5° C (97.7°-100° F) Heat loss: from evaporation, conduction, convection, radiation	Subnormal (preterm birth, infection, low environmental temperature, inadequate clothing, dehydration) Increased (infection, high environmental temperature, excessive clothing, proximity to heating unit or in direct sunshine, chemical dependence, diarrhea and dehydration) Temperature not stabilized by 6-8 hr after birth (if mother received magnesium sulfate, newborn less able to conserve heat by vasoconstriction; maternal analgesics possibly reducing thermal stability in newborn)
Observe and monitor respiratory rate and effort:			
Observe respirations when infant is at rest Observe respiratory effort Count respirations for full minute	40/min Tendency to be shallow and irregular in rate, rhythm, and depth when infant is awake	30-60/min Short periodic breathing episodes and no evidence of respiratory distress or apnea (>20 sec); periodic breathing First period (reactivity): 50-60/min Second period: 50-70/min Stabilization (1-2 days): 30-40/min Crackles (fine)	Apneic episodes: >20 sec (preterm infant: rapid warming or cooling of infant; CNS or blood glucose instability) Bradypnea: <25/min (maternal narcosis from analgesics or anesthetics, birth trauma) Tachypnea: >60/min (RDS, transient tachypnea of the newborn, congenital diaphragmatic hernia)
Auscultate breath sounds	Crackles may be heard after birth No adventitious sounds audible on inspiration and expiration		Breath sounds: Crackles (coarse), rhonchi, wheezing
Listen for sounds audible without stethoscope	Breath sounds: bronchial; loud, clear		Expiratory grunt (narrowing of bronchi) Distress evidenced by nasal flaring, grunting, retractions, labored breathing Stridor (upper airway occlusion)

TABLE 24-3 Physical Assessment of Newborn—cont'd

AREA ASSESSED AND APPRAISAL PROCEDURE	NORMAL FINDINGS: AVERAGE FINDINGS	NORMAL FINDINGS: NORMAL VARIATIONS	DEVIATIONS FROM NORMAL RANGE: POSSIBLE PROBLEMS (ETIOLOGY)
Obtain blood pressure (BP) (usually not done in normal term infant)			
Check oscillometric monitor BP cuff: BP cuff width affects readings, use appropriate-size cuff and palpate brachial, popliteal, or posterior tibial pulse (depending on measurement site)	60-80/40-50 mm Hg (approximate ranges) At birth Systolic: 60-80 mm Hg Diastolic: 40-50 mm Hg At 2 weeks Systolic: 68-88 mm Hg Diastolic: 40-60 mm Hg	Variation with change in activity level: awake, crying, sleeping	Difference between upper and lower extremity pressures (coarctation of aorta) Hypotension (sepsis, hypovolemia) Hypertension (coarctation of aorta, renal involvement, thrombus)
Weight			
Put cloth or paper protective liner in place and adjust scale to 0 g or pounds and ounces Weigh at same time each day Protect newborn from heat loss	Female: 3400 g (7.5 lb) Male: 3500 g (7.7 lb) Regaining of birth weight within first 2 weeks	2500-4000 g (5.5-8.8 lb) Acceptable weight loss: 10% or less in first 3-5 days Second baby weighing more than first (on average)	Weight ≤2500 g (preterm, small for gestational age, rubella syndrome) Weight ≥4000 g (large for gestational age, maternal diabetes, heredity—normal for these parents) Weight loss more than 10% to 15% (growth failure, dehydration); assess breastfeeding success

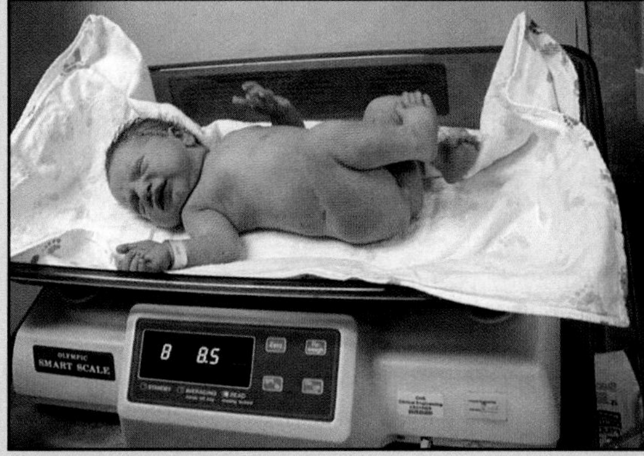

Weighing the infant. The nurse never leaves the infant alone on a scale. The scale is covered to protect against cross-infection. (Courtesy Wendy and Marwood Larson-Harris, Roanoke, VA.)

AREA ASSESSED AND APPRAISAL PROCEDURE	NORMAL FINDINGS: AVERAGE FINDINGS	NORMAL FINDINGS: NORMAL VARIATIONS	DEVIATIONS FROM NORMAL RANGE: POSSIBLE PROBLEMS (ETIOLOGY)
Length			
Measure length from top of head to heel; measuring is difficult in term infant because of presence of molding, incomplete extension of knees	50 cm (19.7 in)	45-55 cm (17.7-21.7 in)	<45 cm (17.7 in) or >55 cm (21.7 in) (chromosomal abnormality, heredity—normal for these parents); some syndromes present shorter than average limb length (skeletal dysplasias, achondroplasia)

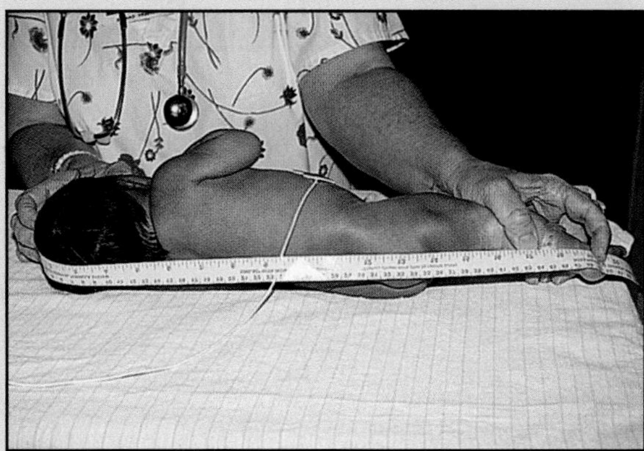

Measuring length crown to heel. To determine total length, include length of legs. If measurements are taken before the infant's initial bath, wear gloves. (Courtesy Marjorie Pyle, RNC, Lifecircle, Costa Mesa, CA.)

Continued

TABLE 24-3 Physical Assessment of Newborn—cont'd

AREA ASSESSED AND APPRAISAL PROCEDURE	NORMAL FINDINGS: AVERAGE FINDINGS	NORMAL FINDINGS: NORMAL VARIATIONS	DEVIATIONS FROM NORMAL RANGE: POSSIBLE PROBLEMS (ETIOLOGY)
Head Circumference			
Measure head at greatest diameter: occipitofrontal circumference May need to remeasure on second or third day after resolution of molding and caput succedaneum	33-35 cm (13-13.8 in) Circumference of head and chest approximately the same for first 1 or 2 days after birth; chest rarely measured on routine basis	32-36.8 cm (12.6-14.5 in)	Microcephaly, head ≤32 cm: (maternal rubella, toxoplasmosis, cytomegalovirus, fused cranial sutures [craniosynostosis]) Hydrocephaly: sutures widely separated, circumference ≥4 cm more than chest circumference (infection) Increased intracranial pressure (hemorrhage, space-occupying lesion)
	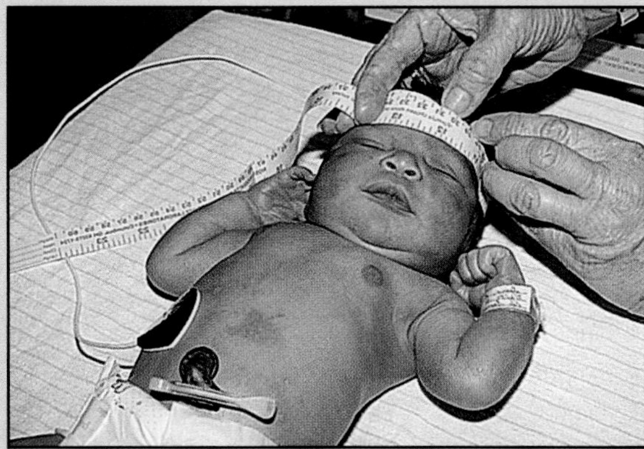 Measuring head circumference. (Courtesy Marjorie Pyle, RNC, Lifecircle, Costa Mesa, CA.)		
Chest Circumference			
Measure at nipple line	2-3 cm (0.8-1.2 in) less than head circumference; average 30-33 cm (11.8-13 in)	≤30 cm	Prematurity
	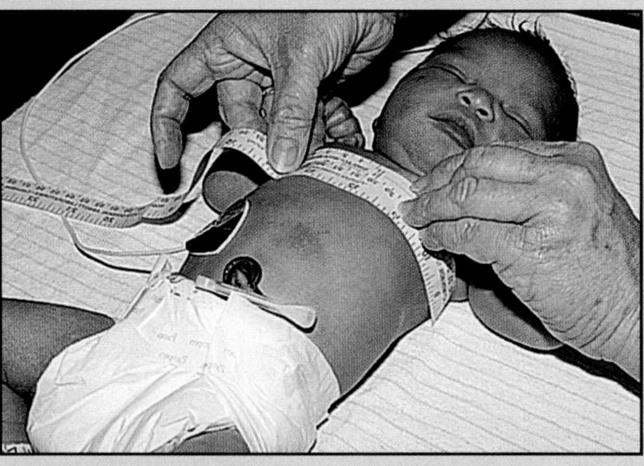 Measuring chest circumference. (Courtesy Marjorie Pyle, RNC, Lifecircle, Costa Mesa, CA.)		
Skin			
Check color Inspect and palpate Inspect semi-naked newborn in well-lighted, warm area without drafts; natural daylight best Inspect newborn when quiet and alert	Generally pink Varies with ethnic origin, skin pigmentation beginning to deepen right after birth in basal layer of epidermis Acrocyanosis common after birth	Mottling Harlequin sign Plethora Telangiectases ("stork bites" or capillary hemangiomas) (see Fig. 23-6, *A*) Erythema toxicum/neonatorum ("newborn rash") (see Fig. 23-6, *B*) Milia Petechiae over presenting part Ecchymoses from forceps in vertex births or over buttocks, genitalia, and legs in breech births	Dark red (preterm, polycythemia) Gray (hypotension, poor perfusion) Pallor (cardiovascular problem, CNS damage, blood dyscrasia, blood loss, twin-to-twin transfusion, infection) Cyanosis (hypothermia, infection, hypoglycemia, cardiopulmonary diseases, neurologic or respiratory malformations) Generalized petechiae (clotting factor deficiency, infection) Generalized ecchymoses (hemorrhagic disease)
Observe for jaundice	None at birth	Physiologic jaundice in up to 60% of term infants in first week of life	Jaundice within first 24 hr (increased hemolysis, Rh isoimmunization, ABO incompatibility)

TABLE 24-3 Physical Assessment of Newborn—cont'd

AREA ASSESSED AND APPRAISAL PROCEDURE	NORMAL FINDINGS: AVERAGE FINDINGS	NORMAL FINDINGS: NORMAL VARIATIONS	DEVIATIONS FROM NORMAL RANGE: POSSIBLE PROBLEMS (ETIOLOGY)
Observe for birthmarks or bruises: Inspect and palpate for location, size, distribution, characteristics, color, if obstructing airway or oral cavity		Mongolian spot (see Fig. 23-5) in infants of African-American, Asian, and Native-American origin	Hemangiomas Nevus flammeus: port-wine stain Nevus vasculosus: strawberry mark Cavernous hemangioma
Check skin condition: Inspect and palpate for intactness, smoothness, texture, edema, pressure points if ill or immobilized	Edema confined to eyelid (result of eye prophylaxis) Opacity: few large blood vessels visible indistinctly over abdomen	Slightly thick; superficial cracking, peeling, especially of hands, feet No visible blood vessels, a few large vessels clearly visible over abdomen Some fingernail scratches	Edema on hands, feet; pitting over tibia; periorbital (overhydration; hydrops) Texture thin, smooth, or of medium thickness; rash or superficial peeling visible (preterm, postterm) Numerous vessels very visible over abdomen (preterm) Texture thick, parchment-like; cracking, peeling (postterm) Skin tags, webbing Papules, pustules, vesicles, ulcers, maceration (impetigo, candidiasis, herpes, diaper rash)
Weigh infant routinely	Dehydration: loss of weight best indicator	Normal weight loss after birth: up to 10% of birth weight	
Gently pinch skin between thumb and forefinger over abdomen and inner thigh to check for turgor	After pinch released, skin returns to original state immediately		Loose, wrinkled skin (prematurity, postmaturity, dehydration: fold of skin persisting after release of pinch) Tense, tight, shiny skin (edema, extreme cold, shock, infection)
Note presence of subcutaneous fat deposits (adipose pads) over cheeks, buttocks		Variation in amount of subcutaneous fat	Lack of subcutaneous fat, prominence of clavicle or ribs (preterm, malnutrition)
Check for vernix caseosa: Observe color, amount, and odor before bath	Whitish, cheesy, odorless	Usually more found in creases, folds	Absent or minimal (postmature infant) Abundant (preterm) Green color (possible in utero release of meconium or presence of bilirubin) Odor (possible intrauterine infection)
Assess lanugo: Inspect for this fine, downy hair, amount and distribution	Over shoulders, pinnae of ears, forehead	Variation in amount	Absent (postmature) Abundant (preterm, especially if lanugo abundant, long, and thick over back)
Head			
Palpate skin	(See "Skin")	Caput succedaneum, possibly showing some ecchymosis (see Fig. 23-10, *A*)	Cephalhematoma (see Fig. 23-10, *B*) Subgaleal hemorrhage (see Fig. 23-10 *C*)
Inspect shape, size	Making up one fourth of body length Molding (see Fig. 23-9)	Slight asymmetry from intrauterine position Lack of molding (preterm, breech presentation, cesarean birth)	Severe molding (birth trauma) Indentation (fracture from trauma)
Palpate, inspect, and note size and status of fontanels (open vs. closed)	Anterior fontanel 5-cm diamond, increasing as molding resolves Posterior fontanel triangle, smaller than anterior	Variation in fontanel size with degree of molding Difficulty in feeling fontanels possible because of molding	Fontanels: Full, bulging (tumor, hemorrhage, infection) Large, flat, soft (malnutrition, hydrocephaly, delayed bone age, hypothyroidism) Depressed (dehydration)
Palpate sutures	Palpable and separated sutures	Possible overlap of sutures with molding	Sutures: Widely spaced (hydrocephaly) Premature closure (fused) (craniosynostosis)
Inspect pattern, distribution, amount of hair; feel texture	Silky, single strands lying flat; growth pattern toward face and neck	Variation in amount	Fine, wooly (preterm) Unusual swirls, patterns, or hairline; or coarse, brittle (endocrine or genetic disorders)
Eyes			
Check placement on face	Eyes and space between eyes each one third the distance from inner to outer canthus	Epicanthal folds: characteristic in some ethnicities	Epicanthal folds when present with other signs (chromosomal disorders such as Down, cri du chat syndromes)

Continued

TABLE 24-3 Physical Assessment of Newborn—cont'd

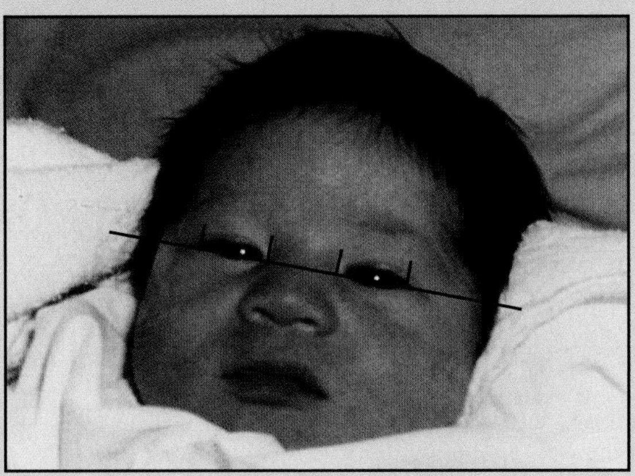

Eyes. In pseudostrabismus, inner epicanthal folds cause the eyes to appear misaligned; however, corneal light reflexes are perfectly symmetric. Eyes are symmetric in size and shape and are well placed.

AREA ASSESSED AND APPRAISAL PROCEDURE	NORMAL FINDINGS: AVERAGE FINDINGS	NORMAL FINDINGS: NORMAL VARIATIONS	DEVIATIONS FROM NORMAL RANGE: POSSIBLE PROBLEMS (ETIOLOGY)
Check for symmetry in size, shape	Symmetric in size, shape		
Check eyelids for size, movement, blink	Blink reflex	Edema if eye prophylaxis drops or ointment instilled	
Assess for discharge	None No tears	Some discharge if silver nitrate used Occasional presence of tears	Discharge: purulent (infection) Chemical conjunctivitis from eye medication is common—requires no treatment
Evaluate eyeballs for presence, size, shape	Both present and of equal size, both round, firm	Subconjunctival hemorrhage	Agenesis or absence of one or both eyeballs Lens opacity or absence of red reflex (congenital cataracts, possibly from rubella, retinoblastoma [cat's-eye reflex]) Lesions: coloboma, absence of part of iris (congenital) Pink color of iris (albinism) Jaundiced sclera (hyperbilirubinemia)
Check pupils	Present, equal in size, reactive to light		Pupils: unequal, constricted, dilated, fixed (intracranial pressure, medications, tumor)
Evaluate eyeball movement	Random, jerky, uneven, focus possible briefly, following to midline	Transient strabismus or nystagmus until third or fourth month	Persistent strabismus Doll's eyes (increased intracranial pressure) Sunset (increased intracranial pressure)
Assess eyebrows: amount of hair, pattern	Distinct (not connected in midline)		Connection in midline (Cornelia de Lange syndrome)
Nose			
Observe shape, placement, patency, configuration	Midline Some mucus but no drainage Preferential nose breather Sneezing to clear nose	Slight deformity (flat or deviated to one side) from passage through birth canal	Copious drainage (rarely congenital syphilis); blockage membranous or bone with cyanosis at rest and return of pink color with crying (choanal atresia) Malformed (congenital syphilis, chromosomal disorder) Flaring of nares (respiratory distress)
Ears			
Observe size, placement on head, amount of cartilage, open auditory canal	Correct placement line drawn through inner and outer canthi of eyes reaching to top notch of ears (at junction with scalp) Well-formed, firm cartilage	Size: small, large, floppy Darwin tubercle (nodule on posterior helix)	Agenesis Lack of cartilage (preterm) Low placement (chromosomal disorder, intellectual disability, kidney disorder) Preauricular tag or sinus Size: possibly overly prominent or protruding ears

TABLE 24-3 **Physical Assessment of Newborn—cont'd**

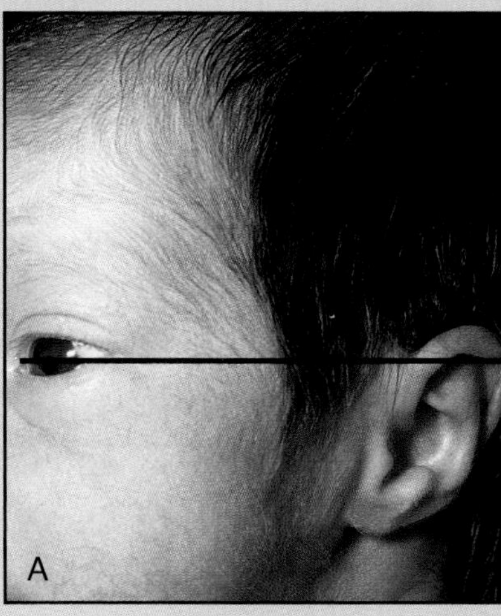

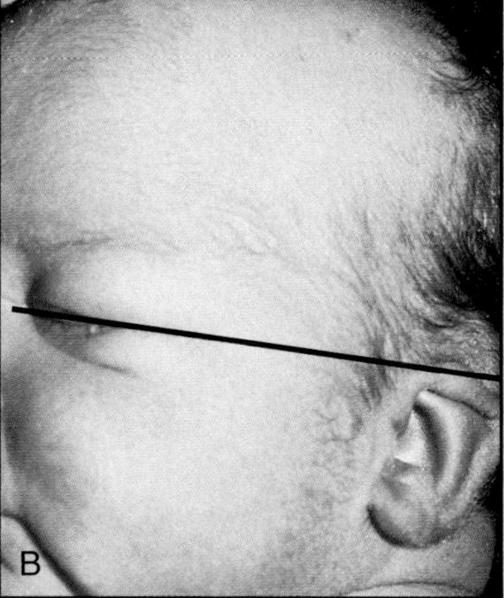

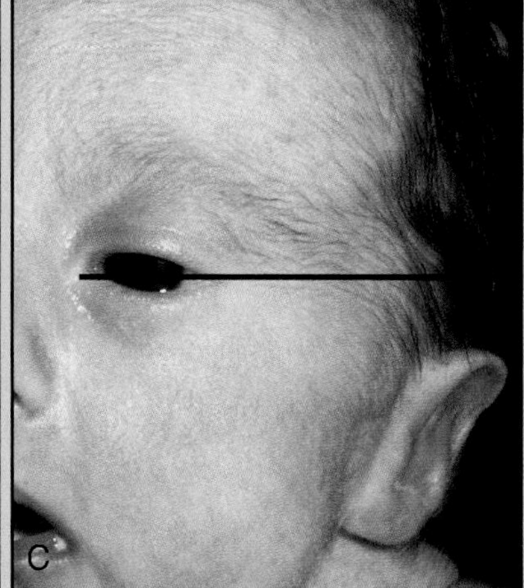

Placement of ears on the head in relation to a line drawn from the inner to the outer canthus of the eye. **A,** Normal position. **B,** Abnormally angled ear. **C,** True low-set ear. (Courtesy Mead Johnson Nutritionals, Evansville, IN.)

AREA ASSESSED AND APPRAISAL PROCEDURE	NORMAL FINDINGS: AVERAGE FINDINGS	NORMAL FINDINGS: NORMAL VARIATIONS	DEVIATIONS FROM NORMAL RANGE: POSSIBLE PROBLEMS (ETIOLOGY)
Assess hearing	Responds to voice and other sounds	State (e.g., alert, asleep) influencing response	Lack of response to loud noise should *not* imply deafness
Perform universal newborn hearing screening to identify deficits (see Fig. 24-11)	Both ears pass		One or both ears fail
Facies			
Observe overall appearance and symmetry of face	Rounded and symmetric; influenced by birth type, molding, or both	Positional deformities	Usually accompanied by other features such as low-set ears, other structural disorders (hereditary, chromosomal aberration)
Mouth			
Inspect and palpate Assess buccal mucosa Dry or moist Pink Status intact Assess lips for color, configuration, movement	Symmetry of lip movement	Transient circumoral cyanosis	Gross anomalies in placement, size, shape (cleft lip or palate [or both], gums) Cyanosis, circumoral pallor (respiratory distress, hypothermia) Asymmetry in movement of lips (seventh cranial nerve paralysis)
Check gums	Pink gums	Inclusion cysts (Epstein pearls—Bohn nodules, whitish, hard nodules on gums or roof of mouth)	Teeth: predeciduous or deciduous (hereditary)
Assess tongue for color, mobility, movement, size	Tongue not protruding, freely movable, symmetric in shape, movement Sucking pads inside cheeks	Short lingual frenulum (ankyloglossia)	Macroglossia (preterm, chromosomal disorder) Thrush: white plaques on cheeks or tongue that bleed if touched *(Candida albicans)*
Assess palate (soft, hard): Arch Uvula	Soft and hard palates intact Uvula in midline	Anatomic groove in palate to accommodate nipple, disappearance by 3 to 4 yr of age Epstein pearls	Cleft hard or soft palate
Assess chin	Distinct chin		Micrognathia—recessed chin with prominent overbite (Pierre Robin or other syndrome)
Evaluate saliva for amount, character	Mouth moist, pink		Excessive salivation and choking or turning blue (esophageal atresia, tracheoesophageal fistula)
Check reflexes: Rooting Sucking Extrusion	Reflexes present	Reflex response dependent on state of wakefulness and hunger	Absent (preterm)
Neck			
Inspect and palpate for movement, flexibility, masses, bruising	Short, thick, surrounded by skin folds; no webbing		Webbing (Turner syndrome)

Continued

TABLE 24-3 Physical Assessment of Newborn—cont'd

AREA ASSESSED AND APPRAISAL PROCEDURE	NORMAL FINDINGS: AVERAGE FINDINGS	NORMAL FINDINGS: NORMAL VARIATIONS	DEVIATIONS FROM NORMAL RANGE: POSSIBLE PROBLEMS (ETIOLOGY)
Check sternocleidomastoid muscles, movement and position of head	Head held in midline (sternocleidomastoid muscles equal), no masses Freedom of movement from side to side and flexion and extension, no movement of chin past shoulder	Transient positional deformity apparent when newborn is at rest: passive movement of head possible	Restricted movement, holding of head at angle (torticollis [wryneck], opisthotonos) Absence of head control (preterm birth, Down syndrome, hypotonia [spinal muscular atrophy])
Assess trachea for position and thyroid gland	Thyroid not palpable		Masses (enlarged thyroid) Distended veins (cardiopulmonary disorder) Skin tags
Chest			
Inspect and palpate			
Shape	Almost circular, barrel shaped	Tip of sternum possibly prominent	Bulging of chest, unequal movement (pneumothorax, pneumomediastinum) Malformation (funnel chest—pectus excavatum)
Observe respiratory movements	Symmetric chest movements, chest and abdominal movements synchronized during respirations	Occasional retractions, especially when crying	Retractions with or without respiratory distress (preterm, RDS) Paradoxic breathing
Evaluate clavicles	Clavicles intact		Fracture of clavicle (trauma); crepitus
Assess ribs	Rib cage symmetric, intact; moves with respirations		Poor development of rib cage and musculature (preterm)
Assess nipples for size, placement, number	Nipples prominent, well formed; symmetrically placed		Nipples Supernumerary, along nipple line Malpositioned or widely spaced
Check breast tissue	Breast nodule: approximately 6 mm in term infant	Breast nodule: 3-10 mm Secretion of witch's milk	Lack of breast tissue (preterm)
Auscultate: Heart sounds and rate and breath sounds (see "Vital Signs")			Sounds: bowel sounds may be heard in diaphragmatic hernia (see "Abdomen")
Abdomen			
Inspect and palpate umbilical cord	Two arteries, one vein Whitish gray Definite demarcation between cord and skin, no intestinal structures within cord Dry around base, drying Odorless Cord clamp in place for 24 to 48 hr	Reducible umbilical hernia	One artery (renal anomaly) Meconium stained (intrauterine distress) Bleeding or oozing around cord (hemorrhagic disease) Redness or drainage around cord (infection, possible persistence of urachus) Hernia: herniation of abdominal contents through cord opening (e.g., omphalocele); defect covered with thin, friable membrane, possibly extensive
Inspect size of abdomen and palpate contour	Rounded, prominent, dome shaped because abdominal musculature not fully developed Liver possibly palpable 1-2 cm (0.4-0.8 in) below right costal margin No other masses palpable No distention Few visible veins on abdominal surface	Some diastasis recti (separation) of abdominal musculature	Gastroschisis: herniation of abdominal contents to the side or above the cord, contents not covered by membranous tissue and may include liver Distention at birth: ruptured viscus, genitourinary masses or malformations: hydronephrosis, teratomas, abdominal tumors Mild (overfeeding, high gastrointestinal tract obstruction) Marked (lower gastrointestinal tract obstruction, anorectal malformation, anal stenosis), often with bilious emesis Intermittent or transient (overfeeding) Partial intestinal obstruction (stenosis of bowel) Visible peristalsis (obstruction) Malrotation of bowel or adhesions Sepsis (infection)
Auscultate bowel sounds and note number, amount, and character of stools	Sounds present within minutes after birth in healthy term infant Meconium stool passing within 24-48 hr after birth		Scaphoid, with bowel sounds in chest and severe respiratory distress (congenital diaphragmatic hernia)

TABLE 24-3 **Physical Assessment of Newborn—cont'd**

AREA ASSESSED AND APPRAISAL PROCEDURE	NORMAL FINDINGS: AVERAGE FINDINGS	NORMAL FINDINGS: NORMAL VARIATIONS	DEVIATIONS FROM NORMAL RANGE: POSSIBLE PROBLEMS (ETIOLOGY)
Assess color		Linea nigra possibly apparent and caused by hormone influence during pregnancy	
Observe movement with respiration	Respirations primarily diaphragmatic, abdominal and chest movement synchronous		Decreased or absent abdominal movement with breathing (phrenic nerve palsy, congenital diaphragmatic hernia)
Genitalia			
Female (see Fig. 23-7, A)			
Inspect and palpate			
General appearance		Increased pigmentation caused by pregnancy hormones	Ambiguous genitalia—wide variation (small phallus not well distinguished from enlarged clitoris)
Clitoris	Usually edematous		Virilized female—extremely large clitoris (congenital adrenal hyperplasia)
Labia majora	Usually edematous, covering labia minora in term newborns	Edema and ecchymosis after breech birth Some vernix caseosa between labia possible	
Labia minora	Possible protrusion over labia majora		Enlarged clitoris with urinary meatus on tip, absent scrotum, micropenis, fused labia Stenosed meatus Labia majora widely separated and labia minora prominent (preterm)
Discharge	Smegma	Blood-tinged discharge from pseudo-menstruation caused by pregnancy hormones	Fecal discharge (fistula)
Vagina	Open orifice Mucoid discharge Hymenal/vaginal tag		Absence of vaginal orifice
Urinary meatus	Beneath clitoris, difficult to see		Bladder exstrophy (bladder outside abdominal cavity and turned inside out)
Check urination	Void within 24 hr; voiding 2-6 times per 24 hr for first 1-2 days; voiding 6-8 times per 24 hr by day 4 or 5	Rust-stained urine (uric acid crystals)	No void within first 24 hours (renal agenesis; Potter syndrome)
Male (see Fig. 23-7, B)			
Inspect and palpate			
General appearance		Increased size and pigmentation caused by pregnancy hormones, (wide variation in size of genitalia)	Ambiguous genitalia Micropenis
Penis			
Urinary meatus appearance	Foreskin covers glans (if uncircumcised), meatus at tip of penis		Urinary meatus not on tip of glans penis (hypospadias, epispadias, foreskin may be retracted or absent)
Prepuce (foreskin)—do not forcibly retract foreskin if uncircumcised	Prepuce covering glans penis and not retractable	Prepuce removed if circumcised	Round meatal opening
Scrotum: Rugae (wrinkles)	Large, edematous, pendulous in term infant; covered with rugae	Scrotal edema and ecchymosis if breech birth Hydrocele, small, noncommunicating	Scrotum smooth and testes undescended (preterm, cryptorchidism) Bifid scrotum Hydrocele Inguinal hernia
Testes	Palpable on each side	Bulge palpable in inguinal canal	Undescended (preterm)
Check urination	Voiding within 24 hr, stream adequate; voiding 2-6 times per 24 hr for first 1-2 days; voiding 6-8 times per 24 hr by day 4 or 5	Rust-stained urine (uric acid crystals)	No void in first 24 hr (renal agenesis; Potter syndrome)
Check reflexes:			
Cremasteric	Testes retracted, especially when newborn is chilled		

Continued

TABLE 24-3 **Physical Assessment of Newborn—cont'd**

AREA ASSESSED AND APPRAISAL PROCEDURE	NORMAL FINDINGS: AVERAGE FINDINGS	NORMAL FINDINGS: NORMAL VARIATIONS	DEVIATIONS FROM NORMAL RANGE: POSSIBLE PROBLEMS (ETIOLOGY)
Extremities			
Make a general check: Inspect and palpate Degree of flexion Range of motion Symmetry of motion Muscle tone	Assuming of position maintained in utero Attitude of general flexion Full range of motion, spontaneous movements	Transient positional deformities	Limited motion (malformations) Poor muscle tone (preterm, maternal medications, CNS anomalies)
Check arms and hands: Inspect and palpate Color Intactness Appropriate placement	Longer than legs in newborn period Contours and movements symmetric	Slight tremors sometimes apparent Some acrocyanosis	Asymmetry of movement (fracture/crepitus, brachial nerve trauma, malformations) Asymmetry of contour (malformations, fracture) Amelia or phocomelia (teratogens) Palmar creases Simian line with short, incurved little fingers (Down syndrome)
Count number of fingers	Five on each hand Fist often clenched with thumb under fingers		Webbing of fingers: syndactyly Absence or excess of fingers Strong, rigid flexion; persistent fists; positioning of fists in front of mouth constantly (CNS disorder) Yellowed nailbeds (meconium staining)
Evaluate joints Shoulder Elbow Wrist Fingers	Full range of motion, symmetric contour		Increased tonicity, clonus, prolonged tremors (CNS disorder)
Check reflexes			
Palmar grasp	Infant's fingers tightly flex around examiner's finger when palm is stimulated	May occur spontaneously when sucking	Weak or absent reflexes can indicate CNS depression
Plantar grasp	Infant's toes flex and curl around examiner's finger when sole of foot at base of toes is stimulated		
Check legs and feet: Inspect and palpate Color Intactness Length in relation to arms and body and to each other	Appearance of bowing because lateral muscles more developed than medial muscles	Feet appearing to turn in but can be easily rotated externally, positional defects tending to correct while infant is crying Acrocyanosis	Amelia, phocomelia (chromosomal defect, teratogenic effect) Temperature of one leg differing from that of the other (circulatory deficiency, CNS disorder)
Number of toes	Five on each foot		Webbing, syndactyly (chromosomal defect) Absence or excess of digits (chromosomal defect, familial trait)
Femur Head of femur as legs are flexed and abducted, placement in acetabulum (see Fig. 23-12)	Intact femur		Femoral fracture (difficult breech birth) Developmental dysplasia of the hip (DDH)
Major gluteal folds	Major gluteal folds even		Gluteal folds uneven: DDH
Soles of feet	Soles well lined (or wrinkled) over two thirds of foot in term infants Plantar fat pad giving flat-footed effect		Soles of feet: Few creases (preterm) Covered with creases (postmature) Congenital clubfoot
Evaluate joints Hip Knee Ankle Toes	Full range of motion, symmetric contour		Hypermobility of joints (Down syndrome)
Check reflexes (see Table 23-4)			Asymmetric movement (trauma, CNS disorder)

TABLE 24-3 **Physical Assessment of Newborn—cont'd**

AREA ASSESSED AND APPRAISAL PROCEDURE	NORMAL FINDINGS: AVERAGE FINDINGS	NORMAL FINDINGS: NORMAL VARIATIONS	DEVIATIONS FROM NORMAL RANGE: POSSIBLE PROBLEMS (ETIOLOGY)
Back			
Assess anatomy:			
Inspect and palpate			
Spine	Spine straight and easily flexed Infant able to raise and support head momentarily when prone	Temporary minor positional deformities, correction with passive manipulation	Limitation of movement (fusion or deformity of vertebra) Spina bifida cystica (meningocele, myelomeningocele)
Shoulders Scapulae Iliac crests Base of spine—pilonidal dimple or sinus	Shoulders, scapulae, and iliac crests lining up in same plane		Pigmented nevus with tuft of hair, location anywhere along the spine often associated with spina bifida occulta Sinus (opening to spinal cord)
Check reflexes (spinal related)			
Test trunk incurvation reflex	Trunk flexed and pelvis swings to stimulated side	May not be apparent in first few days but is usually present in 5-6 days	If transverse lesion is present, no response below lesion; absence of response: central nervous system abnormality or CNS depression
Test magnet reflex	Lower limbs extend as pressure applied to feet with legs in semiflexed position	Weak or exaggerated response with breech presentation	Absence: suggestive of CNS damage or malformation
Anus			
Inspect and palpate Placement Patency Test for sphincter response (active "wink" reflex)	One anus with good sphincter tone Passage of meconium within 24 hr after birth Anal "wink" present, anal opening patent	Passage of meconium within 48 hr of birth	Imperforate anus without fistula Rectal atresia and stenosis Absence of anal opening; drainage of fecal material from vagina in female or urinary meatus in male (rectal fistula) or along perineal raphe (midline area between base of penis and anus)—anorectal malformation
Observe for the following: Abdominal distention Passage of meconium from anal opening Fecal drainage from perineum, penis, vagina			
Stools			
Observe frequency, color, consistency	Meconium followed by transitional and soft yellow stool		No stool (obstruction) Frequent watery stools (infection, phototherapy)

Postterm or Postmature Infant

Infants born of a gestation that extends beyond 42 weeks are considered to be postterm, regardless of birth weight. Some infants are appropriate for gestational age, but show the characteristics of progressive placental dysfunction. These infants are labeled as postmature and are likely to have little if any vernix caseosa, absence of lanugo, abundant scalp hair, and long fingernails. The skin is often cracked, parchment-like, and desquamating. A common finding in postmature infants is a wasted physical appearance that reflects intrauterine deprivation. Depletion of subcutaneous fat gives them a thin, elongated appearance. The little vernix caseosa that remains in the skinfolds may be stained deep yellow or green, which is usually an indication of meconium in the amniotic fluid.

There is a significant increase in fetal and neonatal mortality in postmature infants compared with those born at term. They are especially prone to fetal distress associated with the decreasing efficiency of the placenta, macrosomia, and meconium aspiration syndrome. The greatest risk occurs during the stresses of labor and birth, particularly in infants of primigravidas, or women giving birth to their first child. Close surveillance with fetal assessment and possible induction of labor is usually recommended when a pregnancy is postterm.

Immediate Interventions

Changes can occur quickly in newborns immediately after birth. Assessment must be followed by implementing appropriate care.

Airway Maintenance

Generally the healthy term infant born vaginally has little difficulty clearing the airway. Most secretions are moved by gravity and brought by the cough reflex to the oropharynx to be drained or swallowed or wiped away. If the infant has excess mucus in the respiratory tract, the mouth and nasal passages can be gently suctioned with a bulb syringe (see Teaching for Self-Management: Suctioning with a Bulb Syringe and Fig. 24-3). Routine chest percussion and suctioning of healthy term or late preterm infants are avoided; evidence is insufficient to support anything other than gentle nasopharyngeal and oropharyngeal suctioning to clear

NURSING CARE PLAN

The Normal Newborn

NURSING DIAGNOSIS	EXPECTED OUTCOME	NURSING INTERVENTIONS	RATIONALES
Ineffective Airway Clearance related to excess mucus production or improper positioning	Neonate's airway remains patent; breath sounds are clear, and no respiratory distress is evident.	Assess respiration and auscultate lungs. Observe for signs of respiratory distress.	To identify potential problems with blocked airway
		Teach parents that gagging, coughing, and sneezing are normal neonatal responses.	To assist neonate in clearing airways
		Teach parents feeding techniques that prevent overfeeding and distention of abdomen and to burp neonate frequently.	To prevent regurgitation and aspiration
		Position neonate on back when sleeping.	To prevent suffocation
		Suction mouth and nasopharynx with bulb syringe as needed; clean nares of crusted secretions.	To clear airway and prevent aspiration and airway obstruction
		Teach parents how to use bulb syringe and how to relieve airway obstruction.	To clear airway
Risk for Imbalanced Body Temperature related to larger body surface relative to mass	Neonate's temperature remains in range of 36.5° to 37.5° C (97.7° to 99.5° F).	Maintain neutral thermal environment.	To identify any changes in neonate's temperature that may be related to other causes
		Monitor neonate's axillary temperature frequently.	To identify any changes promptly and to prevent hypothermia and cold stress
		Bathe neonate efficiently when temperature is stable, using warm water, drying carefully, and avoiding exposing neonate to drafts.	To avoid heat loss from evaporation and convection
		Report any alterations in temperature findings promptly.	To assess for signs of infection or hypoglycemia and facilitate prompt treatment
Risk for Infection related to immature immunologic defenses and environmental exposure	Neonate will be free from signs of infection.	Review maternal record for evidence of any risk factors.	To ascertain whether neonate is predisposed to infection
		Monitor temperature and other vital signs.	To identify early possible evidence of infection, especially temperature instability
		Have all care providers, including parents, perform proper hand hygiene before handling newborn.	To protect newborn from infection
		Provide prescribed eye prophylaxis.	To prevent infection
		Keep genital area clean and dry using proper cleansing techniques.	To prevent skin irritation, cross-contamination, and infection
		Keep umbilical stump clean and dry.	To promote drying and to minimize chance of infection
		If infant is circumcised, keep site clean and apply diaper loosely.	To prevent infection and trauma
		Teach parents to keep neonate away from crowds and environmental irritants.	To reduce potential sources of infection
Risk for Injury related to sole dependence on caregiver	Neonate remains free of injury.	Monitor environment for hazards such as sharp objects (e.g., long fingernails, caregiver's jewelry).	To prevent injury
		Handle neonate gently and support head, ensure use of car seat by parents, teach parents to avoid placing neonate on high surfaces unsupervised, and to supervise pet and sibling interactions with neonate.	To prevent injury
		Assess neonate frequently for any evidence of jaundice, and teach parents to monitor for jaundice.	To identify rising bilirubin levels, treat promptly, and prevent complications such as acute bilirubin encephalopathy and kernicterus

NURSING CARE PLAN—cont'd

The Normal Newborn

NURSING DIAGNOSIS	EXPECTED OUTCOME	NURSING INTERVENTIONS	RATIONALES
Readiness for Enhanced Family Coping related to anticipatory guidance regarding responses to neonate's crying	Parents will verbalize their understanding of methods of coping with neonate's crying and describe increased success in interpreting neonate's cries.	Alert parents to crying as neonate's form of communication and that cries can be differentiated to indicate hunger, wetness, pain, and loneliness.	To provide reassurance that crying is not indicative of neonate's rejection of parents and that parents will learn to interpret different cries of their child
		Teach parents normal patterns of infant crying and alert them to the danger of shaking a baby.	To provide anticipatory guidance and to prevent injury to the infant
		Differentiate self-consoling behaviors from fussing or crying.	To give parents concrete examples of interventions
		Discuss methods of consoling the crying neonate, such as changing diapers, talking softly to neonate, holding neonate's arms close to body, swaddling, picking neonate up, rocking, using pacifier, feeding, or burping.	To provide anticipatory guidance and promote parental confidence

secretions. The nurse should auscultate the infant's chest with a stethoscope to determine if crackles or inspiratory stridor is present. Fine crackles may be auscultated for several hours after birth, especially in neonates born by cesarean. If the bulb syringe does not clear mucus interfering with respiratory effort, mechanical suction may be used.

TEACHING FOR SELF-MANAGEMENT

Suctioning with a Bulb Syringe

- The bulb syringe should always be kept in the infant's crib.
- The mouth is suctioned first to prevent the infant from inhaling pharyngeal secretions by gasping as the nares are touched.
- The bulb is compressed (see Fig. 24-3) and the tip is inserted into one side of the mouth. The center of the infant's mouth is avoided because the gag reflex can be stimulated.
- The nasal passages are suctioned one nostril at a time.
- When the infant's cry does not sound as though it is through mucus or a bubble, suctioning can be stopped.

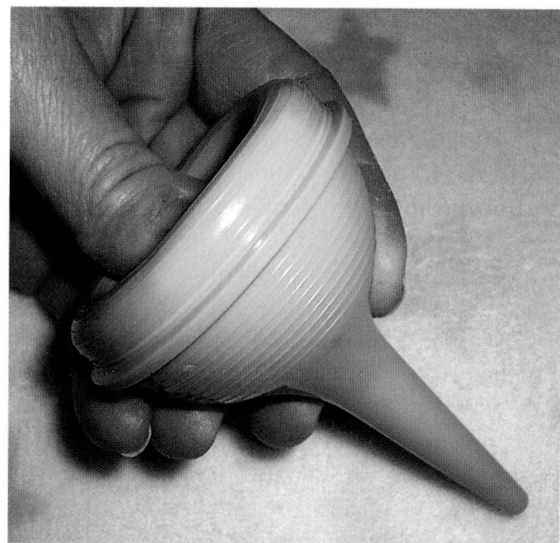

FIG 24-3 Bulb syringe. Bulb is compressed before inserting tip into mouth. (Courtesy Cheryl Briggs, RNC, Annapolis, MD.)

If the newborn has an obstruction that is not cleared with suctioning, the neonatal or pediatric care provider should be notified. Further investigation must occur to determine if a mechanical defect (e.g., tracheoesophageal fistula or choanal atresia [see Chapter 36]) is causing the obstruction.

Deeper suctioning may be needed to remove mucus from the newborn's nasopharynx or posterior oropharynx. However, this type of suctioning should be performed only after an assessment of the risks involved.

Maintaining an Adequate Oxygen Supply

Four conditions are essential for maintaining an adequate oxygen supply:

- A clear airway
- Effective establishment of respirations
- Adequate circulation, adequate perfusion, and effective cardiac function
- Adequate thermoregulation

Newborns who encounter respiratory problems are likely to exhibit signs and symptoms that indicate some degree of distress. Preterm infants are at greatest risk for respiratory distress (see the Signs of Potential Complications box; see also Chapter 34).

SIGNS OF POTENTIAL COMPLICATIONS

Abnormal Newborn Breathing

- Bradypnea (≤30 respirations/min)
- Tachypnea (≥60 respirations/min)
- Abnormal breath sounds: coarse or fine crackles, wheezes, expiratory grunt
- Respiratory distress: nasal flaring, retractions, stridor, gasping, chin tug
- Seesaw or paradoxical respirations
- Skin color: cyanosis, mottling
- Pulse oximetry value: <95%

Maintaining Body Temperature

Effective neonatal care includes maintenance of a neutral thermal environment (see Chapter 23). Cold stress increases the need for oxygen and can deplete glucose stores. The infant can react to exposure to cold by increasing the respiratory rate and can become cyanotic.

The ideal method for promoting warmth and maintaining neonatal body temperature is early skin-to-skin contact (SSC) with the mother. The naked infant is placed prone directly on the mother's chest; both mother and infant are then covered with a warm blanket and a cap is placed on the infant's head. Early SSC has distinct short- and long-term benefits including temperature stabilization, reduced crying, improved breastfeeding initiation and duration, and maternal attachment (Moore, Anderson, Bergman, & Dowswell, 2012). Other interventions to promote warmth include drying and wrapping the newborn in warmed blankets immediately after birth, keeping the head well covered, and keeping the ambient temperature of the nursery or mother's room at 22° to 26° C (72° to 78° F) (American Academy of Pediatrics [AAP] & ACOG, 2012).

If the infant does not remain skin-to-skin with the mother during the first 1 to 2 hours after birth, the nurse places the thoroughly dried infant under a radiant warmer or in a warm incubator until the body temperature stabilizes. The infant's skin temperature is used as the point of control in a warmer with a servo-controlled mechanism. The control panel is usually maintained between 36° and 37° C (96.8° and 98.6° F). This setting should maintain the healthy term newborn's skin temperature at approximately 36.5° to 37° C (97.7° to 98.6° F). A thermistor probe (automatic sensor) is usually placed on the upper quadrant of the abdomen immediately below the right or left costal margin (never over a bone). A reflector adhesive patch can be used over the probe to provide adequate warming. This probe is designed to detect minor temperature changes resulting from external environmental factors or neonatal factors (peripheral vasoconstriction, vasodilation, or increased metabolism) before a dramatic change in core body temperature develops. The servo-controller adjusts the temperature of the warmer to maintain the infant's skin temperature within the preset range. The sensor needs to be checked periodically to make sure it is securely attached to the infant's skin. The axillary temperature of the newborn is checked every hour (or more often as needed) until the newborn's temperature stabilizes. The length of time to stabilize and maintain body temperature varies; each newborn should therefore be allowed to achieve thermal regulation as necessary, and care should be individualized.

During all procedures, heat loss must be avoided or minimized for the newborn; therefore, examinations and activities are performed with the newborn under a heat panel. The initial bath is postponed until the newborn's skin temperature is stable and can adjust to heat loss from a bath. Even a healthy term infant can become hypothermic. Inadequate drying and wrapping immediately after birth, a cold birthing room, or birth in a car on the way to the hospital can cause the newborn's temperature to fall below the normal range (hypothermia). The hypothermic infant should be warmed gradually because rapid warming can cause apneic spells and acidosis. Therefore, the warming process is monitored to progress slowly over 2 to 4 hours.

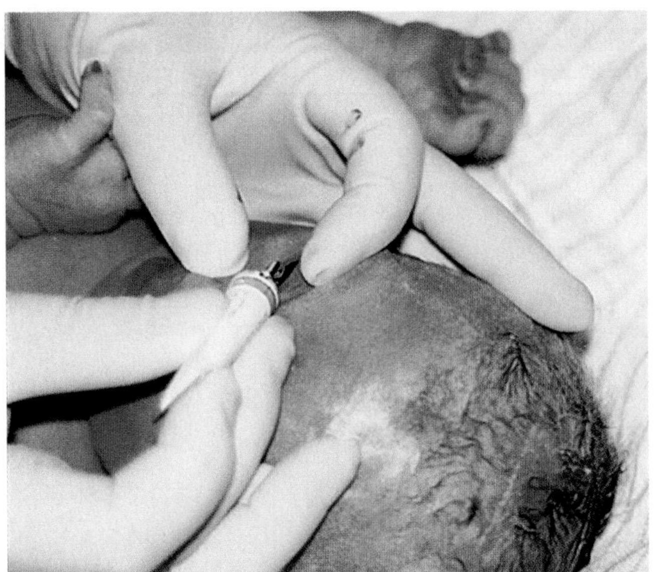

FIG 24-4 Instillation of medication into eye of newborn. Thumb and forefinger are used to open the eye; medication is placed in the lower conjunctiva from the inner to the outer canthus. (Courtesy Marjorie Pyle, Lifecircle, Costa Mesa, CA.)

Eye Prophylaxis

The U.S. Preventive Services Task Force (USPSTF, 2011) and the Canadian Paediatric Society Infectious Diseases and Immunization Committee (2002) recommend instilling a prophylactic agent in the eyes of all neonates to prevent ophthalmia neonatorum or neonatal conjunctivitis, which is an inflammation caused by sexually transmitted bacteria acquired during passage through the mother's birth canal. Prophylactic medication is targeted primarily toward preventing infection from *Neisseria gonorrhoeae.* Without prompt treatment this infection can lead to blindness (Smith, 2012) (Fig. 24-4). Erythromycin 0.5% ophthalmic ointment, tetracycline 1% ointment, and silver nitrate 1% solution are considered effective as preventive medications, although silver nitrate and tetracycline are not available in the United States (Canadian Paediatric Society Infectious Diseases and Immunization Committee, 2002; USPSTF, 2011). In some countries, 2.5% povidone-iodine solution is used, although this is not currently approved for use in the United States. Eye prophylaxis is usually administered within the first hour after birth. It may be delayed up to 2 hours until after the first breastfeeding so that eye contact and parent-infant attachment and bonding are facilitated. Eye prophylaxis for every newborn is mandated by law in the majority of U.S. states without regard to the mode of birth. In some states parents may refuse eye prophylaxis by signing a form that becomes part of the newborn record (Dekker, 2012).

Topical antibiotics such as erythromycin are not effective in treating chlamydial conjunctivitis; systemic treatment is needed. A 14-day course of oral erythromycin or an oral sulfonamide may be given for chlamydial conjunctivitis (AAP Committee on Infectious Diseases, 2012).

Vitamin K Prophylaxis

Administering vitamin K intramuscularly is routine in the newborn period in the United States and Canada. A single

MEDICATION GUIDE

Eye Prophylaxis: Erythromycin Ophthalmic Ointment, 0.5%, and Tetracycline Ophthalmic Ointment, 1%

Action
These antibiotic ointments are both bacteriostatic and bactericidal *caused by Neisseria gonorrhoeae.*

Indication
These medications are applied to prevent ophthalmia neonatorum in newborns of mothers who are infected with *Neisseria gonorrhoeae*. Eye prophylaxis for ophthalmia neonatorum is required by law in all U.S. states and in some Canadian provinces.

Neonatal Dosage
Apply a 1- to 2-cm ribbon of ointment to the lower conjunctival sac of each eye; can also be used in drop form

Adverse Reactions
Can cause chemical conjunctivitis that lasts 24 to 48 hours; vision can be blurred temporarily

Nursing Considerations
Administer within 1 to 2 hours of birth. Wear gloves. Cleanse the eyes if necessary before administration. Open the eyes by putting a thumb and finger at the corner of each lid and gently pressing on the periorbital ridges. Squeeze the tube and spread the ointment from the inner canthus of the eye to the outer canthus. Do not touch the tube to the eye. After 1 minute excess ointment may be wiped off. Observe eyes for irritation. Explain the treatment to the parents.

intramuscular (IM) injection of 0.5 to 1 mg of vitamin K is given soon after birth to prevent hemorrhagic disease of the newborn. In the United States, administration can be delayed until after the first breastfeeding in the birthing room (AAP & ACOG, 2012). In Canada, newborns should receive the injection within 6 hours after birth when the infant is stable and there has been opportunity for interaction with the parents (McMillan & Canadian Paediatric Society Fetus and Newborn Committee, 2014). Vitamin K is synthesized by intestinal flora, which are not present at birth. The introduction of bacteria begins with the first feedings, and by the age of 7 days, healthy newborns are able to produce their own vitamin K.

Promoting Parent-Infant Interaction

Today's birthing practices promote the family as the focus of care. Parents generally desire to share in the birth process and have early contact with their infants. The infant can be put to breast soon after birth. Early contact between mother and newborn can be important in developing future relationships; it also has a positive effect on the initiation and duration of breastfeeding. Rooming-in during the hospital stay promotes parent-infant interaction. Early mother-infant contact produces physiologic benefits for the mother and neonate. Maternal levels of oxytocin and prolactin rise with early breastfeeding. The process of developing active immunity begins as the infant ingests antibodies from the mother's colostrum.

MEDICATION GUIDE

Vitamin K: Phytonadione (AquaMEPHYTON, Konakion)

Action
This intervention provides vitamin K because the newborn does not have the intestinal flora to produce this vitamin in the first week after birth. It also promotes formation of clotting factors (II, VII, IX, X) in the liver.

Indication
Vitamin K is used for preventing and treating hemorrhagic disease in the newborn.

Neonatal Dosage
Administer a 0.5-mg (0.25-ml) dose to newborns weighing less than 1500 g and a 1-mg (0.5-ml) dose to newborns weighing more than 1500 g) intramuscularly soon after birth; the injection can be delayed until after initial breastfeeding.* Vitamin K is never administered by the intravenous (IV) route for the prevention of hemorrhagic disease of the newborn except in some cases of a preterm infant who has no muscle mass. In such instances the medication is diluted and given over 10 to 15 minutes while closely monitoring the infant with a cardiorespiratory monitor. Rapid IV administration of vitamin K can cause cardiac arrest.

Adverse Reactions
Edema, erythema, and pain at the injection site occur rarely; hemolysis, jaundice, and hyperbilirubinemia have been reported, particularly in preterm infants.

Nursing Considerations
Follow the procedure for intramuscular injection on (see Fig. 24-15).

**Administration may be delayed up to 6 hours in Canada.*
Data from American Academy of Pediatrics Committee on Fetus and Newborn (2003, reaffirmed 2009). Controversies concerning vitamin K and the newborn. *Pediatrics, 112*(1 Pt 1), 191-192. McMillan, D. & Canadian Paediatric Society Fetus and Newborn Committee. (1997, reaffirmed 2014). Routine administration of vitamin K to newborns. *Paediatrics and Child Health, 2*(6), 429-431.

CARE MANAGEMENT: FROM 2 HOURS AFTER BIRTH UNTIL DISCHARGE

Depending on the model of care delivery, the mother/baby nurse or newborn nursery nurse is responsible for ongoing assessment and care of the newborn. Astute assessment skills and appropriate interventions promote positive outcomes, especially for newborns who experience any problems before going home. Newborn care is family centered—the nurse provides education and support for the new parents throughout the hospital stay and assists them in preparing for discharge from the birthing facility.

Common Newborn Problems

Birth Injuries

Birth trauma includes any physical injury sustained by a newborn during labor and birth. Although most injuries are minor and resolve during the neonatal period without treatment, some types of trauma require intervention; a few are serious enough to be fatal. (See Chapter 35 for more information on birth injuries.)

Retinal and subconjunctival hemorrhages result from rupture of capillaries caused by increased pressure during birth. These hemorrhages usually clear within 5 days and present no further problems. Parents need explanation and reassurance that these injuries are harmless.

Erythema, ecchymoses, petechiae, abrasions, lacerations, or edema of the buttocks and extremities can be present. Localized discoloration can appear over the presenting part as a result of forceps- or vacuum-assisted birth. Ecchymoses and edema can appear anywhere on the body. Petechiae (pinpoint hemorrhagic areas) acquired during birth can extend over the upper trunk and face. These lesions are benign if they disappear within 2 or 3 days of birth and no new lesions appear. Ecchymoses and petechiae can be signs of a more serious disorder, such as thrombocytopenic purpura. To differentiate hemorrhagic areas from a skin rash or discolorations, the nurse attempts to blanch the skin by pressing with two fingers, lifting the fingers off the skin, and waiting for the return of blood. Petechiae and ecchymoses will not blanch because extravasated blood remains within the tissues, whereas skin rashes and discolorations will blanch.

Trauma to the presenting fetal part can occur during labor and birth. Caput succedaneum and cephalhematoma are discussed in Chapter 23 (see Fig. 23-10). Forceps injury and bruising from the vacuum cup occur at the site of application of the instruments. A forceps injury commonly produces a linear mark across both sides of the face in the shape of forceps blades. The affected areas are kept clean to minimize the risk for infection. These injuries usually resolve spontaneously within several days with no specific therapy.

Bruises over the face can be the result of face presentation (Fig. 24-5). In a breech presentation, bruising and swelling may be seen over the buttocks or genitalia (see Fig. 23-8). The skin over the entire head can be ecchymotic and covered with petechiae caused by a tight nuchal cord. If the hemorrhagic areas do not disappear spontaneously in 2 days or if the infant's condition changes, the primary health care provider is notified.

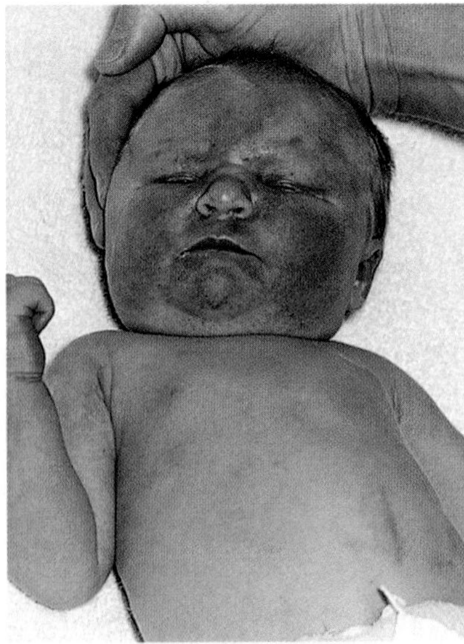

FIG 24-5 Marked bruising on the entire face of an infant born vaginally after face presentation. Less severe ecchymoses were present on the extremities. Phototherapy was required for treatment of jaundice resulting from the breakdown of accumulated blood. (From O'Doherty, N. [1986]. *Neonatology: Micro atlas of the newborn.* Nutley, NJ: Hoffman-La Roche.)

Accidental lacerations can be inflicted with a scalpel during a cesarean birth. These cuts can occur on any part of the body but are most often found on the scalp, buttocks, and thighs. They are usually superficial and need only to be kept clean. If skin closure is needed, an adhesive substance or strips may be applied. Sutures are rarely needed.

Physiologic Problems

Jaundice

Assessment and Screening. A majority of newborn infants experience some level of jaundice due to hyperbilirubinemia during the first few days of life, usually occurring after 24 hours. In most cases it is *physiologic jaundice,* caused by increased levels of unconjugated bilirubin; physiologic jaundice is usually self-limiting and requires no treatment. It peaks at about 3 to 5 days and resolves after 1 to 2 weeks. In some cases phototherapy is needed to lower bilirubin levels to within an acceptable range. Physiologic jaundice must be differentiated from pathologic jaundice, which is associated with higher levels of unconjugated bilirubin. This type of jaundice can appear in the first 24 hours and often requires phototherapy to resolve (see Chapter 23). Jaundice can also be associated with breastfeeding (see Chapter 25).

Every newborn should be assessed for jaundice at least every 8 to 12 hours; this can be easily done when vital signs are assessed. To differentiate cutaneous jaundice from normal skin color, the nurse applies pressure with a finger over a bony area (e.g., the nose, forehead, sternum) for several seconds to empty all the capillaries in that spot, then releases the pressure by lifting the finger. If jaundice is present, the blanched area will appear yellowish before the capillaries refill. The conjunctival sacs and buccal mucosa also are assessed, especially in darker-skinned infants. Assessing for jaundice in natural light is recommended because artificial lighting and reflection from nursery walls can distort the actual skin color.

Visual assessment of jaundice alone does not provide an accurate assessment of the level of serum bilirubin, especially in dark-skinned newborns (Burgos, Flaherman, & Newman, 2012). A more accurate noninvasive assessment of hyperbilirubinemia is accomplished using transcutaneous bilirubinometry [TcB] (Fig. 24-6). TcB devices allow for repetitive estimations

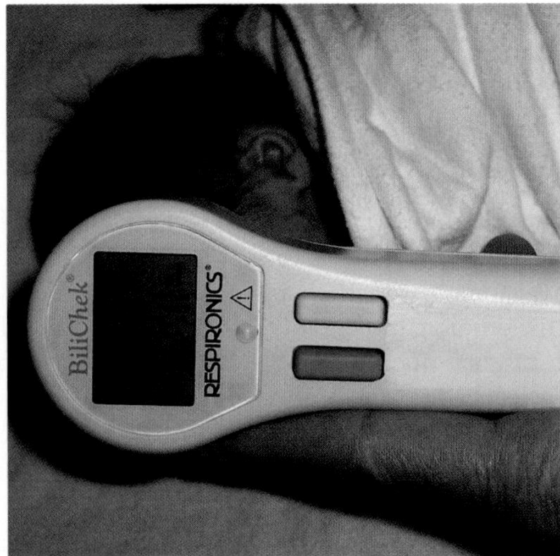

FIG 24-6 Transcutaneous monitoring of bilirubin with a transcutaneous bilirubinometry (TcB) monitor. (Courtesy Cheryl Briggs, RNC, Annapolis, MD.)

of bilirubin and work well on both dark- and light-skinned infants. TcB levels demonstrate linear correlation with serum determinations of bilirubin levels in full-term infants (Dijk & Hulzebos, 2012; Maisels, DeRidder, Kring, & Balasubramaniam, 2009). TcB monitors can be used to screen for clinically significant jaundice and decrease the need for serum bilirubin measurements.

If an infant appears jaundiced in the first 24 hours of life, a TcB or total serum bilirubin (TSB) level should be measured and results interpreted based on the newborn's age in hours according to the hour-specific nomogram for infants born at 35 weeks of gestation or later (AAP Subcommittee on Hyperbilirubinemia, 2004). Repeat testing is based on the risk level (low, intermediate, or high), the age of the neonate, and the progression of jaundice.

In an effort to prevent severe hyperbilirubinemia and the neurologic complications of acute bilirubin encephalopathy and kernicterus, the AAP and the Canadian Paediatric Society recommend routine screening of all newborns before hospital discharge using TcB or serum bilirubin measurement (AAP Subcommittee on Hyperbilirubinemia, 2004; Barrington, Sankaran, & Canadian Paediatric Society Fetus and Newborn Committee, 2011). In general, if the TcB level is greater than 12 mg/dl, a serum bilirubin check is done and levels are interpreted according to the hour-specific nomogram (AAP Subcommittee on Hyperbilirubinemia, 2004) (Fig. 24-7). A tool at www.bilitool.org facilitates calculating the risk for neonatal hyperbilirubinemia.

Infants in the lower risk category are less likely to develop hyperbilirubinemia. However, the AAP warns that all infants should be considered as being at potential risk for hyperbilirubinemia, even if they were identified as being in the low risk category. This means that all newborns should be followed after hospital discharge for the development of unexpected jaundice and that parents should be given printed and oral information about newborn jaundice (Bromiker, Bin-Nun, Schimmel, et al., 2012; Maisels et al., 2009).

Adequate feeding is essential in preventing hyperbilirubinemia. Newborns should breastfeed early (within 1 to 2 hours after birth) and often (at least 8 to 12 times/24 hours) (AAP Section on Breastfeeding, 2012; AAP Subcommittee on Hyperbilirubinemia, 2004). Colostrum acts as a laxative to promote stooling, which helps rid the body of bilirubin. Formula-fed infants should be fed after birth when their physiologic status has stabilized and thereafter at least every 3 to 4 hours.

Routine assessment of risk factors for severe hyperbilirubinemia is advised. The most common risk factors include gestational age less than 38 weeks, exclusive breastfeeding (especially in association with breastfeeding difficulties and excessive weight loss), significant jaundice in a sibling, isoimmune or other hemolytic disease (e.g., glucose-6-phosphate dehydrogenase [G6PD] deficiency), cephalhematoma, significant bruising, and East Indian race (AAP Subcommittee on Hyperbilirubinemia, 2004).

Close follow-up of infants at risk for hyperbilirubinemia is essential; parents should be educated and encouraged to

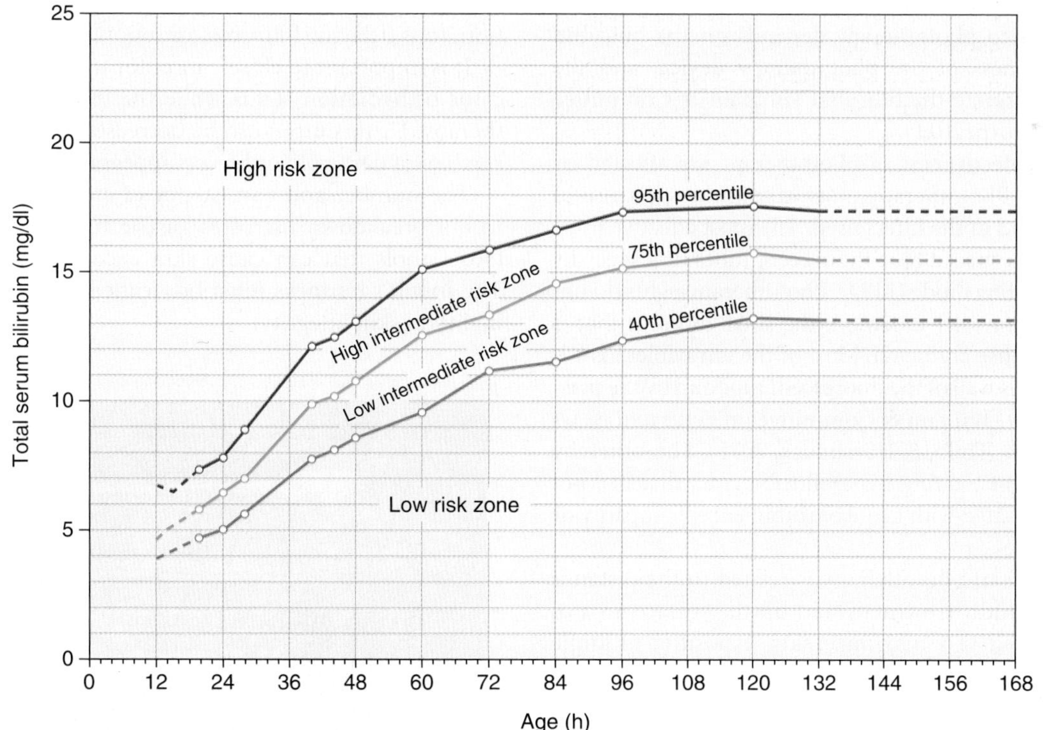

FIG 24-7 Nomogram for designation of risk in 2840 well newborns at 36 or more weeks of gestational age with birth weight of 2000 g or more or 35 or more weeks of gestational age with birth weight of 2500 g or more based on the hour-specific serum bilirubin values. (This nomogram should not be used to represent the natural history of neonatal hyperbilirubinemia.) (From Bhutani, V., Johnson, L., & Sivieri, E.M. [1999]. Predictive ability of a predischarge hour-specific serum bilirubin for subsequent significant hyperbilirubinemia in healthy term and near-term newborns. *Pediatrics, 103*[1], 6-14.)

follow postdischarge recommendations (AAP Subcommittee on Hyperbilirubinemia, 2004). Follow-up should occur 48 to 72 hours after discharge from the birthing facility or sooner based on the length of stay and presence of risk factors for hyperbilirubinemia (Burgos et al., 2012).

Therapy for Hyperbilirubinemia. The decision to treat an infant for hyperbilirubinemia is based on total serum bilirubin levels, the infant's gestational age, and the presence of risk factors. Using a nomogram that plots bilirubin levels according to gestational age, the provider determines the appropriate management plan (Maisels, 2010). The AAP provides guidelines that provide direction for health care providers in determining the need for phototherapy or exchange transfusion (AAP Committee on Hyperbilirubinemia, 2004).

The goal of treatment of hyperbilirubinemia is to help reduce the newborn's serum levels of unconjugated bilirubin. There are two ways to reduce unconjugated bilirubin levels: phototherapy and exchange blood transfusion. Phototherapy is the most common treatment. Exchange transfusion is used to treat those infants whose levels of serum bilirubin are rising rapidly despite the use of intensive phototherapy.

Phototherapy. The purpose of phototherapy is to reduce the level of circulating unconjugated bilirubin or keep it from increasing. Phototherapy uses light energy to change the shape and structure of unconjugated bilirubin, converting it into a conjugated form that can be excreted through urine and stool. Phototherapy is delivered through lamp, blanket, pad, or cover-body devices. The severity of the newborn's hyperbilirubinemia determines the type of phototherapy device and strength of light, duration of treatment, and venue (hospital or home). The neonate's response to phototherapy depends on the bilirubin level, the effectiveness of the phototherapy device, and the infant's ability to excrete the bilirubin (Bhutani & Committee on Fetus and Newborn, 2011).

The dose and effectiveness of phototherapy are affected by the source of light. Phototherapy units vary in the spectrum of light they deliver and in the filters used. The most effective therapy is achieved with special blue fluorescent tubes or a specially designed light-emitting diode (LED). Phototherapy lights do not emit significant ultraviolet radiation; the small amount that is emitted does not cause erythema. Most of the ultraviolet light is absorbed by the glass wall of the fluorescent tube and by the plastic cover of the light (Bhutani & Committee on Fetus and Newborn, 2011; Kamath, Thilo, & Hernandez, 2011). Phototherapy is usually effective in treating hyperbilirubinemia that has not reached levels associated with acute bilirubin encephalopathy or kernicterus.

The effectiveness of phototherapy is related to the distance between the light and the neonate and on the surface area of skin that is exposed. To maximize skin exposure, multiple devices may be used simultaneously. For example, a neonate may be placed under a phototherapy lamp while also lying on a fiberoptic pad or LED mattress (Bhutani & Committee on Fetus and Newborn, 2011).

During phototherapy using a lamp, the infant, wearing only a diaper, is placed under a bank of lights approximately 45 to 50 cm from the light source. Phototherapy can be used for the infant in an incubator (Fig. 24-8) or in an open crib. The distance varies according to unit protocol and type of light used. The irradiance of the light is monitored routinely with a radiometer, with measurements at several sites over the neonate's body surface during treatment to ensure efficacy of therapy (Bhutani & Committee on Fetus and Newborn, 2011).

Within 4 to 6 hours after initiation of phototherapy, the bilirubin level should begin to decrease. Phototherapy is used until the infant's serum bilirubin level decreases to within an acceptable range. The decision to discontinue therapy is based on the observation of a definite downward trend in the bilirubin values.

When a phototherapy lamp is used, the infant's eyes must be protected by an opaque mask to prevent retinal damage. The eye shield should cover the eyes completely but not occlude the nares. Before the mask is applied, the infant's eyes should be closed gently to prevent excoriation of the corneas. The mask should be removed periodically and during infant feedings so that the eyes can be assessed and cleansed with water and the parents can have visual contact with the infant.

Phototherapy can cause changes in the infant's temperature, depending partially on the bed used—bassinet, incubator, or radiant warmer. When under a phototherapy light, infants are usually clothed only with a diaper. The infant's temperature should be closely monitored. Phototherapy lights can increase the rate of insensible water loss, which contributes to fluid loss and dehydration. Therefore, the infant must be adequately hydrated. Hydration maintenance in the healthy newborn is accomplished through breastfeeding or infant formula. Feedings of glucose water or plain water have no advantage or benefit because these liquids do not promote excretion of bilirubin in the stools and can actually perpetuate enterohepatic circulation, thus delaying bilirubin excretion.

It is important to closely monitor urinary output as an indicator of hydration status while the infant is receiving phototherapy. Urine output can be decreased or unaltered; the urine can have a dark gold or brown appearance.

The number and consistency of stools are monitored. Bilirubin breakdown increases gastric motility, which results in loose stools that can cause skin excoriation and breakdown. The infant's buttocks must be cleaned after each stool to help maintain skin integrity.

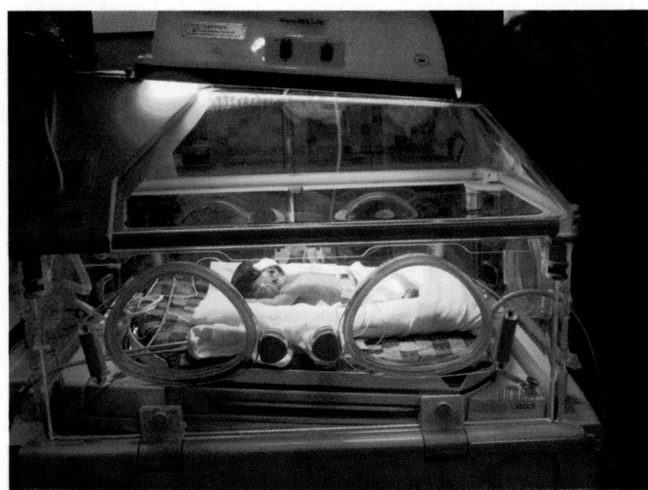

FIG 24-8 Infant under phototherapy lights while in incubator. (Courtesy Cheryl Briggs, RNC, Annapolis, MD.)

SAFETY ALERT

No ointments, creams, or lotions should be applied to the newborn's skin during phototherapy because they can absorb heat and cause burns.

If the infant is under phototherapy lights, maximizing skin exposure to the light is important. Infants need to be turned at least every 2 to 3 hours. A fine maculopapular rash can appear during phototherapy, but this condition is transient. In rare instances there can be bullous eruptions or the development of bronze baby syndrome in which the skin appears grayish brown. Researchers are investigating the potential long-term effects of phototherapy (e.g., retinal damage, malignant melanoma), although the evidence has yet to be evaluated (Bhutani & Committee on Fetus and Newborn, 2011; Xiong, Qu, Cambier, & Mu, 2011).

In addition to phototherapy lights, other systems are used for phototherapy. A bassinet system provides special blue light above and beneath the infant. Another phototherapy device is a fiberoptic blanket that is connected to a light source. The blanket is flexible and can be placed around the infant's torso or underneath the infant in the bassinet. There are also bilirubin beds with LED lights in a pad that covers the surface of the bassinet (Fig. 24-9). The LEDs do not produce heat and can be used with radiant warmers. These devices are usually less effective when used alone as compared with conventional phototherapy lights. They can be very useful in combination with overhead phototherapy lights. In certain instances the infant's bilirubin levels increase rapidly and intensive phototherapy is required; this situation involves the use of a combination of conventional lights and fiberoptic blankets to maximize bilirubin reduction. Although fiberoptic lights do not produce heat as do conventional lights, staff should ensure that a covering pad is placed between the infant's skin and the fiberoptic device to prevent skin burns, especially in preterm infants. The newborn can remain in the mother's room in an open crib or in her arms during treatment. The use of eye patches depends on whether the devices are used alone or in combination with phototherapy lights.

Home Phototherapy. The use of home phototherapy should be reserved for healthy term infants with bilirubin levels in the "optional phototherapy" range according to the nomogram. The concern is that home phototherapy units do not provide the same level of irradiance or body surface coverage as phototherapy devices used in the hospital (AAP Committee on Hyperbilirubinemia, 2004).

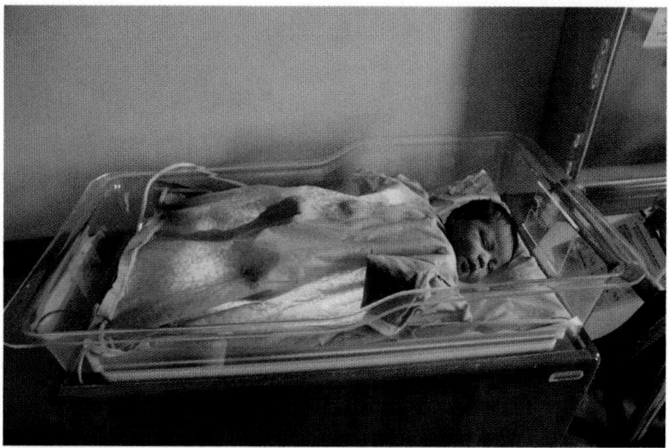

FIG 24-9 Infant receiving phototherapy using bilirubin bed. (Courtesy Cheryl Briggs, RNC, Annapolis, MD.)

Phototherapy and Parent-Infant Interaction. The traditional use of phototherapy raises concerns related to psychobehavioral issues, including parent-infant separation, potential social isolation, decreased sensorineural stimulation, altered biologic rhythms, altered feeding patterns, and activity changes. Parental anxiety can be greatly increased, particularly at the sight of the newborn with eyes covered and under special lights. The interruption of breastfeeding for phototherapy is a potential deterrent to successful maternal-infant attachment and interaction. Because research has demonstrated that bilirubin catabolism occurs primarily within the first few hours after initiating phototherapy, there is increased support for the removal of the infant from treatment for feeding and holding. Intermittent phototherapy can be just as effective as continuous therapy when used correctly. The benefits of stopping phototherapy for short periods so parents can feed and hold the newborn should be carefully considered by the health care team and the parents.

Follow-Up. Close follow-up is needed for infants who have been treated for hyperbilirubinemia. Repeat testing of serum bilirubin levels and follow-up visits with the pediatric health care provider are expected. Some institutions or third-party providers pay for a home visit to evaluate the infant's condition and to monitor the mother's health. When follow-up serum bilirubin levels are needed after discharge from the hospital, a health care technician or nurse may draw the blood for the specimen or the parents may take the baby to a laboratory to have blood drawn for a serum bilirubin. In some cases parents take the newborn to an outpatient clinic or physician's office to be evaluated.

Exchange Transfusion. When phototherapy is not effective in reducing serum bilirubin levels or with severe hyperbilirubinemia such as in hemolytic disease, **exchange transfusion** may be needed. This procedure is done in an intensive care setting. The infant's blood is replaced with a combination of blood products such as red blood cells (RBCs) mixed with 5% albumin or fresh frozen plasma (Kaplan, Wong, Sibley, & Stevenson, 2011) (see Chapter 36).

Hypoglycemia. **Hypoglycemia** in a term infant during the early newborn period is defined as a blood glucose concentration less than adequate to support neurologic, organ, and tissue function; however, there is a lack of consensus among experts regarding the precise level at which this concentration occurs. Similarly, there is no consensus about when to screen for hypoglycemia or the level at which treatment should be instituted (Adamkin & Committee on Fetus and Newborn, 2011). Hypoglycemia that warrants treatment is usually defined as blood glucose levels less than 40 mg/dl, although some experts recommend treatment for levels less than 50 mg/dl (McGowan, Rozance, Price-Douglas, & Hay, 2011).

Bedside glucose monitoring is performed using reagent test strips with or without a reflectance colorimeter. Because of variations in devices and operator techniques, it is recommended that any level less than 45 mg/dl should be followed up with a serum glucose level (Kalhan & Devaskar, 2011).

At birth, the maternal source of glucose is cut off when the umbilical cord is clamped. Most healthy term newborns experience a transient decrease in glucose levels to as low as 30 mg/dl during the first 1 to 2 hours after birth, with a subsequent mobilization of free fatty acids and ketones to help maintain adequate glucose levels (Blackburn, 2013). Infants who are asphyxiated or have other physiologic stress can experience hypoglycemia as a result of a decreased glycogen supply, inadequate gluconeogenesis, or overutilization of glycogen stored during fetal life. There is concern about neurologic injury as a result of severe or prolonged hypoglycemia, especially in combination with ischemia (Kalhan & Devaskar, 2011).

There is no need to routinely assess glucose levels of healthy term infants. Adequate feeding helps these neonates maintain normal glucose levels.

Glucose levels should be measured in neonates at 34 weeks of gestation or more if risk factors or clinical manifestations of hypoglycemia are present. Infants considered to be at risk for hypoglycemia include those who are SGA or LGA, infants of mothers with diabetes, and late preterm infants. The frequency of glucose testing is determined by the risk factors for each individual newborn. All at-risk infants should be fed within the first hour, with glucose testing done 30 minutes after feeding. For at least the first 24 hours after birth, late preterm and SGA neonates should be fed every 2 to 3 hours, with glucose levels measured before each feeding. LGA infants and infants of mothers with diabetes should have glucose screening before feedings for at least the first 12 hours after birth; further testing is done if glucose levels are less than 45 mg/dl (Adamkin & Committee on Fetus and Newborn, 2011).

Glucose testing should be done on any infant with clinical signs of hypoglycemia. The clinical signs of hypoglycemia can be transient or recurrent and include jitteriness, lethargy, poor feeding, abnormal cry, hypotonia, temperature instability (hypothermia), respiratory distress, apnea, and seizures (Kalhan & Devaskar, 2011). It is important to remember that hypoglycemia can be present in the absence of clinical manifestations.

Late preterm infants are at increased risk for hypoglycemia. They have decreased glycogen stores and lack hepatic enzymes for gluconeogenesis and glycogenolysis. Their hormonal regulation and insulin secretion are immature. The increased risk of cold stress and feeding difficulties adds to the risk for hypoglycemia (Cooper et al., 2012).

The at-risk asymptomatic neonate with glucose levels less than 25 mg/dl in the first 4 hours or less than 35 mg/dl from 4 to 24 hours of age should be fed. Glucose testing should be repeated 1 hour after feeding. If levels remain low despite feeding, IV dextrose is warranted. In such infants the treatment should be aimed at maintaining the blood glucose levels greater than 45 mg/dl. For the neonate with clinical signs of hypoglycemia, regardless of cause or age, IV dextrose infusion is usually recommended. For any infant with hypoglycemia, follow-up glucose testing at specified intervals is needed until glucose levels are stable (Adamkin & Committee on Fetus and Newborn, 2011; McGowan et al., 2011).

Hypocalcemia. Hypocalcemia is defined as serum calcium levels of less than 7.8 to 8 mg/dl in term infants and slightly lower (7 mg/dl) in preterm infants. Hypocalcemia is common in critically ill neonates but also can occur in infants of mothers with diabetes or in those who had perinatal asphyxia or trauma and in low-birth-weight and preterm infants. Infants born to mothers treated with anticonvulsants during pregnancy also are at risk (Rigo, Mohamed, & De Curtis, 2011). Early-onset hypocalcemia usually occurs within the first 24 to 48 hours after birth. Signs of hypocalcemia include jitteriness, high-pitched cry, irritability, apnea, intermittent cyanosis, abdominal distention, and laryngospasm, although some hypocalcemic infants are asymptomatic. Jitteriness is a symptom of both hypoglycemia and hypocalcemia; therefore, hypocalcemia must be considered if the therapy for hypoglycemia proves ineffective.

In most instances early-onset hypocalcemia is self-limiting and resolves within 1 to 3 days. Treatment usually includes early feeding of an appropriate source of calcium such as fortified human milk or preterm infant formula (Jones, Hayes, Starbuck, & Porcelli, 2011).

Laboratory and Diagnostic Tests

Because newborns experience many transitional events in the first 28 days of life, laboratory samples are often collected to determine adequate physiologic adaptation and to identify disorders that can adversely affect the child's life beyond the neonatal period. Blood samples for most laboratory tests can be obtained from the neonate with a heel puncture, also known as a *heelstick.* Tests commonly performed other than blood glucose and bilirubin levels include newborn screening tests and serum drug levels. Standard laboratory values for a term newborn are listed in Table 24-4.

TABLE 24-4 Standard Laboratory Values in a Term Neonate

HEMATOLOGY		VALUES
Hemoglobin (g/dl)		14 to 24
Hematocrit (%)		44 to 64
Red blood cells (RBCs)/μL		4.8×10^6 to 7.1×10^6
Reticulocytes (%)		1.8 to 4.6
Fetal hemoglobin (% of total)		50 to 70
Platelet count/mm^3		150,000 to 300,000
White blood cells (WBCs)/μL		9000 to 30,000
Bilirubin, total (mg/dl)*	24 hr	2 to 6
	48 hr	6 to 7
	3 to 5 days	4 to 6
Serum glucose (mg/dl)	<1 day	40 to 60
	>1 day	50-90
Arterial blood gases	pH	7.35-7.45
	Pco_2	35 to 45 mm Hg
	Po_2	60 to 80 mm Hg
	HC03	18-26 mEq/L
	Base excess	(-5) to (+5)
	O_2 saturation	92-94%

dl, Deciliter; *μL,* microliter; *Pco_2,* partial pressure of carbon dioxide; *Po_2,* partial pressure of oxygen.

*Bilirubin levels should be interpreted according to the hour-specific nomogram (AAP Subcommittee on Hyperbilirubinemia, 2004).

Data from American Academy of Pediatrics (AAP) Subcommittee on Hyperbilirubinemia. (2004). Clinical practice guideline: Management of hyperbilirubinemia in the newborn infant 35 or more weeks of gestation. *Pediatrics, 114* (1), 297-316; Blackburn, S.T. (2013). *Maternal, fetal, and neonatal physiology* (4th ed.). Maryland Heights, MO: Elsevier Saunders; Pagana, K.D., & Pagana, T.J. (2011). *Mosby's diagnostic and laboratory test reference* (11th ed.). St. Louis: Mosby; Wood, A.M., & Jones, M.D. (2011). Acid-base homeostasis and oxygenation. In S. L. Gardner, B. S. Carter, M. Enzman-Hines, & J.A. Hernandez (Eds.), *Merenstein & Gardner's handbook of neonatal intensive care* (7th ed.). St Louis: Mosby.

Universal Newborn Screening

Mandated by U.S. law, newborn genetic screening is an important public health program aimed at early detection of genetic diseases that result in severe health problems if not treated early. The universal screening program is state-based and involves a variety of components including education, screening, follow-up, treatment, and a system for monitoring and evaluation. The U.S. Department of Health and Human Services (USDHHS) Discretionary Advisory Committee on Heritable Disorders in Newborns and Children (2013) recommends screening for 31 core disorders and 26 secondary disorders. The core disorders include hemoglobinopathies (e.g., sickle cell disease), inborn errors of metabolism (e.g., phenylketonuria [PKU], galactosemia), severe combined immunodeficiency, and critical congenital heart disease (Howell, Terry, Tait, et al., 2012). The majority of disorders included in the screening are not symptomatic at birth. Individual states select additional disorders to include in the screening. The most current list is available through the National Newborn Screening and Genetics Resource Center (NNSGRC) at http://genes-r-us.uthscsa.edu/sites/genes-r-us/files/nbsdisorders.pdf. In Canada, universal newborn screening policies and practices are varied. Individual provinces in Canada determine the disorders included in newborn screening; however, all provinces screen for PKU and congenital hypothyroidism (Wilson, Kennedy, Potter, et al., 2010).

Capillary blood samples are obtained from newborn infants using a heelstick; blood is collected on a special filter paper and sent to a designated state laboratory for analysis (Fig. 24-10). Samples are usually collected in the hospital after 24 hours of age and before discharge; testing may be delayed for sick or preterm infants or those born outside the hospital (ACOG Committee on Genetics, 2011). The screening test should be repeated at age 1 to 2 weeks if the initial specimen was obtained when the infant was younger than 24 hours.

The American College of Medical Genetics (2009) recommends that states retain the residual dried blood filter spots. These blood samples are useful for future testing and research purposes. However, ethical concerns are related to the need for parental consent to retain blood samples and use them for biomedical research. Nurses need to be aware of policies and procedures regarding retention and use of newborn screening samples in the state where they practice so they are able to provide information to parents (Tluczek & De Luca, 2013).

Families should be educated about universal newborn screening during the prenatal period (ACOG Committee on Genetics, 2011). However, this is not common practice; newborn screening is not usually discussed with parents prior to birth. This may be related to the fact that in the majority of states informed consent is not required for newborn screening (Tarini & Goldenberg, 2012). In many cases discussion about newborn screening occurs in the hospital setting at the time of blood sample collection. Nurses can provide education for parents regarding the purpose of the screening, the procedure for blood sampling, when to expect results, and the importance of follow-up (Araia, Wilson, Chakraborty, et al., 2012; Tluczek & De Luca, 2013).

COMMUNITY ACTIVITY

Visit the National Newborn Screening and Genetics Resource Center (NNSGRC) website (http://genes-r-us.uthscsa.edu). Review the information for parents and family about resources, disorders tested, and screening programs.

At the NNSGRC website, visit the newborn screening program site for your state. What types of disorders are including in newborn screening? Does your state require newborn hearing screening? Review the information for parents about diagnostic testing and community support services.

Newborn Hearing Screening. Hearing loss is the most commonly diagnosed genetic disorder of all the core conditions in the universal screening program (Howell et al., 2012). The Joint Committee on Infant Hearing (2007) recommends routine hearing screening for all newborns before hospital discharge or no later than 1 month of age. The Canadian Paediatric Society recommends hearing screening for all newborns (Patel, Feldman, & Canadian Paediatric Society Community Paediatrics Committee, 2014). Through early hearing detection and intervention (EHDI) programs, the outcome for infants who are deaf or hard of hearing can be maximized.

Using noninvasive technology, newborn hearing screening provides information about the pathways from the external ear to the cerebral cortex. Two tests commonly are used to assess

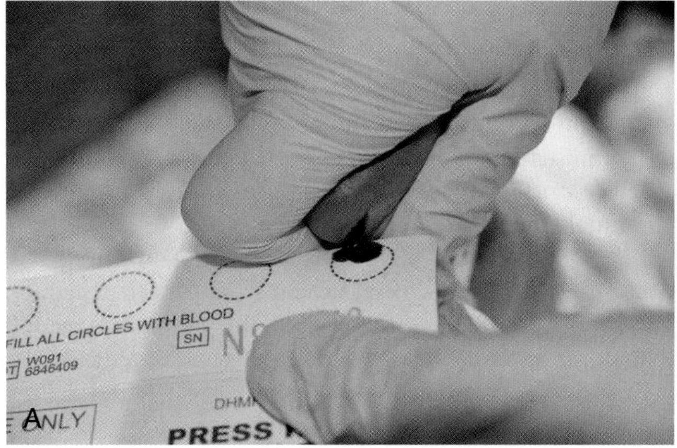

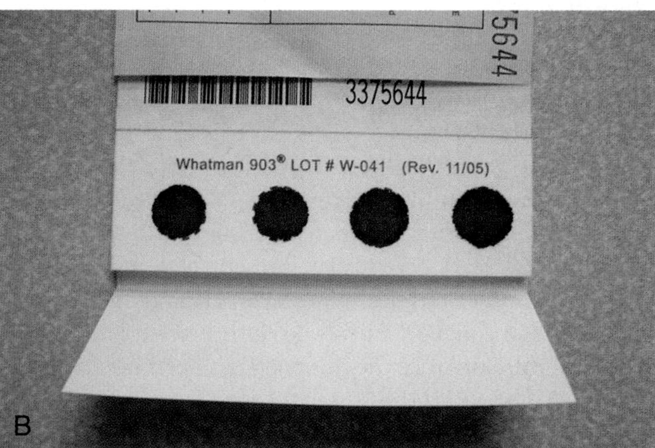

FIG 24-10 **A,** Nurse obtaining blood sample from newborn's heel for universal screening. Sample is applied to filter paper. **B,** All four circles must be filled in completely. (Courtesy Cheryl Briggs, RNC, Annapolis, MD.)

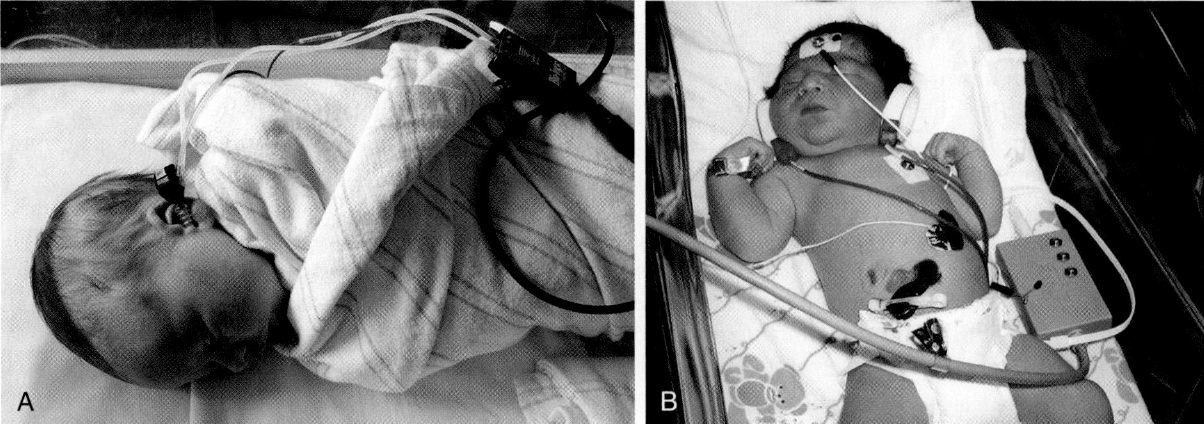

FIG 24-11 Newborn hearing screening. **A,** Evoked otoacoustic emissions (EOAE) test. **B,** Auditory brain response (ABR) test. (**A,** Courtesy Julie and Darren Nelson, Loveland, CO. **B,** Courtesy Dee Lowdermilk, Chapel Hill, NC.)

hearing function in the newborn. Initial screening is done with the evoked otoacoustic emissions (EOAE) test. The auditory brainstem response (ABR) test is used as follow-up if the initial screening is abnormal. Neither test is definitive in diagnosing hearing loss; they are used to determine whether further, more accurate hearing testing is needed through audiologic evaluation. For the EOAE test, a soft rubber earpiece that makes a soft clicking noise is placed in the baby's outer ear (Fig. 24-11, *A*). A healthy ear will "echo" the click sound back to a microphone inside the earpiece. The ABR test is performed by attaching sensors to the baby's forehead and behind each ear. An earphone is placed in the baby's outer ear and sends a series of quiet sounds into the sleeping baby's ear (see Fig. 24-11, *B*). The sensors measure the responses of the baby's acoustic nerve. The responses are recorded and stored in a computer.

Newborns who do not pass the initial screening test should have the hearing screening test repeated as part of follow-up care. If the infant still does not pass, a comprehensive audiologic evaluation should be done by 3 months of age. Regardless of the outcome of hearing testing, all infants should have regular and ongoing surveillance of developmental, hearing, and speech-language skills through regular well-child visits beginning at the age of 2 months so that any hearing loss can be promptly identified and treated (Joint Committee on Infant Hearing, 2007).

Screening for Critical Congenital Heart Disease (CCHD). CCHD was added to the uniform screening panel in the United States in 2011 and is endorsed by the AAP (AAP Section on Cardiology and Cardiac Surgery Executive Committee, 2012). The noninvasive screening test is performed using pulse oximetry to measure oxygen saturation for the purpose of detecting hypoxemia. Pulse oximetry testing can detect some critical congenital heart defects that present with hypoxemia in the absence of other physical symptoms. Hypoxemia can be the first sign that a congenital heart defect is present and other symptoms can develop once the newborn has been discharged. Screening is performed at 24 to 48 hours of age. Oxygen saturation is measured in the right hand and one foot. A "passing" result is oxygen saturation of greater than 95% in either extremity, with a less than 3% absolute difference between the upper and lower extremity readings. Immediate evaluation is needed if the oxygen saturation is less than 90%. The baby is evaluated for hemodynamic stability and hypoxemia; an echocardiogram is usually performed (AAP Section on Cardiology and Cardiac Surgery Executive Committee, 2012).

Collection of Specimens

Ongoing evaluation and screening of a newborn often requires obtaining blood by heelstick or venipuncture or the collection of a urine specimen. Laboratory tests may be ordered routinely (e.g., newborn screening) or for a specific purpose as directed by the health care provider.

Heelstick. Most blood specimens are drawn by laboratory technicians. Nurses, however, may be required to perform heelsticks to obtain blood for glucose monitoring, newborn screening, or other tests.

Blood samples should be collected in a manner that minimizes pain and trauma to the infant and maximizes the accuracy of test results. If a laboratory technician is collecting the specimen, the nurse assists as needed to maximize safety and infant comfort.

It is helpful to warm the heel before the sample is taken; application of heat for 5 to 10 minutes helps dilate the vessels in the area. A cloth soaked with warm water and wrapped loosely around the foot provides effective warming (Fig. 24-12, *A*). Disposable heel warmers are available from a variety of companies but should be used with care to prevent burns. Nurses should wear gloves when collecting any specimen. The nurse cleanses the area with an appropriate skin antiseptic, restrains the infant's foot with a free hand, and then punctures the site. A spring-loaded automatic puncture device causes less pain and requires fewer punctures than a manual lance blade.

The most serious complication of an infant heelstick is necrotizing osteochondritis resulting from lancet penetration of the bone. To prevent this problem, the puncture is made at the outer aspect of the heel and penetrates no deeper than 2.4 mm. To identify the appropriate puncture site, the nurse draws an imaginary line from between the fourth and fifth toes and parallel to the lateral aspect of the foot to the heel, where the puncture is made; a second line can be drawn from the great toe to the medial aspect of the heel (see Fig. 24-12, *B*). Repeated trauma

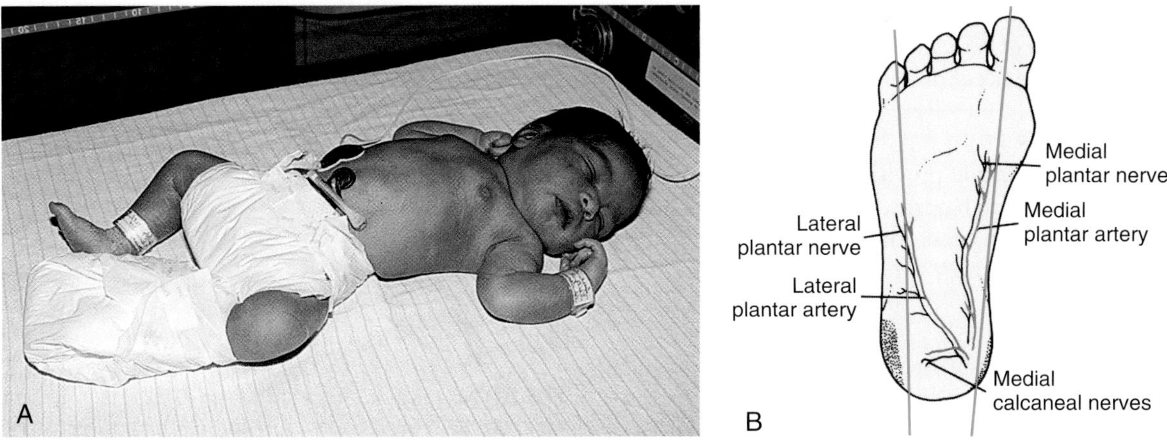

FIG 24-12 Heelstick. **A,** Newborn with foot wrapped for warmth to increase blood flow to extremity before heelstick. **B,** Heelstick sites *(shaded areas)* on infant's foot for obtaining samples of capillary blood. (**A,** Courtesy Marjorie Pyle, RNC, Lifecircle, Costa Mesa, CA.)

to the walking surface of the heel can cause fibrosis and scarring that can lead to problems with walking later in life.

After the specimen has been collected, gentle pressure is applied with a dry gauze pad. No further skin cleanser should be applied because it will cause the site to continue to bleed. The site is then covered with an adhesive bandage. The nurse safely disposes of equipment used, reviews the laboratory requisition for correct identification, and checks the specimen for accurate labeling and routing.

A heelstick is traumatic for the infant and causes pain. After several heelsticks, infants have been observed to withdraw their feet when they are touched. The nurse can reduce procedural pain using a variety of nonpharmacologic techniques including allowing the mother to hold the neonate skin to skin, using nonnutritive sucking with or without oral sucrose, or swaddling the neonate (see later discussion of neonatal pain) (McNair, Yeo, Johnston, & Taddio, 2013). To reassure the infant and promote feelings of safety, the neonate should be cuddled and comforted when the procedure is complete and appropriate pain management measures taken to minimize the pain.

Venipuncture. Occasionally laboratory tests are ordered that require larger samples of blood than can be collected with a heelstick. Venous blood samples can be drawn from antecubital, saphenous, superficial wrist, and rarely, scalp veins. When venipuncture is required, positioning of the needle is extremely important. A 23- or 25-gauge butterfly needle or hypodermic needle with a syringe is used (Fig. 24-13). Patience is required during the procedure because the blood return in small veins is slow and consequently the small needle must remain in place longer than a larger needle. A tourniquet is optional but can help increase blood flow with venipuncture. The infant is carefully restrained during the procedure to prevent injury. If venipuncture or arterial puncture is performed for blood gas studies, crying, fear, and agitation will affect the values; therefore, every effort must be made to keep the infant quiet during the procedure. Pressure must be maintained over an arterial or femoral vein puncture with a dry gauze square for 3 to 5 minutes to prevent bleeding from the site.

For an hour after any venipuncture, the nurse observes the infant frequently for evidence of bleeding or hematoma formation at the puncture site. The infant is cuddled and comforted when the procedure is completed, and appropriate pain management measures are taken. The nurse assesses and documents the infant's tolerance of the procedure.

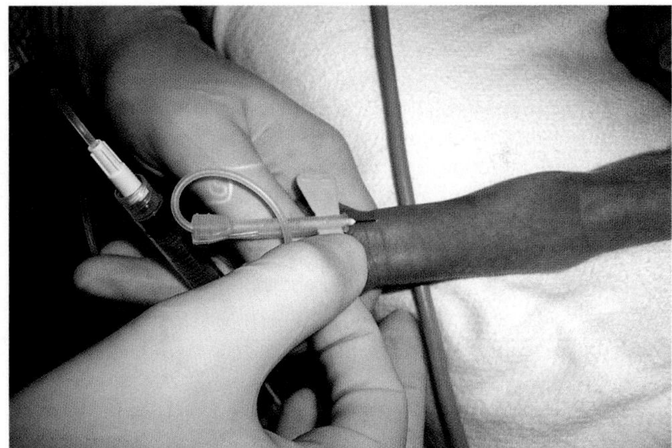

FIG 24-13 Venipuncture using a butterfly needle. (Courtesy Cheryl Briggs, RNC, Annapolis, MD.)

Urine Specimen. Analysis of urine is a valuable laboratory tool for infant assessment; the way in which the specimen is collected can influence the results. The urine sample should be fresh and analyzed within 1 hour of collection. A urine collection bag is often used to obtain a specimen.

Interventions

Protective Environment

The provision of a protective environment is basic to the care of the newborn. The construction, maintenance, and operation of nurseries in accredited hospitals are monitored by national professional organizations such as the AAP, The Joint Commission (TJC), the Occupational Safety and Health Administration (OSHA), and local or state governing bodies. In addition, hospital personnel develop their own policies and procedures for protecting the newborns under their care. Prescribed standards cover areas such as environmental factors, measures to control infection, and safety factors.

Current health care trends and the focus on nonseparation of mothers and babies (rooming-in) have prompted some hospitals to abandon having a separate newborn nursery. In the mother/baby model of care, the infant stays in the mother's room, which reduces the need for a separate nursery.

Environmental Factors

Environmental factors include provision of adequate lighting, elimination of potential fire hazards, safety of electrical appliances, adequate ventilation, and controlled temperature and humidity (AAP & ACOG, 2012).

Infection Control Factors

Measures to control infection in newborn nurseries include adequate floor space to permit the positioning of bassinets at least 3 feet apart in all directions, hand hygiene facilities, and areas for cleaning and storing equipment and supplies. Only specified personnel directly involved in the care of mothers and infants are allowed in these areas, thereby reducing the opportunities for the transmission of pathogenic organisms.

SAFETY ALERT

Proper hand hygiene is essential to prevent the spread of health care–associated infection. Personnel should wash hands with soap and water or use an alcohol-based handrub in accordance with hospital infection control policies. Hand hygiene should be performed before and after touching the infant, before an invasive procedure or medication administration, after contact with potentially contaminated objects (e.g., computer keyboards, telephone, countertop surfaces), and after removing sterile or nonsterile gloves (World Health Organization [WHO], 2009).

Health care workers must wear gloves when handling infants until blood and amniotic fluid have been removed from the skin, when drawing blood (e.g., heelstick), when caring for a fresh wound (e.g., circumcision), and during diaper changes.

Visitors such as siblings and grandparents are expected to perform hand hygiene before having contact with infants or equipment. Individuals with infectious conditions are excluded from contact with newborns or must take special precautions when working with infants. This group includes people with upper respiratory tract infections, gastrointestinal tract infections, and infectious skin conditions.

Preventing Infant Abduction

Nurses discuss infant security precautions with the mother and her family because infant abductions are an ongoing concern. In 1999 The Joint Commission issued a sentinel alert and called for a management plan to address infant security (The Joint Commission, 1999). As a result, many units have special limited-entry systems. Nurses teach mothers and their families to check the identity of any person who comes to remove the baby from their room. Personnel usually wear picture identification badges. On some units all staff members wear matching scrubs or special badges. Other units use closed-circuit television, computer monitoring systems, fingerprint identification pads, or infant bracelet security systems (Fig. 24-14) that alarm if the newborn is separated from the mother or is taken outside the boundaries of the unit. Nurses and new parents must work together to ensure the safety of newborns in the hospital environment (Hiner, Pyka, Burks, et al., 2012).

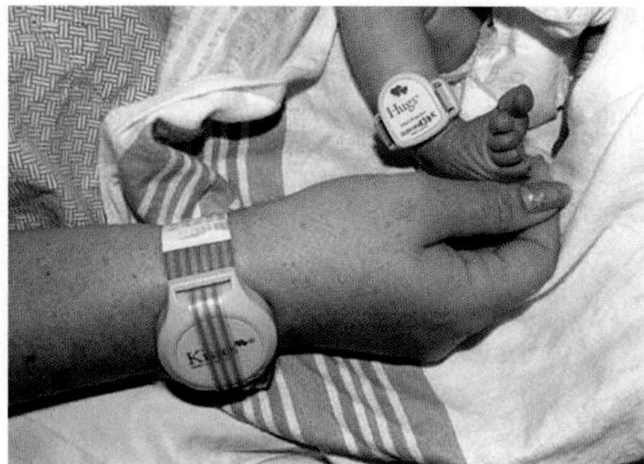

FIG 24-14 Mother and infant wear electronic bracelets as part of an infant security system. (Courtesy Shannon Perry, Phoenix, AZ.)

SAFETY ALERT

Nurses play a critical role in educating parents about measures to prevent infant abduction. Parents should be instructed how to identify legitimate hospital personnel, to never leave the newborn in the hospital room without direct supervision, and to request a second staff member to verify the identity of any questionable person who wants to take the baby from the mother's room. Parents should be instructed to use caution when posting photos of the new baby on the Internet and publishing public notices about the birth (AAP & ACOG, 2012).

Preventing Newborn Falls

Newborn infants are at risk for injury as a result of falling. Although newborn falls are likely underreported, it is estimated that approximately 600 to 1600 falls occur each year in U.S. hospitals (Helsey, McDonald, & Stewart, 2010). Most falls occur when the mother falls asleep while holding the newborn in her bed or in a reclining chair, although some falls occur at birth or when the infant is transported. Infants who fall, even from low level surfaces such as beds or chairs, are at risk of sustaining head injury that can include skull fracture. Parents may hesitate to report falls due to feelings of guilt and fear of reproach from staff members (Paul, Goodman, Remorino, & Bolger, 2011).

Nurses can help prevent newborn falls by identifying risk factors such as maternal medications (e.g., opioids) that cause drowsiness and can increase the risk of the mother falling asleep while holding the infant. Parents should be instructed to place their newborn in the supine position in the bassinet for sleep. Although bed-sharing is a controversial topic because some believe it promotes bonding, parents need to be aware of potential risks related to this practice. Infants should not be placed on couches or armchairs, whether or not a parent is present (Matteson, Henderson-Williams, & Nelson, 2013). Some hospitals ask parents and staff to sign an infant safety pledge to promote client safety; staff members conduct hourly rounds to monitor for fall risks (Galuska, 2011). Newborns are always transported in their bassinets and are never carried outside the mother's room. Educating parents using a nonjudgmental approach may increase the likelihood that a parent will report a newborn fall (Paul et al., 2011).

Therapeutic and Surgical Procedures

Intramuscular Injection. Newborns routinely receive IM injections before discharge. A single dose of vitamin K is

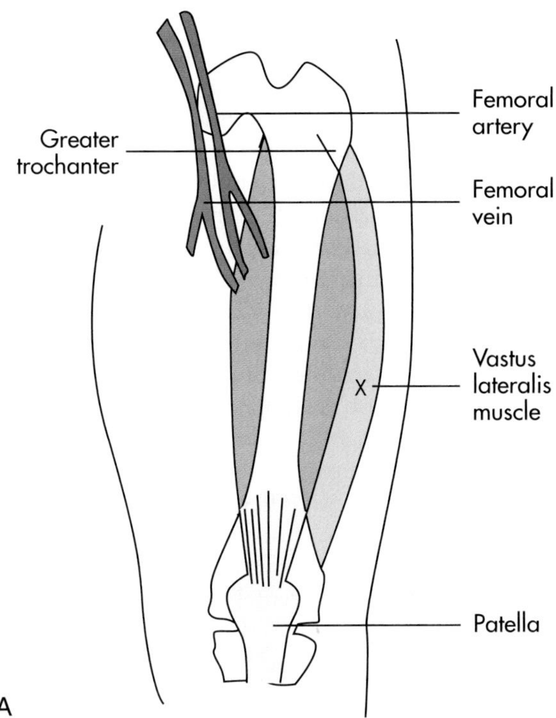

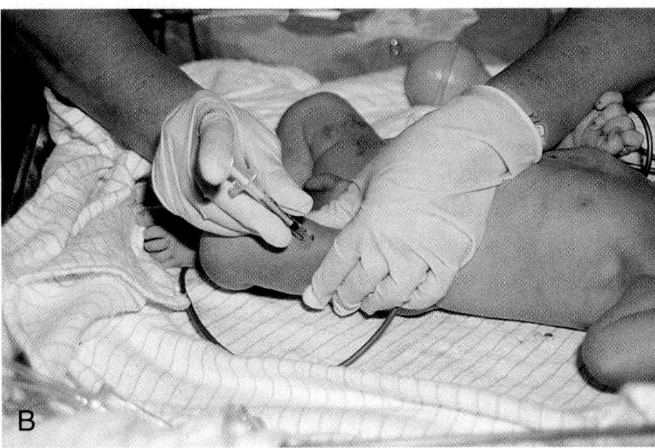

FIG 24-15 Intramuscular injection. **A,** Acceptable intramuscular injection site for newborn infant. *X,* injection site. **B,** Infant's leg stabilized for intramuscular injection. Nurse is wearing gloves to give injection. (**B,** Courtesy Marjorie Pyle, Lifecircle, Costa Mesa, CA.)

administered shortly after birth and hepatitis B (Hep B) vaccine is administered before discharge. Under specific circumstances, other IM injections may be ordered, such as a dose of HepB immune globulin for infants born to mothers who are positive for HepB.

Selection of the appropriate equipment and site for IM injection is important. In most cases a 25-gauge, ⅝-inch needle is used. Injections must be given in muscles large enough to accommodate the medication, and major nerves and blood vessels must be avoided. The muscles of newborns may not tolerate more than 0.5 ml per IM injection. The preferred injection site for newborns is the vastus lateralis (Fig. 24-15). The dorsogluteal muscle is very small, poorly developed, and dangerously close to the sciatic nerve, which occupies a proportionately larger area in infants than in older children. Therefore, it is not recommended as an injection site in small children. The newborn's deltoid muscle has an inadequate amount of muscle for IM administration. A key factor in preventing and minimizing local reaction to IM injections is adequate deposition of the medication deep within the muscle; therefore, muscle size, needle length, and amount of medication injected should be carefully considered.

The nurse wears nonsterile gloves when administering an injection. The neonate's leg should be stabilized. The nurse cleanses the injection site with an appropriate skin antiseptic and then stabilizes the infant's muscle between the thumb and forefinger. The needle is inserted into the vastus lateralis at a 90-degree angle. The medication is injected slowly. After the medication is injected, the nurse withdraws the needle quickly and places a dry gauze pad over the site, applying gentle pressure to minimize pain and bleeding.

The nurse comforts the infant after an injection and discards equipment properly. Needles are never recapped but are properly discarded in an appropriate safety container. The name of the medication, date and time, amount, route, and site of injection are documented in the newborn's record.

MEDICATION GUIDE

Hepatitis B Vaccine (Recombivax HB, Engerix-B)

Action

Hepatitis B (HepB) vaccine induces protective antihepatitis B antibodies in 95% to 99% of healthy infants who receive the recommended three doses. The duration of protection of the vaccine is unknown.

Indication

HepB vaccine is for immunizing against infection caused by all known subtypes of hepatitis B virus (HBV).

Neonatal Dosage

The usual dosage is Recombivax HB 5 mcg/0.5 ml or Engerix-B 10 mcg/0.5 ml intramuscularly at birth, at 1 to 2 months, and at 6-18 months.

Adverse Reactions

Common adverse reactions are rash, fever, erythema, swelling, and pain at the injection site.

Nursing Considerations

- Parental consent must be obtained before administration. Follow proper procedure for administration of intramuscular (IM) injection (see Fig. 24-15). If infant also needs hepatitis B immune globulin (HBIg), use separate sites for the two injections.
- For infants of mothers with negative HepB status, administer HepB vaccine before discharge from birthing facility.
- For infants born to hepatitis B surface antigen (HBsAg)–positive mothers, administer HepB vaccine and HBIg within 12 hours after birth.
- For infants born to mothers whose HepB status is unknown:
  - ≤2000 g: administer HepB vaccine and HBIG within 12 hours after birth
  - ≥2000 g: administer HepB vaccine within 12 hours; if mother's HepB results are positive, give HBIG by 1 week of age

Data from Centers for Disease Control and Prevention (CDC). (2014). Advisory Committee on Immunization Practices recommended immunization schedule for persons aged 0 through 18 years—United States, 2014. *MMWR Morbidity and Mortality Weekly Report, 63*(5), 108-109.

Immunizations. Hepatitis B (HepB) vaccination is recommended for all infants before discharge (see Medication Guide: Hepatitis B). Prior to administering the vaccine, the nurse obtains parental consent and notes the mother's HepB status. Infants at highest risk for contracting HepB are those born to women who have HepB or whose HepB status is unknown. If the mother is positive for HepB, the infant should receive the HepB vaccine and HepB immune globulin (HBIG) within 12 hours after birth (see Medication Guide: Hepatitis B Immune Globulin (Centers for Disease Control and Prevention [CDC], 2014).

MEDICATION GUIDE

Hepatitis B Immune Globulin

Action
Hepatitis B immune globulin (HBIG) provides a high titer of antibody to hepatitis B surface antigen (HBsAg).

Indication
The HBIG vaccine provides prophylaxis against infection in infants born of HBsAg-positive mothers.

Neonatal Dosage
Administer one 0.5-ml dose intramuscularly within 12 hours of birth.

Adverse Reactions
Hypersensitivity may occur.

Nursing Considerations
The HBIG vaccine must be given within 12 hours of birth. Follow proper procedure for administration of intramuscular injection (see Fig. 24-15). (See guidelines for administration in Medication Guide: Hepatitis B Vaccine.) The HBIG vaccine can be given at the same time as the HepB vaccine but at a different site. Document the date, time, and site of injection, as well as the lot number and expiration date of the vaccine, according to agency policy.

Data from Centers for Disease Control and Prevention (CDC). (2014). Advisory Committee on Immunization Practices recommended immunization schedule for persons aged 0 through 18 years—United States, 2014. *MMWR Morbidity and Mortality Weekly Report, 63*(5), 108-109.

Circumcision

Policies and Recommendations. Circumcision is the removal of all or part of the foreskin (prepuce) of the penis. Usually it is performed during the first few days of life but is sometimes done at a later time for preterm or ill neonates or for religious or cultural reasons.

The CDC reports that rates of newborn circumcision performed in U.S. hospitals peaked at 64.5% in 1981, dropping to a low of 55.4 in 2007. Rates increased slightly to 58.3% in 2010 (Owings, Uddin, & Williams, 2013).

Changes in recommendations from the AAP regarding newborn male circumcision (NMC) have likely influenced U.S. circumcision rates. The AAP policy on circumcision that was issued in 1999 and reaffirmed in 2005 recognized potential benefits of NMC, although the AAP did not deem them sufficient to recommend routine newborn circumcision (AAP Task Force on Circumcision, 2005). In 2012 the AAP issued a new policy statement regarding newborn male circumcision. The policy states: "Evaluation of current evidence indicates that the health benefits of newborn male circumcision outweigh the risks and that the procedure's benefits justify access to this procedure for families who choose it" (AAP Task Force on Circumcision, 2012, p. 585). The health benefits of NMC cited by AAP include prevention of urinary tract infection in male infants younger than 1 year, reduced risk for penile cancer, and reduced risk for heterosexual acquisition of sexually transmitted infections, particularly HIV (AAP Task Force on Circumcision, 2012). In spite of the new evidence, AAP does not recommend the practice of routine newborn circumcision.

The Canadian Paediatric Society does not support routine newborn circumcision. They recommend that parents should be informed of the current state of medical knowledge about the benefits and harm related to circumcision. The Society acknowledges that parental decisions may "ultimately be based on personal, religious, and cultural factors" (Outerbridge & Canadian Paediatric Society Fetus and Newborn Committee, 1996).

The World Health Organization (WHO) (2012) recognizes male circumcision as an important intervention in reducing the risk for heterosexually acquired HIV in men. The organization recommends early infant circumcision for newborn males weighing more than 2500 grams and without medical contraindication (WHO & Jhpiego, 2010).

Even with the change in AAP policy on NMC, newborn male circumcision remains a controversial topic. Opponents of circumcision feel that the procedure is unnatural and unnecessary and that it violates basic human rights. They cite concerns about acute pain; risks related to acute complications such as hemorrhage, infection, and penile injury (removal of excessive skin, damage to the meatus or glans); and long-term implications such as adverse effects on sexual function and pleasure. Websites such as www.intactamerica.org discourage parents from circumcising their newborn sons.

Parental Decision. Circumcision is a matter of personal parental choice. Parents usually decide to have their newborn circumcised for one or more of the following reasons: hygiene, religious conviction, tradition, culture, or social norms. Cost and insurance coverage are considerations in the parents' decision-making process. Parents need to make an informed choice regarding newborn circumcision based on the most current evidence and recommendations. Health care providers and nurses who care for childbearing families can help parents make an informed choice about newborn circumcision by providing factual, unbiased, evidence-based information. They can provide opportunities for discussion about the benefits and risks of the procedure.

Expectant parents need to begin learning about circumcision during the prenatal period, but circumcision often is not discussed with the parents. In many instances it is only when the mother is being admitted to the hospital or birthing unit that she is first confronted with the decision regarding circumcision. Because the stress of the intrapartum period makes this a difficult time for parental decision making, this is not an ideal time to broach the topic of circumcision and expect a well-informed decision.

Circumcision requires informed consent. Although the health care provider who will perform the procedure is legally responsible for educating parents about newborn circumcision so they can make an informed decision, nurses are often involved in discussions on this topic and should provide parents with current evidence-based information.

Procedure. Circumcision is not performed immediately after birth because of the danger of cold stress and decreased clotting factors but is usually done in the hospital before discharge. The circumcision of a Jewish male infant is commonly performed on the eighth day after birth at home in a ceremony called a *bris*. This timing is logical from a physiologic standpoint because clotting factors decrease somewhat immediately after birth and do not return to prebirth levels until the end of the first week.

Feedings may be withheld up to 2 to 3 hours before the circumcision to prevent vomiting and aspiration, although in some hospitals, infants are allowed to breastfeed until they are taken to the nursery for the procedure. To prepare the infant for the circumcision, he is positioned on a plastic restraint form (Fig. 24-16) and the penis is cleansed with soap and water or an antiseptic solution such as povidone-iodine. The infant is draped to provide warmth and a sterile field, and the sterile equipment is readied for use.

In the hospital setting newborn circumcision is usually performed using the Gomco (Yellen) or Mogen clamp or the PlastiBell device. The technique is usually based on health care provider training and preference. The procedure takes only a few minutes to perform. Use of the Gomco or Mogen clamp involves surgical removal of the foreskin. The clamp technique minimizes blood loss (Fig. 24-17). After the circumcision is completed, a small petrolatum gauze dressing is applied to the penis for the first 24 hours; thereafter, parents are instructed to apply petrolatum to keep the penis from adhering to the diaper (Association of Women's Health, Obstetric and Neonatal Nurses [AWHONN], 2013).

With the PlastiBell technique, the plastic bell is first fitted over the glans, a suture is tied around the rim of the bell, and excess foreskin is cut away. The plastic rim remains in place for about a week; it falls off after healing has taken place, usually within 5 to 7 days (Fig. 24-18). Petrolatum or dressings are not applied to the penis following circumcision with the PlastiBell (AWHONN, 2013).

Procedural Pain Management. Circumcision is painful. The pain is characterized by both physiologic and behavioral

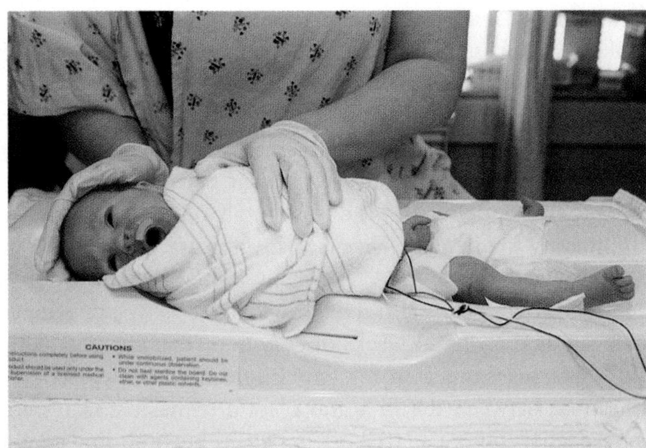

FIG 24-16 Positioning of infant in Circumstraint. (Courtesy Paul Vincent Kuntz, Texas Children's Hospital, Houston, TX.)

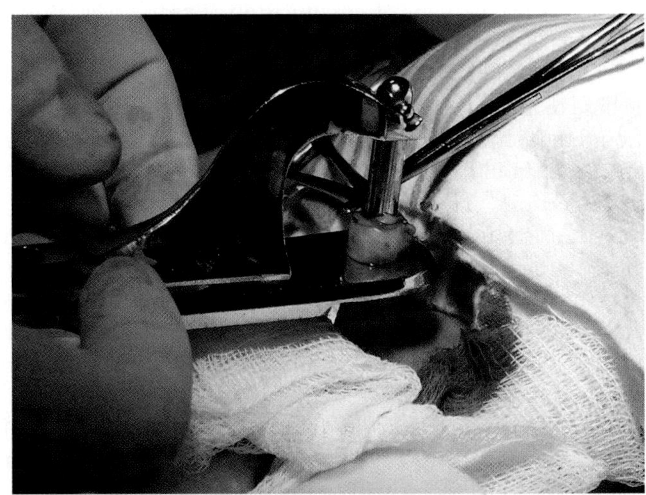

FIG 24-17 Circumcision with the Gomco (Yellen) clamp. After hemostasis occurs, the foreskin (over the metal dome) is cut away. (Courtesy Cheryl Briggs, RNC, Annapolis, MD.)

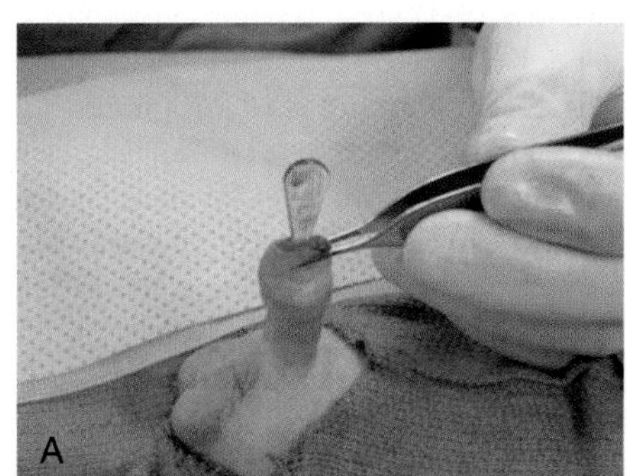

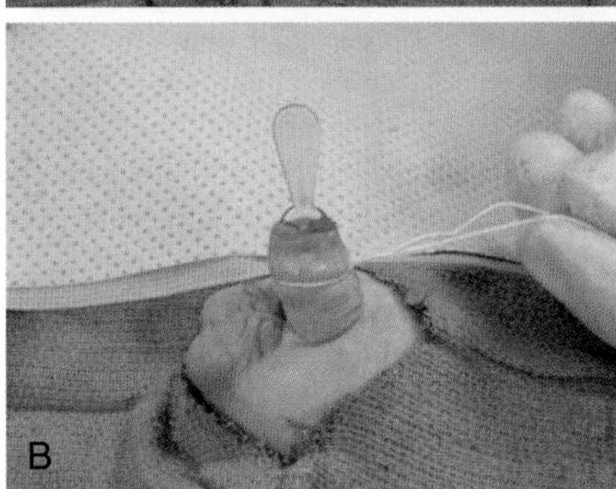

FIG 24-18 The PlastiBell technique. **A,** The PlastiBell is placed over the glans inside the prepuce. **B,** A string is then tied around the prepuce and positioned in the groove of the bell. The excess foreskin is trimmed and the handle is broken off the bell. The foreskin remnant and bell are expected to slough in 1 to 2 weeks. (From Holcomb, G.W., Murphy, J.P., Ostlie D.J. (2014). *Ashcraft's pediatric surgery* [6th ed.]. Philadelphia, Elsevier.)

changes in the infant (see discussion that follows). Four types of anesthesia and analgesia are used for newborn circumcision: ring block, dorsal penile nerve block (DPNB), topical anesthetic such as eutectic mixture of local anesthetic (EMLA) (prilocaine-lidocaine) or LMX4 (4% lidocaine), and concentrated oral sucrose. Nonpharmacologic methods such as nonnutritive sucking and swaddling can be used to enhance pain management.

The Cochrane group exploring pain relief for neonatal circumcision found that DPNB was the most effective intervention for decreasing the pain of circumcision (Brady-Fryer, Wiebe, & Lander, 2004). A DPNB includes subcutaneous injections of buffered lidocaine at the 2 o'clock and 10 o'clock positions at the base of the penis. A ring block is the subcutaneous injection of buffered lidocaine on each side of the penile shaft. The circumcision should not be performed for at least 5 minutes after these injections.

EMLA cream can be applied to the penis at least 1 hour before the circumcision. The area where the prepuce attaches to the glans is well coated with 1 g of the cream and then covered with a transparent occlusive dressing or finger cot. Just before the procedure, the cream is removed. Blanching or redness of the skin can occur.

After the circumcision the infant is comforted until he is quiet. If the parents were not present during the procedure, the infant is returned to them. The infant can be fussy for several hours and can have disturbed sleep-wake states and disorganized feeding behaviors. Some infants will go into a deep sleep after circumcision until they are awakened for feeding. Liquid acetaminophen 10 to 15 mg/kg may be administered orally after the procedure and repeated every 4-6 hours (as ordered by the health care provider) for a maximum of 30 to 45 mg/kg/24 hours (Zeltzer & Krane, 2011).

Care of the Newly Circumcised Infant. Postcircumcision protocols vary. In many settings the circumcision site is assessed for bleeding every 15 to 30 minutes for the first hour and then hourly for the next 4 to 6 hours. The nurse monitors the infant's urinary output, noting the time and amount of the first voiding after the circumcision.

If bleeding occurs from the circumcision site, the nurse applies gentle pressure with a folded sterile gauze pad. A hemostatic agent such as Gelfoam® powder or sponge can be applied to help control bleeding. If bleeding is not easily controlled, a blood vessel may need to be ligated. In this event, one nurse notifies the physician and prepares the necessary equipment (i.e., circumcision tray and suture material) while another nurse maintains intermittent pressure until the physician arrives.

Nurses provide education for parents related to care of the circumcised infant, which includes observing for complications such as bleeding or infection (see Teaching for Self-Management: Care of the Circumcised Newborn at Home). Parents need support and encouragement as they perform postcircumcision care. Newborns typically cry when the diaper is changed and when petrolatum gauze is removed and reapplied. This can make new parents feel anxious because they do not want to inflict pain on the infant. Nurses can inform parents that the discomfort is usually temporary and will soon subside. Additionally, nurses can teach parents a variety of nonpharmacologic comfort measures.

TEACHING FOR SELF-MANAGEMENT

Care of the Circumcised Newborn at Home

- Wash hands before touching the newly circumcised penis.

Check for Bleeding

- Check circumcision site for bleeding with each diaper change.
- If bleeding occurs, apply gentle pressure with a folded sterile gauze square. If bleeding does not stop with pressure, notify primary health care provider.

Observe for Urination

- Check to see that the infant urinates after being circumcised.
- Infant should have a wet diaper 2 to 6 times per 24 hours the first 1 to 2 days after birth and then at least 6 to 8 times per 24 hours after 3 to 4 days.

Keep Area Clean

- Change the diaper and inspect the circumcision at least every 4 hours.
- Wash the penis gently with warm water to remove urine and feces. Apply petrolatum to the glans with each diaper change (omit petrolatum if a PlastiBell was used). Do not use baby wipes because they can contain alcohol.
- Do not wash the penis with soap until the circumcision is healed (5 to 6 days).
- Apply the diaper loosely over the penis to prevent pressure on the circumcised area.

Check for Infection

- The glans penis is dark red after circumcision and then becomes covered with yellow exudate in 24 hours, which is normal and will persist for 2 to 3 days. Do not attempt to remove it.
- Redness, swelling, discharge, or odor indicates infection. Notify the pediatric health care provider if you think the circumcision area is infected.

Provide Comfort

- Circumcision is painful. Handle the area gently.
- Provide comfort measures such as holding the baby skin-to-skin, cuddling, swaddling, or rocking.

Neonatal Pain

Neonatal Responses to Pain

There is clear evidence that neonates can feel pain, despite previous thinking that the immaturity of the nervous system prevented or blunted pain sensation and that neonates were incapable of remembering painful experiences. Pain in the neonate and pain in later life can be qualitatively different, but research has substantiated that newborns do experience pain (Blackburn, 2013).

Pain has physiologic and psychologic components. Its psychologic component and the diffuse total body response to pain exhibited by the neonate led many health care providers in the past to believe that infants, especially preterm infants, do not experience pain. The central nervous system is well developed, however, as early as 24 weeks of gestation. The peripheral and spinal structures that transmit pain information are present and functional between the first and second trimesters. The pituitary-adrenal axis is also well developed at this time, and a fight-or-flight reaction is observed in response to the catecholamines released in response to stress.

The physiologic response to pain in neonates can be life threatening. Pain response can decrease tidal volume, increase demands on the cardiovascular system, increase metabolism, and cause neuroendocrine imbalance. The hormonal-metabolic response to pain in a term infant has greater magnitude and shorter duration than in adults. The newborn's sympathetic response to pain is less mature and therefore less predictable than an adult's.

Pain response is influenced by a variety of factors such as characteristics of the painful stimulus, gestational age, biologic factors, and behavioral state. The source, location, and timing of the pain affect the response; newborns respond differently to acute pain than to prolonged or recurrent pain. Pain perception and stress can be greater in preterm infants, although they often display less vigorous pain responses than term infants (Maxwell, Malavolta, & Fraga, 2013). There can be genetic differences in pain responses related to the amounts and types of neurotransmitters and receptors available to mediate pain. The behavioral state of the neonate also affects the pain response. Those who are more awake tend to have more robust pain responses than those in sleep states (Gardner, Enzman-Hines, & Dickey, 2011).

The most common behavioral sign of pain is a vocalization or crying, ranging from a whimper to a distinctive high-pitched, shrill cry. Facial expressions include grimacing, eye squeeze, brow contraction, deepened nasolabial furrows, a taut and quivering tongue, and an open mouth (Fig. 24-19) (Box 24-4). The infant will flex and adduct the upper body and lower limbs in an attempt to withdraw from the painful stimulus. The preterm infant has a lower than normal threshold for initiation of this response (Gardner et al., 2011).

Pain can result in significant changes in heart rate, blood pressure (increased or decreased), intracranial pressure, vagal tone, respiratory rate, and oxygen saturation. Neonates respond to painful stimuli with release of epinephrine, norepinephrine, glucagon, corticosterone, cortisol, 11-deoxycorticosterone, lactate, pyruvate, and glucose (Blackburn, 2013).

Assessment of Neonatal Pain

In assessing pain the nurse needs to consider the health of the neonate, the type and duration of the painful stimulus, environmental factors, and the infant's state of alertness. For example, severely compromised neonates may be unable to generate a pain response although they are, in fact, experiencing pain.

Every neonate should have an initial pain assessment as well as a pain management plan. The National Association of Neonatal Nurses (NANN) developed practice guidelines stating that all nurses who care for newborns should have education and competency validation in pain assessment. Pain should be assessed and documented on a regular basis (Walden & Gibbins, 2008).

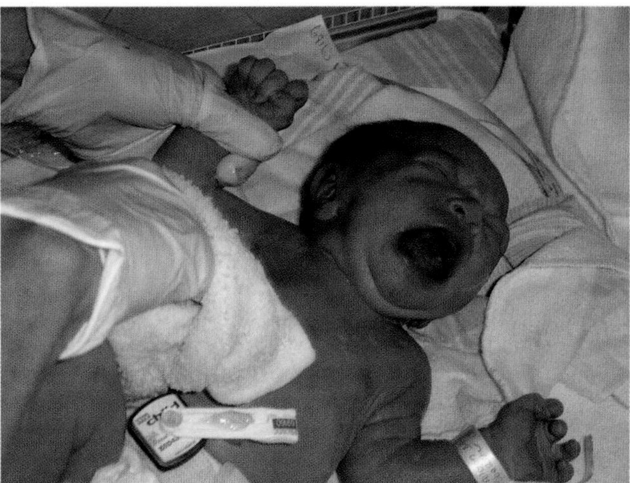

FIG 24-19 Signs of discomfort: note eye squeeze, brow bulge, nasolabial furrow, and wide-spread mouth. (Courtesy Kathryn Alden, Chapel Hill, NC.)

BOX 24-4 Manifestations of Acute Pain in the Neonate

Physiologic Responses

- Vital signs
  - Increased heart rate
  - Increased blood pressure
  - Rapid, shallow respirations
- Oxygenation
  - Decreased transcutaneous oxygen saturation ($tcPo_2$)
  - Decreased arterial oxygen saturation (Sao_2)
- Skin
  - Pallor or flushing
  - Diaphoresis
  - Palmar sweating
- Laboratory evidence of metabolic or endocrine changes
  - Hyperglycemia
  - Lowered pH
  - Elevated corticosteroids
- Other observations
  - Increased muscle tone
  - Dilated pupils
  - Decreased vagal nerve tone
  - Increased intracranial pressure

Behavioral Responses

- Vocalizations
  - Crying
  - Whimpering
  - Groaning
- Facial expression
  - Grimaces
  - Brow furrowed
  - Chin quivering
  - Eyes tightly closed
  - Mouth open and squarish
- Body movements and posture
  - Limb withdrawal
  - Thrashing
  - Rigidity
  - Flaccidity
  - Fist clenching
- Changes in state
  - Changes in sleep-wake cycles
  - Changes in feeding behavior
  - Changes in activity level
  - Fussiness, irritability
  - Listlessness

Data from Blackburn, S. (2013). *Maternal, fetal, and neonatal physiology: A clinical perspective* (4th ed.). St. Louis: Mosby; Gardner, S.L., Enzman-Hines, M., & Dickey, L.A. (2011). Pain and pain relief. In S.L. Gardner, B.S. Carter, M. Enzman-Hines, & J.A. Hernandez (Eds.), *Merenstein & Gardner's handbook of neonatal intensive care* (7th ed.). St. Louis: Mosby.

TABLE 24-5 CRIES Neonatal Postoperative Pain Scale*

	0	1	2
Crying	No	High pitched	Inconsolable
Requires oxygen for saturation >95%	No	<30%	>30%
Increased vital signs	Heart rate and blood pressure equal to or less than preoperative state	Heart rate and blood pressure <20% of preoperative state	Heart rate and blood pressure >20% of preoperative state
Expression	None	Grimace	Grimace and grunt
Sleepless	No	Wakes at frequent intervals	Constantly awake

Coding Tips for Using CRIES

Crying	The characteristic cry of pain is high pitched. If no cry or cry that is not high pitched, score 0. If cry is high pitched but infant is easily consoled, score 1. If cry is high pitched and infant is inconsolable, score 2.
Requires oxygen for saturation >95%	Look for changes in oxygenation. Infants experiencing pain manifest decreases in oxygenation as measured by total carbon dioxide or oxygen saturation. (Consider other causes of changes in oxygenation, such as atelectasis, pneumothorax, oversedation.) If no oxygen is required, score 0. If <30% oxygen is required, score 1. If >30% oxygen is required, score 2.
Increased vital signs	Note: Measure blood pressure last because this may wake the infant, causing difficulty with other assessments. Use baseline preoperative parameters from a nonstressed period. Multiply baseline heart rate (HR) × 0.2; then add this to baseline HR to determine the HR that is 20% over baseline. Do likewise for blood pressure (BP). Use mean BP. If HR and BP are both unchanged or less than baseline, score 0. If HR or BP is increased but increase is <20% of baseline, score 1. If either one is increased >20% over baseline, score 2.
Expression	The facial expression most often associated with pain is a grimace. This may be characterized by brow lowering, eyes squeezed shut, deepening of the nasolabial furrow, open lips and mouth. If no grimace is present, score 0. If grimace alone is present, score 1. If grimace and noncry vocalization grunt are present, score 2.
Sleepless	This is scored based on the infant's state during the hour preceding this recorded score. If the child has been continuously asleep, score 0. If he or she has awakened at frequent intervals, score 1. If he or she has been awake constantly, score 2.

*Neonatal pain assessment tool developed at the University of Missouri—Columbia.
From Krechel, S.W., & Bildner, J. (1995). CRIES: A new neonatal postoperative pain measurement score. Initial testing of validity and reliability. *Paediatric Anaesthesia, 5*(1), 53-61.

Pain assessment tools include:

- Neonatal Infant Pain Scale (NIPS) (Lawrence, Alcock, McGrath, et al., 1993)
- Premature Infant Pain Profile (PIPP) (Stevens, Johnston, Petryshen, & Taddio, 1996)
- Neonatal Pain Agitation and Sedation Scale (NPASS) (Hummel, Puchalski, Creech, & Weiss, 2008)

A pain assessment tool used by nurses in some neonatal intensive care units (NICUs) is CRIES (Krechel & Bildner, 1995) (Table 24-5). This tool was developed for use by nurses who work with preterm and term infants. CRIES is an acronym for the physiologic and behavioral indicators of pain used in the tool: ***c***rying, ***r***equiring increased oxygen, ***i***ncreased vital signs, ***e***xpression, and ***s***leeplessness. Each indicator is scored from 0 to 2. The total possible pain score, which represents the worst pain, is 10. A pain score greater than 4 should be considered significant. This tool can be used on infants between 32 weeks of gestation and 20 weeks after birth.

Healthy term newborns are exposed to fewer sources of pain than preterm infants in an NICU where painful procedures are inherent to care management. Even in low risk newborns, nurses need to assess for signs of discomfort as part of routine assessments and especially during and after routine procedures such as heelsticks, injections, and circumcisions (Maxwell et al., 2013).

Management of Neonatal Pain

The goals of the management of neonatal pain are to (1) minimize the intensity, duration, and physiologic cost of the pain and (2) maximize the neonate's ability to cope with and recover from the pain. Nonpharmacologic and pharmacologic strategies are used. It is important to note that despite research evidence, policies, and standards of practice focused on assessing and managing pain in newborns, acute infant pain remains undermanaged and, in some cases, unmanaged (Gardner et al., 2011).

Nonpharmacologic Management. A variety of nonpharmacologic pain management techniques are used with neonates. Nurses and parents may combine two or more techniques as they seek to promote infant comfort and reduce pain.

One of the most common measures is swaddling or snugly wrapping the infant with a blanket. Swaddling limits the neonate's boundaries, aids in self-regulation, and reduces

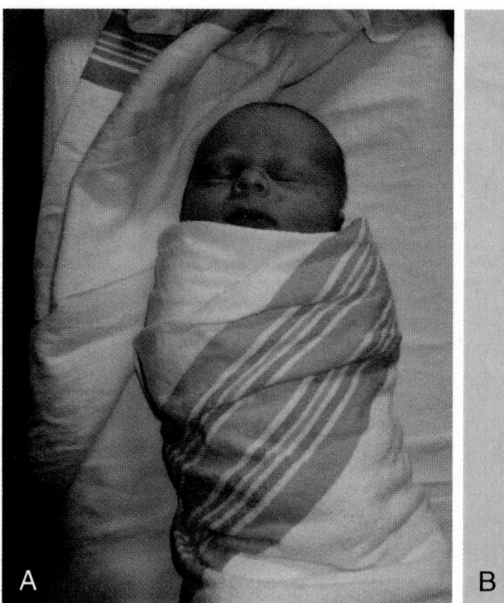

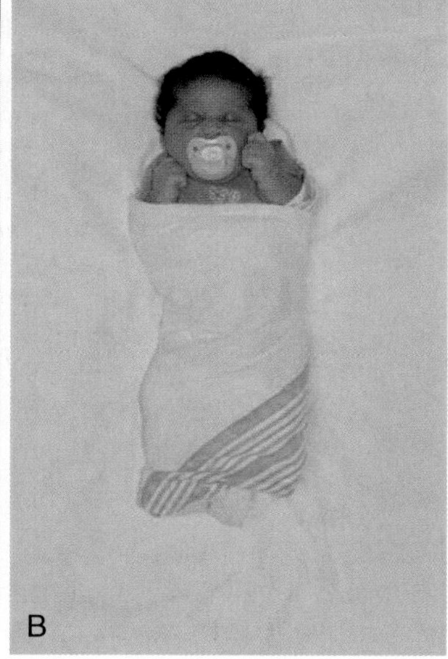

FIG 24-20 **A,** Newborn is swaddled with arms extended. **B,** Newborn is swaddled with arms flexed. (**A,** Courtesy Jennifer and Travis Alderman, Durham, NC. **B,** Courtesy Cheryl Briggs, RNC, Annapolis, MD.)

physiologic and behavioral stress resulting from acute pain (Riddell, Racine, Turcotte, et al., 2012). Swaddling is popular among nurses and parents as a comfort measure for calming a fussy baby and for promoting sleep. However, it is important that it is done properly. Safe swaddling involves wrapping the infant snugly in a blanket with the arms extended legs flexed, and hips in neutral position without rotation (Fig. 24-20, *A*) (AAP, 2014). In the early newborn period, nurses often swaddle infants with the arms flexed (Fig. 24-20, *B*).

SAFETY ALERT

Swaddling an infant tightly with legs extended is associated with increased risk for hip dislocation (developmental dysplasia of the hip [DDH]). The correct way to swaddle an infant is with the hips in slight flexion and abducted and allowing freedom of movement of the knees. It is important that the blanket is not wrapped too tightly as it can cause overheating or respiratory compromise. There should be space for 2 to 3 adult fingers between the infant's chest and the swaddle. A swaddled infant should be lying on his or her back. Swaddling is not recommended after approximately 2 months of age when the infant is capable of rolling over (AAP, 2014).

Other nonpharmacologic pain relief measures are used by nurses and parents. Facilitated tucking, a hand-swaddling technique in which the care provider holds the neonate in a flexed, side-lying position, is effective for reducing pain and distress in preterm infants (Riddell et al., 2012).

Nonnutritive sucking (NNS) on a pacifier is a common comfort measure used with newborns. Oral sucrose in small amounts given with a syringe with or without a pacifier for sucking is safe and effective in reducing neonatal pain during painful procedures such as venipunctures or heelsticks (Cignacco, Sellam, Stoffel, et al. 2012; Kassab, Roydhouse, Fowler, & Foureur, 2012; Riddell et al., 2012; Stevens, Yamada, Lee, & Ohlsson, 2013). Oral sucrose and NNS used in combination before or during a painful procedure can help reduce discomfort (Liaw, Zeng, Yang, et al., 2011; Naughton, 2013).

Skin-to-skin contact with the mother who holds the infant prone on her chest, also known as *kangaroo care,* during a painful procedure can help reduce pain (Johnston, Campbell-Yeo, Fernandes, et al., 2014; Kostandy, Anderson, & Good, 2013; Riddell et al., 2012). Breastfeeding or breast milk helps reduce pain during heel lancing and blood collection (Academy of Breastfeeding Medicine, 2010; Shah, Herbozo, Aliwalas, & Shah, 2012).

Distraction with visual, oral, auditory, or tactile stimulation can be helpful in term neonates or older infants (see Evidence-Based Practice box). *Sensorial saturation* uses multiple senses to diminish minor pain. This technique involves speaking softly to the infant, massaging the face, and providing oral sucrose solution on the tongue (Bellieni, Tei, Coccina, & Buonocore, 2012).

Other nonpharmacologic measures for reducing pain in newborns include touch, massage, rocking, holding, and environmental modification (e.g., low noise and lighting). Combining two or more nonpharmacologic methods can result in more effective pain reduction (Gabriel, de Mendoza, Figeuroa, et al., 2013).

Pharmacologic Management. Pharmacologic agents are used to alleviate pain associated with procedures. Local anesthesia is routinely used during procedures such as circumcision and chest tube insertion. Topical anesthesia is used for circumcision, lumbar puncture, venipuncture, and heelsticks. Nonopioid analgesia (oral liquid acetaminophen) is effective for mild to moderate pain from inflammatory conditions. Morphine and fentanyl are the most widely used opioid analgesics for pharmacologic management of neonatal pain. Continuous or bolus IV infusion of opioids provides effective and safe pain control. Other methods for managing neonatal pain are epidural infusion, local and

EVIDENCE-BASED PRACTICE

Nonpharmacologic Pain Relief for Newborns

Ask the Question

For term newborns, which complementary or alternative pain relief interventions are effective for minor painful procedures, such as heelstick?

Search for the Evidence

Search Strategies

English language research-based publications on newborn, pain, breastfeeding, heelstick, and sucrose were included.

Databases Used

Cochrane Collaborative Database, National Guideline Clearinghouse (AHRQ), CINAHL, PubMed, and UpToDate

Critical Appraisal of the Evidence

- Pain scores in newborns assess physical changes to determine pain levels. Term newborns have lower pain scores during minor painful procedures when they use sucking-related interventions and are held and rocked. Preterm newborns 30 to 36 weeks benefit from kangaroo care (being held skin-to-skin prone on caregiver's chest), sucking-related interventions, and swaddling (Riddell, Racine, Turcotte, et al., 2012).
- Breastfeeding is the first choice for single painful procedures for the multisensorial and synergistic comfort it brings. It also provides the parents a caregiving role (Academy of Breastfeeding Medicine [ABM] Protocol Committee, 2010).
- Skin-to-skin contact, along with 24% sucrose or 25% to 50% glucose administered via pacifier, dropper, syringe, or finger provide significant pain relief (ABM, 2010; Kassab, Roydhouse, Fowler, & Foureur, 2012).
- Preterm babies are at risk for more painful procedures. If breastfeeding is not possible, sucking-related interventions with sucrose decrease pain scores. However, there is concern that prolonged sucrose exposures in premature infants can lead to delays in motor skills and attention scores (ABM Protocol Committee, 2010).
- For term infants, sensorial saturation uses multiple senses to diminish minor pain. A protocol of simultaneously massaging the infant's face, speaking to the infant, and instilling a sweet solution into the infant's mouth is more effective for relieving pain than the sweet solution alone (Bellieni, Tei, Coccina, & Buonocore, 2012).

Apply the Evidence: Nursing Implications

- Nonpharmacologic pain relief methods for newborns use the gate-control theory to distract the newborn's attention by using strong single or multisensorial stimulation. Warmth, touch, auditory and visual attention, and sucking a sweet solution decrease pain scores.
- Sensorial saturation can be easily accomplished in the nursery. Parents who are taught this technique become active participants in their newborn's procedural care. However, they need clear education that using sucrose is not an appropriate long-term strategy for use at home.
- Although skin-to-skin contact, breastfeeding, and human milk are not well researched as pain relief interventions for preterm newborns, the ABM recommends that parents be allowed to try these measures (ABM Protocol Committee, 2010).
- Comfort measures usually work best when initiated a few minutes before the procedure to allow the newborn time to relax and reorganize (Kassab et al., 2012).
- Procedures other than single heelsticks or needlestick should be evaluated for pharmacologic analgesia. Sucrose is not sufficient pain relief for circumcisions.

Quality and Safety Competencies: Evidence-Based Practice*

Knowledge

Describe how the strength and relevance of available evidence influences the choice of interventions in provision of client-centered care.

Multisensorial stimulation that includes sucrose and sucking works best for pain relief.

Skills

Participate in structuring the work environment to facilitate integration of new evidence into standards of practice.

Parents can learn skills to manage their newborn's pain.

Attitudes

Value the need for continuous improvement in clinical practice based on new knowledge.

Nurses can explain to parents the evidence for pain relief in newborns.

References

Academy of Breastfeeding Medicine (ABM) Protocol Committee. (2010). Clinical protocol #23: Non-pharmacologic management of procedure-related pain in the breastfeeding infant. *Breastfeeding Medicine, 5*(6), 315–319.

Bellieni, C. V., Tei, M., Coccina, F., & Buonocore, G. (2012). Sensorial saturation for infants' pain. *Journal of Maternal, Fetal, and Neonatal Medicine, 25*(Suppl 1), 79–81.

Kassab, M. I., Roydhouse, J. K., Fowler, C., & Foureur, M. (2012). The effectiveness of glucose in reducing needle-related procedural pain in infants. *Journal of Pediatric Nursing, 27*(1), 3–17.

Riddell, R. P., Racine, N. M., Turcotte, K., et al. (2012). Non-pharmacological management of infant and young child procedural pain. *Evidence-Based Child Health, 7*(6), 1905–2121.

Pat Mahaffee Gingrich

*Adapted from QSEN at www.qsen.org.

regional nerve blocks, and intradermal or topical anesthetics (Gardner et al., 2011).

Promoting Parent-Infant Interaction

Nurses play an important role in promoting early social interaction between parents and their newborn infant. From birth throughout the hospital stay, nurses assess attachment behaviors (see Chapter 22) and provide support and education to parents as they become acquainted with the neonate. Nurses working in outpatient settings or home care provide follow-up assessments and care related to parent-child interactions. By teaching parents to recognize infant cues and respond appropriately, the nurse facilitates development of the parents' confidence in meeting the needs of their newborn (see Teaching for Self-Management: Helping Parents Recognize, Interpret, and Respond to Newborn Behaviors).

The sensitivity of the parent to the social responses of the infant is basic to the development of a mutually satisfying

TEACHING FOR SELF-MANAGEMENT

Helping Parents Recognize, Interpret, and Respond to Newborn Behaviors

Learning to read a baby's body language can enable parents to be more effective in preventing and solving problems around the infant's sleeping, eating, and crying and enhances parent-infant interaction. Nurses can teach new parents the following:

1. **Identify three newborn "zones," traditionally referred to as *newborn states.***
- "Resting zone": also known as *sleep states*
  - *Still/deep sleep:* Baby is completely still. Breathing is regular. No spontaneous activity. No movement of eyes, and eyelids stay shut. No vocalizing. Muscles are totally relaxed.
  - *Active/light sleep:* Baby may wiggle or vocalize. Eyes may flash open. Baby may make sucking movements—but still be asleep.
- "Ready zone": *alert state*
  - Baby's eyes are bright. Baby can focus on an object or person. Baby reacts to stimulation. Motor activity is minimal.
- "Rebooting zone": *fussy/crying state*
  - Baby's motor activity increases and is jerky. Baby is less responsive and moves from fussing to crying.

2. **Identify signs of stress.**
- When babies are stressed or overstimulated, they show changes in their body and behavior. These changes are called *SOSs* (Signs of Over-Stimulation), traditionally referred to as a baby's *stress response.*
  - *Body SOSs:* changes in color (becoming more red or pale); changes in breathing (becoming more irregular or choppy); changes in movement (becoming jerky or having more tremors)
  - *Behavioral SOSs:* "spacing out" (going from an alert state to a drowsy state); "switching off" (gaze aversion, or looking away from parent); "shutting down" (going from drowsy to a sleep state)
- When baby shows an SOS, parents should *decrease* stimulation and *increase* support by doing one or several of the following:
  - Quiet one's voice.
  - Glance away from baby.
  - Encourage baby to suck a finger or mother's breast.
  - Swaddle baby.
  - Place baby skin-to-skin.

3. **Help baby sleep well.**
- Distinguish active/light sleep from still/deep sleep.
- Parent's care:
  - *Prepare baby to sleep:* swaddling may help; feed in quiet, dark room at night and active, light environment during day.
  - *Get baby to sleep:* put baby down for sleep while he or she is still awake.
  - *Help baby stay asleep:* don't pick up during active/light sleep.
  - After breastfeeding is well established, notice when sleeping baby moves into active/light sleep. Wait and see if baby will transition from active/light sleep back to deep/still sleep—and sleep a bit longer.

4. **Help baby eat well.**
- Recognize early signs of hunger during the first few weeks: wiggling, making sucking movements, bringing hand to mouth.
- Notice if a fragile baby "spaces out" or "shuts down" when trying to eat. Bring this baby skin-to-skin and decrease stimulation before resuming feeding.
- If a parent needs to wake a fragile or small baby to eat, do so from active/light sleep, not from still/deep sleep.

5. **Help crying baby: consider what "TO DO."**
- T: *Talk* quietly to baby in sing-song voice.
- O: *Observe* to see if baby takes self-calming actions: brings his or her hand to his or her mouth, making sucking movements, or moves into the fencing reflex position.
- DO: *Bring* baby's hands to his or her chest; encourage sucking; make gentle "shooshing" sounds; swaddle baby; and/or bring baby skin-to-skin.

6. **Play with baby so he or she can learn and grow.**
- Demonstrate baby's ability to look at a parent's face, watch a toy move, or turn to parent's voice.
- Watch for an SOS during play. If an SOS occurs, decrease stimulation and increase support as described previously.
- Observe baby's developing process of interaction: first, getting quiet and still; second, turning toward parent; third, turning toward and looking at parent.
- Reinforce benefits of sensitive, face-to-face parent interaction with baby.

Data from Tedder, J.L. (2008). Give them the HUG: An innovative approach to helping parents understand the language of their newborn. *Journal of Perinatal Education, 17*(2), 14-20; Tedder, J.L. H.U.G.: *Help-understanding-guidance for young families.* Available at www.hugyourbaby.org.

parent-child relationship. Sensitivity increases over time as parents become more aware of their infant's social capabilities. In supporting parents, nurses need to consider cultural beliefs and traditions that influence parenting behaviors and infant care practices (see Cultural Considerations box).

The activities of daily care during the neonatal period are the best times for infant and family interactions. While caring for their newborn, the mother and father (or other family member) can talk to the infant, play baby games, caress and cuddle the baby, and perhaps use infant massage. Feeding is an optimal time for interaction because the infant is usually awake and alert, at least at the beginning of the feeding. Too much stimulation should be avoided after feeding and before a sleep period. In Figure 24-21 a great-grandmother and infant are shown engaging in arousal, imitation of facial expression, and smiling. Older children's contact with a newborn is encouraged and supervised based on the developmental level of the child (Fig. 24-22). Parents often keep memento books that record the birth, the hospital stay, and their infant's progress. Other parents create blogs to share their development as a family.

Discharge Planning and Parent Education

Infant care activities can cause anxiety for new parents. Support from nurses can be an important factor in determining whether new parents seek and accept help in the future. It is best for the nurse to avoid trying to cover all the content about newborn care at one time because the parents can be overwhelmed by too much information and become more anxious. Instead, parent education should occur throughout the hospital stay. However, because hospital stays after birth are relatively short, teaching all the content that is necessary can be a challenge for the nurse. As a result, many institutions have developed home visitation programs that take the necessary teaching to the new parents, although the hospital nurse still provides most of the essential information about newborn care. Printed materials about newborn care are provided to parents. In addition, nurses can direct parents to reliable websites for information on infant care (e.g., www.healthychildren.org).

CULTURAL CONSIDERATIONS

Cultural Beliefs and Practices Related to Infant Care

Nurses working with childbearing families from other cultures and ethnic groups must be aware of cultural beliefs and practices that are important to individual families. People with a strong sense of heritage may hold on to traditional health beliefs long after adopting other U.S. lifestyle practices. These health beliefs can involve practices regarding the newborn. For example, some Asians, Hispanics, Eastern Europeans, and Native Americans delay breastfeeding until the mother's milk is "in" (day 3 or 4) because they believe that colostrum is "bad." Some Hispanics and African-Americans place a belly band over the infant's umbilicus. In some Hispanic cultures, infants wear a special bracelet to help protect them from the evil eye (mal de ojo) (see photo). The birth of a male child is generally preferred by Asians and Eastern Indians, and some Asians and Haitians delay naming their infants. Families of Hindu heritage name the baby on the 11th day during a "cradle ceremony." Some women from India keep the cord of a male infant as a good omen that will ward off evil and will bring them more male infants in the future. The practice of skin-to-skin contact after birth may conflict with cultural beliefs about thermoregulation; some women from Africa prefer that the newborn is wrapped prior to being placed on the mother's chest. On the other hand, women from Mexico are wrapped in warm blankets after birth and wrap the newborn inside their blankets. Cultural beliefs influence when the newborn is taken out of the house, such as after the cord falls off, or after the mother's confinement period is over (approximately 30 days after birth). Weighing the infant can raise concerns for some women such as those from rural India, who may believe that frequent weighing will slow the infant's growth.

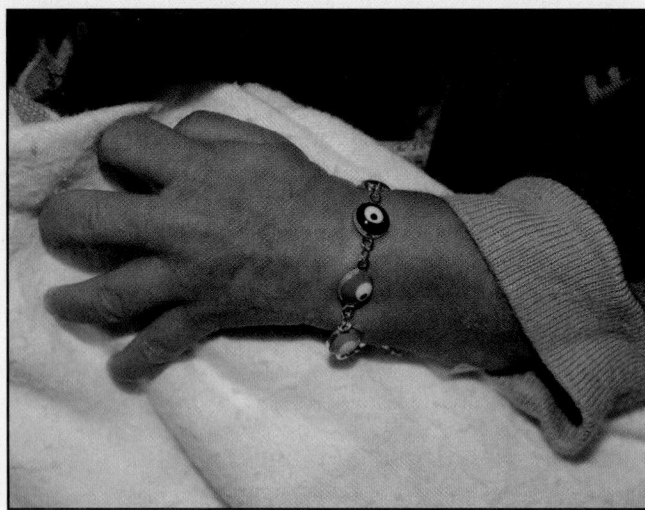

Newborn wearing "evil eye" bracelet. (Courtesy Cheryl Briggs, RNC, Annapolis, MD.)

Data from Giger, J. N. (2013). *Transcultural nursing* (6th ed.). St. Louis: Mosby; Purnell, L. D. (2014). *Culturally competent health care* (3rd ed.). Philadelphia: F.A. Davis.

To set priorities for teaching, the nurse follows parental cues. Knowledge deficits or gaps should be identified before beginning to teach. Normal growth and development and the changing needs of the infant (e.g., for personal interaction and stimulation, growth milestones, exercise, injury prevention, and social contacts), as well as the topics that follow, should be included during discharge planning with parents. Safety issues should be addressed (see Teaching for Self-Management: Infant Safety).

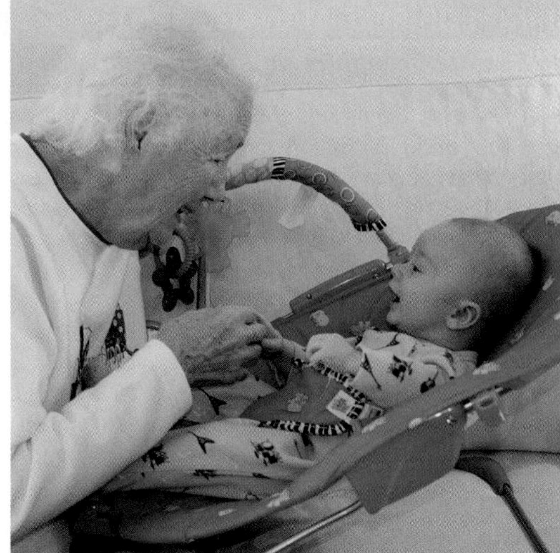

FIG 24-21 Great-grandmother and infant enjoying social interaction. (Courtesy Freida Belding, Bird City, KS.)

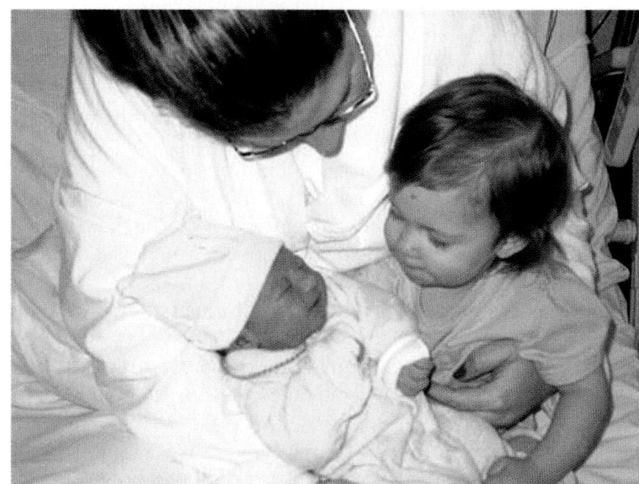

FIG 24-22 Mother supervising contact of older sibling with newborn. (Courtesy Rebekah Vogel, Fort Collins, CO.)

Temperature

Parents need to understand practical information related to thermoregulation. The nurse discusses the following topics in parent teaching:

- The causes of changes in body temperature (e.g., overwrapping, cold stress with resultant vasoconstriction, or minimal response to infection) and the body's response to extremes in environmental temperature
- Ways to promote normal body temperature, such as dressing the infant appropriately for the environmental air temperature and protecting the infant from exposure to direct sunlight
- Use of warm wraps or extra blankets in cold weather
- Technique for taking the newborn's axillary temperature, and normal values for axillary temperature
- Signs to be reported to the primary health care provider such as high or low temperatures with accompanying fussiness, lethargy, irritability, poor feeding, and excessive crying

TEACHING FOR SELF-MANAGEMENT

Infant Safety

- Always lay the baby flat in bed (in the bassinet or crib) on his or her back for sleep, for naps, and at night. Do not place your infant on the abdomen for sleep.
- Room-sharing, but not bed-sharing, is recommended during the early weeks.
- Never put your baby on a cushion, pillow, beanbag, or waterbed to sleep. Your baby may suffocate.
- There should be no bumper pads, blankets, stuffed toys, or other soft objects in the baby's crib because of the risk for suffocation.
- Do not cover the baby with blankets or quilts; dress the baby in light sleep clothing such as a sleep sack or one-piece sleeper.
- Check your baby's crib for safety. Slats should be no more than 2¼ inches apart. The space between the mattress and sides should be less than 2 fingerwidths. The bedposts should have no decorative knobs.
- The crib mattress should be firm and should fit snugly against the crib rails.
- Do not use a crib with drop rails.
- Never leave your baby alone on a bed, couch, or table. Even newborns can move enough to eventually reach the edge and fall off.
- When using an infant carrier, place the carrier on the floor in a place where you can see the baby. It should never be on a high place, such as a table, sofa, or store counter.
- Infant carriers do not keep your baby safe in a car. Always place your baby in an approved car safety seat when traveling in a motor vehicle (car, truck, bus, or van). Car safety seats are recommended for travel on trains and airplanes as well. Use the car safety seat for *every* ride. Your baby should be in a rear-facing infant car safety seat from birth until age 2 years or until exceeding the car seat's limits for height and weight. The car safety seat should be in the back seat of the car (see Fig. 24-24). This precaution is especially important in vehicles with front passenger air bags because when air bags inflate, they can be fatal for infants and toddlers. If an infant must ride in the front seat, disable the air bag.
- When bathing your baby, never leave him or her alone. Newborns and infants can drown in 1 to 2 inches of water.
- Be sure that your hot water heater is set at 49° C (120° F) or less. Always check bath water temperature with your elbow before putting your baby in the bath.
- Do not tie anything around your baby's neck. Pacifiers, for example, tied around the neck with a ribbon or string can strangle your baby.
- Keep the crib or playpen away from window blind and drapery cords; your baby could strangle on them.
- Keep the crib and playpen well away from radiators, heat vents, and portable heaters. Linens in the crib or playpen can catch fire if they come into contact with these heat sources.
- Install smoke detectors on every floor of your home. Check them once a month to be sure they are working properly. Change batteries twice a year.
- Avoid exposing your baby to cigarette or cigar smoke in your home or other places. Passive exposure to tobacco smoke greatly increases the likelihood that your infant will have respiratory symptoms and illnesses.
- Be gentle with your baby. Do not pick your baby up or swing your baby by the arms or throw him or her up in the air. Never shake the baby.

Data from American Academy of Pediatrics (AAP) Task Force on Sudden Infant Death Syndrome. (2011). SIDS and other sleep-related infant deaths: Expansion of recommendations for a safe infant sleeping environment. *Pediatrics, 128*(5):e1341-e1367; National Institute of Child Health and Human Development. (2013). *Safe to sleep public education campaign.* Bethesda, MD: Author. National Highway Traffic Safety Administration (NHTSA) Parents Central. (2012). *From car seats to car keys: Keeping kids safe.* Washington, DC: Author.

Respirations

The nurse provides information to parents regarding the normal characteristics of newborn respirations, emergency procedures, and measures to protect the infant. It is helpful to discuss signs of respiratory infection and to offer suggestions related to care of the infant who experiences symptoms. The following points are included in teaching about respirations:

- Normal variations in the rate and rhythm of respirations
- Reflexes such as sneezing to clear the airway
- Use of the bulb syringe
- Steps to take if the infant appears to be choking
- The need to protect the infant from:
  - Exposure to people with upper respiratory tract infections and respiratory syncytial virus
  - Exposure to secondhand tobacco smoke
  - Suffocation from loose bedding, water beds, and beanbag chairs; drowning (in bath water); entrapment under excessive bedding or in soft bedding; anything tied around the infant's neck; poorly constructed playpens, bassinets, or cribs
- Sleep position—on back when put to sleep; room sharing but not bed sharing is recommended during the early weeks
- Avoid the use of baby powder or corn starch; these substances can cause lung irritation
- Notify the health care provider if the infant develops symptoms such as difficulty breathing or swallowing, nasal congestion, excess drainage of mucus, coughing, sneezing, decreased interest in feeding, or fever.
- If the infant has a respiratory illness such as the "common cold," the following suggestions can be helpful:
  - Feed smaller amounts more often to prevent overtiring the infant.
  - Hold the baby in an upright position to feed.
  - For sleeping, raise the infant's head and chest by raising the mattress 30 degrees (do *not* use a pillow).
  - Avoid drafts; do not overdress the baby.
  - Use only medications prescribed by a pediatric health care provider. Do not use over-the-counter medications without provider approval.
  - Use nasal saline drops in each nostril and suction well with bulb syringe to decrease and relieve secretions.

Feeding Patterns

Nurses instruct parents about infant feeding and provide assistance based on whether they have chosen breastfeeding or formula feeding. Feeding patterns and practices for newborns are discussed in Chapter 25.

Elimination

Awareness of the normal elimination patterns of newborns helps parents recognize problems related to voiding or stooling. The following points are included in teaching about elimination:

- Color of normal urine and number of voidings to expect each day: at least two to six for the first 1 to 3 days; then a minimum of six to eight voidings per day thereafter. Urine should be pale yellow (like lemonade).
- Changes to be expected in the color and consistency of the stool (i.e., meconium to transitional to soft yellow or golden yellow) and the number of bowel movements, plus the odor of stools for breastfed or bottle-fed infants (see Box 23-1).
- Formula-fed infants may have as few as one stool every other day after the first few weeks of life; stools are pasty to semi-formed.
- Breastfed infants should have at least three stools every 24 hours for the first few weeks. The stools are looser and resemble mustard mixed with cottage cheese; the odor is less offensive than stools of infants who are formula fed.

Safe Sleeping, Positioning, and Holding

The AAP recommends placing the infant in the supine position for sleep during the first year of life to prevent sudden infant death syndrome (SIDS). Infants should lie on a firm surface, specifically on a firm crib mattress covered by a fitted sheet. Soft materials such as bumper pads, comforters, quilts, pillows, sheepskins, or stuffed toys should not be placed in the crib. Room sharing but not bed sharing is recommended during infant sleep; bed sharing can increase the risk of suffocation and falls. Infants may be brought into the parent's bed for comforting or for breastfeeding but should be returned to the crib or bassinet before the parent goes to sleep (AAP Task Force on Sudden Infant Death Syndrome [SIDS], 2011) (see Teaching for Self-Management: Infant Safety).

Parent education prior to hospital discharge should include specific information about safe sleep practices. The Safe to Sleep campaign from the National Institute of Child Health and Human Development (2013) provides materials for health care professionals and parents. The educational resources are designed to reach culturally diverse audiences with messages about promoting a safe sleep environment and preventing SIDS (see www.nichd.nih.gov/sts/Pages/default.aspx).

To help remind parents about safe sleep, some hospitals post a laminated safe sleep card in the newborn's bassinet. Using the mnemonic ABC developed by FirstCandle.com, a nonprofit organization that promotes safe sleeping practices, the message is, "I sleep safest Alone, on my Back, in my Crib" (Hitchcock, 2012).

Anatomically, the infant's shape—a barrel chest and flat, curveless spine—facilitates the infant to roll from the side to the prone position; therefore, the side-lying position for sleep is not recommended. When the infant is awake, "tummy time" can be provided under parental supervision so the infant can begin to develop appropriate muscle tone for eventual crawling; placing the infant prone at intervals when awake aids in preventing a misshapen head (positional plagiocephaly).

Care must be taken to prevent the infant from rolling off flat, unguarded surfaces. When an infant is on such a surface, the parent or nurse who must turn away from the infant even for a moment should always keep one hand placed securely on the infant.

The infant is always held securely with the head supported because newborns are unable to maintain an erect head posture for more than a few moments. Figure 24-23 illustrates various positions for holding an infant with adequate support.

CLINICAL REASONING CASE STUDY

Safe Infant Sleep Practices

The mother/baby nurse is teaching the new parents about safe sleep practices for their healthy term newborn son. The grandmother is listening and insists that all her babies slept most soundly when they were on their "tummies." The mother proudly shows the nurse a photo of the baby's nursery at home, including an antique crib with colorful fabric covered bumper pads and a matching fluffy quilt. There are several stuffed animals in the crib. What information should the nurse provide related to safety concerns for the newborn?

1. Evidence—Is there sufficient evidence to draw conclusions about the safety of the sleep environment in terms of preventing sudden infant death syndrome or infant injury?
2. Assumptions—What assumptions can be made about the following factors related to safe infant sleep?
   a. Infant positioning for sleep
   b. Risk for suffocation
   c. Risk for injury
3. What implications and priorities for nursing care can be drawn at this time?
4. Does the evidence objectively support your conclusion?

Rashes

Diaper Rash. The majority of infants develop a diaper rash at some time. This dermatitis or skin inflammation appears as redness, scaling, blisters, or papules. Various factors contribute to diaper rash including infrequent diaper changes, diarrhea, use of plastic pants to cover the diaper, a change in the infant's diet such as when solid foods are added, or when breastfeeding mothers eat certain foods.

Parents are instructed in measures to help prevent and treat diaper rash. Diapers should be checked often and changed as soon as the infant voids or stools. Plain water with mild soap, if needed, is used to cleanse the diaper area; if baby wipes are used, they should be unscented and contain no alcohol. The infant's skin should be allowed to dry completely before applying another diaper. Exposing the buttocks to air can help dry up diaper rash. Because bacteria thrive in moist, dark areas, exposing the skin to dry air decreases bacterial proliferation. Zinc oxide ointments can be used to protect the infant's skin from moisture and further excoriation (AWHONN, 2013).

Although diaper rash can be alarming to parents and annoying to babies, most cases resolve within a few days with simple home treatments. There are instances when diaper rash is more serious and requires medical treatment.

The warm, moist atmosphere in the diaper area provides an optimal environment for *Candida albicans* growth; dermatitis appears in the perianal area, inguinal folds, and lower abdomen. The affected area is intensely erythematous with a sharply demarcated, scalloped edge, often with numerous satellite lesions that extend beyond the larger lesion (AWHONN, 2013). Therapy consists of applications of an anticandidal ointment,

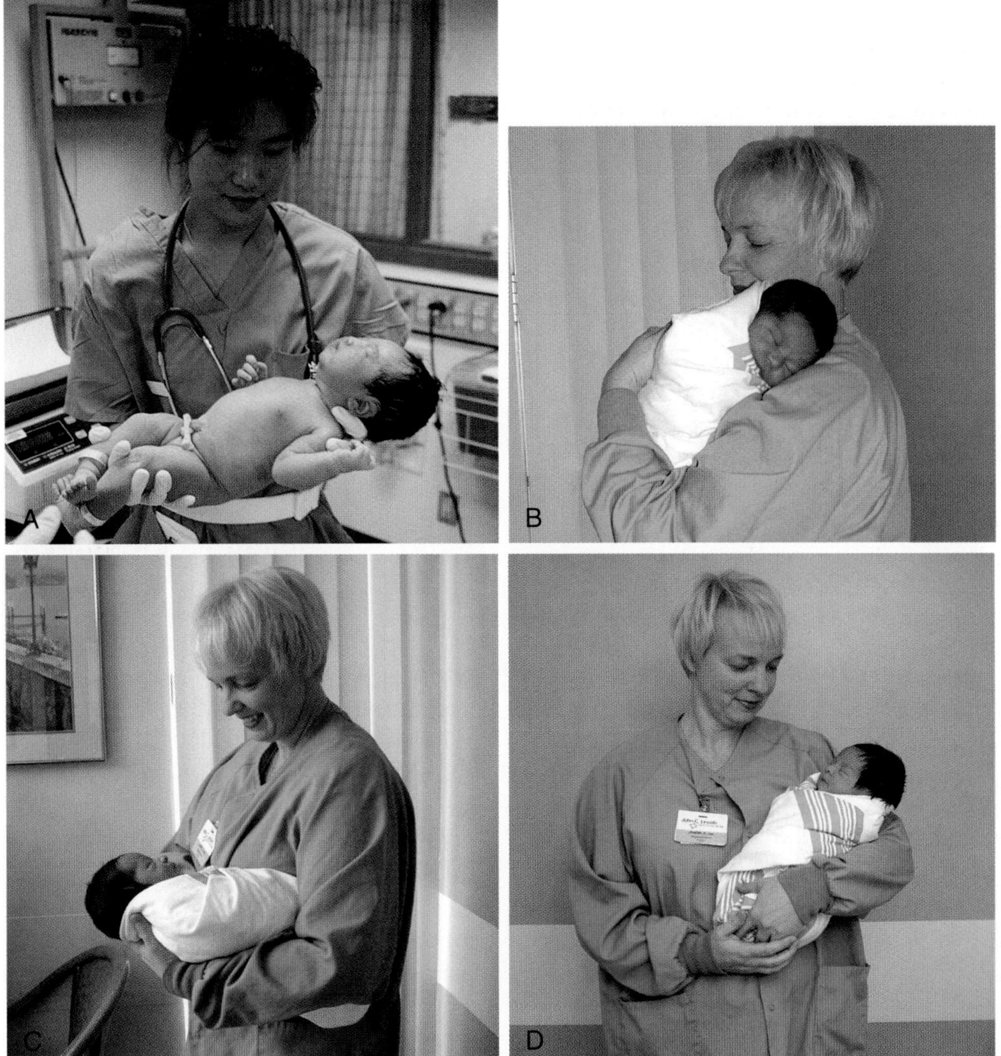

FIG 24-23 Holding the baby securely with support for head. **A,** Holding infant while moving infant from scale to bassinet. Baby is undressed to show posture. **B,** Holding baby upright in "burping" position. **C,** "Football" (under the arm) hold. **D,** Cradling hold. (**A,** Courtesy Kim Molloy, Knoxville, IA. **B, C,** and **D,** Courtesy Julie Perry Nelson, Loveland, CO.)

such as clotrimazole or miconazole, with each diaper change. Sometimes the infant is given an oral antifungal preparation such as nystatin or fluconazole to eliminate any gastrointestinal source of infection.

Other Rashes. A rash on the cheeks can result from the infant's scratching with long unclipped fingernails or from rubbing the face against the crib sheets, particularly if regurgitated stomach contents are not washed off promptly. The newborn's skin begins a natural process of peeling and sloughing after birth. Dry skin may be treated with an emollient applied once or twice daily (AWHONN, 2013). Newborn rash, erythema toxicum, is a common finding (see Fig. 23-6, *B*) and needs no treatment.

Clothing

Parents commonly ask how warmly they should dress their infant. A simple suggestion is to dress the child for the environment as they dress themselves, adding no more than one layer more than they would be wearing as adults. Overheating should be avoided (AAP Task Force on Sudden Infant Death Syndrome, 2011). A cap or bonnet is needed to protect the scalp and minimize heat loss if the weather is cool or to protect against sunburn. Wrapping the infant snugly in a blanket maintains body temperature and promotes a feeling of security. Overdressing in warm temperatures can cause discomfort, as can underdressing in cold weather. Parents are encouraged to dress the infant at all times in flame-retardant clothing. The eyes should be shaded if it is sunny and hot. Infant sunglasses are available to protect the infant's eyes when outdoors (Fig. 24-24).

Car Seat Safety

Infants should travel only in federally approved rear-facing safety seats secured in the rear seat using the vehicle safety belt (Fig. 24-25). To secure the infant in the rear-facing car safety seat, shoulder harnesses are placed in the slots at or below the level of the infant's shoulders. The harness is snug, and the retainer clip is placed at the level of the infant's armpits as opposed to on the abdomen or neck area.

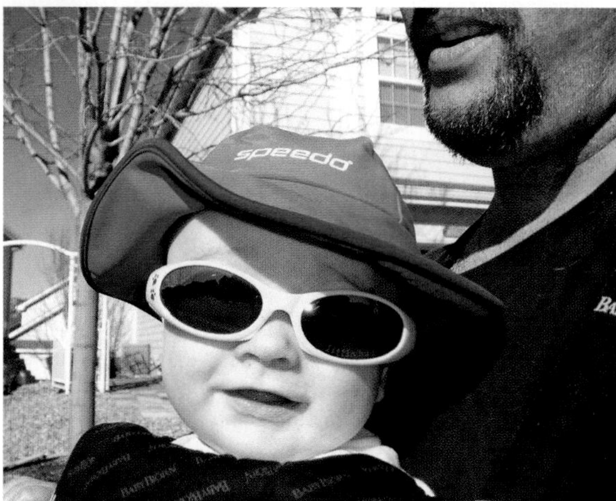

FIG 24-24 Sunglasses protect the infant's eyes. (Courtesy Julie Perry Nelson, Loveland, CO.)

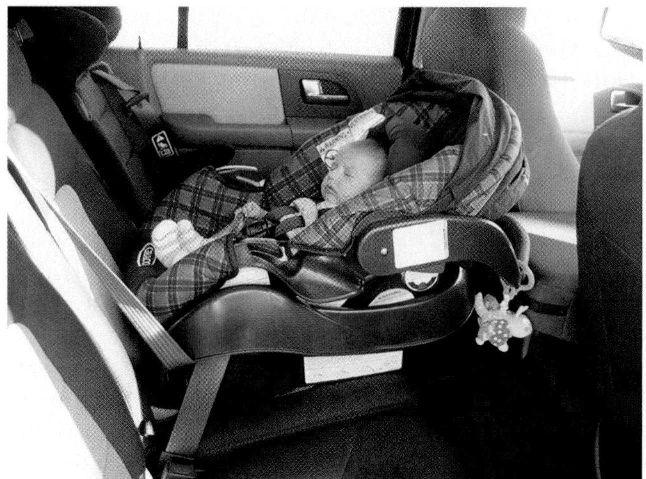

FIG 24-25 Rear-facing car seat in rear seat of car. Infant is placed in seat when going home from the hospital. (Courtesy Brian and Mayannyn Sallee, Anchorage, AK.)

SAFETY ALERT

Infants and toddlers should use a rear-facing car seat until the age of 2 years or for as long as possible up to the weight and height limit for their particular car seat. The safest area of the car is the back seat. A car safety seat that faces the rear gives the best protection for an infant's disproportionately weak neck and heavy head. In this position the force of a frontal crash is spread over the head, neck, and back; the back of the car safety seat supports the spine (AAP, 2012; National Highway Traffic Safety Administration [NHTSA], 2012).

In cars equipped with front air bags, rear-facing infant seats should never be placed in the front seat. Serious injury can occur if the air bag inflates because these types of infant seats fit close to the dashboard. If the infant must ride in the front seat, the air bag must be turned off. For cars with side air bags, parents should read the vehicle owner's manual for information about placement of car seats next to a side air bag (AAP, 2012; NHTSA, 2012).

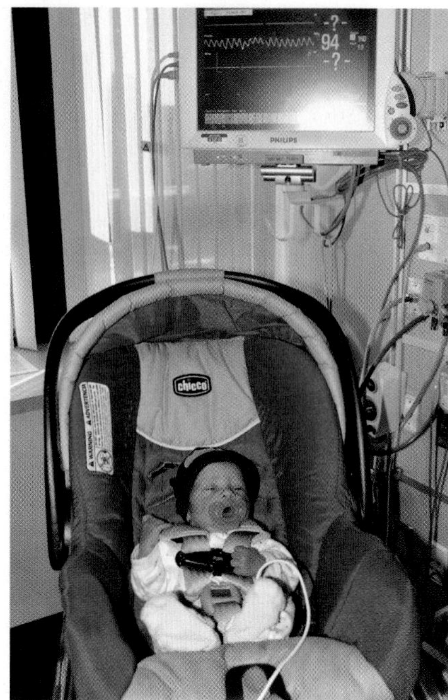

FIG 24-26 Infant Car Seat Challenge: testing is done before discharge from the birthing facility. Preterm infant is in car seat with pulse oximetry monitoring. (Courtesy Cheryl Briggs, RNC, Annapolis, MD.)

Infants are positioned at a 45-degree angle in a car seat to prevent slumping and subsequent airway obstruction. Many seats allow for adjustment of the seat angle. For seats that are not adjustable, a tightly rolled newspaper, a solid-core Styrofoam roll, or a firm roll of fabric can be placed under the car safety seat to place the infant at a 45-degree angle (Bull, Engle, & AAP Committee on Injury, Violence, and Poison Prevention & Committee on Fetus and Newborn, 2009).

Before discharge from the birth institution, infants born at less than 37 weeks of gestation should be observed in a car seat (preferably their own) for at least 90 to 120 minutes or a period of time equal to the length of the car ride home. This is known as the Infant Car Seat Challenge. The infant is monitored for apnea, bradycardia, and a decrease in oxygen saturation (Fig. 24-26). If the infant exhibits any of these clinical signs, travel home should be in a Federal Motor Vehicle Safety Standard 213 (FMVSS 213)–approved car bed (Bull et al., 2009).

SAFETY ALERT

If the parents do not have a car safety seat, arrangements should be made to make an appropriate seat available for purchase, loan, or donation. Parents need to be cautioned about purchasing a secondhand car safety seat without knowing its history. They should never use a car seat that was involved in a moderate to severe crash, is too old, has visible cracks, does not have a label with the model number and manufacture date, does not come with instructions, is missing parts, or was recalled (AAP, 2012).

Nonnutritive Sucking

Sucking is the infant's chief pleasure. However, sucking needs may not be satisfied by breastfeeding or bottle-feeding alone.

In fact, sucking is such a strong need that infants who are deprived of sucking, such as those with a cleft lip, will suck on their tongues. Several benefits of nonnutritive sucking have been demonstrated, such as an increased weight gain in preterm infants, increased ability to maintain an organized state, and decreased crying.

There is compelling evidence that pacifiers help prevent SIDS. The AAP Task Force on Sudden Infant Death Syndrome (2011) suggests that parents consider offering a pacifier for naps and bedtime. The pacifier should be used when the infant is placed supine for sleep, and it should not be reinserted once the infant falls asleep. No infant should be forced to take a pacifier. Pacifiers are to be cleaned often and replaced regularly and should not be coated with any type of sweet solution. Pacifier use for breastfeeding infants should be delayed for 3 to 4 weeks to ensure that breastfeeding is well established.

Problems arise when parents are concerned about the sucking of fingers, thumb, or pacifier and try to restrain this natural tendency. Before giving advice, nurses should investigate the parents' feelings and base the guidance they give on the information solicited. For example, some parents see no problem with the infant sucking on a thumb or finger but find the use of a pacifier objectionable. In general, either practice need not be restrained unless thumb sucking or pacifier use persists past 4 years of age or past the time when the permanent teeth erupt. Parents are advised to consult with their pediatric health care provider or pediatric dentist about this topic.

A parent's excessive use of the pacifier to calm the infant should also be explored, however. Placing a pacifier in the infant's mouth as soon as the infant begins to cry can reinforce a pattern of distress and relief.

SAFETY ALERT

If parents choose to let their infant use a pacifier, they need to be aware of certain safety considerations before purchasing one. A homemade or poorly designed pacifier can be dangerous because the entire object can be aspirated if it is small or a portion can become lodged in the pharynx. Improvised pacifiers, such as those made from a padded nipple, also pose dangers because the nipple can separate from the plastic collar and be aspirated. Safe pacifiers are made of one piece that includes a shield or flange large enough to prevent entry into the mouth and a handle that can be grasped (Fig. 24-27).

Bathing and Umbilical Cord Care

Bathing. Bathing serves several purposes. It provides opportunities for (1) cleansing the skin, (2) observing the infant's condition, (3) promoting comfort, and (4) parent-child-family interaction.

An important consideration in skin cleansing is the preservation of the skin's acid mantle, which is formed from the uppermost horny layer of the epidermis, sweat, superficial fat, metabolic products, and external substances such as amniotic fluid and microorganisms. To protect the newborn's skin it is best to use a cleanser with a neutral pH and preferably without preservatives or with preservatives recognized as safe and well tolerated in neonates. Antimicrobial cleansers should not be used (AWHONN, 2013).

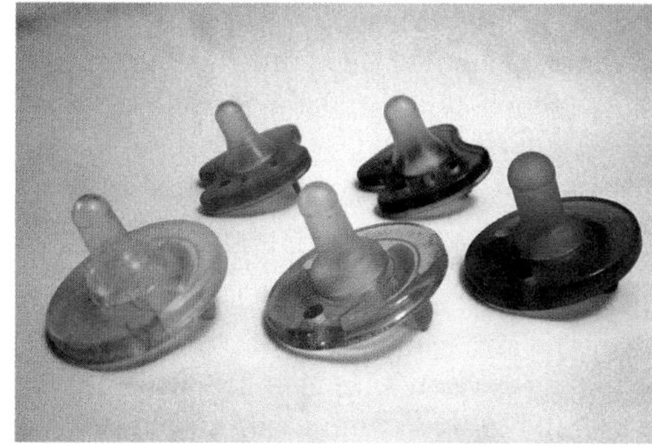

FIG 24-27 Safe pacifiers for term and preterm infants. Note one-piece construction, easily grasped handle, and large shield with ventilation holes. (Courtesy Julie Perry Nelson, Loveland, CO.)

The latest neonatal skin care guidelines from AWHONN (2013) indicate that bathing should be performed according to agency protocols using sponge bathing, immersion, or *swaddled bathing*. Sponge baths are usually given until the infant's umbilical cord falls off and the umbilicus is healed. However, bathing the newborn by immersion has been found to allow less heat loss and provoke less crying. It has not been shown to increase the risk of bacterial colonization of the cord (AWHONN). *Swaddled bathing* is a type of immersion bathing in which the newborn is swaddled in a blanket or towel and immersed in a tub of warm water. One body part at a time is unwrapped and washed (AWHONN).

Ideally the initial bath is delayed for at least 2 hours after birth until the neonate has reached thermal and cardiorespiratory stability. This bath should be quick (5 to 10 minutes) and can be performed at the mother's bedside or in the nursery. Tap water and a minimal amount of pH neutral or slightly acidic cleanser are recommended. Following the bath the infant should be immediately dried, diapered, and wrapped in warm blankets; a cap is placed on the head. Ten minutes later, the newborn is dressed, wrapped in warm blankets, and the cap is changed (AWHONN, 2013).

A daily bath is not necessary for achieving cleanliness and can do harm by disrupting the integrity of the newborn's skin; cleansing the perineum after a soiled diaper and daily cleansing of the face are usually sufficient. In general, infants should not be bathed more frequently than every other day; the hair should be shampooed once or twice a week (AWHONN, 2013).

The infant bath time provides a wonderful opportunity for parent-infant social interaction (Fig. 24-28). While bathing the baby, parents can talk to the infant, caress and cuddle the infant, and engage in arousal and imitation of facial expressions and smiling. Parents can pick a time for the bath that is easy for them and when the baby is awake, usually before a feeding.

Umbilical Cord Care. The goal of cord care is to prevent or decrease the risk for hemorrhage and infection. The umbilical cord stump is an excellent medium for bacterial growth and can easily become infected. Hospital protocol determines the technique for routine cord care. AWHONN (2013) recommendations for cord care include cleaning the cord with water (using cleanser sparingly if needed to remove debris) during the initial bath. Evidence does not support the routine use of antiseptic or antimicrobial preparations for cord care (AWHONN; Lund & Durand, 2011).

The plastic cord clamp that was applied at birth is removed once the stump has dried (Fig. 24-29), typically in 24 to 48 hours. The stump and base of the cord should be assessed for edema, redness, and purulent drainage with each diaper change. The area should be kept clean and dry and open to air or loosely covered with clothing. If soiled, the area is cleansed with plain water and dried thoroughly. The diaper is folded down and away from the stump (AWHONN, 2013). The umbilical cord begins to dry, shrivel, and blacken by the second or third day of life. The stump deteriorates through the process of dry gangrene; therefore, odor alone is not a positive indicator of omphalitis (infection of the umbilical stump). Cord separation time is influenced by several factors, including type of cord care, type of birth, and other perinatal events. The average cord separation time is 10 to 14 days, although it can take up to 3 weeks. Some dried blood may be seen in the umbilicus at separation (Fig. 24-30). Parents are instructed in appropriate home cord care (per pediatric health care practitioner or institution protocol) and the expected time of cord separation.

See Teaching for Self-Management: Home Care for information regarding bathing, skin care, cord care, nail care, and dressing the infant.

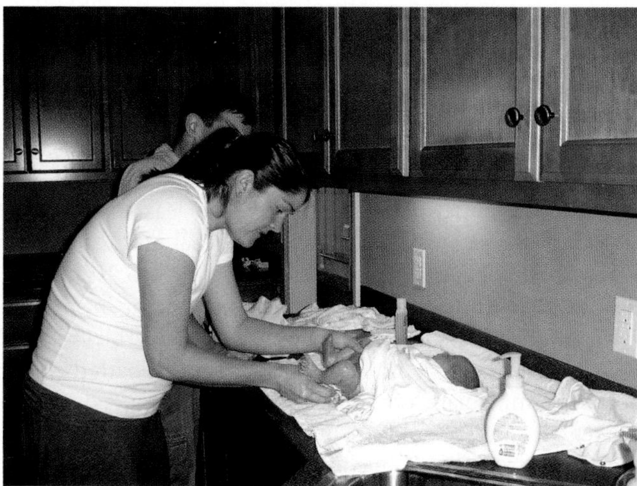

FIG 24-28 Mother and father giving newborn a sponge bath at home. (Courtesy Kathryn Alden, Chapel Hill, NC.)

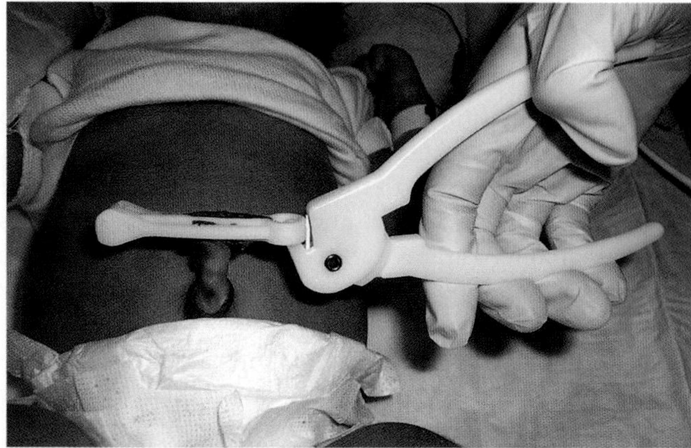

FIG 24-29 With special tool, nurse removes clamp after cord dries (approximately 24 to 48 hours after birth). (Courtesy Cheryl Briggs, RNC, Annapolis, MD.)

Infant Follow-up Care

Follow-up care after hospital discharge usually occurs within 72 hours at the clinic or health care provider's office. This is especially important for breastfed newborns for monitoring their weight and hydration status. When infants are discharged at less than 48 hours of age, home care follow-up is an essential component of care. Home care may be provided either by a nurse as part of the routine follow-up care of infants or through a visiting nurse or community health nurse referral service.

Cardiopulmonary Resuscitation

All personnel working with infants must have current infant cardiopulmonary resuscitation (CPR) certification. Parents should receive instruction in relieving airway obstruction and CPR. Classes are often offered in hospitals and clinics during the prenatal period or to parents of newborns. Such instruction is especially important for parents whose infants were preterm or have a history of cardiac or respiratory problems. Some grandparents take CPR classes. Babysitters should also learn CPR.

Practical Suggestions for the First Weeks at Home

Numerous changes occur during the first weeks of parenthood. Care management should be directed toward helping parents

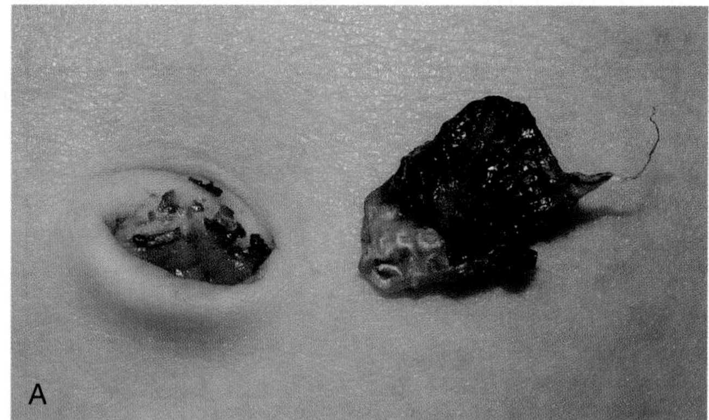

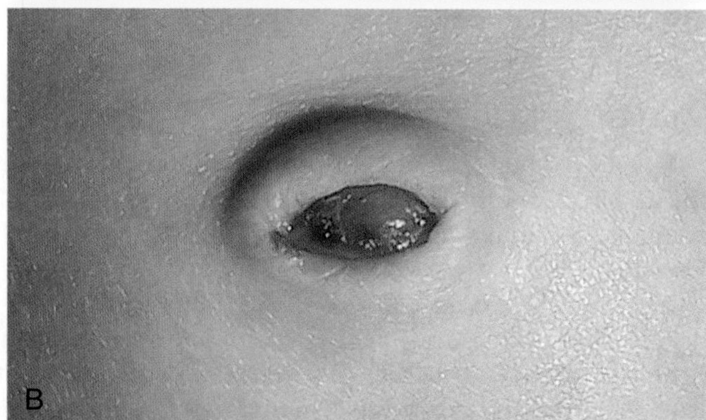

FIG 24-30 Cord separation. A, Cord separated with some dried blood still in the umbilicus. B, Umbilicus cleansed and beginning to heal. (Courtesy Cheryl Briggs, RNC, Annapolis, MD.)

TEACHING FOR SELF-MANAGEMENT

Home Care: Bathing, Cord Care, Skin Care, and Nail Care

Timing

- Newborns do not need a bath every day. Every 2 or 3 days is often enough.
- Fit bath time into the family's schedule.
- Give a bath at any time convenient to you but not immediately after a feeding period because the increased handling can cause regurgitation.

Prevent Heat Loss

- The temperature of the room should be 26°-27° C (79-81° F) and the bathing area should be free of drafts (close the door in the room where the bath is performed).
- The water temperature should be between 38° C and 40° C (100° F to <104° F). A water thermometer is useful for determining appropriate water temperature.
- Control heat loss during the bath to conserve the infant's energy. Bathe the infant quickly; with a sponge bath expose only a portion of the body at a time; and dry thoroughly.

Gather Supplies and Clothing Before Starting

- Tub for water placed in a safe place on a sturdy surface
- Towels for drying the infant and a clean washcloth
- Mild cleanser with a neutral pH and preferably with no preservatives
- Diaper
- Clothing suitable for wearing indoors: shirt; stretch suit or nightgown optional
- Cotton balls
- Receiving blanket

Bathe the Baby

- Take the infant to the bathing area when all supplies are ready.
- Never leave the infant alone on bath table or in the bathwater, not even for a second! If you have to leave, take the infant with you or place the infant back into the crib.
- Test the temperature of the water. Do not hold the infant under running water—the water temperature can change, and the infant can be scalded or chilled rapidly. For immersion bathing (tub bath), carefully lower the infant into the tub; the head and neck should be above the water. The tub should be filled with enough water to keep the baby's shoulders covered; this helps reduce heat loss. First wash the baby's face with a soft washcloth and plain water. Then proceed to wash the rest of the body, going from top to bottom.
- If sponge bathing is to be performed, undress the baby and wrap in a towel with the head exposed. Uncover and gently wash one part of the body at a time, taking care to keep the rest of the baby covered as much as possible to prevent heat loss.
- Begin by washing the baby's face with water; do not use soap on the face. Cleanse the eyes from the inner canthus outward using separate parts of a clean washcloth for each eye. For the first 2 to 3 days, a discharge can result from the reaction of the conjunctiva to the substance (erythromycin) used as a prophylactic measure against infection. Any discharge should be considered abnormal and reported to the pediatric health care provider.
- Cleanse the ears and nose with twists of moistened cotton or a corner of the washcloth. Do not use cotton-tipped swabs because they can cause injury. The areas behind the ears need daily cleansing.
- Wash between the skinfolds. Place your hand under the baby's shoulders and lift gently to expose the neck, lift the chin, and wash the neck, taking care to cleanse between the skinfolds.
- Wash the genital area last.
- If the hair is to be washed, begin by wrapping the infant in a towel with the head exposed. Hold the infant in a football position (under the arm) with one hand, using the other hand to wash the hair. Wash the scalp with water and shampoo that is mild for the eyes and safe for babies. Massage the scalp gently, rinse well, and dry thoroughly. A blow dryer is never used on an infant because the temperature is too hot for a baby's skin.

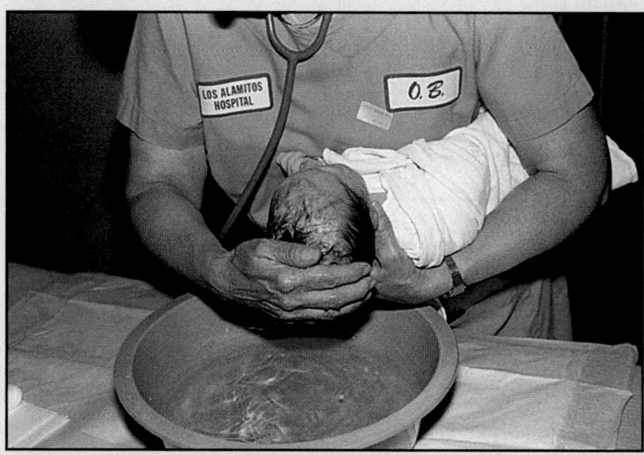

Wash hair with baby wrapped to limit heat loss. (Courtesy Marjorie Pyle, RNC, Lifecircle, Costa Mesa, CA.)

Skin Care

- If the skin appears dry or cracking, apply an emollient (lotion) once or twice daily. Check with your pediatric health care provider about the type of emollient to use.
- The fragile skin can be injured by too vigorous cleansing. If stool or other debris has dried and caked on the skin, soak the area to remove it. Do not attempt to rub it off because abrasion can result. Cleanse gently using a mild cleanser and pat dry.
- Babies are very prone to sunburn and should be kept out of direct sunlight. Use of sunscreens should be discussed with the health care provider. For infants younger than 6 months, sunscreen is applied to areas not covered by protective clothing or shade such as the face and backs of the hands.
- Babies often develop rashes that are normal. Neonatal acne resembles pimples and can appear at 2 to 4 weeks of age, resolving without treatment by 6 to 8 months. Heat rash is common in warm weather, which appears as a fine red rash around creases or folds where the baby sweats.

Cord Care

- Cleanse with plain water around base of the cord where it joins the skin. Notify the health care provider of any odor, discharge, or skin inflammation (redness) around the cord. The clamp is removed by the nurse when the cord is dry (approximately 24 to 48 hours after birth). Keep the diaper folded down so that it does not cover the cord. A wet or soiled diaper will slow or prevent drying of the cord and foster infection. When the cord drops off after 10 to 14 days, a few small drops of blood may be seen. If there is active bleeding, notify the pediatric health care provider.

Nail Care

- Do not cut fingernails and toenails immediately after birth. The nails have to grow out far enough from the skin so that the skin is not cut by mistake. If the baby scratches himself or herself, apply loosely fitted mitts over each of the baby's hands.

Continued

TEACHING FOR SELF-MANAGEMENT—cont'd

Home Care: Bathing, Cord Care, Skin Care, and Nail Care

Do so as a last resort, however, because it interferes with the baby's ability for self-consolation sucking on thumb or finger. When the nails have grown, the fingernails and toenails can be trimmed with manicure scissors or clippers; nails should be cut straight across. The ideal time to trim the nails is when the infant is sleeping. Soft emery boards may be used to file the nails. Nails should be kept short.

Genital Care

- Cleanse the genitalia of infants daily and after voiding or stooling using disposable diaper wipes or soft cloths and water (with gentle cleanser if needed). For girls, the genitalia are cleansed by gently separating the labia and gently washing from the pubic area to the anus. For uncircumcised boys, wash and rinse the penis with soap and warm water. Do not attempt to retract the foreskin. The health care provider will inform you when the foreskin can safely be retracted. By age 3 years in the majority of boys, the foreskin can be retracted easily without causing pain or trauma. For others, the foreskin is not retractable until adolescence. As soon as the foreskin is partly retractable and the child is old enough, he can be taught self-care. Once healed, the circumcised penis does not require any special care other than cleansing with diaper changes.
- The infant's skin should be allowed to dry completely before applying another diaper.
- Exposing the buttocks to air can help dry up diaper rash. Because bacteria thrive in moist dark areas, exposing the skin to dry air decreases bacterial proliferation. Zinc oxide ointments can be used to protect the infant's skin from moisture and further excoriation.

Data from American Academy of Pediatrics. (2013). *Baby 0-12 mos.* Available at www.healthychildren.org/english/ages-stages/baby/bathing-skin-care/Pages/default.aspx; Association of Women's Health, Obstetric and Neonatal Nursing (AWHONN). (2013). *Neonatal skin care* (3rd ed.). Washington, DC: Author.

cope with infant care, role changes, altered lifestyle, and changes in family structure resulting from the addition of a new baby.

Parents must be helped to anticipate events during the transition from birthing facility to home. This is especially important for first-time parents. Even the simplest strategies can provide enormous support. Printed materials reinforcing education topics are helpful, as is a list of available community resources and websites that provide reliable information about child care. Classes in the prenatal period or during the postpartum stay are helpful. Instructions for the first days at home include relevant topics such as activities of daily living, dealing with visitors, and activity and rest.

Interpretation of Crying and Use of Quieting Techniques. Crying is an infant's first social communication. Some babies cry more than others, but all babies cry. They cry to communicate that they are hungry, uncomfortable, wet, ill, or bored and sometimes for no apparent reason at all. The longer parents are around their infants, the easier it becomes to interpret the meaning of infant cries and to respond appropriately. Many infants have a fussy period during the day, often in the late afternoon or early evening when everyone is naturally tired. Environmental tension adds to the length and intensity of crying spells. Babies also have periods of vigorous crying when no comforting can help. These periods of crying can last for long stretches until the infants seem to cry themselves to sleep. The nurse informs new parents that time and infant maturation will take care of these types of cries. Many hospitals distribute a DVD on infant crying to new parents. The Period of PURPLE Crying is an example (Box 24-5). It is intended to help parents understand that crying is normal and help them cope with infant crying. If parents have greater understanding of infant crying, they may be less likely to inflict harm such as occurs with shaken-baby syndrome.

Nurses should instruct new parents about strategies to calm a crying or fussy baby. Certain types of sensory stimulation can calm and quiet infants and help them get to sleep. Important characteristics of this sensory stimulation—whether tactile, vestibular, auditory, or visual—appear to be that the stimulation is mild, slow, rhythmic, and consistently and regularly presented. Tactile simulation can include skin-to-skin contact, warmth, patting, and back rubbing. Swaddling provides widespread and constant tactile stimulation and a sense of security. Vestibular stimulation is especially effective and can be accomplished by mild rhythmic movement such as rocking or by holding the infant upright, as on the parent's shoulder. Some infants respond to being held in a body carrier. Rhythmic sounds can provide auditory stimulation; parents can use devices that provide white noise or sounds resembling the mother's heartbeat.

Recognizing Signs of Illness. In addition to explaining the need for well-baby follow-up visits, the nurse should discuss with parents the signs of illness in newborns (see Teaching for Self-Management: Signs of Illness). Of particular importance is the parents' assessment of jaundice in newborns discharged early. Parents should be advised to call their pediatric care provider immediately if they notice increasing jaundice or signs of illness.

BOX 24-5 The *Period of PURPLE Crying*

The *Period of PURPLE Crying* is a program to educate new parents about infant crying and the dangers of shaking a baby. Each letter in the acronym *PURPLE* represents key concepts:

P = Peak of crying. Your baby may cry more each week—the most in month 2, then less in months 3 to 5.
U = Unexpected. Crying can come and go and you don't know why.
R = Resists soothing. Your baby may not stop crying no matter what you try.
P = Pain-like face. Crying babies may look like they are in pain, even when they are not.
L = Long lasting. Crying can last as much as 5 hours a day, or more.
E = Evening. Your baby may cry more in the later afternoon and evening.

From Barr, RG and Barr, M: *The period of PURPLE crying.* Available at www.PURPLEcrying.info.

TEACHING FOR SELF-MANAGEMENT

Signs of Illness

Notify the pediatric health care provider if any of these signs occur:

- Fever: temperature greater than 38° C (100.4° F) axillary; also a continual rise in temperature (Note: Tympanic [ear] thermometers are not recommended for infants younger than 3 months.)
- Hypothermia: temperature less than 36.5° C (97.7° F) axillary
- Poor feeding or little interest in food: refusal to eat for two feedings in a row
- Vomiting: more than one episode of forceful vomiting or frequent vomiting (over a 6-hour period)
- Diarrhea: two consecutive green, watery stools (Note: Stools of breastfed infants are normally looser than stools of formula-fed infants. Diarrhea leaves a water ring around the stool, whereas breastfed stools do not.)
- Decreased bowel movement: in a breastfed infant, fewer than three stools per day; in a formula-fed infant, less than one stool every other day
- Decreased urination: fewer than six to eight wet diapers per day after 3 to 4 days of age
- Breathing difficulties: labored breathing with flared nostrils or absence of breathing for more than 15 seconds (Note: A newborn's breathing is normally irregular and between 30 to 40 breaths/min. Count the breaths for a full minute.)
- Cyanosis (bluish skin color) whether accompanying a feeding or not
- Lethargy: sleepiness, difficulty waking, or periods of sleep longer than 6 hours (most newborns sleep for short periods, usually from 1 to 4 hours, and wake to be fed)
- Inconsolable crying (attempts to quiet not effective) or continuous high-pitched cry
- Bleeding or purulent (yellowish) drainage from umbilical cord or circumcision; foul odor or redness at the site
- Drainage from the eyes

KEY POINTS

- Assessment of the newborn requires data from the prenatal, intrapartal, and postnatal periods.
- The immediate assessment of the newborn includes Apgar scoring and a general evaluation of physical status.
- Knowledge of biologic and behavioral characteristics is essential for guiding assessment and interpreting data.
- Gestational age assessment provides important information for predicting risks and guiding care management.
- Nursing care immediately after birth includes maintaining an open airway, preventing heat loss, and promoting parent-infant interaction.
- Providing a protective environment is a key responsibility of the nurse and includes such measures as careful identification procedures, support of physiologic functions, and ways to prevent infection.
- The newborn has social and physical needs.
- Newborns require careful assessment for physiologic and behavioral manifestations of pain.
- Nonpharmacologic and pharmacologic measures are used to reduce infant pain.
- Before hospital discharge, nurses provide anticipatory guidance for parents regarding feeding and elimination patterns; positioning and holding; comfort measures; car seat safety; bathing, skin care, cord care, and nail care; and signs of illness.
- All parents should have instruction in infant CPR.

REFERENCES

Academy of Breastfeeding Medicine (ABM) Protocol Committee. (2010). ABM clinical protocol #23: Non-pharmacologic management of procedure-related pain in the breastfeeding infant. *Breastfeeding Medicine*, *5*(6), 315–319.

Adamkin, D. H., & Committee on Fetus and Newborn (2011). Clinical report—Postnatal glucose homeostasis in late-preterm and term infants. *Pediatrics*, *127*(3), 575–579.

American Academy of Pediatrics (AAP). (2014). *Swaddling: Is it safe?* Elk Grove Village, IL: Author.

American Academy of Pediatrics (AAP). (2012). *Car seats: Information for families.* Elk Grove Village, IL: Author.

American Academy of Pediatrics (AAP) Committee on Infectious Diseases. (2012). *Red book: 2012 report of the committee on infectious diseases* (29th ed.). Elk Grove Village, IL: Author.

American Academy of Pediatrics (AAP) Section on Breastfeeding. (2012). Breastfeeding and the use of human milk—Policy statement. *Pediatrics*, *129*(3), e827–e841.

American Academy of Pediatrics (AAP) Section on Cardiology and Cardiac Surgery Executive Committee. (2012). Endorsement of Health and Human Services recommendation for pulse oximetry screening for critical congenital heart disease. *Pediatrics*, *129*(1), 190–192.

American Academy of Pediatrics (AAP) Subcommittee on Hyperbilirubinemia. (2004). Clinical practice guideline: Management of hyperbilirubinemia in the newborn infant 35 or more weeks of gestation. *Pediatrics*, *114*(1), 297–316.

American Academy of Pediatrics (AAP) Task Force on Circumcision. (1999, reaffirmed 2005). Circumcision policy statement. *Pediatrics*, 103(3), 686–693.

American Academy of Pediatrics (AAP) Task Force on Circumcision. (2012). Circumcision policy statement. *Pediatrics*, *130*(3), 585–586.

American Academy of Pediatrics (AAP) Task Force on Sudden Infant Death Syndrome. (2011). SIDS and other sleep-related infant deaths: Expansion of recommendations for a safe infant sleeping environment. *Pediatrics*, *128*(5), e1341–e1367.

American Academy of Pediatrics (AAP) & American College of Obstetricians and Gynecologists (ACOG). (2012). *Guidelines for perinatal care* (7th ed.). Elk Grove Village, IL: Author.

American College of Medical Genetics. (2009). *Position statement on importance of residual newborn screening dried blood spots.* Available at www.acmg.net/StaticContent/NewsReleases/Blood_Spot_Position_Statement2009.pdf.

American College of Obstetricians and Gynecologists (ACOG) Committee on Genetics. (2011). Committee opinion no. 481: Newborn screening. *Obstetrics and Gynecology*, *117*(3), 762–765.

American College of Obstetricians and Gynecologists (ACOG) Committee on Obstetric Practice. (2006, reaffirmed 2010). Committee opinion no. 333: The Apgar score. *Obstetrics and Gynecology*, *107*(5), 1209–1212.

American College of Obstetricians and Gynecologists (ACOG) Committee on Obstetric Practice & Society for Maternal-Fetal Medicine. (2013). Committee opinion no. 579: Definition of term pregnancy. *Obstetrics and Gynecology*, *122*(5), 1139–1140.

Araia, M. H., Wilson, B. J., Chakraborty, P., et al. (2012). Factors associated with knowledge of and satisfaction with newborn screening education: A survey of mothers. *Genetics in Medicine*, *14*(12), 963–970.

Association of Women's Health, Obstetric and Neonatal Nurses (AWHONN). (2013). *Neonatal skin care: Evidence-based clinical practice guideline* (3rd ed.). Washington, DC: Author.

Ballard, J., Khoury, J., Wedig, K., et al. (1991). New Ballard score, expanded to include extremely premature infants. *Journal of Pediatrics*, *119*(3), 417–423.

Barrington, K. J., Sankaran, K., & Canadian Paediatric Society Fetus and Newborn Committee. (2007, reaffirmed 2011). Guidelines for detection, management, and prevention of hyperbilirubinemia in term and late preterm newborn infants. *Paediatrics and Child Health*, *12*(Suppl B), 1B–12B.

Bellieni, C. V., Coccina, F., & Buonocore, G. (2012). Sensorial stimulation for infants' pain. *Journal of Maternal-Fetal and Neonatal Medicine*, *25*(S1), 79–81.

Bhutani, V. K., & Committee on Fetus and Newborn (2011). Phototherapy to prevent severe neonatal hyperbilirubinemia in the newborn infant 35 or more weeks of gestation. *Pediatrics*, *128*(4), e1046–e1052.

Blackburn, S. T. (2013). *Maternal, fetal, and neonatal physiology: A clinical perspective* (4th ed.). St. Louis: Saunders.

Brady-Fryer, B., Wiebe, N., & Lander, J. (2004). Pain relief for neonatal circumcision. *The Cochrane Database of Systematic Reviews*, *2004*, 3, CD004217.

Bromiker, R., Bin-Nun, A., Schimmel, M. S., et al. (2012). Neonatal hyperbilirubinemia in the low-intermediate-risk category on the bilirubin nomogram. *Pediatrics*, *130*(3), e470–e475.

Brown, V. D., & Landers, S. (2011). Heat balance. In S. L. Gardner, B. S. Carter, M. Enzman-Hines, & J. A. Hernandez (Eds.), *Merenstein & Gardner's handbook of neonatal intensive care* (7th ed.). St. Louis: Mosby.

Bull, M., Engle, W. A., & American Academy of Pediatrics (AAP) Committee on Injury, Violence, and Poison Prevention, and Committee on Fetus and Newborn (2009). Safe transportation of preterm and low birth weight infants at hospital discharge. *Pediatrics*, *123*(5), 1424–1429.

Burgos, A. E., Flaherman, V. J., & Newman, T. B. (2012). Screening and follow-up for neonatal hyperbilirubinemia: A review. *Clinical Pediatrics (Philadelphia)*, *51*(1), 7–16.

Canadian Paediatric Society (CPS) Infectious Diseases and Immunization Committee. (2002). Recommendations for prevention of neonatal ophthalmia. *Paediatrics and Child Health*, *7*(7), 480–488.

Centers for Disease Control and Prevention (CDC). (2014). Advisory Committee on Immunization Practices recommended immunization schedule for persons aged 0 through 18 years—United States, 2014. *MMWR Morbidity and Mortality Weekly Report*, *63*(5), 108–109.

Cignacco, E. L., Sellam, G., Stoffel, L., et al. (2012). Oral sucrose and "facilitated tucking" for repeated pain relief in preterms: A randomized control trial. *Pediatrics*, *129*(2), 299–308.

Cooper, B. M., Holditch-Davis, D., Verklan, M. T., et al. (2012). Newborn clinical outcomes of the AWHONN late preterm infant research-based practice project. *Journal of Obstetric, Gynecologic and Neonatal Nursing*, *41*(6), 774–785.

Craighead, D. V. (2012). Early term birth: Understanding the health risks to infants. *Nursing for Women's Health*, *16*(2), 136–145.

Dekker, R. (2012). Is erythromycin eye ointment always necessary for newborns? *Evidence Based Birth*. Available at http://evidencebasedbirth.com/is-erythromycin-eye-ointment-always-necessary-for-newborns.

Dijk, P., & Hulzebos, C. (2012). An evidence-based review on hyperbilirubinemia. *Acta Paediatrica*, *101*(Suppl 464), 3–10.

Gabriel, M. A. M., de Mendoza, B. R. H., Figeuroa, L. J., et al. (2013). Analgesia with breastfeeding in addition to skin-to-skin contact during heel prick. *Archives of Disease in Childhood. Fetal and Neonatal Edition*, *98*(6), F499–F503.

Galuska, L. (2011). Prevention of in-hospital newborn falls. *Nursing for Women's Health*, *15*(1), 59–61.

Gardner, S. L., Enzman-Hines, M., & Dickey, L. A. (2011). Pain and pain relief. In S. L. Gardner, B. S. Carter, M. Enzman-Hines, & J. A. Hernandez (Eds.), *Merenstein & Gardner's handbook of neonatal intensive care* (7th ed.). St. Louis: Mosby.

Gardner, S. L., & Hernandez, J. A. (2011). Initial nursery care. In S. L. Gardner, B. S. Carter, M. Enzman-Hines, & J. A. Hernandez (Eds.), *Merenstein & Gardner's handbook of neonatal intensive care* (7th ed.). St. Louis: Mosby.

Helsey, L., McDonald, J. V., & Stewart, V. T. (2010). Addressing in-hospital falls of newborn infants. *The Joint Commission Journal on Quality and Patient Safety*, *36*(7), 327–333.

Hiner, J., Pyka, J., Burks, C., et al. (2012). Preventing infant abductions: An infant security program transitioned into an interdisciplinary model. *Journal of Perinatal and Neonatal Nursing*, *26*(1), 47–56.

Hitchcock, S. (2012). Endorsing safe infant sleep. *Nursing for Women's Health*, *16*(5), 387–396.

Howell, R. R., Terry, S., Tait, V. F., et al. (2012). CDC grand rounds: Newborn screening and improved outcomes. *MMWR Morbidity and Mortality Weekly Report*, *61*(21), 390–393.

Hummel, P., Puchalski, M., Creech, S. D., & Weiss, M. G. (2008). Clinical reliability and validity of the N-PASS: Neonatal pain, agitation, and sedation scale with prolonged pain. *Journal of Perinatology*, *28*(1), 55–60.

Johnston, C., Campbell-Yeo, M., Fernandes, A., et al. (2014). Skin-to-skin care for procedural pain neonates. *The Cochrane Database of Systematic Reviews, 2014*, *1*, CD008435.

Joint Committee on Infant Hearing. (2007). Year 2007 position statement: Principles and guidelines for early hearing detection and intervention programs. *Pediatrics*, *120*(4), 898–921.

Jones, J. E., Hayes, R. D., Starbuck, A. L., & Porcelli, P. J. (2011). Fluid and electrolyte management. In S. L. Gardner, B. S. Carter, M. Enzman-Hines, & J. A. Hernandez (Eds.), *Merenstein & Gardner's handbook of neonatal intensive care* (7th ed.). St. Louis: Mosby.

Kalhan, S. C., & Devaskar, S. U. (2011). Disorders of carbohydrate metabolism. In R. J. Martin, A. A. Fanaroff, & M. C. Walsh (Eds.), *Fanaroff & Martin's neonatal-perinatal medicine* (9th ed.). St. Louis: Mosby.

Kamath, B. C., Thilo, E. H., & Hernandez, J. A. (2011). Jaundice. In S. L. Gardner, B. S. Carter, M. Enzman-Hines, & J. A. Hernandez (Eds.), *Merenstein & Gardner's handbook of neonatal intensive care* (7th ed.). St. Louis: Mosby.

Kaplan, M., Wong, R. J., Sibley, E., & Stevenson, D. K. (2011). Neonatal jaundice and liver disease. In R. J. Martin, A. A. Fanaroff, & M. C. Walsh (Eds.), *Fanaroff & Martin's neonatal-perinatal medicine* (9th ed.). St. Louis: Mosby.

Kassab, M. I., Roydhouse, J. K., Fowler, C., & Foureur, M. (2012). The effectiveness of glucose in reducing needle-related procedural pain in infants. *Journal of Pediatric Nursing*, *27*(1), 3–17.

Kattwinkel, J., Perlman, J. M., Aziz, K., et al. (2010). Part 15: Neonatal resuscitation: 2010 American Heart Association guidelines for cardiopulmonary resuscitation and emergency cardiovascular care. *Circulation*, *122*(Suppl 3), S909–S919.

Kenney, P. M., Hoover, D., Williams, L. C., & Iskersky, V. (2011). Cardiovascular diseases and surgical interventions. In S. L. Gardner, B. S. Carter, M. Enzman-Hines, & J. A. Hernandez (Eds.), *Merenstein & Gardner's handbook of neonatal intensive care* (7th ed.). St. Louis: Mosby.

Kostandy, R., Anderson, G. C., & Good, M. (2013). Skin-to-skin contact diminishes pain from hepatitis B vaccine injection in healthy full-term infants. *Neonatal Network, 32*(4), 274–280.

Krechel, S., & Bildner, J. (1995). CRIES: a new neonatal postoperative pain measurement score—Initial testing of validity and reliability. *Paediatric Anaesthesia, 5*(1), 53–61.

Lawrence, J., Alcock, D., McGrath, P., et al. (1993). The development of a tool to assess neonatal pain. *Neonatal Network, 12*(6), 59–66.

Liaw, J., Zeng, W., Yang, L., et al. (2011). Nonnutritive sucking and oral sucrose relieve neonatal pain during intramuscular injection of hepatitis vaccine. *Journal of Pain Symptom Management, 42*(6), 918–930.

Lindstrom, K., Lindblad, F., & Hjern, A. (2011). Preterm birth and attention-deficit/hyperactivity disorder. *Pediatrics, 127*(5), 858–865.

Lund, C. H., & Durand, D. J. (2011). Skin and skin care. In S. L. Gardner, B. S. Carter, M. Enzman-Hines, & J. A. Hernandez (Eds.), *Merenstein & Gardner's handbook of neonatal intensive care* (7th ed.). St. Louis: Mosby.

Maisels, M. J. (2010). Screening and early postnatal management strategies to prevent hazardous hyperbilirubinemia in newborns of 35 or more weeks of gestation. *Seminars in Fetal and Neonatal Medicine, 15*(3), 129–135.

Maisels, M. J., Deridder, J. M., Kring, E. A., & Balasubramaniam, M. (2009). Routine transcutaneous bilirubin measurement with clinical risk factors improve the prediction of subsequent hyperbilirubinemia. *Journal of Perinatology, 29*(9), 612–617.

Martin, J. A., Hamilton, B. E., Ventura, S. J., et al. (2013). Births: Final data for 2011. *National Vital Statistics Reports, 62*(1), 1–69.

Matteson, T., Henderson-Williams, A., & Nelson, J. (2013). Preventing in-hospital newborn falls. *MCN: The American Journal of Maternal/Child Nursing, 38*(6), 359–366.

Maxwell, L. G., Malavolta, C. P., & Fraga, M. V. (2013). Assessment of pain in the neonate. *Clinics in Perinatology, 40*(3), 457–469.

McGowan, J. E., Rozance, P. J., Price-Douglas, W., & Hay, W. W. (2011). Glucose homeostasis. In S. L. Gardner, B. S. Carter, M. Enzman-Hines, & J. A. Hernandez (Eds.), *Merenstein & Gardner's handbook of neonatal intensive care* (7th ed.). St. Louis: Mosby.

McMillan, D., & Canadian Paediatric Society (CPS) Fetus and Newborn Committee. (1997, reaffirmed 2014). Routine administration of vitamin K to newborns. *Paediatrics and Child Health,* 2(6), 429–431.

McNair, C., Yeo, M. C., Johnston, C., & Taddio, A. (2013). Nonpharmacologic management of pain during common needle puncture procedures in infants: Current evidence and practical considerations. *Clinics in Perinatology, 40*(3), 493–508.

Moore, E. R., Anderson, G. C., Bergman, N., & Dowswell, T. (2012). Early skin-to-skin contact for mothers and their healthy newborn infants. *The Cochrane Database of Systematic Reviews, 5,* CD003519.

National Highway Traffic Safety Administration (NHTSA) Parents Central. (2012). *From car seats to car keys: Keeping kids safe.* Washington, DC: Author. Available at www.safercar.gov/parents/Home.htm.

National Institute of Child Health and Human Development (NICHD). (2013). *Safe to sleep public education campaign.* Bethesda, MD: Author.

Naughton, K. A. (2013). The combined use of sucrose and nonnutritive sucking for procedural pain in both term and preterm neonates. *Advances in Neonatal Care, 13*(1), 9–19.

Niermeyer, S., & Clarke, S. B. (2011). Delivery room care. In S. L. Gardner, B. S. Carter, M. Enzman-Hines, & J. A. Hernandez (Eds.), *Merenstein & Gardner's handbook of neonatal intensive care* (7th ed.). St. Louis: Mosby.

Outerbridge, E., & Canadian Paediatric Society Fetus and Newborn Committee (1996). Neonatal circumcision revisited. *Canadian Medical Association Journal, 154*(6), 769–780.

Owings, M., Uddin, S., & Williams, S. (2013). Trends in circumcision for male newborns in U.S. hospitals: 1979-2010. *Health E-stat.* Available at www.cdc.gov/nchs/data/hestat/circumcision_2013/circumcision_2013.htm.

Patel, H., Feldman, M., & Canadian Paediatric Society (CPS) Community Paediatrics Committee. (2011, reaffirmed 2014). Universal newborn hearing screening. *Paediatrics and Child Health, 16*(5), 301–305.

Paul, S. P., Goodman, A., Remorino, R., & Bolger, S. (2011). Newborn falls in-hospital: Time to address the issue. *Practising Midwife, 14*(4), 29–32.

Phillips, R. M., Goldstein, M., Hougland, K., et al. (2013). Multidisciplinary guidelines for the care of late preterm infants. *Journal of Perinatology, 33*(S2), S5–S22.

Reddy, U. M., Bettegowda, V. R., Dias, T., et al. (2011). Term pregnancy: A period of heterogeneous risk for infant mortality. *Obstetrics and Gynecology, 117*(6), 1279–1287.

Riddell, R. P., Racine, N. M., Turcotte, K., et al. (2012). Non-pharmacological management of infant and young child procedural pain. *Evidence-Based Child Health, 7*(6), 1905–2121.

Rigo, J., Mohamed, M. W., & De Curtis, M. (2011). Disorders of calcium, phosphorus, and magnesium metabolism. In R. J. Martin, A. A. Fanaroff, & M. C. Walsh (Eds.), *Fanaroff and Martin's neonatal-perinatal medicine: Diseases of the fetus and infant* (9th ed.). St. Louis: Mosby.

Sengupta, S., Carrion, V., Shelton, J., et al. (2013). Adverse neonatal outcomes associated with early-term birth. *JAMA Pediatrics, 167*(11), 1053–1059.

Shah, P. S., Herbozo, C., Aliwalas, L. L., & Shah, V. S. (2012). Breastfeeding or breast milk for procedural pain in neonates. *The Cochrane Database of Systematic Reviews, 2012, 12,* CD004950.

Smith, J. B. (2012). Routine newborn care. In C. A. Gleason, & S. U. Devaskar (Eds.), *Avery's diseases of the newborn* (9th ed.). Philadelphia: Saunders.

Stevens, B., Johnston, C., Petryshen, P., & Taddio, A. (1996). Premature infant pain profile: Development and initial validation. *Clinical Journal of Pain, 12*(1), 13–22.

Stevens, B., Yamada, J., Lee, G. Y., & Ohlsson, A. (2013). Sucrose for analgesia in newborn infants undergoing painful procedures. *The Cochrane Database of Systematic Reviews, 2013, 1,* CD001069.

Tarini, B. A., & Goldenberg, A. J. (2012). Ethical issues and newborn screening in the genomics era. *Annual Review of Genomics and Human Genetics, 13,* 381–393.

The Joint Commission. (1999). *Sentinel event alert: Infant abductions, preventing future occurrences.* Available at www.jointcommission.org/assets/1/18/SEA_9.pdf.

Tluczek, A., & De Luca, J. M. (2013). Newborn screening policy and practice issues for nurses. *Journal of Obstetric, Gynecologic and Neonatal Nursing, 42*(6), 718–727.

United States Department of Health and Human Services (USDHHS) Discretionary Advisory Committee on Heritable Disorders in Newborns and Children. (2013). *Recommended uniform screening panel.* Available at www.hrsa.gov/advisorycommittees/mchbadvisory/heritabledisorders/recommendedpanel/index.html.

United States Preventive Services Task Force (USPSTF). (2011). *Ocular prophylaxis for gonococcal ophthalmia neonatorum.* Available at www.uspreventiveservicestaskforce.org/uspstf10/gonoculproph/gonocupsum.htm.

Walden, M., & Gibbins, S. (2008). *Pain assessment & management guideline for practice* (2nd ed.). Glenview, IL: National Association of Neonatal Nurses.

Wilson, K., Kennedy, S. J., Potter, B. K., et al. (2010). Developing a national newborn screening strategy for Canada. *Health Law Review, 18*(2), 31–39.

World Health Organization (WHO) & Jhpiego. (2010). *Manual for early infant male circumcision under local anesthesia.* Geneva, Switzerland: WHO. Available at http://whqlibdoc.who.int/publications/2010/9789241500753_eng.pdf?ua=1.

World Health Organization (WHO). (2012). *Voluntary medical male circumcision for HIV prevention*. Available at www.who.int/hiv/topics/malecircumcision/fact_sheet/en/index.htl.

World Health Organization (WHO). (2009). *WHO guidelines on hand hygiene in health care: A summary*. Geneva, Switzerland: WHO Press.

Xiong, T., Qu, Y., Cambier, S., & Mu, D. (2011). The side effects of phototherapy for neonatal jaundice: What do we know? What should we do? *European Journal of Pediatrics, 170*(10), 1247–1255.

Zeltzer, L. K., & Krane, E. J. (2011). Pediatric pain management. In R. M. Kliegman, B. F. Stanton, J. W. St. Geme, III, et al. (Eds.), *Nelson textbook of pediatrics* (19th ed.). Philadelphia: Saunders.

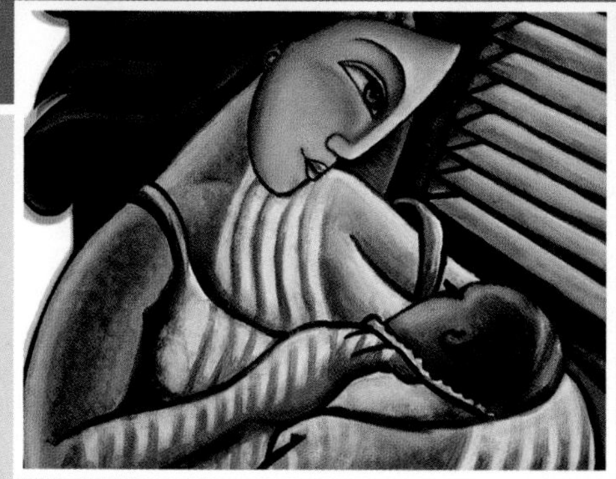

CHAPTER 25

Newborn Nutrition and Feeding

Kathryn R. Alden

http://evolve.elsevier.com/Lowdermilk/MWHC/

LEARNING OBJECTIVES

- Describe current recommendations for infant feeding.
- Explain the nurse's role in helping families choose an infant feeding method.
- Discuss benefits of breastfeeding for infants, mothers, families, and society.
- Describe nutritional needs of infants.
- Describe anatomic and physiologic aspects of breastfeeding.
- Recognize newborn feeding-readiness cues.
- Explain maternal and infant indicators of effective breastfeeding.
- Examine nursing interventions to facilitate and promote successful breastfeeding.
- Analyze common problems associated with breastfeeding and interventions to help resolve them.
- Compare powdered, concentrated, and ready-to-use forms of commercial infant formulas.
- Develop a teaching plan for the formula-feeding family.

Good nutrition in infancy fosters optimal growth and development. Infant feeding is more than providing nutrition; it is an opportunity for social, psychologic, and even educational interaction between parent and infant. It can establish a basis for developing good eating habits that last a lifetime.

Through preconception and prenatal education and counseling nurses play an instrumental role in helping parents make an informed decision about infant feeding. Scientific evidence is clear that human milk provides the best nutrition for infants, and parents should be strongly encouraged to choose breastfeeding (American Academy of Pediatrics [AAP] Section on Breastfeeding, 2012). Although many consider commercial infant formula to be equivalent to breast milk, this belief is erroneous. Human milk is the gold standard for infant nutrition. It is species specific, uniquely designed to meet the needs of human infants. The composition of human milk changes to meet the nutritional needs of growing infants. It is highly complex, with antiinfective and nutritional components combined with growth factors, enzymes that aid in digestion and absorption of nutrients, and fatty acids that promote brain growth and development. Infant formulas are usually adequate in providing nutrition to maintain infant growth and development within normal limits, but they are not equivalent to human milk.

Breastfeeding is defined as the transfer of human milk from the mother to the infant; the infant receives milk directly from the mother's breast. *Exclusive breastfeeding* means that the infant receives no other liquid or solid food (AAP Section on Breastfeeding, 2012). If the infant is fed expressed breast milk from the mother or a donor milk bank, it is called *human milk feeding*.

Whether the parents choose breastfeeding, human milk feeding, or formula feeding, nurses provide support and ongoing education. Parent education and care management are necessarily based on current research findings and standards of practice. Nurses and lactation consultants (who are most often nurses) provide education, assistance, and support for mothers, infants, and families prior to discharge from the birthing facility. After discharge nurses and lactation consultants in primary care and community health settings provide ongoing support and assistance to promote optimal feeding practices and positive health outcomes.

This chapter focuses on meeting nutritional needs for normal growth and development from birth to 6 months, with emphasis on the neonatal period when feeding practices and patterns are established. Breastfeeding and formula feeding are addressed. Information on breastfeeding is focused on the direct transfer of milk from mother to infant.

RECOMMENDED INFANT NUTRITION

The American Academy of Pediatrics (AAP) recommends exclusive breastfeeding for the first 6 months of life and that breastfeeding continues as complementary foods are introduced. Breastfeeding should continue for 1 year and thereafter as desired by the mother and her infant (AAP Section on Breastfeeding, 2012). According to the World Health Organization (WHO, 2013), infants should be exclusively breastfed for 6 months, receive safe and nutritionally adequate complementary foods beginning at 6 months, and continue breastfeeding until age 2 or beyond.

Exclusive breastfeeding for the first 6 months of life is also recommended by other professional health care organizations such as the American Academy of Family Physicians (AAFP, 2012), Academy of Breastfeeding Medicine (ABM Board of Directors, 2008), the American College of Obstetricians and Gynecologists (ACOG Committee on Health Care for Underserved Women and Committee on Obstetric Practice, 2007), and the American Dietetic Association (ADA, 2009). The Association of Women's Health, Obstetric and Neonatal Nurses (AWHONN, 2007) actively supports breastfeeding as the ideal form of infant nutrition and provides guidelines for nurses in promoting breastfeeding and supporting breastfeeding families.

Breastfeeding Rates

Breastfeeding rates in the United States have risen steadily over the past decade. The Centers for Disease Control and Prevention (CDC, 2014) reported that the U.S. breastfeeding initiation rate in 2011 was 79%, which is the highest ever reported. The 6-month breastfeeding rate was 49%, and the 12-month rate was 27%. The rate of exclusive breastfeeding at 3 months was 40.7% and at 6 months, 18.8%. The increase in breastfeeding rates may be related to the increase in the percentage of facilities with at least 90% of mothers and newborns having skin-to-skin contact after birth and in the percentage of facilities with at least 90% of mothers and newborns rooming-in. Early skin-to-skin contact, which places the neonate directly on the mother's chest after birth, fosters the initiation of breastfeeding during the first hour. Rooming-in helps mothers to establish breastfeeding and to learn to recognize infant hunger cues (CDC).

In spite of the increases in breastfeeding rates, the United States continues to fall short of the *Healthy People 2020* goals of 81% of infants ever breastfed, 60.6% breastfeeding at 6 months, and 34.1% at 12 months. Goals for exclusive breastfeeding are 46.2% through 3 months and 25.5% through 6 months (U.S. Department of Health and Human Services [USDHHS], 2010b).

Trends remain unchanged in breastfeeding rates among minority groups in the United States. The lowest breastfeeding rates are among non-Hispanic black women (Allen, Li, Scanlon, et al., 2013; Jensen, 2012), although the overall percentage of non-Hispanic black women who breastfeed has increased in recent years from 47.4% in 2000 to 58.9% in 2008 (Allen et al.) The minority group most likely to breastfeed is Hispanic women.

Historically, breastfeeding rates have been lower among women participating in the Special Supplemental Nutrition Program for Women, Infants, and Children (WIC). However, that trend appears to be changing as breastfeeding rates in this population of women increased from 63.1% in 2010 to 67.1% in 2012 (Johnson, Thorn, McGill, et al., 2013).

Benefits of Breastfeeding

Extensive evidence exists concerning the health benefits of breastfeeding and human milk for infants, with some of the benefits extending into adulthood (Table 25-1). These benefits are optimized when infants are breastfed exclusively and when the duration of breastfeeding is increased (Mass, 2011). The evidence supporting breastfeeding as the ideal form of infant nutrition is so strong that health care professionals may need to present information about it from two perspectives: benefits of and risks of not breastfeeding (Spatz & Lessen, 2011).

Breastfeeding is associated with health benefits for mothers (see Table 25-1). The benefits are increased with the number of children who were breastfed and the total length of time of lactation.

The psychologic benefits for mothers include enhanced bonding and attachment. For many women breastfeeding is associated with a sense of empowerment in the ability to provide nutrition for the infant.

Breastfeeding is convenient. The milk is ready to feed and at the proper temperature. In most cases there is no need for bottles or other equipment.

The economic benefits of breastfeeding affect families, employers, insurers, and the entire nation. Because infant formula is expensive, breastfeeding represents a significant savings for families. It reduces health care costs and decreases employee absenteeism. It has been estimated that the United States could save $13 billion per year, and more than 900 infant deaths could be prevented if 90% of infants were breastfed exclusively for 6 months (Bartick & Reinhold, 2010).

TABLE 25-1 Benefits of Breastfeeding

BENEFITS FOR THE INFANT	BENEFITS FOR THE MOTHER	BENEFITS TO FAMILIES AND SOCIETY

• Reduced risk for:
  • Nonspecific gastrointestinal infections
  • Celiac disease
  • Childhood inflammatory bowel disease
  • Necrotizing enterocolitis in preterm infants
  • Clinical asthma, atopic dermatitis, and eczema
  • Lower respiratory tract infection
  • Otitis media
  • SIDS
  • Obesity in adolescence and adulthood
  • Types 1 and 2 diabetes
  • Acute lymphocytic and myeloid leukemia
• Enhanced neurodevelopmental outcomes, especially in preterm infants
	• Decreased postpartum bleeding and more rapid uterine involution
	• Reduced risk for:
	  • Ovarian cancer and breast cancer (primarily premenopausal)
	  • Type 2 diabetes
	  • Hypertension, hypercholesterolemia, and cardiovascular disease
	  • Rheumatoid arthritis
	• Unique bonding experience
	• Increased maternal role attainment
		• Convenient; ready to feed
		• No bottles or other necessary equipment
		• Less expensive than infant formula
		• Reduced annual health care costs
		• Less parental absence from work because of ill infant
		• Reduced environmental burden related to disposal of formula packaging and equipment

SIDS, Sudden infant death syndrome.
Data from American Academy of Pediatrics Section on Breastfeeding. (2012). Breastfeeding and the use of human milk—Policy statement. *Pediatrics, 129*(3), e827-e841; Ip, S., Chung, M., Raman, G., et al. (2009). A summary of the Agency for Healthcare Research and Quality's evidence report on breastfeeding in developed countries. *Breastfeeding Medicine, 4*(Suppl 1), S17-S30; Stuebe, A. (2009). The risks of not breastfeeding for mothers and infants. *Reviews in Obstetrics and Gynecology, 2*(4), 222-231.

Breastfeeding has environmental benefits. It reduces the waste that is deposited in landfills, including formula packaging, bottles, nipples, and other equipment. There is no need for fuel to prepare or transport human milk, which saves energy resources (USDHHS, 2011).

CHOOSING AN INFANT FEEDING METHOD

For most women there is a clear choice to either breastfeed or formula feed. In some cases women decide to combine breastfeeding and formula feeding. However, this practice can be associated with a shorter duration of breastfeeding (Holmes, Auinger, & Howard, 2011). Some women want their infants to receive breast milk but prefer not to feed directly from their breasts. These women express their milk and bottle feed it to their infants.

Breastfeeding

Women most often choose to breastfeed because they are aware of the benefits to the infant (Nelson, 2012). This reinforces the importance of prenatal education about the numerous benefits of breastfeeding.

Breastfeeding is a natural extension of pregnancy and childbirth; it is much more than simply a means of supplying nutrition. Many women seek the unique bonding experience between mother and infant that is characteristic of breastfeeding.

Women tend to select the same method of infant feeding for each of their children. If the first child was breastfed, subsequent children will likely also be breastfed.

Partner and family support is a major factor in the mother's decision to breastfeed. Women who perceive their partners to prefer breastfeeding are more likely to breastfeed. Women are more likely to breastfeed successfully when partners and family members are positive about breastfeeding and have the skills to support it.

Cultural factors influence infant feeding decisions. For example, in the Hispanic culture breastfeeding is the norm, whereas formula feeding is more common among African-American families.

The decision to breastfeed exclusively is related to the mother's knowledge about the health benefits to the infant and her comfort level with breastfeeding in social settings (Stuebe & Bonuck, 2011). The likelihood that women will breastfeed exclusively may be greater if they made the decision during pregnancy (Tenfelde, Finnegan, & Hill, 2011).

There appears to be a relationship between maternal weight and infant feeding decisions. Women who are overweight or obese are less likely to breastfeed than women who are underweight or of average weight (Mehta, Siega-Riz, Herring, et al., 2011).

Other factors influence decisions about infant nutrition. Social and systemic factors create obstacles or barriers to breastfeeding among women in the United States. These include a lack of broad social support for breastfeeding and the widespread marketing by infant formula companies. In addition, there is a lack of prenatal breastfeeding education for expectant parents and insufficient training and education of health care professionals about breastfeeding. There is a lack of support for breastfeeding mothers during the first 2 to 3 weeks after birth, when they are most likely to encounter difficulties. In some institutions the policies and practices do not support exclusive breastfeeding (Mass, 2011).

A major obstacle for women is employment and the need to return to work after birth (Mass, 2011). Other common barriers include lack of comfort or uneasiness with breastfeeding, pain, lifestyle incompatibility, discomfort with public breastfeeding, and a lack of formal support (Nelson, 2012).

Formula Feeding

Parents who choose to formula feed often make this decision without complete information and understanding of the benefits of breastfeeding. Even women who are educated about the advantages of breastfeeding may still decide to formula feed. Cultural beliefs and myths and misconceptions about breastfeeding influence women's decision making. Many women see bottle feeding as more convenient or less embarrassing than breastfeeding. Some view formula feeding as a way to ensure that the father, other family members, and daycare providers can feed the baby. Some women lack confidence in their ability to produce breast milk of adequate quantity or quality. Women who have had previous unsuccessful breastfeeding experiences may choose to formula feed subsequent infants. Some women see breastfeeding as incompatible with an active social life, or they think that it will prevent them from going back to work. Modesty issues and societal barriers exist against breastfeeding in public. A major barrier for many women is the influence of family and friends (Nelson, 2012).

Contraindications to Breastfeeding

Breastfeeding is contraindicated in a few circumstances. Newborns who have galactosemia should not receive human milk. Breastfeeding is contraindicated for mothers who are positive for human T-cell lymphotropic virus types I or II and those with untreated brucellosis. Women should not breastfeed if they have active tuberculosis (TB) or if they have active herpes simplex lesions on the breasts. However, neither of these conditions precludes a mother from expressing milk for her infant. Women with active TB can breastfeed when they have been treated for at least 2 weeks and are deemed noninfectious. Varicella that occurs 5 days before or 2 days after birth and acute H1N1 infection require temporary separation of mother and infant. In both instances it is safe for infants to receive expressed milk (AAP Section on Breastfeeding, 2012).

In the United States maternal human immunodeficiency virus (HIV) infection is considered a contraindication for breastfeeding (AAP Section on Breastfeeding, 2012). However, this is not true in other countries. In developing countries where HIV is prevalent, the benefits of breastfeeding for infants outweigh the risk of contracting HIV from infected mothers (WHO, 2013).

CULTURAL INFLUENCES ON INFANT FEEDING

Cultural beliefs and practices are significant influences on infant feeding methods. Although recognized cultural norms exist, one cannot assume that generalized observations about any cultural group hold true for all members of that group. Many regional and ethnic cultures are found within the United States. Dealing effectively with these groups requires that nurses are knowledgeable and sensitive to the cultural factors influencing infant feeding practices.

In general people who have immigrated to the United States from poorer countries often choose to formula feed their infants because they believe it is a better, more "modern" method or because they want to adapt to U.S. culture and perceive that formula feeding is the custom. Hispanic women who are more acculturated may be less likely to breastfeed and, if they do, tend to breastfeed for a shorter duration (Ahluwalia, D'Angelo, Morrow, & McDonald, 2012).

Breastfeeding beliefs and practices vary across cultures. For example, among the Muslim culture, breastfeeding for 24 months is customary. Before the first feeding rubbing a small piece of softened date on the newborn's palate is a ritual. Because of the cultural emphasis on privacy and modesty, Muslim women may choose to bottle feed formula or expressed breast milk while in the hospital.

Because of beliefs about the harmful nature or inadequacy of colostrum, some cultures apply restrictions on breastfeeding for a period of days after birth. Such is the case for many cultures in southern Asia, the Pacific Islands, and parts of sub-Saharan Africa. Before the mother's milk is deemed to be "in," babies are fed prelacteal food such as honey or clarified butter in the belief that these substances will help clear out meconium. Other cultures begin breastfeeding immediately and offer the breast each time the infant cries.

A common practice among Mexican women is *las dos cosas* ("both things"). This refers to combining breastfeeding and commercial infant formula. It is based on the belief that by combining the two methods, the mother and infant receive the benefits of breastfeeding, and the infant receives the additional vitamins from infant formula (Bartick & Reyes, 2012). This practice can result in problems with milk supply and babies refusing to latch on to the breast, which can lead to early termination of breastfeeding.

Cultural expectations influence breastfeeding patterns and behaviors. In many Western cultures, women are more likely to try to "schedule" feeding sessions. This is in contrast to more frequent breastfeeding in some developing countries where mothers "wear" their babies close against their bodies as they go about daily activities. Those babies have constant or frequent access to the breast to feed on demand (Mohrbacher, 2013).

Some cultures have specific beliefs and practices related to the mother's intake of foods that foster milk production. Korean mothers often eat seaweed soup and rice to enhance milk production. Hmong women believe that boiled chicken, rice, and hot water are the only appropriate nourishments during the first postpartum month. The balance between energy forces, hot and cold, or yin and yang is integral to the diet of the lactating mother. Hispanics, Vietnamese, Chinese, East Indians, and Arabs often use this belief in choosing foods. "Hot" foods are considered best for new mothers. This belief does not necessarily relate to the temperature or spiciness of foods. For example, chicken and broccoli are considered "hot," whereas many fresh fruits and vegetables are considered "cold." Families often bring desired foods into the health care setting.

NUTRIENT NEEDS

Fluids

During the first 2 days of life the fluid requirement for healthy infants (more than 1500 g) is 60 to 80 ml of water per kilogram of body weight per day. From days 3 to 7 the requirement is 100 to 150 ml/kg/day; from day 8 to day 30 it is 120 to 180 ml/kg/day (Dell, 2011). In general, neither breastfed nor formula-fed infants need to be given water, not even those living in very hot climates. Breast milk contains 87% water, which easily meets fluid requirements. Feeding water to infants can decrease caloric consumption at a time when they are growing rapidly.

Infants have room for little fluctuation in fluid balance and should be monitored closely for fluid intake and water loss. They lose water through excretion of urine and insensibly through respiration. Under normal circumstances they are born with some fluid reserve, and some of the weight loss during the first few days is related to fluid loss. However, in some cases they do not have this fluid reserve, possibly because of inadequate maternal hydration during labor or birth.

Energy

Infants require adequate caloric intake to provide energy for growth, digestion, physical activity, and maintenance of organ metabolic function. Energy needs vary according to age, maturity level, thermal environment, growth rate, health status, and activity level. For the first 3 months the infant needs 110 kcal/kg/day. From 3 months to 6 months the requirement is 100 kcal/kg/day. This level decreases slightly to 95 kcal/kg/day from 6 to 9 months and increases to 100 kcal/kg/day from 9 months to 1 year (AAP Committee on Nutrition, 2009).

Human milk provides an average of 67 kcal/100 ml or 20 kcal/oz. The fat portion of the milk provides the greatest amount of energy. Infant formulas simulate the caloric content of human milk. Usually a standard formula contains 20 kcal/oz, although the composition differs among brands.

Carbohydrate

According to the Institute of Medicine (IOM, 2005), the recommended adequate intake (AI) for carbohydrate in the first 6 months of life is 60 g/day and 95 g/day for the second 6 months. Because newborns have only small hepatic glycogen stores, carbohydrates should provide at least 40% to 50% of the total calories in the diet. Moreover, newborns may have a limited ability to carry out *gluconeogenesis* (the formation of glucose from amino acids and other substrates) and *ketogenesis* (the formation of ketone bodies from fat), the mechanisms that provide alternative sources of energy.

As the primary carbohydrate in human milk and commercially prepared infant formula, lactose is the most abundant carbohydrate in the diet of infants up to age 6 months. Lactose provides calories in an easily available form. Its slow breakdown and absorption also increase calcium absorption. Corn syrup solids or glucose polymers are added to infant formulas to supplement the lactose in the cow's milk and thereby provide sufficient carbohydrates.

Oligosaccharides, another form of carbohydrate found in breast milk, are critical in the development of microflora in the intestinal tract of the newborn. These prebiotics promote an acidic environment in the intestines, preventing the growth of gram-negative and other pathogenic bacteria, thus increasing the infant's resistance to gastrointestinal (GI) illness.

Fat

Fats provide a major energy source for infants, supplying as much as 50% of the calories in breast milk and formula. The recommended AI of fat for infants younger than 6 months is 31 g/day (IOM, 2005). The fat content of human milk is composed of lipids, triglycerides, and cholesterol; cholesterol is an essential element for brain growth. Human milk contains the essential fatty acids (EFAs) linoleic acid and linolenic acid and the long-chain polyunsaturated fatty acids arachidonic acid (ARA) and docosahexaenoic acid (DHA). Fatty acids are important for growth, neurologic development, and visual function. Cow's milk contains fewer of the EFAs and no polyunsaturated fatty acids. Most formula companies add DHA to their products, although there is a lack of evidence supporting the benefit (Lawrence & Lawrence, 2011b). Modified cow's milk is used in most infant formulas, but the milk fat is removed, and another fat source such as corn oil, which the infant can digest and absorb, is added in its place. If whole milk or evaporated milk without added carbohydrate is fed to infants, the resulting fecal loss of fat (and therefore loss of energy) can be excessive because the milk moves through the infant's intestines too quickly for adequate absorption to take place. This can lead to poor weight gain.

Protein

High-quality protein from breast milk, infant formula, or other complementary foods is necessary for infant growth. The protein requirement per unit of body weight is greater in the newborn period than at any other time of life. For infants younger than 6 months the recommended AI for protein is 9.1 g/day (IOM, 2005).

Human milk contains the two proteins whey and casein in a ratio of approximately 70:30 compared with the ratio of 20:80 in most cow's milk–based formulas (Blackburn, 2013). This whey-to-casein ratio in human milk makes it more easily digestible and produces the soft stools seen in breastfed infants. The primary whey protein in human milk is α-lactalbumin; this protein is high in essential amino acids needed for growth. The whey protein lactoferrin in human milk has iron-binding capabilities and bacteriostatic properties, particularly against gram-positive and gram-negative aerobes, anaerobes, and yeasts. The casein in human milk enhances the absorption of iron, thus preventing iron-dependent bacteria from proliferating in the GI tract (Lawrence & Lawrence, 2011a). The amino acid components of human milk are uniquely suited to the newborn's metabolic capabilities. For example, cystine and taurine levels are high, whereas phenylalanine and methionine levels are low.

Vitamins

With the exception of vitamin D, human milk contains all of the vitamins required for infant nutrition, with individual variations based on maternal diet and genetic differences. Vitamins are added to cow's-milk formulas to resemble levels found in breast milk. Although cow's milk contains adequate amounts of vitamins A and B complex, vitamin C (ascorbic acid), vitamin E, and vitamin D must be added.

Vitamin D facilitates intestinal absorption of calcium and phosphorus, bone mineralization, and calcium resorption from bone. According to the AAP, all infants who are breastfed or partially breastfed should receive 400 International Units of vitamin D daily, beginning the first few days of life. Nonbreastfeeding infants and older children who consume less than 1 quart per day of vitamin D–fortified milk should also receive 400 International Units of vitamin D each day (Wagner, Grier, & AAP Section on Breastfeeding and Committee on Nutrition, 2008).

Vitamin K, required for blood coagulation, is produced by intestinal bacteria. However, the gut is sterile at birth, and a few days are required for intestinal flora to become established and produce vitamin K. To prevent hemorrhagic problems in the newborn an injection of vitamin K is given at birth to all newborns in the United States and Canada, regardless of feeding method (AAP Section on Breastfeeding, 2012; McMillan & Canadian Paediatric Society Fetus and Newborn Committee) (1997, reaffirmed 2014).

The breastfed infant's vitamin B_{12} intake depends on the mother's dietary intake and stores. Mothers who are on strict vegetarian (vegan) diets and those who consume few dairy products, eggs, or meat are at risk for vitamin B_{12} deficiency. Mothers who have had bariatric surgery are also at risk for vitamin B_{12} deficiency. Breastfeeding infants may need vitamin B_{12} supplements in these instances.

Minerals

The mineral content of commercial infant formula is designed to reflect that of breast milk. Unmodified cow's milk is much higher in mineral content than human milk, which also makes it unsuitable for infants during the first year of life. Minerals are typically highest in human milk during the first few days after birth and decrease slightly throughout lactation.

The ratio of calcium to phosphorus in human milk is 2:1, an optimal proportion for bone mineralization. Although cow's milk is high in calcium, the calcium-to-phosphorus ratio is low, resulting in decreased calcium absorption. Consequently young infants fed unmodified cow's milk are at risk for hypocalcemia, seizures, and tetany. The calcium-to-phosphorus ratio in commercial infant formula is between that of human milk and cow's milk.

Iron levels are low in all types of milk; however, iron from human milk is better absorbed than iron from cow's milk, iron-fortified formula, or infant cereals. Breastfed infants draw on iron reserves deposited in utero and benefit from the high lactose and vitamin C levels in human milk that facilitate iron absorption. Full-term infants have enough iron stores from the mother to last for the first 4 months. After 4 months of age, infants who are exclusively breastfed are at risk for iron deficiency. The AAP recommends giving exclusively breastfed infants an iron supplement (1 mg/kg/day) beginning at 4 months and continuing until the infant is consuming iron-containing complementary foods such as iron-fortified cereals. Infants who are partially breastfed should receive the same iron supplement if more than half of their daily feedings consist of human milk and they are not consuming iron-rich foods. Formula-feeding infants should receive an iron-fortified commercial infant formula until 12 months of age. Infants younger than 1 year should never be fed whole milk (Baker, Greer, & AAP Committee on Nutrition, 2010).

Fluoride levels in human milk and commercial formulas are low. This mineral, which is important in preventing dental caries, can cause spotting of the permanent teeth (fluorosis) in excess amounts. Experts recommend that no fluoride supplements are given to infants younger than 6 months. From 6 months to 3 years, fluoride supplements are based on the concentration of fluoride in the water supply (AAP Section on Breastfeeding, 2012).

ANATOMY AND PHYSIOLOGY OF LACTATION

Anatomy of the Lactating Breast

Each female breast is composed of approximately 15 to 20 segments (lobes) embedded in fat and connective tissues and well supplied with blood vessels, lymphatic vessels, and nerves (Fig. 25-1). Within each lobe is glandular tissue consisting of alveoli, the milk-producing cells, surrounded by myoepithelial cells that contract to send the milk forward to the nipple during milk ejection. Each nipple has multiple pores that transfer milk to the suckling infant. The ratio of glandular to adipose tissue in the lactating breast is approximately 2:1 compared with a 1:1 ratio in the nonlactating breast. Within each breast is a complex, intertwining network of milk ducts that transport milk from the alveoli to the nipple. The milk ducts dilate and expand at milk ejection (Fig. 25-2).

The size and shape of the breast are not accurate indicators of its ability to produce milk. Although nearly every woman can lactate, a small number have insufficient mammary gland development to breastfeed their infants exclusively. Typically these women experience few breast changes during puberty or early pregnancy. In some cases they are still able to produce some breast milk, although the quantity is not likely to be sufficient to meet the nutritional needs of the infant. These mothers can offer supplemental nutrition to support optimal infant growth.

Because of the effects of estrogen, progesterone, human placental lactogen, and other hormones of pregnancy, changes occur in the breasts in preparation for lactation. Breasts increase in size due to growth of glandular and adipose tissue. Blood flow to the breasts nearly doubles during pregnancy. Sensitivity of the breasts increases, and veins become more prominent. The nipples become more erect, and the areolae darken. Nipples and areolae enlarge. Around week 16 of gestation the alveoli begin producing prepartum milk, or *colostrum*. Montgomery glands on the areola enlarge. The oily substance secreted by these sebaceous glands helps provide protection against the mechanical stress of sucking and invasion by pathogens. The odor of the secretions can be a means of communication with the infant.

Lactogenesis

After the mother gives birth a precipitous fall in progesterone triggers the release of prolactin from the anterior pituitary gland. During pregnancy prolactin prepares the breasts to secrete milk and during lactation to synthesize and secrete milk. Prolactin levels are highest during the first 10 days after birth, gradually declining over time but remaining above baseline levels for the duration of lactation. Prolactin is produced in response to infant suckling and emptying of the breasts (Fig. 25-3, *A*). Milk production is a supply-meets-demand system (i.e., as milk is removed

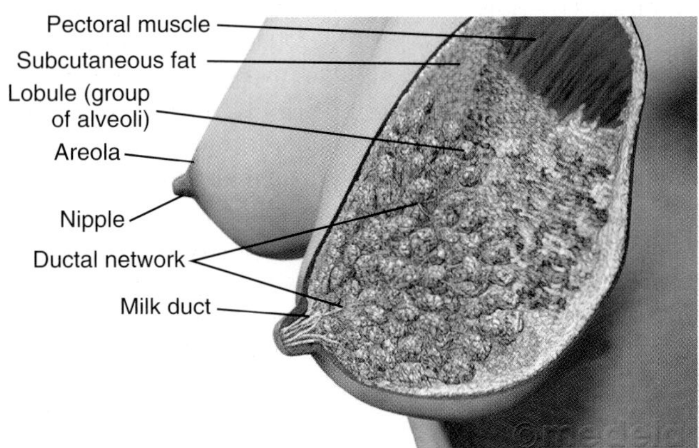

FIG 25-1 Anatomy of the lactating breast. (Courtesy Medela, Inc., McHenry, IL.)

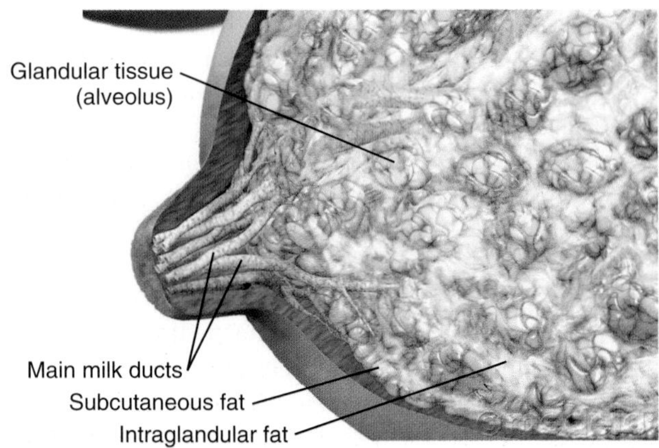

FIG 25-2 Enhanced view of milk glands and ducts. (Courtesy Medela, Inc., McHenry, IL.)

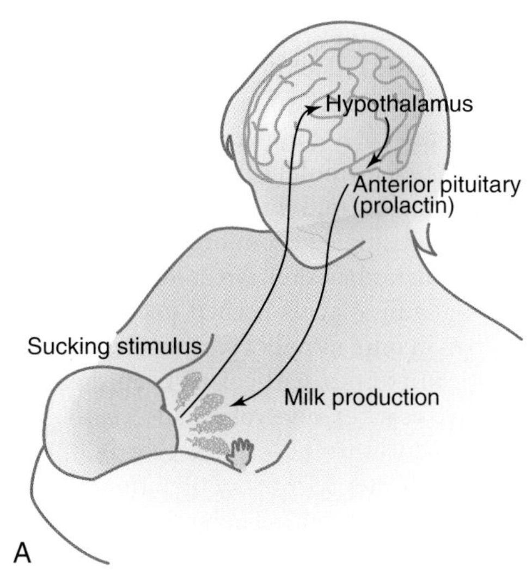

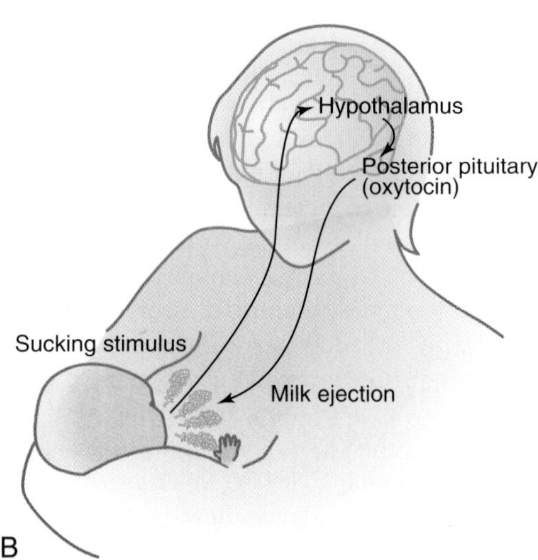

FIG 25-3 Maternal breastfeeding reflexes. **A,** Milk production. **B,** Milk ejection (let-down).

from the breast, more is produced). Incomplete removal of milk from the breasts can lead to decreased milk supply.

Oxytocin is essential to lactation. As the nipple is stimulated by the suckling infant, the posterior pituitary is prompted by the hypothalamus to produce oxytocin. This hormone is responsible for the milk ejection reflex (MER), or let-down reflex (see Fig. 25-3, *B*). The myoepithelial cells surrounding the alveoli respond to oxytocin by contracting and sending the milk forward through the ducts to the nipple. The MER is triggered multiple times during a feeding session. Thoughts, sights, sounds, or odors that the mother associates with her baby (or other babies) such as hearing the baby cry can trigger the MER. Many women report a tingling "pins and needles" sensation in the breasts as milk ejection occurs, although some mothers can detect milk ejection only by observing the sucking and swallowing of the infant. The MER also can occur during sexual activity because oxytocin is released during orgasm. The reflex can be inhibited by fear, stress, and alcohol consumption.

Oxytocin is the same hormone that stimulates uterine contractions during labor. Consequently, the MER can be triggered during labor, as evidenced by leakage of colostrum. This reflex readies the breasts for immediate feeding by the infant after birth. Oxytocin has the important function of contracting the mother's uterus after birth to control postpartum bleeding and promote uterine involution. Thus mothers who breastfeed are at decreased risk for postpartum hemorrhage. Uterine contractions that occur with breastfeeding are often painful during and after feeding for the first 3 to 5 days. These afterpains are more common in multiparas and tend to resolve completely within 1 week after birth.

Prolactin and oxytocin have been called the "mothering hormones" because they affect the postpartum woman's emotions and her physical state. Many women report feeling thirsty or very relaxed during breastfeeding, probably as a result of these hormones.

The nipple-erection reflex is an important part of lactation. When the infant cries, suckles, or rubs against the breast, the nipple becomes erect, which aids in the propulsion of milk through the ducts to the nipple pores. Nipple sizes, shapes, and ability to become erect vary with individuals. Some women have flat or inverted nipples that do not become erect with stimulation; these women likely need assistance with effective latch. Their infants should not be offered bottles or pacifiers until breastfeeding is well established.

Uniqueness of Human Milk

Human milk is the ideal food for human infants. It is a dynamic substance with a composition that changes to meet the changing nutritional and immunologic needs of the growing infant. Breast milk is specific to the needs of each infant; for example, the milk produced by mothers of preterm infants differs in composition from that of mothers who give birth at term.

Human milk contains immunologically active components that provide some protection against a broad spectrum of bacterial, viral, and protozoal infections. The major immunoglobulin (Ig) in human milk is secretory IgA; IgG, IgM, IgD, and IgE are also present. Human milk also contains T and B lymphocytes, epidermal growth factor, cytokines, interleukins, bifidus factor, complement (C3 and C4), and lactoferrin, all of which have a specific role in preventing localized and systemic bacterial and viral infections (Lawrence & Lawrence, 2011a).

Human milk composition and volumes vary according to the stage of lactation. In lactogenesis stage I, beginning at approximately 16 to 18 weeks of pregnancy, the breasts prepare for milk production by producing prepartum milk, or colostrum. Stage II of lactogenesis begins with birth as progesterone levels drop sharply when the placenta is removed. For the first 2 to 3 days after birth, the baby receives colostrum, a clear, yellowish fluid that is rich in antibodies and higher in protein but lower in fat than mature milk. The high protein level of colostrum facilitates binding of bilirubin, and the laxative action of colostrum promotes early passage of meconium. Colostrum is important in establishing normal *Lactobacillus bifidus* flora in the infant's digestive tract. It gradually changes to transitional milk. By 3 to 5 days after birth the woman experiences a noticeable increase in milk production. This is often referred to as *the milk coming in*. Breast milk continues to change in composition for approximately 10 days, when the mature milk is established. This is stage III of lactogenesis (Lawrence & Lawrence, 2011a).

The composition of human milk changes over time as the infant grows and develops. Fat is the most variable component of human milk with changes in concentration over a feeding, over a 24-hour period, and across time. Variations in fat content exist between breasts and among individuals (Lawrence & Lawrence, 2011a). During each feeding the concentration of fat gradually increases from the lower fat foremilk to the richer hindmilk. The hindmilk contains the denser calories from fat necessary for ensuring optimal growth and contentment between feedings. Because of this changing composition of human milk during each feeding, breastfeeding the infant long enough to supply a balanced feeding is important.

Milk production gradually increases as the baby grows. Infants have fairly predictable growth spurts (at approximately 10 days, 3 weeks, 6 weeks, 3 months, and 6 months), when more frequent feedings stimulate increased milk production. These growth spurts usually last 24 to 48 hours, after which the infants resume their usual feeding pattern as the mother's milk supply increases.

CARE MANAGEMENT

Supporting Breastfeeding Mothers and Infants

The key to encouraging mothers to breastfeed is education and anticipatory guidance, beginning as early as possible during and even before pregnancy. Each encounter with an expectant mother is an opportunity to educate, dispel myths, clarify misinformation, and address concerns. Prenatal education and preparation for breastfeeding influence feeding decisions, breastfeeding success, and the amount of time that women breastfeed. Prenatal preparation ideally includes the father of the baby, partner, or another significant support person and provides information about benefits of breastfeeding and how he or she can participate in infant care and nurturing.

Connecting expectant mothers with women from similar backgrounds who are breastfeeding or have successfully breastfed is often helpful. Nursing mothers' support groups such as La Leche League provide information about breastfeeding along with opportunities for breastfeeding mothers to interact with one another and share concerns (Fig. 25-4). Community-based peer counseling programs such as those instituted by the Special Supplemental Nutrition Program for Women, Infants, and Children (WIC) are beneficial (Chapman & Perez-Escamilla, 2012 ; Wambach, Aaronson, Breedlove, et al., 2011).

For women with limited access to health care, the postpartum period may provide the first opportunity for education about breastfeeding. Even women who have indicated the desire to formula feed can benefit from information about the benefits of breastfeeding. Offering these women the chance to try breastfeeding with the assistance of a nurse or lactation consultant can influence a change in infant feeding practices.

Promoting feelings of competence and confidence in the breastfeeding mother and reinforcing the unequaled contribution she is making toward the health and well-being of her infant are the responsibility of the nurse and other health care professionals. The first 2 weeks of breastfeeding can be the most challenging as mothers are adjusting to life with a newborn, the baby is learning to latch on and feed effectively, and the mother may be experiencing nipple or breast discomfort. This is a time when support is critical. Primiparous women are most likely to experience early breastfeeding problems, which often result in less exclusive breastfeeding and shorter duration of breastfeeding (Chantry, 2011). Anticipatory guidance during the prenatal period and especially during the hospital stay after birth can provide the mother with information and increase her confidence in her ability to successfully breastfeed her infant. New mothers need access to lactation support following discharge through primary care offices or outpatient lactation services. Peer support is also helpful.

The most common reasons for breastfeeding cessation are insufficient milk supply, painful nipples, and problems getting the infant to feed (Lauwers & Swisher, 2011; Lawrence & Lawrence, 2011a; Wagner, Chantry, Dewey, & Nommsen-Rivers, 2013). Early and ongoing assistance and support from health care professionals to prevent and address problems with breastfeeding can help promote a successful and satisfying breastfeeding experience for mothers and infants. Many health care agencies have certified lactation consultants on staff. These health care professionals, who are usually nurses, have specialized training and experience in helping breastfeeding mothers and infants.

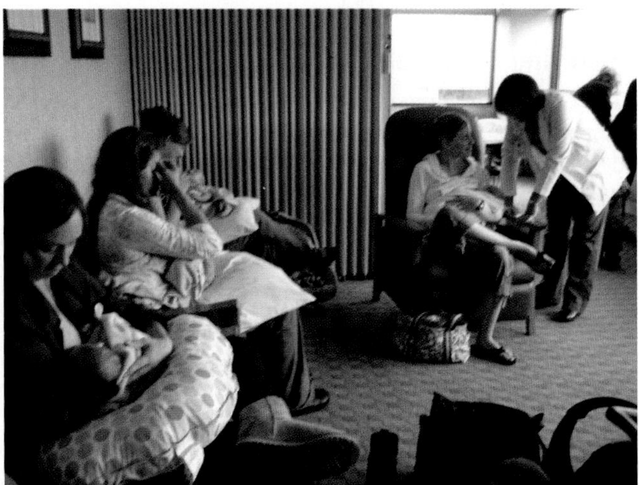

FIG 25-4 Breastfeeding mothers support group with lactation consultant. (Courtesy Shannon Perry, Phoenix, AZ.)

The U.S. Breastfeeding Committee (USBC, 2010a) has identified key competencies for health care professionals related to breastfeeding care and services. The competencies include knowledge, skills, and attitudes to promote and support breastfeeding. The USBC identifies specific competencies for those who provide more "hands-on" care (e.g., nurses and lactation consultants). The competencies are to "assist in early initiation of breastfeeding, assess the lactating breast, perform an infant feeding observation, recognize normal and abnormal infant feeding patterns, and develop and appropriately communicate a breastfeeding care plan" (USBC, 2010a, p. 5).

All parents are entitled to a birthing environment in which breastfeeding is promoted and supported. The Baby-Friendly Hospital Initiative (BFHI), sponsored by the WHO and UNICEF, was founded in 1991 to encourage institutions to offer optimal levels of care for lactating mothers. When a hospital achieves the "Ten Steps to Successful Breastfeeding for Hospitals," it is recognized as a Baby-Friendly hospital (Box 25-1). As of December 2013, 172 hospitals and birthing centers in the United States were designated as Baby-Friendly (Baby-Friendly USA, 2013), although many hospitals and birthing facilities are working toward the designation. Approximately 7% of live births in the United States occur at Baby-Friendly facilities (CDC, 2013). More than 20,000 facilities in more than 150 countries have achieved Baby-Friendly status (BFUSA). The Breastfeeding Committee for Canada (2014) reported that 7 hospitals or birthing centers and 17 community health services have achieved Baby-Friendly designation. Women are more likely to achieve their goals for exclusive breastfeeding if they give birth in facilities where all or most of the 10 steps are in place (Perrine, Scanlon, Li, et al., 2012).

The Joint Commission (TJC) issued a set of Perinatal Core Measures that includes exclusive breast milk feeding. In implementing the core measures, hospitals strive to improve their adherence to

BOX 25-1 10 Steps to Successful Breastfeeding for Hospitals

1. Have a written breastfeeding policy that is communicated routinely to all health care staff.
2. Train all health care staff in skills necessary to implement this policy.
3. Inform all pregnant women about the benefits and management of breastfeeding.
4. Help mothers initiate breastfeeding within ½ hour of birth.
5. Show mothers how to breastfeed and maintain lactation, even if they should be separated from their infants.
6. Give newborn infants no food or drink other than breast milk unless medically indicated.
7. Practice rooming-in (i.e., allow mothers and infants to remain together 24 hours a day).
8. Encourage breastfeeding on demand.
9. Give no artificial teats or pacifiers (also called dummies or soothers) to breastfeeding infants.
10. Foster the establishment of breastfeeding support groups and refer mothers to them on discharge from the hospital or clinic.

From Baby-Friendly USA (BFHI USA). (2012). *The ten steps to successful breastfeeding.* Available at www.babyfriendlyusa.org/about-us/baby-friendly-hospital-initiative/the-ten-steps.

evidence-based best practices that can result in increased rates of exclusive breastfeeding (TJC, 2012; USBC, 2010b). Care management of the breastfeeding mother and infant requires that nurses and other health care professionals are knowledgeable about the benefits and basic anatomic and physiologic aspects of breastfeeding. They also need to know how to help the mother with feedings and discuss interventions for common problems. Ongoing support of the mother enhances her self-confidence and promotes a satisfying and successful breastfeeding experience. Mothers should be encouraged to ask for help with breastfeeding, especially while they are in the hospital. Primiparas are likely to need the most assistance and in many facilities are routinely seen by lactation consultants.

The mother needs to understand infant behaviors in relation to breastfeeding and recognize signs that the baby is ready to feed. Infants exhibit **feeding-readiness cues** or early signs of hunger. Instead of waiting to feed until the infant is crying in a distraught manner or withdrawing into sleep, the mother should attempt to breastfeed when the baby exhibits feeding cues (see Evidence-Based Practice box):

- Hand-to-mouth or hand-to-hand movements
- Sucking motions
- Rooting reflex—infant moves toward whatever touches the area around the mouth and attempts to suck
- Mouthing

EVIDENCE-BASED PRACTICE

Maternal Feeding Styles and Childhood Obesity

Ask the Question

Does caregiver responsiveness to infant feeding cues have an effect on obesity in early childhood and beyond?

Search for the Evidence

Search Strategies English language research-based publications on infant, feeding, satiety, breastfeeding, overweight, obesity were included.

Databases Used Cochrane Collaborative Database, National Guideline Clearinghouse (AHRQ), CINAHL, PubMed, and UpToDate

Critical Appraisal of the Evidence

- Childhood obesity can have its roots in the feeding patterns established in infancy. This research field for primary prevention of obesity is new, and many infant feeding studies are in the pipeline.
- Overfeeding can impair the infant's ability to self-regulate. Infants whose caregivers are responsive to an infant's hunger and satiety (full) cues are significantly less likely to be overweight (DiSantis, Hodges, Johnson, & Fisher, 2011).
- Discordant responsiveness occurs when the caregiver perceives that the infant cannot recognize hunger or satiety. Restrictive feeding style is associated with maternal fear of causing obesity. Pressuring feeding style is associated with caregiver concern that the infant has poor appetite and will be underweight (Gross, Mendelsohn, Fierman, & Messito, 2011).
- Low-income, food-insecure mothers are more likely to be discordant, either restrictive or pressuring, than food-secure mothers (Gross, Mendelsohn, Fierman, et al., 2012). Authoritative parenting style is associated with pressuring to eat (Collins, Duncanson, & Burrows, 2014).

Apply the Evidence: Nursing Implications

- Parental education in infant hunger and satiety cues should ideally begin in prenatal education classes, and be reinforced intensively during the postpartum period. The nurse should point out the infant cues, and praise the parents for appropriate responsiveness.
- Videos and printed material, as well as warm lines, should be made available to new parents. Specific suggestions as to how much formula to feed initially and as the infant grows, and how voiding and stool patterns and weight gain reflect adequate nutrition can provide education guidelines.
- Assessing for familial and cultural beliefs enables the nurse to address parental and extended family concerns. The nurse can address how the new mother might respond to well-meaning but incorrect comments from family and strangers.
- Education regarding the various newborn cries and their possible reasons can reassure parents and their extended families that feeding should not be the first and only option.
- Breastfed infants are less likely to be overfed than infants who are formula fed.
- Nurses can advocate on a local and national level to eliminate food insecurity.

Quality and Safety Competencies: Evidence-Based Practice*

Knowledge

Describe EBP to include the components of research evidence, clinical expertise, and client/family values.

Parental education about correctly interpreting infant feeding cues can help to prevent overfeeding and childhood obesity.

Skills

Read original research and evidence reports related to area of practice.

As a new topic this field of research is still developing tools to measure infant feeding cues and caregiver responsiveness, and will soon begin to develop interventions for clinical trials.

Attitudes

Appreciate the importance of regularly reading relevant professional journals.

As further research is published, systematic analyses and clinical guidelines may emerge as to the best interventions for healthy habits in infancy.

References

Collins, C., Duncanson, K., & Burrows, T. (2014). A systematic review investigating associations between parenting style and child feeding behaviours. *Journal of Human Nutrition and Diet*, Jan 6, 2014 (Epub ahead of print).

DiSantis, K. I., Hodges, E. A., Johnson, S. L., & Fisher, J. O. (2011). The role of responsive feeding in overweight during infancy and toddlerhood: A systematic review. *International Journal of Obesity (London)*, *35*(4), 480–492.

Gross, R. S., Mendelsohn, A. L., Fierman, A. H., & Messito, M. J. (2011). Maternal controlling feeding styles during early infancy. *Clinical Pediatrics (Philadelphia)*, *50*(12), 1125–1133.

Gross, R. S., Mendelsohn, A. L., Fierman, A. H., et al. (2012). Food insecurity and obesogenic maternal infant feeding styles and practices in low-income families. *Pediatrics*, *130*(2), 254–261.

Pat Mahaffee Gingrich

*Adapted from QSEN at www.qsen.org/.

Babies normally consume small amounts of milk with feedings during the first 3 days of life. As the baby adjusts to extrauterine life and the digestive tract is cleared of meconium, milk intake increases from 15 to 30 ml per feeding in the first 24 hours to 60 to 90 ml by the end of the first week.

In the postpartum period interventions focus on helping the mother and the newborn initiate successful breastfeeding. An important goal is to build maternal confidence in breastfeeding. Interventions to promote successful breastfeeding include educating and assisting mothers and their partners with basics such as latch and positioning, signs of adequate feeding, and self-care measures such as prevention of engorgement. It is important to provide the parents with a list of resources that they can contact after discharge from the birthing facility.

The ideal time to begin breastfeeding is within the first hour after birth. Newborns without complications should be allowed to remain in direct skin-to-skin contact with the mother until the baby is able to breastfeed for the first time (AAP Section on Breastfeeding, 2012). This is true both for mothers who gave birth by cesarean and for those who gave birth vaginally. Early skin-to-skin contact is associated with higher rates of exclusive breastfeeding and increased duration of breastfeeding (Augustin, Donovan, Lozano, et al., 2013; Moore, Anderson, Bergman, et al., 2012; Suzuki, 2013).

Routine procedures such as vitamin K injection, eye prophylaxis, weighing, and bathing should be delayed until the neonate has completed the first feeding (AAP Section on Breastfeeding, 2012).

Positioning

For the initial feedings it can be advantageous to encourage and assist the mother to breastfeed in a semi-reclining position with the newborn lying prone, skin-to-skin on the mother's bare chest. Her body supports the baby. The mother is more relaxed, nipple pain is reduced or eliminated, and she has more freedom of movement to use her hands. The baby is able to use inborn reflexes to latch onto the breast and feed effectively. This approach to breastfeeding is based on the concept of "biological nurturing" (Colson, 2010, 2012).

The four traditional positions for breastfeeding are the football or clutch hold (under the arm), modified cradle, cross-cradle or across the lap, cradle, and side-lying (Fig. 25-5). The mother should be encouraged to use the position that most easily facilitates latch while allowing maximal comfort. The football or clutch hold is often recommended for early feedings because the mother can see the baby's mouth easily as she guides the infant onto the nipple.

Mothers who gave birth by cesarean often prefer the football or clutch hold. The modified cradle or across-the-lap hold works well for early feedings, especially with smaller babies. The side-lying position allows the mother to rest while breastfeeding. Women with perineal pain and swelling often prefer this position. Cradling is the most common breastfeeding position for infants who have learned to latch easily and feed effectively. Before discharge from the birth institution the nurse can help the mother try all of the positions so she will be confident in trying these positions at home.

During breastfeeding the mother should be as comfortable as possible. After arranging for privacy, the nurse might suggest that she empty her bladder and attend to other needs before starting a feeding session. The nurse who is assisting with breastfeeding should be at the mother's eye level. The mother holds the infant securely at the level of the breast, supported by firm pillows or folded blankets, facing toward her. The baby's mouth is directly in front of the nipple. The mother should support the baby's neck and shoulders with her hand and not push on the occiput. The baby's body is held in alignment (ears, shoulders, and hips are in a straight line) during latch and feeding.

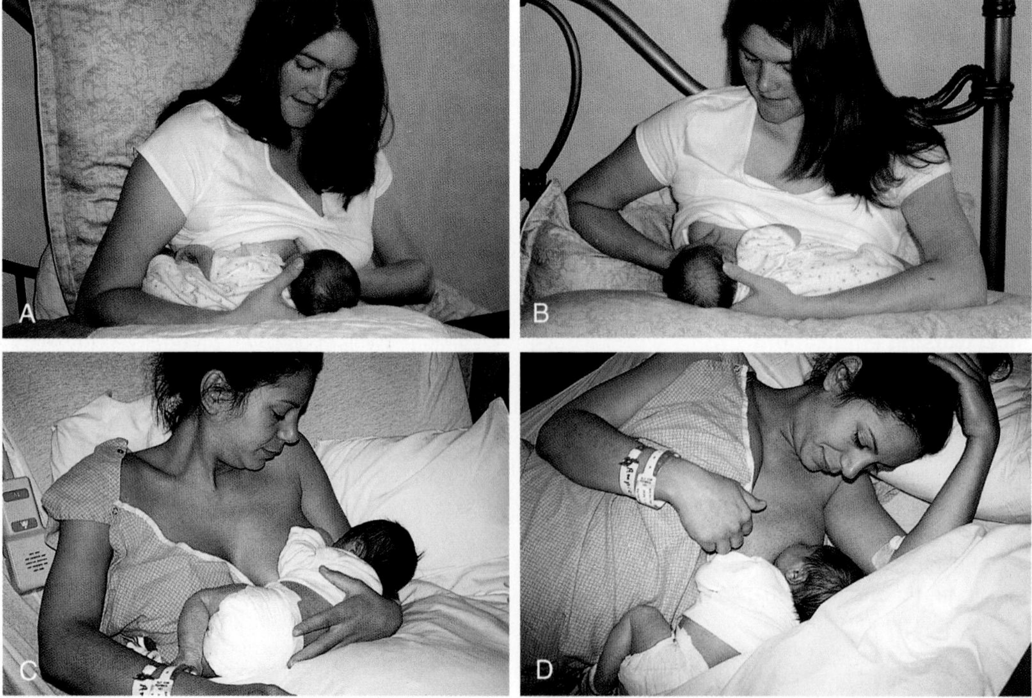

FIG 25-5 Breastfeeding positions. **A,** Football or clutch (under the arm) hold. **B,** Across the lap (modified cradle). **C,** Cradling. **D,** Lying down. (**A** and **B,** Courtesy Kathryn Alden, Chapel Hill, NC; **C** and **D,** courtesy Marjorie Pyle, RNC, Lifecircle, Costa Mesa, CA.)

Latch

Latch, or latch-on, is defined as placement of the infant's mouth over the nipple, areola, and breast, making a seal between the mouth and breast to create adequate suction for milk removal. In preparation for latch during early feedings the mother should manually express a few drops of colostrum or milk and spread it over the nipple. This action lubricates the nipple and entices the baby to open the mouth as the milk is tasted.

To facilitate latch the mother supports her breast in one hand with the thumb on top and four fingers underneath at the back edge of the areola. The breast is compressed slightly with the fingers parallel to the infant's lips, as one might compress a large sandwich in preparing to take a bite, so an adequate amount of breast tissue is taken into the mouth with latch. Most mothers need to support the breast during feeding for at least the first days until the infant is adept at feeding.

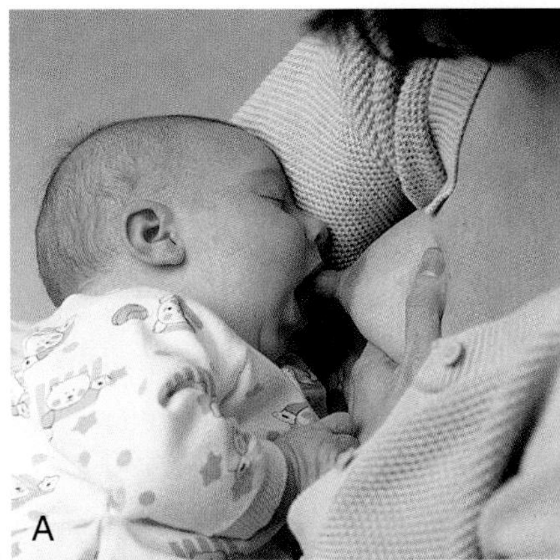

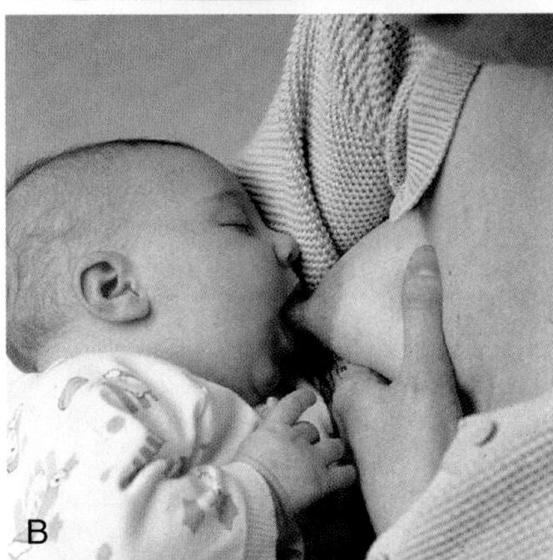

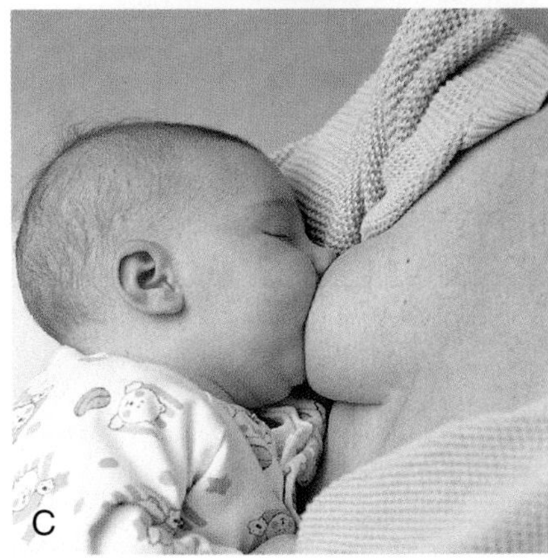

FIG 25-6 Latch. **A,** Mother tickles baby's lips with nipple until he or she opens wide. **B,** Once baby's mouth is opened wide, she quickly "hugs" baby to breast. **C,** Baby should have as much areola (dark area around nipple) in his or her mouth as possible, not just the nipple. (Courtesy Medela, Inc., McHenry, IL.)

The mother holds the baby close to the breast with the infant's mouth directly in front of the nipple. The infant who is displaying the rooting reflex with the mouth opening widely may easily latch on. If the infant is not readily opening the mouth, the mother tickles the baby's lips with her nipple, stimulating the mouth to open. When the mouth is open wide and the tongue is down, the mother quickly "hugs" the baby to the breast, bringing him or her onto the nipple (Fig. 25-6). The amount of areola in the baby's mouth with correct latch depends on the size of the baby's mouth and the size of the areola and nipple. If breastfeeding is painful, the baby likely has not taken enough of the breast into the mouth, and the tongue is pinching the nipple.

Mothers may also use the *asymmetric latch technique*. When the baby's mouth opens widely, the mother moves the baby in toward her body so the chin and lower mandible make contact with the breast first, followed by the top lip. When the baby is latched on, the nose is tilted slightly away from the mother's breast, and the chin is pressed into the underside of the breast. The infant's mouth placement is asymmetric on the areola; the lower part is covered by the baby's mouth, but the top is clearly visible above the top lip.

Once the infant is latched on and sucking, there are signs that the feeding is going well. These include (1) the mother reports a firm tugging sensation on her nipple but feels no pinching or pain; (2) the baby sucks with cheeks rounded, not dimpled; (3) the baby's jaw glides smoothly with sucking; and (4) swallowing is usually audible. Sucking creates a vacuum in the intraoral cavity as the breast is compressed between the tongue and the palate. When the infant is latched on and sucking correctly, breastfeeding is not painful. If she feels pinching or pain after the initial sucks or does not feel a strong tugging sensation on the nipple, the latch and positioning are evaluated. Any time the signs of adequate latch and sucking are not present, the baby should be taken off the breast, and latch attempted again. To prevent nipple trauma as the baby is taken off the breast, the mother is instructed to break the suction by inserting a finger in the side of the baby's mouth between the gums and leaving it there until the nipple is completely out of the mouth (Fig. 25-7) (see Nursing Care Plan).

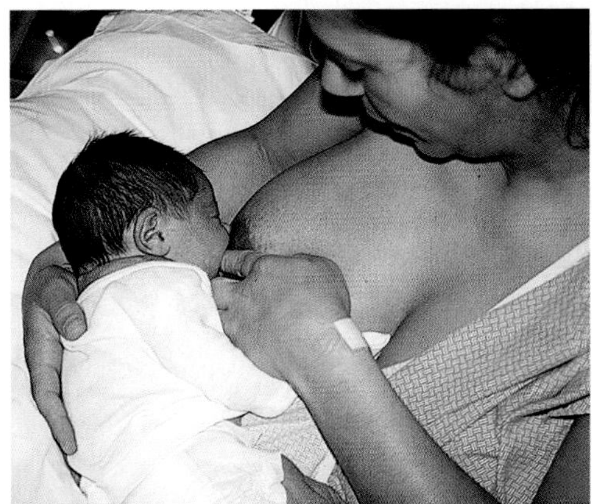

FIG 25-7 Removing infant from breast by inserting a finger to break suction. (Courtesy Marjorie Pyle, RNC, Lifecircle, Costa Mesa, CA.)

NURSING CARE PLAN

Breastfeeding and Infant Nutrition

NURSING DIAGNOSIS	EXPECTED OUTCOMES	NURSING INTERVENTIONS	RATIONALES
Ineffective Breastfeeding related to knowledge deficit of the mother as evidenced by ongoing incorrect latch technique	Mother will demonstrate correct latch technique. Infant will latch correctly and suck with gliding jaw movements and audible swallowing. Mother will report "tugging" but no nipple pain with infant suckling. Mother will express increased satisfaction with breastfeeding, and neonate will exhibit satisfaction of hunger and sucking needs.	Assess mother's knowledge and motivation for breastfeeding.	To provide starting point for teaching
		Observe breastfeeding session at least once each shift.	To provide baseline assessment for positive reinforcement and problem identification
		Describe and demonstrate ways to stimulate sucking reflex, various positions for breastfeeding, use of pillows during session, and how to facilitate a comfortable and effective latch.	To promote maternal and neonatal comfort and effective latch
		Monitor position of infant's mouth on areola and position of head and body.	To give positive reinforcement for correct latch position or to correct poor latch position
		Teach mother ways to stimulate neonate to maintain an awake state by diapering, unwrapping, massaging, or burping.	To complete breastfeeding session thoroughly and satisfactorily
Ineffective Infant Feeding Pattern related to inability to coordinate sucking and swallowing	Neonate will coordinate sucking and swallowing to accomplish effective feeding pattern.	Assess for factors that can contribute to ineffective sucking and swallowing.	To provide basis for plan of care
		Teach mother to observe feeding-readiness cues.	To enhance effective feeding
		Modify feeding methods as needed.	To maintain hydration status and nutritional requirements
		Promote calm, relaxed atmosphere.	To provide pleasant breastfeeding experience for mother and neonate
		Refer to lactation consultant.	To provide specialized support
Anxiety related to ineffective infant feeding pattern	Mother will report decrease in anxiety level and express satisfaction with breastfeeding.	Assess mother's feelings and anxieties about breastfeeding.	To identify specific concerns
		Monitor maternal anxiety level during feeding sessions.	To provide basis for care planning
		Provide education about breastfeeding.	To help mother increase her knowledge about breastfeeding and improve her confidence
		Provide positive reinforcement for feeding pattern improvement.	To decrease anxiety
		Monitor weight, intake, and output of neonate.	To provide information regarding effective feeding
		Enlist assistance of support persons.	To provide positive feedback for increasing skill
		Provide information for lactation support.	To decrease anxiety after discharge
		Initiate follow-up (telephone calls, follow-up with health care provider, outpatient lactation consultant) as needed.	To assess progress, detect problems, and provide support

The nurse should observe at least one feeding every 8 to 12 hours while the mother and newborn are in the hospital (Holmes, McLeod, & Bunik, 2013). Using a standard breastfeeding scoring tool such as the LATCH (Jenson, Wallace, & Kelsay, 1994) to document observations provides consistency in assessment criteria. With the LATCH assessment tool, each letter represents a scored item: *L*atch, *A*udible swallowing, *T*ype of nipple, *C*omfort level of the mother, and *H*old (positioning). During the feeding assessment the nurse can provide education about breastfeeding, help with feeding techniques, and offer support. If the mother's partner or other family members are present, the nurse can include them in the teaching and demonstrate how they can help the mother and provide support.

Milk Ejection or Let-down

As the baby begins sucking on the nipple, the milk ejection, or let-down, reflex is stimulated (see Fig. 25-3, *B*). The following signs indicate that milk ejection has occurred:

- The mother may feel a tingling sensation in the nipples and breasts, although many women never feel when milk ejection (let-down) occurs.
- The baby's suck changes from quick, shallow sucks to a slower, more drawing sucking pattern.
- Audible swallowing is present as the baby sucks.
- In the early days the mother feels uterine cramping and can have increased lochia during and after feedings.
- The mother feels relaxed or drowsy during feedings.
- The opposite breast may leak.

Frequency of Feedings

Feeding patterns vary because every mother-infant dyad is unique. Breastfeeding frequency is influenced by a variety of factors, including the infant's age, weight, maturity level, stomach capacity and gastric emptying time, and the storage capacity of the breast (i.e., the milk available when the breast is full).

Newborns need to breastfeed at least 8 to 12 times in a 24-hour period (AAP Section on Breastfeeding, 2012). Some infants breastfeed every 2 to 3 hours throughout a 24-hour period. Others cluster-feed, breastfeeding every hour or so for three to five feedings and then sleeping for 3 to 4 hours between clusters. During the first 24 to 48 hours after birth most babies do not awaken this often to feed. Parents need to understand that they should awaken the baby to feed at least every 3 hours during the day and at least every 4 hours at night. (Feeding frequency is determined by counting from the beginning of one feeding to the beginning of the next.) Once the infant is feeding well and gaining weight adequately, going to demand feeding is appropriate, in which case the infant determines the frequency of feedings. (With demand feeding the infant should still receive at least eight feedings in 24 hours.).

> **SAFETY ALERT**
>
> Nurses should caution parents against attempting to place newborn infants on strict feeding schedules. Strict scheduling of feedings (forcing the baby to wait for a set amount of time before feeding) can result in failure to meet the nutritional needs of infants.

Infants should be fed whenever they exhibit feeding cues. Keeping the baby close is the best way to observe and respond to these cues. Newborns should remain with mothers during the recovery period after birth and room-in during the hospital stay. At home babies should be kept nearby so parents can observe signs that the baby is ready to feed. The mother and breastfeeding infant should sleep in proximity (in the same room but not in the same bed) to promote breastfeeding (AAP Section on Breastfeeding, 2012).

Duration of Feedings. The duration of breastfeeding sessions varies greatly because the timing of milk transfer differs for each mother-baby pair. The average time for early feedings is 30 to 40 minutes or approximately 15 to 20 minutes per breast. As infants grow they become more efficient at breastfeeding, and consequently the length of feedings decreases. The amount of time an infant spends breastfeeding is not a reliable indicator of the amount of milk the infant consumes because some of the time at the breast is spent in nonnutritive sucking.

In the early days after birth the mother may be instructed to feed on the first breast until the neonate falls asleep and try to wake the baby and offer the second breast. Some mothers prefer one-sided nursing, which means that the baby nurses only one breast at each feeding. The first breast offered should be alternated at each feeding to ensure that each breast receives equal stimulation and emptying.

Instead of instructing mothers to feed for a set number of minutes, nurses should teach them to look for signs that the baby has finished feeding (e.g., the baby's sucking and swallowing pattern has slowed, the breast is softened, the baby appears content and may fall asleep or release the nipple).

If a baby seems to be feeding effectively and urine output and bowel movements are adequate but the weight gain is not satisfactory, the mother may be switching to the second breast too soon. Feeding on the first breast until it softens ensures that the baby receives the higher-fat hindmilk, which usually results in increased weight gain.

INDICATORS OF EFFECTIVE BREASTFEEDING

One of the most common concerns of breastfeeding mothers is how to determine if the baby is getting enough milk. In the newborn period, when breastfeeding is becoming established, parents should be taught about the signs that breastfeeding is going well. Awareness of these signs helps them recognize when problems arise so they can seek appropriate assistance (Box 25-2).

During the early days of breastfeeding, keeping a feeding diary can be helpful. This involves recording the time and length of feedings and infant urine output and bowel movements. The data from the diary provide evidence of the effectiveness of breastfeeding and are useful to health care providers in assessing adequacy of feeding. Parents are instructed to take this feeding diary to the follow-up visit with the infant's health care provider.

The infant's output is highly indicative of feeding adequacy. It is important that parents are aware of the expected changes in the characteristics of urine output and bowel movements during the early newborn period. As the volume of breast milk increases, urine becomes more dilute and should be light yellow; dark, concentrated urine can be associated with inadequate intake and possible

BOX 25-2 Signs of Effective Breastfeeding

Mother
- Onset of copious milk production (milk is "in") by day 3 or 4
- Firm tugging sensation on nipple as infant sucks but no pain
- Uterine contractions and increased vaginal bleeding while feeding (first week or less)
- Feels relaxed and drowsy while feeding
- Increased thirst
- Breasts soften or feel lighter while feeding
- With milk ejection (let-down), can feel warm rush or tingling in breasts, leaking of milk from opposite breast

Infant
- Latches without difficulty
- Has bursts of 15 to 20 sucks/swallows at a time
- Audible swallowing is present
- Easily releases breast at end of feeding
- Infant appears content after feeding
- Has at least three substantive bowel movements and six to eight wet diapers every 24 hours after day 4

dehydration. (Note: Infants with jaundice often have darker urine as bilirubin is excreted.) Infants should have at least six to eight sufficiently wet diapers (light yellow urine) every 24 hours after day 4. The first 1 to 2 days after birth newborns pass meconium stools, which are greenish black, thick, and sticky. By day 2 or 3 the stools become greener, thinner, and less sticky. If the mother's milk has come in by day 3 or 4, the stools start to appear greenish yellow and are looser. By the end of the first week breast milk stools are yellow, soft, and seedy (they resemble a mixture of mustard and cottage cheese). If an infant is still passing meconium stool by day 3 or 4, breastfeeding effectiveness and milk transfer should be assessed.

Infants should have at least three stools (quarter-size or larger) per day for the first month. Some babies stool with every feeding. The stooling pattern gradually changes; breastfed infants can continue to stool more than once per day or they may stool only every 2 or 3 days. As long as the baby continues to gain weight and appears healthy, this decrease in the number of bowel movements is normal.

Supplements, Bottles, and Pacifiers

Unless a medical indication exists, no supplements should be given to breastfeeding infants (AAP Section on Breastfeeding, 2012). With sound breastfeeding knowledge and practice, supplements are rarely needed. Early supplementation by hospital staff undermines a new mother's confidence and models behavior that is counterproductive to establishing breastfeeding.

When supplementation is deemed necessary, giving the baby expressed breast milk is best. If the mother is not able to provide the milk, the recommended alternative is pasteurized donor milk from a milk bank. However, in many cases donor milk is not readily accessible and a commercial infant formula is used. Before supplementation it is important to perform a careful evaluation of the mother-infant dyad.

Possible indications for supplementary feeding include infant factors such as hypoglycemia, dehydration, weight loss of more than 7% associated with delayed lactogenesis, delayed passage of bowel movements or meconium stool continued to day 5, poor milk transfer, or hyperbilirubinemia (ABM Protocol Committee, 2009).

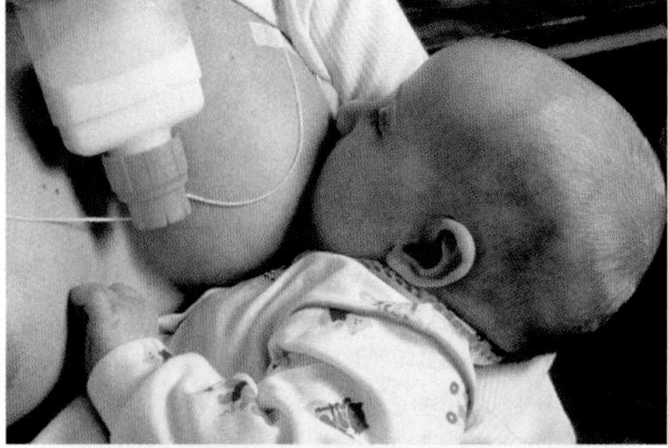

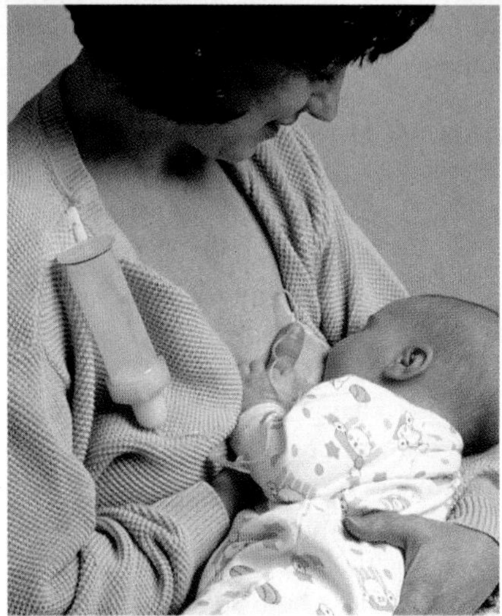

FIG 25-8 Supplemental nursing device. (Courtesy Medela, Inc, McHenry, IL.)

Maternal indications for possible supplementation include delayed lactogenesis and intolerable pain during feedings. Women who have had previous breast surgery such as augmentation or reduction may need to provide supplementary feedings for their infants (ABM Protocol Committee, 2009).

Newborns can become confused going from breast to bottle or bottle to breast when breastfeeding is first being established. Breastfeeding and bottle feeding require different oral motor skills. It is best to avoid bottles until breastfeeding is well established, usually after 3 or 4 weeks.

If supplemental feeding is needed, nurses or lactation consultants can help parents use supplemental nursing devices. This allows the baby to be supplemented with expressed breast milk or infant formula while still breastfeeding (Fig. 25-8). Infants can also be fed with a spoon, dropper, cup, or syringe. If parents choose to use bottles, a slow-flow nipple is recommended. Although some parents combine breastfeeding and bottle feeding, some infants never take a bottle and go directly from the breast to a cup.

Because of the correlation between pacifier use and a decreased risk of sudden infant death syndrome (SIDS), experts recommend pacifier use for healthy term infants at nap or sleep time, but only after breastfeeding is well established at about 3 or 4 weeks of age (AAP Section on Breastfeeding, 2012).

Special Considerations

Sleepy Baby

Some babies need to be awakened for feedings for the first few days after birth. If the infant is awakened from a sound sleep, attempts at feeding may be unsuccessful. Babies are more likely to feed if they are awakened from a light or active sleep state. Signs that the infant is in this sleep state are movements of the eyelids, body movements, and making sounds while sleeping. Unwrapping the baby, changing the diaper, sitting the baby upright, talking to him or her with variable pitch, gently massaging his or her chest or back, and stroking the palms or soles may bring the baby to an alert state. It is helpful to place the sleepy baby skin-to-skin with the mother; she can move the infant to the breast when feeding-readiness cues are apparent.

Fussy Baby

Babies sometimes awaken from sleep crying frantically. Although they are hungry, they cannot focus on feeding until they are calmed. Parents can swaddle the baby, hold him or her close, talk soothingly, and allow him or her to suck on a clean finger until calm enough to latch on to the breast. Placing the baby skin-to-skin with the mother can be very effective in calming a fussy infant. Fussiness during feeding can be the result of birth injury such as bruising of the head or fractured clavicle. Changing the feeding position can help alleviate this problem.

Infants who were suctioned extensively or intubated at birth can demonstrate an aversion to oral stimulation. The baby may scream and stiffen if anything approaches the mouth. Parents need to spend time holding and cuddling the baby before attempting to breastfeed.

An infant can become fussy and appear discontented when sucking if the nipple does not extend far enough into the mouth. The feeding can begin with well-organized sucks and swallows, but the infant soon begins to pull off the breast and cry. The mother should support her breast throughout the feeding so the nipple stays in the same position as the feeding proceeds and the breast softens.

Fussiness can be related to GI distress (e.g., cramping, gas pains, gastroesophageal reflux). It can occur in response to an occasional feeding of infant formula, or it can be related to something the mother has ingested, although most women are able to eat a normal diet without causing GI distress to the breastfeeding infant. Persistent crying or refusing to breastfeed can indicate illness. Parents are instructed to notify the health care provider if either circumstance occurs.

Some mothers find that their babies are less fussy when placed in a sling or carrier. Some slings make it easy to breastfeed without removing the baby from the sling (Fig. 25-9).

Slow Weight Gain

Newborn infants typically lose 5% to 6% of body weight after birth before they begin to gain weight. Weight loss of more than 7% in a breastfeeding infant during the first 3 days of life needs to be investigated (Lauwers & Swisher, 2011). After the early milk has transitioned to mature milk, infants should gain approximately 110 to 200 g (3.9 to 7 oz) per week or 20 to 28 g (0.7 to 1 oz) per day for the first 3 months. (Breastfed infants usually do not gain weight as quickly as formula-fed infants.)

Parents are taught the warning signs of ineffective breastfeeding, including inadequate weight gain, minimal output, and feeding constantly. If any of these warning signs is present, the parent should notify the health care provider.

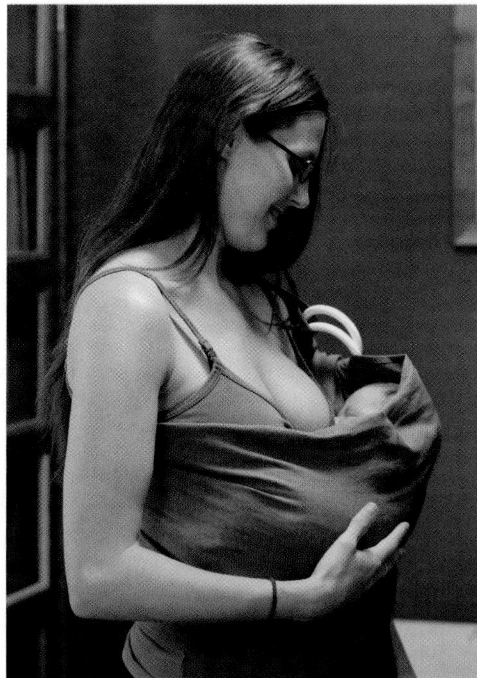

FIG 25-9 Baby breastfeeding while in sling. (Courtesy Julie Perry Nelson, Loveland, CO.)

At times slow weight gain is related to inadequate breastfeeding. Feedings can be short or infrequent, or the infant can be latching incorrectly or sucking ineffectively or inefficiently. Other possibilities are illness or infection; malabsorption; or circumstances that increase the baby's energy needs such as congenital heart disease, cystic fibrosis, or simply being small for gestational age. Slow weight gain must be differentiated from failure to thrive; this can be a serious problem that warrants medical intervention.

Maternal factors can be the cause of slow weight gain. The mother can have a problem with inadequate emptying of the breasts, pain with feeding, or inappropriate timing of feedings. Inadequate glandular breast tissue or previous breast surgery can affect milk supply. Severe intrapartum or postpartum hemorrhage (Sheehan syndrome), illness, or medications can decrease milk supply. Stress and fatigue also negatively affect milk production (Lauwers & Swisher, 2011; Lawrence & Lawrence, 2011a).

In most instances the solution to slow weight gain is to increase feeding frequency and to improve the feeding technique. Positioning and latch are evaluated, and adjustments are made. Adding a feeding or two in a 24-hour period can help. If the problem is a sleepy baby, parents are instructed in waking techniques.

Using alternate breast massage during feedings can help increase the amount of milk going to the infant. With this technique the mother massages her breast from the chest wall to the nipple whenever the baby has sucking pauses. This technique also can increase the fat content of the milk, which aids in weight gain.

When babies are calorie deprived and need supplementation, they can receive expressed breast milk or formula with a supplemental nursing device (see Fig. 25-8), spoon, cup, syringe, or bottle. In most cases supplementation is necessary only for a short time until the baby gains weight and is feeding adequately.

Jaundice

Chapter 23 and Chapter 36 discuss jaundice (hyperbilirubinemia) in the newborn in detail. Breastfeeding infants can develop *early-onset jaundice* or *breastfeeding-associated jaundice,* which is associated with insufficient feeding and infrequent stooling. Colostrum has a natural laxative effect and promotes early passage of meconium. Bilirubin is excreted from the body primarily through the intestines. Infrequent stooling allows bilirubin in the stool to be resorbed into the infant's system, thus increasing bilirubin levels (Blackburn, 2013). To prevent early-onset, breastfeeding-associated jaundice, newborns should be breastfed frequently during the first several days of life. Increased frequency of feedings is associated with decreased bilirubin levels.

To treat early-onset jaundice, breastfeeding is evaluated in terms of frequency and length of feedings, positioning, latch, and milk transfer. Factors such as a sleepy or lethargic infant or maternal breast engorgement can interfere with effective breastfeeding and should be corrected. If the infant's intake of milk needs to be increased, a supplemental feeding device can deliver additional breast milk or formula while the infant is nursing. Bilirubin levels are closely monitored.

Late-onset jaundice or *breast milk jaundice* affects a small number of breastfed infants and develops between 5 and 10 days of age. Affected infants typically thrive, gain weight, and stool normally; all pathologic causes of jaundice have been ruled out. In the presence of other risk factors, hyperbilirubinemia can be severe enough to require phototherapy. In most cases of breast milk jaundice no intervention is necessary. Some health care providers recommend temporary interruption of breastfeeding for 12 to 24 hours to allow bilirubin levels to decrease, although this approach is not preferred (Blackburn, 2013; Lawrence & Lawrence, 2011a).

Any breastfeeding infant who develops jaundice should be evaluated carefully for weight loss greater than 7%, decreased milk intake, infrequent stooling (fewer than three stools per day), and decreased urine output (fewer than four to six wet diapers per day). Bilirubin levels should be assessed by serum testing or transcutaneous monitoring (see Chapter 24).

Preterm Infants

Human milk is the ideal food for preterm infants, with benefits that are unique and in addition to those received by term healthy infants. Breast milk enhances retinal maturation in the preterm infant and improves neurocognitive outcomes; it also decreases the risk of sepsis and necrotizing enterocolitis. Greater physiologic stability occurs with breastfeeding compared to bottle feeding (AAP Section on Breastfeeding, 2012; Lawrence & Lawrence, 2011a).

Initially preterm milk contains higher concentrations of energy, protein, sodium, chloride, potassium, iron, and magnesium than term milk. It is more similar to term milk by approximately 4 to 6 weeks. Depending on gestational age and physical condition, many preterm infants are capable of breastfeeding for at least some feedings each day. Mothers of preterm infants who are not able to breastfeed their infants should begin pumping their breasts as soon as possible after birth with a hospital-grade electric pump (Fig. 25-10). Pumping frequency depends on the mother's breastfeeding goals but may be recommended 8 to 10 times every 24 hours to establish the milk supply. These women are taught proper handling and storage of breast milk to minimize bacterial contamination and growth. Kangaroo care (skin-to-skin contact) is encouraged until the baby is able to breastfeed and while breastfeeding is established because it enhances milk production (Lauwers & Swisher, 2011; Meier, Patel, Bigger, et al., 2013).

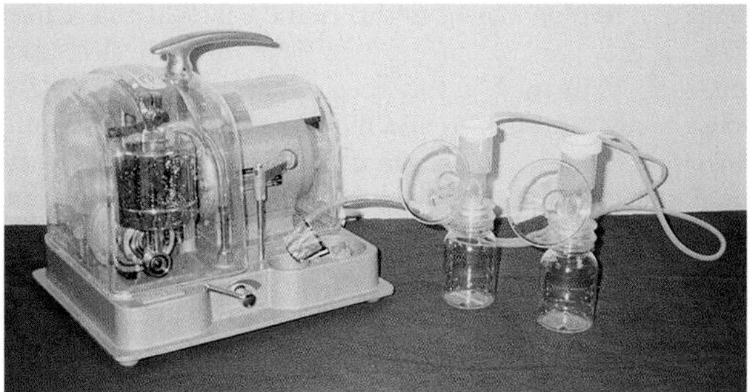

FIG 25-10 Hospital-grade electric breast pump. (Courtesy Kathryn Alden, Chapel Hill, NC.)

Mothers of preterm infants often receive specific emotional benefits in breastfeeding or providing breast milk for their babies. They find rewards in knowing that they can provide the healthiest nutrition for the infant and believe that breastfeeding enhances feelings of closeness to the infant.

Late Preterm Infants

Neonates born at 34 0/7 to 36 6/7 weeks of gestation are categorized as *late preterm infants.* These newborns are at risk for feeding difficulties because of their low energy stores and high energy demands. Additionally, they are more prone to hypothermia, hypoglycemia, and hyperbilirubinemia (ABM Protocol Committee, 2011a; Cooper, Holditch-Davis, Verklan, et al., 2012). They tend to be sleepy, with minimal and short wakeful periods. Late preterm infants often tire easily while feeding and have a weak suck and low tone; these factors can contribute to inadequate milk intake resulting in dehydration and poor weight gain (Meier, Patel, Wright, & Engstrom, 2013b). This predisposes mothers to delayed onset of lactogenesis II and inadequate milk supply.

Goals of care are to nourish the infant and protect the mother's milk supply. A lactation consultant should be involved in planning and providing appropriate care that usually includes milk expression with a hospital-grade pump and supplementation of the infant with expressed breast milk or infant formula (Meier et al., 2013).

Early and extended skin-to-skin contact promotes breastfeeding and helps prevent hypothermia. Because these infants are more prone to positional apnea than term infants, mothers are advised to use the clutch (under the arm or football) or cross-cradle hold for feeding, and avoid flexing the head, which can impede breathing. When supplementation is needed, expressed breast milk is the optimal supplement. Due to their weak suck, many infants are fed with a bottle, although in some cases a supplemental feeding device can be used (see Fig. 25-8) (Lanese & Cross, 2013; Meier, Patel, Wright, & Engstrom, 2013).

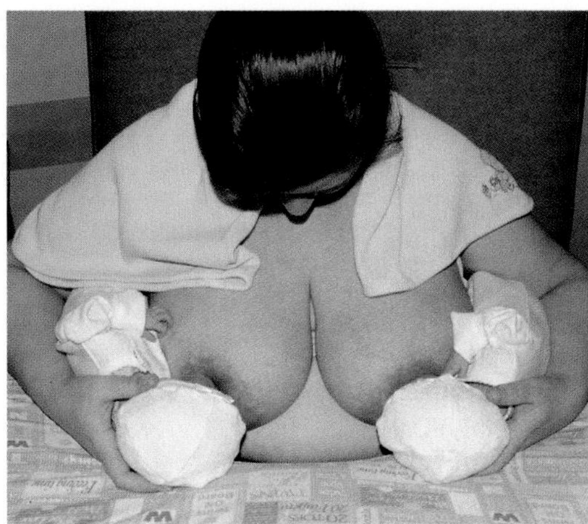

FIG 25-11 Breastfeeding twins. (Courtesy Cheryl Briggs, RNC, Annapolis, MD.)

Breastfeeding Multiple Infants

Breastfeeding is especially beneficial to twins, triplets, and other higher-order multiples because of the immunologic and nutritional advantages and the opportunity for the mother to interact with each baby frequently. Most mothers are capable of producing an adequate milk supply for multiple infants. Parenting multiples can be overwhelming; mothers and their husbands or partners need extra support and help to learn how to manage feedings (Fig. 25-11). Parents of multiples can find breastfeeding information and support through groups such as La Leche League International (www.lalecheleague.org/nb/nbmultiples.html).

Expressing and Storing Breast Milk

Breast milk expression is a common practice, typically performed to obtain breast milk for someone other than the mother to feed to the baby. It is most often associated with maternal employment. In some situations expression of breast milk is necessary or desirable such as when engorgement occurs, when the mother's nipples are sore or damaged, when the mother and baby are separated as in the case of a preterm infant who remains in the hospital after the mother is discharged, or when the mother leaves the infant with a caregiver and will not be present for feeding. Some women express milk to have an emergency supply. Some women choose to pump exclusively, providing breast milk for their infants but never allowing the baby to suckle at the breast. Because pumping and hand expression are rarely as efficient as a baby in removing milk from the breast, the milk supply is never judged based solely on the volume expressed. Milk volume can be more accurately assessed using prefeeding and postfeeding infant weights, also known as *test weights* (Lauwers & Swisher, 2011).

Hand Expression

All mothers should be instructed in hand expression. This simple technique can actually be more effective than an electric breast pump for expressing colostrum, which tends to be thicker than mature milk (Flaherman, Gay, Scott, et al., 2012; Morton, Hall, & Pessl, 2013-2014). Hand expression during the first 3 days after birth can have a positive effect on milk production during the early weeks. Morton and colleagues report that combining hand expression and hands-on pumping (breast massage before and during pumping) with the use of an electric breast pump can increase milk production and enhance fat content and caloric value of milk (Morton, Wong, Hall, et al., 2012). A video of hand expression of breast milk is available at http://newborns.stanford.edu/Breastfeeding/HandExpression.html.

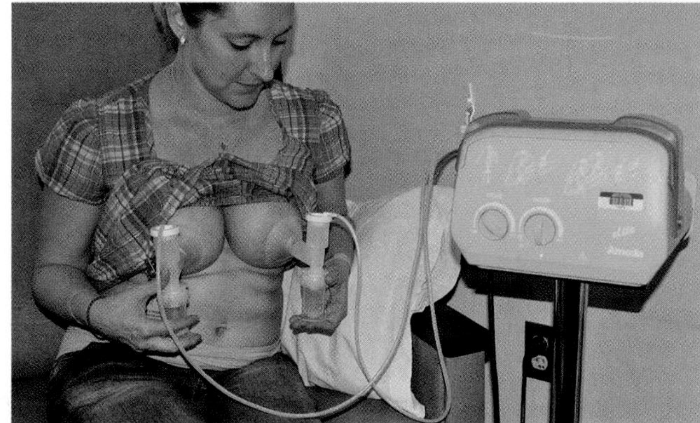

FIG 25-12 Bilateral breast pumping. (Courtesy Cheryl Briggs, RNC, Annapolis, MD.)

Mechanical Milk Expression (Pumping)

For most women recommendations are to initiate pumping only after the milk supply is well established and the infant is latching and breastfeeding well. However, when breastfeeding is delayed after birth such as when babies are ill or preterm, mothers should begin pumping with an electric breast pump as soon as possible and continue to pump regularly until the infant is able to breastfeed effectively. Early pumping may be initiated if the baby is too sleepy to feed effectively or if there are issues with latching or milk transfer. Milk expression is essential to maintaining milk supply if breastfeeding is interrupted. Double pumping (pumping both breasts at the same time) saves time and can stimulate the milk supply more effectively than single pumping (Fig. 25-12).

The amount of milk obtained when pumping depends on the type of pump being used, the time of day, the time since the baby breastfed, the mother's milk supply, how practiced she is at pumping, and her comfort level (pumping is uncomfortable for some women). Breast milk can vary in color and consistency, depending on the time of day, the age of the baby, and foods the mother has eaten.

Types of Pumps. Many types of breast pumps are available, varying in price and effectiveness. Before purchasing or renting a breast pump, the mother will benefit from counseling by a nurse or lactation consultant to determine which pump best suits her needs. The flange (funnel-shaped device that fits over the nipple or areola) should fit the nipple to prevent nipple pain, trauma, and possible reduction in milk supply. Mothers are advised to use the lowest suction setting on electric pumps, increasing gradually if needed. Breast massage before and during pumping can increase the amount of milk obtained (Lauwers & Swisher, 2011).

Manual or hand pumps are the least expensive and can be the most appropriate when portability and quietness of operation are important. These pumps are most often used by mothers who are pumping for an occasional bottle (Fig. 25-13).

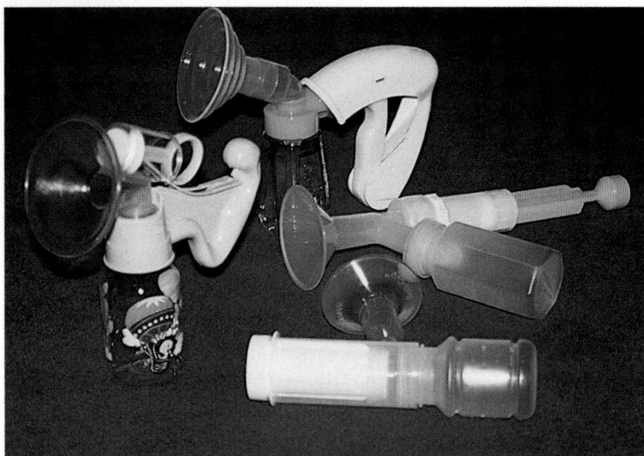

FIG 25-13 Manual breast pumps. (Courtesy Marjorie Pyle, RNC, Lifecircle, Costa Mesa, CA.)

Full-service electric pumps, or hospital-grade pumps (see Figs. 25-10 and 25-12), most closely duplicate the sucking action and pressure of the breastfeeding infant. When breastfeeding is delayed after birth (e.g., preterm or ill newborn) or when the mother and baby are separated for lengthy periods, these pumps are most appropriate. Because hospital-grade breast pumps are very heavy and expensive, portable versions of these pumps are available to rent for home use.

Electric self-cycling double pumps are efficient and easy to use. They are designed for working mothers. Some of these pumps come with carry bags containing coolers to store pumped milk.

Smaller electric or battery-operated pumps are typically used when pumping is performed occasionally, but some models are satisfactory for working mothers or others who pump on a regular basis.

Storage of Breast Milk

Mothers who express and feed breast milk to their infants need to be educated about safe practices for handling, storing, and feeding. Attention to hand hygiene and proper cleaning of equipment can reduce the risk of bacterial contamination. This is especially important when mothers are providing milk for preterm or ill neonates (Labiner-Wolfe & Fein, 2013; Meier, Patel, Bigger, et al., 2013). Guidelines for storing expressed breast milk for a healthy term infant are listed in the Teaching for Self-Management box: Breast Milk Storage Guidelines for Home Use for Term Infants).

The preferred containers for long-term storage of breast milk have hard sides such as hard plastic or glass with an airtight seal. Flexible polyethylene bags are not recommended for long-term milk storage (>72 hours) because there is a greater chance of leakage, puncture, and loss of immune cells (Lauwers & Swisher, 2011).

Maternal Employment

Returning to work after birth is associated with a decrease in the duration of breastfeeding. Women who return to work often face workplace challenges in breastfeeding such as lack of flexibility in work schedules, inadequate breaks to allow time for pumping, lack of privacy, lack of space for pumping, and lack of support from supervisors or coworkers. Mothers in educational

TEACHING FOR SELF-MANAGEMENT

Breast Milk Storage Guidelines for Home Use for Term Infants

- Before expressing or pumping breast milk, wash your hands.
- Containers for storing milk should be washed in hot, soapy water and rinsed thoroughly; they can also be washed in a dishwasher. If the water supply may not be clean, boil containers after washing. Plastic bags designed specifically for breast milk storage can be used for short-term storage (<72 hours).
- Write the date of expression on the container before storing milk. A waterproof label is best.
- Store milk in serving sizes of 2 to 4 ounces to prevent waste.
- Storing breast milk in the refrigerator or freezer with other food items is acceptable.
- You can combine milk from pumping sessions in the same day; cool freshly expressed milk before adding it to the refrigerated container. Do not add warm milk to a container of refrigerated milk.
- When storing milk in a refrigerator or freezer, place containers in the middle or back of the freezer, not on the door.
- When filling a storage container that will be frozen, fill only three quarters full, allowing space at the top of the container for expansion.
- To thaw frozen breast milk, place container in the refrigerator for gradual thawing or under warm, running water for quicker thawing. Never boil or microwave.
- Milk thawed in the refrigerator can be stored for 24 hours.
- Thawed breast milk should never be refrozen.
- Shake milk container before feeding baby and test the temperature of the milk on the inner aspect of your wrist.
- Any unused milk left in the bottle after feeding is discarded.

LOCATION OF STORAGE	TEMPERATURE	RECOMMENDED SAFE DURATION FOR STORAGE
Room temperature	16-29° C (60-85° F)	3-4 hours optimal 6-8 hours acceptable*
Refrigerator	4° C (39° F) or lower	72 hours optimal 5-8 days acceptable*
Freezer	Less than −4° C (24° F)	6 months optimal 12 months acceptable

*Under very clean conditions.

Modified from Academy of Breastfeeding Medicine Protocol Committee. (2010). ABM clinical protocol no. 8: Human milk storage information for home use for full-term infants. *Breastfeeding Medicine, 5*(3), 127-130.

SAFETY ALERT

Breast milk is never thawed or heated in a microwave oven. Microwaving does not heat evenly and can cause encapsulated boiling bubbles to form in the center of the liquid, which may not be detected when drops of milk are checked for temperature. Babies have sustained severe burns to the mouth, throat, and upper GI tract as a result of microwaved milk. In addition, microwaving significantly decreases the antiinfective properties and vitamin C content. The safety of low-temperature microwaving is questionable (ABM Protocol Committee, 2010; Lawrence & Lawrence, 2011a).

settings face similar challenges. Issues that can affect continued breastfeeding while working include fatigue, child care concerns, competing demands, and household responsibilities.

Employed mothers can continue breastfeeding with appropriate guidance and support. They are encouraged to set realistic goals for employment and breastfeeding, with accurate information regarding the costs, risks, and benefits of available feeding options. Women need information about planning for their return to work; nurses and lactation consultants can provide guidance. Websites such as www.workandpump.com include information about choosing pumps and other supplies, making a plan for breastfeeding and expressing milk, and preparing for their return to work.

Women who are able to breastfeed their infants during the workday tend to breastfeed longer. With increasing numbers of women having the option of working from home, this situation is becoming more common. In some settings mothers are able to breastfeed during the workday, either by going to an on-site daycare center or by having a friend or relative bring the baby to her for some feedings. Many working mothers pump their milk while they are at work and save the milk for later feedings. Working mothers who are unable to pump or breastfeed their infants during the workday have the shortest duration of breastfeeding.

Because women are a significant proportion of the workforce, many companies make provisions for breastfeeding women returning to work. The Affordable Care Act (USDHHS, 2010a) mandates that employers provide accommodations for breastfeeding mothers, specifically reasonable breaks during the workday and a non-bathroom space for milk expression until the child's first birthday. Breastfeeding programs typically include on-site lactation rooms (Fig. 25-14) and education and consulting services. Some employers provide on-site child care and high-quality breast pumps for their employees (Marinelli, Moren, Taylor, & Academy of Breastfeeding Medicine, 2013). Workplace support for breastfeeding mothers has improved significantly in recent years. However, further efforts are needed to educate employers about the importance of supporting their breastfeeding employees. Employers need to realize that breastfeeding programs can provide short- and long-term cost savings with significant health benefits for mothers, infants, and families. The Health Resources and Services Administration offers a free toolkit for employers: the "Business Case for Breastfeeding" outlines steps that employers can take to support breastfeeding employees (www.womenshealth.gov/breastfeeding/programs/business-case/tool-kit.cfm://aks/hrsa/gov).

Weaning

Weaning is initiated when babies are introduced to foods other than breast milk and concludes with the last breastfeeding. Gradual weaning over weeks or months is easier for mothers and infants than abrupt weaning. Abrupt weaning is likely to be distressing for mother and baby and physically uncomfortable for the mother because it can cause engorgement and mastitis (Mohrbacher, 2013).

Weaning is initiated by either the infant or the mother. With infant-led weaning the infant moves at his or her own pace in omitting feedings, which usually facilitates a gradual decrease in the mother's milk supply. Mother-led weaning means that the mother decides which feedings to drop. This approach is most easily undertaken by omitting the feeding of least interest to the baby or the one through which the infant is most likely to sleep. Every few days thereafter the mother drops another feeding until the infant is gradually weaned from the breast (Lauwers & Swisher, 2011).

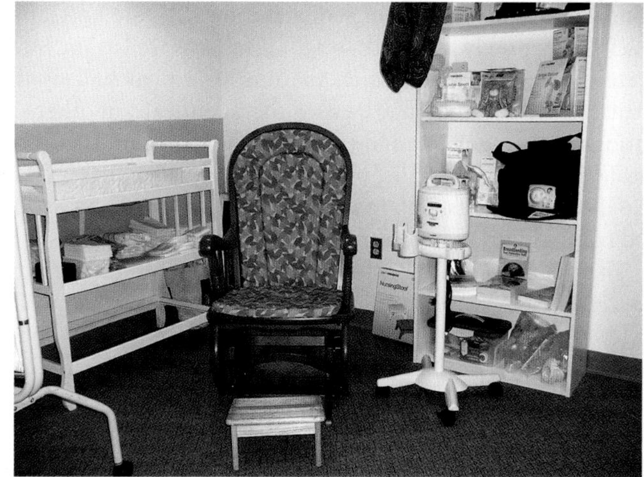

FIG 25-14 Lactation room. Note breast pump, rocking chair, nursing foot stool, changing table, books, and supplies. (Courtesy Cheryl Briggs, RNC, Annapolis, MD.)

Infants can be weaned directly from the breast to a cup. Bottles are usually offered to infants younger than 6 months. If the infant is weaned before 1 year of age, the infant should receive iron-fortified formula instead of cow's milk (AAP Section on Breastfeeding, 2012).

If abrupt weaning is necessary, breast engorgement can occur. To relieve the discomfort the mother can take mild analgesics such as ibuprofen, wear a supportive bra, apply ice packs or cabbage leaves to the breasts, and pump small amounts if needed. When possible it is best to avoid pumping because the breasts should remain full enough to promote a decrease in the milk supply (Lauwers & Swisher, 2011).

Weaning is often a very emotional time for mothers; many believe that it is the end to a special, satisfying relationship with the infant and benefit from time to adapt to the changes. Sudden weaning can evoke feelings of guilt and disappointment. Some women go through a grieving period after weaning. Nurses and others can help the mother by discussing other ways to continue this nurturing relationship with the infant such as skin-to-skin contact while bottle feeding or holding and cuddling the baby. Support from the father or partner and other family members is essential at this time.

Milk Banking

The AAP recommends pasteurized donor milk for preterm infants if the mother's own milk is not available despite substantial lactation support (AAP Section on Breastfeeding, 2012). The value of donor milk is emphasized by the ABM in their recommendation of pasteurized donor milk for the healthy term and preterm infant when the mother's milk is not available (ABM Protocol Committee, 2009).

For infants who cannot be breastfed but who also cannot survive except on human milk, banked donor milk is critically important. Because of the antiinfective and growth-promoting properties of human milk and its superior nutrition, processed donor milk is used in some neonatal intensive care units, primarily for severely low birth weight infants as well as for other preterm or sick infants when the mother's own milk is not available. Donor milk may be used therapeutically in other situations such as for infants with short gut syndrome, formula intolerance, metabolic disorders, or congenital anomalies. It is also used for infants with IgA deficiency who are not breastfed, and older children or adults with IgA deficiency.

The Human Milk Banking Association of North America (HMBANA) (www.hmbana.org) has established annually reviewed guidelines for the operation of not-for-profit donor human milk banks (HMBANA, 2013). Interestingly, there is no federal oversight or regulation of milk banking in the United States. However, some states have laws and regulations that specify how donor milk is to be procured, processed, and distributed (Landers & Hartmann, 2012). Currently there are 16 HMBANA milk banks in the United States and Canada, with more in various stages of planning and development (Updegrove, 2013). The milk banks collect, screen, process, and distribute the milk donated by lactating mothers. All donors are screened both by interview and serologically for communicable diseases. Donor milk is stored frozen until it is heat processed to kill potential pathogens; it is then refrozen for storage until it is dispensed for use. The heat processing adds a level of protection for the recipient that is not possible with any other donor tissue or organ. Banked milk is dispensed only by prescription. A per-ounce fee is charged by the bank to pay for the processing costs, but the HMBANA guidelines prohibit payment to donors (Landers & Hartmann).

COMMUNITY ACTIVITY

The Human Milk Banking Association of North America is a non-profit organization that provides donor milk that has been safely pasteurized and tested. It is dispensed only by hospital purchase order or health care provider prescription. Go to the website: www.hmbana.org and read about how milk is processed. Also explore how a woman can become a milk donor. Examine websites that offer milk sharing via the Internet: Eats on Feets (www.eatsonfeets.org) and Human Milk for Human Babies (http://hm4hb.net). What is the process for procuring human milk? What is the cost? What information is available about potential risks?

Milk Sharing

Some mothers acquire donor milk for their babies through Internet-based milk sharing or community sharing of donor human milk (see Community Activity box). The U.S. Food and Drug Administration (FDA, 2010) issued a warning regarding this practice, recommending that potential users should consult a health care provider before obtaining milk from a source other than the baby's own mother. They warn individuals against feeding donor milk procured directly from individuals or through the Internet, citing safety risks including exposing the infant to infectious diseases or chemical contaminants in donor milk. Samples of milk purchased through the Internet have been shown to have high overall bacterial growth and contamination with pathogenic bacteria; this is likely related to improper techniques for collecting, storing, and shipping the milk (Keim, Hogan, McNamara, et al., 2013).

SAFETY ALERT

Nurses and lactation consultants should be aware of the safety concerns associated with Internet-based or community milk sharing. Parents who indicate an interest in obtaining donor human milk for their infant should be directed to one of the HMBANA milk banks and should be cautioned about the safety risks associated with feeding donor milk from an alternative source.

Care of the Mother

Nutrition. In general the breastfeeding mother should eat a healthy, well-balanced diet. Caloric intake during lactation should be sufficient to achieve the goal of balancing energy intake and expenditure. Most women are able to achieve that balance by adding 450 to 500 calories per day (AAP Section on Breastfeeding, 2012). Even with the increased caloric intake, women who are breastfeeding tend to lose weight more quickly than those who are formula feeding (Lawrence & Lawrence, 2011a).

Medications or diets that promote weight loss are not recommended for breastfeeding mothers. Rapid loss of large amounts of weight can be detrimental, given that fat-soluble contaminants to which the mother has been exposed are stored in body fat reserves and these can be released into the breast milk. Another potential consequence of weight loss is reduced milk production. For most women a weight loss of 1 to 2 kg (2.2 to 4.4 lb) per month is safe; however, if weight loss exceeds this amount, careful evaluation of infant weight and feeding pattern is recommended. The mother's diet is also evaluated.

No specific foods that the breastfeeding mother must consume or avoid have been identified. In most cases the woman can consume a normal diet, according to her personal preferences and cultural practices. Women may be told to continue taking their prenatal vitamins as long as they are breastfeeding.

It is recommended that breastfeeding mothers consume 200 to 300 mg of the omega-3 long-chain polyunsaturated fatty acids (docosahexaenoic acid [DHA]) daily. A DHA supplement and a multivitamin may be needed for women who are undernourished and those on vegan diets (AAP Section on Breastfeeding, 2012).

Mothers are encouraged to drink fluids in response to thirst (women often report feeling thirsty when they are breastfeeding). It can be helpful for the mother to know that if her urine appears light yellow (like lemonade), she is probably consuming adequate fluids. Excessive consumption of water or other fluids by the mother does not increase milk supply, and overhydration can actually decrease milk production.

Rest. The breastfeeding mother should rest as much as possible, especially in the first 1 or 2 weeks after birth. Fatigue, stress, and worry can negatively affect milk production and ejection (let-down). The nurse can encourage the mother to sleep when the baby sleeps. Breastfeeding in a side-lying position promotes rest for the mother. The father or partner, grandparents, other relatives, and friends can help with household chores and caring for other children.

Breast Care. The breastfeeding mother's normal routine bathing is all that is necessary to keep her breasts clean. Soap can have a drying effect on nipples; therefore, the mother should

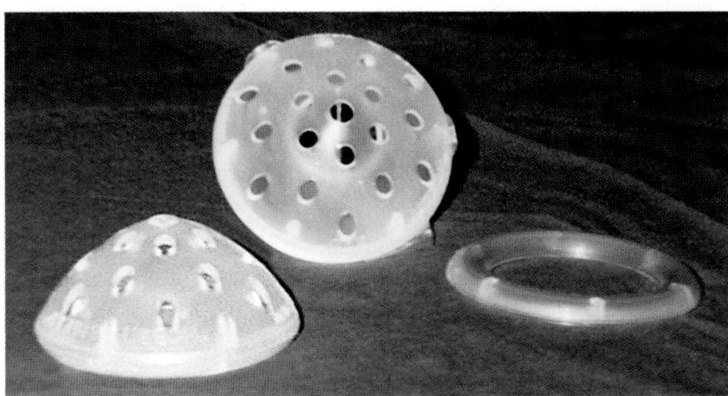

FIG 25-15 Breast shells.

avoid washing the nipples with soap. Breast creams should not be used routinely because they can block the natural oil secreted by the Montgomery glands on the areola.

The mother with flat or inverted nipples may benefit from wearing breast shells in her bra, although there is a lack of evidence to support the effectiveness of doing so. It is thought that these hard plastic devices exert mild pressure around the base of the nipple to encourage nipple eversion. Breast shells are also useful for sore nipples to keep the mother's bra or clothing from touching the nipples (Fig. 25-15).

If a mother needs breast support, she will likely be uncomfortable unless she wears a bra because otherwise the ligament that supports the breast (Cooper ligament) will stretch and be painful. Bras should fit well and provide nonbinding support. Underwire or improperly fitting bras can cause clogged milk ducts.

If milk leakage between feedings is a problem, mothers can wear breast pads (disposable or washable) inside the bra. Plastic-lined breast pads are not recommended because they trap moisture and can contribute to sore nipples. Pads should be changed when they are damp.

Breastfeeding and Contraception. Although breastfeeding confers a period of infertility, it is not considered an effective method of contraception unless the mother is strictly following guidelines for the lactational amenorrhea method of contraception (see Chapter 8). Breastfeeding delays the return of ovulation and menstruation; however, ovulation can occur before the first menstrual period after birth.

The contraceptives least likely to affect breastfeeding and milk production are the nonhormonal methods such as the lactational amenorrhea method, natural family planning, barrier methods (diaphragm/cap, spermicides, condoms), and intrauterine devices.

Hormonal contraceptives containing estrogen, including combined estrogen-progesterone pills or injectables, are not recommended for breastfeeding mothers because of the potential for reducing milk supply. Progestin-only contraceptives (pill, injection, or implant) are better options for breastfeeding mothers, although their use is not recommended during the first 6 weeks after birth (Lawrence & Lawrence, 2014) (see Chapter 8).

Breastfeeding During Pregnancy. Breastfeeding women who become pregnant can continue to breastfeed if there are no medical contraindications (e.g., risk of preterm labor). For pregnant women who are breastfeeding, adequate nutrition is especially important to promote normal fetal growth.

Nipple tenderness associated with early pregnancy can cause discomfort when breastfeeding the older child. The taste and composition of breast milk are altered during pregnancy, which can prompt some children to self-wean (Lawrence & Lawrence, 2011a).

When the baby is born, colostrum is produced. The practice of breastfeeding a newborn and an older child is called tandem nursing. The nurse should remind the mother always to feed the infant first to ensure that he or she is receiving adequate nutrition. The supply-meets-demand principle works in this situation, just as with breastfeeding multiples.

Breastfeeding After Breast Surgery. Previous breast surgery can affect the ability to produce breast milk and transfer it to the infant. Surgical procedures can damage nerves and interrupt milk ducts. Before undergoing breast surgery all women should discuss their lactation potential with their surgeon.

Women who have had augmentation mammoplasty (breast implants) may be able to breastfeed successfully. Many women have breast augmentation surgery purely for cosmetic reasons. However, if the procedure was done because of hypoplastic or asymmetric breasts or for breast reconstruction following cancer surgery, there can be concerns about adequate milk production. Submuscular implants are less likely to cause these problems; implants placed through periareolar incisions are more likely to result in breastfeeding problems. Large implants can impede milk flow by compressing milk ducts. Women who have had hyaluronic acid injections for breast enhancement can safely breastfeed (Smith & Heads, 2013).

Reduction mammoplasty causes problems with milk production and transfer because of interference with milk ducts, removal of glandular tissue, and nerve damage (Newton, 2012). Even so, many women are still able to breastfeed while also supplementing with infant formula or banked donor milk.

! NURSE ALERT

Women may not self-report breast augmentation or reduction mammoplasty. If surgical scars are present on the breast, the nurse should inquire about the type of surgery and the reason it was performed. Mothers with a history of breast surgery should be informed about the risk of interference with milk production and transfer. They are instructed to monitor their infants carefully for signs of adequate feeding.

It is possible for some women with a history of breast cancer to breastfeed. However, treatment for breast cancer (surgery, radiation, chemotherapy) can result in reduced milk supply or absence of lactation in the affected breast.

Breastfeeding and Obesity. Women who are overweight or obese are more likely to experience delayed onset of lactogenesis stage II and reduced milk production compared with women of average weight. There is some evidence that breastfeeding duration may be shorter among this population of mothers (Lepe, Bacardí Gascón, Castañeda-González, et al., 2011; Turcksin, Bel, Galjaard, & Devlieger, 2012; Wojcicki, 2011).

For women who have had bariatric surgery and plan to breastfeed, it is important to know when the surgery was performed. Nutrient and weight losses tend to stabilize approximately 12 to 18 months following the procedure. If the mother is consuming at least 1800 kcal/day and her weight has stabilized, her milk supply may be adequate. Breastfeeding mothers who have had a malabsorptive procedure such as a Roux-en-Y gastric bypass should take daily dietary supplements, including a prenatal vitamin, vitamin B_{12}, iron with vitamin C (to maximize absorption), and calcium (Lamb, 2011; La Leche League International, 2012). It is important to monitor infant weight gain. Vitamin B_{12} deficiency or decreased milk production can cause failure to thrive. In addition, vitamin B_{12} deficiency can result in infant anemia, developmental delays, and neurologic problems (Lamb, 2011).

Medications, Alcohol, Smoking, and Caffeine. Although much concern exists about the compatibility of drugs and breastfeeding, few drugs are absolutely contraindicated during lactation (Sachs & Committee on Drugs, 2013). Considerations in evaluating the safety of a specific medication during breastfeeding include the pharmacokinetics of the drug in the maternal system and the absorption, metabolism, distribution, storage, and excretion in the infant. The gestational and chronologic age of the infant, body weight, and breastfeeding pattern are also considered. In general, any medication that is given to an infant routinely is safe for a mother who is breastfeeding. The benefits of breastfeeding should be weighed against any risks of the medication to the infant (Sachs et al.).

MEDICATION ALERT

Breastfeeding mothers should be cautioned about taking any medications except those that are deemed essential. They are advised to check with their health care provider before taking any medication.

Information about the safety of medications and breastfeeding can be accessed through the Drugs and Lactation Database (LactMed), a website provided by National Library of Medicine: http://toxnet.nlm.nih.gov/cgi-bin/sis/htmlgen?LACT. The AAP recommends that providers consult this resource for the most current evidence-based information about specific medications for breastfeeding mothers (Sachs et al., 2013).

Breastfeeding should be discontinued temporarily when the mother undergoes imaging procedures that use radiopharmaceuticals. Mothers are advised to pump and discard milk for a period of time based on the properties of the specific radioactive agent (Sachs et al., 2013).

Drugs that are associated with adverse effects on the breastfeeding infant include antimetabolite and cytotoxic medications and drugs of abuse such as cocaine, heroin, amphetamines, and phencyclidine.

Women who have been stable on a methadone maintenance program should be allowed to breastfeed. Their infants may have decreased severity of neonatal abstinence symptoms when they are receiving breast milk (Lawrence & Lawrence, 2011a).

Pain in postpartum breastfeeding mothers is most safely managed with nonopioid analgesics such as ibuprofen. When opioid analgesia is used, breastfeeding infants are at risk of sedation and sucking difficulties. Parenteral doses of morphine or butorphanol are preferred over meperidine. Oral hydrocodone is often used; however, frequent administration and doses greater than 10 mg can result in neonatal sedation (Montgomery, Hale, & Academy of Breastfeeding Medicine, 2012). Oxycodone is considered less desirable because relatively high amounts are transferred to the nursing infant and can lead to central nervous system depression (Sachs et al., 2013).

As the use of antidepressant, antianxiety, and mood stabilizing medications rises among childbearing women, there are increasing concerns about the effects of these medications on breastfeeding infants. There is a lack of evidence about the long-term effects on infants and children. Medications that are not recommended while breastfeeding include citalopram, diazepam, escitalopram, fluoxetine, lithium, nortriptyline, sertraline, and venlafaxine because of the high levels excreted in breast milk and potential risks to the infant (Sachs et al., 2013) (see also Chapter 31).

Although there is no standard recommendation about avoiding alcohol use when breastfeeding, it is important for mothers to be aware of potential risks. The AAP Section on Breastfeeding (2012) recommends that alcohol intake by breastfeeding women should be minimal. Intake of alcohol should be limited to occasional consumption of less than 0.5 g/kg of body weight (e.g., 8 oz wine or 2 beers). Alcohol passes freely from the blood into breast milk, with peak levels occurring in 30 to 60 minutes on an empty stomach and 60 to 90 minutes when consumed with food. The MER and milk production can be adversely affected by maternal alcohol intake. If a breastfeeding mother chooses to have one or two drinks, she should not breastfeed for at least 2 hours. Contrary to popular belief, pumping and discarding milk do not accelerate removal of alcohol from the milk (Lawrence & Lawrence, 2011a). Some mothers use test strips for alcohol content of breast milk; however, there is a lack of evidence to support the accuracy or reliability of these strips.

Smoking by breastfeeding mothers should be strongly discouraged (AAP Section on Breastfeeding, 2012). It can impair milk production; it also exposes the infant to the risks of secondhand smoke. Nicotine is transferred to the infant in breast milk, whether the mother smokes or uses a nicotine patch, although the effect on the infant is uncertain. Lactating mothers who continue to smoke should be advised not to smoke within 2 hours before breastfeeding and never to smoke in the same room with the infant.

Moderate intake of caffeine by breastfeeding mothers appears to pose no risk to normal full-term infants. Minimal amounts of caffeine pass through to the infant in the breast milk. However, caffeine accumulates in infants, especially if they are preterm (Lawrence & Lawrence, 2011a).

Herbal Preparations. Herbs and herbal preparations such as teas are often recommended for breastfeeding women, especially when there is a need to increase milk supply. Although these herbal preparations may seem to be effective for some women, the recommendations are based on anecdotal information. There is a lack of evidence related to the prevalence, effectiveness, and safety of herbs during breastfeeding (Budzynska, Gardner, Dugoua, et al., 2012). Herbals are not regulated by the FDA because they are considered dietary supplements. Consequently there is a lack of quality control; unknown additives in and unknown side effects from herbal preparations can be harmful to the infant. Although some herbs may be considered safe, others contain pharmacologically active compounds that can have unfavorable effects. A thorough maternal history should include the use of any herbal remedies. Each remedy should then be evaluated for its compatibility with breastfeeding. LactMed provides information about the safety of herbal preparations and breastfeeding. Additionally, regional poison control centers can provide information on the active properties of herbs (Lawrence & Lawrence, 2011a; Sachs et al., 2013).

Common Concerns of the Breastfeeding Mother. The breastfeeding mother can experience some common problems. In most cases these complications are preventable if the mother receives appropriate education about breastfeeding. Early recognition and prompt resolution of these problems are important to prevent interruption of breastfeeding and to promote the mother's comfort and sense of well-being. Emotional support provided by the nurse or lactation consultant is essential to help allay the mother's frustration and anxiety and prevent early cessation of breastfeeding.

Engorgement. *Engorgement* is a common response of the breasts to the sudden change in hormones and the onset of significantly increased milk volume. It usually occurs 3 to 5 days after birth when the milk "comes in." As milk production rapidly increases, the volume can exceed the storage capacity of the alveoli in the breasts. If milk is not removed, the alveoli become distended, causing impairment of capillary blood flow surrounding the alveolar cells. As the blood vessels become more congested, fluid leaks into the surrounding tissue, resulting in edema. The milk ducts can be compressed by the tissue edema so milk cannot flow easily from the breasts. The breasts can become firm, tender, and hot and can appear shiny and taut. The areolae are firm, and the nipples can flatten, making it difficult for the infant to latch on to the breast (see Clinical Reasoning Case Study). Because back pressure on full milk glands inhibits milk production, if milk is not removed from the breasts, the milk supply can diminish.

CLINICAL REASONING CASE STUDY

Breastfeeding: Engorgement

The nurse on the mother/baby unit is caring for Johanna, a 37-year-old primipara who gave birth to a baby girl by emergency cesarean 3 days ago. During the morning assessment the nurse observes that Johanna's breasts are engorged. She sent the baby to the nursery during the night for feeding because she was exhausted. The engorgement seems to have happened overnight while Johanna was sleeping.

1. Evidence—Does the nurse have enough evidence at this time to draw conclusions about the engorgement and feeding issues facing this mother and infant?
2. Assumptions—What assumptions can be made about the following issues?
   a. The need to relieve the engorgement
   b. Johanna's understanding of milk production
   c. The infant's ability to feed effectively
   d. Johanna's commitment to breastfeeding
3. What implications and priorities for nursing care can be identified at this time?
4. Does the evidence objectively support your conclusion?

When engorgement occurs it is a temporary condition that is usually resolved within 24 hours. The mother is instructed to feed every 2 hours, softening at least one breast and pumping the other breast as needed to soften it. Pumping during engorgement does not cause a problematic increase in milk supply.

A variety of interventions are used to treat engorgement, although there is a lack of research evidence confirming the effectiveness of any specific intervention. Frequently used treatments for engorgement include the use of cold (ice packs, gel packs, cold compresses) after breastfeeding, chilled cabbage leaves, warmth (warm compresses, warm showers) before breastfeeding, antiinflammatory medications, breast massage, and pumping.

To reduce swelling of breast tissue surrounding the milk ducts, ice packs are often recommended in a 15- to 20-minutes-on, 45-minutes-off rotation between feedings. The ice packs should cover both breasts. Large bags of frozen peas make easy packs and can be refrozen between uses.

Fresh, raw cabbage leaves placed over the breasts between feedings can help relieve engorgement. It is thought that the effect of the cabbage leaves is related to the coolness of the leaves and phytoestrogens within them. They are washed, dried, chilled in the refrigerator or freezer, crushed slightly to break up the veins in the leaves, and then placed over the breasts for 15 to 20 minutes (Fig. 25-16). This treatment can be repeated for two or three sessions. Frequent application of cabbage leaves can decrease milk supply. Cabbage leaves should not be used if the mother is allergic to cabbage or develops a skin rash.

Antiinflammatory medications such as ibuprofen can help reduce the pain and swelling associated with engorgement. Ibuprofen also helps reduce fever and aching in the breasts that are often associated with engorgement.

Because heat increases blood flow, its application to an already congested breast is usually counterproductive. However, occasionally standing in a warm shower starts the milk leaking, or the mother may be able to manually express enough milk to soften the areola sufficiently to allow the baby to latch and breastfeed.

As a result of engorgement, excessive intravenous fluids during labor, or oxytocin for labor induction or augmentation, the nipple and areola can become distended, making it difficult for the newborn to latch successfully. A technique called *reverse pressure softening* manually displaces the areolar interstitial fluid

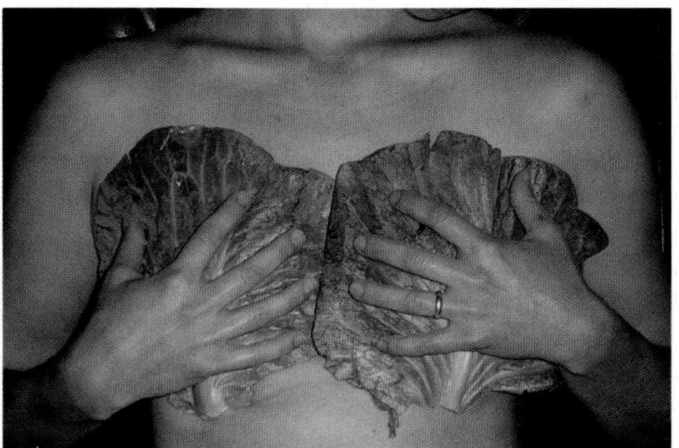

FIG 25-16 Cabbage leaves to treat engorgement. (Courtesy Kathryn Alden, Chapel Hill, NC.)

inward, softening the areola and making it easier for the infant's mouth to grasp the nipple and areola with latch (Lauwers & Swisher, 2011).

Sore Nipples. Mild nipple tenderness during the first few days of breastfeeding is common. Severe soreness or painful, abraded, cracked, or bleeding nipples are not normal and most often result from poor positioning, incorrect latch, improper suck, or infection. Severe nipple pain can be related to vasospasm or Raynaud's phenomenon (Lawrence & Lawrence, 2011a). The key to preventing sore nipples is correct breastfeeding technique. Limiting the time at the breast does not prevent sore nipples. They are often the result of the mother allowing the baby to latch on to the breast before the mouth is open wide.

For the first few days after birth the mother can experience some mild discomfort with the infant's initial sucks. This should quickly dissipate as the milk begins to flow and acts as a lubricant. To make the initial sucks less painful the mother can express a few drops of colostrum or milk to moisten the nipple and areola before latch. If the mother continues to experience nipple pain or discomfort after the first few sucks, the nurse or lactation consultant helps her evaluate the latch and baby's position at the breast. If the nipple pain continues, the mother needs to remove the baby from the breast, breaking suction with her finger in the baby's mouth (see Fig. 25-7). Repositioning the mother or infant can be helpful in resolving the nipple discomfort. The mother then proceeds to attempt latch again, making sure that the baby's mouth is open wide before latching him or her on to the breast (see Fig. 25-6).

The nurse or lactation consultant can assess the infant's suck by inserting a clean, gloved finger into the mouth and stimulating the infant to suck. If the tongue is not extruding over the lower gum and the mother reports pain or pinching with sucking, the baby may have *ankyloglossia*, which is a short or tight frenulum (commonly known as tongue-tie). In some instances this condition is corrected surgically to free the tongue for less painful, more effective breastfeeding (Lawrence & Lawrence, 2011a).

The treatment for sore nipples is first to identify the cause and then attempt to correct the problem. Early assessment and intervention are essential to increase the likelihood that the mother will continue to breastfeed. Once the problem is identified and corrected, sore nipples should heal within a few days, even though the baby continues to breastfeed regularly. When sore nipples occur, the woman is advised to start the feeding on the least sore nipple. It is important to assess the nipples for cracking or other damage to the skin integrity, which increases the risk of infection. If there is any break in the skin, the mother is advised to wipe the nipples with water after feeding to remove the baby's saliva. A thin coating of a topical antibiotic may help reduce the risk of infection and promote healing (the antibiotic cream or ointment should be removed before breastfeeding). Sore nipples should be open to air as much as possible. To promote comfort, breast shells may be worn inside the bra; these devices allow air to circulate while keeping clothing off sore nipples (see Fig. 25-15).

Rapid healing of sore nipples is critical to relieve the mother's discomfort, maintain breastfeeding, and prevent mastitis. Although numerous creams, ointments, gels, and gel pads have been used to treat sore nipples, there is a lack of conclusive evidence related to the effectiveness of any particular method. However, because they have not been shown to cause harm, many health care professionals recommend their use. Some women report increased comfort for sore nipples with the application of purified lanolin or hydrogel pads. If nipples are extremely sore or damaged and if the mother cannot tolerate breastfeeding, she may need to use an electric breast pump for 24 to 48 hours to allow the nipples to begin healing before resuming breastfeeding. She should use a pump that effectively empties the breasts (see Figs. 25-10 and 25-12).

The mother who has a sudden onset of sore nipples or experiences sore nipples after days or weeks of comfortable breastfeeding likely has some type of nipple infection, most often bacterial or fungal (candidiasis). Other possible causes are skin problems such as psoriasis, allergic reactions, or vasospasm. Careful assessment and referral for treatment are needed.

Insufficient Milk Supply. A major reason that women stop breastfeeding is perceived or actual insufficient milk supply (Brand, Kothari, & Stark, 2011; Lauwers & Swisher, 2011). Careful evaluation of the mother-infant dyad is needed, including assessment of infant weight gain or loss, feeding technique, and milk transfer and consideration of possible medical causes for low supply (e.g., medications, glandular insufficiency, previous breast surgery). Stress and fatigue can cause decreased milk production.

Interventions for increasing milk supply are based on causative factors. In many cases the mother is told to spend time with the baby skin to skin, increase feeding frequency, express milk using an electric pump, rest as much as possible, consume a healthy diet, and reduce stress. If nonpharmacologic measures to increase milk supply are not effective, galactogogues (medications or other substances that are believed to increase milk supply) may be recommended. Mothers often use herbal galactagogues such as fenugreek, blessed thistle, goat's rue, and shatavari to increase milk production. However, there is a lack of evidence to support the use of these substances (Sachs & Committee on Drugs, 2013).

Pharmaceutical galactogogues must be prescribed by the health care provider. Metoclopramide and domperidone are the most commonly prescribed medications; both are dopamine antagonists typically used to treat gastroesophageal reflux. It is thought that they increase prolactin levels, which enhances milk production. There is a lack of evidence to support the use of these medications in breastfeeding women (Sachs et al., 2013).

MEDICATION ALERT

Metoclopramide clearance in neonates is prolonged, which increases the risk of conditions resulting from overdose such as methemoglobinemia. Mothers are at risk for adverse reactions to metoclopramide including depression, suicidal ideation, and GI disturbances (Sachs et al., 2013).

Domperidone is often prescribed for lactating women in Canada and other countries (Flanders, Lowe, Kramer, et al., 2012), although it is not available in the United States except through some compounding pharmacies (ABM Protocol Committee, 2011b; Lauwers & Swisher, 2011). The FDA has issued a warning against the use of domperidone, stating that "the importation of this drug presents a public health risk and violates the Federal Food, Drug, and Cosmetic Act (the Act)" (FDA, 2012).

Plugged Milk Ducts. A milk duct can become plugged or clogged, causing an area of the breast to become swollen and tender. This area typically does not empty or soften with feeding or pumping. A small white pearl may be visible on the tip of the nipple; this pearl is the curd of milk blocking the flow. The mother is afebrile and has no generalized symptoms.

Plugged milk ducts are most often the result of inadequate removal of milk from the breast, which can be caused by clothing that is too tight, a poorly fitting or underwire bra, or always using the same position for feeding. Application of warm compresses to the affected area and to the nipple before feeding helps promote emptying of the breast and release of the plug.

Frequent feeding is recommended, with the baby beginning the feeding on the affected side to foster more complete emptying. The mother is advised to massage the affected area while the infant nurses or while she is pumping. Varying feeding positions and feeding without wearing a bra may be useful in resolving a plugged duct. Plugged milk ducts can increase susceptibility to breast infection. For recurrent plugged ducts, taking lecithin, a fat emulsifier, may be useful (Lawrence & Lawrence, 2011a).

Mastitis. Although the term mastitis means inflammation of the breast, it is most often used to refer to infection of the breast. It is characterized by the sudden onset of influenza-like symptoms, including fever, chills, body aches, and headache. The woman usually has localized breast pain and tenderness and a hot, reddened area on the breast. Mastitis most commonly occurs in the upper outer quadrant of the breast; one or both breasts can be affected. Most cases occur during the first 6 weeks of breastfeeding, although mastitis can occur at any time (Lawrence & Lawrence, 2011a).

Certain factors can predispose a woman to mastitis. Inadequate emptying of the breasts is common; this can be related to engorgement, plugged ducts, a sudden decrease in the number of feedings, abrupt weaning, or wearing underwire bras. Sore, cracked nipples can lead to mastitis by providing a portal of entry for causative organisms (*Staphylococcus, Streptococcus,* and *Escherichia coli* are most common). Stress, fatigue, maternal illness, ill family members, breast trauma, and poor maternal nutrition also are predisposing factors for mastitis (Lauwers & Swisher, 2011; Lawrence & Lawrence, 2011a). Breastfeeding mothers should be taught the signs of mastitis before they are discharged from the hospital after birth, and they need to know to call the health care provider promptly if the symptoms occur. Treatment includes antibiotics such as cephalexin or dicloxacillin for 10 to 14 days and analgesic and antipyretic medications such as ibuprofen. The mother is advised to rest as much as possible and breastfeed or pump frequently, striving to empty the affected side adequately. Warm compresses to the breast before feeding or pumping can be useful. Adequate fluid intake and a balanced diet are important for the mother with mastitis (Lauwers & Swisher, 2011).

Complications of mastitis include breast abscess, chronic mastitis, and fungal infections of the breast. Most complications can be prevented by early recognition and treatment (see Chapter 34).

Follow-Up After Discharge

Problems with sore nipples, engorgement, and jaundice are likely to occur after discharge from the birth institution. The nurse educates the mother about potential problems she may encounter once she is home. She should be given a list of resources for help with breastfeeding concerns. Community resources for breastfeeding mothers include lactation consultants in hospitals, primary care offices, or private practice; nurses in pediatric or obstetric offices; support groups such as La Leche League; and peer counseling programs (e.g., those offered through WIC). The Internet has many websites containing current and correct information about breastfeeding (e.g., www.breastfeeding.com). The National Breastfeeding Helpline (1-800-994-9662) through the Office of Women's Health provides breastfeeding information and counseling by English- and Spanish-speaking counselors.

Telephone follow-up by nurses or lactation consultants in hospitals, birth centers, clinics, or offices within the first day or two after discharge can help identify problems and offer needed advice and support. Breastfeeding infants should be seen by a health care provider at 3 to 5 days of age and again at 2 to 3 weeks to assess weight gain and offer encouragement and support to the mother (AAP Section on Breastfeeding, 2012).

FORMULA FEEDING

Parent Education

The majority of infants receives at least some amount of commercial infant formula during their first year of life. Some parents choose formula feeding instead of breastfeeding; others combine the two methods. If the infant is weaned from breastfeeding before the first birthday, iron-fortified infant formula should be given (AAP Section on Breastfeeding, 2012).

It is important for nurses and other health care professionals to be intentional about providing education for parents related to formula preparation, feeding, and common problems they can encounter. Because of the lack of clear information about the practical aspects of formula feeding, parents often rely on advice from friends and family. If that advice is incorrect and the parents use unsafe practices for formula preparation and feeding, the infant is at risk for foodborne illness and burns (see Teaching for Self-Management box: Formula Preparation and Feeding).

Readiness for Feeding

Ideally the first feeding of formula is given after the neonate's initial transition to extrauterine life. Feeding-readiness cues include stability of vital signs, effective breathing pattern, presence of bowel sounds, an active sucking reflex, and signs described earlier for breastfed infants.

Feeding Patterns

In the first 24 to 48 hours of life a newborn typically consumes 15 to 30 ml of formula at a feeding. Intake gradually increases during the first week of life. Most newborns are drinking 90 to 150 ml at a feeding by the end of the second week or sooner. The newborn infant should be fed at least every 3 to 4 hours, even if it is necessary to wake him or her for the feedings; however, rigid feeding schedules are not recommended. The infant showing an adequate weight gain can be allowed to sleep at night and be fed only on awakening. Most newborns need six to eight feedings in

24 hours; the number of feedings decreases as the infant matures and consumes more at each feeding. By 3 to 4 weeks after birth a fairly predictable feeding pattern has usually developed. Scheduling feedings arbitrarily at predetermined intervals may not meet a newborn's needs, but initiating feedings at convenient times often moves the feedings to times that work for the family.

Mothers usually notice increases in the infant's appetite at the age of approximately 10 days, 3 weeks, 6 weeks, 3 months, and 6 months. These appetite spurts correspond to growth spurts. Mothers should increase the amount of formula per feeding by approximately 30 ml to meet the baby's needs at these times.

Feeding Technique

Infants should be held for all feedings. During feedings parents are encouraged to sit comfortably, holding the infant close in a semi-upright position with good head support. Feedings provide opportunities to bond with the baby through touching, talking, singing, or reading to the infant. Parents should consider feedings a time of peaceful relaxation with the infant. Mothers who bottle feed should be encouraged to spend some time with their newborns in skin-to-skin contact.

> **SAFETY ALERT**
>
> A bottle should never be propped with a pillow or other inanimate object and left with the infant. This practice can result in choking, and it deprives the infant of important interaction during feeding. Moreover, propping the bottle has been implicated in causing nursing-bottle caries or decay of the first teeth resulting from continuous bathing of the teeth with carbohydrate-containing fluid as the infant sporadically sucks the nipple.

Newborns must learn to coordinate sucking, swallowing, and breathing as they feed. The typical fast flow of milk from bottles can create difficulty for an infant trying to learn to feed. A slow-flow nipple is often used for the first few weeks.

Traditionally parents are told to position the infant in a semi-reclining position and to hold the bottle so that fluid fills the nipple and none of the air in the bottle is allowed to enter it (Fig. 25-17, *A*). A more physiologic approach to bottle feeding is called *paced bottle feeding*. With this method of feeding the bottle is held at more of a horizontal angle; when the baby pauses between bursts of sucking, the parent withdraws the nipple, allowing it to rest on the baby's lip until he or she is ready to resume sucking (Lauwers & Swisher, 2011). This position slows the flow of milk from the bottle so the infant is more in control. Paced bottle feeding works well for infants who are primarily breastfeeding but are occasionally fed from a bottle.

If the infant falls asleep or ceases to suck, it usually indicates that he or she has consumed enough formula to feel satiated. Teach parents to look for these cues and avoid overfeeding, which can contribute to obesity.

Instruct parents to observe the infant for signs of stress during feeding, including turning the head, arching the back, choking, sputtering, changing color, moving the arms, and tensing fists (Lauwers & Swisher, 2011). When these signs occur, the parent should stop feeding and attempt to calm the infant before resuming. The signs can indicate that the infant is finished with the feeding and does not want to drink any more.

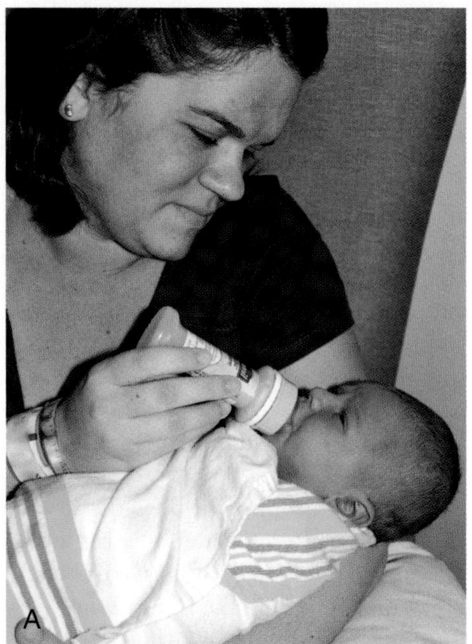

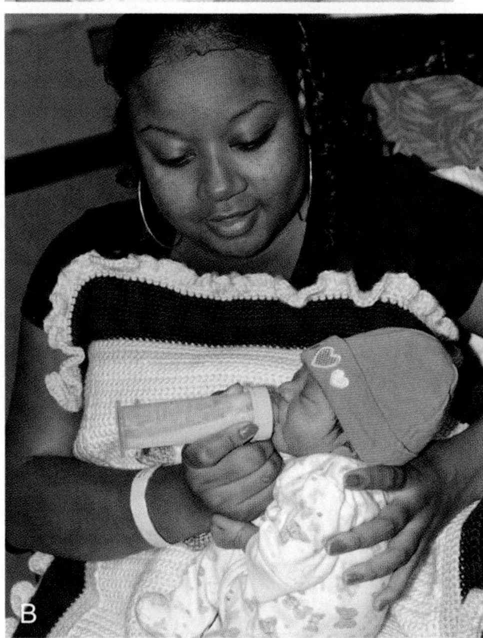

FIG 25-17 **A,** Bottle feeding: traditional technique with infant semi-reclining **B,** Paced bottle feeding: infant is more upright. (Courtesy Cheryl Briggs, RNC, Annapolis, MD.)

Most infants swallow air when fed from a bottle and need a chance to burp several times during a feeding. Parents are taught various positions that can be used for burping (Fig. 25-18).

Common Concerns

Parents need to know what to do if the infant spits up. They may need to decrease the amount of feeding or feed smaller amounts more frequently. Burping the infant several times during a feeding such as when the infant's sucking slows down or stops can decrease spitting. Holding the baby upright for 30 minutes after feeding and avoiding bouncing or placing him or her on the abdomen soon after the feeding is finished also can help. Spitting can be a result of overfeeding, or it can be symptomatic of gastroesophageal reflux. Parents should report vomiting one third or more of the feeding at most feeding sessions or projectile vomiting to the health care

TEACHING FOR SELF-MANAGEMENT

Formula Preparation and Feeding

Formula Preparation

- Using warm soapy water, wash your hands, arms, and under your nails; rinse well. Clean and sanitize the surface where you will be preparing the bottles.
- Thoroughly wash bottles, nipples, rings, caps, can opener, and other preparation utensils in hot soapy water and rinse thoroughly. Squeeze water through nipples to make sure that the holes are open.
- Place bottles, nipples, rings, and caps in a pot and cover with water; boil for 5 minutes; remove items from pot with sanitized tongs and allow them to air dry. (Do this before using items the first time; thereafter you can continue to do this or place items in the dishwasher.)
- Note the expiration date on the formula container. It should be used before the expiration date. Any unopened expired formula should be returned to the place of purchase.
- Read the label on the container of formula and mix it exactly according to the directions.
- Mix formula with tap water deemed safe by the local health department. Allow cold water to run for 2 minutes before collecting it. Then bring it to a rolling boil and continue boiling for 1 to 2 minutes. If using bottled water, make sure that it is labeled as "sterile"; unsterile bottled water must be boiled. After boiling allow water to cool before mixing the formula but not for longer than 30 minutes.
- If using a can of ready-to-feed or concentrated formula, wash the top of the can with hot soapy water and rinse well. Shake the can before opening.
- Mixing formula
    - Ready-to-feed: No mixing is needed; do not add water. Pour desired amount of formula into clean bottle; add nipple and ring.
    - Concentrate: Pour desired amount of formula into clean bottle and add equal amount of cooled boiled water. Add nipple and ring and shake well.
    - Powder: When first opening the container of powder, write the date on the lid. Using the scoop from the container, add 1 scoop of powdered formula for each 2 ounces of boiled, cooled water in a clean bottle. For example, if 6 ounces of water is in the bottle, add three scoops of powder. Add nipple and ring and shake well.
- If preparing multiple bottles at the same time, place nipple right side up on each bottle and cover with a clean nipple cap. Use bottles within 48 hours.
- Opened cans of ready-to-feed or concentrated formula should be covered and refrigerated. Any unused portions must be discarded after 48 hours.
- Bottles or cans of unopened formula can be stored at room temperature.
- If the formula is refrigerated, warm it by placing the bottle in a pan of hot water. Never use a microwave to warm any food to be given to a baby. Test the temperature of the formula by letting a few drops fall on the inside of your wrist. If the formula feels comfortably warm to you, the temperature is correct.

Feeding Techniques and Tips

- Newborns should be fed at least every 3 to 4 hours and should never go longer than 4 hours without feeding until a satisfactory pattern of weight gain is established. This period can be as long as 2 weeks. If a baby cries or fusses between feedings, check to see if the diaper should be changed and if the baby needs to be picked up and cuddled. If the baby continues to cry and acts hungry, feed him or her. Babies do not get hungry on a regular schedule.
- Infants gradually increase the amount of milk they drink with each feeding. The first day or so most newborns consume 15 to 30 ml (0.5 to 1 ounce) with each feeding. This amount increases as the infant grows. If any formula remains in the bottle as the feeding ends, it must be thrown away because saliva from the baby's mouth can cause the formula to spoil.
- Keep a feeding diary, writing down the amount of formula the infant drinks with each feeding for the first week or so. Also record the number of the baby's wet diapers and bowel movements. Take this diary with you to the baby's first follow-up visit with the primary health care provider.
- For feeding hold the infant close in a semi-reclining position. Talk to him or her during the feeding. This time is ideal for social interaction and cuddling.
- Place the nipple in the infant's mouth on the tongue. It should touch the roof of the mouth to stimulate the baby's sucking reflex. Hold the bottle like a pencil. Keep it tipped so the nipple stays filled with milk and the baby does not suck in air.
- Taking a few sucks and then pausing briefly before continuing to suck again is normal for infants. Some infants take longer to feed than others. Be patient. Keep the baby awake; encouraging sucking may be necessary. Moving the nipple gently in the infant's mouth may stimulate sucking.
- Another technique that can be used for bottle feeding is *paced bottle feeding.* The infant is placed in a more upright position, and the bottle is held at a more horizontal angle. When the baby pauses between bursts of sucking, withdraw the nipple and allow it to rest on the baby's lip until he or she is ready to resume sucking. This slows the flow of milk from the bottle so the infant is more in control. Paced bottle feeding works well for infants who are primarily breastfeeding but are occasionally fed from a bottle.
- Newborns are apt to swallow air when sucking. Give the infant opportunities to burp several times during a feeding. As he or she gets older, you will know better when to stop for burping.
- After the first 2 or 3 days the stools of a formula-fed infant are yellow and soft but formed. The infant may have a stool with each feeding in the first 2 weeks, although this amount can decrease to one or two stools each day. It is not abnormal for formula-fed infants to have a stool every other day.

Safety Tips

- Infants should be held and never left alone while feeding. Never prop the bottle. The infant might inhale formula or choke on any that was spit up. Infants who fall asleep with a propped bottle of milk or juice can be prone to cavities when the first teeth come in.
- Know how to use the bulb syringe and help an infant who is choking.

Data from World Health Organization & Food and Agriculture Organization of the United Nations. (2007). *Safe preparation, storage, and handling of powdered infant formula: Guidelines.* Geneva: World Health Organization. U.S. Department of Agriculture. (2008). *Infant nutrition and feeding.* Washington, DC; USDA.

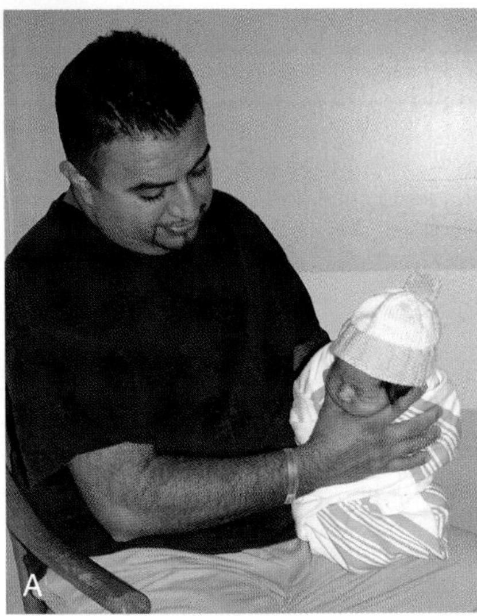

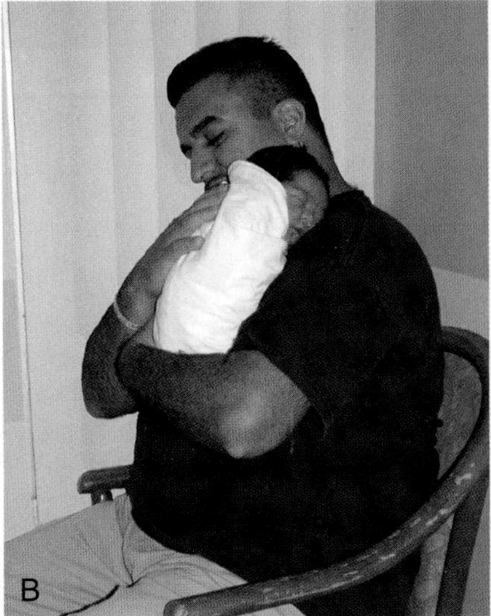

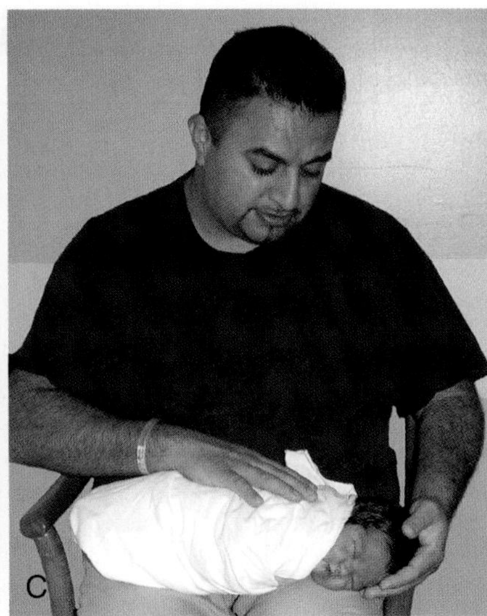

FIG 25-18 Positions for burping an infant. **A,** Sitting. **B,** On shoulder. **C,** Across lap. (Courtesy Julie Perry Nelson, Loveland, CO.)

provider and should be cautioned to refrain from changing the infant's formula without consulting the health care provider.

Bottles and Nipples

Various brands and styles of bottles and nipples are available. Most babies feed well with any bottle and nipple. The bottles, nipples, rings, and caps should be washed in warm soapy water, using a bottle and nipple brush to facilitate thorough cleansing. They should be placed in boiling water for 5 minutes and allowed to air dry; this should be done at least before the first use and thereafter unless they are cleaned in a dishwasher (see Teaching for Self-Management box: Formula Preparation and Feeding). Boiling of feeding equipment is recommended if the infant has oral thrush.

Infant Formulas

Commercial Formulas

Commercial infant formulas are designed to resemble human milk as closely as possible, although none has ever duplicated it. The exact composition of infant formula varies with the manufacturer, but all must meet specific standards.

Infants who are not breastfed should be given commercial iron-fortified formulas. Families with limited income may be eligible for services through the WIC program, which provides iron-fortified infant formula.

The most widely used commercially prepared formulas are cow's milk–based formulas that have been modified to closely resemble the nutritional content of human milk. The caloric content of standard infant formula is 20 kcal/oz. These formulas are altered from cow's milk by removing butterfat, decreasing the protein content, and adding vegetable oil and carbohydrate. Regardless of the commercial brand, the standard cow's milk–based formulas have essentially the same compositions of vitamins, minerals, protein, carbohydrates, and essential amino acids, with minor variations such as the source of carbohydrate; nucleotides to enhance immune function; and long-chain polyunsaturated fatty acids (DHA and ARA), which are thought to improve visual and cognitive function. Furthermore, the FDA regulates the manufacture of infant formula in the United States to ensure product safety. Standard cow's milk-based formulas are sold as low-iron and iron-fortified formulas; however, only the iron-fortified formulas meet infants' requirements.

Four main categories of commercially prepared infant formulas are available: (1) cow's milk-based formulas; (2) soy-based formulas, commonly used for children who are lactose or cow's milk-protein intolerant; (3) casein- or whey-hydrolysate formulas, used primarily for children who cannot tolerate or digest cow's milk- or soy-based formulas; and (4) amino acid formulas, used for infants with multiple food protein intolerances.

The AAP Committee on Nutrition indicates that few solid indications exist for the use of soy protein-based formulas instead of cow's milk-based formulas (Bhatia, Greer, & AAP Committee on Nutrition, 2008). Soy-based formulas are recommended for infants with galactosemia and congenital lactase deficiency; infants with secondary lactase deficiency may benefit as well. Infants with documented IgE allergies caused by cow's milk should be fed an extensively hydrolyzed protein formula. Soy protein-based formulas have not been proven to be effective against colic or in the prevention of allergy in healthy or high-risk infants.

Alternate milk sources such as goat's milk; skim or low-fat milk; condensed milk; or raw, unpasteurized milk from any animal source should not be fed to infants because they are inadequate to support growth and can contain excess protein or an inadequate calcium-to-phosphorus ratio, which can cause seizures.

SAFETY ALERT

Because of concerns about potential harmful effects of bisphenol A (BPA), parents should be cautioned about using hard plastic polycarbonate baby bottles or containers. BPA is a chemical that is used to harden plastics, prevent bacterial contamination of foods, and prevent can rusting. It is in many food and liquid containers, including baby bottles. The AAP (2012) recommends avoiding clear plastic bottles or containers imprinted with the recycling number 7 and the letters PC and purchasing bottles that are certified or identified as BPA-free. Glass bottles are an alternative, but parents must be aware of the risk for injury if the bottle is dropped or broken. Because heat can cause the release of BPA from plastic, polycarbonate bottles should never be boiled, heated in the microwave, or washed in a dishwasher (AAP, 2012).

Formula Preparation

Commercial formulas are available in three forms: powder, concentrate, and ready to feed. All forms are equivalent in terms of nutritional content, but they vary considerably in cost.

- Ready-to-feed formula is the most expensive but the easiest to use. The desired amount is poured into the bottle. The opened can is refrigerated safely for 48 hours. This type of formula can be purchased in individual disposable bottles for the most convenient feeding.
- Concentrated formula is less expensive than ready to feed. It is diluted with equal parts of water and can be stored in the refrigerator for 48 hours after opening.
- Powdered formula is the least expensive. It is easily mixed by using one scoop for every 60 ml of water.

The commercial infant formula must include label directions for preparation and use of the formula with pictures and symbols for the benefit of individuals who cannot read. Some manufacturers translate the directions into languages such as Spanish, French, Vietnamese, Chinese, and Arabic to prevent misunderstanding and errors in formula preparation.

SAFETY ALERT

An important aspect to impress on families is that the proportions must not be altered (i.e., neither diluted to extend the amount of formula nor concentrated to provide more calories). The newborn's kidneys are immature; giving the infant overly concentrated formula can provide protein and minerals in amounts that exceed the excretory ability of the kidneys. In contrast, if the formula is diluted too much (sometimes done to save money), the infant does not consume sufficient calories to grow appropriately.

The water used to mix either powdered or concentrated liquid formula need not contain any fluoride, especially in the first 6 months of life. Excess fluoride can permanently stain the teeth once they appear.

Sterilization of formula rarely is recommended when families have access to a safe public water supply. Instead formula is prepared with attention to cleanliness. When water from a private well is used, parents should be advised to contact the health department to have a chemical and bacteriologic analysis of the water performed before using the water in formula preparation. The presence of nitrates, excess fluoride, or bacteria can be harmful to the infant.

It is usually safe to mix infant formula with cold tap water that has been boiled for 1 to 2 minutes and allowed to cool. Bottled water that is labeled as "sterile" is safe for mixing formula. However, nonsterile bottled water should be boiled for 1 to 2 minutes and cooled.

If the conditions in the home appear unsanitary, the nurse should recommend the use of ready-to-feed formula or teach the mother to sterilize the formula. The two traditional methods for sterilization are terminal heating and the aseptic method. In the terminal heating method the prepared formula is placed in the bottles, which are topped with the nipples placed upside down and covered with the caps and sealed loosely with the rings. The bottles are then boiled together in a water bath for 25 minutes. In the aseptic method the bottles, rings, caps, nipples, and any other necessary equipment such as a funnel are boiled separately, after which the formula is poured into the bottles. Instructions for formula preparation and feeding are provided in the Teaching for Self-Management box: Formula Preparation and Feeding.

Vitamin and Mineral Supplementation

Commercial iron-fortified formula has all of the nutrients that infants need for the first 6 months of life. After 6 months fluoride supplementation is recommended based on levels in the water supply.

Weaning

The bottle-fed infant gradually learns to use a cup, and the parents find that they are preparing fewer bottles. The bottle feeding before bedtime is often the last one to remain. Babies have a strong need to suck, and the baby who has the bottle taken away too early or abruptly compensates with nonnutritive sucking on his or her fingers, thumb, a pacifier, or even the tongue. Therefore, weaning from a bottle should be attempted gradually because the baby has learned to rely on the comfort that sucking provides.

Complementary Feeding: Introducing Solid Foods

Complementary feedings are defined as foods or liquids given to the infant in addition to breast milk or formula. The AAP Committee on Nutrition (2009) recommends introducing solid foods after 4 months of age and preferably after 6 months of age. The AAP Section on Breastfeeding (2012) recommends waiting until 6 months. Traditionally the recommended first foods were single-grain cereals, followed by vegetables and fruits. However, there is a lack of evidence to support any particular order as having advantages for infants. Breastfeeding infants in particular can benefit from a source of iron such as iron-fortified cereal or meat. New foods should be introduced slowly to assess for any allergic reaction or intolerance. It is best to offer no more than three new foods per week. Fruits and vegetables should be offered to infants daily starting at 6 to 8 months. Fruit juices are not recommended before 6 months of age because it is possible that the infant who drinks juice will consume less breast milk or formula. Consumption of low-nutrient foods such as fatty or sugary foods or restaurant foods should be limited.

In spite of the recommendations from the AAP, many parents begin complementary feedings earlier than 4 months. They need to be informed that the infant receives the right balance of nutrients from breast milk or formula during the first 4 to 6 months. The notion that the feeding of solids helps the infant sleep through the night is not true. Parents should not put cereal into the infant's bottle. Introduction of solid foods before the infant is 4 to 6 months of age can result in overfeeding and decreased intake of breast milk or formula.

Cultural beliefs and traditions affect complementary feeding practices. First foods given to infants vary widely. For example, first foods for Egyptian infants include bread soaked in milk and tea or yogurt sweetened with honey. Chinese and Vietnamese infants are sometimes fed prechewed rice paste, rice, or sweetened porridge.

Nurses and other health care professionals educate parents regarding complementary feedings. This most often occurs during well-baby supervision visits with the pediatric health care provider. Early feeding practices have implications for long-term dietary patterns; therefore, it is essential to teach parents about proper nutrition.

KEY POINTS

- Human breast milk is species-specific and is the recommended form of infant nutrition. It provides immunologic protection against many infections and diseases.
- Breast milk changes in composition with each stage of lactogenesis, during each feeding, and as the infant grows.
- During the prenatal period expectant parents should be informed of the benefits of breastfeeding for infants, mothers, families, and society.
- Infants should be breastfed within the first hour after birth and at least 8 to 12 times every 24 hours thereafter.
- Parents should be taught to recognize the signs of effective breastfeeding.
- Breast milk production is based on a supply-meets-demand principle: the more the infant nurses, the greater the milk supply.
- Infants go through predictable growth spurts.
- Sore nipples are most often caused by incorrect latch.
- Commercial infant formulas provide satisfactory nutrition for most infants.
- Infants should be held for feedings.
- Parents should be instructed about the types of infant formulas, proper preparation for feeding, and correct feeding technique.
- Solid (complementary) foods should be introduced at about 6 months of age.
- Unmodified cow's milk is inappropriate for infants less than 1 year of age.
- Nurses must be knowledgeable about feeding methods and provide education and support for families.

REFERENCES

Academy of Breastfeeding Medicine (ABM) Board of Directors. (2008). Position on breastfeeding. *Breastfeeding Medicine*, *3*(4), 267–270.

Academy of Breastfeeding Medicine (ABM) Protocol Committee. (2009). ABM clinical protocol #3: Hospital guidelines for the use of supplementary feedings in the healthy term breastfed infant. *Breastfeeding Medicine*, *4*(3), 175–182.

Academy of Breastfeeding Medicine (ABM) Protocol Committee. (2010). ABM clinical protocol #8: Human milk storage information for home use for full-term infants. *Breastfeeding Medicine*, *5*(3), 127–130.

Academy of Breastfeeding Medicine (ABM) Protocol Committee. (2011a). ABM clinical protocol #10: Breastfeeding the late preterm infant. *Breastfeeding Medicine*, *5*(3), 127–130.

Academy of Breastfeeding Medicine (ABM) Protocol Committee. (2011b). ABM clinical protocol #9: Use of galactogogues in initiating or augmenting the rate of maternal milk secretion. *Breastfeeding Medicine*, *6*(1), 41–49.

Ahluwalia, I. B., D'Angelo, D., Morrow, B., & McDonald, J. A. (2012). Association between acculturation and breastfeeding among Hispanic women: Data from the Pregnancy Risk Assessment and Monitoring System. *Journal of Human Lactation*, *28*(2), 167–173.

Allen, J. A., Li, R., Scanlon, K. S., et al. (2013). Progress in increasing breastfeeding and reducing racial/ethnic differences—United States, 2000-2008. *MMWR Morbidity and Mortality Weekly Report*, *62*(5), 77–80.

American Academy of Family Physicians (AAFP). (2012). *Breastfeeding policy statement*. Available at www.aafp.org/online/en/home/policy/policies/b/breastfeedingpolicy.html.

American Academy of Pediatrics (AAP). (2012). *Ages and stages: Baby bottles and bisphenol A (BPA)* Available at www.healthychildren.org/English/ages-stages/baby/feeding-nutrition/pages/Baby-Bottles-And-Bisphenol-A-BPA.

American Academy of Pediatrics (AAP) Committee on Nutrition. (2009). *Pediatric nutrition handbook* (6th ed.). Elk Grove Village, IL: AAP.

American Academy of Pediatrics (AAP) Section on Breastfeeding. (2012). Breastfeeding and the use of human milk—policy statement. *Pediatrics*, *129*(3), e827–e841.

American College of Obstetricians and Gynecologists (ACOG) Committee on Health Care for Underserved Women and Committee on Obstetric Practice. (2007). Breastfeeding: Maternal and infant aspects. *ACOG Clinical Review*, *12*(1), 1S–16S.

American Dietetic Association (ADA). (2009). Position of the American Dietetic Association: Promoting and supporting breastfeeding. *Journal of the American Dietetic Association*, *109*(11), 1926–1942.

Association of Women's Health, Obstetric and Neonatal Nurses (AWHONN). (2007). *Breastfeeding and the role of the nurse in the promotion of breastfeeding*. Washington, DC: AWHONN.

Augustin, A. L., Donovan, K., Lozano, E. A., et al. (2013). Still nursing at 6 months: A survey of breastfeeding mothers. *MCN: The American Journal of Maternal/Child Nursing*, *39*(1), 50–55.

Baby-Friendly, U.S.A., & BFUSA (2013). *Baby-Friendly hospitals and birth centers*. Available at www.babyfriendlyusa.org/eng/03.html.

Baker, R. D., Greer, F. R., & American Academy of Pediatrics (AAP) Committee on Nutrition. (2010). Clinical report: Diagnosis and prevention of iron-deficiency and iron-deficiency anemia in infants and young children (0-3 years of age). *Pediatrics*, *126*(5), 1–11.

Bartick, M., & Reinhold, A. (2010). The burden of suboptimal breastfeeding in the United States: A pediatric cost analysis. *Pediatrics*, *125*(5), e1048–e1056.

Bartick, M., & Reyes, C. (2012). Las dos cosas: An analysis of attitudes of Latina women on non-exclusive breastfeeding. *Breastfeeding Medicine*, *7*(1), 19–24.

Bhatia, J., Greer, F., & American Academy of Pediatrics (AAP) Committee on Nutrition. (2008). Use of soy protein-based formulas in infant feeding. *Pediatrics*, *121*(5), 1062–1068.

Blackburn, S. T. (2013). *Maternal, fetal, and neonatal physiology* (4th ed.). St. Louis: Mosby.

Brand, E., Kothari, C., & Stark, M. A. (2011). Factors related to breastfeeding discontinuation between hospital discharge and 2 weeks' postpartum. *Journal of Perinatal Education*, *20*(1), 36–44.

Breastfeeding Committee for Canada. (2014). *Baby-Friendly initiative in Canada: Status report*. Available at http://breastfeedingcanada.ca/documents/BFI%20Status%20Report%202014%20with%20WHO%20Country%20report.pdf.

Budzynska, K., Gardner, Z. E., Dugoua, J., et al. (2012). Systematic review of breastfeeding and herbs. *Breastfeeding Medicine*, *7*(6), 489–503.

Centers for Disease Control and Prevention (CDC). (2014). *Breastfeeding report card—United States*. Available at www.cdc.gov/breastfeeding/pdf/2014BreastfeedingReportCard.pdf.

Chantry, C. J. (2011). Supporting the 75%: Overcoming barriers after breastfeeding initiation. *Breastfeeding Medicine*, *6*(5), 337–339.

Chapman, D. J., & Perez-Escamilla, R. (2012). Breastfeeding among minority women: Moving from risk factors to interventions. *Advances in Nutrition*, *3*(1), 95–104.

Colson, S. (2010). What happens to breastfeeding when mothers lie back? *Clinical Lactation*, *1*(1), 11–14.

Colson, S. (2012). The laid-back breastfeeding revolution. *Midwifery Today*, *101*, 9–11 and 66.

Cooper, B. M., Holditch-Davis, D., Verklan, M. T., et al. (2012). Newborn clinical outcomes of the AWHONN late preterm infant research-based practice project. *Journal of Obstetric, Gynecologic and Neonatal Nursing*, *41*(6), 774–785.

Dell, K. M. (2011). Fluid, electrolytes, and acid-base homeostasis. In R. J. Martin, A. A. Fanaroff, & M. C. Walsh (Eds.), *Fanaroff and Martin's neonatal-perinatal medicine: Diseases of the fetus and infant* (9th ed.). St. Louis: Mosby.

Flaherman, V. J., Gay, B., Scott, C., et al. (2012). Randomised control trial comparing hand expression with breast pumping for mothers of term newborns feeding poorly. *Archives of Diseases of Children. Fetal and Neonatal Edition, 97*(1), F18–F23.

Flanders, D., Lowe, A., Kramer, M., et al. (2012). *A consensus statement on the use of domperidone to support lactation.* Canadian Lactation Consultant Association. Available at www.ilca.org/i4a/pages/index.cfm?pageid=3520.

Holmes, A. V., Auinger, P., & Howard, C. R. (2011). Combination feeding of breast milk and formula: Evidence for shorter breast-feeding duration from the National Health and Nutrition Examination Survey. *Journal of Pediatrics, 159*(2), 186–191.

Holmes, A. V., McLeod, A. Y., & Bunik, M. (2013). ABM clinical protocol #5: Peripartum breastfeeding management for the healthy mother and infant at term, revision 2013. *Breastfeeding Medicine, 8*(6), 469–473.

Human Milk Banking Association of North America (HMBANA). (2013). *Guidelines for the establishment and operation of a donor human milk bank.* Ft. Worth, TX: HMBANA.

Institute of Medicine. (2005). *Dietary reference intakes for energy, carbohydrate, fiber, fatty acids, cholesterol, protein, and amino acids.* Washington, DC: National Academies Press.

Jensen, E. (2012). Participation in the Supplemental Nutrition Program for Women, Infants, and Children (WIC) and breastfeeding: National, regional, and state level analyses. *Maternal and Child Health Journal, 16*(3), 624–631.

Jenson, D., Wallace, S., & Kelsay, P. (1994). LATCH: A breastfeeding charting system and documentation tool. *Journal of Obstetric, Gynecologic and Neonatal Nursing, 23*(1), 27–32.

Johnson, B., Thorn, B., McGill, B., et al. (2013). *WIC participant and program characteristics 2012.* Alexandria, VA: U.S. Department of Agriculture, Food and Nutrition Service.

Keim, S. A., Hogan, J. S., McNamara, K. A., et al. (2013). Microbial contamination of human milk purchased via the internet. *Pediatrics, 132*(5), e1227–e1235.

Labiner-Wolfe, J., & Fein, S. B. (2013). How US mothers store and handle their expressed breast milk. *Journal of Human Lactation, 29*(1), 54–58.

La Leche League International. (2012). Bariatric surgery and lactation. In *The Breastfeeding Answer Book* Update.

Lamb, M. (2011). Weight-loss surgery and breastfeeding. *Clinical Lactation, 2*(2-3), 17–21.

Landers, S. L., & Hartmann, B. T. (2012). Donor human milk banking and the emergence of milk sharing. *Pediatric Clinics of North America, 60*(1), 247–260.

Lanese, M. G., & Cross, M. (2013). Breastfeeding a preterm infant. In R. Mannel, P. J. Martens, & M. Walker (Eds.), *Core curriculum for lactation consultant practice* (3rd ed.). Burlington, MA: Jones and Bartlett.

Lauwers, J., & Swisher, A. (2011). *Counseling the nursing mother: A lactation consultant's guide* (5th ed.). Sudbury, MA: Jones and Bartlett.

Lawrence, R. M., & Lawrence, R. A. (2011a). *Breastfeeding: A guide for the medical profession* (7th ed.). St. Louis: Mosby.

Lawrence, R. M., & Lawrence, R. A. (2011b). Breastfeeding: More than just good nutrition. *Pediatrics in Review, 32*(7), 267–280.

Lawrence, R. M., & Lawrence, R. A. (2014). The breast and the physiology of lactation. In R. K. Creasy, R. Resnik, J. D. Iams, et al. (Eds.), *Creasy & Resnik's maternal-fetal medicine* (7th ed.). Philadelphia: Elsevier Saunders.

Lepe, M., Bacardí Gascón, M., Castañeda-González, et al. (2011). Effect of maternal obesity on lactation: Systematic review. *Nutrición Hospitalaria, 26*(6), 1266–1269.

Marinelli, K. A., Moren, K., Taylor, J. S., & Academy of Breastfeeding Medicine (ABM). (2013). Breastfeeding support for mothers in workplace employment or educational settings: Summary statement. *Breastfeeding Medicine, 8*(1), 137–142.

Mass, S. B. (2011). Supporting breastfeeding in the United States: The Surgeon General's call to action. *Current Opinions in Obstetrics and Gynecology, 23*(6), 460–464.

McMillan, D., & Canadian Paediatric Society (CPS) Fetus and Newborn Committee (1997). Routine administration of vitamin K to newborns. Reaffirmed 2014 *Paediatrics and Child Health, 2*(6), 429–431. Available at www.cps.ca/documents/position/administration-vitamin-K-newborns.

Mehta, U. J., Siega-Riz, A. M., Herring, A. H., et al. (2011). Maternal obesity, psychological factors, and breastfeeding duration. *Breastfeeding Medicine, 6*(6), 369–376.

Meier, P. P., Patel, A. L., Bigger, H. R., et al. (2013). Supporting breastfeeding in the neonatal intensive care unit: Rush Mother's Milk Club as a case study of evidence-based care. *Pediatric Clinics of North America, 60*(1), 209–226.

Meier, P. P., Patel, A. L., Wright, K., & Engstrom, J. L. (2013). Management of breastfeeding during and after the maternity hospitalization for late preterm infants. *Clinics in Perinatology, 40*(4), 689–705.

Mohrbacher, N. (2013). Breastfeeding and growth: Birth through weaning. In R. Mannel, P. J. Martens, & M. Walker (Eds.), *Core curriculum for lactation consultant practice* (3rd ed.). Burlington, MA: Jones and Bartlett.

Montgomery, A., Hale, T. W., & The Academy of Breastfeeding Medicine (ABM). (2012). ABM protocol #15: Analgesia and anesthesia for the breastfeeding mother, revised 2012. *Breastfeeding Medicine, 7*(6), 547–553.

Moore, E. R., Anderson, G. C., Bergman, N., et al. (2012). Early skin-to-skin contact for mothers and their healthy newborn infants. *The Cochrane Database of Systematic Reviews, 2012*, 5, CD003519.

Morton, J., Hall, J. Y., & Pessl, M. (2013-2014). Five steps to improve bedside breastfeeding care. *Nursing for Women's Health, 17*(6), 478–488.

Morton, J., Wong, R. J., Hall, J. Y., et al. (2012). Combining hand techniques with electric pumping increases the caloric content of milk in mothers of preterm infants. *Journal of Perinatology, 32*(10), 791–796.

Nelson, A. M. (2012). A meta-synthesis related to infant feeding decision making. *MCN: The American Journal of Maternal/Child Nursing, 37*(4), 247–252.

Newton, E. R. (2012). Lactation and breastfeeding. In S. G. Gabbe, J. R. Niebyl, J. L. Simpson, et al. (Eds.), *Obstetrics: Normal and problem pregnancies* (6th ed.). Philadelphia: Saunders.

Perrine, C. G., Scanlon, K. S., Li, R., et al. (2012). Baby-friendly hospital practices and meeting exclusive breastfeeding intention. *Pediatrics, 130*(1), 1–7.

Sachs, H. C., & Committee on Drugs (2013). The transfer of drugs and therapeutics into human breast milk: An update on selected topics. *Pediatrics, 132*(3), e796–e809.

Smith, A., & Heads, J. (2013). Breast pathology. In R. Mannel, P. J. Martens, & M. Walker (Eds.), *Core curriculum for lactation consultant practice* (3rd ed.). Burlington, MA: Jones and Bartlett.

Spatz, D. L., & Lessen, R. (2011). *The risks of not breastfeeding: Position statement.* Morrisville, NC: International Lactation Consultant Association.

Stuebe, A. M., & Bonuck, K. (2011). What predicts intent to breastfeed exclusively? Breastfeeding knowledge, attitudes, and beliefs in a diverse urban population. *Breastfeeding Medicine, 6*(6), 413–420.

Suzuki, S. (2013). Effect of early skin-to-skin contact on breastfeeding. *Journal of Obstetrics and Gynaecology, 33*(7), 695–696.

Tenfelde, S., Finnegan, L., & Hill, P. D. (2011). Predictors of breastfeeding exclusivity in a WIC sample. *Journal of Obstetric, Gynecologic, and Neonatal Nursing, 40*(2), 179–189.

The Joint Commission (TJC). (2012). *Specifications manual for Joint Commission national quality core measures, version 2013 A1.* Washington, DC: The Joint Commission. Available at https://manual.jointcommission.org/releases/TJC2013A/MIF0170.html.

Turcksin, R., Bel, S., Galjaard, S., & Devlieger, R. (2012). Maternal obesity and breastfeeding intention, initiation, intensity and duration: A systematic review. *Maternal and Child Nutrition*. Epub ahead of print.

Updegrove, K. H. (2013). Donor human milk banking: Growth, challenges, and the role of HMBANA. *Breastfeeding Medicine, 8*(5), 435–437.

U.S. Breastfeeding Committee (USBC). (2010a). *Core competencies in breastfeeding care and services for all health care professionals* (rev. ed.). Washington, DC: USBC.

U.S. Breastfeeding Committee (USBC). (2010b). *Implementing the Joint Commission perinatal care core measure on exclusive breast milk feeding* (rev. ed.). Washington, DC: USBC.

U.S. Department of Health and Human Services (USDHHS). (2010a). *Affordable Care Act: About the law.* Available at www.hhs.gov/healthcare/rights/index.html.

U.S. Department of Health and Human Services (USDHHS). (2010b). *Healthy People 2020.* Washington, DC: USDHHS.

U.S. Department of Health and Human Services (USDHHS). (2011). *The Surgeon General's call to action to support breastfeeding.* Washington, DC: USDHHS.

U.S. Food and Drug Administration (FDA). (2010). *Use of donor milk.* Available at www.fda.gov/ScienceResearch/SpecialTopics/PediatricTherapeuticsResearch/ucm235203.htm.

U.S. Food and Drug Administration (FDA). (2012). *Import alert 61-07.* Available at www.accessdata.fda.gov/cms_ia/importalert_166.html.

Wagner, E. A., Chantry, C. J., Dewey, K. G., & Nommsen-Rivers, L. A. (2013). Breastfeeding concerns at 3 and 7 days postpartum and feeding status at 2 months. *Pediatrics, 132*(4), e865–e875.

Wagner, C., Grier, F., & American Academy of Pediatrics (AAP) Section on Breastfeeding, and Committee on Nutrition (2008). Prevention of rickets and vitamin D deficiency in infants, children and adolescents. *Pediatrics, 122*(5), 1142–1152.

Wambach, K. A., Aaronson, L., Breedlove, G., et al. (2011). A randomized control trial of breastfeeding support and education for adolescent mothers. *Western Journal of Nursing Research, 33*(4), 486–505.

Wojcicki, J. M. (2011). Maternal prepregnancy body mass index and initiation and duration of breastfeeding: A review of the literature. *Journal of Women's Health, 20*(3), 341–347.

World Health Organization (WHO). (2013). *Essential nutrition actions: Improving maternal, newborn, infant and young child health and nutrition.* Geneva, Switzerland: Author.

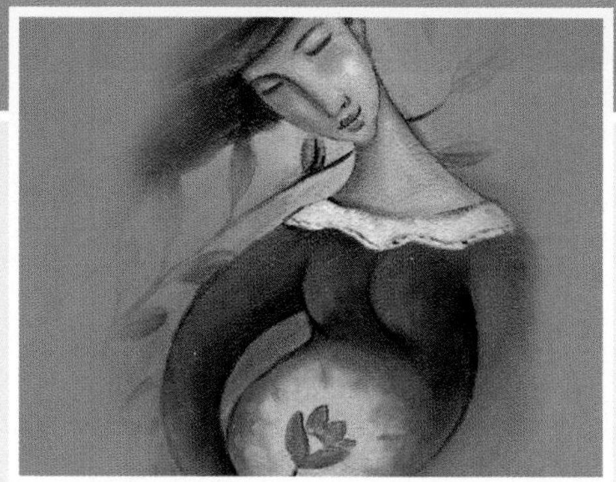

CHAPTER 26

Assessment of High Risk Pregnancy

Janet A. Tucker

http://evolve.elsevier.com/Lowdermilk/MWHC/

LEARNING OBJECTIVES

- Explore biophysical, psychosocial, sociodemographic, and environmental influences on high risk pregnancy.
- Examine risk factors identified through history, physical examination, and diagnostic techniques.
- Differentiate among screening and diagnostic techniques, including when they are used in pregnancy and for what purposes.
- Discuss psychologic considerations for the woman and her family experiencing a high risk pregnancy.
- Develop a teaching plan to explain screening and diagnostic techniques and implications of findings to women and their families.

In the most recent year for which figures are available, nearly 4 million births occurred in the United States (Martin, Hamilton, & Osterman, et al., 2013). Many of these were the result of pregnancies considered to be *high risk* because the life or health of the mother, fetus, or newborn was jeopardized by circumstances coincidental with or unique to the pregnancy. Care of these high risk clients requires the combined efforts of medical and nursing personnel. Factors associated with a diagnosis of a high risk pregnancy are identified in this chapter. Diagnostic techniques often used to monitor the maternal-fetal unit at risk also are described.

ASSESSMENT OF RISK FACTORS

Pregnancies can be designated as high risk for any of several undesirable outcomes. In the past risk factors were evaluated only from a medical standpoint. Therefore, only adverse medical, obstetric, or physiologic conditions were considered to place the woman at risk. Today a more comprehensive approach to high risk pregnancy is used, and the factors associated with high risk childbearing are grouped into broad categories based on threats to health and pregnancy outcome. Categories of risk include biophysical, psychosocial, sociodemographic, and environmental (Box 26-1). Risk factors are interrelated and cumulative in their effects.

Biophysical risks include factors that originate within the mother or fetus and affect the development or functioning of either one or both. Examples include genetic disorders, nutritional and general health status, and medical or obstetric-related illnesses. Box 26-2 lists common risk factors for several pregnancy-related problems.

Psychosocial risks consist of maternal behaviors and adverse lifestyles that have a negative effect on the health of the mother or fetus. These risks may include emotional distress, disturbed interpersonal relationships, inadequate social support, and unsafe cultural practices.

Sociodemographic risks arise from the mother and her family. These risks may place the mother and fetus at risk. Examples include lack of prenatal care, low income, marital status, and ethnicity (see Box 26-1).

Environmental factors include hazards in the workplace and the woman's general environment and may include environmental chemicals (e.g., lead, mercury), anesthetic gases, and radiation (Chambers & Scialli, 2014; Cunningham, Leveno, Bloom, et al., 2014).

ANTEPARTUM TESTING

Standard prenatal tests that are done for all pregnant women are discussed in Chapter 14 and listed in Table 14-1. This chapter concentrates on the testing that is done for high risk pregnancies rather than for those considered routine. Antepartum testing has two major goals. The first is to identify fetuses at risk for injury caused by acute or chronic interruption of oxygenation so permanent injury or death might be prevented. The second goal is to identify appropriately oxygenated fetuses so unnecessary intervention can be avoided (Miller, Miller, & Tucker, 2013). In most cases monitoring begins by 32 to 34 weeks of gestation and continues regularly until birth. Assessment tests should be selected on the basis of their effectiveness, and the results must be interpreted in light of the complete clinical

BOX 26-1 Categories of High Risk Factors

Biophysical Factors

Genetic considerations. Genetic factors may interfere with normal fetal or neonatal development, result in congenital anomalies, or create difficulties for the mother. These factors include defective genes, transmissible inherited disorders and chromosomal anomalies, multiple pregnancy, large fetal size, and ABO incompatibility.

Nutritional status. Adequate nutrition, without which fetal growth and development cannot proceed normally, is one of the most important determinants of pregnancy outcome. Conditions that influence nutritional status include the following: young age; three pregnancies in the previous 2 years; tobacco, alcohol, or drug use; inadequate dietary intake because of chronic illness or food fads; inadequate or excessive weight gain; and hematocrit value less than 33%.

Medical and obstetric disorders. Complications of current and past pregnancies, obstetric-related illnesses, and pregnancy losses put the woman at risk (see Box 26-2).

Psychosocial Factors

Smoking. A strong, consistent, causal relationship has been established between maternal smoking and reduced birth weight. Risks include low-birth-weight infants, higher neonatal mortality rates, increased rates of miscarriage, and increased incidence of premature rupture of membranes. These risks are aggravated by low socioeconomic status, poor nutritional status, and concurrent use of alcohol.

Caffeine. Birth defects in humans have not been related to caffeine consumption. However, pregnant women who consume more than 200 mg of caffeine daily (equivalent to about 12 ounces of coffee per day) may be at increased risk for miscarriage or giving birth to infants with intrauterine growth restriction.

Alcohol. Although the exact effects of alcohol in pregnancy have not been quantified and its mode of action is largely unexplained, it exerts adverse effects on the fetus, resulting in fetal alcohol syndrome, fetal alcohol effects, learning disabilities, and hyperactivity.

Drugs. The developing fetus may be affected adversely by drugs through several mechanisms. They can be teratogenic, cause metabolic disturbances, produce chemical effects, or cause depression or alteration of central nervous system function. This category includes medications prescribed by a health care provider or bought over the counter, and commonly abused drugs such as heroin, cocaine, and marijuana. (See Chapter 31 for more information about drug and alcohol abuse.)

Psychologic status. Childbearing triggers profound and complex physiologic, psychologic, and social changes, with evidence to suggest a relationship between emotional distress and birth complications. This risk factor includes conditions such as specific intrapsychic disturbances and addictive lifestyles; a history of child or spouse abuse; inadequate support systems; family disruption or dissolution; maternal role changes or conflicts; noncompliance with cultural norms; unsafe cultural, ethnic, or religious practices; and situational crises.

Sociodemographic Factors

Low income. Poverty underlies many other risk factors and leads to inadequate financial resources for food and prenatal care, poor general health, increased risk of medical complications of pregnancy, and greater prevalence of adverse environmental influences.

Lack of prenatal care. Failure to diagnose and treat complications early is a major risk factor arising from financial barriers or lack of access to care; depersonalization of the system resulting in long waits, routine visits, variability in health care personnel, and unpleasant physical surroundings; lack of understanding of the need for early and continued care or cultural beliefs that do not support the need; and fear of the health care system and its providers.

Age. Women at both ends of the childbearing age spectrum have an increased incidence of poor outcomes; however, age may not be a risk factor in all cases. Physiologic and psychologic risks should be evaluated.

Adolescents. More complications are seen in young mothers (younger than 15 years) and in pregnancies occurring less than 6 years after menarche. Complications include anemia, preeclampsia, prolonged labor, and contracted pelvis and cephalopelvic disproportion. The fetus has a greatly increased risk of low birth weight and of dying during the first year of life. Long-term social implications of early motherhood are lower educational attainment, lower income, increased dependence on government support programs, higher divorce rates, and higher parity.

Mature mothers. The risks to older mothers are not from age alone but from other considerations such as number and spacing of previous pregnancies, genetic disposition of the parents, medical history, lifestyle, nutrition, and prenatal care. The increased likelihood of chronic diseases and complications that arise from more invasive medical management of a pregnancy and labor combined with demographic characteristics put an older woman at risk. Conditions more likely to be experienced by mature women include chronic hypertension and preeclampsia, diabetes, prolonged labor, cesarean birth, placenta previa, placental abruption, and death. Her fetus is at greater risk for low birth weight and macrosomia, chromosomal abnormalities, congenital malformations, and neonatal death.

Parity. The number of previous pregnancies is a risk factor associated with age and includes all first pregnancies, especially a first pregnancy at either end of the childbearing age continuum. The incidence of preeclampsia and dystocia is increased with a first birth.

Marital status. The increased mortality and morbidity rates for unmarried women, including an increased risk for preeclampsia, are often related to inadequate prenatal care and a young childbearing age.

Residence. The availability and quality of prenatal care vary widely with geographic residence. Women in metropolitan areas have more prenatal visits than those in rural areas who have fewer opportunities for specialized care and consequently a higher incidence of maternal mortality. Health care in the inner city, where residents are usually poorer and begin childbearing earlier and continue longer, may be of lower quality than in a more affluent neighborhood.

Ethnicity. Although ethnicity by itself is not a major risk, race is associated with some poor pregnancy outcomes. Non-Caucasian women are more than three times as likely as Caucasian women to die of pregnancy-related causes. African-American babies have the highest rates of prematurity and low birth weight, with the infant mortality rate among African-Americans being more than double that among Caucasians.

Environmental Factors

Various environmental substances can affect fertility and fetal development, the chance of a live birth, and the child's subsequent mental and physical development. Environmental influences include infections, radiation, chemicals such as mercury and lead, therapeutic drugs, illicit drugs, industrial pollutants, cigarette smoke, stress, and diet. Paternal exposure to mutagenic agents in the workplace has been associated with an increased risk of miscarriage.

BOX 26-2 Specific Pregnancy Problems and Related Risk Factors

Polyhydramnios
Poorly controlled diabetes mellitus
Fetal congenital anomalies (e.g., gastrointestinal obstruction, twin-twin transfusion syndrome)

Intrauterine Growth Restriction
Maternal Causes
Hypertensive disorders
Diabetes
Chronic renal disease
Collagen vascular disease
Thrombophilia
Cyanotic heart disease
Poor weight gain
Smoking, alcohol use, illicit drug use
Living at a high altitude

Fetoplacental Causes
Chromosomal abnormalities
Congenital malformations
Intrauterine infection
Genetic syndromes (e.g., trisomy 13 and trisomy 18)
Abnormal placental development

Oligohydramnios
Renal agenesis (Potter syndrome)
Premature rupture of membranes
Prolonged pregnancy
Uteroplacental insufficiency
Severe intrauterine growth restriction (IUGR)
Maternal hypertensive disorders

Chromosomal Abnormalities
Advanced maternal age
Parental chromosomal rearrangements
Previous pregnancy with autosomal trisomy
Abnormal ultrasound findings during the current pregnancy (e.g., fetal structural anomalies, IUGR, amniotic fluid volume abnormalities)
Increased risk, as calculated from noninvasive screening results (e.g., nuchal translucency and maternal serum analytes)

Data from Baschat, A., Galan, H., & Gabbe, S. (2012). Intrauterine growth restriction. In S. Gabbe, J. Niebyl, & J. Simpson (Eds.), *Obstetrics: Normal and problem pregnancies* (6th ed.). Philadelphia: Saunders; Gilbert, W. (2012). Amniotic fluid disorders. In S. Gabbe, J. Niebyl, & J. Simpson (Eds.), *Obstetrics: Normal and problem pregnancies* (6th ed.). Philadelphia: Saunders; Simpson, J., Richards, D., Otano, L., et al. (2012). Prenatal genetic diagnosis. In S. Gabbe, J. Niebyl, & J. Simpson (Eds.), *Obstetrics: Normal and problem pregnancies* (6th ed.). Philadelphia: Saunders.

picture. Box 26-3 lists common maternal and fetal indications for antepartum testing that are supported by available evidence (Miller et al.).

The remainder of this chapter describes maternal and fetal assessment tests that are often used to monitor high risk pregnancies.

BIOPHYSICAL ASSESSMENT

Daily Fetal Movement Count

Assessment of fetal activity by the mother is a simple yet valuable method for monitoring the fetus's condition. The daily fetal movement count (DFMC) (also called *kick count*) can be assessed at home and is noninvasive, inexpensive, and simple to understand and usually does not interfere with a daily routine. It is frequently used to monitor the fetus in pregnancies complicated by conditions that may affect fetal oxygenation (see Box 26-2). The presence of movements is generally a reassuring sign of fetal health. During the third trimester the fetus makes about 30 gross body movements each hour. The mother is able to recognize 70% to 80% of these movements (Greenberg, Druzin, & Gabbe, 2012).

BOX 26-3 Common Maternal and Fetal Indications for Antepartum Testing

Diabetes
Chronic hypertension
Preeclampsia
Fetal growth restriction
Multiple gestation
Oligohydramnios
Preterm premature rupture of membranes
Late term or postterm gestation
Previous stillbirth
Decreased fetal movement
Systemic lupus erythematosus
Renal disease
Cholestasis of pregnancy

From Miller, L., Miller, D., & Tucker, S. (2013). *Mosby's pocket guide to fetal monitoring: A multidisciplinary approach* (7th ed.). St. Louis: Mosby.

Several different protocols are used for counting. One recommendation is to count once a day for 60 minutes (Fig. 26-1 is an example of a form used to record fetal kick counts). Other common recommendations are that mothers count fetal activity two or three times daily (e.g., after meals or before bedtime) for 2 hours or until 10 movements are counted or all fetal movements in a 12-hour period each day until a minimum of 10 movements are counted. Except for establishing a very low number of daily fetal movements or a trend toward decreased motion, the clinical value of the absolute number of fetal movements has not been established, other than in the situation in which fetal movements cease entirely for 12 hours (the so-called *fetal alarm signal*). A count of fewer than 3 fetal movements within 1 hour warrants further evaluation by a nonstress test (NST) or a contraction stress test and a complete or modified biophysical profile (see later discussion). Women should be taught the significance of the presence or absence of fetal movements, the procedure for counting, how to record findings on a daily fetal movement record, and when to notify the health care provider.

SAFETY ALERT

In assessing fetal movements it is important to remember that they are usually not present during the fetal sleep cycle; they may be reduced temporarily if the woman is taking depressant medication, drinking alcohol, or smoking a cigarette. They do not decrease as the woman nears term. Obesity decreases perception of fetal movements and consequently the ability of the mother to count them.

Ultrasonography

Diagnostic ultrasonography is an important, safe technique in antepartum fetal surveillance. It is considered by many to be the most valuable diagnostic tool used in obstetrics (Richards, 2012). It provides critical information to health care providers regarding fetal activity and gestational age, normal versus abnormal fetal growth curves, fetal and placental anatomy, fetal well-being, and visual assistance with which invasive tests can be performed more safely (Richards; Simpson, Richards, Otano, & Driscoll, 2012).

Fetal Movement Chart

This chart will help to keep track of your baby's well-being. Carefully count the number of movements your baby makes during the same hour every evening, when babies are typically most active. For example, between 9 and 10 p.m.

If your baby has not moved for 12 hours, please contact 602.406.3521. Be sure to bring this chart with you when visiting your doctor.

Daily Chart of Baby Kicks

DAYS OF WEEK	MONDAY	TUESDAY	WEDNESDAY	THURSDAY	FRIDAY	SATURDAY	SUNDAY
DATE							
KICKS							
DATE							
KICKS							
DATE							
KICKS							
DATE							
KICKS							
DATE							
KICKS							
DATE							
KICKS							
DATE							
KICKS							
DATE							
KICKS							
DATE							
KICKS							

Fetal movement (kick count) chart. Courtesy of St. Joseph's Hospital and Medical Center, Phoenix, AZ.

FIG 26-1 Fetal movement (kick count) chart. (Courtesy St. Joseph Hospital and Medical Center, Phoenix, AZ.)

Sound is a form of wave energy that causes small particles in a medium to oscillate. The frequency of sound, which refers to the number of peaks or waves that move over a given point per unit of time, is expressed in hertz (Hz). Sound with a frequency of one cycle, or one peak per second, has a frequency of 1 Hz. When directional beams of sound strike an object, an echo is returned. The time delay between the emission of the sound and the return and direction of the echo is noted. From these data the distance and location of an object can be calculated. Ultrasound is sound frequency higher than that detectable by humans (greater than 20,000 Hz). Ultrasound images are a reflection of the strength of the sending beam, the strength of the returning echo, and the density of the medium (e.g., muscle [uterus], bone, tissue [placenta], fluid, or blood) through which the beam is sent and returned.

An ultrasound examination can be performed either abdominally or transvaginally during pregnancy. Ultrasound scans produce a two- or three-dimensional view of the area being examined and can be used to create pictorial images (Fig. 26-2, *A* and *B*). Box 26-4 explains the differences in these scans and the views they produce.

Abdominal ultrasonography is more useful after the first trimester when the pregnant uterus becomes an abdominal organ. During the procedure the woman should have a full bladder to displace the uterus upward to provide a better image of the fetus. Transmission gel or paste is applied to the woman's abdomen to enhance the transmission and reception of the sound waves before a transducer is moved over the skin. She is positioned with small pillows under her head and knees. The display panel is positioned so the woman or her partner (or both) can observe the images on the screen if they desire.

Transvaginal ultrasonography, in which the probe is inserted into the vagina, allows pelvic anatomic features to be evaluated in greater detail and intrauterine pregnancy to be diagnosed earlier. A transvaginal ultrasound examination is well tolerated by most pregnant women because it removes the need

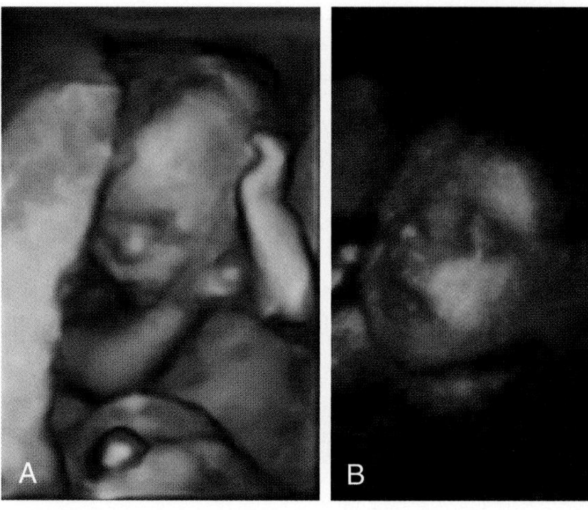

FIG 26-2 Fetus seen on three-dimensional ultrasound. **A,** View of fetus at 15 weeks and 3 days of gestation. **B,** Close-up view of fetal face later in pregnancy. (**A,** Courtesy Christina and Eva Gardner, Marion, AR; **B,** courtesy Margaret Spann, New Johnsonville, TN.)

BOX 26-4 Types of Ultrasound Scans

Two-Dimensional (2D)
- Sound waves are sent straight down from the ultrasound transducer.
- The image produced includes only two dimensions (length and width), so it appears flat.
- The image is viewed in black, white, or shades of gray.
- This is the standard medical scan used in pregnancy.

Three-Dimensional (3D)
- Sound waves are sent out at different angles. The returning echoes are processed by a computer program, which adds a third dimension (depth) to the 2D scan, producing a 3D image.
- The image is usually displayed in sepia tones rather than in black and white.
- This scan can be used for diagnostic or management purposes. Viewing certain anomalies using a 3D scan provides further information that assists in planning for care at birth and for the neonate. These images are also often requested by pregnant women and families simply for their own enjoyment.

Four-Dimensional (4D)
- This scan adds a fourth dimension (time) to the 3D scan.
- The images produced are recorded and played back in succession. As the image is continuously updated, the fetus is viewed in real time.

for a full bladder. It is especially useful in obese women whose thick abdominal layers cannot be penetrated adequately with an abdominal approach. A transvaginal ultrasound may be performed with the woman in a lithotomy position or with her pelvis elevated by towels, cushions, or a folded pillow. This pelvic tilt is optimal to image the pelvic structures. A protective cover such as a condom, the finger of a clean surgical glove, or a special probe cover provided by the manufacturer is used to cover the transducer probe. The probe is lubricated with a water-soluble gel and placed in the vagina either by the examiner or by the woman herself. During the examination the position of the probe or the tilt of the examining table may be changed so the complete pelvis is in view. The procedure is not physically painful, although the woman feels pressure as the probe is moved. Transvaginal ultrasonography is optimally used in the first trimester to detect ectopic pregnancies, monitor the developing embryo, help identify abnormalities, and help establish gestational age. In some instances it may be used along with abdominal scanning to evaluate preterm labor in second- and third-trimester pregnancies.

Levels of Ultrasonography

The American College of Obstetricians and Gynecologists (ACOG, 2009) describes three levels of ultrasonography:

- *Standard* (also called basic) examinations are used most frequently and can be performed by ultrasonographers or other health care professionals, including nurses, who have had special training. Indications for standard ultrasonography are described in detail in the next section. In the second and third trimesters a standard ultrasound examination is used to evaluate fetal presentation, amniotic fluid volume (AFV), cardiac activity, placental position, fetal growth parameters, and number of fetuses. It is also used to perform an anatomic survey of the fetus.
- *Limited* examinations are performed for specific indications such as identifying fetal presentation during labor or estimating AFV. These examinations are usually performed by the woman's physician in the office or the labor and birth unit.
- *Specialized* (also called detailed) or *targeted* examinations are performed if a woman is suspected of carrying an anatomically or physiologically abnormal fetus. Indications for this comprehensive examination include abnormal history or laboratory findings or the results of a previous standard or limited ultrasound examination. Specialized ultrasonography is performed by highly trained and experienced personnel.

Indications for Use

Major indications for obstetric sonography are listed by trimester in Table 26-1. During the first trimester ultrasound examination is performed to obtain information regarding the number, size, and location of gestational sacs; the presence or absence of fetal cardiac and body movements; the presence or absence of uterine abnormalities (e.g., bicornuate uterus or fibroids) or adnexal masses (e.g., ovarian cysts or an ectopic pregnancy); and pregnancy dating.

During the second and third trimesters information regarding the following conditions is sought: fetal viability, number, position, gestational age, growth pattern, and anomalies; amniotic fluid volume; placental location and condition; presence of uterine fibroids or anomalies; presence of adnexal masses; and cervical length.

Ultrasonography provides earlier diagnoses, allowing therapy to be instituted earlier in the pregnancy, thereby decreasing the severity and duration of morbidity, both physical and emotional, for the family. For instance, early diagnosis of a fetal anomaly gives the family choices such as intrauterine surgery or other therapy for the fetus, termination of the pregnancy, or preparation for the care of an infant with a disorder.

TABLE 26-1 Major Uses of Ultrasonography During Pregnancy

FIRST TRIMESTER	SECOND TRIMESTER	THIRD TRIMESTER
Confirm pregnancy	Establish or confirm dates	Confirm gestational age
Confirm viability	Confirm viability	Confirm viability
Determine gestational age	Detect polyhydramnios, oligohydramnios	Detect macrosomia
Rule out ectopic pregnancy	Detect congenital anomalies	Detect congenital anomalies
Detect multiple gestation	Detect intrauterine growth restriction (IUGR)	Detect IUGR
Determine cause of vaginal bleeding	Assess placental location	Determine fetal position
Use for visualization during chorionic villus sampling	Use for visualization during amniocentesis	Detect placenta previa or placental abruption
Detect maternal abnormalities such as bicornuate uterus, ovarian cysts, fibroids		Use for visualization during amniocentesis, external version
		Biophysical profile
		Amniotic fluid volume assessment
		Doppler flow studies
		Detect placental maturity

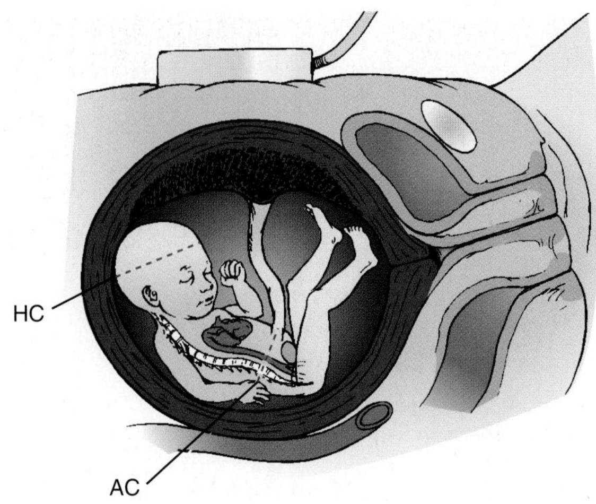

FIG 26-3 Appropriate planes of sections *(dotted lines)* for head circumference *(HC)* and abdominal circumference *(AC)*.

Fetal Heart Activity. Fetal heart activity can be demonstrated by about 6 weeks of gestation using transvaginal ultrasound. When the fetus is in a favorable position, good views of the fetal cardiac anatomy are possible in most women at 13 weeks of gestation (Richards, 2012). Fetal death can be confirmed by lack of heart motion along with the presence of fetal scalp edema and maceration and overlap of the cranial bones.

Gestational Age. Gestational dating by ultrasonography is indicated for conditions such as uncertain dates for the last normal menstrual period, recent discontinuation of oral contraceptives, a bleeding episode during the first trimester, uterine size that does not agree with dates, and other high risk conditions. In fact, growing evidence suggests that pregnancies should be dated by an ultrasound performed before 22 weeks of gestation rather than by menstrual dates because the ultrasound dating is more accurate than even "sure" menstrual dates (Richards, 2012). A standard set of measurements has been accepted as being the most useful for determining gestational age: the crown-rump length (after 10 weeks), the biparietal diameter (BPD) (after 12 weeks), the femur length (after 12 weeks), the head circumference, and the abdominal circumference (Fig. 26-3). An ultrasound examination performed for pregnancy dating between 14 and 22 weeks of gestation is comparable to one performed during the first trimester in terms of accuracy. However, after that time ultrasound dating is less reliable because of variability in fetal size (Richards).

Fetal Growth. Fetal growth is determined by both intrinsic growth potential and environmental factors. Conditions that require ultrasound assessment of fetal growth include poor maternal weight gain or pattern of weight gain, previous pregnancy with intrauterine growth restriction (IUGR), chronic infections, ingestion of drugs (tobacco, alcohol, and over-the-counter and street drugs), maternal diabetes, hypertension, multifetal pregnancy, and other medical or surgical complications.

Serial evaluations of BPD, limb length, and abdominal circumference can allow differentiation among size discrepancies resulting from inaccurate dates, true IUGR, and macrosomia. IUGR may be symmetric (the fetus is small in all parameters) or asymmetric (head and body growth do not match). Symmetric IUGR reflects a chronic or long-standing insult and may be caused by low genetic growth potential, intrauterine infection, chromosomal anomaly, maternal undernutrition, or heavy smoking. Asymmetric growth suggests an acute or late-occurring deprivation such as placental insufficiency resulting from hypertension, renal disease, or cardiovascular disease. Reduced fetal growth is still one of the most frequent conditions associated with stillbirth. Macrosomic infants (those weighing 4000 g or more) are at increased risk for traumatic injury and asphyxia during birth. Macrosomia also may be characterized as symmetric or asymmetric.

Fetal Anatomy. Anatomic structures that can be identified by ultrasonography (depending on the gestational age) include the following: head (including ventricles and blood vessels), neck, spine, heart, stomach, small bowel, liver, kidneys, bladder, and limbs. Ultrasonography permits the confirmation of normal anatomy and detection of major fetal malformations. The presence of an anomaly may influence the location of birth (e.g., a subspecialty center versus a basic care center) and the method of birth (vaginal versus cesarean) to optimize neonatal outcomes. For example, plans are often made for a fetus with a condition that will require immediate surgery to be born in or near a hospital able to provide that care rather than in a small community hospital that is totally unequipped to meet the newborn's needs.

The number of fetuses and their presentations can be assessed by ultrasonography, allowing plans for therapy and mode of birth to be made in advance.

Fetal Genetic Disorders and Physical Anomalies. A prenatal screening technique called *nuchal translucency* (NT) screening uses ultrasound measurement of fluid in the nape of the fetal neck between 10 and 14 weeks of gestation to identify possible fetal abnormalities (Fig. 26-4). A fluid collection greater than 3 mm is considered abnormal. When combined with low maternal serum marker levels, elevated NT indicates a possible increased risk of certain chromosomal abnormalities in the fetus, including trisomies 13, 18, and 21. An elevated NT alone indicates an increased risk of fetal cardiac disease. If the NT is

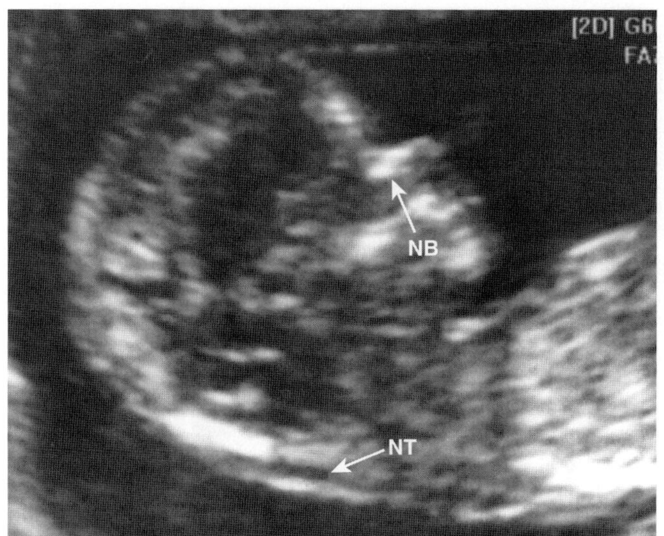

FIG 26-4 Midsagittal view of a 12-week fetus showing the nuchal translucency *(NT)* and nasal bone *(NB)*. (From Gabbe, S., Niebyl, J., & Simpson, J. [2012]. *Obstetrics: Normal and problem pregnancies* [6th ed.]. Philadelphia: Saunders.)

abnormal, diagnostic genetic testing is recommended (ACOG, 2009; Gilbert, 2011).

Other ultrasound findings, including the presence or absence (and length, if present) of a nasal bone, short femur or humerus, echogenic intracardiac focus, echogenic bowel, and pyelectasis (enlargement of the renal pelvis, the part of the kidney that collects urine), have been associated with trisomy 21 (Down syndrome) in the fetus. These findings are considered soft markers only; they are not diagnostic for the anomaly. Women in whom these soft markers are found who are at low risk to have a fetus with trisomy 21 should receive expert counseling about the advisability of further diagnostic testing (Simpson et al., 2012).

Placental Position and Function. The pattern of uterine and placental growth and the fullness of the maternal bladder influence the apparent location of the placenta by ultrasonography. During the first trimester differentiation between the endometrium and small placenta is difficult. By 14 to 16 weeks the placenta is clearly defined, but if it is seen to be low lying, its relationship to the internal cervical os can sometimes be altered dramatically by varying the fullness of the maternal bladder. In approximately 4% to 6% of all pregnancies in which ultrasound scanning is performed during the second trimester, the placenta seems to be overlying the os. However, most cases of placenta previa diagnosed during the second trimester resolve by term, primarily because of the elongation of the lower uterine segment as pregnancy advances. Therefore, if placenta previa is diagnosed during the second trimester, repeated ultrasounds should be performed as pregnancy progresses until the placenta moves well away from the cervical os or it becomes clear that the previa will persist (Francois & Foley, 2012; Richards, 2012).

Another use for ultrasonography is grading of placental aging. Calcium and fibrin deposits in an aging placenta result in intervillous hemorrhagic infarcts. Also as blood vessels in the placenta age and thicken, oxygen transport is affected. However, whether these placental changes adversely affect fetal outcomes in postterm pregnancies is unknown, given that most fetuses continue to grow (Gilbert, 2011).

Adjunct to Other Invasive Tests. The safety of amniocentesis is increased when the positions of the fetus, placenta, and pockets of amniotic fluid can be identified accurately. Ultrasound scanning has reduced risks previously associated with amniocentesis, such as fetomaternal hemorrhage from a pierced placenta. Percutaneous umbilical blood sampling and chorionic villus sampling also are guided by ultrasonography to identify the cord and chorion frondosum accurately.

Fetal Well-being. Physiologic parameters of the fetus that can be assessed with ultrasound scanning include AFV, vascular waveforms from the fetal circulation, heart motion, fetal breathing movements (FBMs), fetal urine production, and fetal limb and head movements. Assessment of these parameters, alone or in combination, yields a fairly reliable picture of fetal well-being. The significance of these findings is discussed in the following sections.

Doppler Blood Flow Analysis. One of the major advances in perinatal medicine is the ability to study blood flow in the fetus and placenta noninvasively using ultrasound. Doppler blood flow analysis is a helpful tool in the management of pregnancies at risk because of maternal hypertension and diabetes mellitus, IUGR, multiple fetuses, and preterm labor because it provides an indication of fetal adaptation and reserve.

When a sound wave is reflected from a moving target, a change occurs in the frequency of the reflected wave relative to the transmitted wave, called the *Doppler effect.* An ultrasound beam scattered by a group of red blood cells (RBCs) is an example of this effect. The velocity of the RBCs can be determined by measuring the change in the frequency of the sound wave reflected off the cells (Fig. 26-5).

The shifted frequencies can be displayed as a plot of velocity versus time, and the shape of these waveforms can be analyzed to give information about blood flow and resistance in a given circulation. Velocity waveforms from the umbilical and uterine arteries, reported as systolic/diastolic (S/D) ratios, can be first detected at 15 weeks of pregnancy. Because of the progressive decline in resistance in both the umbilical and uterine arteries, this ratio normally decreases as pregnancy advances. Findings of absent or reversed end-diastolic blood flow and S/D ratios greater than 3 indicate placental vascular disease. IUGR may result from this placental insufficiency. In addition to IUGR, abnormal elevations in the S/D ratio are seen in hypertensive disorders of pregnancy or other causes of uteroplacental insufficiency (Baschat, Galan, & Gabbe, 2012; Gilbert, 2011). In postterm pregnancies evaluated by Doppler umbilical flow studies, an elevated S/D ratio indicates a poorly perfused placenta. Abnormal results also are seen with certain chromosomal abnormalities (trisomy 13 and 18) in the fetus and lupus erythematosus in the mother. Exposure to nicotine from maternal smoking also has been reported to increase the S/D ratio (see Fig. 26-5).

Amniotic Fluid Volume. Abnormalities in AFV are frequently associated with fetal disorders. Subjective determinants of oligohydramnios (decreased fluid) include the absence of fluid pockets in the uterine cavity and the impression of crowding of small fetal parts. An objective criterion of decreased AFV is met if the deepest vertical pocket of fluid measured in two perpendicular planes is less than 2 cm (Kaimal, 2014). Increased amniotic fluid is called polyhydramnios or sometimes

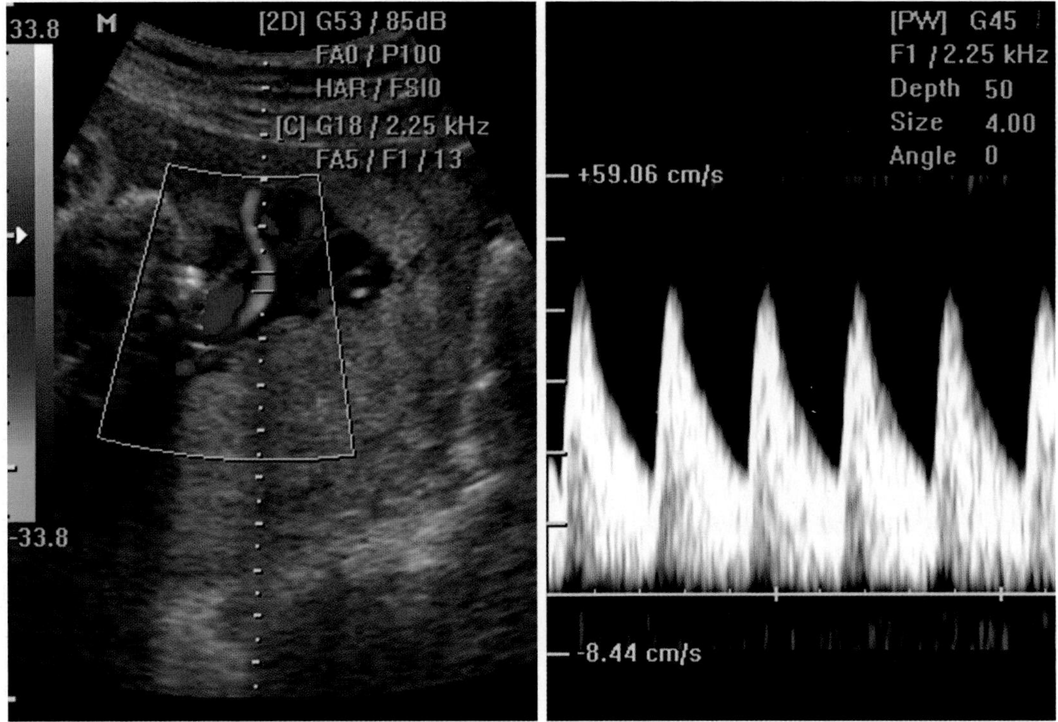

FIG 26-5 Color and spectral Doppler evaluation of the umbilical artery. In the left panel the coiling arteries and vein are shown. *Red* indicates flow toward the transducer, and *blue* is flow away. The sample gate for the pulse Doppler is superimposed. On the right is the result of the pulse Doppler, depicting a normal flow velocity waveform. (From Gabbe, S., Niebyl, J., & Simpson, J. [2012]. *Obstetrics: Normal and problem pregnancies* [6th ed.]. Philadelphia: Saunders.)

just *hydramnios*. Subjective criteria for polyhydramnios include multiple large pockets of fluid, the impression of a floating fetus, and free movement of fetal limbs. Polyhydramnios is usually objectively defined as pockets of amniotic fluid measuring more than 8 cm (Gilbert, 2012).

The total AFV can be evaluated by a method in which the vertical depths (in centimeters) of the largest pocket of amniotic fluid in all four quadrants surrounding the maternal umbilicus are totaled, providing an amniotic fluid index (AFI). A normal AFI is 10 cm or greater, with the upper range of normal around 25 cm. AFI values between 5 and 10 cm are considered to be low normal, whereas an AFI of less than 5 cm indicates oligohydramnios. With polyhydramnios the AFI is greater than 25 cm (Miller et al., 2013). Oligohydramnios is associated with congenital anomalies (e.g., renal agenesis [Potter syndrome]) and growth restriction. Polyhydramnios is associated with neural tube defects (NTDs), obstruction of the fetal gastrointestinal tract, multiple fetuses, and fetal hydrops.

Biophysical Profile. Real-time ultrasound permits detailed assessment of the physical and physiologic characteristics of the developing fetus and cataloging of normal and abnormal biophysical responses to stimuli. The biophysical profile (BPP) is a noninvasive dynamic assessment of a fetus that is based on acute and chronic markers of fetal disease. The BPP includes AFV, FBMs, fetal movements, and fetal tone determined by ultrasound and fetal heart rate (FHR) reactivity determined by means of the NST. Therefore, the BPP can be considered a physical examination of the fetus, including determination of vital signs. FHR reactivity, FBMs, fetal movement, and fetal tone reflect current central nervous system (CNS) status, whereas the AFV demonstrates the adequacy of placental function over a longer period of time (Miller et al., 2013). BPP scoring and management are detailed in Tables 26-2 and 26-3.

TABLE 26-2 Scoring the Biophysical Profile

BIOPHYSICAL VARIABLE	SCORE 2	SCORE 0
Fetal breathing movements	At least one episode of fetal breathing movements of at least 30-second duration in a 30-minute observation	Absent fetal breathing movements or less than 30 seconds of sustained fetal breathing movements in 30 minutes
Fetal movements	At least three trunk/limb movements in 30 minutes	Fewer than three episodes of trunk/limb movements in 30 minutes
Fetal tone	At least one episode of active extension with return to flexion of fetal limb or trunk; opening and closing of hand considered normal tone	Absence of movement or slow extension/flexion
Amniotic fluid index (AFI)	AFI >5 cm or at least one pocket >2 cm	AFI ≤5 cm and no single pocket >2 cm
Nonstress test	Reactive	Nonreactive

From Miller, L., Miller, D., & Tucker, S. (2013). *Mosby's pocket guide to fetal monitoring: A multidisciplinary approach* (7th ed.). St. Louis: Mosby.

The BPP is used frequently in the late second and the third trimester for antepartum fetal testing because it is a reliable predictor of fetal well-being. A BPP of 8 or 10 with a normal AFV is considered normal. Advantages of the test include excellent sensitivity and a low false-negative rate (Miller et al., 2013).

TABLE 26-3 Biophysical Profile Management

SCORE	INTERPRETATION	MANAGEMENT
10	Normal; low risk for chronic asphyxia	Repeat testing at weekly to twice-weekly intervals.
8	Normal; low risk for chronic asphyxia	Repeat testing at weekly to twice-weekly intervals.
6	Suspect chronic asphyxia	If ≥36-37 weeks of gestation or <36 weeks with positive testing for fetal pulmonary maturity, consider delivery; if <36 weeks and/or fetal pulmonary maturity testing negative, repeat biophysical profile in 4 to 6 hours; deliver if oligohydramnios is present.
4	Suspect chronic asphyxia	If ≥36 weeks of gestation, deliver; if <32 weeks of gestation, repeat score.
0-2	Strongly suspect chronic asphyxia	Extend testing time to 120 minutes; if persistent score ≤4, deliver, regardless of gestational age.

Modified from Manning, F.A., Harman, C.R., Morrison, I., et al. (1990). Fetal assessment based on fetal biophysical profile scoring. *American Journal of Obstetrics and Gynecology, 162*(3), 703-700. Mannin, F.A. (1992). Biophysical profile scoring. In J. Nijhuis (Ed.), *Fetal behavior*. New York: Oxford University Press.

One limitation of the test is that if the fetus is in a quiet sleep state, the BPP can require a long period of observation. Also unless the ultrasound examination is videotaped, it cannot be reviewed (Greenberg et al., 2012).

Modified Biophysical Profile. The modified BPP (mBPP) is being used increasingly as a way to shorten the testing time required for the complete BPP by assessing the components that are most predictive of perinatal outcome. The mBPP combines the NST, which assesses the current fetal condition, with measurement of the quantity of amniotic fluid, an indicator of placental function over a longer period of time. The AFI (rather than the AFV) is often used to measure the amount of amniotic fluid present. Desired test results are a reactive NST and a normal AFI. An AFI greater than 5 is generally considered normal (Greenberg et al., 2012; Miller et al., 2013).

Nursing Role

Although a growing number of nurses perform ultrasound scans and BPPs in certain centers, the main roles of nurses are counseling and educating women about the procedure. Ultrasound is widely used and in fact is considered a standard part of current prenatal care. Unlike many diagnostic tests, most women look forward to and enjoy their prenatal ultrasound. Exposure to diagnostic ultrasonography during pregnancy appears to be safe for the fetus (Richards, 2012).

Nonmedical Ultrasounds

Three- and four-dimensional ultrasonography for nonmedical purposes has become increasingly popular with pregnant women and their families. Although insurance does not cover the cost, women can have ultrasound images made of the fetus, just as professional photographs are often taken of infants and children. Both the American Institute of Ultrasound in Medicine (AIUM) and the ACOG have published statements that strongly discourage this practice. Although ultrasonography is considered safe, exposure of the fetus to high-frequency soundwaves without a clear medical indication for doing so should be avoided. In addition, casual ultrasonography performed by people who are not qualified health care professionals could give false reassurance to women or result in the discovery of abnormalities in settings that are not conducive to discussion and follow-up of findings (ACOG, 2009; AIUM, 2012; Richards, 2012). Helping the expectant family to understand the role of ultrasound beyond providing a picture of the baby is a component of prenatal education.

CLINICAL REASONING CASE STUDY

Nonmedical Use of Ultrasound

Alicia is a 24-year-old G2 P1 0 0 1 at 19 weeks of gestation. She presents at the maternal-fetal medicine clinic for a targeted ultrasound. Her primary obstetrician suspected a ventricular septal defect in the fetal heart during Alicia's ultrasound in his office last week. As you are taking a history prior to her ultrasound, Alicia says, "There is a new ultrasound business right near my house that advertises walk-in appointments and nice framed 3D pictures. Will I get a 3D picture of her face today? Why couldn't I have just gone to that place?"

1. Evidence—Is there sufficient evidence that Alicia needs a specific type of ultrasound performed by a maternal fetal medicine specialist?
2. Assumptions—Describe an underlying assumption about each of the following types of ultrasound examinations performed during pregnancy.
   a. Standard or basic examination
   b. Limited examination
   c. Specialized or targeted examination
   d. Nonmedical examination
3. What implications and priorities for nursing care can be drawn at this time?
4. Does the evidence objectively support your conclusion?

Magnetic Resonance Imaging

Magnetic resonance imaging (MRI) is a noninvasive radiologic technique used for obstetric and gynecologic diagnosis. Similar to computed tomography (CT), MRI provides excellent pictures of soft tissue. Unlike CT, ionizing radiation is not used. Therefore, vascular structures within the body can be visualized and evaluated without injecting an iodinated contrast medium, thus eliminating any known biologic risk. Similar to sonography, MRI is noninvasive and can provide images in multiple planes, but no interference occurs from skeletal, fatty, or gas-filled structures, and imaging of deep pelvic structures does not require a full bladder.

With MRI the examiner can evaluate fetal structure (CNS, thorax, abdomen, genitourinary tract, musculoskeletal system) and overall growth, the placenta (position, density, and presence of gestational trophoblastic disease), and the quantity of amniotic fluid. Maternal structures (uterus, cervix, adnexa, and pelvis), the biochemical status (pH, adenosine triphosphate content) of tissues and organs, and soft-tissue, metabolic, or functional anomalies can also be evaluated.

The woman is placed on a table in the supine position with one hip elevated if possible and moved into the bore of the main magnet, which is similar in appearance to a CT scanner. Depending on the reason for the study the procedure may take from 20 to 60 minutes, during which time the woman must be perfectly still except for short breaks. Because of the long time needed to produce MRIs, the fetus will probably move, which will obscure anatomic details. The only way to ensure that this problem does not occur is to administer a sedative to the mother, but this approach should be reserved for selected cases in which visualization of fetal detail is critical.

MRI has little effect on the fetus. Concerns that the FHR or fetal movement will decrease have not been supported.

BIOCHEMICAL ASSESSMENT

Biochemical assessment involves biologic examination (e.g., of chromosomes in exfoliated cells) and chemical determinations (e.g., lecithin/sphingomyelin [L/S] ratio, or phosphatidylglycerol [PG]) (Table 26-4). Procedures used to obtain the needed specimens include amniocentesis, percutaneous umbilical blood sampling, chorionic villus sampling, and maternal sampling (Box 26-5).

TABLE 26-4 Summary of Biochemical Monitoring Techniques

TEST	POSSIBLE FINDINGS	CLINICAL SIGNIFICANCE
Maternal Blood		
Coombs test	Titer of 1:8 and increasing	Significant Rh incompatibility
Cell-free DNA screening	> normal amount of DNA from specific chromosomes	Fetus with trisomy 13, 18, or 21
AFP	See AFP later in table	
Amniotic Fluid Analysis		
Lung profile:		Fetal lung maturity
L/S ratio	2:1	
Phosphatidylglycerol	Present	
LBC	≥50,000/μL	
Creatinine	>2 mg/dl	Gestational age >36 weeks
Lipid cells	>10%	Gestational age >35 weeks
AFP	High levels after 15 weeks of gestation	Open neural tube or other defect
Osmolality	Declines after 20 weeks of gestation	Advancing gestational age
Genetic disorders: Sex-linked, Chromosomal, Metabolic	Dependent on cultured cells for karyotype and enzymatic activity	Counseling possibly required

AFP, Alpha-fetoprotein; *L/S*, lecithin/sphingomyelin; *LBC*, lamellar body count.

BOX 26-5 Fetal Rights

Amniocentesis, percutaneous umbilical blood sampling (PUBS), and chorionic villus sampling (CVS) are prenatal tests used for diagnosing fetal defects in pregnancy. They are invasive and carry risks to the mother and fetus. A consideration of induced abortion is linked to the performance of these tests because no treatment for genetically affected fetuses has been developed; therefore, the issue of fetal rights is a key ethical concern in prenatal testing for fetal defects.

Amniocentesis

Amniocentesis is performed to obtain amniotic fluid, which contains fetal cells. Under direct ultrasonographic visualization, a needle is inserted transabdominally into the uterus, amniotic fluid is withdrawn into a syringe, and the various assessments are performed (Fig. 26-6). Amniocentesis is possible after week 14 of pregnancy, when the uterus becomes an abdominal organ and sufficient amniotic fluid is available for testing. Indications for the procedure include prenatal diagnosis of genetic disorders or congenital anomalies (NTDs in particular), assessment of pulmonary maturity, and (rarely) diagnosis of fetal hemolytic disease.

Complications in the mother and fetus occur in less than 1% of cases and include the following:

Maternal: leakage of amniotic fluid, hemorrhage, fetomaternal hemorrhage with possible maternal Rh isoimmunization, infection, labor, placental abruption, inadvertent damage to the intestines or bladder, and amniotic fluid embolism (anaphylactoid syndrome of pregnancy)

Fetal: death, hemorrhage, infection (amnionitis), and direct injury from the needle

Many of the complications have been minimized or eliminated by using ultrasonography to direct the procedure.

SAFETY ALERT

Because of the possibility of fetomaternal hemorrhage, administering Rh_0D immune globulin to the woman who is Rh negative is standard practice after an amniocentesis.

Indications for Use

Genetic Concerns. Historically prenatal assessment of genetic disorders focused on women older than 35 years (Box 26-6), women with a previous child with a chromosomal abnormality, or a family history of chromosomal anomalies. Inherited errors of metabolism (such as Tay-Sachs disease), hemophilia, thalassemia, and other disorders for which marker genes are known also can be detected by prenatal screening. Fetal cells can be cultured for karyotyping of chromosomes (see Chapter 3). Karyotyping also permits determination of fetal gender, which is important if an X-linked disorder (occurring almost always in a male fetus) is suspected.

Biochemical analysis of enzymes in amniotic fluid can detect inborn errors of metabolism or fetal structural anomalies. For example, alpha-fetoprotein (AFP) levels in amniotic fluid are assessed as a follow-up for elevated levels in maternal serum. High AFP levels in amniotic fluid help confirm the diagnosis of an NTD such as spina bifida or anencephaly or an abdominal wall defect such as omphalocele. The elevation results from the increased leakage of cerebrospinal or abdominal fluid into the amniotic fluid through the closure defect.

Fetal Maturity. Late in pregnancy accurate assessment of fetal lung maturity is possible by examining amniotic fluid to determine the L/S ratio or for the presence of PG. However, because both of these tests require considerable time, technical expertise, and cost to perform, they are generally used as primary tests only in special clinical circumstances. They may also be used as secondary tests if simpler and less expensive automated tests indicate lung immaturity (Mercer, 2014).

Until recently the TDx FLM assay and a subsequent modification, the TDx FLM II assay, were used as primary tests for fetal lung maturity. These assays determined the surfactant-to-albumin (S/A) ratio. However, they are no longer available for use in the United States. Instead, the lamellar body count (LBC) has become the primary test for determining fetal lung maturity.

Lamellar bodies are surfactant-containing particles secreted by type II pneumocytes. The number of lamellar bodies found in the amniotic fluid increases with the onset of functional fetal pulmonary maturity. The LBC compares favorably with the L/S ratio and the PG test in predicting fetal lung maturity. The automated test is simple to perform, and almost all hospital laboratories have the equipment used to perform it (Mercer, 2014) (see Table 26-4).

Fetal Hemolytic Disease. In the past amniocentesis was used for identification and follow-up of fetal hemolytic disease in cases of isoimmunization. Amniocentesis is now performed for this reason only in rare circumstances because of the availability of noninvasive testing. Doppler velocimetry of the fetal middle cerebral artery has become the method of choice to monitor accurately and noninvasively for fetal anemia in isoimmunized pregnancies (Moise, 2012).

Chorionic Villus Sampling

The combined advantages of earlier diagnosis and rapid results have made chorionic villus sampling (CVS) a popular technique for genetic studies in the first trimester. Indications for CVS are similar to those for amniocentesis, although CVS cannot be used for maternal serum marker screening because no fluid is obtained. CVS performed in the second trimester carries no greater risk of pregnancy loss than amniocentesis and is considered equal to amniocentesis in diagnostic accuracy. When performed after the first trimester, the procedure is better known as *late CVS* or *placental biopsy* (Simpson et al., 2012).

CVS can be performed in the first or second trimester, ideally between 10 and 13 weeks of gestation, and involves the removal of a small tissue specimen from the fetal portion of the placenta (Figs. 26-7 and 26-8). Because chorionic villi originate in the zygote, this tissue reflects the genetic makeup of the fetus (Gilbert, 2011).

CVS procedures can be accomplished transcervically or transabdominally. In transcervical sampling a sterile catheter is introduced into the cervix under continuous ultrasonographic guidance, and a small portion of the chorionic villi is aspirated with a syringe. The aspiration cannula and obturator must be placed at a suitable site, and rupture of the amniotic sac must be avoided (see Fig. 26-7). The transcervical procedure is contraindicated if a cervical infection such as chlamydia or herpes is present (Gilbert, 2011).

If the abdominal approach is used, an 18- or 20-gauge spinal needle with stylet is inserted under sterile conditions through the abdominal wall into the chorion frondosum under ultrasound guidance. The stylet is then withdrawn, and the chorionic tissue is aspirated into a syringe (see Fig. 26-8).

BOX 26-6 Elimination of Maternal Age as an Indication for Invasive Prenatal Diagnosis

Maternal age of 35 years and older has been a standard indication for invasive prenatal testing since 1979. However, because most genetically abnormal children are born to parents of varying ages who have no history of abnormality, genetic screening is now recommended for all women, regardless of age (Gilbert, 2011). The American College of Obstetricians and Gynecologists (ACOG) published guidelines in 2007 (and reaffirmed them in 2011) stating that no specific age should be used as a threshold for invasive or noninvasive screening. Furthermore, all women, regardless of age, should have the option of invasive testing without first having screening (ACOG, 2011).

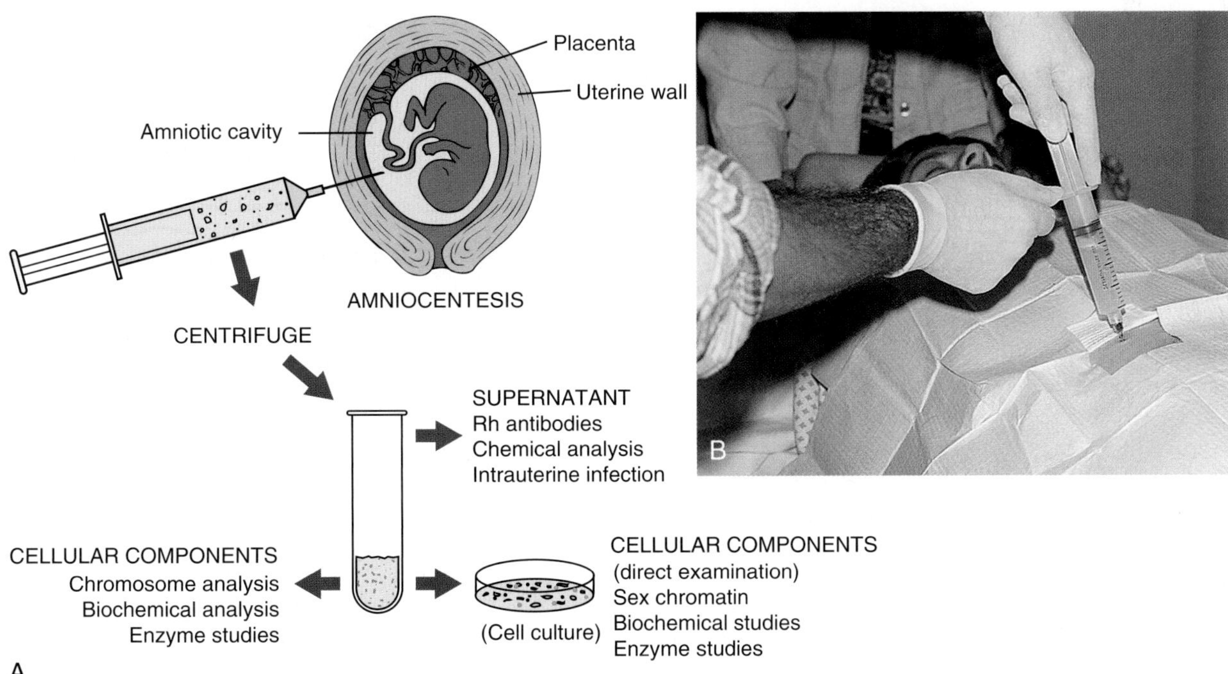

FIG 26-6 A, Amniocentesis and laboratory use of amniotic fluid aspirant. B, Transabdominal amniocentesis. (B, Courtesy Marjorie Pyle, RNC, Lifecircle, Costa Mesa, CA.)

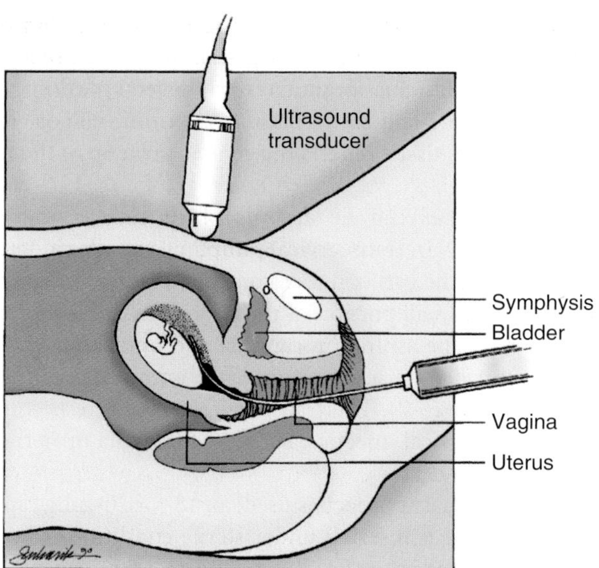

FIG 26-7 Transcervical chorionic villus sampling. (From Gabbe, S., Niebyl, J., & Simpson, J. [2012]. *Obstetrics: Normal and problem pregnancies* [6th ed.]. Philadelphia: Saunders.)

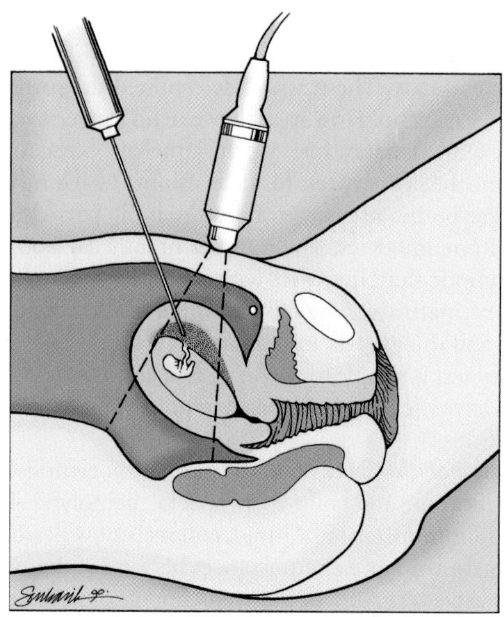

FIG 26-8 Transabdominal chorionic villus sampling. (From Gabbe, S., Niebyl, J., & Simpson, J. [2012]. *Obstetrics: Normal and problem pregnancies* [6th ed.]. Philadelphia: Saunders.)

CVS is a relatively safe procedure. The incidence of IUGR, placental abruption, and preterm birth is no higher in women undergoing CVS than would be expected in the general population. In the early 1990s there was controversy concerning an increased risk for fetal limb reduction defects associated with CVS. However, the consensus of further studies is that when CVS is performed after 9 completed weeks of gestation, the risk for limb reduction defects is no higher than it is in the general population (Simpson et al., 2012).

SAFETY ALERT

Because of the possibility of fetomaternal hemorrhage, women who are Rh negative should receive Rh_oD immune globulin after CVS to prevent isoimmunization, regardless of whether the procedure is performed transcervically or transabdominally, unless the fetus is known to be Rh negative (Simpson et al., 2012).

Use of amniocentesis and CVS is declining because of advances in noninvasive screening techniques. These techniques include measurement of NT, maternal serum screening tests in the first and second trimesters, and ultrasonography in the second trimester. A recently available assessment method, cell-free deoxyribonucleic acid (DNA) screening, can be performed as early as 10 weeks of gestation, therefore providing mothers information sooner in the pregnancy to aid in decision making regarding further testing (see later discussion and the Evidence-Based Practice box).

Percutaneous Umbilical Blood Sampling

Direct access to the fetal circulation during the second and third trimesters is possible through percutaneous umbilical blood sampling (PUBS) (also called *cordocentesis*). PUBS can be used for fetal blood sampling and transfusion. However, PUBS has been replaced in many centers by placental biopsy because it is a safer, easier, and faster alternative. Improvements in cytogenetic and molecular diagnostic testing have decreased the need for fetal blood samples. Many tests that were once performed using fetal blood can now be done using DNA-based analysis of chorionic villi (Simpson et al., 2012).

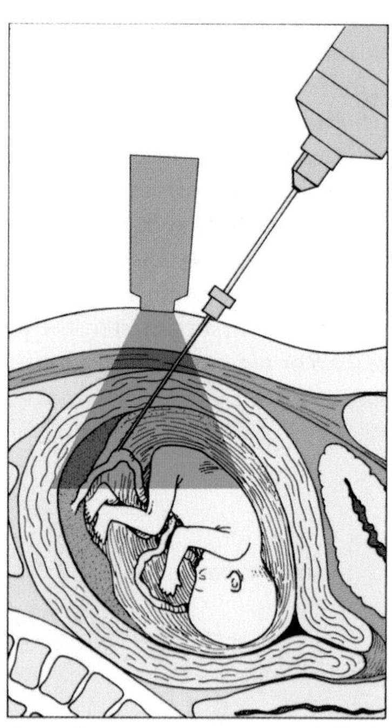

FIG 26-9 Technique for percutaneous umbilical blood sampling guided by ultrasound.

PUBS involves the insertion of a needle directly into a fetal umbilical vessel, preferably the vein, under ultrasound guidance. Ideally the umbilical cord is punctured near its insertion into the placenta (Figs. 26-9 and 26-10). At this point the cord is well anchored and will not move, and the risk of maternal blood contamination (from the placenta) is slight. Generally a small amount of blood is removed and tested immediately by the Kleihauer-Betke procedure (Apt test) to ensure that it is fetal in origin (Simpson et al., 2012). The most common genetic indication for the use of PUBS is evaluation of mosaic results

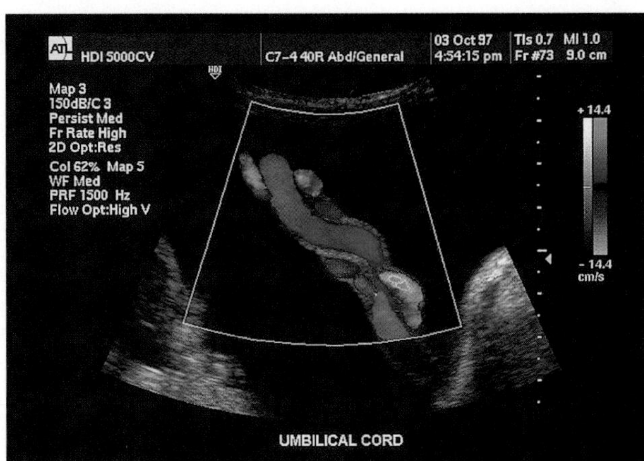

FIG 26-10 Umbilical cord as seen on ultrasound at 26 weeks of gestation. (Courtesy Advanced Technology Laboratories, Bothell, WA.)

found on amniocentesis or CVS, when a sample of fetal blood is required to determine the specific mutation. PUBS is also used to assess for fetal anemia, infection, and thrombocytopenia (Wapner, 2014). Complications that can occur include loss of the pregnancy, hematomas, bleeding from the puncture site in the umbilical cord, transient fetal bradycardia, and fetomaternal hemorrhage. Maternal complications are rare but include hemorrhage and transplacental hemorrhage (Simpson et al., 2012).

In fetuses at risk for isoimmune hemolytic anemia, PUBS permits precise identification of fetal blood type and RBC count and may prevent the need for further intervention. If the fetus is positive for the presence of maternal antibodies, a direct blood test can confirm the degree of anemia resulting from hemolysis. Intrauterine transfusion of severely anemic fetuses can be performed 4 to 5 weeks earlier than through the intraperitoneal route.

Follow-up includes continuous FHR monitoring for 1 to 2 hours after the procedure. Women should also be taught to count fetal movements at home (Gilbert, 2011) (see previous discussion and Fig. 26-1).

Maternal Assays

Alpha-Fetoprotein

Maternal serum alpha-fetoprotein (AFP) levels are used as a screening tool for NTDs in pregnancy. Through this technique approximately 80% to 85% of all open NTDs and open abdominal wall defects can be detected early. Screening is recommended for all pregnant women.

The cause of NTDs is not well understood, but 95% of all affected infants are born to women with no family history of similar anomalies (Wapner, 2014). The defect occurs in approximately 1 in 1000 live births. Risk factors for NTDs include a history of this disorder in a prior pregnancy, folic acid deficiency, pregestational diabetes, and teratogen exposure (e.g., valproic acid [Depakote], carbamazepine [Tegretol]) (Wolf, 2014).

AFP is produced in the fetal gastrointestinal tract and liver, and increasing levels are detectable in the serum of pregnant women from 14 to 34 weeks of gestation. Although amniotic fluid AFP measurement is diagnostic for NTD, maternal serum AFP is a screening tool only. Maternal serum AFP (MSAFP) screening can be performed with reasonable reliability any time between 15 and 20 weeks of gestation (16 to 18 weeks being ideal) (Wapner, 2014).

Once the maternal level of AFP is determined, it is compared with normal values for each week of gestation. Values also should be correlated with maternal age, weight, race, presence of a multifetal pregnancy, and whether the woman has insulin-dependent diabetes. Until recently, an amniocentesis to obtain fluid for determining amniotic fluid AFP and acetylcholinesterase levels was recommended as standard follow-up testing when the AFP level in maternal serum was found to be elevated. A targeted ultrasound performed by an experienced sonographer, however, has since been shown to be as sensitive and specific for identifying NTDs as the amniotic fluid AFP and acetylcholinesterase measurements, which require invasive testing via amniocentesis (Wapner, 2014).

Multiple Marker Screens

Screening to detect fetal chromosomal abnormalities, particularly trisomy 21 (Down syndrome) is available, beginning in the first trimester of pregnancy at 11 to 14 weeks of gestation (Cunningham et al., 2014). This first-trimester screen includes measurement of two maternal biochemical markers, pregnancy-associated placental protein (PAPP-A) and human chorionic gonadotropin (hCG) or the free beta-human chorionic gonadotropin (β-hCG) subunit, and evaluation of fetal nuchal translucency (NT), or a combination of both. In the presence of a fetus with trisomy 21, hCG levels are higher than normal in the first trimester, whereas PAPP-A levels are lower than normal. First-trimester screening using PAPP-A and hCG or β-hCG levels has been shown to be as accurate for detecting fetuses with trisomy 21 as triple screening in the second trimester (Cunningham et al., 2014; Wapner, 2014). Another biochemical marker that can be measured during the first trimester, at 8 to 10 weeks of gestation, is a disintegrin and metalloproteinase 12 (ADAM 12), a glycoprotein that is synthesized by the placenta and secreted throughout pregnancy. Decreased levels of ADAM 12 are found in women carrying a fetus with trisomy 21 (Wapner).

About one third of all fetuses with an increased NT have a chromosomal abnormality; half of these are trisomy 21. Combining the serum marker and NT values results in the detection of Down syndrome in 79% to 87% of cases. These results are comparable to those obtained with quad screening (see discussion following) in the second trimester (Cunningham et al., 2014).

Assessment of the fetal nasal bone by ultrasound during the first trimester provides another way to predict trisomy 21. The nasal bone cannot be identified on ultrasound in about one third to one quarter of fetuses who have trisomy 21 (Wapner, 2014).

In the second trimester triple screening and quad screening are available to screen for fetuses with trisomy 21 and trisomy 18. The triple-marker screen, performed at 16 to 18 weeks of gestation, measures the levels of three maternal serum markers: MSAFP, unconjugated estriol, and hCG. In the presence of a fetus with trisomy 21 the MSAFP and unconjugated estriol levels are low, whereas the hCG level is elevated. Low values in all three markers are associated with trisomy 18 (Cunningham et al., 2014).

The quad screen adds an additional marker, a placental hormone called inhibin A, to increase the accuracy of screening for Down syndrome in women less than 35 years of age.

EVIDENCE-BASED PRACTICE

Cell-Free Fetal DNA Testing for Trisomies

Ask the Question

For women at risk for trisomies or sex chromosome aneuploidies, is there a noninvasive screening test?

Search for the Evidence

Search Strategies English language research-based publications since 2011 on noninvasive prenatal screening, cell-free fetal DNA, trisomy, and aneuploidy were included.

Databases Used Cochrane Collaborative Database, National Guideline Clearinghouse (AHRQ), CINAHL, PubMed, UpToDate, and the professional websites for ACOG and AWHONN

Critical Appraisal of the Evidence

In the past, women at risk for genetic abnormality had the option of screening of maternal blood for serum analytes ("triple screen"), with or without ultrasound for nuchal translucency, an early visible marker for trisomy 21. These combinations had a detection rate ranging from 50% to 95% (Gregg, Gross, Best, et al., 2013). More diagnostic testing, such as chorionic villus sampling and amniocentesis, are definitive but invasive.

- Introduced as a noninvasive pregnancy screening test, cell-free fetal DNA (cffDNA) testing isolates fetal DNA fragments from maternal blood to determine sex and screen for trisomies 21, 18, and 13 with an excellent negative predictive value, high detection rate, and a lower false-positive rate (Mersy, Smits, van Winden, et al., 2013).
- In addition, testing for sex chromosome aneuploidies, such as Turner (45X) and Klinefelter (45XXY), is available at some laboratories (Gregg et al., 2013). Knowing the sex early can also assist in screening for sex chromosome–linked diseases, such as hemophilia and Duchenne muscular dystrophy (Colmant, Morin-Surroca, Fuchs, et al., 2013).
- Offered at 10 to 20 weeks of gestation, cffDNA has limited sensitivity in the presence of a high body mass index. In addition, it may reflect placental DNA, which may have mosaicism and differ from the true fetal karyotype. A "vanishing twin" may confound the results. For these reasons professional recommendations advocate that in the event of abnormal cffDNA results, direct fetal DNA sampling using invasive techniques be used for confirmation (Gregg et al., 2013; Langlois, Brock, Genetics Committee et al., 2013).
- First-trimester ultrasound is still the gold standard for identifying nuchal translucency, multiple fetuses, placental abnormalities, and congenital abnormalities. Maternal blood test for alpha-fetoprotein, although variable in sensitivity, is still recommended at 15 to 20 weeks of gestation as a screening test for open neural tube defects (Gregg et al., 2013).

Apply the Evidence: Nursing Implications

- Earlier screening for trisomies provides pregnant women with either earlier reassurance of a normal fetus or earlier chance to adjust to abnormality. The timing allows for the option for a less risky first trimester termination.
- Pretest counseling recommendations include the benefits and limitations of cffDNA testing. This includes the recommendation for further diagnostic testing using invasive techniques, prior to any irrevocable obstetric decisions (Gregg et al., 2013; Langlois et al., 2013).
- Women and families may need help sorting out the bewildering array of tests available during pregnancy. Tests are only useful if they provide usable information, so health care providers should have knowledge and information ready to assist clients for all possible test result outcomes.
- This test may help women avoid routine invasive procedures, a cost savings. However, cffDNA is expensive, running up to $2,000 or more. As with all new tests, much research and discussion are needed regarding cost analysis, appropriate population, and economic justice.
- Ethical debates will undoubtedly multiply with the eventual availability of more prenatal genetic testing, including whole-genome sequencing.

Quality and Safety Competencies: Evidence-Based Practice (EBP)*

Knowledge

Describe how the strength and relevance of available evidence influences the choice of interventions in provision of client-centered care.

Health care teams use systematic analysis and professional recommendations to address the meaning of changing prenatal testing options.

Skills

Participate in structuring the work environment to facilitate integration of new evidence into standards of practice.

Pretest counseling provides appropriate and realistic expectations for pregnant women and their families.

Attitudes

Value the concept of EBP as integral to determining best clinical practices.

EBP guides prenatal testing practice so that women get meaningful, actionable, and affordable testing.

DNA, Deoxyribonucleic acid.

References

Colmant, C., Morin-Surroca, M., Fuchs, F., et al. (2013). Non-invasive prenatal testing for fetal sex determination: Is ultrasound still relevant? *European Journal of Obstetrical, Gynecological and Reproductive Biology, 171*(2), 197–204.

Gregg, A. R., Gross, S. J., Best, R. G., et al. (2013). American College of Medical Genetics and Genomics statement on noninvasive prenatal screening for fetal aneuploidy. *Genetics in Medicine, 15*(5), 395–398.

Langlois, S., Brock, J. A., Genetics Committee, et al. (2013). Current status of non-invasive prenatal detection of Down syndrome, trisomy 18, and trisomy 13 using cell-free DNA in maternal plasma. *Journal of Obstetrics and Gynaecology of Canada, 5*(2), 177–181.

Mersy, E., Smits, L. J., van Winden, L. A., et al. (2013). Noninvasive detection of fetal trisomy 21: A systematic review and report of quality and outcomes of diagnostic accuracy studies performed between 1997 and 2012. *Human Reproduction Update, 19*(4), 318–329.

Pat Mahaffee Gingrich

*Adapted from QSEN at www.qsen.org.

DNA, Deoxyribonucleic acid.

Elevated inhibin A levels indicate the possibility of Down syndrome (Cunningham et al., 2014; Wapner, 2014). The addition of inhibin A to the other three markers increases the detection rate for Down syndrome to about 75% in women who are less than 35 years old and to more than 80% in women 35 years of age or older (Simpson et al., 2012). Similar to triple marker screening, the optimal time to perform the quad screen is between 16 and 18 weeks of gestation (Wapner).

The ability of multiple marker tests to detect chromosomal abnormalities depends on the accuracy of gestational age assessment. These tests are screening procedures only and are not diagnostic. A positive screening test result indicates an increased risk but is not diagnostic of trisomy 21 or another chromosome abnormality. Women with positive screening results should be offered diagnostic testing by amniocentesis or CVS for fetal karyotyping (Cunningham et al., 2014).

Coombs' Test

The indirect Coombs' test is a screening tool for Rh incompatibility. If the maternal titer for Rh antibodies is greater than 1:8, amniocentesis for determination of bilirubin in amniotic fluid is indicated to establish the severity of fetal hemolytic anemia. However, middle cerebral artery Doppler studies to determine the degree of fetal hemolysis have almost entirely replaced serial amniocentesis (see earlier discussion) (Moise, 2012). The Coombs' test can also detect other antibodies that may place the fetus at risk for incompatibility with maternal antigens.

Cell-Free DNA Screening in Maternal Blood

A screening method for noninvasive prenatal genetic diagnosis (noninvasive prenatal testing [NIPT]) is now available for use in the clinical setting. Cell-free DNA screening already provides a definitive diagnosis noninvasively for fetal Rh status, fetal gender, and certain paternally transmitted single gene disorders (Cunningham et al., 2014; Simpson et al., 2012).

The method works by amplifying cell-free DNA. If the fetus has a normal karyotype, the amount of DNA is consistent with the known standard for the normal amount. For example, if more than the expected amount of chromosome 21 DNA is detected, it can then be assumed that the fetus is contributing the extra amount and therefore has trisomy 21. The same is true for trisomies 13 and 18. The test cannot actually distinguish fetal from maternal DNA, but it can accurately predict the fetal status by measuring the amount of DNA circulating in maternal blood and comparing it with known standards. The cell-free DNA screen in combination with ultrasound does not provide a definitive diagnosis for all cases of fetal trisomy 21. Women who have a positive cell-free circulating DNA test without confirming ultrasound findings or a negative blood screen with abnormal ultrasound findings require invasive diagnostic testing such as amniocentesis or CVS for a definitive diagnosis (Palomaki, Kloza, Lambert-Messerlian, et al., 2011) (see Evidence-Based Practice box).

Circulating cell-free DNA studies for the detection of fetal chromosomal abnormalities can be performed as early as 10 weeks of gestation. The test is offered to women considered to be at risk for chromosomal abnormalities, including those with advanced maternal age, screen-positive maternal serum screens, or ultrasound abnormalities. Women who have previously given birth to a child with a chromosomal abnormality are also candidates for the screen (Cunningham et al., 2014). It is simple to perform; a sample of maternal blood is obtained by venipuncture and sent to a commercial laboratory. Results are usually available in about 10 business days. The screen has been shown to be 98% effective at detecting trisomy 21 and 99% effective at detecting trisomy 13 or 18. In less than 1% of cases no result is available because not enough DNA was retrieved to perform the screen (Palomaki et al., 2011; Palomaki, Deciu, Kloza, et al., 2012).

FETAL CARE CENTERS

With developing technology, diagnosis and subsequent treatment options exist for some fetal anomalies. Fetal care centers have evolved in response to the need to provide diagnostic and therapeutic options as well as support services for families with a fetal anomaly diagnosis (ACOG, 2011). ACOG and the American Academy of Pediatrics (AAP) recommend that these families have access to support services such as genetic counseling, social work, chaplain services, a palliative care team, and ethics consultation because of the complex emotional stressors they face. Care coordination is critical for the successful management of high risk pregnancies. The majority of fetal care centers has a staff member, often a nurse, who coordinates care and assists the family in navigating multiple appointments with obstetric and pediatric providers.

ANTEPARTUM ASSESSMENT USING ELECTRONIC FETAL MONITORING

Indications

First- and second-trimester antepartum assessment is directed primarily at the diagnosis of fetal anomalies. The goal of third-trimester testing is to determine whether the intrauterine environment continues to support the fetus. The testing is often used to determine the timing of childbirth for women at risk for uteroplacental insufficiency (UPI). Gradual loss of placental function results first in inadequate nutrient delivery to the fetus, leading to IUGR. Subsequently, respiratory function also is compromised, resulting in fetal hypoxia. Evidence-based recommendations for condition-specific testing schemes in cases of identified risk factors have been difficult to develop and often do not exist. There is no ideal single test or testing strategy for all high risk pregnancies (Greenberg et al., 2012).

However, there is evidence to support antepartum assessment using electronic fetal monitoring in pregnancies complicated by the risk factors listed in Box 26-7. Currently the NST and the mBPP are the primary methods used for antepartum fetal evaluation in high risk women at most sites. The complete BPP and the contraction stress test are used for follow-up evaluation in women who have a persistently nonreactive NST or mBPP. Traditionally testing has begun at 32 to 34 weeks of gestation, with earlier initiation of testing recommended for women with multiple high risk conditions. Testing is usually performed once or twice weekly (Greenberg et al., 2012).

Nonstress Test

The nonstress test (NST) is the most widely applied technique for antepartum evaluation of the fetus. The basis for the NST is that the normal fetus produces characteristic heart rate patterns in response to fetal movement, uterine contractions, or stimulation. In the term fetus, accelerations are associated with movement more than 85% of the time (Greenberg et al., 2012). The most common reason for the absence of FHR accelerations is the quiet fetal sleep state. However, medications such as narcotics, barbiturates, and beta-blockers; maternal smoking; and the presence of fetal malformations can also adversely affect the test (Gilbert, 2011; Greenberg et al.). The NST can be performed easily and quickly in an outpatient setting because it is noninvasive, easy to perform and interpret, and relatively inexpensive and has no known contraindications. Disadvantages include the requirement for twice-weekly testing and a high false-positive rate. The test also is slightly less sensitive in detecting fetal compromise than the contraction stress test or the BPP (Greenberg et al.; Miller et al., 2013).

BOX 26-7 Indications for Fetal Assessment Using Electronic Fetal Monitoring

- Diabetes
- Hypertension
- Intrauterine growth restriction
- Multiple gestation
- Oligohydramnios
- Intrahepatic cholestasis
- Renal disease
- Decreased fetal movement
- Previous fetal death
- Postterm pregnancy
- Systemic lupus erythematosus

Data from Greenberg, M., Druzin, M., & Gabbe, S. (2012). Antepartum fetal evaluation. In S. Gabbe, J. Niebyl, & J. Simpson (Eds.), *Obstetrics: Normal and problem pregnancies* (6th ed.). Philadelphia: Saunders.

Procedure

The woman is seated in a reclining chair (or in semi-Fowler position) with a slight lateral tilt to optimize uterine perfusion and prevent supine hypotension. The FHR is recorded with a Doppler transducer, and a tocodynamometer is applied to detect uterine contractions or fetal movements. The tracing is observed for signs of fetal activity and a concurrent acceleration of FHR. If evidence of fetal movement is not apparent on the tracing, the woman may be asked to depress a button on a handheld event marker connected to the monitor when she feels fetal movement. The movement is then noted on the tracing. Because almost all accelerations are accompanied by fetal movement, the movements need not be recorded for the test to be considered reactive. The test is usually completed within 20 to 30 minutes, but more time may be required if the fetus must be awakened from a sleep state.

Care providers sometimes suggest that the woman drink orange juice or be given glucose to increase her blood sugar level and thereby stimulate fetal movements. Although this practice is common, there is no evidence that it increases fetal activity (Greenberg et al., 2012).

Vibroacoustic stimulation (see later discussion) is often used to stimulate fetal activity if the initial NST result is nonreactive and thus possibly shortens the time required to complete the test (Greenberg et al., 2012).

Interpretation

NST results are either reactive (Fig. 26-11) or nonreactive (Fig. 26-12). Box 26-8 lists criteria for both results.

A nonreactive test requires further evaluation. The testing period is often extended, usually for an additional 20 minutes, with the expectation that the fetal sleep state will change and the test will become reactive. During this time vibroacoustic stimulation (see later discussion) may be used to stimulate fetal activity. If the test does not meet the criteria after 40 minutes, a BPP usually is performed. Once NST testing is initiated, it is usually repeated once or twice weekly for the remainder of the pregnancy (Greenberg et al., 2012).

Vibroacoustic Stimulation

Vibroacoustic stimulation (also called the *fetal acoustic stimulation test [FAST]*) is another method of testing antepartum FHR response. This test is generally performed in conjunction

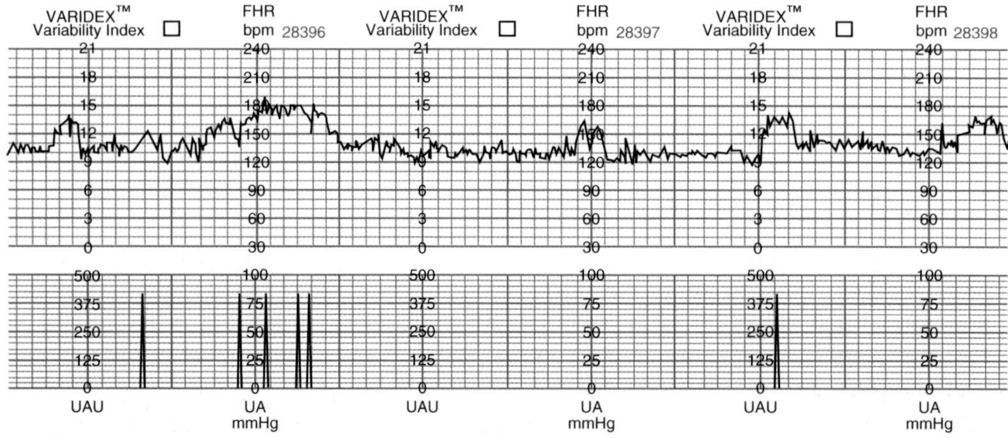

FIG 26-11 Reactive nonstress test. (From Gabbe, S., Niebyl, J., & Simpson, J. [2012]. *Obstetrics: Normal and problem pregnancies* [6th ed.]. Philadelphia: Saunders.)

with the NST and uses a combination of sound and vibration to stimulate the fetus. Whether the acoustic or the vibratory component alters the fetal state is unclear. The fetus is monitored for 5 minutes before stimulation to obtain a baseline FHR. If the fetal baseline pattern is nonreactive, the sound source (usually a laryngeal stimulator) is then activated for 3 seconds on the maternal abdomen over the fetal head. The desired result is a reactive NST, which usually occurs within 3 minutes of stimulation. The accelerations produced may have a significant increase in duration (Fig. 26-13). The test may be repeated at 1-minute intervals up to 3 times when no response is noted. Further evaluation is needed with BPP or contraction stress test if the pattern remains nonreactive (Greenberg et al., 2012).

BOX 26-8 Interpretation of the Nonstress Test

Reactive test: Two accelerations in a 20-minute period, each lasting at least 15 seconds and peaking at least 15 beats/min above the baseline. (Before 32 weeks of gestation, an acceleration is defined as a rise of at least 10 beats/min lasting at least 10 seconds from onset to offset; see Fig. 26-11.)

Nonreactive test: A test that does not demonstrate at least two qualifying accelerations within a 20-minute window (see Fig. 26-12)

From Miller, L., Miller, D., & Tucker, S. (2013). *Mosby's pocket guide to fetal monitoring: A multidisciplinary approach* (7th ed.). St. Louis: Mosby.

Contraction Stress Test

The contraction stress test (CST) or *oxytocin challenge test (OCT)* was the first widely used electronic fetal assessment test. It was devised as a graded stress test of the fetus, and its purpose was to identify the jeopardized fetus that was stable at rest but showed evidence of compromise after stress. Uterine contractions decrease uterine blood flow and placental perfusion. If this decrease is sufficient to produce hypoxia in the fetus, a deceleration in FHR results.

! NURSING ALERT

In a healthy fetoplacental unit uterine contractions do not usually produce late decelerations, whereas if underlying UPI exists, contractions produce late decelerations.

The CST provides an earlier warning of fetal compromise than the NST and produces fewer false-positive results. However, the CST is more time consuming and expensive than the

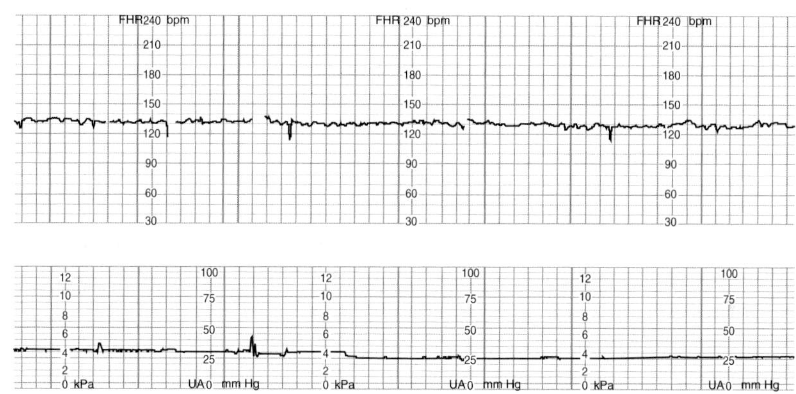

FIG 26-12 Segment of nonreactive nonstress test in term pregnancy. The lack of accelerations meeting minimum criteria continued for 40 minutes. (From Miller, L., Miller, D., & Tucker, S. [2013]. *Mosby's pocket guide to fetal monitoring: A multidisciplinary approach* [7th ed.]. St. Louis: Mosby.)

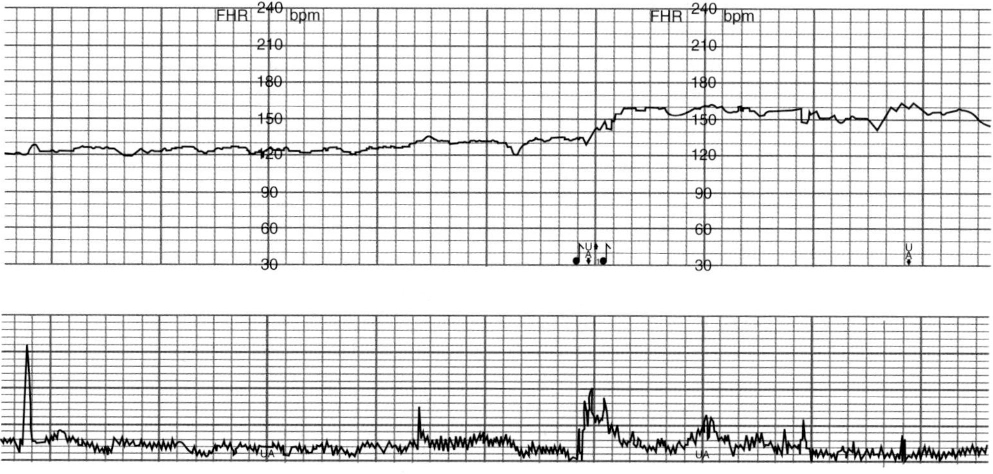

FIG 26-13 Reactive nonstress test after vibroacoustic stimulation. The stimulus was applied at the point marked by the musical notes. A sustained fetal heart rate acceleration was produced. *FHR,* Fetal heart rate. (From Gabbe, S., Niebyl, J., & Simpson, J. [2012]. *Obstetrics: Normal and problem pregnancies* [6th ed.]. Philadelphia: Saunders.)

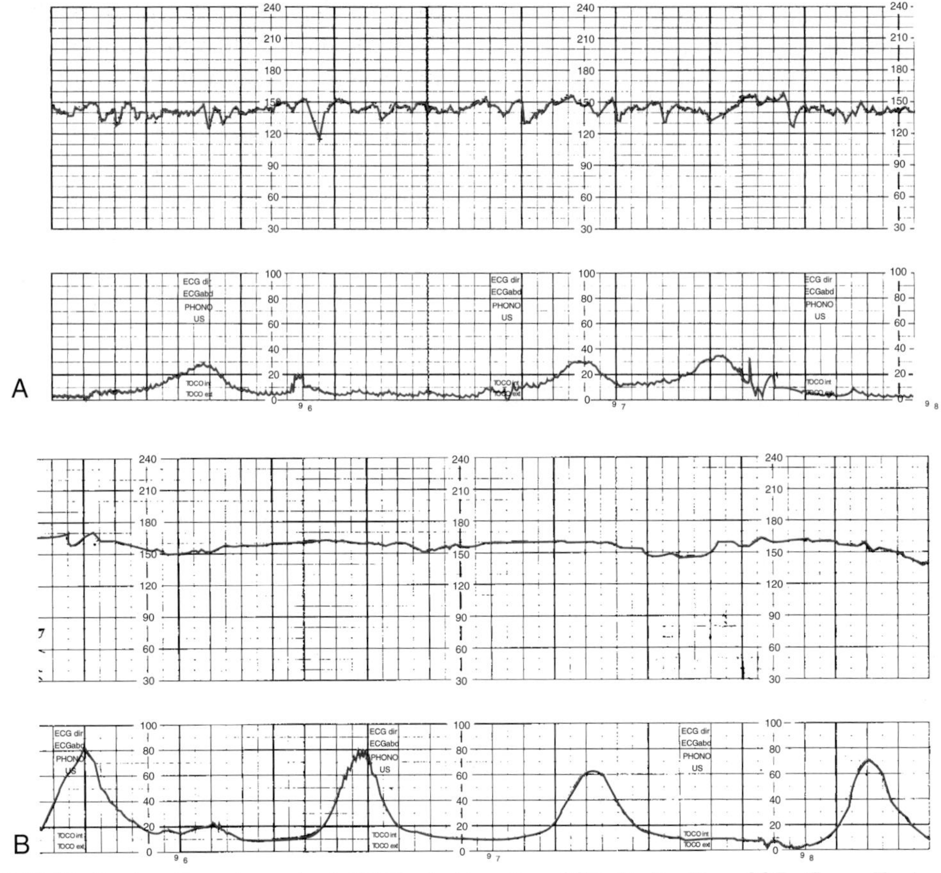

FIG 26-14 Contraction stress test (CST). **A**, Negative CST. **B**, Positive CST. (From Tucker, S. [2004]. *Pocket guide to fetal monitoring and assessment* [5th ed.]. St. Louis: Mosby.)

NST. It is also an invasive procedure if oxytocin stimulation is required. In general, the CST cannot be performed on women who should not give birth vaginally at the time the test is done. Absolute contraindications for the CST are the following: preterm labor, placenta previa, vasa previa, reduced cervical competence, multiple gestations, and previous classic incision for cesarean birth (Miller et al., 2013). Because of these disadvantages, the CST is used infrequently.

Procedure

The woman is placed in semi-Fowler position or sits in a reclining chair with a slight lateral tilt to optimize uterine perfusion and avoid supine hypotension. She is monitored electronically with the fetal ultrasound transducer and uterine tocodynamometer. The tracing is observed for 10 to 20 minutes for baseline rate and variability and the possible occurrence of spontaneous contractions. The two methods of CST are the nipple-stimulated contraction test and the more commonly used oxytocin-stimulated contraction test.

Nipple-Stimulated Contraction Test. Several methods of nipple stimulation have been described. In one approach the woman applies warm, moist washcloths to both breasts for several minutes. She is then asked to massage one nipple for 10 minutes. Massaging the nipple causes a release of oxytocin from the posterior pituitary. An alternative approach is for her to massage one nipple through her clothes for 2 minutes, rest for 5 minutes, and repeat the cycles of massage and rest as necessary to achieve adequate uterine activity. When adequate contractions or hyperstimulation (defined as uterine contractions lasting more than 90 seconds or five or more contractions in 10 minutes) occur, stimulation should be stopped.

Oxytocin-Stimulated Contraction Test. Exogenous oxytocin also can be used to stimulate uterine contractions. An intravenous (IV) infusion is begun, and a dilute solution of oxytocin (e.g., 30 units in 500 ml of fluid) is infused into the tubing of the main IV line through a piggyback port and delivered by an infusion pump to ensure an accurate dose. One method of oxytocin infusion is to begin at 0.5 milliunits/min and double the dose every 20 minutes until three uterine contractions of moderate intensity, each lasting 40 to 60 seconds, are observed within a 10-minute period. These criteria for contractions were selected to approximate the stress experienced by the fetus during the first stage of labor (Greenberg et al., 2012).

Interpretation

CST results are negative, positive, equivocal, suspicious, or unsatisfactory. If no late decelerations are observed with the contractions, the findings are considered negative (Fig. 26-14, *A*). Repetitive late decelerations render the test results positive (see Fig. 26-14, *B*). Table 26-5 lists criteria for each possible test result and the clinical significance of each.

The desired CST result is negative because it has consistently been associated with good fetal outcomes. The likelihood of fetal death occurring within 1 week of a negative CST is less than 1 in 1000 (Greenberg et al., 2012). Positive CST results

TABLE 26-5 Interpretation of the Contraction Stress Test

INTERPRETATION	CLINICAL SIGNIFICANCE
Negative	
At least three uterine contractions in a 10-minute period, with no late or significant variable decelerations	Usually resume routine weekly testing schedule
Positive	
Late decelerations occur with 50% or more of contractions, even if there are fewer than three contractions in 10 minutes	Usually warrants hospital admission for further evaluation and/or delivery
Suspicious or Equivocal	
Prolonged, variable, or late decelerations occurring with less than 50% of the contractions	Repeat testing next day
Equivocal-Hyperstimulatory	
Decelerations that occur in the presence of contractions more frequent than every 2 minutes or lasting longer than 90 seconds	Repeat testing next day
Unsatisfactory	
Failure to produce three contractions within a 10-minute window or inability to trace the fetal heart rate	Repeat test next day

From Miller, L., Miller, D., & Tucker, S. (2013). *Mosby's pocket guide to fetal monitoring: A multidisciplinary approach* (7th ed.). St. Louis: Mosby.

have been associated with intrauterine fetal death, late FHR decelerations in labor, IUGR, and meconium-stained amniotic fluid. A positive CST result usually leads to hospitalization for further close observation or birth. Unsatisfactory, suspicious, and equivocal tests must be repeated within 24 hours (Miller et al., 2013).

PSYCHOLOGIC CONSIDERATIONS RELATED TO HIGH RISK PREGNANCY

Once a pregnancy has been identified as high risk, the pregnant woman and her fetus are monitored carefully throughout the remainder of the pregnancy. All women who undergo antepartum assessments are at risk for real and potential problems and may feel anxious. In most instances the tests are ordered because of suspected fetal compromise, deterioration of a maternal condition, or both. In the third trimester, pregnant women are most concerned about protecting themselves and their fetuses and consider themselves most vulnerable to outside influences. The label of *high risk* often increases this sense of vulnerability.

When a woman is diagnosed with a high risk pregnancy, she and her family will likely experience stress related to the diagnosis. The woman may exhibit various psychologic responses, including anxiety, low self-esteem, guilt, frustration, and inability to function. A high risk pregnancy can also affect parental attachment, accomplishment of the tasks of pregnancy, and family adaptation to the pregnancy. If the woman is fearful for her well-being, she may continue to feel ambivalent about the pregnancy or may not accept its reality. She may not be able to complete preparations for the baby or go to childbirth classes if she is placed on restricted activity at home or hospitalized. The family may become frustrated because they cannot engage in activities that prepare them for parenthood. The nurse can help the woman and her family regain control and balance in their lives by providing support and encouragement, information about the pregnancy problem and its management, and opportunities to make as many choices as possible about the woman's care.

NURSES' ROLE IN ASSESSMENT AND MANAGEMENT OF THE HIGH RISK PREGNANCY

Nursing interventions for all pregnant women include education, anticipatory planning, counseling for family adaptation, assessment, and planning of appropriate interventions. Providing care to women facing a high risk pregnancy draws on nurses' unique knowledge in understanding the physiologic and psychosocial needs when a pregnancy is complicated by a maternal or fetal issue. Along with receiving a diagnosis of a maternal or fetal health concern, mothers may experience loss and grief, increased stress, uncertainty, information needs, and decision-making dilemmas (Lalor, Begley, & Galavan, 2009).

High risk pregnancies are often accompanied by additional testing and procedures. In these situations the nurse's role is one of educator and supporter as women undergo procedures such as ultrasonography, MRI, CVS, PUBS, and amniocentesis. In some instances the nurse may assist the physician with the test or procedure. When educating the woman and her family, the nurse must explain the purpose of each test, how it is performed, and the difference between screening and diagnostic tests. The nurse must also be aware of potential moral and ethical implications associated with certain tests. For example, women and their families may need to make a decision about pregnancy termination based on test results.

In many settings nurses actually perform tests such as NSTs, CSTs, and BPPs; conduct an initial assessment; and begin necessary interventions for nonreassuring results. Nurses who perform these tests have had additional education and training and function under guidance of established protocols and in collaboration with obstetric providers. Client teaching, which is an integral component of this role, involves preparing the woman for the test, interpreting the findings, and providing psychosocial support when needed.

Women with high risk pregnancies will likely receive many different services from multiple care providers. For all childbearing families effective care management requires that disciplines cooperate, communicate, and collaborate to provide care that promotes the best possible outcomes for mothers and babies. This coordination of care is even more essential in meeting the needs of families who are dealing with the additional stressors associated with a high risk pregnancy (Barron, 2014).

KEY POINTS

- A high risk pregnancy is one in which the life or well-being of the mother or infant is jeopardized by a biophysical or psychosocial disorder coincident with or unique to pregnancy.
- Biophysical, sociodemographic, psychosocial, and environmental factors place the pregnancy and fetus or neonate at risk.
- Biophysical assessment techniques include DFMCs, ultrasonography, and MRI.
- Biochemical monitoring techniques include amniocentesis, PUBS, CVS, MSAFP, multiple marker screens, and cell-free DNA screening in maternal blood.
- Fetal care centers have evolved in response to the need to provide diagnostic and therapeutic options as well as care coordination and other support services for families with a fetal anomaly diagnosis.
- Reactive NSTs and negative CSTs suggest fetal well-being.
- Most assessment tests have some degree of risk for the mother and fetus and usually cause some anxiety for the woman and her family.
- The nurse's roles in assessment and management of the high risk pregnancy are primarily those of educator and support person.

REFERENCES

American College of Obstetricians and Gynecologists (ACOG). (2007). *Screening for fetal chromosomal abnormalities. Practice bulletin no. 77*. Washington, DC: ACOG.

American College of Obstetricians and Gynecologists (ACOG). (2009). *Ultrasonography in pregnancy. Practice bulletin no. 101*. Washington, DC: ACOG.

American College of Obstetricians and Gynecologists (ACOG). (2011). Maternal-fetal intervention and fetal care centers. *Obstetrics and Gynecology, 118*(2 Pt 1), 405–410.

American Institute of Ultrasound in Medicine (AIUM). (2012). *Prudent use in pregnancy*. Laurel, MD: AIUM.

Barron, M. L. (2014). Antenatal care. In K. Rice Simpson, & P. Creehan (Eds.), *AWHONN's perinatal nursing* (4th ed.). Philadelphia: Lippincott Williams & Wilkins.

Baschat, A., Galan, H., & Gabbe, S. (2012). Intrauterine growth restriction. In S. Gabbe J. Niebyl, & J. Simpson (Eds.), *Obstetrics: Normal and problem pregnancies* (6th ed.). Philadelphia: Saunders.

Chambers, C., & Scialli, A. R. (2014). Teratogenesis and environmental exposure. In R. K. Creasy, R. Resnik, J. D. Iams, et al. (Eds.), *Creasy and Resnik's maternal-fetal medicine: Principles and practice* (7th ed.). Philadelphia: Saunders.

Cunningham, F., Leveno, K., Bloom, S., et al. (2014). *Williams obstetrics* (24th ed.). New York: McGraw-Hill Education.

Francois, K., & Foley, M. (2012). Antepartum and postpartum hemorrhage. In S. Gabbe, J. Niebyl, & J. Simpson (Eds.), *Obstetrics: Normal and problem pregnancies* (6th ed.). Philadelphia: Saunders.

Gilbert, E. (2011). *Manual of high risk pregnancy & delivery* (5th ed.). St. Louis: Mosby.

Gilbert, W. (2012). Amniotic fluid disorders. In S. Gabbe, J. Niebyl, & J. Simpson (Eds.), *Obstetrics: Normal and problem pregnancies* (6th ed.). Philadelphia: Saunders.

Greenberg, M., Druzin, M., & Gabbe, S. (2012). Antepartum fetal evaluation. In S. Gabbe, J. Niebyl, & J. Simpson (Eds.), *Obstetrics: Normal and problem pregnancies* (6th ed.). Philadelphia: Saunders.

Kaimal, A. J. (2014). Assessment of fetal health. In R. K. Creasy, R. Resnik, J. D. Iams, et al. (Eds.), *Creasy and Resnik's maternal-fetal medicine: Principles and practice* (7th ed.). Philadelphia: Saunders.

Lalor, J., Begley, C., & Galavan, E. (2009). Recasting hope: A process of adaptation following fetal anomaly diagnosis. *Social Science & Medicine, 68*(3), 462–472.

Martin, J., Hamilton, B., Osterman, M., et al. (2013). Births: Final data for 2012. *National Vital Statistics Reports, 62*(9), 1–87.

Mercer, B. M. (2014). Assessment and induction of fetal pulmonary maturity. In R. K. Creasy, R. Resnik, J. D. Iams, et al. (Eds.), *Creasy and Resnik's maternal-fetal medicine: Principles and practice* (7th ed.). Philadelphia: Saunders.

Miller, L., Miller, D., & Tucker, S. (2013). *Mosby's pocket guide to fetal monitoring: A multidisciplinary approach* (7th ed.). St. Louis: Mosby.

Moise, K. (2012). Red cell alloimmunization. In S. Gabbe, J. Niebyl, & J. Simpson (Eds.), *Obstetrics: Normal and problem pregnancies* (6th ed.). Philadelphia: Saunders.

Palomaki, G. E., Deciu, C., Kloza, E. M., et al. (2012). DNA sequencing of maternal plasma reliably identifies trisomy 18 and trisomy 13 as well as Down syndrome: An international collaborative study. *Genetics in Medicine, 14*(3), 296–305.

Palomaki, G. E., Kloza, E. M., Lambert-Messerlia, G. M., et al. (2011). DNA sequencing of maternal plasma to detect Down syndrome: An international clinical validation. *Genetics in Medicine, 13*(11), 913–920.

Richards, D. (2012). Obstetrical ultrasound: Imaging, dating, and growth. In S. Gabbe, J. Niebyl, & J. Simpson (Eds.), *Obstetrics: Normal and problem pregnancies* (6th ed.). Philadelphia: Saunders.

Simpson, J., Richards, D., Otano, L., & Driscoll, D. (2012). Prenatal genetic diagnosis. In S. Gabbe, J. Niebyl, & J. Simpson (Eds.), *Obstetrics: Normal and problem pregnancies* (6th ed.). Philadelphia: Saunders.

Wapner, R. J. (2014). Prenatal diagnosis of congenital disorders. In R. K. Creasy, R. Resnik, J. D. Iams, et al. (Eds.), *Creasy and Resnik's maternal-fetal medicine: Principles and practice* (7th ed.). Philadelphia: Saunders.

Wolf, R. B. (2014). Skeletal imaging. In R. K. Creasy, R. Resnik, J. D. Iams, et al. (Eds.), *Creasy and Resnik's maternal-fetal medicine: Principles and practice* (7th ed.). Philadelphia: Saunders.

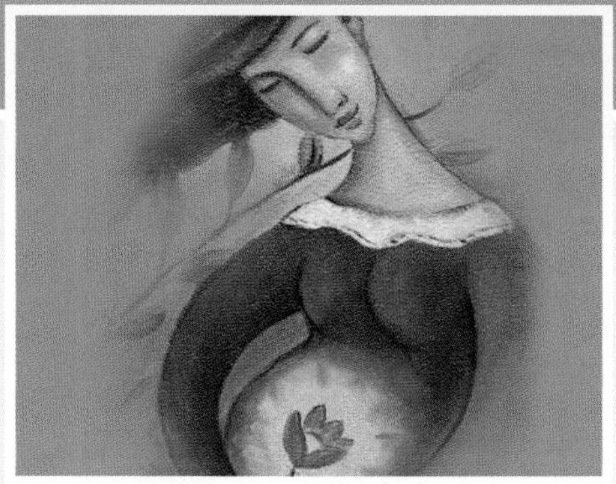

CHAPTER 27

Hypertensive Disorders

Dusty Dix

http://evolve.elsevier.com/Lowdermilk/MWHC/

LEARNING OBJECTIVES

- Differentiate among gestational hypertension, preeclampsia, and chronic hypertension.
- Describe etiologic theories and pathophysiology of preeclampsia.
- Compare care management of women with mild or severe gestational hypertension and preeclampsia with or without severe features.
- Describe appropriate nursing actions during and after an eclamptic seizure.
- Discuss the preconception, antepartum, intrapartum, and postpartum management of the woman with chronic hypertension.

Pregnancy-associated hypertensive disorders develop during pregnancy, labor, or after birth. These disorders include gestational hypertension and preeclampsia–eclampsia. Chronic hypertensive disorders precede pregnancy. Women with chronic hypertension can also develop superimposed preeclampsia. The classification, pathophysiologic changes, assessment, and management of pregnancy-associated hypertensive disorders are discussed in this chapter, with a primary focus on preeclampsia. The care of women with hypertensive disorders during the perinatal period requires a collaborative effort. Care management is directed toward early detection, thorough assessment, and timely intervention.

SIGNIFICANCE AND INCIDENCE

Hypertensive disorders are common medical complications of pregnancy, occurring in approximately 5% to 10% of all pregnancies. The incidence varies among hospitals, regions, and countries (Sibai, 2012). Hypertensive disorders are a major cause of perinatal morbidity and mortality worldwide, primarily related to uteroplacental insufficiency and premature birth (Backes, Markham, Moorehead, et al., 2011; Sibai). Perinatal outcomes are worse in women who have severe essential hypertension, early gestational hypertension, and preeclampsia with severe features (Duley, 2011). Preeclampsia is a significant risk factor for intrauterine growth restriction (IUGR) and fetal demise. The rate of stillbirth in women who have preeclampsia with severe features is 21 per 1000 (Backes et al., 2011).

In the United States and Canada hypertensive disorders are one of the top causes of maternal morbidity and mortality, related to renal failure, coagulopathy, cardiac or liver failure, placental abruption, seizures, and stroke (Duley, 2011; Harvey & Sibai, 2013). Of maternal deaths worldwide, 10% to 15% can be attributed to preeclampsia and eclampsia (Uzan, Carbonnel, Piconne, et al., 2011). Preeclampsia accounts for more than 50,000 maternal deaths worldwide each year. According to the World Health Organization, approximately one woman dies every 7 minutes from complications related to preeclampsia (Romero-Arauz, Morales-Borrego, García-Espinosa, & Peralta-Pedrero, 2012).

CLASSIFICATION

The classification of hypertensive disorders in pregnancy is confusing because standard definitions are not used consistently by all health care providers. The classification system most commonly used in the United States is based on recommendations from the American College of Obstetricians and Gynecologists (ACOG) (2002) and the National High Blood Pressure Education Program Working Group on High Blood Pressure in Pregnancy (Working Group) (2000). More recently, the ACOG convened a task force of experts in the management of hypertension in pregnancy. The Task Force on Hypertension in Pregnancy chose to continue use of this classification system, although it modified some of the system components (ACOG, 2013). The current classification system is summarized in Table 27-1.

Gestational Hypertension

Gestational hypertension is the onset of hypertension without proteinuria or other systemic findings diagnostic for preeclampsia after week 20 of pregnancy (ACOG, 2013). Hypertension is defined as a systolic blood pressure (BP) greater than

TABLE 27-1 Classification of Hypertensive States of Pregnancy

TYPE	DESCRIPTION
Gestational Hypertensive Disorders	
Gestational hypertension	Development of hypertension after week 20 of pregnancy in a previously normotensive woman without proteinuria or other systemic findings (see description of Preeclampsia below)
Preeclampsia	Development of hypertension and proteinuria in a previously normotensive woman after 20 weeks of gestation or in the early postpartum period. In the absence of proteinuria, the development of new-onset hypertension with the new onset of any of the following: thrombocytopenia, renal insufficiency, impaired liver function, pulmonary edema, or cerebral or visual symptoms
Eclampsia	Development of convulsions or coma not attributable to other causes in a preeclamptic woman
Chronic Hypertensive Disorders	
Chronic hypertension	Hypertension in pregnant woman present before pregnancy
Superimposed preeclampsia	Chronic hypertension in association with preeclampsia

Data from American College of Obstetricians and Gynecologists (ACOG). (2013). Executive summary: Hypertension in pregnancy. *Obstetrics and Gynecology, 122*(5), 1122-1131.

140 mm Hg or a diastolic BP greater than 90 mm Hg. The hypertension should be recorded on two occasions at least 4 hours apart after 20 weeks of gestation in a woman with a previously normal blood pressure (ACOG, 2013). Only one pressure (either systolic or diastolic) needs to be elevated to meet the definition of hypertension (Harvey & Sibai).

The definitions of gestational hypertension are the same as the definitions for blood pressure readings for preeclampsia (Table 27-2). Gestational hypertension does not persist longer than 12 weeks postpartum and usually resolves during the first postpartum week (Harvey & Sibai, 2013). Some women who are initially thought to have gestational hypertension are eventually diagnosed with chronic hypertension instead. Others go on to develop proteinuria or other systemic findings, thereby changing their diagnosis to preeclampsia.

Preeclampsia

Preeclampsia is a pregnancy-specific condition in which, traditionally, hypertension and proteinuria develop after 20 weeks of gestation in a woman who previously had neither condition. The signs and symptoms of preeclampsia also can develop for the first time during the postpartum period. The recent ACOG Task Force on Hypertension in Pregnancy eliminated proteinuria as a requirement for the diagnosis of preeclampsia (see Evidence-Based Practice box). Although proteinuria may still be used to diagnose preeclampsia, it is often difficult to collect a 24-hour urine sample for accurate measurement in a timely manner. In the absence of proteinuria preeclampsia may be defined as hypertension along with either thrombocytopenia, impaired liver function, the new development of renal insufficiency, pulmonary edema, or new-onset cerebral or visual disturbances (see Table 27-2) (ACOG, 2013). Table 27-3 lists common laboratory changes that occur in preeclampsia.

TABLE 27-2 Diagnostic Criteria for Preeclampsia and Preeclampsia with Severe Features

	PREECLAMPSIA	SEVERE FEATURES OF PREECLAMPSIA
Component		
Hypertension	Blood pressure (BP) reading ≥140/90 mm Hg × 2, at least 4 hours apart after 20 weeks of gestation in a previously normotensive woman	BP reading ≥160/110 mm Hg × 2, at least 4 hours apart while the client is on bed rest (unless antihypertensive therapy has already been initiated)
Proteinuria	Proteinuria of ≥300 mg in a 24-hr specimen Protein/creatinine ratio ≥0.3 (with each measured as mg/dl) ≥1+ on dipstick (used only if quantitative methods are not available	Massive proteinuria (>5 g in a 24-hr specimen) is no longer used as a diagnostic criterion
Thrombocytopenia	Platelet count <100,000/μL	Platelet count <100,000/μL
Impaired liver function	Elevated blood levels of liver transaminases to twice the normal concentration	Abnormally elevated blood concentrations of liver enzymes to twice the normal concentration; severe persistent epigastric or right upper quadrant pain unresponsive to medication and not accounted for by alternative diagnoses, or both
Renal insufficiency	New development of serum creatinine >1.1 mg/dl or a doubling of the serum creatinine concentration in the absence of other renal disease	Progressive renal insufficiency (serum creatinine concentration >1.1 mg/dl or a doubling of the serum creatinine concentration in the absence of other renal disease
Pulmonary edema		Present
Cerebral or visual disturbances		New onset

Modified from American College of Obstetricians and Gynecologists (ACOG). (2013). Executive summary: Hypertension in pregnancy. *Obstetrics and Gynecology, 122*(5), 1122-1131.

Eclampsia

Eclampsia is the onset of seizure activity or coma in a woman with preeclampsia who has no history of preexisting pathology that can result in seizure activity (Harvey & Sibai, 2013; Markham & Funai, 2014). In developed countries eclampsia occurs in approximately 1 of 2000 births (Duley, 2011). Although eclamptic seizures can occur before, during, or after birth, approximately 50% of cases occur during the antepartum period (Poole, 2014).

Chronic Hypertension

Chronic hypertension is defined as hypertension that is present before the pregnancy (ACOG, 2013). Hypertension initially diagnosed during pregnancy that persists longer than 12 weeks postpartum is also classified as chronic hypertension (Harvey & Sibai, 2013).

TABLE 27-3 Common Laboratory Changes in Preeclampsia

	NORMAL NONPREGNANT	PREECLAMPSIA	HELLP
Hemoglobin, hematocrit	12-16 g/dl, 37%-47%	May ↑	↓
Platelets (cells/mm³)	150,000-400,000/mm³	<100,000/mm³	<100,000/mm³
Prothrombin time (PT), partial thromboplastin time (PTT)	12-14 sec, 60-70 sec	Unchanged	Unchanged
Fibrinogen	200-400 mg/dl	300-600 mg/dl	↓
Fibrin split products (FSPs)	Absent	Absent or present	Present
Blood urea nitrogen (BUN)	10-20 mg/dl	↑	↑
Creatinine	0.5-1.1 mg/dl	>1.1 mg/dl	↑
Lactate dehydrogenase (LDH)*	45-90 units/l	↑	↑ (>600 units/L)
Aspartate aminotransferase (AST)	4-20 units/l	Elevated	↑ (>70 units/L)
Alanine aminotransferase (ALT)	3-21 units/l	Elevated	↑
Creatinine clearance	80-125 ml/min	130-180 ml/min	↓
Burr cells or schistocytes	Absent	Absent	Present
Uric acid	2-6.6 mg/dl	>5.9 mg/dl	>10 mg/dl
Bilirubin (total)	0.1-1 mg/dl	Unchanged or ↑	↑ (>1.2 mg/dl)

*LDH values differ according to the test or assays being performed.

Data from American College of Obstetricians and Gynecologists (ACOG). (2002). *Diagnosis and management of preeclampsia and eclampsia.* ACOG practice bulletin no. 33. Washington, DC: ACOG; ACOG. (2013). Executive summary: Hypertension in pregnancy. *Obstetrics & Gynecology, 122*(5), 1122-1131; Dildy, G. (2004). Complications of preeclampsia. In G. Dildy, M. Belfort, G. Saade, et al. (Eds.), *Critical care obstetrics* (4th ed.). Malden, MA: Blackwell Science; Harvey, C., & Sibai, B. (2013). Hypertension in pregnancy. In N.H. Troiano, C.J. Harvey, & B.F. Chez (Eds.), *AWHONN's high risk and critical care obstetrics* (3rd ed.). Philadelphia: Lippincott Williams & Wilkins.

Chronic Hypertension with Superimposed Preeclampsia

Women with chronic hypertension may develop superimposed preeclampsia. This condition, which is associated with adverse maternal or fetal outcomes, can be difficult to diagnose (ACOG, 2013).

PREECLAMPSIA

Etiology

Preeclampsia is a condition unique to human pregnancy. It occurs in approximately 2% to 7% of healthy nulliparous pregnant women and much more frequently in women with multifetal gestation, a history of preeclampsia, chronic hypertension, and preexisting diabetes (Sibai, 2012).

Common risk factors associated with the development of preeclampsia are listed in Box 27-1. The strongest risk factors are a first pregnancy when the woman is younger than 19 or older than 40 years of age, a first pregnancy with a new partner, and a history of preeclampsia with severe features (Gilbert, 2011). Pregnancy-onset snoring may also be a risk factor for gestational hypertension and preeclampsia (O'Brien, Bullough, Owusu, et al., 2012).

BOX 27-1 Common Risk Factors for Preeclampsia

- Primigravida younger than 19 or older than 40 years
- Preeclampsia with severe features in a previous pregnancy
- Family history (mother or sister) of preeclampsia
- Paternal history (partner previously fathered a preeclamptic pregnancy in another woman)
- African descent
- Multifetal gestation
- Maternal infection/inflammation in current pregnancy (i.e., urinary tract infection, periodontal disease)
- Preexisting medical or genetic conditions
  - Chronic hypertension
  - Renal disease
  - Pregestational diabetes mellitus
  - Connective tissue disease (i.e., systemic lupus erythematosus, rheumatoid arthritis)
  - Thrombophilia (i.e., antiphospholipid antibody syndrome, protein C or S deficiency, factor V Leiden mutation)
  - Obesity

From Gilbert, E.S. (2011). *Manual of high risk pregnancy and delivery* (ed. 5). St. Louis: Mosby; Harvey, C., & Sibai, B. (2013). Hypertension in pregnancy. In N. Troiano, C. Harvey, & B. Chez (Eds.), *AWHONN's high risk and critical care obstetrics* (3rd ed.). Philadelphia: Lippincott Williams & Wilkins.

The cause of preeclampsia is unknown. Many theories have been suggested to explain its etiology. Theories include abnormal trophoblast invasion, immunologic response to partially foreign genetic placental and fetal tissue, stimulation of the inflammatory system by cardiovascular changes of pregnancy, various dietary deficiencies, and genetic abnormalities (Harvey & Sibai, 2013).

Pathophysiology

Preeclampsia is a progressive disorder, with the placenta as the root cause. Therefore, the disease begins to resolve after the placenta has been expelled. Current thought is that the pathologic changes that occur in the woman with preeclampsia are caused by disruptions in placental perfusion and endothelial cell dysfunction (ACOG, 2013; Gilbert, 2011; Harvey & Sibai, 2013; Sibai, 2012). These changes develop early in pregnancy, long before the signs and symptoms of preeclampsia become evident (Eiland, Nzerue, & Faulkner, 2012; Markham & Funai, 2014). Normally in pregnancy the spiral arteries in the uterus widen from thick-walled muscular vessels to thinner, saclike vessels with much larger diameters. This change increases the capacity of the vessels, allowing them to handle the increased blood volume of pregnancy. Because this vascular remodeling does not occur or only partially develops in women with preeclampsia, decreased placental perfusion and hypoxia result (Harvey & Sibai).

Placental ischemia is thought to cause endothelial cell dysfunction by stimulating the release of a substance that is toxic to endothelial cells. This anomaly causes generalized vasospasm, which results in poor tissue perfusion in all organ systems, increased peripheral resistance and BP, and increased endothelial cell permeability, leading to intravascular protein and fluid loss and ultimately to less plasma volume. The main pathogenic factor is not an increase in BP but poor perfusion as a result

EVIDENCE-BASED PRACTICE

What's Up with Preeclampsia?

Ask the Question

For pregnant women what are the new best practices for identifying and treating preeclampsia?

Search for the Evidence

Search Strategies English language research-based publications since 2012 on preeclampsia and gestational hypertension were included.

Databases Used Cochrane Collaborative Database, National Guideline Clearinghouse (AHRQ), CINAHL, PubMed, UpToDate, and the professional websites for ACOG and AWHONN

Critical Appraisal of the Evidence

Risk factors for preeclampsia include young or old age, nulliparity, smoking, unmarried status, African-American, multiple fetuses, chronic hypertension, diabetes, and history of preeclampsia.

Recent research has also found the following to be risk factors for preeclampsia:

- For women with normal prepregnancy weight, excessive (>10) increase in body mass index (BMI) during pregnancy is associated with increased risk for preeclampsia. For overweight and obese women, even moderate BMI increase (5-10) can increase risk (Swank, Caughey, Farinelli, et al., 2014).
- Higher levels of C-reactive protein, an indicator of general inflammation, are associated with an increased risk for preeclampsia, especially with elevated BMI (Rebelo, Schlussel, Vaz, et al., 2013).
- Low levels of placental growth factor, an angiogenic factor, when detected before 35 weeks of gestation, is a secondary marker for placental dysfunction and is highly sensitive for preeclampsia (Chappell, Duckworth, Seed, et al., 2013).
- Psychosocial stress and chronic hypertension each increase risk for preeclampsia. When paired, their additive effect can increase the risk up to 20-fold (Yu, Zhang, Wang, et al., 2013).
- Preeclampsia is more likely to occur when birth occurs during the colder months of the year (Beltran, Wu, & Laurent, 2013).

The American College of Obstetricians and Gynecologists (ACOG) Task Force on Hypertension in Pregnancy (2013) has issued the following guideline changes for diagnosis and treatment of preeclampsia:

- Although proteinuria may still be used for diagnosis, a massive amount (greater than 5 g in a 24-hour urine collection) is no longer considered to be a severe feature of preeclampsia. Routine screening, beyond an appropriate medical history, is not recommended.
- Vitamins C and E to prevent preeclampsia do not prevent preeclampsia.
- Daily low-dose aspirin can help high risk women.
- Antihypertensives (labetalol or hydrazaline) are useful for severe hypertension.
- Magnesium sulfate is used for seizure prevention but not as an antihypertensive agent.

Apply the Evidence: Nursing Implications

- Preconception counseling for modifiable risk factors, such as smoking and weight gain, can decrease preeclampsia risk. When possible, planning a pregnancy to give birth during warm months may be preferable.
- Physical activity has a protective effect against preeclampsia (Kasawar, do Nascimento, Costa, et al., 2012).
- Teaching stress management techniques for lifelong and pregnancy stress is important, especially in the presence of chronic hypertension.
- In addition to assessing blood pressure, alert nurses are often the first to note subtle clinical changes indicating preeclampsia, such as sudden weight gain, edema, headache, oliguria, right-sided pain, and fetal distress.
- In the event of emergent hypertensive crisis, nurses must be familiar and proficient with assessments, including reflexes and fetal monitoring; must understand medications; and must be proactive in environmental alteration, such as limiting visitors and lowering lights and sound in the room.

Quality and Safety Competencies: Evidence-Based Practice (EBP)*

Knowledge

Describe reliable sources for locating evidence reports and clinical practice guidelines.

Use of high-level evidence guides the comprehensive prepregnancy and prenatal care of women at risk for preeclampsia.

Skills

Locate evidence reports related to clinical practice topics and guidelines.

Relevant systematic reviews and professional guidelines provide recommendations for improving outcomes by identifying women at risk for preeclampsia and educating clients about prevention and treatment.

Attitudes

Value the concept of EBP as integral to determining best clinical practices.

An evidence base guides practice and fosters client confidence and efficacy.

References

ACOG Task Force on Hypertension in Pregnancy (2013). *Hypertension in pregnancy.* Available at www.acog.org/Resources_And_Publications/Task_Force_and_Work_Group_Reports/Hypertension_in_Pregnancy.

Beltran, A. J., Wu, J., & Laurent, O. (2013). Associations of meteorology with adverse pregnancy outcomes: A systematic review of preeclampsia, preterm birth and birth weight. *International Journal of Research in Public Health, 11*(1), 91–172.

Chappell, L. C., Duckworth, S., Seed, P. T., et al. (2013). Diagnostic accuracy of placental growth factor in women with suspected preeclampsia: A prospective multicenter study. *Circulation, 128*(19), 2121–2131.

Kasawar, K. T., do Nascimento, S. L., Costa, M. L., et al. (2012). Exercise and physical activity in the prevention of pre-eclampsia: Systematic review. *Acta Obstetricia et Gynecologica Scandinavica, 91*(10), 1147–1157.

Rebelo, F., Schlussel, M. M., Vaz, J. S., et al. (2013). C-reactive protein and later preeclampsia: Systematic review and meta-analysis taking into account the weight status. *Journal of Hypertension, 31*(1), 16–26.

Swank, M. L., Caughey, A. B., Farinelli, C. K., et al. (2014). The impact of change in pregnancy body mass index on the development of gestational hypertensive disorders. *Journal of Perinatology, 34*(3), 181–185.

Yu, Y., Zhang, S., Wang, G., et al. (2013). The combined association of psychosocial stress and chronic hypertension with preeclampsia. *American Journal of Obstetrics and Gynecology, 209*(5), 438.e1–e.12.

Pat Mahaffee Gingrich

*Adapted from QSEN at www.qsen.org.

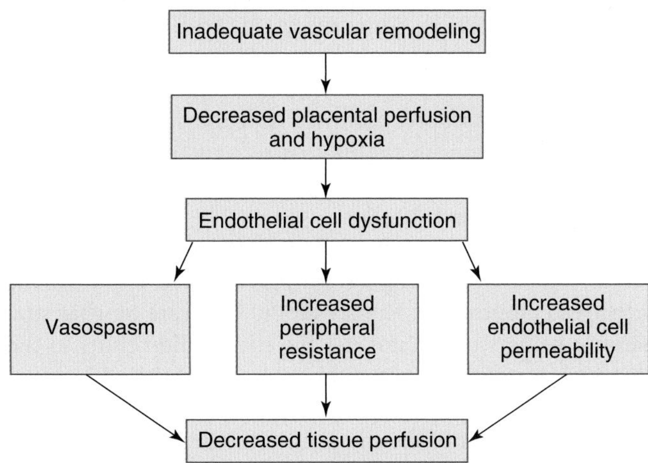

FIG 27-1 Etiology of preeclampsia: disruptions in placental perfusion and endothelial cell dysfunction. (Data from Gilbert E. [2011]. *Manual of high risk pregnancy and delivery* [5th ed.]. St. Louis: Mosby; Harvey, C., & Sibai, B. [2013]. Hypertension in pregnancy. In N. Troiano, C. Harvey, & B. Chez [Eds.], *AWHONN's high risk and critical care obstetrics* [3rd ed]. Philadelphia: Wolters Kluwer/Lippincott Williams & Wilkins; Markham, K. B., & Funai, E. F. [2014]. Pregnancy-related hypertension. In R. K. Creasy, R. Resnik, J. D. Iams, et al. [Eds.], *Creasy and Resnik's maternal-fetal medicine: Principles and practice* [7th ed.]. Philadelphia: Saunders.)

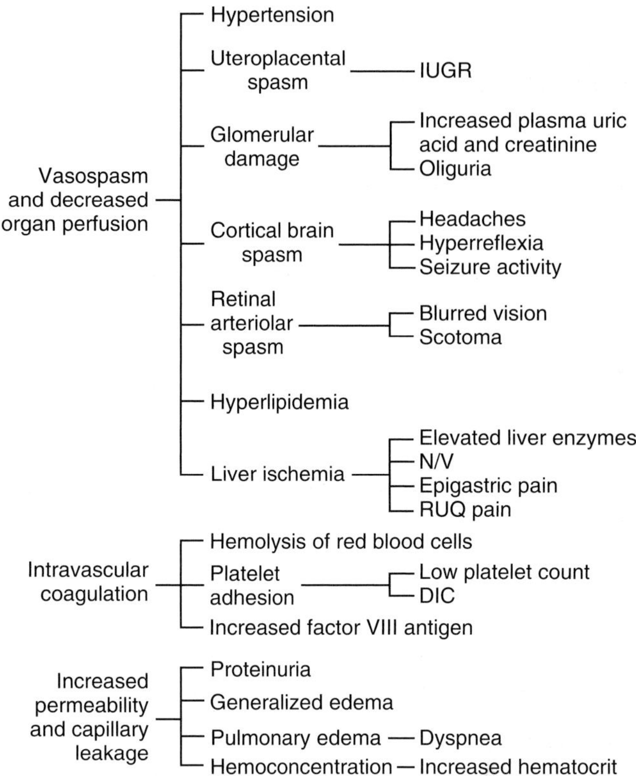

FIG 27-2 Consequences of endothelial cell dysfunction. *DIC,* Disseminated vascular coagulation; *IUGR,* intrauterine growth restriction, *N/V,* nausea/vomiting; *RUQ,* right upper quadrant. (From Gilbert, E. [2011]. *Manual of high risk pregnancy & delivery* [5th ed.]. St. Louis: Mosby.)

of vasospasm and reduced plasma volume (Fig. 27-1) (Gilbert 2011; Markham & Funai, 2014). Figure 27-2 demonstrates how endothelial cell dysfunction causes many of the common signs and symptoms of preeclampsia.

Reduced kidney perfusion decreases the glomerular filtration rate and can lead to degenerative glomerular changes and oliguria. Pathologic changes in the endothelial cells of the glomeruli (glomerular endotheliosis) are uniquely characteristic of preeclampsia. Protein, primarily albumin, is lost in the urine. Uric acid clearance is decreased, but serum uric acid levels increase. Sodium and water are retained. Acute tubular necrosis and renal failure may occur (Gilbert, 2011; Poole, 2014).

Plasma colloid osmotic pressure decreases as serum albumin levels decrease. Intravascular volume is reduced as fluid moves out of the intravascular compartment, resulting in hemoconcentration, increased blood viscosity, and tissue edema. The hematocrit value increases as fluid leaves the intravascular space. Arteriolar vasospasm can lead to endothelial damage and increased capillary permeability, predisposing the woman to pulmonary edema (see Fig. 27-2) (Gilbert, 2011; Poole, 2014).

Decreased liver perfusion can lead to impaired liver function and elevated liver enzyme levels. If hepatic edema and subcapsular hemorrhage develop, the woman may complain of epigastric or right upper quadrant pain. Hemorrhagic necrosis in the liver can result in a subcapsular hematoma, which is a rare occurrence (Gilbert, 2011; Poole, 2014). Rupture of a subcapsular hematoma is a life-threatening complication and a surgical emergency (see Fig. 27-2).

Neurologic complications associated with preeclampsia include cerebral edema and hemorrhage and increased central nervous system (CNS) irritability. CNS irritability manifests as headaches, hyperreflexia, positive ankle clonus, and seizures. Arteriolar vasospasms and decreased blood flow to the retina can lead to visual disturbances such as scotoma (dim vision or blind or dark spots in the visual field) and blurred or double vision (Gilbert, 2011; Poole, 2014).

Traditionally preeclampsia was considered to primarily affect the woman, causing hypertension, proteinuria, and perhaps associated multisystem dysfunction. However, it is now recognized that preeclampsia can also greatly affect the fetus, resulting in fetal growth restriction, decreased amniotic fluid volume, abnormal fetal oxygenation, low birth weight, and preterm birth (Sibai, 2012).

HELLP Syndrome

HELLP syndrome is a laboratory diagnosis for a variant of severe preeclampsia that involves hepatic dysfunction, characterized by hemolysis *(H),* elevated liver enzymes *(EL),* and low platelet *(LP)* count. It is not a separate illness. Specific laboratory findings are needed to diagnose HELLP syndrome and distinguish it from other serious diseases that share the same signs and symptoms. HELLP syndrome occurs in 0.5% to 0.9% of all pregnancies—10% to 20% of women with preeclampsia with severe features develop it (Harvey & Sibai, 2013). Table 27-3 lists laboratory changes that occur in HELLP syndrome. Traditionally it was not diagnosed unless all three laboratory abnormalities were present. Currently, however, women who develop only one or two of the diagnostic laboratory values are being diagnosed with incomplete HELLP, partial HELLP, or the ELLP syndrome (Harvey & Sibai).

The pathophysiologic changes of HELLP syndrome occur as a result of arteriolar vasospasm, endothelial cell dysfunction with fibrin deposits, and adherence of platelets in blood vessels. Red blood cells are damaged as they pass through narrowed blood vessels and become hemolyzed, resulting in a decreased red blood cell and platelet count, as well as hyperbilirubinemia. Endothelial damage and fibrin deposits in the liver lead to impaired liver function and can cause hemorrhagic necrosis. Liver enzymes are elevated when hepatic tissue is damaged (Gilbert, 2011).

HELLP syndrome usually develops during the antepartum period. The clinical presentation is often nonspecific. Most women with the disorder report a history of malaise, influenza-like symptoms, and epigastric or right upper quadrant abdominal pain. Symptoms tend to worsen at night and improve during the daytime. HELLP syndrome can progress rapidly (Harvey & Sibai, 2013).

! NURSING ALERT

An extremely important point to understand is that many women with HELLP syndrome may not have signs or symptoms of severe features of preeclampsia. For example, although most women have hypertension, BP may be only mildly elevated in 15% to 50% of cases. Proteinuria may be absent. As a result, women with HELLP syndrome are often misdiagnosed with a variety of other medical or surgical disorders (Sibai, 2012).

HELLP syndrome occurs more often in Caucasian women than in women of other races. A diagnosis of HELLP syndrome is associated with an increased risk for maternal death and adverse perinatal outcomes, including pulmonary edema, acute renal failure, disseminated intravascular coagulopathy (DIC), placental abruption, liver hemorrhage or failure, acute respiratory distress syndrome (ARDS), sepsis, and stroke. The reported perinatal mortality rate ranges from 7.4% to 34%, with a maternal mortality rate of approximately 1% (Sibai, 2012). The rate of preterm birth in women with HELLP syndrome is approximately 70%, with 15% occurring before 28 weeks of gestation. Most of the perinatal deaths occur before 28 weeks of gestation in association with placental abruption or severe fetal growth restriction (Sibai).

CARE MANAGEMENT

Identifying and Preventing Preeclampsia

Numerous clinical trials have examined various interventions to prevent preeclampsia, including protein or salt restriction; zinc, magnesium, fish oil, or vitamins C and E supplementation; use of diuretics or other antihypertensive medications or heparin; and bed rest. All of these interventions demonstrated minimal to no benefit in preventing or reducing the severity of preeclampsia (Sibai, 2012). However, low-dose aspirin (60 to 80 mg) has been found to reduce preeclampsia and adverse outcomes in selected high risk women. It is recommended that daily low-dose aspirin therapy be initiated late in the first trimester for women who have a history of early-onset preeclampsia and subsequent preterm birth at less than 34 weeks of gestation or a history of preeclampsia in more than one previous pregnancy (ACOG, 2013).

No reliable test that can be used as a routine screening tool for predicting preeclampsia has yet been developed. However, the search for biomarkers that can identify individual women who will develop hypertension during pregnancy is ongoing (Harvey & Sibai, 2013). For example, the tyrosine kinase (sFLt) and serum placental growth factor (PIGF) ratio at 22 to 26 weeks of gestation was shown in one study to be highly predictive of early-onset preeclampsia. An abnormal uterine artery Doppler velocimetry in the first or second trimester of pregnancy has also been suggested as a good screening test to predict preeclampsia (Gilbert, 2011).

Although research offers future promise, much work remains before a screening test for preeclampsia is available for widespread clinical use. Nurses should be aware of what strategies are being studied and use the most valid results so they can counsel pregnant women about evidence-based interventions. Meanwhile, early prenatal care to identify women at risk and early detection of the disease are the best ways to care for women who have or may develop preeclampsia.

Assessment and Nursing Diagnoses

Accurate measurement of BP is essential for the early detection of hypertensive disorders. Personnel caring for pregnant women need to be consistent in taking and recording BP measurements in a standardized manner. Both the National High Blood Pressure Education Program and the American Heart Association (AHA) have published extensive recommendations for accurately measuring BP (National High Blood Pressure Education Program, 2000; Pickering, Hall, Appel, et al., 2005;). Box 27-2 provides detailed instructions for measurement.

Assessment for edema is another component of the physical examination, although the presence of edema is no longer included in the definition of preeclampsia. Edema is assessed for distribution, degree, and pitting. Dependent edema is edema of the lowest or most dependent parts of the body, where hydrostatic pressure is greatest. If a pregnant woman is ambulatory, the edema may first be evident in the feet and ankles. If she is confined to bed, it is more likely to occur in the sacral region. Pitting edema leaves a small

BOX 27-2 Blood Pressure Measurement

- Measure blood pressure with the woman seated (ambulatory) or in the lateral recumbent position with the arm at heart level. Neither the woman nor the health care provider should talk while the blood pressure is being measured.
- After positioning, allow the woman at least 10 minutes of quiet rest before the blood pressure measurement to encourage relaxation.
- Instruct the woman to refrain from tobacco or caffeine use 30 minutes before the blood pressure measurement.
- Use the right arm each time.
- Support the arm in a horizontal position at heart level.
- Use the proper-size cuff (cuff should cover approximately 80% of the upper arm or be 1½ times the length of the upper arm).
- Maintain a slow, steady deflation rate.
- Take the average of two readings at least 6 hours apart to minimize recorded blood pressure variations across time.
- Use the Korotkoff phase V (disappearance of sound) for recording the diastolic value.
- Use accurate equipment. The mercury sphygmomanometer is the most accurate device.
- If interchanging manual and electronic devices, use caution in interpreting different blood pressure values.

Data from Peters, R. (2008). High blood pressure in pregnancy. *Nursing for Women's Health, 12*(5), 412-421.

depression or pit after finger pressure is applied to the swollen area (Fig. 27-3). The pit, which is caused by movement of fluid to adjacent tissue away from the point of pressure, normally disappears within 10 to 30 seconds. Although the amount of edema is difficult to quantify, the method shown in Figure 27-4 may be used to record relative degrees of edema formation.

Deep tendon reflexes (DTRs) reflect the balance between the cerebral cortex and spinal cord. They are evaluated as a baseline and to detect any changes. The biceps and patellar reflexes are assessed and the findings recorded (Fig. 27-5 and Table 27-4). To elicit the biceps reflex, the examiner strikes a downward blow over the thumb, which is situated over the biceps tendon (see Fig. 27-5, *A*). Normal response is flexion of the arm at the elbow, described as a 2+ response. The patellar reflex is elicited with the woman's legs hanging freely over the end of the examining table or with the woman lying on her side with the knee slightly flexed (see Fig. 27-5, *D*). The patellar tendon (inferior to the patella) is tapped with a percussion hammer. Normal response is the extension or kicking out of the leg.

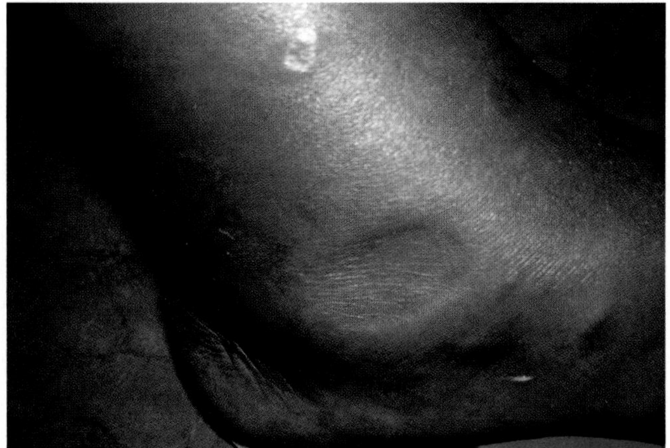

FIG 27-3 Pitting edema. (Courtesy Shannon Perry, Phoenix, AZ.)

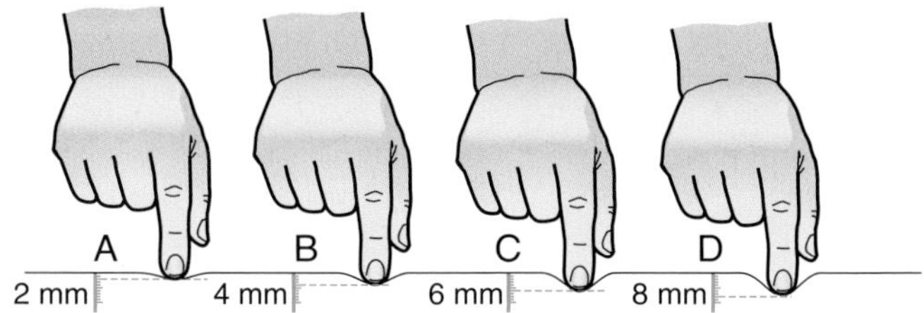

FIG 27-4 Assessment of pitting edema of lower extremities. A, +1; B, +2; C, +3; D, +4.

To assess for clonus (hyperactive reflexes) at the ankle joint, the examiner supports the leg with the knee flexed (see Fig. 27-5, *F*). With one hand the examiner sharply dorsiflexes the foot, maintains the position for a moment, and then releases the foot. Normal (negative clonus) response is elicited when no rhythmic oscillations (jerks) are felt while the foot is held in dorsiflexion. When the foot is released, no oscillations are seen as the foot drops to the plantar-flexed position. Abnormal (positive clonus) response is recognized by rhythmic oscillations of one or more "beats" felt when the foot is in dorsiflexion and seen as the foot drops to the plantar-flexed position.

The presence of proteinuria is ideally determined by evaluation of a 24-hour urine collection. In a 24-hour specimen, proteinuria is defined as a concentration at or greater than 300 mg. Although proteinuria may still be used to define preeclampsia, studies have shown little relationship between the degree of proteinuria in women with preeclampsia and pregnancy outcome. Therefore, massive proteinuria (greater than 5 g) is not considered to be a severe feature of preeclampsia. Because a 24-hour collection to measure the quantity of protein and creatinine clearance is more reflective of true renal status, it is preferred over dipstick testing, which should not be used for diagnosis of preeclampsia if at all possible (ACOG, 2013). Alkaline, concentrated, or dilute urine can yield a false reading.

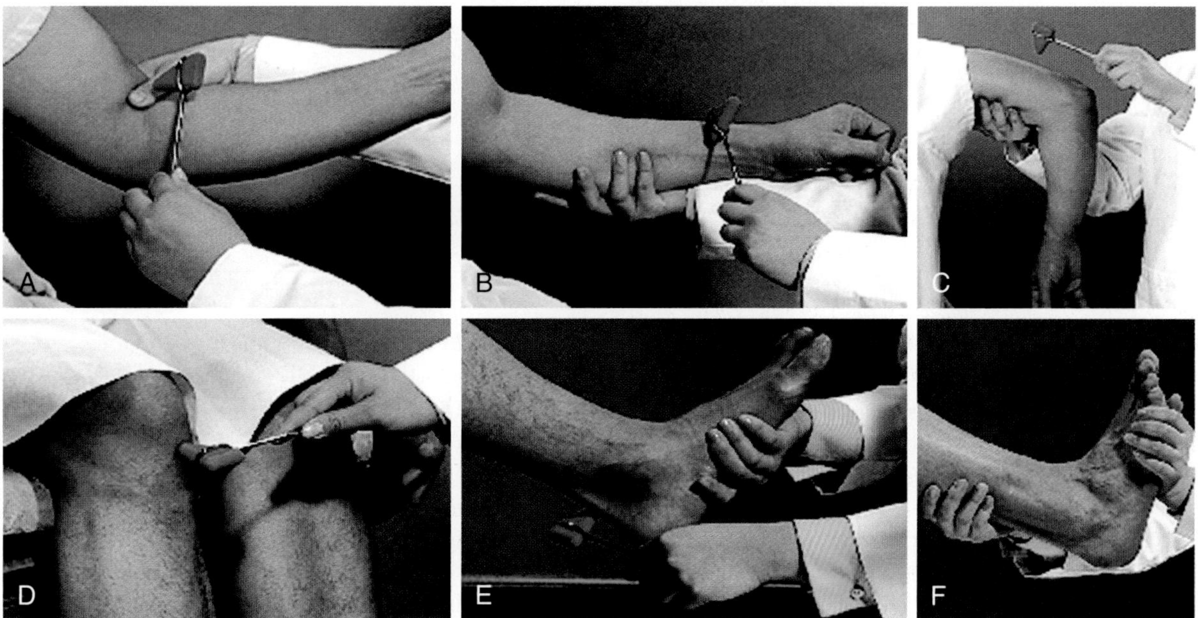

FIG 27-5 Location of tendons for evaluation of deep tendon reflexes. **A**, Biceps. **B**, Brachioradial. **C**, Triceps. **D**, Patellar. **E**, Achilles, **F**, Evaluation of ankle clonus. (From Seidel, H., Ball, J., Dains, J., et al. [2011]. *Mosby's guide to physical examination* [7th ed.]. St. Louis: Mosby.)

TABLE 27-4 Assessing Deep Tendon Reflexes

GRADE	DEEP TENDON REFLEX RESPONSE
0	No response
1+	Sluggish or diminished
2+	Active or expected response
3+	More brisk than expected, slightly hyperactive
4+	Brisk, hyperactive, with intermittent or transient clonus

From Seidel, H., Ball, J., Dains, J., et al. (2011). *Mosby's guide to physical examination* (7th ed.). St. Louis: Mosby.

Urine contaminated with bacteria, blood, and amniotic fluid also can yield a false positive for proteinuria. Therefore, to ensure accurate results, proteinuria should be determined using only a urine specimen that has been collected by either a thorough clean-catch midstream technique or catheterization (Gilbert, 2011).

During the examination the woman is evaluated for signs and symptoms considered to be severe features of preeclampsia such as severe headaches (usually frontal), epigastric pain (heartburn), right upper quadrant abdominal pain, or visual disturbances such as scotoma, photophobia, or double vision.

Nursing diagnoses for the woman with preeclampsia may include the following:

- *Anxiety* related to
  - Preeclampsia and its effects on woman and infant
- *Deficient Knowledge* related to
  - Management of preeclampsia (diet, medications, activity restriction, plans for labor and birth)
- *Disabled Family Coping* related to
  - Restricted activity and concern over a high risk pregnancy
  - Financial concerns
- *Powerlessness* related to
  - Inability to prevent or control condition and outcomes
- *Risk for Injury* to mother related to
  - Hypertension
  - Central nervous system (CNS) irritability secondary to cerebral edema
  - Vasospasm
  - Decreased renal perfusion
- *Risk for Injury* to fetus related to
  - Disruption of oxygen transfer from environment to fetus
  - Intrauterine growth restriction (IUGR)
  - Placental abruption
  - Preterm birth

Interventions

Mild Gestational Hypertension and Preeclampsia Without Severe Features

In the past, both gestational hypertension and preeclampsia were usually described as either "mild" or "severe." Because preeclampsia is a dynamic disease process, this practice is no longer recommended. A diagnosis of "mild preeclampsia" applies only at the time it is made. Women must be evaluated frequently to determine if the disease has progressed to the point that severe features are present (see Table 27-2) (ACOG, 2013).

The goals of therapy for women with mild gestational hypertension and preeclampsia without severe features are to ensure maternal safety and to deliver a healthy newborn as close to term as possible. Prior to 37 gestational weeks, care management is expectant with close monitoring of the maternal and fetal status. Women with mild gestational hypertension or preeclampsia can be safely managed at home, provided they have frequent maternal and fetal evaluation (Gilbert, 2011; Sibai, 2012). Vaginal birth by induction of labor, preceded by cervical ripening (if necessary), is recommended at 37 gestational weeks. At this gestational age the risks to the fetus outweigh any potential benefits of continuing the pregnancy (ACOG, 2013; Backes et al., 2011; Sibai, 2012).

Criteria for home management include BP less than 150/100 mm Hg and no increase in proteinuria if they have no symptoms, a normal platelet count, and normal liver enzymes (Sibai, 2012). Successful home care requires the woman to be well educated about preeclampsia and highly motivated to follow the plan of care (see Teaching for Self-Management: Assessing and Reporting Clinical Signs of Preeclampsia). All teaching should include the woman and her family, and time must be allowed for them to absorb information, ask questions, and voice concerns. Methods for enhancing learning include visual aids, DVDs or Internet videos, handouts, and demonstrations with return demonstrations. Furthermore, the effects of illness, language, age, cultural beliefs, and support systems must be considered.

TEACHING FOR SELF-MANAGEMENT

Assessing and Reporting Clinical Signs of Preeclampsia

- Take your blood pressure as directed. Always sit to take your blood pressure and use your right arm each time for consistent and accurate readings. Support your arm on a table in a horizontal position at heart level.
- Report to your health care provider immediately any increase in your blood pressure.
- Dipstick test your clean-catch urine sample as directed to assess proteinuria.
- Report to your health care provider if proteinuria is 1+ or more or if you have a decrease in urine output.
- Assess your baby's activity daily. Decreased activity (four or fewer movements per hour) may indicate fetal compromise and should be reported.
- Be sure to keep your scheduled prenatal appointments so that any changes in your or your baby's condition can be detected.
- Keep a daily log or diary of your assessments for your home health care nurse, or take it with you to your next prenatal visit.
- Report to your health care provider immediately any headache, dizziness, or blurred vision.

Maternal and Fetal Assessment

Initial maternal laboratory evaluation for women with preeclampsia without severe features includes measurement of serum creatinine, platelet count, liver enzymes, and a 24-hour urine protein assessment. Thereafter, the platelet count and liver enzymes should be assessed weekly. Women are also evaluated for signs or symptoms of severe features such as severe headaches, blurred or double vision, mental confusion, right upper quadrant or epigastric pain, nausea or vomiting, shortness of breath, and decreased urinary output (ACOG, 2013; Sibai, 2012). BP should be monitored twice weekly and proteinuria assessed weekly (ACOG).

Fetal evaluation generally includes daily fetal movement counts and nonstress testing or a biophysical profile once or twice weekly until birth. (See Chapter 26 for more information on fetal assessment tests.) Ultrasound evaluation of amniotic fluid status and determination of estimated fetal weight are performed at the time preeclampsia is diagnosed and serially thereafter, depending on findings (Sibai, 2012).

Activity Restriction. Complete or partial bed rest for the duration of the pregnancy is still recommended frequently by health care providers. However, no evidence has been found that this practice improves pregnancy outcome. Moreover, prolonged bed rest is known to increase the risk of thrombophlebitis (Sibai, 2012). Other adverse physiologic outcomes related to complete bed rest include cardiovascular deconditioning; diuresis with accompanying fluid, electrolyte, and weight loss; muscle atrophy; and psychologic stress. These changes begin on the first day of bed rest and continue for the duration of therapy. Therefore, restricted activity rather than complete bed rest is recommended (ACOG, 2013; Sibai).

Women with preeclampsia generally feel reasonably well; therefore, boredom from activity restriction is common. Diversionary activities, including television and computer or smart phone use, visits from friends, and a comfortable and convenient environment are ways to cope with the boredom. Participation in online prenatal classes also may be possible. Gentle exercise (e.g., range-of-motion exercises, stretching, Kegel exercises, pelvic tilts) is important in maintaining muscle tone, blood flow, regular bowel function, and a sense of well-being (see Teaching for Self-Management: Coping with Activity Restriction).

A high risk pregnancy can be very stressful for a woman and her family. Family stressors include separation from family members when hospitalized, need for activity restriction, financial concerns, ability to manage the household, family activities, and child care. The family needs to use coping mechanisms and support systems to help them through this crisis. An excellent web-based support group for pregnant women on restricted activity is Sidelines (www.sidelines.org) (Gilbert, 2011). Relaxation techniques also may help reduce stress and prepare the woman for labor and birth.

Diet. Women with preeclampsia can have a regular diet with adequate protein (60 to 70 g), calcium (1200 mg), 600 mcg of folic acid, and adequate zinc (11 to 12 mg) and sodium (1.5 g). Adequate fluid intake (six to eight 8-ounce glasses of water per day) is encouraged to enhance renal perfusion and bowel function (Gilbert, 2011; Otten, Helwig, & Meyers, 2006) (see Teaching for Self-Management: Diet for Preeclampsia).

TEACHING FOR SELF-MANAGEMENT

Coping with Activity Restriction

At Home

- Clarify with your health care provider: What is bed rest? Question your activity level, positioning, bathroom privileges, children's visits, activities, personal hygiene, mobility, diet, and visitors.
- Have your computer, tablet, or smart phone available at your bedside. These devices can be used to communicate with friends, conduct business, and shop as necessary. Also use your computer or smart phone to communicate with Internet support groups and obtain information.
- Have a television and DVD player to watch television programs or movies (can also watch on computer or tablet) and a radio, CD player, or MP3 player to listen to music.
- Delegate responsibilities to family members or friends as much as possible (i.e., attend to the laundry, pick up groceries, drop off and pick up dry cleaning, meet repair people, attend to child care, organize meals).
- Have these available for use on your bed or couch:
  - Eggcrate mattress
  - Pillows and more pillows (body pillow)
- Keep a big trash basket near your bed and daytime resting place.
- Place a box or crate near the bed/sofa to store items such as:
  - Post-it Notes
  - Cups with lids and flexible straws
  - Paper plates
  - Plastic forks, spoons, and knives
  - Baby monitor or walkie-talkies
  - Wet wipes
  - Notebook to record questions for providers, telephone numbers, to-do lists
  - Envelopes and stationery
  - Take-out menus
  - Reading materials
  - Books
  - Audio books
  - Magazines
- Stock a mini-refrigerator or cooler with water or other beverages or healthy snacks.
- Plan for family time—visits and interaction, particularly with small children (see the Teaching for Self-Management box: Activities for Children of Women on Activity Restriction in Chapter 32).
- Explore your interest in a new hobby.
  - Work crossword or jigsaw puzzles.
  - Learn to embroider, smock, crochet, or knit.
  - Do mending or sewing.
- Do craft projects; make something for the baby.
- Identify relaxation exercises and activities (music) and implement.
- Arrange to have a facial, manicure/pedicure, neck massage, or other special treat when you need a lift.

In the Hospital

- Clarify with your health care provider: What is bed rest? Question your activity level, positioning, bathroom privileges, children's visits, activities, personal hygiene, mobility, diet, and visitors.
- In addition to survival tips for the home, the following may be useful in the hospital setting:
  - Bring your own pillow, shampoo, and conditioner.
  - Have a wheelchair for outside visits or visiting other antepartal women if allowed.
  - If possible bring a laptop computer or a tablet so you can watch movies or television programs if Internet access is available.
  - Ask friends to bring healthy food and snacks rather than flowers when visiting.
  - Explore your interest in handheld games.
  - Work with staff regarding scheduling (e.g., obstetrics provider examinations, vital signs, nursing assessments).
  - Bring earplugs to block the hospital noise.
  - Ask for a room with a view.
  - Have a large calendar and clock for easy viewing. Record significant events on the calendar.

TEACHING FOR SELF-MANAGEMENT

Diet for Preeclampsia

- Eat a nutritious, balanced diet (60 to 70 g protein, 1200 mg calcium, 600 mcg folic acid, 11 to 12 mg zinc, and 1.5 g sodium). Consult with registered dietitian on the diet best suited for you.
- Salt foods to taste. Limiting excessively salty foods (luncheon meats, pretzels, chips, pickles, and sauerkraut) will likely be necessary to meet the recommended sodium intake of 1.5 g/day.
- Eat foods with roughage (whole grains, raw fruits, and vegetables).
- Drink six to eight 8-ounce glasses of water per day.
- Avoid alcohol and tobacco and limit caffeine intake.

Severe Gestational Hypertension and Preeclampsia with Severe Features

Women with severe gestational hypertension are at greater risk for pregnancy complications than are women who have preeclampsia without severe features. Therefore, these women should be managed as if they have preeclampsia with severe features. Women diagnosed with severe gestational hypertension or preeclampsia with severe features should be hospitalized immediately for a thorough evaluation of maternal-fetal status (Sibai, 2012). These women are placed on magnesium sulfate to prevent eclamptic seizures. Maternal assessments include monitoring BP, urine output, and cerebral status as well as for the presence of epigastric pain, tenderness, labor, or vaginal bleeding (Sibai). Laboratory evaluation includes a platelet count, liver enzymes, and serum creatinine (see Table 27-3). Fetal assessment includes continuous electronic fetal heart rate monitoring, a biophysical profile, and ultrasound evaluation of fetal growth and amniotic fluid (Sibai). If evidence of fetal growth restriction is found, umbilical artery Doppler velocimetry is recommended (ACOG, 2013; Sibai).

After this initial assessment period a multidisciplinary plan of care is developed with the woman and her family. The goals of care management are to ensure maternal safety, assess the degree of maternal and fetal risk, formulate a plan for giving birth, and prevent eclampsia and other serious complications such as placental abruption, HELLP syndrome, fetal growth restriction, and fetal demise. If the pregnancy has reached 34 weeks of gestation or more, it is recommended that birth be expedited soon after maternal stabilization has been achieved (ACOG, 2013). At or beyond 34 weeks of gestation, the risks of continuing the pregnancy are considered greater than the risks of preterm birth (Backes et al., 2011; Sibai, 2012).

Expectant Management. Women who are less than 34 0/7 weeks of gestation and have no indication for giving birth immediately may be candidates for expectant management. These women should be hospitalized at a tertiary care facility that is able to provide both maternal and neonatal intensive care. Care management decisions should be made in consultation with a perinatologist (a maternal fetal medicine specialist), and client and family counseling by a neonatologist should be provided (ACOG, 2013; Sibai, 2012).

Expectant management includes the use of oral antihypertensive medications to maintain a BP less than 160/110 mm Hg. Management also includes ongoing maternal and fetal assessment for indicators of worsening condition. Corticosteroids (betamethasone) are ordered to enhance fetal lung maturation for gestations less than 34 weeks. The dose is 12.5 mg intramuscularly, repeated in 24 hours. Optimal benefit begins 24 hours after the first dose is administered and lasts for 7 days (see Medication Guide: Antenatal Glucocorticoid Therapy with Betamethasone or Dexamethasone in Chapter 32) (ACOG, 2013; Gilbert, 2011; Sibai, 2012). Most women managed expectantly develop a maternal or fetal indication for giving birth within 2 weeks, although some are able to continue their pregnancies safely for several more weeks. Immediate birth is indicated if any of the following complications are present: uncontrollable severe hypertension, eclampsia, pulmonary edema, placental abruption, DIC, evidence of nonreassuring fetal status, or intrapartum fetal demise (ACOG; Sibai).

CLINICAL REASONING CASE STUDY

Severe Preeclampsia

Karen is a 30-year-old G1 P0 who is currently 32 weeks of gestation. At 28 weeks of gestation Karen developed preeclampsia. Since then Karen has been home on modified bed rest. A home health nurse visits her twice a week and calls her daily.

Today when the home health nurse visits, Karen tells her, "I have a terrible headache and hardly slept at all last night." When asked about other symptoms Karen replies, "My vision is blurry, I'm seeing spots, and my stomach hurts." Karen's blood pressure is 154/100, she has pitting edema in her legs, and her first voided urine this morning tested 3+ for protein. The nurse calls Karen's physician, who decides to admit her to the labor and birth unit immediately. At the hospital Karen continues to complain of a severe headache and seeing spots. Physical assessment reveals a blood pressure of 160/110 and 4+ deep tendon reflexes with 3 beats of ankle clonus. The electronic fetal monitor reveals minimal variability and late decelerations.

1. Evidence—Is there sufficient evidence to draw conclusions about Karen's diagnosis?
2. Assumptions—Describe the rationale for each of the following:
   a. Karen's probable diagnosis
   b. Signs and symptoms associated with this diagnosis
   c. Laboratory values associated with this diagnosis
   d. Risks associated with the diagnosis
3. What implications and priorities for nursing care can be drawn at this time?
4. Does the evidence objectively support your conclusion?

Intrapartum Care. Intrapartum nursing care is directed toward the early identification of fetal heart rate (FHR) abnormalities and the prevention of maternal complications. Continuous FHR and uterine contraction monitoring are initiated and the woman is assessed for signs of placental abruption such as a tense, tender uterus. Maternal evaluation also includes assessment of the central nervous, cardiovascular, pulmonary, hepatic, and renal systems. Vital signs and assessments are performed as ordered and per hospital policy. Client and family education and supportive measures are also initiated (Gilbert, 2011; Poole, 2014) (see Nursing Care Plan).

The woman with preeclampsia with severe features is maintained on bed rest with the side rails up in a quiet, darkened environment. Emergency drugs, oxygen, and suction equipment should be checked and readily available (Box 27-3). To reduce the risk of pulmonary edema, total

NURSING CARE PLAN

Preeclampsia with Severe Features

NURSING DIAGNOSIS	EXPECTED OUTCOME	INTERVENTIONS	RATIONALES
Risk for Injury to woman and fetus related to CNS irritability (seizures)	Woman will show diminished signs of CNS irritability (e.g., DTRs ≤2+, absence of clonus) and have no seizure activity.	Establish baseline data (e.g., DTRs, clonus).	To use as basis for evaluating effectiveness of treatment
		Administer IV magnesium sulfate per physician's orders.	To decrease hyperreflexia and minimize risk of seizure activity
		Monitor maternal vital signs, level of consciousness, FHR, urine output, DTRs, IV flow rate, and serum levels of magnesium sulfate.	To assess for and prevent magnesium sulfate toxicity (e.g., drowsiness, lethargy, slurred speech, loss of DTRs, depressed respirations, cardiac arrest)
		Have calcium gluconate or calcium chloride on the unit.	To be available if needed as an antidote for magnesium sulfate toxicity
		Maintain a quiet, darkened environment.	To avoid stimuli that may precipitate seizure activity
Ineffective Peripheral Tissue Perfusion related to preeclampsia secondary to arteriolar vasospasm	Woman will exhibit signs of adequate tissue perfusion (i.e., adequate urine output and normal FHR tracing).	Administer IV magnesium sulfate per physician order.	To relax vasospasms and increase renal perfusion
		Place woman on bed rest in side-lying position.	To maximize uteroplacental blood flow, reduce blood pressure, and promote diuresis
		Monitor FHR tracing for rate, baseline variability, and absence of late decelerations.	To assess for evidence of adequate uteroplacental oxygenation
Other Possible Nursing Diagnoses			
Risk for Excess Fluid Volume related to increased sodium retention secondary to administration of magnesium sulfate	Woman will exhibit signs of normal fluid volume (i.e., balanced intake and output, normal serum creatinine levels, normal breath sounds), adequate oxygenation (i.e., normal respirations; full orientation to person, time, and place), normal range of cardiac output (i.e., normal pulse rate and rhythm), and fetal well-being (i.e., adequate fetal movement, normal FHR and pattern).	Monitor woman for signs of fluid volume excess (increased edema, decreased urine output, elevated serum creatinine level, weight gain, dyspnea, crackles).	To detect potential complications
Risk for Impaired Gas Exchange related to pulmonary edema secondary to increased vascular resistance		Monitor woman for signs of impaired gas exchange (increased respirations, dyspnea, altered blood gases, hypoxemia).	To detect potential complications
Risk for Decreased Cardiac Output related to use of antihypertensive drugs		Monitor woman for signs of decreased cardiac output (altered pulse rate and rhythm).	To detect potential complications
Risk for Injury to Fetus related to uteroplacental insufficiency secondary to use of antihypertensive medications		Monitor fetus for abnormal signs (decreased fetal activity, abnormal FHR or pattern).	To prevent complications
		Record findings and report signs of increasing problems to physician.	To enable timely interventions

CNS, Central nervous system; *DTR,* deep tendon reflex; *FHR,* fetal heart rate; *IV,* intravenous.

intravenous (IV) and oral fluids should not exceed 125 ml/hr. Intensive hemodynamic monitoring with a pulmonary artery (Swan-Ganz) catheter to evaluate central venous and pulmonary artery pressures is not a routine standard of care. It is indicated only in selected women, such as those with oliguria unresponsive to a fluid challenge (Markham & Funai, 2014; Poole, 2014).

Magnesium Sulfate. Magnesium sulfate is the drug of choice for preventing and treating seizure activity (eclampsia). It is almost always administered intravenously as a secondary infusion (piggyback) by a volumetric infusion pump. Per protocol or health care provider's order, an initial loading dose of 4 to 6 g of magnesium sulfate is infused over 15 to 30 minutes. This dose is followed by a maintenance dose of magnesium sulfate that is diluted in an IV solution (e.g., 40 g of magnesium sulfate in 1000 ml of lactated Ringer's solution [1 g = 25 ml]) and administered by an infusion pump at 2 to 3 g/hr. This dose should maintain a therapeutic serum magnesium level of 4 to 7 mEq/L. Contrary to popular belief, magnesium sulfate has little effect on maternal BP when administered in this fashion (Markham & Funai, 2014; Poole, 2014).

Magnesium sulfate is rarely given intramuscularly because the absorption rate cannot be controlled, injections are painful, and tissue necrosis may occur. However, the intramuscular (IM) route may be used in low-resource settings or with some women who are being transported to a tertiary care center. The IM dose is a 10-g loading dose (administered as two separate injections of 5 g in each buttock). The maintenance dosage is 5 g administered every 4 hours in alternating buttocks (Harvey & Sibai, 2013). Local anesthetic can be added to the solution to reduce injection pain. The Z-track technique should be used for the deep IM injection, followed by gentle massage at the site.

BOX 27-3 Hospital Precautionary Measures

- Environment
  - Quiet
  - Nonstimulating
  - Lighting subdued
- Seizure precautions
  - Suction equipment tested and ready to use
  - Oxygen administration equipment tested and ready to use
  - Call button within easy reach
- Emergency medications available on the unit
  - Hydralazine
  - Labetalol
  - Nifedipine
  - Magnesium sulfate
  - Calcium gluconate or calcium chloride
- Emergency birth pack easily accessible

It is unclear how magnesium sulfate works to prevent and treat eclamptic seizures. It may cause vasodilation in the peripheral and cerebral circulation, prevent or decrease cerebral edema, or function as a central anticonvulsant (Harvey & Sibai, 2013). Because magnesium is excreted in the urine, accurate recordings of maternal urine output must be obtained. If renal function declines, not all of the magnesium sulfate will be excreted adequately, resulting in magnesium toxicity. Common side effects of magnesium sulfate are a feeling of warmth, flushing, diaphoresis, and burning at the IV site. Symptoms of magnesium toxicity include absent deep tendon reflexes, respiratory depression, blurred vision, slurred speech, severe muscle weakness, and cardiac arrest (Harvey & Sibai). Blood can be drawn to determine the serum magnesium level if toxicity is suspected (Box 27-4).

MEDICATION ALERT

High serum levels of magnesium can cause relaxation of smooth muscle, such as the uterus. However, when administered as a 4- to 6-g loading dose followed by a 1- to 2-g/hr maintenance dose, magnesium sulfate has not been shown to significantly affect the need for oxytocin (Pitocin) stimulation of labor. Other than a brief period of uterine muscle relaxation during and immediately after administration of the loading dose, no evidence of decreased uterine contractility has been observed (Cunningham, Leveno, Bloom, et al., 2014).

BOX 27-4 Care of the Woman with Preeclampsia Receiving Magnesium Sulfate

Client and Family Teaching

- Explain technique, rationale, and reactions to expect
  - Route and rate
  - Purpose of "piggyback" infusion
- Reasons for use
  - Tailor information to woman's readiness to learn
  - Explain that magnesium sulfate is used to prevent disease progression.
  - Explain that magnesium sulfate is used to prevent seizures, *not* to decrease blood pressure.
- Reactions to expect from medication
  - Initially the woman appears flushed and feels hot, sedated, and nauseated. She may experience burning at the IV site, especially during the bolus.
  - Sedation continues.
- Monitoring to anticipate
  - *Maternal:* blood pressure, pulse, respiratory rate, DTRs, level of consciousness, urine output (indwelling catheter), presence of headache, visual disturbances, epigastric pain
  - *Fetal:* FHR and activity

Administration

- Verify physician's order.
- Position woman in side-lying position.
- Prepare solution and administer with an infusion control device (pump).
- Piggyback a solution of 40 g of magnesium sulfate in 1000 ml lactated Ringer's solution using an infusion control device at the ordered rate: loading dose—initial bolus of 4 to 6 g over 15 to 30 min; maintenance dose—2 g/hr, according to unit protocol or specific physician's order

Maternal and Fetal Assessments

Vital signs and assessments are performed as ordered by the health care provider and per hospital protocol.

- Monitor blood pressure, pulse, and respiratory rate every 15 to 30 minutes, depending on the woman's condition.
- Monitor FHR and contractions continually.
- Monitor intake and output, DTRs, presence of headache, visual disturbances, level of consciousness, and epigastric pain at least hourly.
- Restrict hourly fluid intake to a total of no more than 125 ml/hr; urinary output should be at least 25 to 30 ml/hr.

Reportable Conditions

- Blood pressure: systolic ≥160 mm Hg or diastolic ≥110 mm Hg
- Respiratory rate: <12 breaths/min
- Urinary output <25 to 30 ml/hr
- Presence of headache, visual disturbances, decrease in level of consciousness, or epigastric pain
- Increasing severity or loss of DTRs, increasing edema
- Any abnormal laboratory values (magnesium level; platelet count; creatinine clearance; levels of uric acid, AST, ALT, prothrombin time, partial thromboplastin time, fibrinogen, fibrin split products)
- Any other significant change in maternal or fetal status

Emergency Measures

- Keep emergency drugs and intubation equipment immediately available.
- Keep the side rails up.
- Keep the lights dimmed, and maintain a quiet environment.

Documentation

- All of the above

ALT, Alanine aminotransferase; *AST,* aspartate aminotransferase; *DTRs,* deep tendon reflexes; *FHR,* fetal heart rate; *IV,* intravenous.

MEDICATION ALERT

If magnesium toxicity is suspected, prompt actions are needed to prevent respiratory or cardiac arrest. The magnesium infusion should be discontinued immediately. Calcium gluconate or calcium chloride (antidotes for magnesium sulfate) can be given intravenously (Cunningham et al., 2014).

The effect of magnesium sulfate on FHR baseline variability is controversial. Because fetal levels of magnesium approximate those of the mother, fetal sedation is possible. However, absent or minimal baseline variability should not be assumed to be the result of magnesium sulfate therapy until other causes of fetal hypoxemia have been ruled out (Poole, 2014). Neonatal serum magnesium levels are almost identical to those of the mother (Markham & Funai, 2014).

SAFETY ALERT

Magnesium sulfate is considered a high-alert medication because it can cause client harm when administered incorrectly. Measures to improve the safe use of this medication include developing detailed policies, procedures, protocols, and standing orders as well as thorough client assessment and documentation. *Never* abbreviate magnesium sulfate as $MgSO_4$ anywhere in the medical record (Institute for Safe Medication Practices [ISMP], 2012).

Control of Blood Pressure. Antihypertensive medications are indicated when the systolic BP exceeds 160 mm Hg or the diastolic BP exceeds 110 mm Hg. Maternal risks associated with severe hypertension include left ventricular failure, cerebral hemorrhage, and placental abruption. To maintain uteroplacental perfusion, antihypertensive therapy must not decrease the arterial pressure too much or too rapidly. Hydralazine (Apresoline), labetalol (Trandate), and nifedipine (Procardia) are effective drugs for treating hypertension intrapartum. They may also be used during pregnancy or in the postpartum period for BP control (ACOG, 2013; Gilbert, 2011; Harvey & Sibai, 2013). Table 27-5 compares antihypertensive agents commonly used to treat hypertension in pregnancy.

Postpartum Care. Throughout the postpartum period the woman needs careful assessment of her vital signs, intake and output, DTRs, and level of consciousness. The magnesium sulfate infusion is continued after birth for seizure prophylaxis as ordered, usually for 12 to 24 hours. Assessments for effects and side effects continue until the medication is discontinued. Given that magnesium sulfate potentiates the action of narcotics, CNS depressants, and calcium channel blockers, these medications must be administered with caution. The signs and symptoms of preeclampsia usually resolve within 48 hours after birth. Clinical signs that demonstrate resolution of preeclampsia include diuresis and decreased edema (Gilbert, 2011).

TABLE 27-5 Pharmacologic Control of Hypertension in Pregnancy

ACTION	TARGET TISSUE	MATERNAL EFFECTS	FETAL EFFECTS	NURSING ACTIONS
Hydralazine (Apresoline, Neopresol)				
Arteriolar vasodilator	Peripheral arterioles: to decrease muscle tone, decrease peripheral resistance; hypothalamus and medullary vasomotor center for minor decrease in sympathetic tone	Headache, flushing, palpitations, tachycardia, some decrease in uteroplacental blood flow, increase in heart rate and cardiac output, increase in oxygen consumption, nausea and vomiting	Tachycardia; late decelerations and bradycardia if maternal diastolic pressure <90 mm Hg	Assess for effects of medication; alert woman (family) to expected effects of medication; assess blood pressure frequently because precipitous drop can lead to shock and perhaps placental abruption; if giving multiple doses, wait at least 20 minutes after the first dose is given to administer an additional dose to allow time to assess the effects of the initial dose; assess urinary output; maintain bed rest in lateral position with side rails up; use with caution in presence of maternal tachycardia
Labetalol Hydrochloride (Normodyne, Trandate)				
Combined alpha- and beta-blocking agent causing vasodilation without significant change in cardiac output	Peripheral arterioles (see *Hydralazine*)	Minimal: flushing, tremulousness, orthostatic hypotension; minimal change in pulse rate	Minimal, if any	See *Hydralazine;* less likely to cause excessive hypotension and tachycardia; less rebound hypertension than hydralazine Do not use in women with asthma or heart failure. Do not exceed 80 mg in a single dose.
Methyldopa (Aldomet)				
Maintenance therapy if needed: 250-500 mg orally every 8 hr (α_2-receptor agonist)	Postganglionic nerve endings: interferes with chemical neurotransmission to reduce peripheral vascular resistance; causes CNS sedation	Sleepiness, postural hypotension, constipation; rare: drug-induced fever in 1% of women and positive Coombs' test result in 20% of women	After 4 months of maternal therapy, positive Coombs' test result in infant	See *Hydralazine*
Nifedipine (Adalat, Procardia)				
Calcium channel blocker	Arterioles: to reduce systemic vascular resistance by relaxation of arterial smooth muscle	Headache, flushing; may interfere with labor	Minimal	See *Hydralazine* Avoid concurrent use with magnesium sulfate because skeletal muscle blockade can result. Do not administer sublingually.

CNS, Central nervous system.

The nurse should assess the postpartum woman regularly for any symptoms of preeclampsia such as headaches, visual disturbances, or epigastric pain. Some women develop signs and symptoms of preeclampsia for the first time after giving birth. Women who develop hypertension and severe features of preeclampsia such as headaches or blurred vision or severe hypertension should be placed on IV magnesium sulfate for seizure prophylaxis. Nonsteroidal antiinflammatory pain medications should be used with caution when hypertension persists for more than 1 day after birth because these agents can contribute to an increase in BP. Women should be taught to contact their health care provider or return to the hospital immediately if they develop headaches, visual disturbances, or epigastric pain after discharge (ACOG, 2013; Sibai, 2012).

Because preeclampsia is a major cause of intrauterine growth restriction and preterm birth, the baby may be cared for in a neonatal intensive care unit (NICU) (Backes et al., 2011; Uzan et al., 2011). Nursing care that facilitates bonding and attachment while the infant is in the NICU includes providing the family with photographs of the infant, keeping the family informed of the infant's status, encouraging the father to visit the NICU, and taking the woman to the NICU by wheelchair after her condition has stabilized (Poole, 2014).

Most women with gestational hypertension become normotensive during the first week after giving birth. On the other hand, hypertension may take longer to resolve in women with preeclampsia. For women with gestational hypertension, preeclampsia, or superimposed preeclampsia, it is recommended that BP be monitored in the hospital or that equivalent outpatient surveillance be performed for at least 72 hours after birth. The BP should then be rechecked at 7 to 10 days postpartum, or earlier in women who are symptomatic. Women with a BP of 150/100 mm Hg or higher (on two occasions that are 4 to 6 hours apart) should be placed on an antihypertensive medication, often labetalol or nifedipine (ACOG, 2013). If this is the case, the BP needs to be checked frequently either at home or at the health care provider's office. Within a few weeks after birth antihypertensive medications often can be discontinued.

Future Health Care

Women with preeclampsia with severe features have a significantly increased risk of developing preeclampsia in a future pregnancy, especially those who had early-onset (diagnosed during the second trimester) preeclampsia. Even if these women remain normotensive in a subsequent pregnancy, they may have a greater likelihood of an adverse pregnancy outcome such as preterm birth, small for gestational age infant, and perinatal death (Sibai, 2012).

Ideally, women who have had preeclampsia in a previous pregnancy should receive counseling during a preconception visit before the next planned pregnancy. At this visit the previous pregnancy history should be reviewed and the prognosis for the upcoming pregnancy discussed. Potential lifestyle modifications such as weight loss and increased physical activity should be encouraged. The current status of any chronic medical conditions, such as diabetes or chronic hypertension, should be assessed, so that they are brought into the best control possible before the upcoming pregnancy. Current medications should be reviewed and their administration modified if necessary for the upcoming pregnancy. If the woman has given birth to a preterm infant during a preeclamptic pregnancy or has had preeclampsia in more than one prior pregnancy, the use of low-dose aspirin during the upcoming pregnancy should be suggested (ACOG, 2013).

Women with preeclampsia (especially early-onset and preeclampsia with severe features) also have an increased risk of developing chronic hypertension and cardiovascular disease later in life. It is believed that preeclampsia does not cause cardiovascular disease but rather that preeclampsia and cardiovascular disease share common risk factors. Further research is needed to determine how to take advantage of this information relating preeclampsia to cardiovascular disease later in life. For now, women should be educated about lifestyle changes (maintaining a healthy weight, increasing physical activity, and avoiding smoking) that may decrease the risk for developing future health problems (ACOG, 2013; Sibai, 2012).

Eclampsia

Eclampsia is usually preceded by premonitory signs and symptoms, including persistent headache, blurred vision, severe epigastric or right upper quadrant abdominal pain, and altered mental status. However, convulsions can appear suddenly and without warning in a seemingly stable woman with only minimal BP elevations (Sibai, 2012). The convulsions that occur in eclampsia are frightening to observe. Tonic contraction of all body muscles (seen as arms flexed, hands clenched, legs inverted) precedes the tonic-clonic convulsion. During this stage muscles alternately relax and contract. Respirations are halted and then begin again with long, deep, stertorous inhalations. Hypotension follows, and muscular twitching, disorientation, and amnesia persist for a while after the convulsion. The woman may also vomit or be incontinent of urine or stool.

Immediate Care. Nursing actions during a convulsion are directed toward ensuring a patent airway and client safety (see Emergency box).

It is important to note the time of onset and duration of the seizure. Call for help but do not leave the bedside. Make certain that the side rails on the bed are raised; pad them with a folded blanket or pillow if possible. Women with eclampsia have been known to sustain fractures from falling out of bed during the seizure. Immediately after the convulsion, lower the head of the bed and turn the woman onto her side. This helps prevent aspiration of vomitus (Gilbert, 2011).

Nursing actions after a convulsion are directed toward maternal stabilization. First assess the status of the woman's airway, breathing, and pulse. Suction secretions from her glottis to clear the airway, insert an oral airway, and administer oxygen at 10 L/min by face mask. If an IV infusion is not in place, start one with an 18-gauge needle. If an IV line was in place before the seizure, it may have infiltrated and will need to be restarted immediately. As soon as IV access is obtained, administer magnesium sulfate as ordered (Gilbert, 2011).

If eclampsia develops after initiating magnesium sulfate therapy, additional magnesium sulfate should be administered. Magnesium sulfate is the drug of choice for treating eclamptic seizures and preventing repeated seizures. One of its advantages over other antiseizure medications such as diazepam (Valium)

EMERGENCY

Eclampsia

Tonic-Clonic Convulsion Signs

- Stage of invasion: 2-3 seconds, eyes fixed, twitching of facial muscles
- Stage of contraction: 15-20 seconds, eyes protrude and are bloodshot, all body muscles in tonic contraction
- Stage of convulsion: muscles relax and contract alternately (clonic), respirations halted; then begin again with long, deep, stertorous inhalation; coma ensues

Intervention

- Keep airway patent: turn head to one side, place pillow under one shoulder or back if possible.
- Call for assistance. Do not leave the bedside.
- Raise side rails and pad them with a folded blanket or pillow if possible.
- Observe and record convulsion activity.

After Convulsion

- Do not leave the woman unattended until fully alert.
- Observe for postconvulsion confusion, coma, and incontinence.
- Use suction as needed.
- Apply a pulse oximetry monitor.
- Administer oxygen via nonrebreather face mask at 10 L/min.
- Start intravenous fluids and monitor for potential fluid overload.
- Give magnesium sulfate or other anticonvulsant drug as ordered.
- Insert an indwelling urinary catheter.
- Monitor blood pressure, pulse, and respirations frequently until stabilized.
- Monitor fetal and uterine status.
- Expedite laboratory work as ordered to monitor kidney and liver function, coagulation system, and drug levels.
- Provide hygiene and a quiet environment.
- Support the woman and her family and keep them informed.
- Be prepared to assist with birth when the woman is in stable condition.

is that it reduces the risk of aspiration because it does not depress the gag reflex (Harvey & Sibai, 2013).

After the woman is stabilized, assess uterine activity, cervical status, and fetal status. During a convulsion the uterus becomes hypercontractile and hypertonic. As a result, the membranes may have ruptured or the cervix may have dilated rapidly, and birth may be imminent (Poole, 2014). The FHR tracing may demonstrate bradycardia, late decelerations, minimal baseline variability, or any combination. These findings usually resolve soon after the convulsion ends and the woman's hypoxia is corrected (Sibai, 2012).

SAFETY ALERT

Immediately after a seizure a woman may be very confused and combative. Restraints may be necessary temporarily. Several hours may be needed for the woman to regain her usual level of mental functioning.

After stabilizing the woman and fetus, a decision is made regarding the timing and method of birth. Eclampsia alone is not an indication for immediate cesarean birth. The route of birth (induction of labor versus cesarean birth) depends on maternal and fetal condition, fetal gestational age, presence of labor, and the cervical Bishop score (ACOG, 2013; Sibai, 2012).

Regional anesthesia is not recommended for eclamptic women with coagulopathy or a platelet count less than 50,000/mm^3 (Sibai, 2012).

Chronic Hypertension

An increasing number of women who give birth have chronic hypertension, which affects approximately 4% to 5% of all pregnancies (Gilbert, 2011). Non-Hispanic black women are much more likely to have a pregnancy complicated by chronic hypertension than are women of other races or ethnicities (Martin, Hamilton, Sutton, et al., 2012). In addition to race, other risk factors for chronic hypertension in pregnancy are older age and obesity. As more women delay childbearing and are obese, the number of pregnancies complicated by chronic hypertension can be expected to increase (Sibai, 2012).

More than 90% of women with chronic hypertension have primary or essential hypertension. In the remaining 10% the hypertension is secondary to a medical condition such as renal or collagen disease (Harvey & Sibai, 2013). Chronic hypertension in pregnancy is associated with maternal complications such as superimposed preeclampsia, stroke, acute kidney injury, heart failure, placental abruption, and death. Fetal risks include IUGR, death, and preterm birth (Cunningham et al., 2014; Sibai, 2012).

Ideally the management of chronic hypertension in pregnancy begins before conception. An evaluation of the cause and severity of the hypertension and the presence of any target organ damage (e.g., heart, eye, and kidney) is performed. Moreover, the woman should be encouraged to make lifestyle changes prior to conception such as smoking and alcohol cessation, participating in aerobic exercise, and losing weight if indicated. A diet that includes a maximum of 2.4 g sodium per day is recommended (Gilbert, 2011). These lifestyle modifications should continue throughout the pregnancy.

Based on the BP and presence of target organ damage, women with chronic hypertension are classified as either low or high risk for pregnancy complications. Antihypertensive medications are frequently discontinued before pregnancy in women with low risk chronic hypertension. This decreases the risk of fetal exposure to some medications (e.g., angiotensin-converting enzyme [ACE] inhibitors) that can be teratogenic (Harvey & Sibai, 2013). For women who persistently have BP readings of 160/105 mm Hg or higher, antihypertensive therapy is suggested. Labetalol (Trandate), nifedipine (Procardia), or methyldopa (Aldomet) are the medications most commonly recommended (see Table 27-5). If antihypertensive therapy is necessary, the BP should be maintained between 120 and 160 mm Hg systolic and 80 to 105 mm Hg diastolic (ACOG, 2013).

Women with chronic hypertension who are considered high risk are monitored closely, and the route and timing of birth depend on the maternal and fetal status. After giving birth the woman should be monitored closely for complications such as pulmonary edema, hypertensive encephalopathy, and renal failure. Women with chronic hypertension can breastfeed if they desire. All antihypertensive medications are present to some degree in breast milk. Levels of methyldopa in breast milk appear to be low and are considered safe. Labetalol also has a low concentration in breast milk. Little is known about the transfer of calcium channel blockers such as nifedipine in breast milk, but no apparent side effects have been noted in infants (Sibai, 2012).

COMMUNITY ACTIVITY

- Visit the National Women's Health Resource Center website at www.healthywomen.org. Select health topics, and under Health Center click on Heart Health. Review any featured articles about hypertension. Go to the Related Conditions link and click on High Blood Pressure. Review client information about definition of high blood pressure, diagnosis, treatment, prevention, facts to know, questions to ask, key Q&A, organizations, and support. Read any related article about pregnancy and high blood pressure.
- Visit the Sister to Sister/The Women's Heart Health Foundation website at www.sistertosister.org. Select Heart Facts and click on Pregnancy Complications. Review client information about preeclampsia. Select Healthy Living, Health Tools, and My Heart Health links and review the information.

Evaluate the information you located on these websites for use with various client populations.

KEY POINTS

- Hypertensive disorders during pregnancy are a leading cause of maternal and perinatal morbidity and mortality worldwide.
- The cause of preeclampsia is unknown, and there are no known reliable tests for predicting women at risk for developing preeclampsia.
- Preeclampsia is a multisystem disease, and the pathologic changes are present long before clinical manifestations such as hypertension become evident.
- HELLP syndrome, which is usually diagnosed during the third trimester, is a variant of preeclampsia, not a separate illness.
- Magnesium sulfate, the anticonvulsant of choice for preventing or controlling eclamptic seizures, requires careful monitoring of reflexes, respirations, and renal function.
- Women with preeclampsia (especially early-onset and preeclampsia with severe features) have an increased risk of developing chronic hypertension and cardiovascular disease later in life.
- The intent of emergency interventions for eclampsia is to prevent self-injury, enhance oxygenation, reduce aspiration risk, and establish control with magnesium sulfate.

REFERENCES

American College of Obstetricians and Gynecologists (ACOG). (2002). *Diagnosis and management of preeclampsia and eclampsia: ACOG practice bulletin no. 33.* Washington, DC: ACOG.

American College of Obstetricians and Gynecologists (ACOG). (2013). Executive summary: Hypertension in pregnancy. *Obstetrics and Gynecology, 122*(5), 1122–1131.

Backes, C., Markham, K., Moorehead, P., et al. (2011). Maternal preeclampsia and neonatal outcomes. *Journal of Pregnancy.* Published online 2011, April 4. Article ID 214365, 7 pages. doi: 10.1155/2011/214365.

Cunningham, F., Leveno, K., Bloom, S., et al. (2014). *Williams obstetrics* (24th ed.). New York: McGraw-Hill Education.

Duley, L. (2011). Pre-eclampsia, eclampsia, and hypertension. *Clinical Evidence* (Online) 1402. Published online 2011, February 14.

Eiland, E., Nzerue, C., & Faulkner, M. (2012). Preeclampsia 2012. *Journal of Pregnancy.* Published online 2012, July 11. Article ID 586578, 7 pages. doi: 10.1155/2012/586578.

Gilbert, E. (2011). *Manual of high risk pregnancy and delivery* (5th ed.). St. Louis: Mosby.

Harvey, C., & Sibai, B. (2013). Hypertension in pregnancy. In N. Troiano, C. Harvey, & B. Chez (Eds.), *AWHONN's high risk and critical care obstetrics* (3rd ed.). Philadelphia: Wolters Kluwer/Lippincott Williams & Wilkins.

Institute for Safe Medication Practices (ISMP). (2012). *ISMP's list of high-alert medications.* Available at www.ismp.org.

Markham, K. B., & Funai, E. F. (2014). Pregnancy-related hypertension. In R. K. Creasy, R. Resnik, J. D. Iams, et al. (Eds.), *Creasy and Resnik's maternal-fetal medicine: Principles and practice* (7th ed.). Philadelphia: Saunders.

Martin, J., Hamilton, B., Sutton, P., et al. (2012). Births: Final data for 2010. *National Vital Statistics Reports, 61*(1), 1–100.

National High Blood Pressure Education Program. (2000). *Working group report on high blood pressure in pregnancy.* NIH Pub. No. 00–3029. Bethesda, MD: National Institutes of Health, National Heart, Lung, and Blood Institute.

O'Brien, L. M., Bullough, A. S., & Owusu, J. T. (2012). Pregnancy-onset habitual snoring, gestational hypertension, and preeclampsia: Prospective cohort study. *American Journal of Obstetrics and Gynecology, 207*(6), 487–489.

Otten, J. J., Helwig, J. P., & Meyers, L. D. (Eds.), (2006). *Dietary reference intakes: The essential guide to nutrient requirements.* Washington, DC: National Academies Press.

Pickering, T., Hall, J., Appel, L., et al. (2005). Recommendations for blood pressure measurement in humans and experimental animals. Part I: Blood pressure measurement in humans: A statement for professionals from the subcommittee of professional and public education of the American Heart Association Council on High Blood Pressure Research. *Hypertension, 45*(1), 142–161.

Poole, J. H. (2014). Hypertensive disorders of pregnancy. In K. Rice Simpson, & P. Creehan (Eds.), *AWHONN's perinatal nursing* (4th ed.). Philadelphia: Lippincott Williams & Wilkins.

Romero-Arauz, J. F., Morales-Borrego, E., García-Espinosa, M., & Peralta-Pedrero, M. L. (2012). Clinical guideline: Preeclampsia-eclampsia. *Revista Medica del Instituto Mexicano del Seguro Social, 50*(5), 569–579 (Article in Spanish. Abstract in English).

Sibai, B. (2012). Hypertension. In S. Gabbe, J. Niebyl, & J. Simpson (Eds.), *Obstetrics: Normal and problem pregnancies* (6th ed.). Philadelphia: Saunders.

Uzan, J., Carbonnel, M., Piconne, O., et al. (2011). Pre-eclampsia: Pathophysiology, diagnosis, and management. *Vascular Health and Risk Management, 7*, 467–474.

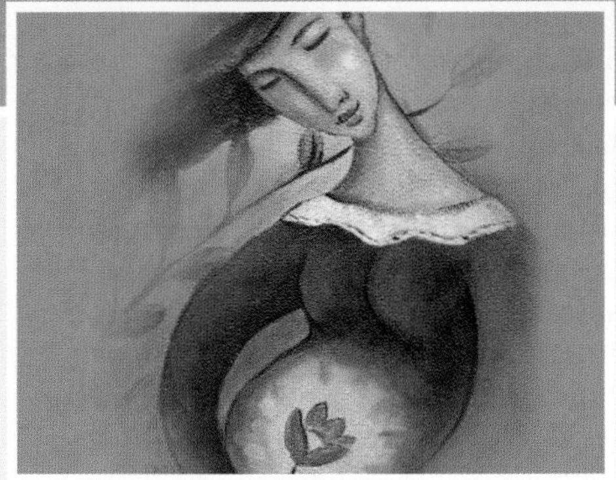

CHAPTER 28

Hemorrhagic Disorders

Kitty Cashion

http://evolve.elsevier.com/Lowdermilk/MWHC/

LEARNING OBJECTIVES

- Differentiate among causes of early pregnancy bleeding, including miscarriage, ectopic pregnancy, cervical insufficiency, and hydatidiform mole.
- Discuss signs and symptoms, possible complications, and management of miscarriage, ectopic pregnancy, cervical insufficiency, and hydatidiform mole.
- Compare and contrast placenta previa and placental abruption in relation to signs and symptoms, complications, and management.
- Discuss the diagnosis and management of disseminated intravascular coagulation.

Bleeding in pregnancy may jeopardize maternal and fetal well-being. Maternal blood loss decreases oxygen-carrying capacity, which places the woman at increased risk for hypovolemia, anemia, infection, and preterm labor and adversely affects oxygen delivery to the fetus. Fetal risks from maternal hemorrhage include blood loss or anemia, hypoxemia, hypoxia, anoxia, and preterm birth. Hemorrhagic disorders in pregnancy are medical emergencies. The incidence and type of bleeding vary by trimester. Ruptured ectopic pregnancy and abruptio placentae (placental abruption) have the highest incidence of maternal mortality. Prompt assessment and intervention by the health care team are essential to save the lives of both the woman and her fetus.

EARLY PREGNANCY BLEEDING

Bleeding during early pregnancy is alarming to the woman and of concern to health care providers. The common bleeding disorders of early pregnancy include miscarriage (spontaneous abortion), cervical insufficiency, ectopic pregnancy, and hydatidiform mole (molar pregnancy).

Miscarriage (Spontaneous Abortion)

A pregnancy that ends as a result of natural causes before 20 weeks of gestation is defined as a **miscarriage (spontaneous abortion)**. This 20-week marker has traditionally been considered to be the point of viability, when a fetus may survive in an extrauterine environment. A fetal weight less than 500 g also may be used to define an abortion (Cunningham, Leveno, Bloom, et al., 2014). The term *miscarriage* rather than *abortion* is used throughout this discussion because it is more appropriate to use with clients. Abortion may be perceived as an insensitive term by families who are grieving a pregnancy loss. Therapeutic or elective induced abortion is discussed in Chapter 8.

Incidence and Etiology

Approximately 10% to 15% of all clinically recognized pregnancies end in miscarriage (Simpson & Jauniaux, 2012). The majority—greater than 80% of miscarriages—are early pregnancy losses, occurring before 12 weeks of gestation (Cunningham et al., 2014). Of all clinically recognized first-trimester losses, 25% result from chromosomal abnormalities (Cunningham et al.). Other possible causes of early miscarriage include endocrine imbalance (as in women who have luteal phase defects, hypothyroidism, or insulin-dependent diabetes mellitus with high blood glucose levels in the first trimester), immunologic factors (e.g., antiphospholipid antibodies), systemic disorders (e.g., lupus erythematosus), and genetic factors. Infections are not a common cause of early miscarriage (Cunningham et al.), but there is an increased risk for a spontaneous abortion with varicella infection in the first trimester (Gilbert, 2011).

A late miscarriage, sometimes called a second-trimester loss, occurs between 12 and 20 weeks of gestation. Risk factors for a second-trimester loss include race, ethnicity, poor outcomes in previous pregnancies, and extremes of maternal age. Other factors associated with an increased risk for miscarriage are severe dietary deficiencies, morbid obesity, regular or heavy alcohol use, and excessive (about 500 mg daily) caffeine intake. Bleeding during the first trimester is also a significant risk factor (Cunningham et al., 2014). Some of these risk factors cannot be modified, but correction of maternal disorders, a healthy lifestyle, adequate early prenatal care, and treatment of pregnancy complications can do much to prevent other causes of miscarriage.

Types

The types of miscarriages include threatened, inevitable, incomplete, complete, and missed. All types of miscarriage can recur in subsequent pregnancies. All types except the threatened miscarriage can lead to infection (Fig. 28-1).

Clinical Manifestations

Signs and symptoms of miscarriage depend on the duration of pregnancy. The presence of uterine bleeding, uterine contractions, or abdominal pain is an ominous sign during early pregnancy and must be considered a threatened miscarriage until proven otherwise.

If miscarriage occurs before the sixth week of pregnancy, the woman may report what she believes is a heavy menstrual flow. Miscarriage that occurs between weeks 6 and 12 of pregnancy causes moderate discomfort and blood loss. After week 12, miscarriage is typified by severe pain, similar to that of labor, because the fetus must be expelled. Diagnosis of the type of miscarriage is based on the signs and symptoms present (Table 28-1).

Symptoms of a *threatened* miscarriage (see Fig. 28-1, *A*) include spotting of blood but with the cervical os closed. Mild uterine cramping may be present.

Inevitable (see Fig. 28-1, *B*) and *incomplete* (see Fig. 28-1, *C*) miscarriages involve a moderate to heavy amount of bleeding with an open cervical os. Tissue may be present with the bleeding. Mild to severe uterine cramping may be present. An inevitable miscarriage is often accompanied by rupture of membranes (ROM) and cervical dilation. Passage of the products of conception occurs. An incomplete miscarriage involves the expulsion of the fetus with retention of the placenta.

In a *complete* miscarriage (see Fig. 28-1, *D*), the cervix has already closed after all fetal tissue was expelled. Slight bleeding may occur and mild uterine cramping may be present, as well.

The term *missed* miscarriage (see Fig. 28-1, *E*) refers to a pregnancy in which the fetus has died but the products of conception are retained in utero for up to several weeks. It may be diagnosed by ultrasonic examination after the uterus stops increasing in size or even decreases in size. There may be no bleeding or cramping, and the cervical os remains closed.

Recurrent (habitual) early miscarriage is three or more spontaneous pregnancy losses before 20 weeks of gestation. The most widely accepted causes of recurrent miscarriage are parental chromosomal abnormalities, antiphospholipid antibody syndrome, and certain uterine abnormalities (Cunningham et al., 2014).

The evaluation of couples experiencing recurrent pregnancy loss usually includes karyotyping of both partners and miscarriage specimens and assessment of the placenta; evaluating the woman's uterine cavity; and testing the woman for antiphospholipid antibody syndrome and thyroid disease. Evaluation should also address the psychological response to this diagnosis because women and their partners often report feelings of guilt, anxiety, and depression. Thus couples experiencing recurrent pregnancy loss should be screened for depression and post-traumatic stress disorder (Rink & Lockwood, 2014).

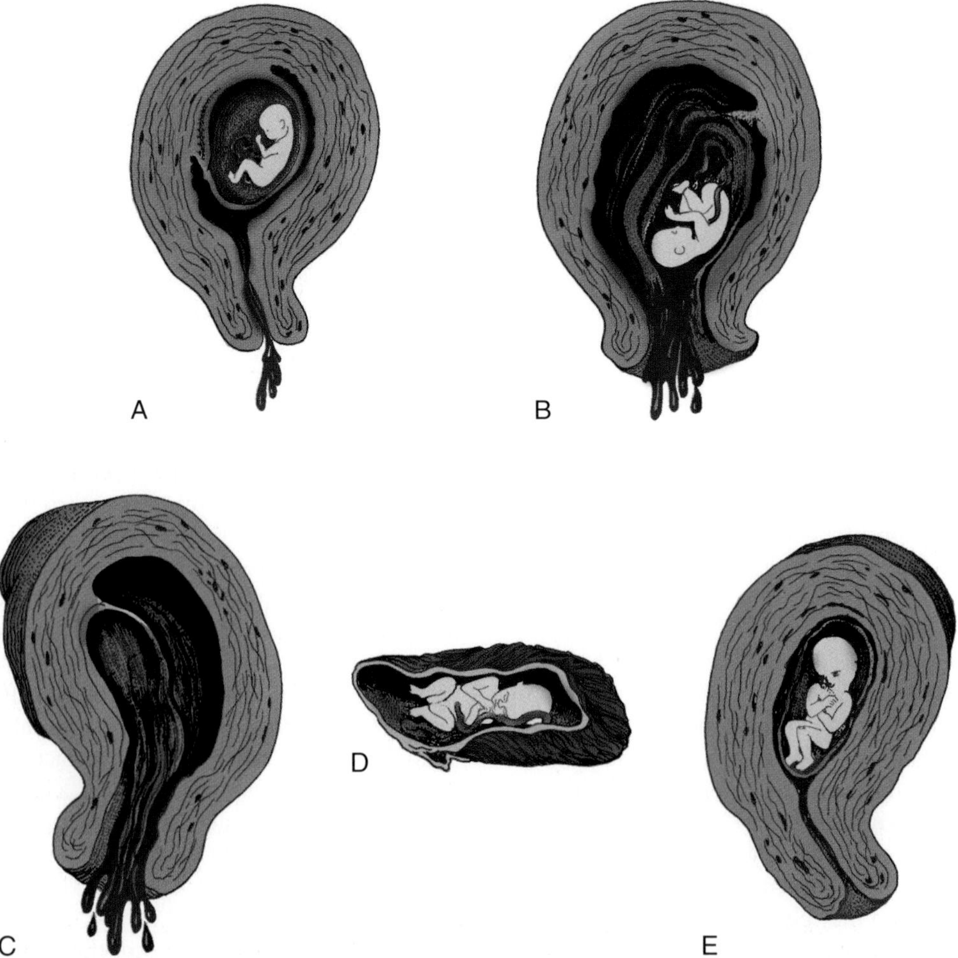

FIG 28-1 Miscarriage. **A**, Threatened. **B**, Inevitable. **C**, Incomplete. **D**, Complete. **E**, Missed.

Miscarriages can become septic, although this is uncommon. Symptoms of a septic miscarriage include fever and abdominal tenderness. Vaginal bleeding, which may be slight to heavy, is usually malodorous.

CARE MANAGEMENT

Assessment and Nursing Diagnoses

Whenever a woman has vaginal bleeding early in pregnancy, a thorough assessment should be performed. The data to be collected include pregnancy history, vital signs, type and location of pain, quantity and nature of bleeding, and emotional status. Laboratory tests may include evaluation of human chorionic gonadotropin (β-hCG) - (pregnancy), hemoglobin level (anemia), and white blood cell count (infection).

The following nursing diagnoses are appropriate for the woman experiencing a miscarriage:

- *Anxiety* related to
  - unknown outcome and unfamiliarity with medical procedures
- *Deficient Fluid Volume* related to
  - excessive bleeding secondary to miscarriage
- *Acute Pain* related to
  - uterine contractions
- *Situational Low Self-Esteem* related to
  - inability to carry a pregnancy successfully to term gestation
- *Risk for Infection* related to
  - surgical treatment
  - dilated cervix

Initial Care. Management depends on the classification of the miscarriage and on signs and symptoms (see Table 28-1). Traditionally, threatened miscarriages have been managed

TABLE 28-1 Assessing Miscarriage and the Usual Management

TYPE OF MISCARRIAGE	AMOUNT OF BLEEDING	UTERINE CRAMPING	PASSAGE OF TISSUE	CERVICAL DILATION	MANAGEMENT
Threatened	Slight, spotting	Mild	No	No	Bed rest is often ordered but has not proven to be effective in preventing progression to actual miscarriage. Repetitive transvaginal ultrasounds and assessment of human chorionic gonadotropin (hCG) and progesterone levels may be done to determine if the fetus is still alive and in the uterus. Further treatment depends on whether progression to actual miscarriage occurs.
Inevitable	Moderate	Mild to severe	No	Yes	Bed rest if no pain, bleeding, or infection If rupture of membranes (ROM), pain, bleeding, or infection is present, then prompt termination of pregnancy is accomplished usually by dilation and curettage.
Incomplete	Heavy, profuse	Severe	Yes	Yes, with tissue in cervix	May or may not require additional cervical dilation before curettage Suction curettage may be performed.
Complete	Slight	Mild	Yes	No (cervix has already closed after tissue passed)	No further intervention may be needed if uterine contractions are adequate to prevent hemorrhage and no infection is present. Suction curettage may be performed to ensure no retained fetal or maternal tissue
Missed	None, spotting	None	No	No	If spontaneous evacuation of the uterus does not occur within 1 month, pregnancy is terminated by method appropriate to duration of pregnancy. Blood clotting factors are monitored until uterus is empty. Disseminated intravascular coagulation (DIC) and incoagulability of blood with uncontrolled hemorrhage may develop in cases of fetal death after the twelfth week, if products of conception are retained for longer than 5 weeks. May be treated with dilation and curettage or misoprostol (Cytotec) given orally or vaginally
Septic	Varies, usually malodorous	Varies	Varies	Yes, usually	Immediate termination of pregnancy by method appropriate to duration of pregnancy Cervical culture and sensitivity studies are performed, and broad-spectrum antibiotic therapy (e.g., ampicillin) is started. Treatment for septic shock is initiated if necessary.
Recurrent (generally defined as three or more consecutive miscarriages)	Varies	Varies	Yes	Yes, usually	Varies; depends on type Prophylactic cerclage may be performed if cervical insufficiency is the cause. Tests of value include karyotyping of both partners and miscarriage specimens and assessment of the placenta; evaluating the woman's uterine cavity; and testing the woman for antiphospholipid antibody syndrome and thyroid disease.

Data from Cunningham, F., Leveno, K., Bloom, S., et al. (2014). *William's obstetrics* (24th ed.). New York: McGraw-Hill Medical; Gilbert, E. (2011). *Manual of high risk pregnancy & delivery* (5th ed.). St. Louis: Mosby; Rink, B.D., & Lockwood, C.J. (2014). Recurrent pregnancy loss. In R.K. Creasy, R. Resnik, J.D. Iams, et al. (Eds.), *Creasy and Resnik's maternal-fetal medicine: Principles and practice* (7th ed.). Philadelphia: Saunders.

expectantly with supportive care. However, there are no proven effective therapies for this condition. Bed rest, although often prescribed, does not prevent progression to actual miscarriage. Repetitive transvaginal ultrasounds and measurement of human chorionic gonadotropin (hCG) and progesterone levels may be performed to determine if the fetus is alive and within the uterus (Cunningham et al., 2014).

Follow-up treatment depends on whether the threatened miscarriage progresses to actual miscarriage or symptoms subside and the pregnancy remains intact. If bleeding and infection do not occur, expectant management is a reasonable option. In approximately half of all threatened miscarriages managed in this way, the pregnancy continues (Cunningham et al., 2014).

Once the cervix begins to dilate, the pregnancy cannot continue and miscarriage becomes inevitable. If all the products of conception are passed, no surgical intervention is necessary. If heavy bleeding, excessive cramping, or infection is present, however, the remaining embryonic, fetal, or placental tissue must be removed from the uterus, usually by suction curettage. In women who are clinically stable, expectant management to allow spontaneous resolution of an incomplete miscarriage is another treatment option (Cunningham et al., 2014; Gilbert, 2011).

Most missed miscarriages eventually end spontaneously. Women may be offered expectant management at the time the pregnancy loss is diagnosed. Expectant management results in eventual spontaneous miscarriage in 16% to 76% of cases (Gilbert, 2011).

Medical management is another treatment option if bleeding and infection are not present. Prostaglandin medications (e.g., misoprostol [Cytotec]) may be given and are usually effective in completing the miscarriage within 7 days (Cunningham et al., 2014). If medical management is chosen, nursing care is similar to the care for any woman whose labor is induced (see Chapter 32). Special care may be needed for management of side effects of prostaglandin, such as nausea, vomiting, and diarrhea. If the products of conception are not passed completely, the woman may be prepared for manual or surgical evacuation of the uterus.

A third management option, and one that is often chosen, is **dilation and curettage (D&C),** a surgical procedure in which the cervix is dilated if necessary and a curette is inserted to scrape the uterine walls and remove uterine contents. Uterine contents may also be removed by suction curettage, using a catheter attached to an electric-powered vacuum source (Cunningham et al., 2014). Pain relief during a D&C is usually achieved by administering analgesics or sedatives intravenously or orally (conscious sedation). A paracervical block using a local anesthetic may also be administered (Cunningham et al.). Before a surgical procedure is performed, a full history should be obtained and general and pelvic examinations conducted. General preoperative and postoperative care is appropriate for the woman requiring surgical intervention for miscarriage. The nurse reinforces explanations, answers any questions or concerns, and prepares the woman for surgery.

After evacuation of the uterus, oxytocin is often given to prevent hemorrhage. For excessive bleeding after the miscarriage, ergot products such as ergonovine (Methergine) or a prostaglandin derivative such as methylcarboprost tromethamine (Hemabate) may be given to contract the uterus. (See the Medication Guide: Drugs Used to Manage Postpartum Hemorrhage in Chapter 33). Antibiotics are given as necessary. Analgesics, such as antiprostaglandin agents (e.g., nonsteroidal antiinflammatory drugs [NSAIDs]), may decrease discomfort from cramping. Transfusion therapy may be required for shock or anemia. The woman who is Rh negative and is not isoimmunized is given $Rh_0(D)$ immune globulin (Cunningham et al., 2014).

Psychosocial aspects of care focus on what the pregnancy loss means to the woman and her family. Grief from perinatal loss is complex and unique to each individual. Explanations are provided regarding the nature of the miscarriage, expected procedures, and possible future implications for childbearing.

As with other fetal or neonatal losses, the woman should be offered the option of seeing the products of conception. She may also want to know what the hospital does with the products of conception or whether she needs to make a decision about final disposition of fetal remains.

Follow-up Care. The woman will likely be discharged home within a few hours after a D&C or as soon as her vital signs are stable, vaginal bleeding remains minimal, and she has recovered from anesthesia. Discharge teaching emphasizes the need for rest. If significant blood loss has occurred, iron supplementation may be ordered. Teaching includes information about normal physical findings, such as cramping, type and amount of bleeding, resumption of sexual activity, and family planning (see Teaching for Self-Management: Discharge Teaching for the Woman After Early Miscarriage).

TEACHING FOR SELF-MANAGEMENT

Discharge Teaching for the Woman After Early Miscarriage

- Clean the perineum after each voiding or bowel movement and change perineal pads often.
- Shower (avoid tub baths) for 2 weeks.
- Avoid tampon use, douching, and vaginal intercourse for 2 weeks.
- Notify your physician if an elevated temperature or a foul-smelling vaginal discharge develops.
- Eat foods high in iron and protein to promote tissue repair and red blood cell replacement.
- Seek assistance from support groups, clergy, or professional counseling as needed.
- Allow yourself (and your partner) to grieve the loss before becoming pregnant again.

Frequently the woman and her partner want to know when she should attempt to become pregnant again. Discuss with them the importance of completely resolving the loss before attempting another pregnancy (Gilbert, 2011). Follow-up care should assess the woman's emotional as well as physical recovery. Referrals to local support groups are provided as needed. Share Pregnancy and Infant Loss Support, Inc. (www.nationalshare.org) is an excellent online resource for families who have experienced an early pregnancy loss.

Follow-up telephone calls after a loss are important. The woman may appreciate a telephone call on what would have been her due date. These calls provide opportunities for the woman to ask questions, seek advice, and receive information to help process her grief.

Cervical Insufficiency

One cause of late miscarriage is cervical insufficiency, which has traditionally been defined as passive and painless dilation of the cervix leading to recurrent preterm births during the second trimester in the absence of other causes. It was believed that these criteria defined women whose early births were caused solely by structural weakness of cervical tissue that could be corrected surgically by cerclage placement. Measurement of cervical length has been used as a way to diagnose cervical insufficiency. However, it is now known that an abnormally short cervix identified during the second trimester can also represent an early step in the process of preterm labor (see Evidence-Based Practice). Therefore, the challenge is to identify women who have cervical changes because of impaired cervical strength before conception or in early pregnancy rather than when they are beginning the process of preterm labor. However, assessment of cervical function to diagnose or rule out cervical insufficiency can be done only during pregnancy (Berghella & Iams, 2014).

EVIDENCE-BASED PRACTICE

Interventions for Short Cervix

Ask the Question

For pregnant women in the second trimester with short cervix and previous preterm birth, what interventions can protect against preterm birth?

Search for the Evidence

Search Strategies English language research-based publications since 2011 on antenatal, short cervix, preterm, cerclage, pessary, and progesterone were included.

Databases Used Cochrane Collaborative Database, National Guideline Clearinghouse (AHRQ), CINAHL, PubMed, UpToDate, and the professional websites for ACOG and AWHONN

Critical Appraisal of the Evidence

Normally the cervix remains thick until the end of pregnancy. If the cervix is short (less than 25 mm), there is a risk for premature cervical opening. Sometimes called "cervical insufficiency," often the first symptom is pregnancy loss in the second trimester. Women with a history of second-trimester loss and preterm birth should have their cervix measured via ultrasound. To prevent preterm birth, three options provide additional mechanical support.

- **Cerclage:** First used in 1902, a cervical suture is placed surgically to tie the cervix closed and clipped at term. Metaanalysis of 12 trials found that compared with no treatment, cerclage decreased preterm births. However, there were no differences in perinatal morbidity or mortality. Cesarean births were more likely in the cerclage group (Alfirevic, Stampalija, Roberts, & Jorgensen, 2012).
- **Pessaries:** Used for centuries to support a prolapsed uterus, pessaries are rings inserted into the vagina that distribute the weight of the uterus away from the cervix and obstruct the internal cervical os. When women with short cervices began using pessaries midpregnancy, they experienced significantly less preterm birth, less use of tocolytic medications, and fewer neonatal intensive care admissions (Abdel-Aleem, Shaaban, & Abdel-Aleem, 2013).
- **Progesterone:** This essential hormone of pregnancy maintenance can be given by oral, vaginal, or intramuscular route. Metaanalysis of trials for women with a short cervix showed that those who received progesterone vaginally had significantly less incidence of preterm birth. Their babies had less morbidity and mortality, respiratory distress syndrome, neonatal intensive care admissions, and need for mechanical ventilation compared with women who were treated with a placebo (Romero, Nicolaides, Conde-Aqudelo, et al., 2012).
- **Comparisons:** A systematic analysis found no difference between cerclage and progesterone in preventing preterm birth in women with short cervix, previous preterm birth, and singleton pregnancy (Conde-Aqudelo et al., 2013). A comparison of 142 women with short cervix, history of previous preterm birth and single pregnancy who were treated with either cerclage (U.S.), vaginal progesterone (UK), and cervical pessary (Spain) found no differences in preterm births, perinatal losses, or neonatal morbidity (Alfirevic, Owen, Carreras Moratonas, et al., 2013). Client preferences may guide available method selection.

Apply the Evidence: Nursing Implications

Cerclage is a surgical procedure, requiring skill, sterile technique, and fetal monitoring. Anesthesia is usually spinal, epidural, or general. For this reason it is usually day surgery, done in proximity to a hospital setting. Clients may be NPO prior to surgery and need rest afterward. Surgery can be stressful, invasive, and expensive.

Vaginal progesterone may cause minor irritation and must be administered every day. Oral progesterone may have side effects of sleepiness, headache, and fatigue. Intramuscular progesterone is given weekly.

Pessaries can increase vaginal discharge and may need to be repositioned for comfort. Despite these side effects, most women were satisfied with this method (Abdel-Aleem et al., 2013).

The risk of very preterm birth and perinatal loss is frightening, and much clinical decision making is based on client history of prior pregnancy loss. Clients frequently carry guilt or anxiety about something they did or didn't do into the current pregnancy. The nurse can explore their understanding and feelings about prior losses and their current pregnancy.

Because the cervix provides protection against pathogens, couples may be instructed to avoid intercourse until 1 week after a cerclage placement and to use condoms thereafter. Clients and partners need pictures, literature, websites, and warm lines to call with questions.

Quality and Safety Competencies: Evidence-Based Practice*

Knowledge

Describe how the strength and relevance of available evidence influences the choice of interventions in provision of client-centered care.

The nurse should be able to explain the pathophysiology of short cervix and treatments for prevention of preterm birth to the client and partner.

Skills

Participate in structuring the work environment to facilitate integration of new evidence into standards of practice.

Client-centered care includes providing a team approach to treatment of short cervix, including psychosocial counseling for anxiety and previous perinatal loss.

Attitudes

Value the need for continual improvement in clinical practice based on new knowledge.

Continued

EVIDENCE-BASED PRACTICE—cont'd

Interventions for Short Cervix

Creating an accepting and caring environment enables honest communication between the client and the health care team about intensely personal reproductive and sexual issues.

References

Abdel-Aleem, H., Shaaban, O. M., & Abdel-Aleem, M. A. (2013). Cervical pessary for preventing preterm birth. In *The Cochrane Database of Systematic Reviews 2013* (p. 5). Chichester, UK: John Wiley & Sons.

Alfirevic, Z., Owen, J., Carreras Moratonas, E., et al. (2013). Vaginal progesterone, cerclage or cervical pessary for preventing preterm birth in asymptomatic singleton pregnant women with a history of preterm birth and a sonographic short cervix. *Ultrasound in Obstetrics and Gynecology, 41*(2), 146–151.

Alfirevic, Z., Stampalija, T., Roberts, D., & Jorgensen, A. L. (2012). Cervical stitch (cerclage) for preventing preterm birth in singleton pregnancy. In *The Cochrane Database of Systematic Reviews 2012* (p. 4). Chichester, UK: John Wiley & Sons.

Conde-Aqudelo, A., Romero, R., Nicolaides, K., et al. (2008). Vaginal progesterone vs. cervical cerclage for the prevention of preterm birth in women with sonographic short cervix, previous preterm birth, and singleton pregnancy: A systematic review and indirect comparison metaanalysis. *American Journal of Obstetrics and Gynecology, 208*(1), 42e1–42e18.

Romero, R., Nicolaides, K., Conde-Aqudelo, A., et al. (2012). Vaginal progesterone in women with an asymptomatic sonographic short cervix in the midtrimester decreases preterm delivery and neonatal morbidity: A systematic review and metaanalysis of individual patient data. *American Journal of Obstetrics and Gynecology, 206*(2), 124e1–124e19.

Pat Mahaffee Gingrich

*Adapted from QSEN at www.qsen.org.

Etiology

Cervical insufficiency may be either acquired or congenital. Congenital risk factors for cervical insufficiency include collagen disorders, uterine anomalies, and ingestion of diethylstilbestrol (DES) by the woman's mother while pregnant with the woman. Because DES has not been used since the early 1970s, however, it is now rare to encounter women who have this risk factor (Berghella & Iams, 2014). A risk factor for acquired cervical insufficiency is a history of previous cervical trauma resulting from lacerations during childbirth or mechanical dilation of the cervix during gynecologic procedures. Women who have had prior cervical surgery such as a biopsy in which a large cone specimen was removed or destroyed are also at risk for cervical insufficiency (Berghella & Iams; Ludmir & Owen, 2012).

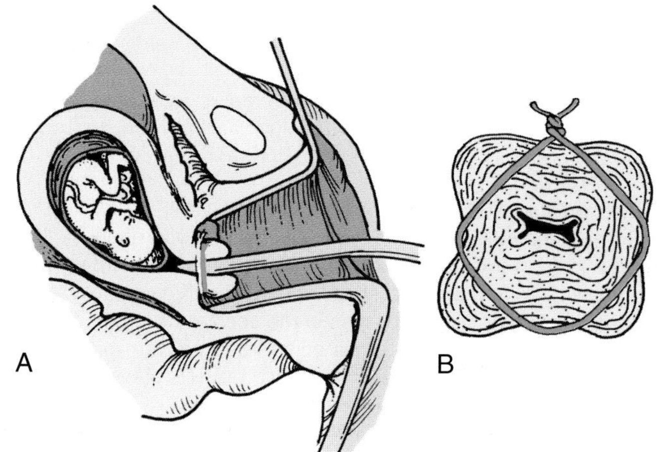

FIG 28-2 **A**, Cerclage correction of premature dilation of the cervical os. **B**, Cross-sectional view of closed internal os.

Diagnosis

Cervical insufficiency is a clinical diagnosis, made by a thorough obstetric history along with speculum and digital pelvic examinations and a transvaginal ultrasound examination. Speculum and digital examinations allow identification of an opening at the internal cervical os, prolapsed fetal membranes, or both. A vaginal ultrasound examination will reveal an abnormally short (<25 mm) cervix. Often the short cervix is accompanied by *cervical funneling* (beaking), effacement of the internal cervical os, although the external cervical os remains closed (Berghella & Iams, 2014; Cunningham et al., 2014; Ludmir & Owen, 2012).

CARE MANAGEMENT

Cervical **cerclage** placement has been the treatment of choice for women with cervical insufficiency due to cervical weakness. Indications for cerclage placement are a poor obstetric history (three or more previous early preterm births or second-trimester losses), a short (<25 mm) cervical length identified on transvaginal ultrasound, and an open cervix found on digital or speculum examination (Berghella & Iams, 2014). The McDonald technique is often the procedure of choice because of its proven effectiveness and ease of placement and removal. In this procedure a suture is placed around the cervix beneath the mucosa to constrict the internal os of the cervix (Fig. 28-2) (Cunningham et al., 2014).

A cerclage may be placed either prophylactically or as a therapeutic or rescue procedure after cervical change has been identified (Berghella & Iams, 2014; Cunningham et al., 2014). A prophylactic, or history-indicated, cerclage is usually placed at 12 to 14 weeks of gestation. An ultrasound-indicated cerclage may be placed therapeutically at 14 to 23 weeks of gestation in women with a singleton pregnancy and a history of a prior preterm birth if a short (<25 mm) cervix is identified on vaginal ultrasound. Finally, a rescue cerclage may be placed between 16 and 23 weeks of gestation in women who are found to have cervical change (>1 cm dilated or prolapsed membranes) on physical examination. The cerclage is removed if preterm premature rupture of membranes or advanced preterm labor that puts pressure on the stitch occurs. If the pregnancy progresses without further complications, the cerclage is removed when the woman reaches 36 weeks of gestation (Berghella & Iams).

In women with an extremely short cervix such as those who were exposed prenatally to DES, who have a history of a large cone biopsy, or who have had a failed vaginal cerclage, an

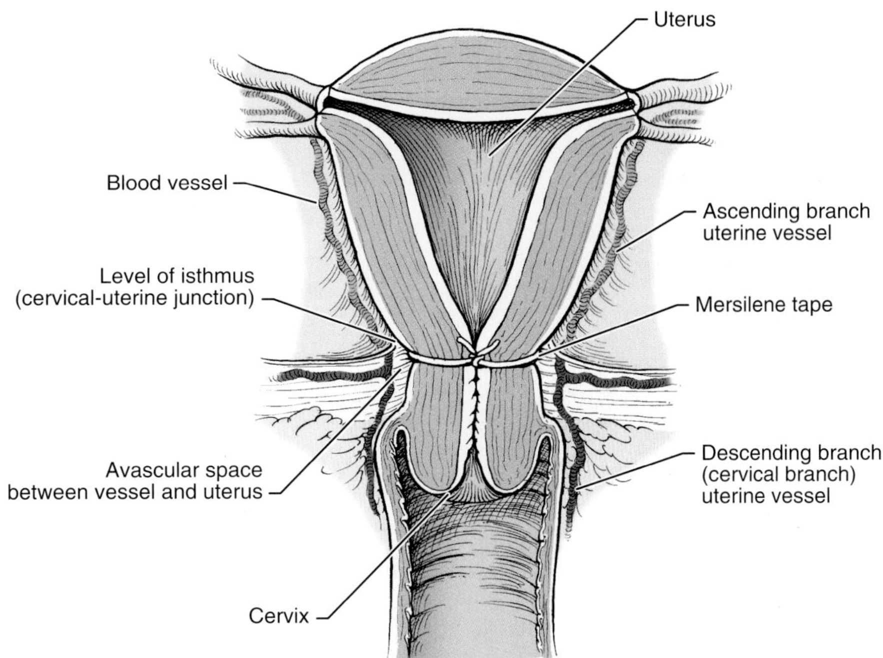

FIG 28-3 Abdominal cerclage. Surgical placement of circumferential Mersilene tape around uterine isthmus and median to uterine vessel. Knot is tied anteriorly. (From: S. Gabbe, J. Niebyl, & J. Simpson [Eds.]. (2012). *Obstetrics: Normal and problem pregnancies* [6th ed.]. Philadelphia: Saunders.)

abdominal cerclage may be performed instead. This procedure is usually done at 11 to 13 weeks of gestation by means of a laparotomy. Suture (Mersilene tape) is placed at the junction of the lower uterine segment and the cervix (Fig. 28-3). Cesarean birth is necessary following an abdominal cerclage, and the suture is left in place if future pregnancies are desired. Although the procedure is usually done during pregnancy, it has been performed between pregnancies with subsequent positive pregnancy outcomes (Ludmir & Owen, 2012).

The nurse assesses the woman's feelings about her pregnancy and her understanding of cervical insufficiency. Evaluating the woman's support systems is also important. Because the diagnosis of cervical insufficiency is usually not made until the woman has lost one or more pregnancies, she may feel guilty or to blame for this impending loss. Assessing for previous reactions to stresses and appropriateness of coping responses is therefore important. The woman needs the support of both her health care providers and her family.

Follow-up Care

The woman will likely be on bed rest for a least a few days immediately following cerclage placement. She will also probably be advised to avoid sexual intercourse, at least until after a postoperative check. Thereafter, decisions about physical activity and lifestyle changes are individualized, based on the status of the woman's cervix, as determined by digital and ultrasound examination (Ludmir & Owen, 2012). The woman must understand the need for close observation and supervision for the remainder of the pregnancy. Additional instruction includes the need to watch for and report signs of preterm labor, rupture of membranes, and infection. Finally, the woman should know the signs that would warrant an immediate return to the hospital, including strong contractions less than 5 minutes apart, preterm premature rupture of membranes, severe perineal pressure, and an urge to push. If management is unsuccessful and the fetus is born before viability, appropriate grief support should be provided. If the fetus is born prematurely, appropriate anticipatory guidance and support will be necessary. (See Chapter 34 for information on high risk newborns and Chapter 37 for information on perinatal loss and grief.)

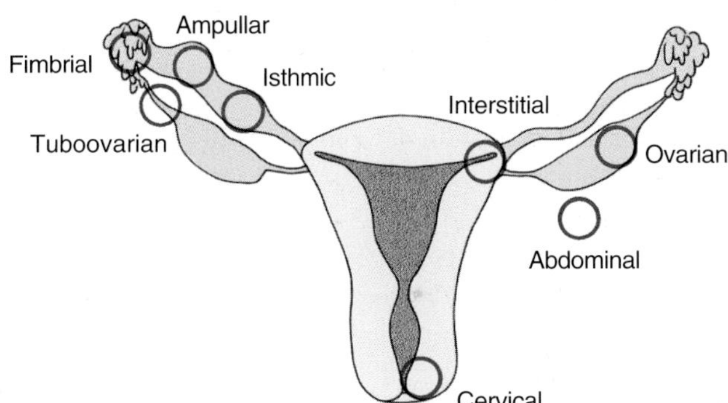

FIG 28-4 Sites of implantation of ectopic pregnancies. Order of frequency of occurrence is ampulla, isthmus, interstitium, fimbria, tuboovarian ligament, ovary, abdominal cavity, and cervix (external os).

Ectopic Pregnancy

Incidence and Etiology

An ectopic pregnancy is one in which the fertilized ovum is implanted outside the uterine cavity (Fig. 28-4). One to two percent of all first-trimester pregnancies in the United States are ectopic, and these account for 6% of all pregnancy-related maternal deaths. Women are less likely to have a successful subsequent pregnancy after an ectopic pregnancy (Cunningham et al., 2014). Ectopic pregnancy is also a leading cause of infertility.

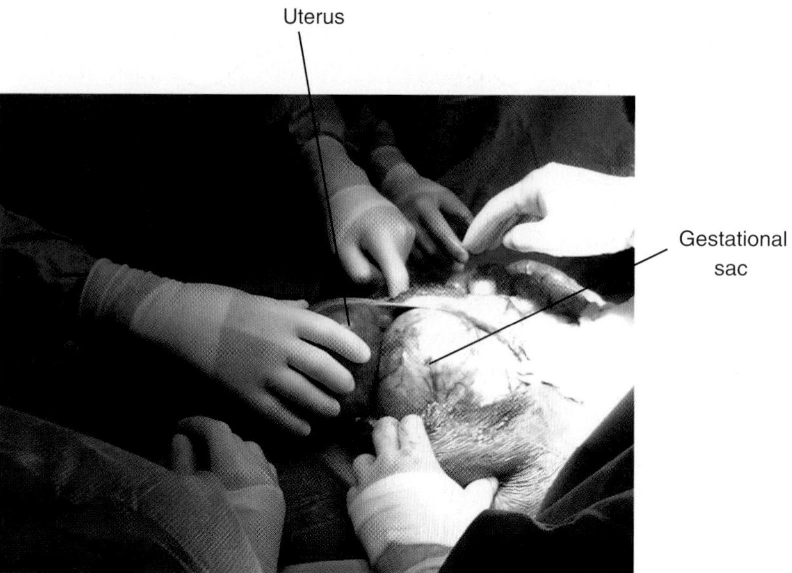

FIG 28-5 Ectopic pregnancy, abdominal, diagnosed on a routine ultrasound at 25 weeks of gestation. Note that the gestational sac is clearly outside the uterus. The placenta was attached to the right uterine tube and right ovary. (Courtesy Danielle L. Tate, MD, Memphis, TN.)

Ectopic pregnancies are often called *tubal pregnancies* because at least 90% are located in the uterine tube (American Society for Reproductive Medicine [ASRM], 2013). Although they are much less common, ectopic pregnancies can also occur in the abdominal cavity, on an ovary, or on the cervix. Of all tubal ectopic pregnancies, approximately 80% are located in the ampulla, or largest portion of the tube (ASRM).

More than 100,000 ectopic pregnancies are reported each year in the United States. The actual number is certainly much larger, however, because only surgically managed cases are reported (ASRM, 2013). Some of the increased incidence is likely because of improved diagnostic techniques, such as more sensitive β-hCG measurement and transvaginal ultrasound, resulting in the identification of more cases. Other causes for the rise include an increased incidence of sexually transmitted infections, tubal infection and damage, popularity of contraceptive methods that predispose failures to be ectopic (e.g., the intrauterine device [IUD]), use of tubal sterilization methods that increase the chance of ectopic pregnancy, increased use of assisted reproductive techniques, and increased use of tubal surgery (Cunningham et al., 2014; Gilbert, 2011).

Ectopic pregnancy is classified according to site of implantation (e.g., tubal, ovarian, or abdominal). The uterus is the only organ capable of containing and sustaining a term pregnancy. Only approximately 5% of abdominal pregnancies reach viability. Surgery to remove the embryo or fetus is usually performed as soon as an abdominal pregnancy is identified, however, because of the high risk for hemorrhage at any time during the pregnancy (Fig. 28-5) (Cunningham et al., 2014; Gilbert, 2011). The chance of fetal survival in an abdominal pregnancy depends on gestational age at birth. The risk for fetal deformity in an abdominal pregnancy is high as a result of pressure deformities caused by oligohydramnios. The most common problems include facial or cranial asymmetry, various joint deformities, limb deficiency, and central nervous system anomalies (Cunningham et al.; Gilbert).

Clinical Manifestations

Most cases of ectopic (tubal) pregnancy are diagnosed before rupture based on the three most classic symptoms: (1) abdominal pain, (2) delayed menses, and (3) abnormal vaginal bleeding (spotting) that occurs approximately 6 to 8 weeks after the last normal menstrual period (Gilbert, 2011). Abdominal pain occurs in almost every case. It usually begins as a dull, lower quadrant pain on one side. The discomfort can progress from a dull pain to a colicky pain when the tube stretches, to sharp, stabbing pain (Cunningham et al., 2014; Gilbert). It progresses to a diffuse, constant, severe pain that is generalized throughout the lower abdomen (Gilbert). Up to 90% of women with an ectopic pregnancy report a period that is delayed 1 to 2 weeks or is lighter than usual, or an irregular period. Mild to moderate dark red or brown intermittent vaginal bleeding occurs in up to 80% of women (Gilbert).

If the ectopic pregnancy is not diagnosed until after rupture has occurred, referred shoulder pain may be present in addition to generalized, one-sided, or deep lower quadrant acute abdominal pain. Referred shoulder pain results from diaphragmatic irritation caused by blood in the peritoneal cavity. The woman may exhibit signs of shock, such as faintness and dizziness, related to the amount of bleeding in the abdominal cavity and not necessarily related to obvious vaginal bleeding. An ecchymotic blueness around the umbilicus (Cullen sign), indicating hematoperitoneum, may also develop in an undiagnosed, ruptured intraabdominal ectopic pregnancy.

Diagnosis

The differential diagnosis of ectopic pregnancy involves consideration of numerous disorders that share many signs and symptoms. Many of these women go to the emergency department experiencing first-trimester bleeding or pain. Miscarriage, ruptured corpus luteum cyst, appendicitis, salpingitis, ovarian cysts, torsion of the ovary, and urinary tract infection are possible diagnoses. The key to early detection of ectopic pregnancy is having a high index of suspicion for this condition. *Every* woman with abdominal pain, vaginal spotting or bleeding, and a positive pregnancy test should undergo screening for ectopic pregnancy.

The most important screening tools for ectopic pregnancy are quantitative β-hCG levels and transvaginal ultrasound examination. When β-hCG levels are greater than 1500 to 2000 milli-International Units/ml, a normal intrauterine pregnancy should be visible on transvaginal ultrasound. Therefore, if β-hCG levels are greater than 1500 milli-International Units/ml but no intrauterine pregnancy is seen on transvaginal ultrasound, an ectopic pregnancy is very likely. β-hCG levels will probably be redrawn every 48 hours to determine if the pregnancy is viable. A transvaginal ultrasound may also be repeated to determine if the pregnancy is inside the uterus. Sometimes the location of an ectopic pregnancy will be visible on transvaginal ultrasound (Cunningham et al., 2014; Gilbert, 2011).

Another laboratory test that can be ordered to determine if the pregnancy is developing normally is a progesterone level. A progesterone level greater than 25 ng/ml almost always rules out the presence of an ectopic pregnancy. However, a progesterone level less than 5 ng/ml suggests either an ectopic pregnancy or an abnormal intrauterine pregnancy (Cunningham et al., 2014).

The woman should also be assessed for the presence of active bleeding, which is associated with tubal rupture. If internal bleeding is present, assessment may reveal vertigo, shoulder pain, hypotension, and tachycardia. A vaginal examination should be performed only once, and then with great caution. Approximately 20% of women with a tubal pregnancy have a palpable mass on examination. Rupturing the mass is possible during a bimanual examination; thus a gentle touch is critical.

CARE MANAGEMENT

Medical Management

Approximately 40% of women diagnosed with ectopic pregnancy are appropriate candidates for medical management, which involves giving methotrexate to dissolve the tubal pregnancy (ASRM, 2013). Methotrexate is an antimetabolite and folic acid antagonist that destroys rapidly dividing cells. It is classified as a hazardous drug and can cause serious toxic side effects even when given in low doses. These side effects can cause safety risks for health care providers if the drug is not handled appropriately. Additionally, the Institute for Safe Medication Practices considers methotrexate to be a high-alert drug (Box 28-1) (National Institute for Occupational Safety and Health, 2012; Shastay & Paparella, 2010).

Methotrexate therapy avoids surgery and is a safe, effective, and cost-effective way of managing many cases of tubal pregnancy. The woman must be hemodynamically stable and have normal liver and kidney function to be eligible for methotrexate therapy. The best results following methotrexate therapy are usually obtained if the mass is unruptured and measures less than 3.5 cm in diameter by ultrasound, if no fetal cardiac activity is noted on ultrasound, and if the initial serum β-hCG level is less than 1000 milli-International Units/L (Cunningham et al., 2014). The woman must also be willing to comply with posttreatment lifestyle restrictions and monitoring. She is informed of how the medication works, possible side effects, general self-care guidelines, and the importance of follow-up care (see Teaching for Self-Management: Teaching for Women Receiving Methotrexate Therapy).

BOX 28-1 Methotrexate Administration

- Obtain the woman's height and weight. These measurements are used to calculate her body surface area in order to determine the correct dose of methotrexate, so they must be accurate.
- The standard dose of methotrexate used to treat ectopic pregnancy is 50 mg/m^2 given intramuscularly, although it may also be ordered as 1 mg/kg.
- The dose of methotrexate should be prepared in the hospital pharmacy under a biologic safety cabinet. Syringe(s) containing the methotrexate should be dispensed from the pharmacy no more than three quarters full without a needle attached in a sealed plastic bag.
- Don two pairs of gloves before removing the syringe(s) from the sealed plastic bag.
- Remove the syringe cap and replace with an appropriate needle for intramuscular injection.
- Do not expel air from the syringe or prime the needle because these actions could aerosolize the methotrexate.
- Check the client's identity and the medication and dosage before injecting the methotrexate. Another nurse should also perform an independent check before the injection is given.
- Dispose of any items worn or used to prepare, dispense, or administer the methotrexate injection in a waste container designated specifically for hazardous drugs.
- Wash your hands thoroughly after removing gloves.

Data from Shastay, A., & Paparella, S. (2010). Ectopic pregnancies and methotrexate: Are you prepared to manage this hazardous drug? *Journal of Emergency Nursing, 36*(1), 57-59.

TEACHING FOR SELF-MANAGEMENT

Teaching for Women Receiving Methotrexate Therapy

- Explain that methotrexate dissolves ectopic (tubal) pregnancies by destroying rapidly dividing cells.
- Explain that urine contains levels of drug metabolite that could be considered toxic for approximately 72 hours after receiving methotrexate. The levels are highest during the first 8 hours after treatment. Teach the woman to avoid getting urine on the toilet seat and to double flush the toilet (with the lid down) after urinating. Also explain that her stools may contain residual drug for up to 7 days.
- Inform the woman of possible side effects. Gastric distress, nausea and vomiting, stomatitis, and dizziness are common. Rare side effects include severe neutropenia, reversible hair loss, and pneumonitis.
- Advise the woman to:
  - Avoid foods and vitamins containing folic acid.
  - Avoid "gas-forming" foods.
  - Avoid sun exposure.
  - Avoid sexual intercourse until the beta-human chorionic gonadotropin (β-hCG) level is undetectable.
  - Keep all scheduled follow-up appointments.
  - Contact her health care provider immediately if she has severe abdominal pain, which may be a sign of impending or actual tubal rupture.

Data from American Society for Reproductive Medicine (ASRM). (2013). Medical treatment of ectopic pregnancy: A committee opinion. *Fertility and Sterility, 100*(3), 638-644; Shastay, A., & Paparella, S. (2010). Ectopic pregnancies and methotrexate: Are you prepared to manage this hazardous drug? *Journal of Emergency Nursing, 36*(1), 57-59.

SAFETY ALERT

Women receiving methotrexate to treat an ectopic pregnancy should not take any analgesic stronger than acetaminophen. Stronger analgesics can mask symptoms of tubal rupture.

Surgical Management

Surgical management depends on the location and cause of the ectopic pregnancy, the extent of tissue involvement, and the woman's desires regarding future fertility. One option is removal of the entire tube (salpingectomy). If the tube has not ruptured and the woman desires future fertility, salpingostomy may be performed instead. In this procedure an incision is made over the pregnancy site in the tube and the products of conception are gently and very carefully removed. The incision is not sutured but left to close by secondary intention instead, given that this method results in less scarring.

If surgery is planned, general preoperative and postoperative care is appropriate for the woman with an ectopic pregnancy. Before surgery, vital signs (pulse, respirations, and blood pressure [BP]) are assessed every 15 minutes or as needed, according to the severity of the bleeding and the woman's condition. Preoperative laboratory tests include determination of blood type and Rh factor, complete blood cell count, and serum quantitative β-hCG level. Ultrasonography is used to confirm an extrauterine pregnancy. Blood replacement may be necessary. The nurse verifies the woman's Rh and antibody status and administers $Rh_0(D)$ immune globulin postoperatively if appropriate.

Follow-Up Care

Women who have received methotrexate therapy have their β-hCG level measured weekly to make certain that it continues to drop steadily until it becomes undetectable. Complete resolution of an ectopic pregnancy usually occurs in 2 to 3 weeks but can require as long as 6 to 8 weeks (ASRM, 2013).

Whether treated medically or surgically, the woman and her family should be encouraged to share their feelings and concerns related to the loss. Future fertility should be discussed. A contraceptive method should be used for at least three menstrual cycles to allow time for the woman's body to heal (Gilbert, 2011). *Every* woman who has been diagnosed with an ectopic pregnancy should be instructed to contact her health care provider as soon as she suspects that she might be pregnant because of the increased risk for recurrent ectopic pregnancy. These women may need referral to grief or infertility support groups. In addition to the loss of the current pregnancy, they are faced with the possibility of future pregnancy losses or infertility. (See Chapter 37 for information on perinatal loss and grief.)

Hydatidiform Mole (Molar Pregnancy)

Hydatidiform mole (molar pregnancy) is a benign proliferative growth of the placental trophoblast in which the chorionic villi develop into edematous, cystic, avascular transparent vesicles that hang in a grapelike cluster. Hydatidiform mole is a gestational trophoblastic disease (GTD). GTD is a group of pregnancy-related trophoblastic proliferative disorders without a viable fetus that are caused by abnormal fertilization. In addition to hydatidiform mole, GTD includes invasive mole and choriocarcinoma (DiGiulio, Wiedaseck, & Monchek, 2012).

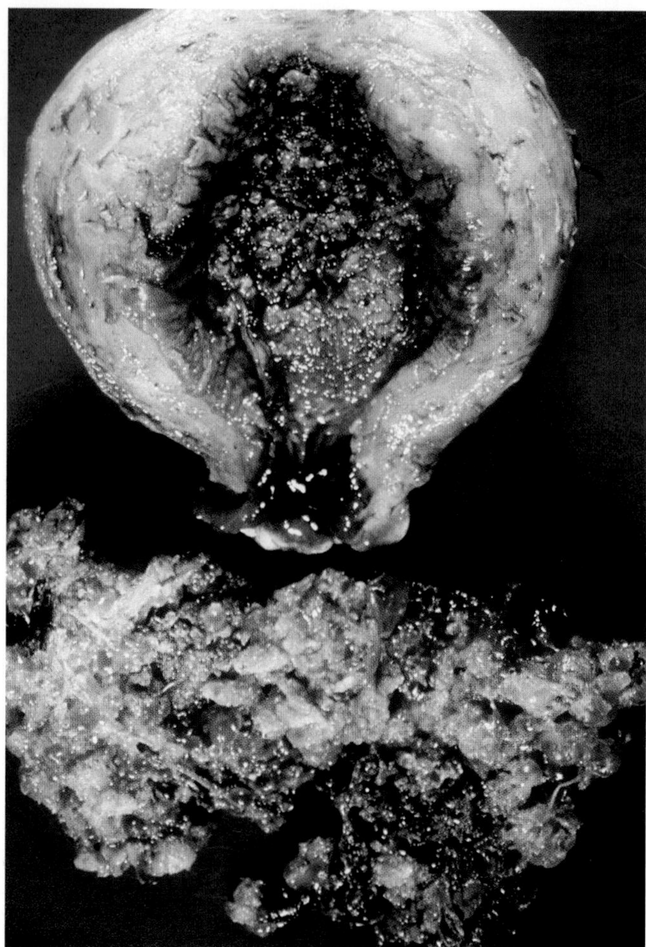

FIG 28-6 Gross specimen in a woman treated for complete hydatidiform mole with primary hysterectomy. (Courtesy John Soper, MD.) (From DiSaia, P., & Creasman, W. [2007]: *Clinical gynecologic oncology* [7th ed.]. Philadelphia: Mosby.)

Incidence and Etiology

Hydatidiform mole occurs in 1 in 1000 pregnancies in the United States (Cohn, Ramaswamy, & Blum, 2014). The cause is unknown, although it may be related to an ovular defect or a nutritional deficiency. Women at increased risk for hydatidiform mole formation are those who have had a prior molar pregnancy and those who are in their early teens or older than 40 years of age (DiGiulio et al., 2012).

Types

A hydatidiform mole may be further categorized as a complete or partial mole. The complete mole results from fertilization of an egg in which the nucleus has been lost or inactivated. The nucleus of a sperm (23,X or 23,Y) duplicates itself (resulting in the diploid number 46,XX or 46,XY) because the ovum has no genetic material or the material is inactive. It is also possible for an "empty" egg to be fertilized by two normal sperm, thereby producing either a 46,XX or 46,XY genotype (Moore, 2014). The mole resembles a bunch of white grapes. The hydropic (fluid-filled) vesicles grow rapidly, causing the uterus to be larger than expected for the duration of the pregnancy. The complete mole contains no fetus, placenta, amniotic membranes, or fluid (Fig. 28-6). Maternal blood has no placenta to receive it; therefore, hemorrhage into the uterine cavity and

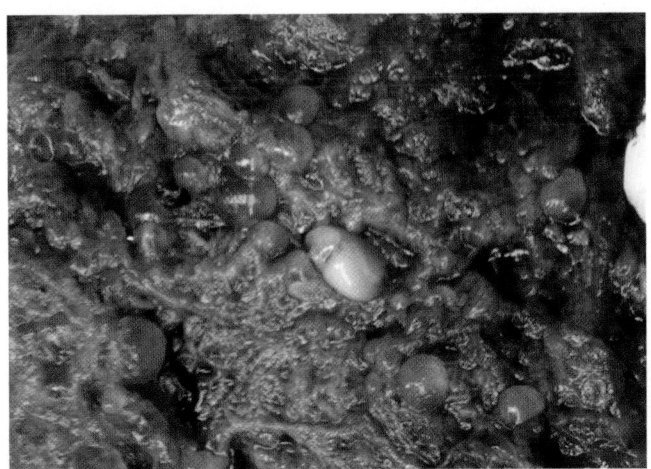

FIG 28-7 Partial hydatidiform mole. (Courtesy Norman L. Meyer, MD, PhD, Memphis, TN.)

vaginal bleeding occur. Approximately 15% to 20% of women with a complete mole have evidence of persistent GTD (Cunningham et al., 2014).

In a partial mole one apparently normal ovum is fertilized by two or more sperm. Triploidy (69XXY) or quadraploidy (92XXXY) genotypes then result (Moore, 2014). Partial moles often have embryonic or fetal parts and an amniotic sac (Fig. 28-7). Congenital anomalies are usually present. The risk of persistent GTD is much less than with a complete mole. If persistent GTD does occur, it is usually not a choriocarcinoma (Cunningham et al., 2014).

Clinical Manifestations

In the early stages the clinical manifestations of a complete hydatidiform mole cannot be distinguished from those of normal pregnancy. Later, vaginal bleeding occurs in almost 95% of cases. The vaginal discharge may be dark brown (resembling prune juice) or bright red and either scant or profuse. It may continue for only a few days or intermittently for weeks. Early in pregnancy the uterus in approximately one half of affected women is significantly larger than expected from menstrual dates. The percentage of women with an excessively enlarged uterus increases as length of time since the last menstrual period increases. Approximately 25% of affected women have a uterus smaller than would be expected from menstrual dates.

Anemia from blood loss, excessive nausea and vomiting (hyperemesis gravidarum), and abdominal cramps caused by uterine distention are relatively common findings. Women may also pass vesicles, which are frequently avascular edematous villi, from the uterus. Preeclampsia occurs in approximately 70% of women with large, rapidly growing hydatidiform moles and occurs earlier than usual in the pregnancy. If preeclampsia is diagnosed before 24 weeks of gestation, hydatidiform mole should be suspected and ruled out. Hyperthyroidism is another serious complication of hydatidiform mole. Usually treatment of the hydatidiform mole restores thyroid function to normal. Partial moles cause few of these symptoms and may be mistaken for an incomplete or missed miscarriage (DiGiulio et al., 2012; Markham & Funai, 2014; Moore, 2014; Nader, 2014).

Diagnosis

Transvaginal ultrasound and serum hCG levels are used for diagnosis. Transvaginal ultrasound is the most accurate tool for diagnosing a hydatidiform mole. A characteristic pattern of multiple diffuse intrauterine masses, often called a *snowstorm pattern,* is seen in place of, or along with, an embryo or a fetus. The trophoblastic tissue secretes the hCG hormone. In a molar pregnancy, hCG levels are persistently high or rising beyond 10 to 12 weeks of gestation, the time they would begin to decline in a normal pregnancy (Cohn et al., 2014; Gilbert, 2011; Moore, 2014).

CARE MANAGEMENT

Surgical Management

Although most moles abort spontaneously, suction curettage offers a safe, rapid, and effective method of evacuating a hydatidiform mole if necessary (Cunningham et al., 2014; Gilbert, 2011). Induction of labor with oxytocic agents or prostaglandin is not recommended because of the increased risk of embolization of trophoblastic tissue. Postevacuation administration of $Rh_0(D)$ immune globulin to women who are Rh negative is necessary to prevent isoimmunization (Gilbert).

Nursing Interventions

The nurse provides the woman and her family with information about the disease process, the necessity for a long course of follow-up, and the possible consequences of the disease. The nurse also helps the woman and her family cope with the pregnancy loss and recognize that the pregnancy was not normal. In addition, the woman and her family are encouraged to express their feelings, and information is provided about local support groups or counseling resources as needed. Internet resources such as Share: Pregnancy and Infant Loss Support, Inc., at www.nationalshare.org and the International Society for the Study of Trophoblastic Disease at www.isstd.org may also be useful. Explanations about the importance of postponing a subsequent pregnancy and contraceptive counseling are provided to emphasize the need for consistent and reliable use of the method chosen.

> **! NURSING ALERT**
>
> To avoid confusion in regard to rising levels of hCG that are normal in pregnancy but could indicate GTD, pregnancy should be avoided during the follow-up assessment period. Any contraceptive method except an intrauterine device (IUD) is acceptable. Oral contraceptives are preferred because they are highly effective. Injectable medroxyprogesterone acetate is a practical option for women who have difficulty complying with the daily dosing required for oral contraceptive use.

Follow-Up Care

Follow-up care includes frequent physical and pelvic examinations along with weekly measurements of the β-hCG level until the level decreases to normal and remains normal for 3 consecutive weeks. Monthly measurements are then taken for 6 months. The follow-up assessment period usually continues for a year. During that time a rising β-hCG level and an enlarging uterus may indicate GTD (see Chapter 11 for further discussion) (DiGiulio et al., 2012; Gilbert, 2011).

COMMUNITY ACTIVITY

Talk with someone who has experienced an early pregnancy loss, either a miscarriage, an ectopic pregnancy, or a hydatidiform mole. What helpful things did her health care providers say or do at the time of the loss? What things did they say or do that were not helpful? Are there things that she wishes had been done or said differently? Which of her suggestions do you think would be helpful to people experiencing a different kind of loss?

LATE PREGNANCY BLEEDING

The major causes of bleeding in late pregnancy are placenta previa and premature separation of the placenta (abruptio placentae, or placental abruption). Rapid assessment for and diagnosis of the cause of bleeding are essential to reduce maternal and perinatal morbidity and mortality (Table 28-2).

Placenta Previa

Because of advances in ultrasonography, especially transvaginal ultrasound, and an increased understanding of the changing relationship between the placenta and the internal cervical os as pregnancy progresses, definitions and classifications of placenta previa have changed. In placenta previa the placenta is implanted in the lower uterine segment such that it completely or partially covers the cervix or is close enough to the cervix to cause bleeding when the cervix dilates or the lower uterine segment effaces (Fig. 28-8) (Hull & Resnik, 2014). When transvaginal ultrasound is used, the placenta is classified as a *complete placenta previa* if it totally covers the internal cervical os. In a *marginal placenta previa* the edge of the placenta is seen on transvaginal ultrasound to be 2.5 cm or closer to the internal cervical os. When the exact relationship of the placenta to the internal cervical os has not been determined or in the case of apparent placenta previa in the second trimester, the term *low-lying placenta* is used (Hull & Resnik).

TABLE 28-2 Summary of Findings: Placental Abruption and Placenta Previa

	PLACENTAL ABRUPTION			
FINDINGS	GRADE 1 MILD SEPARATION (10%-20%)	GRADE 2 MODERATE SEPARATION (20%-50%)	GRADE 3 SEVERE SEPARATION (>50%)	PLACENTA PREVIA
Physical and Laboratory Findings				
Bleeding, external, vaginal	Minimal	Absent to moderate	Absent to moderate	Minimal to severe and life threatening
Total amount of blood loss	<500 ml	1000-1500 ml	>1500 ml	Varies
Color of blood	Dark red	Dark red	Dark red	Bright red
Shock	Rare; none	Mild shock	Common, often sudden, profound	Uncommon
Coagulopathy	Rare, none	Occasional DIC	Frequent DIC	None
Uterine tonicity	Normal	Increased, may be localized to one region or diffuse over uterus, uterus fails to relax between contractions	Tetanic, persistent uterine contractions, boardlike uterus	Normal
Tenderness (pain)	Usually absent	Present	Agonizing, unremitting uterine pain	Absent
Ultrasonographic Findings				
Location of placenta	Normal, upper uterine segment	Normal, upper uterine segment	Normal, upper uterine segment	Abnormal, lower uterine segment
Station of presenting part	Variable to engaged	Variable to engaged	Variable to engaged	High, not engaged
Fetal position	Usual distribution*	Usual distribution*	Usual distribution*	Commonly transverse, breech, or oblique
Gestational or chronic hypertension	Usual distribution*	Commonly present	Commonly present	Usual distribution*
Fetal effects	Normal fetal heart rate and pattern	Abnormal fetal heart rate and pattern	Abnormal fetal heart rate and pattern; fetal death can occur	Normal fetal heart rate and pattern

DIC, Disseminated intravascular coagulation.
*Usual distribution refers to the expected variations of incidence seen when there is no concurrent problem.

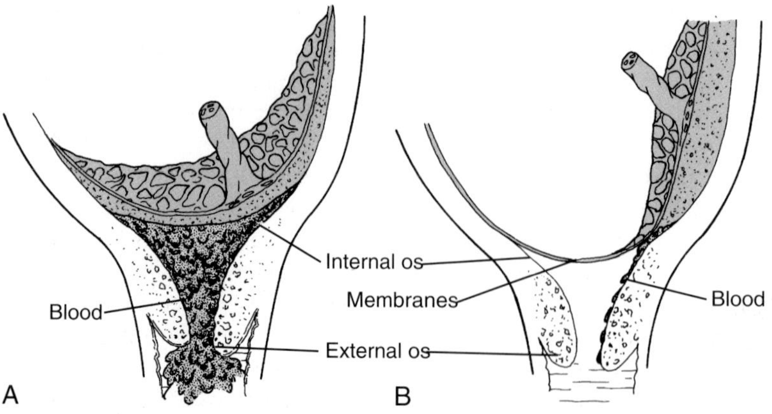

FIG 28-8 Types of placenta previa. **A**, Complete. **B**, Marginal.

Incidence and Etiology

Placenta previa affects approximately 1 in 200 pregnancies at term. Some evidence suggests that the incidence of placenta previa is increasing, perhaps as a result of more cesarean births. In addition to a history of previous cesarean birth, other risk factors for placenta previa include advanced maternal age (more than 35 to 40 years of age), multiparity, history of prior suction curettage, and smoking (Hull & Resnik, 2014). Living at a higher altitude is also a risk factor for placenta previa. Like cigarette smoking, a higher altitude causes a decrease in uteroplacental oxygenation and thus a need for increased placental surface area. Placenta previa also occurs more frequently in women carrying male fetuses. A possible explanation for this is that placental sizes are larger in pregnancies involving male fetuses (Francois & Foley, 2012). Multiple gestation is also a risk factor for placenta previa because of the larger placental area in these pregnancies (Cunningham et al., 2014). Women who had placenta previa in a previous pregnancy are more likely than others to develop the problem in a subsequent pregnancy, perhaps as a result of a genetic predisposition. Previous cesarean birth and curettage in the past for miscarriage or induced abortion are risk factors for placenta previa because both result in endometrial damage and uterine scarring (Francois & Foley; Hull & Resnik).

Clinical Manifestations

Placenta previa is typically characterized by painless bright red vaginal bleeding during the second or third trimester. In the past, placenta previa was usually diagnosed after an episode of bleeding. Currently, however, most cases are diagnosed by ultrasound before significant vaginal bleeding occurs. This bleeding is associated with the disruption of placental blood vessels that occurs with stretching and thinning of the lower uterine segment (Francois & Foley, 2012). The initial bleeding is usually a small amount and stops as clots form. It can recur, however, at any time (Gilbert, 2011).

Vital signs may be normal, even with heavy blood loss, because a pregnant woman can lose up to 40% of her blood volume without showing signs of shock. Clinical presentation and decreasing urinary output may be better indicators of acute blood loss than vital signs alone. The fetal heart rate (FHR) is normal unless a major detachment of the placenta occurs.

Abdominal examination usually reveals a soft, relaxed, nontender uterus with normal tone. The presenting part of the fetus usually remains high because the placenta occupies the lower uterine segment. Thus the fundal height is often greater than expected for gestational age. Because of the abnormally located placenta, fetal malpresentation (breech and transverse or oblique lie) is common.

Maternal and Fetal Outcomes

The major maternal complication associated with placenta previa is hemorrhage. Another serious complication is development of an abnormal placental attachment (e.g., *placenta accreta, increta,* or *percreta*) (see Chapter 33). If excessive bleeding cannot be controlled, hysterectomy may be necessary (Cunningham et al., 2014; Hull & Resnik, 2014). Because most women with placenta previa give birth by cesarean, surgery-related trauma to structures adjacent to the uterus and anesthesia complications are also possible. In addition, blood transfusion reactions, anemia, thrombophlebitis, and infection may occur.

The greatest risk of fetal death is caused by preterm birth. Other fetal risks include stillbirth, malpresentation, and fetal anemia. Intrauterine growth restriction (IUGR) has also been associated with placenta previa. This association can be related to poor placental exchange (Gilbert, 2011). The incidence of fetal anomalies is increased in pregnancies complicated by placenta previa (Cunningham et al., 2014).

Diagnosis

All women with painless vaginal bleeding after 20 weeks of gestation should be assumed to have a placenta previa until proven otherwise. A transabdominal ultrasound examination should be performed initially followed by a transvaginal scan, unless the transabdominal ultrasound clearly shows that the placenta is not located in the lower uterine segment. A transvaginal ultrasound is better than a transabdominal scan for accurately determining placental location (Hull & Resnik, 2014). If ultrasonographic scanning reveals a normally implanted placenta, a speculum examination may be performed to rule out local causes of bleeding (e.g., cervicitis, polyps, carcinoma of the cervix), and a coagulation profile is obtained to rule out other causes of bleeding.

CARE MANAGEMENT

Once placenta previa has been diagnosed, a management plan is developed. The woman will be managed either expectantly or actively, depending on the gestational age, amount of bleeding, and fetal condition.

Potential nursing diagnoses include:

- *Decreased Cardiac Output* related to:
  - excessive blood loss secondary to placenta previa
- *Deficient Fluid Volume* related to:
  - excessive blood loss secondary to placenta previa
- *Ineffective Peripheral Tissue Perfusion* related to:
  - hypovolemia and shunting of blood to central circulation
- *Anxiety* related to:
  - maternal condition and pregnancy outcome
- *Grieving* related to:
  - actual or perceived threat to self, pregnancy, or infant

Expectant Management. Expectant management (observation and bed rest) is implemented if the fetus is at less than 36 weeks of gestation and has a normal FHR tracing, the bleeding is mild (<250 ml) and stops, and the woman is not in labor. The purpose of expectant management is to allow the fetus time to mature (Gilbert, 2011). The woman will initially be hospitalized in a labor and birth unit for continuous FHR and contraction monitoring. Large-bore intravenous (IV) access should be initiated immediately. Initial laboratory tests include hemoglobin, hematocrit, platelet count, and coagulation studies. A "type and screen" blood sample should be maintained at all times in the hospital's transfusion services department to allow for immediate crossmatch of blood component therapy if necessary. If the woman is at less than 34 weeks of gestation, antenatal corticosteroids should be administered (Francois & Foley, 2012; Gilbert).

If the bleeding stops, the woman will most likely be placed on bed rest with bathroom privileges and limited activity (e.g., able to use the bathroom, shower, and move around her hospital room for 15 to 30 minutes at a time, four times a day). No vaginal or rectal examinations are performed, and the woman is placed on "pelvic rest" (nothing in the vagina). Ultrasound examinations may be performed every 2 to 3 weeks. Fetal surveillance may include a nonstress test (NST) or biophysical profile (BPP) once or twice weekly. Bleeding is assessed by checking the amount of blood on perineal pads, bed pads, and linens. Serial laboratory values are evaluated for decreasing hemoglobin and hematocrit levels and changes in coagulation values. The woman should also be monitored for signs of preterm labor. Magnesium sulfate can be given for tocolysis if uterine contractions are identified (Francois & Foley, 2012; Gilbert, 2011).

The woman with placenta previa should always be considered a potential emergency because massive blood loss with resulting hypovolemic shock can occur quickly if bleeding resumes. The possibility always exists that she will require an emergency cesarean for birth. Placenta previa in a preterm gestation may be an indication for transfer to a tertiary-care perinatal center, given that a neonatal intensive care unit may be necessary for care of the preterm infant. Also because many community hospitals are not prepared to perform emergency surgery 24 hours per day, 7 days per week, transfer to a tertiary-care center may be necessary to ensure constant access to cesarean birth.

Home Care. Sometimes women with placenta previa are discharged from the hospital before giving birth to be managed at home. The woman's condition should be stable, and she should have experienced no vaginal bleeding for at least 48 hours before discharge (Hull & Resnik, 2014). A candidate for home care must meet other strict criteria as well. She should be willing and able to comply with activity restrictions (bed rest with bathroom privileges and pelvic rest), live within 20 minutes of the hospital, and have access to a telephone, close supervision by family or friends in the home, and constant access to transportation (Francois & Foley, 2012). If bleeding resumes, she needs to return to the hospital immediately. She must also be able to keep all appointments for fetal testing, laboratory assessments, and prenatal care. Visits by a perinatal home care nurse may be arranged.

If hospitalization or home care with activity restriction is prolonged, the woman can have concerns about her work- or family-related responsibilities or become bored with inactivity. She should be encouraged to participate in her own care and decisions about care as much as possible. Providing diversionary activities or encouraging her to participate in activities she enjoys and can perform during bed rest are necessary. Participating in a support group made up of other women on bed rest while hospitalized or online if at home may be a helpful coping mechanism (see Teaching for Self-Management: Coping with Activity Restriction in Chapter 27).

Active Management. If the woman definitely has placenta previa and she is at or beyond 36 weeks of gestation, birth is appropriate. If bleeding is excessive or continues or there are concerns about the condition of the fetus, immediate birth is indicated, regardless of gestational age (Hull & Resnik, 2014). All women whose placenta lies within 2 cm of the cervix, as documented by a transvaginal ultrasound performed late in the third trimester, should give birth by cesarean. However, an asymptomatic woman whose placenta clearly lies more than 2 cm from the cervical os can safely be allowed to labor (Francois & Foley, 2012; Hull and Resnik).

If cesarean birth is planned, the nurse continually assesses maternal and fetal status while preparing the woman for surgery. Maternal vital signs are assessed frequently for decreasing BP, increasing pulse rate, changes in level of consciousness, and oliguria. Fetal assessment is maintained by continuous electronic fetal monitoring (EFM) to assess for signs of hypoxia.

Blood loss may not stop with the birth of the infant. The large vascular channels in the lower uterine segment may continue to bleed because of that segment's diminished muscle content. The natural mechanism to control bleeding so characteristic of the upper part of the uterus—the interlacing muscle bundles, the "living ligature" contracting around open vessels—is absent in the lower part of the uterus. Postpartum hemorrhage may therefore occur even if the fundus is contracted firmly (see Chapter 33).

Emotional support for the woman and her family is extremely important. The actively bleeding woman is concerned not only for her own well-being but also for that of her fetus. All procedures should be explained, and a support person should be present. The woman should be encouraged to express her concerns and feelings. If the woman and her support person or family desire pastoral support, the nurse can notify the hospital chaplain service or provide information about other supportive resources.

CLINICAL REASONING CASE STUDY

Third-Trimester Vaginal Bleeding

Crystal is a 41-year-old G5 P2 1 1 4 (one set of twins) who presents to the emergency department with heavy vaginal bleeding. She has had no prenatal care but is approximately 33 weeks of gestation by her LMP. Crystal said, "I was fine when I went to bed last night. In the middle of the night I woke up and found a huge puddle of blood in my bed. I called the ambulance right away and they brought me here." During her medical screening exam you learn that Crystal has had one cesarean birth (with her twins) and a D&C after a miscarriage 5 years ago. She also smokes 1 pack of cigarettes per day.

1. Evidence—Is there sufficient evidence to determine the cause of Crystal's bleeding?
2. Assumptions—Describe an underlying assumption about each of the following issues:
   a. Possible diagnoses for Crystal
   b. Diagnostic tests necessary to determine the cause of Crystal's bleeding
   c. Inpatient and outpatient management options for Crystal
3. What implications and priorities for nursing care can be drawn at this time?
4. Does the evidence objectively support your conclusion?

D&C, Dilation and curettage; *LMP,* last menstrual period.

Premature Separation of the Placenta (Abruptio Placentae [Placental Abruption])

Premature separation of the placenta, or abruptio placentae, is the detachment of part or all of a normally implanted placenta from the uterus (Fig. 28-9). Separation occurs in the area of the decidua basalis after 20 weeks of gestation and before the birth of the infant.

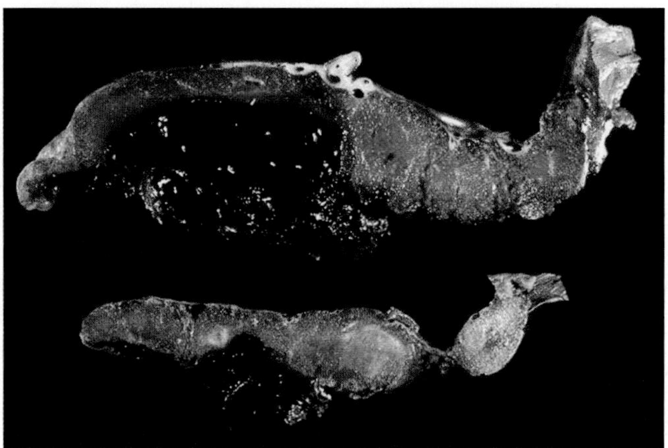

FIG 28-9 Placental abruption. Premature separation of normally implanted placenta. A large retroplacental clot is present. (From Creasy, R., Resnik, R., Iams, J., et al. [2009]. *Creasy & Resnik's maternal-fetal medicine: Principles and practice* [6th ed.]. Philadelphia: Saunders.)

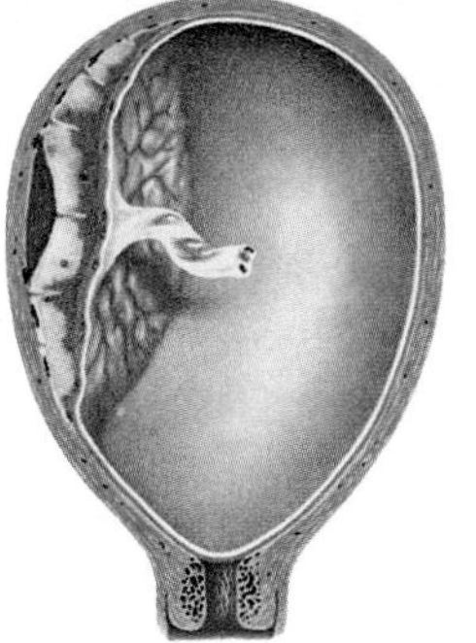

Partial separation
(concealed hemorrhage)

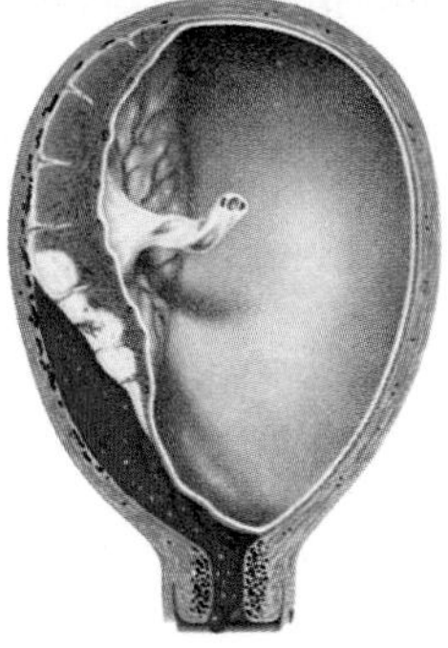

Partial separation
(apparent hemorrhage)

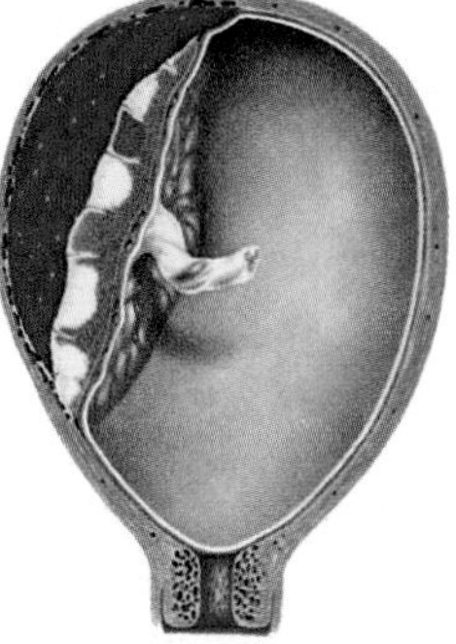

Complete separation
(concealed hemorrhage)

FIG 28-10 Placental abruption, showing partial and complete placental separation.

Incidence and Etiology

Placental abruption is a serious complication that accounts for significant maternal and fetal morbidity and mortality. Approximately 1 in 75 to 1 in 226 pregnancies is complicated by placental abruption. The range in incidence likely reflects both variable criteria for diagnosis and an increased recognition of milder forms of abruption. Approximately one third of all antepartum bleeding is caused by placental abruption (Francois & Foley, 2012).

Maternal hypertension, whether chronic or pregnancy related, is the most consistently identified risk factor for abruption. Cocaine use is also a risk factor because it causes vascular disruption in the placental bed. Blunt external abdominal trauma, most often the result of motor vehicle accidents (MVAs) or maternal battering, is another frequent cause of placental abruption (Cunningham et al., 2014; Francois & Foley, 2012). Other risk factors include cigarette smoking, a history of abruption in a previous pregnancy, and preterm premature rupture of membranes (preterm PROM). There has been great interest in a possible association between thrombophilic disorders and abruption. However, both retrospective and prospective studies of women with the factor V Leiden mutation have shown no increase in risk for abruption (Hull & Resnik, 2014). Abruption is more likely to occur in twin gestations than in singletons (Francois & Foley). Women who have had two previous abruptions have a recurrence risk of 25% in the next pregnancy (Hull & Resnik).

Classification

The most common classification of placental abruption is according to type and severity. This classification system is summarized in Table 28-2.

Clinical Manifestations

The separation may be partial or complete, or only the margin of the placenta may be involved. Bleeding from the placental site may dissect (separate) the membranes from the decidua basalis and flow out through the vagina (70% to 80%), it may remain concealed (retroplacental hemorrhage) (10% to 20%), or both (Fig. 28-10) (Francois & Foley, 2012; Gilbert, 2011). Clinical symptoms vary with degree of separation (see Table 28-2). If cesarean birth is performed, blood clots may be noted on entry into the uterus. A blood clot often will be attached to the posterior surface of the placenta (referred to as a retroplacental clot) (see Fig. 28-9).

Classic symptoms of placental abruption include vaginal bleeding, abdominal pain, and uterine tenderness and contractions (Cunningham et al., 2014; Hull & Resnik, 2014). Bleeding may result in maternal hypovolemia (i.e., shock, oliguria, anuria) and coagulopathy. Mild to severe uterine hypertonicity is present. Pain is mild to severe and localized over one region of the uterus or diffuse over the uterus with a boardlike abdomen.

Extensive myometrial bleeding damages the uterine muscle. If blood accumulates between the separated placenta and the uterine wall, it may produce a couvelaire uterus. The uterus appears purple or blue, rather than its usual "bubblegum pink" color, and contractility is lost. Shock may occur and is out of proportion to blood loss. Laboratory findings include a positive Apt test result (blood in the amniotic fluid); a decrease in hemoglobin and hematocrit levels, which may appear later; and a decrease in coagulation factor levels. Clotting defects (e.g., disseminated intravascular coagulation [DIC]) may be present when more than 50% of the placental surface area abrupts (Francois and Foley, 2012). A Kleihauer-Betke (KB) test may be ordered to determine the presence of fetal-to-maternal bleeding (transplacental hemorrhage), although it is of no diagnostic value. The KB test may be useful, however, to guide $Rh_o(D)$ immune globulin therapy in Rh-negative women who have had an abruption (Hull & Resnik, 2014).

Maternal and Fetal Outcomes

The mother's prognosis depends on the extent of placental detachment, overall blood loss, degree of coagulopathy present, and the time that passes between placental detachment and birth. Maternal complications are associated with the abruption or its treatment. Hemorrhage, hypovolemic shock, hypofibrinogenemia, and thrombocytopenia are associated with severe abruption. Renal failure and pituitary necrosis may result from ischemia. In rare cases, women who are Rh negative can become sensitized if fetal-to-maternal hemorrhage occurs and the fetal blood type is Rh positive.

Fetal complications, which include IUGR and preterm birth, are related to the severity and timing of the hemorrhage. The size of the hemorrhage is related to fetal survival. Large (>60 ml) hemorrhages are associated with 50% or higher fetal mortality (Francois & Foley, 2012). Risks for neurologic defects, cerebral palsy, and death from sudden infant death syndrome are greater in newborns following placental abruption (Cunningham et al., 2014; Francois & Foley).

Diagnosis

Placental abruption is primarily a clinical diagnosis. Although ultrasound can be used to rule out placenta previa, it cannot detect all cases of abruption. A retroplacental mass may be detected with ultrasonographic examination, but negative findings do not rule out a life-threatening abruption. In fact, at least 50% of abruptions cannot be identified on ultrasound (Hull & Resnik, 2014). Hypofibrinogenemia and evidence of DIC support the diagnosis, but many women with placental abruption do not develop coagulopathy. The diagnosis of abruption is confirmed after birth by visual inspection of the placenta. Adherent clot on the maternal surface of the placenta and depression of the underlying placental surface are usually present (see Fig. 28-9) (Francois & Foley, 2012; Gilbert, 2011).

Placental abruption should be highly suspected in the woman who experiences a sudden onset of intense, usually localized, uterine pain, with or without vaginal bleeding. Initial assessment is much the same as for placenta previa. Physical examination usually reveals abdominal pain, uterine tenderness, and contractions. The fundal height may be measured over time because an increasing fundal height indicates concealed bleeding. Approximately 60% of live fetuses exhibit abnormal FHR patterns, and elevated uterine resting tone may also be noted on the monitor tracing (Francois & Foley, 2012). Coagulopathy, as evidenced by abnormal clotting studies (fibrinogen, platelet count, partial thromboplastin time [PTT], fibrin split products), may be present if a large or complete abruption has occurred.

CARE MANAGEMENT

Expectant Management. Management depends on the severity of blood loss and fetal maturity and status. If the fetus is between 20 and 34 weeks of gestation and both the woman and fetus are stable, expectant management can be implemented. The woman is monitored closely because the abruption may extend at any time. The fetus is assessed regularly for evidence of appropriate growth because there is risk for IUGR. In addition, assessments of fetal well-being (e.g., NST and BPP) are performed regularly. See Chapter 26 for further discussion of these tests. Corticosteroids are given to accelerate fetal lung maturity (Hull & Resnik, 2014).

Active Management. Immediate birth is the management of choice if the fetus is at term gestation or if the bleeding is moderate to severe and the mother or fetus is in jeopardy. At least one large-bore (16- to 18-gauge) IV line should be started. Maternal vital signs are monitored frequently to observe for signs of declining hemodynamic status, such as increasing pulse rate and decreasing BP. Serial laboratory studies include hematocrit or hemoglobin determinations and clotting studies. Continuous EFM is mandatory. An indwelling catheter is inserted for continuous assessment of urine output, an excellent indirect measure of maternal organ perfusion. Blood and fluid volume replacement may be necessary, along with administering blood products to correct any coagulation defects.

Although vaginal birth is usually preferable, cesarean birth may become necessary. Cesarean birth should not be attempted when a woman has severe and uncorrected coagulopathy because it can result in uncontrollable bleeding (Francois & Foley, 2012).

Nursing care of women experiencing moderate to severe abruption is demanding because it requires constant close monitoring of the maternal and fetal condition. Information about placental abruption, including the cause, treatment, and expected outcome, is given to the woman and her family. Emotional support is also extremely important because the woman and her family may be experiencing fetal loss in addition to the woman's critical illness.

Cord Insertion and Placental Variations

When fetal vessels lie over the cervical os, the condition is termed vasa previa. In vasa previa the vessels are implanted into the fetal membranes rather than into the placenta. Usually these vessels are protected only by the membranes (not by Wharton's jelly); thus they are at risk for rupture or compression. Vasa previa is rare, affecting between 1 in 1275 and 1 in 8333 pregnancies (Hull & Resnik, 2014). There are two variations of vasa previa. In both situations artificial or spontaneous rupture of the membranes or traction on the cord may rupture one or more of the fetal vessels. As a result the fetus may rapidly bleed to death (Francois & Foley, 2012; Sosa, 2014). Risk factors for vasa previa include low-lying placentas, pregnancies resulting from assisted reproductive technology, and multiple gestations (Francois & Foley).

One variation of vasa previa, *velamentous insertion of the cord*, occurs when the cord vessels begin to branch at the membranes and then course onto the placenta (Fig. 28-11). The other variant of vasa previa occurs when the placenta has divided into two or more lobes rather than remaining as a single mass. This is known as a *succenturiate* placenta (Fig. 28-12). Fetal vessels then run between the lobes of the placenta. The vessels collect at the periphery, and the main trunks eventually unite to form the vessels of the cord. During the third stage of labor one or more of the separate lobes may remain attached to the decidua basalis, preventing uterine contraction and increasing the risk of postpartum hemorrhage.

Another placental variation is *Battledore* (marginal) insertion of the cord (Fig. 28-13). This variation also increases the

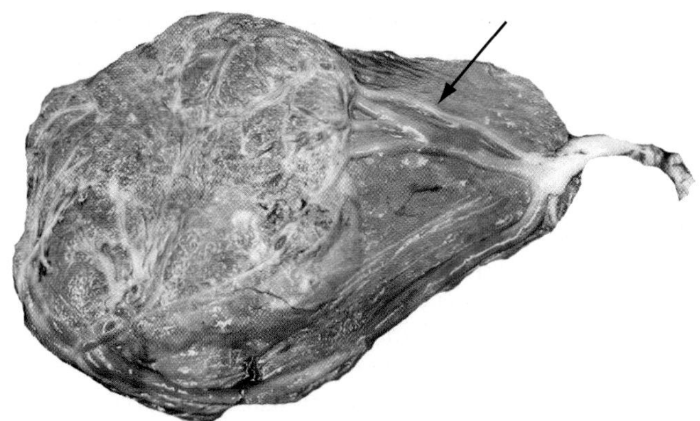

FIG 28-11 Vasa previa (velamentous insertion of cord). *Arrow* shows velamentous cord insertion in the placenta. (From Creasy, R., Resnik, R., Iams, J., et al. [2009]. *Creasy & Resnik's maternal-fetal medicine: Principles and practice* [6th ed.]. Philadelphia: Saunders.)

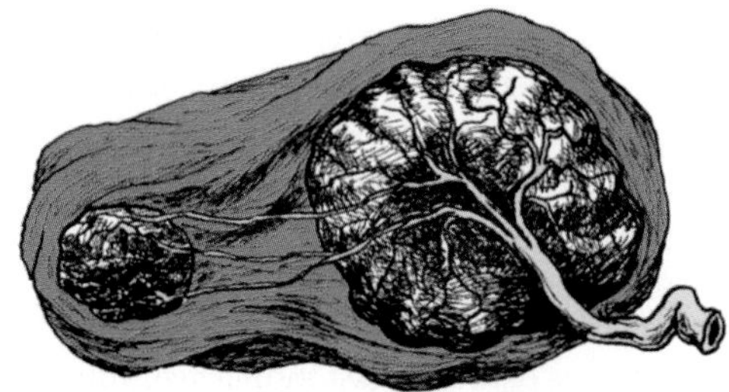

FIG 28-12 Vasa previa (succenturiate placenta).

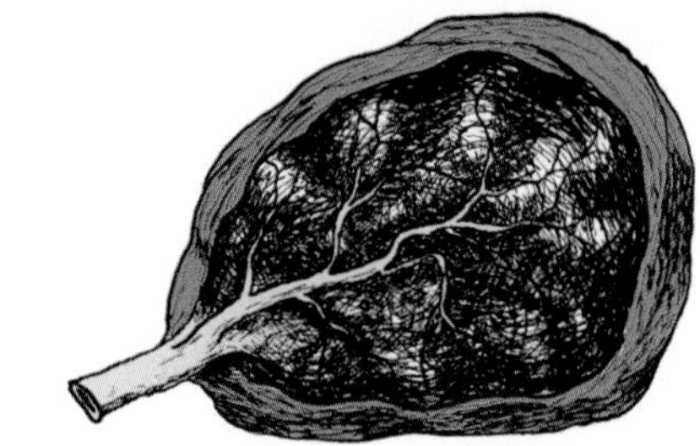

FIG 28-13 Battledore (marginal) cord insertion.

risk of fetal hemorrhage, especially after marginal separation of the placenta.

Clotting Disorders in Pregnancy

Normal Clotting

Normally a delicate balance (homeostasis) exists between the opposing hemostatic and fibrinolytic systems. The hemostatic system stops the flow of blood from injured vessels, first by a platelet plug, which is followed by the formation of a fibrin clot. The coagulation process involves an interaction of the coagulation factors that constantly circulate in the bloodstream in which each factor sequentially activates the factor next in line, the "cascade effect" sequence. The fibrinolytic system is the process through which the fibrin clot is split into fibrinolytic degradation products and circulation is restored.

Clotting Problems

Disseminated Intravascular Coagulation. Disseminated intravascular coagulation (DIC), or consumptive coagulopathy, is a pathologic form of clotting that is diffuse and consumes large amounts of clotting factors, causing widespread external bleeding, internal bleeding, or both and clotting (Cunningham et al., 2014). DIC is never a primary diagnosis. Instead it results from some event that triggered the clotting cascade, either extrinsically, by the release of large amounts of tissue thromboplastin, or intrinsically, by widespread damage to vascular integrity.

In the obstetric population, DIC is most often triggered by the release of large amounts of tissue thromboplastin, which occurs in placental abruption (the most common cause of severe consumptive coagulopathy in obstetrics) and in the retained dead fetus syndrome and amniotic fluid embolus (anaphylactoid syndrome of pregnancy). Severe preeclampsia, HELLP (*H*emolysis, *E*levated *L*iver enzymes, and *L*ow *P*latelet count) syndrome, and gram-negative sepsis are examples of conditions that can trigger DIC because of widespread damage to vascular integrity (Cunningham et al., 2014; Gilbert, 2011). DIC is an overactivation of the clotting cascade and the fibrinolytic system, resulting in depletion of platelets and clotting factors, which causes the formation of multiple fibrin clots throughout the body's vasculature, even in the microcirculation. Blood cells are destroyed as they pass through these fibrin-choked vessels. Thus DIC results in a clinical picture of clotting, bleeding, and ischemia (Cunningham et al.). Clinical manifestations and laboratory test results are summarized in Box 28-2.

BOX 28-2 Clinical Manifestations and Laboratory Screening Results for Women with Disseminated Intravascular Coagulation

Possible Physical Examination Findings

- Spontaneous bleeding from gums, nose
- Oozing, excessive bleeding from venipuncture site, intravenous access site, or site of insertion of urinary catheter
- Petechiae (e.g., on the arm where blood pressure cuff was placed)
- Other signs of bruising
- Hematuria
- Gastrointestinal bleeding
- Tachycardia
- Diaphoresis

Laboratory Coagulation Screening Test Results

- Platelets—decreased
- Fibrinogen—decreased
- Factor V (proaccelerin)—decreased
- Factor VIII (antihemolytic factor)—decreased
- Prothrombin time—prolonged
- Activated partial thromboplastin time—prolonged
- Fibrin degradation products—increased
- D-dimer test (specific fibrin degradation fragment)—increased
- Red blood smear—fragmented red blood cells

Data from Cunningham, F., Leveno, K., Bloom, S., et al. (2014). *Williams obstetrics* (24th ed.). New York: McGraw-Hill Education. Labelle, C., & Kitchens, C. (2005). Disseminated intravascular coagulation: Treat the cause, not the lab values, *Cleveland Clinic Journal of Medicine, 72*(5), 377–397.

CARE MANAGEMENT

Medical management in all cases of DIC involves correction of the underlying cause (e.g., removal of the dead fetus, treatment of existing infection or of preeclampsia or eclampsia, or removal of an abrupted placenta). Volume expansion, rapid replacement of blood products and clotting factors, optimization of oxygenation, achievement of normal body temperature, and continued reassessment of laboratory parameters are the usual forms of treatment. Vitamin K administration, recombinant activated factor VIIa, fibrinogen concentrate, and hemostatic agents should be considered as additional therapies (Francois & Foley, 2012).

Nursing Interventions

Nursing interventions include assessment for signs of bleeding (see Box 28-2) and complications from the administration of blood and blood products, administering fluid or blood replacement as ordered, cardiac and hemodynamic monitoring, and protecting the woman from injury. Because renal failure is one consequence of DIC, urinary output is closely monitored by using an indwelling catheter. Urinary output must be maintained at more than 30 ml/hr (Gilbert, 2011). Vital signs are assessed frequently. If DIC develops before birth, continuous electronic fetal monitoring is necessary. The woman should be maintained in a side-lying tilt to maximize blood flow to the uterus. Oxygen may be administered through a nonrebreather face mask at 10 L/min or per hospital protocol or physician order. DIC usually is "cured" with the birth and as coagulation abnormalities resolve.

The woman and her family will be anxious and concerned about her condition and prognosis. The nurse offers explanations about care and provides emotional support to the woman and her family through this critical time.

KEY POINTS

- Blood loss during pregnancy should always be regarded as a warning sign until the cause is determined.
- Some miscarriages occur for unknown reasons, but fetal or placental maldevelopment and maternal factors account for many others.
- The type of miscarriage and signs and symptoms direct care management.
- Cervical insufficiency may be treated with a cerclage placed cervically or abdominally; the woman is instructed on recognizing the warning signs of preterm labor, preterm premature rupture of membranes, and infection.
- Ectopic pregnancy is a significant cause of maternal morbidity and mortality.
- Hydatidiform mole is a gestational trophoblastic disease (GTD). GTD is a group of pregnancy-related trophoblastic proliferative disorders without a viable fetus that are caused by abnormal fertilization.
- Placenta previa and placental abruption are differentiated by type of bleeding, uterine tonicity, and presence or absence of pain.
- Management of late-pregnancy bleeding requires immediate evaluation; care is based on gestational age, amount of bleeding, and fetal condition.
- DIC is a pathologic form of clotting that causes widespread bleeding and clotting. It is never a primary diagnosis but always results from some event that triggered the clotting cascade.

REFERENCES

American Society for Reproductive Medicine (ASRM). (2013). Medical treatment of ectopic pregnancy: A committee opinion. *Fertility and Sterility, 100*(3), 638–644.

Berghella, V., & Iams, J. D. (2014). Cervical insufficiency. In R. K. Creasy, R. Resnik, J. D. Iams, et al. (Eds.), *Creasy and Resnik's maternal-fetal medicine: Principles and practice* (7th ed.). Philadelphia: Saunders.

Cohn, D., Ramaswamy, B., & Blum, K. (2014). Malignancy and pregnancy. In R. K. Creasy, R. Resnik, J. D. Iams, et al. (Eds.), *Creasy and Resnik's maternal-fetal medicine: Principles and practice* (7th ed.). Philadelphia: Saunders.

Cunningham, F., Leveno, K., Bloom, S., et al. (2014). *Williams obstetrics* (24th ed.). New York: McGraw-Hill Education.

DiGiulio, M., Wiedaseck, S., & Monchek, R. (2012). Understanding hydatidiform mole. *MCN: The American Journal of Maternal/Child Nursing, 37*(1), 30–34.

Francois, K., & Foley, M. (2012). Antepartum and postpartum hemorrhage. In S. Gabbe, J. Niebyl, & J. Simpson (Eds.), *Obstetrics: Normal and problem pregnancies* (6th ed.). Philadelphia: Saunders.

Gilbert, E. (2011). *Manual of high risk pregnancy & delivery* (5th ed.). St. Louis: Mosby.

Hull, A. D., & Resnik, R. (2014). Placenta previa, placenta accreta, abruptio placentae, and vasa previa. In R. K. Creasy, R. Resnik, J. D. Iams, et al. (Eds.), *Creasy and Resnik's maternal-fetal medicine: Principles and practice* (7th ed.). Philadelphia: Saunders.

Ludmir, J., & Owen, J. (2012). Cervical insufficiency. In S. Gabbe, J. Niebyl, & J. Simpson (Eds.), *Obstetrics: Normal and problem pregnancies* (6th ed.). Philadelphia: Saunders.

Markham, K. B., & Funai, E. F. (2014). Pregnancy-related hypertension. In R. K. Creasy, R. Resnik, J. D. Iams, et al. (Eds.), *Creasy and Resnik's maternal-fetal medicine: Principles and practice* (7th ed.). Philadelphia: Saunders.

Moore, T. R. (2014). Placenta and umbilical cord imaging. In R. K. Creasy, R. Resnik, J. D. Iams, et al. (Eds.), *Creasy and Resnik's maternal-fetal medicine: Principles and practice* (7th ed.). Philadelphia: Saunders.

Nader, S. (2014). Thyroid disease and pregnancy. In R. K. Creasy, R. Resnik, J. D. Iams, et al. (Eds.), *Creasy and Resnik's maternal-fetal medicine: Principles and practice* (7th ed.). Philadelphia: Saunders.

National Institute for Occupational Safety and Health (NIOSH). (2012). *NIOSH list of antineoplastic and other hazardous drugs in healthcare settings*. Available at www.cdc.gov/niosh/topics/hazdrug.

Rink, B. D., & Lockwood, C. J. (2014). Recurrent pregnancy loss. In R. K. Creasy, R. Resnik, J. D. Iams, et al. (Eds.), *Creasy and Resnik's maternal-fetal medicine: Principles and practice* (7th ed.). Philadelphia: Saunders.

Shastay, A., & Paparella, S. (2010). Ectopic pregnancies and methotrexate: Are you prepared to manage this hazardous drug? *Journal of Emergency Nursing, 36*(1), 57–59.

Simpson, J., & Jauniaux, E. (2012). Pregnancy loss. In S. Gabbe, J. Niebyl, & J. Simpson (Eds.), *Obstetrics: Normal and problem pregnancies* (6th ed.). Philadelphia: Saunders.

Sosa, M. E. B. (2014). Bleeding in pregnancy. In K. Rice Simpson, & P. Creehan (Eds.), *AWHONN's perinatal nursing* (4th ed.). Philadelphia: Lippincott Williams & Wilkins.

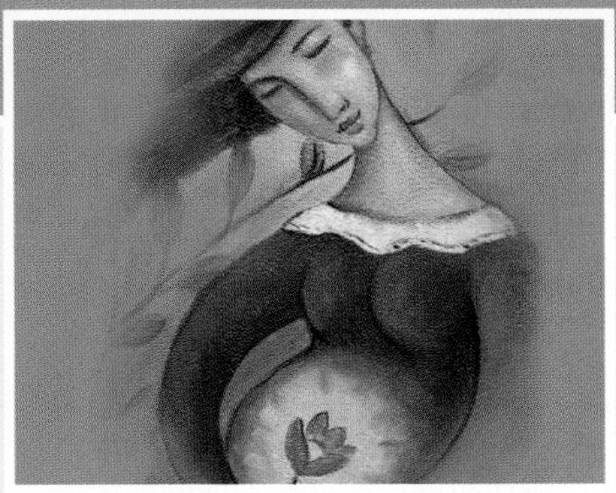

CHAPTER 29

Endocrine and Metabolic Disorders

Jo M. Kendrick

http://evolve.elsevier.com/Lowdermilk/MWHC/

LEARNING OBJECTIVES

- Differentiate the types of diabetes mellitus and their respective risk factors in pregnancy.
- Compare insulin requirements during pregnancy, postpartum, and with lactation.
- Identify maternal and fetal risks or complications associated with diabetes in pregnancy.
- Develop a plan of care for the pregnant woman with pregestational or gestational diabetes.
- Explain the effects of hyperemesis gravidarum on maternal and fetal well-being.
- Discuss management of the woman with hyperemesis gravidarum.
- Explain the effects of thyroid disorders on pregnancy.
- Compare the management of a pregnant woman with hyperthyroidism with one who has hypothyroidism.
- Discuss care management for the woman with phenylketonuria during the perinatal period.
- Examine the effects of maternal phenylketonuria on pregnancy outcome.

This chapter discusses the care of women for whom pregnancy represents a significant risk because it is superimposed on an endocrine or metabolic disorder. Specific disorders covered include diabetes mellitus, hyperemesis gravidarum, hyper- and hypothyroidism, and phenylketonuria. Providing safe and effective care for women with these disorders and their fetuses is a challenge. Although unique needs related to the specific endocrine or metabolic condition are present, these women also experience the feelings, needs, and concerns associated with a normal pregnancy. The primary objective of nursing care is to achieve optimal outcomes for both the pregnant woman and the fetus. With the active participation of well-motivated women in the treatment plan and careful management from a multidisciplinary health care team, positive outcomes are often possible.

DIABETES MELLITUS

Worldwide, the incidence of diabetes mellitus is growing at a rapid rate, mostly because of increases in overweight, obesity, and physical inactivity. An estimated 347 million people are now diabetic, and the disease is expected to become the seventh leading cause of death worldwide by 2030 (World Health Organization [WHO], 2013). In 2012 an estimated 29.1 million people in the United States (9.3% of the total population) had diabetes. Of these, 8.1 million were undiagnosed (Centers for Disease Control and Prevention [CDC], 2014). If this trend continues, it is predicted that by 2050 as many as 1 in 3 adults in the United States will have diabetes. The prevalence of diabetes among women of childbearing age is increasing in the United States, which will greatly affect the care of mothers and children for years to come (Moore, Hauguel-DeMouzon, & Catalano, 2014).

Diabetes mellitus is the most common endocrine disorder associated with pregnancy, occurring in approximately 4% to 14% of pregnant women (Gilbert, 2011). The perinatal mortality rate for well-managed pregnancies complicated by diabetes, excluding major congenital malformations, is approximately the same as for any other pregnancy (Landon, Catalano, & Gabbe, 2012). The key to an optimal pregnancy outcome is strict maternal glucose control before conception and throughout the gestational period. Consequently, for women with diabetes, much emphasis is placed on preconception counseling.

Pregnancy complicated by diabetes is still considered high risk. It is most successfully managed by a multidisciplinary approach involving the obstetrician, perinatologist, internist or endocrinologist, ophthalmologist, nephrologist, neonatologist, nurse, nutritionist or dietitian, and social worker. A favorable outcome also requires commitment and active participation by the pregnant woman and her family.

Pathogenesis

Diabetes mellitus refers to a group of metabolic diseases characterized by hyperglycemia resulting from defects in insulin secretion, insulin action, or both (American Diabetes Association [ADA], 2013a). Insulin, produced by the beta cells in the islets of Langerhans in the pancreas, regulates blood glucose levels by enabling glucose to enter adipose and muscle cells, where it is used for energy. When insulin is insufficient or ineffective in promoting glucose uptake by the muscle and adipose cells, glucose accumulates in the bloodstream, and hyperglycemia results. Hyperglycemia causes hyperosmolarity of the blood, which attracts intracellular fluid into the vascular system, resulting in cellular dehydration and expanded blood volume. Consequently, the kidneys function to excrete large volumes of urine (polyuria) in an attempt to regulate excess vascular volume and to excrete the unusable glucose (glycosuria). Polyuria, along with cellular dehydration, causes excessive thirst (polydipsia).

The body compensates for its inability to convert carbohydrate (glucose) into energy by burning proteins (muscle) and fats. However, the end products of this metabolism are ketones and fatty acids, which, in excess quantities, produce ketoacidosis and acetonuria. Weight loss occurs as a result of the breakdown of fat and muscle tissue. This tissue breakdown causes a state of starvation that compels the individual to eat excessive amounts of food (polyphagia).

Over time, diabetes causes significant changes in the microvascular and macrovascular circulations. These structural changes affect a variety of organ systems, particularly the heart, the eyes, the kidneys, and the nerves. Complications resulting from diabetes include premature atherosclerosis, retinopathy, nephropathy, and neuropathy.

Diabetes may be caused either by impaired insulin secretion, when the beta cells of the pancreas are destroyed by an autoimmune process, or by inadequate insulin action in target tissues at one or more points along the metabolic pathway. Both of these conditions are commonly present in the same person, and determining which, if either, abnormality is the primary cause of the disease is difficult (ADA, 2013a). For additional information on diabetes, visit the American Diabetes Association (ADA)'s website at www.diabetes.org.

Classification

The current classification system includes four groups: type 1 diabetes, type 2 diabetes, other specific types (e.g., diabetes caused by genetic defects in beta cell function or insulin action, disease or injury of the pancreas, or drug-induced diabetes), and gestational diabetes mellitus (GDM) (ADA, 2013b; Moore et al., 2014).

Type 1 diabetes includes cases that are caused primarily by pancreatic islet beta cell destruction and that are prone to ketoacidosis. People with type 1 diabetes usually have an abrupt onset of illness at a young age and an absolute insulin deficiency. Type 1 diabetes includes cases thought to be caused by an autoimmune process and those for which the cause is unknown (ADA, 2013b; Landon et al., 2012).

Type 2 diabetes is the most prevalent form of the disease and includes individuals who have insulin resistance and usually relative (rather than absolute) insulin deficiency. Although type 2 diabetes was once believed to affect mostly older individuals, increasing numbers of children and adolescents have been diagnosed with the disorder since the early 1990s (Moore et al., 2014). Specific causes of type 2 diabetes are unknown at this time. It often goes undiagnosed for years because hyperglycemia develops gradually and is often not severe enough for the person to recognize the classic signs of polyuria, polydipsia, and polyphagia. Most people who develop type 2 diabetes are obese or have an increased amount of body fat distributed primarily in the abdominal area. Other risk factors for the development of type 2 diabetes include aging, a sedentary lifestyle, family history and genetics, puberty, hypertension, and prior gestational diabetes. Type 2 diabetes often has a strong genetic predisposition (ADA, 2013b; Moore et al.).

Pregestational diabetes mellitus is the label sometimes given to type 1 or type 2 diabetes that existed before pregnancy.

The traditional definition of GDM is carbohydrate intolerance with the onset or first recognition occurring during pregnancy (American College of Obstetricians and Gynecologists [ACOG], 2013). This definition is appropriate whether or not management includes medication in addition to dietary changes or the diabetes persists after pregnancy. It does not exclude the possibility that the glucose intolerance preceded the pregnancy or that medication might be required for optimal glucose control (Landon et al., 2012). The ADA has adopted a new definition for gestational diabetes that excludes women with overt diabetes (type 1 or type 2) that is diagnosed during pregnancy. This definition for GDM is simply diabetes diagnosed during pregnancy that is clearly not overt (preexisting) diabetes (ADA, 2013a).

Classification of Diabetes in Pregnancy

Dr. Priscilla White, a physician who worked with pregnant women with diabetes during the 1940s, developed a system specifically to further classify diabetes in this group of women (Table 29-1). White's system was based on age at diagnosis, duration of illness, and presence of end-organ, especially eye and kidney, involvement (Landon et al., 2012; Moore et al., 2014). Her classification system has been modified through the years, changing her original definitions and adding increasing complexity, which has resulted in confusion (Sacks & Metzger, 2013). It is still frequently used, however, to assess maternal and fetal risk.

A new system has since been developed by the ADA that further classifies type 1 and type 2 diabetes as (a) without vascular complications and (b) with vascular complications that are specified. This distinction is important, because perinatal risk increases with vascular complications regardless of the duration of illness. Only women whose glucose intolerance was diagnosed during pregnancy but who do not meet the criteria defining type 1 or type 2 diabetes are included in the gestational diabetes category. It has been suggested that White's modified classification system be replaced by the new ADA system in clinical practice (Sacks & Metzger, 2013).

Metabolic Changes Associated with Pregnancy

Normal pregnancy is characterized by complex alterations in maternal glucose metabolism, insulin production, and metabolic homeostasis. During normal pregnancy adjustments in maternal metabolism allow for adequate nutrition for the mother and the developing fetus. Glucose, the primary fuel used by the fetus, is transported across the placenta through the process of carrier-mediated facilitated diffusion, meaning that the glucose levels in the fetus are directly proportional to maternal levels. Although glucose crosses the placenta, insulin does not. Around the tenth week of gestation the fetus begins to secrete its own insulin at levels adequate to use the glucose obtained from the mother. Therefore, as maternal glucose levels rise, fetal glucose levels are increased, resulting in increased fetal insulin secretion.

During the first trimester of pregnancy the pregnant woman's metabolic status is significantly influenced by the rising levels of estrogen and progesterone. These hormones stimulate the beta cells in the pancreas to increase insulin production, which promotes increased peripheral use of glucose and decreased blood glucose, with fasting levels being reduced by approximately 10% (Fig. 29-1, *A*). At the same time, an increase in tissue glycogen stores and a decrease in hepatic glucose production occur, which further encourage lower fasting glucose levels. As a result of these normal metabolic changes of pregnancy, women with insulin-dependent diabetes are prone to hypoglycemia during the first trimester.

During the second and third trimesters, pregnancy exerts a "diabetogenic" effect on the maternal metabolic status. Because of the major hormonal changes, decreased tolerance to glucose, increased insulin resistance, decreased hepatic glycogen stores, and increased hepatic production of glucose occur. Rising levels of human chorionic somatomammotropin, estrogen, progesterone, prolactin, cortisol, and insulinase increase insulin resistance through their actions as insulin antagonists. Insulin resistance is a glucose-sparing mechanism that ensures an abundant supply of glucose for the fetus. Maternal insulin requirements gradually increase from approximately 18 to 24 weeks of gestation to approximately 36 weeks of gestation. Maternal insulin requirements may double or quadruple by the end of the pregnancy (see Fig. 29-1, *B* and *C*).

At birth, expulsion of the placenta prompts an abrupt drop in levels of circulating placental hormones, cortisol, and insulinase (see Fig. 29-1, *D*). Maternal tissues quickly regain their prepregnancy sensitivity to insulin. For the nonbreastfeeding mother the prepregnancy insulin-carbohydrate balance usually returns in approximately 7 to 10 days (see Fig. 29-1, *E*). Lactation uses maternal glucose; therefore, the breastfeeding mother's insulin requirements remain lower during lactation. On completion of weaning the mother's prepregnancy insulin requirement is reestablished (see Fig. 29-1, *F*).

TABLE 29-1 White's Classification of Diabetes in Pregnancy (Modified)

Gestational Diabetes	
Class A_1	Woman has two or more abnormal values on OGTT with normal fasting blood sugar. Blood glucose levels are diet controlled.
Class A_2	Woman was not known to have diabetes before pregnancy but requires medication for blood glucose control.
Pregestational Diabetes	
Class B	Onset of disease occurs after age 20 and duration of illness <10 years.
Class C	Onset of disease occurs between 10 and 19 years of age or duration of illness for 10 to 19 years or both.
Class D	Onset of disease occurs at <10 years of age or duration of illness >20 years or both.
Class F	Client has developed diabetic nephropathy.
Class R	Client has developed retinitis proliferans.
Class T	Client has had a renal transplant.

OGTT, Oral glucose tolerance test.

Data from Landon, M., Catalano, P., & Gabbe, S. (2012). Diabetes mellitus complicating pregnancy. In S. Gabbe, J. Niebyl, & J. Simpson (Eds.), *Obstetrics: Normal and problem pregnancies* (6th ed.). Philadelphia: Saunders; Moore, T.R., Hauguel-deMouzon, S., & Catalano, P. (2014). Diabetes in pregnancy. In R.K. Creasy, R. Resnik, J.D. Iams, et al., (Eds.), *Creasy and Resnik's maternal-fetal medicine: Principles and practice* (7th ed.). Philadelphia: Saunders.

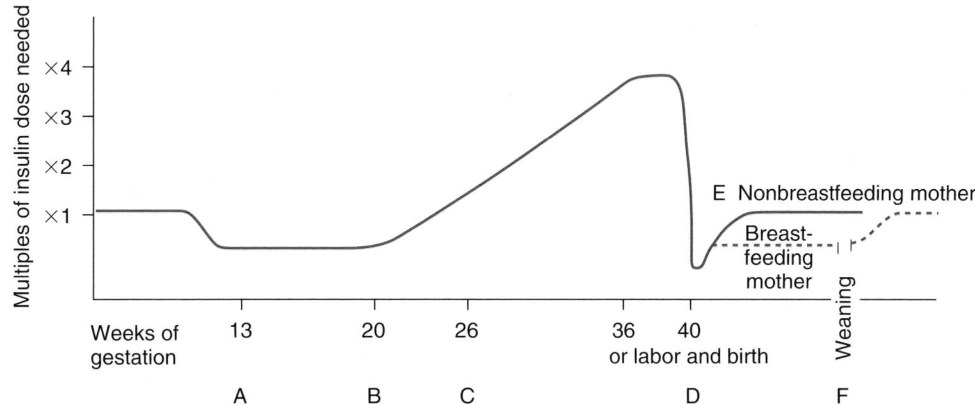

FIG 29-1 Changing insulin needs during pregnancy. *A,* First trimester: Insulin need is reduced because of increased insulin production by pancreas and increased peripheral sensitivity to insulin; nausea, vomiting, and decreased food intake by mother and glucose transfer to embryo or fetus contribute to hypoglycemia. *B,* Second trimester: Insulin needs begin to increase as placental hormones, cortisol, and insulinase act as insulin antagonists, decreasing insulin's effectiveness. *C,* Third trimester: Insulin needs may double or even quadruple but usually level off after 36 weeks of gestation. *D,* Day of birth: Maternal insulin requirements decrease dramatically to approach prepregnancy levels. *E,* Breastfeeding mother maintains lower insulin requirements, as much as 25% less than those of prepregnancy; insulin needs of nonbreastfeeding mother return to prepregnancy levels in 7 to 10 days. *F,* Weaning of breastfeeding infant causes mother's insulin needs to return to prepregnancy levels.

PREGESTATIONAL DIABETES MELLITUS

Only about 10% of pregnancies complicated by diabetes occur in women who have preexisting disease (Landon et al., 2012). Women who have pregestational diabetes mellitus can have either type 1 or 2 diabetes, which may be complicated by vascular disease, retinopathy, nephropathy, or other diabetic complications. Type 2 is a more common diagnosis than type 1. Almost all women with pregestational diabetes are insulin dependent during pregnancy. According to White's classification system, these women fall into classes B through T (see Table 29-1).

The diabetogenic state of pregnancy imposed on the compromised metabolic system of the woman with pregestational diabetes has significant implications. The normal hormonal adaptations of pregnancy affect glycemic control, and pregnancy may accelerate the progress of vascular complications.

During the first trimester, when maternal blood glucose levels are normally reduced and the insulin response to glucose is enhanced, glycemic control may be improved. The insulin dose for the woman with well-controlled diabetes may have to be reduced to prevent hypoglycemia. Nausea, vomiting, and cravings typical of early pregnancy result in dietary fluctuations that influence maternal glucose levels and may necessitate a reduction in the insulin dose.

Because insulin requirements steadily increase after the first trimester, the insulin dose must be adjusted accordingly to prevent hyperglycemia. Insulin resistance begins as early as 14 to 16 weeks of gestation and continues to rise until it stabilizes during the last few weeks of pregnancy.

COMMUNITY ACTIVITY

Visit the March of Dimes website at www.marchofdimes.com. Review the information specifically intended for women with gestational diabetes and preexisting diabetes. Read the section on preconception, "Baby makes three. Are you ready?" Determine the helpfulness of this information for your clients. Develop a teaching plan for a woman with pregestational diabetes based on the information you decided would be useful.

Preconception Counseling

Preconception counseling is recommended for all women of reproductive age who have diabetes because it is associated with less perinatal mortality and fewer preterm births and congenital anomalies (Moore et al., 2014). Under ideal circumstances, women with pregestational diabetes are counseled before conception to plan the optimal time for pregnancy, establish glycemic control before conception, and diagnose any vascular complications of diabetes. However, estimates indicate that less than 20% of women with diabetes in the United States participate in preconception counseling (Landon et al., 2012).

The woman's partner should be included in the counseling to assess the couple's level of understanding related to the effects of pregnancy on the diabetic condition and of the potential complications of pregnancy as a result of diabetes. The couple should also be informed of the anticipated alterations in management of diabetes during pregnancy and the need for a multidisciplinary team approach to health care. Financial implications of diabetic pregnancy and other demands related to frequent maternal and fetal surveillance should be discussed. In addition, medications the woman is currently taking must be assessed for safety during pregnancy. Medications that carry risk for adverse maternal or fetal outcomes should be changed to ones that are safer but equally effective. Preconception counseling should also include discussion of microvascular and macrovascular complications that carry significant risk for maternal morbidity and mortality during pregnancy such as coronary artery disease and renal insufficiency. Renal transplantation may be necessary prior to conception. Contraception is another important aspect of preconception counseling to assist the couple in planning effectively for pregnancy. They should be encouraged to use reliable contraception until glycemic control is optimal.

Maternal Risks and Complications

Although maternal morbidity and mortality rates have improved significantly, the pregnant woman with diabetes remains at risk for the development of complications during pregnancy. Poor glycemic control around the time of conception and in the early weeks of pregnancy is associated with an increased incidence of miscarriage. Women with good glycemic control before conception and in the first trimester are no more likely to miscarry than women who do not have diabetes (Moore et al., 2014).

Poor glycemic control later in pregnancy, particularly in women without vascular disease, increases the rate of fetal macrosomia. Macrosomia has been defined as a birth weight more than 4000 to 4500 g or greater than the 90th percentile. It occurs in approximately 40% of pregestational diabetic pregnancies and up to 50% of pregnancies complicated by GDM (Landon et al., 2012). Infants born to women with diabetes tend to have a disproportionate increase in shoulder, trunk, and chest size. Because of this tendency the risk for shoulder dystocia is greater in these babies than in other macrosomic infants. Therefore, women with diabetes face an increased likelihood of cesarean birth because of failure of fetal descent or labor progress or of operative vaginal birth (birth involving the use of episiotomy, forceps, or vacuum extractor) (Moore et al., 2014).

Women with preexisting diabetes are at risk for several obstetric and medical complications, including hypertension, preeclampsia, cesarean birth, preterm birth, and maternal mortality. In general, the risk of developing these complications increases with the duration and severity of the woman's diabetes. For example, more than one third of women who have had diabetes for more than 20 years develop preeclampsia. Women with nephropathy and hypertension in addition to diabetes are also increasingly likely to develop preeclampsia. Poor glycemic control at the beginning of pregnancy is also related to the development of preeclampsia. The rate of hypertensive disorders in all types of pregnancies complicated by diabetes is 15% to 30%. Chronic hypertension occurs in 10% to 20% of all pregnant women with diabetes and in up to 40% of women who have preexisting renal or retinal vascular disease (Moore et al., 2014).

Hydramnios (polyhydramnios) frequently develops during the third trimester of pregnancy in women with diabetes. Its cause is unknown. One theory is that hydramnios in women with diabetes is caused by an increased glucose concentration in amniotic fluid resulting from maternal and fetal hyperglycemia, which induces fetal polyuria. The complications most frequently associated with hydramnios (usually defined as an amniotic fluid index [AFI] greater than 25 cm) are placental abruption, uterine dysfunction, and postpartum hemorrhage (Cunningham, Leveno, Bloom, et al., 2014).

Infections are more common and more serious in pregnant women with diabetes than in those without the disease. Disorders of carbohydrate metabolism alter the normal resistance of the body to infection. The inflammatory response, leukocyte function, and vaginal pH are all affected. Vaginal infections, particularly monilial vaginitis, are more common. Urinary tract infections (UTIs) are also more prevalent. Infection is serious because it causes increased insulin resistance and may result in ketoacidosis.

Ketoacidosis (accumulation of ketones in the blood resulting from hyperglycemia and leading to metabolic acidosis) occurs most often during the second and third trimesters, when the diabetogenic effect of pregnancy is greatest. When the maternal metabolism is stressed by illness or infection, the woman is at increased risk for diabetic ketoacidosis (DKA). DKA can also be caused by poor compliance with treatment or the onset of previously undiagnosed diabetes (Moore et al., 2014). The use of beta-mimetic drugs such as terbutaline (Brethine) for tocolysis to treat preterm labor or corticosteroids given to enhance fetal lung maturation may also contribute to the risk for hyperglycemia and subsequent DKA (Mercer, 2014; Simhan, Berghella, & Iams, 2014).

DKA may occur with blood glucose levels barely exceeding 200 mg/dl, compared with 300 to 350 mg/dl in the nonpregnant state. In response to stress factors such as infection or illness, hyperglycemia occurs as a result of increased hepatic glucose production and decreased peripheral glucose use. Stress hormones, which act to impair insulin action and further contribute to insulin deficiency, are released. Fatty acids are mobilized from fat stores to enter the circulation. As they are oxidized, ketone bodies are released into the peripheral circulation. The woman's buffering system is unable to compensate, and metabolic acidosis develops. The excessive blood glucose and ketone bodies result in osmotic diuresis with subsequent loss of fluid and electrolytes, volume depletion, and cellular dehydration. DKA is a medical emergency. Prompt treatment is necessary to prevent maternal coma or death. Ketoacidosis occurring at any time during pregnancy can lead to intrauterine fetal death. The incidence of DKA has decreased in recent years because of advances in clinical management and blood glucose monitoring (Inturrisi, Lintner, & Sorem, 2013). Currently it affects only about 1% to 2% of pregnant women with diabetes. The rate of intrauterine fetal demise (IUFD) with DKA, formerly approximately 35%, is now 10% or less (Moore et al., 2014) (Table 29-2).

TABLE 29-2 Differentiation of Hypoglycemia (Insulin Shock) and Hyperglycemia (Diabetic Ketoacidosis)

CAUSES	ONSET	SYMPTOMS	INTERVENTIONS
Hypoglycemia (insulin shock)			
Excess insulin Insufficient food (delayed or missed meals) Excessive exercise or work Indigestion, diarrhea, vomiting	Rapid (regular insulin) Gradual (modified insulin or oral hypoglycemic agents)	Irritability Hunger Sweating Nervousness Personality change Weakness Fatigue Blurred or double vision Dizziness Headache Pallor; clammy skin Shallow respirations Rapid pulse Laboratory values Urine: Negative for sugar and acetone Blood glucose: less than 70 mg/dl	Check blood glucose level when symptoms first appear. If blood glucose is less than 70 mg/dl, eat 2-4 glucose tablets or gel (8-16 g carbohydrate) immediately. Recheck blood glucose level in 15 minutes. If glucose level is still less than 70 mg/dl, eat 2-4 additional glucose tablets. Recheck blood glucose level in 15 minutes. If glucose level is still less than 70 mg/dl, notify health care provider immediately. If woman is unconscious, administer 50% dextrose IV push, 5% to 10% dextrose in water IV drip, or 1 mg glucagon intramuscularly. Obtain blood and urine specimens for laboratory testing.
Hyperglycemia (DKA)			
Insufficient insulin Excess or wrong kind of food Infection, injuries, illness Emotional stress Insufficient exercise	Slow (hours to days)	Thirst Nausea or vomiting Abdominal pain Constipation Drowsiness Dim vision Increased urination Headache Flushed, dry skin Rapid breathing Weak, rapid pulse Acetone (fruity) breath odor Laboratory values Urine: Positive for sugar and acetone Blood glucose: greater than 200 mg/dl	Notify primary health care provider. Administer insulin in accordance with blood glucose levels. Give IV fluids such as normal saline solution or one-half normal saline solution; potassium when urinary output is adequate; bicarbonate for pH <7. Monitor laboratory testing of blood and urine.

DKA, Diabetic ketoacidosis; *IV*, intravenous.

The risk of hypoglycemia (a less than normal amount of glucose in the blood) is also increased during pregnancy. Early in pregnancy, when hepatic production of glucose is diminished and peripheral use of glucose is enhanced, hypoglycemia occurs frequently, often during sleep. Later in pregnancy it may also result as insulin doses are adjusted to maintain euglycemia (a normal blood glucose level). Women with a prepregnancy history of severe hypoglycemia are at increased risk for severe hypoglycemia during gestation. Hypoglycemic episodes do not appear to have significant damaging effects on fetal well-being (see Table 29-2).

Fetal and Neonatal Risks and Complications

From the moment of conception the infant of a woman with diabetes faces an increased risk of complications that may occur during the antepartum, intrapartum, or neonatal periods. Infant morbidity and mortality rates associated with diabetic pregnancy are significantly reduced with strict control of maternal glucose levels before and during pregnancy.

Despite improvements in the care of pregnant women with diabetes, the perinatal mortality rate is three times higher for women with diabetes than for women who do not have this disease. Major causes of perinatal mortality are congenital malformations, respiratory distress syndrome, and extreme prematurity. IUFD (sometimes called *stillbirth*) remains a major concern. Approximately 4% of all stillbirths occur in women whose pregnancies are complicated by preexisting diabetes. Poor glycemic control is the most consistent finding in women who had a stillbirth. In addition to hyperglycemia, other causes of stillbirth include congenital abnormalities, placental insufficiency or fetal growth restriction, macrosomia or polyhydramnios, or obstructed labor (intrapartum stillbirth) (Reddy & Spong, 2014).

Hyperglycemia during the first trimester of pregnancy, when organs and organ systems are forming, is the main cause of diabetes-associated birth defects. Anomalies commonly seen in infants born to women with diabetes affect primarily the cardiovascular system and the central nervous system (CNS) (Moore et al., 2014) (see Chapter 35).

The fetal pancreas begins to secrete insulin at 10 to 14 weeks of gestation. The fetus responds to maternal hyperglycemia by secreting large amounts of insulin (hyperinsulinism). Insulin acts as a growth hormone, causing the fetus to produce excess stores of glycogen, protein, and adipose tissue and leading to increased fetal size, or macrosomia. Birth injuries are more common in infants born to mothers with diabetes compared with mothers who do not have diabetes, and macrosomic fetuses have the highest risk for this complication. Common birth injuries associated with diabetic pregnancies include brachial plexus palsy, facial nerve injury, humerus or clavicle fracture, and cephalhematoma. Most of these injuries are associated with difficult vaginal birth and shoulder dystocia (Moore et al., 2014).

Hypoglycemia at birth is also a risk for infants born to mothers with diabetes (for further discussion of neonatal complications related to maternal diabetes, see Chapter 35).

CARE MANAGEMENT

Assessment and Nursing Diagnoses

When a pregnant woman with diabetes initiates prenatal care, a thorough evaluation of her health status is completed. At the initial visit a complete physical examination is performed to assess the woman's health status. In addition to the routine prenatal examination, specific efforts are made to assess the effects of the diabetes, especially retinopathy, nephropathy, peripheral and autonomic neuropathy, peripheral vascular and cardiac involvement (Gilbert, 2011).

Routine prenatal laboratory tests are performed, and baseline renal function may be assessed with a 24-hour urine collection for total protein excretion and creatinine clearance. Urinalysis and culture are performed to assess for the presence of a UTI, which is common in diabetic pregnancy. Because of the risk of coexisting thyroid disease, thyroid function tests may also be performed (see later discussion of thyroid disorders). The glycosylated hemoglobin A_{1c} level may be measured to assess recent glycemic control. With prolonged hyperglycemia some of the hemoglobin remains saturated with glucose for the life of the red blood cell (RBC). Therefore, a test for glycosylated hemoglobin provides a "diabetic report card," an evaluation of glycemic control over the previous 4 to 6 weeks. Hemoglobin A_{1c} levels greater than 6 indicate elevated glucose levels during the previous 4 to 6 weeks (Gilbert, 2011). Fasting blood glucose or random (1 to 2 hours after eating) glucose levels may be assessed during antepartum visits (Fig. 29-2).

Self-monitoring blood glucose records should be reviewed at every prenatal visit. Accuracy of reporting should be reviewed periodically by accessing the meter memory and addressed if falsification of blood glucose results is detected. Most meters can be downloaded using manufacturer software but this cannot replace logging, which affords more information for both the health care provider and the woman.

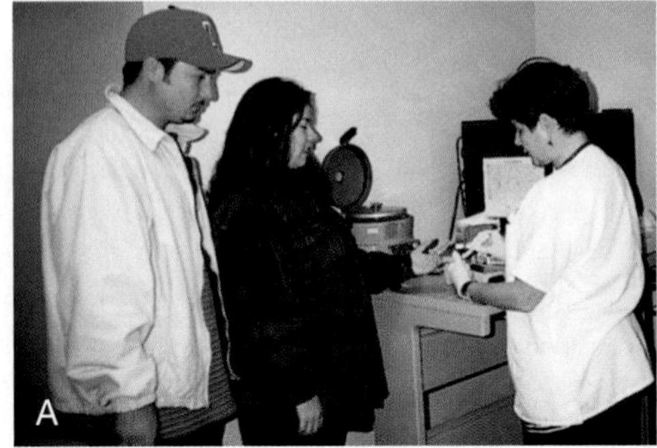

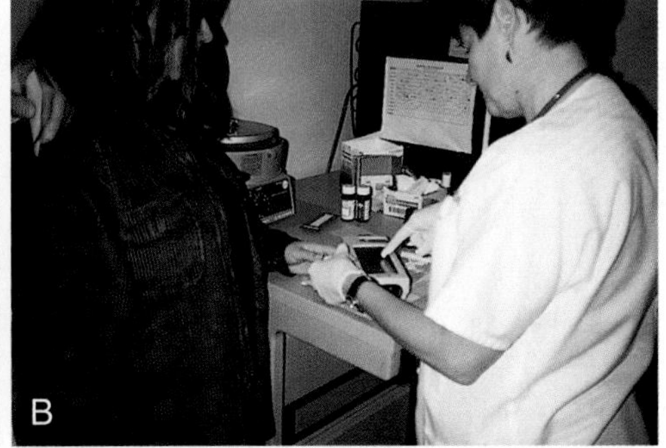

FIG 29-2 **A,** Clinic nurse collects blood to determine glucose level. **B,** Nurse interprets glucose value displayed by monitor. (Courtesy Dee Lowdermilk, UNC Ambulatory Care Clinics, Chapel Hill, NC.)

Potential nursing diagnoses for the woman with pregestational diabetes include the following:

- *Deficient Knowledge* related to
  - diabetic pregnancy, management, and potential effects on pregnant woman and fetus
  - insulin administration and its effects
  - hypoglycemia and hyperglycemia
  - diabetic diet
- *Anxiety, Grieving, Powerlessness, Disturbed Body Image, Situational Low Self-Esteem, Spiritual Distress, Ineffective Role Performance, Interrupted Family Processes* related to
  - stigma of being labeled "diabetic"
  - effects of diabetes and its potential sequelae on the pregnant woman and the fetus
- *Risk for Injury* to fetus related to
  - disruption of oxygen transfer from environment to fetus
  - birth trauma
- *Risk for Injury* to mother related to
  - improper insulin administration
  - hypoglycemia and hyperglycemia
  - cesarean or operative vaginal birth
  - postpartum infection

Interventions

Antepartum

Because of her high risk status, a woman with pregestational diabetes is monitored much more frequently and thoroughly than other pregnant women. During the first and second trimesters of pregnancy, her routine prenatal care visits are scheduled every 1 to 2 weeks. In the last trimester she will likely be seen 1 or 2 times each week. In the past, routine hospitalization for management of the diabetes, such as for insulin dose changes, was common. With the availability of improved home glucose monitoring and the growing reluctance of third-party payers to reimburse for hospitalization, pregnant women with diabetes generally now are managed as outpatients. Some client and family education and maternal and fetal assessment may be performed in the home, depending on the woman's insurance coverage and care provider preference.

Achieving and maintaining constant euglycemia is the primary goal of medical therapy. Blood glucose levels should be in the range of 60 to 99 mg/dl before meals and 100 to 129 mg/dl when measured 1 hour after a meal (ADA, 2013a). Postmeal glucose levels at 2 hours should be no higher than 120 mg/dl (Landon et al., 2012) (Table 29-3). (Euglycemia is achieved through a combination of diet, insulin, and exercise. Providing the woman with the knowledge, skill, and motivation she needs to achieve and maintain excellent blood glucose control is the primary nursing goal.

TABLE 29-3 Target Blood Glucose Levels During Pregnancy

TIME OF DAY	TARGET PLASMA GLUCOSE LEVEL (mg/dl)
Premeal or fasting	60-99
Postmeal (1 hr)	100-129
Postmeal (2 hr)	≤120

Data from American Diabetes Association (ADA). (2013). Standards of medical care in diabetes—2013. *Diabetes Care, 36*(Suppl 1), S11-S65; Landon, M., Catalano, P., & Gabbe, S. (2012). Diabetes mellitus complicating pregnancy. In S. Gabbe, J. Niebyl, & J. Simpson (Eds.), *Obstetrics: Normal and problem pregnancies* (6th ed.). Philadelphia: Saunders.

Achieving euglycemia requires commitment on the part of the woman and her family to make the necessary lifestyle changes, which can sometimes seem overwhelming. Maintaining tight blood glucose control necessitates that the woman follow a consistent daily schedule. She must get up and go to bed, eat, exercise, and take insulin at the same time each day. Blood glucose measurements are taken frequently to determine how well the major components of therapy (diet, insulin, and exercise) are working together to control blood glucose levels. The pregnant woman with diabetes should wear a medical identification bracelet at all times and carry insulin, syringes or pens, blood glucose meter, and glucose tablets with her whenever she is away from home.

Because the woman with pregestational diabetes is at increased risk for infections, eye problems, and neurologic changes, foot and general skin care are important. A daily bath that includes thorough perineal and foot care is important. For dry skin, lotions, creams, or oils can be applied. Tight clothing should be avoided. Shoes or slippers that fit properly should be worn at all times and are best worn with socks or stockings. Feet should be inspected regularly; toenails should be cut straight across, and professional help should be sought for any foot problems. Extremes of temperature should be avoided.

Diet. The woman with pregestational diabetes has usually had nutrition counseling regarding managing her diabetes. However, because pregnancy produces special nutritional concerns and needs, the woman must be educated to incorporate these changes into dietary planning. The woman who has "controlled" her diabetes for several years may find it difficult to adjust to the changes in her insulin and dietary needs mandated by pregnancy. Nutritional counseling is usually provided by a registered dietitian. Counseling should address general nutrition principles appropriate for all pregnant women as well as diabetes-specific nutritional needs.

Dietary management during diabetic pregnancy must be based on blood glucose levels. The diet is individualized to allow for increased fetal and metabolic requirements, with consideration of such factors as prepregnancy weight and dietary habits, overall health, ethnic background, lifestyle, stage of pregnancy, knowledge of nutrition, and insulin therapy. The dietary goals are to provide weight gain consistent with a normal pregnancy, prevent ketoacidosis, and minimize wide fluctuation of blood glucose levels.

For women with a BMI of 22 to 27, dietary counseling includes advice to consume about 35 kcal/kg of ideal body weight per day (Landon et al., 2012). In contrast, for obese women with a BMI of 30 or greater, experts recommend that the caloric intake total 25 kcal/kg of actual weight per day or less (Moore et al., 2014). The average diet includes 2200 calories (first trimester) to 2500 calories (second and third trimesters). Total calories may be distributed among three meals and one evening snack or, more commonly, three meals and two or three snacks. Meals should be eaten on time and never skipped. Going more than 4 hours without food intake increases the risk for episodes of hypoglycemia. Snacks must be planned carefully in accordance with insulin therapy to prevent fluctuations in blood glucose levels. A large bedtime snack of at least 25 g of complex carbohydrate with some protein or fat is recommended to help prevent hypoglycemia and starvation ketosis during the night (Moore et al.).

The ideal diet is composed of 55% carbohydrate, 20% protein, and 25% fat, with less than 10% as saturated fat (Cunningham, et al., 2014) (see Teaching for Self-Management: Dietary Management for Pregnant Women with Diabetes). Simple carbohydrates are limited. Complex carbohydrates that are high in fiber content are recommended because the starch and protein in such foods help regulate the blood glucose level by more sustained glucose release (Gilbert, 2011; Moore et al., 2014).

TEACHING FOR SELF-MANAGEMENT

Dietary Management for Pregnant Women with Diabetes

- Follow the prescribed diet plan.
- Eat a well-balanced diet, including daily food requirements for a normal pregnancy.
- Divide daily food intake among three meals and two or three snacks, depending on individual needs.
- Eat a substantial bedtime snack to prevent a severe drop in blood glucose level during the night.
- Take daily vitamins and iron as prescribed by the health care provider.
- Avoid foods high in refined sugar.
- Eat consistently each day; never skip meals or snacks.
- Eat foods high in dietary fiber.
- Avoid alcohol and nicotine; limit caffeine.
- Avoid excessive use of nonnutritive sweeteners.

Exercise. Although studies have shown that exercise enhances the use of glucose and decreases insulin need in women without diabetes, data regarding exercise in women with pregestational diabetes are limited. Any prescription of exercise during pregnancy for women with diabetes should be given by the primary health care provider and monitored closely to prevent complications. Regular exercise may be contraindicated in women with diabetes who also have uncontrolled hypertension, advanced retinopathy, or severe autonomic or peripheral neuropathy (Gilbert, 2011).

When exercise is prescribed by the health care provider as part of the treatment plan, specific instructions are given to the woman. Aerobic exercise with resistance training for at least 30 minutes most days of the week is the best type of exercise (Gilbert, 2011). Other exercises that may be recommended are non–weight-bearing activities such as arm exercises or use of a recumbent bicycle. The best time for exercise is after meals, when the blood glucose level is rising. To monitor the effect of insulin on blood glucose levels the woman can measure her blood glucose before, during, and after exercise. The onset of hypoglycemia may be delayed in women with pregestational diabetes, so blood glucose should be monitored for several hours after exercising. Exercising with another person is prudent for safety reasons. Women should be advised to avoid exercise if they have positive urine ketones or a blood glucose greater than 250 mg/dl because hyperglycemia and ketosis can worsen with physical activity.

SAFETY ALERT

Uterine contractions may occur during exercise. The woman should be advised to stop exercising immediately if they are detected, drink two to three glasses of water, and lie down on her side for an hour. If the contractions continue, she should contact her health care provider.

Insulin Therapy. Adequate insulin is the primary factor in the maintenance of euglycemia during pregnancy, thus ensuring proper glucose metabolism of the woman and fetus. Insulin requirements during pregnancy change dramatically as the pregnancy progresses, necessitating frequent adjustments in the dose. In the first trimester, from weeks 3 to 7 of gestation, insulin requirements are increased, followed by a decrease between weeks 7 and 15 of gestation. The commonly prescribed insulin dose is 0.7 units/kg in the first trimester for women with type 1 diabetes. During the second and third trimesters, because of insulin resistance, the dose must be increased significantly to maintain target glucose levels. Insulin requirements normally peak at 36 weeks of gestation and drop significantly after that (Moore et al., 2014).

For the woman with type 1 pregestational diabetes who has typically been accustomed to one injection per day of intermediate-acting insulin, multiple daily injections of mixed insulin are a new experience. The woman with type 2 diabetes previously treated with oral hypoglycemics is faced with the task of learning to self-administer injections of insulin. The nurse is instrumental in educating and supporting women with pregestational diabetes in regard to insulin administration and adjustment of the insulin dose to maintain euglycemia (see Teaching for Self-Management: Self-Administration of Insulin and Box 29-1).

TEACHING FOR SELF-MANAGEMENT

Self-Administration of Insulin

Procedure for Mixing NPH (Intermediate-Acting) and Rapid-Acting Insulin

- Wash hands thoroughly and gather supplies. Be sure the insulin syringe corresponds to the concentration of insulin you are using.
- Check the insulin bottle to be certain it is the appropriate type, and check the expiration date.
- Gently rotate (do not shake) the insulin vial to mix the insulin.
- Wipe off the rubber stopper of each vial with alcohol.
- Draw into syringe the amount of air equal to total dose.
- Inject air equal to NPH dose into NPH vial. Remove syringe from vial.
- Inject air equal to rapid-acting insulin dose into vial and leave syringe in the vial.
- Invert insulin bottle and withdraw insulin dose.
- Without adding more air to NPH vial, carefully withdraw NPH dose.

Procedure for Self-Injection of Insulin

- Select proper injection site.
- Injection site should be clean. No need to use alcohol. If alcohol is used, let it dry before injecting.
- Puncture the skin at a 90-degree angle.
- Slowly inject the insulin.
- As you withdraw the needle, cover the injection site with sterile gauze and apply gentle pressure to prevent bleeding.
- Record insulin dose and time of injection.

Since 1982 most insulin preparations have been produced by inserting portions of deoxyribonucleic acid (DNA) ("recombinant DNA") into special laboratory-cultivated bacteria or yeast cells. The cells then produce synthetic human insulin (Humulin), which is less likely to cause antibody formation than animal-derived (beef or pork) insulin. More recently insulin products called *insulin analogues,* in which the structure differs slightly from human insulin, have been produced. This small alteration in insulin structure results in changes in the onset and peak of action of the medication. The most commonly used insulin preparations include rapid acting, short acting, intermediate acting, and long acting (Landon et al., 2012) (Table 29-4). Mixtures of short- and intermediate-acting insulins in several proportions are also available but usually are not in the correct percentages to be effective in pregnancy. Therefore, they are rarely used.

BOX 29-1 Helpful Hints for Using Insulin

- The most common type of insulin used during pregnancy is a biosynthetic human insulin (Humulin) made by programming *Escherichia coli* bacteria to produce insulin.
- Insulin is classified either as rapid acting, short acting, intermediate acting, or long acting (see Table 29-4).
- Unused vials of insulin should be stored in the refrigerator until reaching their expiration date. Insulin should not be frozen. Vials currently in use can be stored at room temperature for up to a month. They should not be left in a car or exposed to extreme heat as in the sun.
- Regular insulin can be mixed with NPH insulin in the same syringe. Lispro insulin can also be mixed in a syringe with NPH insulin. Once mixed, the syringe can be used immediately or stored for future use. If it is used later, the syringe should be rotated 20 times before injection.
- Glargine insulin is usually administered at bedtime. It cannot be mixed with any other insulin in the same syringe. Prepared syringes are stable for 2 weeks in the refrigerator.
- Insulin may be administered by pen injector, jet injector, or insulin pump, in addition to syringe.
- The abdomen is the preferred injection site because insulin is best absorbed there. Other possible injection sites are the upper outer arm (not the deltoid area), the thighs, and the buttocks.
- Each injection should be given 2 inches from the previous injection in one quadrant before moving to another quadrant.

Lispro (Humalog) and aspart (NovoLog) are commonly prescribed rapid-acting insulins with a shorter duration of action than regular insulin. They are preferred for use during pregnancy (Landon et al., 2012). Advantages of rapid-acting insulins include convenience because they are injected immediately before mealtime, produce less hyperglycemia after meals, and cause fewer hypoglycemic episodes in some people. Because their effects last only 3 to 5 hours, most clients require a longer-acting insulin in addition to the rapid-acting insulin to maintain optimal blood glucose levels (Gilbert, 2011; Landon et al.) (see Table 29-4).

Glargine (Lantus) is long-acting insulin lasting approximately 24 hours. Small amounts of glargine insulin are released slowly, with no pronounced peak. This preparation is most often used with women who have insulin-resistant diabetes (type 2) requiring high doses of long-acting insulin. Glargine insulin is combined with rapid-acting insulin to prevent hypoglycemia. Glargine insulin is not approved for use in pregnancy but appears to be safe. When it is administered with rapid- or short-acting insulin, unpredictable spikes in insulin levels and resulting hypoglycemia appear to occur less often (Landon et al., 2012) (see Table 29-4).

Most women with insulin-dependent diabetes are managed with three or four injections per day (Landon et al., 2012). An insulin regimen that works well for pregnancy is to administer short-acting insulin before each meal and longer-acting insulin at bedtime. This regimen, referred to as *basal/bolus insulin,* provides a more physiologic profile (Gilbert, 2011; Landon et al.). Basal, or long-acting insulin, provides glucose control between meals and reduces hepatic glucose production. Bolus, or prandial insulin (rapid or short acting), provides coverage for glucose with meals (Gilbert). The ratio of basal to bolus is usually 50/50 or 40/60 in pregnancy (Landon et al.).

Continuous subcutaneous insulin infusion (CSII) systems are used increasingly during pregnancy. The insulin pump is designed to mimic more closely the function of the pancreas in secreting insulin (Fig. 29-3). This portable battery-powered device is worn similar to a pager during most daily activities. The pump infuses rapid-acting insulin (usually lispro or aspart) (Landon et al., 2012) at a set basal rate. It has the capacity to deliver up to 24 different basal rates in 24 hours although only three or four rates are necessary to provide individualized

TABLE 29-4 Common Insulin Preparations

TYPE OF INSULIN	EXAMPLES GENERIC (TRADE) NAME	ONSET OF ACTION	PEAK OF ACTION	DURATION OF ACTION
Rapid acting	Lispro (Humalog)	15 min	30-90 min	4-5 hr
	Aspart (NovoLog)	15 min	1-3 hr	3-5 hr
Short acting	Humulin R	30 min	2-4 hr	5-7 hr
	Novolin R	30 min	2.5-5 hr	6-8 hr
Intermediate acting	Humulin NPH	1-2 hr	6-12 hr	18-24 hr
	Novolin N	1.5 hr	4-20 hr	24 hr
	Humulin Lente	1-3 hr	6-12 hr	18-24 hr
	Novolin L	2.5 hr	7-15 hr	22 hr
Long acting	Humulin Ultralente	4-6 hr	8-20 hr	>36 hr
	Glargine (Lantus)	1 hr	None	24 hr

L, Lente; *NPH (or N),* neutral protamine Hagedorn; *R,* regular.

Data from Landon, M.B., Catalano, P.M., & Gabbe, S.G. (2012). Diabetes mellitus complicating pregnancy. In S. Gabbe, J. Niebyl, & J.L. Simpson (Eds), *Obstetrics: Normal and problem pregnancies* (6th ed.). Philadelphia: Saunders.

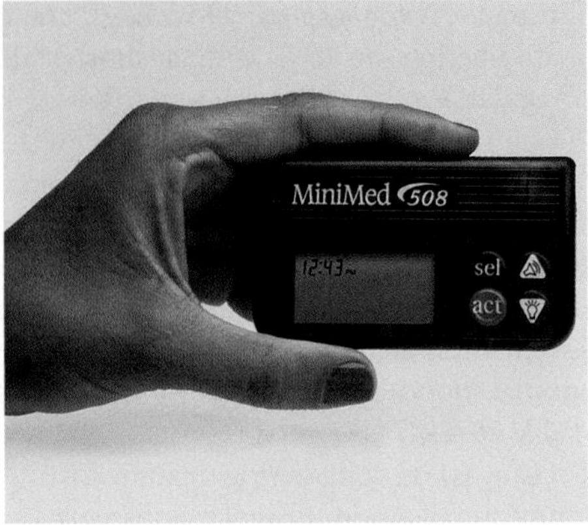

FIG 29-3 Insulin pump shows basal rate for pregnant women with diabetes. (Courtesy MiniMed, Inc., Sylmar, CA.)

glycemic control. The pump also delivers bolus doses of insulin before meals to control postprandial blood glucose levels or to correct elevations in blood glucose. A fine-gauge plastic catheter is inserted into subcutaneous tissue, usually in the abdomen, and attached to the pump syringe by connecting tubing. The subcutaneous catheter and connecting tubing are changed every 2 to 3 days. Although the insulin pump is convenient and generally provides good glycemic control, complications such as pump failure, precipitation of insulin inside the pump mechanism, abscess formation, and poor uptake from the infusion site still can occur. To safely use the pump during pregnancy, the woman must monitor her blood glucose levels frequently and be able to count carbohydrates appropriately. Therefore, use of the insulin pump requires a knowledgeable, motivated woman; skilled health care providers; and prompt 24-hour availability of emergency assistance (Gilbert, 2011).

Self-Monitoring of Blood Glucose (SMBG). Blood glucose testing at home using a glucose meter is considered the standard of care for monitoring blood glucose levels during pregnancy. It provides the most important tool available to the woman to assess her degree of glycemic control. The newer meters are calibrated to provide plasma (rather than whole blood) glucose values. The nurse must be knowledgeable about the specific glucose meter that the woman uses in order to troubleshoot problems, assess accuracy of technique, and determine accuracy of reported results. To perform blood glucose monitoring a drop of blood is obtained and placed on a test strip. Most glucose meters allow the user to obtain the blood sample from the forearm or palm rather than a finger. Fingersticks are recommended during pregnancy, however, because use of other sites can affect the accuracy of results. After a specified amount of time the glucose level is displayed by the meter (see Teaching for Self-Management: Self-Monitoring of Blood Glucose). Blood glucose levels are routinely measured at various times throughout the day such as before breakfast, lunch, and dinner; 1 to 2 hours after each meal; at bedtime; and in the middle of the night if nighttime insulin is being adjusted. When any adjustment in the insulin dose or diet is made, more frequent measurement of blood glucose is warranted. If nausea, vomiting, or diarrhea occurs or if infection is present, the woman is asked to monitor her blood glucose levels more closely than usual.

TEACHING FOR SELF-MANAGEMENT

Self-Monitoring of Blood Glucose (SMBG)

- Gather supplies, check expiration date, and read instructions on testing materials. Prepare glucose meter for use according to the manufacturer's directions.
- Wash hands in warm water (warmth increases circulation).
- Select site on side of any finger (all fingers should be used in rotation).
- Pierce site with lancet (may use automatic spring-loaded, puncturing device). Cleaning the site with alcohol is not necessary.
- Drop hand down to side; with other hand gently squeeze finger from hand to fingertip.
- Allow blood to be drawn into glucose test strip.
- Record results displayed.
- Repeat as instructed by the health care provider and as needed for signs of hypoglycemia or hyperglycemia.

Target levels of blood glucose during pregnancy are lower than nonpregnant values (see Table 29-3). Acceptable fasting levels are generally between 60 and 99 mg/dl, and peak (1 hour) postmeal levels should be between 100 and 129 mg/dl (ADA, 2013a). Two-hour postmeal levels should be 120 mg/dl or less (Landon et al., 2012). The woman should be told to report recurrent episodes of hypoglycemia (less than 70 mg/dl) and hyperglycemia (more than 200 mg/dl) to her health care provider so adjustments in diet or insulin therapy can be made.

Pregnant women with diabetes are much more likely to develop hypoglycemia than hyperglycemia. Most episodes of mild or moderate hypoglycemia can be treated with oral intake of 15 g of carbohydrate, preferably in the form of commercial glucose tablets (Gilbert, 2011) (see Teaching for Self-Management: Treatment for Hypoglycemia). If severe hypoglycemia occurs and the woman experiences a decrease in or loss of consciousness or an inability to swallow, she will require a parenteral injection of glucagon or intravenous (IV) glucose. Because hypoglycemia can develop rapidly and impaired judgment can be associated with even moderate episodes, family members, friends, and work colleagues must be able to recognize signs and symptoms quickly and initiate proper treatment if necessary.

Some women with long-term pregestational diabetes develop hypoglycemia unawareness, a condition in which early symptoms of hypoglycemia are not recognized. Women with hypoglycemia unawareness should test their blood glucose levels more frequently, especially during the night, in order to detect hypoglycemia earlier. Glycemic thresholds in women with hypoglycemia unawareness should be higher than for other women with diabetes in order to avoid dangerous hypoglycemia. The threshold for recognition of hypoglycemia should be determined at the first prenatal visit so that individual guidelines for hypoglycemia can be determined and the woman and her family educated.

Hyperglycemia is less likely than hypoglycemia to occur, although it can rapidly progress to DKA, which is associated with an increased risk of fetal death (Landon et al., 2012). Women and family members should be particularly alert for signs and symptoms of hyperglycemia when infections or other illnesses occur (see Teaching for Self-Management: What to Do When Illness Occurs).

TEACHING FOR SELF-MANAGEMENT

Treatment for Hypoglycemia

- Be familiar with signs and symptoms of hypoglycemia (nervousness, headache, fatigue, shaking, irritability, tachycardia, hunger, blurred vision, sweaty skin, tingling of mouth or extremities).
- Check blood glucose level immediately when hypoglycemic symptoms occur.
- If blood glucose is less than 70 mg/dl, immediately eat 2 to 4 glucose tablets or gel (8-16 g carbohydrate). If glucose tablets or gel are not available, then other simple carbohydrates (15 g) can be eaten instead. Examples are:
  - ½ cup (4 oz) unsweetened orange juice
  - ½ cup (4 oz) regular (not diet) soda
  - 5 or 6 hard candies
  - 1 cup (8 oz) skim milk
- Rest for 15 minutes, and then recheck blood glucose.
- If glucose level is greater than 70 mg/dl, eat a meal to stabilize the sugar level.
- If glucose level is still less than 70 mg/dl, eat 2 to 4 additional glucose tablets.
- Wait 15 minutes, and then recheck blood glucose. If the level is still less than 70 mg/dl, notify your health care provider immediately.
- If nausea related to hypoglycemia prevents ingestion of carbohydrate, inject 0.15 mg glucagon intramuscularly. This will elevate the blood glucose enough to allow eating.

TEACHING FOR SELF-MANAGEMENT

What to Do When Illness Occurs

- Be sure to take insulin even if unable to eat or appetite is less than normal. (Insulin needs are increased with illness or infection.)
- Call the health care provider and relay the following information:
  - Symptoms of illness (e.g., nausea, vomiting, diarrhea)
  - Elevated temperature
  - Most recent blood glucose level
  - Urine ketones
  - Time and amount of last insulin dose
- Increase oral intake of fluids to prevent dehydration.
- Rest as much as possible.
- If you are unable to reach your health care provider and blood glucose exceeds 200 mg/dl with moderate urine ketones present, seek emergency treatment at the nearest health care facility. Do not attempt to self-treat for this condition.

Urine Testing. Urine testing for glucose is not beneficial during pregnancy. Because of the lowered renal threshold for glucose, the degree of glycosuria does not accurately reflect the blood glucose level. However, urine testing for ketones continues to have a place in diabetes management. Monitoring for urine ketones may detect inadequate caloric or carbohydrate intake or skipped meals or snacks. Testing may also be performed when illness occurs or when the blood glucose level is greater than 200 mg/dl (Gilbert, 2011).

Complications Requiring Hospitalization. Occasionally hospitalization is necessary to regulate insulin therapy and stabilize glucose levels. Infection, which can lead to hyperglycemia and DKA, is an indication for hospitalization, regardless of gestational age. Hospitalization during the third trimester for close maternal and fetal observation may be indicated for women whose diabetes is poorly controlled. In addition, women with diabetes are more likely than women who do not have diabetes to also have preexisting hypertension or develop preeclampsia, which may necessitate hospitalization (Gilbert, 2011).

Fetal Surveillance. Diagnostic techniques for fetal surveillance are often performed to assess fetal growth and well-being. The goals of fetal surveillance are to detect fetal compromise as early as possible and prevent IUFD or unnecessary preterm birth.

Early in pregnancy the estimated date of birth is determined. A baseline sonogram is obtained during the first trimester to assess gestational age. Follow-up ultrasound examinations are usually performed during the pregnancy (as often as every 3 to 4 weeks) to monitor fetal growth; estimate fetal weight; and detect hydramnios, macrosomia, and congenital anomalies.

Because the fetus of a woman with diabetes is at increased risk for neural tube defects such as spina bifida, anencephaly, or microcephaly, measurement of maternal serum alpha-fetoprotein is performed between 15 and 20 weeks of gestation (ideally between 16 and 18 weeks of gestation) (Wapner, 2014). In addition, a detailed ultrasound study to examine the fetus for neural tube defects and other anomalies should be performed between 18 and 20 weeks of gestation (Moore et al., 2014).

Ultrasound measurement of the fetal nuchal translucency (NT) in conjunction with maternal serum screening late in the first trimester (between 11 and 14 weeks of gestation) has been found to increase the detection of heart defects and other anomalies in women with pregestational diabetes (Miller, de Veciana, Turan, et al., 2013). Fetal echocardiography may be performed between 20 and 22 weeks of gestation to detect cardiac anomalies, especially in women who had less than desirable glucose control early in pregnancy, as demonstrated by a hemoglobin A_{1c} level greater than 6% at the first prenatal visit (Gilbert, 2011; Moore et al., 2014). Some practitioners repeat this fetal surveillance test at 34 weeks of gestation. Doppler studies of the umbilical artery may be performed in women with vascular disease to detect placental compromise.

Most fetal surveillance measures are concentrated in the third trimester, when the risk of fetal compromise is greatest. The goals of antepartum testing during the third trimester are to monitor fetal growth and ensure fetal well-being. Pregnant women should be taught how to make daily fetal movement counts, beginning at 28 weeks of gestation (see Chapter 26) (Moore et al., 2014).

The nonstress test (NST) is the preferred primary method to evaluate fetal well-being. It is usually begun by 32 weeks of gestation and performed at least twice weekly. If the NST is nonreactive, a biophysical profile or contraction stress test will be performed. Testing often begins earlier, between 28 and 32 weeks of gestation, in women who have vascular disease or poor glucose control (Landon et al., 2012) (see Chapter 26).

Determination of Birth Date and Mode of Birth. The optimal time for birth is between 39 and 40 weeks of gestation, as long as good metabolic control is maintained and parameters of antepartum fetal surveillance remain within normal limits. Reasons to proceed with birth before term include poor metabolic control, coexisting hypertension, and nonreassuring responses to fetal testing (Moore et al., 2014).

Many practitioners plan for elective labor induction between 38 and 40 weeks of gestation.

To confirm fetal lung maturity an amniocentesis should be performed when birth will occur before 38 weeks of gestation. For the pregnancy complicated by diabetes, fetal lung maturation is best predicted by the amniotic fluid phosphatidylglycerol (greater than 3%). If the fetal lungs are still immature, birth should be postponed until 40 weeks of gestation as long as fetal assessment test results remain reassuring. After that time, however, the benefits of conservative management are outweighed by the increasing risk of fetal compromise if the pregnancy is allowed to continue. Birth, despite poor fetal lung maturity, may be necessary when testing suggests fetal compromise or worsening maternal condition, such as deteriorating renal function or severe preeclampsia (Moore et al., 2014).

Although vaginal birth is expected for most women with pregestational diabetes, the cesarean rate for these women is as high as 80% (Cunningham et al., 2014). The American College of Obstetricians and Gynecologists (ACOG) recommends that cesarean birth be considered when the estimated fetal weight is expected to be greater than 4500 g in an attempt to reduce the risk of shoulder dystocia. This recommendation may reduce the risk of shoulder dystocia to some degree for an individual woman, but the benefit to a larger group of women is unclear (Moore et al., 2014). Fetal distress and induction failures before term also contribute to the high rate of cesarean birth in these women (Gilbert, 2011).

Intrapartum

During the intrapartum period the woman with pregestational diabetes must be monitored closely to prevent complications related to dehydration, hypoglycemia, and hyperglycemia. An IV line is inserted for infusion of a maintenance fluid. Initially this infusion will be either normal saline or lactated Ringer's solution. Once active labor begins or glucose levels fall below 70 mg/dl, a piggybacked pump-controlled infusion of a solution containing 5% dextrose should be added. The dextrose provides the energy (calories) necessary for the woman to accomplish the work and manage the stress of labor and birth. Most commonly, insulin is administered by continuous infusion, piggybacked into the main IV line. Only rapid- or short-acting insulin can be administered intravenously. Insulin may also be given intermittently by subcutaneous injection as needed to maintain glucose levels within the target range. Determinations of blood glucose levels are made every hour, and fluids and insulin are adjusted to maintain the blood glucose level between 90 and 110 mg/dl (Moore et al., 2014). Maintaining this target glucose level is essential because hyperglycemia during labor can cause metabolic problems in the neonate, particularly hypoglycemia (Landon et al., 2012).

During labor continuous fetal heart monitoring is necessary. The woman should assume an upright or side-lying position during labor to prevent supine hypotension caused by a large fetus or polyhydramnios. Labor, whether spontaneous or induced, is allowed to progress as long as expected rates of cervical dilation and fetal descent are maintained, and fetal well-being is evident. Failure to progress in labor may indicate a macrosomic infant and cephalopelvic disproportion, necessitating a cesarean birth. The woman is observed and treated during labor for complications of diabetes such as hyperglycemia, ketosis, and ketoacidosis. During second-stage labor, shoulder dystocia may occur with the birth of a macrosomic infant (see Chapter 35). A neonatologist, pediatrician, or neonatal nurse practitioner will likely be present at the birth to initiate assessment and neonatal care.

If a cesarean birth is planned, it should be scheduled in the early morning to facilitate glycemic control. Women should take their full dose of insulin the night before surgery. No morning insulin is given on the day of surgery, and the woman is given nothing by mouth. Epidural anesthesia is recommended because hypoglycemia can be detected earlier if the woman is awake. After surgery, glucose levels should be monitored carefully.

Postpartum

During the first 24 hours postpartum, insulin requirements decrease substantially because the major source of insulin resistance, the placenta, has been removed. Women with type 1 diabetes usually only require 50% to 60% of their pregnancy insulin dose on the first postpartum day, provided they are eating a full diet (Gilbert, 2011). Women who give birth by cesarean may need an IV infusion of glucose and insulin until they resume a regular diet (Moore et al., 2014). A subcutaneous dose of insulin should be given at least an hour before discontinuing IV insulin.

After birth, several days may be required to reestablish carbohydrate homeostasis (see Fig. 29-1, *D* and *E*). Blood glucose levels are carefully monitored in the postpartum period and the insulin dose is adjusted appropriately. The woman who has insulin-dependent diabetes must realize the importance of eating on time even if the baby needs feeding or other pressing demands exist. Women with type 2 diabetes may resume taking their prepregnancy oral hypoglycemics if these medications are compatible with breastfeeding and provide adequate glycemic control.

Possible postpartum complications include preeclampsia or eclampsia, hemorrhage, and infection. Hemorrhage is a possibility if the mother's uterus was overdistended (hydramnios, macrosomic fetus) or overstimulated (oxytocin induction). Postpartum infections such as endometritis are more likely to occur in women with diabetes than in women who do not have diabetes.

Mothers are encouraged to breastfeed. In addition to the advantages of maternal satisfaction and pleasure, breastfeeding has an antidiabetogenic effect for the children of women with diabetes and for women with gestational diabetes. Breastfed infants of women with diabetes are also less likely to become obese (Moore et al., 2014). These benefits are important because a child born to a mother with type 2 diabetes has a 70% chance of also developing type 2 diabetes later in life (Gilbert, 2011).

Insulin requirements in breastfeeding women may be one half of prepregnancy levels because of the carbohydrate used in human milk production. Because glucose levels are lower than normal, breastfeeding women are at increased risk for hypoglycemia, especially in the early postpartum period and after breastfeeding sessions, particularly after late-night nursing (Gilbert, 2011; Moore et al., 2014). Breastfeeding mothers with diabetes may be at increased risk for mastitis and yeast infections of the breast. The insulin dose, which is decreased during lactation, must be recalculated at weaning (see Fig. 29-1, *F*).

The mother may have early breastfeeding difficulties. Poor metabolic control may delay lactogenesis and contribute to decreased milk production (Moore et al., 2014). Initial contact with and opportunity to breastfeed the infant may be delayed for mothers who gave birth by cesarean or if infants are placed in neonatal intensive care units or special care nurseries for observation during the first few hours after birth. Support and assistance from nursing staff and lactation specialists can facilitate the mother's early experience with breastfeeding and encourage her to continue.

The new mother needs information about family planning and contraception. Although family planning is important for all women, it is essential for the woman with diabetes in order to safeguard her own health and promote optimal outcomes in future pregnancies. The risks and benefits of contraceptive methods should be discussed with the mother and her partner before discharge from the hospital. Barrier methods are often recommended as safe, inexpensive options that have no inherent risks for women with diabetes. An intrauterine device (IUD) may also be used without concerns about an increased risk of infection (Landon et al., 2012).

Use of oral contraceptives by women with diabetes is controversial because of the possible increased risk of thromboembolic and vascular complications and the effect on carbohydrate metabolism (Landon et al., 2012). In nonsmoking women who are less than 35 years old and do not have vascular disease, combination low-dose oral contraceptives may be prescribed. Progestin-only oral contraceptives also may be used because they do not significantly affect glucose levels (Cunningham et al., 2014). Close monitoring of blood pressure and lipid levels is necessary to detect complications (Landon et al., 2012).

Opinion is divided about the use of long-acting parenteral progestins, such as Depo-Provera. Some health care providers recommend their use, particularly in women who are noncompliant with daily dosing oral contraceptives. In contrast, other health care providers believe this method may adversely affect glycemic control. In addition, although Depo-Provera may lower serum triglyceride and high-density lipoprotein (HDL) cholesterol levels, it does not lower total cholesterol or low-density lipoprotein (LDL) levels. For this reason it is not recommended as a first-choice method for contraception for women with diabetes (Landon et al., 2012). Implants that contain only progesterone (e.g., Implanon, Nexplanon) can be used by many women with diabetes because they do not significantly affect glucose levels (Cunningham et al., 2014).

Transdermal (patch) and transvaginal (vaginal ring) are newer contraceptive options, particularly effective in women who prefer weekly or every-third-week dosing, respectively. For women weighing more than 90 kg (198 lb) the contraceptive failure rate with transdermal administration is higher than in normal-weight women. Therefore, this method is contraindicated in obese women. In addition, women who choose the patch as their contraceptive method may be at risk for developing thromboembolic disease (Cunningham et al., 2014).

The risks associated with pregnancy increase with the duration and severity of diabetes. In addition, pregnancy may contribute to the vascular changes associated with diabetes. This information needs to be thoroughly discussed with the woman and her partner. Sterilization is often recommended for the woman who has completed her family, who has poor metabolic control, or who has significant vascular problems. Vasectomy for the partner is very effective and is safer than surgical sterilization in the woman with diabetes.

GESTATIONAL DIABETES MELLITUS

Gestational diabetes mellitus (GDM) complicates approximately 7% of all pregnancies (a range of 1% to 14%, depending on the population and the type of diagnostic test used) and accounts for 200,000 cases per year (ADA, 2013b). It occurs more often now worldwide than in the past, probably because of increasing rates of overweight and obesity (ACOG, 2013). According to White's classification system, women with GDM fall into classes A_1 and A_2 (see Table 29-1). It is more likely to occur among Hispanic, African-American, Native-American, Asian, and Pacific Islander women than Caucasians and is likely to recur in future pregnancies; the risk for development of overt diabetes later in life is also increased (ACOG). This tendency is especially true of women whose GDM is diagnosed early in pregnancy (Landon et al., 2012). Classic risk factors for GDM include a family history of diabetes and a previous pregnancy that resulted in an unexplained stillbirth or the birth of a malformed or macrosomic fetus. Other risk factors for GDM include obesity, hypertension, glycosuria, and maternal age older than 25 years. However, more than half of all women diagnosed with GDM do not have these risk factors (Landon et al.).

Although most women are screened for GDM between 24 and 28 weeks of gestation, those with strong risk factors should be screened earlier in pregnancy. Women with morbid obesity, a strong family history of diabetes, a history of GDM in a previous pregnancy, or a history of giving birth to a macrosomic stillborn infant or an infant weighing more than 4500 g are candidates for early screening. If the early screening results are normal, they should be rescreened at 24 to 28 weeks of gestation (Landon et al., 2012).

GDM is usually diagnosed during the second half of pregnancy. As fetal nutrient demands rise during the late second and the third trimesters, maternal nutrient ingestion induces greater and more sustained levels of blood glucose. At the same time maternal insulin resistance is also increasing because of the insulin-antagonistic effects of the placental hormones, cortisol, and insulinase. Consequently maternal insulin demands rise as much as threefold. Most pregnant women are capable of increasing insulin production to compensate for insulin resistance and maintain euglycemia. However, when the pancreas is unable to produce sufficient insulin or the insulin is not used effectively, GDM can result.

Fetal Risks

No increase in the incidence of birth defects has been found among infants of women who develop GDM after the first trimester because the critical period of organ formation has already passed by that time (Moore et al., 2014). Obesity

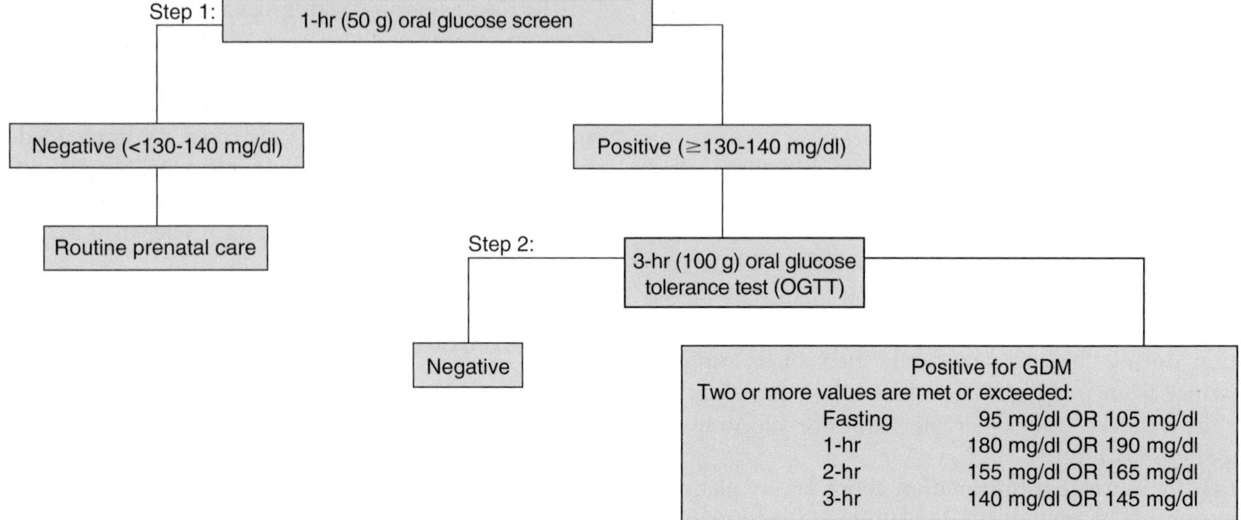

FIG 29-4 Two-step method for diagnosing gestational diabetes mellitus (GDM), recommended by the American College of Obstetricians and Gynecologists (ACOG). Data from American College of Obstetricians and Gynecologists (ACOG). (2013). *Gestational diabetes mellitus.* ACOG practice bulletin no. 137. Washington, DC: ACOG.

(BMI >30) also contributes to congenital defects even in the absence of GDM. As with pregestational diabetes, infants born to women with GDM are at risk for macrosomia and associated risks for birth trauma and electrolyte imbalances including neonatal hypoglycemia

CARE MANAGEMENT

Screening for Gestational Diabetes Mellitus

All pregnant women not known to have pregestational diabetes should be screened for GDM by history, clinical risk factors, or laboratory screening of blood glucose levels (ACOG, 2013). Based on history and clinical risk factors, some women are at low risk for developing GDM; therefore, glucose testing for this population may not be cost-effective. This group includes normal-weight women younger than 25 years of age who have no family history of diabetes, are not members of an ethnic or a racial group known to have a high prevalence of the disease, and have no history of abnormal glucose tolerance or adverse obstetric outcomes usually associated with GDM. However, only 10% of pregnant women meet all of these criteria (ACOG).

Two different blood glucose screening methods for GDM are used in the United States. The ACOG still recommends the two-step screening method that has been used for many years. The first step is a screen consisting of a 50-g oral glucose load followed by a plasma glucose measurement 1 hour later. The woman need not be fasting when the screen is done. A glucose value of 130 to 140 mg/dl is considered a positive screen. An initial positive screening result is followed by step 2, a 3-hour (100-g) oral glucose tolerance test (OGTT) on another day. The ACOG recommends use of the two-step screening procedure because there is no evidence that the one-step method leads to clinically significant improvement in maternal or newborn outcomes. Use of the one-step method does, however, significantly increase health care costs because more women will be diagnosed with GDM and thus will require more visits, tests, and procedures than pregnant women who do not have this disease (ACOG, 2013).

The OGTT is administered after an overnight fast and at least 3 days of unrestricted diet (at least 150 g of carbohydrate) and physical activity. The woman is instructed to avoid caffeine because it increases glucose levels and to abstain from smoking for 12 hours before the test. The 3-hour OGTT requires a fasting blood glucose level, which is drawn before giving a 100-g glucose load. Blood glucose levels are then drawn 1, 2, and 3 hours later. The woman is diagnosed with GDM if two or more values are met or exceeded (ACOG, 2013). Two different sets of glucose values are commonly used to diagnose GDM following the 100-g OGTT (Fig. 29-4). At this time, use of one set of glucose values cannot be clearly recommended over the other. Therefore, providers are urged to select one set of blood glucose values and use it consistently in their practice (ACOG).

An international consensus group, the International Association of Diabetes and Pregnancy Study Groups (IADPSG),

CLINICAL REASONING CASE STUDY

Screening for Gestational Diabetes Mellitus (GDM)

Kelly is a 30-year-old G1 P0 African-American woman who is obese. Both her mother and maternal grandmother have been diagnosed with type 2 diabetes. Kelly failed her 50-g oral glucose screen, which was performed at 26 weeks of gestation, with a value of 160 mg/dl. She reported to her health care provider's office one week later to have a 3-hour OGTT done. Kelly's test results from the 3-hour OGTT were fasting blood glucose (FBS), 96 mg/dl; 1 hour, 182 mg/dl; 2 hour, 161 mg/dl; 3 hour, 138 mg/dl.

1. Evidence—Is there sufficient evidence at this time to determine if Kelly has gestational diabetes (GDM)?
2. Assumptions—Describe an underlying assumption regarding the following interventions for the management of GDM:
   a. Medical nutrition therapy (diet)
   b. Insulin
   c. Oral hypoglycemic agents
3. What implications and priorities for nursing care can be drawn at this time?
4. Does the evidence objectively support your conclusion?

consisting of representatives from multiple obstetric and diabetic organizations including the ADA, recommends a different (one-step) method of screening and diagnosis. Increasing rates of obesity and diabetes have resulted in more women of childbearing age with type 2 diabetes, many of whom are undiagnosed when they become pregnant. The IADPSG recommends that high risk women be tested for overt diabetes at their initial prenatal visit using standard criteria for diagnosis (ADA, 2013b). If the tests done early in pregnancy for overt diabetes are normal, a 75-g OGTT diagnostic test is administered between 24 and 28 weeks of gestation. The 75-g OGTT requires a fasting blood glucose level, which is drawn before giving the glucose load. Blood glucose levels are then drawn 1 and 2 hours later. A diagnosis of GDM is made if only one glucose value is exceeded (Fig. 29-5). The one-step method of screening and diagnosis significantly increases the incidence of GDM. The ACOG does not recommend this method (ACOG, 2013; ADA 2013b). However, some practitioners in the United States are using the IADPSG recommendations for screening and diagnosing GDM (ADA, 2013b) (see Evidence-Based Practice box).

EVIDENCE-BASED PRACTICE

Debating Gestational Diabetes Diagnosis

Ask the Question

For pregnant women with hyperglycemia, at what level do diagnosis and treatment for gestational diabetes become most beneficial for the baby?

Search for the Evidence

Search Strategies English language research-based publications since 2011 on gestational diabetes screening or diagnosis, hyperglycemia, ADA, ACOG, and NIH were included.

Databases Used Cochrane Collaborative Database, National Guideline Clearinghouse (AHRQ), CINAHL, PubMed, UpToDate, and the professional websites for ACOG, ADA, and AWHONN

Toward a Diagnosis of Gestational Diabetes Mellitus

Background:

- High serum glucose in pregnancy is associated with complications such as preeclampsia, macrosomia, operative vaginal birth, shoulder dystocia, birth injury, cesarean birth, neonatal hypoglycemia, need for neonatal intensive care, respiratory distress, and jaundice. A commonly accepted method of diagnosing gestational diabetes mellitus (GDM) has been a nonfasting glucose challenge at 24-28 weeks of gestation (Moyer, 2014). For a 50-g glucose challenge test, the most common cutoff was 140 mg/dl, a level that was associated with macrosomia and gestational hypertension (Prutsky, Domecq, Sunderesh, et al., 2013). An elevated result triggered a fasting 2- or 3-hour oral glucose tolerance test (OGTT). A second abnormal result resulted in diagnosis of GDM. Using this approach, about 5% to 6% of pregnant women received treatment, including diet, exercise, glucose monitoring, and possibly metformin.

Conflicting Guidelines:

- ACOG: In 2006 at least nine different criteria were used to identify gestational diabetes, using 50-100 g of glucose as the challenge. The American College of Obstetrics and Gynecology (ACOG) approach used two-step screening, clinical criteria, and history. Critics of this approach questioned its reliance on maternal, rather than newborn, outcomes; its acceptance of clinical criteria or history alone for diagnosis; and its ambiguous screening cutoffs (Ryan, 2013).
- ADA: In 2008 the International Association of Diabetes in Pregnancy Study Group (IADPSG) set out to identify levels at which treatment would benefit the baby. They proposed a one-step approach, consisting of a 75-g OGTT. Abnormal levels were set based on their association with macrosomia and cord blood C-peptide, a marker for fetal insulin levels. One abnormal result was enough to trigger diagnosis of GDM. This approach is estimated to identify GDM in nearly 18% of all pregnant women. The American Diabetes Association (ADA) endorsed this approach (Ryan, 2013).

NIH Consensus Conference:

- Criticism of the one-step approach includes reliance on just one abnormal result and the unintended consequences of labeling women with GDM: increase in cesarean birth and possibly labor induction, additional fetal assessments, more intensive newborn assessments, significantly increased client costs, life disruptions, and psychologic stress. To resolve the differences between the ACOG and ADA approaches, the National Institutes of Health (NIH) convened a Consensus Conference. The NIH statement found some advantages for convenience of diagnosis within the context of one visit; however, there was insufficient evidence of clear improvement in client outcomes to recommend the one-step approach. Therefore, the NIH group recommended continuing the current two-step approach and called for further targeted research (Vandorsten, Dodson, Espeland, et al., 2013).

Quality and Safety Competencies: Evidence-Based Practice (EBP)*

Knowledge

Describe reliable sources for locating evidence reports and clinical practice guidelines.

The nurse working with pregnant women needs to understand evolving professional recommendations.

Skills

Locate evidence reports related to clinical practice topics and guidelines.

Relevant systematic reviews and professional guidelines provide recommendations for improving perinatal outcomes.

Attitudes

Value the concept of EBP as integral to determining best clinical practices.

EBP represents the best practice and its use fosters client confidence and efficacy.

References

Moyer, V. A. (2014). Screening for gestational diabetes mellitus: U.S. Preventive Services Task Force recommendation statement. *Annals of Internal Medicine, 160*(6), 414–420.

Ryan, E. A. (2013). Clinical diagnosis of gestational diabetes. *Clinical Obstetrics and Gynecology, 56*(4), 774–787.

Prutsky, G. J., Domecq, J. P., Sundaresh, V., et al. (2013). Screening for gestational diabetes: A systematic review and meta-analysis. *Journal of Clinical Endocrinology and Metabolism, 98*(11), 4311–4318.

Vandorsten, J. P., Dodson, W. C., Espeland, M. A., et al. (2013). NIH consensus development conference: Diagnosing gestational diabetes mellitus. *NIH Consensus State of the Science Statements, 29*(1), 1–31.

Pat Mahaffee Gingrich

*Adapted from QSEN at www.qsen.org.

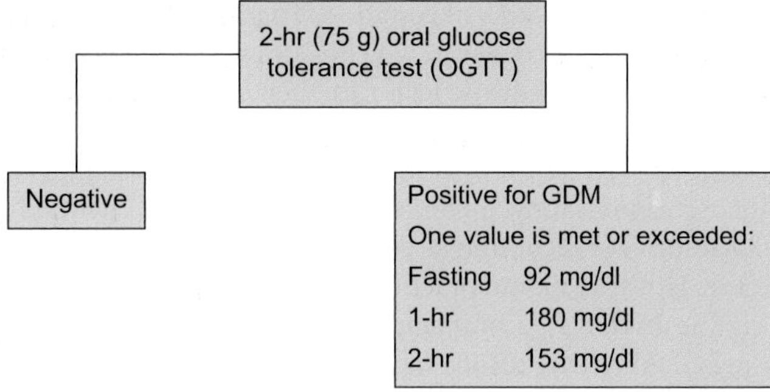

FIG 29-5 One-step method for diagnosing gestational diabetes mellitus (GDM), recommended by the International Association of Diabetes in Pregnancy Study Groups (IADPSG). Data from American Diabetes Association (ADA) (2013). Position statement: Diagnosis and classification of diabetes mellitus. *Diabetes Care*, *36*(Suppl 1), S67-S74.

Nursing diagnoses and expected outcomes of care for women with GDM are basically the same as those for women with pregestational diabetes except that the time frame for planning may be shortened with GDM because the diagnosis is usually made later in pregnancy (see Nursing Care Plan).

Interventions

Antepartum

When the diagnosis of GDM is made, treatment begins immediately, allowing little or no time for the woman and her family to adjust to the diagnosis before they are expected to participate in the treatment plan. With each step of the treatment plan the nurse and other health care providers should educate the woman and her family, providing detailed and comprehensive explanations to ensure understanding, participation, and

NURSING CARE PLAN

The Pregnant Woman with Gestational Diabetes

NURSING DIAGNOSIS	EXPECTED OUTCOME	INTERVENTIONS	RATIONALES
Deficient Knowledge related to gestational diabetes as evidenced by the woman's questions and concerns	The woman will be able to verbalize important information regarding gestational diabetes, its management, and potential effects on the pregnancy and fetus.	Assess woman's current knowledge base regarding the disease process, management, effects on pregnancy and fetus, and potential complications.	To provide database for further teaching
		Explain pathophysiologic aspects of diabetes, its effects on pregnancy and fetus, and potential complications.	To promote compliance with treatment plan
		Explain principles of diabetic diet and have woman plan her meals for 1 day following these principles.	To promote self-management and compliance with treatment plan
		Demonstrate procedure for blood glucose monitoring and obtain return demonstration.	To establish woman's comfort and competence with procedure
		Demonstrate procedure for insulin administration, should this become necessary, and obtain return demonstration.	To establish woman's comfort and competence with procedure
		Explain importance of correctly taking oral hypoglycemic medication (right dose, right time), should this become necessary.	To promote self-management and compliance with treatment plan
		Review signs and symptoms of hypoglycemia and hyperglycemia and appropriate interventions for both.	To promote prompt recognition of complications and self-management
		Provide contact numbers for health care team for prompt interventions and answers to questions on ongoing basis.	To promote comfort
		Review expected plan of care.	To allay anxiety and enlist cooperation of woman in her care
Risk for Fetal Injury related to elevated maternal glucose levels	The fetus will remain free of injury and be born at term in a healthy state.	Assess woman's current diabetic control.	To identify risk for fetal macrosomia
		Monitor fundal height during each prenatal visit.	To identify appropriate fetal growth
		Assess fetal movement and heart rate during each prenatal visit and perform fetal assessment tests as ordered during the third trimester.	To assess fetal well-being
Anxiety related to threat to maternal and fetal well-being as evidenced by the woman's verbal expressions of concern	The woman will identify sources of anxiety and report feeling less anxious.	Through therapeutic communication promote open relationship with woman.	To promote trust
		Listen to woman's feelings and concerns.	To assess for any misconception or misinformation that may be contributing to anxiety
		Review potential dangers by providing factual information.	To correct any misconceptions or misinformation
		Encourage woman to share concerns with her health care team.	To promote collaboration in her care

adherence to the necessary interventions. Potential complications should be discussed, and the need for maintaining euglycemia throughout the remainder of the pregnancy reinforced. Knowing that GDM typically disappears when the pregnancy is over may be reassuring for the woman and her family.

As with pregestational diabetes, the aim of therapy in women with GDM is strict blood glucose control. Fasting blood glucose levels should range from 60 to 99 mg/dl, and 1-hour postprandial values between 100 and 129 mg/dl (ADA, 2013a). Postmeal glucose levels at 2 hours should be no higher than 120 mg/dl (Landon et al., 2012) (see Table 29-3).

Diet. Dietary modification is the mainstay of treatment for GDM. The woman with GDM is placed on a standard diet for women with diabetes. The usual prescription is 30 kcal/kg/day based on a normal preconception weight. For obese women the usual prescription is up to 25 kcal/kg/day, which translates into 1500 to 2000 kcal/day. Carbohydrate intake is restricted to approximately 50% of caloric intake (Moore et al., 2014). Dietary counseling by a registered dietitian is recommended.

Exercise. There are few published studies on the benefits of exercise in women with GDM. In adults who are not pregnant, exercise increases lean muscle mass and improves sensitivity to insulin. Therefore, a moderate exercise program is recommended for overweight or obese women with GDM in order to improve blood sugar control and facilitate weight loss (ACOG, 2013).

Self-Monitoring of Blood Glucose. Blood glucose monitoring is necessary to determine whether euglycemia can be maintained by diet and exercise. Women are instructed to monitor their blood sugar daily. The frequency and timing of blood glucose monitoring should be individualized for each woman. A typical schedule for monitoring blood glucose is on rising in the morning, 1 or 2 hours after breakfast, before and after lunch, before dinner, and at bedtime (Moore et al., 2014). Women with GDM usually perform self-monitoring at home with a review of their results at prenatal visits to determine the effectiveness of diet and exercise. If glycemic thresholds are not met, then pharmacologic intervention is indicated.

Pharmacologic Therapy. Approximately 25% of women with GDM require insulin during the pregnancy to maintain satisfactory blood glucose levels, despite compliance with the prescribed diet (Landon et al., 2012). In contrast to women with insulin-dependent diabetes, women with GDM are managed initially with diet and exercise alone. If fasting plasma glucose levels are persistently greater than 95 mg/dl, 1-hour postmeal levels are persistently greater than 140 mg/dl, or 2-hour postmeal levels are persistently greater than 120 mg/dl, insulin therapy is begun (ACOG, 2013).

For the past several years oral hypoglycemic therapy has been used as an alternative to insulin in women with GDM who require medication in addition to diet for blood glucose control. Women who are unable or unwilling to take insulin by injection or are cognitively impaired also may be candidates for oral hypoglycemic medication.

Glyburide is the oral agent most frequently prescribed. The fact that only minimal amounts of glyburide cross the placenta to the fetus makes it a good drug for use during pregnancy (Moore et al., 2014). Several studies have shown that glyburide controls blood glucose levels as well as insulin does in women with GDM. Furthermore, research revealed no increase in hypoglycemia or macrosomia in neonates whose mothers took glyburide. However, in one study neonates born to women taking glyburide were found to be more likely to experience birth injury or require phototherapy. Glyburide may not work as well in women who are obese or who experienced higher levels of hyperglycemia early in pregnancy (Landon et al., 2012). Studies have shown that glyburide should be taken at least 30 minutes (preferably 1 hour) before a meal so its peak effect covers the 2-hour postmeal blood glucose level. Because episodes of hypoglycemia can occur between meals, women taking glyburide should always carry their glucose meter with them, along with glucose tablets or gel (Moore et al.).

Metformin is another oral hypoglycemic agent sometimes used in the management of GDM. Although metformin crosses the placenta, it does not appear to be teratogenic. However, glyburide may be better than metformin at controlling blood glucose levels in women with GDM because glyburide causes the maternal pancreas to produce more insulin, whereas metformin decreases hepatic glucose production and increases peripheral sensitivity to insulin (Landon et al., 2012).

Fetal Surveillance. Women with GDM whose blood glucose levels are well controlled by diet are at low risk for an IUFD. Therefore, antepartum fetal testing is not performed routinely in these women unless they also have hypertension, a history of a prior stillbirth, or suspected macrosomia. Women with these complications or those who require insulin for blood glucose control may have twice-weekly NSTs beginning at 32 weeks of gestation. Women with uncomplicated GDM begin fetal testing at 40 weeks of gestation. In general, women with well-controlled GDM can continue pregnancy until 40 weeks of gestation and the spontaneous onset of labor. However, fetal growth should be monitored carefully because the risk for macrosomia as the pregnancy approaches 40 weeks of gestation is apparently increased (Landon et al., 2012).

Intrapartum

During the labor and birth process blood glucose levels are monitored hourly to maintain levels at 80 to 110 mg/dl. Levels within this range decrease the incidence of neonatal hypoglycemia. Infusing rapid-acting insulin intravenously may be necessary during labor to maintain the desired blood glucose levels. However, it is usually possible to maintain excellent glucose control in women with GDM during labor by avoiding the use of IV fluids containing dextrose (Moore et al., 2014). If glucose-containing solutions are given, they should be administered by an infusion device so that inadvertent boluses are avoided. Although GDM is not an indication for cesarean birth, this procedure may be necessary in the presence of preeclampsia or macrosomia.

Postpartum

Although most women with GDM return to normal glucose levels after childbirth, up to one third will be found to have diabetes or impaired glucose metabolism when they are screened postpartum. It is estimated that 15% to 50% of women who have had GDM will develop type 2 diabetes later in life (ACOG, 2013).

The ACOG recommends assessing all women who had GDM for carbohydrate intolerance with a 75-g, 2-hr OGTT or a fasting plasma glucose level at 6 to 12 weeks postpartum. The optimal frequency of subsequent testing has not been established. However, the ADA recommends repeat testing at least every 3 years for women with a history of GDM and normal postpartum glucose testing results (Landon et al., 2012). Obesity is a major risk factor for the later development of diabetes. Women with a history of GDM, particularly those who are overweight, should be encouraged to make lifestyle changes that include weight loss and exercise to reduce this risk (Gilbert, 2011). Children born to women with GDM are also at risk for becoming obese in childhood or adolescence (Landon et al., 2012).

Low-dose oral contraceptives may be safely used by women with a history of GDM. The rate of subsequent diabetes in these women is no different from that in women without a history of GDM who use low-dose oral contraceptives. Women who are also obese or have hypertension or high lipid levels in addition to a history of GDM should use a contraceptive method without the potential for causing cardiovascular side effects. For these women, the intrauterine device is a good option (Cunningham et al., 2014).

HYPEREMESIS GRAVIDARUM

Nausea and vomiting complicate 50% to 80% of all pregnancies, typically beginning at 4 to 10 weeks of gestation. These symptoms are usually confined to the first 20 weeks of gestation (Kelly & Savides, 2014). Although nausea and vomiting are distressing, they are typically benign, with no significant metabolic alterations or risks to the mother or fetus.

The cause of nausea and vomiting in pregnancy is not well understood, although it may involve relaxation of the smooth muscle of the stomach and increasing levels of estrogen and human chorionic gonadotropin (hCG). Gastric dysrhythmias, reduced gastric motility, and gastroesophageal reflux may also contribute to nausea and vomiting during pregnancy. Some authorities have suggested that nausea and vomiting are evolutionary adaptations that occur during pregnancy in order to protect the woman and fetus from potentially harmful foods. Pregnancies complicated by nausea and vomiting generally have a more favorable outcome than those without these symptoms (Gordon, 2012; Kelly & Savides, 2014).

When vomiting during pregnancy becomes excessive enough to cause weight loss, electrolyte imbalance, nutritional deficiencies, and ketonuria, the disorder is termed hyperemesis gravidarum. This disorder occurs in approximately 0.5% of all live births. Hyperemesis gravidarum usually begins during the first trimester, but approximately 10% of women with the disorder continue to have symptoms throughout the pregnancy (Kelly & Savides, 2014). Hyperemesis gravidarum is the second most common reason for hospitalization during pregnancy in the United States (Summers, 2012).

Risk factors for hyperemesis include clinical hyperthyroid disorders, prepregnancy psychiatric diagnosis, previous pregnancy complicated by hyperemesis gravidarum, molar pregnancy, multiple gestation with a male and female fetus, diabetes, and gastrointestinal disorders (Cappell, 2012). For unknown reasons women carrying a female fetus are more likely than those carrying a male fetus to develop hyperemesis (Kelly & Savides, 2014). A family history of hyperemesis may also be present (Gilbert, 2011). Women 30 years of age and older and women who smoke have a lower risk for hyperemesis (Tamay & Kuscu, 2011).

Severe but rare maternal complications of hyperemesis gravidarum include esophageal rupture, pneumomediastinum, and deficiencies of vitamin K and thiamine with resulting Wernicke encephalopathy (CNS involvement) (Kelly & Savides, 2014).

Infants born to women who had poor pregnancy weight gain because of hyperemesis may be small for gestational age, have a low birth weight, or be born prematurely. They may also have 5-minute Apgar scores less than 7 (Kelly & Savides, 2014).

Etiology

Psychosocial, cultural, and psychogenic, as well as physiologic, factors may play a part in the development of hyperemesis gravidarum for some women (Tamay & Kusco, 2011). Conflicting feelings regarding prospective motherhood, body changes, and lifestyle alterations may contribute to episodes of vomiting, particularly if these feelings are excessive or unresolved. Women with associated psychosocial factors usually improve dramatically while in the hospital but may resume vomiting after discharge.

Clinical Manifestations

The woman with hyperemesis gravidarum usually has significant weight loss and dehydration. She may have dry mucous membranes, decreased BP, increased pulse rate, and poor skin turgor. Frequently she is unable to keep down even clear liquids taken by mouth. Laboratory tests may reveal electrolyte imbalances.

CARE MANAGEMENT

Assessment

Whenever a pregnant woman has nausea and vomiting, the first priority is a thorough assessment to determine the severity of the problem. In most cases the woman should be told to come immediately to the health care provider's office or the emergency department because the severity of the illness is often difficult to determine by telephone conversation.

The assessment should include frequency, severity, and duration of episodes of nausea and vomiting. If the woman reports vomiting, the assessment should also include the approximate amount and color of the vomitus. Other symptoms such as diarrhea, indigestion, and abdominal pain or distention also are identified. The woman is asked to report any precipitating factors relating to the onset of her symptoms. Any pharmacologic or nonpharmacologic treatment measures used should be recorded. Prepregnancy weight and documented weight gain or loss during pregnancy are important to note.

The woman's weight and vital signs are measured, and a complete physical examination is performed, with attention to signs of fluid and electrolyte imbalance and nutritional status. The most important initial laboratory test to be obtained is a determination of ketonuria. Other laboratory tests that may be ordered are a urinalysis, a complete blood cell count, electrolytes, liver enzymes, and bilirubin levels. These tests help rule out underlying diseases such as gastroenteritis, pyelonephritis, pancreatitis, cholecystitis, peptic ulcer, and hepatitis (Cunningham et al., 2014). Because of the recognized association between hyperemesis gravidarum and hyperthyroidism, thyroid levels may also be measured (Nader, 2014).

Psychosocial assessment includes asking the woman about anxiety, fears, and concerns related to her own health and the effects on pregnancy outcome. Family members should be assessed both for anxiety and their role in providing support for the woman.

Potential nursing diagnoses for women experiencing hyperemesis gravidarum include:

- *Deficient Fluid Volume* related to excessive vomiting as evidenced by fluid and electrolyte imbalance
- *Imbalanced Nutrition: Less Than Body Requirements*, related to nausea and persistent vomiting as evidenced by weight decrease as compared with prepregnant weight
- *Anxiety* related to effects of hyperemesis on fetal well-being as evidenced by woman's statements of concern

Interventions

Initial Care

Initially the woman who is unable to keep down clear liquids by mouth requires IV therapy for correction of fluid and electrolyte imbalances. In the past women requiring IV therapy were admitted to the hospital. However, today they may be and often are successfully managed at home, even if on enteral therapy. Medications may be used if nausea and vomiting are uncontrolled. The ACOG recommends the use of pyridoxine (vitamin B_6), either alone or in combination with doxylamine (Unisom) as initial medical management because these medications are considered to be both safe and effective (Gordon, 2012).

Other frequently prescribed drugs include promethazine (Phenergan), chlorpromazine (Thorazine), prochlorperazine (Compazine), and trimethobenzamide (Tigan). These medications demonstrated benefit clinically, but their safety in pregnancy has not been proven. Metoclopramide (Reglan) accelerates gastric emptying and corrects gastric dysrhythmias. It has been demonstrated in some small studies to be both safe and effective. Ondansetron (Zofran) and droperidol (Inapsine) have been used to treat postoperative nausea and vomiting but their use in pregnancy has not been well studied (Kelly & Savides, 2014).

Corticosteroids (methylprednisolone [Medrol] or hydrocortisone) may be prescribed for women who do not respond well to the medications previously discussed. These medications have not been proven to treat hyperemesis effectively in all women, however. Because exposure to corticosteroids may increase the risk of facial clefting, they should be used with caution and avoided if possible during the first trimester, when organs and organ systems are developing (Kelly & Savides, 2014).

Finally, enteral or parenteral nutrition may be used as a last resort in women who are nonresponsive to other medical therapies (Kelly & Savides, 2014). Because of potential risks, parenteral therapy should only be used after multiple medical management and enteral tube feeding attempts have been unsuccessful (Gordon, 2012).

Nursing Interventions. Nursing care of the woman with hyperemesis gravidarum involves implementing the medical plan of care, whether it is given in the hospital or home setting. Interventions may include initiating and monitoring IV therapy, administering drugs and nutritional supplements, and monitoring the woman's response to interventions. The nurse observes her for any signs of complications such as metabolic acidosis (secondary to starvation), jaundice, or hemorrhage and alerts the health care provider should these occur. Monitoring includes assessing the woman's nausea, retching without vomiting, and vomiting, given that these symptoms, although related, are separate. Intake and output, including the amount of emesis, should be measured accurately and recorded. Oral hygiene while the woman is receiving nothing by mouth and after episodes of vomiting helps lessen associated discomforts. Assistance with positioning and providing a quiet, restful environment that is free from odors may increase her comfort.

Once the vomiting has stopped, feedings are started in small amounts at frequent intervals. In the beginning limited amounts of oral fluids and bland foods such as crackers, toast, or baked chicken are offered. The diet progresses slowly as tolerated until the woman is able to consume a nutritionally sound diet. Because sleep disturbances may accompany hyperemesis gravidarum, promoting adequate rest is important. The nurse can help coordinate treatment measures and periods of visitation to provide opportunity for rest periods.

Follow-Up Care

Most women are able to take nourishment by mouth after several days of treatment. They should be encouraged to eat small, frequent meals and foods that sound appealing (e.g., nongreasy, dry, sweet, and salty foods). In many instances women discover that foods they normally like have no appeal at all during this time. (See Teaching for Self-Management: Diet for Hyperemesis for more suggestions.) Many pregnant women find exposure to cooking odors nauseating. Having other family members cook may lessen the woman's nausea and vomiting, even if only

TEACHING FOR SELF-MANAGEMENT

Diet for Hyperemesis

- Avoid an empty stomach. Eat frequently, at least every 2 to 3 hours. Separate liquids from solids and alternate every 2 to 3 hours.
- Eat a high-protein snack at bedtime.
- Eat dry, bland, low-fat, and high-protein foods. Cold foods may be better tolerated than those served at a warm temperature.
- In general, eat what sounds good to you rather than trying to balance your meals.
- Follow the salty and sweet approach; even so-called junk foods are okay.
- Eat protein after sweets.
- Dairy products may stay down more easily than other foods.
- If you vomit even when your stomach is empty, try sucking on a Popsicle.
- Try ginger tea. Peel and finely dice a knuckle-sized piece of ginger and place it in a mug of boiling water. Steep for 5 to 8 minutes and add brown sugar to taste.
- Try warm ginger ale (with sugar, not artificial sweetener) or water with a slice of lemon.
- Drink liquids from a cup with a lid.

temporarily. The woman is counseled to contact her health care provider immediately if the nausea and vomiting recur.

The woman with hyperemesis gravidarum needs calm, compassionate, and sympathetic care, with recognition that the manifestations of hyperemesis can be physically and emotionally debilitating to her and stressful for her family. Irritability, tearfulness, and mood changes are often consistent with this disorder. Fetal well-being is the woman's primary concern. The nurse can provide an environment conducive to discussion of concerns and help the woman identify and mobilize sources of support. The family should be included in the plan of care whenever possible. Their participation may help alleviate some of the emotional stress associated with this disorder.

THYROID DISORDERS

Hyperthyroidism

Hyperthyroidism in pregnancy is rare. The incidence varies, occurring in approximately 2 to 17 of every 1000 births (Cunningham et al., 2014). In 90% to 95% of pregnant women it is caused by Graves' disease (Nader, 2014). Clinical manifestations of hyperthyroidism include heat intolerance, diaphoresis, fatigue, anxiety, emotional lability, and tachycardia. Many of these symptoms also occur with pregnancy; thus the disorder can be difficult to diagnose. Signs that may help differentiate hyperthyroidism from normal pregnancy changes include weight loss, goiter, and a pulse rate greater than 100 beats/minute (Nader). Laboratory findings typically include elevated free thyroxine (T_4) and triiodothyronine (T_3) levels and greatly suppressed thyroid-stimulating hormone (TSH) levels (Nader). Moderate and severe hyperthyroidism must be treated during pregnancy. Untreated or inadequately treated women have an increased risk of miscarriage, preterm birth, and giving birth to stillborn infants or infants with goiter, hyperthyroidism, or hypothyroidism. However, most neonates born to women with hyperthyroidism have normal thyroid function. Women with hyperthyroidism are at increased risk for developing severe preeclampsia and heart failure (Cunningham et al.; Nader).

The primary treatment of hyperthyroidism during pregnancy is drug therapy. The medications most often prescribed in the United States are propylthiouracil (PTU) or methimazole (MM). Both drugs are effective at controlling symptoms, but both have potentially dangerous maternal and fetal side effects. PTU can cause hepatic toxicity serious enough to require liver transplantation. When taken during the first trimester of pregnancy, MM can cause choanal atresia or esophageal atresia, facial anomalies, and developmental delay in exposed fetuses. Although the likelihood of maternal and fetal side effects from both drugs is low, a panel convened by the U.S. Food and Drug Administration (FDA) and the American Thyroid Association recommended that PTU be used only in the first trimester of pregnancy or by women who are intolerant of or allergic to MM. Women requiring drug therapy for hyperthyroidism should be switched to MM for the remainder of pregnancy (Mestman, 2012; Nader, 2014).

The usual starting dose of PTU is 100 to 150 mg three times a day. For MM the initial dose is generally 20 mg/day. Women usually show clinical improvement (weight gain and less tachycardia) within 2 to 6 weeks after beginning therapy. Once clinical improvement occurs, the dose of PTU or MM may be cut in half. If symptoms worsen, the medication dosage is doubled (Mestman, 2012). During therapy thyroid test results are used to taper the drug to the smallest effective dose to prevent development of unnecessary fetal or neonatal hypothyroidism. In many women the medication can be discontinued by 32 to 36 weeks of gestation. PTU readily crosses the placenta and may cause fetal hypothyroidism, which is characterized by goiter, bradycardia, and intrauterine growth restriction (IUGR) (Nader, 2014).

Both medications work well in and are well tolerated by most women. The most common maternal side effects of both PTU and MM are pruritus and skin rash. Other possible side effects include drug-related fever, bronchospasm, migratory polyarthritis, a lupus-like syndrome, and cholestatic jaundice (Mestman, 2012; Nader, 2014). The most severe side effect is agranulocytosis, which occurs rarely and usually develops only in older women and in those taking high doses of the drug. Symptoms of agranulocytosis are fever and unexpected sore throat, which should be reported immediately to the health care provider; also the woman should stop taking the medication (Mestman; Nader). Beta-adrenergic blockers such as propranolol (Inderal) may be used in severe hyperthyroidism to control maternal symptoms, especially elevated heart rate. However, long-term use of these medications is not recommended because of the potential for IUGR, bradycardia, and hypoglycemia (Nader).

! NURSING ALERT

A serious but uncommon complication of undiagnosed or partially treated hyperthyroidism is thyroid storm, which can occur in response to stress such as labor and vaginal birth, infection, preeclampsia, or surgery. A woman with this emergency disorder may have fever, restlessness, tachycardia, vomiting, hypotension, or stupor. Prompt treatment is essential. IV fluids and oxygen are administered, along with high doses of PTU. After administration of PTU, iodide is given. Other medications include antipyretics, dexamethasone, and beta-blockers (Cunningham et al., 2014; Nader, 2014).

After birth, women taking either PTU or MM who choose to breastfeed should be informed that the medications do appear in small amounts in breastmilk (Lawrence & Lawrence, 2011). However, they do not appear to adversely affect the neonate's thyroid function. The woman should take her antithyroid medication just after breastfeeding, thus allowing a 3- to 4-hour period before nursing again (Mestman, 2012; Nader, 2014).

Radioactive iodine must not be used in diagnosis or treatment of hyperthyroidism in pregnancy because therapeutic doses given to treat maternal thyroid disease may also destroy the fetal thyroid (Cunningham et al., 2014).

In severe cases surgical treatment of hyperthyroidism, subtotal thyroidectomy, can be performed during pregnancy. Surgery is best performed during the early second trimester of pregnancy when the risk for teratogenesis and preterm labor is lower, although it can be done during the first or third trimester if necessary. Surgery is usually reserved for women with severe disease, those for whom drug therapy proves toxic, and those who are unable to follow the prescribed medical regimen. Risks associated with the surgery are hypoparathyroidism, recurrent laryngeal nerve paralysis, and anesthesia-related complications (Nader, 2014).

Hypothyroidism

Hypothyroidism occurs in two to three pregnancies per 1000. Because severe hypothyroidism is often associated with infertility and an increased risk of miscarriage, it is not often seen during pregnancy (Cunningham et al., 2014). Although iodine deficiency is rare in the United States, it is a common cause of maternal, fetal, and neonatal hypothyroidism in the rest of the world (Nader, 2014). Adult hypothyroidism is usually caused by glandular destruction by autoantibodies, most commonly because of Hashimoto's thyroiditis. Characteristic symptoms of hypothyroidism include weight gain, lethargy, decrease in exercise capacity, and cold intolerance. Women who are moderately symptomatic can also develop constipation, hoarseness, hair loss, brittle nails, and dry skin. Laboratory values in pregnancy include elevated levels of TSH, with or without low T_4 levels (Nader).

Pregnant women with untreated hypothyroidism are at increased risk for miscarriage, preeclampsia, gestational hypertension, placental abruption, preterm birth, and stillbirth. Infants born to mothers with hypothyroidism may also be of low birth weight (Cunningham et al., 2014; Nader, 2014). These outcomes can be improved with early treatment (Nader).

Thyroid hormone supplements are used to treat hypothyroidism. Levothyroxine (e.g., T_4 [Synthroid]) is most often prescribed during pregnancy. The usual beginning dosage is 0.1 to 0.15 mg/day, with adjustment by 25 to 50 mcg every 4 to 6 weeks as necessary based on the maternal TSH level (Cunningham et al., 2014; Nader, 2014). The aim of drug therapy is to maintain the TSH level at the lower end of the normal range for pregnant women. Women with little or no functioning thyroid tissue require higher doses of levothyroxine. In addition, as pregnancy progresses, increased doses of thyroid hormone are usually required. This increased demand during pregnancy is probably related to increased estrogen levels (Cunningham et al.; Nader).

MEDICATION ALERT

If taking iron supplementation, pregnant women should be told to take levothyroxine at a different time of day, at least 4 hours apart, from their iron tablets because ferrous sulfate decreases absorption of T_4 (Nader, 2014).

The fetus depends on maternal thyroid hormones until approximately 18 weeks of gestation, when fetal production begins. Normal maternal T_4 levels early in pregnancy are important for proper fetal brain development. Studies have shown that even mild maternal hypothyroidism during the first trimester has been associated with long-term neuropsychologic damage in their children. More research needs to be conducted on this topic (Mestman, 2012).

Nursing Interventions

Education of the pregnant woman with thyroid dysfunction is essential to promote compliance with the plan of treatment. Important points to discuss with the woman and her family include the disorder and its potential effect on her, her family, and her fetus; the medication regimen and possible side effects; the need for continuing medical supervision; and the importance of adherence.

The woman often needs the nurse's help to cope with the discomforts and frustrations associated with symptoms of the disorder. For example, a woman with hyperthyroidism who has nervousness and hyperactivity along with weakness and fatigue can benefit from suggestions to channel excess energies into quiet diversional activities such as reading or crafts. Discomfort associated with hypersensitivity to heat (hyperthyroidism) or cold intolerance (hypothyroidism) can be minimized by appropriate clothing and regulation of environmental temperatures and by avoiding temperature extremes.

Nutrition counseling with a registered dietitian may provide guidance in selecting a well-balanced diet. The woman with hyperthyroidism who has increased appetite and poor weight gain and the hypothyroid woman who has anorexia and lethargy need counseling to ensure adequate intake of nutritionally sound foods to meet both maternal and fetal needs.

MATERNAL PHENYLKETONURIA

Phenylketonuria (PKU), a recognized cause of cognitive impairment, is an inborn error of metabolism caused by an autosomal recessive trait that creates a deficiency in the enzyme phenylalanine hydrolase. Absence of this enzyme impairs the body's ability to metabolize the amino acid phenylalanine found in all protein foods. Consequently, toxic accumulation of phenylalanine in the blood occurs, which interferes with brain development and function. Individuals with this disorder also have hypopigmentation of hair, eyes, and skin because phenylalanine inhibits melanin production. PKU affects 1 in every 10,000 to 15,000 Caucasian newborns (Cunningham et al., 2014).

PKU was the first inborn error of metabolism to be universally screened in the United States. Since 1961 all newborns have been tested soon after birth for this disorder. Prompt diagnosis and therapy with a phenylalanine-restricted diet significantly decrease the incidence of cognitive impairment (Aminoff & Douglas, 2014). The special diet should be followed indefinitely because individuals who do not continue phenylalanine restriction have been reported to have significantly lower IQs (Cunningham et al., 2014).

The keys to the prevention of fetal anomalies caused by maternal PKU are the identification of women in their reproductive years with the disorder and dietary compliance for women who are diagnosed. Screening for undiagnosed homozygous maternal PKU at the first prenatal visit may be warranted, especially in individuals with a family history of the disorder, with low intelligence of uncertain origin, or who have given birth to microcephalic infants. Ideally women with PKU begin dietary phenylalanine restriction before conception and continue it throughout pregnancy (Aminoff & Douglas, 2014). The dietary modification normally excludes all high-protein foods such as meat, milk, eggs, and nuts and wheat products, making it very similar to a vegan diet (Feillet & Agostoni, 2010; Gilbert, 2011). Phenylalanine levels are monitored at least once and preferably twice a week throughout pregnancy (Gilbert). Experts recommend that maternal phenylalanine levels be less than 6 mg/dl for at least 3 months before conception and range between 2 and 6 mg/dl throughout pregnancy. These levels are associated with a decrease in fetal sequelae (Cunningham et al., 2014; Gilbert). High maternal phenylalanine levels are associated with microcephaly, cognitive impairment, and congenital heart defects in their children (Aminoff & Douglas; Cunningham et al.). Ultrasound examinations are used for fetal surveillance beginning in the first trimester. A spontaneous vaginal birth is anticipated.

Women with PKU should be advised against breastfeeding because their milk contains a high concentration of phenylalanine (Aminoff & Douglas, 2014). If these women choose to breastfeed despite the risk, their phenylalanine blood levels must be monitored closely. Infants diagnosed with PKU can usually be breastfed safely if the mother does not also have PKU because human breast milk is a relatively low-phenylalanine food (Pollard, 2012). If infants with PKU are breastfed, the amount of human breast milk ingested daily may be monitored so phenylalanine levels do not get too high. Another strategy is to alternate human breast milk feedings with products that contain little or no phenylalanine (Pollard).

KEY POINTS

- In pregnant women with pregestational diabetes, lack of glycemic control before conception and in the first trimester of pregnancy may be responsible for fetal congenital malformations.
- For pregnant women who have diabetes and are insulin dependent, insulin requirements increase as the pregnancy progresses and may quadruple by term as a result of insulin resistance created by placental hormones, insulinase, and cortisol. After birth, levels decrease dramatically; breastfeeding affects insulin needs.
- Poor glycemic control before and during pregnancy in women who have diabetes can lead to maternal complications such as miscarriage, infection, and dystocia (difficult labor) caused by fetal macrosomia.
- Careful glucose monitoring, insulin administration when necessary, and dietary counseling are used to create a normal intrauterine environment for fetal growth and development in the pregnancy complicated by diabetes mellitus.
- Because GDM is asymptomatic in most cases, all women who are not known to have pregestational diabetes undergo routine screening by history, clinical risk factors, or laboratory assessment of blood glucose levels during pregnancy. Two different methods for diagnosing GDM are currently used.
- The woman with hyperemesis gravidarum may have significant weight loss and dehydration. Management focuses on restoring fluid and electrolyte balance and preventing recurrence of nausea and vomiting.
- Thyroid dysfunction, hyperthyroidism or hypothyroidism, during pregnancy requires close monitoring of thyroid hormone levels to regulate therapy and prevent fetal insult.
- High levels of phenylalanine in the maternal bloodstream cross the placenta and are teratogenic to the developing fetus. Damage can be prevented or minimized by dietary restriction of phenylalanine before and during pregnancy.

REFERENCES

American College of Obstetricians and Gynecologists (ACOG). (2013). *Gestational diabetes mellitus.* ACOG practice bulletin no. 137. Washington, DC: ACOG.

American Diabetes Association (ADA). (2013a). Standards of medical care in diabetes—2013. *Diabetes Care, 36*(Suppl 1), S11–S65.

American Diabetes Association (ADA). (2013b). Position statement: Diagnosis and classification of diabetes mellitus. *Diabetes Care, 36*(Suppl 1), S67–S74.

Aminoff, M. J., & Douglas, V. C. (2014). Neurologic disorders. In R. K. Creasy, R. Resnik, J. D. Iams, et al. (Eds.), *Creasy and Resnik's maternal-fetal medicine: Principles and practice* (7th ed.). Philadelphia: Saunders.

Cappell, M. (2012). Hepatic and gastrointestinal diseases. In S. Gabbe, J. Niebyl, & J. Simpson (Eds.), *Obstetrics: Normal and problem pregnancies* (6th ed.). Philadelphia: Saunders.

Centers for Disease Control and Prevention (CDC). (2014). *National diabetes statistics report, 2014.* Available at www.cdc.gov/diabetes/pubs/statsreport14/nati.

Cunningham, F., Leveno, K., Bloom, S., et al. (2014). *Williams obstetrics* (24th ed.). New York: McGraw-Hill Education.

Feillet, F., & Agostoni, C. (2010). Nutritional issues in treating phenylketonuria. *Journal of Inherited Metabolic Disease, 33*(6), 659–664.

Gilbert, E. (2011). *Manual of high risk pregnancy & delivery* (5th ed.). St. Louis: Mosby.

Gordon, M. C. (2012). Maternal physiology. In S. Gabbe, J. Niebyl, & J. Simpson (Eds.), *Obstetrics: Normal and problem pregnancies* (6th ed.). Philadelphia: Saunders.

Inturrisi, M., Lintner, N. C., & Sorem, K. (2013). Diabetic ketoacidosis and continuous insulin infusion management in pregnancy. In N. Troiano, C. Harvey, & B. Chez (Eds.), *AWHONN's high risk and critical care obstetrics* (3rd ed.). Philadelphia: Wolters Kluwer/Lippincott Williams & Wilkins.

Kelly, T. F., & Savides, T. J. (2014). Gastrointestinal disease in pregnancy. In R. K. Creasy, R. Resnik, J. D. Iams, et al. (Eds.), *Creasy and Resnik's maternal-fetal medicine: Principles and practice* (7th ed.). Philadelphia: Saunders.

Landon, M., Catalano, P., & Gabbe, S. (2012). Diabetes mellitus complicating pregnancy. In S. Gabbe, J. Niebyl, & J. Simpson (Eds.), *Obstetrics: Normal and problem pregnancies* (6th ed.). Philadelphia: Saunders.

Lawrence, R. M., & Lawrence, R. A. (2011). *Breastfeeding: A guide for the medical profession* (7th ed.). St. Louis: Mosby.

Mercer, B. M. (2014). Assessment and induction of fetal pulmonary maturity. In R. K. Creasy, R. Resnik, J. D. Iams, et al. (Eds.), *Creasy and Resnik's maternal-fetal medicine: Principles and practice* (7th ed.). Philadelphia: Saunders.

Mestman, J. (2012). Thyroid and parathyroid diseases in pregnancy. In S. Gabbe, J. Niebyl, & J. Simpson (Eds.), *Obstetrics: Normal and problem pregnancies* (6th ed.). Philadelphia: Saunders.

Miller, J., de Veciana, M., Turan, S., et al. (2013). First trimester detection of fetal anomalies in pregestational diabetes using nuchal translucency, ductus venosus Doppler, and maternal glycosylated hemoglobin. *American Journal of Obstetrics and Gynecology, 208*(5), 385.e1–385.e8.

Moore, T. R., Hauguel-deMouzon, S., & Catalano, P. (2014). Diabetes in pregnancy. In R. K. Creasy, R. Resnik, J. D. Iams, et al. (Eds.), *Creasy and Resnik's maternal-fetal medicine: Principles and practice* (7th ed.). Philadelphia: Saunders.

Nader, S. (2014). Thyroid disease and pregnancy. In R. K. Creasy, R. Resnik, J. D. Iams, et al. (Eds.), *Creasy and Resnik's maternal-fetal medicine: Principles and practice* (7th ed.). Philadelphia: Saunders.

Pollard, M. (2012). *Evidence-based care for breastfeeding mothers: A resource for midwives and allied healthcare professionals.* New York: Routledge.

Reddy, U. M., & Spong, C. Y. (2014). Stillbirth. In R. K. Creasy, R. Resnik, J. D. Iams, et al. (Eds.), *Creasy and Resnik's maternal-fetal medicine: Principles and practice* (7th ed.). Philadelphia: Saunders.

Sacks, D. A., & Metzger, B. E. (2013). Classification of diabetes in pregnancy: Time to reassess the alphabet. *Obstetrics and Gynecology, 121*(2), 345–348.

Simhan, H. N., Berghella, V., & Iams, J. D. (2014). Preterm labor and birth. In R. K. Creasy, R. Resnik, J. D. Iams, et al. (Eds.), *Creasy and Resnik's maternal-fetal medicine: Principles and practice* (7th ed.). Philadelphia: Saunders.

Summers, A. (2012). Emergency management of hyperemesis gravidarum. *Emergency Nurse, 20*(4), 24–28.

Tamay, A., & Kuscu, N. (2011). Hyperemesis gravidarum: Current aspect. *Journal of Obstetrics and Gynaecology, 31*(8), 708–712.

Wapner, R. J. (2014). Prenatal diagnosis of congenital disorders. In R. K. Creasy, R. Resnik, J. D. Iams, et al. (Eds.), *Creasy and Resnik's maternal-fetal medicine: Principles and practice* (7th ed.). Philadelphia: Saunders.

World Health Organization (WHO). (2013). 10 facts about diabetes. Available at www.who.int/features/factfiles/diabetes/facts/en/.

30 CHAPTER

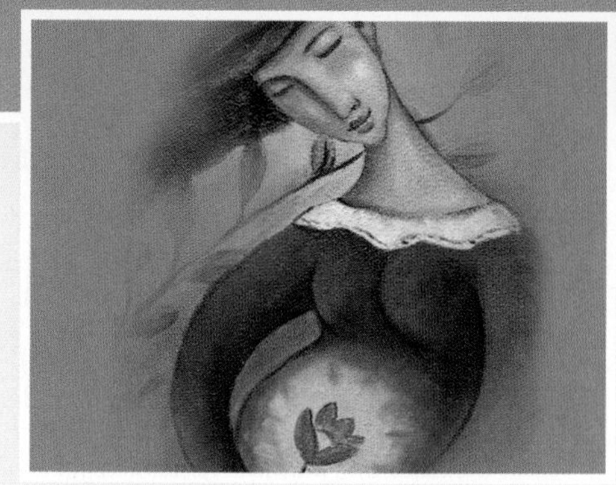

Medical-Surgical Disorders

Kristen S. Montgomery

http://evolve.elsevier.com/Lowdermilk/MWHC/

LEARNING OBJECTIVES

- Describe the management of selected cardiovascular disorders in pregnant women.
- Identify nursing interventions for a pregnant woman with a cardiovascular disorder.
- Discuss anemia during pregnancy.
- Explain the care of pregnant women with pulmonary disorders.
- Examine the effect of a gastrointestinal disorder on gastrointestinal function during pregnancy.
- Identify the effects of neurologic disorders on pregnancy.
- Describe the care of women whose pregnancies are complicated by autoimmune disorders.
- Differentiate signs and symptoms and management during pregnancy of urinary tract infections.
- Explain the basic principles of care for a pregnant woman who is having surgery.
- Discuss the implications of trauma in regard to mother and fetus.
- Identify priorities in assessment and stabilization measures for the pregnant trauma victim.

For most women, pregnancy represents a normal part of life. This chapter discusses the care of women for whom pregnancy represents a significant risk because it is superimposed on a preexisting medical condition. Care of women with normal pregnancies who develop medical or surgical problems that could happen to anyone at any time of life but occur during pregnancy is also discussed. With the active participation of well-motivated women in the treatment plan and careful management from a multidisciplinary health care team, positive pregnancy outcomes are often possible in both of these situations.

This chapter focuses on cardiovascular disorders, along with selected hematologic, respiratory, integumentary, neurologic, autoimmune, gastrointestinal, and urinary tract diseases. Care of the pregnant woman undergoing surgery or experiencing trauma also is discussed.

CARDIOVASCULAR DISORDERS

During a normal pregnancy the maternal cardiovascular system undergoes many changes that place a physiologic strain on the heart (see Chapter 13). The major cardiovascular changes that occur during a normal pregnancy and affect the woman with cardiac disease are increased intravascular volume, decreased systemic vascular resistance, cardiac output changes occurring during labor and birth, and the intravascular volume changes that occur just after childbirth. These physiologic changes are present during pregnancy and continue for a few weeks after birth. The normal heart can compensate for the increased workload so that pregnancy, labor, and birth are generally well tolerated, but the diseased heart is hemodynamically challenged.

If the cardiovascular changes are not well tolerated, cardiac failure can develop during pregnancy, labor, or the postpartum period. In addition, if myocardial disease develops, valvular disease exists, or a congenital heart defect is present, *cardiac decompensation* (inability of the heart to maintain a sufficient cardiac output) may occur.

About 1% of pregnancies are complicated by serious heart disease. The risk of maternal morbidity and mortality ranges from low to high, depending on the cardiac defect (Roos-Hesselink, Ruys, & Johnson, 2013). The rates of congenital heart disease and mitral valve disease are increasing in women of childbearing age, whereas the incidence of rheumatic fever has diminished. The presence of a maternal congenital cardiac defect increases the risk to the fetus for a congenital heart defect from 1% to about 4% to 6% (Roos-Hesselink et al.). A perinatal mortality of up to 50% is anticipated with persistent cardiac decompensation. Box 30-1 lists maternal cardiac disease risk groups.

The degree of disability experienced by the woman with cardiac disease is often more important in the treatment and prognosis of cardiac disease complicating pregnancy than is the diagnosis of cardiovascular disease. The New York Heart

BOX 30-1 Maternal Cardiac Disease Risk Groups

Group I (Mortality Rate <1%)
Atrial septal defect
Ventricular septal defect (uncomplicated)
Patent ductus arteriosus
Pulmonic and tricuspid disease
Biosynthetic valve prosthesis (porcine and human allograft)
Tetralogy of Fallot (corrected)
Mitral stenosis (New York Heart Association [NYHA] classes I and II)

Group II (Mortality Rate 5%-15%)
Mitral stenosis (NYHA classes III and IV or with atrial fibrillation)
Aortic stenosis
Coarctation of aorta (uncomplicated)
Uncorrected tetralogy of Fallot
Previous myocardial infarction
Marfan syndrome with normal aorta
Artificial heart valve

Group III (Mortality Rate 25%-50%)
Pulmonary hypertension
Coarctation of the aorta (complicated)
Endocarditis
Marfan syndrome with aortic involvement
Eisenmenger syndrome

Data from Gaddipati, S., & Troiano, N.H. (2013). Cardiac disorders in pregnancy. In N.H. Troiano, C.J. Harvey, & B.F. Chez (Eds.), *AWHONN's high risk and critical care obstetrics* (3rd ed.). Philadelphia: Lippincott Williams & Wilkins.

Association's (NYHA) functional classification of organic heart disease is a widely accepted standard:

- Class I: asymptomatic without limitation of physical activity
- Class II: symptomatic with slight limitation of activity
- Class III: symptomatic with marked limitation of activity
- Class IV: symptomatic with inability to carry on any physical activity without discomfort

No classification of heart disease can be considered rigid or absolute, but the NYHA classification offers a basic practical guide for treatment, assuming that frequent prenatal visits, good client cooperation, and appropriate obstetric care occur. The functional classification may change for the pregnant woman because of the hemodynamic changes that occur in the cardiovascular system during pregnancy. A 30% to 45% increase in cardiac output occurs compared with nonpregnancy resting values, with most of the increase in the first trimester and the peak at 20 to 26 weeks of gestation (Blanchard & Daniels, 2014). The functional classification of the disease is determined at 3 months and again at 7 or 8 months of gestation. Pregnant women may progress from class I or II to III or IV during the pregnancy as cardiac output increases and more stress is placed on the heart. Women with cyanotic congenital heart disease do not fit into the NYHA classification because their exercise-induced symptoms have causes unrelated to heart failure.

A diagnosis of cardiac disease depends on the history, physical examination, radiographic and electrocardiographic findings, Holter monitoring, and, if indicated, ultrasonographic results. Most diagnostic studies are noninvasive and can be safely performed during pregnancy. The differential diagnosis of heart disease also involves ruling out respiratory problems and other potential causes of chest pain.

The maternal mortality rate in women with cardiac events is higher than that for abortion, genital tract sepsis, and hemorrhage (Easterling & Stout, 2012). The highest risk of complications or death occurs in women with pulmonary hypertension, complicated coarctation of the aorta, and Marfan syndrome with aortic involvement (Roos-Hesselink et al., 2013).

Cardiac diseases vary in their effect on pregnancy depending on whether they are acute or chronic conditions. The following discussion focuses on selected congenital and acquired cardiac conditions and other cardiac disorders. A review of the care of the pregnant woman who has had a heart transplant concludes this section.

Congenital Cardiac Disease

Septal Defects

Atrial Septal Defect. Atrial septal defect (ASD) (an abnormal opening between the atria), one of the causes of a left-to-right shunt, is one of the most common congenital defects seen during pregnancy. This defect may go undetected because the woman usually is asymptomatic. The pregnant woman with an ASD will most likely have an uncomplicated pregnancy. Some women may have right-sided heart failure or arrhythmias as the pregnancy progresses as a result of increased plasma volume (Gaddipati & Troiano, 2013). The risk for congenital heart disease to the fetus of a woman with ASD is 4% to 10% (Tomlinson, 2011).

Ventricular Septal Defect. Ventricular septal defect (VSD) (an abnormal opening between the right and left ventricles), another cause of a left-to-right shunt, is usually diagnosed and corrected early in life. As a result, a VSD is not very common in pregnancy. Women with small, uncomplicated VSDs usually do not have pregnancy complications. For women with a large VSD, there is a higher risk for arrhythmias, heart failure, and pulmonary hypertension. Medical management includes rest and decreased physical activity, as well as administration of anticoagulants, if indicated (Gaddipati & Troiano, 2013). The risk for a congenital heart defect to the fetus of a woman with VSD is 6% to 10% (Tomlinson, 2011).

Patent Ductus Arteriosus. Patent ductus arteriosus (PDA) is another cause of a left-to-right shunt that is usually diagnosed and corrected during infancy. Possible complications of a PDA include those of VSD as well as endocarditis and pulmonary emboli. Medical management is the same as for VSD (Blanchard & Daniels, 2014).

Acyanotic Lesions

Coarctation of the Aorta. Coarctation of the aorta (localized narrowing of the aorta near the insertion of the ductus) is an example of an acyanotic congenital heart lesion. If at all possible the lesion should be corrected surgically before pregnancy (Blanchard & Daniels, 2014; Roos-Hesselink et al., 2013). However, pregnancy is usually relatively safe for the woman with uncomplicated, uncorrected coarctation. Maternal mortality is about 3% for uncorrected defects (Blanchard & Daniels). Complications include hypertension, congestive heart failure, infective endocarditis, cerebrovascular accident (stroke), aortic dissection, aneurysm, and rupture (Blanchard & Daniels; Easterling & Stout, 2012). The mainstays of treatment for uncorrected coarctation of the aorta during pregnancy are rest and antihypertensive medications, preferably beta-adrenergic blocking agents. Vaginal birth is preferable, with epidural anesthesia and shortening of the second stage with vacuum extraction or use of forceps, if necessary. Beta-blockers should be continued throughout labor. Because of the risk of endocarditis, antibiotic prophylaxis is recommended at birth (see later discussion).

Cyanotic Lesions

Tetralogy of Fallot. Tetralogy of Fallot is by far the most common cyanotic heart disease observed during pregnancy (Roos-Hesselink et al., 2013). Components of tetralogy of Fallot include a VSD, pulmonary stenosis, overriding aorta, and right ventricular hypertrophy, leading to a right-to-left shunt. Women with tetralogy of Fallot are encouraged to have surgical repair before conception because pregnancy does not pose a significant risk once the VSD and pulmonary stenosis have been repaired. Women with uncorrected tetralogy of Fallot, however, experience more right-to-left shunting during pregnancy, resulting in reduced blood flow through the pulmonary circulation and increasing hypoxemia, which can cause syncope or death (Gaddipati & Troiano, 2013). Maintenance of venous return in women with uncorrected tetralogy of Fallot is critical. Therefore, the most dangerous time for these women is the late third trimester of pregnancy and the early postpartum period, when venous return is reduced by the large pregnant uterus and by peripheral venous pooling after birth. Use of pressure-graded support hose is recommended. Blood loss during birth may also adversely affect venous return; thus blood volume must be adequately maintained. Prophylactic antibiotics should be given during the intrapartum period (Blanchard & Daniels, 2014).

Acquired Cardiac Disease

Mitral Valve Stenosis

Mitral valve stenosis (narrowing of the opening of the mitral valve caused by stiffening of valve leaflets, which obstructs blood flow from the left atrium to the left ventricle) is the characteristic lesion resulting from rheumatic heart disease (RHD) (Tomlinson, 2011). As the mitral valve narrows, dyspnea worsens, occurring first on exertion and eventually at rest. A tight stenosis plus the increase in blood volume and cardiac output of normal pregnancy may cause pulmonary edema, atrial fibrillation, right-sided heart failure, infective endocarditis, pulmonary embolism, and massive hemoptysis (Blanchard & Daniels, 2014; Cunningham, Leveno, Bloom, et al., 2014). Maternal mortality is related to functional capacity. Almost all maternal deaths related to mitral stenosis occur in women who are classified as NYHA class III or class IV (Cunningham et al.).

Pharmacologic treatment for women with a history of rheumatic heart disease may include diuretics such as furosemide (Lasix) to prevent pulmonary edema and beta-blockers or calcium channel blockers to prevent tachycardia (Easterling & Stout, 2012). A combination of drugs will most likely be needed. Cardioversion may be needed for new-onset atrial fibrillation. Women who have chronic atrial fibrillation may require digoxin and beta-blockers or calcium channel blockers to control the heart rate. In addition, anticoagulant therapy may be needed to prevent embolism (Blanchard & Daniels, 2014). About 25% of women with mitral valve stenosis experience cardiac failure for the first time during pregnancy (Cunningham et al., 2014).

Care of the woman with mitral stenosis typically is managed by reducing her activity, restricting dietary sodium, and monitoring weight. The pregnant woman with mitral stenosis should be assessed clinically for symptoms and with echocardiograms to monitor the atrial and ventricular size, as well as heart valve function. Prophylaxis for intrapartum endocarditis and pulmonary infections may be provided for women at high risk (Blanchard & Daniels, 2014; Easterling & Stout, 2012) (Box 30-2).

During labor adequate pain control is required to prevent tachycardia. Epidural analgesia for labor is preferred (Tomlinson, 2011). Laboring and birthing in the lateral decubitus position are desirable. The lithotomy position, with the woman supine and her feet in stirrups, is an invitation to pulmonary edema (Blanchard & Daniels, 2014). Shortening the second stage of labor by vacuum- or forceps-assisted birth is also important to decrease the cardiac workload. Even with close monitoring, the woman with moderate to severe mitral stenosis is at risk for pulmonary edema, right-sided heart failure, and hypotension. Central hemodynamic monitoring may be necessary for some women during labor, birth, and the postpartum period because fluid shifts can place the woman at risk for pulmonary edema.

For women with NYHA class III or IV cardiac disease, percutaneous balloon mitral valvuloplasty can be performed, but this procedure should be considered only when symptoms cannot be controlled by standard means. Mitral balloon valvuloplasty is optimally performed after the first trimester to decrease radiation risks to the fetus. This relatively safe nonsurgical procedure is now performed more frequently during pregnancy than surgical valvotomy (Blanchard & Daniels, 2014). The balloon procedure is just as successful as surgical repair and is associated with less maternal and fetal morbidity and mortality (Cunningham et al., 2014).

BOX 30-2 Prophylaxis for Bacterial Endocarditis During Labor and Birth

High Risk Clients

In active labor: ampicillin 2 g IV or IM plus gentamicin 1.5 mg/kg (not to exceed 120 mg)

6 hours later: ampicillin 1 g IV or IM or amoxicillin 1 g PO

Penicillin-Allergic Clients

In active labor: vancomycin 1 g IV over 1-2 hr plus gentamicin as above

Moderate Risk Clients

In active labor: amoxicillin 2 g PO or ampicillin 2 g IV or IM

Penicillin-Allergic Clients

In active labor: vancomycin 1 g IV over 1-2 hr

IM, Intramuscular; *IV,* intravenous; *PO,* by mouth.
Data from Dajani, D.A., Taubert, K.A., Wilson, W., Bolger, A.F., Bayer, A., et al. (1997). Prevention of bacterial endocarditis: Recommendations by the American Heart Association. *JAMA* 96, 358-366.

Mitral Valve Prolapse

Mitral valve prolapse (MVP) is a fairly common, usually benign, condition. More specific echocardiographic diagnostic criteria have resulted in significantly reduced prevalence estimates for MVP (perhaps 1% of the female population) than previously thought (Blanchard & Daniels, 2014). The mitral valve leaflets prolapse into the left atrium during ventricular systole, allowing some backflow of blood. Midsystolic click and late systolic murmur are hallmarks of this syndrome. Most cases are asymptomatic. A few women have atypical chest pain (sharp and located in the left side of the chest) that occurs at rest and does not respond to nitrates. They may also have anxiety, palpitations, dyspnea on exertion, and syncope. If women are symptomatic, beta-blocking drugs are given to relieve chest pain and palpitations and reduce the risk of life-threatening arrhythmias (Cunningham et al., 2014). If symptoms are unusually severe, thyroid function should also be checked (Blanchard & Daniels, 2014). Pregnancy and its associated hemodynamic changes may alter or alleviate the murmur and click of MVP, as well as symptoms (Cunningham et al.; Easterling & Stout, 2012). Antibiotic prophylaxis for bacterial endocarditis is no longer recommended for women with uncomplicated mitral valve prolapse. Pregnancy, labor, and birth are usually safe and well tolerated (Blanchard & Daniels; Cunningham et al.).

Aortic Stenosis

Aortic stenosis (narrowing of the opening of the aortic valve leading to an obstruction to left ventricular ejection) is rarely encountered as a complication of pregnancy because most women who develop this condition do so after their childbearing years are over. In the past, the maternal mortality rate was reported to be as high as 17%, but it has decreased over the past several decades (Easterling & Stout, 2012). Medical management is similar to that for mitral stenosis.

Ischemic Heart Disease

Myocardial Infarction

Myocardial infarction (MI) (an acute ischemic event) is a rare event in women of childbearing age, usually occurring in the third trimester, with a maternal mortality rate of 5% to 8% (Tomlinson, 2011). When MI occurs *peripartum* (period of time that extends from the last month of pregnancy through the first few months postpartum), the mortality approaches 20%. MI is estimated to occur in only 1 in 10,000 women during pregnancy and usually in women more than 33 years of age (Blanchard & Daniels, 2014). Increasing age, chronic hypertension, diabetes, hypertensive disorders of pregnancy, thrombophilias, and postpartum infection are risk factors. Many of these factors are related to obesity so it is anticipated that the incidence of MI will rise because increasing numbers of women are obese (Tomlinson). Women with an MI intrapartum are likely to also have preeclampsia with severe features or eclampsia. Antepartal or postpartal MIs are most likely related to diabetes, coronary artery disease, and lipid disorders (Martin, Hill, & Foley, 2012). Women who have MIs during pregnancy or the postpartum period should be assessed for thrombophilias (deficiency of proteins involved in coagulation inhibition), such as antiphospholipid antibody.

Medical management for pregnant women after MI is the same as for nonpregnant women and includes the administration of oxygen, aspirin, beta-blockers, nitrates, and heparin. Women who have had symptomatic cardiac disease during the pregnancy should continue cardiac medications and receive oxygen during labor. Because pain can lead to tachycardia and increased cardiac demand, pain control during labor is crucial (Martin et al., 2012). The side-lying position is preferred to avoid pressure on the vena cava. Vaginal birth is preferable, with avoidance of maternal pushing and a vacuum- or forceps-assisted birth (Easterling & Stout, 2012).

Other Cardiac Diseases and Conditions

Primary Pulmonary Hypertension

Women with primary pulmonary hypertension (PPH) have constriction of the arteriolar vessels in the lungs, leading to an increase in the pulmonary artery pressure. As a result of this pathology, there is right ventricular hypertension, right ventricular hypertrophy and dilation, and right ventricular failure with tricuspid regurgitation and systemic congestion. The major physiologic difficulty in PPH is maintaining blood flow to the lungs. Any event that significantly decreases venous return to the heart, such as hypotension, impairs the ability of the right ventricle to pump blood through the pulmonary vessels with their high, fixed vascular resistance. Because hypotension can occur quickly and is often unresponsive to medical therapy, it must be avoided at all costs (Blanchard & Daniels, 2014).

Symptoms may be nonspecific, such as fatigue and shortness of breath. Dyspnea on exertion is the most common symptom (Cunningham et al., 2014).

PPH is diagnosed by electrocardiography. Although cardiac catheterization remains the standard procedure for measuring pulmonary artery pressures, noninvasive echocardiography is often used to provide an estimate of these pressures (Cunningham et al., 2014). Mortality rates reported during pregnancy are as high as 50%, so pregnancy is not advised in women with this condition (Blanchard & Daniels, 2014). The most dangerous times for women with this condition are the intrapartal and early postpartal periods because of increases in cardiac output and fluid shifts (Roos-Hesselink et al., 2013).

Medical management of women with PPH during pregnancy includes limiting activity and avoiding supine positioning (Roos-Hesselink et al., 2013). Diuretics, supplemental oxygen, and vasodilator medications also will be ordered. During labor and birth hypotension must be avoided by carefully establishing epidural analgesia and preventing blood loss (Cunningham et al., 2014).

Marfan Syndrome

Marfan syndrome is an autosomal dominant genetic disorder characterized by generalized weakness of the connective tissue, resulting in joint deformities, ocular lens dislocation, and weakness of the aortic wall and root. Associated cardiovascular changes include mitral valve prolapse, mitral regurgitation, aortic regurgitation, aortic root dilation, and possible dissection or rupture of the aortic root (Roos-Hesselink et al., 2013).

The majority of deaths from Marfan syndrome are caused by aortic dissection and rupture. Excruciating chest pain is the most common symptom of aortic dissection. Aortic dissection most often occurs in the third trimester or postpartum. Overall the maternal mortality rate associated with Marfan syndrome is greater than 50%. However, it is significantly increased if the aortic root diameter measures more than 4 cm (Easterling & Stout, 2012). Preconception genetic counseling is recommended to make women aware of the risks of pregnancy with this condition. Because the condition is inherited, each child born to a woman with Marfan syndrome has a 50% chance of having the disorder (Blanchard & Daniels, 2014; National Marfan Association, 2013). Baseline data should be gathered about the aortic root before pregnancy or at the first prenatal visit by noninvasive imaging with transesophageal echocardiography, computed tomography (CT), or magnetic resonance imaging (MRI).

Management during pregnancy includes restricted activity and use of beta-blockers; surgery may be indicated in some women (Roos-Hesselink et al., 2013). Vaginal birth is considered safe for women with aortic root diameters less than 4 cm. Some authorities, however, recommend that women with larger aortic root diameters give birth by elective cesarean because of concerns about increased pressure in the aorta during labor (Roos-Hesselink et al.).

Infective Endocarditis

Infective endocarditis is inflammation of the innermost lining—the endocardium—of the heart, caused by invasion of microorganisms. In the United States, women at greatest risk to develop infective endocarditis are those who have congenital heart lesions, degenerative valve disease, or intracardiac devices or who use drugs intravenously (Cunningham et al., 2014). Bacterial endocarditis, leading to incompetence of heart valves and thus congestive heart failure and cerebral emboli, can result in death. Treatment is with antibiotics. Prophylactic treatment with antibiotics is used only for women at highest risk for this condition.

Eisenmenger Syndrome

Eisenmenger syndrome is a right-to-left or bidirectional shunting that can occur either at the atrial or the ventricular level of the heart and is combined with elevated pulmonary vascular resistance (Roos-Hesselink et al., 2013). The syndrome is associated with high mortality (50% in mothers and 50% in fetuses). Because of the risk for poor pregnancy outcomes, pregnancy should be avoided by women with Eisenmenger syndrome (Gaddipati & Troiano, 2013).

In women who become pregnant despite the risks, physical activity is strictly limited. Hospitalization may be necessary to provide optimal care, which includes oxygen administration, rest, and fetal monitoring. During labor and birth, intrathecal or epidural morphine sulfate is recommended to maintain hemodynamic stability. Hypotension must be avoided at all costs because it results in more right-to-left shunting (Blanchard & Daniels, 2014; Easterling & Stout, 2012). Pulse oximetry is a useful assessment tool to guide the treatment plan during labor and birth. Cesarean birth should be performed only for obstetric indications and avoided whenever possible (Roos-Hesselink et al., 2013).

Peripartum Cardiomyopathy

Peripartum cardiomyopathy (PCM) is congestive heart failure with cardiomyopathy. The classic criteria for the diagnosis of PCM include development of congestive heart failure in the last month of pregnancy or within the first 5 postpartum months, absence of heart disease before the last month of pregnancy, a left ventricular ejection fraction (EF) of less than 45%, and, most important, lack of another cause for heart failure. The cause of the disease is unknown. The U.S. incidence is 1 in 3000 to 4000 live births (Blanchard & Daniels, 2014).

Associated risk factors for PCM include maternal age older than 35 years, multifetal gestation, preeclampsia, gestational hypertension, multiparity, African descent, and prolonged tocolytic therapy. Maternal mortality has been reported with rates as high as 56%, but more recent data have indicated a lower rate, more likely around 9% (Martin et al., 2012). Clinical findings are those of congestive heart failure (left ventricular failure). Clinical manifestations include dyspnea, fatigue, and edema, as well as radiologic findings of cardiomegaly.

Medical management of PCM includes a regimen used for congestive heart failure: diuretics, sodium and fluid restriction, afterload-reducing agents, and digoxin. Anticoagulation may be necessary if the cardiac chambers are significantly dilated and contract poorly because of the increased risk for clot formation. During labor epidural anesthesia is often used for pain control to decrease the cardiac workload and reduce tachycardia. Cesarean birth should be performed only for obstetric indications (Easterling & Stout, 2012).

In half of all women with PCM, left ventricular dysfunction resolves within 6 months. These women generally do well. If left ventricular dysfunction does not resolve within 6 months, however, approximately 85% of women with PCM will die in the next 4 to 5 years. Death is usually the result of progressive congestive heart failure, arrhythmia, or thromboembolism (Easterling & Stout, 2012). The recurrence rate for cardiomyopathy in a subsequent pregnancy is high—anywhere from 20% to 50%. The risk of recurrence is increased in women who did not have complete recovery of left ventricular function after the initial episode of PCM (Blanchard & Daniels, 2014).

Valve Replacement

Pregnant women with mechanical or bioprosthetic heart valves require specialized care for this high risk situation. The primary medical management, anticoagulation, is both controversial and complicated. A high risk for thromboembolism exists because of the hypercoagulability of pregnancy. At the same time, the use of anticoagulants during pregnancy presents the possibility of maternal and fetal hemorrhage. Some oral anticoagulants pose a significant risk to the fetus for abnormalities and intracranial hemorrhage. Prosthetic heart valve thrombosis is a life-threatening emergency during pregnancy and requires clot removal surgery, which carries a high mortality rate (Roos-Hesselink et al., 2013).

Women with bioprosthetic heart valves usually do not require anticoagulation during pregnancy. This type of valve is an ideal replacement for women of childbearing age. A disadvantage of this valve, however, is premature failure, which may occur within 10 to 15 years of placement. Premature valve failure may be exacerbated by pregnancy (Tomlinson, 2011).

The recommendations for pregnant women with mechanical prosthetic valves who need anticoagulation therapy include several different treatment regimens. Because the most effective and safest management has not been determined through controlled trials, the decision regarding choice of therapy should be made between the physician and the woman, who should be fully informed about the potential risks of the various options to her and her unborn child. One option is to use subcutaneous heparin for the first 12 weeks of gestation. Warfarin (Coumadin) then is used until week 35 of gestation, followed by a return to heparin (intravenous) until after the birth. If prothrombin time (PT) results are reported in international normalized ratio (INR) values, then the desired range is between 2.5 and 3.5 (Tomlinson, 2011). A second option is to use warfarin for the entire pregnancy up to 35 weeks of gestation followed by intravenous heparin until labor begins. Data are inconclusive regarding the use of low-molecular-weight heparin (Lovenox). Anticoagulation therapy should be discontinued during active labor and resumed in the postpartum period. Warfarin does not adversely affect breastfeeding.

Heart Transplantation

Increasing numbers of heart recipients are successfully completing pregnancies. It is recommended that pregnancy be avoided for at least 1 year after the transplant (Blanchard & Daniels, 2014). Before conception the woman should be assessed for quality of ventricular function and potential rejection of the transplant. She also should be considered to be stabilized on her immunosuppressant regimen. Women who have no evidence of rejection and have normal cardiac function at the beginning of the pregnancy appear to do well during pregnancy, labor, and birth. Risks to the woman include hypertension, preeclampsia, preterm birth, and mild rejection episodes (Martin et al., 2012).

CARE MANAGEMENT

The presence of cardiac disease is a significant influencing factor in the decision-making process for or against becoming pregnant. Couples planning a pregnancy must understand the risks involved in their situation. If the pregnancy is unplanned, the nurse should explore the couple's desire to continue the pregnancy in light of the risks involved. Pregnancy termination is one option, depending on the severity of the cardiac defect. The family may need further information to make an informed decision regarding the future of the pregnancy.

Assessment and Nursing Diagnoses

The pregnant woman with a cardiac disorder is in a high risk situation. She requires detailed assessment throughout the peripartum period to determine the potential for optimal maternal health and a viable fetus. Her care will be provided by a multidisciplinary team, including a cardiologist, obstetrician, perinatologist, and registered nurse experienced in the care of women with high risk pregnancies. If she chooses to continue the pregnancy, the woman's condition may be assessed as often as weekly. For additional information on cardiac disease, visit the American Heart Association's website at www.americanheart.org.

Potential nursing diagnoses include:

- *Fear* related to
  - increased peripartum risk
- *Risk for Ineffective Coping/Compromised Family Coping* related to
  - woman's cardiac condition
  - changes in role performance
- *Ineffective Peripheral Tissue Perfusion* related to
  - hypotensive syndrome
- *Activity Intolerance* related to
  - cardiac condition
- *Deficient Knowledge* related to
  - cardiac condition
  - pregnancy and how it affects cardiac condition
  - medication: dosages and possible side effects
  - requirements to alter self-care activities
- *Self-Care Deficit* (Bathing, Dressing, Toileting) related to
  - fatigue or activity intolerance
  - need for bed rest
- *Impaired Home Maintenance* related to
  - woman's confinement to bed and/or limited activity level

COMMUNITY ACTIVITY

- Identify a major medical center near where you live. Check to see if they offer maternity services. If they do, see if they have information related to high risk pregnancies and the staff available to care for them. Maternal-fetal medicine physicians (perinatologists) are physicians who specialize in high risk maternal care. Determine how many providers are at the facility and what types of resources they offer online for women with a high risk pregnancy. Also find out if the hospital offers high risk neonatal care. Many infants born to women with medical complications need to be cared for in a neonatal intensive care unit (NICU). Review the website for information on what the NICU is like and resources to support the family with an infant in the NICU.
- Review the local newspaper or community websites to determine if there are support groups in your area for women with high risk pregnancies. Also check online sites because many women connect with online communities when they are pregnant.

Interventions

Antepartum

Therapy for the pregnant woman with heart disease is focused on minimizing stress on the heart, which intensifies as cardiac output increases. Cardiac output begins to rise significantly early in pregnancy and probably peaks somewhere between 25 and 30 weeks of gestation (Gordon, 2012). Factors that increase the risk of cardiac decompensation are avoided. The workload of the cardiovascular system is reduced by appropriate treatment of any coexisting emotional stress, hypertension, anemia, hyperthyroidism, or obesity.

Signs and symptoms of cardiac decompensation are taught at the first prenatal visit and reviewed at each subsequent visit (see the Signs of Potential Complications box).

SIGNS OF POTENTIAL COMPLICATIONS

Cardiac Decompensation

Pregnant Woman: Subjective Symptoms

- Increasing fatigue or difficulty breathing, or both, with her usual activities
- Feeling of smothering
- Frequent cough
- Palpitations; feeling that her heart is "racing"
- Generalized edema: swelling of face, feet, legs, fingers (e.g., rings do not fit anymore)

Nurse: Objective Signs

- Irregular, weak, rapid pulse (≥100 beats/min)
- Progressive, generalized edema
- Crackles at base of lungs after two inspirations and exhalations that do not clear after coughing
- Orthopnea; increasing dyspnea
- Rapid respirations (≥25 breaths/min)
- Moist, frequent cough
- Cyanosis of lips and nailbeds

Infections are treated promptly because respiratory, urinary, or gastrointestinal (GI) tract infections can complicate the condition by accelerating the heart rate and by direct spread of organisms (e.g., streptococci) to the heart structures. The woman should notify her physician at the first sign of infection or exposure to an infection. Vaccination against influenza and pneumococci can be given (Easterling & Stout, 2012).

Nutrition counseling is necessary, optimally with the woman's family present. The pregnant woman needs a well-balanced diet with iron and folic acid supplementation, high protein levels, and adequate calories to gain weight. Iron supplements tend to cause constipation, so the woman should increase her intake of fluids and fiber. A stool softener may also be prescribed. It is important that the woman with a cardiac disorder avoid straining during defecation, thus causing the Valsalva maneuver (forced expiration against a closed airway, which when released, causes blood to rush to the heart and overload the cardiac system). Sodium restriction may be necessary. The woman's intake of potassium may be monitored to prevent hypokalemia, especially if she is taking diuretics. Depending on the specific cardiac condition, some women may be limited in their total daily fluid intake. A referral to a registered dietitian may be necessary for a nutritional plan of care.

Cardiac medications are prescribed as needed, with attention to fetal well-being. The hemodynamic changes that occur during pregnancy, such as increased plasma volume and increased renal clearance of drugs, can alter the amount of medication needed to establish and maintain a therapeutic drug level. Therefore, monitoring drug levels during pregnancy is crucial to maintain effective therapy for the woman while minimizing risk to the fetus. Table 30-1 lists information on medications that are often used to treat cardiac disorders during pregnancy.

Anticoagulant therapy may be prescribed during pregnancy for several conditions, such as recurrent venous thrombosis, pulmonary embolus, rheumatic heart disease, prosthetic valves, or cyanotic congenital heart defects. If anticoagulant therapy is required during pregnancy a number of various regimens may be recommended (see the section on valve disorders for more discussion of anticoagulant therapy). The nurse should be aware of the goals of therapy and monitor

TABLE 30-1 Selected Drugs Used in Treatment of Cardiac Disorders in the Pregnant Woman

GENERIC (TRADE) NAME	USE IN PREGNANCY	POTENTIAL SIDE EFFECTS
Digoxin (Lanoxin)	Maternal and fetal arrhythmias, heart failure	No evidence for unfavorable side effects on the fetus
Procainamide (Procanbid, Pronestyl)	Maternal and fetal arrhythmias	Limited data; no fetal side effects reported
Verapamil (Calan, Isoptin)	Maternal and fetal arrhythmias	Limited data; other than one case of fetal death of uncertain cause, no adverse fetal or newborn effects reported
B-Blockers (a class of drugs)	Hypertension, maternal arrhythmias, myocardial ischemia, mitral stenosis, hypertrophic cardiomyopathy, hyperthyroidism, Marfan syndrome	Fetal bradycardia, low placental weight, possible IUGR, hypoglycemia; no information on carvedilol
Heparin	Anticoagulation	None reported
Warfarin (Coumadin)	Anticoagulation	Crosses placenta; fetal hemorrhage, embryopathy, CNS abnormalities
Diuretics (a class of drugs)	Hypertension, congestive heart failure	Hypovolemia leads to reduced uteroplacental perfusion, fetal hypoglycemia, thrombocytopenia, hyponatremia, hypokalemia; thiazide diuretics can inhibit labor and suppress lactation
Lidocaine (Xylocaine)	Local anesthesia, maternal arrhythmias	No evidence for unfavorable fetal effects; high serum levels may cause CNS depression at birth
Quinidine (Quinidex)	Maternal and fetal arrhythmias	Minimal oxytocic effect, high dosages may cause premature labor or miscarriage; transient neonatal thrombocytopenia and damage to eighth cranial nerve reported
Nifedipine (Procardia, Adalat)	Hypertension, tocolysis	Fetal distress related to maternal hypotension reported
ACE inhibitors (a class of drugs)	Hypertension	Oligohydramnios, IUGR, prematurity, neonatal hypotension, renal failure, anemia, death, skull ossification defect, limb contractures, patent ductus arteriosus
Sodium nitroprusside	Hypertension, aortic dissection	Limited data; potential thiocyanate fetal toxicity, fetal mortality reported in animals

ACE, Angiotensin-converting enzyme; *CNS,* central nervous system; *IUGR,* intrauterine growth restriction.
From Blanchard, D.G., & Daniels, L.B. (2014). Cardiac diseases. In R.K. Creasy, R. Resnik, J.D. Iams, et al. (Eds.), *Creasy and Resnik's maternal-fetal medicine: Principles and practice* (7th ed.). Philadelphia: Saunders.

the PT and INR accordingly. The woman may need to learn to self-administer injectable agents such as heparin or low-molecular-weight heparin. A woman taking warfarin (Coumadin) requires specific nutritional teaching to avoid foods high in vitamin K, such as raw, dark green leafy vegetables, which counteract the effects of warfarin. In addition, she will require a folic acid supplement.

Tests for fetal maturity and well-being and placental sufficiency may be necessary. Other therapy is directly related to the functional classification of heart disease. The nurse must reinforce the need for close medical supervision (see the Nursing Care Plan).

Heart Surgery During Pregnancy. Ideally surgery to correct a cardiac lesion should be performed prior to pregnancy. In some women, however, cardiac disease is diagnosed for the first time during pregnancy. The maternal mortality risk does not increase, but there is a fetal mortality risk of 10% to 15% if heart surgery is performed, especially if cardiopulmonary bypass is used. If possible, surgery should be postponed until the third trimester of pregnancy, when the risk to the fetus is considerably decreased (Blanchard & Daniels, 2014).

Intrapartum

For all pregnant women the intrapartum period is the one that causes the most apprehension in clients and caregivers. The woman with impaired cardiac function has additional reasons to be anxious because labor and giving birth place an additional burden on her already compromised cardiovascular system.

Assessments include the routine assessments for all laboring women, as well as for cardiac decompensation. In addition, arterial blood gases (ABGs) may be needed to assess for adequate oxygenation. A pulmonary artery catheter may be inserted to monitor hemodynamic status accurately during labor and birth. Electrocardiographic monitoring and continuous monitoring of blood pressure and oxygen saturation (pulse oximetry) are usually instituted for the woman, and continuous fetal heart rate monitoring is used to monitor the fetus.

Nursing care during labor and birth focuses on promoting cardiac function. Minimize anxiety by maintaining a calm atmosphere in the labor and birth rooms. Provide anticipatory guidance by keeping the woman and her family informed of labor progress and events that can occur, as well as answering any questions. Support the woman's childbirth preparation method to the degree it is feasible for her cardiac condition. Nursing techniques that promote comfort, such as back massage, also are used.

Cardiac function is supported by keeping the woman's head and shoulders elevated and body parts resting on pillows. The side-lying position usually facilitates positive hemodynamics during labor. Discomfort is relieved with medication and supportive care. Physiologically the ideal labor for a woman with heart disease is one that is short and pain free. Therefore, use of epidural anesthesia is encouraged, although care must be taken to avoid hypotension, a common side effect of regional anesthesia (Easterling & Stout, 2012; Gaddipati & Troiano, 2013).

> **! NURSING ALERT**
>
> A pulse rate of 100 beats/minute or greater or a respiratory rate of 25 breaths/minute or greater is a concern. Check the respiratory status frequently for developing dyspnea, coughing, or crackles at the base of the lungs. Note the color and temperature of the skin as well. Pale, cool, clammy skin may indicate cardiac shock.

> **LEGAL TIP: Cardiac and Metabolic Emergencies**
>
> The management of emergencies such as maternal cardiopulmonary distress or arrest or maternal metabolic crisis should be documented in policies, procedures, and protocols. Any independent nursing actions appropriate to the emergency should be clearly identified.

Beta-adrenergic agents such as terbutaline (Brethine) are associated with various side effects, including tachycardia, irregular pulse, myocardial ischemia, and pulmonary edema. Therefore, these medications should not be used in women with known or suspected heart disease (Gilbert, 2011; Simhan, Berghella, & Iams, 2014; Simhan, Iams, & Romero, 2012). A synthetic oxytocin (Syntocinon) can be used to induce labor. This drug does not appear to cause significant coronary artery constriction in doses prescribed for labor induction or control of postpartum uterine atony. Cervical ripening agents containing prostaglandin are usually tolerated well but should be used cautiously.

If there are no obstetric problems, vaginal birth is recommended and may be accomplished with the woman in the side-lying position to facilitate uterine perfusion. If the supine position is used, position a pad under one hip to displace the uterus laterally and minimize the danger of supine hypotension. Have the woman flex her knees and place her feet flat on the bed. To prevent compression of popliteal veins and an increase in blood volume in the chest and trunk as a result of the effects of gravity, do not use stirrups. Open-glottis pushing is recommended. The woman should avoid the Valsalva maneuver when pushing in the second stage of labor because it reduces diastolic ventricular filling and obstructs left ventricular outflow. Mask oxygen is important. Episiotomy and vacuum extraction or outlet forceps can be used to decrease the length of the second stage of labor and decrease the heart's workload during that time. Cesarean birth is not routinely recommended for women who have cardiovascular disease because of the risks of dramatic fluid shifts, sustained hemodynamic changes, and increased blood loss.

According to the American Heart Association, prophylactic antibiotics to prevent infective endocarditis are recommended only for those women considered to be at the highest risk. Women who should receive prophylactic antibiotics include those with a prosthetic heart valve, a history of infective endocarditis, unrepaired congenital heart disease or a congenital heart defect repaired with prosthetic material or with residual defects at or adjacent to the repair site, or cardiac transplant recipients who develop cardiac valvulopathy (Blanchard & Daniels, 2014) (see Box 30-2). Oxytocin is usually given immediately after birth to prevent hemorrhage. Ergot products (e.g., methylergonovine [Methergine]) should not be used because they increase blood pressure. Fluid balance should be maintained and blood loss replaced. If tubal sterilization after vaginal birth is desired, surgery can be delayed for several days if necessary, until the woman is hemodynamically near normal, afebrile, nonanemic, and able to ambulate normally (Cunningham et al., 2014).

Postpartum

Monitoring for cardiac decompensation in the postpartum period is essential. The first 24 to 48 hours after birth are the most hemodynamically difficult for the woman. Hemorrhage or infection, or both, may worsen the cardiac condition. The woman with a cardiac disorder may continue to require a pulmonary artery catheter and ABG monitoring.

NURSING CARE PLAN

The Pregnant Woman with Heart Disease

NURSING DIAGNOSIS	EXPECTED OUTCOME	NURSING INTERVENTIONS	RATIONALES
Activity Intolerance related to effects of pregnancy on the woman with rheumatic heart disease with mitral valve stenosis	Woman will verbalize a plan to change lifestyle throughout pregnancy so as to reduce the risk of cardiac decompensation.	Assist the woman in identifying factors that decrease activity tolerance and explore extent of limitations.	To establish a baseline for evaluation
		Help the woman develop an individualized program of activity and rest, taking into account the living and working environment, as well as support of family and friends.	To maintain sufficient cardiac output
		Teach the woman to monitor physiologic responses to activity (e.g., pulse rate, respiratory rate) and reduce activity that causes fatigue or pain.	To maintain sufficient cardiac output and prevent potential injury to the fetus
		Enlist the woman's family and friends to assist her in pacing activities and to provide support in performing role functions and self-management activities that are too strenuous.	To increase the chances of compliance with activity restrictions
		Suggest that the woman maintain an activity log that records activities, time, duration, intensity, and physiologic response.	To evaluate effectiveness of and adherence to the activity program
		Discuss various quiet diversional activities that the woman can or may perform.	To decrease the potential for boredom during rest periods
Risk for Ineffective Therapeutic Regimen Management related to the woman's first pregnancy and perceived sense of wellness	Woman will participate in an effective therapeutic regimen for pregnancy complicated by heart disease.	Identify factors such as insufficient knowledge about the effect of cardiac disease on pregnancy that might inhibit the woman from participating in a therapeutic regimen.	To promote early interventions, such as teaching about the importance of rest
		Teach the woman and her family about factors such as lack of rest or not taking prescribed medications that might adversely affect the pregnancy.	To provide information and promote empowerment over the situation
		Encourage expression of feelings about the disease and its potential effect on the pregnancy.	To promote a sense of trust
		Identify resources in the community.	To provide a shared sense of common experiences and sources of assistance if needed to fulfill personal, family, and home responsibilities
		Encourage the woman to verbalize her plan for carrying out the regimen of care.	To evaluate the effects of teaching

NURSING CARE PLAN—cont'd

The Pregnant Woman with Heart Disease

NURSING DIAGNOSIS	EXPECTED OUTCOME	NURSING INTERVENTIONS	RATIONALES
Decreased Cardiac Output related to increased circulatory volume secondary to pregnancy and cardiac disease	Woman will exhibit signs of adequate cardiac output (i.e., normal pulse and blood pressure; normal heart and breath sounds; normal skin color, tone, and turgor; normal capillary refill; normal urine output; no evidence of edema).	Reinforce the importance of activity and rest cycles.	To prevent cardiac complications
		Reinforce the importance of the frequent visit schedule to the caregiver.	To provide adequate surveillance of the high risk pregnancy
		Teach the woman and her family members the signs of cardiac decompensation.	To provide information about when to contact the health care provider
		Teach the woman to lie on her side.	To increase uteroplacental blood flow
		Teach the woman to elevate her legs while sitting.	To promote venous return
		Monitor intake and output and check for edema.	To assess for renal complications or venous return problems
		Monitor the fetal heart rate and fetal activity and perform a nonstress test as indicated.	To assess fetal status and detect uteroplacental insufficiency

SAFETY ALERT

The immediate postbirth period is hazardous for a woman whose heart function is compromised. Cardiac output increases rapidly as extravascular fluid is remobilized into the vascular compartment. At the moment of birth, intraabdominal pressure is reduced dramatically; pressure on veins is removed, the splanchnic vessels engorge, and blood flow to the heart is increased.

Care in the postpartum period is tailored to the woman's functional capacity. Postpartum assessment of the woman with cardiac disease includes vital signs, oxygen saturation levels, lung and heart auscultation, presence and degree of edema, amount and character of bleeding, uterine tone and fundal height, urinary output, pain (especially chest pain), the activity-rest pattern, dietary intake, mother-infant interactions, and emotional state. The head of the bed is elevated, and the woman is encouraged to lie on her side. Bed rest may be ordered, with or without bathroom privileges. Progressive ambulation may be permitted as tolerated. The nurse may help the woman meet her grooming and hygiene needs and other activities. Bowel movements without stress or strain are promoted with stool softeners, diet, and fluids.

The woman may need a family member to help care for the infant. Breastfeeding is not contraindicated, but some women with heart disease (particularly those with life-threatening disease) may be unable to breastfeed. The woman who chooses to breastfeed will need the support of her family and the nursing staff to be successful. For example, she may need assistance in positioning herself or the infant for feeding. To further conserve the woman's energy, the infant can be given to the mother and taken from her after the feeding. Most medications used to manage cardiac disorders are compatible with breastfeeding. Thiazide diuretics, however, may suppress lactation (Blanchard & Daniels, 2014). Because diuretics can cause neonatal diuresis that can lead to dehydration, lactating women must be monitored closely to determine if medication doses can be reduced and still be effective.

If the woman is unable to breastfeed and her energies do not allow her to bottle feed the infant, the baby can be kept at the bedside so she can look at and touch her baby to establish an emotional bond with a low expenditure of energy. The infant should be held at the mother's eye level and near her lips and brought to her fingers. At the same time, involving the mother passively in her infant's care helps the mother feel vitally important—as she is—to the infant's well-being (e.g., "You can offer something no one else can: you can provide your baby with your sounds, touch, and rhythms that are so comforting"). Perhaps the woman can be encouraged to make a tape recording of her talking, singing, or whispering, which can be played for the baby in the nursery to help the infant feel her presence and be in contact with her voice. This also enhances maternal-infant bonding.

Preparation for discharge is carefully planned with the woman and family. Provision of help for the woman in the home by relatives, friends, and others must be addressed. If necessary, the nurse refers the family to community resources (e.g., for assistance with household activities). Rest and sleep periods, activity, and diet must be planned. The couple may need information about reestablishing sexual relations and contraception or sterilization.

Women with congenital heart disease should be offered contraceptive counseling. In general, the complications associated with pregnancy are usually greater than the risks associated with any form of contraception (Easterling & Stout, 2012). Women at particular risk for thromboembolism should avoid combined estrogen-progestin oral contraceptives, but progestin-only pills may be used. Parenteral progestins (e.g., medroxyprogesterone [Depo-Provera]) are safe and effective. However, they cause irregular bleeding, which may be problematic for women on anticoagulant therapy. An intrauterine device (IUD) may be used by some women with congenital heart lesions. Although a theoretic risk exists for developing endocarditis, the actual risk for women using an IUD is probably very minimal (Easterling & Stout).

Monitoring for cardiac decompensation continues through the first few weeks after birth because of hormonal shifts that affect hemodynamics. Maternal cardiac output is usually stabilized by 2 weeks postpartum (Easterling & Stout, 2012).

Men and women with congenital heart disease are at increased risk for having children who also have congenital heart disease. The risk for affected mothers is greater, approximately two to more than three times that of affected fathers. Children born with congenital heart disease to parents with congenital heart defects appear to inherit the risk for a defect in general rather than for a specific defect (Easterling & Stout, 2012). Therefore, preconception counseling and genetic counseling before a subsequent pregnancy are essential.

OTHER MEDICAL DISORDERS IN PREGNANCY

Anemia

Anemia is a common medical disorder of pregnancy, affecting from 20% to 52% of women (Kilpatrick, 2014). Anemia results in a reduction of the oxygen-carrying capacity of the blood. Because the oxygen-carrying capacity of the blood is decreased, the heart tries to compensate by increasing the cardiac output. This effort increases the workload of the heart and stresses ventricular function. Therefore, anemia that occurs with any other complication (e.g., preeclampsia) may result in congestive heart failure.

An indirect index of the oxygen-carrying capacity is the packed red blood cell (RBC) volume, or hematocrit level. The normal hematocrit range in nonpregnant women is 37% to 47%. However, normal values for pregnant women with adequate iron stores may be as low as 33%. According to the Centers for Disease Control and Prevention (CDC), anemia in pregnancy is defined as hemoglobin less than 11 g/dl in the first and third trimesters and less than 10.5 g/dl in the second trimester (Kilpatrick, 2014). A hemoglobin level less than 6 to 8 mg/dl is considered severe anemia (Blackburn, 2013).

When a woman has anemia during pregnancy, the loss of blood at birth, even if minimal, is not well tolerated. She is at an increased risk for requiring blood transfusions. Women with anemia have a higher incidence of puerperal complications, such as infection, than postpartum women with normal hematologic values.

Care of the anemic pregnant woman requires that the health care provider distinguish between the normal physiologic anemia of pregnancy and disease states. The majority of cases of anemia in pregnancy are caused by iron deficiency. The other types include a considerable variety of acquired and hereditary anemias, such as folic acid deficiency, sickle cell anemia, and thalassemia.

Iron Deficiency Anemia

Iron deficiency anemia is the most common anemia of pregnancy. It is diagnosed by checking the woman's serum ferritin level in addition to her hemoglobin and hematocrit levels. The serum ferritin level reflects iron reserves (Samuels, 2012). A serum ferritin value less than 12 mcg/l in the presence of a low hemoglobin value indicates iron deficiency anemia (Blackburn, 2013). There appears to be an association between maternal iron deficiency anemia, especially severe anemia, and preterm birth and low-birth-weight infants, although whether these poor pregnancy outcomes are caused by iron deficiency anemia is uncertain (Samuels). Usually even the fetus of an anemic woman will receive adequate iron stores from the mother, at the cost of further depleting the mother's iron level (Blackburn).

Generally iron deficiency anemia is preventable or easily treated with iron supplements. Because of the increased amounts of iron needed for fetal development and maternal stores, pregnant women are often encouraged to take prophylactic iron supplementation (Blackburn, 2013; Gilbert, 2011). Most women with iron deficiency anemia can absorb as much iron as they need by taking one 325-mg tablet of ferrous sulfate twice each day (Samuels, 2012). Some pregnant women cannot tolerate the prescribed oral iron because of nausea and vomiting associated with the pregnancy and as a side effect of iron therapy. In such cases they may be given parenteral iron therapy by intramuscular or intravascular injection. Women who are severely anemic may require blood transfusions (Samuels).

Teach the importance of iron supplements for preventing or treating iron deficiency anemia. In addition, teach dietary ways to decrease the GI side effects of iron therapy (see Teaching for Self-Management: Iron Supplementation in Chapter 15).

Folate Deficiency Anemia

Folate is a water-soluble vitamin found naturally in dark green leafy vegetables, citrus fruits, eggs, legumes, and whole grains. Even in well-nourished women, folate deficiency is common. Poor diet, cooking with large volumes of water, and increased alcohol use may contribute to folate deficiency. During pregnancy the need for folate increases, both because of fetal demands and because it is less well absorbed from the GI tract during gestation.

Folic acid is the form of the vitamin used in vitamin supplements. The recommended daily intake of folic acid for nonpregnant women is 400 mcg. Pregnant women need 50% more, or 600 mcg/day (Otten, Helwig, & Meyers, 2006). Since 1998 the U.S. Food and Drug Administration (FDA) has required the addition of folic acid to cereals, pasta, breads, and other foods that are labeled "enriched." However, the amount added is small, and most pregnant women need a supplement. Both prescription and nonprescription prenatal vitamins contain more than this amount of folic acid and should be sufficient to prevent and treat folate deficiency. Women at particular risk for folate deficiency include those who have significant hemoglobinopathies, take an anticonvulsant medication, or are pregnant with a multifetal gestation. These women require larger doses of folic acid (Samuels, 2012).

Folate deficiency is the most common cause of megaloblastic anemia during pregnancy, but a vitamin B_{12} deficiency must also be considered. Vitamin B_{12} deficiency in pregnant women is seen much more often than in the past because of the increasing number of women who become pregnant after undergoing bariatric surgery. Megaloblastic anemia rarely occurs before the third trimester of pregnancy (Kilpatrick, 2014; Samuels, 2012). Women with megaloblastic anemia caused by folic acid deficiency have the usual presenting symptoms and signs of anemia: pallor, fatigue, and lethargy, as well as glossitis and skin roughness, which are associated specifically with megaloblastic anemia (Kilpatrick). Folate deficiency usually improves rapidly with folic acid therapy. It rarely occurs in the fetus and is not a significant cause of perinatal morbidity. Iron deficiency often occurs along with folate deficiency (Samuels).

Sickle Cell Hemoglobinopathy

Sickle cell hemoglobinopathy is a disease caused by the presence of abnormal hemoglobin in the blood. Sickle cell trait (SA hemoglobin pattern) is sickling of the RBCs but with a normal RBC life span. Most people with sickle cell trait are asymptomatic. Approximately 1 in 12 African-American adults in the United States has sickle cell trait (Samuels, 2012). Women with sickle cell trait require genetic counseling and partner testing to determine their risk of producing children with sickle cell trait or disease.

Women with sickle cell trait usually do well in pregnancy. However, they are at increased risk for preeclampsia, intrauterine fetal death, preterm birth and low-birth-weight infants, and postpartum endometritis. They are also at increased risk for urinary tract infections (UTIs) and may be deficient in iron (Kilpatrick, 2014; Samuels, 2012).

Sickle cell anemia (sickle cell disease) is a recessive, hereditary, familial hemolytic anemia that affects people of African or Mediterranean ancestry. These individuals usually have abnormal hemoglobin types (SS or SC). The average life span of RBCs in a person with sickle cell anemia is only 5 to 10 days, in comparison to the 120-day life span of a normal RBC. Sickle cell anemia occurs in 1 in 708 African-Americans in the United States (Samuels, 2012). People with sickle cell anemia have recurrent attacks (crises) of fever and pain, most often in the abdomen, joints, or extremities, although virtually all organ systems can be affected. These attacks are attributed to vascular occlusion when RBCs assume a characteristic sickled shape. Crises are usually triggered by dehydration, hypoxia, or acidosis (Samuels).

Women with sickle cell anemia require genetic counseling before pregnancy. All children born to a woman with sickle cell anemia will be affected in some way by the disease. The woman's partner must be tested to determine the couple's risk of producing children with sickle cell disease rather than sickle cell trait. Women with sickle cell anemia are at risk for poor pregnancy outcomes, including miscarriage, IUGR, and stillbirth. Although maternal mortality is rare, maternal morbidity is significant and includes an increased risk for preeclampsia and infection, particularly in the urinary tract and in the lungs. The frequency of painful crises also appears to be increased during pregnancy (Samuels, 2012).

The woman is monitored carefully during pregnancy for the development of a UTI or preeclampsia. In addition, she will have serial ultrasound examinations to monitor fetal growth and will likely have antepartum fetal testing performed regularly during the third trimester. Infections are treated aggressively with antibiotics. If crises occur they are managed with analgesia, oxygen, and hydration.

If no complications occur, pregnancy can continue until term. Intrapartum, women with sickle cell disease should be encouraged to labor in a side-lying position. They may require supplemental oxygen. Adequate hydration should be maintained while preventing fluid overload. Conduction anesthesia (e.g., epidural or combined spinal epidural anesthesia) is recommended because it provides excellent pain relief. Vaginal birth is preferred. Cesarean birth should be performed only for obstetric indications (Samuels, 2012).

SAFETY ALERT

Women with sickle cell anemia are not iron deficient. Therefore, routine iron supplementation, even that found in prenatal vitamins, should be avoided because these women can develop iron overload (Samuels, 2012).

Thalassemia

Thalassemia is a relatively common anemia in which an insufficient amount of hemoglobin is produced to fill the RBCs. Thalassemia is a hereditary disorder that involves the abnormal synthesis of the alpha or beta chains of hemoglobin. Beta thalassemia is the more common variety in the United States and usually occurs in people of Mediterranean, North African, Middle Eastern, and Asian descent (Kilpatrick, 2014).

Beta thalassemia minor is the heterozygous form of this disorder. People with heterozygous beta thalassemia are carriers of the disorder and are usually asymptomatic (Samuels, 2012). They may be mildly anemic but are usually healthy otherwise. Women whose pregnancies are complicated by beta thalassemia minor generally do not experience associated maternal or infant complications if their condition is stable (Blackburn, 2013) and do not require antepartum fetal testing. Iron therapy should only be prescribed for women who are iron deficient, although folic acid supplementation is recommended for all women with beta thalassemia minor (Samuels).

The homozygous form of beta thalassemia is known as thalassemia major, or Cooley's anemia. Persons with this form of the disease usually have hepatosplenomegaly and bone deformities caused by massive marrow tissue expansion. These individuals usually die of infection or cardiovascular complications fairly early in life. If women live to reach childbearing age, infertility is common. If women with this disorder do become pregnant, they usually experience severe anemia and congestive heart failure, although successful full-term pregnancies have been reported. Women with beta thalassemia major are managed much like those with sickle cell anemia during pregnancy (Samuels, 2012).

Pulmonary Disorders

As pregnancy advances and the uterus presses on the thoracic cavity, a woman may have increased respiratory difficulty. This difficulty is compounded by pulmonary disease.

Asthma

Asthma is a chronic inflammatory disorder involving the tracheobronchial airways, with increased airway responsiveness to a variety of stimuli. It is characterized by periods of exacerbations and remissions. Exacerbations are usually triggered by stimuli such as allergens, upper respiratory infection, medications (i.e., aspirin, beta-blockers), environmental pollutants, occupational exposures, exercise, cold air, or emotional stress (Gibson & Powrie, 2011). In many cases the actual cause may be unknown, although a family history of allergy is common in people with asthma. In response to stimuli, there is widespread but reversible narrowing of the hyperreactive airways, making it difficult to breathe. The clinical manifestations are expiratory wheezing, productive cough, thick sputum, dyspnea, or any combination.

Asthma may be the most common potentially serious medical condition to complicate pregnancy. It affects approximately 4% to 8% of all pregnancies. The prevalence and morbidity rates are increasing, although the asthma-related mortality has dropped in recent years (Whitty & Dombrowski, 2014).

The effect of pregnancy on asthma is unpredictable. In one large study 23% of women with asthma improved during pregnancy, whereas 30% became worse (Whitty & Dombrowski, 2014). If asthma worsens, the more severe symptoms usually occur between 17 and 24 weeks of gestation (Gilbert, 2011). Asthma appears to be associated with preterm birth, preeclampsia, small for gestational age fetuses, IUGR, and an increased rate of cesarean birth (Whitty & Dombrowski, 2014).

The ultimate goal of asthma therapy in pregnancy is maintaining adequate oxygenation of the fetus by preventing hypoxic episodes in the mother. Achieving this goal requires monitoring lung function objectively (e.g., peak expiratory flow rate and forced expiratory volume in 1 second), avoiding or controlling asthma triggers (e.g., dust mites, animal dander, pollen, wood smoke), educating clients about the importance of controlling asthma during pregnancy, and drug therapy. Current drug therapy for asthma emphasizes treatment of airway inflammation to decrease airway hyperresponsiveness and prevent asthma symptoms. Decreasing airway inflammation with inhaled corticosteroids is the preferred treatment for managing persistent asthma during pregnancy (Whitty & Dombrowski, 2014).

During pregnancy women with poorly controlled asthma may benefit from ultrasound examinations and antenatal testing. Because asthma has been associated with IUGR and preterm birth, accurate pregnancy dating should be established by a first-trimester ultrasound if possible. Evaluation of fetal activity and growth by serial ultrasound examinations may be considered for women who have suboptimally controlled asthma or moderate to severe asthma (beginning at 32 weeks of gestation) and after recovery from a severe asthma exacerbation. All women with asthma should be encouraged to attend to fetal activity (see Chapter 26 for information on daily fetal movement counts) (Whitty & Dombrowski, 2014). Acute exacerbations may require albuterol, steroids, aminophylline, beta-adrenergic agents, and oxygen. Women with severe exacerbations unresponsive to treatment may require intubation and mechanical ventilation (Whitty & Dombrowski, 2012).

Although asthma exacerbations during labor are very rare, medications for asthma are continued during labor and the postpartum period. Women who have received systemic corticosteroids during the previous 4 weeks should be given stress doses of corticosteroids during labor and for the first 24 hours after birth (Whitty & Dombrowski, 2012). Pulse oximetry should be instituted during labor. Epidurals are recommended for pain relief. Morphine and meperidine are histamine-releasing narcotics and should be avoided. Fentanyl may be used as an alternative for pain relief because it is less likely to cause histamine release (Gibson & Powrie, 2011).

During the postpartum period women who have asthma are at increased risk for hemorrhage. If excessive bleeding occurs, prostaglandin (PG)E_1 or E_2 can be given, although the woman's respiratory status should be monitored (Whitty & Dombrowski, 2012). Because carboprost (15-methyl $PGF_{2\alpha}$ [Hemabate]) and ergonovine and methylergonovine can cause bronchospasm, their use should be avoided (Cunningham et al., 2014). In general, only small amounts of asthma medications enter breast milk; therefore, their use is not considered a contraindication to breastfeeding. However, in sensitive individuals theophylline in breast milk can cause vomiting, feeding difficulties, jitteriness, and cardiac arrhythmias in neonates (Whitty & Dombrowski, 2012). The woman usually returns to her prepregnancy asthma status within 3 months after giving birth.

Cystic Fibrosis

Cystic fibrosis is a common autosomal recessive genetic disorder in which the exocrine glands produce excessive viscous secretions, which causes problems with both respiratory and digestive functions. Most people with cystic fibrosis have chronic obstructive pulmonary disease, pancreatic exocrine insufficiency, and elevated levels of sweat electrolytes. Morbidity and mortality are usually caused by progressive chronic bronchial pulmonary disease (Whitty & Dombrowski, 2014).

Because the gene for cystic fibrosis was identified in 1989, data can be collected for the purpose of genetic counseling for couples regarding carrier status. In the United States, approximately 4% of the Caucasian population are carriers of the cystic fibrosis gene. Cystic fibrosis occurs in 1 in 3200 Caucasian live births (Whitty & Dombrowski, 2014). People with cystic fibrosis live longer than in the past because of earlier diagnosis and advances in antibiotic therapy and nutritional support. More than 40% of all individuals in the United States with cystic fibrosis are more than 18 years old (Whitty & Dombrowski, 2014). Men tend to live a little longer (median age of survival is 29.6 years) compared with women, whose median age of survival is 27.3 years. Although most men with cystic fibrosis are infertile, women with the disease are often fertile and thus able to become pregnant (Whitty & Dombrowski, 2012).

In women with good nutrition, mild obstructive lung disease, and minimal lung impairment, pregnancy is tolerated well (Whitty & Dombrowski, 2012). In women with severe disease the pregnancy is often complicated by chronic hypoxemia and frequent pulmonary infections. Risk factors that may predict a poor pregnancy outcome are poor prepregnancy nutritional status, significant pulmonary disease with hypoxemia, pulmonary hypertension, liver disease, and diabetes mellitus. The incidence of preterm birth, IUGR, and uteroplacental insufficiency is increased (Whitty & Dombrowski, 2014).

Care of the pregnant woman with cystic fibrosis requires a team effort. Ideally the woman should lose or gain weight to reach 90% of her ideal body weight before becoming pregnant. A weight gain of 11 to 12 kg (24 to 26 lb) is recommended during pregnancy. Women who are unable to achieve the recommended weight gain through oral supplements may require nasogastric tube feedings at night. Pancreatic insufficiency may put the woman at risk for malnutrition because she cannot meet the increased nutritional requirements of pregnancy. If malnutrition is severe, parenteral hyperalimentation may be necessary. Fat-soluble vitamins may not be well absorbed, resulting in deficiency in those nutrients. Throughout pregnancy frequent monitoring of the woman's weight, blood glucose, hemoglobin, total protein, serum albumin, prothrombin time, and fat-soluble vitamins A and E is suggested. Pancreatic enzymes should be adjusted as necessary (Whitty & Dombrowski, 2014).

Women with cystic fibrosis are followed closely with serial pulmonary function testing. Test results are used both to guide management and to predict pregnancy outcome. Inhaled recombinant human deoxyribonuclease I may be given to improve lung function by decreasing sputum viscosity. Inhaled 7% saline also produces both short- and long-term benefits (Cunningham et al., 2014). Early detection and treatment of infection are critical. Management of infection includes IV antibiotics along with chest physical therapy and bronchial drainage (Whitty & Dombrowski, 2012).

Fetal assessment is essential, given that the fetus is at risk for uteroplacental insufficiency, which can result in IUGR. Maternal nutritional status and weight gain during pregnancy significantly affect fetal growth. Fundal height should be measured routinely, and ultrasound examinations performed to evaluate fetal growth and amniotic fluid volume. Fetal movement counts are often recommended, starting at 28 weeks of gestation. Nonstress tests (NSTs) should be initiated at 32 weeks of gestation or sooner if evidence of fetal compromise exists (see Chapter 26 for more information on fetal assessment tests) (Whitty & Dombrowski, 2012).

During labor increased cardiac output stresses the cardiovascular system and can lead to cardiopulmonary failure in the woman with pulmonary hypertension or cor pulmonale. These women are also more likely to develop right-sided heart failure. Epidural or local analgesia is the preferred analgesic for birth, with vaginal birth recommended. Cesarean birth should be reserved for obstetric indications. If general anesthesia is needed for cesarean birth, anticholinergic medications should not be given before surgery because they tend to promote airway drying (Whitty & Dombrowski, 2014).

Breastfeeding appears to be safe as long as the sodium content of the milk is not abnormal (Lawrence & Lawrence, 2011). Pumping and discarding the milk are continued until the sodium content has been determined. Milk samples should be tested periodically for sodium, chloride, and total fat, and the infant's growth pattern should be monitored.

Acute Respiratory Distress Syndrome

Acute respiratory distress syndrome (ARDS), or shock lung, occurs when the lungs are unable to maintain levels of oxygen and carbon dioxide within normal limits. Severe hypoxemia, in spite of high levels of inspired oxygen, is accompanied by an increase in pulmonary capillary permeability, a decrease in lung volume, and shunting of blood.

ARDS is not specific to pregnancy; it can also result from trauma, pneumonia, sepsis, aspiration of gastric contents, fat emboli, acute pancreatitis, and drug overdose. When ARDS is associated with pregnancy, the precipitating factors can also be amniotic fluid embolism, air embolism, tocolytic therapy, asthma, thromboembolism, disseminated intravascular coagulopathy, pyelonephritis, preeclampsia, eclampsia, severe hemorrhage, blood transfusion reactions, or peripartum cardiomyopathy (Gibson & Powrie, 2011).

An initial intervention is to find and correct the underlying cause, if possible. To provide the best fetal environment, early intubation and mechanical ventilation are recommended. With severe lung injury, positive end-expiratory pressure (PEEP) may be necessary. Sedatives may be prescribed for intubation and ventilation. The administration of vasoactive agents, inotropic agents, and corticosteroids may be necessary. Maintaining fluid balance is a challenge and a key component of management. For the woman who is hypovolemic, administration of blood may help increase cardiac output. For the woman who is hypervolemic, diuretics may be necessary to maintain adequate cardiac output. Whether birth of the fetus improves maternal oxygenation remains controversial (Cunningham et al., 2014).

The postpartum incidence of ARDS is affected not by the method of birth but by the amount of trauma occurring during pregnancy and birth. ARDS can also occur after miscarriage or therapeutic abortion.

Laboratory results are important in identifying the origin of acute pulmonary problems. Chest radiographs can indicate the presence of infiltrates in the lungs, and ABGs identify the status of acid-base balance. The priority assessments are vital signs, oxygen saturation levels, and signs and symptoms of thrombophlebitis and hemorrhage. During the postpartum period, apprehension, distended neck veins, cyanosis, diaphoresis, or pallor may indicate hypoxemia. Mental confusion or disorientation also may be noted.

The pulse rate increases to compensate for respiratory insufficiency of any origin. The severity of the pulmonary problem increases as the pulse rate increases. An initial increase in blood pressure occurs as cardiac output increases in an attempt to supply the tissue with oxygen. When lung damage is severe, blood pressure decreases.

Respiratory changes are the most important indicators of ARDS. The rate and depth of respirations, respiratory pattern, symmetry of chest movement, and use of accessory muscles should be noted; therefore, observation of respiratory characteristics after activity is important.

! NURSE ALERT

If there is any indication of abnormality, respirations are counted for a full minute; an error in rate of plus or minus four respirations per minute may be highly significant.

On auscultation, crackles, rhonchi, wheezes, or a pleural friction rub should be reported, especially when they are present after an earlier assessment with normal findings. The pregnant woman should be positioned for breathing comfort. Oxygen and emergency equipment should be available. The woman should be reassured and coached in relaxation techniques to lessen her anxiety.

Although they are usually younger and healthier than most adults who develop ARDS, pregnant women with this condition still experience mortality rates of 25% to 40%. With pulmonary injury, the clinical condition is determined by the degree of damage, the ability to compensate for it, and the stage of the disease. Ideally, lung injury will be detected at an early stage and the underlying disease process promptly identified and treated. At present, there are no long term follow-up studies on pregnant women who recovered from respiratory distress syndrome. Nonpregnant clients have been reported to require several years to recover normal lung function (Cunningham et al., 2014).

Integumentary Disorders

Dermatologic disorders induced by pregnancy include melasma (chloasma), vascular "spiders," palmar erythema, and striae gravidarum (see Chapter 13). A number of chronic skin disorders may complicate pregnancy. These disorders may be present prior to pregnancy or appear for the first time during pregnancy. The course of these disorders varies during pregnancy. Acne, for example, may improve. Psoriasis is unpredictable during pregnancy, but postpartum flares are common. Lesions from neurofibromatosis may increase in size and number during pregnancy (Cunningham et al., 2014). Explanation, reassurance, and commonsense measures should suffice for normal skin changes. In contrast, disease processes during and soon after pregnancy may be extremely difficult to diagnose and treat.

SAFETY ALERT

Isotretinoin (Accutane), commonly prescribed for cystic acne, is highly teratogenic. There is a risk for craniofacial, cardiac, and central nervous system (CNS) malformations in exposed fetuses. This drug should not be taken during pregnancy.

Pruritus is a major symptom in several pregnancy-related skin diseases. *Pruritus gravidarum,* generalized itching without the presence of a rash, develops in up to 14% of pregnant women. It is often limited to the abdomen and is usually caused by skin distention and development of striae. Pruritus gravidarum is associated with twin gestation, fertility treatment, diabetes, and nulliparity. It is not associated with poor perinatal outcomes. It is treated symptomatically with skin lubrication, topical antipruritics, and oral antihistamines. Ultraviolet light and careful exposure to sunlight decrease itching. Pruritus gravidarum usually disappears shortly after birth but can recur in approximately half of all subsequent pregnancies (Rapini, 2014).

Another common pregnancy-specific cause of pruritus is pruritic urticarial papules and plaques of pregnancy (PUPPP) (Fig. 30-1), also known as polymorphic eruption of pregnancy. PUPPP classically appears in primigravidas during the third trimester. The lesions usually appear first on the abdomen but can spread to the arms, thighs, back, and buttocks. PUPPP almost always causes pruritus, and the itching is severe in 80% of cases. It is associated with increased maternal weight gain, an increased rate of twin gestation, hypertension, and induction of labor. It is not, however, associated with poor maternal or fetal outcomes. Therefore, the goal of therapy is simply to relieve maternal discomfort. Antipruritic topical medications, topical steroids, and oral antihistamines usually provide relief. Women with severe symptoms may require oral prednisone. PUPPP usually resolves before birth or within several weeks after birth.

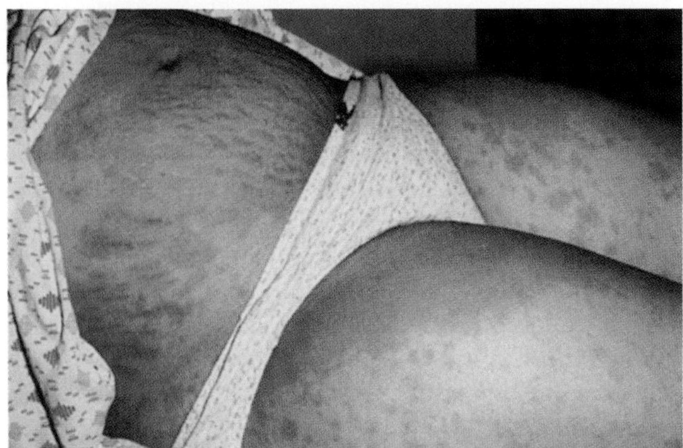

FIG 30-1 Pruritic urticarial papules and plaques of pregnancy (PUPPP). Lesions commonly begin in the abdominal striae. Confluent, erythematous urticarial papules and plaques are seen on the thighs in this woman. (From R.K. Creasy, R. Resnik, J.D. Iams, et al. [Eds.]. [2014]. *Creasy and Resnik's maternal-fetal medicine: Principles and practice* [7th ed.]. Philadelphia: Saunders.)

It rarely persists or begins after birth. PUPPP does not usually recur in subsequent pregnancies (Kroumpouzos, 2012; Rapini, 2014).

Intrahepatic cholestasis of pregnancy (ICP) is a liver disorder unique to pregnancy that is characterized by generalized pruritus. The itching commonly affects the palms and soles but can occur on any part of the body and is usually worse at night. No skin lesions are present. Women with ICP have elevated serum bile acids and elevated liver function tests. Jaundice may be present. Up to one half of women with ICP develop dark urine and light-colored stools. The cause of ICP is unknown, but approximately half of women have a family history of the disorder. ICP occurs more frequently during the winter months. A geographic variance in the prevalence of the disease also exists. ICP occurs most often in Southeast Asia, Chile, Bolivia, and Scandinavia, although it is seen less frequently now in Chile and in Scandinavia than in the past (Cappell, 2012; Williamson, Mackillop, & Heneghan, 2014).

The major fetal complications associated with ICP are asphyxial events, meconium staining, stillbirth, and preterm birth. The cause of these complications is likely related to increased levels of fetal serum bile acids. Treatment consists of giving ursodeoxycholic acid, which effectively controls the pruritus and laboratory abnormalities associated with ICP, and continued monitoring of liver function tests and bile acid levels (Cappell, 2012; Williamson et al., 2014). Antepartum fetal testing is essential. If liver function tests do not improve, induction of labor is considered at 36 to 37 weeks of gestation if the fetal lungs are mature. Symptoms usually disappear and laboratory abnormalities resolve within 2 to 4 weeks postpartum. ICP can recur in subsequent pregnancies, however, or with oral contraceptive use (Cappell).

Neurologic Disorders

The pregnant woman with a neurologic disorder must deal with potential teratogenic effects of prescribed medications, changes of mobility during pregnancy, and impaired ability to care for the baby. The nurse should be aware of all medications the woman is taking and the associated potential for producing congenital anomalies. As the pregnancy progresses, the woman's center of gravity shifts and causes balance and gait changes. The nurse should advise the woman of these expected changes and suggest safety measures as appropriate. Family and community resources may be needed to assist in providing infant care for the neurologically impaired woman.

Epilepsy

Epilepsy (often called *seizure disorder*) is a disorder of the brain that causes recurrent seizures and is the most common major neurologic disorder accompanying pregnancy. Less than 1% of all pregnant women have a seizure disorder (Aminoff & Douglas, 2014). Seizure disorders are either acquired (less than 15% of all cases) or idiopathic (more than 85% of all cases), which means that a specific cause for the seizures cannot be identified. The majority of women with a seizure disorder who become pregnant have an uneventful pregnancy with an excellent outcome (Samuels & Niebyl, 2012).

Women with epilepsy should receive preconception counseling if at all possible. A detailed history of medication use and seizure frequency should be obtained. If the woman has frequent seizures before conception, she is likely to continue this pattern during pregnancy; therefore, achieving effective seizure control is extremely important before conception, even if changing medications is required (Samuels & Niebyl, 2012).

Infants born to women taking anticonvulsant medications have an increased incidence of congenital anomalies, including cleft lip and palate, congenital heart disease, and neural tube defects (NTDs). These anomalies are often related to the dose, type, and number of anticonvulsant medications taken (Aminoff & Douglas, 2014; Samuels & Niebyl, 2012). However, epilepsy itself can be associated with an increased risk of fetal malformations (Aminoff & Douglas).

SAFETY ALERT

Carbamazepine (Tegretol) and valproate (Depakote) should be avoided if possible during pregnancy because their use is associated with NTDs in the fetus.

Several anticonvulsant medications have been developed for use during the 2000s. More information is needed regarding the fetal effects of these medications. Any anticonvulsant medication required to achieve good seizure control in a woman with epilepsy should be used, however, regardless of the increased risk of fetal anomalies because the most important goal during pregnancy is to prevent seizures (Samuels & Niebyl, 2012).

Pregnant women with epilepsy are advised to take a folic acid supplement of 4 mg daily, which may decrease the incidence of NTDs. They are also encouraged to take a prenatal vitamin containing vitamin D daily because anticonvulsant medications can interfere with production of the active form of this vitamin (Samuels & Niebyl, 2012).

During pregnancy only one anticonvulsant medication—at the lowest dose level that is effective at keeping the woman seizure free—should be prescribed. The increase in plasma volume that is a normal pregnancy change can affect drug metabolism and distribution. Therefore, blood levels of anticonvulsant medications should be checked and drug dosages adjusted as necessary (Aminoff & Douglas, 2014; Samuels & Niebyl, 2012). With client cooperation and close monitoring, most women with epilepsy should experience no change or even have fewer seizures during pregnancy. An increase in seizure frequency is usually related either to noncompliance with taking prescribed anticonvulsant medications or to sleep deprivation (Samuels & Niebyl).

In addition to congenital anomalies, the fetus of a woman with epilepsy is also at risk for IUGR. Determining an accurate gestational age as early as possible is important. This information decreases any confusion later in pregnancy in regard to fetal growth issues. Maternal serum screening around 16 weeks of gestation and ultrasound examination at 18 to 22 weeks of gestation should be performed to assess for the presence of an NTD or other fetal anomalies. Nonstress testing later in pregnancy is not necessary, unless the woman has other medical or obstetric factors that increase the risk for stillbirth (Samuels & Niebyl, 2012).

Managing anticonvulsant therapy during prolonged labor is challenging. During labor, absorption of medications given orally is unpredictable, especially if vomiting occurs. Women who are maintained on phenytoin (Dilantin) or phenobarbital may be given these medications parenterally during labor. No parenteral form of carbamazepine has been developed. Oral administration of carbamazepine may be attempted, but if the woman experiences a seizure or a preseizure aura, she may be given phenytoin intravenously instead to carry her through labor. Vaginal birth is preferred (Samuels & Niebyl, 2012).

After birth the levels of anticonvulsant medications must be monitored frequently for the first few weeks because they can rise rapidly. If medication dose levels were increased during pregnancy, they will need to be decreased quickly to prepregnancy levels. All of the major anticonvulsant medications are found in breast milk, but the use of these medications is not a contraindication to breastfeeding. However, topiramate has been associated with neonatal weight loss; thus it probably should not be prescribed if the woman is breastfeeding (Aminoff & Douglas, 2014; Samuels & Niebyl, 2012). Neonatal sedation may be a side effect of carbamazepine, primidone (Mysoline), and phenobarbital (Samuels & Niebyl).

During the neonatal period infants can have a hemorrhagic disorder associated with exposure to anticonvulsant medications in utero, which causes vitamin K deficiency. Some authorities recommend giving vitamin K daily during the last few weeks of pregnancy to women taking anticonvulsant medications, but this practice is not considered the standard of care (Samuels & Niebyl, 2012).

All methods of contraception can be used by women with an idiopathic seizure disorder. However, commonly prescribed anticonvulsant medications such as carbamazepine, primidone, phenobarbital, and phenytoin reduce the effectiveness of oral contraceptives. Therefore, use of other contraceptive methods, such as the intrauterine device or hormonal implants, should be considered (Cunningham et al., 2014). Valproic acid and the newer anticonvulsant medications have not been reported to cause oral contraceptive failure (Aminoff & Douglas, 2014). In planning for future childbearing, couples should be informed that children born to women with a seizure disorder of unknown cause have a four times greater chance of developing an idiopathic seizure disorder compared with the general population. Epilepsy in the father does not appear to increase a child's risk for developing a seizure disorder (Samuels & Nieby, 2012).

Multiple Sclerosis

Multiple sclerosis (MS), a patchy demyelinization of the spinal cord and CNS, may be a viral disorder. It occurs equally in men and women. Onset of symptoms, which include weakness of one or both lower extremities, visual complaints, and loss of coordination, is subtle and usually occurs between the ages of 20 and 40 years. The disease is characterized by exacerbations and remissions. Pregnancy does not seem to worsen the disease (Samuels & Niebyl, 2012).

Remissions during pregnancy are common. If an exacerbation occurs, it is more likely to do so during the third trimester of pregnancy or postpartum. Treatment may include corticosteroids and immunosuppressive agents. Several drugs and biopharmaceuticals are available for treating MS. Their use in pregnancy has been limited; thus few data and no controlled studies are available. However, many consist of molecules that are too large to cross the placenta. Therefore, they may be acceptable for use during pregnancy. They do not appear to be associated with anomalies (Samuels & Niebyl, 2012). Interferon is also sometimes used to treat MS relapses during pregnancy and postpartum. Its safety for use during pregnancy has not been established, although in theory it should not cross the placenta because of its large molecular size (Stuart & Bergstrom, 2011).

Women who have become paraplegic with MS are more likely to develop UTIs during pregnancy but may feel no symptoms. Therefore, they should be screened routinely. Women who have become paraplegic or have lumbosacral lesions as a result of MS may have little pain during labor. Determining when labor begins may be difficult for them. Uterine contractions occur normally, but these women may have difficulty pushing effectively during the second stage of labor. Therefore, vacuum- or forceps-assisted birth may be necessary (Samuels & Niebyl, 2012). Epidural anesthesia can be used during labor (Stuart & Bergstrom, 2011).

Depression is common among women with MS; thus they should be assessed frequently for evidence of postpartum depression. Breastfeeding is encouraged, although medications that are Lactation Risk Category L5 should not be prescribed. Intravenous immunoglobulin (IVIG) is considered safe for use during lactation; no adverse effects in infants have been reported. All hormonal contraceptives may be used by women with MS (Stuart & Bergstrom, 2011).

Bell Palsy

Bell palsy is an acute idiopathic facial paralysis. The cause is unknown, but it may be related to the reactivation of herpes simplex virus infection or acute human immunodeficiency virus type 1 (HIV-1) retroviral infection. Bell palsy occurs fairly often, especially in women of reproductive age. An association between Bell palsy and pregnancy was first cited by Bell in 1830. Pregnant women are affected four times more often than nonpregnant women. Women who develop Bell palsy during pregnancy have an increased risk for gestational hypertension or preeclampsia as well (Cunningham et al., 2014).

The clinical manifestations of Bell palsy include the sudden development of a unilateral facial weakness, with maximal weakness within 48 hours after onset, pain surrounding the ear, difficulty closing the eye on the affected side, hyperacusis (abnormal acuteness of the sense of hearing), and occasionally a loss of taste (Aminoff & Douglas, 2014; Cunningham et al., 2014).

No effects of maternal Bell palsy have been observed in infants. Maternal outcome is generally good unless a complete block in nerve conduction occurs. Steroid therapy is the only medical treatment that has been shown to influence the outcome of Bell palsy. To be effective, treatment should begin within the first 3 to 5 days after the paralysis develops (Aminoff & Douglas, 2014). Supportive care includes prevention of injury to the constantly exposed cornea, facial muscle massage, careful chewing and manual removal of food from inside the affected cheek, and reassurance. Although 80% of affected men and nonpregnant women recover to a satisfactory level within a year, only approximately half of women who develop the disorder during pregnancy do so (Cunningham et al., 2014).

Autoimmune Disorders

Autoimmune disorders make up a large group of diseases that disrupt the function of the immune system of the body. In these types of disorders the body's immune system is unable to distinguish "self" from "nonself." As a result, antibodies develop that attack its normally present antigens, causing tissue damage. Autoimmune disorders can occur during pregnancy because a large percentage of women with an autoimmune disease are women of childbearing age (Gilbert, 2011). Common autoimmune diseases include systemic lupus erythematosus, myasthenia gravis, antiphospholipid syndrome, rheumatoid arthritis, and systemic sclerosis (Chin & Branch, 2012; Cunningham et al., 2014).

Systemic Lupus Erythematosus

Systemic lupus erythematosus (SLE) is a chronic, multisystem inflammatory disease that affects the skin, joints, kidneys, lungs, nervous system, liver, and other body organs. The exact cause is unknown but probably involves the interaction of immunologic, environmental, hormonal, and genetic factors. SLE is the most common serious autoimmune disease affecting women of reproductive age. It occurs two to four times more often in African-American and Hispanic women than in Caucasian women and is nine times more common in women than in men. Most cases of SLE occur in adolescence or young adulthood (Chin & Branch, 2012; Lockshin, Salmon, & Erkan, 2014).

Common symptoms, including myalgias, fatigue, weight change, and fevers, occur in nearly all women with SLE at some time during the course of the disease. Although a diagnosis of SLE is suspected based on clinical signs and symptoms, it is confirmed by laboratory testing that demonstrates the presence of circulating autoantibodies. As is the case with other autoimmune diseases, SLE is characterized by a series of exacerbations (flares) and remissions (Chin & Branch, 2012; Lockshin et al., 2014).

Pregnancy probably does not increase the likelihood of serious SLE flares (Lockshin et al., 2014). However, it appears that disease activity at the beginning of pregnancy is an important predictor of exacerbations during pregnancy. Therefore, women are advised to wait until they have been in remission for at least 6 months before attempting to become pregnant (Chin & Branch, 2012; Gilbert, 2011). In addition to exacerbations, other maternal risks include an increased rate of miscarriage, nephritis, preeclampsia, possible need to give birth at a preterm gestation, and an increased risk of cesarean birth. Fetal risks include stillbirth, IUGR, and preterm birth (Chin & Branch).

Medical therapy during pregnancy is kept to a minimum in women who are in remission or who have a mild form of SLE. Occasional doses of nonsteroidal antiinflammatory drugs (NSAIDs) can be given to treat arthralgia. Low-dose aspirin can be used throughout pregnancy (Cunningham et al., 2014). Glucocorticoids such as prednisone are often used to treat SLE during pregnancy, either as maintenance therapy or short-term treatment for flares. There is a small risk of fetal cleft lip and palate if glucocorticoids are used during early pregnancy. Prolonged use of this group of medications also increases the risks for bone demineralization, gestational diabetes, preeclampsia, premature rupture of membranes, and IUGR. Given the significant risks associated with long-term glucocorticoid use, hydroxychloroquine, an antimalarial drug, may be the best medication for maintenance SLE therapy during pregnancy. It significantly reduces SLE disease activity but appears to cause no adverse effects on the fetus (Chin & Branch, 2012).

Prenatal care otherwise focuses on close monitoring to detect common pregnancy complications such as hypertension, proteinuria, and IUGR. Ultrasound examinations are performed frequently to monitor fetal growth. Fetal assessment tests, including daily fetal movement counts and weekly or twice-weekly NSTs and amniotic fluid volume assessments or biophysical profiles, likely begin at 30 to 32 weeks of gestation (see Chapter 26). More frequent ultrasound examinations and fetal testing are necessary if the woman develops an SLE flare, antiphospholipid syndrome, hypertension, proteinuria, or evidence of IUGR (Chin & Branch, 2012).

Women with SLE can develop an exacerbation during labor. Any maintenance medications should be continued throughout the intrapartum period or resumed immediately postpartum at the last pregnancy dose. Even if a flare does not occur, all women who have received chronic glucocorticoid therapy (20 mg or more of prednisone daily for at least 3 weeks) need larger (stress) doses of steroids during labor (Chin & Branch, 2012). Vaginal birth is preferred, but cesarean birth is common because of maternal and fetal complications.

Close monitoring of all women with SLE should continue after birth. Women who have more severe SLE manifestations or who had an SLE exacerbation during pregnancy are at greatest risk to experience a postpartum flare (Chin & Branch, 2012).

Women with SLE and chronic vascular or renal disease should limit their number of pregnancies because of maternal complications associated with the illness and increased adverse perinatal outcomes. If desired, the safest time for tubal sterilization is during the postpartum period or when the disease is in remission (Cunningham et al., 2014). Estrogen-containing oral contraceptives may increase the risk of thromboembolism (Gilbert, 2011). Progestin-only implants and injections provide effective contraception with no known effects on lupus flares (Cunningham et al.). Barrier methods, in addition to progestin-only contraceptive options, are the least risky forms of contraception for women with SLE (Gilbert). Evidence does not support concerns regarding an increased risk of infection when IUDs are prescribed for women receiving immunosuppressive therapy (Cunningham et al.).

Myasthenia Gravis

Myasthenia gravis (MG), an autoimmune motor (muscle) end-plate disorder that involves acetylcholine use, affects the motor function at the myoneural junction. Muscle weakness results, particularly of the eyes, face, tongue, neck, limbs, and respiratory muscles. In addition, women may experience ptosis, diplopia, and dysphagia. Women are affected twice as often as men, and the incidence peaks between the ages of 20 and 30 years (Denney, Porter, & Branch, 2011). Because the greatest period of risk is during the first year after diagnosis, pregnancy should probably be avoided until symptomatic improvement occurs (Cunningham et al., 2014). The response of women with MG to pregnancy is unpredictable; remission, exacerbation, or continued stability during pregnancy can occur.

Pregnancy does not appear to affect the overall course of MG, but as the uterus enlarges respirations may be compromised. Also the normal fatigue experienced by many pregnant women may be tolerated poorly by those with MG (Cunningham et al., 2014). Treatment during pregnancy is the same as for nonpregnant women. Usual medications include glucocorticoids and acetylcholinesterase inhibitors. Monitoring blood glucose values is important because hyperglycemia may result from corticosteroid therapy. Thymectomy may result in remission of the disease but is best performed before or after pregnancy, if at all possible. For severe weakness, plasmapheresis or IVIG therapy may be needed (Aminoff & Douglas, 2014).

Because MG does not affect smooth muscle, most women usually tolerate labor well. Vaginal birth is desired, but vacuum or forceps assistance may be required because of muscle weakness. Oxytocin may be given, but all medications that cause muscular relaxation should be avoided if at all possible. Narcotics must be used cautiously because they may cause respiratory depression, and women with MG are already at risk for respiratory muscle weakness. Regional analgesia is preferred (Aminoff & Douglas, 2014; Cunningham et al., 2014). After birth, women must be carefully supervised because relapses often occur during the puerperium.

SAFETY ALERT

Magnesium sulfate must not be administered to women with MG because it inhibits the release of acetylcholine and can trigger myasthenic crisis.

Approximately 10% to 15% of neonates born to women with MG develop neonatal myasthenia. This transient disorder results from the transfer of maternal antibody against acetylcholine receptors across the placenta. Symptoms, including a poor cry, respiratory difficulties, weakness in suckling, a weak Moro reflex, and feeble limb movements, usually appear within the first 72 hours after birth. Neonatal myasthenia can be treated with anticholinesterase medications and usually resolves by 6 weeks after birth (Aminoff & Douglas, 2014).

Gastrointestinal Disorders

Compromise of GI function during pregnancy is a concern. Obvious physiologic alterations, such as the greatly enlarged uterus, and less apparent changes, such as hormonal differences and hypochlorhydria (deficiency of hydrochloric acid in the stomach's gastric juice), require understanding for proper diagnosis and treatment. Gallbladder disease and inflammatory bowel disease are examples of GI disorders that may occur during pregnancy.

Cholelithiasis and Cholecystitis

Cholelithiasis (the presence of gallstones in the gallbladder) occurs more often in women than in men. Its incidence increases during pregnancy, probably because of increased hormone levels and pressure from the enlarged uterus that interferes with the normal circulation and drainage of the gallbladder. Most gallstones are asymptomatic during pregnancy. Usually the first symptom of cholelithiasis is biliary colic, epigastric or right upper quadrant pain that can radiate to the back or shoulders (Cappell, 2012; Williamson et al., 2014). Pain may occur spontaneously or after eating a high-fat meal. Approximately two thirds of clients with biliary colic have recurrent attacks (Cappell). Multiparity and prepregnancy obesity are risk factors for cholelithiasis (Williamson et al.).

Cholecystitis (inflammation of the gallbladder) is usually caused when a gallstone obstructs a cystic duct. As in biliary colic that occurs with cholelithiasis, epigastric or right upper quadrant pain is present, but the pain is usually more severe and prolonged. Nausea, vomiting, and fever may also be present. Acute cholecystitis is the third most common indication for nonobstetric surgical intervention in pregnancy, occurring in about 4 cases per 10,000 pregnancies (Cappell, 2012).

Often gallbladder surgery is postponed until the puerperium. The woman can usually be managed conservatively for the remainder of the pregnancy (see Teaching for Self-Management: Nutritional Counseling for the Pregnant Woman with Cholelithiasis or Cholecystitis). However, women with recurrent biliary colic or acute cholecystitis generally require immediate cholecystectomy. Although the second trimester has traditionally been considered the safest time for this surgery, it is increasingly performed at any time during pregnancy because of improved surgical techniques and outcomes. Both laparoscopic and open cholecystectomy procedures are acceptable during pregnancy (Cappell, 2012; Cunningham et al., 2014). Preoperative care includes IV fluids, discontinuing oral intake, analgesia, and usually antibiotics (Cappell).

TEACHING FOR SELF-MANAGEMENT

Nutritional Counseling for the Pregnant Woman with Cholelithiasis or Cholecystitis

- Assess your diet for foods that cause discomfort and flatulence, and omit foods that trigger episodes.
- Reduce dietary fat intake to 40 to 50 g/day.
- Limit protein to 10% to 12% of total calories.
- Choose foods so that most of the calories come from carbohydrates.
- Prepare food without adding fats or oils as much as possible.
- Avoid fried foods.

Inflammatory Bowel Disease

Inflammatory bowel disease refers to ulcerative colitis and Crohn disease. It is relatively common in young women, so these disorders are seen during pregnancy. The incidence of an inflammatory bowel disease flare is not increased in pregnancy and no evidence suggests that pregnancy significantly affects either ulcerative colitis or Crohn disease (Cunningham et al., 2014; Kelly & Savides, 2014). In general, infants born to mothers with inflammatory bowel disease have a higher risk for preterm birth, low birth weight, and being small for gestational age. However, these infants do not have an increased risk for congenital anomalies (Kelly & Savides). Active disease early in pregnancy increases the risk for a poor pregnancy outcome (Cunningham et al.).

Treatment of inflammatory bowel disease is usually the same for the pregnant woman as it is for the nonpregnant woman. Discontinuing her prepregnancy medications can cause the woman to have a relapse or disease flare. The medications 5-aminosalicylates, prednisone, and 6-mercaptopurine or azathioprine are often prescribed for treatment of inflammatory bowel disease. Occasionally biologic agents such as infliximab also are ordered. Antibiotics such as metronidazole and ciprofloxacin may also be necessary from time to time. These drugs appear to be safe for use during pregnancy (Kelly & Savides, 2014). Folic acid supplementation is especially important because of problems with intestinal malabsorption. Calcium supplementation is also necessary because osteoporosis is common. Some women may require parenteral nutrition (Cunningham et al., 2014). Surgery during pregnancy is done for emergencies such as intestinal obstruction, perforation, abscess, or fulminant colitis. In these situations, surgery is required for the mother's health (Kelly & Savides).

Urinary Tract Infections

UTIs are a common medical complication of pregnancy, occurring in approximately 20% of all pregnancies. They are also responsible for 10% of all hospitalizations during pregnancy (Duff, 2014). UTIs include asymptomatic bacteriuria, cystitis, and pyelonephritis. They are usually caused by coliform organisms that are a normal part of the perineal flora. By far the most common cause is *Escherichia coli,* a gram-negative bacterium responsible for 85% of cases. Another gram-negative bacterium that causes UTIs is *Klebsiella pneumoniae.* The gram-positive organisms group B streptococci, enterococci, and staphylococci account for approximately 3% to 7% of all infections (Gilbert, 2011).

Asymptomatic Bacteriuria

Asymptomatic bacteriuria refers to the persistent presence of bacteria within the urinary tract of women who have no symptoms. A clean-voided urine specimen containing more than 100,000 organisms per milliliter is diagnostic. If asymptomatic bacteriuria is not treated, up to 40% of infected women will subsequently develop symptomatic infection during the pregnancy. Therefore, the American College of Obstetricians and Gynecologists (ACOG) recommends that all women be screened for asymptomatic bacteriuria at their first prenatal visit (Colombo, 2012). Asymptomatic bacteriuria has been associated with preterm birth and low-birth-weight infants, (American Academy of Pediatrics [AAP] & ACOG, 2012; Cunningham et al., 2014).

Asymptomatic bacteriuria should be treated with an antibiotic. Antibiotics that are often prescribed include amoxicillin, ampicillin, cephalexin (Keflex), ciprofloxacin (Cipro), levofloxacin (Levaquin), nitrofurantoin (Macrodantin), and trimethoprim-sulfamethoxazole (Bactrim DS). Several different regimens, including single-dose or 3-, 7-, and 10-day treatment may be used (Cunningham et al., 2014). A repeat urine culture is usually ordered 1 to 2 weeks after completing therapy because approximately 15% of women do not respond to therapy or have a reinfection (Colombo, 2012). Women who have persistent or frequent recurrences of bacteriuria may be placed on suppressive therapy, often nitrofurantoin each night at bedtime, for the remainder of the pregnancy (Cunningham et al.).

Cystitis

Cystitis (bladder infection) is characterized by dysuria, urgency, and frequency, along with lower abdominal or suprapubic pain. Usually white blood cells, as well as bacteria, are found in the urine. Microscopic or gross hematuria also may be present. Typically, symptoms are confined to the bladder rather than becoming systemic. Cystitis is usually uncomplicated but it may lead to ascending UTI if untreated. Approximately 40% of pregnant women with pyelonephritis experienced symptoms of bladder infection before developing pyelonephritis (Cunningham et al., 2014).

Cystitis is often treated with a 3-day course of antibiotic therapy, which is usually 90% effective in curing the infection. Antibiotics often prescribed include amoxicillin, ampicillin, cephalexin (Keflex), ciprofloxacin (Cipro), levofloxacin (Levaquin), nitrofurantoin (Macrodantin), and trimethoprim-sulfamethoxazole (Bactrim DS) (Cunningham et al., 2014). Phenazopyridine (Pyridium), a urinary analgesic, is often prescribed along with an antibiotic for relief of symptoms caused by irritation of the urinary tract. Although phenazopyridine is effective at relieving dysuria, urgency, and frequency, women should be taught that the medication colors urine and tears orange. Therefore, they should be instructed to avoid wearing contact lenses while taking this medication and warned that it will stain underwear.

CLINICAL REASONING CASE STUDY

Urinary Tract Infection

Emily is a 23-year-old G1 P0 who has her initial prenatal visit at 8 weeks of gestation. She is complaining of urinary frequency and burning with urination. During the visit a routine urine sample is collected and sent to the lab. Emily declines antibiotics because she wants to be sure she really has an infection, choosing to wait on the lab results. Two days later Emily receives a call at work from her health care provider, telling her that she needs to pick up a prescription for an antibiotic because her lab results indicated that she has a urinary tract infection (UTI). Emily asks, "Is the antibiotic okay for the baby? I thought medications should be avoided in the first trimester."

1. Evidence—Is there sufficient evidence to determine the type of UTI that Emily has?
2. What assumptions can be made about the following issues:
   a. Risks associated with UTI during pregnancy
   b. Management plan for treating UTI during pregnancy
3. What are the priorities for nursing care at this time?
4. Does the evidence objectively support your conclusion?

Pyelonephritis

Renal infection (pyelonephritis) is the most common serious medical complication of pregnancy and the leading cause of septic shock during pregnancy (Cunningham et al., 2014). The most common maternal complications associated with pyelonephritis include anemia, septicemia, transient renal dysfunction, and pulmonary insufficiency. Women with pyelonephritis can develop urosepsis, sepsis syndrome, and renal dysfunction. In addition, pulmonary injury resembling ARDS can occur in pregnant women with acute pyelonephritis, most likely the result of damage to alveolar tissue caused by the release of endotoxins from gram-negative bacteria (Colombo, 2012; Cunningham et al.). Recurrent pyelonephritis is thought to cause fetal death and IUGR. Acute pyelonephritis is associated with preterm labor (Colombo).

Pyelonephritis develops most often during the second trimester of pregnancy and is usually caused by the *E. coli* organism. Infection develops only in the right kidney in at least half of all cases. The onset of pyelonephritis is often abrupt, with fever, shaking chills, and aching in the lumbar area of the back. Anorexia and nausea and vomiting also can be present. Usually one or both costovertebral angles are tender to palpation (Duff, 2014).

Women diagnosed with pyelonephritis are usually admitted to the hospital immediately. Treatment with IV antibiotics is started as soon as urine and blood samples for culture and sensitivity have been collected (Cunningham et al., 2014). Given the high resistance of *E. coli* to ampicillin, cephalexin (Keflex), and cefazolin (Ancef), these medications are not recommended. Ceftriaxone (Rocephin) is often prescribed because it provides excellent coverage against many of the organisms that commonly cause pyelonephritis (Duff, 2014). The woman must be monitored closely for the possible development of sepsis (Cunningham et al., 2014). A woman with mild to moderate disease (low-grade fever, normal or slightly elevated white blood cell count, and no nausea or vomiting) may be treated with oral antibiotics as an outpatient (Duff, 2014).

Clinical symptoms generally resolve within a couple of days after antibiotic therapy is begun. The antibiotic may need to be changed based on the results of the initial culture and sensitivity testing, or if the woman has not responded to therapy within 48 hours (Gilbert, 2011). Most women become afebrile within 72 hours. If no clinical improvement is seen within 48 to 72 hours, an ultrasound should be performed to assess for a urinary tract obstruction. Once the woman is afebrile, she will be changed from IV to oral antibiotics (Cunningham et al., 2014).

Usually antibiotic therapy is continued for 7 to 14 days after the woman is discharged from the hospital. A urine culture will likely be repeated 1 to 2 weeks after antibiotic therapy has been completed. Recurrent infection develops in 30% to 40% of women after completion of treatment for pyelonephritis. Therefore, urine cultures should be obtained each trimester for the remainder of the pregnancy. Many women are maintained on a prophylactic antibiotic (often nitrofurantoin once or twice daily) for the remainder of the pregnancy (Colombo, 2012; Cunningham et al., 2014).

Nursing Interventions

Nurses are often responsible for teaching pregnant women about taking medications safely and effectively. This education is especially important in regard to antibiotics because this type of medication is so often misused by the general public. The woman should be instructed to finish the entire course of prescribed antibiotic therapy rather than stopping the medication as soon as she feels better. Failure to do so can lead to the creation of additional drug-resistant organisms. Antibiotics should be taken on time and around the clock so that medication levels in the body remain constant. Finally, many women will develop a yeast infection while taking antibiotics because the medication kills normal flora in the genitourinary tract as well as pathologic organisms. Therefore, they should be encouraged to include yogurt, cheese, or milk containing active acidophilus cultures in their diet while on antibiotics.

Women should also be taught simple ways to prevent UTIs. See Teaching for Self-Management: Prevention of Genital Tract Infections in Chapter 7 for several suggestions.

SURGERY DURING PREGNANCY

The need for abdominal surgery occurs as frequently among pregnant women as among nonpregnant women of comparable age. However, pregnancy may make the diagnosis more difficult. An enlarged uterus and displaced internal organs may make abdominal palpation more difficult, alter the position of an affected organ, or change the usual signs and symptoms associated with a particular disorder. The most common surgical emergency during pregnancy is appendicitis (Cappell, 2012).

Appendicitis

Appendicitis occurs approximately once in 1000 pregnancies. The incidence is 30%, 45%, and 25% in the first, second, and third trimesters, respectively (Mahomed, 2011). The diagnosis of appendicitis is often delayed because the usual signs and symptoms mimic some normal changes of pregnancy such as nausea and vomiting and increased white blood cell (WBC) count. As pregnancy progresses, the appendix is pushed upward and to the right from its usual anatomic location (see Fig. 13-14) (Cunningham et al., 2014). Because of these changes, rupture of the appendix and the subsequent development of peritonitis occur in up to 25% of pregnant women with appendicitis (Cappell, 2012).

The most common symptom of appendicitis in pregnant women is right lower quadrant abdominal pain, regardless of gestational age. Nausea and vomiting are often present, but loss of appetite is not a reliable indicator of appendicitis. Fever, tachycardia, a dry tongue, and localized abdominal tenderness are commonly found in nonpregnant people with appendicitis, but they are less likely indicators for the disorder in pregnant women. Because of the physiologic increase in WBCs that occurs in pregnancy, this test is not helpful in making the diagnosis. A urinalysis and a chest x-ray should be performed to rule out UTI and right lower lobe pneumonia, given that both of these conditions can cause lower abdominal pain (Kelly & Savides, 2014). Appendicitis can also be confused with other disorders such as cholecystitis, preterm labor, pyelonephritis, or placental abruption (abruptio placentae) (Cunningham et al., 2014).

Radiologic imaging is necessary if appendicitis is suspected after history, physical examination, and laboratory studies have been completed. Although CT is the imaging test of choice in nonpregnant clients because it is highly accurate, the use of ultrasound during pregnancy is preferred to avoid fetal exposure to radiation from CT (Cappell, 2012). MRI may be used if appendicitis has not been confirmed by other imaging techniques (Cappell; Kelly & Savides, 2014).

Prompt surgical intervention to remove the appendix is still the standard treatment (Kelly & Savides, 2014). Laparoscopic surgery may be performed during the first and second trimesters of pregnancy if the appendix has not ruptured or the diagnosis is uncertain. Antibiotics are often administered for uncomplicated appendicitis and are definitely necessary if rupture, abscess, or peritonitis has occurred. Clindamycin and gentamicin are often prescribed because they are considered both effective and safe. The maternal mortality rate from ruptured appendix is about 4%. The fetal mortality rate from ruptured appendix is much higher, more than 30% (Cappell, 2012).

CARE MANAGEMENT

Initial assessment of the pregnant woman requiring surgery focuses on her presenting signs and symptoms. A thorough history and physical examination are performed. Laboratory testing includes, at a minimum, a complete blood count with differential and a urinalysis. Additional laboratory and other diagnostic tests may be necessary to reach a diagnosis. In addition, fetal heart rate (FHR) and activity, along with uterine activity, should be monitored, and constant vigilance for symptoms of impending obstetric complications maintained. The extent of presurgery assessment is determined by the immediacy of surgical intervention and the specific disorder that requires surgery.

Hospital Care

When surgery becomes necessary during pregnancy, the woman and her family are concerned about the effects of the procedure and medication on fetal well-being and the course of pregnancy. An important aspect of preoperative nursing care is encouraging the woman to express her fears, concerns, and questions.

Preoperative care for a pregnant woman differs from that for a nonpregnant woman in one significant aspect: the presence of at least one other person, the fetus. Continuous FHR and uterine contraction monitoring should be performed if the fetus is considered viable. Procedures such as preparation of the operative site and time of insertion of IV lines and urinary retention catheters vary with the physician and the facility. However, in every instance there is a total restriction of solid foods and liquids or a clear specification of the type, amount, and time at which clear liquids may be taken before surgery. Some bowel preparation such as clear liquids and laxatives may be required before surgery. Food by mouth is restricted for several hours before a scheduled procedure. Even if she has had nothing by mouth—but more important, if surgery is unexpected—the woman is in danger of vomiting and aspirating, and special precautions are taken before anesthetic is administered (e.g., administering an antacid).

Intraoperatively perinatal nurses may collaborate with the surgical staff to increase their knowledge about the special needs of pregnant women undergoing surgery. One intervention to improve fetal oxygenation is positioning the woman on the operating table with a lateral tilt to avoid compression of the maternal vena cava. Continuous FHR and uterine contraction monitoring during surgery may be performed if the fetus is considered viable. Monitoring may be accomplished by using sterile Aquasonic gel and a sterile sleeve for the transducer. During abdominal surgery uterine contractions may be palpated manually. However, many practitioners simply monitor for the FHR and presence of uterine contractions before and after the procedure.

In the immediate recovery period general observations and care pertinent to postoperative recovery are initiated. Frequent assessments are carried out for several hours after surgery. Whether the woman is cared for in the surgical postanesthesia recovery area or in a labor and birth unit, continuous fetal and uterine monitoring will likely be initiated or resumed because of the potential risk for preterm labor. Tocolysis may be necessary if preterm labor occurs (see Chapter 32).

Home Care

Plans for the woman's return home and for convalescent care should be completed as early as possible before discharge. Depending on her insurance coverage, nursing care may be provided through a home health agency. If not, the woman and other support individuals must be taught necessary skills and procedures, such as wound care. Ideally the woman and other caregivers should have opportunities for supervised practice before discharge so that they can feel comfortable with their knowledge and ability before being totally responsible for providing care. Box 30-3 lists information that should be included in discharge teaching for the postoperative client. The woman also may need referrals to various community agencies for evaluation of the home situation, child care, home health care, and financial or other assistance.

TRAUMA DURING PREGNANCY

Trauma remains a common complication during pregnancy because most pregnant women in the United States continue their usual activities. Approximately 30,000 pregnant women in the United States experience treatable injuries each year because of trauma (Mozurkewich & Pearlman, 2012).

BOX 30-3 Discharge Teaching for Home Care After Surgery

- Care of incision site
- Diet and elimination related to gastrointestinal (GI) function
- Signs and symptoms of developing complications: wound infection, thrombophlebitis, pneumonia
- Equipment needed and technique for assessing temperature
- Recommended schedule for resumption of activities of daily living
- Treatments and medications ordered
- List of resource individuals and their telephone numbers
- Schedule of follow-up visits

If birth has not occurred:

- Assessment of fetal activity (kick counts)
- Signs of preterm labor

Significance

Approximately 1 in 12 pregnancies are complicated by physical trauma (Mendez-Figueroa, Dahike, Vrees, & Rouse, 2013). As pregnancy progresses the risk of trauma increases because more cases of trauma are reported in the third trimester than earlier in gestation. Most maternal injuries are a result of motor vehicle accidents (MVAs) and falls (Robbins, Martin, & Wilson, 2014), and most maternal deaths are caused by MVAs (Ruth & Miller, 2013). Serious injuries are more likely to occur in an MVA if the woman is not wearing a seat belt with a shoulder harness and is ejected from the vehicle. Therefore, to improve chances of survival for mother and fetus, pregnant women should wear properly positioned restraints at all times when in a motor vehicle (see Fig. 14-17). However, approximately one third of pregnant women do not wear seat belts because of discomfort, inconvenience, or fears of hurting the baby. Other sources of trauma include intimate partner violence, assaults, and suicide attempts (Robbins et al.).

Trauma is the leading cause of death among women of childbearing age. It is also the leading cause of nonobstetric maternal death in the United States (Mendez-Figueroa et al., 2013; Ruth & Miller, 2013). Fetal morbidity and mortality are also significantly affected by maternal trauma. In fact, trauma causes fetal death more often than maternal death (Gilbert, 2011). Fetal death rates related to maternal trauma are reported to be as high as 65% (Ruth & Miller), and this information is probably underreported (Mozurkewich & Pearlman, 2012). Fortunately most trauma injuries during pregnancy are minor and have no effect on pregnancy outcome. However, each case must be evaluated carefully because pregnancy can mask signs of severe injury.

The effect of trauma on pregnancy is influenced by the length of gestation, type and severity of the trauma, and degree of disruption of uterine and fetal physiologic features. Trauma increases the incidence of preterm labor and birth, placental abruption, and fetal or neonatal death (Robbins et al., 2014). Other common fetal effects of trauma include premature rupture of membranes (PROM), fetomaternal transfusion, skull injuries, and hypoxia because of maternal respiratory compromise (Gilbert, 2011).

Special considerations for mother and fetus are necessary when trauma occurs during pregnancy because of the physiologic alterations that accompany pregnancy and because of the presence of the fetus.

Maternal Physiologic Characteristics

Optimal care for the pregnant woman after trauma depends on understanding the physiologic state of pregnancy and its effects on trauma. The pregnant woman's body exhibits responses different from those of a nonpregnant person to the same traumatic insults. Because of this, management strategies must be adapted for appropriate resuscitation, fluid therapy, positioning, assessments, and most other interventions. Significant maternal adaptations and the relation to trauma are summarized in Table 30-2.

The uterus and bladder are confined to the bony pelvis during the first trimester of pregnancy and are at reduced risk for injury in cases of abdominal trauma. After pregnancy progresses beyond the fourteenth week, the uterus becomes an abdominal organ, and the risk for injury in cases of abdominal trauma increases. During the second and third trimesters, the distended bladder becomes an abdominal organ and is at

TABLE 30-2 Maternal Adaptations During Pregnancy and Relation to Trauma

SYSTEM	ALTERATION	CLINICAL RESPONSES
Respiratory	↑ Oxygen consumption	↑ Risk of acidosis
	↑ Tidal volume	↑ Risk of respiratory mismanagement
	↓ Functional residual capacity	
	Chronic compensated alkalosis	↓ Blood-buffering capacity
	↓ $PaCO_2$	
	↓ Serum bicarbonate	
Cardiovascular	↑ Circulating volume, 1600 ml	Can lose 1000 ml blood
	↑ CO	No signs of shock until blood loss >30% total blood volume
	↑ Heart rate	
	↓ SVR	↓ Placental perfusion in supine position
	↓ Arterial blood pressure	
	Heart displaced upward to left	Point of maximal impulse, fourth intercostal space
Renal	↑ Renal plasma flow	
	Dilation of ureters and urethra	↑ Risk of stasis, infection
	Bladder displaced forward	↑ Risk of bladder trauma
Gastrointestinal	↓ Gastric motility	↑ Risk of aspiration
	↑ Hydrochloric acid production	
	↓ Competency of gastroesophageal sphincter	Passive regurgitation of stomach acid if head lower than stomach
Reproductive	↑ Blood flow to organs	Source of ↑ blood loss
	Uterine enlargement	Vena caval compression in supine position
Musculoskeletal	Displacement of abdominal viscera	↑ Risk of injury, altered rebound response
	Pelvic venous congestion	Altered pain referral
	Cartilage softened	↑ Risk of pelvic fracture Center of gravity changed
	Fetal head in pelvis	↑ Risk of fetal injury
Hematologic	↑ Clotting factors	↑ Risk of thrombus formation
	↓ Fibrinolytic activity	

CO, Cardiac output; *$PaCO_2$,* arterial partial pressure of carbon dioxide; *SVR,* systemic vascular resistance.

increased risk for injury and rupture. Bowel injuries occur less often during pregnancy because of the protection provided by the enlarged uterus.

The elevated levels of progesterone that accompany pregnancy relax smooth muscle and profoundly affect the GI tract. GI motility decreases, with a resultant increased time required for gastric emptying, whereas the production of hydrochloric acid increases in the last trimester, and the gastroesophageal sphincter relaxes (Ruth & Miller, 2013). Because of these changes, airway management of the unconscious pregnant woman is critical.

! NURSING ALERT

The unconscious pregnant woman is at increased risk for regurgitation of gastric contents and aspiration whenever her head is positioned lower than her stomach or if abdominal pressure is applied.

A pregnant woman has decreased tolerance for hypoxia and apnea because of her decreased functional residual capacity and increased renal loss of bicarbonate. Acidosis develops more quickly in the pregnant than in the nonpregnant state.

Cardiac output increases 30% to 50% over prepregnancy values and is position dependent in the third trimester. Because of compression of the inferior vena cava and descending aorta by the pregnant uterus, cardiac output decreases dramatically if the woman is placed in the supine position. Therefore, the supine position must be avoided, even in women with cervical spine injuries. It is a primary priority that lateral uterine displacement be accomplished without any head movement. As soon as the neck is immobilized, the stretcher should be tilted laterally (Mozurkewich & Pearlman, 2012; Ruth & Miller, 2013).

Circulating blood volume increases 40% to 50% during gestation. As a result, significant intraabdominal or intrauterine blood loss can occur with only minimal changes in vital signs (Robbins et al., 2014). By the time maternal tachycardia and hypotension, which are considered hallmark symptoms of blood loss, are evident, massive hemorrhage has likely already occurred (Ruth & Miller, 2013).

Fetal Physiologic Characteristics

Perfusion of the uterine arteries, which provide the primary blood supply to the uteroplacental unit, depends on adequate maternal arterial pressure because these vessels lack autoregulation. Therefore, maternal hypotension decreases uterine and fetal perfusion. Maternal shock results in splanchnic and uterine artery vasoconstriction, which decreases blood flow and oxygen transport to the fetus. Electronic fetal monitoring (EFM) tracings can assist in evaluating maternal status after trauma. They reflect fetal cardiac responses to hypoxia and hypoperfusion, including tachycardia or bradycardia, minimal or absent baseline variability, and late decelerations.

Careful monitoring of fetal status assists greatly in maternal assessment because the fetal monitor tracing serves as an "oximeter" of internal maternal well-being. Hypoperfusion may be present in the pregnant woman before the onset of clinical signs of shock. The EFM tracings show the first signs of maternal compromise, such as when maternal heart rate, blood pressure (BP), and color appear normal, yet the EFM printout shows signs of fetal hypoxia (Miller, Miller, & Tucker, 2013).

Mechanisms of Trauma

Blunt Abdominal Trauma

Blunt abdominal trauma is most commonly the result of MVAs but also may be the result of battering or falls. Maternal and fetal mortality and morbidity rates are directly correlated with whether the mother remains inside the vehicle or is ejected. Maternal death is usually the result of a head injury or exsanguination from a major vessel rupture. Serious retroperitoneal hemorrhage after lower abdominal and pelvic trauma is reported more frequently during pregnancy. Serious maternal abdominal injuries are usually the result of splenic rupture or liver or renal injury.

When the mother survives, placental abruption is the most common cause of fetal death (Gilbert, 2011). Placental separation is thought to be a result of deformation of the elastic myometrium around the relatively inelastic placenta. Shearing of the placental edge from the underlying decidua basalis results and is worsened by the increased intrauterine pressure resulting from the impact. It is critical that all pregnant victims be carefully evaluated for signs and symptoms of placental abruption after even minor blunt abdominal trauma.

! NURSING ALERT

Signs and symptoms of placental abruption include uterine tenderness or pain, uterine irritability, uterine contractions, vaginal bleeding, leaking of amniotic fluid, or a change in FHR characteristics.

Pelvic fracture may result from severe injury and may produce bladder trauma or retroperitoneal bleeding with the two-point displacement of pelvic bones that usually occurs. One point of displacement is commonly at the symphysis pubis, and the second point is posterior because of the structure of the pelvis. Careful evaluation for clinical signs of internal hemorrhage is indicated.

Direct fetal injury as a complication of trauma during pregnancy most often involves the fetal skull and brain. Most commonly this injury accompanies maternal pelvic fracture in late gestation, after the fetal head becomes engaged. When the force of the impact is great enough to fracture the maternal pelvis, the fetus often sustains a skull fracture. Evaluation for fetal skull fracture or intracranial hemorrhage is indicated.

Uterine rupture as a result of trauma is rare, occurring in less than 1% of severe cases. Rupture is more likely to occur in a previously scarred uterus. When uterine rupture occurs it is usually associated with a direct blow delivered with substantial force (Cunningham et al., 2014). Traumatic uterine rupture almost always results in fetal death. Maternal death occurs less frequently, in about 30% of cases (Ruth & Miller, 2013).

Penetrating Abdominal Trauma

Bullet and stab wounds are the most frequent causes of penetrating abdominal trauma in pregnant women. When the uterus sustains penetrating wounds, the fetus is more likely than the mother to be seriously injured. The enlarged uterus may protect other maternal organs, particularly the bowel, but the fetus is more vulnerable (Robbins et al., 2014).

Numerous factors determine the extent and severity of maternal and fetal injury from a bullet wound, including size and velocity of the bullet, anatomic region penetrated, angle of entry, path of the bullet, organs damaged, gestational age, and exit wound. Once the bullet enters the body, it may ricochet several times as it encounters organs or bone, or it may sever a large blood vessel. During the second half of pregnancy the fetus usually sustains a direct injury from the bullet. Gunshot wounds require surgical exploration to determine the extent of injury and repair damage as needed.

Stab wounds are limited by the length and width of the penetrating object and are usually confined to the pathway of the weapon. Maternal and fetal injury is less if the stab wound is located in the upper abdomen and from movement of the penetrating object from above the head downward toward the abdomen than from movement of the penetrating object from the ground upward toward the lower abdomen. Stab wounds usually require surgical exploration to clean out debris, determine extent of injury, and repair damage.

Thoracic Trauma

Thoracic trauma is reported to produce 25% of all trauma deaths. Pulmonary contusion results from nearly 75% of blunt thoracic trauma and is a potentially life-threatening condition. Pulmonary contusion can be difficult to recognize, especially if flail chest also is present or if there is no evidence of thoracic injury. Pulmonary contusion should be suspected in cases of thoracic injury, especially after blunt acceleration or deceleration trauma, such as that occurring when a rapidly moving vehicle crashes into an immovable object.

Penetrating wounds into the chest can result in pneumothorax or hemothorax. This type of injury is usually caused by an MVA that results in impalement by the steering column or a loose article in the vehicle that became a projectile with the force of impact. Stab wounds into the chest also may occur as a result of violence.

CARE MANAGEMENT

Immediate Stabilization

Immediate priorities for stabilization of the pregnant woman after trauma should be identical to those of the nonpregnant trauma client. Pregnancy should not result in any restriction of the usual diagnostic, pharmacologic, or resuscitative procedures or maneuvers (AAP & ACOG, 2012). The initial response of many trauma team members when caring for the pregnant woman is to assess fetal status first because of the concern for a healthy neonate. Instead the trauma team should follow a methodic evaluation of maternal status to ensure complete assessment and stabilization of the mother. Fetal survival depends on maternal survival, and stabilizing the mother improves the chance of fetal survival.

SAFETY ALERT

Priorities of care for the pregnant woman after trauma must be to resuscitate the woman and stabilize her condition first and then to consider fetal needs.

Primary Survey

The systematic evaluation begins with a primary survey and the initial CABDs of resuscitation: *c*ompressions, *a*irway, *b*reathing, and *d*efibrillation. Increased oxygen needs during gestation necessitate a rapid response. The presence of a cervical spine injury is always assumed.

SAFETY ALERT

Hyperextension of the neck is avoided; instead jaw thrust is used to establish an airway for the trauma victim.

Once an airway is established, assessment should focus on adequacy of oxygenation. The chest wall is observed for movement. If breathing is absent, ventilations and endotracheal intubation are initiated. Supplemental oxygen should be administered with a tight-fitting, nonrebreathing face mask at 10 to 12 L/min to maintain adequate oxygen availability to the fetus. The chest wall is assessed for penetrating chest wound or flail chest. Breathing with a flail chest is rapid and labored; chest wall movements are uncoordinated and asymmetric; crepitus from bony fragments may be palpated.

Rapid placement of two large-bore (14- to 16-gauge) IV lines is necessary in the majority of seriously injured women. It is important to place the lines while veins are still distended. Cardiac arrest during the immediate stabilization period is usually the result of profound hypovolemia, necessitating massive fluid resuscitation. Infusion of crystalloids such as Ringer's solution or normal saline solution should be given as a 3:1 ratio; that is, 3 ml of crystalloid replacement to 1 ml of the estimated blood loss is given over the first 30 to 60 minutes of acute resuscitation. Because of the 50% increase in blood volume during pregnancy, published formulas for nonpregnant adults used for estimating crystalloid and blood replacement to counter blood loss must be adjusted upward for pregnancy. When severe hemorrhage exists, transfusion with fresh frozen plasma, platelets, and packed red blood cells at a 1:1:1 ratio lowers the rate of coagulopathy and may improve survival (Mendez-Figueroa et al., 2013).

Replacement of red blood cells and other blood components is anticipated, and blood is drawn for type, crossmatch, complete blood cell count, and platelet count. Infusion of type-specific whole blood or packed red blood cells is usually necessary to improve fetal oxygenation status and replace blood loss. During an extreme emergency, type O Rh-negative blood may be administered without matching.

Administering vasopressor drugs to treat maternal hypotension should be avoided if possible. These medications may significantly reduce uterine blood flow and thus decrease oxygen delivery to the fetus. In addition, their use does not address the cause of the hypovolemia (Ruth & Miller, 2013).

After 20 weeks of gestation venous return to the heart is best accomplished by positioning the uterus to one side to eliminate the weight of the uterus compressing the inferior vena cava or the descending aorta. This facilitates efforts to establish the forward flow of blood through resuscitation and stabilization. If a lateral position is not possible because of resuscitative efforts or cervical spine immobilization, the uterus can be manually deflected, or a wedge should be inserted underneath one side of the backboard or stretcher.

Cardiopulmonary Resuscitation of the Pregnant Woman

Trauma, cardiac abnormalities, embolism, magnesium overdose, sepsis, intracranial hemorrhage, anesthetic complications, eclampsia, and uterine rupture are the most common causes of cardiac arrest in a pregnant woman (Robbins et al., 2014). Special modifications are necessary when cardiopulmonary resuscitation (CPR) is performed during the second half of pregnancy. In nonpregnant women chest compressions produce a cardiac output of only about 30% of normal. Cardiac output in pregnant women may be even less as a result of aortocaval compression caused by the gravid uterus. Therefore, uterine displacement during resuscitation efforts is critical (Cunningham et al., 2014). The uterus may be displaced laterally either manually or by placing a wedge, rolled blanket, or towel under one of the woman's hips. If defibrillation is needed, the paddles must be placed one rib interspace higher than usual because the heart is displaced slightly by the enlarged uterus (see the Emergency box).

EMERGENCY

Cardiopulmonary Resuscitation for the Pregnant Woman

Assessment

- Determine unresponsiveness and no breathing or no normal breathing.
- Activate emergency medical system and get AED if available.
- Return to victim and check for pulse.
- Begin chest compressions if no pulse is felt.

Compressions

- Position the woman on a flat, firm surface with her uterus displaced to the left with a wedge (e.g., a rolled towel placed under her hip) or manually or place her in a left lateral position.
- Begin chest compressions at a rate of 100/minute. Push hard and push fast! At the end of each compression allow the chest to recoil (reexpand) completely.
- Chest compressions may be performed slightly higher on the sternum if the uterus is enlarged enough to displace the diaphragm into a higher position.
- After five cycles of 30 compressions and two breaths (or approximately 2 minutes), check for a pulse. If no pulse is present, continue CPR.

Airway

- Open airway using head tilt-chin lift maneuver.

Breathing

- Deliver breaths using a face mask or bag-mask device if possible.
- Deliver each breath over 1 second, watching for chest rise.
- Deliver breaths using a ratio of 30 chest compressions to 2 breaths.

Defibrillation

- Use an AED according to standard protocol to analyze heart rhythm and deliver shock if indicated.

AED, Automated external defibrillator; *CPR,* cardiopulmonary resuscitation
Data from Vanden Hoek, T.L., Morrison, L.J., Shuster, M., et al. (2010). Part 12: Cardiac arrest in special situations: 2010 American Heart Association guidelines for cardiopulmonary resuscitation and emergency cardiovascular care science. *Circulation, 122*(Suppl 3), S829-S861.

Complications, including laceration of the liver, rupture of the spleen or uterus, hemothorax, hemopericardium, or fracture of ribs or sternum may be associated with CPR on a pregnant woman. Fetal complications, including cardiac arrhythmia or asystole related to maternal defibrillation and medications and CNS depression related to antiarrhythmic drugs and inadequate uteroplacental perfusion, with possible fetal hypoxemia and acidemia, also may occur.

If the resuscitation is successful, the woman must be monitored carefully afterward. She remains at increased risk for recurrent cardiac arrest and arrhythmias (e.g., ventricular tachycardia, supraventricular tachycardia, bradycardia). Therefore, her cardiovascular, pulmonary, and neurologic status should be assessed continually. If the pregnancy remains intact, uterine activity and resting tone must be monitored. Fetal status and gestational age should also be determined and used in decision making regarding continuation of the pregnancy or the timing and route of birth.

Another common reason for performing CPR on a pregnant woman is airway obstruction caused by choking. Clearing an airway obstruction is usually accomplished by performing abdominal thrusts. However, during the second and third trimesters, chest thrusts rather than abdominal thrusts should be used (see the Emergency box and Fig. 30-2).

EMERGENCY

Relief of Foreign Body Airway Obstruction

If the pregnant woman is unable to speak or cough, perform chest thrusts. Stand behind her and place your arms under her armpits to encircle her chest. Press backward with quick thrusts until the foreign body is expelled (see Fig. 30-2). If the woman becomes unconscious, carefully support her to the ground, immediately activate EMS, and begin CPR.

EMS, Emergency medical services; *CPR,* cardiopulmonary resuscitation. Data from Berg, R.A., Hemphill, R., Abella, B.S., et al. (2010). Part 5: Adult basic life support: 2010 American Heart Association guidelines for cardiopulmonary resuscitation and emergency cardiovascular care science. *Circulation, 122*(Suppl 3), S685-S705.

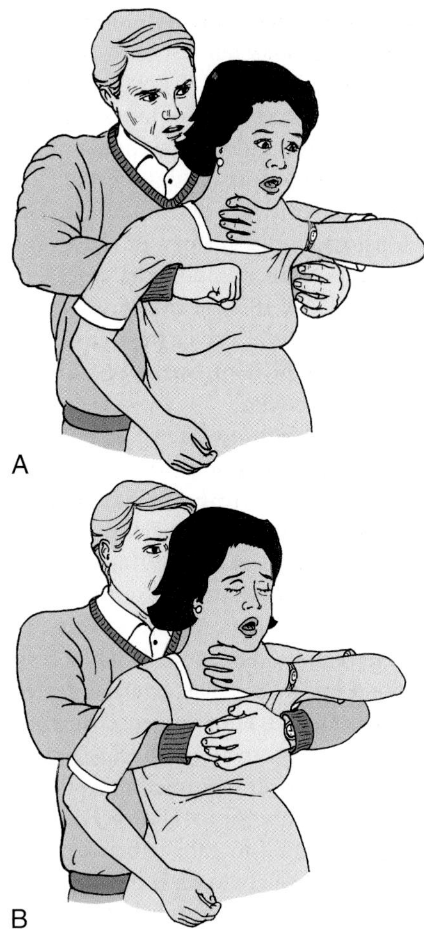

FIG 30-2 Clearing airway obstruction in woman in late stage of pregnancy. **A,** Standing behind victim, place your arms under woman's armpits and across chest. Place thumb side of your clenched fist against middle of sternum, and place other hand over fist. **B,** Perform backward chest thrusts until foreign body is expelled or woman becomes unconscious (see Emergency box: Relief of Foreign Body Airway Obstruction). (Data from Berg, R.A., Hemphill, R., Abella, B.S., et al. (2010). Part 5: Adult basic life support: 2010 American Heart Association guidelines for cardiopulmonary resuscitation and emergency cardiovascular care science. *Circulation, 122*(Suppl 3), S685-S705.)

Secondary Survey

After immediate resuscitation and successful stabilization measures, a more detailed *secondary survey* of the mother and fetus should be accomplished. A complete physical assessment including all body systems is performed.

The maternal abdomen should be evaluated carefully because a large percentage of serious injuries involve the uterus, intraperitoneal structures, and the retroperitoneum. The greatest clinical concern after severe abdominal trauma is placental abruption because as many as 40% of these women have an abruption. If placental abruption occurs, the associated fetal mortality rate can be as high as 50% to 80% (Mozurkewich & Pearlman, 2012). Assessments should focus on recognition of this complication, with careful evaluation of fetal monitor tracings, uterine tenderness, labor, or vaginal bleeding. Ultrasound examination may be performed to determine gestational age, viability of the fetus, and placental location. However, ultrasound studies cannot exclude placental abruption. Most cases of abruption that occur as a result of trauma are associated with relatively minor injuries (Robbins et al., 2014).

If trauma is the result of a penetrating wound, the woman should be completely undressed and carefully examined for all entrance and exit wounds. Focused abdominal ultrasound for trauma (FAST) and CT are commonly used to assess the likelihood of intraabdominal bleeding. Peritoneal lavage is less frequently used because of the availability of FAST, but it can be performed on hemodynamically unstable women to rule out bleeding or gross visceral perforation. Under direct visualization the peritoneum is incised, and a peritoneal dialysis catheter is positioned. If aspiration yields free-flowing blood, the test is considered positive. If not, 1 L of saline is infused into the peritoneal cavity. The recovered lavage fluid is then examined for evidence of blood, bile, or bowel contents. Exploratory laparotomy is recommended if active hemorrhage or bowel perforation is suspected (Robbins et al., 2014).

Exploratory laparotomy is necessary after a gunshot wound to explore the abdominal cavity for organ damage and to repair any damage, with careful examination of all organs, the entire bowel, and posterior vessels. If uterine injury is found, a careful evaluation of the risks and benefits of cesarean birth is quickly accomplished. A cesarean birth is desirable if the fetus is alive and near term and may be necessary for the preterm fetus because of the high incidence of fetal injury in these cases. The fetus usually tolerates surgery and anesthesia if adequate uterine perfusion and oxygenation are maintained. Tetanus prophylaxis guidelines are not changed by pregnancy.

Trauma may affect numerous systems in the maternal body and may affect more than the pregnancy. External signs of maternal trauma should suggest the possibility of internal trauma. Back and neck pain suggest spine injury, abrasions on the chest suggest chest injury, and limb pain and malposition suggest limb fractures. If head injury results in nonresponsiveness, suspect spinal, thoracic, and abdominal injuries. Hypovolemic shock can occur with internal hemorrhage, fracture of long bones, ruptured liver or spleen, hemothorax, or arterial dissection.

All female trauma victims of childbearing age should be considered pregnant until proven otherwise. Determination of the health history and a history of the events preceding the trauma are important components of care. If the pregnant woman was involved in an MVA, it should be determined whether she was the driver or a passenger and if she was ejected from the vehicle or used a restraining device and remained within the vehicle.

Electronic Fetal Monitoring. External FHR and contraction monitoring is recommended after blunt trauma in a viable gestation for a minimum of 4 hours, regardless of injury severity. Fetal monitoring should be initiated soon after the woman is stable (Cunningham et al., 2014; Robbins et al., 2014). Continuous EFM may show early signs of placental abruption, including a change in baseline rate, loss of accelerations, or the presence of late decelerations, especially when accompanied by absent or minimal variability. The external device to monitor uterine activity, the tocodynamometer, is unable to measure pressures, so the pattern made with this device shows the frequency and duration of contractions only. Palpation is required to evaluate the intensity of contractions and the uterine resting tone. It is important to palpate between contractions to verify that the uterus is well relaxed. If the uterus does not relax between contractions, placental abruption could be present.

The exact duration of FHR and contraction monitoring required after blunt abdominal trauma are not known. Monitoring should be continued indefinitely if uterine contractions, abnormal FHR characteristics, vaginal bleeding, uterine tenderness or irritability, serious maternal injury, or ruptured membranes are present (Cunningham et al., 2014). Most physicians recommend continuous monitoring for at least 24 hours because most serious complications appear to develop soon after the traumatic event (Robbins et al., 2014).

> **LEGAL TIP: Care of the Pregnant Woman Involved in a Minor Trauma Situation**
>
> After minor trauma the pregnant woman may be discharged after an adequate period of EFM that demonstrates a normal (category I) tracing (see Chapter 18) and absence of uterine contractions. However, clear instructions must be given for immediate return if vaginal bleeding, leaking of amniotic fluid, decreased fetal movement, or severe abdominal pain occurs.

Fetomaternal Hemorrhage. The potential for fetomaternal hemorrhage exists after trauma. Hemorrhage can lead to fetal anemia, distress, or even death. If the pregnant trauma victim is Rh negative, fetomaternal hemorrhage can result in sensitization and hemolytic disease of the neonate. The Kleihauer-Betke assay is often performed in women following blunt abdominal trauma to estimate the amount of fetal blood within the maternal circulation. Because most cases have less than 30 ml of hemorrhage, however, Kleihauer-Betke test results seldom alter management (Cunningham et al., 2014; Robbins et al., 2014). Usually the routine administration of 300 mcg of Rh_o(D) immune globulin is sufficient to protect almost all Rh-negative pregnant trauma clients from isoimmunization (Mozurkewich & Pearlman, 2012).

Ultrasound. Ultrasonography after trauma is not as sensitive as EFM for diagnosing placental abruption. Ultrasound may be useful to help establish gestational age, locate the placenta, evaluate cardiac activity (to determine whether the fetus is alive), and determine amniotic fluid volume. It also may be used to evaluate the presence of intraabdominal fluid that would suggest the presence of intraabdominal hemorrhage.

Radiation Exposure. If the pregnant woman has sustained serious injuries, any necessary radiographic examination should be performed, regardless of fetal exposure. If radiographic examination would be performed for the nonpregnant trauma victim, it also should be performed for the pregnant woman. Abdominal or pelvic CT scanning can be used to visualize extraperitoneal and retroperitoneal structures and the genitourinary tract. Radiation exposure of less than 5 rads has not been associated with fetal abnormalities or pregnancy loss, and the radiation level associated with abdominal or pelvic CT scans is far below this amount (Robbins et al., 2014). Blunt head trauma and loss of consciousness necessitate skull films and CT assessment with neurosurgical consultation. MRI also can safely be used to assess injuries because it does not produce ionizing radiation (Robbins et al.).

Perimortem Cesarean Birth. In the presence of multisystem trauma, perimortem cesarean birth may be indicated. Removal of the stressor of pregnancy early in the process of resuscitation may increase the chance for an intact neonatal outcome and also improve maternal resuscitative efforts (Robbins et al., 2014). Therefore, a cesarean birth should be performed after 4 minutes of resuscitative efforts if there is no spontaneous return of circulation (Mozurkewich & Pearlman, 2012; Robbins et al., 2014; Ruth & Miller, 2013). It should be emphasized that perimortem cesarean birth is rarely successful, especially when the maternal arrest is related to trauma (Ruth & Miller).

KEY POINTS

- The normal hemodynamic values are significantly altered as a result of pregnancy.
- The stress of the normal maternal adaptations to pregnancy on a heart whose function is already taxed may cause cardiac decompensation.
- Maternal morbidity and mortality are significant risks in a pregnancy complicated by mitral stenosis.
- Anemia, a common medical disorder of pregnancy, affects at least 20% of pregnant women.
- Asthma is a common medical condition to complicate pregnancy, and the prevalence and morbidity from this disorder are increasing.
- Pruritus is a common symptom in pregnancy-specific inflammatory skin diseases.

- A pregnant woman with epilepsy should take only one anticonvulsant medication at the lowest dose level that is effective at keeping her seizure free.
- Autoimmune disorders can occur during pregnancy because a large percentage of people with an autoimmune disorder are women of childbearing age. Common autoimmune diseases include SLE and MG.
- Cholecystitis and cholelithiasis are common GI problems in pregnancy.
- UTIs are a common medical complication of pregnancy.
- Pyelonephritis is the most common serious medical complication of pregnancy and the leading cause of septic shock during pregnancy.
- In the pregnant woman, an enlarged uterus, displaced internal organs, and altered laboratory values may confuse the diagnosis when the need for immediate abdominal surgery occurs.
- Perioperative care for a pregnant woman differs from that for a nonpregnant woman in one significant aspect: the presence of at least one other person, the fetus.
- The active roles assumed by most pregnant women today place them at risk for vehicular crashes, falls, violence, and other injuries.
- Pregnancy does not limit or restrict resuscitative, diagnostic, or pharmacologic treatment after trauma.
- Fetal survival depends on maternal survival. After trauma the first priority, before consideration of fetal concerns, is to resuscitate and stabilize the mother.
- Optimal care for the pregnant victim of trauma depends on knowledge of the physiologic state of pregnancy.
- Minor trauma can be associated with major complications for the pregnancy, including placental abruption, fetomaternal hemorrhage, preterm labor and birth, and fetal death.
- Trauma from accidents is the most common cause of death in women of childbearing age.
- In the case of a cardiac arrest in a pregnant woman, the standard advanced cardiac life support guidelines should be implemented with a few slight modifications: the uterus must be displaced to the left, and the defibrillation paddles should be placed one rib interspace higher.

REFERENCES

American Academy of Pediatrics (AAP) & American College of Obstetricians and Gynecologists (ACOG). (2012). *Guidelines for perinatal care* (7th ed.). Washington, DC: ACOG.

Aminoff, M. J., & Douglas, V. C. (2014). Neurologic disorders. In R. K. Creasy, R. Resnik, J. D. Iams, et al. (Eds.), *Creasy and Resnik's maternal-fetal medicine: Principles and practice* (7th ed.). Philadelphia: Saunders.

Blackburn, S. (2013). *Maternal, fetal, and neonatal physiology: A clinical perspective* (4th ed.). St. Louis: Saunders.

Blanchard, D. G., & Daniels, L. B. (2014). Cardiac diseases. In R. K. Creasy, R. Resnik, J. D. Iams, et al. (Eds.), *Creasy and Resnik's maternal-fetal medicine: Principles and practice* (7th ed.). Philadelphia: Saunders.

Cappell, M. (2012). Hepatic and gastrointestinal diseases. In S. Gabbe, J. Niebyl, & J. Simpson (Eds.), *Obstetrics: Normal and problem pregnancies* (6th ed.). Philadelphia: Saunders.

Chin, J. R., & Branch, D. W. (2012). Collagen vascular diseases. In S. Gabbe, J. Niebyl, & J. Simpson (Eds.), *Obstetrics: Normal and problem pregnancies* (6th ed.). Philadelphia: Saunders.

Colombo, D. (2012). Renal disease. In S. Gabbe, J. Niebyl, & J. Simpson (Eds.), *Obstetrics: Normal and problem pregnancies* (6th ed.). Philadelphia: Saunders.

Cunningham, F., Leveno, K., Bloom, S., et al. (2014). *Williams obstetrics* (24th ed.). New York: McGraw-Hill Education.

Denney, J. M., Porter, T. F., & Branch, D. W. (2011). Autoimmune diseases. In D. James, P. Steer, C. Weiner, & B. Gonik (Eds.), *High risk pregnancy: Management options* (4th ed.). Philadelphia: Saunders.

Duff, P. (2014). Maternal and fetal infections. In R. K. Creasy, R. Resnik, J. D. Iams, et al. (Eds.), *Creasy and Resnik's maternal-fetal medicine: Principles and practice* (7th ed.). Philadelphia: Saunders.

Easterling, T., & Stout, K. (2012). Heart disease. In S. Gabbe, J. Niebyl, J. Simpson, et al. (Eds.), *Obstetrics: Normal and problem pregnancies* (6th ed.). Philadelphia: Saunders.

Gaddipati, S., & Troiano, N. (2013). Cardiac disorders in pregnancy. In N. Troiano, C. Harvey, & B. Chez (Eds.), *AWHONN's high risk and critical care obstetrics* (3rd ed.). Philadelphia: Wolters Kluwer/Lippincott Williams & Wilkins.

Gibson, P. S., & Powrie, R. (2011). Respiratory diseases. In D. James, P. Steer, C. Weiner, & B. Gonik (Eds.), *High risk pregnancy: Management options* (4th ed.). Philadelphia: Saunders.

Gilbert, E. (2011). *Manual of high risk pregnancy & delivery* (5th ed.). St. Louis: Mosby.

Gordon, M. (2012). Maternal physiology. In S. Gabbe, J. Niebyl, J. Simpson, et al. (Eds.), *Obstetrics: Normal and problem pregnancies* (6th ed.). Philadelphia: Saunders.

Kelly, T. F., & Savides, T. J. (2014). Gastrointestinal disease in pregnancy. In R. K. Creasy, R. Resnik, J. D. Iams, et al. (Eds.), *Creasy and Resnik's maternal-fetal medicine: Principles and practice* (7th ed.). Philadelphia: Saunders.

Kilpatrick, S. J. (2014). Anemia and pregnancy. In R. K. Creasy, R. Resnik, J. D. Iams, et al. (Eds.), *Creasy and Resnik's maternal-fetal medicine: Principles and practice* (7th ed.). Philadelphia: Saunders.

Kroumpouzos, G. (2012). Skin disease in pregnancy and puerperium. In S. Gabbe, J. Niebyl, J. Simpson, et al. (Eds.), *Obstetrics: Normal and problem pregnancies* (6th ed.). Philadelphia: Saunders.

Lawrence, R. A., & Lawrence, R. M. (2011). *Breastfeeding: A guide for the medical profession* (7th ed.). St. Louis: Mosby.

Lockshin, M. D., Salmon, J. E., & Erkan, D. (2014). Pregnancy and rheumatic diseases. In R. K. Creasy, R. Resnik, J. D. Iams, et al. (Eds.), *Creasy and Resnik's maternal-fetal medicine: Principles and practice* (7th ed.). Philadelphia: Saunders.

Mahomed, K. (2011). Abdominal pain. In D. James, P. Steer, C. Weiner, & B. Gonik (Eds.), *High risk pregnancy: Management options* (4th ed.). Philadelphia: Saunders.

Martin, S., Hill, A. J., & Foley, M. (2012). Cardiac disease. In J. Queenan, C. Lockwood, & C. Spong (Eds.), *Queenan's management of high-risk pregnancy: An evidenced-based approach* (6th ed.). Hoboken, NJ: Wiley.

Mendez-Figueroa, H., Dahike, J. D., Vrees, R. A., & Rouse, D. J. (2013). Trauma in pregnancy: An updated systematic review. *American Journal of Obstetrics and Gynecology, 209*(1), 1-10.

Miller, L., Miller, D., & Tucker, S. (2013). *Mosby's pocket guide to fetal monitoring: A multidisciplinary approach* (7th ed.). St. Louis: Mosby.

Mozurkewich, E., & Pearlman, M. (2012). Trauma and related surgery in pregnancy. In S. Gabbe, J. Niebyl, J. Simpson, et al. (Eds.), *Obstetrics: Normal and problem pregnancies* (6th ed.). Philadelphia: Saunders.

National Marfan Association. (2013). *Frequently asked questions on Marfan syndrome*. Available at www.marfan.org/marfan/2448/Pregnancy-and-Reproduction.

Otten, J. J., Helwig, J. P., & Meyers, L. D. (Eds.). (2006). *Dietary reference intakes: The essential guide to nutrient requirements*. Washington, DC: National Academies Press.

Rapini, R. (2014). The skin and pregnancy. In R. K. Creasy, R. Resnik, J. D. Iams, et al. (Eds.), *Creasy and Resnik's maternal-fetal medicine: Principles and practice* (7th ed.). Philadelphia: Saunders.

Robbins, K. S., Martin, S. R., & Wilson, W. C. (2014). Intensive care considerations for the critically ill parturient. In R. K. Creasy, R. Resnik, J. D. Iams, et al. (Eds.), *Creasy and Resnik's maternal-fetal medicine: Principles and practice* (7th ed.). Philadelphia: Saunders.

Roos-Hesselink, J. W., Ruys, P. T. E., & Johnson, M. R. (2013). Pregnancy in adult congenital heart disease. *Current* Cardiology Reports, *15*(9), 401.

Ruth, D., & Miller, R. S. (2013). Trauma in pregnancy. In N. Troiano, C. Harvey, & B. Chez (Eds.), *AWHONN's high risk and critical care obstetrics* (3rd ed.). Philadelphia: Wolters Kluwer/Lippincott Williams & Wilkins.

Samuels, P. (2012). Hematologic complications of pregnancy. In S. Gabbe, J. Niebyl, & J. Simpson (Eds.), *Obstetrics: Normal and problem pregnancies* (6th ed.). Philadelphia: Saunders.

Samuels, P., & Niebyl, J. (2012). Neurologic disorders. In S. Gabbe, J. Niebyl, & J. Simpson (Eds.), *Obstetrics: Normal and problem pregnancies* (6th ed.). Philadelphia: Saunders.

Simhan, H. N., Berghella, V., & Iams, J. D. (2014). Preterm labor and birth. In R. K. Creasy, R. Resnik, J. D. Iams, et al. (Eds.), *Creasy and Resnik's maternal-fetal medicine: Principles and practice* (7th ed.). Philadelphia: Saunders.

Simhan, H., Iams, J., & Romero, R. (2012). Preterm birth. In S. Gabbe, J. Niebyl, & J. Simpson (Eds.), *Obstetrics: Normal and problem pregnancies* (6th ed.). Philadelphia: Saunders.

Stuart, M., & Bergstrom, L. (2011). Pregnancy and multiple sclerosis. *Journal of Midwifery & Women's Health, 56*(1), 41–47.

Tomlinson, M. (2011). Cardiac disease. In D. James, P. Steer, C. Weiner, & B. Gonik (Eds.), *High risk pregnancy: Management options* (4th ed.). Philadelphia: Saunders.

Whitty, J., & Dombrowski, M. (2012). Respiratory diseases in pregnancy. In S. Gabbe, J. Niebyl, & J. Simpson (Eds.), *Obstetrics: Normal and problem pregnancies* (6th ed.). Philadelphia: Saunders.

Whitty, J. E., & Dombrowski, M. P. (2014). Respiratory diseases in pregnancy. In R. K. Creasy, R. Resnik, J. D. Iams, et al. (Eds.), *Creasy and Resnik's maternal-fetal medicine: Principles and practice* (7th ed.). Philadelphia: Saunders.

Williamson, C., Mackillop, L., & Heneghan, M. A. (2014). Diseases of the liver, biliary system, and pancreas. In R. K. Creasy, R. Resnik, J. D. Iams, et al. (Eds.), *Creasy and Resnik's maternal-fetal medicine: Principles and practice* (7th ed.). Philadelphia: Saunders.

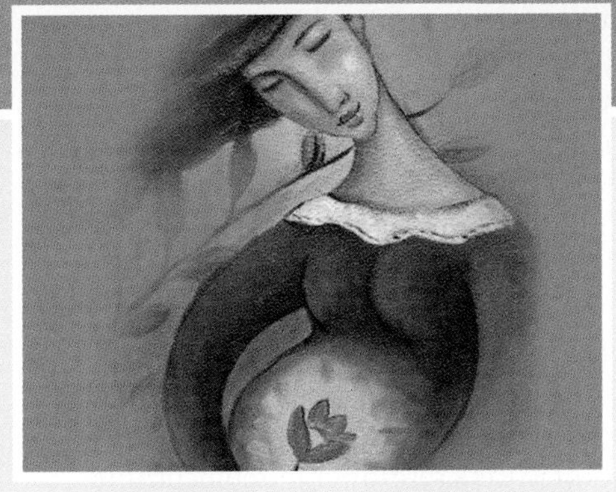

CHAPTER 31

Mental Health Disorders and Substance Abuse

Jan Sherman

http://evolve.elsevier.com/Lowdermilk/MWHC/

LEARNING OBJECTIVES

- Describe mental health disorders occurring in the perinatal period, including mood disorders, anxiety disorders, post-traumatic stress disorder, and bipolar disorder.
- Compare postpartum blues, postpartum depression, and postpartum psychosis including risk factors, assessment, and management.
- Evaluate the role of the nurse in caring for women with mental health disorders during pregnancy and the postpartum period.
- Examine substance abuse during pregnancy, including prevalence, barriers to treatment, legal considerations, and commonly abused drugs.
- Discuss the care of pregnant women who use, abuse, or are dependent on alcohol or illicit or prescription drugs.

This chapter covers the most common maternal mental health disorders: perinatal mood disorders, anxiety disorders, postpartum depression, and postpartum psychosis, which usually manifests as bipolar disorder. Issues related to substance abuse during pregnancy also are discussed.

MENTAL HEALTH DISORDERS DURING PREGNANCY

Management of mental health disorders takes place primarily in community settings. Compared with births in the general non–mentally ill population, women with mental illness who give birth have a higher risk of obstetric complications (Thornton, Guendelman, & Hosang, 2009). However, mentally ill women who are treated are at lower risk than women who are not treated.

Perinatal mental illness has been recognized and discussed throughout history. In the 19th century, medical interest in perinatal mental illness accelerated, along with more general interest in severe mental illness (O'Hara & Wisner, 2014).

Women are at the greatest risk for developing a psychiatric disorder between the ages of 18 and 45 years—the childbearing years. Women who have serious mental disorders may be engaging in sexual activities that can result in pregnancy. The pregnant woman may have a history of disorder in mood, anxiety, substance use, schizophrenia, personality, or development. Assessment throughout pregnancy and the postpartum period is critical to the mother's and the baby's health. With a history or current symptoms of mental illness, referral to a mental health care provider for evaluation is recommended. Mental health disorders have implications for the pregnant woman, the fetus, the newborn, and the entire family.

Perinatal Mood Disorders

Although the general public commonly uses the term *depression*, the term connotes a range of disorders that are collectively termed mood disorders (Yonkers, Vigod, & Ross, 2011). **Perinatal mood disorders (PMDs)** are a set of disorders that can occur any time during pregnancy as well as in the first year postpartum and can include depression, anxiety, obsessive-compulsive disorder, post-traumatic stress disorder (PTSD), and postpartum psychosis.

Depression *during* pregnancy is a major risk factor for postpartum depression (PPD). Postpartum depression has been associated with negative effects on child development, including a difficult infant and childhood temperament, attachment insecurity, and increased risk of developmental delay and lower IQ scores. A substantial rate of suicide occurs postpartum, because maternal suicide accounts for up to 20% of postpartum deaths in depressed women (Wisner, Sit, Altemus, et al., 2012).

Prevalence

Perinatal mental health problems are common worldwide. Clinical depression is common among reproductive-age women and is a leading cause of disability in U.S. women each year. Between 14% and 23% of pregnant women will experience depression symptoms during pregnancy. An estimated 5% to 25% of women will have PPD. In high-income countries, about 10% of pregnant women and 13% of women who have just given birth experience a mental disorder, primarily depression or anxiety. Depression accounts for $30 to $50 billion in lost productivity and direct medical costs in the United States each year. Higher rates of common perinatal mental disorders have also been seen among women from low- and lower-middle-income countries (American Academy of Pediatrics [AAP] & American College of Obstetricians and Gynecologists [ACOG], 2012, Rahman, Fisher, Bower, et al., 2013).

Studies have shown that untreated maternal depression can negatively affect an infant's cognitive, neurologic, and motor skill development. A mother's untreated depression can also negatively affect older children's mental health and behavior. During pregnancy depression can lead to preeclampsia, preterm birth, and low birth weight (AAP & ACOG, 2012; ACOG, 2010; Mikacich, 2014).

Diagnosis

A mood disorder that emerges during childbearing requires a thorough medical and family history, review of systems, and complete physical examination. The use of prescribed and over-the-counter medications as well as commonly abused substances must be assessed. Thyroid abnormalities and anemia, which are common in childbearing women, should be ruled out (AAP & ACOG, 2012; Yonkers et al., 2011).

To be diagnosed with major depression, at least five of the following signs or symptoms must be present nearly every day: depressed mood, often with spontaneous crying; markedly diminished interest in all activities; insomnia or hypersomnia; weight changes (increases or decreases); psychomotor retardation or agitation; fatigue or loss of energy; feelings of worthlessness or inappropriate guilt; diminished ability to concentrate; and suicidal ideation with or without a suicidal plan (American Psychiatric Association [APA], 2013). The 10-item Edinburgh Postnatal Depression Scale (see later discussion) accurately identifies depression in pregnant and postpartum women (Sadock, Sadock, & Ruiz, 2009).

! NURSING ALERT

Diagnostic assessment for depression in pregnant women is difficult because many of the symptoms of pregnancy mimic depression. Critical cues are the presence of psychologic symptoms, a suicide plan, and major disruptions in sleep pattern. Risk factors for developing depression in pregnancy include a prior history in self or family, a lack of social support, stressful life events, partner discord, and history of premenstrual syndrome (PMS).

CARE MANAGEMENT

Medical management of depression is usually a combination of antidepressants and cognitive-behavioral therapy (CBT) or interpersonal psychotherapy (IPT). For mild cases of depression in pregnant women, psychotherapy is the treatment of choice as the initial intervention. Both IPT and CBT are time-limited treatments (usually 10 to 12 sessions) that focus on present problems and encourage the woman to regain control over her mood and functioning. Short-term therapies, such as CBT, may be delivered by psychiatrists and non-physician professionals such as psychologists, psychiatric nurse clinical specialists or practitioners, or licensed clinical social workers (Guille, Newman, Fryml, et al., 2013; Wisner et al., 2012).

Self-help strategies such as exercise, respite from caregiving, self-help groups, and making time for one's self can be helpful.

Antidepressant Medications. It is estimated that more than 6% of women are prescribed an antidepressant at some point during pregnancy (Ray & Stowe, 2014). No consensus exists regarding safety in the use of antidepressant medications by pregnant women. To date, the U.S. Food and Drug Administration (FDA) has not approved any psychotropic medication for use during pregnancy. None of these medications is rated as an FDA Category A drug (controlled studies show no risk to the fetus) (see Box 31-1 for FDA pregnancy risk categories of most common antidepressant medications). The commonly used antidepressant drugs are often divided into four groups: selective serotonin reuptake inhibitors (SSRIs), serotonin/norepinephrine reuptake inhibitors (SNRIs), tricyclic antidepressants (TCAs), and monoamine oxidase inhibitors (MAOIs). The most common antidepressants are listed in Table 31-1.

Because the majority of women are not aware of their pregnancy until at least 6 weeks of gestation, psychotropic medications may not be discontinued until after the period of greatest potential risk to the fetus has passed. Risk-benefit analyses of depression treatment options should consider the potential risks that can accrue if depressive episodes go untreated in the pregnant woman. Risks include severe psychologic distress, suicide, financial hardships, and inability to plan for transition to parenthood. Most women who discontinue antidepressant medications relapse during pregnancy. The majority of relapses occurs in the first trimester, and relapse is more prevalent in women with

BOX 31-1 FDA Pregnancy Risk Categories

Category A
Adequate and well-controlled studies have failed to demonstrate a risk to the fetus in the first trimester of pregnancy (and there is no evidence of risk in later trimesters).

Category B
Animal reproduction studies have failed to demonstrate a risk to the fetus and there are no adequate and well-controlled studies in pregnant women.

Category C
Animal reproduction studies have shown an adverse effect on the fetus and there are no adequate and well-controlled studies in humans, but potential benefits may warrant use of the drug in pregnant women despite potential risks.

Category D
There is positive evidence of human fetal risk based on adverse reaction data from investigational or marketing experience or studies in humans, but potential benefits may warrant use of the drug in pregnant women despite potential risks.

Category X
Studies in animals or humans have demonstrated fetal abnormalities and/or there is positive evidence of human fetal risk based on adverse reaction data from investigational or marketing experience, and the risks involved in use of the drug in pregnant women clearly outweigh potential benefits.

Category N
FDA has not classified drug

FDA, U.S. Food and Drug Administration.
From www.drugs.com. (2014). *FDA categories A,B,C,D,X,N explained.* Available at www.drugs.com/pregnancy-categories.html.

histories of chronic depression. Because randomized clinical trial data regarding the relative safety of available psychotropic medications are unavailable, clinical decision making is complicated.

Concerns regarding the safety of antidepressant medications are common (Ray & Stowe, 2014). However, untreated depression can also cause adverse effects on the developing fetus and neonate, such as preterm birth, small head circumference, and low Apgar scores. For women with a diagnosis of major depression, treatment with antidepressants is appropriate. Use of antidepressants, including SSRIs, is indicated for vegetative signs accompanying a major depressive episode (MDE) that do not resolve with supportive interventions. There is a lack of definitive evidence to demonstrate a statistically significant association between fetal exposure to anti-depressant medications and congenital abnormalities, although isolated cases have been reported (Box 31-2). Reports have linked third-trimester

TABLE 31-1 Antidepressant Medications

	PREGNANCY RISK CATEGORY*	LACTATION RISK CATEGORY*
Selective Serotonin Reuptake Inhibitors (SSRIs)		
Citalopram (Celexa)	C	L3
Escitalopram (Lexapro)	C	L3 in older infants
Fluoxetine (Prozac)	C	L2 in older infants; L3 in neonates
Fluvoxamine (Luvox)	C	L2
Paroxetine (Paxil)	D	L2
Sertraline (Zoloft)	C	L2
Serotonin/Norepinephrine Reuptake Inhibitors (SNRIs)		
Bupropion (Wellbutrin) IR & SR	B	L3
Maprotiline (Ludiomil)	B	L3
Mirtazapine (Remeron)	C	L3
Trazodone (Desyrel)	C	L2
Venlafaxine (Effexor)	C	L3
Tricyclic Antidepressants (TCAs)		
Amitriptyline (Elavil)	D	L2
Amoxapine (Asendin)	C	L2
Clomipramine (Anafranil)	C	L2
Desipramine (Norpramin)	C	L2
Doxepin (Sinequan)	C	L5
Imipramine (Tofranil)	D	L2
Nortriptyline (Pamelor)	D	L2
Monoamine Oxidase Inhibitors (MAOIs)		
Phenelzine (Nardil)	C	Unknown
Tranylcypromine (Parnate)	C	Unknown

B = Animal studies have not shown fetal risk, but no controlled studies in pregnant women *or* animal studies showed adverse effect that was not confirmed in controlled studies in women in first trimester—no risk in later trimesters.
C = Animal studies show adverse effects on fetus, but no controlled studies in pregnant women *or* no studies available.
D = Positive evidence of human fetal risk.
L2 = Drug studied in limited number of breastfeeding women without an increase in adverse effects in infant *or* risk is remote.
L3 = No controlled studies in breastfeeding women *or* studies show minimal nonthreatening adverse effects.
L5 = Contraindicated because studies have shown significant and documented risk to infant.
IR, Intermediate release; *SR*, sustained release.
*From Hale, T. (2012). *Medications and mother's milk* (15th ed.). Amarillo, TX: Pharmasoft; Schatzberg, A., Cole, J.O., DeBattista, C. (Eds.). (2010). *Manual of clinical psychopharmacology* (7th ed.). Arlington, VA: American Psychiatric Publishing.

BOX 31-2 SSRIs: Effects on Pregnancy and Birth Defects

Intrauterine Fetal Demise and Miscarriage
Studies to support an association between miscarriage rates and antidepressant use have inadequate control for confounding variables related to the depressive disorder. There is no evidence that the rate of stillbirths is increased during antidepressant treatment (Wisner, Sit, Altemus, et al., 2012).

Physical Malformations
The majority of studies does not demonstrate an association between tricyclic antidepressants (TCAs) and birth defects. Similarly, studies of first-trimester selective serotonin reuptake inhibitor (SSRI) exposure do not demonstrate consistent data to support a risk for structural malformations (Wisner et al., 2012).

Persistent Pulmonary Hypertension of the Newborn (PPHN)
Grigoriadis, VonderPorten, and Ross (2014) found that the risk of PPHN seems to be increased for infants exposed to SSRIs in late pregnancy. A significant relation for exposure to SSRIs in early pregnancy was not evident.

Poor Neonatal Adaptation Syndrome
Infants who are exposed in late pregnancy to SSRI or serotonin/norepinephrine reuptake inhibitors (SNRIs) have a 10% to 30% rate of poor neonatal adaptation syndrome, which often is proven to be associated with low systemic levels of the antidepressants. Although most signs of this neonatal syndrome resemble neonatal withdrawal from opioids, benzodiazepines, and ethanol, in some cases SSRI withdrawal is associated with respiratory failure that necessitates short-term respiratory support, which is unique to the SSRIs and SNRIs (Ornoy & Koren, 2013).

Neonatal Seizures
Hayes, Wu, Shelton, et al. (2013) found that third-trimester SSRI use is associated with infant convulsions within the first 14 days of life.

Cardiac Defects
The association of SSRI use and neonatal cardiac defects, in particular septal defects, has been of concern. However, Margulis, Abou-Ali, Strazzeri, et al. (2013) found no association between maternal use of SSRIs in early pregnancy and cardiac malformations or septal defects.

Data from Grigoriadis, S., VonderPorten, E.H., & Ross, L.E. (2014). Prenatal exposure to antidepressants and persistent pulmonary hypertension of the newborn: Systematic review and meta-analysis. *British Medical Journal,* 348:f6932; Hayes, R.M., Wu, P., Shelton, R.C., et al. (2012). Maternal antidepressant use and adverse outcomes: A cohort study of 228,876 pregnancies. *American Journal of Obstetrics and Gynecology, 207*(1), 49.e1-49.e9; Margulis, A.V., Abou-Ali, A., Strazzeri, M.M., et al. (2013). Use of selective serotonin reuptake inhibitors in pregnancy and cardiac malformations: A propensity-score matched cohort in CPRD. *Pharmacoepidemiology and Drug Safety, 22*(9), 942-951; Ornoy, A., & Koren, G. (2014). Selective serotonin reuptake inhibitors in human pregnancy: On the way to resolving the controversy. *Seminars in Fetal & Neonatal Medicine, 19*(3), 188-194; Wisner, K.L., Sit, D.K.Y., Altemus, M., et al. (2012). Mental health and behavioral disorders in pregnancy. In S.G. Gabbe, J.R. Niebyl, J.L. Simpson, et al. (Eds.), *Obstetrics: Normal and problem pregnancies* (6th ed.). Philadelphia: Saunders.

use of SSRIs by pregnant women to a constellation of neonatal signs that include continuous crying, irritability, jitteriness, and restlessness; shivering; fever; tremors; hypertonia or rigidity; tachypnea or respiratory distress; feeding difficulty; sleep disturbance; hypoglycemia; and seizures. The onset of these signs ranged from several hours to several days after birth and usually resolved within 1 to 2 weeks (Hudak, Tan, & AAP, 2012). Paroxetine has been associated with ventricular septal defects for first-trimester exposure; venlafaxine has been associated with a poor neonatal adaptation syndrome and mirtazapine with greater risk of preterm birth (Sadock et al., 2009).

Although less information is known regarding the use of SSRIs during pregnancy compared with the use of TCAs, this class of drugs is emerging as first-line agents in treatment (Ray & Stowe, 2014). They are relatively safe and carry fewer side effects than the TCAs. However, if an SSRI is taken with dextromethorphan, an agent found in cough syrup, the combination could trigger the serotonin syndrome (e.g., mental status changes, agitation, hyperreflexia, shivering, and diarrhea). The most frequent side effects with the SSRIs are gastrointestinal (GI) disturbances (e.g., nausea and diarrhea), headache, and insomnia. SSRIs also can inhibit specific P-450 isoenzymes, resulting in a marked elevation in drug concentration and a reduction in drug clearance.

The TCAs cause many central nervous system (CNS) and peripheral nervous system side effects. In overdose, these medications can cause death. A common CNS effect is sedation. Other side effects include weight gain, tremors, grand mal seizures, nightmares, agitation or mania, and extrapyramidal side effects. Anticholinergic side effects include dry mouth, blurred vision (usually temporary), difficulty voiding, constipation, sweating, and difficulty with orgasm.

The use of MAOIs during pregnancy is contraindicated because of the risk for fetal growth restriction. In animals hypertension with subsequent placental hypoperfusion and complications with anesthesia during labor have been reported (Sadock et al., 2009).

Nursing Interventions

Nursing strategies include educating the woman about depression as an illness and the plan of care, including medications. For the woman who refuses medications during pregnancy, the nurse should discuss alternative treatments and respect her choice. The nurse also can be effective by maintaining a caring relationship, which includes being hopeful. The nurse can ask about a time when the woman was coping well and how she was able to combat the depression then.

ANXIETY DISORDERS

Anxiety disorders are the most common psychiatric disorders, and some (e.g., panic disorder, generalized anxiety disorder, PTSD, agoraphobia) are twice as likely to be diagnosed in women compared with men. Anxiety and stress during pregnancy are associated with miscarriage, preterm birth, and birth complications, although a direct causal relationship has not been established (Glover, 2014).

Anxiety disorders are characterized by prominent symptoms of anxiety that impair functioning. Examples are obsessive-compulsive disorder (OCD), PTSD, generalized anxiety disorder, panic disorder, agoraphobia, and other phobias (Wisner et al., 2012).

Diagnosis

Panic attacks are characterized by brief (5 to 15 minutes), intense episodes of fear or discomfort. Panic attacks occur in a variety of anxiety disorders, as well as in healthy individuals exposed to acute stress. Symptoms include palpitations, sweating, shortness of breath, choking, nausea, abdominal discomfort, dizziness, unsteadiness, numbness or tingling, chills, hot flashes, or a fear of dying or losing control (Wisner et al., 2012).

Panic disorder is diagnosed if panic attacks are recurrent or associated with a continuing fear of future attacks, which results in anxiety between attacks. The most disabling consequence of panic disorder, agoraphobia, occurs in 30% to 40% of women with untreated panic disorder. Individuals with agoraphobia restrict their activities outside the home or insist on being accompanied by another individual due to fear of having a panic attack where help is unavailable (Wisner et al., 2012).

Generalized anxiety disorder is characterized by excessive worrying about multiple problems. The issues of concern to people with generalized anxiety disorder are realistic but the level of worry is much more intense than appropriate. For example, a woman might worry for hours about whether a friend received a thank-you note for a baby shower gift (Wisner et al., 2012). The pregnant woman also may have persistent thoughts that something is wrong with the fetus.

Individuals with generalized anxiety disorder often have physical symptoms associated with worrying, such as muscle tension, fatigue, headache, nausea, diarrhea, or abdominal pain. To meet criteria for the disorder, individuals must have significant impairment of functioning and anxiety for at least 6 months (Wisner et al., 2012).

PTSD can occur as a result of rape or intimate partner violence (see Chapter 5). Symptoms include reexperiencing the traumatic event, persistent avoidance of stimuli, and numbing, as well as difficulty sleeping, irritability or angry outbursts, difficulty concentrating, hypervigilance, and exaggerated startle response. Nurses can support the healing process of individuals with PTSD by being alert to what the woman is experiencing during pregnancy and labor.

If the current pregnancy is a result of rape, the woman may be extremely ambivalent about the baby. If the rape occurred some time ago, the whole experience of pregnancy with prenatal visits and physical examinations can trigger memories of the original trauma. She may avoid prenatal care because of the anxiety triggered by bodily touch and vaginal examinations. Some pregnant women with PTSD may feel more comfortable with a female nurse-midwife or a female physician. Giving birth can trigger memories of being out of control, and she may lose contact with reality. The nurse can verbalize understanding of the anxiety and orient the woman to current reality by saying, "You're having an examination to make sure the baby is okay," or, "You're in labor preparing to give birth to your baby. I am your nurse. You're in the hospital. I will check on you frequently. You are safe here." Treatment usually includes psychotherapy and referral to support groups.

CARE MANAGEMENT

When anxiety substantially impairs work, family, or social adjustment, mental health evaluation is indicated and treatment is appropriate. Generalized anxiety disorder responds to a variety of antidepressant medications as well as cognitive therapy (Wisner et al., 2012). Cognitive therapy, a time-limited, structured psychotherapy, also is for panic disorder. Panic disorder responds to most antidepressant medications, which are first-line therapies for this disorder (Wisner et al., 2012). Benzodiazepines are also effective but can be associated with abuse and physical dependence in some women. Prenatal benzodiazepine exposure increases the risk of oral cleft. Maternal benzodiazepine use shortly before birth is associated with floppy infant syndrome (ACOG, 2008).

Note that most of the antianxiety medications are FDA Category D (evidence of human fetal risk) or Category X (demonstrated fetal abnormalities and use is contraindicated) (Table 31-2). However, benzodiazepines should not be abruptly discontinued during pregnancy, and they should be tapered sufficiently before the birth to limit neonatal withdrawal syndrome.

OCD is effectively treated with SSRIs. A behavioral therapy technique, exposure and response prevention, is also effective for OCD (Wisner et al., 2012). PTSD is partially responsive to antidepressant medication, but cognitive therapy with exposure is more effective. The first-line medication treatment for social phobia is SSRIs; cognitive therapy also can be very helpful. Specific phobias are most effectively treated with focused desensitization psychotherapy rather than medication (Wisner et al., 2012).

A risk-to-benefit evaluation for treatments during pregnancy must be individualized for the pregnant woman with anxiety disorder, which, like an MDE, can have a negative effect on pregnancy outcome. If psychotherapy treatment is refused, not available, or ineffective, pharmacologic treatment should be considered (Wisner et al., 2012).

TABLE 31-2 Antianxiety Medications

ANTIANXIETY MEDICATIONS	PREGNANCY RISK CATEGORY*	LACTATION RISK CATEGORY*
Alprazolam (Xanax)	D	L3
Buspirone (BuSpar)	C	L3
Chlordiazepoxide (Librium)	D	L3
Clonazepam (Klonopin)	C	L3
Clorazepate (Tranxene)	D	L3
Diazepam (Valium)	D	L3; L4 if used chronically
Flurazepam (Dalmane)	X	L3
Lorazepam (Ativan)	D	L3
Midazolam (Versed)	D	L3
Temazepam (Restoril)	X	L3
Triazolam (Halcion)	X	L3

C = Animal studies show adverse effects on fetus, but no controlled studies in pregnant women *or* no studies available.
D = Positive evidence of human fetal risk.
X = Contraindicated because studies have shown significant and documented risk to fetus.
L3 = No controlled studies in breastfeeding women *or* studies show minimal adverse effects.
L4 = Possibly hazardous.
*From Hale, T. (2012). *Medications and mother's milk* (15th ed.). Amarillo, TX: Pharmasoft; Schatzberg, A., Cole, J.O., DeBattista, C. (Eds.). (2010). *Manual of clinical psychopharmacology* (7th ed.). Arlington, VA: American Psychiatric Publishing.

Nursing Interventions

Nursing strategies to reduce anxiety include empowerment through education; sensory interventions such as music therapy and aromatherapy; medication (see Table 31-2); behavioral interventions such as breathing exercises, progressive muscle relaxation, and guided imagery; and cognitive strategies such as encouraging positive self-talk and questioning negative thinking.

Nurses should educate women about the dangers of benzodiazepines during pregnancy, assess for use during pregnancy, and help pregnant women find other ways to handle their anxiety and insomnia, or refer them to a psychiatrist who specializes in psychiatric disorders in pregnancy.

Special Considerations for Medications During Pregnancy

Even though the basic rule is to avoid administering any medication to a pregnant woman, particularly during the first trimester, decisions about the use of medications during pregnancy should be made jointly by the woman, her partner, and her health care providers. If the woman is stable and appears likely to remain well while not taking medication, then discontinuation before pregnancy is a viable option. For those women with a history of relapse after medication discontinuation, remaining on the drug during pregnancy is advised. There is a lack of conclusive evidence that antipsychotic medications (either typical or atypical) are teratogenic (Sadock et al., 2009).

Although a pregnant woman should be receiving the lowest therapeutic dose, psychotropic medications may have to be increased over the course of pregnancy to maintain adequate therapeutic serum concentrations and response (Sadock et al., 2009). Administering psychotherapeutic medications at or near birth can cause a baby to be overly sedated at birth and require ventilatory support or to be physically dependent on the drug and require detoxification and treatment of a withdrawal syndrome (see Chapter 35).

If a woman becomes psychotic during pregnancy, it is usually either because she has stopped taking mood stabilizers or antipsychotics or because she has a history of schizophrenia. Psychosis is a medical emergency. To treat a psychotic state, antipsychotic medication or electroconvulsive therapy (ECT) can be used (Sadock et al., 2009). Lithium is currently considered the first-line medication for the treatment of psychosis during pregnancy (Roy & Payne, 2009).

Most of the mood-stabilizing medications such as lithium carbonate, carbamazepine (Tegretol), gabapentin (Neurontin), lamotrigine (Lamictal), and valproic acid (Depakote) are Category D (see Table 31-3 for FDA categories of mood stabilizers). In women with preexisting illness, there is a high recurrence of mania during pregnancy that can present as psychosis; thus maintenance on lithium is important to deter the development of adverse effects in the mother and infant. Mood stabilizers are often taken over the life span by women with bipolar disorder. Women with this disorder should receive preconception counseling. Those who have experienced a single manic episode

TABLE 31-3 Mood Stabilizers

MOOD STABILIZERS	PREGNANCY RISK CATEGORY*	LACTATION RISK CATEGORY*
Carbamazepine (Tegretol XR)	C	L2
Clonazepam (Klonopin)	C	L3
Gabapentin (Neurontin)	C	L3
Lamotrigine (Lamictal)	C	L3
Lithium carbonate (Eskalith)	C	L4
Topiramate (Topamax)	C	L3
Valproic acid (Depakene, Depakote, Depakote ER)	D	L2

C = Animal studies show adverse effects on fetus, but no controlled studies in pregnant women *or* no studies available.
D = Positive evidence of human fetal risk.
L2 = Drug studied in limited number of breastfeeding women without an increase in adverse effects in infant *or* risk is remote.
L3 = No controlled studies in breastfeeding women *or* studies show minimal nonthreatening adverse effects.
L4 = Possibly hazardous.
*From Hale, T. (2012). *Medications and mother's milk* (15th ed.). Amarillo, TX: Pharmasoft; Schatzberg, A., Cole, J.O., DeBattista, C. (Eds.). (2010). *Manual of clinical psychopharmacology* (7th ed.). Arlington, VA: American Psychiatric Publishing.

may elect to have the medication tapered gradually and make an attempt to have a lithium-free pregnancy or, if indicated, reinstitute the lithium after the first trimester.

If the pregnant woman is receiving pharmacologic treatment, the nurse must make sure that she is being treated by a psychiatrist or an advanced practice psychiatric nurse. No woman should withdraw abruptly from any psychotropic medication because of the risk of withdrawal symptoms.

POSTPARTUM MOOD DISORDERS

The weeks after birth are a time of vulnerability to psychologic complications for many women, causing significant distress for the mother, disrupting family life, and, if prolonged, negatively affecting the child's emotional and social development. Preexisting mood and anxiety disorders are particularly likely to recur or worsen during these weeks. Such conditions can interfere with attachment to the newborn and family integration, and some may threaten the safety and well-being of the mother, the newborn, and other children. Because birth is usually thought to be a happy event, a new mother's emotional distress can puzzle and immobilize family and friends. When she most needs the caring attention of loved ones, they may either criticize or withdraw because of their anxiety. Nurses can offer anticipatory guidance, assess the mental health of new mothers, offer therapeutic interventions, and make referrals when necessary. Failure to do so can result in tragic consequences. In the rarest of cases, a disturbed mother may kill her infant, other family members, or herself.

Mood disorders are the predominant mental health disorder in the postpartum period (APA, 2013). Up to 85% of women experience a mild depression or "baby blues" after the birth of a child; however, the woman's functioning is usually not impaired. Baby blues are characterized by mood swings, feelings of sadness and anxiety, crying, difficulty sleeping, and loss of appetite. The symptoms resolve within a few days, and treatment is not needed (Paschetta, Berrisford, Coccia, et al., 2014).

Postpartum Depression

Serious depression, experienced by 10% to 15% of postpartum women, can eventually incapacitate them to the point of being unable to care for themselves or their babies (Sadock et al., 2009). **Postpartum depression** affects women from all cultures, although the manifestations vary.

The *Diagnostic and Statistical Manual of Mental Disorders, fifth edition (DSM-V)* contains the official guidelines for the assessment and diagnosis of psychiatric illness (APA, 2013). However, specific criteria for PPD are not listed. Instead, women must meet the criteria for an MDE and the criteria for the *peripartum-onset* specifier. The diagnosis of PPD is therefore an MDE with an onset in pregnancy or within 4 weeks of childbirth (APA). The following discussion focuses on the postpartum onset.

The cause of PPD can be biologic, psychologic, situational, or multifactorial. Estrogen fluctuations and postpartum hypogonadism (the change from the high levels of estrogen and progesterone at the end of pregnancy to the much lower levels of both hormones that are present after birth) are important etiologic factors. Women at greatest risk for PPD are those with a history of anxiety or depression and especially those who had a previous episode of major depressive disorder (MDD) in the past, including during or after pregnancy (Cunningham, Leveno, Bloom, et al., 2014; Davey, Tough, Adair, & Benzies, 2011). Other risk factors include younger age, unintended pregnancy, personal history of severe premenstrual dysphoria, family history of mood disorder, unmarried status, marital discord, lack of social support, socioeconomic deprivation, lower education, substance abuse, and stressful life events in the previous year (Cunningham et al.; Le Strat, Dubertret, & Le Foll, 2011). Women facing multiple or severe psychosocial problems or chronic interpersonal difficulties are at increased risk for an MDE.

Poor nutrition may also contribute to the pathogenesis of an MDE. Folate and vitamin B_{12} are needed for the synthesis of serotonin and other neurotransmitters. Marginal or low folate also increases the likelihood of a poor response to antidepressant medication as well as the potential for relapse in people who initially responded well to pharmacologic therapy (Wisner et al., 2012).

Complications of pregnancy and birth increase the risk for PPD (Blom, Jansen, Verhulst, et al., 2010). Having a preterm, low-birth-weight, and ill neonate is associated with higher rates of PPD (Vigod, Villegas, Dennis, & Ross, 2010). Women who are victims of intimate partner violence are at increased risk for PPD (Beydoun, Beydoun, Kaufman, et al., 2012; Cerulli, Talbor, Tang, & Chaudron, 2011; Woolhouse, Gartland, Hegarty, et al., 2012). Cultural practices can positively or negatively affect the development of PPD. Common risk factors for PPD are listed in Box 31-3.

Paternal Postpartum Depression

Often women are not alone in their experience of PPD; new fathers may have PPD as well. The incidence is unclear, with reports varying from 10% to more than 50% (Letourneau,

BOX 31-3 Risk Factors for Postpartum Depression

- Prenatal anxiety or depression
- History of major depressive episode
- History of postpartum depression
- Life stress
- Major life event (e.g., moving, job loss)
- Lack of social support
- Unmarried
- Marital relationship problems
- Intimate partner violence
- Thyroid imbalance
- Diabetes: type 1, type 2, or gestational
- Mothers who have undergone infertility treatment
- Complicated pregnancy or birth
- Complications of breastfeeding
- Preterm or ill infant
- Mothers of multiples
- Postpartum blues
- Low socioeconomic status
- Unintended pregnancy

Data from Beck, C. (2002). Revision of the postpartum depression predictors inventory. *Journal of Obstetric, Gynecologic, and Neonatal Nursing, 31*(4), 394-402; Beck, C. (2001). Predictors of postpartum depression: An update. *Nurse Researcher, 50*(5), 275-282; Postpartum Support International. (2014). Depression during pregnancy and postpartum. Available at www.postpartum.net/get-the-facts/depression-during-pregnancy-postpartum.aspx.

Tryphonopoulos, Duffett-Leger, et al., 2012; Paulson & Bazemore, 2010). The best predictor of paternal depression is having a partner with PPD. Men may not exhibit classic symptoms of PPD but are likely to display fatigue, frustration, anger, irritability, indecisiveness, and withdrawal from social situations (Paulson & Bazemore).

Postpartum Depression Without Psychotic Features

PPD is an intense and pervasive sadness with severe and labile mood swings; it is more serious and persistent than postpartum blues. Intense fears, anger, anxiety, and despondency that persist past the baby's first few weeks are not a normal part of postpartum blues. These symptoms rarely disappear without outside help (Sadock et al., 2009). Most of these mothers seek help only after reaching a "crisis point."

The symptoms of postpartum major depression do not differ from those of nonpostpartum mood disorders except that the mother's ruminations of guilt and inadequacy feed her worries about being an incompetent and inadequate parent. In PPD there can be loss of appetite or odd food cravings (often sweet desserts) and binges with abnormal appetite and weight gain. New mothers report an increased yearning for sleep, sleeping heavily but awakening instantly with any infant noise, and an inability to go back to sleep after infant feedings. Determining difficulty falling asleep is a relevant screening question to ascertain risk for PPD.

A distinguishing feature of PPD is irritability. These episodes of irritability can flare up with little provocation, and they sometimes escalate to violent outbursts or dissolve into uncontrollable sobbing. Many of these outbursts are directed against significant others (e.g., "He never helps me") or the baby (e.g., "She cries all the time, and I feel like hitting her"). Women with postpartum MDEs often have severe anxiety, panic attacks, and spontaneous crying long after the usual duration of baby blues.

Many women feel especially guilty about having depressive feelings at a time when they believe they should be happy. They can be reluctant to discuss their symptoms or their negative feelings toward the infant. A prominent feature of PPD is rejection of the infant, often caused by abnormal jealousy. The mother can be obsessed by the notion that the baby will take her place in her partner's affections. Attitudes toward the infant can include disinterest, annoyance with care demands, and blaming because of her lack of maternal feeling. When observed, she can appear awkward in her responses to the baby. Obsessive thoughts about harming the infant are very frightening to her. Often she does not share these thoughts because of embarrassment; when she does, other family members become very frightened.

Medical Management. The natural course is one of gradual improvement over the 6 months after birth. However, supportive treatment alone is not effective for major PPD. Antidepressant medication along with some form of psychotherapy is used to treat severe depression during or after pregnancy. Often an SSRI is prescribed initially. If symptoms improve during a 6-week trial period, the medication should be continued for at least 6 months to prevent relapse. If response to the medication is less than optimal, another SSRI can be prescribed instead (Cunningham et al., 2014) (see Tables 31-1, 31-2, and 31-3). Alternative therapies such as herbs, dietary supplements, massage, aromatherapy, and acupuncture may be helpful. Psychotherapy focuses on the woman's fears and concerns regarding her new responsibilities and roles and monitoring for suicidal or homicidal thoughts. Support groups and marital counseling can be helpful. For some women, hospitalization is necessary.

Postpartum Depression with Psychotic Features

The most severe of the perinatal mood disorders, **postpartum psychosis,** is rare, affecting approximately 0.1% to 0.2% of postpartum women (Sadock et al., 2009).

Episodes of postpartum psychosis are typified by auditory or visual hallucinations, paranoid or grandiose delusions, elements of delirium or disorientation, and extreme deficits in judgment accompanied by high levels of impulsivity that can contribute to increased risks of suicide or infanticide (in 5% of psychotic women) (Sadock et al., 2009). Characteristically, the woman begins to complain of fatigue, insomnia, and restlessness and can have episodes of tearfulness and emotional lability. Complaints regarding the inability to move, stand, or work also are common. Later, suspiciousness, confusion, incoherence, irrational statements, and obsessive concerns about the baby's health and welfare can be present. Delusions are present in 50% of women with postpartum psychosis, and hallucinations occur in approximately 25% of women with this disorder. Auditory hallucinations that command the mother to kill the infant can occur in severe cases. When delusions are present, they are often related to the infant. The mother may think the infant is possessed by the devil, has special powers, or is destined for a terrible fate. Grossly disorganized behavior can be manifested as a disinterest in the infant or an inability to provide care. Some women will insist that something is wrong with the baby or accuse nurses or family members of hurting or poisoning their child.

> **! NURSING ALERT**
>
> Nurses are advised to be alert for mothers who are agitated, overactive, confused, complaining, or suspicious.

Postpartum psychosis is most commonly associated with the diagnosis of bipolar disorder (or manic-depressive disorder). Rates of postpartum relapse in women with bipolar disorder range from 32% to 67%. Perinatal episodes of the disorder tend to be depressive and are more likely to recur in subsequent pregnancies. Postpartum psychosis tends to show onset within 2 weeks postpartum; however, it can present later in the course of the illness as a depression (Sadock et al., 2009).

Postpartum psychosis is defined by the presence of one or more episodes of abnormally elevated energy levels, cognition, and mood and one or more depressive episodes. The elevated moods are clinically referred to as *mania.* Clinical manifestations of a manic episode include at least three of the following: grandiosity, decreased need for sleep, pressured speech, flight of ideas, distractibility, psychomotor agitation, and excessive involvement in pleasurable activities without regard for negative consequences (APA, 2013). While in a manic state mothers need constant supervision when caring for their infant. Usually, however, they are too preoccupied to provide child care. Individuals who experience manic episodes also commonly experience depressive episodes or symptoms or mixed episodes, in which features of both mania and depression are present at the same time. These episodes are usually separated by periods of "normal" mood, but in some individuals, depression and mania may rapidly alternate. These rapid changes in mood are known as *rapid cycling.*

Medical Management. Postpartum psychosis carries a relatively good prognosis with early detection and aggressive treatment; however, if left untreated, it can progress to the second postpartum year and become more refractory to treatment (Sadock et al., 2009). Postpartum psychosis is a psychiatric emergency, and the mother will probably need inpatient psychiatric care. Antipsychotics (Table 31-4) and mood stabilizers (see Table 31-3) such as lithium are the treatments of choice. Antidepressants should be used very cautiously in treating postpartum psychosis, even when depressive symptoms are present, because of the risk for precipitating rapid cycling. Because of potential risks to the breastfeeding infant, informed consent regarding the risks and benefits of exposing the newborn to a psychotropic agent and maternal mental illness must be discussed and documented (see additional discussion of lactation and psychotropic medications later in this chapter). ECT, especially when bilaterally administered, has also been shown to be highly effective in the treatment of postpartum psychosis. It is usually advantageous for the mother to have contact with her baby if she so desires, but visits must be closely supervised. Psychotherapy is indicated after the period of acute psychosis has passed.

Even though the prevalence of PPD is fairly well established, some women are unlikely to seek help from a mental health care provider. This can be related to social stigma of mental illness, cultural beliefs, lack of knowledge, or fear of child custody implications (Yonkers et al., 2011).

TABLE 31-4 Antipsychotic Medications

ANTIPSYCHOTIC MEDICATIONS	PREGNANCY RISK CATEGORY*	LACTATION RISK CATEGORY*
Traditional Antipsychotics		
Chlorpromazine (Thorazine)	C	L3
Fluphenazine (Prolixin)	C	L3
Haloperidol (Haldol)	C	L2
Perphenazine (Trilafon)	C	L3
Thioridazine (Mellaril)	C	L4
Thiothixene (Navane)	C	L4
Trifluoperazine (Stelazine)	Unknown	Unknown
Atypical Antipsychotics		
Aripiprazole (Abilify)	C	L3
Clozapine (Clozaril)	C	L3
Loxapine (Loxitane)	C	L4
Olanzapine (Zyprexa)	C	L2
Quetiapine (Seroquel)	C	L4
Risperidone (Risperdal)	C	L3
Ziprasidone (Geodon)	C	L4

C = Animal studies show adverse effects on fetus, but no controlled studies in pregnant women *or* no studies available.
L2 = Drug studied in limited number of breastfeeding women without an increase in adverse effects in infant *or* risk is remote.
L3 = No controlled studies in breastfeeding women *or* studies show minimal nonthreatening adverse effects.
L4 = Possibly hazardous.
*From Hale, T. (2012). *Medications and mother's milk* (15th ed.). Amarillo, TX: Pharmasoft; Schatzberg, A., Cole, J.O., & DeBattista, C. (Eds.). (2010). *Manual of clinical psychopharmacology* (7th ed.). Arlington, VA: American Psychiatric Publishing.

CARE MANAGEMENT

Primary health care providers usually recognize severe PPD or postpartum psychosis but may miss milder forms. Even if it is recognized, the woman may be treated inappropriately or subtherapeutically. Identification and treatment of maternal depression must be continued beyond the immediate postpartum period to prevent negative effects of maternal depression on the children of these mothers. To recognize symptoms of PPD as early as possible, the nurse should be an active listener and demonstrate a caring attitude. Nurses cannot depend on women to volunteer unsolicited information about their depression or ask for help. Examples of ways to initiate conversation include the following: "Now that you've had your baby, how are things going for you? Have you had to change many things in your life since having the baby?" and "How much time do you spend crying?" If the nurse assesses that the new mother is depressed, she or he must ask if the mother has thought about hurting herself or the baby. The woman may be more willing to answer honestly if the nurse says, "Many women feel depressed after having a baby, and some feel so badly that they think about hurting themselves or the baby. Have you had these thoughts?" (see Nursing Care Plan).

NURSING CARE PLAN

Postpartum Depression

NURSING DIAGNOSIS	EXPECTED OUTCOME	INTERVENTIONS	RATIONALES
Risk for Injury to the woman and/or newborn related to woman's emotional state and/or treatment	The mother and newborn will remain free of injury. The woman's family will verbalize understanding of the need for maternal and infant supervision and have a plan to provide that supervision.	Assess the postpartum woman for risk factors for depression (before discharge).	To determine if she is at risk and in need of prompt interventions or referral
		Provide information about signs of postpartum depression (PPD) to woman and family.	To promote prompt recognition of problems
		Observe maternal-infant interactions before discharge.	To determine appropriateness
		Maintain frequent contact with woman by telephone calls and home visits after discharge.	To determine if further interventions are necessary
		Counsel woman and family to contact health care provider if behaviors indicating depression, such as crying, increase.	To provide prompt care and referral if necessary and avoid injury to newborn and mother
		Provide opportunities for woman and family to verbalize feelings and concerns in a nonjudgmental setting.	To promote a trusting relationship
		Assess woman for any suicidal thoughts or plans.	To provide for safety of woman and infant
		Assist family to develop a plan for maternal and infant supervision.	To provide for safety of woman and infant
		Provide information about community resources for assistance.	To ensure care if woman is unable to care for herself or infant
		Reinforce teaching or refer breastfeeding mother to lactation consultant.	To obtain information regarding effects of antidepressant and antipsychotic medications
Disabled Family Coping related to postpartum maternal depression as evidenced by family members' denial of woman's illness	Family will identify positive coping mechanisms and initiate a plan to cope with the woman's depression.	Provide opportunity for family and significant others to verbalize feelings and concerns.	To establish a trusting relationship
		Give information regarding postpartum depression to the family.	To clarify any misconceptions or misinformation
		Assist family to identify positive coping mechanisms that have been effective during past crises.	To promote active participation in care
		Assist family to identify community sources of support.	To provide additional resources as needed
		Refer family to mental health care provider as needed.	To provide further expertise from a mental health professional
Risk for Impaired Parenting related to inability of mother to attach to infant	Woman demonstrates appropriate attachment behaviors in infant interactions. Woman expresses satisfaction with infant.	Observe maternal-infant interactions.	To assess quality of interactions and to determine need for interventions
		Encourage the woman to express her anxiety, fears, or other feelings.	To allow woman to ventilate her concerns and have them accepted
		Encourage the woman to have as much contact with the infant as possible.	To minimize separation and to promote attachment
		Encourage family participation in care of infant.	To promote attachment
		Demonstrate infant care and explain infant behaviors.	To enhance mother's care abilities and understanding of infant's abilities
		Make referrals as needed to community resources.	To assist the woman in developing parenting skills or promoting confidence in infant care

> **! NURSING ALERT**
>
> Because mothers with PPD with psychotic features can harm their infants, extra caution is needed in assessment and intervention. The nurse needs to ask specifically if the mother has had thoughts about harming her baby.

Screening for Postpartum Depression

When PPD is identified early it is highly treatable. Screening for depression during pregnancy and the postpartum period aids in prevention and early intervention for depressive symptoms. There are no national guidelines for depression screening during pregnancy and after birth. The American College of Obstetricians and Gynecologists (ACOG) Committee on Obstetric Practice (2010) and the Agency for Healthcare Research and Quality (AHRQ, 2013) cite a lack of sufficient evidence to warrant firm recommendations for universal screening of postpartum women, although they recognize there are benefits to screening. The U.S. Preventive Services Task Force (USPSTF, 2009) recommends screening of adults for depression, including during pregnancy and the postpartum period.

Postpartum nurses can screen for PPD before women are discharged from the birth setting. Although this identifies some who are at risk, it is important that follow-up screening is also done. PPD is most likely to occur around 4 weeks after birth. Follow-up assessments for risks and signs of PPD can be done by primary care providers during pediatric care visits for the infant and during postpartum follow-up visits for the mother. The American Academy of Pediatrics (AAP) recommends maternal depression screening at the infant's 1-, 2-, and 4-month visits (Earls & AAP Committee on Psychosocial Aspects of Child and Family Health, 2010). Women with a positive screen should be referred appropriately for evaluation and treatment.

In perinatal populations the most widely used and validated tools are the Edinburgh Postnatal Depression Scale (EPDS) and the Postpartum Depression Screening Scale (PDSS). Both are brief, self-report questionnaires specifically developed for use with perinatal women, which take between 5 and 10 minutes to complete (Milgrom & Gemmill, 2014).

The EPDS tool asks the woman to respond to 10 statements about the common symptoms of depression. The woman is asked to choose the response that is closest to describing how she has felt for the past week. A maximum score on the EPDS is 30; women with scores of 12 or higher may possibly have depression and need further assessment. One item on the tool addresses suicidal thoughts; responses to this item should be carefully examined (Cox, Holden, & Sagovsky, 1987).

The PDSS is a 35-item Likert response scale that assesses for seven dimensions of depression: sleeping or eating disturbances, anxiety or insecurity, emotional lability, mental confusion, loss of self, guilt or shame, and suicidal thoughts (Beck, 2008a, 2008b; Myers, Aubuchon-Endsley, & Bastian, 2013). Both published tools are designed to be used by nurses and other health care professionals to elicit information from the woman during an interview to assess risk. Areas assessed include the predictors of depression as listed in Box 31-3.

In addition, a simple two-item tool has been shown to be effective in identifying women at risk for PPD. If the woman answers yes to either of the two questions, the screen is considered to be positive. The questions are as follows: "Over the past 2 weeks have you ever felt down, depressed, or hopeless?" and "Over the past 2 weeks have you felt little interest or pleasure in doing things?" (Earls & AAP Committee on Psychosocial Aspects of Child and Family Health, 2010).

If PPD screening results are positive or if the woman's self-report shows signs that she might be depressed, a formal screening is needed to determine the urgency of the referral and the type of provider. Also important is the need to assess the woman's family because they may be able to offer valuable information, as well as need to express how they have been affected by the woman's emotional disorder.

Interventions

Nursing Care on the Postpartum Unit

The postpartum nurse observes the new mother carefully for any signs of tearfulness and conducts further assessments as necessary. Nurses must discuss PPD to prepare new parents for potential problems in the postpartum period and discuss ways to help prevent PPD (see Teaching for Self-Management: Preventing Postpartum Depression and Chapters 21 and 22). The family must be able to recognize the symptoms and know where to go for help. Printed materials that explain what the woman can do to prevent depression can be used as part of discharge education (Logsdon, Tomasulo, Eckert, et al., 2012).

> **TEACHING FOR SELF-MANAGEMENT**
>
> ***Preventing Postpartum Depression***
>
> - Share knowledge about postpartum emotional problems with close family and friends.
> - At least once each day or every other day, purposely relax for 15 minutes: deep breathing, meditating, taking a hot bath.
> - Take care of yourself: eat a balanced diet.
> - Exercise on a regular basis, at least 30 minutes a day.
> - Sleep as much as possible; make a promise to yourself to try to sleep when the baby sleeps.
> - Get out of the house: try to leave home for 30 minutes a day; take a walk outdoors or walk at the mall.
> - Share your feelings with someone close to you; don't isolate yourself at home with the TV.
> - Don't overcommit yourself or feel like you need to be a superwoman. Ask for help from family and friends.
> - Don't place unrealistic expectations on yourself; no mother is perfect!
> - Be flexible with your daily activities.
> - Go to a new mothers' support group: for example, take a postpartum exercise class or attend a breastfeeding support group.
> - Don't be ashamed of having emotional problems after your baby is born. It happens to approximately 15% of women.

Women are often discharged before the blues or depression occurs. If the postpartum nurse is concerned about the mother, a mental health consult should be requested before the mother leaves the hospital. Routine instructions regarding PPD should be given to the person who comes to take the woman home; for example, "If you notice that your wife [or partner] is upset or crying a lot, please call the postpartum care provider immediately—don't wait for the routine postpartum appointment." (See Teaching for Self-Management: Signs of Postpartum Blues, Depression, and Psychosis.)

TEACHING FOR SELF-MANAGEMENT

Signs of Postpartum Blues, Depression, and Psychosis

- Baby blues (these should go away in a few days or a week):
  - Sad, anxious, or overwhelmed feelings
  - Crying spells
  - Loss of appetite
  - Difficulty sleeping
- Postpartum depression (can begin any time in the first year):
  - Same signs as baby blues, but they last longer and are more severe
  - Thoughts of harming yourself or your baby
  - Not having any interest in the baby
- Postpartum psychosis:
  - Seeing or hearing things that are not there
  - Feelings of confusion
  - Rapid mood swings
  - Trying to hurt yourself or your baby
- When to call your health care provider:
  - The baby blues continue for more than 2 weeks
  - Symptoms of depression get worse
  - Difficulty performing tasks at home or at work
  - Inability to care for yourself or your baby
  - Thoughts of harming yourself or your baby

Data from U.S. Department of Health and Human Services Office of Women's Health. (2009). *Depression during and after pregnancy*. Available at www.womenshealth.gov/publications/our-publications/fact-sheet/depression-pregnancy.pdf.

Nursing Care in the Home and Community

Postpartum home visits can reduce the incidence of or complications from depression. A brief home visit or phone call at least once a week until the new mother returns for her postpartum visit may save the life of a mother and her infant; however, home visits may not be feasible or available. Supervision of the mother with emotional complications can become a prime concern. Because depression can greatly interfere with her mothering functions, family and friends may need to participate in the infant's care. This is a time for the extended family and friends to determine what they can do to help; the nurse can work with them to ensure adequate supervision and their understanding of the woman's mental illness.

When the woman has PPD, a partner often reacts with confusion, shock, denial, and anger and feels neglected and blamed. The nurse can provide nonjudgmental opportunities for the partner to verbalize feelings and concerns, help the partner identify positive coping strategies, and be a source of encouragement for the partner to continue supporting the woman. Suggestions for partners of women with PPD include helping around the house, setting limits with family and friends, going with her to appointments with the health care provider, educating himself or herself, writing down concerns and questions to take to the primary care provider or therapist, and just being with her—sitting quietly, hugging her, and demonstrating concern and compassion. Both the woman and her partner need an opportunity to express their needs, fears, thoughts, and feelings in a nonjudgmental environment.

Even if the woman is severely depressed, hospitalization can be avoided if adequate resources can be mobilized to ensure safety for mother and infant. The nurse in home health care needs to make frequent phone calls or home visits for assessment and counseling. Community resources that may be helpful are temporary child care or foster care, homemaker service, Meals on Wheels, parenting guidance centers, mother's-day-out programs, and telephone support groups such as Postpartum Support International (http://postpartum.net) and Depression After Delivery (www.depressionafterdelivery.com).

Referral

Women with moderate to severe cases of PPD should be referred to a mental health professional such as a psychiatric nurse practitioner or psychiatrist for evaluation and therapy. Inpatient psychiatric hospitalization may be necessary. This decision is made when the safety of the mother or children is threatened.

Providing Safety

If delusional thinking about the baby is suspected, the nurse asks, "Have you thought about hurting your baby?" When depression is suspected, the nurse asks, "Have you thought about hurting yourself?" Four criteria can be used to measure the seriousness of a suicidal plan: method, availability, specificity, and lethality. Has the woman specified a method? Is the method of choice available? How specific is the plan? If the method is concrete and detailed, with access to carry it out at hand, the suicide risk increases. How lethal is the method? The most lethal method is shooting, with hanging a close second. The least lethal is slashing one's wrists.

! NURSING ALERT

Suicidal thoughts or attempts are among the most serious symptoms of PPD and require immediate assessment and intervention.

Psychiatric Hospitalization

Women with postpartum psychosis have a psychiatric emergency and must be referred immediately to a psychiatric health care provider who is experienced in working with women with PPD, can prescribe medication and other forms of therapy, and can assess the need for hospitalization.

LEGAL TIP: Commitment for Psychiatric Care

If a woman with PPD is experiencing active suicidal ideation or harmful delusions about the baby and is unwilling to seek treatment, legal intervention may be necessary to commit the woman to an inpatient setting for treatment.

If allowed within the inpatient psychiatric setting, the reintroduction of the baby to the mother can occur at the mother's own pace. A schedule is set for increasing the number of hours the mother cares for the baby over several days, culminating in the infant's staying overnight in the mother's room. This method allows the mother to experience meeting the infant's needs and giving up sleep for the baby, a situation difficult for new mothers even under ideal conditions. The mother's readiness for discharge and caring for the baby is assessed. Her interactions with her baby are carefully supervised and guided. A postpartum nurse is often asked to assist the psychiatric nursing staff in assessment of the mother-infant interactions.

Nurses should observe the mother for signs of bonding with the baby. Attachment behaviors are defined as eye-to-eye contact; physical contact that involves holding, touching, cuddling, and talking to the baby and calling the baby by name; and the initiation of appropriate care. A staff member is assigned to observe the baby at all times. Praise and encouragement are used to bolster the mother's self-esteem and self-confidence.

Psychotropic Medications

If the woman with PPD is not breastfeeding, in most cases antidepressants can be prescribed without special precautions. A variety of medications can be prescribed for these women, including TCAs, SSRIs, SNRIs, MAOIs, mood stabilizers, and antipsychotic medications.

MAOIs may be used for women with major depression who are not responsive to other medications and for women with panic disorder and bipolar disorder. Hypertensive crisis is the main reason that MAOIs are not prescribed more frequently than other psychotropic medications. The woman should be taught to watch for signs of hypertensive crisis—a throbbing occipital headache, stiff neck, chills, nausea, flushing, retroorbital pain, apprehension, pallor, sweating, chest pain, and palpitations. This crisis is brought on by the woman taking any of a large variety of over-the-counter medications or eating foods that contain tyramine, which normally is broken down by the enzyme *monoamine oxidase* (Hadley, Albanese, & Rochester, 2012).

MEDICATION ALERT

People taking MAOIs must be taught to totally avoid medications and foods that contain tyramine. Pseudoephedrine-containing medications, aged cheese, red wine, fava or Italian green beans, brewer's yeast, smoked fish, chicken or beef livers, and preserved meats are examples of tyramine-containing substances (Hadley, Albanese, & Rochester, 2012).

The woman taking mood stabilizers (see Table 31-3) must be taught about the many side effects, and especially for those taking lithium, the need to have serum lithium levels determined every 6 months. Women with severe psychiatric syndromes such as schizophrenia, bipolar disorder, or psychotic depression will probably require antipsychotic medications (see Table 31-4). Most of these medications can cause sedation and orthostatic hypotension—both of which can interfere with the mother being able to care safely for her baby. They also can cause peripheral nervous system (PNS) effects such as constipation, dry mouth, blurred vision, tachycardia, urinary retention, weight gain, and agranulocytosis. CNS effects may include akathisia, dystonias, parkinsonian-like symptoms, tardive dyskinesia (irreversible), and neuroleptic malignant syndrome (potentially fatal). Medication education is especially important when caring for women who are taking antipsychotic medications. The nurse should use discretion in selecting the content to be shared because of the women's altered thought processes and the large number of side/toxic effects. The nurse may choose to do more extensive education with a close family member. The newer, atypical antipsychotic medications such as aripiprazole, olanzapine, quetiapine, risperidone, and ziprasidone are usually safer and have fewer side effects than the older, more traditional antipsychotics. Their safety in breastfeeding women, however, has not been established.

Psychotropic Medications and Lactation

Use of any psychotropic medication in a breastfeeding mother is done with consideration of risks and benefits. The risk of not treating the mother versus not breastfeeding the infant prompts providers to prescribe medications that reduce maternal symptoms without harming the infant. Concerns about many psychotropic drugs are related to the long-term use and potential effects on the infant (Lawrence & Lawrence, 2011).

Factors that affect the passage of a medication through breast milk include the size of the molecule, the solubility in lipids and water, the protein-binding capacity, the drug's pH, and the rate of diffusion. Infant factors to consider relate to the gestational and chronologic age of the infant, weight, health, and frequency and amount of feeding (Lawrence & Lawrence, 2011). To minimize the infant's exposure to maternal medication, the mother should avoid breastfeeding when the blood levels of the medication are peaking.

SSRIs are the most common treatment for PPD; they are also prescribed for anxiety disorders. Research has shown that the majority of the SSRIs taken by breastfeeding mothers pass through the milk to the infant in small amounts and have no untoward effects on the infant (Kendall-Tackett & Hale, 2010). Paroxetine (Paxil), sertraline (Zoloft), and nortriptyline (Pamelor) provide less infant exposure than fluoxetine (Prozac) and citalopram (Celexa). All breastfeeding mothers who take SSRIs should be taught to monitor their infants for signs of irritability, poor feeding, and alterations in sleep pattern (Hudak et al., 2012; Kendall-Tackett & Hale).

CLINICAL REASONING CASE STUDY

Postpartum Depression

Cara, 37, gave birth to a 7 lb, 6 oz boy 4 weeks ago. She has been diagnosed with postpartum depression, and an SSRI (paroxetine [Paxil]) medication has been prescribed. Cara is breastfeeding and has concerns about taking the medication.

1. Evidence—Is there sufficient evidence regarding the safety of psychotropic medications and lactation?
2. Assumptions—What assumptions can be made about the following?
   a. Lactation risk categories of SSRI medications
   b. Timing of feeding and medication administration
   c. Risks of discontinuing medications while breastfeeding
3. What is the nursing priority in this situation?
4. Does the evidence objectively support your conclusion?

SSRI, Selective serotonin reuptake inhibitor.

Benzodiazepines, mood stabilizers, and antipsychotic medications are used frequently in the treatment of postpartum psychiatric disorders despite the lack of research in this population. No long-term effects have been reported in exclusively breastfed infants whose mothers were taking benzodiazepines on a regular basis. The shorter-acting agents (alprazolam [Xanax], lorazepam [Ativan]) are favored over those with longer half-lives (clonazepam [Klonopin], diazepam [Valium]) (Lawrence & Lawrence, 2011).

Mood-stabilizing medications are present in the breast milk of women who take these drugs. Lithium has been the most extensively studied. Lithium has been linked to several serious adverse effects in breastfeeding infants, including hypotonia, hypothermia, cyanosis, and electrocardiogram abnormalities. Therefore, its use is not recommended in breastfeeding mothers. Valproic acid (Depakote) and carbamazepine (Tegretol) are considered reasonably safe while breastfeeding, although careful monitoring for infant hepatotoxicity is recommended. The benefits of breastfeeding and the potential risks must be carefully considered before using lithium or other mood stabilizers.

In summary, all psychotropic medications studied to date are excreted in breast milk. The best psychotropic medications for breastfeeding women are those with the greatest documentation of prior use, lower FDA risk category, few or no metabolites, and fewer side effects.

When breastfeeding women have emotional complications and need psychotropic medications, referral to a mental health care provider who specializes in postpartum disorders is preferred. The woman should be informed of the risks and benefits to her and her infant of the medications to be taken. Depressed women will need the nurse to reinforce the importance of taking antidepressants as ordered. Because antidepressants usually do not exert any significant effect for approximately 2 weeks and usually do not reach full effect for 4 to 6 weeks, many women discontinue taking the medication on their own. Client and family teaching should reinforce the need for taking medications until therapeutic effects are present and for as long as prescribed by the health care provider.

A complete guide to breastfeeding and drug compatibility can be found at the Drugs and Lactation Database (LactMed; http://toxnet.nlm.nih.gov/cgi-bin/sis/htmlgen?LACT). This is a peer-reviewed and fully referenced database of drugs to which breastfeeding mothers may be exposed. Among the data included are maternal and infant levels of drugs, possible effects on breastfed infants and on lactation, and alternate drugs to consider.

Other Treatments for PPD

Other treatments for PPD include hormone therapy (often combined with antidepressant medication), complementary or alternative therapies, and ECT. Complementary and alternative medicine (CAM) therapies are increasingly being used by people with psychiatric disorders. Several commonly used CAM therapies (bright light therapy, exercise, massage, repetitive transcranial magnetic stimulation, and acupuncture) are considerations in the treatment of perinatal depression. A number of these treatments may be reasonable to consider for women during pregnancy or postpartum, but the safety and efficacy of these relative to standard treatments must still be systematically determined (Deligiannidis & Freeman, 2014; Manber, 2010).

ECT may be used for women with PPD who have not improved with antidepressant therapy. Psychotherapy in the form of group therapy or individual (interpersonal) therapy has been used with positive results alone and in conjunction with antidepressant therapy; however, more studies are needed to determine what types of professional supports are most effective. Repetitive transcranial magnetic stimulation is a new therapy for PPD, but more studies need to be done to demonstrate the efficacy (Garcia, Flynn, Pierce, & Caudle, 2010). Alternative therapies may be used alone but often are used with other treatments for PPD. Safety and efficacy studies of these alternative therapies are needed to ensure that care and advice are based on evidence.

! NURSING ALERT

St. John's wort is often used to treat depression. It has not been proven safe for women who are breastfeeding.

PERINATAL SUBSTANCE ABUSE

Large numbers of women of childbearing age abuse potentially addictive and mood-altering drugs. Use of cocaine, marijuana, diazepam, opioids (including morphine, heroin, codeine, meperidine, methadone, and oxycodone), other prescription drugs, and approximately 150 other substances can lead to chemical dependency. Chemical dependency is a chronic, relapsing, and progressive disease. Without treatment or participation in recovery activities, it can progress and result in disability or premature death.

Pregnant women who abuse drugs can display warning signs such as receiving no prenatal care, late entry into care, or sporadic care, with multiple missed appointments. They may also show evidence of poor nutrition, have frequent encounters with law enforcement officials, or engage in marital and family disputes.

Dual diagnosis, which is very common, is the coexistence of **substance abuse** and another psychiatric disorder. Mood and anxiety disorders are the psychiatric disorders that are most commonly seen along with substance abuse in women. The psychiatric illness usually occurs before substance use begins (Wisner et al., 2012).

Drugs that affect the mother can also affect the fetus in multiple ways either directly or indirectly. Early in gestation drugs can cause significant teratogenic effects. During the fetal period, after major structural development is complete, drugs exert more subtle effects, including abnormal growth and maturation, alterations in neurotransmitters and their receptors, and brain organization. These are considered to be the direct effects of drugs (Behnke, Smith, Committee on Substance Abuse, & Committee on Fetus and Newborn, 2013). Drugs that exert a pharmacologic effect on the mother can indirectly affect the fetus. Indirect effects include altered delivery of nutrition to the fetus, either because of placental insufficiency or altered maternal health behaviors attributable to the mother's addiction.

Maternal factors such as decreased access/compliance with health care, increased exposure to violence, and increased risk of mental illness and infection can also indirectly place the fetus at risk (Behnke et al., 2013).

Prevalence

Because many pregnant women are reluctant to reveal their use of substances or the extent of their use, data on prevalence are highly variable. Approximately 15% of all pregnant women have a substance-abuse problem (Gilbert, 2011). Blinded urine drug screens conducted at hospitals across the United States revealed that similar rates of substance use during pregnancy occurred in women of different ages, races, and social classes, although the specific substances used differed by race and social class. African-American and poor women were more likely to use illicit substances, particularly cocaine, whereas Caucasian and educated women were more likely to use alcohol, although poly-substance abuse was common (Wisner et al., 2012). National surveys have found that among pregnant women, those who are younger generally report more abuse of substances than their older counterparts. In one study pregnant women ages 15 to 17 had rates of illicit drug use (15.8%) that were similar to women of the same age who were not pregnant (13%) (National Institute of Drug Abuse [NIDA], 2011a).

Barriers to Treatment

Many pregnant women who are substance abusers do not receive treatment for their addictions. Social stigma, labeling, and guilt are significant barriers to receiving necessary care. Women often do not seek help because of the fear of losing custody of their child or children or criminal prosecution. Pregnant women who abuse substances commonly have little understanding of the ways in which these substances affect them, their pregnancies, and their babies. In many instances pregnant mothers who use psychoactive substances receive negative feedback from society and health care providers, who not only may condemn them for endangering the life of the fetus but may also even withhold support as a result. Barriers within the drug treatment system can also deter these women from receiving the help they need. Traditionally substance-abuse treatment programs have not addressed issues that affect pregnant women such as concurrent need for obstetric care and child care for other children. Long waiting lists and lack of health insurance present further barriers to treatment. Pregnant women with co-occurring substance abuse and psychiatric disorders face unique barriers because of the social stigma attached to both conditions and insufficient knowledge and training to manage coexisting disorders.

Legal Considerations

Practitioners should be aware that laws in some states consider in utero drug exposure to be a form of child abuse or neglect under civil child-welfare statutes. Health care providers may be required to report positive drug test results in pregnant women or their newborns to the state's child protection agency (AAP & ACOG, 2012). States vary in their requirements for the evidence of drug exposure to the fetus or newborn to report a case to the child welfare system. Legally mandated testing and reporting can potentially place the provider in an adversarial relationship with the client (AAP & ACOG).

Commonly Abused Drugs

Tobacco

Tobacco is a legal substance that can be addicting or harmful to the pregnant woman, fetus, and newborn. Fetal tobacco exposure is well known to be a risk factor for low birth weight and intrauterine growth restriction (IUGR). Decreasing birth weight is related to the number of cigarettes smoked. Multiple studies have demonstrated a clear association between maternal smoking and perinatal morbidity and mortality. Maternal complications related to smoking include placenta previa, placental abruption, preterm premature rupture of membranes, and ectopic pregnancy. Fetal and neonatal risks related to maternal tobacco use include IUGR, low birth weight, perinatal mortality, and sudden infant death syndrome. Children born to mothers who smoke during pregnancy are at increased risk of asthma, infantile colic, and childhood obesity (AAP & ACOG, 2012).

Alcohol

Alcohol continues to be one of the most widely abused substances during pregnancy, and its effects on fetal development and infant outcomes have been well studied. Data from prenatal clinics and postnatal studies suggest that 20% to 30% of women drink at some time during pregnancy (National Institute on Alcohol Abuse and Alcoholism [NIAAA], 2010; Substance Abuse and Mental Health Services Administration [SAMSHA], 2012).

Alcohol is a known teratogen. It easily crosses the placenta to the fetus. A significant concentration of the drug can be identified in the amniotic fluid as well as in maternal and fetal blood (Behnke et al., 2013). Ethanol has direct teratogenic effects during the embryonic and fetal stages of development. It also causes altered neurotransmitter levels in the brain, altered brain morphology and neuronal development, and hypoxia (Behnke et al.).

Prenatal exposure to alcohol is probably the most common preventable cause of cognitive disability in the United States. Children exposed to binge drinking are 1.7 times more likely to be intellectually impaired and 2.5 times more likely to demonstrate delinquent behavior than children who were not exposed to alcohol (AAP & ACOG, 2012). Disorders associated with prenatal alcohol exposure include fetal alcohol syndrome (FAS), alcohol-related birth defects (ARBDs), and alcohol-related neurodevelopmental disorder. See Chapter 35 for information on newborn consequences of prenatal alcohol exposure.

Marijuana

Marijuana, a substance derived from the cannabis plant, is the most common illicit drug used in the United States. It is usually rolled into a cigarette and smoked but also may be mixed into food and eaten. Although the federal government considers marijuana a Schedule I substance (having no medicinal uses and high risk for abuse), two states have legalized marijuana for adult recreational use, and 23 states and the District of Columbia have passed laws allowing its use as a treatment for certain medical conditions (NIDA, 2014; ProCon.org, 2014).

Unlike other drugs, the placenta appears to limit fetal exposure to marijuana. The adverse effects of marijuana on the fetus are thought to be attributable to complex pharmacologic actions on developing systems, altered uterine blood flow, and altered maternal health behaviors (Behnke et al., 2013).

Cocaine

Cocaine is a powerfully addictive stimulant drug made from the leaves of the coca plant. It is one of the oldest known psychoactive substances. Cocaine is a Schedule II drug, which means that it has high potential for abuse but can also be administered for legitimate medical purposes, such as local anesthesia for some eye, ear, and throat surgeries.

Cocaine is generally sold on the street as a fine, white crystalline powder and is also known as "coke," "C," "snow," "flake," or "blow." It can be snorted, smoked, or injected. The term "crack," which is the street name given to freebase cocaine, refers to the crackling sound heard when the mixture is smoked.

Pregnant cocaine users have an increased incidence of miscarriage, preterm labor, and placental abruption. They may give birth to infants who are small for gestational age. Intrauterine fetal demise (IUFD, stillborn) is also a risk. Because cocaine easily crosses both the placenta and the blood-brain barrier, it can cause significant teratogenic effects in the developing fetus (Behnke et al., 2013).

Methamphetamine

Methamphetamine is a relatively cheap and highly addictive stimulant that affects the CNS. It was developed early in the 20th century from its parent drug, amphetamine, and was used originally in nasal decongestants and bronchial inhalers (NIDA, 2013). Methamphetamine is classified by the U.S. Drug Enforcement Administration as a Schedule II stimulant, which makes it legally available only through a nonrefillable prescription. Medically it may be indicated for the treatment of attention deficit hyperactivity disorder (ADHD) and as a short-term component of weight-loss treatments.

Methamphetamine is a white, odorless, bitter-tasting crystalline powder that easily dissolves in water or alcohol. It is also called "meth," "chalk," "ice," and "crystal" as well as many other terms.

Methamphetamine readily crosses the placenta and the blood-brain barrier and stimulates the CNS. Maternal risks associated with its use include preterm birth and placental abruption. Fetal effects include small size, lethargy, and heart and brain abnormalities (NIDA, 2013).

Opioids

Opioids are a class of natural, endogenous, and synthetic compounds. Morphine is one of many naturally occurring opioids. Codeine, heroin, hydromorphone (Dilaudid), fentanyl (Sublimaze), and methadone are examples of synthetic opioids (Hudak et al., 2012). Opioids act by attaching to specific proteins called opioid receptors, which are found in the brain, spinal cord, GI tract, and other organs in the body. When these drugs attach to their receptors, they reduce the perception of pain. In addition, opioids produce a euphoric response because these drugs also affect the brain regions involved in reward. Opioids rapidly cross the placenta, with drug equilibration between the mother and the fetus (Behnke et al., 2013).

Prescription Drug Abuse

Psychotherapeutic medications such as stimulants, sleeping pills, tranquilizers, and pain relievers are used by an estimated 2% of American women. Such medications can bring relief from undesirable conditions such as insomnia, anxiety, and pain. Because the medications have mind-altering capacity, misuse can produce psychologic and physical dependency in the same manner as illicit drugs. Prescription drug abuse is the intentional use of a medication without a prescription; in a way other than as prescribed; or for the experience or feeling it causes. Prescription drug abuse remains a significant problem in the United States (NIDA, 2011b).

CARE MANAGEMENT

Screening

All pregnant women should be screened at their first prenatal visit regarding their past and present use of tobacco, alcohol, and other drugs, including the recreational use of prescription and over-the-counter medications as well as herbal remedies. Substance use information can be obtained by interview or use of a standardized screening tool. The overall approach and emotional tone of the clinician is more important than the specific wording or content used. Women are more likely to report substance use when asked in a nonjudgmental manner by an empathic interviewer and within the context of general health questions (AAP & ACOG, 2012).

Information about drug use should be obtained by first asking about the woman's intake of over-the-counter and prescribed medications. Next her use of legal drugs such as caffeine, nicotine, and alcohol should be determined. Finally she should be questioned about her use of illicit drugs such as cocaine, heroin, and marijuana. The approximate frequency and amount should be documented for each drug used (Seidel, Ball, Dains, et al., 2011).

Use of validated screening questionnaires, along with the assurance of confidentiality, improves client-provider communication and can increase the truthfulness of client responses (AAP & ACOG, 2012).The *4Ps Plus* is a screening tool designed specifically to identify pregnant women who need in-depth assessment (Box 31-4). It consists of five questions and takes less than a minute to complete. Because women frequently deny or greatly underreport usage when asked about drug or alcohol consumption during pregnancy, asking about substance use before pregnancy is often an effective screening method (Wisner et al., 2012).

Toxicologic testing is often performed to screen for illicit drug use. Because positive test results have implications for clients beyond their health, informed consent should be obtained before testing is done. The legal implications of testing and the need for consent from the mother can vary among states; therefore, health care providers should be aware of local laws and legislative changes that can influence regional practice (AAP & ACOG, 2012).

BOX 31-4 Screening with the *4Ps Plus*

Parents: Did either of your parents ever have a problem with alcohol or drugs?
Partner: Does your partner have a problem with alcohol or drugs?
Past: Have you ever had any beer or wine or liquor?
Pregnancy: In the month before you knew you were pregnant, how many cigarettes did you smoke? In the month before you knew you were pregnant, how much beer, wine, or liquor did you drink?

From Chasnoff, I.J., Hung, W.C. (1999). *The 4Ps plus.* Chicago: NTI Publishing.

Several biologic specimens can be used to screen for drug exposure. The three specimens most commonly used to establish drug exposure during the prenatal and perinatal periods are urine, meconium, and hair; however, none is accepted as a gold standard. Other specimens such as umbilical cord tissue, cord blood, human milk, and amniotic fluid may also be used for testing (Behnke et al., 2013; Hudak et al., 2012).

Urine has been the most frequently tested biologic specimen because of its ease of collection. Both maternal and neonatal urine can be tested for the presence of several drugs. Urine testing identifies only recent drug use, because threshold levels of drug metabolites generally can be detected in urine only for several days. Therefore, false-negative urine test results can occur in the presence of significant intrauterine drug exposure. Urine is a good medium for detecting marijuana, nicotine, opiate, cocaine, and amphetamine exposure (Behnke et al., 2013; Hudak et al., 2012).

Drugs become trapped within the hair, so it can be analyzed to determine past drug use over a longer period. Hair is useful in detecting nicotine, opiate, cocaine, and amphetamine exposure. Both maternal and neonatal hair samples can be tested (Behnke et al., 2013; Hudak et al., 2012).

Umbilical cord tissue and meconium can also be analyzed to determine past drug use over a longer period of time. Both substances can be used to assess fetal exposure to amphetamines, opiates, cocaine, cannabinoids, and alcohol (Behnke et al., 2013; Hudak et al., 2012). Umbilical cord tissue has the additional benefit of availability at the time of birth. Therefore, results from umbilical cord tissue testing may be available more rapidly than those obtained from meconium testing, because meconium may not be passed by the neonate for several days after birth (Montgomery, Plate, Alder, et al., 2006; United States Drug Testing Laboratories, Inc. [USDTL], 2012b).

A 6-inch segment of the umbilical cord is required for testing (USDTL, 2012a). Collection instructions can be found at www.usdtl.com/cordstat.html.

Assessment

Because substance-abusing pregnant women are at risk for a variety of infections and medical conditions, a comprehensive medical history should be obtained, and a complete physical examination performed. Laboratory assessments likely include screening for syphilis, hepatitis B and C, and human immunodeficiency virus (HIV). A complete blood count and a skin test to screen for tuberculosis may also be ordered. In addition, the woman may be tested for other common sexually transmitted infections such as gonorrhea and chlamydia (Wisner et al., 2012). Initial and serial ultrasound studies are usually performed to determine gestational age because the woman may have had amenorrhea as a result of her drug use or have no idea when her last menstrual period occurred.

Interventions

Medical Management

The information gained by toxicologic testing should be used to assist the pregnant woman or new mother to receive the treatment she needs and not as a vehicle for punishment (AAP & ACOG, 2012). Intervention with the pregnant substance abuser begins with education about specific effects on pregnancy, the fetus, and the newborn for each drug used. Consequences of perinatal drug use should be clearly communicated, and abstinence recommended as the safest course of action unless the woman is abusing opioids. Women are often more receptive to making lifestyle changes during pregnancy than at any other time in their lives. The casual, experimental, or recreational drug user is frequently able to achieve and maintain sobriety when she receives education, support, and continued monitoring throughout the remainder of the pregnancy. Periodic screening throughout pregnancy of women who have admitted to drug use may help them to continue abstinence.

It is difficult to estimate the full extent of the consequences of maternal drug abuse and to determine the specific hazard of a particular drug to the fetus. Multiple factors can have consequences and all interact to affect maternal, fetal, and child outcomes (NIDA, 2010). These factors include:

- The number and amount of all drugs abused, including nicotine
- The extent of prenatal care
- Possible neglect or abuse of the child
- Exposure to violence in the environment
- Socioeconomic conditions
- Maternal nutrition
- Other health conditions
- Exposure to sexually transmitted diseases

Treatment for substance abuse is individualized for each woman, depending on the type of drug used and the frequency and amount of use. Research has shown the value of evidence-based treatments in changing drug abuse and addiction behaviors in pregnant women. One recommended treatment is contingency management, in which participants are given incentives, such as small cash amounts, privileges, or prizes, for maintaining abstinence. Compared to a standard treatment condition, motivational incentive approaches appear to increase treatment retention and prolong abstinence in pregnant women with cocaine, opiate, and nicotine dependence (AAP & ACOG, 2012).

Women are more likely to attempt to stop smoking during pregnancy than at any other time in their lives. Quitting before conception is ideal, but even quitting before 16 weeks of gestation significantly decreases the adverse risks. Smoking-cessation programs during pregnancy are effective and should be offered to all pregnant smokers. These programs should continue throughout the postpartum period as well, because many women resume smoking after the birth (Gilbert, 2011; Wisner et al., 2012). The USPSTF (2009) found inadequate evidence to evaluate the safety or efficacy of pharmacotherapy (e.g., nicotine replacement therapy) during pregnancy.

The 5 A's Intervention was developed by the U.S. Public Health Service and is a best-practice guideline supported by the ACOG and the National Cancer Institute. The intervention is designed to take about 5 to 15 minutes and should be implemented with every client who is smoking or who has recently quit (see Box 4-12) (Agency for Healthcare Research and Quality [AHRQ], 2012). For more information on smoking cessation, visit the American Lung Association website at www.lungusa.org or the CDC website at www.cdc.gov/tobacco/data_statistics/fact_sheets/cessation/quitting/index.htm.

Detoxification, short-term inpatient or outpatient treatment, long-term residential treatment, aftercare services, and self-help support groups are all possible options for alcohol and drug abuse rehabilitation. Women for Sobriety may be a more helpful organization for women than Alcoholics Anonymous or Narcotics Anonymous, which were originally developed for male substance abusers. In general long-term treatment of any sort is becoming increasingly difficult to obtain, particularly for women who lack insurance coverage. Although some programs allow a woman to keep her children with her at the treatment facility, far too few of them are available to meet the demand.

COMMUNITY ACTIVITY

Look in your local phone book's yellow pages or go online to find an "open" (one that welcomes visitors) twelve-step meeting in your community. Alcoholics Anonymous, Narcotics Anonymous, and Cocaine Anonymous are all examples of twelve-step recovery groups. Attend an open meeting held by one of these groups. Discuss your experience with your clinical group. Did pregnant women or new mothers attend the meeting? What was your impression of the meeting format and the discussion that occurred? Did you notice anything at the meeting that surprised you? Do you think that attending twelve-step meetings would be helpful for pregnant women or new mothers attempting to achieve and maintain sobriety? Give reasons to support your answer to the last question.

Women should be advised to remain abstinent from alcohol consumption during pregnancy because there is no known safe threshold for use. Health care providers should advise women that low-level consumption of alcohol in early pregnancy is not an indication for pregnancy termination. However, women who have already consumed alcohol during a current pregnancy should be advised to stop to minimize further risk (AAP & ACOG, 2012).

Pregnant women requiring withdrawal from alcohol should be admitted for inpatient management. Alcohol withdrawal treatment during pregnancy consists of the administration of benzodiazepines, commonly chlordiazepoxide (Librium), diazepam (Valium), lorazepam (Ativan), and oxazepam (Serax). Disulfiram (Antabuse) is teratogenic; therefore, its use in aversion therapy is contraindicated during pregnancy. Four medications are approved by the FDA for treating alcohol dependence, but their use during pregnancy has been limited. Acute management of alcohol withdrawal also includes thiamine replacement and maintenance of adequate hydration and electrolyte balance (Wisner et al., 2012).

Pregnant women who use cocaine should be advised to stop using immediately. These women need a great deal of assistance such as an alcohol and drug treatment program, individual or group counseling, and participation in self-help support groups to accomplish this major lifestyle change successfully.

Methamphetamines are stimulants with vasoconstrictive characteristics similar to those of cocaine and are used similarly. As is the case with cocaine users, methamphetamine users are urged to immediately stop all use during pregnancy. Because methamphetamine users are extremely psychologically addicted, the rate of relapse is very high.

The most effective treatments for methamphetamine addiction at this time are behavioral therapies, such as cognitive-behavioral and contingency-management interventions. There are currently no medications that counteract the specific effects of methamphetamine or that prolong abstinence from and reduce the abuse of methamphetamine (NIDA, 2013).

Research is under way to develop pharmacologic treatments for methamphetamine addiction. One approach targets the activity of glial cells. A drug called AV411 (ibudilast) that suppresses the neuroinflammatory actions of glial cells has been shown to inhibit methamphetamine self-administration in rats and is now being fast-tracked in clinical trials to establish its safety and effectiveness in humans with methamphetamine addiction (NIDA, 2013).

Another treatment option is using the body's immune system to neutralize methamphetamine in the bloodstream before it reaches the brain. This approach includes injecting a user with antimethamphetamine antibodies or with vaccines that stimulate the body to produce its own such antibodies. Researchers have also begun a clinical trial to establish the safety of an antimethamphetamine monoclonal antibody known as mAb7F9 in human methamphetamine users (NIDA, 2013).

Opioids are highly addictive and may require prolonged treatment. Maintenance programs with methadone can sustain opioid concentrations in the mother and fetus to minimize opioid craving and prevent fetal stress. Methadone maintenance treatment (MMT) has been used in opioid-dependent pregnant women for many years and is considered the standard of care for pregnant women who are dependent on heroin or other narcotics (Kraft & van der Anker, 2012; Wisner et al., 2012).

Opioid replacement therapy has been shown to decrease opioid and other drug abuse; reduce criminal activity; improve individual functioning; and decrease rates of infections such as hepatitis B and C, HIV, other sexually transmitted infections, and tuberculosis. In addition, opioid replacement therapy is associated with reduced fetal exposure to illicit drug use and improved neonatal outcomes. However, 30% to 80% of infants exposed to opioids, including methadone or buprenorphine, in utero require treatment for neonatal abstinence syndrome (NAS). Neither the incidence nor the severity of NAS correlates directly with the maternal medication dose at birth (see Chapter 35) (Wisner et al., 2012).

Buprenorphine, a synthetic opioid, has been found to be equally effective and as safe as methadone in the adult outpatient treatment of opioid dependence. Buprenorphine, either alone (Subutex) or in combination with naloxone (Suboxone), is used as both a first-line treatment of heroin addiction and a replacement drug for methadone (Hudak et al., 2012).

Nursing Interventions

Although substance abusers can be difficult to care for at any time, they are often particularly challenging during the intrapartum and postpartum periods because of manipulative and demanding behavior. Typically these women display poor control over their behavior and a low threshold for pain. Increased dependency needs and lack of involvement with infant care may also be apparent.

Nurses must understand that substance abuse is an illness and that these women deserve to be treated with patience, kindness, consistency, and firmness when necessary (Box 31-5). Even women who are actively abusing drugs experience pain during labor and after giving birth and may need both pharmacologic and nonpharmacologic interventions. Developing a standardized plan of care so clients have limited opportunities to play staff members against one another is helpful. Mother-infant attachment should be promoted by identifying the woman's strengths and reinforcing positive maternal feelings

BOX 31-5 Dealing with Pregnant Substance Abusers

Realize that the decision to become and remain sober can *only* be made by the substance abuser.
Understand that nurses do not have the power to cure anyone. They only serve as educators, supporters, and advocates.
Educate yourself about the effects of drug use in general and its effect on pregnancy and the newborn specifically.
Treat substance abusers with the same respect and consideration that you show other people.
Become familiar with your local treatment centers. Learn which of them accept pregnant women. Keep an up-to-date list of groups meeting in your community.
Remember that there are no "hopeless cases." It is *never* too late to quit!
Practice patience and persistence. It may take months or years to see the effects of your work.

and behaviors. Staffing should be sufficient to ensure strict surveillance of visitors and prevent unsupervised drug use.

Advice regarding breastfeeding must be individualized. Although all abused substances appear in breast milk, some in greater amounts than others, breastfeeding is definitely contraindicated in women who use amphetamines, alcohol, cocaine, heroin, or marijuana. However, methadone use is not a contraindication to breastfeeding. The baby's nutrition and safety needs are of primary importance in this consideration. For some women a desire to breastfeed can provide strong motivation to achieve and maintain sobriety.

Smoking can interfere with the let-down reflex. Women who smoke and breastfeed should avoid smoking for 2 hours before a feeding to minimize the amount of nicotine in the milk and improve the milk-ejection reflex. All smokers should be discouraged from smoking in the same room with the infant because exposure to secondhand smoke can increase the likelihood that the infant will experience behavioral and respiratory health problems.

Follow-Up Care

Before a known substance abuser is discharged with her baby, the home situation must be assessed to determine that the environment is safe and that someone will be available to meet the infant's needs if the mother is unable to do so. The social services department of the birthing facility is usually involved in interviewing the mother before discharge to ensure that the infant's needs will be met. Family members or friends are sometimes asked to become actively involved with the mother and infant after discharge. A home care or public health nurse may be asked to make home visits to assess the mother's ability to care for the baby and provide guidance and support. If serious questions about the infant's well-being exist, the case is likely to be referred to the state child protective services agency for further action.

KEY POINTS

- Because pregnant women may have a history of mental disorder or substance abuse, careful assessment is extremely important at the first and each subsequent prenatal and postpartum visit.
- Mood disorders account for most mental health disorders in the postpartum period.
- Psychotherapy is the first-line treatment option for women with mild to moderate peripartum depression.
- Antidepressant medications are the usual treatment for PPD; however, specific precautions are needed for breastfeeding women.
- Treatment of peripartum onset of anxiety disorders requires a combination of medication, education, supportive measures, and psychotherapy.
- Treatment of both depression and anxiety is critical to improving mental health.
- Peripartum depression with suicidal or homicidal intent or plan as well as peripartum depression with psychotic features is a psychiatric emergency. Immediate evaluation by a mental health professional is warranted.
- Identification of women at greatest risk for substance abuse during pregnancy and depression in the postpartum period can be facilitated by use of various screening tools.
- Alcohol abuse during pregnancy is the leading cause of cognitive disability in the United States, and it is entirely preventable.
- Treatment programs must start with an understanding that substance abuse in women is a complex problem surrounded by multiple individual, familial, and social issues that require many levels of intervention and treatment.

REFERENCES

Agency for Healthcare Research and Quality (AHRQ). (2012). *Five major steps to intervention (the "5 A's")*. Rockville, MD: AHRQ. Available at www.ahrq.gov/professionals/clinicians-providers/guidelines-recommendations/tobacco/5steps.html.

Agency for Healthcare Research and Quality (AHRQ). (2013). *Efficacy and safety of screening for postpartum depression*. Available at http://effectivehealthcare.ahrq.gov/index.cfm/search-for-guides-reviews-and-reports/?productid=1438&pageaction=displayproduct.

American Academy of Pediatrics (AAP) & the American College of Obstetricians and Gynecologists (ACOG). (2012). *Guidelines for perinatal care* (7th ed.). Elk Grove Village, IL, and Washington, DC: Authors.

American College of Obstetricians and Gynecologists (ACOG). (2008). Use of psychiatric medications during pregnancy and lactation ACOG practice bulletin no. 92. *Obstetrics and Gynecology*, *111*(4), 1001–1020.

American College of Obstetricians and Gynecologists Committee on Obstetric Practice (ACOG). (2010). Committee opinion no. 453: Screening for depression during and after pregnancy. *Obstetrics and Gynecology*, *115*(2, Part 1), 394–395.

American Psychiatric Association (APA). (2013). *Diagnostic and statistical manual of mental disorders*. 5th ed., text rev. Washington, DC: American Psychiatric Publishing.

Beck, C. (2008a). State of the science on postpartum depression: What nurse researchers have contributed—part 1. *MCN: The American Journal of Maternal/Child Nursing, 33*(2), 122–126.

Beck, C. (2008b). State of the science on postpartum depression: What nurse researchers have contributed—part 2. *MCN: The American Journal of Maternal/Child Nursing, 33*(3), 151–156.

Behnke, M., Smith, V. C., & Committee on Substance Abuse, & Committee on Fetus and Newborn (2013). Prenatal substance abuse: Short- and long-term effects on the exposed fetus. *Pediatrics, 131*(3), e1009–e1024.

Beydoun, H. A., Beydoun, M. A., Kaufman, J. S., et al. (2012). Intimate partner violence against adult women and its association with major depressive disorder, depressive symptoms and postpartum depression: A systematic review and meta-analysis. *Social Science & Medicine, 75*(6), 959–975.

Blom, E. A., Jansen, P. W., Verhulst, F. C., et al. (2010). Perinatal complications increase the risk of postpartum depression: The generation R study. *British Journal of Obstetrics and Gynaecology, 117*(11), 1390–1398.

Cerulli, C., Talbor, N. L., Tang, W., & Chaudron, L. H. (2011). Co-occurring intimate partner violence and mental health diagnoses in perinatal women. *Journal of Women's Health, 20*(12), 1797–1803.

Cox, J. L., Holden, J. M., & Sagovsky, R. (1987). Detection of postnatal depression: Development of the 10-item Edinburgh Postnatal Depression Scale. *British Journal of Psychiatry, 150*, 782–786.

Cunningham, F., Leveno, K., Bloom, S. et al. (2014). *Williams obstetrics* (24th ed.). New York: McGraw-Hill Education.

Davey, H. L., Tough, S. C., Adair, C. E., & Benzies, K. M. (2011). Risk factors for sub-clinical and major postpartum depression among a community cohort of Canadian women. *Maternal and Child Health Journal, 15*(7), 866–875.

Deligiannidis, K. M., & Freeman, M. P. (2014). Complementary and alternative medicine therapies for perinatal depression. *Best Practice & Research. Clinical Obstetrics & Gynaecology, 28*(1), 85–95.

Earls, M. F., & American Academy of Pediatrics (AAP) Committee on Psychosocial Aspects of Child and Family Health (2010). Incorporating recognition and management of perinatal and postpartum depression into pediatric practice. *Pediatrics, 126*(5), 1032–1039.

Garcia, K. S., Flynn, P., Pierce, K. J., & Caudle, M. (2010). Repetitive transcranial magnetic stimulation treats postpartum depression. *Brain Stimulation, 3*(1), 36–41.

Gilbert, E. (2011). *Manual of high risk pregnancy and delivery* (5th ed.). St. Louis: Mosby.

Glover, V. (2014). Maternal depression, anxiety and stress during pregnancy and child outcome; What needs to be done. *Best Practice & Research. Clinical Obstetrics & Gynaecology, 28*(1), 25–35.

Guille, C., Newman, R., Fryml, L. D., et al. (2013). Management of postpartum depression. *Journal of Midwifery & Women's Health, 58*(6), 632–642.

Hadley, D. E., Albanese, W. P., & Rochester, C. D. (2012). Psychiatric drug interactions explored. *Pharmacy Practice News*. February 2012. Available at www.pharmacypracticenews.com/download/ppn0212_ER_WM.pdf.

Hudak, M. L., Tan, R. C., & American Academy of Pediatrics (AAP) Committee on Drugs and Committee on Fetus and Newborn (2012). Neonatal drug withdrawal. *Pediatrics, 129*(2), e540–e560.

Kendall-Tackett, K., & Hale, T. W. (2010). Review: The use of antidepressants in pregnant and breastfeeding women: A review of recent studies. *Journal of Human Lactation, 26*(2), 187–195.

Kraft, W. K., & van den Anker, J. N. (2012). Pharmacologic management of the opioid neonatal abstinence syndrome. *Pediatric Clinics of North America, 59*(5), 1147–1165.

Lawrence, R. A., & Lawrence, R. M. (2011). *Breastfeeding: A guide for the medical profession* (7th ed.). St. Louis: Mosby.

Le Strat, Y., Dubertret, C., & Le Foll, B. (2011). Prevalence and correlates of major depressive episode in pregnant and postpartum women in the United States. *Journal of Affective Disorders, 135*(1-3), 128–138.

Letourneau, N., Tryphonopoulos, P. D., Duffett-Leger, L., et al. (2012). Support intervention needs and preferences of fathers affected by postpartum depression. *Journal of Perinatal & Neonatal Nursing, 26*(1), 69–80.

Logsdon, M. C., Tomasulo, R., Eckert, D., et al. (2012). Identification of mothers at risk for postpartum depression by hospital-based perinatal nurses. *MCN: The American Journal of Maternal/Child Nursing, 37*(4), 218–225.

Manber, R., Schnyer, R. N., Lyell, D., et al. (2010). Acupuncture for depression during pregnancy: A randomized controlled trial. *Obstetrics and Gynecology, 115*(3), 511.

Mikacich, J. (2014). Drawing out postpartum depression. Available at www.acog.org/About_ACOG/ACOG_Departments/District_Newsletters/District_IX/December_2012/Drawing_out_postpartum_depression.

Milgrom, J., & Gemmill, A. W. (2014). Screening for perinatal depression. *Best Practice & Research. Clinical Obstetrics & Gynaecology, 28*(1), 13–23.

Montgomery, D., Plate, C., Alder, S. C., et al. (2006). Testing for fetal exposure to illicit drugs using umbilical cord tissue vs meconium. *Journal of Perinatology, 26*(1), 11–14.

Myers, E. R., Aubuchon-Endsley, N., & Bastian, L. A. (2013). *Efficacy and safety of screening for postpartum depression.* Comparative effectiveness review 106. Rockville, MD: Agency for Healthcare Research and Quality.

National Institute on Alcohol Abuse and Alcoholism. (2010). *Fetal alcohol exposure.* Available at www.niaaa.nih.gov/alcohol-health/fetal-alcohol-exposure.

National Institute of Drug Abuse (NIDA). (2010). *Cocaine: Abuse and addiction.* Available at www.drugabuse.gov/publications/research-reports/cocaine-abuse-addiction/what-are-effects-maternal-cocaine-use.

National Institute of Drug Abuse (NIDA). (2011a). *Topics in brief: Prenatal exposure to drugs of abuse.* Available at www.drugabuse.gov/publications/topics-in-brief/prescription-drug-abuse.

National Institute of Drug Abuse (NIDA). (2011b). *Topics in brief: Prescription drug abuse.* Available at www.drugabuse.gov/publications/topics-in-brief/prenatal-exposure-to-drugs-abuse.

National Institute of Drug Abuse (NIDA). (2013). *Methamphetamine: Abuse and addiction.* Available at www.drugabuse.gov/publications/research-reports/methamphetamine-abuse-addiction/what-methamphetamine.

National Institute of Drug Abuse (NIDA). (2014). *Drug facts: Marijuana.* Available at www.drugabuse.gov/publications/drugfacts/marijuana.

O'Hara, M. W., & Wisner, K. L. (2014). Perinatal mental illness: Definition, description, aetiology. *Best Practice & Research. Clinical Obstetrics & Gynaecology, 28*(1), 3–12.

Paschetta, E., Berrisford, G., Coccia, F., et al. (2014). Perinatal psychiatric disorders: An overview. *American Journal of Obstetrics and Gynecology, 210*(6), 501–509, e6.

Paulson, J. F., & Bazemore, S. D. (2010). Prenatal and postpartum depression in fathers and its association with maternal depression: A meta-analysis. *Journal of the American Medical Association, 303*(19), 1961–1969.

ProCon.org. (2014). 23 Legal Medical Marijuana States and DC. Available at http://medicalmarijuana.procon.org/view.resource.php?resourceID=000881.

Rahman, A., Fisher, J., Bower, P., et al. (2013). Interventions for common perinatal mental disorders in women in low-and middle-income countries: A systematic review and meta-analysis. *Bulletin of the World Health Organization, 91*(8), 593–601.

Ray, S., & Stowe, Z. N. (2014). The use of antidepressant medication in pregnancy. *Best Practice & Research. Clinical Obstetrics & Gynaecology, 28*(1), 71–83. Available at www.bestpracticeobgyn.com/article/S1521-6934%2813%2900136-3/abstract.

Roy, P., & Payne, J. (2009). Treatment of bipolar disorder during and after pregnancy. In C. Zarate, & K. Husseini (Eds.), *Bipolar depression: Molecular neurobiology, clinical diagnosis and pharmacotherapy*. Cambridge, MA: Birkhauser.

Sadock, B., Sadock, V., & Ruiz, P. (2009). (9th ed.) *Kaplan & Sadock's comprehensive textbook of psychiatry*. (Vol. 2) Philadelphia: Lippincott Williams & Wilkins.

Seidel, H., Ball, J., Dains, J., et al. (2011). *Mosby's guide to physical examination* (7th ed.). St. Louis: Mosby.

Substance Abuse and Mental Health Services Administration (SAMHSA). (2012). *Results from the 2010 National Survey on Drug Use and Health: Summary of National Findings*. Available at www.samhsa.gov/data/NSDUH/2k10NSDUH/2k10Results.htm#3.1.3.

Thornton, D., Guendelman, S., & Hosang, N. (2009). Obstetric complications in women with diagnosed mental illness: The relative success of California's county mental health system. *Health Services Research*, *45*(1), 246–264.

United States Drug Testing Laboratories, Inc. (2012a). *CordStat*. Available at www.usdtl.com/cordstat.html.

United States Drug Testing Laboratories, Inc. (2012b). *MecStat*. Available at www.usdtl.com/mecstat.html.

U.S. Preventive Services Task Force (USPSTF). (2009). *Screening for depression in adults*. Rockville, MD: Agency for Healthcare Research and Quality. Available at www.ahrq.gov/CLINIC/uspstf/uspsaddepr.htm.

Vigod, S. N., Villegas, L., Dennis, C. L., & Ross, L. E. (2010). Prevalence and risk factors for postpartum depression among women with preterm and low-birth-weight infants: A systematic review. *British Journal of Obstetrics and Gynaecology*, *117*(5), 540–550.

Wisner, K. L., Sit, D. K. Y., Altemus, M., et al. (2012). Mental health and behavioral disorders in pregnancy. In S. G. Gabbe, J. R. Niebyl, J. L. Simpson, et al. (Eds.), *Obstetrics: Normal and problem pregnancies* (6th ed.). Philadelphia: Saunders.

Woolhouse, H., Gartland, D., Hegarty, K., et al. (2012). Depressive symptoms and intimate partner violence in the 12 months after childbirth: A prospective pregnancy cohort study. *British Journal of Obstetrics and Gynaecology*, *119*(3), 315–323.

Yonkers, K. A., Vigod, S., & Ross, L. E. (2011). Diagnosis, pathophysiology, and management of mood disorders in pregnant and postpartum women. *Obstetrics and Gynecology*, *117*(4), 961–977.

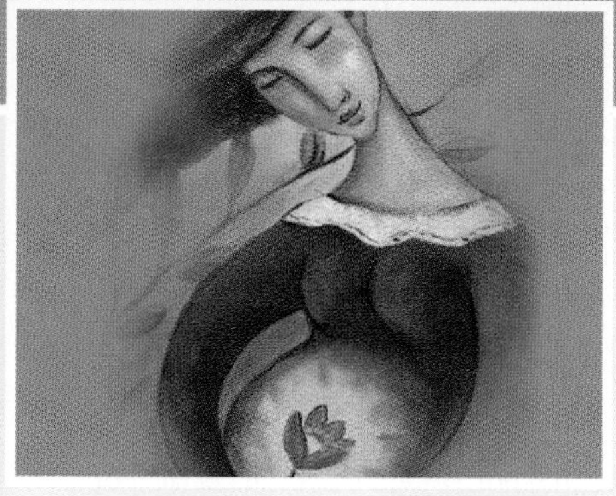

CHAPTER 32

Labor and Birth Complications

Deborah R. Bambini

http://evolve.elsevier.com/Lowdermilk/MWHC/

LEARNING OBJECTIVES

- Differentiate between preterm birth and low birth weight.
- Describe the criteria for very preterm, early preterm, and late preterm and the implications of each.
- Discuss major risk factors associated with preterm labor.
- Analyze current interventions to prevent spontaneous preterm birth.
- Discuss the use of tocolytics and antenatal glucocorticoids for management of preterm labor.
- Design a nursing care plan for women with preterm premature rupture of membranes (preterm PROM).
- Explain the care of a woman with postterm pregnancy.
- Explain the challenge of caring for obese women during labor and birth.
- Summarize the nursing care for a trial of labor, the induction and augmentation of labor, forceps- and vacuum-assisted birth, cesarean birth, and vaginal birth after a cesarean birth (VBAC).
- Discuss obstetric emergencies and their appropriate management.

When complications arise during labor and birth, risk for perinatal morbidity and mortality increases. Some complications are anticipated, especially if the woman is identified to be at high risk during the antepartum period; other complications are unexpected or unforeseen. It is crucial for nurses to understand the normal birth process to prevent and detect deviations from normal labor and birth and to promptly implement nursing measures when complications arise. Optimal care of the laboring woman, fetus, and family experiencing complications is possible only when the nurse and other members of the obstetric team use their knowledge and skills in a concerted effort to provide competent and compassionate care. This chapter focuses on the problems of preterm labor and birth, dystocia, obesity, postterm pregnancy, and obstetric emergencies.

PRETERM LABOR AND BIRTH

Preterm labor is generally diagnosed clinically as regular contractions along with a change in cervical effacement or dilation or both or presentation with regular uterine contractions and cervical dilation of at least 2 cm. **Preterm birth** is any birth that occurs between 20 0/7 and 36 6/7 weeks of gestation (American College of Obstetricians and Gynecologists [ACOG], 2012). The preterm birth rate for all races in the United States has dropped each year since 2008, reaching 11.55% in 2012, the most recent year for which data are available (Martin, Hamilton, Osterman, et al., 2013a). This decline was largely the result of three major practice changes: (1) improved fertility practices that reduced the risk for higher-order multiple gestations; (2) limiting scheduled births at less than 39 weeks of gestation to only those with valid indications; and (3) increased use of strategies to prevent recurrent preterm birth (Simhan, Iams, & Romero, 2012).

Preterm births are categorized as *very preterm* (<32 weeks of gestation), *moderately preterm* (32 to 34 weeks of gestation), and *late preterm* (34 to 36 weeks of gestation). The degree of risk for an infant born prematurely is directly related to the degree of prematurity. About 75% of all preterm births in the United States are categorized as late preterm. Late preterm infants are at increased risk for early death and long-term health problems when compared with infants who are born full term. Although late preterm babies do experience significant problems, the great majority of infant deaths and the most serious morbidity occur among the infants who are born before 32 weeks of gestation (very preterm birth) (Simhan, Berghella, & Iams, 2014). The very preterm birth rate in the United States was approximately 1.93% in 2012 (Martin et al., 2013a).

The World Health Organization estimates that 9.6% (almost 13 million) of all births worldwide in 2005 were preterm. The rate of preterm birth is highest in Africa and North America and lowest in Europe (Simhan et al., 2012). The incidence of preterm birth varies with race. In the United States, non-Hispanic black women have the highest rate, followed by Hispanic women. Non-Hispanic white women have the lowest rate of preterm birth. Although the rate of preterm birth for non-Hispanic black women reached a record low of 16.53% in 2012, this rate is still far higher than for non-Hispanic white women (Martin et al., 2013a).

Preterm Birth Versus Low Birth Weight

Although they have distinctly different meanings, the terms *preterm birth* or *prematurity* and *low birth weight* were often interchanged in the past. Preterm birth describes length of gestation (i.e., less than 37 0/7 weeks regardless of the weight of the infant), whereas low birth weight describes only weight at the time of birth (i.e., 2500 g or less). Because birth weight was far easier to determine than gestational age, in many settings and publications low birth weight was used as a substitute term for preterm birth. Preterm birth, however, is a more dangerous health condition for an infant because less time in the uterus correlates with immaturity of body systems. Low-birth-weight babies can be, but are not necessarily, preterm; low birth weight can be caused by conditions other than preterm birth, such as **intrauterine growth restriction (IUGR),** a condition of inadequate fetal growth not necessarily correlated with initiation of labor. Pregnant women who have various complications of pregnancy that interfere with uteroplacental perfusion, such as gestational hypertension or poor nutrition, may give birth to a baby at term who is low birth weight because of IUGR. However, infants born at a preterm gestation can weigh more than 2500 g at birth. Currently, thanks to advances in pregnancy dating, outcomes related to gestational age can increasingly be distinguished from outcomes related to birth weight. Therefore, use of birth weight as a substitute for gestational age in developed countries is no longer considered acceptable (Simhan et al., 2014).

Spontaneous Versus Indicated Preterm Birth

Preterm births are divided into two categories: spontaneous and indicated. Spontaneous preterm births occur following an early initiation of the labor process in the apparent absence of maternal or fetal illness and make up nearly 75% of all preterm births in developed countries. Conditions such as preterm labor with intact membranes and preterm PROM often result in preterm birth (Simhan et al., 2014). Box 32-1 lists risk factors for the development of spontaneous preterm labor.

Indicated preterm births occur as a means to resolve maternal or fetal risk related to continuing the pregnancy. About 25% of all preterm births in the United States are indicated because of medical or obstetric conditions that affect the mother, the fetus, or both. An increase in the number of indicated preterm births between 34 and 36 weeks of gestation accounts for much of the rise in late preterm births (Simhan et al., 2012). Box 32-2 lists common causes of indicated preterm births. The remainder of this section deals with spontaneous preterm labor and birth.

Causes of Spontaneous Preterm Labor and Birth

Causes of preterm labor and birth are multifactorial (Flood & Malone, 2012). Infection is the only factor shown to be definitely associated with preterm labor. When bacterial cervical or urinary tract infections are present, the risk of preterm birth increases. Women in spontaneous preterm labor with intact membranes commonly have organisms that are normally found in the lower genital tract present in their amniotic fluid, placenta, and membranes (Simhan et al., 2014). Clinical and laboratory evidence of infection are more common when birth occurs earlier than 30 to 32 weeks of gestation rather than closer to term. Intraabdominal infections (e.g., appendicitis) also have been related to preterm birth (Simhan et al., 2012). Women with periodontal disease have been shown to have an increased risk for preterm birth. However, the risk is not reduced by periodontal care, suggesting that the link between periodontal disease and preterm birth is not a cause-and-effect relationship (Simhan et al., 2012).

Another proposed cause of preterm labor and birth is bleeding at the site of placental implantation in the uterus in the first or second trimester of pregnancy. The resulting uteroplacental ischemia or hemorrhage at the decidual layer of the placenta may somehow activate the preterm labor process. Intrauterine inflammation is associated with infection, uterine vascular compromise, and decidual hemorrhage and can contribute to preterm labor. Maternal and fetal stress, uterine overdistention,

BOX 32-1 Risk Factors for Spontaneous Preterm Labor

- History of previous spontaneous preterm birth
- Nonwhite race
- Genital tract colonization and infection
- Multifetal gestation
- Second-trimester bleeding
- Low prepregnancy weight

Data from Simhan, H.N., Berghella, V., & Iams, J.D. (2014). Preterm labor and birth. In R.K. Creasy, R. Resnik, J.D. Iams, et al. (Eds.), *Creasy and Resnik's maternal-fetal medicine: Principles and practice* (7th ed.). Philadelphia: Saunders; Simhan, H., Iams, J., & Romero, R. (2012). Preterm birth. In S. Gabbe, J. Niebyl, & J. Simpson (Eds.), *Obstetrics: Normal and problem pregnancies* (6th ed.). Philadelphia: Saunders.

BOX 32-2 Common Causes of Indicated Preterm Birth

- Preexisting or gestational diabetes
- Chronic hypertension
- Preeclampsia
- Obstetrical disorders or risk factors in the current or a previous pregnancy
- Previous cesarean birth via a classic uterine incision
- Placental disorders
- Medical disorders
- Seizures
- Thromboembolism
- Maternal HIV or active herpes infection
- Obesity
- Advanced maternal age
- Fetal disorders
- Chronic (IUGR) or acute (abnormal NST or BPP) fetal compromise
- Excessive or inadequate amount of amniotic fluid
- Congenital fetal abnormalities

BPP, Biophysical profile; *HIV*, human immunodeficiency virus; *IUGR*, intrauterine growth restriction; *NST*, nonstress test.
Data from Simhan, H., Iams, J., & Romero, R. (2012). Preterm birth. In S. Gabbe, J. Niebyl, & J. Simpson (Eds.), *Obstetrics: Normal and problem pregnancies* (6th ed.). Philadelphia: Saunders.

allergic reaction, and a decrease in progesterone are other factors that can play a part in initiating preterm labor. It is becoming increasingly clear that preterm labor is caused by multiple pathologic processes that eventually result in uterine contractions, cervical changes, and rupture of membranes (Buhimschi & Norman, 2014; Simhan et al., 2014).

Predicting Spontaneous Preterm Labor and Birth

Risk Factors

Predicting those at risk for preterm labor and birth includes identification of risk factors. In addition to the risk factors listed in Box 32-1, poverty; lack of education; living in a disadvantaged neighborhood, state, or region; and lack of access to prenatal care also have been identified as risk factors. The risk for preterm birth also appears to be genetically related. For example, women whose sisters gave birth prematurely are also more likely to do so, and the grandparents of women who give birth prematurely are more likely to have been born prematurely themselves than the grandparents of women who give birth at term (Simhan et al., 2014). Researchers have developed a variety of other risk scoring systems; however, no risk scoring system has thus far been successful in lowering the preterm birth rate (DeFranco, Lewis, & Odibo, 2013).

Cervical Length

One possible predictor of preterm labor is endocervical length. Changes in cervical length occur before uterine activity, so cervical measurement can identify women in whom the labor process has begun. However, because preterm cervical shortening occurs over a period of weeks, neither digital nor ultrasound cervical examination is very sensitive at predicting imminent preterm birth. Women whose cervical length is greater than 30 mm are unlikely to give birth prematurely even if they have symptoms of preterm labor (Simhan et al., 2012; Simhan et al., 2014).

Fetal Fibronectin Test

Fetal fibronectin (fFN) has been studied extensively and is marketed in the United States as a diagnostic test for preterm labor. fFN is a glycoprotein "glue" found in plasma and produced during fetal life. It normally appears in cervical and vaginal secretions early in pregnancy and then again in late pregnancy. The test is performed by collecting fluid from the woman's vagina using a swab during a speculum examination. The presence of fFN during the late second and early third trimesters of pregnancy may be related to placental inflammation, which is thought to be one cause of spontaneous preterm labor. The presence of fFN alone is not very sensitive as a predictor of preterm birth, however. Often the test is used to predict who will *not* go into preterm labor, because preterm labor is very unlikely to occur in women with a negative result (Simhan et al., 2014).

A combined approach to predicting preterm birth has been found to increase sensitivity and negative predictive value. Combining the evaluation of fFN levels and ultrasound measurement of cervical length was found to increase the ability to identify those at risk for preterm labor within the next 7 days as well as better identify those at low risk (DeFranco et al., 2013).

CARE MANAGEMENT

Assessment

DeFranco, Lewis, and Odibo (2013) reported that 30.2% of women who experienced preterm labor signs ultimately experienced preterm birth, whereas Simhan, Iams, and Romero (2012) state that at least 50% of all women who ultimately give birth prematurely have no identifiable risk factors. Therefore, it is important that all women be educated about preterm labor, not only in early pregnancy but also in the preconception period.

Nursing assessment for factors that contribute to this risk begins early in pregnancy and continues throughout the prenatal period. The onset of preterm labor is often insidious and can be easily mistaken for normal discomforts of pregnancy. Nursing diagnoses, expected outcomes of care, and evidence-based interventions are established for each woman based on her assessment findings (see the Nursing Care Plan).

NURSING CARE PLAN

Preterm Labor

NURSING DIAGNOSIS	EXPECTED OUTCOME	NURSING INTERVENTIONS	RATIONALES
Deficient Knowledge related to recognition of preterm labor	Woman and partner describe signs and symptoms of preterm labor.	Assess what woman and partner know about preterm labor and birth and how to recognize its presence.	To identify areas of deficit
		Discuss signs and symptoms that serve as warning signs of preterm labor so that woman or her partner has adequate information.	To identify problems early
		Provide written supplemental materials that include a list of warning signs and instructions regarding what to do if any of listed signs occur.	Couple can reinforce and review learning and act swiftly and appropriately should a sign occur
		Discuss and demonstrate how to assess and time contractions.	To provide needed skills to assess signs of labor

Continued

NURSING CARE PLAN—cont'd

Preterm Labor

NURSING DIAGNOSIS	EXPECTED OUTCOME	NURSING INTERVENTIONS	RATIONALES
Risk for Injury (maternal/fetal) related to recurrence of preterm labor	Woman demonstrates ability to assess self for signs of recurring labor; maternal-fetal well-being is maintained.	Teach woman and partner how to monitor uterine contraction activity daily.	To provide immediate evidence of worsening condition
		Instruct woman and partner to report rupture of membranes, vaginal bleeding, cramping, pelvic pressure, or low backache to appropriate health care resource immediately.	Because such symptoms can be signs of labor
		Have woman monitor her weight, diet, fluid intake, and vital signs on a daily basis.	To evaluate for potential problems
		Have woman limit activities to those recommended in restricted activity plan.	To decrease likelihood of onset of labor
		Encourage woman to use side-lying position when reclining.	To enhance placental perfusion
		Teach woman signs and symptoms of thrombophlebitis, and encourage gentle exercise of lower extremities.	Because pregnancy and limited activity increase risk for clot formation
		Counsel couple to abstain from sexual intercourse and nipple stimulation if symptoms of preterm labor occur.	Because such activities may stimulate uterine contractions
		Encourage woman to practice relaxation techniques.	To decrease uterine tone and decrease anxiety and stress
		Teach woman to take tocolytic or other medications per physician's orders.	To inhibit uterine contractions
		Teach woman and partner about and have them report any medication side effects immediately.	To prevent medication-induced complications
		Have family arrange for alternative strategies in carrying out woman's usual roles and functions.	To decrease stress and limit temptations to increase activity
		If small children are part of household, encourage family to make alternative arrangements for child care.	To enhance woman's adherence to her restricted activity protocol
Anxiety related to preterm labor and potential birth of premature neonate	Feeling and symptoms of anxiety are reduced.	Provide calm, soothing atmosphere, and encourage family to provide emotional support.	To facilitate coping
		Encourage verbalization of fears.	To decrease intensity of emotional response
		Involve woman and family in home management of her condition.	To promote greater sense of control
		Help woman identify and use appropriate coping strategies and support systems.	To reduce fear and anxiety
		Explore use of desensitization strategies such as progressive muscle relaxation, visual imagery, or thought stopping.	To reduce fear-related emotions and related physical symptoms
		Provide information about online support groups.	To reduce fear and anxiety
Deficient Diversional Activity related to modified bed rest	Woman will verbalize diminished feelings of boredom.	Assist woman to creatively explore personally meaningful activities that can be pursued from the bed.	To ensure activities that have meaning, purpose, and value to individual
		Maintain emphasis on personal choices of woman.	Because doing so promotes control and minimizes imposition of routines by others
		Evaluate support and system resources that are available in environment.	To assist in providing diversional activities
		Explore ways for woman to remain an active participant in home management and decision making.	To promote control
		Engage support of family and friends in carrying out chosen activities and making necessary environmental alterations.	To ensure success
		Encourage woman to use Internet to communicate with other women on bed rest.	To obtain support and share feelings
		Teach woman about stress management and relaxation techniques.	To help manage tension of confinement

EVIDENCE-BASED PRACTICE

Magnesium Sulfate for Neuroprotection Against Cerebral Palsy

Ask the Question

For women anticipating preterm birth, can any prenatal treatment protect the premature newborn from cerebral palsy?

Search for the Evidence

Search Strategies English language research-based publications since 2011 on magnesium sulfate, neuroprotection, preterm, premature were included.

Databases Used Cochrane Collaborative Database, National Guideline Clearinghouse (AHRQ), CINAHL, PubMed, UpToDate, and the professional websites for ACOG and AWHONN

Critical Appraisal of the Evidence

Among the many challenges for a premature baby is the risk of cerebral palsy, the most common motor disability in children. Alert clinicians noticed that newborns whose mothers had been given magnesium sulfate for tocolysis or preeclampsia were less likely to have cerebral palsy. Further research confirmed its benefit and safety.

- Magnesium sulfate facilitates vasodilation, reduces inflammation, and reduces calcium uptake into cells. It may delay cellular injury or death and increases blood flow to the brain (Merrill, 2013).
- Although magnesium sulfate is no longer recommended for stopping preterm labor, the American College of Obstetricians and Gynecologists (ACOG) and the Society for Maternal-Fetal Medicine (SMFM) (2013) still recommend magnesium sulfate for neuroprotection against cerebral palsy in women anticipating preterm birth at less than 32 weeks of gestation. In addition, they recommend the short-term use (up to 48 hours) from 24 to 34 weeks of gestation to allow for the administration of betamethasone for lung maturity.
- Study protocols are in place for ongoing research into the advisability of using neuroprotective magnesium sulfate for later gestational age, up to 34 weeks (Crowther, Middleton, Wilkinson, et al., 2013).
- Administering magnesium sulfate requires intravenous infusion and close monitoring for 24 hours, often in a hospital setting. A cost-effectiveness analysis reveals that giving neuroprotective magnesium sulfate to clients with threatened preterm birth saves $1.5 million for every case of cerebral palsy that is averted (Bickford, Magee, Mitton, et al., 2013).

Apply the Evidence: Nursing Implications

- Magnesium sulfate should be given in settings where staff are familiar with its use, monitoring is available, and emergency resuscitation and ventilation equipment is available.
- Typical use in women in active preterm labor or with preterm premature rupture of membranes is a 4-g loading dose given over 30 to 60 minutes, followed by the maintenance dose of 1 g/hr, given until birth or for up to 24 hours, whichever comes first. Other tocolytics are discontinued.
- Prior to the loading dose, the nurse obtains baseline vital signs and patellar reflexes. These are repeated at 10 minutes after initiation and at the end of the loading dose. During the maintenance dose, vitals are repeated hourly, reflexes every 2 hours, and continuous electronic fetal monitoring is recommended.
- Signs of magnesium toxicity include decrease in respirations of 4 breaths per minute from baseline rate or to less than 12 per minute; systolic blood pressure drop of 15 mm Hg from baseline; diminished reflexes; decreased urinary output; or fetal heart rate abnormalities. If these are noted, the nurse should stop the infusion and notify the health care provider. Calcium gluconate should be available nearby as an antidote.
- To improve safety, the infusion should be given via infusion device in prepackaged concentrations clearly labeled as loading and maintenance doses, and double-checked by another nurse.
- Neonatal hypermagnesemia, although rare, can present as apnea, respiratory depression, lethargy, poor feeding, and hyporeflexia. Neonatal resuscitation should be available.

Quality and Safety Competencies: Safety*

Knowledge

Discuss effective strategies to reduce reliance on memory.

Clearly labeled standardized packaging of magnesium sulfate doses prevents medication errors.

Skills

Demonstrate effective use of technology and standardized practices that support safety and quality.

Standardized protocols and administering magnesium sulfate in facilities familiar with its use and equipped with adequate emergency equipment improve client safety.

Attitudes

Appreciate the cognitive and physical limits of human performance.

Having another nurse double-check bags and infusion timing prevents client injury.

References

American College of Obstetricians and Gynecologists (ACOG) Committee on Obstetric Practice & Society for Maternal-Fetal Medicine (SMFM). (2013). Committee opinion no. 573: Magnesium sulfate use in obstetrics. *Obstetrics and Gynecology, 122*(3), 727–728.

Bickford, C. D., Magee, L. A., Mitton, C., et al. (2013). Magnesium sulphate for fetal neuroprotection: A cost-effectiveness analysis. *BioMed Central (BMC) Health Services Research, 13*, 527.

Crowther, C. A., Middleton, P. F., Wilkinson, D., et al. (2013). Magnesium sulphate at 30 to 34 weeks' gestational age: Neuroprotection trial (MAGENTA)—Study protocol. *BioMed Central (BMC)Pregnancy Childbirth, 13*, 91.

Merrill, L. (2013). Magnesium sulfate during anticipated preterm birth for infant neuroprotection. *Nursing for Women's Health, 17*(1), 44–50.

Pat Mahaffee Gingrich

*Adapted from QSEN at www.qsen.org.

Interventions

Prevention

Primary prevention strategies that address risk factors associated with preterm labor and birth are less costly in human and financial terms than the high-tech and often lifelong care required by preterm infants and their families. Programs aimed at health promotion and disease prevention that encourage healthy lifestyles for the population in general and women of childbearing age in particular should be developed. Preconception counseling and care for women, especially those with a history of preterm birth, can identify correctable risk factors and provide a means to encourage women to participate in health-promoting activities. Smoking cessation, for example, has been shown to prevent preterm labor and birth.

Preterm birth can be prevented in some women by administering prophylactic progesterone supplementation. Daily vaginal suppositories or creams and weekly intramuscular injections of 17-alpha hydroxyprogesterone caproate have been shown to decrease the rate of preterm birth by about 40% in women with a history of prior preterm birth or with a short (less than 20-mm length) cervix before 25 weeks of gestation. Supplementation begins at 16 weeks and continues until 36 weeks of gestation. Progesterone supplementation does not affect the rate of preterm birth in women with multiple gestations. Exactly how progesterone works to prevent preterm birth is unclear (Simhan et al., 2012; Simhan et al., 2014).

Early Recognition and Diagnosis

Although preterm birth is often not preventable, early recognition of preterm labor is still essential to implement interventions that have been demonstrated to reduce neonatal morbidity and mortality. These interventions include (Simhan et al., 2012):

- Transferring the mother before birth to a hospital equipped to care for her preterm infant
- Giving antibiotics during labor to prevent neonatal group B streptococci infection
- Administering glucocorticoids to women in labor to prevent or reduce neonatal and infant morbidity and mortality from health problems including respiratory distress syndrome, intraventricular hemorrhage, and necrotizing enterocolitis
- Administering magnesium sulfate to women giving birth before 32 weeks of gestation to reduce the incidence of cerebral palsy in their infants

Although maternal transport helps ensure a better health outcome for the mother and the baby, it also has a downside. Women may be transported to tertiary centers far from home, making visits by family and friends difficult and increasing the anxiety levels of the woman and her family. Attention to the needs of the woman and her family before, during, and after the transport is essential to comprehensive nursing care (see Chapter 34).

BOX 32-3 Signs and Symptoms of Preterm Labor

Uterine Activity
- Uterine contractions occurring more frequently than every 10 minutes persisting for 1 hour or more
- Uterine contractions may be painful or painless

Discomfort
- Lower abdominal cramping similar to gas pains; may be accompanied by diarrhea
- Dull, intermittent low back pain (below the waist)
- Painful, menstrual-like cramps
- Suprapubic pain or pressure
- Pelvic pressure or heaviness; feeling that "baby is pushing down"
- Urinary frequency

Vaginal Discharge
- Change in character or amount of usual discharge: thicker (mucoid) or thinner (watery), bloody, brown or colorless, increased amount, odor
- Rupture of amniotic membranes

Because more than half of preterm births occur in women without obvious risk factors, it is essential that all pregnant women are taught the symptoms of preterm labor (Box 32-3). The nurse caring for women in a prenatal setting should educate them about about how to recognize signs of preterm labor and then assess for these symptoms at each prenatal visit. Women also must be taught the significance of these symptoms of preterm labor and what to do should they occur (see Teaching for Self-Management: What to Do if Symptoms of Preterm Labor Occur).

TEACHING FOR SELF-MANAGEMENT

What to Do if Symptoms of Preterm Labor Occur

- Empty your bladder.
- Drink two to three glasses of water or juice.
- Lie down on your side for 1 hour.
- Palpate for contractions.
- If symptoms continue, call your health care provider or go to the birthing facility.
- If symptoms go away, resume light activity, but not what you were doing when the symptoms began.
- If symptoms return, call your health care provider or go to the birthing facility.
- If any of the following symptoms occur, call your health care provider or go to the birthing facility immediately:
  - Uterine contractions every 10 minutes or less for 1 hour or more
  - Vaginal bleeding
  - Smelly vaginal discharge
  - Fluid leaking from the vagina

In particular, client education regarding any symptoms of uterine contractions or cramping between 20 0/7 and 36 6/7 weeks of gestation must emphasize that these symptoms are not just normal discomforts of pregnancy but indications of possible preterm labor (Fig. 32-1). Waiting too long to see a health care provider could result in inevitable preterm birth without sufficient time to implement the interventions that have been shown to improve infant outcomes (see preceding discussion).

As mentioned, the diagnosis of preterm labor is based on three major diagnostic criteria:

- Gestational age between 20 0/7 and 36 6/7 weeks
- Uterine activity (e.g., regular contractions)
- Progressive cervical change (e.g., effacement of 80%, or cervical dilation of 2 cm or greater)

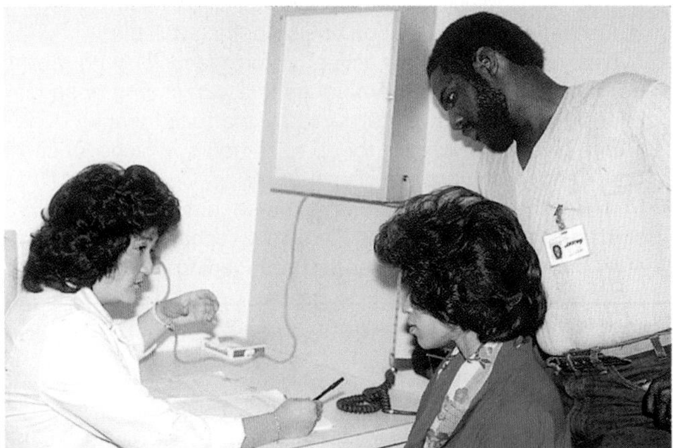

FIG 32-1 A nurse teaching a couple signs and symptoms of preterm labor. (Courtesy Marjorie Pyle, RNC, Lifecircle, Costa Mesa, CA.)

If the presence of fFN is used as another diagnostic criterion, a sample of cervical and vaginal secretions for testing should be obtained before an examination for cervical changes because the lubricant used to examine the cervix can reduce the accuracy of the test for fFN. The presence of vaginal bleeding or ruptured membranes or a history of intercourse within the past 24 hours also can reduce the accuracy of the test results.

The pregnant woman at 30 weeks of gestation with an irritable uterus but no documented cervical change is not in preterm labor, although she should be carefully evaluated during follow-up care to determine whether she has progressed to active preterm labor (e.g., effacement, dilation, or both). Misdiagnosis of preterm labor can lead to inappropriate use of pharmacologic agents that can be dangerous to the health of the woman, the fetus, or both (ACOG, 2012).

Lifestyle Modifications

Activity Restriction. Activity restriction, including bed rest and limited work, is commonly prescribed to prevent preterm birth. Bed rest, however, is not a benign intervention, and no evidence has been published in the literature to support its effectiveness in reducing preterm birth rates (Simhan et al., 2012; Simhan et al., 2014). Therefore, bed rest should not be routinely recommended (ACOG, 2012). Many health care providers recommend only modified bed rest.

 **COMMUNITY FOCUS**

Identify a website intended for pregnant women who are on activity restriction for preterm labor. What criteria did you use to evaluate the website to determine the quality of the information provided? List at least three suggestions found on the website that would be helpful for women on activity restriction and their families.

Restriction of Sexual Activity. Restriction of sexual activity is frequently recommended for women at risk for preterm birth. This intervention has not been shown to be effective at preventing preterm birth. However, sexual abstinence has not been studied in women with specific risk factors for preterm birth, such as a short cervix. Therefore, more research is indicated (Simhan et al., 2014).

Home Care. Home care of the woman at risk for preterm birth is a challenge for the nurse, who must assist the woman and her family in dealing with the many difficulties faced by families in which one member is unable to fulfill usual role responsibilities.

The woman's environment can be modified for convenience by using tables and storage units around her bed or daytime resting place to keep essential items within reach (e.g., cell or smart phone, television, radio, MP3 player, CD player, computer with Internet access, snacks, books, magazines, newspapers, and items for hobbies) (Fig. 32-2). Ensuring that the bed or couch is near a window and the bathroom is also helpful. Covering the bed with an eggcrate mattress can relieve discomfort. Women often find that a daily schedule of smaller, more frequent meals, activities (e.g., paying bills, planning and helping with meal preparation, hobbies), limited naps, and hygiene and grooming (e.g., shower, dressing in street clothes, applying makeup) reduces boredom and helps them maintain control and normalcy. See Teaching for Self-Management: Activities for Children of Women on Activity Restriction for additional ideas and suggestions. Also see Teaching for Self-Management: Coping with Activity Restriction in Chapter 27 for more information. With modified bed rest, women are usually allowed bathroom privileges for toileting and showering and can be up to the table for meals.

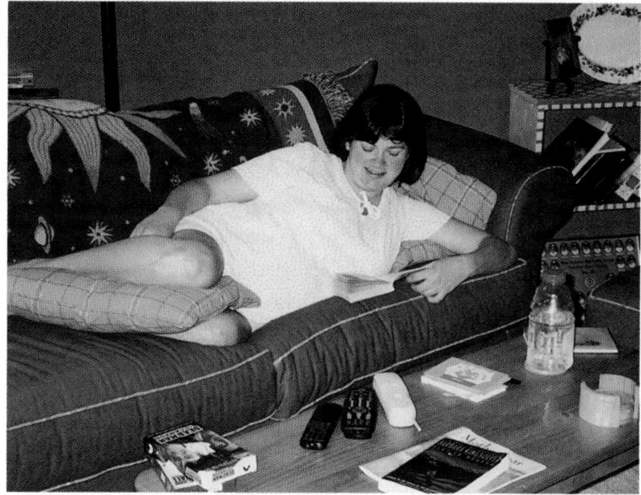

FIG 32-2 Woman at home on restricted activity for preterm labor prevention. Note how she has arranged her daytime resting area so that needed items are close at hand. (Courtesy Amy Turner, Cary, NC.)

TEACHING FOR SELF-MANAGEMENT

Activities for Children of Women on Activity Restriction

- Schedule brief play periods throughout the day.
- Keep a few favorite toys in a box or basket close to the bed or couch.
- Read to the children.
- Put puzzles together.
- Watch videos or play video games (remote control for television is ideal).
- Play card or board games.
- Color in coloring books.
- Cut out pictures from magazines and paste them on cardboard.
- Play bed basketball with a soft (sponge) ball or rolled up sock and a trash can or empty laundry basket.

Suppression of Uterine Activity

Tocolytics are medications given to arrest labor after uterine contractions and cervical change have occurred. No medications that have been approved for use as tocolytics by the U.S. Food and Drug Administration (FDA) are currently available in the United States. Ritodrine (Yutopar) was approved but has been withdrawn from the U.S. market. However, it is still used as a tocolytic in other countries. Drugs marketed for other purposes, such as treatment of asthma or hypertension or as antiinflammatory or analgesic agents, are used on an "off-label" basis (i.e., drugs known to be effective for a specific purpose, although not specifically developed and tested for this purpose) to suppress preterm labor (Simhan et al., 2014). No tocolytic has been shown to reduce the rate of preterm birth. Rather, the rationale for giving these medications is to delay birth long enough to allow time for maternal transport and for corticosteroids to reach maximum benefit to reduce neonatal morbidity and mortality. Studies of individual drugs used for tocolysis rarely contain information about whether delaying birth improved infant outcomes (Simhan et al., 2012). Selecting the appropriate tocolytic medication requires consideration of each drug's effectiveness, risks, and side effects. Important contraindications exist to the use of all tocolytics. Maternal and fetal contraindications to tocolytic therapy are listed in Box 32-4. Box 32-5 describes nursing care for women receiving tocolytic therapy.

Magnesium sulfate is the most commonly used tocolytic agent because maternal and fetal or neonatal adverse reactions are less common than with the beta-adrenergic agonists. Clinicians are familiar with its use as a treatment of preeclampsia and believe it is safer to use when compared with the beta-adrenergic agonists. However, although magnesium sulfate is still frequently used, its effectiveness as a tocolytic is not supported by the literature (see the Medication Guide: Tocolytic Therapy for Preterm Labor) (Simhan et al., 2012; Simhan et al., 2014).

BOX 32-4 Contraindications to Tocolysis

Maternal
- Preeclampsia with severe features or eclampsia
- Bleeding with hemodynamic instability
- Contraindications to specific tocolytic medications

Fetal
- Intrauterine fetal demise
- Lethal fetal anomaly
- Nonreassuring fetal status
- Chorioamnionitis
- Preterm premature rupture of membranes (preterm PROM)

Data from American College of Obstetricians and Gynecologists. (ACOG). (2012). *Management of preterm labor.* ACOG practice bulletin no. 127. Washington, DC: ACOG.

BOX 32-5 Nursing Care for the Woman Receiving Tocolytic Therapy

- Explain the purpose and side effects of the tocolytic medication(s) to the woman and her family.
- Position the woman on her side to enhance placental perfusion and reduce pressure on the cervix.
- Monitor maternal vital signs including lung sounds and respiratory effort, fetal heart rate and pattern, and labor status according to hospital protocol and professional standards.
- Assess the mother and fetus for signs of adverse reactions related to the tocolytic medication(s) being administered (see the Medication Guide: Tocolytic Therapy for Preterm Labor).
- Determine maternal fluid balance by measuring the daily weight and intake and output.
- Limit fluid intake to 2500 to 3000 ml/day, especially if a beta-adrenergic agonist or magnesium sulfate is being administered.
- Provide psychosocial support and opportunities for the woman and family to express feelings and concerns.
- Offer comfort measures as needed.
- Encourage diversional activities and relaxation techniques.

SAFETY ALERT

Because magnesium sulfate depresses the function of the central nervous system (CNS), it is essential that the nurse frequently assesses the woman's respiratory status, deep tendon reflexes, and level of consciousness to identify signs that the serum level of magnesium sulfate is reaching toxic levels.

Beta$_2$-adrenergic agonists (e.g., ritodrine and terbutaline [Brethine]) have been widely used as tocolytics. They have many maternal and fetal adverse reactions, however, including beta$_1$-stimulated cardiopulmonary (e.g., tachycardia) effects and beta$_2$-stimulated metabolic (e.g., hyperglycemia) effects. Therefore, beta$_2$-adrenergic agonists are increasingly being replaced by medications that are safer and have fewer adverse reactions. They should not be used in women with known or suspected heart disease, preeclampsia with severe features or eclampsia, pregestational or gestational diabetes, or hyperthyroidism (Simhan et al., 2012; Simhan et al., 2014). Use of beta$_2$ -adrenergic agonists is also contraindicated in women with migraine headaches (Gilbert, 2011).

Terbutaline, the most commonly administered beta-adrenergic agonist used for tocolysis, relaxes uterine smooth muscle by stimulating beta$_2$-receptors in the uterine smooth muscle. Terbutaline is often given subcutaneously to facilitate maternal transfer to a tertiary center or to initiate tocolytic therapy while another agent with a slower onset of action is administered concurrently. Additionally, a subcutaneous injection of 0.25 mg may be given to suppress uterine tachysystole during labor induction or augmentation or to suppress contractions prior to cesarean birth. Long-term oral or subcutaneous administration (e.g., terbutaline pump) as maintenance therapy to suppress preterm labor has not been proven to be effective at reducing prematurity or neonatal morbidity so use of the drug for this purpose is not recommended (Gilbert, 2011; Simhan et al., 2012; Simhan et al., 2014) (see Medication Guide: Tocolytic Therapy for Preterm Labor).

Nifedipine (Adalat, Procardia), a calcium channel blocker, is a tocolytic agent that can suppress contractions. It works by preventing calcium from entering smooth muscle cells, thus reducing uterine contractions. Because of its ease of administration and low incidence of significant maternal and fetal side effects, nifedipine's use is increasing (see Medication Guide: Tocolytic Therapy for Preterm Labor) (Simhan et al., 2012; Simhan et al., 2014).

MEDICATION ALERT

Administering nifedipine and magnesium sulfate simultaneously can cause skeletal muscle blockade. In addition, nifedipine should not be given along with or immediately following a beta$_2$-adrenergic agonist (e.g., terbutaline) because of effects on maternal heart rate and blood pressure (Simhan et al., 2012; Simhan et al., 2014).

SAFETY ALERT

Because using a calcium channel blocker can result in orthostatic hypotension and dizziness, it is essential to instruct women to slowly change position from supine to upright and then sit until any dizziness disappears before standing. In addition, it is important to maintain adequate fluid balance to reduce the drop in blood pressure that can occur with the drug-related vasodilation.

Indomethacin (Indocin), a nonsteroidal antiinflammatory drug (NSAID), has been shown in some trials to suppress preterm labor by blocking the production of prostaglandins. Serious maternal side effects are uncommon, and indomethacin is usually well tolerated. However, serious fetal or neonatal side effects have caused major concerns about its use as a tocolytic. Therefore, limiting the use of indomethacin to a period of 48 hours or less in women with preterm labor at less than 32 weeks of gestation is recommended (Simhan et al., 2012; Simhan et al., 2014) (see Medication Guide: Tocolytic Therapy for Preterm Labor).

MEDICATION GUIDE

Tocolytic Therapy for Preterm Labor

MEDICATION AND ACTION	DOSAGE AND ROUTE*	ADVERSE EFFECTS	NURSING CONSIDERATIONS
Magnesium Sulfate			
CNS depressant; Relaxes smooth muscles, including uterus	IV fluid should contain 40 g in 1000 ml, piggyback to primary infusion, and administer using controller pump: Loading dose: 4-6 g over 20-30 minutes Maintenance dose: 1-4 g/hr Use for stabilization only Discontinue within 24-48 hours at the maintenance dose or if intolerable adverse effects occur	**Maternal:** • Hot flushes, sweating, burning at the IV insertion site, nausea and vomiting, dry mouth, drowsiness, blurred vision, diplopia, headache, ileus, generalized muscle weakness, lethargy, dizziness • Hypocalcemia • Dyspnea • Transient hypotension • Some reactions may subside when loading dose is completed **Intolerable:** • Respiratory rate fewer than 12 breaths/minute • Pulmonary edema • Absent DTRs • Chest pain • Severe hypotension • Altered level of consciousness • Extreme muscle weakness • Urine output less than 25-30 ml/hour or less than 100 ml/4 hours • Serum magnesium level of 10 mEq/L (9 mg/dl) or greater **Fetal (uncommon):** Decreased breathing movement Reduced FHR variability Nonreactive NST	Assess woman and fetus to obtain baseline before beginning therapy and then before and after each incremental change; follow frequency of agency protocol. Drug is almost always given IV but can also be administered IM. Monitor serum magnesium levels with higher doses; therapeutic range is between 4 and 7.5 mEq/L or 5-8 mg/dl. Discontinue infusion and notify physician if intolerable adverse effects occur. Ensure that calcium gluconate or calcium chloride is available for emergency administration to reverse magnesium sulfate toxicity. Should not be given to women with myasthenia gravis. Total IV intake should be limited to 125 ml/hr.
Beta-Adrenergic Agonist (Beta-Mimetic)			
Terbutaline (Brethine) Relaxes smooth muscles, inhibiting uterine activity, and causing bronchodilation	Subcutaneous injection of 0.25 mg every 4 hours Treatment should last no longer than 24 hours Discontinue use if intolerable adverse effects occur	**Maternal (most are mild and of limited duration):** • Tachycardia, chest discomfort, palpitations, arrhythmias • Tremors, dizziness, nervousness • Headache • Nasal congestion • Nausea and vomiting • Hypokalemia • Hyperglycemia • Hypotension **Intolerable:** • Tachycardia greater than 130 beats/minute • BP less than 90/60 • Chest pain • Cardiac arrhythmias • Myocardial infarction • Pulmonary edema	Should not be used in women with a history of cardiac disease, pregestational or gestational diabetes, severe gestational hypertension, preeclampsia with severe features or eclampsia, or hyperthyroidism, or with significant hemorrhage. Myocardial infarction leading to death has been reported after use.

Continued

MEDICATION GUIDE—cont'd

Tocolytic Therapy for Preterm Labor

MEDICATION AND ACTION	DOSAGE AND ROUTE*	ADVERSE EFFECTS	NURSING CONSIDERATIONS
Beta-Adrenergic Agonist (Beta-Mimetic)—cont'd		**Fetal:** • Tachycardia • Hyperinsulinemia • Hyperglycemia	Assess woman and fetus according to agency protocol, being alert for adverse effects. Assess maternal glucose and potassium levels before treatment is initiated and periodically during treatment. Significant hyperglycemia (greater than 180 mg/dl) and hypokalemia (less than 2.5 mEq/L) may occur. Notify physician if the woman exhibits the following: Maternal heart rate greater than 130 beats/minute; arrhythmias, chest pain BP less than 90/60 mm Hg Signs of pulmonary edema (e.g., dyspnea, crackles, decreased SaO_2). Fetal heart rate greater than 180 beats/minute. Hyperglycemia occurs more frequently in women who are being treated simultaneously with corticosteroids. Ensure that propranolol (Inderal) is available to reverse adverse effects related to cardiovascular function.
Prostaglandin Synthetase Inhibitors (NSAIDs)			
Indomethacin (Indocin) Relaxes uterine smooth muscle by inhibiting prostaglandins	Loading dose: 50 mg orally, then 25-50 mg orally every 6 hours for 48 hours	**Maternal (common):** • Nausea and vomiting • Heartburn **Less common, but more serious:** • GI bleeding • Prolonged bleeding time • Thrombocytopenia • Asthma in aspirin-sensitive clients **Fetal:** • Constriction of ductus arteriosus • Oligohydramnios, caused by reduced fetal urine production • Neonatal pulmonary hypertension	The long-acting formulations decrease the incidence of adverse effects. Used only if gestational age is less than 32 weeks. Administer for 48 hours or less. Do not use in women with renal or hepatic disease, active peptic ulcer disease, poorly controlled hypertension, asthma, or coagulation disorders. Can mask maternal fever. Assess woman and fetus according to agency policy, being alert for adverse affects. Determine amniotic fluid volume and function of fetal ductus arteriosus before initiating therapy and within 48 hours of discontinuing therapy; assessment is critical if therapy continues for more than 48 hours. Administer with food to decrease GI distress. Monitor for signs of postpartum hemorrhage.
Calcium Channel Blockers			
Nifedipine (Adalat, Procardia) Relaxes smooth muscles including the uterus by blocking calcium entry	Initial dose: 10-20 mg, orally, every 3 to 6 hours until contractions are rare, followed by long-acting formulations of 30 or 60 mg every 8-12 hours for 48 hours while corticosteroids are being given (however, the ideal dose has not been established)	**Maternal (most effects are mild):** • Hypotension • Headache • Flushing • Dizziness • Nausea **Fetal:** • Hypotension (questionable)	Avoid concurrent use with magnesium sulfate because skeletal muscle blockade can result. Should not be given simultaneously with or immediately after terbutaline because of effects on heart rate and blood pressure. Assess woman and fetus according to agency protocol, being alert for adverse effects. Do not use sublingual route of administration.

NOTE: There are variations in recommended administration protocols; always consult agency protocol, which should be evidence based.

BP, Blood pressure; *CNS,* central nervous system; *DTRs,* deep tendon reflexes; *FHR,* fetal heart rate; *GI,* gastrointestinal; *IM,* intramuscular; *IV,* intravenous; *NSAIDs,* nonsteroidal antiinflammatory drugs; *NST,* nonstress test; *SaO_2,* arterial oxygen saturation; *SOB,* shortness of breath.

Data from Gilbert, E. (2011). *Manual of high risk pregnancy & delivery* (5th ed.). St. Louis: Mosby; Simhan, H.N., Berghella, V., & Iams, J.D. (2014). Preterm labor and birth. In R.K. Creasy, R. Resnik, J.D. Iams, et al. (Eds.), *Creasy and Resnik's maternal-fetal medicine: Principles and practice* (7th ed.). Philadelphia: Saunders; Simhan, H., Iams, J., & Romero, R. (2012). Preterm birth. In S. Gabbe, J. Niebyl, & J. Simpson (Eds.), *Obstetrics: Normal and problem pregnancies* (6th ed.). Philadelphia: Saunders.

Promotion of Fetal Lung Maturity

Antenatal glucocorticoids, given as intramuscular (IM) injections to the mother to accelerate fetal lung maturity by stimulating fetal surfactant production, are now considered one of the most effective and cost-efficient interventions for preventing morbidity and mortality associated with preterm labor. Antenatal glucocorticoids have been shown to significantly reduce the incidence of respiratory distress syndrome, intraventricular hemorrhage, necrotizing enterocolitis, and death in neonates, without increasing the risk of infection in either mothers or newborns (Mercer, 2014a). The National Institutes of Health (NIH) consensus panel recommended that all women between 24 and 34 weeks of gestation be given a single course of antenatal glucocorticoids when preterm birth is threatened, unless evidence indicates that glucocorticoids will have an adverse effect on the mother or birth is imminent. In general, women who are candidates for tocolytic therapy are also candidates for antenatal glucocorticoids. The regimen for administration of antenatal glucocorticoids is given in the Medication Guide: Antenatal Glucocorticoid Therapy with Betamethasone or Dexamethasone.

The optimal timing and dosage of antenatal glucocorticoids is still being researched. Repetitive weekly doses may be beneficial but offer potential risks to fetal growth and development. Currently, a single repeat course of antenatal glucocorticoids may be considered if preterm birth threatens again after the initial course has been completed. This rescue course is given identically to the initial course if the initial course was administered more than 2 weeks previously, the gestational age remains less than 32 6/7 weeks, and imminent preterm birth is still considered likely (Mercer, 2014a; Simhan et al., 2014).

MEDICATION GUIDE

Antenatal Glucocorticoid Therapy with Betamethasone or Dexamethasone

Action

Stimulates fetal lung maturation by promoting release of enzymes that induce production or release of lung surfactant. **Note:** The U.S. Food and Drug Administration has not approved these medications for this use (i.e., this is an unlabeled use for obstetrics).

Indication

To prevent or reduce the severity of neonatal respiratory distress syndrome by accelerating lung maturity in fetuses between 24 and 34 weeks of gestation. Infants born to women who received antenatal glucocorticoids are also less likely to experience intraventricular hemorrhage, necrotizing enterocolitis, or neonatal death.

Dosage and Route

- *Betamethasone:* 12 mg intramuscular (IM) for two doses 24 hours apart
- *Dexamethasone:* 6 mg IM for four doses 12 hours apart

Maternal Effects

- Transient (lasting 72 hours) increase in white blood cell (WBC) count
- Hyperglycemia

Fetal Effects

Transient (lasting 72 hours) decrease in fetal breathing and body movements

Nursing Considerations

- Give deep IM in ventral gluteal or vastus lateralis muscle.
- Medication *must* be given by IM injection; oral administration is *not* an acceptable alternative.
- Injection is painful.
- Medication should *not* affect maternal blood pressure.
- Assess blood glucose levels. Women with diabetes whose blood sugars have previously been well controlled may require increased insulin doses for several days.

Data from Simhan, H., Iams, J., & Romero, R. (2012). Preterm birth. In S. Gabbe, J. Niebyl, & J. Simpson (Eds.), *Obstetrics: Normal and problem pregnancies* (6th ed.). Philadelphia: Saunders.

! NURSING ALERT

All women between 24 and 34 weeks of gestation who are at risk for preterm birth within 7 days should receive treatment with a single course of antenatal glucocorticoids (Mercer, 2014a). Because optimal benefit to the fetus begins 24 hours after the first injection, timely administration is essential.

Management of Inevitable Preterm Birth

When preterm birth appears inevitable, magnesium sulfate may be administered to reduce or prevent neonatal neurologic morbidity (e.g., cerebral palsy). Current recommendations are that magnesium sulfate for neuroprotection is given to women who are at least 24 but less than 32 weeks of gestation at the time birth is expected to occur. How magnesium sulfate works to provide neuroprotection is not well understood. Although it is likely that the neuroprotective effects are the result of residual concentrations of the medication in the neonate's system, data are insufficient to determine the precise maternal dose necessary to achieve the benefit (Simhan et al., 2012; Simhan et al., 2014). Currently the dose of magnesium sulfate administered for neuroprotection is the same as that given for tocolysis (see Medication Guide: Tocolytic Therapy for Preterm Labor).

Labor that has progressed to a cervical dilation of 4 cm or more is likely to lead to inevitable preterm birth. If birth appears imminent, preparations to care for a small, immature neonate should be made. Women in preterm labor can rapidly progress to birth, and a very small fetus can be born through a partially dilated cervix. Also malpresentation (e.g., breech presentation) occurs much more frequently in preterm than in term fetuses. Therefore, nurses must be prepared to handle the emergency birth of a preterm infant, from either cephalic or breech presentation, without the woman's primary health care provider being present. Personnel skilled at neonatal resuscitation should be present at the time of birth. Equipment, supplies, and medications used for neonatal resuscitation should be gathered in advance and prepared for immediate use. If birth occurs in a hospital that is not prepared to provide continuing care for a preterm neonate, plans should be made for transfer of the baby to a higher level of care as soon as possible.

Fetal and Early Neonatal Loss

Preterm birth or the presence of congenital anomalies or genetic disorders incompatible with life are major reasons for intrauterine fetal demise (stillbirth) or early neonatal death. In many of these situations the parents will already have been told that the fetus has died or that the baby has a condition that is incompatible with life and will most likely die very soon after birth. Sometimes, however, the fetal death is unexpected, diagnosed only after the woman has been admitted to the labor and birth unit. Whatever the case, labor and birth nurses must be prepared to provide sensitive care to these women and their families (see Chapter 37).

If fetal or early neonatal death is expected, the parents and members of the health care team need to discuss the situation before the birth and decide on a management plan that is acceptable to everyone. Despite counseling about the likelihood of a poor outcome, some parents want "everything possible," including cesarean birth for an abnormal fetal heart rate (FHR) tracing, to be done for the baby. If such intervention is not desired, usually the FHR is not monitored during labor.

Another major decision is whether to attempt neonatal resuscitation and to what lengths. Sometimes the feasibility of neonatal resuscitation cannot be determined until the baby's size and physical appearance have been assessed. If the baby is too small, too immature, or too malformed for effective resuscitation, comfort care can be provided instead. The baby is kept warm and comfortable, either at the mother's bedside or in the nursery, depending on the parents' desires, until death occurs. Parents can choose to view and hold the baby as they wish.

After the birth the woman should be given the opportunity to decide if she wants to stay on the maternity unit or be moved to another hospital unit. She may prefer to be away from the sound of crying babies and exposure to other families who have had healthy infants. However, postpartum care and grief support may not be as good on another hospital unit, where the staff is not experienced in postpartum and bereavement care. Whether death occurs in utero or after birth, parents are faced with the same needs. See Chapter 37 for additional information on dealing with families experiencing a perinatal loss.

PREMATURE RUPTURE OF MEMBRANES

Premature rupture of membranes (PROM) is the spontaneous rupture of the amniotic sac and leakage of amniotic fluid beginning before the onset of labor at any gestational age. Preterm premature rupture of membranes (preterm PROM) (i.e., membrane rupture before 37 0/7 weeks of gestation) is associated with approximately 10% of all preterm births in the United States. Preterm PROM occurs twice as often in African-Americans as in other racial groups. The frequency of preterm PROM appears to have decreased since the 1990s (Mercer, 2012). Preterm PROM most likely results from pathologic weakening of the amniotic membranes caused by inflammation, stress from uterine contractions, or other factors that cause increased intrauterine pressure. Infection of the urogenital tract is a major risk factor associated with preterm PROM (Mercer, 2012, 2014b). Box 32-6 lists other risk factors. PROM or preterm PROM is diagnosed after the woman reports either a sudden gush of fluid or a slow leak of fluid from the vagina.

BOX 32-6 Risk Factors for Preterm Premature Rupture of Membranes (Preterm PROM)

- History of prior preterm birth, especially if associated with preterm PROM
- History of cervical conization or cerclage
- Urinary or genital tract infection
- Short cervical length in the second trimester
- Preterm labor in the current pregnancy
- Uterine overdistention
- Second- and third-trimester bleeding
- Pulmonary disease
- Connective tissue disorders
- Low socioeconomic status
- Low body mass index
- Nutritional deficiencies (copper and ascorbic acid)
- Cigarette smoking

Data from Mercer, B. (2012). Premature rupture of the membranes. In S. Gabbe, J. Niebyl, & J. Simpson (Eds.), *Obstetrics: Normal and problem pregnancies* (6th ed.). Philadelphia: Saunders.

Chorioamnionitis is the most common maternal complication of preterm PROM, making it a major complication of pregnancy (see later discussion). Other less common but serious maternal complications include placental abruption, sepsis, and death (Mercer, 2012, 2014b). Fetal complications from preterm PROM are primarily related to intrauterine infection, cord prolapse, umbilical cord compression associated with oligohydramnios, and placental abruption. Another possible fetal complication when preterm PROM occurs prior to 20 weeks of gestation is pulmonary hypoplasia (Mercer, 2012, 2014b).

CARE MANAGEMENT

Management of PROM is determined for each woman based on an assessment of the estimated risk of maternal, fetal, and neonatal complications if pregnancy is allowed to continue or immediate labor and birth are attempted. At term (at or after 37 0/7 weeks of gestation), because infection is the greatest maternal, fetal, and neonatal risk, birth is the best option. Labor will most likely be induced if it does not begin spontaneously soon after PROM occurs (Mercer, 2012, 2014b).

Active pursuit of labor and birth, rather than expectant management, is recommended for women who experience preterm PROM between 34 and 36 weeks of gestation. Although infants born at this gestational age have a higher risk for complications than babies born at or after 37 0/7 weeks, serious morbidity and mortality is uncommon. Because conservative management at this gestational age prolongs pregnancy by only a few days, significantly increases the risk of chorioamnionitis, and has not been shown to improve neonatal outcomes, immediate birth is considered to be the best management option. If pulmonary maturity can be documented, women with preterm PROM at 32 to 33 weeks gestation may also be offered immediate birth because they have an increased risk for complications with conservative management (Mercer, 2014b).

Preterm PROM before 32 weeks of gestation is usually managed expectantly or conservatively because the risks to the fetus and newborn associated with preterm birth are considered to be greater than the risks of infection. Women will likely be hospitalized in an attempt to prolong the pregnancy and allow additional time for fetal maturation unless intrauterine infection, significant vaginal bleeding, placental abruption, preterm labor, or fetal compromise occurs (Mercer, 2012, 2014b). Nursing support of the woman and her family is critical at this time. They are often anxious about the health of the baby and the woman may fear that she was responsible in some way for the membrane rupture. Other nursing interventions include encouraging expression of feelings and concerns, providing information, and making referrals as needed.

Conservative management of preterm PROM includes fetal assessment by nonstress test (NST) and biophysical profile (BPP). The woman should also be taught how to assess her fetus using daily fetal movement counts (DFMCs) because a slowing of fetal movement is a warning sign of severe fetal compromise. (See Chapter 26 for further discussion of these tests.) In addition, the woman will be monitored for signs of labor, placental abruption, and the development of intrauterine infection. Antenatal glucocorticoids are administered to women who are less than 32 weeks of gestation because they decrease the risk of several neonatal complications. In addition, a 7-day course of broad-spectrum antibiotics (e.g., ampicillin, erythromycin) is administered. Antibiotic treatment has been shown to prolong the time between membrane rupture and birth, decrease maternal chorioamnionitis and postpartum endometritis, and prevent sepsis, pneumonia, and intraventricular hemorrhage in the neonate (Mercer, 2012).

Vigilance for signs of infection is a major part of the client education and nursing care after preterm PROM. The woman must be taught how to keep her genital area clean and that nothing should be introduced into her vagina. Signs of infection (e.g., fever, foul-smelling vaginal discharge, maternal and fetal tachycardia) should be reported immediately. If chorioamnionitis develops, labor is induced. If preterm labor occurs, tocolytic medications may be administered in an attempt to gain time for transporting the woman to a hospital capable of providing care to a preterm infant or for antenatal corticosteroids or antibiotics to reach effective levels (Gilbert, 2011).

CHORIOAMNIONITIS

Chorioamnionitis, bacterial infection of the amniotic cavity, is a major cause of complications for mothers and newborns at any gestational age. It occurs in approximately 1% to 5% of term births but in as many as 25% of preterm births (Duff, 2012). Other terms for this condition include *clinical chorioamnionitis, amnionitis, intrapartum infection, amniotic fluid infection*, and *intraamniotic infection*. Chorioamnionitis is usually diagnosed by the clinical findings of maternal fever, maternal and fetal tachycardia, uterine tenderness, and foul odor of amniotic fluid (Fishman & Gelber, 2012).

Chorioamnionitis most often occurs after membranes rupture or labor begins, as organisms that are part of the normal vaginal flora ascend into the amniotic cavity. Many of the risk factors for chorioamnionitis are associated with a long labor, such as prolonged membrane rupture, multiple vaginal examinations, and use of internal FHR and contraction monitoring modes (Duff, 2014). Other risk factors include young maternal age, low socioeconomic status, nulliparity, and preexisting infections of the lower genital tract (Duff, 2012).

Women with chorioamnionitis can develop bacteremia. They are also more likely to have dysfunctional labor, which can result in the need for cesarean birth (see later discussion). If cesarean birth is necessary, wound infection or pelvic abscess can occur (Duff, 2012).

Neonatal risks include pneumonia, bacteremia, and sepsis. Death is more likely to occur in preterm than in term infants (Duff, 2012). There is increasing evidence that intrauterine infection is associated with increased risks of respiratory distress syndrome, periventricular leukomalacia, and cerebral palsy. It is thought that intrauterine infection leads to fetal infection that eventually produces a fetal inflammatory response syndrome with resulting pulmonary and central nervous system damage (Duff, 2014).

To prevent maternal and neonatal complications, prompt treatment with intravenous (IV) broad-spectrum antibiotics and birth of the fetus are necessary. Ampicillin or penicillin and gentamicin are most often used to treat chorioamnionitis during labor. After cesarean birth, an antibiotic that provides coverage for anaerobic organisms, such as clindamycin (Cleocin) or metronidazole (Flagyl) should be added. One additional dose of a combination of broad-spectrum antibiotics (e.g., ampicillin and gentamicin) given postpartum is usually sufficient treatment for women with chorioamnionitis (Duff, 2014).

The increased use of intrapartum antibiotic prophylaxis during labor in women who are group B streptococci (GBS) positive to prevent neonatal GBS infection has decreased the incidence of chorioamnionitis. Other measures that have proven to be effective in decreasing the frequency of chorioamnionitis are active management of labor (see later discussion), induction of labor rather than expectant management, following rupture of membranes at term, and use of prophylactic antibiotics in selected women with preterm PROM (Duff, 2014).

POSTTERM PREGNANCY, LABOR, AND BIRTH

A **postterm pregnancy** (also sometimes referred to as a *postdates* or *prolonged* pregnancy) is one that has 42 completed weeks of gestation (294 days) or more from the first day of the last menstrual period (LMP) (Cunningham, Leveno, Bloom, et al., 2014). Many pregnancies are misdiagnosed as postterm. The use of first-trimester ultrasound for pregnancy dating has confirmed that the first day of the LMP, traditionally used for pregnancy dating, is much less reliable as a predictor of true gestational age. Therefore, use of the LMP alone for pregnancy dating tends to greatly overestimate the number of postterm gestations (Rampersad & Macones, 2012).

The exact cause of true postterm pregnancy is still unknown. However, it is clear that the timing of labor is determined by complex interactions among the fetus, the placenta and membranes, the uterine myometrium, and the cervix. For example, congenital primary fetal adrenal hypoplasia and placental sulfatase deficiency cause low estrogen production. Low levels of estrogen can result in a decrease in prostaglandin precursors, thereby preventing normal cervical ripening, reducing the formation of oxytocin receptors in the myometrium, and delaying the onset of labor. Although postterm pregnancy is more common in primiparous women, a woman who experiences one postterm pregnancy is more likely to experience it again in subsequent pregnancies (Rampersad & Macones, 2012).

Clinical manifestations of postterm pregnancy include maternal weight loss (more than 1.4 kg [approximately 3 lb]/wk) and decreased uterine size (related to decreased amniotic fluid), meconium in the amniotic fluid, and advanced bone maturation of the fetal skeleton with an exceptionally hard fetal skull (Gilbert, 2011).

Maternal and Fetal Risks

Maternal risks are often related to dysfunctional labor, such as increased risk for perineal injury related to fetal macrosomia. Risk for hemorrhage and infection is higher. Interventions such as induction of labor with prostaglandins or oxytocin, forceps- or vacuum-assisted birth, and cesarean birth are more likely to be necessary. Each of these interventions, of course, carries its own set of risks. The woman also may experience fatigue, physical discomfort, and psychologic reactions such as depression, frustration, and feelings of inadequacy as she passes her estimated date of birth. Relationships with close friends and family members may become strained and the woman's negative feelings about herself may be projected as feelings of resentment toward the fetus (Gilbert, 2011; Rampersad & Macones, 2012).

Another complication associated with postterm pregnancy is abnormal fetal growth. Although the risk of having a small for gestational age (SGA) infant is increased, only 10% to 20% of postterm fetuses are undernourished. Macrosomia (birth weight more than 4000 g) occurs far more often. Macrosomia occurs when the placenta continues to provide adequate nutrients to support fetal growth after 40 weeks of gestation. Macrosomic infants have an increased risk for operative birth and shoulder dystocia, leading to fetal injury (Rampersad & Macones, 2012).

Other fetal risks associated with postterm gestation are related to the intrauterine environment. After 43 to 44 weeks of gestation, the placenta begins to age. Enlarging areas of infarction and increased deposition of calcium and fibrin in its tissue decrease the placenta's reserve and can affect its ability to oxygenate the fetus. Decreased amniotic fluid (less than 400 ml), oligohydramnios, is the complication most frequently associated with postterm pregnancy. Because of the decreased amount of amniotic fluid, there is a potential for cord compression and resulting hypoxemia (Gilbert, 2011). Other potential complications include meconium-stained amniotic fluid and increased chance of meconium aspiration (Rampersad & Macones, 2012).

Postmaturity syndrome occurs in 10% to 20% of neonates born following postterm pregnancies. Postmaturity syndrome is characterized by dry, cracked, peeling skin; long nails; meconium staining of skin, nails, and umbilical cord; and perhaps loss of subcutaneous fat and muscle mass (Gilbert, 2011; Rampersad & Macones, 2012).

CARE MANAGEMENT

The management of postterm pregnancy is controversial. However, because perinatal morbidity and mortality increase greatly after 42 weeks of gestation, pregnancies are usually not allowed to continue after this time. In the United States, most physicians induce labor at 41 weeks of gestation. An alternative approach is to initiate twice-weekly fetal testing at 41 weeks of gestation. The testing generally consists of either a BPP or NST along with an assessment of amniotic fluid volume (see Chapter 26 for discussion of these tests). Evidence is insufficient to determine which of the two management approaches is better (Rampersad & Macones, 2012).

During the postterm period the woman is encouraged to assess fetal activity daily, assess for signs of labor, and keep appointments with her primary health care provider (see Teaching for Self-Management: Postterm Pregnancy). The woman and her family should be encouraged to express their feelings (e.g., frustration, anger, impatience, fear) about the prolonged pregnancy and helped to realize that these feelings are normal. At times the emotional and physical strain of a postterm pregnancy can seem overwhelming. Referral to a support group or another supportive resource may be needed.

TEACHING FOR SELF-MANAGEMENT

Postterm Pregnancy

- Perform daily fetal movement counts.
- Assess for signs of labor.
- Call your primary health care provider if your membranes rupture or if you notice a decrease in or no fetal movement.
- Keep appointments for fetal assessment tests and cervical checks.
- Go to the birthing facility soon after labor begins.

During labor the fetus of a woman with a postterm pregnancy should be continuously monitored electronically for a more accurate assessment of the FHR and pattern. Inadequate fluid volume can lead to compression of the umbilical cord, which results in fetal hypoxia that is reflected in variable or prolonged deceleration patterns. If oligohydramnios is present, an amnioinfusion may be performed to restore amniotic fluid volume to maintain a cushioning of the cord. See Chapter 18 for additional information on amnioinfusion.

CLINICAL REASONING CASE STUDY

Postterm Pregnancy

Angela is a 31-year-old primigravida, presenting to the office for a routine prenatal visit. She is 40 weeks and 2 days of gestation and expresses her concern, stating, "My friends tell me that you'll try to talk me into inducing labor or a cesarean. I want to have my baby naturally! I don't want medications or surgery! This baby will know when he is ready." Angela has a birth plan that you have reviewed with her and plans to have both of her sisters and her husband be a part of the birth.

1. Evidence—Is there sufficient evidence to advise Angela about the best approach at this time?
2. Assumptions—Describe the underlying assumptions about each of the following:
   a. Accuracy of last menstrual period (LMP)
   b. Determination of postterm versus late-term gestation
   c. Physiology underlying the onset of labor
   d. Placental function after 40 weeks
   e. Criteria for determining adequate placental function
   f. Additional risks as gestational age increases
3. What are the implications and priorities for nursing care at this time?
4. Does the evidence objectively support your conclusion?

DYSFUNCTIONAL LABOR (DYSTOCIA)

Dysfunctional labor (dystocia) is defined as a long, difficult, or abnormal labor caused by various conditions associated with the five factors affecting labor. It is estimated that dysfunctional labor occurs in approximately 8% to 11% of all births and it is the most common indication for cesarean birth (Gilbert, 2011). A diagnosis of dysfunctional labor is ultimately responsible for approximately 60% of all cesarean births in the United States (Cunningham et al., 2014). It can be caused by any of the following factors:

- Ineffective uterine contractions or maternal bearing-down efforts (the powers)
- Alterations in the pelvic structure (the passage)
- Fetal causes, including abnormal presentation or position, anomalies, excessive size, and number of fetuses (the passenger)
- Maternal position during labor and birth
- Psychologic responses of the mother to labor related to past experiences, preparation, culture and heritage, and support system

These five factors are interdependent. In assessing the woman for an abnormal labor pattern, the nurse must consider the ways in which these factors interact and influence labor progress. Dysfunctional labor is suspected when there is an alteration in the characteristics of uterine contractions, a lack of progress in the rate of cervical dilation, or a lack of progress in fetal descent and expulsion.

Gilbert (2011) cited several factors that seem to increase a woman's risk for dysfunctional labor including the following:

- Overweight
- Short stature
- Advanced maternal age
- Infertility
- Prior version
- Masculine characteristics
- Uterine abnormalities (e.g., congenital malformations; overdistention, as with multiple gestation or polyhydramnios)
- Malpresentations and positions of the fetus
- Cephalopelvic disproportion (CPD) (or fetopelvic disproportion [FPD])
- Uterine overstimulation with oxytocin
- Maternal fatigue, dehydration and electrolyte imbalance, and fear
- Administration of an analgesic too early in labor or use of continuous epidural analgesia

Abnormal Uterine Activity

Abnormal uterine activity can be further described as being *hypertonic* or *hypotonic*.

Hypertonic Uterine Dysfunction

The woman experiencing hypertonic uterine dysfunction, or primary dysfunctional labor, often is an anxious nullipara who is having frequent and painful contractions that are ineffective in causing cervical dilation or effacement to progress. These contractions usually occur in the latent phase of first-stage labor (cervical dilation of less than 4 cm) and are usually uncoordinated. The force of the contractions may be in the midsection of the uterus rather than in the fundus; therefore, the uterus is unable to apply downward pressure to push the presenting part against the cervix. The uterus may not relax completely between contractions.

Women with hypertonic uterine dysfunction may be exhausted and express concern about loss of control because of the intense pain they are experiencing and the lack of progress. Therapeutic rest, which is achieved with a warm bath or shower and the administration of an analgesic such as morphine to inhibit uterine contractions, reduce pain, and encourage sleep, is usually prescribed to manage hypertonic uterine dysfunction. In the absence of pain, zolpidem (Ambien) may be used to facilitate rest and sleep. After a 4- to 6-hour rest, these women are likely to awaken in active labor with a normal uterine contraction pattern (Gilbert, 2011; Wing & Farinelli, 2012).

Hypotonic Uterine Dysfunction

The second and more common type of uterine dysfunction is hypotonic uterine dysfunction, or secondary uterine inertia. The woman initially makes normal progress into the active phase of first-stage labor but then the contractions become weak and inefficient or stop altogether. The uterus is easily indented, even at the peak of contractions. Intrauterine pressure (IUP) during the contraction (usually less than 25 mm Hg) is insufficient for progress of cervical effacement and dilation. CPD and malposition are common causes of this type of uterine dysfunction.

A woman with hypotonic uterine dysfunction may become exhausted and be at increased risk for infection. Management usually consists of ruling out CPD and assessing the FHR and pattern, characteristics of amniotic fluid if membranes are ruptured, and maternal well-being. An intrauterine pressure catheter (IUPC) may be inserted to accurately evaluate uterine activity. If findings are normal, labor augmentation measures may be implemented (e.g., ambulation, hydrotherapy, rupture of membranes, nipple stimulation, oxytocin infusion).

Secondary Powers

Secondary powers, or bearing-down efforts, are compromised when large amounts of an analgesic are given. Anesthesia can also block the bearing-down reflex and, as a result, alter the effectiveness of voluntary bearing-down efforts. Exhaustion resulting from lack of sleep or long labor and fatigue resulting from inadequate hydration and food intake reduce the effectiveness of the woman's voluntary bearing-down efforts. Maternal position can work against the forces of gravity and decrease the strength and effectiveness of the contractions. Table 32-1 summarizes the characteristics of dysfunctional labor.

Abnormal Labor Patterns

Six abnormal labor patterns were identified and classified by Friedman (1989) in the 1950s according to the nature of cervical dilation and fetal descent. These patterns are (1) prolonged latent phase, (2) protracted active phase dilation, (3) secondary arrest: no change, (4) protracted descent, (5) arrest of descent, and (6) failure of descent. Table 32-2 further describes abnormal labor patterns. These patterns can result from a variety of causes, including ineffective uterine contractions, pelvic contractures, CPD, abnormal fetal presentation

TABLE 32-1 Dysfunctional Labor: Primary and Secondary Powers

PRIMARY POWERS (ABNORMAL UTERINE ACTIVITY)		SECONDARY POWERS
HYPERTONIC UTERINE DYSFUNCTION	**HYPOTONIC UTERINE DYSFUNCTION**	**INADEQUATE VOLUNTARY EXPULSIVE FORCES**
Description		
Usually occurs before 4-cm dilation; cause unknown, may be related to fear and tension	Cause is usually cephalopelvic disproportion or fetal malposition	Involves abdominal and levator ani muscles Occurs in second stage of labor; cause may be related to nerve block anesthetic, analgesia, exhaustion
Change in Pattern of Progress		
Pain out of proportion to intensity of contractions and to effectiveness of contractions in effacing and dilating the cervix Contractions increase in frequency and are uncoordinated Uterus is contracted between contractions, cannot be indented	Contractions decrease in frequency and intensity Uterus easily indented even at peak of contractions Uterus relaxed between contractions (normal)	No voluntary urge to push or bear down or inadequate or ineffective pushing
Potential Maternal Effects		
Loss of control related to intensity of pain and lack of progress Exhaustion Fear regarding unexpected nature of labor	Infection Exhaustion Stress regarding change in progress	Spontaneous vaginal birth prevented; assisted birth likely
Potential Fetal Effects		
Fetal asphyxia with meconium aspiration	Fetal infection Fetal and neonatal death	Fetal asphyxia
Care Management		
Initiate therapeutic rest measures Administer analgesic (e.g., morphine) if membranes are intact and pelvic adequacy is confirmed to relieve pain and permit woman to rest Assist with measures to enhance rest and relaxation (e.g., hydrotherapy, massage, music, distracting activities)	Rule out cephalopelvic disproportion Augment labor with oxytocin (Pitocin) Perform amniotomy Assist with measures to enhance the progress of labor (e.g., position changes, ambulation, hydrotherapy)	Coach woman in bearing down with contractions; assist with relaxation between contractions Position woman in favorable position for pushing Reduce epidural infusion rate Assist with forceps- or vacuum-assisted birth Prepare for cesarean birth if abnormal fetal status occurs

TABLE 32-2 Abnormal Labor Patterns

PATTERN	NULLIPARAS	MULTIPARAS
Prolonged latent phase	>20 hour	>14 hour
Protracted active phase dilation	<1.2 cm/hour	<1.5 cm/hr
Secondary arrest: no change	≥2 hour	≥2 hour
Protracted descent	<1 cm/hour	<2 cm/hour
Arrest of descent	≥1 hour	≥1/2 hour
Failure of descent	No change during deceleration phase and second stage	
Precipitous labor	>5 cm/hour	10 cm/hour

or position, early use of analgesics, nerve block analgesia or anesthesia, and anxiety and stress. Progress in either the first or the second stage of labor can be protracted (prolonged) or arrested (stopped). Abnormal progress can be identified by plotting cervical dilation and fetal descent on a labor graph (partogram) at various intervals after the onset of labor and comparing the resulting curve with the expected labor curve for a nulliparous or multiparous labor. If a woman exhibits an abnormal labor pattern, the primary health care provider should be notified.

Maternal morbidity and mortality from uterine rupture, infection, severe dehydration, and postpartum hemorrhage are higher for women experiencing dysfunctional labor. The fetus is at increased risk for hypoxia. A long and difficult labor also can have an adverse psychologic effect on the mother, father or partner, and family.

Studies done since 2000 indicate that the pattern of labor progression is different from what Friedman observed in the 1950s. In general, modern labor progresses at a slower rate. The active labor phase now lasts twice as long as Friedman described. It is common for more than 2 hours to pass in the active phase of labor without cervical dilation. Maternal characteristics have changed considerably since Friedman's work was published. Women giving birth are older and heavier, and both of these factors are associated with longer labors. Clinical guidelines incorporating this new information must be developed to assist health care providers in managing contemporary labor and birth (Thorp & Laughon, 2014).

Precipitous Labor

Precipitous labor is defined as labor that lasts less than 3 hours from the onset of contractions to the time of birth. This abnormal labor pattern occurs in approximately 2% of all births in the United States. Precipitous birth alone is not usually associated with significant maternal or infant morbidity or mortality (Wing & Farinelli, 2012).

Precipitous labor can result from hypertonic uterine contractions that are tetanic in intensity. Conditions often associated with this type of uterine contraction include placental abruption, uterine tachysystole, and recent cocaine use (Wing & Farinelli, 2012).

Maternal complications can include uterine rupture, lacerations of the birth canal, amniotic fluid embolism (anaphylactoid syndrome of pregnancy), and postpartum hemorrhage. Fetal complications include shoulder dystocia (Wing & Farinelli), hypoxia caused by decreased periods of uterine relaxation between contractions, and, in rare instances, intracranial trauma related to rapid birth (Cunningham et al., 2014).

Women who have experienced precipitous labor often describe feelings of disbelief that their labor began so quickly, alarm that their labor progressed so rapidly, panic about the possibility they would not make it to the hospital in time to give birth, and finally, relief when they arrived at the hospital. In addition, women have expressed frustration when nurses did not believe them when they reported their readiness to push. Progress can be so rapid in some women that they may have difficulty remembering the details of their childbirth. They should be provided with an opportunity to discuss their labor and birth with caregivers.

Alterations in Pelvic Structure

Pelvic Dystocia

Pelvic dystocia can occur whenever there are contractures of the pelvic diameters that reduce the capacity of the bony pelvis, including the inlet, the midpelvis, outlet, or any combination of these planes. Pelvic contractures can be caused by congenital abnormalities, maternal malnutrition, neoplasms, or lower spinal disorders. An immature pelvic size predisposes some adolescent mothers to pelvic dystocia. Pelvic deformities also can be the result of vehicular or other accidents or trauma.

Soft-Tissue Dystocia

Soft-tissue dystocia results from obstruction of the birth passage by an anatomic abnormality other than that involving the bony pelvis. The obstruction can result from placenta previa (low-lying placenta) that partially or completely obstructs the internal cervical os. Other causes, such as leiomyomas (uterine fibroids) in the lower uterine segment, ovarian tumors, and a full bladder or rectum, can prevent the fetus from entering the pelvis. Occasionally cervical edema occurs during labor when the cervix is caught between the presenting part and the symphysis pubis or when the woman begins bearing-down efforts prematurely, thereby inhibiting complete dilation. Sexually transmitted infections (e.g., human papillomavirus) can alter cervical tissue integrity and thus interfere with adequate effacement and dilation.

Fetal Causes

Dystocia of fetal origin can be caused by anomalies, excessive fetal size (macrosomia), malpresentation, malposition, or multifetal pregnancy. Complications associated with dystocia of fetal origin include neonatal asphyxia, fetal injuries or fractures, and maternal vaginal lacerations. Although spontaneous vaginal birth is possible in these instances, a forceps-assisted, vacuum-assisted, or cesarean birth often is necessary.

Anomalies

Gross ascites, large tumors, open neural tube defects (e.g., myelomeningocele), and hydrocephalus are examples of fetal anomalies that can cause dystocia. The anomalies affect the relationship of the fetal anatomy to the maternal pelvic capacity, with the result that the fetus is unable to descend through the pelvis and birth canal.

Cephalopelvic Disproportion

Cephalopelvic disproportion (CPD), also called fetopelvic disproportion (FPD), is disproportion between the size of the fetus and the size of the mother's pelvis. With CPD the fetus cannot fit through the maternal pelvis to be born vaginally. Although CPD is often related to excessive fetal size, or macrosomia (i.e., 4000 g or more), the problem in many cases is malposition of the fetal presenting part rather than true CPD (Wing & Farinelli, 2012). Fetal macrosomia is associated with maternal diabetes mellitus, obesity, multiparity, or the large size of one or both parents. If the maternal pelvis is too small, abnormally shaped, or deformed, CPD can be of maternal origin. In this case, the fetus can be of average size or even smaller. CPD cannot be accurately predicted (Wing & Farinelli).

Malposition

The most common fetal malposition is persistent occipitoposterior position (i.e., right occipitoposterior [ROP] or left occipitoposterior [LOP]; see Chapter 16), occurring in approximately 15% of all labors during the latent phase of the first stage of labor. About 5% of all fetuses are in this position at birth (Gilbert, 2011). Labor, especially the second stage, is prolonged. The woman typically complains of severe back pain from the pressure of the fetal head (occiput) pressing against her sacrum. See Box 19-8 for suggested positions to relieve back pain and encourage rotation of the fetal occiput to an anterior position, which will facilitate birth.

Evidence supports encouraging women whose fetus is in an occipitoposterior position to assume and maintain a Sims position on the same side as the fetal spine as much as possible during labor. There is limited evidence to support the commonly used hands-and-knees position (Desbriere, Blanc, Le Dû, et al., 2013).

Malpresentation

Malpresentation (the fetal presentation is something other than cephalic or head first) is another commonly reported complication of labor and birth. Breech presentation is the most common form of malpresentation, occurring in 3% to 4% of all labors (Lanni & Seeds, 2012). The three types of breech presentation are (Gilbert, 2011) (Fig. 32-3):

- Frank breech (hips flexed, knees extended)
- Complete breech (hips and knees flexed)
- Footling breech (when one foot [single footling] or both feet [double footling] present before the buttocks)

Breech presentations are associated with multifetal gestation, preterm birth, fetal and maternal anomalies, hydramnios, and oligohydramnios. High rates of breech presentation are also noted in fetuses with certain genetic disorders (e.g., trisomies 13, 18, and 21; Potter syndrome [renal agenesis]; and myotonic dystrophy). Fetuses with neuromuscular disorders have a high rate of breech presentation, perhaps because they are less capable of movement within the uterus (Thorp & Laughon, 2014). Diagnosis is made by abdominal palpation (e.g., Leopold maneuvers) and vaginal examination and usually confirmed by ultrasound scan.

During labor the descent of the fetus in a breech presentation may be slow because the breech is not as effective a dilating wedge as is the fetal head. There is risk of prolapse of the cord if the membranes rupture in early labor. The presence of meconium in amniotic fluid is not necessarily a sign of fetal distress because it results from pressure on the fetal abdominal wall as it travels through the birth canal. Assessment of FHR and pattern should be used to determine whether the passage of meconium is an expected finding associated with breech presentation or is an abnormal sign associated with fetal hypoxia. The heart tones of fetuses (FHTs) in a breech position are best heard at or above the umbilicus.

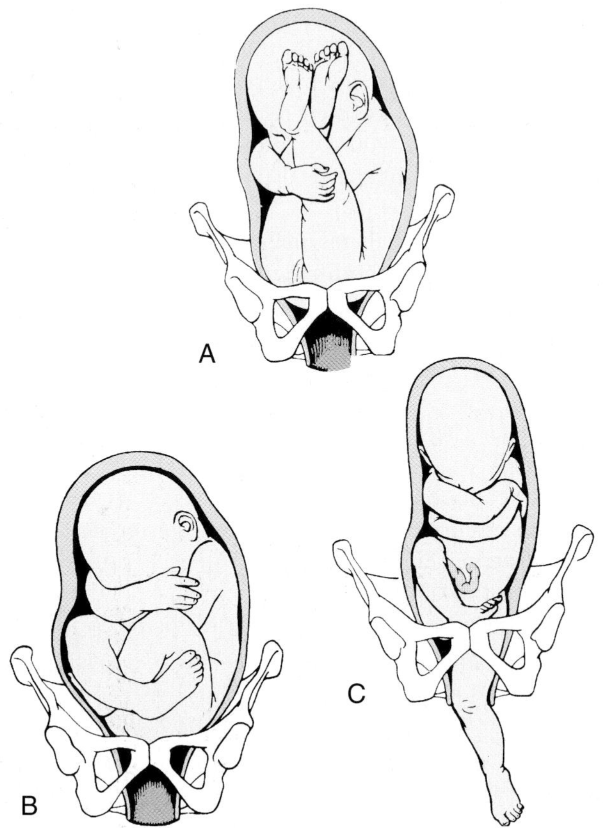

FIG 32-3 Breech presentation. **A,** Frank breech. **B,** Complete breech. **C,** Single footling breech. (From Gilbert, E. [2011]. *Manual of high risk pregnancy & delivery* [5th ed.]. St. Louis: Mosby.)

Vaginal birth is accomplished by mechanisms of labor that manipulate the buttocks and lower extremities as they emerge from the birth canal (Fig. 32-4). Risks associated with vaginal birth from a breech presentation include prolapse of the umbilical cord (especially in single or double footling breech presentations), trapping of the after-coming fetal head (especially with preterm infants), and trauma resulting from extension of the fetal head or nuchal position of the arms. Safe vaginal birth from a breech presentation is largely dependent on the experience, judgment, and skill of the health care provider who assists the birth. Criteria for attempting a vaginal birth from a breech presentation are (Thorp & Laughon, 2014):

- Frank or complete breech presentation
- Estimated fetal weight between 2000 and 3800 g
- Normal (gynecoid) maternal pelvis with adequate measurements
- Flexed fetal head

External cephalic version (ECV) (see later discussion) may be tried to turn the fetus to a vertex presentation. If the attempt at ECV is unsuccessful, the woman usually gives birth by cesarean (Gilbert, 2011).

Face and brow presentations are uncommon and are associated with fetal anomalies, pelvic contractures, and CPD. Spontaneous vaginal birth is possible if the fetus flexes to a vertex presentation, although forceps often are used. Cesarean birth is indicated if the presentation persists, if fetal distress occurs, or if

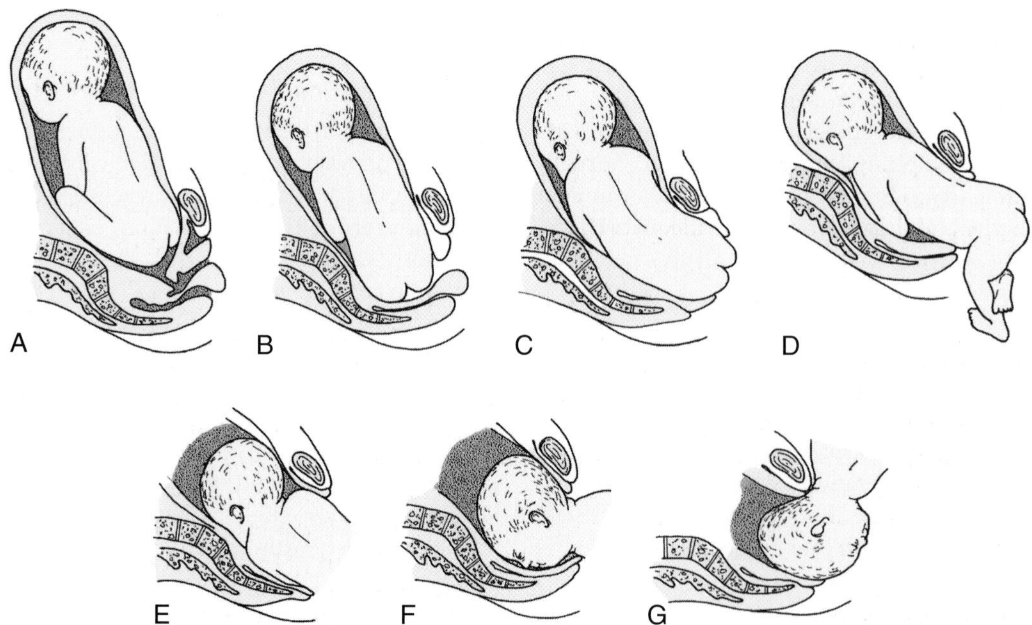

FIG 32-4 Mechanism of labor in breech presentation. **A,** Breech before onset of labor. **B,** Engagement and internal rotation. **C,** Lateral flexion. **D,** External rotation or restitution. **E,** Internal rotation of shoulders and head. **F,** Face rotates to sacrum when occiput is anterior. **G,** Head is born by gradual flexion during elevation of fetal body.

labor stops progressing. Cesarean birth is usually necessary for a fetus in a transverse lie (i.e., shoulder) presentation, although ECV may be attempted after 36 to 37 weeks of gestation (Thorp & Laughon, 2014).

Multifetal Pregnancy

Multifetal pregnancy is the gestation of twins, triplets, quadruplets, or more infants. Twin gestations accounted for more than 3.3% of all live births in the United States in 2012. The rate of triplet or higher-order multiple births in 2012 was 124.4 per 100,000 births, the lowest rate in 18 years (Martin et al., 2013a). The number of multiple-gestation pregnancies rose dramatically in the 1980s and 1990s, most likely due to fertility-enhancing medications and procedures as well as more women older than age 35 continuing childbearing. When compared with younger women, those 35 years and older are naturally more likely to have a multifetal pregnancy. The rate of triplet and higher-order multiple pregnancies has been steadily declining since the all-time high rate of 193.5 per 100,000 births in 1998. This decrease has been attributed to refinements in the treatments used for infertility, particularly limiting the number of embryos transferred during in vitro fertilization (IVF) procedures (Malone & D'Alton, 2014; Newman & Unal, 2012).

Multiple births are associated with more complications (e.g., dysfunctional labor) than singleton births. The higher incidence of fetal and newborn complications and higher risk of perinatal mortality primarily stem from the birth of low-birth-weight infants resulting from preterm birth or IUGR (or both), in part related to placental dysfunction and twin-to-twin transfusion. Fetuses can experience distress and asphyxia during the birth process as a result of cord prolapse and the onset of placental separation with the birth of the first fetus. As a result the risk for long-term problems such as cerebral palsy is higher among infants who were part of a multiple birth.

In addition, fetal complications such as congenital anomalies and abnormal presentations can result in dysfunctional labor and an increased incidence of cesarean birth. For example, in only 40% to 45% of all twin pregnancies do both fetuses present in the vertex position, the most favorable for vaginal birth. In 35% to 40% of the pregnancies, one twin can present in the vertex position and the other in a breech or transverse lie presentation (Bowers, 2014).

The health status of the mother can be compromised by an increased risk for hypertension, anemia, and hemorrhage associated with uterine atony, placental abruption, and multiple or adherent placentas. Duration of the phases and stages of labor can vary from the duration experienced with singleton births.

Teamwork and planning are essential components of the management of labor and birth in multiple pregnancies, especially those of higher-order multiples. The nurse plays a key role in coordinating the activities of many highly skilled health care professionals. Early detection and management of the maternal, fetal, and newborn complications associated with multiple births are essential to achieve a positive outcome for mother and babies. Maternal positioning and active support are used to enhance labor progress and placental perfusion. Stimulation of labor with oxytocin, epidural anesthesia, internal or external version, and forceps and vacuum assistance may be used to accomplish the vaginal birth of twins. Cesarean birth is almost always performed with higher-order multiple births. Each infant has its own team of health care providers present at the birth. Nurses provide important emotional support to women and their families to help reduce anxiety and stress. They explain events as they occur and offer updates on the status of the mother and infants.

Position of the Woman

The functional relationship among the uterine contractions, the fetus, and the mother's pelvis are altered by the maternal position. In addition, the position can provide a mechanical advantage or disadvantage to the mechanisms of labor by altering the effects of gravity and the body-part relationships that are important to the progress of labor. See Box 19-8 for suggested positions to enhance fetal descent.

Discouraging maternal movement or restricting labor to the recumbent or lithotomy position can compromise progress. The incidence of dysfunctional labor in women confined to these positions is increased, resulting in a greater need for augmentation of labor or forceps-assisted, vacuum-assisted, or cesarean birth.

Psychologic Responses

Hormones and neurotransmitters released in response to stress (e.g., catecholamines) can cause dysfunctional labor. Sources of stress vary for each woman, but pain and the absence of a support person are often related to dysfunctional labor. Confinement to bed and restriction of maternal movement can be a source of psychologic stress that compounds the physiologic stress caused by immobility in the unmedicated laboring woman. When anxiety is excessive it can inhibit cervical dilation and result in prolonged labor and increased pain perception. Anxiety also causes increased levels of stress-related hormones (e.g., beta-endorphin, adrenocorticotropic hormone, cortisol, and epinephrine). These hormones act on the smooth muscles of the uterus. Increased levels can cause dysfunctional labor by reducing uterine contractility.

CARE MANAGEMENT

Risk assessment is a continual process in the laboring woman. By reviewing the woman's past labor or labors and observing her physical and psychologic responses to the current labor, any factors that might contribute to dysfunctional labor should be identified. The initial and ongoing physical assessments provide information about maternal well-being; status of labor in terms of the characteristics of uterine contractions and progress of cervical effacement and dilation; fetal well-being in terms of FHR and pattern, presentation, station, and position; and status of the amniotic membranes. Nursing diagnoses that might be identified in women experiencing dystocia include the following:

- *Risk for Injury* to mother or fetus related to
  - interventions implemented for dystocia
- *Powerlessness* related to
  - loss of control
- *Ineffective Coping* related to
  - inadequate support system
  - exhaustion secondary to a prolonged labor process
  - pain

- *Risk for Impaired Parenting* related to
  - separation from infant associated with emergency cesarean birth
  - emotional responses to a traumatic childbirth experience

Nursing diagnoses, expected outcomes of care, and interventions are established for each woman based on assessment findings. Many interventions for dysfunctional labor (e.g., ECV, cervical ripening, induction or augmentation of labor, and operative procedures [forceps- or vacuum-assisted birth, cesarean birth]) are implemented collaboratively with other members of the health care team. Commonly performed interventions are discussed in detail in the Obstetric Procedures section. Nursing interventions are identified with each procedure.

When providing care for a woman who is experiencing labor or birth complications, all members of the health care team are responsible for complying with professional standards of care. This promotes client safety and helps improve outcomes.

OBESITY

Excessive weight is an increasingly serious problem for children, adolescents, and adults living in affluent nations, including the United States, and pregnant women are no exception. The body mass index (BMI) is used to define obesity. People with a BMI of 25 or greater are categorized as overweight, whereas those with a BMI of 30 or greater are considered obese. Individuals with a BMI of 40 or greater are classified as severely obese (Picklesimer & Dorman, 2013).

Obese women are likely to begin pregnancy with preexisting medical conditions such as chronic hypertension and type 2 diabetes. While pregnant, they can develop pregnancy-associated hypertensive disorders, or gestational diabetes may be diagnosed. Obese women also have an increased incidence of a postterm pregnancy. All of these factors can increase the likelihood that labor will be induced. In addition to an increased risk for cesarean birth in general, obese women are also more likely to require emergency cesarean birth. During the postpartum period they are at risk for thromboembolism and wound disruption and infection after cesarean birth (Picklesimer & Dorman, 2013). As the woman's BMI increases, so does the risk for developing these complications (Halloran, Cheng, Wall, et al., 2012).

CARE MANAGEMENT

Nursing care of obese women during labor and birth is challenging for a number of reasons. Sometimes standard furniture such as beds, chairs, and operating tables is simply not large enough to accommodate the woman's size. Extra-large furniture may not fit through a standard doorway, so room renovation can be necessary. Some hospitals have created rooms specifically designed to accommodate obese clients (Fig. 32-5). Continuous external FHR and contraction monitoring can be extremely difficult if not impossible to perform. Special equipment, such as extra-large blood pressure cuffs, is necessary to properly assess the woman's condition.

Even routine procedures require more time and effort to accomplish when a woman is obese. This can slow essential interventions and increase risks to the mother and fetus, such as when an emergency cesarean birth is needed. Establishing IV access, for example, can require multiple attempts, sometimes by multiple people. Mobility is often a problem. Moving the woman from a labor room to the operating room and transferring her from a bed to the operating table can require the assistance of additional personnel or special equipment, especially if regional anesthesia is already in effect. If it is not, surgery can be further delayed by anesthetic complications, such as difficulty establishing an epidural or spinal block or accomplishing endotracheal intubation.

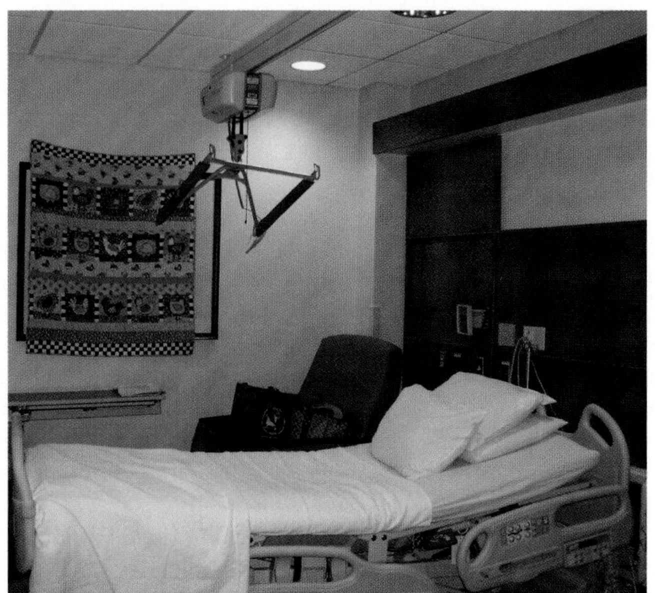

FIG 32-5 Room specifically designed to accommodate obese pregnant clients. Note lift attached to ceiling for use in transferring women from the bed to chairs or stretchers. (Courtesy Dee Lowdermilk, Chapel Hill, NC).

Postoperatively, obese women are at increased risk for thromboembolic complications. In the immediate recovery period, use of thromboembolic stockings (TED hose) and sequential compression device (SCD) boots helps to decrease the risk of thrombus formation. Some women also may be given heparin prophylactically for clot prevention (Simpson & O'Brien-Abel, 2014). In the postpartum period women should also be encouraged to get out of bed and begin ambulating as soon as possible.

Keeping the incision clean and dry to prevent wound infection and promote healing is another postoperative challenge. Many obese women have a pannus (large roll of abdominal fat) that overlies a lower abdominal transverse skin incision made just above the pubic area. The pannus causes the area to remain moist, which encourages infection. Women should be taught to wash the incision with soap and water several times a day, drying the area well afterward. Using a handheld hair dryer on a low setting works well. Sutures or staples used to close the skin incision are generally left in place longer than usual to avoid possible wound disruption when they are removed. Sometimes the skin and subcutaneous layers of the incision are left open to heal by secondary intention to avoid possible dehiscence. If this course of action is chosen, the woman and other family members are taught to perform dressing changes and wound care.

OBSTETRIC PROCEDURES

Version

Version is the turning of the fetus from one presentation to another. It may be performed externally or internally by the health care provider.

External Cephalic Version

External cephalic version (ECV) is used in an attempt to turn the fetus from a breech or shoulder presentation to a vertex presentation for birth. It may be attempted in a labor and birth setting late in gestation. ECV is attempted by the exertion of gentle, constant pressure on the abdomen (Fig. 32-6). Before ECV is attempted, ultrasound scanning is done to:

- Determine the fetal position
- Locate the umbilical cord
- Rule out placenta previa
- Evaluate the adequacy of the maternal pelvis
- Assess the amount of amniotic fluid, the gestational age, and the presence of any anomalies

An NST is performed to confirm fetal well-being, or the FHR and pattern are monitored for a period of time (i.e., 10 to 20 minutes). Informed consent is obtained. A tocolytic agent such as terbutaline often is given to relax the uterus and facilitate the maneuver. Contraindications to ECV include (Thorp & Laughon, 2014):

- Uterine anomalies
- Third-trimester bleeding
- Multiple gestation
- Oligohydramnios
- Evidence of uteroplacental insufficiency
- A nuchal cord (identified by ultrasound)
- Previous cesarean birth or other significant uterine surgery
- Obvious CPD

ECV is most successful in a multiparous woman who has a normal amount of amniotic fluid and whose fetus is not yet engaged in the pelvis (Rosman, Guijt, Vlemmix, et al., 2013). The procedure should be performed in a hospital equipped to provide emergency surgery because 1% to 2% of women who have ECV develop placental abruption or umbilical cord compression requiring immediate cesarean birth (Thorp & Laughon, 2014).

During an attempted ECV the nurse continuously monitors the FHR and pattern, especially for bradycardia and variable decelerations; checks the maternal vital signs; and assesses the woman's level of comfort because the procedure can be painful. After the procedure is completed, the nurse continues to monitor maternal vital signs and uterine activity and assess for vaginal bleeding until the woman's condition is determined to be stable. FHR and pattern monitoring should continue for at least 1 hour. Women who are Rh negative should receive Rh immune globulin because the manipulation can cause fetomaternal bleeding (Thorp & Laughon).

Internal Version

With internal version the fetus is turned by the health care provider, who inserts a hand into the uterus and changes the presentation to cephalic (head) or podalic (foot). Internal version is only rarely used, most often in twin gestations to deliver the second fetus. The safety of this procedure has not been documented; maternal and fetal injury is possible. Cesarean birth is the usual method for managing malpresentation in multifetal pregnancies. The nurse's role is to monitor the status of the fetus and to provide support to the woman.

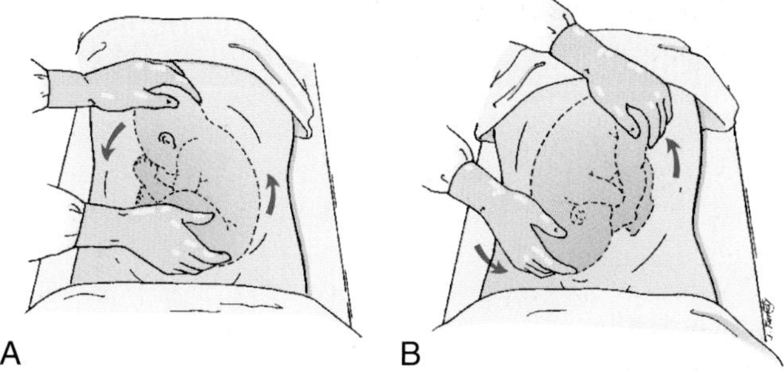

FIG 32-6 External version of fetus from breech to vertex presentation. This must be achieved without force. **A,** Breech is pushed up out of pelvic inlet while head is pulled toward inlet. **B,** Head is pushed toward inlet while breech is pulled upward.

Induction of Labor

Induction of labor is the chemical or mechanical initiation of uterine contractions before their spontaneous onset for the purpose of bringing about birth. Labor may be induced either electively or for indicated reasons. Induction of labor is one of the most commonly performed obstetric procedures in the United States. Approximately 24% of term births (infants born between 37 and 41 weeks of gestation) result from labors that were induced (Hill & Harvey, 2013). It is likely that the rate of elective inductions is increasing more rapidly than the rate of indicated inductions. Additionally, there is concern that elective inductions may increase the risk of cesarean birth, especially among primigravid women and particularly those older than age 35 (Martin, Hamilton, Sutton, et al., 2012; Thorp & Laughon, 2014; Wing & Farinelli, 2012).

Induction of labor is indicated if continuing the pregnancy could be dangerous for either the woman or the fetus, and if no contraindications exist to artificial rupture of the membranes (amniotomy) or augmenting uterine contractions with oxytocin. Prior to labor induction, gestational age should be determined and any potential risks to the maternal-fetal unit evaluated. Women must be fully counseled regarding risks, benefits, and alternatives of labor stimulation methods as part of the process for informed consent (ACOG, 2013a; Thorp & Laughon, 2014). Box 32-7 lists indications and contraindications for labor induction.

Elective Induction of Labor

An elective induction is one in which labor is initiated without a medical indication. Methods to ripen the cervix (e.g., application of prostaglandins or intracervical insertion of a balloon catheter) enhance the likelihood of successful induction. Many elective inductions are purely for the convenience of the woman or her primary health care provider. At times, however, labor may be electively induced to allay maternal fears and anxieties associated with prior perinatal losses or to ensure that experienced multispecialty personnel are available to handle anticipated maternal or neonatal complications immediately

BOX 32-7 Indications and Contraindications for Labor Induction

Maternal Indications
- Hypertensive complications of pregnancy: gestational hypertension, preeclampsia, eclampsia
- Fetal death
- Chorioamnionitis

Fetal Indications
Any condition in which a variety of fetal tests demonstrate significant fetal jeopardy in any of the following situations:
- Diabetes
- Postterm pregnancy, especially when oligohydramnios is present
- Hypertensive complications of pregnancy
- Intrauterine growth restriction
- Isoimmunization
- Chorioamnionitis
- Premature rupture of membranes with established fetal maturity

Contraindications
- Acute, severe fetal distress
- Shoulder presentation (transverse lie)
- Floating fetal presenting part
- Uncontrolled hemorrhage
- Placenta previa
- Previous uterine incision that prohibits a trial of labor

Relative Contraindications
- Grand multiparity (five or more pregnancies that ended after 20 weeks of gestation)
- Multiple gestation
- Suspected cephalopelvic disproportion (CPD)
- Breech presentations
- Inability to adequately monitor the FHR throughout labor

Data from Thorp, J.M., & Laughon, S.K. (2014). Clinical aspects of normal and abnormal labor. In R.K. Creasy, R. Resnik, J.D. Iams, et al. (Eds.), *Creasy and Resnik's maternal-fetal medicine: Principles and practice* (7th ed.). Philadelphia: Saunders.

TABLE 32-3 Bishop Score

	SCORE			
	0	1	2	3
Dilation (cm)	0	1-2	3-4	≥5
Effacement (%)	0-30	40-50	60-70	≥80
Station (cm)	−3	−2	−1, 0	+1, +2
Cervical consistency	Firm	Medium	Soft	Soft
Cervical position	Posterior	Midposition	Anterior	Anterior

Modified from Bishop, E.H. (1964). Pelvic scoring for elective induction. *Obstetrics and Gynecology*, 24(2), 266-268.

following birth (Wing & Farinelli, 2012; Yount & Lassiter, 2013).

The major risks associated with elective labor induction at term are increased rates of cesarean birth, neonatal morbidity, and cost (Wing & Farinelli, 2012). To prevent iatrogenic prematurity, elective induction of labor should not be initiated until the woman reaches 39 completed weeks of gestation (ACOG, 2013a; Swamy, 2012). The American College of Obstetricians and Gynecologists (ACOG) and the American Academy of Pediatrics (AAP) have for many years recommended that elective induction of labor not be initiated until the woman reaches 39 weeks or more of gestation. The National Quality Forum and The Joint Commission have developed perinatal quality measures to monitor appropriate gestational age for elective birth (Simpson, 2011). The March of Dimes and the Association of Women's Health, Obstetric and Neonatal Nurses (AWHONN) have created informational campaigns to educate pregnant women and their families about the dangers of early-term births (visit their websites at www.gothefull40.com and www.marchofdimes.com/pregnancy/getready_atleast39weeks.html) (Craighead, 2012). Birth data from the United States for 2011, the most recent data available, indicate that births at 37 to 38 weeks of gestation have declined, whereas births at 39 weeks of gestation or more are increasing (Martin et al., 2013b).

Chemical, mechanical, physical, and alternative methods are used to ripen the cervix and induce labor. IV oxytocin (Pitocin) and amniotomy are the most common methods used in the United States. Success rates for induction of labor are higher when the condition of the cervix is favorable, or inducible. Cervical ripeness is the most important predictor of successful induction. A rating system such as the Bishop score (Table 32-3) can be used to evaluate inducibility. For example, a score of 8 or more on this 13-point scale indicates that the cervix is soft, anterior, 50% or more effaced, and dilated 2 cm or more and that the presenting part is engaged. When the Bishop score totals 8 or more, induction of labor is usually successful (ACOG, 2013a; Gilbert, 2011; Swamy, 2012). The Bishop score should be documented prior to the use of methods to ripen the cervix or induce labor.

Cervical Ripening Methods

Chemical Agents. Preparations of prostaglandins E_1 (PGE_1) and E_2 (PGE_2) have been shown to be effective when used before induction to "ripen" (soften and thin) the cervix (see Medication Guides: Prostaglandin E_1 [PGE_1]: Misoprostol [Cytotec] and Prostaglandin E_2 [PGE_2]: Dinoprostone [Cervidil Insert; Prepidil Gel]) (Hill & Harvey, 2013). In some cases, women spontaneously begin laboring after the administration of prostaglandin, thereby eliminating the need to administer oxytocin to induce labor. Additional advantages of prostaglandin use for cervical ripening include decreased oxytocin induction time and a decrease in the amount of oxytocin required for successful induction (Gilbert, 2011). PGE_1, although much less expensive and more effective than PGE_2 for inducing labor and birth, is associated with a higher risk for uterine tachysystole with abnormal fetal heart rate and pattern changes and passage of meconium into the amniotic fluid. Most of these adverse outcomes are associated with higher dose protocols (ACOG, 2013a; Wing & Farinelli, 2012). Although the drug's manufacturer has acknowledged for several years that PGE_1 is effective for cervical ripening and labor induction, it has not yet been approved by the FDA for these uses (Thorp & Laughon, 2014; Yount & Lassiter, 2013). PGE_2 in the form of a vaginal insert (dinoprostone [Cervidil]), although more expensive than PGE_1, has the major advantage of easy removal should adverse reactions, including uterine tachysystole, occur (Yount & Lassiter).

MEDICATION GUIDE

Prostaglandin E_1 (PGE_1): Misoprostol (Cytotec)

Action

PGE_1 ripens the cervix, making it softer and causing it to begin to dilate and efface; it stimulates uterine contractions.

Indications

- PGE_1 is used for preinduction cervical ripening (ripen cervix before oxytocin induction of labor when the Bishop score is 4 or less) and to induce labor or abortion (abortifacient agent); it has not yet been approved by the FDA for cervical ripening or labor induction (i.e., this is an unlabeled use for obstetrics).
- It should not be used if the woman has a history of previous cesarean birth or other major uterine surgery.

Dosage and Administration

- Misoprostol is available either as a 100- or a 200-mcg tablet. Therefore, tablets must be broken to prepare the correct dose. This preparation should take place in the pharmacy to ensure accurate doses.
- Recommended initial dose is 25 mcg. Insert intravaginally into the posterior vaginal fornix using the tips of index and middle fingers without the use of a lubricant. Repeat every 4 hours or until an effective contraction pattern is established (three or more uterine contractions in 10 minutes), the cervix ripens (Bishop score of 8 or greater), or significant adverse effects occur.

Adverse Effects

Higher doses (e.g., 50 mcg every 6 hours) are more likely to result in adverse reactions such as nausea and vomiting, diarrhea, fever, uterine tachysystole with or without an abnormal FHR and pattern, or fetal passage of meconium. The risk for adverse reactions is reduced with lower dosages and longer intervals between doses.

Nursing Considerations

- Explain the procedure to the woman and her family; ensure that an informed consent has been obtained as per agency policy.
- Assess the woman and fetus before each insertion and during treatment following agency protocol for frequency. Assess maternal vital signs and health status, FHR and pattern, and status of pregnancy, including indications for cervical ripening or induction of labor, signs of labor or impending labor, and the Bishop score. Recognize that an abnormal FHR and pattern; maternal fever, infection, vaginal bleeding, or hypersensitivity; and regular, progressive uterine contractions contraindicate the use of misoprostol.
- Avoid giving aluminum hydroxide and magnesium-containing antacids along with misoprostol.
- Use with caution in women with renal failure because the medication is eliminated through the kidneys.
- Have the woman void before insertion.
- Assist the woman to maintain a supine position with a lateral tilt or a side-lying position for 30 to 40 minutes after insertion.
- Prepare to (1) swab the vagina to remove unabsorbed medication using a saline-soaked gauze wrapped around fingers or (2) administer terbutaline 0.25 mg subcutaneously if significant adverse effects occur.
- Initiate oxytocin for induction of labor no sooner than 4 hours after the last dose of misoprostol was administered, following agency protocol, if ripening has occurred and labor has not begun.
- Document all assessment findings and administration procedures.

FDA, U.S. Food and Drug Administration; *FHR*, fetal heart rate.

Data from Hill, W., & Harvey, C. (2013). Induction of labor. In N. Troiano, C. Harvey, & B. Chez (Eds.), *AWHONN's high risk and critical care obstetrics* (3rd ed.). Philadelphia: Wolters Kluwer/Lippincott Williams & Wilkins; Moleti, C. (2009). Trends and controversies in labor induction, *MCN: The American Journal of Maternal/Child Nursing, 34*(1), 40-47; Thorp, J.M., & Laughon, S.K. (2014). Clinical aspects of normal and abnormal labor. In R.K. Creasy, R. Resnik, J.D. Iams, et al. (Eds.), *Creasy and Resnik's maternal-fetal medicine: Principles and practice* (7th ed.). Philadelphia: Saunders.

Mechanical and Physical Methods. Mechanical dilators ripen the cervix by stimulating the release of endogenous prostaglandins. Balloon catheters (e.g., Foley catheter) can be inserted through the intracervical canal to ripen and dilate the cervix. The catheter balloon is inflated above the internal cervical os with 30 to 50 ml of sterile water. This process results in pressure and stretching of the lower uterine segment and the cervix, as well as the release of endogenous prostaglandins. It is especially helpful for women who cannot receive exogenous prostaglandins for cervical ripening. The balloon usually falls out within 8 to 12 hours, when cervical dilation reaches approximately 3 cm. Evidence supports the insertion of a balloon catheter as a cervical ripening method because of its low cost compared with prostaglandins, stability at room temperature, and reduced risk for uterine tachysystole with or without fetal heart rate changes (ACOG, 2013a; Hill & Harvey, 2013; Yount & Lassiter, 2013).

Hydroscopic dilators (substances that absorb fluid from surrounding tissues and then enlarge) also can be used for cervical ripening. Laminaria tents (natural cervical dilators made from desiccated seaweed) and synthetic dilators containing magnesium sulfate (Lamicel) are inserted into the endocervix without rupturing the membranes. As they absorb fluid, they expand and cause cervical dilation and the release of endogenous prostaglandins. These dilators are left in place for 6 to 12 hours before being removed to assess cervical dilation. Fresh dilators are inserted if further cervical dilation is necessary. Synthetic dilators swell faster than natural dilators and become larger with less discomfort. When compared with prostaglandins, these mechanical methods achieved a lower rate of birth within 24 hours, but caused no change in the cesarean birth rate. Additionally, they were less likely to cause uterine tachysystole with or without changes in the fetal heart rate (ACOG, 2013a; Thorp & Laughon, 2014).

Hydroscopic dilators compare favorably with prostaglandins in their effectiveness in ripening the cervix but are associated with increased discomfort at insertion and during expansion and a higher incidence of postpartum maternal and newborn infections. They are a reliable alternative when prostaglandins are contraindicated or are unavailable.

Nursing responsibilities for women who have dilators inserted include (Gilbert, 2011):

- Documenting the number of dilators and sponges inserted during the procedure, as well as the number removed
- Assessing for urinary retention, rupture of membranes, uterine tenderness or pain, contractions, vaginal bleeding, infection, and fetal distress

MEDICATION GUIDE

Prostaglandin E_2 (PGE_2): Dinoprostone (Cervidil Insert; Prepidil Gel)

Action

PGE_2 ripens the cervix, making it softer and causing it to dilate and efface; it stimulates uterine contractions. Dinoprostone is the only FDA-approved medication for cervical ripening or labor induction.

Indications

- PGE_2 is used for preinduction cervical ripening (ripen the cervix before oxytocin induction of labor when the Bishop score is 4 or less) and for induction of labor or abortion (abortifacient agent).
- It is not recommended for use if the woman has a history of previous cesarean birth or other major uterine surgery.

Dosage and Route

Cervidil Insert

Dosage is 10 mg of dinoprostone designed to be gradually released (approximately 0.3 mg/hr) over 12 hours. Insert is placed transvaginally into the posterior fornix of the vagina. The insert is removed after 12 hours or at the onset of active labor or earlier if tachysystole or abnormal FHR and patterns occur.

Prepidil Gel

Dosage is 0.5 mg of dinoprostone in a 2.5-ml syringe. Gel is administered through a catheter attached to the syringe into the cervical canal just below the internal cervical os. Dose may be repeated every 6 hours as needed for cervical ripening up to a maximum cumulative dose of 1.5 mg (3 doses) in a 24-hour period.

Adverse Effects

Potential adverse effects include headache, nausea and vomiting, diarrhea, fever, hypotension, uterine tachysystole with or without an abnormal FHR and pattern, or fetal passage of meconium.

Nursing Considerations

- Explain the procedure to the woman and her family. Ensure that an informed consent has been obtained as per agency policy.
- Assess the woman and fetus before each insertion and during treatment following agency protocol for frequency. Assess maternal vital signs and health status, FHR and pattern, and status of pregnancy, including indications for cervical ripening or induction of labor, signs of labor or impending labor, and the Bishop score. Recognize that an abnormal FHR and pattern; maternal fever, infection, vaginal bleeding, or hypersensitivity; and regular, progressive uterine contractions contraindicate the use of dinoprostone.
- Avoid use in women with asthma, glaucoma, and hypotension or hypertension.
- Use with caution if the woman has cardiac, renal, or hepatic disease; anemia; jaundice; diabetes; epilepsy; or genitourinary (GU) infections.
- Bring the gel to room temperature just before administration. Do not force the warming process by using a warm-water bath or other source of external heat such as microwave because heat may cause inactivation.
- Keep the insert frozen until just before insertion. No warming is needed.
- Have the woman void before insertion.
- Assist the woman to maintain a supine position with a lateral tilt or a side-lying position for at least 30 minutes after insertion of the gel or for 2 hours after placement of the insert.
- Allow the woman to ambulate after the recommended period of bed rest and observation.
- Prepare to pull the string to remove the insert and to administer terbutaline 0.25 mg subcutaneously if significant adverse effects occur. There is no effective way to remove the gel from the vagina if uterine tachysystole or abnormal FHR and patterns occur.
- Delay the initiation of oxytocin for induction of labor for 6 to 12 hours after the last instillation of the gel or for 30 to 60 minutes after removal of the insert, or follow agency protocol for induction if ripening has occurred but labor has not begun.
- Document all assessment findings and administration procedures.

FDA, U.S. Food and Drug Administration; *FHR*, fetal heart rate.

Data from Hill, W., & Harvey, C. (2013). Induction of labor. In N. Troiano, C. Harvey, & B. Chez (Eds.), *AWHONN's high risk and critical care obstetrics* (3rd ed.). Philadelphia: Wolters Kluwer/Lippincott Williams & Wilkins; Moleti, C. (2009). Trends and controversies in labor induction, *MCN: The American Journal of Maternal/Child Nursing, 34*(1), 40-47.

Amniotic membrane stripping or sweeping is a method of inducing labor through the release of prostaglandins and oxytocin. The procedure involves separation of the membrane from the wall of the cervix and lower uterine segment by inserting a finger into the internal cervical os and rotating it 360 degrees. Membrane stripping seems to work best when the woman is a primigravida at term with an unripe cervix and with the vertex well applied to the cervix. In some studies it has been associated with shorter pregnancies and a decreased likelihood of progressing past 42 weeks of gestation. The procedure is uncomfortable and increases the risk for infection, rupture of membranes, bleeding, and precipitous labor and birth (Wing & Farinelli, 2012).

Routine membrane stripping is not recommended because there is no evidence that this practice improves maternal or fetal outcome. However, weekly membrane stripping at term shortens the time interval to the onset of spontaneous labor and may decrease the need for labor induction using chemical or mechanical methods. Therefore, membrane stripping may be offered after 39 weeks of gestation to women who wish to hasten the onset of spontaneous labor (Wing & Farinelli, 2012).

Physical methods such as sexual intercourse (prostaglandins in the semen and stimulation of contractions with orgasm), nipple stimulation (release of endogenous oxytocin from the pituitary gland), and walking (gravity applies pressure to the cervix, which stimulates the secretion of endogenous oxytocin) may be used by women to "self-induce" labor in an effort to "get it over with." Breast (nipple) stimulation has been shown to increase the number of women who go into labor within 72 hours, but safety issues associated with this method have not been fully evaluated. Although orgasm does stimulate uterine contractions, there is inadequate evidence to support the belief that sexual intercourse enhances cervical ripening (Thorp & Laughon, 2014). Ambulation is an effective measure to augment labor (Yount & Lassiter, 2013).

Alternative Methods. Various alternative methods have been used by women to stimulate cervical ripening and the onset of labor. For example, blue cohosh and castor oil can be used for their labor stimulation effects, and black cohosh and evening primrose oil can ripen the cervix. Nurses must be knowledgeable about these preparations and ask about their use when assessing women during prenatal visits and on admission during labor. Women may accidentally take too much of the preparation or use it incorrectly. Also these preparations may potentiate the effect of pharmacologic methods to stimulate cervical ripening and uterine contractions, thereby increasing the potential for tachysystole and precipitous labor and birth (Gilbert, 2011; Yount & Lassiter, 2013).

Acupuncture has been used effectively to induce labor and has been found, in several studies, to reduce the duration of labor, the use of oxytocin, and the rate of cesarean birth. Specific points have been identified to stimulate uterine contractions or to facilitate cervical dilation. More than one treatment may be required to establish labor (Gilbert, 2011).

Amniotomy. Amniotomy (i.e., artificial rupture of membranes [AROM]) can be used to induce labor when the condition of the cervix is favorable (ripe) or to augment labor if progress begins to slow. Labor usually begins within 12 hours of AROM. Amniotomy can decrease the duration of labor by up to 2 hours, even without oxytocin administration. However, if amniotomy does not stimulate labor, the resulting prolonged rupture may lead to chorioamnionitis. Variable FHR deceleration patterns can occur as a result of cord compression associated with umbilical cord prolapse or a decreased amount of amniotic fluid. Once an amniotomy is performed, the woman is committed to labor with an unknown outcome for how and when she will give birth. For this reason amniotomy often is used in combination with oxytocin induction.

Before the procedure the woman should be told what to expect. She also should be assured that the actual rupture of the membranes is painless for her and the fetus, although she may experience some discomfort when the Amnihook or other sharp instrument is inserted through the vagina and cervix (Box 32-8). The presenting part of the fetus should be engaged and well applied to the cervix prior to the procedure to prevent cord prolapse (Wing & Farinelli, 2012). The woman should also be free of active infection of the genital tract (e.g., herpes) and should be human immunodeficiency virus (HIV) negative. After rupture the amniotic fluid is allowed to drain slowly. The color, odor, and consistency of the fluid are assessed (i.e., for the presence or absence of meconium or blood). The time of rupture is recorded.

SAFETY ALERT

The FHR is assessed before and immediately after the amniotomy to detect any changes. Transient tachycardia is common. Bradycardia and variable decelerations can indicate cord compression or prolapse.

The woman's temperature should be checked at least every 2 hours after rupture of membranes, more frequently if signs or symptoms of infection are noted. If her temperature is 38° C (100.4° F) or higher, the nurse notifies the primary health care provider. The nurse assesses for other signs and symptoms of infection, such as maternal chills, uterine tenderness on palpation, foul-smelling vaginal drainage, and fetal tachycardia. Comfort measures, such as frequently changing the woman's underpads and perineal cleansing, are implemented.

BOX 32-8 Procedure: Assisting with Amniotomy

Procedure

- Explain to the woman what will be done.
- Assess the fetal heart rate (FHR) and pattern before the procedure begins to obtain a baseline reading.
- Place several underpads under the woman's buttocks to absorb the fluid.
- Position the woman on a padded bedpan, fracture pan, or rolled-up towel to elevate her hips.
- Assist the health care provider who is performing the procedure by providing sterile gloves and lubricant for the vaginal examination.
- Unwrap the sterile package containing an Amnihook or Allis clamp and pass the instrument to the primary health care provider, who inserts it alongside the fingers and then hooks and tears the membranes.
- Reassess the FHR and pattern.
- Assess the color, consistency, and odor of the fluid.
- Assess the woman's temperature every 2 hours or per protocol.
- Evaluate the woman for signs and symptoms of infection.

Documentation

Record the following:

- FHR and pattern before and after the procedure
- Time of rupture
- Color, odor, and consistency of the fluid
- Maternal status (how well procedure was tolerated)

LEGAL TIP: Performing Amniotomy

Performing amniotomy is outside the scope of practice of nurses. In some locations, however, nurses have been asked to perform this procedure. A policy that is consistent with professional standards of care and clearly explains the nurse's role in amniotomy should be in place in all labor and birth areas.

Oxytocin

Oxytocin is a hormone normally produced by the posterior pituitary gland. It stimulates uterine contractions and aids in milk let-down. Synthetic oxytocin (Pitocin) may be used either to induce labor or to augment labor that is progressing slowly because of inadequate uterine contractions. Oxytocin is used in the majority of all births in the United States. It is also the drug most commonly associated with adverse events during labor and birth. The most common errors involving oxytocin administration during labor are dose related.

SAFETY ALERT

Oxytocin is included on the list of high-alert medications designated by the Institute for Safe Medication Practices because it has the potential to cause significant harm when used inappropriately (Institute for Safe Medication Practices [ISMP], 2012).

Oxytocin can present hazards to the mother and fetus. Maternal hazards include placental abruption, uterine rupture, unnecessary cesarean birth due to abnormal FHR and patterns, postpartum hemorrhage, and infection. When placental perfusion is diminished by contractions that are too frequent or prolonged, the fetus can experience hypoxemia and acidemia, which eventually result in late decelerations and minimal or absent baseline variability. The goal of oxytocin use is to produce contractions of normal intensity, duration, and frequency using the lowest dose possible (Simpson, 2011).

The primary health care provider writes the order for the induction or augmentation of labor with oxytocin. The nurse implements the order by initiating the primary IV infusion and administering the oxytocin solution through a secondary line. The nurse's actions related to the assessment and care of a woman whose labor is being induced are guided by hospital protocol and professional standards (Fig. 32-7 and the Medication Guide: Oxytocin [Pitocin]).

The recommended protocol for administering oxytocin is to begin with a starting dose of 1 milliunit/min and to increase by 1 to 2 milliunits/min no more frequently than every 30

MEDICATION GUIDE

Oxytocin (Pitocin)

Action

Oxytocin is a hormone produced in the posterior pituitary gland that stimulates uterine contractions and aids in milk let-down. Pitocin is a synthetic form of this hormone.

Indications

Oxytocin is used primarily for labor induction and augmentation; it is also used to control postpartum bleeding.

Dosage

- The IV solution containing oxytocin should be mixed in a standard concentration. Concentrations often used are 10 units in 1000 ml of fluid, 20 units in 1000 ml of fluid, or 30 units in 500 ml of fluid.
- Oxytocin is administered intravenously through a secondary line connected to the main line at the proximal port (connection closest to the IV insertion site). Oxytocin is always administered by infusion pump.
- Begin oxytocin administration at 1 milliunit/minute. Increase the rate by 1 to 2 milliunits/minute, no more frequently than every 30 to 60 minutes based on the response of the woman and fetus and the progress of labor.
- The goal of oxytocin administration is to produce acceptable uterine contractions as evidenced by:
  - Consistent achievement of 200 to 220 MVUs *or*
  - A consistent pattern of one contraction every 2 to 3 minutes, lasting 80 to 90 seconds, and strong to palpation

Adverse Effects

- Possible maternal adverse effects include uterine tachysystole, placental abruption, uterine rupture, unplanned cesarean birth caused by abnormal FHR and patterns, postpartum hemorrhage, infection, and death from water intoxication (e.g., severe hyponatremia).
- Possible fetal adverse effects include hypoxemia and acidosis, eventually resulting in abnormal FHR and patterns.

Nursing Considerations

- Client and partner teaching and support:
  - Reasons for use of oxytocin (e.g., start or improve labor)
  - Reactions to expect concerning the nature of contractions: the intensity of the contraction increases more rapidly, holds the peak longer, and ends more quickly; contractions come regularly and more often
  - Monitoring to anticipate
- Continue to keep woman and her partner informed regarding progress.
- Remember that women vary greatly in their response to oxytocin; some require only very small amounts of medication to produce adequate contractions, whereas others need larger doses.
- Assessment:
  - Assess fetal status using electronic fetal monitoring; evaluate tracing every 15 minutes and with every change in dose during the first stage of labor and every 5 minutes during the active pushing phase of the second stage of labor.
  - Monitor the contraction pattern and uterine resting tone every 15 minutes and with every change in dose during the first stage of labor and every 5 minutes during the second stage of labor.
  - Monitor blood pressure, pulse, and respirations every 30 to 60 minutes and with every change in dose.
  - Assess intake and output; limit IV intake to 1000 ml in 8 hours; urine output should be 120 ml or more every 4 hours.
  - Perform a vaginal examination as indicated.
  - Monitor for side effects, including nausea, vomiting, headache, and hypotension.
  - Observe emotional responses of the woman and her partner.
- Use a standard definition for uterine tachysystole that does not include an abnormal FHR and pattern or the woman's perception of pain (see Emergency: Uterine Tachysystole with Oxytocin).
- The rate of oxytocin infusion should be continually titrated to the lowest dose that achieves acceptable labor progress. Usually the oxytocin dose can be decreased or discontinued after rupture of membranes and in the active phase of first-stage labor.
- Documentation:
  - The time the oxytocin infusion is begun, and each time the infusion is increased, decreased, or discontinued
  - Assessment data as described above
  - Interventions for uterine tachysystole and abnormal FHR and patterns and the response to the interventions
  - Notification of the primary health care provider and that person's response

FHR, Fetal heart rate; *IV,* intravenous; *MVUs,* Montevideo units.

Data from American College of Obstetricians and Gynecologists (ACOG). (2009, reaffirmed in 2013a). *Induction of labor.* ACOG practice bulletin no. 107. Washington, DC; Clark, S., Simpson, K., Knox, G., et al. (2009). Oxytocin: New perspectives on an old drug, *American Journal of Obstetrics and Gynecology, 200*(1):35, e1-e6; Hill, W., & Harvey, C. (2013). Induction of labor. In N. Troiano, C. Harvey, & B. Chez (Eds.), *AWHONN's high risk and critical care obstetrics* (3rd ed.). Philadelphia: Wolters Kluwer/Lippincott Williams & Wilkins; Mahlmeister, L. (2008). Best practices in perinatal care: Evidence-based management of oxytocin induction and augmentation of labor, *Journal of Perinatal and Neonatal Nursing, 22*(4), 259-263; Simpson, K.R., & O'Brien-Abel, N. (2014). Labor and birth. In K. Rice Simpson, & P. Creehan (Eds.), *AWHONN's perinatal nursing* (4th ed.). Philadelphia: Lippincott Williams & Wilkins; Simpson, K., & Knox, G. (2009). Oxytocin as a high-alert medication: Implications for perinatal patient safety, *MCN: The American Journal of Maternal/Child Nursing, 34*(1), 8-15.

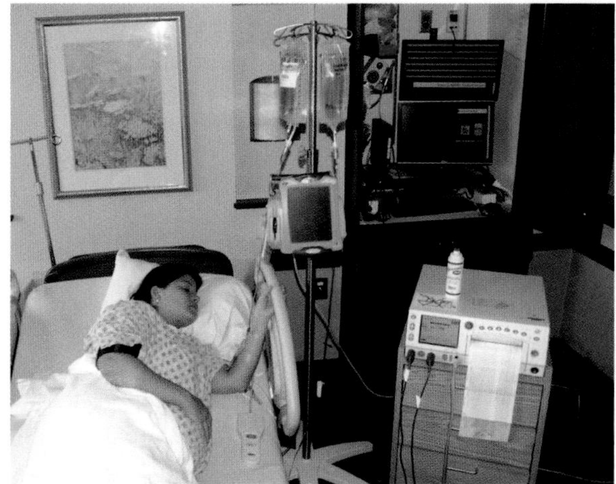

FIG 32-7 Woman in side-lying position receiving oxytocin. (Courtesy Cheryl Briggs, RNC, Annapolis, MD.)

minutes (Simpson, 2011). This recommendation is based on research findings related to the pharmacokinetics of oxytocin. The uterus responds to oxytocin within 3 to 5 minutes of IV administration. The half-life of oxytocin (the time required to metabolize and eliminate half the dose) is approximately 10 to 12 minutes. Approximately 40 minutes is required to reach a steady state of oxytocin (the point in time when the rate of oxytocin administered intravenously equals the rate of oxytocin elimination) and for the full effect of a dosage increment to be reflected in more intense, frequent, and longer contractions (Hill & Harvey, 2013; Simpson) (see Medication Guide: Oxytocin [Pitocin] and Fig. 32-7). Low-dose (physiologic) protocols such as the one described result in decreased risk for oxytocin-induced tachysystole and unnecessary cesarean birth because of abnormal FHR or patterns (Simpson). High-dose protocols, in which the initial dose of oxytocin is larger and the dosage is increased more rapidly, have been found to result in shorter labors, fewer forceps-assisted births, and fewer cesarean births because of dystocia. However, high-dose protocols have been associated with an increased incidence of uterine tachysystole and more cesarean births related to fetal distress (Kunz, Loftus, & Nichols, 2013; Wing & Farinelli, 2012). Some practitioners administer oxytocin in 10-minute pulsed infusions rather than as a continuous infusion. This method, which is more like endogenous secretion of oxytocin than the other approaches, is reported to be effective for labor induction but requires significantly less oxytocin use (Simpson; Wing & Farinelli).

Nursing Interventions. An evidence-based protocol for preparing and administering oxytocin should be established by the obstetric department (physicians, nurses) in each institution. Other safety measures recommended for use of this high-alert drug are using a standard concentration of oxytocin and a standard definition of uterine tachysystole that does not include an abnormal FHR or pattern or the woman's perception of pain. Additionally, standardized treatment of oxytocin-induced uterine tachysystole is recommended (Kunz et al., 2013; Simpson, 2011; Swamy, 2012) (see Emergency box: Uterine Tachysystole with Oxytocin [Pitocin] Infusion).

EMERGENCY

Uterine Tachysystole with Oxytocin (Pitocin) Infusion

Signs
- More than five contractions in 10 minutes *or*
- A series of single contractions lasting >2 minutes *or*
- Contractions of normal duration occurring within 1 minute of each other

Interventions (with Normal [Category I] FHR Tracing)
- Reposition or maintain woman in side-lying position (either side).
- Administer IV fluid bolus with 500 ml lactated Ringer's solution.
- If uterine activity has not returned to normal after 10 minutes, decrease the oxytocin dose by at least half. If uterine activity has not returned to normal after another 10 minutes, discontinue the oxytocin infusion until fewer than five contractions occur in 10 minutes.

Interventions (with Indeterminate [Category II] or Abnormal [Category III] FHR Tracing)
- Discontinue oxytocin infusion immediately.
- Reposition or maintain woman in side-lying position (either side).
- Administer IV fluid bolus with 500 ml lactated Ringer's solution.
- Consider giving oxygen at 10 L/minute if the above interventions do not resolve the indeterminate or abnormal (category II or category III) FHR tracing.
- If no response, consider giving 0.25 mg terbutaline subcutaneously according to unit protocol or standing orders.
- Notify primary health care provider of actions taken and maternal and fetal response.

Resumption of Oxytocin After Resolution of Tachysystole
- If the oxytocin infusion has been discontinued for less than 20 to 30 minutes, resume at no more than one half the rate that caused the tachysystole.
- If the oxytocin infusion has been discontinued for more than 30 to 40 minutes, resume at the initial starting dose.

FHR, Fetal heart rate; *IV,* intravenous.
Data from Simpson, K. (2011). Clinicians' guide to the use of oxytocin for labor induction and augmentation. *Journal of Midwifery & Women's Health, 56*(3), 214-221.

The definition of excessive uterine contractions needs to be standardized. The Eunice Kennedy Shriver National Institute of Child Health and Human Development, along with the ACOG and the Society for Maternal-Fetal Medicine, sponsored a workshop in April 2008 to review definitions, interpretation, and research recommendations for intrapartum fetal monitoring. Workshop participants also recommended standardizing definitions regarding uterine contractions for use in clinical practice. This group defined uterine tachysystole as more than five contractions in 10 minutes, averaged over a 30-minute window. The term tachysystole applies to both spontaneous and stimulated labor. Participants also recommended that use of the terms *hyperstimulation* and *hyperactivity* be abandoned because they are not defined (Macones, Hankins, Spong, et al., 2008).

Augmentation of Labor

Augmentation of labor is the stimulation of uterine contractions after labor has started spontaneously and progress is unsatisfactory. Augmentation is usually implemented to manage hypotonic uterine dysfunction, resulting in a slowing of the labor process (protracted active phase). Common augmentation methods include oxytocin infusion and amniotomy. Noninvasive methods such as emptying the bladder, ambulation and position changes, relaxation measures, nourishment and hydration, and hydrotherapy should be attempted before initiating invasive interventions. The administration procedure and nursing assessment and care measures for augmenting labor with oxytocin are similar to those used for induction of labor with oxytocin (see Medication Guide: Oxytocin [Pitocin]).

Some physicians advocate active management of labor, that is, augmentation of labor to establish efficient labor with the aggressive use of oxytocin so that the woman gives birth within 12 hours of admission to the labor unit. Advocates of active management believe that intervening early (as soon as a nulliparous woman is not dilating her cervix at least 1 cm/hr) with use of higher (pharmacologic) oxytocin doses administered at frequent increment intervals (e.g., a starting dose of 6 milliunits/min with increases of 6 milliunits/min every 15 minutes) shortens labor (Gilbert, 2011).

Additional components of the active management of labor include (1) strict criteria to diagnose that the woman is indeed in active labor with 100% cervical effacement, (2) amniotomy within 1 hour of admission of a woman in labor if spontaneous rupture of the membranes has not occurred, and (3) continuous presence of a personal nurse who provides one-on-one care for the woman while she is in labor. Many U.S. obstetricians emphasize using high-dose oxytocin protocols but do not implement all the other components of active management. At least one review of published studies on the effectiveness of active management of labor protocols concluded that the presence of a personal nurse who provides constant emotional and physical support is the only component associated with shorter labors and lower rates of cesarean birth (Gilbert, 2011).

Operative Vaginal Birth

Operative vaginal births are performed using either forceps or a vacuum extractor. The use of both devices continues to decline. In 2012, less than 4% of all births were accomplished using forceps or vacuum assistance (Martin et al., 2013a). Indications and prerequisites for the use of both instruments are similar. The decision to use forceps or vacuum is based on the experience and personal preference of the physician performing the procedure. There are several types of operative vaginal births (AAP & ACOG, 2012).

Forceps-Assisted Birth

A **forceps-assisted birth** is one in which an instrument with two curved blades is used to assist in the birth of the fetal head. The cephalic-like curve of the forceps commonly used is similar to the shape of the fetal head, with a pelvic curve to the blades conforming to the curve of the pelvic axis. The blades are joined by a pin, screw, or groove arrangement. These locks prevent the forceps from compressing the fetal skull (Fig. 32-8). There are several types of forceps-assisted births, defined primarily by the station and position of the fetal head in relationship to the maternal pelvis (Table 32-4) (AAP & ACOG, 2012).

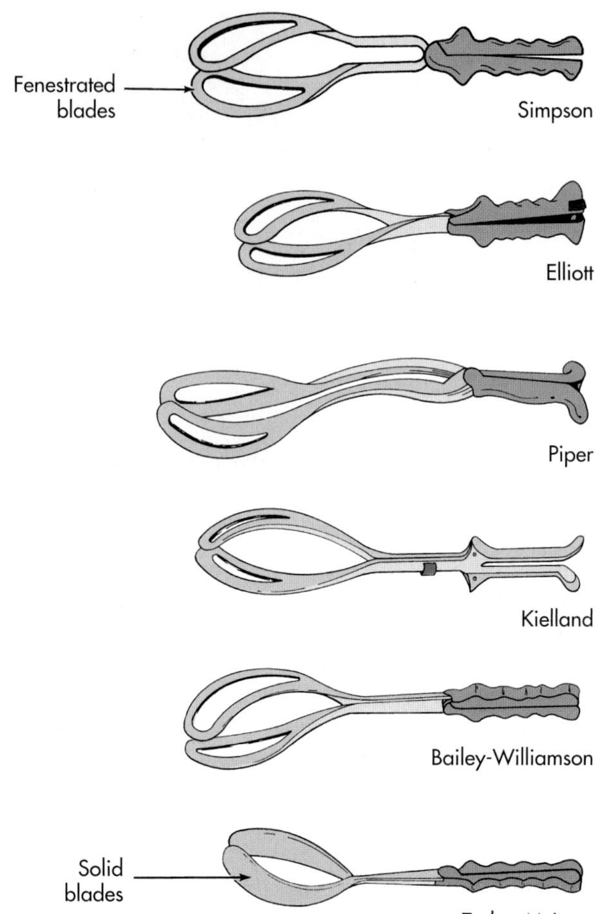

FIG 32-8 Types of forceps. Piper forceps are used to assist delivery of the head in a breech birth.

TABLE 32-4 Definitions for Forceps- and Vacuum-Assisted Births

Outlet	Fetal scalp is visible on the perineum without manually separating the labia
Low	Fetal head is at least at the +2 station
Midpelvis	Fetal head is engaged (no higher than 0 station) but above the +2 station

Data from American Academy of Pediatrics (AAP) and American College of Obstetricians and Gynecologists (ACOG) (2012). *Guidelines for perinatal care* (7th ed.). Washington, DC: ACOG.

Maternal indications for forceps-assisted birth include a prolonged second stage of labor and the need to shorten the second stage of labor for maternal reasons (e.g., maternal exhaustion or maternal cardiopulmonary or cerebrovascular disease) (Nielsen & Galan, 2012). Fetal indications include birth of a fetus in distress or in certain abnormal presentations; arrest of rotation; or extraction of the head in a breech presentation. The use of forceps during birth has been decreasing, replaced by vacuum extraction or cesarean birth (Nielsen & Galan; Thorp & Laughon, 2014).

Certain conditions are required for a forceps-assisted birth to be successful. The woman's cervix must be fully dilated to prevent lacerations and hemorrhage. The bladder should be empty. The presenting part must be engaged—vertex presentation is desired. Membranes must be ruptured so that the position of the fetal head can be precisely determined and

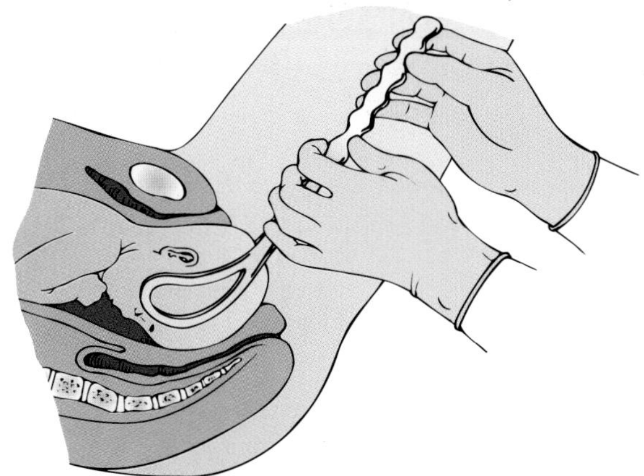

FIG 32-9 Outlet forceps-assisted extraction of the head.

the forceps can firmly grasp the head during birth (Fig. 32-9). In addition, the size of the maternal pelvis must be assessed as adequate for the estimated fetal head circumference and weight.

Medical Management. Both blades are positioned by the physician, and the handles are locked. Traction is usually applied during contractions. The mother may or may not be instructed to push during contractions, depending on physician preference. If a decrease in the fetal heart rate occurs, the forceps are removed and reapplied.

SAFETY ALERT

Because compression of the cord between the fetal head and the forceps will cause a decrease in FHR, the FHR is assessed, reported, and recorded before and after application of the forceps.

Nursing Interventions. When a forceps-assisted birth is deemed necessary, the nurse obtains the type of forceps requested by the physician. The nurse can explain to the mother that the forceps blades fit the same way two tablespoons fit around an egg, with the blades placed in front of the baby's ears.

After birth the mother should be assessed for vaginal or cervical lacerations, urinary retention, and hematoma formation in the pelvic soft tissues, which can result from blood vessel damage. The infant should be assessed for bruising or abrasions at the site of the blade applications, facial palsy resulting from pressure of the blades on the facial nerve, and subdural hematoma. Newborn and postpartum caregivers should be told that a forceps-assisted birth was performed.

Vacuum-Assisted Birth

Vacuum-assisted birth, or vacuum extraction, is a birth method involving the attachment of a vacuum cup to the fetal head, using negative pressure to assist in the birth of the head (Fig. 32-10, *A*). It is generally not used to assist birth before 34 weeks of gestation. Indications for its use are the same as those for outlet forceps. Prerequisites for use include a completely dilated cervix, ruptured membranes, engaged head, vertex presentation, and no suspicion of CPD (Cunningham et al., 2014). The types of vacuum-assisted births are defined the same as for forceps-assisted births—by the station and position of the fetal head in relation to the maternal pelvis (see Table 32-4) (AAP & ACOG, 2012). Advantages of vacuum-assisted compared with forceps-assisted birth are the ease with which the vacuum can be placed and the need for less anesthesia. Also it is far easier to teach and to learn the skills necessary to safely use the vacuum than to gain a similar level of skill with forceps (Thorp & Laughon, 2014).

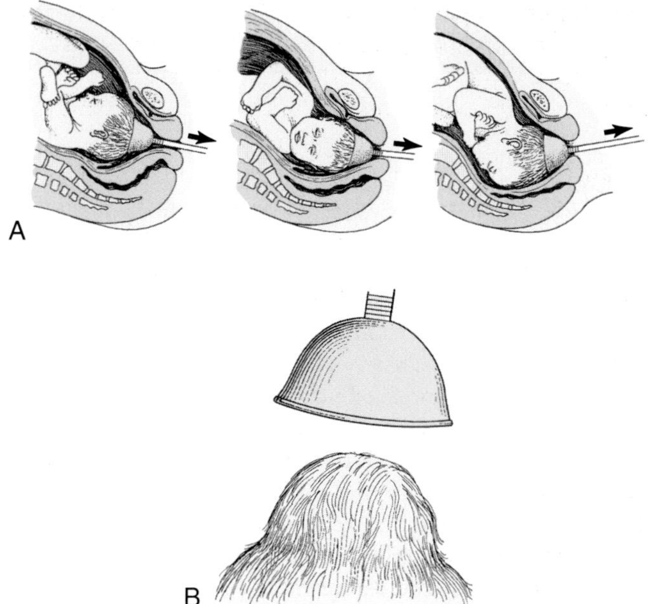

FIG 32-10 Use of vacuum extraction to rotate fetal head and assist with descent. **A,** Arrow indicates direction of traction on the vacuum cup. **B,** Caput succedaneum formed by the vacuum cup.

Medical Management. The vacuum cup is applied to the fetal head by the physician. There are basically two types of vacuum devices. One is a self-contained unit, which allows the physician to both position the cup on the baby's head and generate the desired amount of negative pressure to create a vacuum. When the other type of vacuum device is used, the physician applies the cup to the baby's head, after which the nurse connects the suction tubing attached to the cup to wall suction or a separate hand pump and generates the amount of pressure requested by the physician. With both devices, a caput develops inside the cup as the pressure is initiated (see Fig. 32-10, *B*). The woman is encouraged to push as traction is applied by the physician. The vacuum cup is released and removed after birth of the head. If vacuum extraction is not successful, a forceps-assisted or cesarean birth is usually performed.

Risks to the newborn include cephalhematoma, scalp lacerations, and subdural hematoma. These complications can be reduced by strict adherence to the manufacturer's recommendations for method of application, amount of pressure to be generated, and duration of application. Maternal risks include perineal, vaginal, or cervical lacerations and soft-tissue hematomas.

Nursing Interventions. The nurse provides education and support for the woman who has a vacuum-assisted birth. The nurse can prepare the woman for birth and encourage her to remain active in the birth process by pushing during contractions. The FHR should be assessed frequently during the procedure. Documentation of the procedure in the medical

BOX 32-9 Assisting with Birth by Vacuum Extraction

- Assess the fetal heart rate frequently during the procedure.
- Encourage the woman to push during contractions.
- If responsible for generating pressure for the vacuum, do not exceed the "green zone" indicated on the pump. Verify with the physician the amount of pressure to be generated.
- Document the number of pulls attempted, the maximum pressure used, and any pop-offs that occur.

record is important and is often the nurse's responsibility (Box 32-9). Neonatal caregivers should be told that the birth was vacuum assisted. After birth the newborn is observed for signs of trauma and infection at the application site and for cerebral irritation (e.g., poor sucking or listlessness). The newborn can be at risk for hyperbilirubinemia and neonatal jaundice as bruising resolves. The parents need to be reassured that the caput succedaneum usually disappears in 3 to 5 days (see Fig. 32-10, *B*) (Gilbert, 2011).

Cesarean Birth

Cesarean birth is the birth of a fetus through a transabdominal incision of the uterus. Whether cesarean birth is planned (scheduled) or unplanned, the loss of experiencing a vaginal birth can have a negative effect on a woman's self-concept. An effort is therefore made to maintain the focus on the birth of the baby rather than on the operative procedure.

The purpose of cesarean birth is to preserve the well-being of the mother and her fetus. It may be the best choice for birth when evidence exists of maternal or fetal complications. Since the advent of modern surgical methods and care and the use of antibiotics, maternal and fetal morbidity and mortality have decreased. In addition, incisions are usually made into the lower uterine segment rather than in the muscular body of the uterus, thus promoting more effective healing. However, despite these advances, cesarean birth still poses threats to the health of the mother and infant.

In 2010, the cesarean birth rate in the United States was 32.8%, down from an all-time high of 32.9% in 2009. This was the first decrease in the overall cesarean birth rate since 1996. The cesarean birth rate has remained unchanged at 32.8% in both 2011 and 2012 (Martin et al., 2013a). Despite this recent small decrease, the cesarean birth rate in the United States remains very high. Part of the reason is that a number of common risk factors for cesarean birth are increasing in frequency, especially in developed countries. These factors include fetal macrosomia, advanced maternal age, obesity, gestational diabetes, multifetal pregnancy, and dystocia in nulliparous women (Thorp & Laughon, 2014). In addition, there has been a decline in the number of VBACs and trial of labor after cesarean (TOLACs). Eden and colleagues found that the number of women who were allowed a TOLAC decreased dramatically after 1996, when information about the increased risk for uterine rupture with VBAC was published (Eden, Denman, Emeis, et al., 2012). Limited use of a TOLAC, due in part to concerns about safety and medicolegal considerations, is another reason for the high cesarean birth rate (Martin et al., 2013b).

BOX 32-10 Indications for Cesarean Birth

Maternal

- Specific cardiac disease (e.g., Marfan syndrome, unstable coronary artery disease)
- Specific respiratory disease (e.g., Guillain-Barré syndrome)
- Conditions associated with increased intracranial pressure
- Mechanical obstruction of the lower uterine segment (tumors, fibroids)
- Mechanical vulvar obstruction (e.g., extensive condylomata)
- History of previous cesarean birth

Fetal

- Abnormal fetal heart rate (FHR) or pattern
- Malpresentation (e.g., breech or transverse lie)
- Active maternal herpes lesions
- Maternal human immunodeficiency virus (HIV) with a viral load of more than 1000 copies/ml
- Congenital anomalies

Maternal-Fetal

- Dysfunctional labor (e.g., cephalopelvic disproportion, "failure to progress" in labor)
- Placental abruption
- Placenta previa
- Elective cesarean birth (cesarean on maternal request)

Data from Berghella, V., & Landon, M. (2012). Cesarean delivery. In S. Gabbe, J. Niebyl, & J. Simpson (Eds.), *Obstetrics: Normal and problem pregnancies* (6th ed.). Philadelphia: Saunders; Duff, P. (2014). Maternal and fetal infections. In R.K. Creasy, R. Resnik, J.D. Iams, et al. (Eds.), *Creasy and Resnik's maternal-fetal medicine: Principles and practice* (7th ed.). Philadelphia: Saunders; Thorp, J.M., & Laughon, S.K. (2014). Clinical aspects of normal and abnormal labor. In R.K. Creasy, R. Resnik, J.D. Iams, et al. (Eds.), *Creasy and Resnik's maternal-fetal medicine: Principles and practice* (7th ed.). Philadelphia: Saunders.

Indications

Few absolute indications exist for cesarean birth. Currently most are performed for conditions that might pose a threat to both the mother and the fetus if vaginal birth occurred, such as placenta previa or placental abruption (Campbell, 2011). Box 32-10 lists common indications for cesarean birth.

Elective Cesarean Birth

Elective cesarean birth, sometimes referred to as *cesarean on request* or *cesarean on demand,* refers to a primary cesarean birth without medical or obstetric indication. Reasons given for elective cesarean birth include fear of pain during labor and birth and the mistaken belief that the surgery will prevent future problems with pelvic support, bladder and bowel incontinence, or sexual dysfunction (Ecker, 2013). At this time evidence is insufficient to recommend elective cesarean birth to prevent urinary or fecal incontinence later in life (ACOG, 2013b; Thorp & Laughon, 2014). Although some nulliparous women may fear the pain of labor because of no firsthand experience, multiparous women may request a cesarean birth after a previous traumatic vaginal birth. Other women desire an elective cesarean birth because of the convenience of planning a date, or having control and choice about when to give birth (Ecker).

Only limited data are available comparing cesarean births on request with planned vaginal births (ACOG, 2013b). In a committee opinion (2013b), the ACOG lists potential risks of cesarean birth on request that include a longer hospital stay for the woman, an increased risk of respiratory problems for the baby, and greater complications in subsequent pregnancies, including uterine rupture and placental implantation problems. The ACOG recommends that cesarean birth on request not be performed unless a gestational age of 39 weeks has been accurately determined. Cesarean birth on request is not recommended for women who desire several additional children, because the risks for placenta previa, placenta accreta, and cesarean hysterectomy increase with each cesarean birth (Berghella & Landon, 2012).

Scheduled Cesarean Birth

Cesarean birth is scheduled or planned if:

- Labor and vaginal birth are contraindicated (e.g., complete placenta previa, active genital herpes, positive HIV status with a high viral load)
- Birth is necessary but labor is not inducible (e.g., hypertensive states that cause a poor intrauterine environment that threatens the fetus)
- This course of action has been chosen by the primary health care provider and the woman (e.g., a repeat cesarean birth)

Women who are scheduled for a cesarean birth usually have time to prepare for it psychologically. However, the psychologic responses of these women may differ. Those having a repeat cesarean birth may have disturbing memories of the conditions preceding the initial (primary) cesarean birth and of their experiences in the postoperative recovery period. They may be concerned about the added burdens of caring for the infant and perhaps other children while recovering from surgery. Others may feel glad that they have been relieved of the uncertainty about the date and time of the birth and are free of the pain of labor.

Unplanned Cesarean Birth

The psychosocial outcomes of unplanned or emergency cesarean birth are usually more pronounced and negative when compared with the outcomes associated with a scheduled or planned cesarean birth. Women and their families experience abrupt changes in their expectations for birth, postpartum care, and care of the new baby at home. This can be an extremely traumatic experience for all.

The woman may approach the procedure tired and discouraged after an ineffective and difficult labor. Fear predominates as she worries about her own safety and well-being and that of her fetus. She may be dehydrated, with low glycogen reserves. Because preoperative procedures must be done rapidly, there is often little time for explanation of the procedures and the operation itself. Because maternal and family anxiety levels are high at this time, much of what is said can be forgotten or misunderstood. The woman can experience feelings of anger or guilt in the postpartum period. Fatigue is often noticeable in these women, and they need much supportive care.

Forced Cesarean Birth

A woman's refusal to undergo cesarean birth when indicated for fetal reasons is often described as a *maternal-fetal conflict*. Health care providers are ethically obliged to protect the well-being of mother as well as fetus; a decision for one affects the other. If a woman refuses a cesarean birth that is recommended because of fetal jeopardy, health care providers must make every effort to find out why she is refusing and provide information that may persuade her to change her mind. If the woman continues to refuse surgery, then health care providers must decide if it is ethical to get a court order for the surgery. Every effort, however, should be made to avoid this legal step.

Surgical Techniques

The skin incision will either be vertical, extending from near the umbilicus to the mons pubis or transverse (Pfannenstiel) in the lower abdomen (Fig. 32-11). The transverse incision, sometimes referred to as the "bikini" incision, is performed more often. The type of skin incision is generally determined by the urgency of the surgery and the presence of any prior skin incisions (Berghella & Landon, 2012). The type of skin incision does *not* necessarily indicate the type of uterine incision.

The two main types of uterine incisions are the low transverse (Fig. 32-12, *A*) or vertical incision, which may be either low or classic (see Fig. 32-12, *B* and *C*). Ideally the vertical incision is contained entirely within the lower uterine segment,

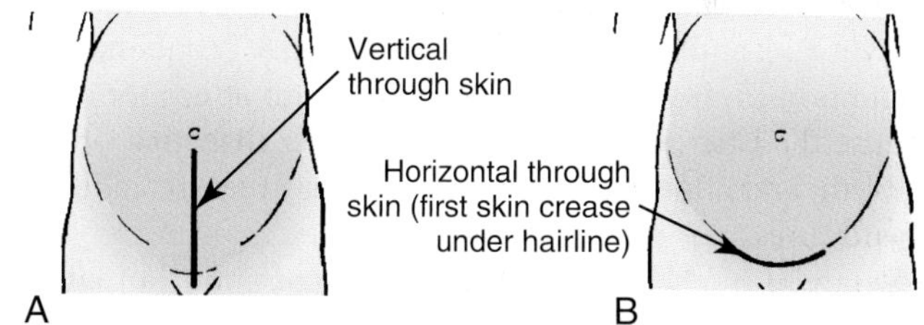

FIG 32-11 Skin incisions for cesarean birth. **A,** Vertical. **B,** Horizontal (Pfannenstiel).

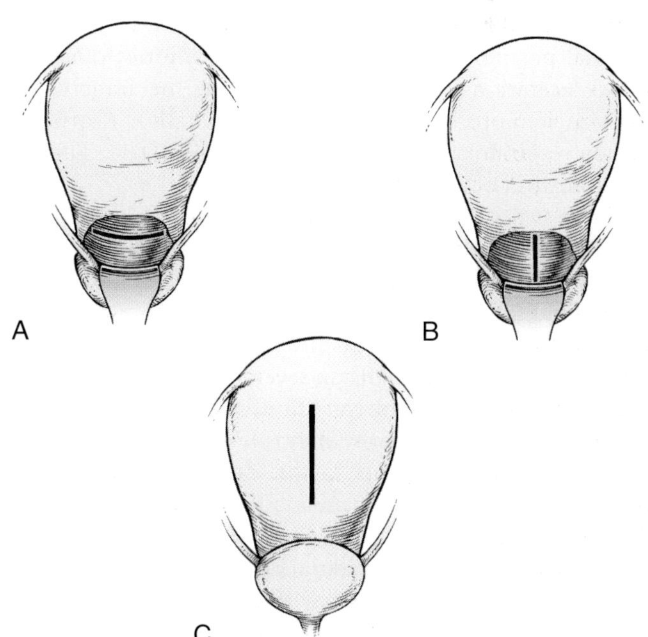

FIG 32-12 Uterine incisions for cesarean birth. **A,** Low transverse incision. **B,** Low vertical incision. **C,** Classic incision. (From Gabbe, S.G., Niebyl, J., Simpson, J., et al. [2012]. *Obstetrics: Normal and problem pregnancies* [6th ed.]. Philadelphia: Saunders.)

but extension into the contractile portion of the uterus (e.g., a classic incision) is common. Indications for a vertical incision include an underdeveloped lower uterine segment, a transverse lie or preterm breech presentation, certain fetal anomalies such as massive hydrocephalus, and an anterior placenta previa (Berghella & Landon, 2012). Because it is associated with a higher incidence of uterine rupture in subsequent pregnancies than is lower-segment cesarean birth, vaginal birth after a classic uterine incision is contraindicated.

The low transverse uterine incision is performed in more than 90% of cesarean births (see Fig. 32-12, *A*). Compared with the vertical incision, the transverse incision is preferred because it does not compromise the upper uterine segment, is easier to perform and repair, and is associated with less blood loss. It also provides for the option of TOLAC and VBAC in subsequent pregnancies (Berghella & Landon, 2012).

Complications and Risks

Possible maternal complications related to cesarean birth include anesthesia events (problems with intubation, drug reactions, aspiration pneumonia), hemorrhage, bowel or bladder injury, amniotic fluid embolism, and air embolism. Possible postpartum complications include atelectasis; endometritis; urinary tract infection; abdominal wound hematoma formation, dehiscence, infection, or necrotizing fasciitis; thromboembolic disease; and bowel dysfunction (Thorp & Laughon, 2014). In addition to these risks, the woman is also at economic risk because the cost of cesarean birth is higher than that of vaginal birth, and a longer recovery period may require additional expenditures.

Cesarean birth is associated with uncommon but significant dangers to the infant. The fetus may be born prematurely if the gestational age has not been accurately determined (iatrogenic prematurity). Fetal asphyxia can occur if the uterus and placenta are poorly perfused as a result of maternal hypotension caused by regional anesthesia (epidural or spinal) or maternal positioning. Fetal injuries (e.g., injuries caused by scalpel lacerations) can also occur during the surgery. The newborn is more likely to require resuscitation efforts and develop respiratory complications (Campbell, 2011; Thorp & Laughon, 2014).

Anesthesia

Spinal, epidural, and general anesthetics are used for cesarean births. Epidural blocks are popular because women want to be awake for and aware of the birth experience. However, the choice of anesthetic depends on several factors. The mother's medical history or present condition, such as a spinal injury, hemorrhage, or coagulopathy, may rule out the use of regional anesthesia. Time is another factor, especially if there is an emergency and the life of the mother or infant is at stake. In an emergency general anesthesia will most likely be used unless the woman already has an epidural block in effect. The woman herself is a factor. Either she may not know all the options or may have fears about having "a needle in her back" or about being awake and feeling pain. She needs to be fully informed about the risks and benefits of the different types of anesthesia so that she can participate in the decision whenever there is a choice.

CARE MANAGEMENT

Prenatal Preparation

A discussion of cesarean birth should be included in all childbirth preparation classes. No woman can be guaranteed a vaginal birth, even if she is in good health and no indication of danger to the fetus exists before the onset of labor. Therefore, every woman needs to be aware of and prepared for the possibility of having a cesarean birth.

Childbirth educators should emphasize the similarities and differences between a cesarean and a vaginal birth. In support of the philosophy of family-centered birth, many hospitals have instituted policies that permit fathers or partners and family members to share in these births as they do in vaginal births. Women who have undergone cesarean birth agree that the continued presence and support of their partners helped them respond more positively to the entire experience. In addition to preparing women for the possibility of cesarean birth, childbirth educators should empower them to believe in their ability to give birth vaginally and to seek care measures during labor that will enhance the progress of their labors and reduce their risk for cesarean birth.

Preoperative Care

Family-centered care is the goal for the woman who is to undergo cesarean birth and for her family. Preparing a woman for cesarean birth is the same as that for other elective or emergency surgery. The primary health care provider discusses, with the woman and her family, the need for the cesarean birth and the prognosis for the mother and infant. A member of the anesthesia care team assesses the woman's cardiopulmonary status and describes the options for anesthesia. Women who are scheduled for an elective cesarean are often told not to eat or drink (remain NPO [nothing by mouth]) for at least 8 hours prior to the surgery. Informed consent is obtained for the procedure.

Blood tests are usually done a day or two before a planned cesarean birth or on admission to the labor and birth unit. Laboratory tests commonly ordered include a complete blood cell count and blood type and Rh status. Maternal vital signs and FHR and pattern are assessed according to hospital protocol until the operation begins. IV fluids are started to maintain hydration and to provide an open line for administering blood or medications if needed. Other preoperative preparations include making sure that an informed consent form has been signed, inserting a retention (Foley) catheter to keep the bladder empty, and administering prescribed preoperative medications. In addition to medications given to prevent aspiration pneumonia, women may also receive prophylactic antibiotics to prevent postoperative infection. In the rare instance that an abdominal-mons shave or a clipping of pubic hair is ordered by the primary health care provider, it is performed in the operating room just prior to making the incision because shaving can result in injury to the skin, thereby increasing the risk for infection. Often, TED hose or SCD boots are placed on the woman's legs to prevent blood clot formation. Removal of contact lenses, dentures, nail polish, and jewelry may be optional, depending on hospital policies and the type of anesthesia used. If the woman wears glasses and is going to be awake, the nurse should make sure her glasses accompany her to the operating room so she can see her infant.

During the preoperative preparation, the support person is encouraged to remain with the woman as much as possible to provide continuing emotional support (if this action is culturally acceptable to the woman and support person). The nurse provides essential information about the preoperative procedures during this time. Although the nursing actions may be carried out quickly if a cesarean birth is unplanned, verbal communication, particularly explanations, is important. Silence can be frightening to the woman and her support person. The nurse's use of touch (if culturally appropriate) can communicate feelings of care and concern for the woman. The nurse can assess the woman's and her partner's perceptions about cesarean birth. As the woman expresses her feelings, the nurse may identify a potential for a disturbance in self-concept during the postpartum period that would need to be addressed. If there is time before the birth, the nurse can teach the woman about postoperative expectations and about pain relief, position changes, leg exercises, coughing, and deep-breathing measures.

Intraoperative Care

Cesarean births occur in operating rooms in the surgical suite or in the labor and birth unit. Staff members from the labor and birth unit may scrub and circulate during the surgery or these functions may be assumed by members of the hospital's surgery staff (Fig. 32-13). If possible, the partner or other support person, who is dressed appropriately for the operating room, accompanies the mother to the operating room and remains close to her for continued comfort and support. In unplanned cesarean birth, the nurse who cared for the woman during labor should be part of the nursing care team in the operating room if possible.

The nurse who is circulating may assist with positioning the woman on the birth (operating) table. It is important to position her so that the uterus is displaced laterally to prevent compression of the inferior vena cava, which causes decreased placental perfusion. This is usually accomplished by placing a wedge under the hip or tilting the table to one side. A retention (Foley) catheter is inserted into the bladder at this time if one is not already in place. The woman's legs should be strapped to the table to ensure proper positioning during the surgery.

As is done in other surgical procedures, a "time out" should be conducted just before the operation begins. This is an opportunity for all members of the surgical team to participate in confirming the woman's identity and the planned procedure(s) to be performed. The circulating nurse is usually responsible for ensuring that the operative consent form has been signed and witnessed and is in the woman's chart. Members of the surgical team confirm that ordered preoperative medications have been given and that blood products, if ordered, are available. Information about drug or other allergies is also shared.

If the partner is not allowed or chooses not to be present, the nurse can stay in communication with him or her and give progress reports whenever possible. If the woman is awake during the birth, the nurse, anesthesia care provider, or both can tell her what is happening and provide support. She may be anxious about the sensations she is experiencing, such as the coldness of solutions used to cleanse the abdomen and pressure or pulling during the actual birth of the infant. She also may be apprehensive because of the bright lights or the presence of unfamiliar equipment and masked and gowned personnel in the room. Explanations can help to decrease her anxiety.

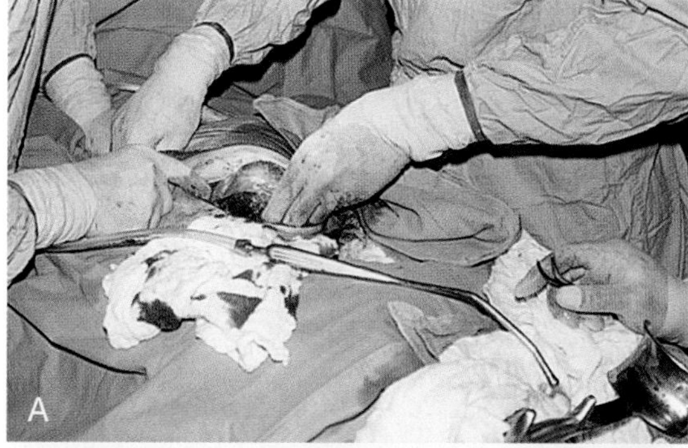

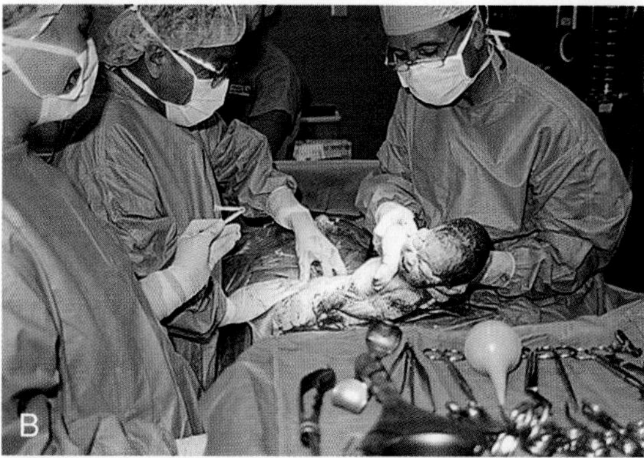

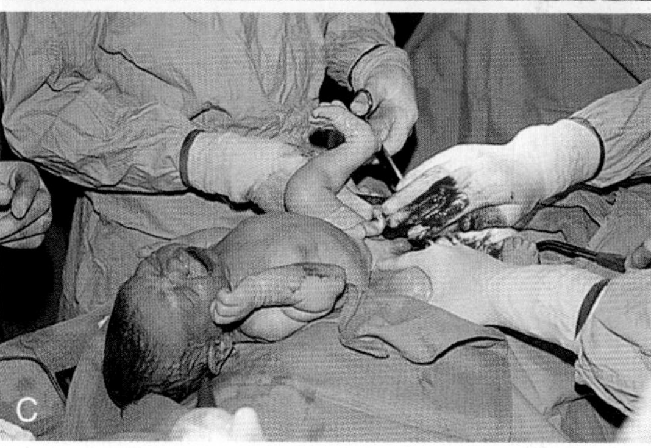

FIG 32-13 Cesarean birth. **A,** "Bikini" incision has been made, the muscle layer is separated, the abdomen is entered, and the uterus has been exposed and incised; suctioning of amniotic fluid continues as head is brought up through the incision. Note small amount of bleeding. **B,** The neonate's birth through the uterine incision is nearly complete. **C,** A quick assessment is performed; note extreme molding of head resulting from cephalopelvic disproportion. (Courtesy Marjorie Pyle, RNC, Lifecircle, Costa Mesa, CA.)

A nurse from the labor and birth unit is usually present to provide care for the infant. In addition, a pediatrician or a nurse team skilled in neonatal resuscitation may also be present for the surgery because these infants are considered to be at risk until evidence of physiologic stability after the birth is observed. A radiant warmer bed with resuscitation equipment is readied before surgery. Personnel who are responsible for care are expert not only in resuscitative techniques but also in their ability to detect normal and abnormal infant responses (AAP & American Heart Association [AHA], 2011). After birth, if the infant's condition permits and the mother is awake, the baby

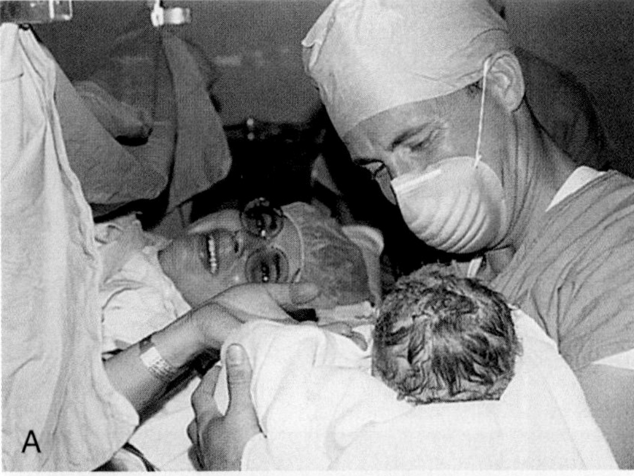

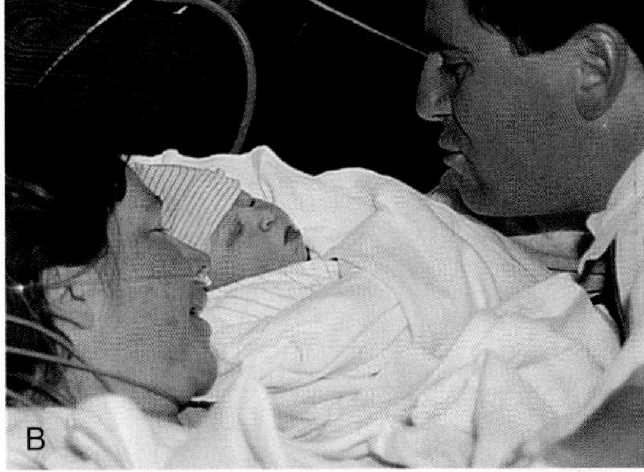

FIG 32-14 **A,** Parents and their newborn. The physician manually removes the placenta, suctions the remaining amniotic fluid and blood from the uterine cavity, and repairs the uterine incision, peritoneum, muscle layer, fatty tissue, and finally the skin, while the new family shares some time together. **B,** Parents become better acquainted with their newborn while mother rests after surgery. (Courtesy Marjorie Pyle, RNC, Lifecircle, Costa Mesa, CA.)

may be placed skin-to-skin on the mother or may be given to the woman's partner to hold (Fig. 32-14). The infant whose condition is compromised is transported after initial stabilization to the newborn nursery or neonatal intensive care unit (NICU) for observation and the implementation of appropriate interventions. In some institutions the partner may accompany the infant; if not, personnel keep the family informed of the infant's progress and parent-infant contacts are initiated as soon as possible.

If family members cannot accompany the woman during surgery, they are directed to the surgical or obstetric waiting room. The physician then reports on the condition of the mother and infant to the family members after the birth is completed. Family members may be allowed to accompany the infant as she or he is transferred to the nursery, giving them an opportunity to see and admire the new baby.

> **LEGAL TIP: Disclosure of Client Information**
> Some mothers or fathers want the privilege of informing family and friends about the sex of the infant (if it was not known before birth) or other information about the birth. Before responding to requests for such information from people waiting outside the birthing area, the nurse should check to see if the mother has given consent for such information to be released and to whom.

Immediate Postoperative Care

Once surgery is completed, the mother is transferred to a postanesthesia recovery area. After a cesarean birth, women have postoperative and postpartum needs that must be addressed. They are surgical clients as well as new mothers. Nursing assessments in this immediate postpartum period follow agency protocol and include degree of recovery from the effects of anesthesia, postoperative and postbirth status, and degree of pain. A patent airway is maintained, and the woman is positioned to prevent possible aspiration. Blood pressure and pulse are assessed at least every 15 minutes for 2 hours. Temperature should be assessed every 4 hours for the first 8 hours after birth and then at least every 8 hours (AAP & ACOG, 2012). The condition of the incisional dressing and the fundus and the amount of lochia are assessed, as well as the IV intake and the urine output through the retention (Foley) catheter. Oxytocin usually is added to at least the first liter of the IV infusion to ensure that the fundus remains firmly contracted, thereby reducing blood loss. The woman is assisted to cough, deep-breathe, turn, and perform leg exercises. She will likely have SCD boots on her legs. Medications for pain relief should be administered before postoperative pain becomes severe.

If the baby is present, the mother and her partner are given some time alone with him or her to facilitate bonding and attachment. The mother may hold her newborn skin-to-skin and initiate breastfeeding. The woman is ready for discharge from the postanesthesia recovery area once her condition is stable and the effects of anesthesia have worn off (i.e., she is alert and oriented and able to feel and move her extremities).

Postoperative Postpartum Care

The attitude of the nurse and other health care team members can influence the woman's perception of herself after a cesarean birth. The caregivers should stress that the woman is a new mother first and a surgical client second. This attitude helps the woman perceive herself as having the same problems and needs as other new mothers, while requiring supportive postoperative care.

The woman's physiologic concerns can be dominated by pain at the incision site and discomfort resulting from intestinal gas. For the first 24 hours following surgery, pain relief may be provided by epidural opioids, patient-controlled analgesia (PCA), or IV or intramuscular injections. The most commonly used analgesics include opioids (e.g., hydromorphone [Dilaudid], morphine sulfate, nalbuphine [Nubain]) and NSAIDs (e.g., ketorolac [Toradol]). If opioids are used, an antiemetic (e.g., metoclopramide [Reglan]) is often administered either as needed by the woman or around the clock as long as the opioid is used. Palpation of the fundus with the possibility of massage should be performed after an analgesic is given to decrease pain. By 24 hours after surgery, women are usually taking oral analgesics. Other comfort measures such as position changes, splinting of the incision with pillows, and relaxation and breathing techniques (e.g., those learned in childbirth classes) may be implemented (see Teaching for Self-Management: Nonpharmacologic Postpartum Pain Relief After Cesarean Birth).

TEACHING FOR SELF-MANAGEMENT

Nonpharmacologic Postpartum Pain Relief After Cesarean Birth

Incisional
- Splint the incision with a pillow when moving or coughing.
- Use relaxation techniques such as music, breathing, and dim lights.

Intestinal Gas
- Walk as often as you can.
- Do not eat or drink gas-forming foods, carbonated beverages, whole milk, or ice.
- Do not use straws for drinking fluids.
- Take antiflatulence medication if prescribed.
- Lie on your left side to expel gas.
- Rock in a rocking chair.

Women are often the best judges of what their bodies need and can tolerate, including the postoperative ingestion of foods and fluids. Some health care providers keep women NPO or allow only "sips and chips" (sips of clear fluids and teaspoons of crushed ice) until bowel sounds return. The diet is then advanced to full liquids. After women are passing flatus they can resume a regular diet (Gilbert, 2011). Because most women have an epidural or spinal anesthetic for surgery, many health care providers allow the early introduction of solid food if desired and tolerated. IV fluids are usually continued until the woman is tolerating fluids orally. Ambulation and rocking in a rocking chair may relieve gas pains. Avoiding gas-forming foods, ice chips, carbonated beverages, and using a straw to drink beverages can help limit gas formation, thereby minimizing the severity of gas pains (see Teaching for Self-Management: Nonpharmacologic Postpartum Pain Relief After Cesarean Birth).

Nursing Interventions

Nurses must be alert to a woman's physiologic needs, managing care to ensure adequate rest and pain relief. Mother-baby care (couplet care) for a cesarean birth mother may have to be modified according to her physical limitations as a surgical client.

Daily care includes perineal care, breast care, and routine hygienic care. The woman may shower after the original incisional dressing is removed, usually on the first postoperative day (if showering is acceptable according to the woman's cultural beliefs and practices). The indwelling (Foley) catheter usually is also removed on the first postpartum day. The woman is encouraged to be out of bed and ambulating several times each day as soon as the urinary catheter is removed. Use of TED hose or SCD boots should continue as long as the woman remains in bed. They may be removed when she begins ambulating. The nurse assesses the woman's vital signs, incision, fundus, and lochia according to hospital policies, procedures, or protocols. Breath sounds, bowel sounds, circulatory status of lower extremities, and urinary and bowel elimination patterns also are assessed. It is important to observe maternal emotional status and progress of attachment to her baby.

SAFETY ALERT

The woman should be taught to seek assistance initially when getting out of bed, especially when an IV line and catheter are still in place. Thereafter, when rising from a supine position, she should sit on the side of the bed first to determine if dizziness will occur, then stand at the bedside, and finally ambulate.

During the postpartum period the nurse provides care that meets the psychologic and teaching needs of women who have had cesarean births. This includes explaining postpartum procedures to help the woman participate in her recovery from surgery. The nurse can also help the woman plan care and visits from family and friends that will allow for adequate rest periods. Providing information on and assistance with infant care can facilitate adjustment to her role as a mother. With adequate support these women can benefit from mother-baby care to facilitate attachment and enhance involvement in newborn care. The woman is supported as she breastfeeds her baby by receiving individualized assistance to comfortably hold and position the baby at her breast. Using the side-lying or football (under the arm or clutch hold) position and supporting the newborn with pillows can enhance comfort and facilitate successful breastfeeding. The partner and other family members can be included in infant teaching sessions and in explanations about the woman's recovery.

SAFETY ALERT

When holding her baby or breastfeeding, a woman may become drowsy and even fall asleep because of the sedation that occurs with the use of analgesics. It is important that someone be with her during these times.

The couple also should be encouraged to express their feelings about the birth experience. Some parents are angry, frustrated, or disappointed that a vaginal birth was not possible. Some women express feelings of low self-esteem or a negative self-image. Others express relief and gratitude that the baby is healthy and safely born. It may be helpful for them to have the nurse who was present during the birth visit and help fill in "gaps" about the experience.

Discharge after cesarean birth is usually by the third postoperative day. The time is often determined by criteria established by the woman's insurance carrier or the federal government (e.g., diagnosis-related groups [DRGs]). The Newborns' and Mothers' Health Protection Act of 1996 provides for a length of stay of up to 96 hours for cesarean births. These criteria may not coincide with the woman's physical or psychosocial readiness for discharge. Some states have added home care provisions for mothers who meet appropriate criteria for discharge and choose to leave sooner than the allowed length of stay. This policy recognizes that home care is less costly than hospital care and in most cases is more beneficial for recovery.

The nurse provides discharge teaching to prepare the woman for self-care and newborn care while trying to ensure that she is comfortable and able to rest. The nurse assesses the woman's information needs and coordinates the health care team's efforts to meet them. Discharge teaching and planning should include information about nutrition; measures to relieve pain and discomfort; exercise and specific activity restrictions; time management that includes periods of uninterrupted rest and sleep; hygiene, breast, and incision care; timing for resumption of sexual activity and contraception; signs of complications (see Teaching for Self-Management: Signs of Postoperative Complications After Discharge Following Cesarean Birth and Teaching for Self-Management: Signs of Postpartum Blues, Depression, and Psychosis in Chapter 31); and infant care. The nurse assesses the woman's need for continued support or counseling to facilitate her emotional recovery from the birth. The woman's family and friends should be educated regarding her needs during the recovery process, and their assistance should be coordinated before discharge. Referral to support groups (e.g., www.birthrites.org) or to community agencies may be indicated to further promote the recovery process. A postdischarge program of telephone follow-up and home visits can facilitate the woman's full recovery after cesarean birth.

TEACHING FOR SELF-MANAGEMENT

Signs of Postoperative Complications After Discharge Following Cesarean Birth

Report the following signs to your health care provider:

- Temperature exceeding 38° C (100.4° F)
- Urination: painful urination, urgency, cloudy urine
- Lochia: heavier than a normal menstrual period, clots, odor
- Cesarean incision: redness, swelling, bruising, foul-smelling discharge or bleeding, wound separation
- Severe, increasing abdominal pain

Trial of Labor

A trial of labor (TOL) is the observance of a woman and her fetus for a reasonable period (e.g., 4 to 6 hours) of spontaneous active labor to assess the safety of vaginal birth for the mother and infant. It may be initiated if the mother's pelvis is of questionable size or shape or if the fetus is in an abnormal presentation or position. By far the most common reason for a TOL is if the woman wishes to have a vaginal birth after a previous cesarean birth. A woman who has had a previous cesarean birth with a low transverse uterine incision may be a candidate for a TOL. Fetal sonography, maternal pelvimetry, or both may be done before a TOL to rule out CPD. During a TOL the woman is evaluated for active labor, including adequate contractions, engagement and descent of the presenting part, and effacement and dilation of the cervix.

The nurse assesses maternal vital signs and FHR and pattern and is alert for signs of potential complications. If complications develop, the nurse is responsible for initiating appropriate actions, including notifying the primary health care provider, and for evaluating and documenting the maternal and fetal responses to the interventions. Nurses must recognize that the woman and her partner are often anxious about maternal and fetal well-being. Supporting and encouraging the woman and her partner and providing information regarding progress can reduce stress and enhance the labor process and facilitate a successful outcome.

Vaginal Birth After Cesarean

Indications for primary cesarean birth, such as dysfunctional labor, breech presentation, or abnormal FHR or patterns, often are nonrecurring. Therefore, a woman who has had a cesarean birth with a low transverse incision may subsequently become pregnant, experience no contraindications to labor and vaginal birth during the pregnancy, and choose to attempt a vaginal birth after cesarean (VBAC). Box 32-11 lists selection criteria suggested by the ACOG for identifying candidates for VBAC.

The overall success rate of VBAC is approximately 60% to 80% (Signore, 2012). The strongest predictors for a successful VBAC are a prior vaginal birth and spontaneous (rather than induced or augmented) labor (ACOG, 2010). Women whose first cesarean birth was performed because of a nonrecurring indication (e.g., breech presentation) also are likely to have a successful VBAC (Berghella & Landon, 2012). Women with the following characteristics are less likely to have a successful VBAC (ACOG, 2010; Eden et al., 2013):

- Recurrent indication (e.g., labor dystocia) for initial cesarean birth
- Increased maternal age
- Non-Caucasian race or ethnicity
- Gestational age >40 weeks
- Maternal obesity (BMI >30)
- Preeclampsia
- Short interpregnancy interval
- Estimated fetal weight >4000 g
- Giving birth at a rural or private hospital

Women who succeed in having a VBAC and thus avoid major abdominal surgery have less hemorrhage, fewer infections, and a shorter recovery period than do women who give birth by repeat cesarean (ACOG, 2010). The major risk associated with VBAC is uterine rupture (see later discussion) (Berghella & Landon, 2012). Other maternal risks include operative injury, blood transfusion, hysterectomy, endometritis, and death (ACOG).

Women are most often the primary decision makers with regard to choice of birth method. During the prenatal period the woman should be given information about VBAC and encouraged to choose it as an alternative to repeat cesarean birth, as long as no contraindications exist. VBAC support groups (e.g., www.vbac.com) and prenatal classes can help prepare the woman psychologically for labor and vaginal birth. Women need to believe not only that their efforts during a TOL will be successful but also that they are fully capable of doing what is necessary to give birth vaginally. They must be given the opportunity to discuss their previous labor experience, including feelings of failure and loss of control, and to express concern they

BOX 32-11 Selection Criteria for Vaginal Birth After Cesarean

- One or two previous low-transverse cesarean births
- Clinically adequate pelvis
- No other uterine scars or history of previous rupture
- Physicians immediately available throughout active labor capable of monitoring labor and performing an emergency cesarean birth if necessary

Data from American College of Obstetricians and Gynecologists (ACOG). (2010). *Vaginal birth after previous cesarean delivery.* ACOG practice bulletin no. 115. Washington, DC: ACOG may have about how they will manage during their upcoming labor and birth. Not everyone is enthusiastic about TOL and VBAC. After being fully informed about the benefits and risks, more than 25% of potential candidates choose to have a repeat cesarean birth instead (Thorp & Laughon, 2014).

If a woman chooses TOL, the nurse is attentive to her psychologic as well as physical needs during the TOL. Anxiety increases the release of catecholamines and can inhibit the release of oxytocin, thus delaying the progress of labor and possibly leading to a repeat cesarean birth. To alleviate such anxiety the nurse can encourage the woman to use breathing and relaxation techniques and to change positions to promote labor progress. The woman's partner can be encouraged to provide comfort measures and emotional support. Collaboration among the woman in labor, her partner, the nurse, and other health care providers often results in a successful VBAC. If a TOL does not result in vaginal birth, the woman will need support and encouragement to express her feelings about having another cesarean birth. It is very important that this outcome not be labeled a failed VBAC.

Since 1996 VBAC rates have been decreasing, with the current rate being less than 10%. Both medical and nonmedical factors have contributed to this decline. In March 2010 the Eunice Kennedy Shriver National Institute of Child Health and Human Development and the National Institutes of Health (NIH) convened a consensus development conference to examine issues related to VBAC. The statement produced by the panel of experts affirmed that TOL is a reasonable option for many women who have had a previous cesarean birth. The experts found, however, that many women who are appropriate candidates for TOL and VBAC do not have access to providers and health care facilities that are able and willing to offer this option (Berghella & Landon, 2012). ACOG continues to recommend that TOL and VBAC be offered only in facilities that have staff immediately available to provide emergency care. Because resources for immediate cesarean birth may not be available in all birthing facilities, the best alternative in some situations may be to refer interested women to other facilities that have the obstetric, anesthetic, pediatric, and surgical staff necessary to offer TOL and VBAC (Berghella & Landon).

OBSTETRIC EMERGENCIES

Meconium-Stained Amniotic Fluid

Meconium-stained amniotic fluid indicates that the fetus has passed meconium (first stool) before birth. Meconium-stained amniotic fluid is green. The consistency of the meconium fluid is often described as either thin (light) or thick (heavy), depending on the amount of meconium present. Three possible reasons for the passage of meconium are (1) it is a normal physiologic function that occurs with maturity (meconium passage being infrequent before weeks 23 or 24, with an increased incidence after 38 weeks) or with a breech presentation; (2) it is the result of hypoxia-induced peristalsis and sphincter relaxation; or (3) it can be a sequel to umbilical cord compression–induced vagal stimulation in mature fetuses.

The major risk associated with meconium-stained amniotic fluid is the development of meconium aspiration syndrome (MAS) in the newborn. MAS causes a severe form of aspiration pneumonia that occurs most often in term or postterm infants who have passed meconium in utero. MAS most likely results from a long-standing intrauterine process, rather than from aspiration immediately following birth as respirations are initiated (see Chapter 34) (Rozance & Rosenberg, 2012).

CARE MANAGEMENT

The presence of a team skilled in neonatal resuscitation is required at the birth of any infant with meconium-stained amniotic fluid. When meconium-stained amniotic fluid is present, the AAP and the American Heart Association's (AHA) Neonatal Resuscitation Program no longer recommends routine suctioning of the newborn's mouth and nose on the perineum (after the head is out but before the rest of the baby is born) followed by endotracheal suctioning after birth. Instead, management of a newborn with meconium-stained amniotic fluid is based only on assessment of the baby's condition at birth. No clinical studies warrant basing tracheal suctioning guidelines simply on meconium consistency (AAP & AHA, 2011). See Emergency: Immediate Management of the Newborn with Meconium-Stained Amniotic Fluid for specific interventions.

EMERGENCY

Immediate Management of the Newborn with Meconium-Stained Amniotic Fluid

Before Birth

- Assess the amniotic fluid for the presence of meconium after rupture of membranes.
- If the amniotic fluid is meconium stained, gather equipment and supplies that might be necessary for neonatal resuscitation.
- Have at least one person capable of performing endotracheal intubation on the baby present at the birth.

Immediately After Birth

- Assess the baby's respiratory efforts, heart rate, and muscle tone.
- Suction only the baby's mouth and nose, using either a bulb syringe or a large-bore suction catheter if the baby has:
    - Strong respiratory efforts
    - Good muscle tone
    - Heart rate >100 beats/minute
- Suction the trachea using an endotracheal tube connected to a meconium aspiration device and suction source to remove any meconium present before many spontaneous respirations have occurred or assisted ventilation has been initiated if the baby has:
    - Depressed respirations
    - Decreased muscle tone
    - Heart rate <100 beats/minute

Data from American Academy of Pediatrics (AAP) & American Heart Association (AHA). (2011). *Textbook of neonatal resuscitation* (6th ed.). Dallas: AHA.

SAFETY ALERT

Every birth should be attended by at least one person whose only responsibility is the baby and who is capable of initiating resuscitation. Either that person or someone else who is immediately available should have the skills required to perform a complete resuscitation, including endotracheal suctioning to remove meconium, if necessary.

Shoulder Dystocia

Shoulder dystocia is an uncommon obstetric emergency that increases the risk for fetal and maternal morbidity and mortality during the attempt to accomplish birth vaginally. Shoulder dystocia is a condition in which the head is born, but the anterior shoulder cannot pass under the pubic arch. It is estimated that 0.34% of all vaginal births are complicated by shoulder dystocia (Leung, Stuart, Suen, et al., 2011). The incidence of shoulder dystocia has increased in recent years, perhaps because of larger birth weights or simply because more attention is now paid to documenting the condition.

Fetopelvic disproportion (FPD) related to excessive fetal size (more than 4000 g) or maternal pelvic abnormalities can cause shoulder dystocia, although up to half of all cases of shoulder dystocia occur with smaller fetuses (Simpson & O'Brien-Abel, 2014; Thorp & Laughon, 2014). Other risk factors for shoulder dystocia include maternal diabetes (risk for macrosomia), a history of shoulder dystocia with a previous birth, and a prolonged second stage of labor. In half of all cases of shoulder dystocia, however, no risk factors are identified (Thorp & Laughon). Shoulder dystocia cannot be accurately predicted or prevented (Simpson & O'Brien-Abel).

Signs that indicate the presence of shoulder dystocia include slowing of the progress of the second stage of labor and formation of a caput succedaneum that increases in size. The nurse should observe for retraction of the fetal head against the perineum immediately following its emergence (turtle sign), an early sign of shoulder dystocia. External rotation does not occur (Simpson & O'Brien-Abel, 2014; Thorp & Laughon, 2014).

Fetal injuries are usually caused either by asphyxia related to the delay in completing the birth or by trauma from the maneuvers used to accomplish the birth. Complications related to trauma include brachial plexus and phrenic nerve injuries and fracture of the humerus or clavicle. The most serious complication is brachial plexus injury (Erb palsy), which occurs in 10% to 20% of infants born following shoulder dystocia. Evidence now exists that brachial plexus injuries can result from intrauterine forces during the second stage of labor rather than from the maneuvers used to accomplish birth (Lanni & Seeds, 2012). If brachial plexus injuries are recognized early and treated properly, 80% to 90% heal completely. Therefore, permanent neurologic injury is rare, occurring in only 1 or 2 of every 10,000 births. The major maternal complications associated with shoulder dystocia are postpartum hemorrhage and rectal injuries (Thorp & Laughon, 2014).

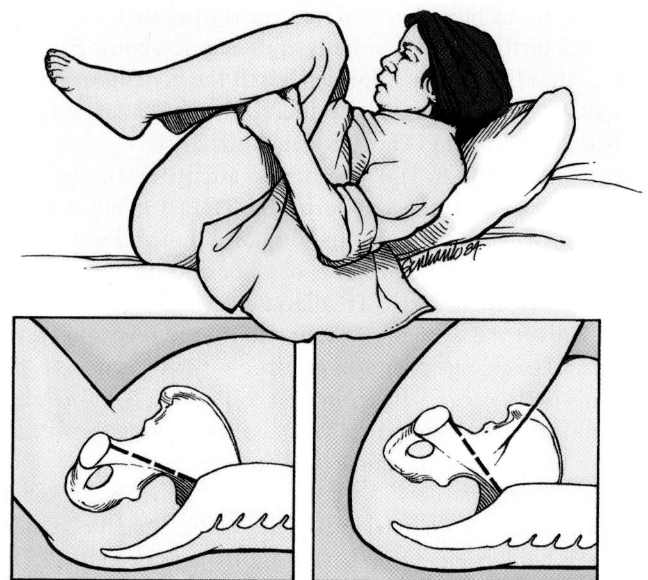

FIG 32-15 McRoberts maneuver. (From Gabbe, S., Niebyl, J., & Simpson, J. [2012]. *Obstetrics: Normal and problem pregnancies* [6th ed.]. Philadelphia: Saunders.)

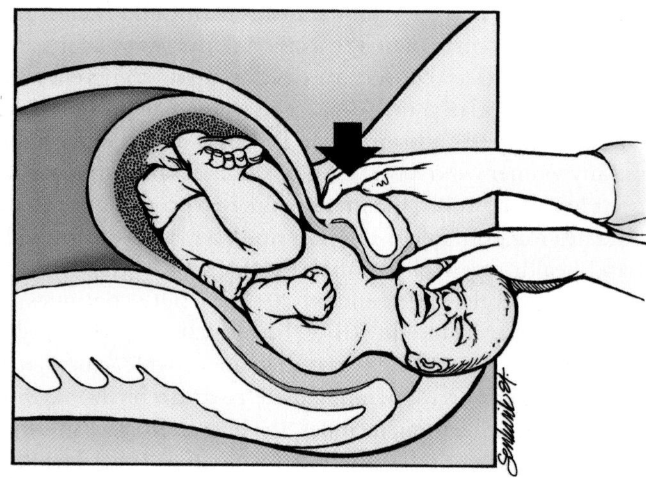

FIG 32-16 Application of suprapubic pressure. (From Gabbe, S., Niebyl, J., & Simpson, J. [2007]. *Obstetrics: Normal and problem pregnancies* [5th ed.]. Philadelphia: Churchill Livingstone.)

CARE MANAGEMENT

Many maneuvers such as suprapubic pressure and maternal position changes have been suggested and tried to free the anterior shoulder, although no particular maneuver has been found to be most effective. The specific method used is less important than is being prepared at every vaginal birth to deal with shoulder dystocia using a planned sequence of interventions if the need arises (Lanni & Seeds, 2012).

In the McRoberts maneuver (Fig. 32-15), the woman's legs are flexed apart, with her knees on her abdomen (Ansell, McAra-Couper, & Smythe, 2012; Lanni & Seeds, 2012). This maneuver causes the sacrum to straighten, and the symphysis pubis to rotate toward the mother's head. The angle of pelvic inclination is decreased, which frees the shoulder. Suprapubic pressure can then be applied to the anterior shoulder (Fig. 32-16) in an attempt to push the shoulder under the symphysis pubis (Rozance & Rosenberg, 2012). The McRoberts maneuver is the preferred method when a woman is receiving epidural anesthesia.

Having the woman move to a hands-and-knees position (the Gaskin maneuver), a squatting position, or lateral recumbent position also has been used to resolve cases of shoulder dystocia. However, the Gaskin maneuver requires that the woman be mobile, with no significant loss of motor function caused by regional anesthesia (Ansell et al., 2012).

Fundal pressure as a method of relieving shoulder dystocia should be avoided. Its use has been associated with neurologic complications (Gilbert, 2011).

When shoulder dystocia is diagnosed, the nurse should stay calm and immediately call for additional assistance (i.e., extra nurses, anesthesia care provider, and neonatal resuscitation

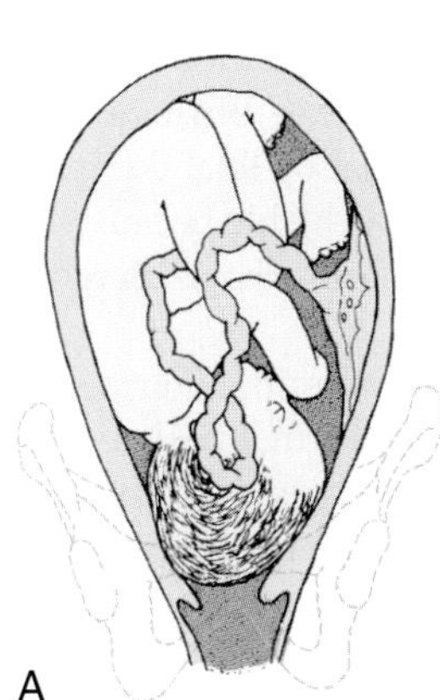

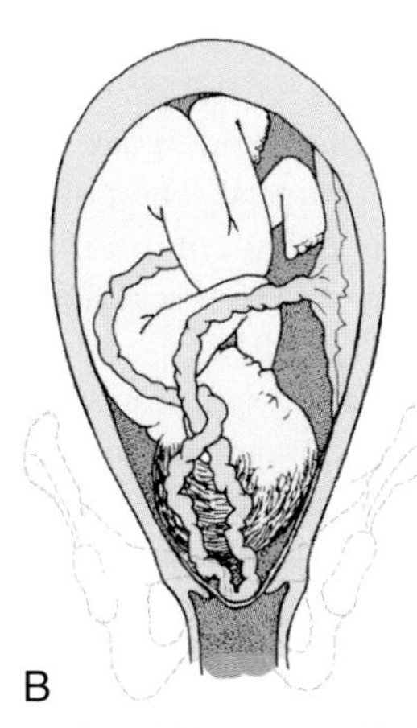

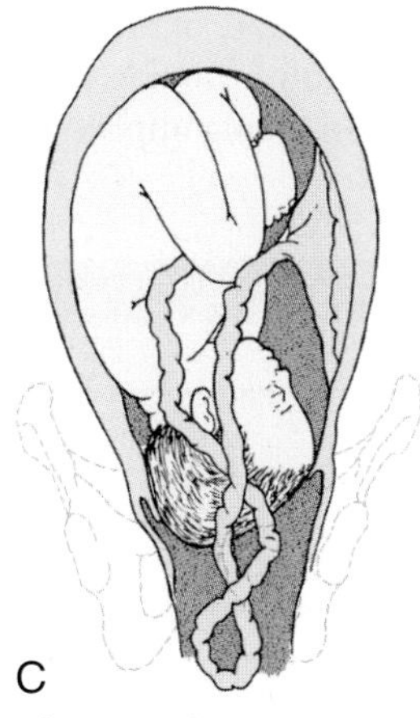

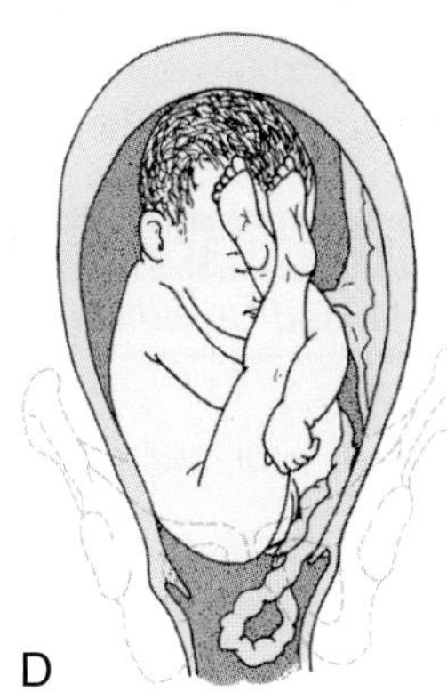

FIG 32-17 Prolapse of umbilical cord. Note pressure of presenting part on umbilical cord, which endangers fetal circulation. **A,** Occult (hidden) prolapse of cord. **B,** Complete prolapse of cord. Note that membranes are intact. **C,** Cord presenting in front of the fetal head may be seen in vagina. **D,** Frank breech presentation with prolapsed cord.

team). The nurse then helps the woman assume the position or positions that may facilitate birth of the shoulders, assists the primary health care provider with these maneuvers and techniques during birth, and documents the maneuvers, including the total amount of time required to resolve the shoulder dystocia. The nurse also provides encouragement and support to reduce anxiety. Newborn assessment should include examination for fracture of the clavicle or humerus as well as brachial plexus injuries and asphyxia (Thorp & Laughon, 2014). Maternal assessment should focus on early detection of hemorrhage and trauma to the vagina, perineum, and rectum.

Prolapsed Umbilical Cord

Prolapse of the umbilical cord occurs when the cord lies below the presenting part of the fetus. Umbilical cord prolapse may be occult (hidden, rather than visible) at any time during labor whether or not the membranes are ruptured (Fig. 32-17, *A* and *B*). It is most common to see frank (visible) prolapse directly after rupture of membranes, when gravity washes the cord in front of the presenting part (see Fig. 32-17, *C* and *D*). Contributing factors include a long cord (longer than 100 cm), malpresentation (breech or transverse lie), or an unengaged presenting part.

If the presenting part does not fit snugly into the lower uterine segment (e.g., as in polyhydramnios), when the membranes rupture, a sudden gush of amniotic fluid may cause the cord to be displaced downward. Similarly the cord may prolapse during amniotomy if the presenting part is high. A small fetus may not fit snugly into the lower uterine segment; as a result, cord prolapse is more likely to occur.

CARE MANAGEMENT

Prompt recognition of a prolapsed umbilical cord is important because fetal hypoxia resulting from prolonged cord compression (i.e., occlusion of blood flow to and from the fetus for more than 5 minutes) usually results in CNS damage or death of the fetus. Pressure on the cord may be relieved by the examiner putting a sterile gloved hand into the vagina and holding the presenting part off the umbilical cord (Fig. 32-18, *A* and *B*). The woman may also be assisted into a position such as a modified Sims (see Fig. 32-18, *C*), Trendelenburg, or knee-chest (see Fig. 32-18, *D*) position, in which gravity keeps the pressure of the presenting part off the cord. If the cervix is fully dilated, a forceps- or vacuum-assisted birth can be performed for the fetus in a cephalic presentation; otherwise, a cesarean birth is likely to be performed. Abnormal FHR and pattern (e.g., bradycardia, absent or minimal variability, and variable or prolonged decelerations), inadequate uterine relaxation, and bleeding also can occur as a result of a prolapsed umbilical cord. (Indications for immediate interventions are presented in Emergency: Prolapsed Umbilical Cord.) Ongoing assessment of the woman and her fetus is critical to determine the effectiveness of each action

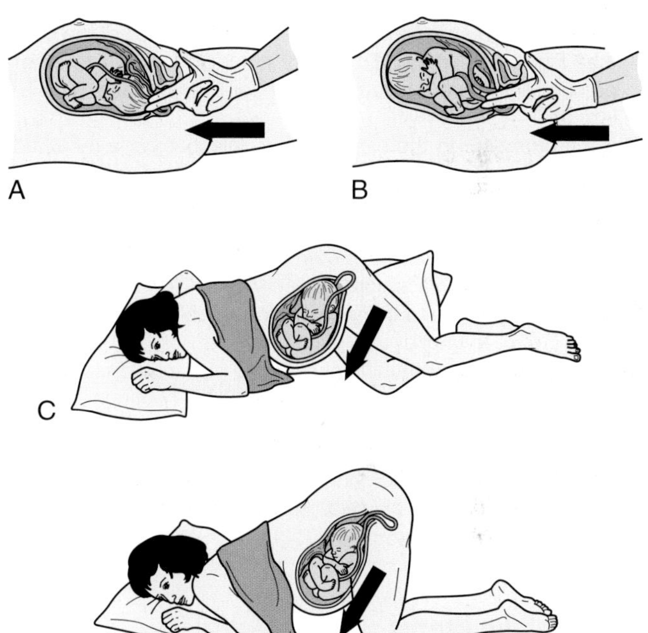

FIG 32-18 Arrows indicate direction of pressure against presenting part to relieve compression of prolapsed umbilical cord. Pressure exerted by examiner's fingers in **A,** vertex presentation, and **B,** breech presentation. **C,** Gravity relieves pressure when woman is in modified Sims position with hips elevated as high as possible with pillows. **D,** Knee-chest position.

taken. The woman and her family are often aware of the seriousness of the situation; therefore, the nurse must provide support by giving explanations for the interventions being implemented and their effect on the status of the fetus.

EMERGENCY

Prolapsed Umbilical Cord

Signs

- Variable or prolonged deceleration during uterine contractions
- Woman reports feeling the cord after membranes rupture
- Cord is seen or felt in or protruding from the vagina

Interventions

- Call for assistance. Do not leave the woman alone.
- Have someone notify the primary health care provider immediately.
- Glove the examining hand quickly and insert two fingers into the vagina to the cervix. With one finger on either side of the cord or both fingers to one side, exert upward pressure against the presenting part to relieve compression of the cord (see Fig. 32-18, *A* and *B*). Do *not* move your hand! Another person may place a rolled towel under the woman's right or left hip.
- Place woman into the extreme Trendelenburg or a modified Sims position (see Fig. 32-18, *C*) or a knee-chest position (see Fig. 32-18, *D*).
- If cord is protruding from vagina, wrap loosely in a sterile towel saturated with warm sterile normal saline solution. Do not attempt to replace cord into cervix.
- Administer oxygen to the woman by nonrebreather mask at 8 to 10 L/minute until birth is accomplished.
- Start intravenous (IV) fluids or increase existing drip rate.
- Continue to monitor fetal heart rate (FHR) continuously, by internal fetal scalp electrode, if possible.
- Explain to woman and support person what is happening and the way it is being managed.
- Prepare for immediate vaginal birth if cervix is fully dilated or cesarean birth if it is not.

Rupture of the Uterus

Uterine rupture, in which there is complete nonsurgical disruption of all uterine layers, is a rare but life-threatening obstetric injury that occurs in 1 of 8000 to 1 in 15,000 births when there is no history of previous uterine scarring (Nikolaou, Kourea, Antonopoulos, et al., 2013). In women with a history of uterine injury, the risk increases to 0.5% if labor occurs spontaneously and 1.5% if it is induced (Kok, Wiersma, Opmeer, et al., 2013). During labor and birth the major risk factor for uterine rupture is a scarred uterus as a result of previous cesarean birth or other uterine surgery. Rupture usually occurs during a TOL for VBAC; symptomatic rupture is rarely observed in planned, repeat cesarean births. The likelihood of uterine rupture depends on the type and location of the previous uterine scar. Uterine rupture occurs most often with a previous classic incision. Other factors that increase the risk for uterine rupture include multiple prior cesarean births, no previous vaginal births, induced or augmented labor, term gestation, multifetal gestation, fetal macrosomia, postcesarean birth infection, and short interpregnancy interval (Berghella & Landon, 2012; Bernstein, Matalon-Grazi, & Rosenn, 2012; Francois & Foley, 2012).

Uterine dehiscence, sometimes called incomplete uterine rupture, is separation of a prior scar. It may go unnoticed unless the woman undergoes a subsequent cesarean birth or other uterine surgery. The potential for maternal or fetal complications as a result of uterine dehiscence is negligible because separation of a prior scar does not result in hemorrhage (Berghella & Landon, 2012).

Signs and symptoms vary with the extent of the uterine rupture. The most common finding is an abnormal FHR tracing, particularly variable or prolonged decelerations or bradycardia. A loss of fetal station also can occur. The woman can experience constant abdominal pain, uterine tenderness, a change in uterine shape, and cessation of contractions (Berghella & Landon, 2012; Francois & Foley, 2012; Holmgren, Scott, Porter, et al., 2012). She may also exhibit signs of hypovolemic shock caused by hemorrhage (i.e., hypotension, tachypnea, pallor, and cool, clammy skin). If the placenta separates, the FHR will be absent. Fetal parts may be palpable through the abdomen.

CARE MANAGEMENT

Prevention is the best treatment. Women who have had a cesarean birth with a classic uterine incision are advised not to labor or attempt vaginal birth in subsequent pregnancies. Those at risk for uterine rupture are assessed closely during labor. Women whose labor is induced with oxytocin or prostaglandin (especially if their previous birth was cesarean) are monitored for signs of uterine tachysystole because this can precipitate uterine rupture. If tachysystole occurs, the oxytocin infusion is discontinued or decreased, and a tocolytic medication may be given to decrease the intensity of the uterine contractions (see Emergency: Uterine Tachysystole with Oxytocin [Pitocin] Infusion). After giving birth, the woman is assessed for excessive bleeding, especially if the fundus is firm and signs of hemorrhagic shock are present.

If rupture occurs, management depends on the severity. A small rupture may be managed with a laparotomy and birth of the infant, repair of the laceration, and blood transfusions, if needed. Hysterectomy may be necessary if the rupture is large and difficult to repair or if the woman is hemodynamically unstable (Francois & Foley, 2012).

The nurse's role can include starting IV fluids, transfusing blood products, administering oxygen, and assisting with preparations for immediate surgery. Supporting the woman's family and providing information about the treatment are important during this emergency. The associated fetal mortality rate is high (approximately 50% to 75%), particularly if the fetus is ejected from the uterus into the abdominal cavity. Maternal morbidity and mortality also can be substantial (Cunningham et al., 2014). Providing information about spiritual support services or suggesting that the family contact their own support system may be warranted.

Amniotic Fluid Embolus

Amniotic fluid embolus (AFE), also known as anaphylactoid syndrome of pregnancy, is a rare but devastating complication of pregnancy characterized by the sudden, acute onset of hypoxia, hypotension, cardiovascular collapse, and coagulopathy. The incidence of AFE in the United States is estimated at

1 in 8000 to 1 in 30,000 births. The true incidence is unknown because of the difficulty in confirming the diagnosis and inconsistent reporting of nonfatal cases (Jones & Clark, 2013).

AFE occurs during labor, during birth, or within 30 minutes after birth. This combination of sudden respiratory and cardiovascular collapse, along with coagulopathy, is similar to that observed in clients with anaphylactic or septic shock. In both conditions a foreign substance is introduced into the circulation, resulting in disseminated intravascular coagulation (DIC), hypotension, and hypoxia (Robbins, Martin, & Wilson, 2014).

In AFE the foreign substance that initiates the condition is presumed to be present in amniotic fluid that is introduced into the maternal circulation. However, the exact factor that initiates AFE has not been identified. In the past, particles of fetal debris (e.g., vernix, hair, skin cells, or meconium) found in amniotic fluid were thought to be responsible for initiating the syndrome; however, fetal debris can be found in the pulmonary circulation of most healthy laboring women. Also fetal debris is identified in only 78% of women diagnosed with AFE. Therefore, AFE is diagnosed clinically (Jones & Clark, 2013; Robbins et al., 2014; Simpson & O'Brien-Abel, 2014). The most recent population-based studies suggest that the U.S. mortality rate has dropped from a reported rate of 61% to a current rate of 22% (Robbins et al.). Neonatal outcome in cases of AFE is poor. If the event occurs before birth, the neonatal survival rate is approximately 80%. However, only half of these fetuses survive neurologically intact (Jones & Clark).

Maternal risk factors for AFE include advanced age; placenta previa or abruption; preeclampsia, eclampsia, and other hypertensive disorders; diabetes; labor induction and forceps-assisted or cesarean birth; and cervical laceration or uterine rupture (Kramer, Rouleau, Liu, et al., 2012). Previously it was thought that the hypertonic uterine contractions that often accompany AFE actually caused the event. Instead, it appears that the physiologic response to AFE produces the hypertonic contractions (Jones & Clark, 2013).

CARE MANAGEMENT

The immediate interventions for AFE are summarized in Emergency: Amniotic Fluid Embolus (Anaphylactoid Syndrome of Pregnancy). Care must be instituted immediately. Cardiopulmonary resuscitation is often necessary. If cardiopulmonary arrest occurs, a perimortem cesarean birth should be considered after 4 minutes of unsuccessful resuscitative efforts, both to improve the chances for optimal fetal survival and to facilitate maternal resuscitation (Robbins et al., 2014). The nurse's immediate responsibility is to assist with the resuscitation efforts.

EMERGENCY

Amniotic Fluid Embolus (Anaphylactoid Syndrome of Pregnancy)

Signs

- Respiratory distress
  - Restlessness
  - Dyspnea
  - Cyanosis
  - Pulmonary edema
  - Respiratory arrest
- Circulatory collapse
  - Hypotension
  - Tachycardia
  - Shock
  - Cardiac arrest
- Hemorrhage
  - Coagulation failure: bleeding from incisions, venipuncture sites, trauma (lacerations); petechiae, ecchymoses, purpura
  - Uterine atony

Interventions

- Oxygenate.
  - Administer oxygen by nonrebreather face mask (8 to 10 L/minute) or resuscitation bag delivering 100% oxygen.
  - Prepare for intubation and mechanical ventilation.
  - Initiate or assist with cardiopulmonary resuscitation. Tilt pregnant woman 30 degrees to her side to displace uterus.
- Maintain cardiac output and replace fluid losses.
  - Position woman onto her side.
  - Administer intravenous (IV) fluids.
  - Administer blood products: packed cells, fresh-frozen plasma.
  - Insert indwelling catheter, and measure hourly urine output.
- Correct coagulation failure.
- Monitor fetal and maternal status.
- Prepare for emergency birth once woman's condition is stabilized.
- Provide emotional support to woman, her partner, and family.

If the woman survives she is usually moved to a critical care unit. Additional interventions include replacing blood and clotting factors and maintaining adequate hydration and blood pressure. The woman is usually placed on mechanical ventilation with continuous hemodynamic monitoring (Robbins et al., 2014).

Support of the woman's partner and family is needed; they will be anxious and distressed. Brief explanations of what is happening are important during the emergency and can be reinforced after the immediate crisis is over. If the woman dies, emotional support and involvement of the perinatal loss support team or other resources for grief counseling are needed. Referral to grief and loss support groups also is appropriate (see Chapter 37). The nursing staff also may need help in coping with feelings and emotions that result from a maternal death.

KEY POINTS

- Preterm birth is any birth that occurs between 20 0/7 and 36 6/7 weeks of gestation.
- Preterm labor is generally diagnosed clinically as regular contractions along with a change in cervical effacement or dilation or both or presentation with regular uterine contractions and cervical dilation of at least 2 cm.
- The incidence of preterm birth varies considerably by race. In the United States, non-Hispanic black women have the highest rate of preterm birth.
- The cause of preterm labor is unknown and is assumed to be multifactorial; therefore, it is not possible to predict with certainty which women will experience preterm labor and birth.

KEY POINTS—cont'd

- Because the onset of preterm labor is often insidious and can be mistaken for normal discomforts of pregnancy, nurses should teach all pregnant women how to detect the early symptoms of preterm labor and to call their primary health care provider when symptoms occur.
- The best reason to use tocolytic therapy is to achieve sufficient time to administer glucocorticoids in an effort to accelerate fetal lung maturity. Additionally, time is allowed for transport of the woman prior to birth to a center equipped to care for preterm infants.
- If fetal or early neonatal death is expected, the parents and members of the health care team need to discuss the situation before the birth and decide on a management plan that is acceptable to everyone.
- Vigilance for signs of infection is an essential component of the care management for women with preterm PROM.
- Dysfunctional labor results from differences in the normal relationships among any of the five factors affecting labor and is characterized by differences in the pattern of progress in labor.
- Obese women are at risk for several pregnancy complications, including cesarean birth. Even routine procedures require more time and effort to accomplish when the client is obese.
- Uterine contractility is increased by the effects of oxytocin and prostaglandin and is decreased by tocolytic agents.
- Labor should not be induced electively until the woman has reached at least 39 weeks of gestation.
- Cervical ripening using chemical or mechanical measures can increase the success of labor induction.
- Expectant parents benefit from learning about operative obstetrics (e.g., forceps-assisted, vacuum-assisted, or cesarean birth) during the prenatal period.
- The basic purpose of cesarean birth is to preserve the well-being of the mother and her fetus.
- Unless contraindicated, vaginal birth is possible after a previous cesarean birth.
- Obstetric emergencies (e.g., meconium-stained amniotic fluid, shoulder dystocia, prolapsed cord, rupture of the uterus, and amniotic fluid embolism) occur rarely but require immediate intervention to preserve the health or life of the mother and fetus or newborn.

REFERENCES

American Academy of Pediatrics (AAP) & American College of Obstetricians and Gynecologists (ACOG). (2012). *Guidelines for perinatal care* (7th ed.). Washington, DC: ACOG.

American Academy of Pediatrics (AAP) & American Heart Association (AHA). (2011). *Textbook of neonatal resuscitation* (6th ed.). Dallas: AHA.

American College of Obstetricians and Gynecologists (ACOG). (2010). *Vaginal birth after a previous cesarean delivery*. ACOG practice bulletin no. 115. Washington, DC: ACOG.

American College of Obstetricians and Gynecologists. (ACOG). (2012). *Management of preterm labor*. ACOG practice bulletin no. 127. Washington, DC: ACOG.

American College of Obstetricians and Gynecologists (ACOG). (2009; reaffirmed in 2013a). *Induction of labor*. ACOG practice bulletin no. 107. Washington, DC: ACOG.

American College of Obstetricians and Gynecologists (ACOG). (2013b). *Cesarean delivery on maternal request*. Committee opinion no. 559. Washington, DC: Author.

Ansell, L., McAra-Couper, J., & Smythe, E. (2012). Shoulder dystocia: A qualitative exploration of what works. *Midwifery*, *28*(4), 521–528.

Berghella, V., & Landon, M. (2012). Cesarean delivery. In S. Gabbe, J. Niebyl, & J. Simpson (Eds.), *Obstetrics: Normal and problem pregnancies* (6th ed.). Philadelphia: Saunders.

Bernstein, S. N., Matalon-Grazi, S., & Rosenn, B. M. (2012). Trial of labor versus repeat cesarean: Are patients making an informed decision? *American Journal of Obstetrics and Gynecology*, *207*(3), 204.e1–204.e6.

Bowers, N. A. (2014). Multiple gestation. In K. Rice Simpson, & P. Creehan (Eds.), *AWHONN's perinatal nursing* (4th ed.). Philadelphia: Lippincott Williams & Wilkins.

Buhimschi, C. S., & Norman, J. E. (2014). Pathogenesis of spontaneous preterm labor. In R. K. Creasy, R. Resnik, J. D. Iams, et al. (Eds.), *Creasy and Resnik's maternal-fetal medicine: Principles and practice* (7th ed.). Philadelphia: Saunders.

Campbell, C. (2011). Elective cesarean delivery: Trends, evidence and implications for women newborns and nurses. *Nursing for Women's Health*, *15*(4), 308–319.

Craighead, D. (2012). Early term birth: Understanding the health risks to infants. *Nursing for Women's Health*, *16*(2), 136–144.

Cunningham, F., Leveno, K., Bloom, S., et al. (2014). *Williams obstetrics* (24th ed.). New York: McGraw-Hill Education.

DeFranco, E. A., Lewis, D. F., & Odibo, A. O. (2013). Improving the screening accuracy for preterm labor: Is the combination of fetal fibronectin and cervical length in symptomatic patients a useful predictor of preterm birth? A systematic review. *American Journal of Obstetrics and Gynecology*, *208*(1), 233.e1–233.e6.

Desbriere, R., Blanc, J., Le Dû, R., et al. (2013). Is maternal posturing during labor efficient in preventing persistent occiput posterior position? A randomized controlled trial. *American Journal of Obstetrics and Gynecology*, *208*(1), 60.e1–60.e8.

Duff, P. (2012). Maternal and perinatal infection—Bacterial. In S. Gabbe, J. Niebyl, & J. Simpson (Eds.), *Obstetrics: Normal and problem pregnancies* (6th ed.). Philadelphia: Saunders.

Duff, P. (2014). Maternal and fetal infections. In R. K. Creasy, R. Resnik, J. D. Iams, et al. (Eds.), *Creasy and Resnik's maternal-fetal medicine: Principles and practice* (7th ed.). Philadelphia: Saunders.

Ecker, J. (2013). Elective cesarean delivery on maternal request. *Journal of the American Medical Association*, *309*(18), 1930–1936.

Eden, K. B., Denman, M. A., Emeis, C. L., et al. (2013). Trial of labor and vaginal delivery rates in women with a prior cesarean. *Journal of Obstetric, Gynecologic and Neonatal Nursing*, *41*(5), 583–598.

Fishman, S. G., & Gelber, S. E. (2012). Evidence for the clinical management of chorioamnionitis. *Seminars in Fetal & Neonatal Medicine*, *17*(1), 46–50.

Flood, K., & Malone, F. D. (2012). Prevention of preterm birth. *Seminars in Fetal & Neonatal Medicine*, *17*(1), 58–63.

Francois, K. E., & Foley, M. R. (2012). Antepartum and postpartum hemorrhage. In S. Gabbe, J. Niebyl, & J. Simpson (Eds.), *Obstetrics: Normal and problem pregnancies* (6th ed.). Philadelphia: Saunders.

Friedman, E. (1989). Normal and dysfunctional labor. In W. Cohen, D. Ackers, & E. Friedman (Eds.), *Management of labor* (6th ed.). Rockville, MD: Aspen.

Gilbert, E. (2011). *Manual of high risk pregnancy & delivery* (5th ed.). St. Louis: Mosby.

Halloran, D. R., Cheng, Y. W., Wall, T. C., et al. (2012). Effect of maternal weight on postterm delivery. *Journal of Perinatology, 32*(2), 85–90.

Hill, W., & Harvey, C. (2013). Induction of labor. In N. Troiano, C. Harvey, & B. Chez (Eds.), *AWHONN's high risk and critical care obstetrics* (3rd ed.). Philadelphia: Wolters Kluwer/Lippincott Williams & Wilkins.

Holmgren, C., Scott, J. R., Porter, T. F., et al. (2012). Uterine rupture with attempted vaginal birth after cesarean delivery: Decision-to-delivery time and neonatal outcome. *Obstetrics and Gynecology, 119*(4), 725–731.

Institute for Safe Medication Practices (ISMP). (2012). *ISMP's list of high-alert medications*. Available at www.ismp.org.

Jones, R., & Clark, S. (2013). Amniotic fluid embolus (anaphylactoid syndrome of pregnancy). In N. Troiano, C. Harvey, & B. Chez (Eds.), *AWHONN's high risk and critical care obstetrics* (3rd ed.). Philadelphia: Wolters Kluwer/Lippincott Williams & Wilkins.

Kok, N., Wiersma, I. C., Opmeer, B. C., et al. (2013). Sonographic measurement of lower uterine segment thickness to predict uterine rupture during a trial of labor in women with previous cesarean section: A meta-analysis. *Ultrasound in Obstetrics & Gynecology, 42*(2), 132–139.

Kramer, M., Rouleau, J., Liu, S., et al. (2012). Amniotic fluid embolism: Incidence, risk factors, and impact on perinatal outcome. *British Journal of Obstetrics and Gynaecology, 119*(7), 874–879.

Kunz, M. K., Loftus, R. J., & Nichols, A. A. (2013). Incidence of uterine tachysystole in women induced with oxytocin. *Journal of Obstetric, Gynecologic and Neonatal Nursing, 42*(1), 12–18.

Lanni, S., & Seeds, J. (2012). Malpresentations and shoulder dystocia. In S. Gabbe, J. Niebyl, & J. Simpson (Eds.), *Obstetrics: Normal and problem pregnancies* (6th ed.). Philadelphia: Saunders.

Leung, T., Stuart, O., Suen, S., et al. (2011). Comparison of perinatal outcomes of shoulder dystocia alleviated by different type and sequence of manoeuvres: A retrospective review. *British Journal of Obstetrics and Gynaecology, 118*(8), 985–990.

Macones, G., Hankins, G., Spong, C., et al. (2008). The 2008 National Institute of Child Health and Human Development workshop report on electronic fetal monitoring: Update on definitions, interpretation, and research guidelines. *Journal of Obstetric, Gynecologic and Neonatal Nursing, 37*(5), 510–515.

Malone, F. D., & D'Alton, M. E. (2014). Multiple gestation: Clinical characteristics and management. In R. K. Creasy, R. Resnik, J. D. Iams, et al. (Eds.), *Creasy and Resnik's maternal-fetal medicine: Principles and practice* (7th ed.). Philadelphia: Saunders.

Martin, J. A., Hamilton, B. E., Osterman, M. J. K., et al. (2013a). Births: Final data for 2012. *National Vital Statistics Reports, 62*(9), 1–87.

Martin, J., Hamilton, B., Sutton, P., et al. (2012). Births: Final data for 2010. *National Vital Statistics Reports, 61*(1), 1–100.

Martin, J. A., Hamilton, B. E., Ventura, S. J., et al. (2013b). Births: Final data for 2011. *National Vital Statistics Reports, 62*(1), 1–70.

Mercer, B. M. (2012). Premature rupture of the membranes. In S. Gabbe, J. Niebyl, & J. Simpson (Eds.), *Obstetrics: Normal and problem pregnancies* (6th ed.). Philadelphia: Saunders.

Mercer, B. M. (2014a). Assessment and induction of fetal pulmonary maturity. In R. K. Creasy, R. Resnik, J. D. Iams, et al. (Eds.), *Creasy and Resnik's maternal-fetal medicine: Principles and practice* (7th ed.). Philadelphia: Saunders.

Mercer, B. M. (2014b). Premature rupture of the membranes. In R. K. Creasy, R. Resnik, J. D. Iams, et al. (Eds.), *Creasy and Resnik's maternal-fetal medicine: Principles and practice* (7th ed.). Philadelphia: Saunders.

Newman, R., & Unal, E. (2012). Multiple gestations. In S. Gabbe, J. Niebyl, & J. Simpson (Eds.), *Obstetrics: Normal and problem pregnancies* (6th ed.). Philadelphia: Saunders.

Nielsen, P., & Galan, H. (2012). Operative vaginal delivery. In S. Gabbe, J. Niebyl, & J. Simpson (Eds.), *Obstetrics: Normal and problem pregnancies* (6th ed.). Philadelphia: Saunders.

Nikolaou, M., Kourea, H. P., Antonopoulos, K., et al. (2013). Spontaneous uterine rupture in a primigravid woman in the early third trimester attributed to adenomyosis: A case report and review of the literature. *The Journal of Obstetrics and Gynaecology Research, 39*(3), 727–732.

Picklesimer, A., & Dorman, K. (2013). Maternal obesity: Effects on pregnancy. In N. Troiano, C. Harvey, & B. Chez (Eds.), *AWHONN's high risk and critical care obstetrics* (3rd ed.). Philadelphia: Wolters Kluwer/Lippincott Williams & Wilkins.

Rampersad, R., & Macones, G. (2012). Prolonged and postterm pregnancy. In S. Gabbe, J. Niebyl, & J. Simpson (Eds.), *Obstetrics: Normal and problem pregnancies* (6th ed.). Philadelphia: Saunders.

Robbins, K. S., Martin, S. R., & Wilson, W. C. (2014). Intensive care considerations for the critically ill parturient. In R. K. Creasy, R. Resnik, J. D. Iams, et al. (Eds.), *Creasy and Resnik's maternal-fetal medicine: Principles and practice* (7th ed.). Philadelphia: Saunders.

Rosman, A. N., Guijt, A., Vlemmix, F., et al. (2013). Contraindications for external cephalic version in breech position at term: A systematic review. *Acta Obstetricia et Gynecologica Scandinavica, 92*(2), 137–142.

Rozance, P., & Rosenberg, A. (2012). The neonate. In S. Gabbe, J. Niebyl, & J. Simpson (Eds.), *Obstetrics: Normal and problem pregnancies* (6th ed.). Philadelphia: Saunders.

Signore, C. (2012). VBAC: What does the evidence show? *Clinical Obstetrics and Gynecology, 55*(4), 961–968.

Simhan, H. N., Berghella, V., & Iams, J. D. (2014). Preterm labor and birth. In R. K. Creasy, R. Resnik, J. D. Iams, et al. (Eds.), *Creasy and Resnik's maternal-fetal medicine: Principles and practice* (7th ed.). Philadelphia: Saunders.

Simhan, H., Iams, J., & Romero, R. (2012). Preterm birth. In S. Gabbe, J. Niebyl, & J. Simpson (Eds.), *Obstetrics: Normal and problem pregnancies* (6th ed.). Philadelphia: Saunders.

Simpson, K. (2011). Clinicians' guide to the use of oxytocin for labor induction and augmentation. *Journal of Midwifery & Women's Health. 56*(3), 214–221.

Simpson, K. R., & O'Brien-Abel, N. (2014). Labor and birth. In K. Rice Simpson, & P. Creehan (Eds.), *AWHONN's perinatal nursing* (4th ed.). Philadelphia: Lippincott Williams & Wilkins.

Swamy, G. K. (2012). Current methods of labor induction. *Seminars in Perinatology, 36*(5), 348–352.

Thorp, J. M., & Laughon, S. K. (2014). Clinical aspects of normal and abnormal labor. In R. K. Creasy, R. Resnik, J. D. Iams, et al. (Eds.), *Creasy and Resnik's maternal-fetal medicine: Principles and practice* (7th ed.). Philadelphia: Saunders.

Wing, D., & Farinelli, C. (2012). Abnormal labor and induction of labor. In S. Gabbe, J. Niebyl, & J. Simpson (Eds.), *Obstetrics: Normal and problem pregnancies* (6th ed.). Philadelphia: Saunders.

Yount, S. M., & Lassiter, N. (2013). The pharmacology of prostaglandins for induction of labor. *Journal of Midwifery & Women's Health, 58*(2), 133–144.

33 CHAPTER

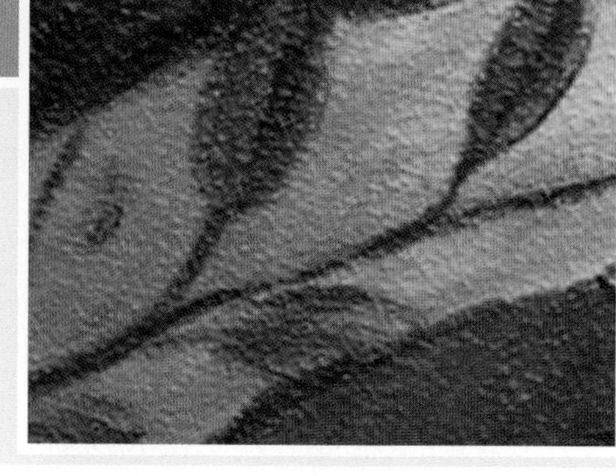

Postpartum Complications

Rhonda K. Lanning

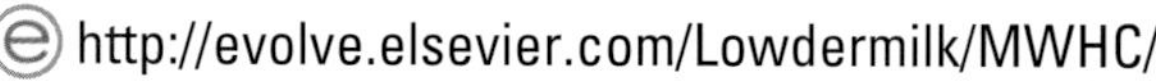

LEARNING OBJECTIVES

- Identify the causes, signs and symptoms, and medical and nursing management of postpartum hemorrhage.
- Describe hemorrhagic shock as a complication of postpartum hemorrhage, including management and hazards of therapy.
- Differentiate the causes of postpartum infection.
- Summarize assessment and care of women with postpartum infection.
- Describe thromboembolic disorders, including incidence, etiology, signs and symptoms, and medical and nursing management.

The postpartum period is a time of change and transition for mothers and newborns. Mothers experience incredible physiologic shifts and emotional adjustments in the hours and days following birth. Perinatal nurses provide education, care, and support for mothers and newborns during this important time. In addition, nurses have the responsibility to pay careful attention to signs and symptoms of complications. The nurse works collaboratively with the health care team to provide safe and effective care to women experiencing postpartum physiologic complications. The nurse's rapid response to complications such as hemorrhage and infection are critical to the well-being of the new mother. This chapter focuses on these two important postpartum complications.

POSTPARTUM HEMORRHAGE

Definition and Incidence

Postpartum hemorrhage (PPH) continues to be a leading cause of maternal morbidity and mortality in the United States and throughout the world (World Health Organization [WHO], 2012). Postpartum hemorrhage is a life-threatening event that can occur with little warning and is often not recognized until the mother has profound symptoms.

PPH is defined as the loss of 500 ml or more of blood after vaginal birth and 1000 ml or more after cesarean birth. Either a 10% change in hematocrit between admission for labor and postpartum or the need for erythrocyte transfusion is also used to define PPH (Francois & Foley, 2012). However, defining PPH clinically can be ambiguous. Diagnosis is often based on subjective observations, with blood loss often being underestimated by as much as 50% (Cunningham, Leveno, Bloom, et al., 2014).

In 2010 The Joint Commission (TJC) issued the *Sentinel Event Alert: Preventing Maternal Death*. It identified the most preventable errors as the following:

- Failure to adequately control blood pressure in hypertensive women
- Failure to adequately diagnose and treat pulmonary edema in women with preeclampsia
- Failure to pay attention to vital signs following cesarean birth
- Hemorrhage following cesarean birth (TJC, 2010)

Postpartum hemorrhage is classified as early or late with respect to the birth. Early, acute, or primary PPH occurs within 24 hours of the birth. Late or secondary PPH occurs more than 24 hours but less than 6 weeks after the birth (Francois & Foley, 2012). Today's health care environment encourages shortened hospital stays after birth, which increases the potential for acute episodes of PPH to occur outside the traditional hospital or birth center setting.

Etiology and Risk Factors

When excessive bleeding is observed, it is important to note the color and consistency of the blood as well as the stage of labor. From birth of the infant until separation of the placenta, the character and quantity of blood passed can suggest excessive bleeding. For example, dark red blood is likely of venous origin, perhaps from varices or superficial lacerations of the birth canal. Bright blood is arterial and can indicate deep lacerations of the cervix. Spurts of blood with clots can indicate partial placental separation. Failure of blood to clot or remain clotted indicates a pathologic condition or coagulopathy such as disseminated intravascular coagulation (DIC) (see Chapter 28).

Excessive bleeding can occur during the period from the separation of the placenta to its expulsion or removal. Commonly such excessive bleeding is the result of incomplete placental separation, undue manipulation of the fundus, or excessive traction on the cord. After the placenta has been expelled or removed, persistent or excessive blood loss usually is the result of uterine atony or prolapse of the uterus into the vagina. Late PPH can be the result of subinvolution of the uterus, endometritis, or retained placental fragments (Francois & Foley, 2012). Predisposing factors for PPH are listed in Box 33-1.

BOX 33-1 Risk Factors and Causes of Postpartum Hemorrhage

Uterine atony
- Overdistended uterus
  - Large fetus
  - Multiple fetuses
  - Hydramnios
  - Distention with clots
- Anesthesia and analgesia
  - Conduction anesthesia
- Previous history of uterine atony
- High parity
- Prolonged labor, oxytocin-induced labor
- Trauma during labor and birth
  - Forceps-assisted birth
  - Vacuum-assisted birth
  - Cesarean birth

Unrepaired lacerations of the birth canal
Retained placental fragments
Ruptured uterus
Inversion of the uterus
Placenta accreta, increta, percreta
Coagulation disorders
Placental abruption
Placenta previa
Manual removal of a retained placenta
Magnesium sulfate administration during labor or the postpartum period
Chorioamnionitis
Uterine subinvolution

Uterine Atony

The greatest risk for early postpartum hemorrhage is during the first hour after birth. During this time, large venous areas are exposed after the placenta separates from the uterine wall. The corpus or body of the uterus is essentially a basket-weave of strong, interlacing smooth muscle bundles through which many large maternal blood vessels pass (see Fig. 4-3). Bleeding is controlled by the contraction of smooth muscle in the uterus. If the uterus is flaccid after detachment of all or part of the placenta, brisk venous bleeding occurs, and normal coagulation of the open vasculature is impaired and continues until the uterine muscle is contracted. This marked hypotonia of the uterus is called uterine atony.

Uterine atony is the leading cause of early PPH. It is associated with high parity, polyhydramnios, fetal macrosomia, and multiple gestations. In such conditions the uterus is "overstretched" and contracts poorly after birth. Other causes of atony include traumatic birth, use of halogenated anesthetic (e.g., halothane), magnesium sulfate, rapid or prolonged labor, chorioamnionitis, use of oxytocin for labor induction or augmentation, and uterine atony in a previous pregnancy (Francois & Foley, 2012).

CLINICAL REASONING CASE STUDY

Postpartum Hemorrhage

You are the mother-baby nurse assigned to Ms. Avery. She is a G6 P5 who gave birth to a 9-lb (4082 kg) baby boy this morning. Ms. Avery had an uncomplicated but precipitous vaginal birth. Perineum is intact. She is breastfeeding. All labs are normal. She is now 5 hours postpartum. A family member calls out from the client's room for assistance. When you walk into the room Ms. Avery is standing up on her way to the bathroom with a large pool of blood on the floor. She states, "I don't know what happened; it all just came when I stood up. I am so dizzy and lightheaded." What do you, as the nurse, do next?

1. Evidence—Is there sufficient evidence to draw conclusions about what the nurse should do?
2. Assumptions—Describe underlying assumptions about each of the following:
   a. Identify risk factors for early postpartum hemorrhage (PPH) and specifically those described for Ms. Avery.
   b. Need for frequent assessments in the early postpartum period
   c. Use of oxytocics for prevention and management of PPH
3. What implications and priorities for nursing care can be made at this time?
4. Does the evidence objectively support your conclusion?

Retained Placenta

When the placenta has not been delivered within 30 minutes after birth despite gentle traction on the umbilical cord and uterine massage, it is described as "retained." Initial management of a retained placenta consists of manual separation and removal by the physician or nurse-midwife (Fig. 33-1). This involves the provider reaching into the uterus and gently separating the placenta from the uterine wall and removing it manually. When the mother has regional anesthesia for labor, supplementary anesthesia is usually not needed. For other women, administration of light nitrous oxide and oxygen inhalation anesthesia or intravenous (IV) pain medications should be considered. A tocolytic medication such as nitroglycerin IV may be given to promote uterine relaxation (Francois & Foley, 2012). After removal of a retained placenta, the woman is at continued risk for PPH and infection.

Fragments of the placenta can remain in the uterus after spontaneous separation of the placenta during the third stage of labor. In this case the woman will have excessive bleeding and the uterus feels boggy (soft) due to uterine atony. Ultrasonography can be used to detect placental fragments. The physician or nurse-midwife may attempt manual exploration to remove the fragments; uterine curettage (removal of uterine contents using a curette or vacuum suction) may be necessary.

In rare instances there is abnormal adherence of the placenta to the myometrium. It is unknown why this occurs, but it is thought to result from zygote implantation in an area of defective endometrium so that no zone of separation exists between the placenta and the decidua. Attempts to remove the placenta in the usual manner are unsuccessful, and laceration or perforation of the uterine wall can result, putting the woman at great risk for severe PPH and infection (Francois & Foley, 2012).

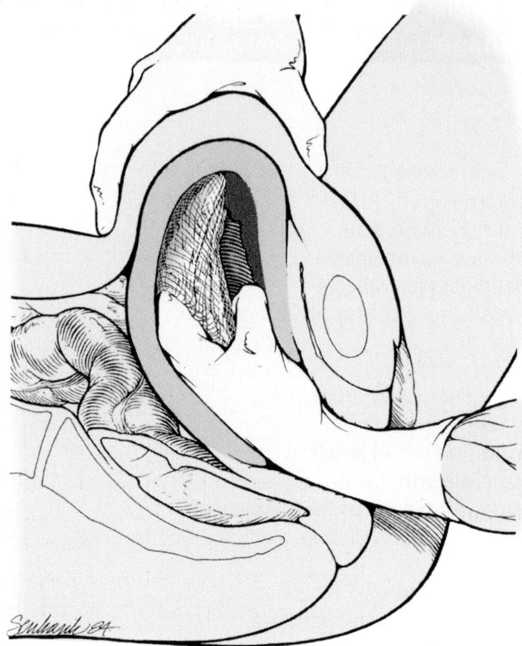

FIG 33-1 Manual uterine exploration. (From Francois, K.E., & Foley, M.R. [2012]. Antepartum and postpartum hemorrhage. In S.G. Gabbe, J.R. Niebyl, J.L. Simpson, et al. [Eds.], *Obstetrics: Normal and problem pregnancies* [6th ed.]. Philadelphia: Saunders.)

Unusual placental adherence can be partial or complete. The following degrees of attachment are recognized:

Placenta accreta—Slight penetration of myometrium
Placenta increta—Deep penetration of myometrium
Placenta percreta—Perforation of uterus

Placenta accreta is most common, with its incidence increasing in association with the rise in cesarean birth rates (Cunningham et al., 2014). Other risk factors include placenta previa, prior uterine surgery, endometrial defects, submucosal fibroids, parity, and maternal age (Francois & Foley, 2012). Placenta accreta can be diagnosed before birth using ultrasound and magnetic resonance imaging (MRI), but often it is not recognized until there is excessive bleeding after birth. Bleeding with complete or total placenta accreta may not occur unless manual removal of the placenta is attempted. With more extensive involvement, bleeding becomes profuse when delivery of the placenta is attempted. Less blood is lost if the diagnosis is made antenatally and no attempt is made to manually remove the placenta. Treatment includes blood component replacement therapy. Hysterectomy can be indicated for all three types of placental adherence if bleeding is uncontrolled (Cunningham et al.).

Lacerations of the Genital Tract

Lacerations of the cervix, vagina, and perineum also are causes of PPH. Hemorrhage related to lacerations should be suspected if bleeding continues despite a firm, contracted uterine fundus. This bleeding can be a slow trickle, an oozing, or frank hemorrhage. Factors that influence the causes and incidence of obstetric lacerations of the lower genital tract include operative birth, precipitous or rapid birth, congenital abnormalities of the maternal soft tissue, and contracted pelvis. Other possible causes of lacerations are size, abnormal presentation and position of the fetus; relative size of the presenting part and the birth canal; previous scarring from infection, injury, or operation; and vulvar, perineal, and vaginal varicosities.

Lacerations of the perineum are the most common of all injuries in the lower portion of the genital tract. These are classified as first, second, third, and fourth degree (see Chapter 19). An episiotomy can extend to become either a third- or fourth-degree laceration.

Prolonged pressure of the fetal head on the vaginal mucosa ultimately interferes with the circulation and may produce ischemic or pressure necrosis. The state of the tissues in combination with the type of birth can result in deep vaginal lacerations, with consequent predisposition to vaginal hematomas.

Cervical lacerations usually occur at the lateral angles of the external os. Most are shallow, and bleeding is minimal. More extensive lacerations may extend into the vaginal vault or into the lower uterine segment.

Lacerations are usually identified and sutured immediately after birth. After the bleeding has been controlled, the care of the woman with lacerations of the perineum is similar to that for women with episiotomies (i.e., analgesia as needed for pain and hot or cold applications as necessary). The need for increased fiber in the diet and increased intake of fluids is emphasized to reduce the risk of constipation. Stool softeners may be used to assist the woman in reestablishing bowel habits without straining and putting stress on the suture lines.

Hematomas

Pelvic hematomas (i.e., a collection of blood in the connective tissue) can be vulvar, vaginal, or retroperitoneal in origin. Vulvar hematomas are the most common. Pain is the most common symptom, and most vulvar hematomas are visible. Vaginal hematomas occur more commonly in association with a forceps-assisted birth, an episiotomy, or primigravidity (Francois & Foley, 2012).

Retroperitoneal hematomas are the least common but life threatening. They are caused by laceration of one of the vessels attached to the hypogastric artery, usually associated with rupture of a cesarean scar during labor. During the postpartum period, if the woman reports persistent perineal or rectal pain or a feeling of pressure in the vagina, a careful examination is made. However, a retroperitoneal hematoma can cause minimal pain and the initial symptoms can be signs of shock (Francois & Foley, 2012).

Hematomas are usually surgically evacuated. Once the bleeding has been controlled, usual postpartum care is provided with careful attention to pain relief, monitoring the amount of bleeding, replacing fluids, and reviewing laboratory results (hemoglobin and hematocrit).

Inversion of the Uterus

Inversion of the uterus (turning inside out) after birth is a rare but potentially life-threatening complication. The incidence of uterine inversion varies from 1 in 2000 to 1 in 20,000 births and differs depending on whether the birth was vaginal or cesarean (Cunningham et al., 2014) and can recur with a subsequent birth. Uterine inversion can be incomplete, complete, or prolapsed. Incomplete inversion cannot be seen; a smooth mass can be palpated through the dilated cervix. In complete inversion, the lining of the fundus crosses through the cervical os and forms a mass in the vagina. Prolapsed inversion of the uterus is obvious—a large, red, rounded mass (perhaps with the placenta attached) protrudes 20 to 30 cm outside the introitus.

Contributing factors to uterine inversion include fundal implantation of the placenta, vigorous fundal pressure, excessive traction applied to the cord, fetal macrosomia, short umbilical cord, tocolysis, prolonged labor, uterine atony, nulliparity, and abnormally adherent placental tissue (Francois & Foley, 2012). The primary presenting signs of uterine inversion are sudden and include hemorrhage, shock, and pain. The uterus is not palpable abdominally. The uterus must be replaced into its proper position by the physician or nurse-midwife.

Prevention—always the easiest, least expensive, and most effective therapy—is especially appropriate for uterine inversion. The umbilical cord should not be pulled unless there are clear signs of placental separation.

Uterine inversion is an emergency situation requiring immediate interventions that include maternal fluid resuscitation, replacement of the uterus within the pelvic cavity, and correction of associated clinical conditions. Tocolytics or halogenated anesthetics may be given to relax the uterus before attempting replacement (Francois & Foley, 2012). Oxytocic agents are administered after the uterus is repositioned; broad-spectrum antibiotics are initiated. The woman's response to treatment is monitored closely to prevent shock or fluid overload. If the uterus has been repositioned manually, care must be taken to avoid aggressive fundal massage.

Subinvolution of the Uterus

Late postpartum bleeding can result from subinvolution of the uterus (delayed return of the enlarged uterus to normal size and function). Recognized causes of subinvolution include retained placental fragments and pelvic infection. Signs and symptoms include prolonged lochial discharge, irregular or excessive bleeding, and sometimes hemorrhage. A pelvic examination usually reveals a larger-than-normal uterus that can be boggy.

Treatment of subinvolution depends on the cause. Ergonovine (Ergotrate) or methylergonovine (Methergine), 0.2 mg every 3 to 4 hours for 24 to 48 hours, is often used. Dilation and curettage (D&C) may be performed to remove retained placental fragments or to debride the placental site. If the cause of subinvolution is infection, antibiotic therapy is needed (Cunningham et al., 2014).

CARE MANAGEMENT

Assessment

Early recognition and treatment of PPH are critical to care management (Fig. 33-2). The first step is to evaluate the contractility of the uterus. If the uterus is hypotonic or boggy, management is directed toward increasing contractility and minimizing blood loss.

If the uterus is firmly contracted and bleeding continues, the source of bleeding still must be identified and treated. Assessment may include visual or manual inspection of the perineum, the vagina, the uterus, the cervix, or the rectum, as well as laboratory studies (e.g., hemoglobin, hematocrit, coagulation studies, platelet count). Treatment depends on the source of the bleeding.

Medical Management

The initial intervention in management of excessive postpartum bleeding due to uterine atony is firm massage of the uterine fundus (see Fig. 21-4). Expression of any clots in the uterus, elimination of bladder distention, and continuous IV infusion of 10 to 40 units of oxytocin added to 1000 ml of lactated Ringer's or normal saline solution also are primary interventions. If the uterus fails to respond to oxytocin, other uterotonic medications are administered. Misoprostol (Cytotec), a synthetic prostaglandin E_1 analog, is often used. An advantage is that it can be given rectally, sublingually, or orally. Methylergonovine may be given intramuscularly to produce sustained uterine contractions. A derivative of prostaglandin $F_2\alpha$ (carboprost tromethamine [Carboprost; Hemabate]) may be given intramuscularly. It can also be given intramyometrially at cesarean birth or intraabdominally after vaginal birth. Prostaglandin E_2 (Dinoprostone) vaginal or rectal suppository can be used for postpartum hemorrhage. (See Medication Guide: Uterotonic Drugs to Manage Postpartum Hemorrhage for a comparison of uterotonic drugs and common dosages used to manage PPH). In addition to the medications used to contract the uterus, rapid administration of crystalloid solutions or blood or blood products or both will be needed to restore the woman's intravascular volume (Francois & Foley, 2012).

> **MEDICATION ALERT**
>
> Use of ergonovine or methylergonovine is contraindicated in the presence of hypertension or cardiovascular disease. Prostaglandin $F_2\alpha$ should not be given to women with a history of asthma as it can cause bronchoconstriction (Francois & Foley, 2012).

Oxygen can be given by nonrebreather face mask to enhance oxygen delivery to the cells. An indwelling urinary catheter is usually inserted to monitor urine output as a measure of intravascular volume. Laboratory studies usually include a complete blood count with platelet count, fibrinogen, fibrin split products, prothrombin time, and partial thromboplastin time. Blood type and antibody screen are done if not previously performed (Cunningham et al., 2014).

If bleeding persists, bimanual compression (Fig. 33-3) may be performed by the obstetrician or nurse-midwife. This procedure involves inserting a fist into the vagina and pressing the knuckles against the anterior side of the uterus, and then placing the other hand on the abdomen and massaging the posterior uterus with it. If the uterus still does not become firm, the health care provider performs manual exploration of the uterine cavity for retained placental fragments.

Surgical Management

If the preceding procedures are ineffective, surgical management is needed. Surgical management options include uterine tamponade (uterine packing or an intrauterine tamponade balloon) (Fig. 33-4), bilateral uterine artery ligation, ligation of utero-ovarian arteries and infundibulopelvic vessels, and

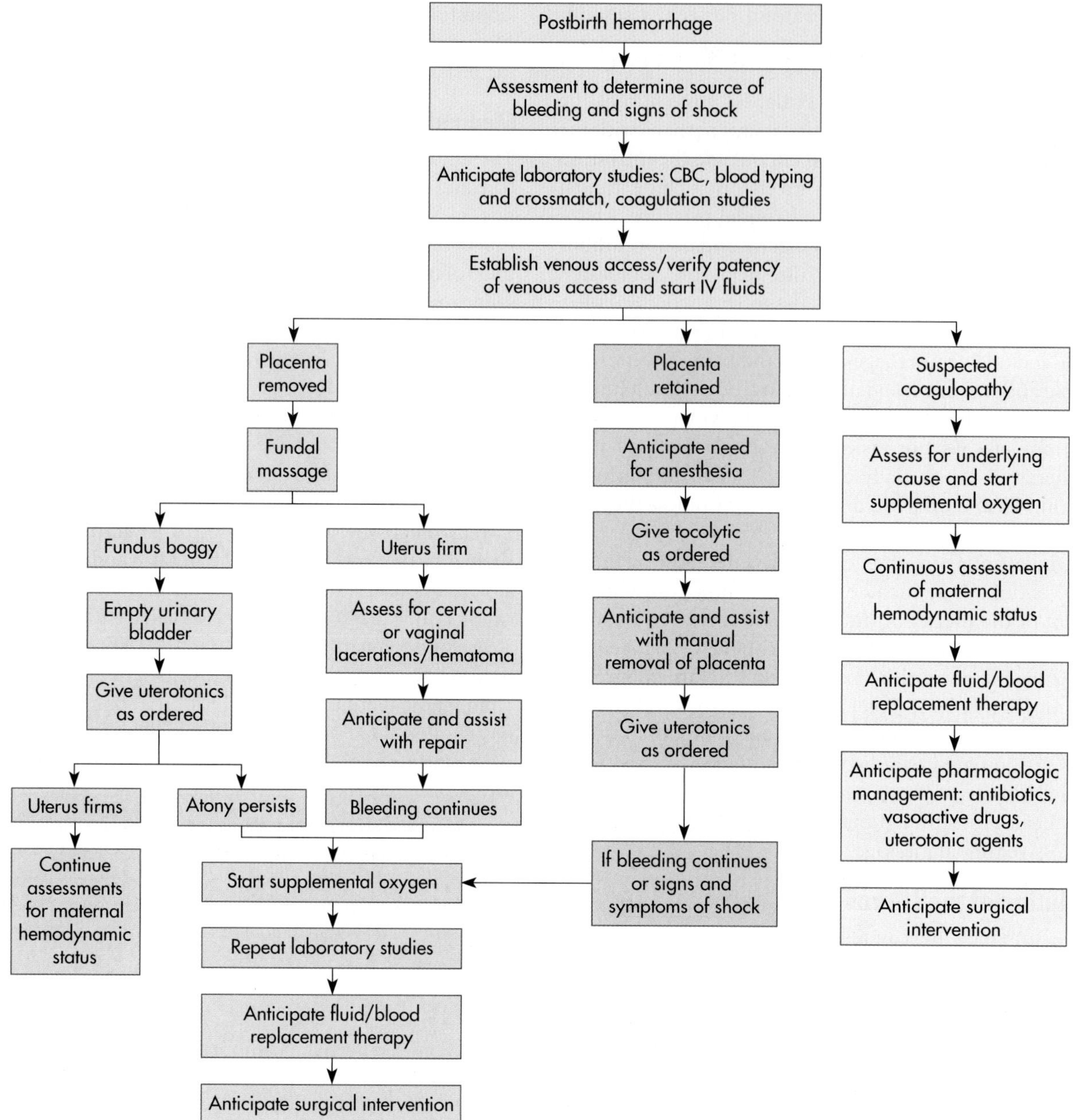

FIG 33-2 Nursing assessments for postpartum bleeding. (Uterotonics are medications to contract the uterus; tocolytics are medications to relax the uterus.) *CBC,* Complete blood count; *IV,* intravenous.

selective arterial embolization. Uterine compression suturing (e.g., B-Lynch or Hayman vertical sutures) may be performed and is sometimes combined with a tamponade balloon (see Fig. 33-4). If other treatment measures are ineffective, hysterectomy likely is needed (Cunningham et al., 2014; Francois & Foley, 2012).

Nursing Interventions

The nurse must be alert to the symptoms of hemorrhage and be prepared to act quickly to minimize blood loss (see Fig. 33-2). Astute assessment of circulatory status can be done with noninvasive monitoring (Box 33-2). Nursing diagnoses, expected outcomes of care, and interventions are based on the cause of PPH as previously discussed (see Nursing Care Plan).

The woman and her family will be anxious about her condition. The nurse can intervene by calmly providing explanations about interventions being performed and the need to act quickly.

Once the woman's condition is stabilized and she has begun the recovery process, preparations for discharge are made. Discharge instructions for the woman who experienced PPH are similar to those for any postpartum woman. In addition, the woman should be told that she will probably feel fatigue, even exhaustion, and will need to limit her physical activities to conserve her strength. She may need instructions about increasing her dietary iron and protein intake and iron supplementation to rebuild lost red blood cell (RBC) volume. She may need assistance with infant care and household activities until she has regained strength. The nurse should assess the mother's anticipated level of support from family and friends and help the mother plan how to ask for help when returning home. Some mothers experiencing a PPH have problems with delayed lactogenesis, insufficient

MEDICATION GUIDE

Uterotonic Drugs to Manage Postpartum Hemorrhage

DRUG	ACTION	SIDE EFFECTS	CONTRAINDICATIONS	DOSAGE AND ROUTE	NURSING CONSIDERATIONS
Oxytocin (Pitocin)	Contraction of uterus; decreases bleeding	Infrequent: water intoxication, nausea and vomiting	None for PPH	10 to 20 units/L up to 80 units/L diluted in lactated Ringer's solution or normal saline at 125 to 200 milliunits/min IV; or 10 to 20 units IM	Continue to monitor vaginal bleeding and uterine tone.
Misoprostol (Cytotec)	Contraction of uterus	Headache, nausea, vomiting, diarrhea, fever, chills	None	600 to 1000 mcg rectally once or 400 mcg sublingually or PO once	Continue to monitor vaginal bleeding and uterine tone.
Methylergonovine (Methergine)	Contraction of uterus	Hypertension, hypotension, nausea, vomiting, headache	Hypertension, preeclampsia, cardiac disease	0.2 mg IM q2-4h up to five doses; may also be given intrauterine or orally	Check blood pressure before giving, and do not give if >140/90 mm Hg; continue monitoring vaginal bleeding and uterine tone.
15-Methylprostaglandin $F_{2}\alpha$ (Prostin/15 m; Carboprost, Hemabate)	Contraction of uterus	Headache, nausea and vomiting, fever, chills, tachycardia, hypertension, diarrhea	Avoid with asthma or hypertension	250 mcg IM or intrauterine injection every q15-90 min up to eight doses	Continue to monitor vaginal bleeding and uterine tone.
Dinoprostone (Prostin E_2)	Contraction of uterus	Headache, nausea and vomiting, fever, chills, diarrhea	Use with caution with history of asthma, hypertension, or hypotension	20 mg vaginal or rectal suppository q2h	Continue to monitor vaginal bleeding and uterine tone.

IM, Intramuscular; *IV,* intravenous; *PO,* by mouth; *PPH,* postpartum hemorrhage.
Data from Francois, K.E., & Foley, M.R. (2012). Antepartum and postpartum hemorrhage. In S.G. Gabbe, J.R. Niebyl, J.L. Simpson, et al. (Eds.), *Obstetrics: Normal and problem pregnancies* (6th ed.). Philadelphia: Saunders; Lyndon, A., Lagrew, D, Shields, L., et al. (Eds.). (2010). *Improving health care response to obstetric hemorrhage.* (California Maternal Quality Care Collaborative Toolkit to Transform Maternity Care). Stanford, CA: California Maternal Quality Care Collaborative (CMQCC). Available at www.cmqcc.org/resource.

milk production, or postpartum depression (PPD). Referrals for home care follow-up or to community resources may be needed, including lactation support or a postpartum doula service.

HEMORRHAGIC (HYPOVOLEMIC) SHOCK

Hemorrhage can result in hemorrhagic (hypovolemic) shock. Shock is an emergency situation in which the perfusion of body organs can become severely compromised and death can occur. Physiologic compensatory mechanisms are activated in response to hemorrhage. The adrenal glands release catecholamines, causing arterioles and venules in the skin, lungs, gastrointestinal tract, liver, and kidneys to constrict. The available blood flow is diverted to the brain and heart and away from other organs, including the uterus. If shock is prolonged, the continued reduction in cellular oxygenation results in an accumulation of lactic acid and acidosis (from anaerobic glucose metabolism). Acidosis (lowered serum pH) causes arteriolar vasodilation; venule vasoconstriction persists. A circular pattern is established (i.e., decreased perfusion, increased tissue anoxia and acidosis, edema formation, and pooling of blood further decrease the perfusion). Cellular death occurs. See Emergency: Hemorrhagic Shock for assessments and interventions for hemorrhagic shock.

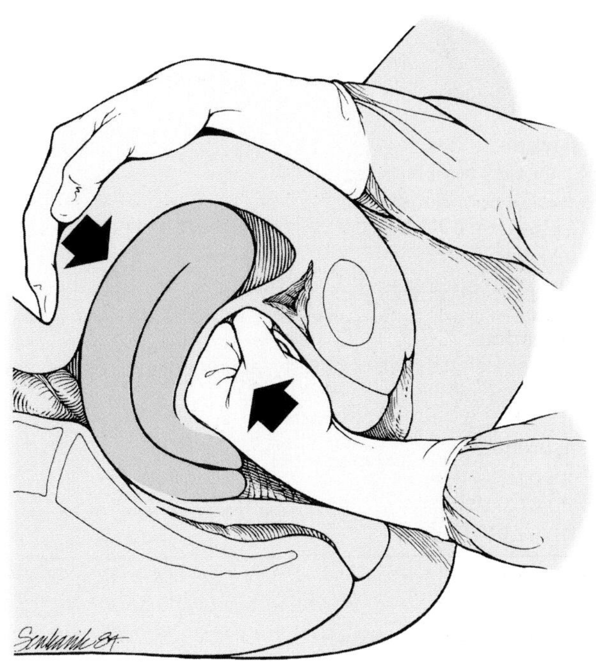

FIG 33-3 Bimanual compression. (From Francois, K.E. & Foley, M.R. [2012]. Antepartum and postpartum hemorrhage. In S.G. Gabbe, J.R. Niebyl, J.L. Simpson, et al. [Eds.], *Obstetrics: Normal and problem pregnancies* [6th ed.]. Philadelphia: Saunders.)

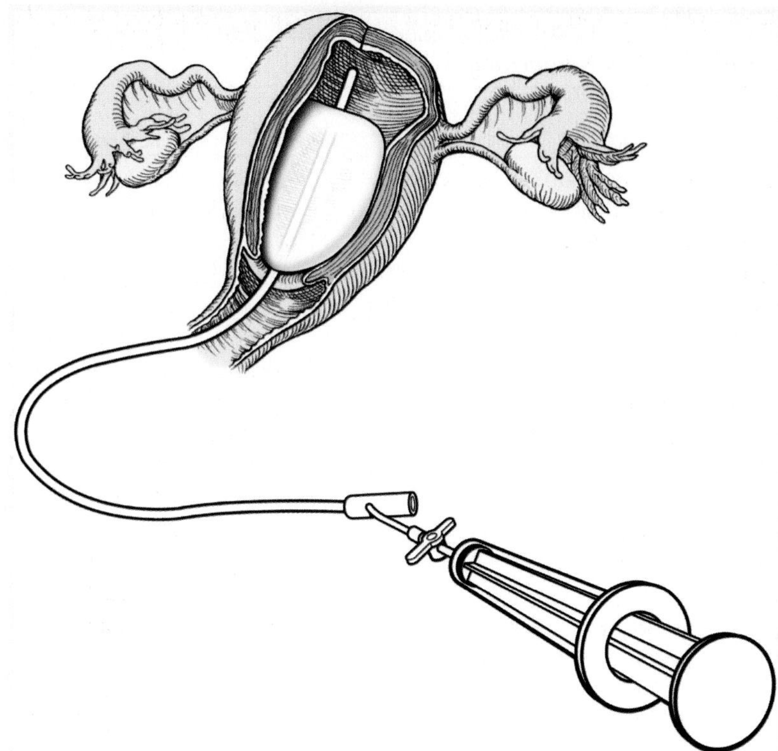

FIG 33-4 Bakri balloon. (From Francois, K.E., & Foley, M.R. [2012]. Antepartum and postpartum hemorrhage. In S.G. Gabbe, J.R. Niebyl, J.L. Simpson, et al. [Eds.], *Obstetrics: Normal and problem pregnancies* [6th ed.], Philadelphia: Saunders.)

BOX 33-2 Noninvasive Assessments of Cardiac Output in Postpartum Women with Excessive Bleeding

Palpation of Pulses (Rate, Quality, Equality)
- Arterial

Auscultation
- Heart sounds/murmurs
- Breath sounds

Inspection
- Skin color, temperature, turgor
- Level of consciousness
- Capillary refill
- Neck veins
- Mucous membranes

Observation
- Presence or absence of anxiety, apprehension, restlessness, disorientation

Measurement
- Blood pressure
- Pulse oximetry
- Urinary output

CARE MANAGEMENT

In order for staff to be best prepared for obstetric hemorrhage, institutions must develop standardized management protocols and regularly conduct emergency drills. The California Maternal Quality Care Collaborative (www.cmqcc.org) has developed best practice approaches that can be adopted by other institutions (Lyndon, Lagrew, Shields, et al., 2010). The use of obstetric rapid response teams and massive transfusion protocols is vital to promoting safe, effective care and improving outcomes.

LEGAL TIP: Standard of Care for Bleeding Emergencies

The standard of care for obstetric emergency situations such as PPH or hypovolemic shock is that provision should be made for the nurse to implement nursing actions independently. Policies, procedures, standing orders or protocols, and clinical guidelines should be established by each health care facility in which births occur and should be agreed on by health care providers involved in the care of obstetric clients.

Medical Management

Vigorous treatment is necessary to prevent adverse outcomes. Management of hypovolemic shock involves restoring circulating blood volume and eliminating the cause of the hemorrhage (e.g., lacerations, uterine atony, or inversion). Critical to successful management of the woman with a hemorrhagic complication is establishment of venous access, preferably with a large-bore IV catheter. Establishing two IV lines facilitates fluid resuscitation. Fluid resuscitation includes administering crystalloids (lactated Ringer's, normal saline solution), colloids (albumin), blood, and blood components. To restore circulating blood volume, a rapid IV infusion of crystalloid solution is given at a rate of 3 ml infused for every 1 ml of estimated blood loss (e.g., 3000 ml infused for 1000 ml of blood loss). Packed red blood cells (RBCs) are usually infused if the woman is still actively bleeding and no improvement in her condition is noted after the initial crystalloid infusion. Infusion of fresh frozen plasma may be needed if clotting factors and platelet counts are below normal values (Cunningham et al., 2014; Francois & Foley, 2012).

Nursing Interventions

Hemorrhagic shock can occur rapidly, but the classic signs of shock may not appear until the postpartum woman has lost 30% to 40% of blood volume. The nurse must continue to reassess the woman's condition as evidenced by the degree of measurable and anticipated blood loss while also mobilizing appropriate resources.

Most interventions are instituted to improve or monitor tissue perfusion. Fluid resuscitation must be monitored carefully because fluid overload can occur. Intravascular fluid overload occurs most often with colloid therapy.

Transfusion reactions can follow administration of blood or blood components, including cryoprecipitates. Even in an emergency, each unit of blood or blood products should be carefully checked per hospital protocol. Complications of fluid or blood replacement therapy include hemolytic reactions, febrile reactions, allergic reactions, circulatory overload, and air embolism.

The nurse continues to monitor the woman's pulse and blood pressure. If invasive hemodynamic monitoring is ordered, the nurse may assist with placement of a central venous pressure (CVP) or pulmonary artery (Swan-Ganz) catheter. Subsequently, the nurse monitors CVP, pulmonary artery pressure, or pulmonary artery wedge pressure as ordered (Gilbert, 2011).

Additional assessments include evaluating skin temperature, color, and turgor and mucous membranes. Breath sounds should be auscultated before fluid volume replacement to provide a baseline for future assessment. The nurse inspects for signs of DIC such as oozing at the sites of incisions or injections and assessment for the presence of petechiae or ecchymosis in areas not associated with surgery or trauma are critical in evaluating for DIC (see Chapter 28).

Oxygen is administered, preferably by a nonrebreather face mask, at 10 to 12 L/min to maintain oxygen saturation. Oxygen saturation should be monitored with a pulse oximeter, although measurements are not always accurate in a client with hypovolemia or decreased perfusion. Level of consciousness is assessed frequently and provides additional indications of blood volume and oxygen saturation (Gilbert, 2011). In early stages of decreased blood flow the woman may report "seeing stars" or feeling dizzy or nauseated. She can become restless and orthopneic. As cerebral hypoxia increases, she can become confused and react slowly to stimuli or not at all. Some women complain of headaches.

Continuous electrocardiographic monitoring may be indicated for the woman who is hypotensive or tachycardic, continues to bleed profusely, or is in shock. A Foley catheter is inserted and a urometer is attached to allow hourly assessment of urine output. The most objective and least invasive assessment of adequate organ perfusion and oxygenation is a urine output of at least 30 ml/hr (Cunningham et al., 2014). Hemoglobin and hematocrit levels, platelet count, and coagulation studies are closely monitored.

EMERGENCY

Hemorrhagic Shock

ASSESSMENTS	CHARACTERISTICS
Respirations	Rapid and shallow
Pulse	Rapid, weak, irregular
Blood pressure	Decreasing (late sign)
Skin	Cool, pale, clammy
Urinary output	Decreasing
Level of consciousness	Lethargy → coma
Mental status	Anxiety → coma
Central venous pressure	Decreased

INTERVENTIONS
- Summon assistance and equipment.
- Start intravenous infusion per standing orders.
- Ensure patent airway; administer oxygen.
- Continue to monitor status.

COAGULOPATHIES

When bleeding is continuous and there is no identifiable source, a coagulopathy can be the cause. The woman's coagulation status must be assessed quickly and continuously. Abnormal results depend on the cause and can include increased prothrombin time, increased partial thromboplastin time, decreased platelets, decreased fibrinogen level, increased fibrin degradation products, and prolonged bleeding time. Causes of coagulopathies can include pregnancy complications such as idiopathic or immune thrombocytopenic purpura, von Willebrand disease, or DIC.

Idiopathic Thrombocytopenic Purpura

Idiopathic or immune thrombocytopenic purpura (ITP) is an autoimmune disorder in which antiplatelet antibodies decrease the life span of the platelets. Thrombocytopenia, capillary fragility, and increased bleeding time are diagnostic findings. ITP can cause severe hemorrhage after cesarean birth or cervical or vaginal lacerations. The incidence of postpartum uterine bleeding and vaginal hematomas is also increased. Neonatal thrombocytopenia can result, but serious bleeding is unusual (Rozance & Rosenberg, 2012).

Medical management focuses on control of platelet stability. If ITP was diagnosed during pregnancy, the woman likely was treated with corticosteroids or IV immunoglobulin. Platelet transfusions are usually given when there is significant bleeding. A splenectomy may be needed if the ITP does not respond to medical management (Cunningham et al., 2014).

von Willebrand Disease

von Willebrand disease (vWD), a type of hemophilia, is probably the most common of all hereditary bleeding disorders. Although vWD is rare, it is among the most common congenital clotting defects in U.S. women of childbearing age. It results from a deficiency or defect in a blood clotting protein called *von Willebrand factor (vWF)*. There are as many as 20 variations of vWD, most of which are inherited as autosomal dominant traits—types I and II are the most common. Symptoms include recurrent bleeding episodes such as nosebleeds or after tooth extraction, bruising easily, prolonged bleeding time (the most important test), factor VIII deficiency (mild to moderate),

NURSING CARE PLAN

Postpartum Hemorrhage

NURSING DIAGNOSIS	EXPECTED OUTCOME	NURSING INTERVENTIONS	RATIONALES
Deficient Fluid Volume related to postpartum hemorrhage	Woman will demonstrate fluid balance as evidenced by stable vital signs, prompt capillary refill time, and balanced intake and output.	Monitor vital signs, oxygen saturation, urine specific gravity, and capillary refill.	To provide baseline data
		Measure and record amount and type of bleeding by weighing and counting saturated pads; if woman is at home, teach her to count pads and save any clots or tissue; if woman is admitted to the hospital, save clots and tissue for further examination.	To estimate type and amount of blood loss for fluid replacement
		Provide quiet environment.	To promote rest and decrease metabolic demands
		Give explanation of all procedures.	To reduce anxiety
		Begin intravenous (IV) access with 18-gauge or larger catheter for infusion of isotonic solution as ordered.	To provide fluid or blood replacement
		Administer medications as ordered, such as oxytocin, misoprostol, methylergonovine, or prostaglandin $F_{2}\alpha$.	To increase contractility of uterus
		Insert indwelling urinary catheter.	To provide most accurate assessment of renal function and hypovolemia
		Prepare for surgical intervention as needed.	To stop source of bleeding
Ineffective Tissue Perfusion related to hypovolemia	Woman will have stable vital signs, oxygen saturation, and arterial blood gases and adequate hematocrit and hemoglobin.	Monitor vital signs, oxygen saturation, arterial blood gases, and hematocrit and hemoglobin.	To assess for hypovolemic shock and decreased tissue perfusion
		Assess capillary refill, mucous membranes, and skin temperature.	To note indicators of vasoconstriction
		Give supplementary oxygen as ordered.	To provide additional oxygenation to tissues
		Suction as needed, and insert oral airway.	To maintain clear, open airway for oxygenation
		Monitor arterial blood gases.	To provide information about acidosis or hypoxia
		Administer sodium bicarbonate if ordered.	To reverse metabolic acidosis
Anxiety related to sudden change in health status	Woman will verbalize that anxious feelings are diminished.	Using therapeutic communication, evaluate woman's understanding of events.	To provide clarification of any misconceptions
		Provide calm, competent attitude and environment	To aid in decreasing anxiety
		Explain all procedures.	To decrease anxiety about unknown
		Allow woman to verbalize feelings.	To permit clarification of information and promote trust
		Continue to assess vital signs or other clinical indicators of hypovolemic shock.	To evaluate if psychologic response of anxiety intensifies physiologic indicators
Risk for Infection related to blood loss and invasive procedures as result of postpartum hemorrhage	Woman will verbalize understanding of risk factors. Woman will demonstrate no signs of infection.	Maintain Standard Precautions and use proper hand hygiene technique when providing care.	To prevent introduction of or spread of infection
		Teach woman to maintain proper hand hygiene (particularly before handling her newborn) and to maintain scrupulous perineal care with frequent change and careful disposal of perineal pads.	To avoid spread of microorganisms
		Monitor vital signs.	To detect signs of systemic infection
		Monitor level of fatigue and lethargy, evidence of chills, loss of appetite, nausea and vomiting, and abdominal pain.	To indicate extent of infection and serve as indicators of status of infection
		Monitor lochia for foul smell.	To indicate status of infection
		Assist with collection of intrauterine cultures or other specimens for laboratory analysis.	To identify specific causative organism
		Monitor laboratory values (i.e., white blood cell [WBC] count, cultures).	For indicators of type and status of infection
		Ensure adequate fluid and nutritional intake.	To promote healthy recovery
		Administer and monitor broad-spectrum antibiotics as ordered.	To prevent or treat infection
		Administer antipyretics as ordered and necessary.	To reduce elevated temperature

and bleeding from mucous membranes. Although factor VIII increases during pregnancy, a risk for PPH still exists as levels of vWF begin to decrease (Cunningham et al., 2014). The woman can be at risk for bleeding for up to 4 weeks after birth.

The treatment of choice is administration of desmopressin, which promotes the release of vWF and factor VIII. It can be given nasally, intravenously, or orally. Transfusion therapy with plasma products that have been treated for viruses and contain factor VIII and vWF also may be used. Concentrates of antihemophiliac factor (Humate-P or Alphanate) can be administered (Cunningham et al., 2014).

VENOUS THROMBOEMBOLIC DISORDERS

Venous thromboembolism (VTE) results from the formation of a blood clot or clots inside a blood vessel and is caused by inflammation (thrombophlebitis) or partial obstruction of the vessel (Fig. 33-5). Three thromboembolic conditions are of concern in the postpartum period:

Superficial venous thrombosis—Involvement of the superficial saphenous venous system

Deep venous thrombosis (DVT)—Occurs most often in the lower extremities; involvement varies but can extend from the foot to the iliofemoral region

Pulmonary embolism (PE)—Complication of DVT occurring when part of a blood clot dislodges and is carried to the pulmonary artery, where it occludes the vessel and obstructs blood flow to the lungs

Incidence and Etiology

The incidence of venous thromboembolism (VTE) is approximately 1 in 1000 pregnancies (Cunningham et al., 2014; Pettker & Lockwood, 2012). VTE can occur in any trimester of pregnancy and in the postpartum period. DVT occurs most often during pregnancy, and PE is more common in the postpartum period. The incidence of VTE in the postpartum period has declined since early ambulation after childbirth has become standard practice. However, PE is a major cause of maternal death (Pettker & Lockwood). The primary causes of thromboembolic disease are venous stasis and hypercoagulation, both of which are present in pregnancy and continue into the postpartum period. Cesarean birth nearly doubles the risk for VTE; therefore, routine preoperative placement of pneumatic compression devices is recommended. Other risk factors include operative vaginal birth; history of venous thrombosis, pulmonary embolism, or varicosities; obesity; maternal age greater than 35; multiparity; and smoking (Pettker & Lockwood).

Clinical Manifestations

Superficial venous thrombosis is the most common form of postpartum thrombophlebitis. It is characterized by pain and tenderness in the lower extremity. Physical examination may reveal warmth; redness; and an enlarged, hardened vein over the site of the thrombosis.

Deep vein thrombosis is more common during pregnancy than in the postpartum period and is characterized by unilateral leg pain, calf tenderness, and swelling. Physical examination may reveal redness and warmth, but women can have a large clot with few symptoms. A positive Homans sign may

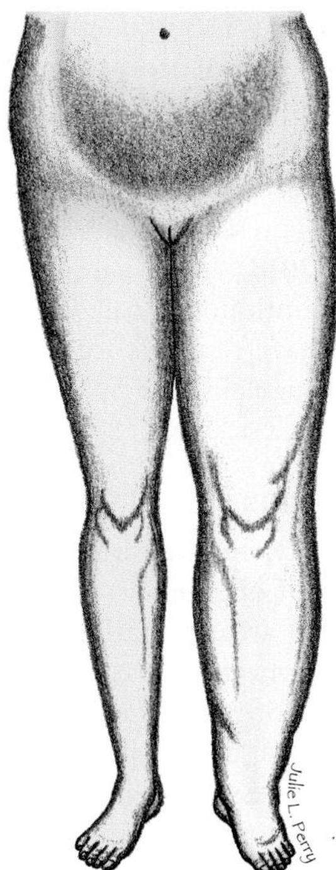

FIG 33-5 Deep venous thrombophlebitis.

be present, but it is usually not performed because more objective tests are needed for diagnosis (Parker & Lockwood, 2012).

Acute pulmonary embolism usually results from dislodged deep vein thrombi. Presenting symptoms are dyspnea and tachypnea (more than 20 breaths/minute). Other signs and symptoms frequently seen include tachycardia (more than 100 beats/minute), apprehension, pleuritic chest pain, cough, hemoptysis, elevated temperature, and syncope (Cunningham et al., 2014; Pettker & Lockwood, 2012).

Physical examination is not a sensitive diagnostic indicator for thrombosis. Venous ultrasonography with or without color Doppler is the most commonly used diagnostic test. MRI and D-dimer assays also may be used (Pettker & Lockwood, 2012). With PE, echocardiographic abnormalities may be seen in right ventricular size or function. Pregnancy limits the usefulness of arterial blood gases and oxygen saturation in diagnosis. A ventilation-perfusion scan, spiral computed tomography scan, magnetic resonance angiography, and pulmonary arteriogram may be used for diagnosis (Pettker & Lockwood).

Medical Management

Superficial venous thrombosis is treated with analgesia (nonsteroidal antiinflammatory agents), rest with elevation of the affected leg, and elastic compression stockings (Cunningham et al., 2014). Heat may also be applied locally.

DVT is initially treated with anticoagulant therapy (usually continuous IV heparin), bed rest with the affected leg elevated, and analgesia. After the symptoms have decreased, the woman may be fitted with elastic compression stockings to wear when she is allowed to ambulate. She is taught how to put on the stockings before getting out of bed. IV heparin therapy continues for 3 to 5 days or until symptoms resolve. Oral anticoagulant therapy (warfarin [Coumadin]) is started during this time and will be continued for about 3 months. In long-term therapy the prothrombin time should be monitored at least monthly in an infant and vitamin K given if necessary (Lawrence & Lawrence, 2011).

Acute PE is an emergent situation that requires prompt treatment. Massive pulmonary emboli can lead to pulmonary hypertension and right ventricular dysfunction; if right ventricular dysfunction is present, mortality can be as high as 25% (Cunningham et al., 2014). Immediate treatment of PE is anticoagulant therapy. Continuous IV heparin therapy is used for PE until symptoms have resolved. Intermittent subcutaneous heparin or oral anticoagulant therapy is often continued for up to 6 months (Pettker & Lockwood, 2012).

Nursing Interventions

In the birthing facility, nursing care of the woman with a thrombosis consists of ongoing assessments: inspecting and palpating the affected area; palpating the peripheral pulses; checking Homans sign; and measuring and comparing leg circumferences. Signs of PE, including chest pain, coughing, dyspnea, and tachypnea, and respiratory status for presence of crackles are also assessed. Laboratory reports are monitored for prothrombin or partial thromboplastin times. The nurse assesses for unusual bleeding. Increased lochia, generalized petechiae, hematuria, or oozing from venipuncture sites should be reported to the provider immediately (James, 2013). In addition, the mother and her family are assessed for their level of understanding about the diagnosis and their ability to cope during the unexpected extended period of recovery.

Interventions include explanations and education about diagnosis and treatment. The woman will need assistance with personal care as long as she is on bed rest; the family should be encouraged to participate in the care if that is what she and they wish. While the woman is on bed rest she should be encouraged to change positions frequently but to avoid placing her knees in a sharply flexed position that could cause pooling of blood in the lower extremities. She also should be cautioned to avoid rubbing the affected area because this action could cause the clot to dislodge. Heparin and warfarin are administered as ordered, and the physician is notified if clotting times are outside the therapeutic level. If the woman is breastfeeding, she is informed that neither heparin nor warfarin is excreted in significant quantities in breast milk (Lawrence & Lawrence, 2011). If the infant has been discharged, the family is encouraged to bring the infant for feedings as permitted by hospital policy; the mother also can express milk to be sent home.

Pain can be managed with a variety of measures. Changing positions, elevating the leg, and applying moist heat may decrease discomfort. It may be necessary to administer analgesics and antiinflammatory medications.

The woman is usually discharged home on oral anticoagulants and will need an explanation of the treatment schedule and possible side effects. If subcutaneous injections are to be given, the woman and family are taught how to administer the medication and about site rotation. They should also be given information about safe care practices to prevent bleeding and injury while she is on anticoagulant therapy (e.g., using a soft toothbrush and an electric razor). She will need information about follow-up with her health care provider to monitor clotting times and regulate the correct dosage of anticoagulant therapy. The woman should also use a reliable form of contraception if taking warfarin because this medication is considered teratogenic (Gilbert, 2011). Oral contraceptives are contraindicated because of the increased risk for thrombosis (Cunningham et al., 2014).

MEDICATION ALERT

Medications containing aspirin are not given to women on anticoagulant therapy because aspirin inhibits synthesis of clotting factors and can lead to prolonged clotting time and increased risk for bleeding.

POSTPARTUM INFECTIONS

Postpartum infection, or *puerperal infection,* is any clinical infection of the genital tract that occurs within 28 days after miscarriage, induced abortion, or birth. The definition used in the United States continues to be the presence of a fever of 38° C (100.4° F) or more on 2 successive days of the first 10 postpartum days (not counting the first 24 hours after birth). In the United States it occurs after approximately 2% of vaginal births and 10% to 15% of cesarean births (Katz, 2012). Other common postpartum infections include wound infections, urinary tract infections (UTIs), and respiratory tract infections. Mastitis, or breast infection, should also be considered as a possible diagnosis among breastfeeding mothers, with symptoms such as fever, malaise, flulike symptoms, and a sore area in a breast (Lawrence & Lawrence, 2011) (Fig. 33-6). (See Chapter 25 for further discussion of mastitis.)

The most common infecting organisms are the numerous streptococcal and anaerobic organisms. *Staphylococcus aureus,* gonococci, coliform bacteria, and clostridia are less common but serious pathogenic organisms that can cause puerperal infection. Postpartum infections are more common in women who have concurrent medical or immunosuppressive conditions or who had a cesarean or other operative birth. Intrapartal factors such as prolonged rupture of membranes, prolonged labor, and intrauterine monitoring of uterine contractions or fetal heart rate and pattern increase the risk for infection (Cunningham

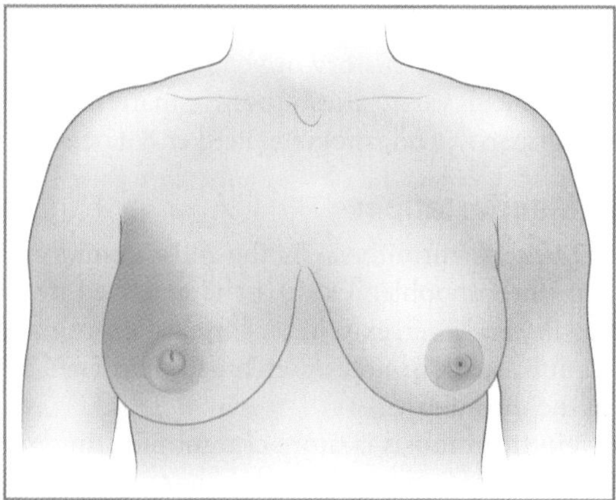

FIG 33-6 Mastitis, right breast, upper quadrant. (In R. K. Creasy, R. Resnik, J. D. Iams, et al. (Eds.), *Creasy and Resnik's maternal-fetal medicine: Principles and practice* (7th ed.). Philadelphia: Saunders.)

et al., 2014). Factors that predispose the woman to postpartum infection are listed in Box 33-3.

Endometritis

Endometritis (infection of the lining of the uterus) is the most common postpartum infection. It usually begins as a localized infection at the placental site (Fig. 33-7) but can spread to the entire endometrium. Incidence is higher after cesarean birth. Signs of endometritis include fever (usually greater than 38° C [100.4° F]), increased pulse, chills, anorexia, nausea, fatigue and lethargy, pelvic pain, uterine tenderness, and foul-smelling, profuse lochia. Leukocytosis and a markedly increased RBC sedimentation rate are typical laboratory findings of postpartum infections. Anemia can also be present. Blood cultures or intracervical or intrauterine bacterial cultures (aerobic and anaerobic) should reveal the offending pathogens within 36 to 48 hours (Cunningham et al., 2014).

Management

Management of endometritis consists of IV broad-spectrum antibiotic therapy (cephalosporins, penicillins, or clindamycin and gentamicin) and supportive care, including hydration, rest, and pain relief. Antibiotic therapy is usually discontinued 24 hours after the woman is asymptomatic. Assessments of lochia, vital signs, and changes in the woman's condition continue during treatment. Comfort measures depend on the symptoms and may include cool compresses, warm blankets, perineal care, and sitz baths. Teaching should include side effects of therapy, prevention of spread of infection, signs and symptoms of worsening condition, adherence to the treatment plan, and the need for follow-up care. Women may need to be encouraged or assisted to maintain mother-infant interactions and breastfeeding.

BOX 33-3 Predisposing Factors for Postpartum Infection

Preconception or Antepartal Factors
- History of previous venous thrombosis, urinary tract infection, mastitis, pneumonia
- Diabetes mellitus
- Alcoholism
- Drug abuse
- Immunosuppression
- Anemia
- Malnutrition

Intrapartal Factors
- Cesarean birth
- Operative vaginal birth
- Prolonged rupture of membranes
- Chorioamnionitis
- Prolonged labor
- Bladder catheterization
- Internal fetal/uterine pressure monitoring
- Multiple vaginal examinations after rupture of membranes
- Epidural analgesia/anesthesia
- Retained placental fragments
- Postpartum hemorrhage
- Episiotomy or lacerations
- Hematomas

Wound Infections

Wound infections are common postpartum infections that often develop after mothers are discharged home. Sites of infection include the cesarean incision and repaired laceration or episiotomy site. Predisposing factors are similar to those for endometritis (see Box 33-3). Signs of wound infection include fever, erythema, edema, warmth, tenderness, pain, seropurulent drainage, and wound separation.

Management

Treatment of wound infections may combine antibiotic therapy with wound debridement. Wounds can be opened and drained. Nursing care includes frequent assessments of the wound and vital signs and wound care. Comfort measures include analgesics, sitz baths, warm compresses, and perineal care. Teaching includes good hygiene techniques (e.g., changing perineal pads front to back, hand hygiene before and after perineal care), self-care measures, and signs of worsening conditions to report to the primary health care provider. The mother is usually discharged to home for self-care or home nursing care after treatment is initiated in the inpatient setting.

Urinary Tract Infections

Urinary tract infections (UTIs) occur in 2% to 4% of postpartum women. Risk factors include urinary catheterization, frequent pelvic examinations, regional (epidural or spinal) anesthesia, genital tract injury, history of UTI, and cesarean birth. Signs and symptoms include dysuria, frequency and urgency, low-grade fever, urinary retention, hematuria, and pyuria. Costovertebral angle tenderness or flank pain can indicate upper UTI. The most common infecting organism is *Escherichia coli*, although other gram-negative aerobic bacilli can cause UTIs.

Management

Medical management for UTIs consists of antibiotic therapy, analgesia, and hydration. Postpartum women are usually treated on an outpatient basis; therefore, teaching should include instructions on how to monitor temperature, bladder function, and appearance of urine. The woman should also be taught about signs of potential complications and the

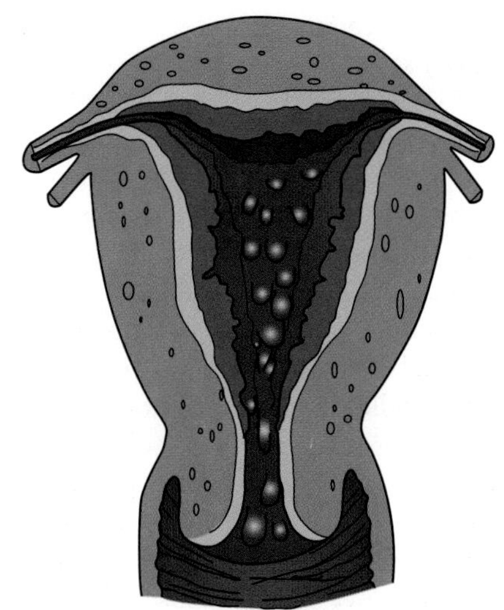

FIG 33-7 Postpartum infection—endometritis.

importance of taking all antibiotics as prescribed. Other suggestions for prevention of UTIs include proper perineal care, wiping from front to back after urinating or having a bowel movement, and increasing fluid intake. Although cranberries and cranberry juice have been widely used for the prevention and treatment of UTIs, the authors of a meta-analysis of 24 studies concluded that the evidence of benefit for drinking cranberry juice to prevent UTIs is small and thus do not recommend it for prevention. Further studies are needed (Jepson, Williams, & Craig, 2012).

CARE MANAGEMENT

Assessment and Nursing Diagnoses

Women who are predisposed to postpartum infection (see Box 33-3) should be assessed carefully. Signs and symptoms associated with postpartum infection were discussed with each infection. Elevation of temperature, redness, and swelling are common signs. The mother may also complain of chills, fever, localized tenderness, or pain. Depending on the type of infection, laboratory tests usually include a complete blood count, venous blood cultures, urine cultures, and uterine tissue cultures. Assessment includes a review of the woman's history, and the laboratory results should be included in the assessment. Nursing diagnoses for women experiencing postpartum infection are listed in Box 33-4.

BOX 33-4 Nursing Diagnoses for Women Experiencing Postpartum Infection

Deficient Knowledge *related to:*
- Cause, management, course of infection
- Transmission and prevention of infection

Impaired Tissue Integrity *related to:*
- Effects of infection process

Acute Pain *related to:*
- Mastitis
- Puerperal infection
- Urinary tract infection

Interrupted Family Processes *related to:*
- Unexpected complication to expected postpartum recovery
- Possible separation from newborn

Risk for Impaired Parenting *related to:*
- Fear of spread of infection to newborn

Interventions

The most effective and least expensive treatment of postpartum infection is prevention. Preventive measures include good prenatal nutrition to reduce risk of anemia and intrapartal hemorrhage. Proper maternal perineal hygiene with thorough hand hygiene is emphasized. Strict adherence to aseptic techniques by all health care personnel caring for women during labor, birth, and the postpartum period is very important. Specific medical, surgical and nursing interventions were discussed with each infection.

Postpartum women are usually discharged to home by 48 hours after birth. This is often before signs of infection are evident. Nurses in birth centers and hospital settings must be able to identify women at risk for postpartum infection and provide anticipatory teaching and counseling before discharge. This teaching should include the signs of infection and when to notify the health care provider. After discharge, telephone follow-up, hotlines, support groups, lactation counselors, home visits by nurses, and teaching materials (videos, written materials) can be used to decrease the risk for postpartum infections. Home care nurses must be able to recognize the signs and symptoms of postpartum infection and then contact the mother's primary health care provider or have her make the contact. Home care nurses must also be able to provide the appropriate nursing care for women who need follow-up care at home.

COMMUNITY ACTIVITY

After giving birth many women are discharged home before an infection can develop. Prepare a "Fact Sheet About Postpartum Infection" that could be distributed to postpartum women on discharge from the hospitals or birth centers in your community. The fact sheet should include a brief summary of the types of common infections, signs and symptoms, ways to help prevent infection, and when to call the health care provider. If your community has a large population of women who do not speak English, consider a fact sheet in Spanish or other language as appropriate.

KEY POINTS

- Postpartum hemorrhage is a major cause of obstetric morbidity and mortality throughout the world and is the leading reason for obstetric intensive care unit admissions.
- Hemorrhagic (hypovolemic) shock is an emergency situation in which the perfusion of body organs can become severely compromised and death can ensue.
- The potential side effects of therapeutic interventions can further compromise the woman with a hemorrhagic disorder.
- Clotting disorders are associated with many obstetric complications.
- Postpartum infection is a major cause of maternal morbidity and mortality throughout the world.
- Postpartum UTIs are common because of trauma experienced during labor.
- Prevention is the most effective and least expensive treatment of postpartum infection.

REFERENCES

Cunningham, F., Leveno, K., Bloom, S., et al. (2014). *Williams obstetrics* (24th ed.). New York: McGraw-Hill.

Francois, K. E., & Foley, M. R. (2012). Antepartum and postpartum hemorrhage. In S. G. Gabbe, J. R. Niebyl, J. L. Simpson, et al. (Eds.), *Obstetrics: Normal and problem pregnancies* (6th ed.). Philadelphia: Saunders.

Gilbert, E. (2011). *Manual of high risk pregnancy & delivery* (5th ed.). St. Louis: Mosby.

James, D. C. (2012). Postpartum care. In K. R. Simpson, & P. A. Creehan (Eds.), *AWHONN's perinatal nursing* (4th ed.). Lippincott Williams & Wilkins.

Jepson, R. G., Williams, G., & Craig, J. C. (2012). Cranberries for preventing urinary tract infections. *The Cochrane Database of Systematic Reviews, 2012, 5*, CD0013321.

Katz, V. (2012). Postpartum care. In S. G. Gabbe, J. R. Niebyl, J. L. Simpson, et al. (Eds.), *Obstetrics: Normal and problem pregnancies* (6th ed.). Philadelphia: Saunders.

Lawrence, R. A., & Lawrence, R. M. (2011). *Breastfeeding: A guide for the medical profession* (7th ed.). St. Louis: Mosby.

Lyndon, A., Lagrew, D., Shields, L., et al. (2010). Improving health care response to obstetric hemorrhage. (California Maternal Quality Care Collaborative Toolkit to Transform Maternity Care). *Stanford, CA: California Maternal Quality Care Collaborative (CMQCC)*. Available at www.cmqcc.org/resource.

Pettker, C. M., & Lockwood, C. J. (2012). Thromboembolic disorders. In S. G. Gabbe, J. R. Niebyl, J. L. Simpson, et al. (Eds.), *Obstetrics: Normal and problem pregnancies* (6th ed.). Philadelphia: Saunders.

Rozance, P. J., & Rosenberg, A. A. (2012). The neonate. In S. G. Gabbe, J. R. Niebyl, J. L. Simpson, et al. (Eds.), *Obstetrics: Normal and problem pregnancies* (6th ed.). Philadelphia: Saunders.

The Joint Commission (2010). *Sentinel event alert, Issue 44: Preventing maternal death.* Available at www.jointcommission.org/sentinel_event_alert_issue_44_preventing_maternal_death.

World Health Organization (2012). *Maternal mortality fact sheet N 348.* Available at www.who.int/mediacentre/factsheets/fs348/en.

34 CHAPTER

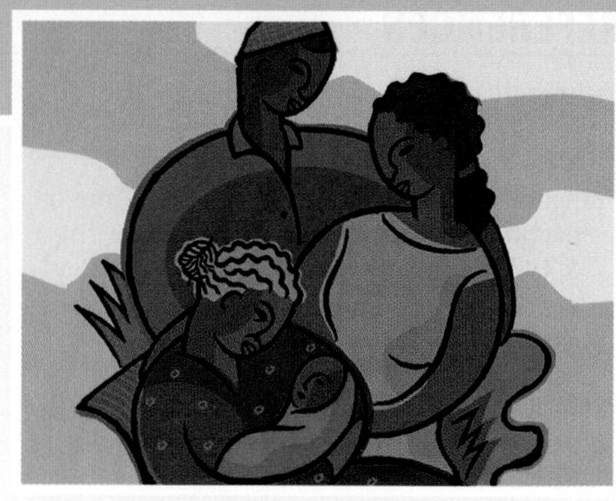

Nursing Care of the High Risk Newborn

Debbie Fraser

http://evolve.elsevier.com/Lowdermilk/MWHC/

LEARNING OBJECTIVES

- Compare characteristics of preterm, late preterm, early term, and postterm neonates.
- Discuss respiratory distress syndrome and the approach to treatment.
- Compare methods of oxygen therapy.
- Analyze appropriate nursing interventions for nutritional care of the preterm infant.
- Discuss the pathophysiology of retinopathy of prematurity, bronchopulmonary dysplasia, patent ductus arteriosus, necrotizing enterocolitis, and intraventricular hemorrhage and the risk factors that predispose preterm infants to these problems.
- Discuss pain assessment and management in the preterm infant.
- Describe the signs and symptoms of perinatal asphyxia.
- Analyze the pathophysiology of meconium aspiration syndrome and its clinical signs.
- Plan developmentally appropriate care for high risk infants.
- Discuss the needs of parents of high risk infants.
- Describe nursing care for late preterm infants and list specific discharge teaching needs for parents of late preterm infants.
- Analyze common problems experienced by small- and large for gestational age infants.
- Evaluate a neonatal transport plan.
- Discuss nursing interventions for families of preterm and high risk infants experiencing anticipatory loss and grief.

Modern technology and expert nursing care have made important contributions to improving the health and overall survival of high risk infants. However, infants who are born considerably before term and survive are particularly susceptible to developing problems related to their preterm birth. These problems can also occur in term and late preterm infants, although not as frequently, and include necrotizing enterocolitis (NEC), bronchopulmonary dysplasia (BPD), intraventricular and periventricular hemorrhage, and retinopathy of prematurity (ROP).

High risk infants are most often classified according to birth weight, gestational age, and predominant pathophysiologic problems (Box 34-1). Intrauterine growth rates differ among infants; factors such as heredity, placental insufficiency, and maternal disease influence intrauterine growth and birth weight. For the high risk infant, an accurate assessment of gestational age (see Chapter 24) is critical in helping the nurse anticipate problems. The response of the preterm, late preterm, or postterm infant to extrauterine life differs from that of the term infant. By understanding the physiologic basis of these differences, the nurse can assess these infants with a keen awareness of the potential problems they are most likely to encounter.

Preterm Infants

The vast majority of high risk infants are those born at less than 37 weeks of gestation: preterm and late preterm infants. The preterm birth rate in the United States showed a fairly steady increase from the early 1980s to 2006. Then, in 2006, the rate began to steadily decline to 11.55% in 2012. The greatest decline (11%) was among late preterm births, which constitute the largest percentage of all preterm births (Martin, Hamilton, Osterman, et al., 2013). This drop may be related to practice-based efforts to reduce elective births prior to 39 weeks of gestation unless there is a medical indication.

At times the nurse is able to anticipate problems, such as when a woman is admitted in preterm labor. At other times the birth of a high risk infant is unanticipated. In either case the personnel and equipment necessary for immediate care of the infant must be available.

Preterm infants are at risk because their organ systems are immature and they lack adequate nutrient reserves. The potential problems and care needs of the preterm infant weighing 2000 g (4.4 lb) differ from those of the term or postterm infant of equal weight. If these infants have physiologic disorders and anomalies as well, they affect the infant's response to treatment. In general, the closer infants are to term in relation to gestational

BOX 34-1 Classification of High Risk Infants

Classification According to Size

Low-birth-weight (LBW) infant: an infant whose birth weight is less than 2500 g (5.5 lb), regardless of gestational age

Very low-birth-weight (VLBW) infant: an infant whose birth weight is less than 1500 g (3.3 lb)

Extremely low-birth-weight (ELBW) infant: an infant whose birth weight is less than 1000 g (2.2 lb)

Appropriate for gestational age (AGA) infant: an infant whose birth weight falls between the 10th and 90th percentiles on intrauterine growth curves

Small for date (SFD) or small for gestational age (SGA) infant: an infant whose rate of intrauterine growth was restricted and whose birth weight falls below the 10th percentile on intrauterine growth curves

Large for gestational age (LGA) infant: an infant whose birth weight falls above the 90th percentile on intrauterine growth curves

Intrauterine growth restriction (IUGR): found in infants whose intrauterine growth is restricted (sometimes used as a more descriptive term for the SGA infant)

Symmetric IUGR: growth restriction in which the weight, length, and head circumference are all affected

Asymmetric IUGR: growth restriction in which the head circumference remains within normal parameters while the birth weight falls below the 10th percentile

Classification According to Gestational Age

- *Preterm (premature):* an infant born before completion of 37 weeks of gestation
- *Late preterm:* an infant born from 34 0/7 through 36 6/7 weeks of gestation
- *Early term:* an infant born from 37 0/7 through 38 6/7 weeks of gestation
- *Full term:* an infant born from 39 0/7 weeks through 40 6/7 weeks of gestation
- *Late term:* an infant born from 41 0/7 through 41 6/7 weeks of gestation
- *Postterm (postmature):* an infant born after 42 weeks of gestation,

Data from American Academy of Pediatrics (AAP) & American College of Obstetricians and Gynecologists (ACOG). (2012). *Guidelines for perinatal care* (7th ed.). Elk Grove Village, IL: Author; American College of Obstetricians and Gynecologists (ACOG). 2013. Committee opinion no. 579: Definition of term pregnancy. *Obstetrics and Gynecology, 122*(5), 1139-1140.

age and birth weight, the easier their adjustment to the external environment.

Preterm, low-birth-weight (LBW), and extremely low-birth-weight (ELBW) infants often require hospitalization beyond the typical 48 hours after birth. Their physiologic immaturity and associated problems can require extensive use of technologic and pharmacologic interventions. The cost of the care of preterm and LBW infants is estimated to be billions of dollars each year and continues to rise as the use of technology increases.

Varying opinions exist about the practical and ethical dimensions of resuscitation of extremely low-birth-weight (ELBW) infants (those infants whose birth weight is 1000 g [2.2 lb] or less). Ethical issues associated with resuscitation of such infants include:

- Should resuscitation be attempted and to what extent should it be continued?
- Who should decide?
- Is the cost of resuscitation justified?
- Do the benefits of technology outweigh the burdens in relation to the quality of life?

Everyone involved (health care providers, nurses, parents, ethicists, clergy, attorneys, etc.) should participate in discussions addressing these controversial questions. Although there are no clear answers, such discussions help clarify the issues and promote family-centered approaches to care. That care can involve sustaining life or providing care and support for a peaceful death. Nurses are key to the care of these infants and their families.

Physiologic Functions

Respiratory Function. The preterm infant is likely to have difficulty making the pulmonary transition from intrauterine to extrauterine life. Numerous problems can affect the respiratory systems of preterm infants:

- Decreased number of functional alveoli
- Deficient surfactant levels
- Smaller lumen in the respiratory system
- Greater collapsibility or obstruction of respiratory passages
- Insufficient calcification of the bony thorax
- Weak or absent gag reflex
- Immature and friable capillaries in the lungs
- Greater distance between functional alveoli and the capillary bed

In combination, these deficits have the potential to severely hinder the preterm infant's respiratory efforts and can produce respiratory distress or apnea. Nurses must be alert to signs of respiratory distress or apnea and ready to intervene to promote adequate oxygenation.

Respiratory difficulty often follows a progressive pattern. Infants normally breathe between 30 and 60 breaths/minute, relying significantly on their abdominal muscles to accomplish this. However, the respiratory rate can increase without a change in rhythm. Early signs of respiratory distress include flaring of the nares and an expiratory grunt. Depending on the cause, retractions can begin as subcostal, suprasternal, or intercostal. If the infant shows increasing respiratory effort (e.g., seesaw breathing patterns, retractions, flaring of the nares, expiratory grunting, and/or apneic spells), this indicates deepening distress. A compromised infant's color progresses from pink to circumoral cyanosis and then to generalized cyanosis.

! NURSING ALERT

Acrocyanosis is a normal finding in the neonate, but central cyanosis indicates an underlying problem that requires immediate evaluation.

Periodic breathing is a respiratory pattern commonly seen in preterm infants. Such infants exhibit 5- to 10-second respiratory pauses followed by 10 to 15 seconds of compensatory rapid respirations. Such periodic breathing should not be confused with *apnea,* which is a 20-second or greater cessation of respiration, or a shorter pause accompanied by bradycardia, cyanosis, or hypotonia (Alvaro, 2012).

Cardiovascular Function. Evaluation of heart rate and rhythm, skin color, blood pressure, perfusion, pulses, oxygen saturation, and acid-base status provides information on cardiovascular status. The nurse must be prepared to intervene if symptoms of hypovolemia, shock, or both are found. These symptoms include hypotension, slow capillary refill (>3 seconds), and continued respiratory distress despite the provision of oxygen and ventilation.

An accurate and timely blood pressure (BP) reading can assist in making an early diagnosis of cardiorespiratory disease and in monitoring the effects of fluid therapy. BP is monitored routinely in the sick neonate by internal or external means. Direct recording with arterial catheters is often used but carries the risks inherent in any procedure in which a catheter is introduced into an artery. An umbilical venous catheter can also be used to monitor the neonate's central venous pressure. Oscillometry (Dinamap) is a noninvasive, effective means for detecting alterations in systemic BP (hypotension or hypertension) and for identifying the need to implement appropriate therapy to maintain cardiovascular function.

Maintaining Body Temperature. Preterm infants are susceptible to temperature instability as a result of numerous factors. Because of their large body surface in relation to their weight, preterm infants are at high risk for heat loss. Other factors that place preterm infants at risk for temperature instability include:

- Minimal insulating subcutaneous fat
- Limited stores of brown fat (an internal source for the generation of heat present in normal term infants)
- Fragile capillaries
- Decreased or absent reflex control of skin capillaries (shiver response)
- Inadequate muscle mass activity (rendering the preterm infant unable to produce his or her own heat)
- Poor muscle tone, resulting in more body surface area being exposed to the cooling effects of the environment
- An immature temperature regulation center in the brain

The goal of thermoregulation is to create a *neutral thermal environment* (NTE), which is the environmental temperature at which oxygen consumption is minimal but adequate to maintain body temperature (Blackburn, 2013). With the knowledge of the four mechanisms of heat transfer (convection, conduction, radiation, and evaporation), the nurse can create an environment for the preterm infant that prevents temperature instability (see Chapter 24). The infant is kept in a radiant warmer bed or in an incubator with control settings to maintain an NTE. Because the preterm infant has few reserves in terms of calories and fat stores, cold sensitivity is a problem. This infant can easily lose heat and develop hypothermia. Physiologically the infant tries to conserve heat and burns more calories, causing the metabolic system to go into overdrive, further stressing the already compromised neonate. This is known as *cold stress.*

A critical nursing role is to prevent or minimize hypothermia and cold stress (see Fig. 23-2) by recognizing the risk factors and using intervention strategies to prevent and treat such stress. Signs of hypothermia and cold stress are listed in Box 34-2.

The nurse should attempt to prevent hyperthermia. Given that overheating produces an increase in oxygen and calorie consumption, the infant is also jeopardized if he or she becomes hyperthermic. The preterm infant is not able to sweat and thus dissipate heat. Overheating can lead to apnea, tachycardia, and eventually bradycardia, as well as consumption of calories that the preterm infant cannot afford to expend (see Box 34-2).

BOX 34-2 Signs of Hypothermia and Hyperthermia

Hypothermia (Cold Stress)

Apnea
Bradycardia
Central cyanosis
Coagulation defects (i.e., pulmonary hemorrhage)
Hypoglycemia
Hypotonia
Hypoxia
Feeding intolerance (abdominal distention, emesis, increased residuals)
Increased metabolic rate
Irritability
Lethargy
Metabolic acidosis
Peripheral vasoconstriction (persistent pulmonary hypertension of the newborn)
Poor weight gain (chronic hypothermia)
Shivering (mature infants in presence of severe hypothermia)
Weak cry or suck

Hyperthermia

Apnea
Central nervous system depression
Dehydration (increased insensible water loss)
Flushed/red skin
Hypernatremia
Irritability
Lethargy
Poor feeding
Seizures
Sweating
Tachycardia
Tachypnea
Warm to touch
Weak or absent cry

Data from Blackburn, S. (2013). *Maternal, fetal, and neonatal physiology: A clinical perspective* (4th ed.). Maryland Heights, MO: Saunders; Brown, V.D., & Landers, S. (2011). Heat balance. In S.L. Gardner, B.S. Carter, M. Enzman-Hines, & J.A. Hernandez (Eds.), *Merenstein & Gardner's handbook of neonatal intensive care* (7th ed.). St. Louis: Mosby.

Central Nervous System Function. The preterm infant's central nervous system (CNS) is susceptible to injury as a result of:

- Birth trauma with damage to immature structures
- Bleeding from fragile capillaries
- An impaired coagulation process, including prolonged prothrombin time
- Recurrent hypoxic and hyperoxic episodes
- Predisposition to hypoglycemia
- Fluctuating systemic BP with concomitant variation in cerebral blood flow and pressure

In the preterm neonate, neurologic function is dependent on gestational age, associated illness factors, and predisposing factors such as intrauterine asphyxia that can cause neurologic damage. Clinical signs of neurologic dysfunction can be subtle, nonspecific, or specific. Five categories of clinical manifestations should be thoroughly evaluated in the preterm infant: seizure activity, hyperirritability, CNS depression, increased intracranial pressure (ICP), and abnormal movements such as decorticate posturing. Primary and tendon reflexes are generally present in preterm infants by 28 weeks of gestation; evaluation of these reflexes should be part of the neurologic examination (see Table 23-4).

The developing nervous system has the ability to reorganize neural connection after injury, meaning that some injuries that would be permanent in adults are not so in infants. Certain neurologic signs appear to be predictive of later abnormalities. These signs include hypotonia, decreased level of activity, weak cry for more than 24 hours, and inability to coordinate suck and swallow. Ongoing assessment and documentation of these neurologic signs are needed for the purpose of discharge teaching and making follow-up recommendations, as well as for their predictive value.

Maintaining Adequate Nutrition. The goal of neonatal nutrition is to promote normal growth and development. However, maintaining adequate nutrition in the preterm infant is complicated by problems with intake and metabolism. Based on the gestational age, the preterm infant often has the following disadvantages with regard to intake: weak or absent suck, swallow, and gag reflexes; difficulty coordinating sucking, swallowing, and breathing; small stomach capacity; and weak abdominal muscles. The preterm infant's metabolic functions are compromised by a limited store of nutrients, a decreased ability to digest proteins or absorb nutrients, and immature enzyme systems.

The nurse must continually assess the infant's ability to consume and digest nutrients. Some preterm infants require gavage or intravenous (IV) feedings instead of oral feedings. An area of research that holds promise for preterm infants is use of minimal enteral nutrition (MEN) that can provide only 1 ml/hr (Anderson, Wood, Keller, & Hay, 2011; de Curtis & Rigo, 2012). These feedings stimulate the gastrointestinal (GI) system with minute amounts of breast milk or formula, usually given via gavage, so that when enteral feedings of greater volume can begin, the GI system is primed for nutrient absorption. They also may help to protect LBW infants from sepsis (Örs, 2013).

Maintaining Renal Function. The preterm infant's immature renal system is unable to adequately excrete metabolites and drugs, concentrate urine, or maintain acid-base, fluid, or electrolyte balance. Therefore, intake and output, as well as specific gravity, must be assessed. Laboratory tests are done to determine acid-base and electrolyte balance. Medication levels are monitored in preterm infants because certain medications can overwhelm the immature system's ability to excrete them.

Maintaining Hematologic Status. The preterm infant is predisposed to hematologic problems because of:

- Increased capillary fragility
- Increased tendency to bleed (prolonged prothrombin time and partial thromboplastin time)
- Slowed production of red blood cells resulting from rapid decrease in erythropoiesis after birth
- Loss of blood due to frequent blood sampling for laboratory tests
- Decreased red blood cell survival related to the relatively larger size of the red blood cell and its increased permeability to sodium and potassium

The nurse assesses such infants for any evidence of bleeding from puncture sites and the GI tract. Infants are examined for signs of anemia (decreased hemoglobin and hematocrit levels, pale skin, increased apnea, lethargy, tachycardia, and poor weight gain). The amount of blood drawn for laboratory testing is closely monitored and recorded.

Resisting Infection. Preterm infants are at increased risk for infection because they have a shortage of stored maternal immunoglobulins, an impaired ability to make antibodies, and a compromised integumentary system (thin skin and fragile capillaries). Preterm infants exhibit various nonspecific signs and symptoms of infection (Box 34-3). Early identification and treatment of sepsis are essential (see Chapter 35). As with all aspects of care, strict attention to hand hygiene is the single most important measure to prevent health care–acquired infections.

BOX 34-3 Signs and Symptoms of Infection

Temperature instability
- Hypothermia
- Hyperthermia

Central nervous system changes
- Lethargy
- Irritability

Changes in color
- Cyanosis, pallor
- Jaundice

Cardiovascular instability
- Poor perfusion
- Hypotension
- Bradycardia/tachycardia

Respiratory distress
- Tachypnea
- Apnea
- Retractions, nasal flaring, grunting

Gastrointestinal problems
- Feeding intolerance
- Vomiting
- Diarrhea
- Glucose instability

Metabolic acidosis

Data from Bodin, M.B. (2014). Immune system. In C. Kenner, & J.W. Lott (Eds.), *Comprehensive neonatal care* (5th ed.). New York: Springer; Edwards, M.S. (2011). Postnatal bacterial infections. In R.J. Martin, A.A. Fanaroff, & M.C. Walsh (Eds.), *Fanaroff & Martin's neonatal-perinatal medicine: Diseases of the fetus and infant* (9th ed.). St. Louis: Mosby.

Growth and Development Potential. Although it is impossible to predict with complete accuracy the growth and development potential of each preterm infant, some findings support an anticipated favorable outcome in the absence of ongoing medical problems that can affect growth, such as BPD, NEC, and CNS problems. The lower the birth weight, the greater the likelihood the infant will experience negative outcomes.

The age of a preterm newborn is corrected by adding the gestational age and the postnatal age. For example, an infant born 4 weeks ago at 32 weeks of gestation would now be considered

36 weeks of age. The infant's corrected age at 6 months after the birth date is then 4 months, and the infant's responses are accordingly evaluated against the norm expected for a 4-month-old. The growth and development milestones (e.g., motor milestones, vocalization, growth) are corrected for gestational age until the child is approximately 2½ years old.

Certain measurable factors predict normal growth and development. The preterm infant experiences catch-up body growth during the first 2 years of life; this is most likely to occur when the infant has a normal birth length (Kliegman, 2011). The head is the first to experience catch-up growth, followed by a gain in weight and height. At the infant's discharge from the hospital, which usually occurs between 36 and 40 weeks of postconception age, the infant should exhibit:

- An ability to raise the head when prone and to hold the head parallel with the body when tested for the head-lag response
- An ability to cry vigorously when hungry
- An appropriate amount and pattern of weight gain according to growth curves
- Neurologic responses appropriate for corrected age

At 39 to 40 weeks of corrected age, the infant should be able to focus on the examiner's or parent's face and to follow with his or her eyes.

Very low-birth-weight (VLBW) (<1500 g [3.3 lb]) survivors are at high risk for neurologic and cognitive disabilities in varying degrees of severity; these include cerebral palsy, borderline intelligence, and learning disabilities (Daily, Carter, & Carter, 2011). Ongoing research focuses on examining other factors including environmental ones that can cause adverse cognitive and neurodevelopmental outcomes for VLBW and ELBW babies as they grow and develop.

CARE MANAGEMENT

The goal of care for the preterm infant is to promote normal growth and development by providing an extrauterine environment that approximates the healthy intrauterine environment. A multidisciplinary team of physicians, nurses, nurse practitioners, infant developmental specialists, and respiratory therapists collaborates to provide the intensive care needed.

The admission of a preterm newborn to the intensive care nursery is usually an emergent situation. A rapid initial evaluation determines the infant's need for lifesaving treatment. Resuscitation is started in the birthing unit, and the newborn's needs for warmth and oxygen are provided for during transfer to the nursery.

Nursing care is focused on the continual assessment and analysis of the infant's physiologic status. Nursing diagnoses and expected outcomes of care such as those in the Nursing Care Plan for the High Risk Infant are identified (see Nursing Care Plan and Clinical Reasoning Case Study). Nurses fulfill many roles in providing the intensive and extended care that these infants require. In addition, they are the support persons and teachers during the first phase of the parents' adjustment to the birth of their preterm infant. Interventions for specific aspects of care including nursing actions are discussed in the following sections.

NURSING CARE PLAN

The High Risk Preterm Newborn

NURSING DIAGNOSIS	EXPECTED OUTCOME	NURSING INTERVENTIONS	RATIONALES
Ineffective Breathing Pattern related to pulmonary and neuromuscular immaturity, decreased energy, fatigue	Infant exhibits adequate oxygenation (i.e., arterial blood gases [ABGs] and acid-base within normal limits [WNL]; oxygen saturation 92% or greater; respiratory rate and pattern WNL; breath sounds clear; absence of grunting and nasal flaring, minimal retractions, skin color WNL).	Position neonate prone or supine, avoiding neck hyperextension.	To promote optimum air exchange. Use a side-lying position after feeding or in cases of excessive mucus production to avoid aspiration.
		Avoid Trendelenburg position.	Can cause increased intracranial pressure and reduce lung capacity
		Suction nasopharynx, trachea, and endotracheal tube as indicated.	To remove mucus
		Avoid oversuctioning.	Can cause bronchospasm, bradycardia, and hypoxia and predispose neonate to intraventricular hemorrhage
		Administer oxygen and monitor neonatal response.	To maintain oxygen saturation
		Maintain a neutral thermal environment.	To conserve oxygen use
		Monitor arterial blood gases, acid-base balance, oxygen saturation, respiratory rate and pattern, breath sounds, and airway patency; observe for grunting, nasal flaring, retractions, and cyanosis.	To detect signs of respiratory distress

NURSING CARE PLAN—cont'd

The High Risk Preterm Newborn

NURSING DIAGNOSIS	EXPECTED OUTCOME	NURSING INTERVENTIONS	RATIONALES
Ineffective Thermoregulation related to immature temperature regulation and minimal subcutaneous fat stores	Infant maintains stable body temperature within normal range for postconceptional age (36.5° to 37.2° C [97.7° to 99° F).	Place neonate in a prewarmed radiant warmer.	To maintain stable temperature
		Place temperature probe on neonatal abdomen.	To control heat levels in radiant warmer
		Take axillary temperature periodically.	To monitor temperature and cross-check functioning of warmer unit
		Avoid infant exposure to cool air and drafts, cold scales, cold stethoscopes, cold examination tables, and prolonged bathing.	To prevent heat loss
		Monitor probe frequently.	Detachment can cause overheating or warmer-induced hyperthermia.
		Transfer infant to a servo-controlled open warmer bed or incubator.	When temperature has stabilized
Risk for Infection related to immature immune system	Infant exhibits no evidence of health-care acquired infection.	Institute scrupulous hand hygiene techniques before and after handling neonate, ensure all supplies and/or equipment are clean before use, and ensure strict aseptic technique with invasive procedures.	To minimize exposure to infective organisms
		Prevent contact with individuals who have communicable infections, and instruct parents in infection-control procedures.	To minimize infection risk
		Administer prescribed antibiotics.	To provide coverage for infection during sepsis workup
		Continually monitor vital signs for stability.	Instability, hypothermia, or prolonged temperature elevations serve as indicators for infection.
Risk for Imbalanced Nutrition: Less Than Body Requirements related to inability to ingest nutrients secondary to immaturity	Infant receives adequate amount of nutrients with sufficient caloric intake to maintain positive nitrogen balance; demonstrates steady weight gain.	Administer parenteral fluid/total parenteral nutrition (TPN) as prescribed.	To provide adequate nutrition and fluid intake
		Monitor for signs of intolerance to TPN.	Can interfere with effective replenishment of nutrients
		Periodically assess readiness for oral feeding (i.e., strong suck, swallow, and gag reflexes).	To provide appropriate transition from TPN to oral feeding as soon as neonate is ready
		Advance volume and concentration of formula when orally feeding per unit protocol.	To avoid overfeeding and feeding intolerance
		If mother desires to breastfeed, demonstrate how to express milk.	To establish and maintain lactation until infant can breastfeed
Risk for Deficient Fluid Volume/Excess Fluid Volume related to immature physiology	Infant exhibits evidence of fluid homeostasis.	Administer parenteral fluids as prescribed and regulate carefully.	To maintain fluid balance
		Avoid hypertonic fluids such as undiluted medications, and concentrated glucose.	To prevent excess solute load on immature kidneys
		Implement strategies (e.g., use of plastic covers and increase of ambient humidity).	To minimize insensible water loss
		Monitor hydration status (i.e., skin turgor, blood pressure, edema, weight, mucous membranes, fontanels, urine specific gravity, electrolytes) and intake and output.	To evaluate for evidence of dehydration or overhydration

Continued

NURSING CARE PLAN—cont'd

The High Risk Preterm Newborn

NURSING DIAGNOSIS	EXPECTED OUTCOME	NURSING INTERVENTIONS	RATIONALES
Risk for Impaired Skin Integrity related to immature skin structure, immobility, or invasive procedures	Infant's skin remains intact, with no evidence of irritation or injury.	Cleanse skin as needed with plain warm water and apply moisturizing agents to skin.	To maintain the skin's acid mantle
		When performing procedures, minimize use of tape and apply a skin barrier between tape and skin; use transparent elastic film for securing central and peripheral lines; use limb electrodes for monitoring or attach with hydrogel and rotate electrodes frequently; remove adhesives with soap and water rather than alcohol or acetone-based adhesive removers.	To minimize skin damage
		Monitor use of thermal devices such as warmers or heating pads carefully.	To prevent burns
		Monitor skin closely for evidence of redness, rash, irritation, bruising, breakdown, ischemia, and infiltration.	To detect and treat potential complications early
Risk for Injury related to increased intracranial pressure (ICP) and intraventricular hemorrhage secondary to immature central nervous system	Infant will exhibit normal ICP with no evidence of intraventricular hemorrhage.	Institute minimum stimulation protocol (i.e., minimal handling, clustering care techniques, avoidance of sudden head movements to one side, undisturbed sleep periods, light variations to simulate day and night, limiting personnel and equipment noise in environment).	To decrease stress responses, which can increase ICP
		Institute ordered pharmacologic and nonpharmacologic pain control methods.	To manage pain and reduce physical stress
		Avoid hypertonic solutions and medications.	To increase cerebral blood flow
		Elevate head of bed 15 to 20 degrees.	To decrease ICP
		Monitor vital signs.	To assess for evidence of ICP
		Recognize signs of overstimulation (i.e., flaccidity, yawning, irritability, crying, staring, active averting).	To stop stimulation to allow rest
Impaired Parenting related to separation and interruption of parent/infant attachment secondary to premature birth	Parents establish contact with neonate; demonstrate competent parenting skills and willingness to care for neonate.	Before parents' first visit to the NICU, prepare them by explaining the neonate's appearance, and the surrounding equipment and its function.	To diminish fear and decrease sense of shock
		Keep parents informed about infant's condition (improvements and setbacks) and important aspects of infant's care; encourage and answer parental questions; actively listen to parents' concerns.	To establish trust, open communication, and caring atmosphere to aid in coping
		Encourage parents to visit the NICU often; to name infant (if that is culturally appropriate); to touch, hold, or caress infant as physical condition permits; to be actively involved in infant's care; and to bring personal items (i.e., clothing, stuffed animals, or pictures of family).	To allow for formation of emotional bond
		Reinforce parents' involvement and praise care endeavors.	To increase self-confidence in their contribution
		Encourage parents to bring other siblings to visit; explain to siblings what they are seeing; encourage siblings to draw pictures or write letters for infant and place in or near infant's crib.	To promote family involvement, help ease sibling fears, and let them contribute to infant's care
		Refer parents to social services as needed.	To ensure comprehensive care
Grieving related to perceived loss of premature infant	Parents express feelings about the potential loss and seek support from staff, family, clergy, and other support systems.	Encourage parents to express feelings about perceived loss of infant.	To reinforce reality and help alleviate guilt
		Encourage parents to use family, friends, clergy, and other support people.	To enhance coping ability
		Plan time on each shift to sit and listen to parents.	To demonstrate concern, empathy, and support
		Inform parents about support groups in the facility and the community.	To encourage parents to use available resources

NICU, Neonatal intensive care unit.

CLINICAL REASONING CASE STUDY

The Preterm Infant

A 1400-g (3-lb) female infant is born at an estimated gestational age of 33 weeks. The parents are very excited about this birth because they have been trying to become pregnant for 6 years. They name the baby Anna. After a brief visit with her parents, Anna is taken to the special care nursery for observation. She is placed on an open-bed warmer to maintain her temperature and is placed on a pulse oximeter and a cardiorespiratory monitor. Anna's oxygen levels are good in room air and she does not require any respiratory support.

1. Evidence—What kinds of initial complications might be expected in an infant born at 33 weeks of gestation?
2. Assumptions—What assumptions can be made about the following?
   a. Anna's expected progress
   b. The possibility of Anna being able to be held by her parents and breastfed
   c. The length of time Anna might be hospitalized
3. What implications and priorities for nursing care can be drawn at this time?
4. Does the evidence objectively support your conclusion?

The nurse uses many technologic support systems to monitor the body responses and maintain the body functions of the infant. Technical skill must be combined with a gentle touch and concern about the traumatic effects of harsh lighting and loud machinery noise. Provision of individualized behavioral and environmental care has been shown to reduce infant stress, conserve energy, and promote better neurobehavioral outcomes (Gardner & Goldson, 2011).

Physical Care

The environmental support measures for the preterm infant typically consist of the following equipment and procedures:

- An incubator or radiant warmer to control body temperature
- Oxygen administration, depending on the infant's cardiopulmonary and circulatory status
- Electronic monitors as needed for the ongoing assessment of respiratory and cardiac functions
- Assistive devices for positioning the infant in neutral flexion and with boundaries
- Clustering of care and minimization of stimulation according to infant cues

Various metabolic support measures that can be instituted consist of the following:

- Parenteral fluids to help support nutrition and maintain normal arterial blood gas (ABG) levels and acid-base balance
- IV access to facilitate the administration of antibiotic therapy if sepsis is a concern
- Blood work to monitor ABG levels, pH, blood glucose levels, electrolytes, and the status of blood cultures

Maintaining Body Temperature

The high risk infant is susceptible to heat loss and its complications. In addition, LBW infants can be unable to increase their metabolic rate because of impaired gas exchange, caloric intake restrictions, or poor thermoregulation. Transepidermal water loss is greater because of skin immaturity in very preterm infants (those at less than 28 weeks of gestation) and can contribute to temperature instability.

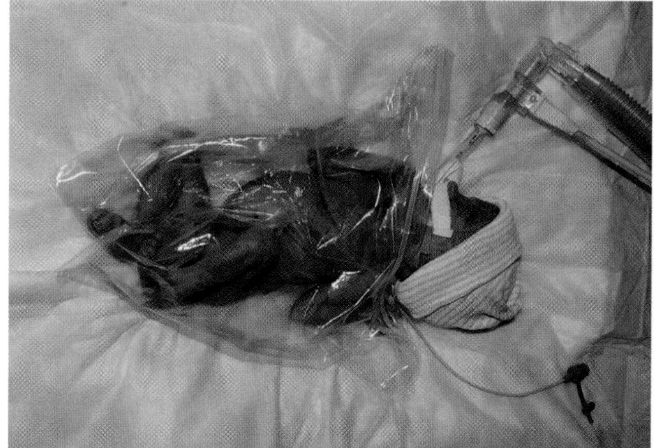

FIG 34-1 Preterm infant in polyethylene bag to protect against heat loss. (Courtesy Cheryl Briggs, RNC, Annapolis, MD.)

The preterm infant should be transferred from the birthing room in a prewarmed incubator; ELBW infants can be placed in a polyethylene bag to decrease heat and water loss (Fig. 34-1). Skin-to-skin contact (kangaroo care) between the stable preterm infant and parent is a viable option for interaction because of the maintenance of appropriate body temperature by the infant (see later in this chapter for further discussion of kangaroo care).

High risk infants are cared for in the thermoneutral environment created by use of an external heat source. A probe to an external heat source supplied by a radiant warmer or a servo-controlled incubator is attached to the infant. The infant acts as a thermostat to regulate the amount of heat supplied by the external source. This idealized environment maintains an infant's normal body temperature between 36.5° and 37.2° C (97.9° F and 99° F). Maintaining a thermoneutral condition in the youngest, most immature infants decreases the need for them to generate additional heat, increasing physiologic stability and decreasing oxygen consumption (Blackburn, 2013; Brown & Landers, 2011).

Care of the Hypothermic Infant. The hypothermic infant can appear pale and mottled; the skin is cool to touch, especially the extremities. Acrocyanosis and respiratory distress can occur as oxygen consumption increases in an effort to generate heat. As hypothermia worsens, the infant can have apnea, bradycardia, and central cyanosis.

When an infant becomes hypothermic, rewarming should begin immediately by providing external heat. However, rapid changes in body temperature can cause apnea and acidosis. For the infant with mild hypothermia, slow rewarming is recommended. External heat sources should be slightly warmer than skin temperature and increased gradually until the infant's temperature is within the range of NTE. For the severely hypothermic infant (body temperature less than 35° C [95° F]), more rapid rewarming is needed. Use of radiant heaters or heated water mattresses helps prevent prolonged metabolic acidosis and hypoglycemia and reduces mortality (Brown & Landers, 2011).

Respiratory Care

Oxygen Therapy. Clinical criteria that indicate the need for oxygen administration include increased respiratory effort, respiratory distress with apnea, tachycardia, bradycardia, and central cyanosis with or without hypotonia. The need for oxygen should be substantiated by biochemical data (arterial oxygen pressure [Pao_2] of less than 60 mm Hg or an oxygen saturation of less than 92%).

Oxygen administered to an infant is warmed and humidified to prevent cold stress and drying of the respiratory mucosa. During the administration of oxygen, the concentration, volume, temperature, and humidity of the gas are carefully controlled. Delivery of oxygen for more than a few minutes requires the use of special equipment (hood, nasal cannula, positive-pressure mask, or endotracheal tube) because the concentration of free-flow oxygen cannot be monitored accurately. Free-flow oxygen into an incubator should not be used because the concentration fluctuates dramatically each time the doors or portholes are opened. The indiscriminate use of oxygen can be hazardous. Possible complications of oxygen therapy include ROP and BPD.

Infants who need oxygen should have their respiratory status assessed at least hourly. This includes a continuous pulse oximetry reading and at least one blood gas measurement. There should also be hourly documentation of pulse oximetry readings as well as the amount of oxygen being administered and the mode of delivery (Gardner, Enzman-Hines, & Dickey, 2011b). Necessary interventions are then determined on the basis of the clinical assessment findings. The interventions ordered are those that can directly manage the underlying disease process and range from hood oxygen administration to ventilator therapy.

Neonatal Resuscitation. In 2010 the American Heart Association (AHA) published neonatal resuscitation guidelines (AHA, 2010). A rapid assessment of infants can identify those who do not require resuscitation: those born at term gestation, with no evidence of meconium or infection in the amniotic fluid; those who are breathing or crying; and those with good muscle tone. If any of these characteristics is absent, the infant should receive the following actions in sequence: (1) initial steps in stabilization: provide warmth by placing the baby under a radiant warmer, position the head to open the airway, clear the airway with a bulb syringe or suction catheter, dry the baby, stimulate breathing, and reposition the baby; (2) ventilation; (3) chest compressions; and (4) administration of epinephrine or volume expansion or both. The decision to move from one category of action to the next is based on the assessment of respirations, heart rate, and color. Rapid decision making is imperative; 30 seconds are allotted for each step. The condition of the infant is reevaluated and the decision made whether to progress to the next step (see Fig. 24-1).

Resuscitation of asphyxiated newborns with 21% oxygen (room air) rather than 100% oxygen is recommended (AHA, 2010). Proponents for room air resuscitation suggest that fewer complications are associated with oxidative stress and hyperoxemia when room air is administered. The 2010 AHA resuscitation standards for neonatal resuscitation indicate that if the infant's condition does not improve within 90 seconds, supplemental oxygen should be provided. The amount of oxygen to use should be determined by the infant's oxygen saturation level and age in minutes. The stated goal is to minimize oxygen free radicals by preventing hyperoxia using supplemental oxygen at levels less than 100% (AHA). A review of several studies indicates that neonatal mortality is reduced by 4% to 5% when room air instead of 100% oxygen is used for neonatal resuscitation (Harach, 2013). Fluctuations in oxygen saturation are also deemed harmful. Experts recommend that oxygen saturations for ELBW infants are maintained between 88% and 93% but definitely not exceeding 95% (Botet, Figueras-Aloy, Miracle-Echegoyen, et al., 2012).

Hood Therapy. A hood can be used to administer oxygen to infants who do not require mechanical pressure support. The hood is a clear plastic cover sized to fit over the head and neck of the infant (Fig. 34-2, *A*). Inside the hood the infant receives a controlled amount of oxygen. The nurse checks the oxygen level at least every hour because the concentration must be adjusted in response to the infant's condition. If the hood is removed for holding, feeding, or suctioning, an alternative source of oxygen must be provided (Gardner et al., 2011b).

Nasal Cannula. Infants requiring low-flow amounts of oxygen can benefit from the use of a nasal cannula (see Fig. 34-2, *B*). These work well for older infants who are recuperating but still require supplemental oxygen. They are the preferred method for home oxygen administration. Nasal cannulas permit the infant to receive an adequate, continuous flow of oxygen while allowing optimal vision, positioning, and parental holding. Infants can breastfeed or bottle feed while receiving oxygen by this method. Nasal cannulas come in various sizes; proper fit is important. The nasal prongs must be inspected and cleaned frequently to make sure they are not partially obstructed by milk or secretions.

Continuous Positive Airway Pressure Therapy. Infants who are unable to maintain an adequate Pao_2 despite the administration

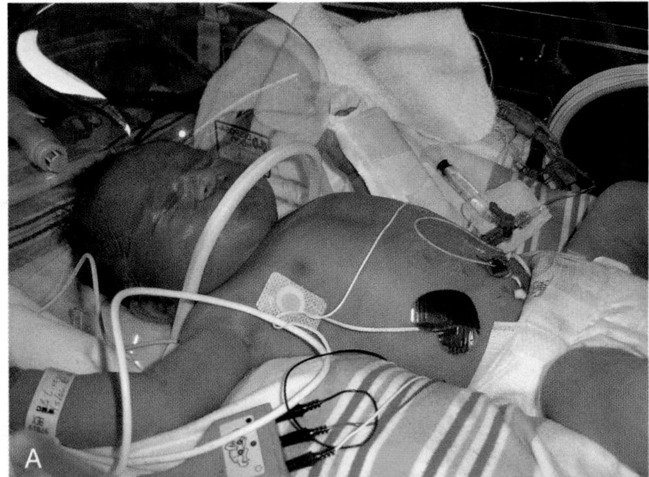

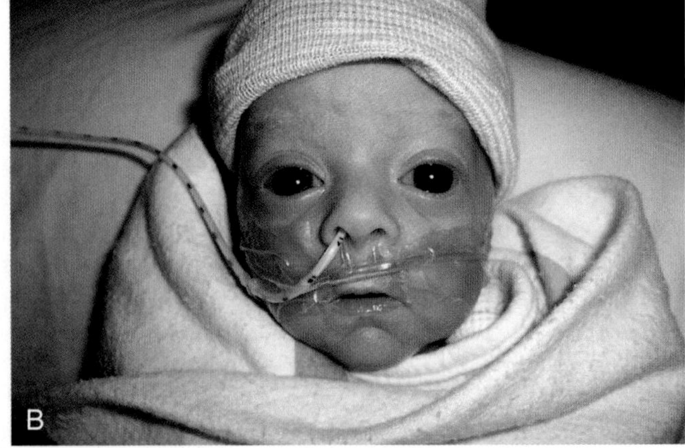

FIG 34-2 A, Infant under oxygen hood. B, Infant with nasal cannula. (A, Courtesy Lauren and Brian LiVecchi, Raleigh, NC; B, courtesy Cheryl Briggs, RNC, Annapolis, MD.)

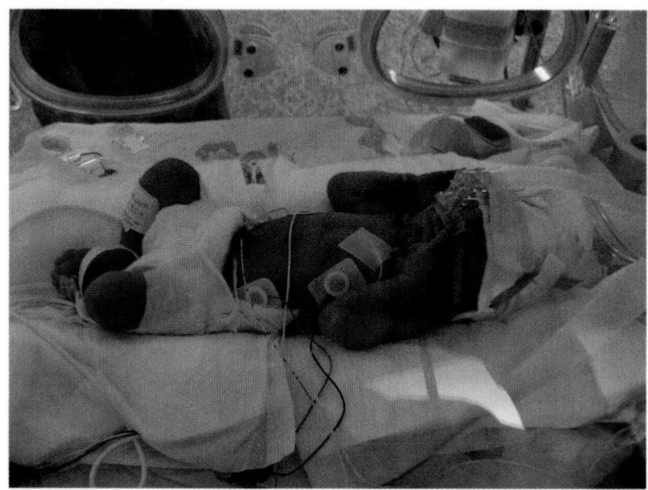

FIG 34-3 Infant receiving ventilatory assistance with nasal continuous positive airway pressure (CPAP). (Courtesy Randi and Jacob Wills, Clayton, NC.)

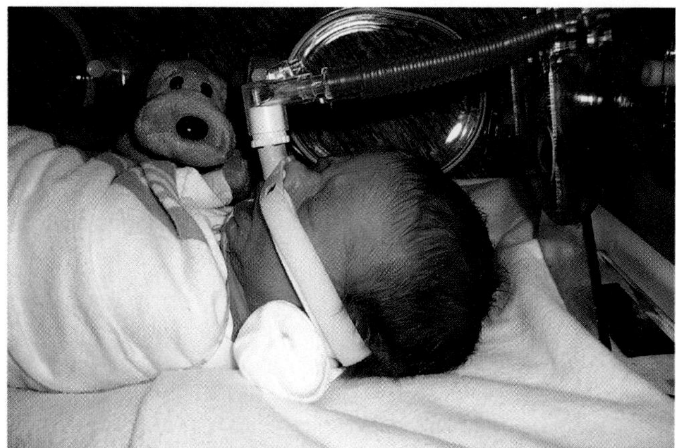

FIG 34-4 Infant intubated and on ventilator. (Courtesy Cheryl Briggs, RNC, Annapolis, MD.)

of oxygen by hood or nasal cannula may require continuous positive airway pressure (CPAP). CPAP infuses oxygen or air under a preset pressure by means of nasal prongs or a face mask (Fig. 34-3). It is often achieved by sending the oxygen bubbling through water to the infant; this is referred to as bubble CPAP. Researchers are investigating whether the work of neonatal breathing is improved with bubble CPAP versus variable-flow devices (Rebello, Yagui, Vale, et al., 2011). In either case, an orogastric tube should be in place for decompression of the stomach during use of nasal prongs. CPAP increases the functional residual capacity, improves the diffusion time of pulmonary gases, including oxygen, and can decrease pulmonary shunting. If implemented early enough, CPAP can preclude the need for mechanical ventilation (Gardner et al., 2011b). CPAP can cause vascular shunting in the pulmonary beds, which can lead to the complications of persistent pulmonary hypertension and severe respiratory distress.

Mechanical Ventilation. Mechanical ventilation must be implemented if other methods of therapy cannot correct abnormalities in oxygenation (Fig. 34-4). Its use is indicated whenever blood gas values demonstrate severe hypoxemia or severe hypercapnia. Intubation and ventilation can be needed for infants who have apnea with bradycardia, ineffective respiratory effort, shock, asphyxia, infection, meconium aspiration syndrome, respiratory distress syndrome (RDS), or congenital defects that affect ventilation (Gardner et al., 2011b). Ventilator settings are determined by the infant's individual needs. The ventilator is set to provide a predetermined amount of oxygen during spontaneous respirations and during mechanical ventilation in the absence of spontaneous respirations. Newer technologies in ventilation allow oxygen to be delivered at lower pressures and in assist modes, thereby preventing the overriding of the infant's spontaneous breathing and providing distending pressures within a physiologic range. Barotrauma and associated complications such as *pneumothorax* (accumulation of air in the pleural space) and *pulmonary interstitial emphysema* (PIE) (free air that accumulates in interstitial tissue) are decreased. See Table 34-1 for a description of the types of mechanical ventilation used in newborns.

TABLE 34-1 Common Methods for Assisted Ventilation in Neonatal Respiratory Distress

METHOD	DESCRIPTION	HOW PROVIDED
Continuous distending pressure—continuous positive airway pressure (CPAP)	Provides constant distending pressure to airway in spontaneously breathing infant	Nasal prongs or nasopharyngeal tubes Face mask Bubble CPAP uses water resistance
Intermittent mandatory ventilation (IMV)	Allows infant to breathe spontaneously at own rate but provides mechanical cycled respirations and pressure at regular preset intervals; infant can maintain asynchronous ventilation efforts, which diminishes effective gas exchange; uses positive end-expiratory pressure (PEEP)	Endotracheal intubation
Synchronized intermittent mandatory ventilation (SIMV)	Mechanically delivered breaths are synchronized to the onset of spontaneous infant breaths; assist or control (A/C) mode facilitates full inspiratory synchrony; involves signal detection of onset of spontaneous respiration from abdominal movement, thoracic impedance, and airway pressure or flow changes; pressure support ventilation provides an inspiratory pressure assist when spontaneous breathing is detected to decrease infant's work of breathing	Patient-triggered infant ventilator with signal detector and A/C mode; endotracheal tube; SIMV, A/C, and pressure support are also referred to as patient-triggered ventilation
Volume guarantee ventilation	Delivers a predetermined volume of gas using an inspiratory pressure that varies according to the infant's lung compliance (often used in conjunction with SIMV)	Volume guarantee ventilator with flow sensor; endotracheal tube
High-frequency oscillation (HFO)	Application of high-frequency, low-volume, sine-wave flow oscillations to airway at rates between 480 and 1200 breaths/minute	Variable-speed piston pump (or loudspeaker, fluidic oscillator); endotracheal tube
High-frequency jet ventilation (HFJV)	Uses a separate, parallel, low-compliant circuit and injector port to deliver small pulses or jets of fresh gas deep into airway at rates between 250 and 900 breaths/minute	May be used alone or with low-rate IMV; endotracheal tube

High-Frequency Ventilation. High-frequency ventilation (HFV) is accomplished through the use of jet ventilators, oscillators, or high-frequency flow interrupters (Gardner et al., 2011b). These methods provide smaller volumes of oxygen at a significantly more rapid rate (more than 300 breaths/minute) than traditional mechanical ventilators. As a result the intrathoracic pressure is decreased and the risk of barotrauma is reduced. HFV is beneficial in treating infants with air leaks, pulmonary hypoplasia, diaphragmatic hernia, and meconium aspiration (Fraser, 2012a).

SAFETY ALERT

Rates of retinopathy of prematurity and bronchopulmonary dysplasia are reduced when arterial oxygen saturation (Sao_2) is kept between 93% and 95%.

Surfactant Administration. Surfactant is a surface-active phospholipid secreted by the alveolar epithelium. Acting much the same as a detergent, this substance reduces the surface tension of fluids that line the alveoli and respiratory passages, resulting in uniform expansion and maintenance of lung expansion at low intraalveolar pressure. Before 34 weeks of gestation, most infants do not produce enough surfactant to survive extrauterine life. As a result, lung compliance is decreased, and inadequate gas exchange occurs as the lungs become atelectatic and require greater pressures to expand.

Surfactant can be administered as an adjunct to oxygen and ventilation therapy. With administration of artificial surfactant, respiratory compliance is improved until the infant can generate sufficient surfactant. Exogenous surfactant is either artificial or natural and is given in several doses through an endotracheal tube. The American Academy of Pediatrics (AAP) recommends the use of surfactant in infants with RDS as soon as possible after birth, especially for ELBW infants and those not exposed to maternal antenatal steroids (Polin, Carlo, & Committee on Fetus and Newborn, 2014). The administration of antenatal steroids to the mother and surfactant replacement has decreased the incidence of RDS and concomitant morbidities. Use of artificial surfactant has been associated with a significantly reduced length of time on ventilators and oxygen therapy, and an increased survival rate in preterm infants (Polin, Carlo, & Committee on Fetus and Newborn). As with any drug therapy, the infant must be monitored for potential side effects such as a patent ductus arteriosus (PDA) and pulmonary hemorrhage (see Medication Guide: Surfactant Replacement).

Additional Therapies

Nitric Oxide Therapy. Inhaled nitric oxide (INO), delivered as a gas, causes potent and sustained pulmonary vasodilation in the pulmonary circulation. Nitric oxide is a colorless, highly diffusible gas that can be administered through the ventilator circuit blended with oxygen. It binds with hemoglobin in red blood cells and is inactivated after metabolism. INO is used to decrease or reverse pulmonary hypertension, pulmonary vasoconstriction, acidosis, and hypoxemia in term and late preterm infants with conditions such as persistent pulmonary hypertension, meconium aspiration syndrome, pneumonia, sepsis, and congenital diaphragmatic hernia. INO therapy can be used in conjunction with surfactant replacement therapy,

MEDICATION GUIDE

Surfactant Replacement

Drug/Source

- Beractant* (Survanta)—Exogenous surfactant from bovine lung extract
- Poractant alpha* (Curosurf)—Modified porcine-derived minced lung extract
- Calfactant* (Infrasurf)—Natural surfactant extracted from calf lung lavage
- Lucinactant (Surfaxin): Synthetic surfactant
- Colfosceril (Exosurf): Synthetic surfactant

Action

These medications provide exogenous surfactant to promote lung maturity.

Indications

Surfactants are used to prevent and treat respiratory distress syndrome (RDS) in preterm infants. The drug should be administered prophylactically to infants less than 30 weeks of gestation with RDS as soon as possible after intubation and initial stabilization. It should be given prophylactically to extremely preterm infants at high risk for RDS, especially if there was no exposure to antenatal steroids. Early rescue surfactant treatment may be given to infants less than 2 hours of age with signs of RDS. Late rescue surfactant treatment may be administered to infants at 4 to 6 hours of age who require mechanical ventilation. Rescue surfactant may be given to infants with hypoxic respiratory failure that results from secondary surfactant deficiency; this includes meconium aspiration syndrome, sepsis or pneumonia, and pulmonary hemorrhage (Polin, Carlo, & Committee on Fetus and Newborn, 2014).

Dosage and Route

Dosage depends on the drug used. Administer via endotracheal tube as a bolus or in smaller amounts, or via infusion into the endotracheal tube through an adaptor port (Polin, Carlo, & Committee on Fetus and Newborn, 2014).

- Beractant* (Survanta)—4 ml/kg
- Poractant alpha* (Curosurf)—2.5 ml/kg
- Calfactant* (Infrasurf)—3 ml/kg
- Lucinactant (Surfaxin) —5.8 ml/kg

Adverse Reactions

Adverse events are most often related to the administration procedure and include oxygen desaturation, transient bradycardia, alterations in blood pressure, and drug reflux.

Nursing Considerations

The nurse observes the infant for changes. Diuresis can occur with improvement. Ventilator settings may need changing as the infant's ability to oxygenate increases.

*Bovine and porcine products can be objectionable to parents because of religious or cultural beliefs (Jewish, Islamic, or Hindu); prior to administering surfactant to infant, informed consent from parents is essential (Gardner et al., 2011b).

Data from Gardner, S., Enzman-Hines, M., & Dickey, L. (2011b). Respiratory diseases. In S. Gardner, B. Carter, M. Enzman-Hines, & J. Hernandez (Eds.), *Merenstein & Gardner's handbook of neonatal intensive care* (7th ed.). St. Louis: Mosby; Polin, R.A., Carlo, W.A., & Committee on Fetus and Newborn. (2014). Surfactant replacement therapy for preterm and term neonates with respiratory distress. *Pediatrics, 133*(1), 156-163.

high-frequency ventilation, or extracorporeal membrane oxygenation (ECMO). In the few studies conducted with human infants, positive results were seen: oxygen saturation improved, and no toxic effects from methemoglobin or increased levels of nitrogen oxide were documented. INO shows much promise in reducing adverse respiratory sequelae of prematurity. Its use has reduced the need for invasive technologies such as ECMO (Gardner et al., 2011b).

Extracorporeal Membrane Oxygenation. ECMO is a very complex and costly treatment that is sometimes used to support life and allow treatment of intractable hypoxemia due to severe cardiac or respiratory failure. This therapy involves a modified heart-lung machine, although in ECMO the heart is not stopped, and blood does not entirely bypass the lungs. Blood is shunted from a catheter in the right atrium or right internal jugular vein by gravity to a servo-regulated roller pump, pumped through a membrane lung, where it is oxygenated, and through a small heat exchanger, where it is warmed, and then returned to the systemic circulation via a major artery such as the carotid artery to the aortic arch. ECMO provides oxygen to the circulation, allowing the lungs to "rest," and decreases pulmonary hypertension and hypoxemia in such conditions as persistent pulmonary hypertension of the newborn, congenital diaphragmatic hernia, sepsis, meconium aspiration, and severe pneumonia. ECMO is contraindicated for preterm infants younger than 34 weeks of gestation because of the anticoagulant therapy required in the pump and circuits, which can increase the potential for intraventricular hemorrhage (Gardner et al., 2011b).

Partial Liquid Ventilation. For infants with severe RDS, the use of partial liquid ventilation (PLV) can improve outcomes. Perfluorocarbon liquid is instilled into the lungs during gaseous (mechanical) ventilation. PLV is beneficial to the surfactant-deficient or immature lung because it reduces or eliminates surface tension, improves oxygenation through the re-creation of a fetal lung environment, and helps reexpand atelectatic areas. The safety and efficacy of PLV are being evaluated in the United States (Gardner et al., 2011b).

Weaning from Respiratory Assistance. The goal of weaning is the withdrawal of all oxygen support. Respiratory assistance is weaned slowly as the infant's status improves. The infant is ready to be weaned from respiratory assistance once the ABG and oxygen saturation levels are maintained within normal limits. A spontaneous, adequate respiratory effort must be present, and the infant must show improved muscle tone during increased activity. Weaning is done in a stepwise and gradual manner. This can consist of the infant being extubated, placed on CPAP, and then weaned to oxygen by means of a hood or nasal cannula. Throughout the weaning process, the infant's oxygen levels are monitored by pulse oximetry, transcutaneous oxygen ($TcPO_2$) monitoring, and blood gas levels. The infant is assessed for signs and symptoms indicating poor tolerance of the process. These include an increased pulse, respiratory distress, or cyanosis, or a combination of these. If these occur, the amount of oxygen being delivered is increased and weaning proceeds more slowly as assessments continue. Underlying causes of intolerance of weaning can be BPD, a PDA, or CNS damage.

Some infants do not tolerate weaning from oxygen therapy before discharge from the hospital. They can require supplementary oxygen at home for weeks or months.

Nutritional Care

It is not always possible to provide enteral (by the GI route) nourishment to a high risk infant. Such infants are often too ill or weak to breastfeed or bottle feed because of respiratory distress or sepsis. Early enteral feeding of the asphyxiated neonate with a low Apgar score also is avoided to prevent bowel necrosis. In such cases, nutrition is provided parenterally. Infants who require parenteral nutrition are likely to have one or more of the following problems:

- Lack of a coordinated suck-and-swallow reflex
- Inability to suck because of a congenital anomaly
- Respiratory distress requiring aggressive ventilator support
- Asphyxiation with a potential for NEC

Type of Nourishment. The type, mode, volume, and schedule of feedings are based on:

- Initially, the birth weight, and then the current weight of the preterm infant
- Pattern of weight gain or loss (infants weighing less than 1500 g (3.3 lb) require more energy for growth and thermoregulation and can gain weight poorly with either breast- or bottle feedings)
- Presence or absence of suck-and-swallow reflex in all infants at less than 35 weeks of gestation
- Behavioral readiness to take oral feedings
- Physical condition, including presence or absence of bowel sounds, abdominal distention, or bloody stools, as well as presence and degree of respiratory distress or apneic episodes
- Residual from previous feeding, if being gavage fed
- Malformations (especially GI defects such as gastroschisis, omphalocele, or esophageal atresia), including the need for a gastrostomy feeding tube
- Renal function, including urinary output and laboratory values (nitrogen balance, electrolyte balance, glucose level); preterm infants are especially susceptible to altered renal function

Human milk is the best source of nutrition for term and preterm infants (AAP Section on Breastfeeding, 2012). Even small preterm infants (32 to 36 weeks) are able to breastfeed if they have adequate sucking and swallowing reflexes and no other contraindications, such as respiratory complications or concurrent illness. Preterm infants who are breastfed rather than bottle fed demonstrate fewer oxygen desaturations, absence of bradycardia, warmer than normal skin temperature, and improved coordination of sucking, swallowing, and breathing (Gardner & Lawrence, 2011). Mothers who wish to breastfeed their preterm infants are encouraged to express their milk using a hospital-grade electric pump until their infants are sufficiently stable to tolerate feeding at the breast, and to continue pumping after feedings until the infant is able to exclusively breastfeed, usually after discharge from the hospital (Meier, Patel, Bigger, et al., 2013). Appropriate guidelines for the storage of expressed mother's milk should be used to decrease the risk of milk contamination and destruction of its beneficial properties (Jones, 2011).

Commercially available preterm formulas are cow's milk based and whey predominant and have a higher concentration of protein, calcium and phosphorus than term formulas to meet the unique needs of the preterm infant (de Curtis & Rigo, 2012). Most preterm formulas are either 22 or 24 cal/oz.

Human milk with fortifier (protein, phosphorus, and calcium) is recommended for LBW preterm infants because it increases weight gain and improves bone mineralization better than nonfortified human milk (Gardner & Lawrence, 2011). Supplementation with iron, vitamin D, and multivitamins may be considered in exclusively breastfed LBW infants.

Weight and Fluid Loss or Gain. The caloric, nutrient, and fluid requirements of high risk infants are greater than those of the healthy term newborn. Premature or dysmature (malnourished) newborns often have limited stores of nutrients and fluids. In addition, symptomatic or asymptomatic hypoglycemia, electrolyte imbalances, or other metabolic disturbances can develop in an infant whose nutritional intake is poor. Such hypoglycemia can cause serious damage to carbohydrate-dependent brain cells.

The infant's weight is measured and recorded daily, and the rate of weight loss or gain is calculated. Further depletion of weight and metabolic stores can occur as a result of one or a combination of the following factors:

- Birth asphyxia
- Increased respirations or respiratory effort
- Patent ductus arteriosus (PDA)
- Hypothermic environment
- Insensible fluid loss caused by evaporation (with radiant heat or phototherapy)
- Vomiting, diarrhea, and dysfunctional absorption from the GI tract
- Growth demands (a preterm infant's growth rate approximates that of fetal growth during the last trimester and is at least two times faster than a term infant's growth rate after birth)
- Inability of the renal system to concentrate urine and maintain an adequate rate of urea excretion, as well as infant's inadequate response to antidiuretic hormone

The high risk newborn is predisposed to weight and fluid losses because of the greater amount of fluid needed to meet the demands of the increased cellular metabolic processes (resulting from stress, repair, or growth). The body weight of preterm infants has higher water content than that of their full-term counterparts (Blackburn, 2013). Most of this water is in the extracellular fluid compartment. Even with the early institution of fluid and nutritional intake, the preterm infant's weight and fluid losses seem exaggerated. Inadequate fluid intake, resulting from either delayed administration or insufficient volume, can further cause weight and fluid losses in the preterm infant.

Insensible water loss (IWL) is an evaporative loss that occurs largely through the skin (70%) and through the respiratory tract (30%). The basal IWL in a term infant is approximately 20 ml/kg/day. It is significantly increased in preterm infants, and especially in ELBW infants with thin, gelatinous skin (Blackburn, 2013). The effects of radiant warmers, incubators, phototherapy, and other factors can increase the IWL. Humidifying the respiratory gases administered can prevent some of this loss.

During the first week of extrauterine life the preterm infant can lose up to 15% of his or her birth weight. In contrast, a weight loss up to 10% is acceptable in a term, appropriate for gestational age (AGA) infant. After the initial week, a preterm infant's loss or gain during each 24-hour period should not exceed 2% of the previous day's weight. (To calculate a weight loss or gain, see Box 34-4.)

BOX 34-4 Calculation of a Weight Loss or Gain

Example 1

Day 1	1750 g (birth weight)	$\frac{70}{1750} = \frac{X}{100}$
Day 3	1680 g 70-g loss	$1750X = 7000$ $1750X\overline{)7000.0}$ = 4.0 X = 4% weight loss

Example 2

Day 3	1680 g	$\frac{40}{1680} = \frac{X}{100}$
Day 4	1720 g 40-g gain	$1680X = 4000$ $1680\overline{)4,000.00}$ = 2.38 X = 2.4% weight gain

Increased stooling or voiding, increased evaporative losses, inadequate volume or incorrect fluid administration, and problems with malabsorption can cause weight loss. Implementation of interventions and frequent assessment of the infant and the environment are necessary to correct the problems. Common interventions include adjusting the incubator temperature; "swamping" or providing high levels of humidity under a cover over the radiant warmer; monitoring and adjusting the volume and type of fluid being administered; assessing the urinary output, including the specific gravity; and assessing the blood glucose levels. Hyperglycemia results in urinary loss of glucose that can cause osmotic diuresis, which increases the risk of dehydration (Yoo, Ahn, Lee, et al., 2013).

If the infant is gaining more than the expected amount of weight, this can be due to overfeeding or fluid retention. The nurse reports and records the findings and continues to assess the infant's fluid status, urinary output, and blood glucose levels. Interventions are determined by the infant's specific disorder and nutritional needs.

Elimination Patterns. The infant's elimination patterns are assessed and documented. This includes the frequency of urination, as well as the amount and color of the urine. The assessment of the infant's bowel movements includes the frequency of stooling and the character of the stool, as well as whether there is constipation, diarrhea, or loss of fats (steatorrhea). The nurse may request guaiac tests to assess for blood in the stool, tests to detect stool-reducing substances, and a pH determination to assess for malabsorption. Infants with unexplained abdominal distention are assessed carefully to rule out the presence of hypomotility obstructions of the GI tract or NEC.

Oral Feeding. Nourishment by the oral route is preferred for the infant who has adequate strength and GI function. The best milk for an infant is from the mother. Breast milk can be fed by breast, bottle, cup, or spoon. Throughout the feeding the nurse assesses the newborn's tolerance of the procedure. Preterm infants can be put to breast for nonnutritive suckling and practice feeds as soon as medically stable. The nurse or lactation consultant assists the mother by providing support and help as necessary when the infant breastfeeds.

The needs of the high risk infant must be considered when determining the type and frequency of the feedings. Many high risk infants cannot suck well enough to breastfeed or bottle feed until they have recovered from their initial illness or matured physically (corrected age more than 32 weeks of gestation). Mothers of high risk infants are encouraged to continue expressing breast milk with a hospital-grade electric pump, especially if theirs is a very premature infant who will not breastfeed for many weeks. Because of the significant breastfeeding attrition rates among these mothers, they need ongoing support and encouragement to continue pumping while their infant is not yet able to nurse. If no breast milk is available (from the mother or a milk bank), commercial formula is used. The calories, protein, and mineral content of commercial formulas vary. The type of nipple selected ("preemie," regular, orthodontic) depends on the infant's ability to suck from the specific type of nipple. The nurse also considers the energy the infant needs to expend in the process. However, the practice of delaying breastfeeding until the baby is able to effectively bottle feed is not evidence-based because studies continue to confirm that breastfeeding is less stressful than bottle feeding (Gardner & Lawrence, 2011).

Overfeeding of the preterm infant should be avoided because this can lead to abdominal distention, with apnea, vomiting, and possibly aspiration of the feeding. The nurse monitors the infant's abdominal girth when distention is obvious.

Gavage Feeding. Gavage feeding is a method of providing nourishment to the infant who is compromised by respiratory distress, the infant who is too immature to have a coordinated suck-and-swallow reflex, or the infant who is easily fatigued by sucking. In gavage feeding, breast milk or commercial infant formula is given to the infant through a nasogastric or orogastric tube (Fig. 34-5). This spares the infant the work of sucking.

Gavage feeding can be done with an intermittently placed tube providing a bolus feeding or continuously through an indwelling catheter. Infants who cannot tolerate large bolus feedings are given continuous feedings. Minimal enteral nutrition can be used to stimulate or prime the GI tract to achieve better absorption of nutrients when bolus or regular intermittent gavage feedings can be given (Blackburn, 2013).

Breast milk or formula can be supplied intermittently via gavage by using a syringe with gravity-controlled flow, or it can be given continuously by using an infusion pump. The type of fluid instilled is recorded with every syringe change. The volume of the continuous feedings is recorded hourly, and the residual gastric aspirate is measured every 2 to 4 hours. Aspirates of less than a 1-hour volume can be re-fed to the infant. For intermittent feedings, residuals of less than 50% of the previous feeding can be re-fed to the infant to prevent the loss of gastric electrolytes. Feeding is usually stopped if the residual is greater than 50% of the feeding or if residuals are increasing and is not resumed until the infant can be assessed for a possible feeding intolerance (Anderson et al., 2011).

The orogastric route for gavage feedings is preferred because most infants are preferential nose breathers. In addition, when indwelling nasogastric tubes are used, there is a risk for necrosis of the nares. However, some infants do not

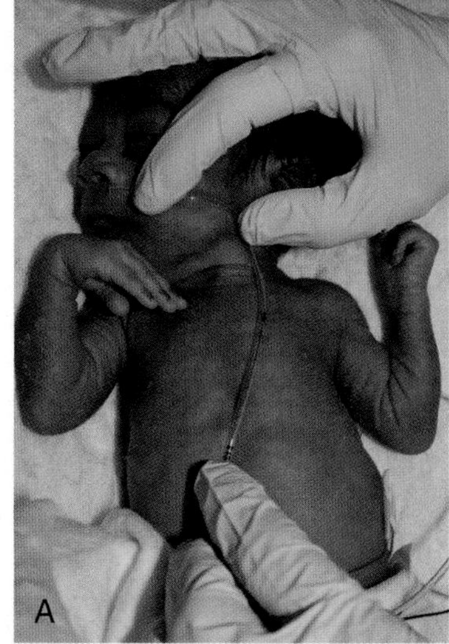

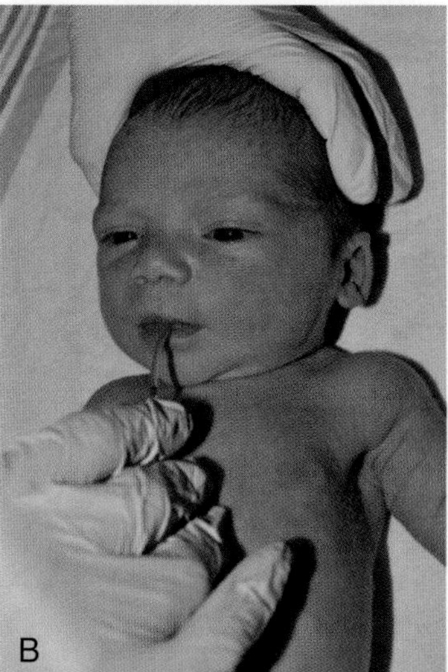

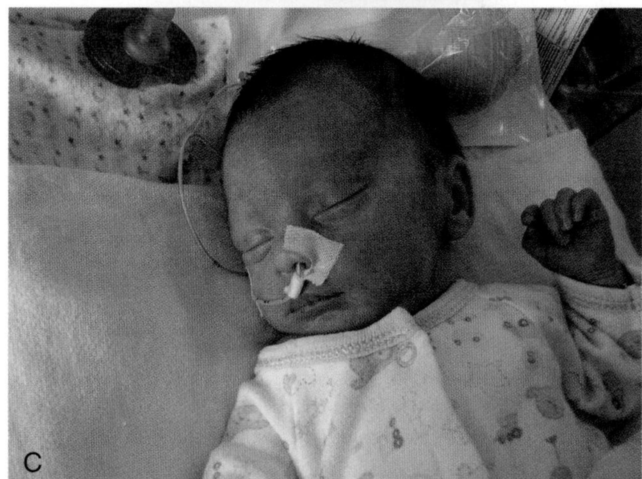

FIG 34-5 Gavage feeding. **A,** Measurement of gavage feeding tube from tip of nose to earlobe and to midpoint between end of xiphoid process and umbilicus. Tape may be used to mark correct length on tube. For accurate measure the infant should be facing up. **B,** Insertion of gavage tube using orogastric route. **C,** Indwelling gavage tube, nasogastric route. After feeding by orogastric or nasogastric tube, infant is propped on right side or placed prone (preterm infant) for 1 hour to facilitate emptying of stomach into small intestine. (**A** and **B,** Courtesy Cheryl Briggs, RNC, Annapolis, MD; **C,** Courtesy Randi and Jacob Wills, Clayton, NC.)

BOX 34-5 Procedure for Inserting a Gavage Feeding Tube

Equipment

- Infant feeding tube
  - For infants less than 1 kg (2.2 lb), size 4 Fr
  - For infants more than 1 kg (2.2 lb), size 5 Fr to 6 Fr
- Stethoscope
- Sterile water (lubricant)
- Syringe: 5 to 10 ml
- Tape, optional transparent dressing
- Gloves

1. Measure the length of the gavage tube from the tip of the nose to the earlobe to the midpoint between the xiphoid process and the umbilicus (see Fig. 34-5, *A*). Mark the tube with indelible ink or a piece of tape.
2. Lubricate the tip of the tube with sterile water and insert gently through the nose or mouth (see Fig. 34-5, *B*) until the predetermined mark is reached. Placement of the tube in the trachea will cause the infant to gag, cough, or become cyanotic.
3. Check correct placement of the tube by:
   a. Pulling back on the plunger to aspirate stomach contents. Lack of stomach aspirate or fluid is not necessarily evidence of improper placement. Aspiration of respiratory secretions can be mistaken for stomach contents; however, the pH of the stomach contents is much lower (more acidic) than the pH of respiratory secretions.
   b. Injecting a small amount of air (1-3 ml) into the tube while listening for gurgling by using a stethoscope placed over the stomach. Ensure that the tube is inserted to the mark; air entering the stomach can be heard even if the tube is positioned above the gastroesophageal (cardiac) sphincter.
   c. Abdominal or chest radiography. This is the only definitive way to verify tube placement.
4. Using tape or a transparent dressing, secure the tube in place and tape it to the cheek to prevent accidental dislodgment and incorrect positioning (see Fig. 34-5, *C*).
   a. Assess the infant's skin integrity before taping the tube.
   b. Edematous or very preterm infants should have a pectin barrier placed under the tape to prevent abrasions, or a hydrocolloid adhesive should be used to prevent epidermal stripping.
5. Tube placement *must* be assessed before each feeding.

tolerate oral tube placement. A small nasogastric feeding tube can be placed in older infants who would otherwise gag or vomit or in ones who are learning to suck. To insert the tube and give the feeding, the nurse should follow the sequence given in Box 34-5.

Gastrostomy Feedings. Gastrostomy feedings are used for infants with neurologic problems or certain congenital malformations that require long-term tube feedings. This involves the surgical placement of a tube through the skin of the abdomen into the stomach. The tube is then taped in an upright position to prevent trauma to the incision site. After the site heals the nurse initiates small bolus feedings per the physician's orders. Feedings by gravity are done slowly over 20- to 30-minute periods. Special care must be taken to prevent rapid bolusing of the fluid because this can lead to abdominal distention, GI reflux into the esophagus, or respiratory compromise. Meticulous skin care at the tube insertion site is necessary to prevent skin breakdown or infection. In addition, intake and output are closely monitored because these infants are prone to diarrhea until regular feedings are established.

Parenteral Nutrition. Supplemental parenteral fluids are indicated for infants who are unable to obtain sufficient fluids or calories by enteral feeding. Some of these infants are dependent on total parenteral nutrition (TPN) for extensive periods. The nurse assesses and documents the following in infants receiving parenteral fluids or TPN:

- Type and infusion rate of the solution
- Functional status of the infusion equipment, including the tubing and infusion pump
- Infusion site for possible complications (phlebitis, infiltration, dislodgment)
- Caloric intake
- Infant's responses to therapy

The physician or nurse practitioner orders TPN per the hospital protocol. These orders must specify the electrolytes and nutrients desired, as well as the volume and rate of infusion. The composition of calories, protein, and fats is calculated on an individual basis.

While caring for the infant receiving parenteral fluids or TPN, the nurse secures and protects the insertion site. Scrupulous hand hygiene is used before handling the TPN tubing or IV sites. Strict sterile technique is implemented for dressing changes (Kilbride, Leick-Rude, Olsen, & Stiens, 2011). The nurse must observe the principles of neonatal skin care. The nurse carefully inspects the infusion site for signs of infiltration and repositions the infant frequently to maintain body alignment and protect the site. Parents need explanations about TPN and the ways in which the IV equipment and solutions affect their infant.

Advancing Infant Feedings. Feedings are advanced as assessment data and the infant's ability to tolerate the feedings warrant. Documentation of a preterm infant's sucking patterns also can be used to determine readiness to nipple feed. Feedings are advanced from passive (parenteral and gavage) to active (bottle- and breastfeeding). At each step the nurse must carefully assess the infant's response to prevent stress to the infant.

The infant receiving nutrition parenterally is gradually weaned off this type of nutrition. To do this the nourishment given by continuous or intermittent gavage feedings is increased and the parenteral fluids are decreased. Even the smallest infant is sometimes given MEN to stimulate the GI system to mature and to enhance caloric intake (Blackburn, 2013).

Feedings are advanced slowly and cautiously because if advanced too rapidly, the infant can develop vomiting (with an attendant risk of aspiration), diarrhea, abdominal distention, and apneic episodes. Rapid advancements in the volume of feeds have been implicated as a risk factor for NEC (Christensen, Lambert, Baer, & Gordon, 2013). Rapid advancement also can cause fluid retention with cardiac compromise or a pronounced diuresis with hyponatremia.

If the infant needs additional calories, a commercial human milk fortifier can be added to the gavaged breast milk, or the number of calories per 30 ml of commercial formula can be increased. Soy and elemental formulas are used only for infants with very special dietary needs, such as allergies to cow's milk or chronic malabsorption. Calories in breast milk can be lost if the cream separates and adheres to the tubing during continuous infusion. This problem is decreased if microbore tubing is used for both continuous and intermittent gavage feedings.

The infant receiving gavage feedings progresses to bottle feeding or breast milk feedings. To do this the gavage feedings are decreased as the infant's ability to suckle breast milk or formula improves. Often during this transition the infant is fed by both bottle or breast and gavage feeding to ensure the intake of both the prescribed volume of food and nutrients. However, when there is an indwelling tube, during breast or bottle feedings, some infants experience increased respiratory effort, so nurses must watch for this. The parents need support during this transition because many families measure their parenting competence by how well they can feed their infant. For breastfed infants, it is important to weigh the infant before and after breastfeeding to determine the infant's intake (Gardner & Lawrence, 2011).

As the time of discharge nears, the appropriate method of feeding and the assessments pertaining to the method (e.g., tolerance of feedings, status of gavage tube placement) are reviewed with the parents. The parents should be encouraged to interact with the infant by talking and making eye contact with the infant during the feeding. This stimulates the psychosocial development of the infant and facilitates bonding and attachment.

Nonnutritive Sucking. If the infant is receiving only parenteral nutrition or gavage feeds, nonnutritive sucking should be encouraged for several reasons (Fig. 34-6). Allowing the infant to suck on a pacifier during gavage or between oral feedings can improve oxygenation. In addition, such nonnutritive sucking can lead to decreased energy expenditure with less restlessness. It also promotes positive weight gain and better sucking skills (Gardner & Lawrence, 2011).

Mothers of preterm infants should be encouraged to allow their infants to start sucking at the breast during kangaroo care (skin-to-skin). In some infants, the suck-and-swallow reflexes are coordinated as early as 32 weeks of gestation. If the neonate is unable to suck, the mother can place the infant near the nipple to encourage nuzzling or licking.

Infants with intrauterine growth restriction (IUGR) can have an age-appropriate sucking reflex but require thermoregulatory support, making it difficult to breastfeed. These infants also may benefit from nonnutritive sucking or nuzzling at the breast for short periods.

Skin Care

The skin of preterm infants is characteristically immature compared with that of full-term infants. Because of its increased sensitivity and fragility, the use of alkaline-based soap that might destroy the acid mantle of the skin is avoided. Vernix caseosa has benefits for the preterm infant's skin. Vernix acts as an epidermal barrier, decreases bacterial contamination of the skin through its antimicrobial peptides and proteins, and decreases transepidermal water loss (Blackburn, 2013). Experts recommend that a validated skin assessment tool such as the Neonatal Skin Condition Score (NSCS) be used once daily to evaluate the high risk infant's skin condition so as to implement interventions aimed at minimizing skin breakdown (Lund & Durand, 2011).

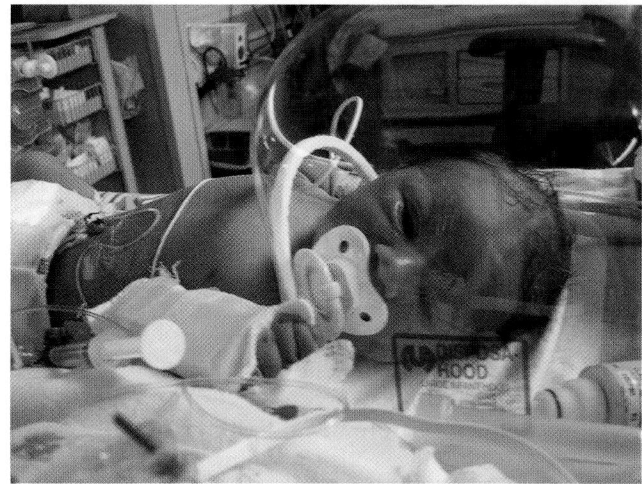

FIG 34-6 Nonnutritive sucking while under oxygen hood. (Courtesy Lauren and Brian LiVecchi, Raleigh, NC.)

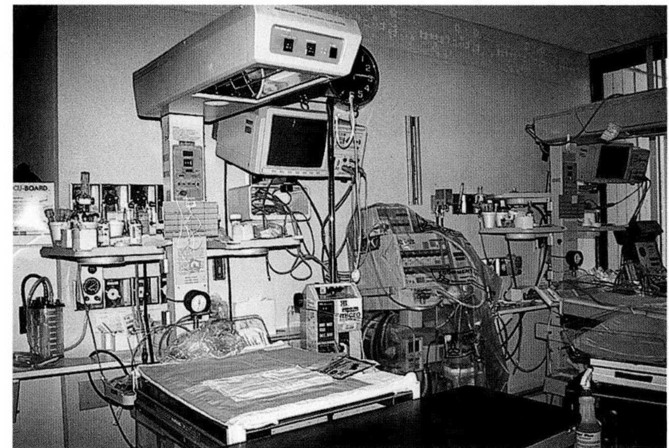

FIG 34-7 Although necessary, neonatal intensive care unit equipment can contribute to significant environmental stimulation. Note bed, wall oxygen attachments, monitor, ventilator, incubator, and pumps, all of which have alarm systems. (Courtesy Marjorie Pyle, RNC, Lifecircle, Costa Mesa, CA.)

Environmental Concerns

Infants in neonatal intensive care units (NICUs) are exposed to high levels of auditory input from the various machine alarms, and this can have adverse effects (Fig. 34-7). In addition, continual noise levels of 45 to 85 decibels (db) are common in NICUs. An incubator alone produces a constant noise level of 60 to 80 db, and each new piece of life-support equipment used adds another 20 db to the background noise. The infant's hearing can be damaged if it is exposed to a constant decibel level of 90 db or frequent decibel swings higher than 110 db. Cochlear damage has been recognized as a side effect of the NICU environment. Hearing losses have been identified in NICU graduates; these losses lead to long-term speech and language deficits. Over time more emphasis has been placed on noise in the NICU and the adverse or long-term effects on neonates (Wachman & Lahav, 2011).

Respiratory equipment or a phototherapy mask can alter the infant's vision, making it difficult to interact with parents and caregivers. The infant may be unable to establish diurnal and nocturnal rhythms because of the continuous exposure to overhead lighting. In addition, sedation or pain medications affect the way in which the infant perceives the environment.

An additional concern in the care of infants is that some drugs used for infant therapy can potentiate environmental hazards. Drugs such as aminoglycosides can potentiate noise-induced hearing loss (Zimmerman & Lahav, 2013). Routine hearing screening should be performed in all infants before discharge, with universal screening completed by no later than the third month of life (AAP Joint Committee on Infant Hearing, 2007).

Research is ongoing to determine the long-term effects of light and noise on the preterm infant (Aita, Johnston, Goulet, et al., 2013). Cycling of light and covering of incubators to reduce direct light hitting the retina are two areas of research. The retina of the immature infant has little protection from the nearly translucent eyelid, thus allowing light to almost constantly penetrate the retina unless it is artificially protected by dimming the lights or using incubator covers. Cycled lighting has been shown to have a positive effect on growth (Morag & Ohlsson, 2011). Light and sound can be adverse stimuli for the preterm infant who is already stressed. Signs of stress include increased metabolic rate, increased oxygen and caloric use, and depression of the immune system. The nurse must monitor the macroenvironment and the microenvironment (unit and immediate environments) for sources of overstimulation. Providing a developmentally supportive environment can lead to decreased complications and length of stay. There are national recommendations for sound and light levels in the NICU.

Nurses can modify the environment to provide a developmentally supportive milieu. In that way the infant's neurobehavioral and physiologic needs can be better met, the infant's developing organization can be supported, and growth and development can be fostered (Legendre, Burtner, Martinez, & Crowe, 2011).

Developmental Care

The goal of developmental care is to support each infant's efforts to become as well organized, competent, and stable as possible. Developmental care includes all care procedures and the physical and social aspects of care in the NICU (Legendre et al., 2011). The caregiver uses the infant's own behavior and physiologic functioning as the basis for planning care and providing interventions. Through caregiver observation, the infant's strengths, thresholds for disorganization, and vulnerable areas can be identified. The family is included in developmental care. Working together, the family and other caregivers provide opportunities to enhance the strengths of the family and the infant and to reduce the stress that is associated with the birth and care of high risk infants.

Reducing light and noise levels by instituting "quiet hours" at regularly scheduled times and positioning are just two ways in which nurses can support infants in their development. Sleep interruptions are minimized, and positioning and bundling the infant help promote self-regulation and prevent disorganization (Allen, 2012; Byrne & Garber, 2013).

Positioning. The motor development of preterm infants permits less flexion than in term infants. Caregivers can provide a variety of positions for infants; side-lying and prone are preferred to supine (but only in the nursery). Body containment with use of blanket rolls, swaddling, holding the infant's arms in a crossed position, and secure holding provide boundaries (Fig. 34-8). Use of facilitated tucking promotes self-regulation during feeding, procedures, and other stressful interventions. The prone position encourages flexion of the extremities; a sling or hip roll assists in maintaining flexion. Keeping the extremities close to the body helps calm the infant and decreases stimulation. Proper body alignment is necessary to prevent developmental problems that can affect the ability to walk as the child matures (Altimier & Phillips, 2013).

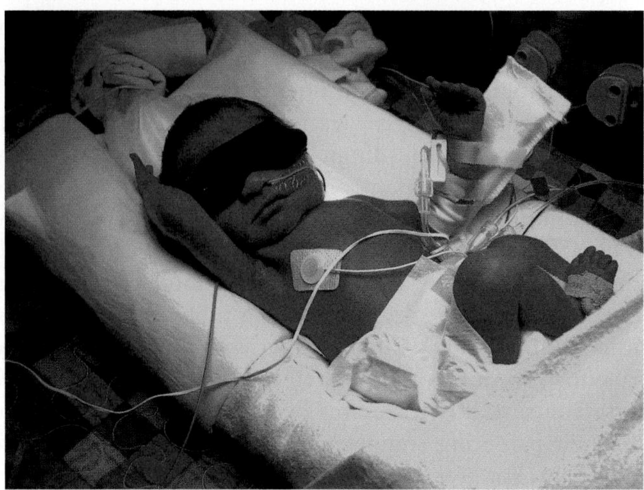

FIG 34-8 Developmental care: positioning of preterm infant using containment while undergoing phototherapy. (Courtesy Randi and Jacob Wills, Clayton, NC.)

Reducing Inappropriate Stimuli. Staff can reduce unnecessary noise by closing doors or portholes on incubators quietly, placing only necessary objects gently on top of incubators, keeping radios at low volume, speaking quietly, and handling equipment noiselessly. Another source is internal noise created by mechanical sources such as CPAP. These noise sources must be considered when thinking about long-term effects on hearing. Earmuffs can be used during scans (Arthurs, Edwards, Austin, et al., 2012).

Infants can be protected from light by dimming the lights during the night, placing a blanket over the incubator, or covering the infant's eyes with a mask. Sleep-wake cycles can be induced with such measures. Infants need periods in which there are no disruptions and sleep can occur. Clustering of care can promote longer uninterrupted periods of sleep (Legendre et al., 2011).

Infant Communication. Infants communicate their needs and ability to tolerate sensory stimulation through physiologic responses. The nurses and parents of high risk infants must therefore be alert to such cues. Although term infants can thrive on stimulation, this same stimulation in high risk infants can provoke physical symptoms of stress and anxiety (Gardner & Goldson, 2011).

Problems with noxious stimuli and barriers to normal contact can cause anxiety and tension. Clues to overstimulation include averting the gaze, hiccupping, gagging, or regurgitating food. Term infants exhibit a startle reflex, and preterm infants move all of their limbs in an uncoordinated fashion in response to noxious stimuli. An irregular respiratory rate or an increased heart rate can develop in severely distressed infants, and they can be unable to regain a calm state.

A relaxed infant state is indicated by stabilization of vital signs, closed eyes, and a relaxed posture. Nonintubated infants may make soothing verbal sounds when they are relaxed. Infants requiring artificial ventilation cannot cry audibly and often show their distress through posturing; they relax once their needs are met. As high risk infants heal and mature, they increasingly respond to stimuli in a self-regulated manner rather than with a dissociated response. Infants who do not show increased self-regulation should be evaluated for a neurologic problem.

Infant Stimulation. The Newborn Individualized Developmental Care and Assessment Program (NIDCAP, 2008) (www.nidcap.com) routinely integrates aspects of neurodevelopmental theory with caregivers' observations, environmental interventions, and parental support. Routine reassessment is built into the program's design. Developmental stimuli may consist of such simple measures as kangaroo care or placing a waterbed mattress on the top of the infant's mattress. The simplest calming technique is for the caregiver to use both hands to contain the infant's extremities close to the body. The care of the infant is organized to allow extended periods of undisturbed rest and sleep. Pain medications or sedatives should be administered consistently per the unit's protocol.

Infants acquire a sense of trust as they learn the feel, sound, and smell of their parents. High risk infants also must learn to trust their caregivers to obtain comfort. However, caregivers in the nursery also can inflict pain as part of the care they must give. For this reason it is important for parents and caregivers to use comforting interventions such as removing painful stimuli, stopping hunger, and changing wet or soiled clothing to foster trust. They can offer nonnutritive sucking or use oral sucrose for pain relief and topical creams before procedures to avoid pain. All these techniques are part of developmental, supportive care (Altimier & Phillips, 2013).

When the infant is ready for stimulation, the nurse has many options. Most infants can tolerate being held, even if only for short periods. Additional ways for the nurse or parents to stimulate infants include cuddling, rocking, singing, talking to the infant, and using music therapy. These activities are beneficial and promote growth and weight gain as well as shorten the length of hospital stay. Stroking the infant's skin during medical therapy can provide tactile stimulation. The caregiver responds to the infant's cues by offering reassurance, providing nonnutritive sucking, stroking the infant's back, and talking to the infant. Infant massage is gaining evidence as a way to promote weight gain (Gardner & Goldson, 2011).

Mobiles and decals that can be changed frequently may be placed within the infant's visual range to stimulate the infant visually. Wind-up musical toys provide rhythmic distractions as long as they are not too loud. If the infant is receiving phototherapy, the protective eyepatches are removed periodically (e.g., during feeding) to allow parent-infant or caregiver-infant interaction.

Kangaroo Care. Although it must be individually adjusted, kangaroo care and short periods of gentle massage can help reduce stress in preterm infants (Fig. 34-9). The parent is bare-chested or may wear a loose-fitting, open-front top that has a modified marsupial-like pocket carrier for the infant. The undressed (except for diaper) infant is placed in a vertical position on the parent's bare chest, which permits direct eye contact, skin-to-skin sensations, and close proximity. Skin-to-skin contact can have a positive healing effect for the mother who had a high risk pregnancy. Additional benefits include early contact with mechanically ventilated infants, maintenance of neonatal thermal stability and oxygen saturation, increased feeding vigor and enhanced breastfeeding, maintenance of organized state, decreased pain perception during painful heelsticks, and minimal untoward effects of being held (Cong, Cusson, Walsh, et al., 2012; Flacking, Ewald, & Wallin, 2011; Jefferies & Canadian Paediatric Society Fetus and Newborn Committee, 2012).

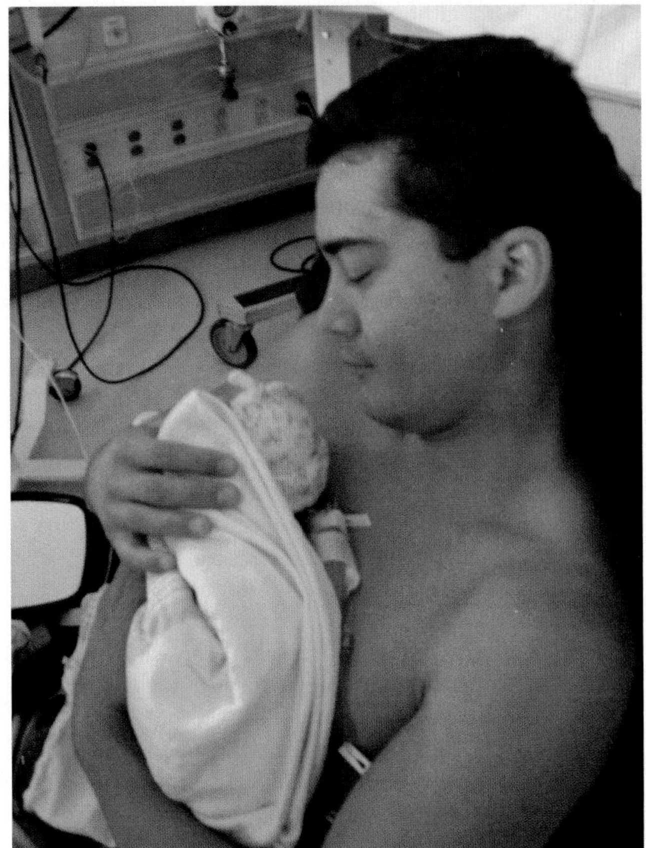

FIG 34-9 Father holding infant in kangaroo care. (Courtesy Randi and Jacob Wills, Clayton, NC.)

Parental Adaptation to a Preterm Infant

Parents of premature infants often have difficulty in bonding and relating to their babies. The need to be empowered to recognize their competence and achieve competence is the basis of the Creating Opportunities for Parent Empowerment (COPE) program. This early educational-behavioral intervention model promotes more positive parent-infant interactions and enhanced ability to read and respond to infant cues (Gooding, Cooper, Blaine, et al., 2011; Siegel, Gardner, & Dickey, 2011).

Parental Tasks. Parents of preterm infants must accomplish numerous psychologic tasks before effective relationships and parenting patterns can evolve. These tasks include the following:

- Experiencing anticipatory grief over the potential loss of an infant. The parent grieves in preparation for the infant's

possible death, although the parent clings to the hope that the infant will survive. This process begins during labor and lasts until the infant dies or shows evidence of surviving. Anticipatory grief occurs when families have knowledge of an impending loss, such as when a baby is admitted to a NICU with problems or when a diagnosis of an anencephalic fetus is made with ultrasonography. The baby is still alive, but the prognosis is poor. Being able to anticipate the loss gives families an opportunity to plan, feel more in control of their situation, and say goodbye in a special way. However, some individuals or family members distance or detach themselves from the experience or from their loved ones as a way of protecting themselves from the pain of loss and grief. How a parent responds to this situation depends on religious, spiritual, and cultural beliefs. These must be considered when planning care. The nurse's role is to advocate for the family so that other health professionals realize that the family is grieving. Being fully present for these families and practicing active listening are important (see Chapter 37).
- The mother's acceptance of her failure to give birth to a healthy full-term infant. Grief and depression typify this phase, which persists until the infant is out of danger and is expected to survive.
- Resuming the process of relating to the infant. As the baby's condition begins to improve and the baby gains weight, is able to breastfeed or bottle feed, and is weaned from the incubator or radiant warmer, the parent can begin the process of developing an attachment to the infant that was interrupted by the infant's critical condition at birth.
- Learning about the ways in which this baby differs in terms of his or her special needs and growth patterns, caregiving needs, and growth and development expectations
- Adjusting the home environment to accommodate the needs of the new infant. Parents are encouraged to limit the number of visitors to minimize exposure of the infant to pathogens. The environmental temperature may have to be altered to optimize conditions for the infant.

Parental Responses. Physical contact with the infant is important to establish early bonding and attachment. If it is not possible for parents to hold the infant, they can touch and stroke the baby as they speak softly (Fig. 34-10). As the infant's condition improves, parents can hold the neonate and provide kangaroo care (see Fig. 34-10). They gradually begin to participate in infant activities, such as feeding, bathing, and changing. Parents go through numerous phases of adjustment as they learn to parent their infant. Nurses facilitate the transition to parenthood through their teaching and support of parental efforts.

Parental Support. The nurse as caregiver, support person, and educator is responsible for shaping the environment and responding with sensitivity to the needs of the parents and infant. Nurses are instrumental in helping parents learn who their infant is and to recognize behavioral cues in his or her development and to use these cues in the care they provide (Gardner & Goldson, 2011).

When a high risk birth is anticipated, the family can be given a tour of the NICU or shown a video to prepare them for the sights and activities of the unit. After an unanticipated preterm birth, the parents can be given a booklet, view a video, or have someone describe what they will see when they go to the unit to see their infant.

As soon as possible, the parents should see and touch their infant so that they can begin to acknowledge the reality of the birth and the infant's true appearance and condition. The premature or sick baby's appearance can be stressful to the parents. They will need encouragement as they begin to accomplish the psychologic tasks imposed by the high risk birth. For the following reasons, a nurse or physician should be present during the parents' first visit:
- To help them "see" the infant rather than focus on the equipment. The importance and purpose of the equipment that surrounds their infant should be explained to them.
- To explain the characteristics normal for an infant of their baby's gestational age; in this way parents do not compare their child with a term, healthy infant
- To encourage the parents to express their feelings about the pregnancy, labor, and birth and the experience of having a high risk infant

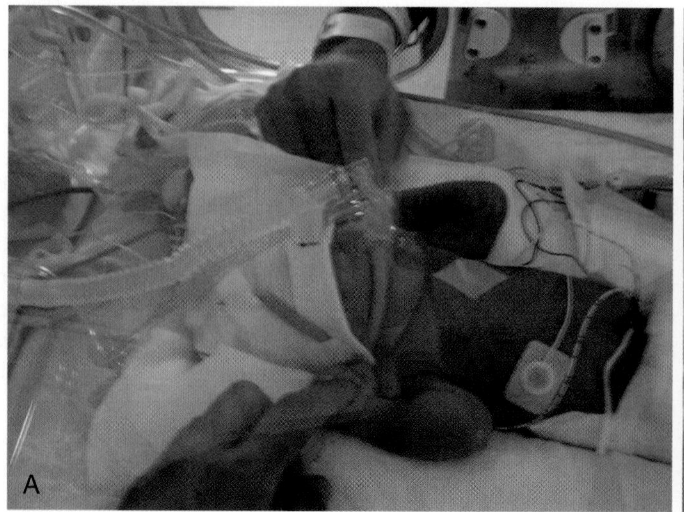

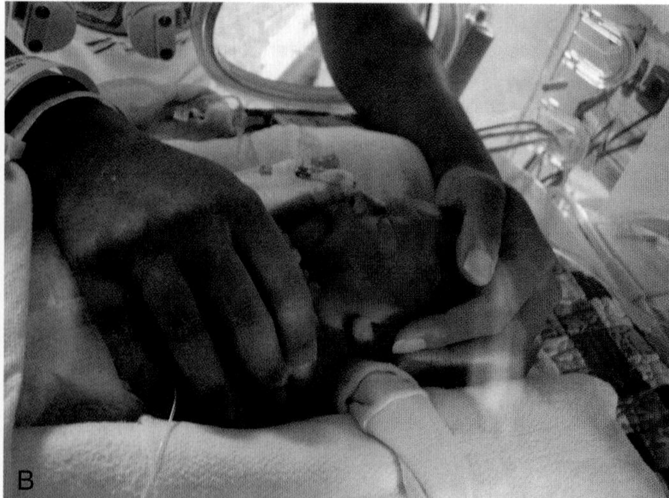

FIG 34-10 A, Mother and father touch preterm infant. B, Mother caresses preterm infant. (Courtesy Randi and Jacob Wills, Clayton, NC.)

- To assess the parents' perceptions of the infant to determine the appropriate time for them to become actively involved in care

When the parents cannot be present physically to visit with the infant, staff members devise appropriate methods to keep them informed and to help them feel connected to the newborn. Examples are daily phone calls, notes written as if by the infant, and photographs of the infant.

The birth of a preterm or high risk infant affects the entire family. Nurses need to consider responses and reactions of grandparents and siblings as they provide family-centered care for the infant and family. Grandparents often experience grief and sadness as they watch their own children experiencing the difficulties and challenges of having a preterm or high risk infant. They worry about the well-being of their grandchild. Siblings also react to the birth of the preterm or high risk infant. If they are old enough to realize that the mother was supposed to be bringing home a new baby, they can be very confused when the baby must remain in the hospital. When possible it can be helpful to allow siblings to visit the new baby in the NICU environment so that they can see the infant (Fig. 34-11). Once the infant is brought home, some children are bewildered and angry at the seemingly disproportionate amount of parental time spent on the newborn. Nurses can facilitate visits by grandparents and siblings while the infant is hospitalized and can help parents anticipate possible reactions of siblings once the baby is discharged.

Some hospitals have support groups for the parents of infants in NICUs. These groups help parents experiencing anxiety and grief by encouraging them to share their feelings. Hospitals may arrange to have an experienced NICU parent make contact with a new group member to provide additional support. The volunteer parents provide support by making hospital visits, phone calls, and home visits. Mothers in particular are prone to post-traumatic stress that can hinder their ability to interact with or care for their infant (Forcada-Guex, Borghini, Pierrehumbert, et al., 2011). They need help in expressing their feelings and, when appropriate, referral for psychologic or family counseling.

Many NICUs use volunteers in varying capacities. After they have gone through the orientation program, volunteers can perform tasks such as holding the infants, stocking bedside cabinets, assembling parent packets, and, in some nurseries, feeding the infants.

Parental Maladaptation. The incidence of physical and emotional abuse is increased in infants who, because of preterm

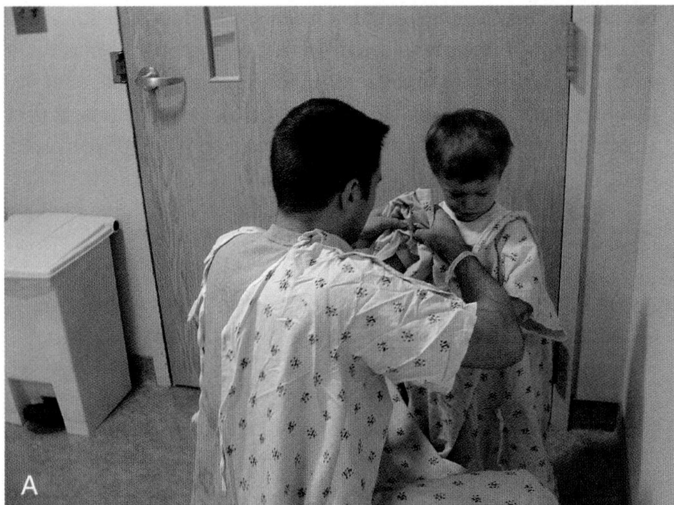

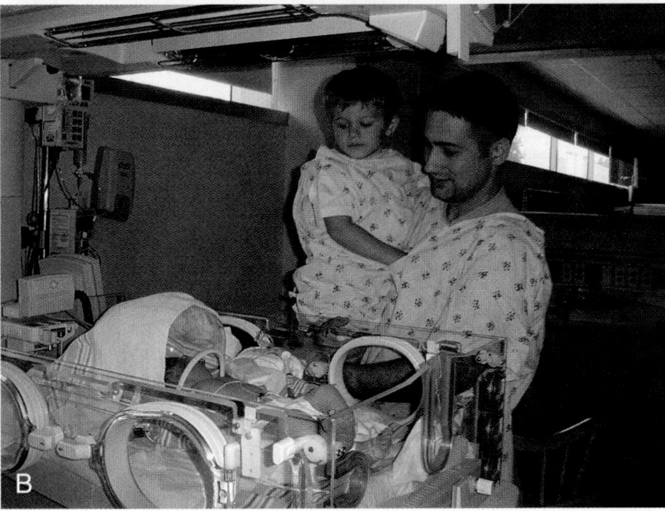

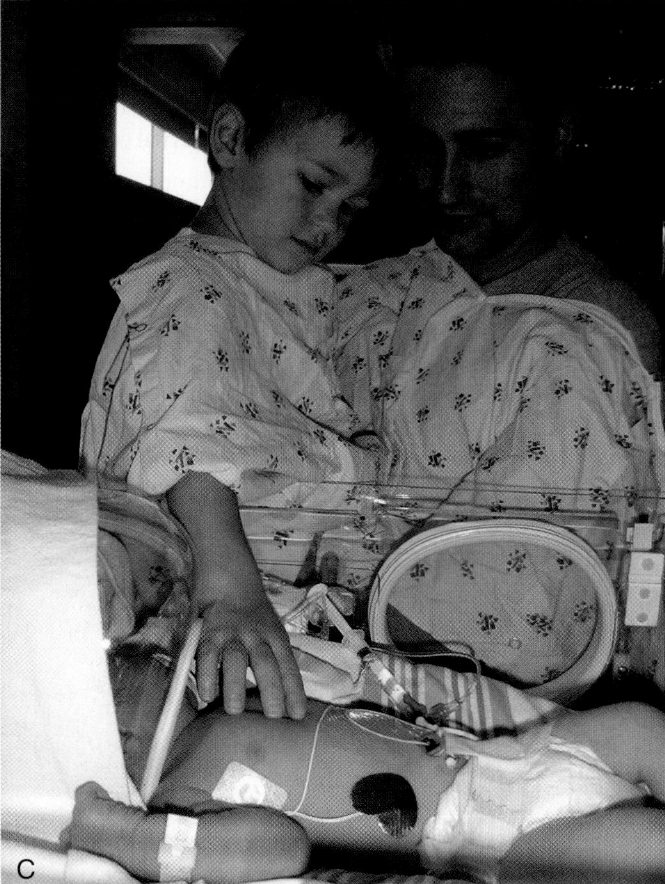

FIG 34-11 Sibling visits newborn in the neonatal intensive care unit. **A,** Father prepares older child for visit. **B,** Sibling observes neonate at a safe distance. **C,** He reaches out to touch the infant. (Courtesy Lauren and Brian LiVecchi, Raleigh, NC.)

birth or high risk condition, are separated from their parents for a time after birth. Physical abuse includes varying degrees of poor nutrition, poor hygiene, and bodily harm. Emotional abuse ranges from subtle disinterest to outright dislike of the infant. Appropriate resources should be made available to assess the parent's feelings regarding the preterm infant's birth. In addition, proper guidance and counseling are made available, including posthospital discharge, to help families adjust to and care for the preterm infant. The ultimate goal is for the family to accept the infant and incorporate this new member into the existing family structure.

Parent Education

The criteria showing an infant's readiness for discharge are that the infant's physiologic condition is stable, the infant is consuming adequate nutrition, and the infant's body temperature is stable. The parents or other caregivers, should demonstrate physical, emotional, and educational readiness to assume responsibility for the total care of the infant. Ideally, the home environment is adequate for meeting the needs of the infant. Resources for parents and health care providers include http://premature-infant.com and www.neonatology.org.

Complications in High Risk Infants

Respiratory Distress Syndrome

Respiratory distress syndrome (RDS) refers to a lung disorder usually affecting preterm infants. Maternal and fetal conditions associated with a decreased incidence and severity of RDS include female sex, African-American race, maternal gestational hypertension, maternal drug abuse, maternal steroid therapy (betamethasone), chronic retroplacental abruption, prolonged rupture of membranes, and IUGR. The incidence and severity of RDS increase as gestational age decreases. Perinatal asphyxia, hypovolemia, male sex, Caucasian race, maternal diabetes (types 1 and 2), second-born twin, familial predisposition, maternal hypotension, cesarean birth without labor, hydrops fetalis, and third-trimester bleeding place an infant at increased risk for RDS. The incidence of RDS in infants weighing less than 1500 g (3.3 lb) is about 45% (Hamvas, 2011).

RDS is caused by a lack of pulmonary surfactant, which leads to progressive atelectasis, loss of functional residual capacity, and ventilation-perfusion imbalance with an uneven distribution of ventilation. This surfactant deficiency can be caused by insufficient surfactant production, abnormal composition and function, disruption of surfactant production, or a combination of these factors. The weak respiratory muscles and an overly compliant chest wall, common among preterm infants, contribute to the sequence of events that occurs. Lung capacity is further compromised by the presence of proteinaceous material and epithelial debris in the airways. The resulting decreased oxygenation, cyanosis, and metabolic or respiratory acidosis can cause the pulmonary vascular resistance (PVR) to be increased. This increased PVR can lead to right-to-left shunting and a reopening of the ductus arteriosus and foramen ovale (Fig. 34-12).

Clinical symptoms of RDS usually appear immediately after or within 6 hours of birth. Physical examination reveals crackles, poor air exchange, pallor, the use of accessory muscles (retractions) and, occasionally, apnea. Radiographic findings

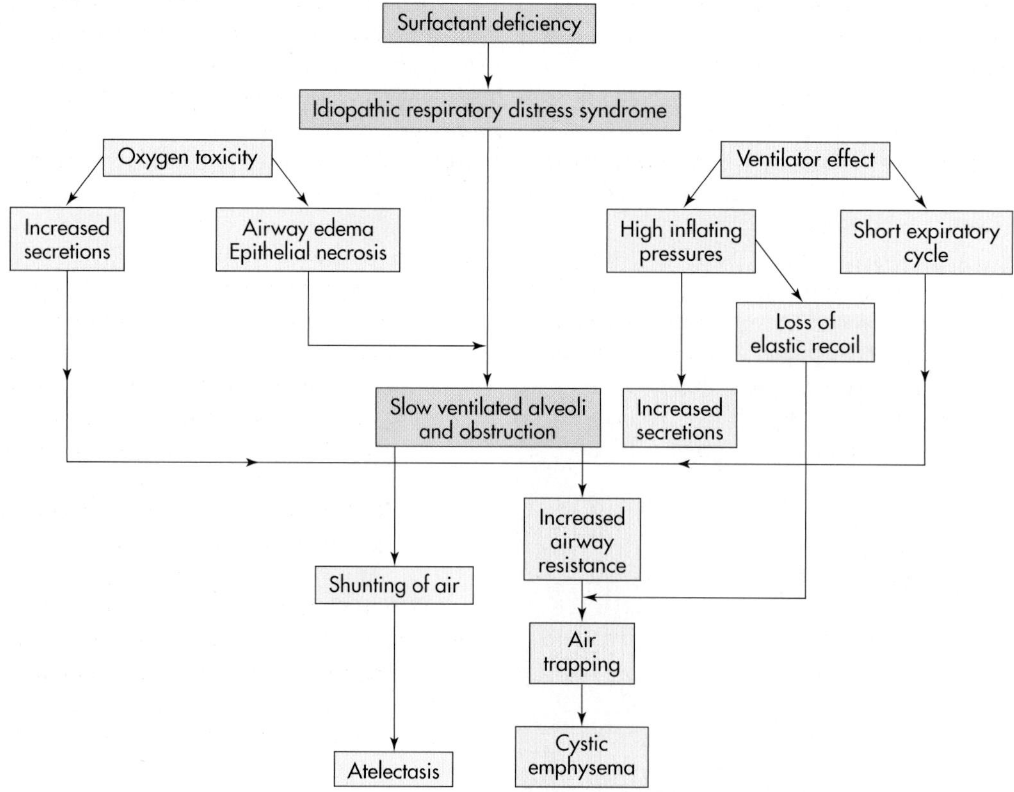

FIG 34-12 Pathogenesis of respiratory distress syndrome (RDS). (From Gardner, S., Enzman-Hines, M., & Dickey, L. [2011]. Respiratory diseases. In S. Gardner, B. Carter, M. Enzman-Hines, & J. Hernandez [Eds.], *Merenstein & Gardner's handbook of neonatal intensive care* [7th ed.]. St. Louis: Mosby.)

include a uniform reticulogranular appearance and air bronchograms (Gardner et al., 2011b; Orlando, 2012). The infant's clinical course is variable, usually with an increased oxygen requirement and increased respiratory effort, atelactasis, loss of functional residual capacity, and worsening of ventilation-perfusion imbalance.

RDS is a self-limiting disease that usually abates after 72 hours. This disappearance of respiratory signs coincides with the production of surfactant in the type 2 cells of the alveoli.

The treatment for RDS is supportive. Adequate ventilation and oxygenation must be established and maintained in an attempt to prevent ventilation-perfusion mismatch and atelectasis. Exogenous surfactant may be administered at birth or shortly after; this has the effect of shortening the typical course of RDS. Positive-pressure ventilation, nasal CPAP, and oxygen therapy may be necessary during the respiratory illness.

The mortality and morbidity rates associated with RDS are attributed to the infant's immature organ systems and the complications associated with the treatment of the disease (Hamvas, 2011). Preventing complications associated with mechanical ventilation is critical. These complications include pulmonary interstitial emphysema, pneumothorax, and chronic lung disease. Acid-base balance is evaluated by monitoring the ABG values (Table 34-2). Pulse oximetry documents trends in oxygenation. Capillary blood gas values indicate the pH and Pco_2 status in infants who are in more stable condition.

The maintenance of an NTE is critical to the care of infants with RDS. Infants with hypoxemia are unable to increase their metabolic rate when they experience cold stress (Hamvas, 2011).

The clinical and radiographic presentation (radiodense lung fields and air bronchograms) of neonatal pneumonia can be similar to that of RDS. Fluid in the minor fissure also can be noted in infants with neonatal pneumonia. Therefore, sepsis evaluation, including blood culture and complete blood count (CBC) with differential, is done in infants with RDS and risk factors to rule out neonatal pneumonia. Occasionally a lumbar puncture is done as part of the sepsis evaluation. Broad-spectrum antibiotics are begun while the results of cultures are awaited.

Fluid and nutrition must be maintained in the critically ill infant with RDS. Parenteral nutrition can be implemented to provide protein and fats to promote a positive nitrogen balance. Daily monitoring of the electrolyte values, urinary output, and weight help evaluate the infant's hydration status.

Frequent blood sampling can make blood transfusions necessary. The critically ill infant usually needs to have a venous hematocrit level of more than 40% to maintain adequate oxygen-carrying capacity (Pranke & Onsten, 2011).

TABLE 34-2 Normal Arterial Blood Gas Values for Neonates

VALUE	RANGE
pH	7.35-7.45
Arterial oxygen pressure (Pao_2)	60-80 mm Hg
Carbon dioxide pressure ($Paco_2$)	35-45 mm Hg
Bicarbonate (HCO_3^-)	18-26 mEq/L
Base excess	(−5) to (+5)
Oxygen saturation	92%-94%

From Wood, A., & Jones, D. (2011). Acid-base homeostasis and oxygenation. In S. Gardner, B. Carter, M. Enzman-Hines, & J. Hernandez (Eds.), *Merenstein & Gardner's handbook of neonatal intensive care* (7th ed.). St. Louis: Mosby.

! NURSING ALERT

When transfusion is needed, the family may request directed donor blood. This donor blood usually is obtained from a family member or close friend of the family who has the same blood type as the infant or a compatible blood type. It may be necessary to notify the infant's family of the potential need for blood transfusion on admission to allow for the processing of directed-donor blood.

Reassuring the family about stringent testing of all blood products can help alleviate some of their anxiety about the transmission of blood-borne pathogens such as human immunodeficiency virus (HIV) and hepatitis B. Because some religions prohibit the use of blood transfusions, it is critical to obtain a complete history from the family, including their religious preference. Alternative strategies for maintaining the infant's hematocrit may be used in these instances.

Retinopathy of Prematurity

Retinopathy of prematurity is a complex multicausal disorder that affects the developing retinal vessels of preterm infants. The normal retinal vessels begin to form in utero at approximately 16 weeks in response to an unknown stimulus. These vessels continue to develop until they reach maturity at approximately 42 to 43 weeks after conception. Once the retina is completely vascularized, the retinal vessels are not susceptible to ROP. The mechanism of injury in ROP is unclear. Oxygen tensions that are too high for the level of retinal maturity initially result in vasoconstriction. After oxygen therapy is discontinued, neovascularization occurs in the retina and vitreous, with capillary hemorrhages, fibrotic resolution, and possible retinal detachment. Scar tissue formation and consequent visual impairment can be mild or severe. The entire disease process in severe cases can take as long as several months to evolve. The infant is examined by an ophthalmologist before discharge, and follow-up examinations are recommended as needed (Fraser, 2012b; Gardner et al., 2011b).

The key to the management of ROP is prevention of preterm birth and early detection. Blood oxygen levels in the preterm infant should be closely monitored and significant fluctuations avoided. Oxygen and ventilator settings should be adjusted to keep oxygen saturations within acceptable levels. Cryotherapy and laser photocoagulation are common treatments for ROP (Gardner et al., 2011b). Researchers are examining the effect of the NICU environment on the development of ROP in relation to light that shines directly through the very thin eyelids of very immature infants. Ambient lighting in the NICU is known to have an effect on the developing eye; although it may not directly cause ROP, it does contribute to other visual problems for the preterm infant. Another potential contributor to ROP is hyperglycemia, which apparently fosters vasoproliferation (Chavez-Valdez, McGowan, Cannon, & Lehmann, 2011).

Bronchopulmonary Dysplasia

Bronchopulmonary dysplasia (BPD) is a chronic pulmonary condition occurring most commonly in preterm infants requiring mechanical ventilation. The etiology of BPD is multifactorial and includes pulmonary immaturity, surfactant deficiency, lung injury and stretch, barotrauma, inflammation caused by oxygen exposure, fluid overload, ligation of a PDA, and a familial predisposition. With the advent of prenatal use of maternal steroids when preterm birth is expected, coupled with use of exogenous surfactant in the neonate, the risk of BPD or chronic lung disease (CLD) has been reduced (Fraser, 2012b).

Clinical signs of BPD include tachypnea, retractions, nasal flaring, increased work of breathing, activity intolerance to handling and feeding, and tachycardia. Infants with BPD can have an increase in ventilatory requirements or are unable to be weaned from the ventilator. Auscultation of the lung fields in affected infants typically reveals crackles, decreased air movement, and occasionally expiratory wheezing. Hypoxia, hypercapnia, and respiratory acidosis are common (Bancalari, 2011).

The treatment for BPD includes oxygen therapy, nutrition, fluid restriction, and medications (diuretics, corticosteroids, and bronchodilators). However, the key to the management of BPD is prevention of prematurity and RDS. Other therapies that can aid in prevention of BPD include antenatal steroids, prophylactic surfactant, avoidance of mechanical ventilation when possible, use of CPAP, gentle ventilation in the delivery room, and administration of vitamin A (Gardner et al., 2011b).

The prognosis for infants with BPD depends on the degree of pulmonary dysfunction and on the infant's overall health status. Oxygen therapy may be continued in the home setting. There is usually progressive normalization of pulmonary function, although abnormalities of small airways can persist. Mortality after hospital discharge is usually due to complications such as respiratory infection (Bancalari & Walsh, 2011).

Patent Ductus Arteriosus

The ductus arteriosus is a normal muscular contractile structure in the fetus connecting the left pulmonary artery and the dorsal aorta, diverting blood to the placenta for gas exchange. The duct constricts after birth as oxygenation, the levels of circulating prostaglandins, and the muscle mass increase. Other factors that promote ductal closure include catecholamines, low pH, bradykinin, and acetylcholine. When the fetal ductus arteriosus fails to close after birth, **patent ductus arteriosus (PDA)** occurs. During the first few days of life when a preterm or sick infant is under stress, the ductus arteriosus can reopen, leading to mottling and cyanosis. It can last only a few minutes until the stress is past, or it can remain open if the infant is quite unstable. The incidence of PDA in infants born at less than 28 weeks of gestation is 70% (Clyman, 2013).

Although a small PDA can be asymptomatic, the clinical presentation in an infant with a significant PDA includes systolic murmur, active precordium, bounding peripheral pulses, tachycardia, tachypnea, crackles, and hepatomegaly. The systolic murmur is heard best at the second or third intercostal space at the upper left sternal border. An increased left ventricular stroke volume causes an active precordium.

Radiographic studies in infants with PDA typically show cardiac enlargement and pulmonary edema. ABGs indicate hypercapnia and metabolic acidosis. Definitive diagnosis is through echocardiography, which can visualize a PDA and measure the amount of blood shunting across the PDA (Kenney, Hoover, Williams, & Iskersky, 2011).

Medical management consists of ventilatory support, fluid restriction, and the administration of indomethacin or ibuprofen (Fraser, 2012b). Ibuprofen and indomethacin inhibit prostaglandin synthesis and cause the PDA to constrict. However, there is some concern that indomethacin reduces blood flow to the brain, kidneys, and GI tract (Clyman, Couto, & Murphy, 2012).

Ventilatory support is adjusted based on the ABG values. Fluid restriction and diuretic therapy are implemented to decrease cardiovascular volume overload. Surgical ligation is done when a PDA is clinically significant and medical management is ineffective.

Nursing management of the infant with PDA focuses on supportive care. The infant needs an NTE, adequate oxygenation, meticulous fluid balance, and parental support.

Germinal Matrix Hemorrhage–Intraventricular Hemorrhage

Germinal matrix hemorrhage–intraventricular hemorrhage (GMH-IVH) is one of the most common types of brain injuries in neonates and is among the most severe from the standpoint of both short- and long-term outcomes. It is the most common type of intracranial hemorrhage, occurring almost exclusively in preterm infants. The risk of GMH-IVH increases with decreasing gestational age. The incidence of GMH-IVH is estimated to be 5% to 11% and has shown a decline in recent years (de Vries, 2011). The decline is attributed to the prenatal use of corticosteroids and postnatal use of surfactant.

The germinal matrix is a loose network of cells abundantly supplied with tiny, fragile, thin-walled vessels. It lies beneath the lining of the lateral ventricles. This area is present and active until 34 to 35 weeks of gestation as a site for production of neurons and glial cells that gradually migrate to the cerebral cortex. The germinal matrix is especially vulnerable to alterations in cerebral blood flow related to blood pressure changes. Hemorrhage occurs when the tiny blood vessels rupture; the hemorrhage can extend into the lateral ventricles, then to the third and fourth ventricles, the subarachnoid space, and even into the white matter of the brain. Large clots can develop and create outflow obstruction from the ventricles (de Vries, 2011).

Infants who experience GMH-IVH are usually less than 34 weeks of gestation with a history of hypoxia, birth asphyxia, RDS, or other events causing impaired venous return or increased venous pressure. In the majority of cases GMH-IVH is diagnosed within the first 3 to 4 days of life. Infants with GMH-IVH can be asymptomatic, develop symptoms gradually, or have an acute catastrophic presentation. Clinical signs suggestive of hemorrhage include decreasing hematocrit, full anterior fontanel, changes in activity level, and decreased muscle tone. With a catastrophic incident, the infant can develop stupor, coma, respiratory distress that progresses to apnea, decerebrate posturing, and seizures; there is a high mortality rate in these cases (Bonifacio, Gonzalez, & Ferriero, 2012).

Morbidity and mortality related to GMH-IVH are based on the severity of the hemorrhage and the associated problems. Small hemorrhages are usually associated with good outcomes and high survival rates. Infants with more severe hemorrhages, posthemorrhagic ventricular dilation, or periventricular leukomalacia have higher mortality rates and greater long-term morbidity. Neurodevelopmental outcomes of GMH-IVH include hydrocephalus, cerebral palsy, developmental delays, learning disorders, and sensory and attention problems (de Vries, 2011).

Care management begins with prevention of preterm birth, birth trauma, and hypoxic-ischemic injury. Antenatal steroids help reduce the risk of GMH-IVH. Prompt and skilled resuscitation at birth minimizes hypoxia and ischemia. Nursing care focuses on recognition of factors that increase the risk of GMH-IVH, interventions to decrease the risk of bleeding, and supportive care to infants who have bleeding episodes. Ongoing assessment of vulnerable infants involves monitoring oxygenation and perfusion and avoiding or minimizing activities that increase cerebral blood flow. If GMH-IVH occurs, care is focused on maintaining oxygenation and perfusion, an NTE, and normoglycemia. The infant is positioned with the head in midline and the head of the bed elevated slightly to prevent or minimize fluctuations in intracranial blood pressure. Rapid infusions of fluids should be avoided. Blood pressure is monitored closely for fluctuations. The use of developmental interventions such as swaddling or containment during painful procedures can help promote greater physiologic stability (Ditzenberger & Blackburn, 2014).

Nursing support for parents includes assessment of their understanding and concerns related to the infant's condition. They need opportunities to discuss their feelings and ask questions about the infant's condition and care as well as the long-term prognosis. Nurses can demonstrate to parents how they can interact with the infant in a developmentally appropriate manner. Nurses can provide anticipatory guidance regarding ways the infant's needs and care will change as he or she matures. For many of these infants a multidisciplinary approach to care is needed to address the neurodevelopmental sequelae of GMH-IVH and to plan for care after hospital discharge (de Vries, 2011).

Necrotizing Enterocolitis

Necrotizing enterocolitis is an acute inflammatory disease of the GI mucosa, commonly complicated by bowel necrosis and perforation. NEC occurs in up to 10% of all LBW infants. More than 90% of cases are preterm infants. Reported mortality rates due to NEC are around 30% (Caplan, 2011).

The exact etiology and pathophysiology of NEC are unclear, although many factors seem to contribute to its development (risk factors are listed in Box 34-6). Three primary conditions appear to be involved in the etiology of NEC. The first is intestinal ischemia that occurs as a result of asphyxia/hypoxia or events that cause a redistribution of blood flow away from the GI tract (e.g., hypotension, hypovolemia, severe stress). A second condition involved in the development of NEC seems to be bacterial colonization of the initially sterile GI tract with harmful organisms prior to the establishment of normal intestinal flora. *Klebsiella, Escherichia coli,* and *Clostridium* are common organisms involved in NEC. A third condition associated with the development of NEC is enteral feeding. The majority of infants with NEC had received some type of enteral feeding. It is thought that the feedings can provide a substrate for bacterial proliferation or that feedings can increase intestinal oxygen demand during absorption and results in tissue hypoxia. Breast milk seems to have a protective effect against the development of NEC—it is rare among infants who are exclusively fed breast milk. The use of probiotics shows promise in reducing the risk of NEC. Use of natural prophylactic probiotics such as *Bifidobacterium infantis* and *Streptococcus thermophilus* to enhance bowel flora appears to decrease the incidence of NEC (AlFaleh & Anabrees, 2014). In addition, MEN can help reduce the risk of NEC.

BOX 34-6 Risk Factors for Necrotizing Enterocolitis

- Asphyxia
- Respiratory distress syndrome
- Umbilical artery catheter
- Exchange transfusion
- Early enteral feedings/hyperosmolar feedings
- Patent ductus arteriosus
- Congenital heart disease
- Myelomeningocele
- Intrauterine growth restriction
- Polycythemia
- Anemia
- Shock
- Gastrointestinal infection

Data from Caplan, M.S. (2011). Neonatal necrotizing enterocolitis: Clinical observations, pathophysiology, and prevention. In R.J. Martin, A.A. Fanaroff, & M.C. Walsh (Eds.), *Fanaroff & Martin's neonatal-perinatal medicine: Diseases of the fetus and infant* (9th ed.). St. Louis: Mosby; Lovvorn, H.N., Glenn, J.B., Pacetti, A.S., & Carter, B.S. (2011). Neonatal surgery. In S.L. Gardner, B.S. Carter, M. Enzman-Hines, & J.A. Hernandez (Eds.), *Merenstein & Gardner's handbook of neonatal intensive care* (7th ed.). St. Louis: Mosby.

The onset of NEC in the term infant usually occurs between 1 and 3 days after birth, but can occur as late as 1 month. In the preterm infant NEC usually occurs within the first 7 days but can be delayed for up to 30 days. The signs of NEC are nonspecific, which is characteristic of many neonatal diseases. Some generalized signs include decreased activity, hypotonia, pallor, recurrent apnea and bradycardia, decreased oxygen saturation values, respiratory distress, metabolic acidosis, oliguria, hypotension, decreased perfusion, temperature instability, and cyanosis. GI symptoms include abdominal distention, increasing or bile-stained residual gastric aspirates, grossly bloody stools, abdominal tenderness, and erythema of the abdominal wall (Caplan, 2011; Lovvorn, Glenn, Pacetti, & Carter, 2011).

A diagnosis is confirmed by a radiographic examination that reveals bowel loop distention, pneumatosis intestinalis (air in the wall of the bowel), pneumoperitoneum, portal air, or a combination of these findings. The abnormal radiographic findings are caused by the bacterial colonization of the GI tract associated with NEC, resulting in ileus. Pneumatosis intestinalis, pneumoperitoneum, and portal air are caused by gas produced by the bacteria that invade the wall of the intestines and escape into the peritoneum and portal system when perforation occurs. The laboratory evaluation in such infants consists of a CBC with differential, coagulation studies, ABG analysis, measurement of serum electrolyte levels, and blood culture. The white blood cell count can be either increased or decreased. The platelet count and coagulation study findings can be abnormal, showing thrombocytopenia and disseminated intravascular coagulation (DIC). Electrolyte levels can be abnormal related to leaking capillary beds and fluid shifts with the infection (Caplan, 2011; Lovvorn et al., 2011).

Management strategies are based on the degree of bowel involvement and the severity of the disease. The goal of treatment is to prevent progression of the NEC, intestinal perforation, and shock.

For the infant with suspected or confirmed NEC, oral or tube feedings are discontinued to rest the GI tract. An orogastric tube is placed and attached to low wall suction to provide gastric decompression. Parenteral therapy (often TPN) is begun. Because NEC is an infectious disease, control of the infection is imperative, with an emphasis on careful hand hygiene before and after infant contact. Antibiotic therapy may be instituted, and surgical resection is performed if perforation or clinical deterioration occurs. Therapy is usually prolonged, and recovery can be delayed by the formation of adhesions, the development of the complications associated with bowel resection, the occurrence of short-bowel syndrome (especially if the ileocecal valve is removed), or the development of intolerance to oral feedings. Some of these infants are candidates for intestinal transplants if they truly have short-bowel syndrome (Caplan, 2011; Lovvorn et al., 2011).

Families need education and support when faced with the crisis of having an infant with NEC. As part of the health care team nurses can help parents understand the severity of the disease, treatment options, and care needed by the infant. When the disease is severe and the prognosis is poor, nurses are instrumental in supporting families with decision making and anticipatory grieving (Gardner & Dickey, 2011; Siegel et al., 2011).

Infant Pain Responses

The physiology of pain and pain assessment in the newborn are discussed in Chapter 24. This discussion focuses on pain assessment and management in the preterm infant.

Pain Assessment

Assessment of pain in the neonate is difficult because evaluation must be based on physiologic changes and behavioral observations. Pain is considered the fifth vital sign, and its assessment is a requirement of The Joint Commission (TJC, 2011). A scale that examines multiple dimensions facilitates accurate assessment of neonatal pain (Gardner, Enzman-Hines, & Dickey, 2011a). Although behaviors such as vocalizations, facial expressions, body movements, and general state are common to all infants, they vary with different situations. Crying associated with pain is more intense and sustained. Facial expression is the most consistent and specific characteristic; scales are available for systematic evaluation of facial features, such as eye squeeze, brow bulge, and open mouth and taut tongue (Prkachin, 2011) (see Fig. 24-19). Most infants respond with increased body movements but can be experiencing pain even when lying quietly with eyes closed. The preterm infant's response to pain can be behaviorally blunted or absent. An infant who receives a muscle-paralyzing agent such as vecuronium is incapable of mounting a behavioral or visible pain response (Box 34-7) yet still feels pain.

! NURSING ALERT

When in doubt about the presence of pain in infants, the nurse should base the need for interventions on the following rule: whatever is painful to an adult or child is painful to an infant unless proved otherwise. The nurse should anticipate pain and intervene promptly, without waiting for physiologic or behavioral signs of pain to appear.

BOX 34-7 Manifestations of Acute Pain in the Neonate

Physiologic Responses

Vital Signs
- Increased heart rate
- Increased blood pressure
- Rapid, shallow respirations

Oxygenation
- Decreased transcutaneous O_2 saturation ($TcPo_2$)
- Decreased arterial O_2 saturation (Sao_2)

Skin
- Pallor or flushing
- Diaphoresis
- Palmar sweating

Other Observations
- Increased muscle tone
- Dilated pupils
- Decreased vagal nerve tone
- Increased intracranial pressure
- Laboratory evidence of metabolic or endocrine changes
  - Hyperglycemia
  - Lowered pH
  - Elevated corticosteroids

Behavioral Responses

Vocalizations: Observe Quality, Timing, and Duration
- Crying
- Whimpering
- Groaning

Facial Expression
- Grimacing
- Brow furrowed
- Chin quivering
- Eyes tightly closed
- Mouth open and squarish

Body Movements and Posture
- Limb withdrawal
- Thrashing
- Rigidity
- Flaccidity
- Fist clenching

Change in State
- Changes in sleep-wake cycles
- Changes in feeding behavior
- Changes in activity level
- Fussiness, irritability
- Listlessness

Adapted from Blackburn, S. (2013). *Maternal, fetal, and neonatal physiology: A clinical perspective* (4th ed.). Maryland Heights, MO: Elsevier; Gardner, S.L., Enzman-Hines, M., & Dickey, L.A. (2011). Pain and pain relief. In S.L. Gardner, B.S. Carter, M. Enzman-Hines, & J.A. Hernandez (Eds.), *Merenstein & Gardner's handbook of neonatal intensive care* (7th ed.). St. Louis: Mosby.

Several tools have been developed for the assessment of pain in the neonate. The CRIES tool is discussed in Chapter 24 (see Table 24-5). Other instruments are the Pain Assessment Tool (PAT) (Hodgkinson, Bear, Thorn, & Van Blaricum, 1994); Scale for Use in Newborns (SUN) (Blauer & Gerstmann, 1998); Behavioral Pain Score (BPS) (Pokela, 1994); Distress Scale for

Ventilated Newborn Infants (DSVNI) (Sparshott, 1995); Neonatal Infant Pain Scale (NIPS) (Lawrence, Alcock, McGrath, et al., 1993); and Premature Infant Pain Profile (PIPP) (Stevens, Johnston, Petryshen, & Taddio, 1996). The PIPP is one of the most widely used scales for preterm infants because it considers behavioral, physiologic, and contextual indicators (Gardner et al., 2011a).

Memory of Pain

Preterm infants are subjected to a variety of repeated noxious stimuli, including multiple heelsticks, venipuncture, endotracheal intubation and suctioning, arterial sticks, chest tube placement, and lumbar puncture. The effects of pain caused by such procedures are not fully known, but researchers have begun to investigate potential consequences. From preliminary reports, it appears that a rewiring of the pain responses occurs in preterm infants who have been subjected to multiple painful treatments early in their lives. The nervous system networks of the preterm infant appear denser and have more branches than those in the average infant, leading to the conclusion that the pain threshold and sensitivity in once preterm infants is heightened for life. There are also changes when the infant has undergone anesthesia (Gardner et al., 2011a).

Consequences of Untreated Pain in Infants

Despite research on the neonate's experience of pain, infant pain remains inadequately managed. This mismanagement is partially due to misconceptions regarding the effects of pain on the neonate, as well as a lack of knowledge of immediate and long-term consequences of untreated pain. Infants respond to noxious stimuli through physiologic indicators (increased heart rate and blood pressure, variability in heart rate and intracranial pressure, and decreases in arterial oxygen saturations and skin blood flow) and behavioral indicators (muscle rigidity, facial expression, crying, withdrawal, and sleeplessness). The physiologic and behavioral indicators, as well as a variety of neurophysiologic responses to noxious stimulation, are responsible for short- and long-term consequences of pain.

Pain Management

The International Evidence-Based Group for Neonatal Pain developed a Consensus Statement for the Prevention and Management of Pain in the Newborn which states that pain must be anticipated and prevented to avoid long-term consequences (Anand and The International Evidence-Based Group for Neonatal Pain, 2001). Nonpharmacologic measures to alleviate pain include repositioning, swaddling, containment, cuddling, rocking, playing music, reducing environmental stimulation, providing tactile comfort measures and nonnutritive sucking, and using oral sucrose. However, nonpharmacologic measures may not be sufficient to decrease physiologic distress, even if behavioral responses such as crying are lessened. In preterm infants additional stimulation such as stroking or environmental light or noise can increase physiologic distress. The effect of the NICU environment must be considered along with other forms of stimuli that can produce stress and pain.

Morphine is the most widely used opioid analgesic for pharmacologic management of neonatal pain, with fentanyl as an effective alternative. Continuous or bolus epidural or IV infusion of opioids provides effective and safe pain control. Other methods are epidural/intrathecal infusion, local and regional nerve blocks, and topical anesthetics, as well as general anesthesia for surgery (Walden, 2014).

Parents are universally concerned that their infants are feeling pain during procedures. Nurses need to address these concerns and encourage the parents to speak with the health care professionals involved. Parents have the right to withhold consent for invasive procedures and are entitled to honest answers from those responsible for the infant's care. When appropriate, they also can help provide comfort measures for the infant. Kangaroo care is one parental intervention that comforts and calms the infant (Cong et al., 2012).

Parents want to know that nurses recognize pain in their infants and that the infants will be comfortable when they (the parents) are not present. They want to know that the nurse will advocate for comfort care for their baby. Although pain is considered a fifth vital sign, it cannot be assessed only at the time of vital signs. There must be ongoing evaluation of the infant's pain level and the effectiveness of comfort measures used. This assessment is not lengthy but can be as simple as walking to the bedside and closely observing the infant's color, posture, movements, and breathing. Pain is a real phenomenon that is preventable in many instances. Pain management is a standard of care, and it is considered unethical not to prevent and effectively treat pain. Another growing area of neonatal nursing is end-of-life and palliative care. Most of this care centers on pain management. Palliative care is really comfort care that supports the needs of the preterm, sick neonate (Walden, 2014).

Late Preterm Infants

Late preterm infants are those born between 34 0/7 and 36 6/7 weeks of gestation (Raju, Higgins, Stark, & Leveno, 2006). Because birth weights of late preterm infants often range from 2000 g (4.4 lb) to 2500 g (5.5 lb) and they appear relatively mature in comparison to the smaller less mature infant, they are often cared for as if they are normal term infants. Risk factors for late preterm infants can easily be overlooked. Compared with term infants, late preterm infants are at increased risk for problems with thermoregulation, hypoglycemia, hyperbilirubinemia, feeding, sepsis, and respiratory function (Hwang, Barfield, Smith, et al., 2013; Phillips, Goldstein, Hougland, et al., 2013). Many of these healthy-appearing infants are admitted directly to postpartum units with their mothers or stay in the NICU only briefly (i.e., less than 24 hours). They are commonly discharged home at 2 to 3 days of age with their mothers. Discharge before 48 hours after birth is not recommended (Phillips et al.).

Recognition of late preterm infants is essential to providing effective care. Initial physical assessment and assessment of gestational age are crucial to identifying these infants. Although the mother's estimated date of birth (EDB) can indicate a longer gestation, infant appearance, behaviors, and/or weight can indicate otherwise. The obstetric estimate of gestational age is usually reliable if it is based on a first-trimester ultrasound. However, if there is a discrepancy between the gestational age based on the obstetric estimate and newborn examination, it is better to rely on the estimate based on the newborn examination. The Association of Women's Health, Obstetric and

TABLE 34-3 Late Preterm Infant Assessment and Interventions

RISK FACTORS	ASSESSMENT	INTERVENTIONS*
Respiratory distress (RD)	Assess for cardinal signs of RD (nasal flaring, grunting, tachypnea, central cyanosis, retractions), for presence of apnea especially during feedings, and for hypothermia and hypoglycemia.	Perform gestational age assessment; observe for signs of RD; monitor oxygenation by pulse oximetry; provide supplemental oxygen judiciously.
Thermal instability	Monitor axillary temperature every 30 minutes immediately after birth until stable, thereafter every 1-4 hours, depending on gestational age and ability to maintain thermal stability.	Provide skin-to-skin care immediately after birth for stable infant; implement measures to prevent excess heat loss (adjust environmental temperature, avoid drafts); bathe only after thermal stability has been maintained for 1 hour.
Hypoglycemia	Monitor for signs and symptoms of hypoglycemia; assess feeding ability (latch, nipple feeding); assess thermal stability, signs and symptoms of RD; monitor bedside glucose in infants with additional risk factors (mother with diabetes, prolonged labor, RD, poor feeding).	Initiate early feedings of human milk or formula; avoid dextrose water or water feedings; provide intravenous dextrose as necessary for hypoglycemia.
Jaundice	Observe for jaundice in first 24 hours; evaluate maternal-fetal history for additional risk factors that may cause increased hemolysis and circulating levels of unconjugated bilirubin (Rh, ABO, spherocytosis, bruising); assess feeding method, voiding, stooling patterns.	Monitor transcutaneous bilirubin, and note risk zone on hour-specific nomogram (see Fig. 24-7).
Feeding problems	Assess suck-swallow and breathing; assess for respiratory distress, hypoglycemia, thermal stability; assess latch-on, maternal comfort with feeding method; weight loss no more than 10% of birth weight.	Initiate early feedings—human milk or formula; ensure maternal knowledge of feeding method and signs of inadequate feeding (sleepiness, lethargy, color changes during feeding, apnea during feeding, decreased or absent urinary output).

*This list is not exhaustive of nursing interventions; additional interventions include those discussed under the care of the high risk infant in this chapter.

Portions adapted from Pappas, B.E., & Robey, D.L. (2015). Care of the late preterm infant. In M.T. Verklan & M. Walden (Eds.), *Core curriculum for neonatal intensive care nursing* (5th ed.). St. Louis: Elsevier; Santa-Donato, A., Medoff-Cooper, B., Bakewell-Sachs, S., et al. (2007). *Late preterm infant assessment guide.* Washington, DC: Association of Women's Health, Obstetric and Neonatal Nurses.

Neonatal Nurses (AWHONN) published evidence-based clinical practice guidelines, the *Assessment and Care of the Late Preterm Infant* (AWHONN, 2010), for the education of perinatal nurses regarding the late preterm infant's risk factors and appropriate care and follow-up (Table 34-3).

Components of nursing care for late preterm infants and their parents are discussed in the following text. Frequent assessment is essential for detecting problems early so that appropriate interventions can be initiated.

Respiratory Distress

Late preterm infants are at increased risk for respiratory problems, including apnea. Close monitoring of respiratory status is essential and any changes are reported promptly to the primary health care provider. An Infant Car Seat Challenge is done prior to discharge (see Chapter 24). Infants may go home on an apnea monitor. If possible, parents should attend an infant cardiopulmonary resuscitation (CPR) class or view a video about infant CPR. To help prevent respiratory infections the nurse should instruct the parents to limit the infant's contact with others outside the home. The nurse should review signs and symptoms of respiratory problems with the parents.

Thermoregulation

Late preterm infants have more difficulty with thermoregulation than term infants, and cold stress is a greater concern. They have less body fat than term infants, a higher ratio of surface area to body weight, decreased glycogen stores, and less mature mechanisms for increasing metabolism for heat. Stores of brown fat are smaller and quickly depleted. Cold stress can quickly lead to hypoglycemia. Nurses must closely monitor body temperature and teach parents to take the infant's temperature. Parents are encouraged to keep a record of this at home and to report high or low temperatures. It is important to remember that temperature instability is often an early sign of neonatal sepsis (Phillips et al., 2013).

Nutrition

Late preterm infants are at greater risk of having breastfeeding difficulties and are more likely to have breastfeeding-associated rehospitalizations than term infants (Radtke, 2011). Feedings should occur at least every 2 to 3 hours and according to infant feeding cues. Late preterm infants eat less than term neonates and have fewer energy reserves to do so. They can have difficulty coordinating sucking, swallowing, and breathing. Breastfeeding can be more problematic if the infant is sleepy and difficult to arouse for feedings. Late preterm infants are prone to early fatigue during feedings and fall asleep before consuming adequate volumes of milk. Nurses should observe at least one feeding every 8 hours. Early and extended skin-to-skin contact promotes breastfeeding. If supplementation is needed, expressed breast milk is the best option. To maximize the milk supply and milk transfer to the infant, mothers should use the electric breast pump after feedings while in the hospital and continue this process at home until the infant is able to successfully remove milk from the breasts and until the milk supply is well established. The mother-baby nurse or lactation consultant can provide instruction and assist breastfeeding mothers with using a breast pump. Mothers also need information regarding safe milk handling and storage guidelines (Jones, 2011). Parents should keep an intake and output record until their health care provider tells them otherwise and should share this record with the health care provider at each visit (Phillips et al., 2013).

Hypoglycemia

Late preterm infants are three times more likely to develop hypoglycemia than term infants (Stuckey-Schrock & Schrock, 2013). Hospital protocols may require routine monitoring of blood glucose until levels are stabilized and the infant is feeding adequately. Although the cut-off value for treatment remains uncertain, blood glucose values of less than 40 or 45 mg/dl, or symptoms of hypoglycemia, should be treated (Blackburn, 2013). Bedside monitoring of blood glucose levels at frequent intervals throughout the late preterm infant's hospital stay is recommended.

Hyperbilirubinemia

Hyperbilirubinemia is more common in late preterm infants because of immaturity of the liver, decreased gastric motility, and increased breakdown of red blood cells (RBCs) (Raju, 2012). They are less able to conjugate and excrete bilirubin. Serum bilirubin levels tend to peak at 5 to 7 days and persist longer than in term infants. Hyperbilirubinemia is the most frequent reason for hospital readmission during the first week of life. Bilirubin levels are closely monitored before discharge, and parents are instructed regarding signs of jaundice and when to notify the health care provider. Follow-up visits soon after hospital discharge are important for monitoring rising bilirubin levels (Phillips et al., 2013; Stuckey-Schrock & Schrock, 2013).

Infection

The immune systems of late preterm infants are immature; thus they are more likely to experience infections. Nurses should assess the late preterm infant for signs and symptoms of infection including temperature instability, lethargy, irritability, poor feeding, or vomiting. Before discharge, nurses provide education for the parents about the common signs and symptoms of infection and when to notify the health care provider.

Postmature Infants

A pregnancy that is prolonged beyond 42 weeks is a *postterm* pregnancy, and the infant who is born is called postterm or *postmature*. Postmaturity can be associated with placental insufficiency, resulting in a fetus that has a wasted appearance (dysmaturity) at birth because of loss of subcutaneous fat and muscle mass. However, not all postterm infants show signs of dysmaturity; some continue to grow in utero and are large at birth. Most postmature infants are oversized but otherwise normal, with advanced development and bone age. A postmature infant has some, but not necessarily all, of the following physical characteristics (McGrath & Hardy, 2011):

- Generally a normal skull, but the reduced dimensions of the rest of the body in the presence of dysmaturity make the skull look inordinately large
- Dry, cracked (desquamating), parchment-like skin at birth
- Firm nails extending beyond the fingertips
- Profuse scalp hair
- Depleted subcutaneous fat layers, leaving the skin loose and giving the infant an "old person" appearance
- Long and thin body
- Absent vernix
- Can have meconium staining (golden yellow to green) of skin, nails, and cord, indicative of a hypoxic episode in utero or a perinatal infection such as listeriosis
- Can have an alert, wide-eyed appearance symptomatic of chronic intrauterine hypoxia

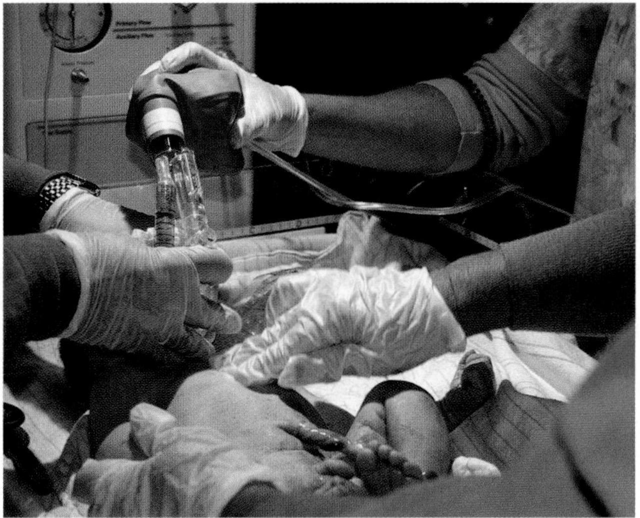

FIG 34-13 Infant being resuscitated at birth. Meconium was present on the abdomen, and umbilical cord. Infant was not breathing, and heart rate was 65 beats/minute at birth. Respirations and heart rate were normal at 2 minutes. (Courtesy Shannon Perry, Phoenix, AZ.)

The perinatal mortality rate is significantly higher in the postmature fetus and neonate. One reason for this is that during labor and birth the increased oxygen demands of the postmature fetus are not fully met. Insufficient gas exchange in the postmature placenta also increases the likelihood of intrauterine hypoxia, which can result in the passage of meconium in utero, thereby increasing the risk for meconium aspiration syndrome (MAS).

Parents may be concerned about the appearance of the postmature infant. Nurses can help them understand reasons for the dry, peeling, skin and other characteristics of postmaturity. Initial bathing should be done with a mild soap. It can be helpful to moisturize the skin with a petrolatum-based ointment. Nurses need to be alert to common problems associated with postmaturity such as meconium aspiration, fetal distress, macrosomia, and birth injury (De los Santos-Garate, Villa-Guillen, Villanueva-Garcia, et al., 2011).

Meconium Aspiration Syndrome

Meconium staining of the amniotic fluid can be indicative of fetal distress, especially in a vertex presentation. It appears in 10% to 15% of all births. Many infants with meconium staining exhibit no signs of depression at birth; approximately 5% of newborns who are exposed to meconium develop MAS (Ambalavanan & Carlo, 2011).

The presence of meconium in the amniotic fluid necessitates careful supervision of labor and close monitoring of fetal well-being. The presence of a team skilled in neonatal resuscitation is required at the birth of any infant with meconium stained amniotic fluid (Fig. 34-13). The mouth and nares of the infant are not routinely suctioned on the perineum before the infant's first breath. However, for infants with meconium staining who are not vigorous, endotracheal suctioning should be performed immediately. Vigorous infants need no special handling (Kattwinkel, AAP, & AHA, 2011).

If the infant is very depressed and the meconium is not removed from the airway at birth, it can migrate down to the terminal airways, causing mechanical obstruction leading to MAS. It also is possible that the fetus aspirated meconium in utero. Such meconium aspiration can cause a chemical pneumonitis. These infants can develop persistent pulmonary hypertension of the newborn, further complicating their management. Infants with MAS who receive surfactant can experience improved oxygenation, decreased severity of respiratory failure, and reduced need for ECMO (Polin, Carlo, & Committee on Fetus and Newborn, 2014). Researchers are examining the use of surfactant lavage in treating meconium aspiration (Choi, Hahn, Lee, et al., 2012).

Persistent Pulmonary Hypertension of the Newborn

The term persistent pulmonary hypertension of the newborn (PPHN) is applied to the combined findings of pulmonary hypertension, right-to-left shunting, and a structurally normal heart. PPHN can occur either as a single entity or as the main component of MAS, congenital diaphragmatic hernia, RDS, hyperviscosity syndrome, or neonatal pneumonia or sepsis. PPHN also is called *persistent fetal circulation* (PFC) because the syndrome includes a reversion to fetal pathways for blood flow (Soltau & Carlo, 2014).

A brief review of the characteristics of fetal blood flow can help in visualizing the problems with PPHN (see Fig. 12-13). In utero, oxygen-rich blood leaves the placenta via the umbilical vein, goes through the ductus venosus, and enters the inferior vena cava. From there it empties into the right atrium and is mostly shunted across the foramen ovale to the left atrium, effectively bypassing the lungs. This blood enters the left ventricle, leaves via the aorta, and preferentially perfuses the carotid and coronary arteries. Thus the heart and brain receive the most oxygenated blood. Blood drains from the brain into the superior vena cava, reenters the right atrium, proceeds to the right ventricle, and exits via the main pulmonary artery. The lungs are a high-pressure circuit, needing only enough perfusion for growth and nutrition. The ductus arteriosus (connecting the main pulmonary artery and the aorta) is the path of least resistance for the blood leaving the right side of the fetal heart, shunting most of the cardiac output away from the lungs and toward the systemic system. This right-to-left shunting is the key to fetal circulation.

After birth, both the foramen ovale and the ductus arteriosus close in response to various biochemical processes, pressure changes within the heart, and dilation of the pulmonary vessels. This dilation allows virtually all of the cardiac output to enter the lungs, become oxygenated, and provide oxygen-rich blood to the tissues for normal metabolism.

PPHN characteristically proceeds into a downward spiral of exacerbating hypoxia and pulmonary vasoconstriction. Prompt recognition and aggressive intervention are required to reverse this process (Orlando, 2012).

The infant with PPHN is typically born at term or post-term and has tachycardia and cyanosis. Management depends on the underlying cause of the persistent pulmonary hypertension. The use of ECMO has improved the chances of survival in these infants (see earlier discussion); however, it is considered a very invasive procedure. Effective use of inhaled nitric oxide (INO) as a pharmacologic intervention has increased. It acts as a vasodilator to decrease the pulmonary hypertension while increasing oxygenation (Bell, 2012). This therapy is proving to work well alone or with high-frequency ventilation. Another pharmacologic treatment is exogenous surfactant because some of these infants appear to be surfactant deficient. Use of environmental strategies such as decreasing adverse stimuli (excessive light and noise) to reduce stress is an area of ongoing research. This intervention is used in conjunction with other therapies.

Another mode of treatment for PPHN and other respiratory disorders of the newborn is high-frequency ventilation, a group of assisted ventilation methods that deliver small volumes of gas at high frequencies and limit the development of high airway pressure, thus reducing barotrauma. High-frequency ventilation decreases carbon dioxide while increasing oxygenation. It can be effectively used in conjunction with INO (Soltau & Carlo, 2014).

It is important to understand that PPHN is considered a cardiovascular and a respiratory problem. The lungs of these infants are healthy, but the hypertension of the cardiovascular system leads to their oxygenation problems.

Other Problems Related to Gestational Age

Small for Gestational Age and Intrauterine Growth Restriction

Infants who are small for gestational age (SGA; e.g., weight is less than the 10th percentile expected at term) and infants who have IUGR (rate of growth does not meet expected growth pattern) are considered high risk. Among these infants perinatal mortality rates are 5 to 20 times greater than for normal term infants (Gardner & Hernandez, 2011).

Various conditions can affect and impede growth in the developing fetus. Conditions occurring in the first trimester that affect all aspects of fetal growth (e.g., infections, teratogens, chromosomal abnormalities) or extrinsic conditions early in pregnancy result in symmetric IUGR (i.e., head circumference, length, and weight, are all less than the 10th percentile). Conditions causing symmetric growth restriction result in an SGA infant, usually with a head circumference that is smaller than that of a term infant and reduced brain capacity. Growth restriction in later stages of pregnancy, as a result of maternal or placental factors, results in asymmetric growth restriction (with respect to gestational age, weight will be less than the 10th percentile, whereas length and head circumference will be greater than the 10th percentile). Infants with asymmetric IUGR have the potential for normal growth and development. There is relative sparing of head and brain growth while weight and somatic organ growth are more seriously altered (Carlo, 2011).

Several physical findings are characteristic of the SGA neonate (Kliegman, 2011):

- Generally a normal skull, but the reduced dimensions of the rest of the body make the skull look inordinately large
- Reduced subcutaneous fat stores
- Loose and dry skin
- Diminished muscle mass, especially over buttocks and cheeks
- Sunken abdomen (scaphoid) as opposed to the well-rounded abdomen seen in normal infants
- Thin, yellowish, dry, and dull umbilical cord (normal cord is gray, glistening, round, and moist)
- Sparse scalp hair
- Wide skull sutures (inadequate bone growth)

Care of the SGA infant is based on the presence of clinical problems and is the same for preterm infants with similar problems. Gas exchange is supported by maintaining a clear airway and preventing cold stress. Hypoglycemia is treated with oral feedings (e.g., breast, formula) or IV dextrose as the infant's condition warrants. An external heat source (radiant warmer or incubator) is used until the infant is able to maintain an adequate body temperature. Nursing support of parents is the same as that given to parents of preterm infants.

Common problems that affect SGA (IUGR) infants are perinatal asphyxia, meconium aspiration, hypoglycemia, polycythemia, and temperature instability.

Perinatal Asphyxia

Commonly IUGR infants have been exposed to chronic hypoxia for varying periods before labor and birth. Labor is a stressor to the normal fetus, but it is an even greater stressor for the growth-restricted fetus. The chronically hypoxic infant is severely compromised even by a normal labor and has difficulty compensating after birth. Appropriate management and resuscitation are essential for these depressed infants.

The birth of SGA babies with perinatal asphyxia can be associated with a maternal history of heavy cigarette smoking; preeclampsia; low socioeconomic status; multifetal gestation; gestational infections such as rubella, cytomegalovirus, and toxoplasmosis; advanced diabetes mellitus; and cardiac problems. The nursing staff must be alert to and prepared for possible perinatal asphyxia during the birth of an infant to a woman with such a history. Sequelae to perinatal asphyxia include MAS (see previous discussion) and hypoglycemia.

Hypoglycemia

All high risk infants have an increased likelihood of developing hypoglycemia (plasma glucose <40 mg/dl) (Armentrout, 2015). Infants who experience physiologic stress can experience hypoglycemia as a result of a decreased glycogen supply, inadequate gluconeogenesis, or overuse of glycogen stored during fetal and postnatal life. Preterm infants can also become hypoglycemic because of inadequate intake and increased metabolic demands as a result of illness. There is insufficient evidence to support the concept that the preterm or high risk infant can tolerate lower levels of serum glucose any better than healthy term infants (Blackburn, 2013) (see Chapter 24 for discussion of hypoglycemia). The SGA infant, like the preterm infant, is at increased risk for hypoglycemia as a result of decreased fetal stores and decreased rate of gluconeogenesis (McGowan, Rozance, Price-Douglas, & Hay, 2011).

Symptoms of hypoglycemia include poor feeding, hypothermia, and diaphoresis. CNS symptoms can include tremors and jitteriness, weak cry, lethargy, floppy posture, convulsions, or coma. Diagnosis is confirmed by blood glucose determinations performed by the laboratory, when suspected, or by point-of-care testing with products such as Accuchek or One-Touch. Blood glucose screening should be done on all high risk infants soon after birth and frequently during the first few hours until glucose levels stabilize.

Polycythemia

Polycythemia or hyperviscosity of the blood is another common problem of the SGA infant. With polycythemia there is an excess in circulating RBC mass. This condition is a result of fetal hypoxia and intrauterine stress that forces the body to produce more RBCs in an attempt to provide oxygen to the developing fetus. Polycythemia is associated with maternal preeclampsia, maternal smoking, maternal diabetes, and delayed cord clamping (Diehl-Jones & Fraser, 2014). With hematocrit greater than 65% or venous hemoglobin greater than 22 g/dl, blood viscosity is increased. This can lead to compromised blood flow and reduced oxygenation of the body organs and increases the risk of neonatal stroke. Many infants with polycythemia are asymptomatic. Others present with plethora, cyanosis, CNS abnormalities (lethargy, jitteriness, seizures), respiratory distress, tachycardia, congestive heart failure, or hypoglycemia. Infants with polycythemia are at increased risk for hyperbilirubinemia. In some cases a partial exchange transfusion to reduce the viscosity of the blood is necessary.

Heat Loss

SGA infants are particularly susceptible to temperature instability as a result of decreased brown fat deposits, decreased adipose tissue, large body surface exposure, and, in many instances, poor flexion, as well as decreased glycogen storage in major organs such as the liver and heart. Therefore, close attention must be given to maintain an NTE. Nursing considerations focus on maintenance of thermoneutrality to promote recovery from perinatal asphyxia because cold stress jeopardizes such recovery.

Large for Gestational Age Infants

The large for gestational age (LGA) infant is defined as weighing 4000 g (8.8 lb) or more at birth. An infant is considered LGA despite gestation when the weight is more than the 90th percentile on growth charts or two standard deviations greater than the mean weight for gestational age. The LGA infant is at greater risk for morbidity than the SGA or preterm infant; such infants have an increased incidence of birth injuries, asphyxia, and congenital anomalies such as heart defects (Carlo, 2011).

All pregnancies of longer than 42 weeks of gestation must be thoroughly evaluated. All large fetuses are monitored during a trial of labor, and preparation is made for a cesarean birth if abnormal fetal heart pattern or poor progress of labor occurs. LGA newborns can be preterm, term, or postterm; they can be infants of mothers with diabetes; or they can be postmature. Each of these problems carries special concerns. Regardless of coexisting potential problems, the LGA infant is at risk by virtue of size alone.

The nurse assesses the LGA infant for hypoglycemia and trauma resulting from vaginal or cesarean birth. Any specific birth injuries are identified and treated appropriately (see Chapter 35).

Discharge Planning

Discharge planning for the high risk newborn begins early in the hospitalization. Throughout the infant's hospitalization the nurse gathers information from the health care team members and the family. This information is used to determine the infant's and family's readiness for discharge. Discharge teaching for the family of a high risk newborn is extensive, requires time and planning, and cannot be adequately accomplished on the day of discharge.

Information is provided about infant care, especially as it pertains to the particular infant's home care needs (e.g., supplemental oxygen, gastrostomy feedings, follow-up medical visits). Parents should be allowed to spend a night or two in a predischarge room providing care for the infant away from the NICU to become better acquainted with the necessary care and to have a time of transition in which questions can be answered regarding home care. Additional parent teaching should include bathing and skin care; requirements for meeting nutritional needs following discharge; safety in the home, including supine sleep position, avoiding exposure to cigarette smoke, prevention of infection (e.g., respiratory syncytial virus [RSV]); and medication administration.

COMMUNITY ACTIVITY

- Visit the March of Dimes website (www.marchofdimes.com/baby/holding-your-baby-close-kangaroo-care.aspx) and explore the resources available for parents of premature infants. Note the list of benefits of skin-to-skin holding. Think about some of the barriers that might prevent parents from holding their premature infant skin-to-skin. How might you overcome some of these barriers?
- Visit www.healthychildren.org, sponsored by the American Academy of Pediatrics. Under the Ages and Stages box, find the section on preemies. Review the information for parents about caring for and bringing home a premature infant. Research the availability of support groups for parents of premature infants in your community.

Durable medical equipment and supplies required for the care of the infant in the home should be delivered to the home before the infant is discharged; parents and care providers should have education in the use of the equipment and ample opportunity to practice. Parents of infants being discharged with special needs such as gavage or gastrostomy feedings, nasal cannula oxygen, tracheostomy, or colostomy should receive several days of thorough education in the procedure before discharge. Preterm infants have a high rate of emergency department visits and readmission to acute care centers; the family absolutely must have a health care provider they can contact for questions regarding infant care and behavior once they are home. Parents should obtain an age-appropriate car seat before the discharge of their infant and demonstrate its correct use. Car seat safety is an essential aspect of discharge planning. Infants who were born at less than 37 weeks of gestation should have an Infant Car Seat Challenge, consisting of a period of observation in an appropriate car seat to monitor for possible apnea, bradycardia, and decreased Sao_2 (Bull, Engle, Committee on Injury, Violence, and Poison Prevention, & Committee on Fetus and Newborn, 2009).

Before discharge all high risk or preterm infants should receive the appropriate immunizations, metabolic screening, hematologic assessment (bilirubin risk as appropriate), and hearing evaluation. Successful discharge of high risk infants to their homes requires a multidisciplinary approach. Medical, nursing, social services, and other professionals (physical therapy, occupational therapy, developmental follow-up specialist) are crucial to the smooth transition of these infants and their families to the home and community. If the infant is transported back to the community hospital that referred either the mother before birth or the infant after birth, interfacility communication is essential to continuity of care.

Instruction in CPR is essential for parents of all infants but especially for those of infants at risk for life-threatening events. Infants considered at risk include those who are preterm, have apnea or bradycardia, or have a tendency to choke. Before taking their infant home, parents must be able to administer CPR. All parents should be encouraged to obtain instruction in CPR at their local Red Cross or other community agency, if it is not provided by the NICU.

Transport to and from a Regional Center

If a hospital is not equipped to care for a high risk mother and fetus or a high risk infant, transfer to a specialized perinatal or tertiary care center is arranged. Maternal transport ideally occurs with the fetus in utero because this has two distinct advantages: (1) the associated neonatal morbidity and mortality are decreased; and (2) infant-parent attachment is supported, thereby avoiding separation of the parents and infant. For a variety of reasons, however, it is not always possible to transport the mother before the birth. These reasons include imminent birth and unanticipated problems; therefore, physicians and nurses in level 1 and 2 facilities must have the skills and equipment necessary for making an accurate diagnosis and implementing emergency interventions to stabilize the infant's condition until transport can occur (Rojas, Shirley, & Rush, 2011). The goal of these interventions is to maintain the infant's condition within the normal physiologic range. Specific attention is given to the following areas:

- Vital signs
- Oxygen and ventilation
- Thermoregulation
- Acid-base balance
- Fluid and electrolyte levels
- Glucose level
- Developmental interventions

Transport teams can include physicians, nurse practitioners, nurses with expertise in neonatal intensive care, and respiratory therapists. The team must have expertise in resuscitation, stabilization, and provision of critical care during the transport, which can occur on the ground or in the air. In a neonatal transport the team should provide information for the parents about the tertiary center. Transport teams can integrate an individual developmental plan of care into their caregiving efforts, thereby initiating multidisciplinary interventions early in the infant's life.

Health care professionals who are responsible for the early stabilization of newborns need specialized training to provide timely, efficient, and effective care. The S.T.A.B.L.E. training program (Box 34-8) is an evidence-based continuing education program that focuses on the postresuscitation and pretransport stabilization of sick neonates (Kendall, Scott, & Karlsen, 2012). It has been endorsed by the March of Dimes and the AAP. Training includes an interactive didactic presentation and a posttest (www.stableprogram.org).

The birth of any high risk infant can cause profound parental stress. Parents may grieve the loss of the ideal infant. They are fearful of the possible eventual outcomes for the infant. They

BOX 34-8 S.T.A.B.L.E. Program on Postresuscitation and Posttransport Stabilization Care of Sick Infants

S—Sugar and safe care (safety, IV fluids, hypoglycemia, hyperglycemia, umbilical catheters)
T—Temperature (hypothermia)
A—Airway (respiratory distress, CPAP, mechanical ventilation, pneumothorax
B—Blood pressure (hypovolemic, cardiogenic, and septic shock)
L—Lab work (lab tests related to infection, sepsis)
E—Emotional support (for parents of infants in NICUs)

CPAP, Continuous positive airway pressure; *IV,* intravenous; *NICU,* neonatal intensive care unit.
Modified from The S.T.A.B.L.E. program. (2013). *S.T.A.B.L.E. program module objectives.* Available at www.stableprogram.org/.

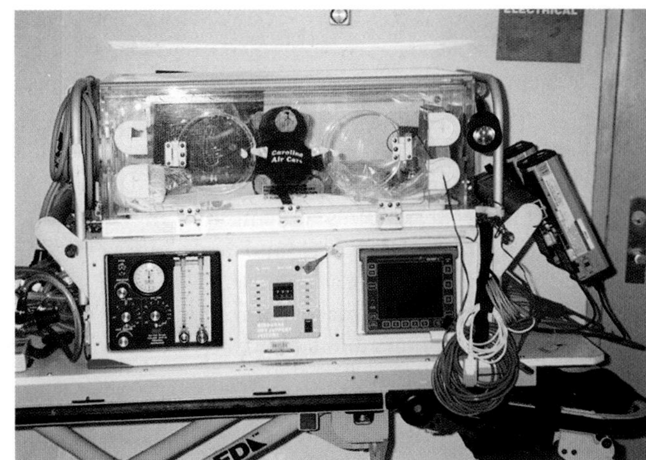

FIG 34-14 Total life support system for transport of high risk newborns. (Courtesy UNC Hospitals, Carolina Air Care, Chapel Hill, NC.)

must deal with the technologic world surrounding their infant, and amid all the equipment, it is sometimes difficult for them to perceive the infant and respond to his or her needs. Parents of high risk infants who have been transported to regional centers therefore need special support. As one way to deal with this problem, many intensive care units provide the family with a handbook or pictures of the tertiary care unit to help them understand what is going on around them. Parents should have the name and telephone number of a contact person at the regional center.

Infants are sometimes transferred back to the referring facility; however, in most cases the infant is discharged home from the tertiary care center. Preterm infants who require thermoregulation and gavage feedings may be cared for in community hospitals closer to home, which allows parents to visit their infant more easily and to work with their personal health care provider on the long-range outcomes for the infant. Specialized incubators make these trips possible (Fig. 34-14). However, parents may express mixed feelings about such return transports and may be reluctant to adapt to a different facility and group of caregivers. To minimize some of these concerns, giving the parents clear information about return transports during the initial discharge planning is important.

Anticipatory Grief

Families experience anticipatory grief when they are told of the impending death of their infant. Anticipatory grief prepares and protects parents who are facing a loss. Parents who have an infant with a debilitating disease (with or without a congenital deformity), but one that may not necessarily threaten the life of the child, also can experience anticipatory grief. An alteration in relationships, a change in lifestyle, and a very real threat to their hopes and dreams for the future can affect the day-to-day interaction of the family with their infant and the staff. Nurses can help facilitate the family's grieving process. If the nurse observes that a family member's daily interactions with the infant change, the nurse should assess the situation and request psychosocial support or intervention by a chaplain or social worker, if necessary.

Loss of an Infant

Parents who know their infant is going to die have a very difficult time. The parents need to direct their attention, energy, and caregiving activities toward the dying infant. However, some parents find it difficult to visit their infant even for short periods once a terminal diagnosis has been made. Grandparents also grieve but often are unsure how to comfort their own child (the infant's parent) during the period of impending death. Health care professionals can help by involving the family in the infant's care, providing privacy, answering questions, and preparing them for the inevitability of the death (see Chapter 37). There is a growing emphasis on hospice and palliative care for infants and their families.

Nurses also experience grief. Many primary staff nurses find themselves grieving as if the infant were their own because they often have worked closely with the infant and family for weeks or even months. Managers and other staff members must acknowledge this grief. Talking about the infant or attending the funeral can help the staff members resolve their feelings about the infant's death.

KEY POINTS

- Preterm infants are at risk for problems stemming from the immaturity of their organ systems.
- Nurses who work with preterm, late preterm, and other high risk infants observe them for respiratory distress and other early symptoms of physiologic disorders.
- The adaptation of parents to preterm, late preterm, or high risk infants differs from that of parents to normal term infants.
- Nurses can facilitate the development of a positive parent-child relationship.
- Nurses' skills in interpreting data, making decisions, and initiating therapy in newborn intensive care units are crucial to ensuring infants' survival.
- Complications of prematurity include respiratory distress syndrome, necrotizing enterocolitis, germinal matrix hemorrhage-intraventricular hemorrhage.

KEY POINTS—cont'd

- Close monitoring of oxygen levels as well as oxygen and ventilator settings can reduce the risk of retinopathy of prematurity.
- Bronchopulmonary dysplasia is a chronic pulmonary condition may require oxygen therapy in the home setting.
- Pain management requires vigilant ongoing assessment, anticipation of painful events, and early interventions to prevent and diminish such a response.
- Nurses need to assess the macroenvironments and microenvironments of the infant and family to create a developmentally positive atmosphere.
- Developmental care is a philosophy that embraces family-centered care and awareness of the effect of environmental stimuli on the physical and psychologic well-being of the infant and family.
- Parents need special instruction (e.g., CPR, oxygen therapy, suctioning, developmental care) before they take home a high risk infant.
- SGA infants are considered at risk because of fetal growth restriction.
- The high incidence of fetal distress among postmature infants is related to the progressive placental insufficiency that can occur in a postterm pregnancy.
- Multidisciplinary health care teams including specially trained nurses transport high risk infants to and from special care units.
- Parents need assistance as they cope with anticipatory grief or loss and grief.

REFERENCES

Aita, M., Johnston, C., Goulet, C., et al. (2013). Intervention minimizing preterm infants' exposure to NICU light and noise. *Clinical Nursing Research, 22*(3), 337–358.

AlFaleh, K., & Anabrees, J. (2014). Probiotics for prevention of necrotizing enterocolitis in preterm infants. *The Cochrane Database of Systematic Reviews 2014, 4*, CD005496.

Allen, K. (2012). Promoting and protecting infant sleep. *Advances in Neonatal Care, 12*(5), 288–291.

Altimier, L., & Phillips, R. M. (2013). The Neonatal Integrative Developmental Care Model: Seven neuroprotective core measures for family-centered developmental care. *Newborn and Infant Nursing Reviews, 13*(1), 9–22.

Alvaro, R. E. (2012). Neonatal apnea. In D. Fraser (Ed.), *Acute respiratory care of the newborn* (3rd ed.). Petaluma, CA: NICU INK Books.

Ambalavanan, N., & Carlo, W. A. (2011). Meconium aspiration. In R. M. Kliegman, B. F. Stanton, J. W. St. Geme, III, et al. (Eds.), *Nelson textbook of pediatrics* (19th ed.). Philadelphia: Elsevier.

American Academy of Pediatrics (AAP) Joint Committee on Infant Hearing. (2007). Year 2007 position statement: Principles and guidelines for early hearing detection and interventions programs. *Pediatrics, 120*(4), 898–921.

American Academy of Pediatrics (AAP) Section on Breastfeeding. (2012). Breastfeeding and the use of human milk. *Pediatrics, 29*(3), e827–e841.

American Heart Association (AHA). (2010). 2010 American Heart Association (AHA) guidelines for cardiopulmonary resuscitation (CPR) and emergency cardiovascular care (ECC) of pediatric and neonatal patients: Pediatric basic life support. *Circulation, 122*(Suppl 3), S862–S875.

Anand, K., & The International Evidence-based Group for Neonatal Pain. (2001). Consensus statement for the prevention and management of pain in the newborn. *Archives of Pediatric and Adolescent Medicine, 155*(2), 173–180.

Anderson, M., Wood, L., Keller, J., & Hay, W. (2011). Enteral nutrition. In S. Gardner, B. Carter, M. Enzman-Hines, & J. Hernandez (Eds.), *Merenstein & Gardner's handbook of neonatal intensive care* (7th ed.). St. Louis: Mosby.

Armentrout, D. (2015). Glucose management. In M. T. Verklan, & M. Walden (Eds.), *Core curriculum for neonatal intensive care nursing* (5th ed.). St. Louis: Elsevier.

Arthurs, O. J., Edwards, A., Austin, T., et al. (2012). The challenges of neonatal magnetic resonance imaging. *Pediatric Radiology, 42*(10), 1183–1194.

Association of Women's Health, Obstetric and Neonatal Nurses (AWHONN). (2010). *Assessment and care of the late preterm infant: Evidence-based clinical practice guidelines.* Washington, DC: Author.

Bancalari, E. (2011). Pathophysiology of bronchopulmonary dysplasia. In R. Polin, W. Fox, & S. Abman (Eds.), *Fetal and neonatal physiology* (4th ed.). Philadelphia: Saunders.

Bancalari, E., & Walsh, M. (2011). Bronchopulmonary dysplasia. In R. Martin, A. Fanaroff, & M. Walsh (Eds.), *Fanaroff and Martin's neonatal-perinatal medicine: Diseases of the fetus and infant* (9th ed.). St. Louis: Mosby.

Bell, S. G. (2012). Neonatal respiratory pharmacotherapy. In D. Fraser (Ed.), *Acute respiratory care of the neonate* (3rd ed.). Petaluma, CA: NICU INK Books.

Blackburn, S. (2013). *Maternal, fetal, and neonatal physiology: A clinical perspective* (4th ed.). St. Louis: Elsevier.

Blauer, T., & Gerstmann, D. (1998). A simultaneous comparison of three neonatal pain scales during common NICU procedures. *Clinical Journal of Pain, 14*(1), 39–47.

Bonifacio, S. L., Gonzalez, F., & Ferriero, D. M. (2012). Central nervous system injury and neuroprotection. In C. A. Gleason, & S. U. Devaskar (Eds.), *Avery's diseases of the newborn* (9th ed.). Philadelphia: Elsevier.

Botet, F., Figueras-Aloy, J., Miracle-Echegoyen, X., et al. (2012). Trends in survival among extremely-low-birth-weight infants (less than 1000g) without significant bronchopulmonary dysplasia. *BMC Pediatrics, 12*, 63.

Brown, V., & Landers, S. (2011). Heat balance. In S. Gardner, B. Carter, M. Enzman-Hines, & J. Hernandez (Eds.), *Merenstein & Gardner's handbook of neonatal intensive care* (7th ed.). St. Louis: Mosby.

Bull, M. J., Engle, W. A., & Committee on Injury, Violence, and Poison Prevention; & Committee on Fetus and Newborn (2009). Safe transportation of preterm and low birth weight infants at hospital discharge. *Pediatrics, 123*(5), 1424–1429.

Byrne, E., & Garber, J. (2013). Physical therapy intervention in the neonatal intensive care unit. *Physical & Occupational Therapy in Pediatrics, 33*(1), 75–110.

Caplan, M. (2011). Neonatal necrotizing enterocolitis: Clinical observations, pathophysiology, and prevention. In R. Martin, A. Fanaroff, & M. Walsh (Eds.), *Fanaroff and Martin's neonatal-perinatal medicine: Diseases of the fetus and infant* (9th ed.). St. Louis: Mosby.

Carlo, W. A. (2011). High-risk infants. In R. M. Kliegman, B. F. Stanton, J. W. St. Geme, III, et al. (Eds.), *Nelson textbook of pediatrics* (19th ed.). Philadelphia: Saunders.

Chavez-Valdez, R., McGowan, J., Cannon, E., & Lehmann, C. U. (2011). Contribution of early glycemic status in the development of severe retinopathy of prematurity in a cohort of ELBW infants. *Journal of Perinatology, 31*(12), 749–756.

Choi, H. J., Hahn, S., Lee, J., et al. (2012). Surfactant lavage therapy for meconium aspiration syndrome: A systematic review and meta-analysis. *Neonatology, 101*(3), 183–191.

Christensen, R. D., Lambert, D. K., Baer, V. L., & Gordon, P. V. (2013). Necrotizing enterocolitis in term infants. *Clinics in Perinatology, 40*(1), 69–78.

Clyman, R. I. (2013). The role of patent ductus arteriosus and its treatments in the development of bronchopulmonary dysplasia. *Seminars in Perinatology, 37*(2), 102–107.

Clyman, R. I., Couto, J., & Murphy, G. M. (2012). Patent ductus arteriosus: Are current neonatal treatment options better or worse than no treatment at all? *Seminars in Perinatology, 36*(2), 123–129.

Cong, X., Cusson, R. M., Walsh, S., et al. (2012). Effects of skin-to-skin on autonomic pain responses in preterm infants. *Journal of Pain, 13*(7), 636–645.

Daily, D., Carter, A., & Carter, B. (2011). Discharge planning and follow-up of the neonatal intensive care unit infant. In S. Gardner, B. Carter, M. Enzman-Hines, & J. Hernandez (Eds.), *Merenstein & Gardner's handbook of neonatal intensive care* (7th ed.). St. Louis: Mosby.

De Curtis, M., & Rigo, J. (2012). The nutrition of preterm infants. *Early Human Development, 88*(Suppl 1), S5–S7.

De Los Santos-Garate, A. M., Villa-Guillen, M., Villanueva-García, D., et al. (2011). Perinatal morbidity and mortality in late-term and post-term pregnancy. NEOSANO perinatal network's experience in Mexico. *Journal of Perinatology, 31*(12), 789–793.

de Vries, L. (2011). Intracranial hemorrhage and vascular lesions. In R. Martin, A. Fanaroff, & M. Walsh (Eds.), *Fanaroff and Martin's neonatal-perinatal medicine: Diseases of the fetus and infant* (9th ed.). St. Louis: Mosby.

Diehl-Jones, W., & Fraser, D. (2014). Hematologic disorders. In M. Verklan, & M. Walden (Eds.), *AWHONN core curriculum for neonatal intensive care nursing* (5th ed.). St. Louis: Saunders.

Ditzenberger, G. R., & Blackburn, S. T. (2014). Neurologic system. In C. Kenner, & J. W. Lott (Eds.), *Comprehensive neonatal care* (5th ed.). New York: Springer.

Flacking, R., Ewald, U., & Wallin, L. (2011). Positive effect of kangaroo mother care on long-term breastfeeding in very preterm infants. *Journal of Obstetric, Gynecologic and Neonatal Nursing, 40*(2), 190–197.

Forcada-Guex, M., Borghini, A., Pierrehumbert, B., et al. (2011). Prematurity, maternal posttraumatic stress and consequences on the mother-infant relationship. *Early Human Development, 87*(1), 21–26.

Fraser, D. (2012a). High-frequency ventilation: The current challenge to neonatal nursing. In D. Fraser (Ed.), *Acute respiratory care of the newborn* (3rd ed.). Petaluma, CA: NICU INK Books.

Fraser, D. (2012b). Complications of positive pressure ventilation. In D. Fraser (Ed.), *Acute respiratory care of the newborn* (3rd ed.). Petaluma, CA: NICU INK Books.

Gardner, S., & Dickey, L. (2011). Grief and perinatal loss. In S. Gardner, B. Carter, M. Enzman-Hines, & J. Hernandez (Eds.), *Merenstein & Gardner's handbook of neonatal intensive care* (7th ed.). St. Louis: Mosby.

Gardner, S., Enzman-Hines, M., & Dickey, L. (2011a). Pain and pain relief. In S. Gardner, B. Carter, M. Enzman-Hines, & J. Hernandez (Eds.), *Merenstein & Gardner's handbook of neonatal intensive care* (7th ed.). St. Louis: Mosby.

Gardner, S., Enzman-Hines, M., & Dickey, L. (2011b). Respiratory diseases. In S. Gardner, B. Carter, M. Enzman-Hines, & J. Hernandez (Eds.), *Merenstein & Gardner's handbook of neonatal intensive care* (7th ed.). St. Louis: Mosby.

Gardner, S., & Goldson, E. (2011). The neonate and the environment: Impact on development. In S. Gardner, B. Carter, M. Enzman-Hines, & J. Hernandez (Eds.), *Merenstein & Gardner's handbook of neonatal intensive care* (7th ed.). St. Louis: Mosby.

Gardner, S., & Lawrence, R. (2011). Breastfeeding the neonate with special needs. In S. Gardner, B. Carter, M. Enzman-Hines, & J. Hernandez (Eds.), *Merenstein & Gardner's handbook of neonatal intensive care* (7th ed.). St. Louis: Mosby.

Gardner, S. L., & Hernandez, J. A. (2011). Initial nursery care. In S. Gardner, B. Carter, M. Enzman-Hines, & J. Hernandez (Eds.), *Merenstein & Gardner's handbook of neonatal intensive care* (7th ed.). St. Louis: Mosby.

Gooding, J., Cooper, L., Blaine, A., et al. (2011). Family support and family-centered care in the neonatal intensive care unit: Origins, advances, impact. *Seminars in Perinatology, 35*(1), 20–28.

Hamvas, A. (2011). Pathophysiology and management of respiratory distress syndrome. In R. Martin, A. Fanaroff, & M. Walsh (Eds.), *Fanaroff and Martin's neonatal-perinatal medicine: Diseases of the fetus and infant* (9th ed.). St. Louis: Mosby.

Harach, T. (2013). Room air resuscitation and targeted oxygenation for infants at birth in the delivery room. *Journal of Obstetric, Gynecologic and Neonatal Nursing, 42*(2), 227–232.

Hodgkinson, K., Bear, M., Thorn, J., & Van Blaricum, S. (1994). Measuring pain in neonates: Evaluating an instrument and developing a common language. *Australian Journal of Advanced Nursing, 12*(1), 17–22.

Hwang, S. S., Barfield, W. D., Smith, R. A., et al. (2013). Discharge timing, outpatient follow-up, and home care of late-preterm and early-term infants. *Pediatrics, 132*(1), 101–108.

Jefferies, A. L., & Canadian Paediatric Society Fetus and Newborn Committee. (2012). Kangaroo care for the preterm infant and family. *Paediatric and Child Health, 17*(3), 141–146.

Jones, F. (2011). *Best practices for expressing, storing and handling human milk* (3rd ed.). Raleigh, NC: Human Milk Banking Association of North America.

Kattwinkel, J., & American Academy of Pediatrics (AAP), & American Heart Association (AHA). (2011). *Textbook of neonatal resuscitation* (6th ed.). Elk Grove Village, IL: American Academy of Pediatrics and American Heart Association.

Kendall, A. B., Scott, P. A., & Karlsen, K. A. (2012). The S.T.A.B.L.E. program: The evidence behind the 2012 update. *Journal of Perinatal and Neonatal Nursing, 26*(2), 147–157.

Kenney, P., Hoover, D., Williams, L., & Iskersky, V. (2011). Cardiovascular diseases and surgical interventions. In S. Gardner, B. Carter, M. Enzman-Hines, & J. Hernandez (Eds.), *Merenstein & Gardner's handbook of neonatal intensive care* (7th ed.). St. Louis: Mosby.

Kilbride, H., Leick-Rude, M., Olsen, S., & Stiens, J. (2011). Total parenteral nutrition. In S. Gardner, B. Carter, M. Enzman-Hines, & J. Hernandez (Eds.), *Merenstein & Gardner's handbook of neonatal intensive care* (7th ed.). St. Louis: Mosby.

Kliegman, R. (2011). Intrauterine growth restriction. In R. Martin, A. Fanaroff, & M. Walsh (Eds.), *Fanaroff and Martin's neonatal-perinatal medicine: Diseases of the fetus and infant* (9th ed.). St. Louis: Mosby.

Lawrence, J., Alcock, D., McGrath, P., et al. (1993). The development of a tool to assess neonatal pain. *Neonatal Network, 12*(6), 59–66.

Legendre, V., Burtner, P., Martinez, K., & Crowe, T. (2011). The evolving practice of developmental care in the neonatal unit: A systematic review. *Occupational Therapy in Pediatrics, 31*(3), 315–338.

Lovvorn, H., Glenn, J., Pacetti, A., & Carter, B. (2011). Neonatal surgery. In S. Gardner, B. Carter, M. Enzman-Hines, & J. Hernandez (Eds.), *Merenstein & Gardner's handbook of neonatal intensive care* (7th ed.). St. Louis: Mosby.

Lund, C., & Durand, D. (2011). Skin and skin care. In S. Gardner, B. Carter, M. Enzman-Hines, & J. Hernandez (Eds.), *Merenstein & Gardner's handbook of neonatal intensive care* (7th ed.). St. Louis: Mosby.

Martin, J. A., Hamilton, B. E., Osterman, M. J., et al. (2013). Births: Final data for 2012. *National Vital Statistics Reports, 62*(9), 1–27.

McGowan, J., Rozance, P., Price-Douglas, W., & Hay, W. (2011). Glucose homeostasis. In S. Gardner, B. Carter, M. Enzman-Hines, & J. Hernandez (Eds.), *Merenstein & Gardner's handbook of neonatal intensive care* (7th ed.). St. Louis: Mosby.

McGrath, J. M., & Hardy, W. (2011). The infant at risk. In S. Mattson, & J. E. Smith (Eds.), *Core curriculum for maternal-newborn nursing* (4th ed.). St. Louis: Saunders.

Meier, P. P., Patel, A. L., Bigger, H. R., et al. (2013). Supporting breastfeeding in the neonatal intensive care unit: Rush mother's milk club as a case study of evidence-based care. *Pediatric Clinics of North America, 60*(1), 209–226.

Morag, I., & Ohlsson, A. (2011). Cycled light in the intensive care unit for preterm and low birth weight infants. *The Cochrane Database of Systematic Reviews* 2011, *1*, CD006982.

NIDCAP Federation International. (2008). Overview: The Newborn Individualized Developmental Care and Assessment Program. Available at www.nidcap.org/nidcap_training.aspx.

Orlando, S. (2012). Pathophysiology of acute respiratory distress. In D. Fraser (Ed.), *Acute respiratory care of the neonate* (3rd ed.). Petaluma, CA: NICU INK Books.

Örs, R. (2013). The practical aspects of enteral nutrition in preterm infants. *Journal of Pediatric and Neonatal Individualized Medicine, 2*(1), 35–40.

Phillips, R. M., Goldstein, M., Hougland, K., et al. (2013). Multidisciplinary guidelines for the care of late preterm infants. *Journal of Perinatology, 33*(Suppl 2), S5–S22.

Pokela, M. (1994). Pain relief can reduce hypoxemia in distressed neonates during routine treatment procedures. *Pediatrics, 93*(3), 379–383.

Polin, R. A., Carlo, W. A., & Committee on Fetus and Newborn (2014). Surfactant replacement therapy for preterm and term neonates with respiratory distress. *Pediatrics, 133*(1), 156–163.

Pranke, P., & Onsten, T. (2011). Umbilical cord blood transfusion and its therapeutic potentialities. In N. Bhattacharya (Ed.), *Regenerative medicine using pregnancy-specific biological substances.* Philadelphia: Springer.

Prkachin, K. (2011). Facial pain expression. *Pain Management, 1*(4), 367–376.

Raju, T. N. (2012). Developmental physiology of late and moderate prematurity. *Seminars in Fetal and Neonatal Medicine, 17*(3), 126–131.

Raju, T., Higgins, R., Stark, A., & Leveno, K. (2006). Optimizing care and outcome for late-preterm (near term) infants: A summary of the workshop sponsored by the National Institute of Child Health and Human Development. *Pediatrics, 118*(3), 1207–1214.

Radtke, J. V. (2011). The paradox of breastfeeding-associated morbidity among late preterm infants. *Journal of Obstetric, Gynecologic and Neonatal Nursing, 40*(1), 9–24.

Rebello, C., Yagui, A., Vale, L., et al. (2011). CPAP with variable flow is comparable with bubble CPAP in preterm infants. *Critical Care, 15*(S2), 1–31.

Rojas, M., Shirley, K., & Rush, M. (2011). Perinatal transport. In S. Gardner, B. Carter, M. Enzman-Hines, & J. Hernandez (Eds.), *Merenstein & Gardner's handbook of neonatal intensive care* (7th ed.). St. Louis: Mosby.

Siegel, R., Gardner, S., & Dickey, L. (2011). Families in crisis: Theoretical and practical considerations. In S. Gardner, B. Carter, M. Enzman-Hines, & J. Hernandez (Eds.), *Merenstein & Gardner's handbook of neonatal intensive care* (7th ed.). St. Louis: Mosby.

Soltau, T. D., & Carlo, W. A. (2014). Respiratory system. In C. Kenner, & J. W. Lott (Eds.), *Comprehensive neonatal nursing care* (5th ed.). New York: Springer.

Sparshott, M. (1995). Assessing the behaviour of the newborn infant. *Paediatric Nursing, 7*(7), 14–16.

Stevens, B., Johnston, C., Petryshen, P., & Taddio, A. (1996). Premature infant pain profile: Development and initial validation. *Clinical Journal of Pain, 12*(1), 13–22.

Stuckey-Schrock, K., & Schrock, S. D. (2013). Head off complications in late preterm infants. *Journal of Family Practice, 62*(4), E3–E8.

The Joint Commission (TJC). (2011). The fifth "vital sign": Complying with the pain management standard PC.01.02.07. *The Source, 9*(11), 1–10.

Wachman, E., & Lahav, A. (2011). The effects of noise on preterm infants in the NICU. *Archives of Disease in Childhood Fetal-Neonatal Edition, 96*(4), F305–F309.

Walden, M. (2014). Pain in the newborn and infant. In C. Kenner, & J. W. Lott (Eds.), *Comprehensive neonatal nursing care* (5th ed.). New York: Springer.

Yoo, H., Ahn, S., Lee, M., et al. (2013). Permissive hyperglycemia in extremely low birth weight infants. *Korean Medical Science, 28*(3), 450–460.

Zimmerman, E., & Lahav, A. (2013). Ototoxicity in preterm infants: Effects of genetics, aminoglycosides, and loud environmental noise. *Journal of Perinatology, 33*(1), 3–8.

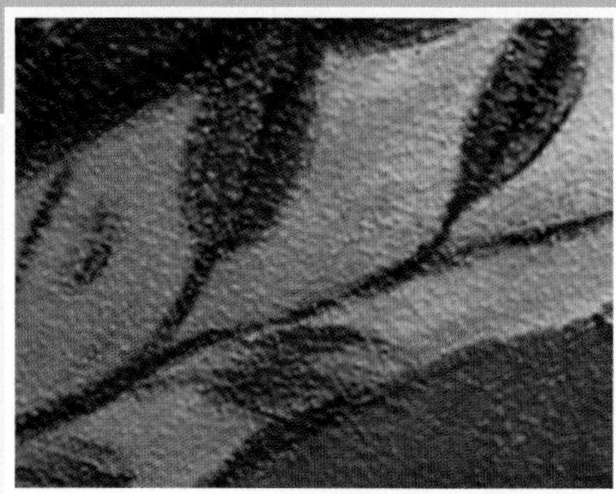

CHAPTER 35

Acquired Problems of the Newborn

Debbie Fraser

http://evolve.elsevier.com/Lowdermilk/MWHC/

LEARNING OBJECTIVES

- Describe assessment and care of infants with soft-tissue, skeletal, and nervous system injuries resulting from birth trauma.
- Develop a plan of care for the neonate of a mother with diabetes.
- Describe in detail the assessment and care of a newborn with a suspected infection.
- Formulate nursing diagnoses for infants and families experiencing common neonatal bacterial and viral infections.
- Interpret the evidence available to guide the care of the infant at risk for group B streptococcal (GBS) sepsis.
- Analyze fetal and neonatal effects of maternal substance abuse during pregnancy.
- Describe concerns for fetal and neonatal well-being related to maternal use of caffeine and selective serotonin reuptake inhibitors.
- Describe the assessment and care of a newborn experiencing drug withdrawal (neonatal abstinence syndrome); include the infant's family.

This chapter deals with acquired problems of the newborn. *Acquired problems* refer to those conditions resulting from environmental rather than genetic factors. The focus is on birth trauma, the infant of a mother with diabetes, neonatal infections, effects of maternal substance abuse on the fetus and neonate, and effects of maternal use of caffeine and antidepressant medications during pregnancy.

BIRTH TRAUMA

Birth trauma or **birth injury** refers to physical injury sustained by a neonate during labor and birth. According to the Agency for Healthcare Research and Quality (AHRQ), the incidence of birth injuries in the United States is 2.19 per 1000 live births, excluding preterm and osteogenesis imperfecta births (AHRQ, 2013). Despite improvements in obstetric techniques; increased use of cesarean surgery for births that would be difficult vaginally; and decreased use of forceps, vacuum extraction, and version and extraction; birth injuries still are an important source of neonatal morbidity. Therefore, the clinician should consider the broad range of birth injuries in the differential diagnosis of neonatal clinical disorders (Mangurten & Puppala, 2011). The nurse's contribution to the welfare of the newborn begins with early observation and accurate documentation. The prompt reporting of signs that indicate deviations from normal permits early initiation of appropriate therapy. In addition, nurses provide essential support and education to parents whose neonates experience birth injury.

In theory, some birth injuries are avoidable, especially with careful assessment of risk factors and appropriate planning for birth. The use of ultrasonography allows antepartum diagnosis of macrosomia, hydrocephalus, and unusual presentations. Elective cesarean birth may be chosen for selected pregnancies to prevent significant birth injury. A small percentage of significant birth injuries are unavoidable despite skilled and competent obstetric care, as in especially difficult or prolonged labor or when the infant is in an abnormal presentation (Mangurten & Puppala, 2011). Some injuries cannot be anticipated until the specific circumstances occur during birth. Emergency cesarean birth can provide last-minute salvage, but in these circumstances the injury may be truly unavoidable. The same injury can be caused in several ways. For example, a cephalhematoma can result from an obstetric technique such as forceps- or vacuum-assisted birth or from pressure of the fetal skull against the maternal pelvis.

Many injuries are minor and resolve readily in the neonatal period without treatment. Other traumas require intervention. A few injuries are considered major trauma and serious enough to be fatal. Major trauma is often the result of instrumentation during birth (forceps or vacuum) and can occur concomitantly with other minor injuries. For example, a neonate who suffers a skull fracture is also likely to have a cephalhematoma (Linder, Linder, Fridman, et al., 2013; van Vleet, 2012).

Several factors predispose an infant to birth injuries. Maternal risk factors include age younger than 16 or older than 35, primigravida, uterine dysfunction that leads to prolonged or precipitous labor, preterm or postterm labor, and cephalopelvic disproportion. Oligohydramnios can increase the likelihood of birth trauma. Injury can result from dystocia caused by fetal

TABLE 35-1 Anatomic Classification of Birth Injuries

SITE OF INJURY	TYPE OF INJURY
Scalp	Caput succedaneum Subgaleal hemorrhage Cephalhematoma
Skull	Linear fracture Depressed fracture Occipital osteodiastasis
Intracranial	Epidural hematoma Subdural hematoma (laceration of falx, tentorium, or superficial veins) Subarachnoid hemorrhage Cerebral contusion Cerebellar contusion Intracerebellar hematoma
Spinal cord (cervical)	Vertebral artery injury Intraspinal hemorrhage Spinal cord transection or injury
Plexus	Erb-Duchenne palsy Klumpke paralysis Total (mixed) brachial plexus injury Horner syndrome Diaphragmatic paralysis Lumbosacral plexus injury
Cranial and peripheral nerve	Radial nerve palsy Medial nerve palsy Sciatic nerve palsy Laryngeal nerve palsy Diaphragmatic paralysis Facial nerve palsy

From Verklan. M., & Lopez, S. (2011). *Neurologic disorders.* In S. Gardner, B. Carter, M. Enzman-Hines, & J. Hernandez (Eds.), *Merenstein & Gardner's handbook of neonatal intensive care* (7th ed.). St Louis: Mosby.

macrosomia, multifetal gestation, abnormal or difficult presentation (not caused by maternal uterine or pelvic conditions), and congenital anomalies. Intrapartum events that can result in scalp injury include the use of internal monitoring of fetal heart rate (FHR) and collection of fetal scalp blood for acid-base assessment. Obstetric birth techniques can cause injury. Forceps- or vacuum-assisted birth and cesarean birth are potential contributory factors. Neonatal risk factors for birth injury include macrosomia, preterm or postterm birth, and congenital anomalies. Often more than one factor is present, and multiple predisposing factors can be related to a single maternal condition (Mangurten & Puppala, 2011; van Vleet, 2012; Verklan & Lopez, 2011).

Birth injuries are usually classified according to their etiology (predisposing factors or mechanisms of injury) or anatomically. Table 35-1 is an example of anatomic classification of birth injuries.

CARE MANAGEMENT

Nurses who perform initial and ongoing assessments of newborns are alert for clinical signs of birth trauma such as bruising; edema; abrasions; or absence, limitation, or asymmetry of movement. There can be immediate evidence of injury following birth or the signs of birth trauma may not appear until later. The neonate can experience impaired mobility, respiratory distress, or acute pain as a result of birth trauma. In some cases, more serious consequences of birth trauma can occur such as seizures or coma.

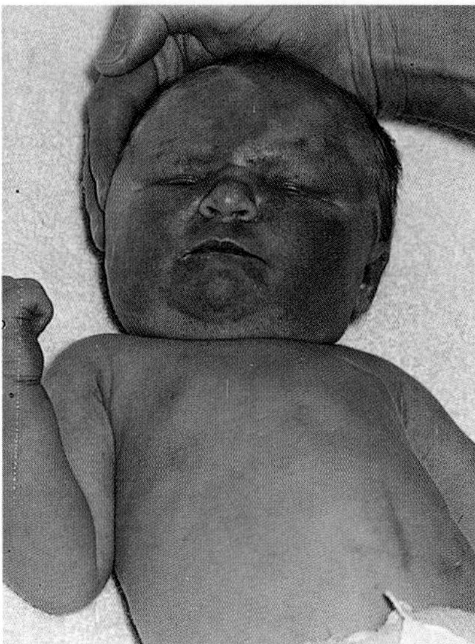

FIG 35-1 Marked bruising on the entire face of an infant born vaginally after face presentation. Less severe ecchymoses were present on the extremities. Phototherapy was required for treatment of jaundice resulting from the breakdown of accumulated blood. (From O'Doherty, N. [1986]. *Neonatology: Micro-atlas of the newborn.* Nutley, NJ: Hoffmann-La Roche.)

Care of the infant with a birth injury is individualized based on the type of injury. Through prompt identification of birth injury and notification of the health care provider, the nurse can proceed as directed with appropriate care measures. Based on the severity of the injury, the newborn may be transferred to the intensive care nursery.

Parents are likely to react to neonatal birth trauma with concern and anxiety. The nurse provides explanations about the type of injury and the treatment plan. Parents may need assistance and support from the nurse as they provide care for the newborn. For example, the nurse can demonstrate how to hold the infant to prevent discomfort from the injury. If the newborn is in the NICU, parents need even greater support from the nursing staff.

Medical and nursing interventions for specific birth injuries are discussed in the following sections.

Soft-Tissue Injuries

Erythema, ecchymoses, petechiae, abrasions, lacerations, and edema of the face, head, buttocks, and extremities can be present. Localized discoloration can appear over presenting or dependent parts. Ecchymoses and edema can appear anywhere on the body and especially on the presenting body part from the application of forceps or vacuum cup. They also can result from manipulation of the infant's body during birth.

Bruises over the face can be the result of face presentation (Fig. 35-1). In a breech presentation, bruising and swelling can occur over the buttocks or genitalia (Fig. 35-2). The skin over the entire head can be ecchymotic and covered with petechiae caused by a tight nuchal cord. Petechiae, or pinpoint hemorrhagic areas, acquired during birth can extend over the upper portion of the trunk and face. These lesions are benign if they

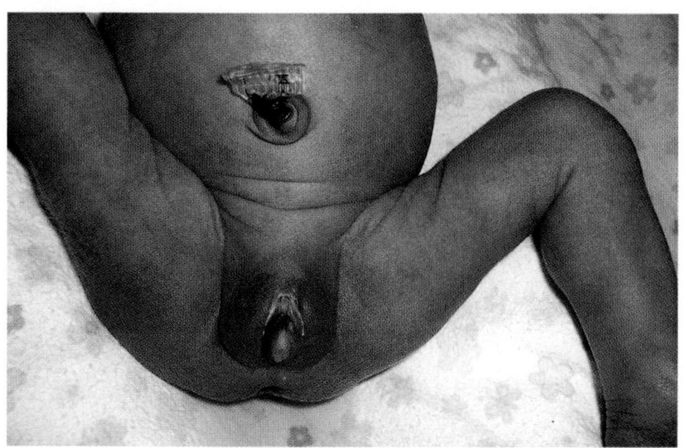

FIG 35-2 Swelling of the genitals and bruising of the buttocks of a preterm infant after a breech birth. Note the position of the infant's legs. (Courtesy Cheryl Briggs, RNC, Annapolis, MD.)

disappear within 2 days of birth and no new lesions appear. Ecchymoses and petechiae can be signs of a more serious disorder, such as thrombocytopenic purpura, if the hemorrhagic areas do not disappear spontaneously in 2 days.

! NURSING ALERT

To differentiate hemorrhagic areas from skin rashes and discolorations such as Mongolian spots, the nurse blanches the skin with two fingers. Because extravasated blood remains within the tissues, petechiae and ecchymoses do not blanch.

Forceps injury occurs at the site of application of the instrument. Forceps injury typically has a linear configuration across both sides of the face, outlining the placement of the forceps. The affected areas are kept clean to minimize the risk of secondary infection. These injuries usually resolve spontaneously within several days with no specific therapy.

Accidental lacerations can be inflicted with a scalpel during cesarean birth or with scissors during an episiotomy. These cuts can occur on any part of the body but most often are found on the scalp, buttocks, and thighs. Usually they are superficial, needing only to be kept clean. Butterfly adhesive strips or topical skin adhesive will usually hold together the edges of more serious lacerations. Rarely are sutures needed.

Two of the most commonly occurring birth injuries are subconjunctival (scleral) and retinal hemorrhages. These injuries result from rupture of capillaries caused by increased intracranial pressure (ICP) during birth. They usually clear within 5 days after birth and present no problems; however, parents need reassurance about their presence.

Caput succedaneum and cephalhematoma are commonly seen in neonates, often as the result of pressure on the fetal head pushing through a dilated cervix (see Fig. 23-10, *A-B*). These are discussed in Chapter 23.

A more serious injury is subgaleal hemorrhage, which is bleeding into the subgaleal compartment (see Fig. 23-10, *C*). The subgaleal compartment is a potential space that contains loosely arranged connective tissue; it is located beneath the galea aponeurosis, the tendinous sheath that connects the frontal and occipital muscles and forms the inner surface of the scalp. The injury occurs as a result of forces that compress and then drag the head through the pelvic outlet (Verklan & Lopez, 2011). This can occur with midforceps birth and vacuum extraction. The bleeding extends beyond bone, often posteriorly into the neck, and continues after birth, with the potential for serious complications such as anemia, hypovolemic shock, or even death. Early detection of the hemorrhage is vital; serial head circumference measurements and inspection of the back of the neck for increasing edema and a firm mass are essential. A boggy scalp, pallor, tachycardia, and increasing head circumference can be early signs of a subgaleal hemorrhage (Mouhayar & Charafeddine, 2012). Another possible early sign of subgaleal hemorrhage is a forward and lateral positioning of the infant's ears because the hematoma extends posteriorly. Infants with risk factors for subgaleal hemorrhage, including those born by forceps- or vacuum-assisted birth, should have their head circumference monitored per unit protocol for up to 48 hours after birth or longer if the head circumference is increasing. Monitoring the infant for changes in level of consciousness and a decrease in hematocrit is also key to early recognition and management. An increase in serum bilirubin levels can be seen as a result of the breakdown of blood cells within the hematoma. Computed tomography (CT) or magnetic resonance imaging (MRI) is useful in confirming the diagnosis. Replacement of lost blood and clotting factors is required in acute cases of hemorrhage. If bleeding continues and the infant's condition deteriorates, neurosurgery may be needed (Mangurten & Puppula, 2011).

Skeletal Injuries

The newborn's immature, flexible skull can withstand considerable deformation (molding) before fracture results (see Fig. 23-9). Substantial force is required to fracture the newborn's skull. Two types of skull fractures typically are identified in the newborn: linear fractures and depressed fractures. The location of the fracture and involvement of underlying structures determine its significance. Linear fractures are most common in the parietal bones, require no treatment, and are usually of no clinical significance. Skull fractures are common in infants with a cephalhematoma (Mangurten & Puppala, 2011).

The soft skull can become indented without laceration of either the skin or the dural membrane. These depressed fractures, or "ping-pong ball" indentations, can occur during difficult births from pressure of the fetal head on the bony pelvis. They also can occur as a result of injudicious application of forceps. A CT scan is done to rule out bone fragments or underlying injury of the brain tissue. Management of depressed skull fractures is controversial; many resolve without intervention. Nonsurgical elevation of the indentation using a manual breast pump or vacuum extractor has been reported. Surgery may be required in the presence of bone fragments or signs of increased intracranial pressure (Basaldella, Marton, Bekelis, & Longatti, 2011).

The clavicle is the bone most often fractured during birth. Generally the break is in the middle third of the bone (Fig. 35-3). Difficult delivery of the shoulders with a vaginal birth or extension of the arms in a breech birth often results in clavicular fracture (Mangurten & Puppala, 2011). Other risk factors include vacuum-assisted birth and birth weight greater than 4000 g (8.8 lb). Limited movement of the arm, crepitus over the bone, and the absence of the Moro reflex on the affected side are

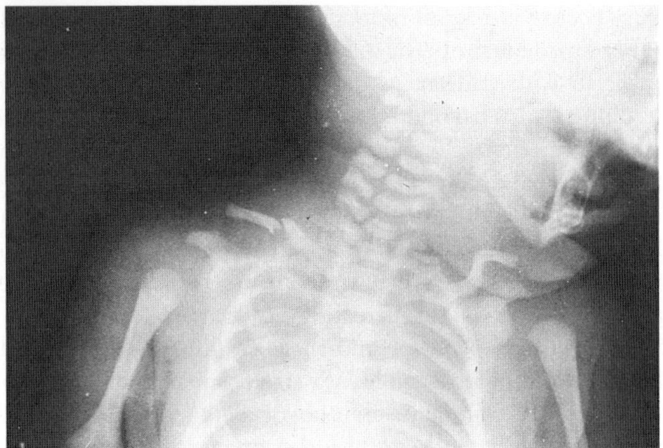

FIG 35-3 Fractured clavicle after shoulder dystocia. (From O'Doherty, N. [1986]. *Neonatology: Micro atlas of the newborn.* Nutley, NJ: Hoffmann-La Roche.)

diagnostic. Except for use of gentle rather than vigorous handling, no accepted treatment for fractured clavicle exists, and the prognosis is good. A sign posted on the bassinet will alert care providers to the need for careful handling. The figure-eight bandage appropriate for an older child should not be used for a newborn.

The humerus and femur can be fractured during a difficult birth. Fractures in newborns generally heal rapidly. Immobilization is accomplished with slings, splints, swaddling, and other devices.

The parents need support in handling these infants because they often are fearful of hurting them. Parents are encouraged to practice handling, changing, and feeding the affected neonate under the guidance of nursing staff prior to hospital discharge. This increases their confidence and knowledge and facilitates attachment. A plan for follow-up therapy is developed with the parents so that the times and arrangements for therapy are acceptable to them.

Peripheral Nervous System Injuries

Brachial plexus injury is the most common type of paralysis associated with a difficult birth, occurring at a rate of 0.6 to 4.6/1000 live births (Fig. 35-4). Approximately 45% of brachial plexus injuries occur with shoulder dystocia (Carlo, 2011a). An increased risk of brachial plexus injury occurs with birth weight greater than 4000 g (8.8 lb), vaginal breech birth, forceps- or vacuum-assisted birth, maternal diabetes, and a prolonged second stage of labor.

Erb-Duchenne paralysis or palsy is the result of injury to the upper plexus involving nerves C5 and C6 caused by stretching or pulling the head away from the shoulder during a difficult birth. The arm hangs limply alongside the body. The shoulder and arm are adducted and internally rotated. The elbow is extended, and the forearm is pronated, with the wrist and fingers flexed; a grasp reflex can be present because finger and wrist movement remains normal (Carlo, 2011a).

Damage to the lower plexus, also known as *Klumpke paralysis or palsy,* is less common. With lower arm paralysis the wrist and hand are flaccid, the grasp reflex is absent, and deep tendon reflexes are present; dependent edema and cyanosis can occur in the affected hand. There can also be a combination of

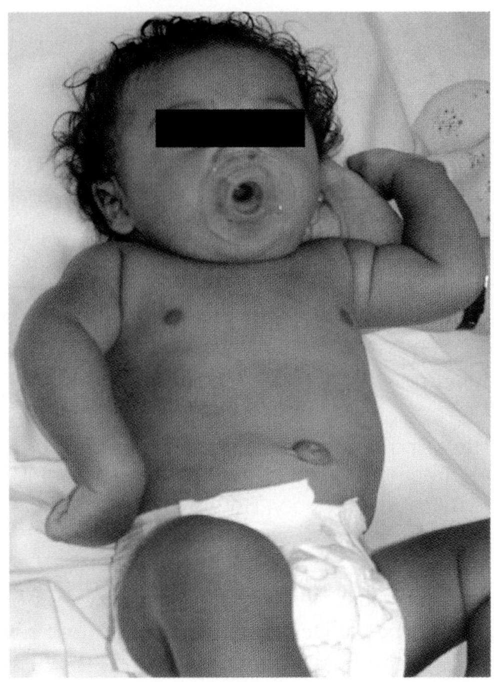

FIG 35-4 Brachial plexus injury (Erb-Duchenne palsy) in newborn infant. The Moro reflex was absent in right upper extremity. Recovery was complete. (From Chung, K.C., Yan, L., & McGillicuddy, J.E. [2012]. *Practical management of pediatric and adult brachial plexus palsies.* Philadelphia: Saunders.)

Erb-Duchenne and Klumpke's paralysis and the entire arm can be paralyzed (Verklan, 2015).

Treatment of brachial plexus injury involves intermittent immobilization across the upper abdomen, proper positioning, and range-of-motion (ROM) exercises. Gentle manipulation and ROM exercises are delayed for 1 week to prevent additional injury to the brachial plexus. Immobilization can be accomplished with a brace or splint or by pinning the infant's sleeve to his or her shirt. Treatment for Klumpke palsy consists of placing the hand in a neutral position, padding the fist, and gently exercising the wrist and fingers (Mangurten & Puppala, 2011).

If edema or hemorrhage is responsible for the paralysis, the prognosis is good, and recovery can be expected in a few weeks. If laceration of the nerves has occurred and healing does not result in return of function within a few months, surgery may be indicated; however, return of function is variable. Full recovery is expected in the majority of infants (Mangurten & Puppala, 2011).

Phrenic nerve injury almost always occurs as a component of brachial plexus injury rather than as an isolated problem. Injury is usually the result of traction on the neck and arm during birth. Injury to the phrenic nerve is usually unilateral, but can be bilateral, and results in diaphragmatic paralysis. Cyanosis and irregular thoracic respirations, with no abdominal movement on inspiration, are characteristic of paralysis of the diaphragm. Neonates with diaphragmatic paralysis usually require mechanical ventilatory support, at least for the first few days after birth, and are at risk of developing pneumonia. In the presence of persistent respiratory distress, diaphragmatic pacing or surgical correction may be necessary (Mangurten & Puppala, 2011).

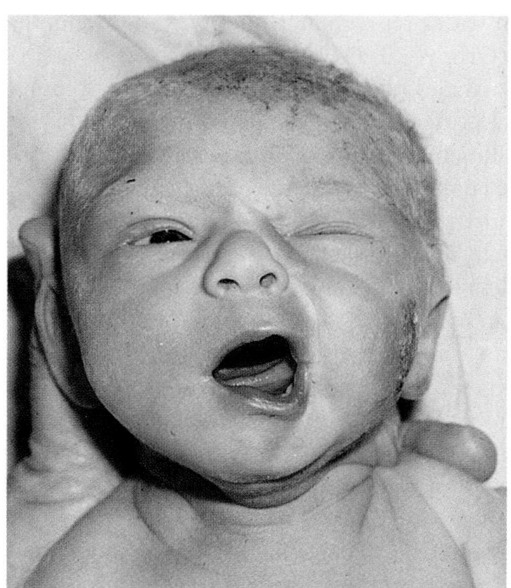

FIG 35-5 Facial paralysis 15 minutes after forceps birth. Absence of movement on affected side is especially noticeable when infant cries. (From O'Doherty, N. [1986]. *Neonatology: Micro atlas of the newborn.* Nutley, NJ: Hoffmann-La Roche.)

Facial paralysis (palsy) (Fig. 35-5) generally is caused by pressure on the facial nerve during birth. Risk factors include a prolonged second stage of labor and forceps-assisted birth. The face on the affected side is flattened and unresponsive to the grimace that accompanies crying or stimulation and the eye remains open on the affected side. Moreover, the forehead does not wrinkle. Usually the infant's face appears distorted, especially when crying. Often the condition is transitory, resolving within hours or days of birth, although total recovery can take weeks or months. Permanent paralysis is rare (Mangurten & Puppala, 2011).

Treatment involves assistance with feeding, prevention of damage to the cornea of the open eye with the application of artificial tears or taping the eye closed, and supportive care of the parents. Feeding can be prolonged, with the milk flowing out the newborn's mouth around the nipple on the affected side. The parents will need understanding and sympathetic encouragement while learning how to feed and care for the infant, as well as how to hold and cuddle the baby (Verklan, 2015).

Central Nervous System Injuries

All types of intracranial hemorrhages (ICH) occur in newborns. ICH as a result of birth trauma is more likely to occur in a large term infant. Risk factors for ICH include vacuum- or forceps-assisted birth, precipitous or prolonged second stage of labor, and increased fetal size (Bode-Jänisch, Bültmann, Hartmann, et al., 2012). In the newborn more than one type of hemorrhage frequently occurs.

Subdural hemorrhage (hematoma), a collection of blood in the subdural space, most often is produced by the stretching and tearing of the large veins in the tentorium of the cerebellum, the dural membrane that separates the cerebrum from the cerebellum. When this type of bleeding occurs, the typical history includes a nulliparous mother, with the total labor and birth occurring in less than 2 or 3 hours; a difficult forceps-assisted birth; or a large for gestational age (LGA) infant. Subdural hematoma occurs less frequently today because of improvements in obstetric care. However, it is especially serious because of its inaccessibility to aspiration by subdural tap. Neonates with subdural hemorrhage usually present with apnea, unequal pupils, tense fontanel, seizures, and even coma (Verklan & Lopez, 2011).

Subarachnoid hemorrhage, a common type of ICH, occurs in term infants as a result of trauma and in preterm infants as a result of hypoxia. Small hemorrhages are the most common. Bleeding is of venous origin, and underlying contusion also can occur. The clinical presentation of hemorrhage in the term infant can vary considerably. In many infants signs are absent and hemorrhaging is diagnosed only because of abnormal findings on lumbar puncture (e.g., red blood cells in the cerebrospinal fluid [CSF]). The initial clinical manifestations of neonatal subarachnoid hemorrhage can be the early onset of alternating depression and irritability, with refractory seizures or apnea. Occasionally the infant appears normal initially, then has seizures on the second or third day of life, followed by no apparent aftereffects (Verklan, 2015).

In general, nursing care of an infant with ICH is supportive and includes monitoring ventilatory and intravenous (IV) therapy, observing and managing seizures, and preventing increased ICP. Minimal handling to promote rest and reduce stress should guide nursing care (Askin & Wilson, 2011).

The most common cause of spinal cord injury in the neonate is a difficult breech birth. Stretching of the spinal cord, usually by forceful longitudinal traction on the trunk while the head is still firmly engaged in the pelvis, is the most common mechanism of injury. Fortunately this injury is rarely seen today because cesarean birth is typically used for breech presentation. However, it can also occur with shoulder dystocia when traction is applied to the head. Brow and face presentations, dystocia, preterm birth, maternal nulliparity, and precipitous birth also have been identified as predisposing factors in spinal cord injury (Mangurten & Puppala, 2011; Verklan & Lopez, 2011).

Clinical manifestations, treatment, and prognosis depend on the severity and location of the injury. Brainstem and high cervical cord injuries are likely to cause stillbirth or rapid death of the neonate. Upper or midcervical lesions may not be recognized at birth but cause death after a few days. Infants can appear normal at birth but show progressive respiratory deterioration and signs of spinal shock including flaccid extremities, diaphragmatic breathing, paralyzed abdominal movements, atonic anal sphincter, and distended bladder. Lower lesions can result in paraplegia and associated complications. Signs of partial spinal cord injuries such as spasticity can be less apparent (Mangurten & Puppala, 2011).

Therapy is supportive and usually unsatisfactory. Infants who survive present a therapeutic challenge that requires combined treatment from many health care providers: pediatrician, neurologist, neurosurgeon, urologist, orthopedist, nurse, physical therapist, and occupational therapist. Parents need to understand fully the implications of severe injury to the spinal cord and the overwhelming implications it presents for the family.

INFANTS OF MOTHERS WITH DIABETES

No single physiologic or biochemical event can explain the diverse clinical manifestations seen in the infants of mothers with diabetes. A better understanding of maternal and fetal metabolism, resulting in stricter control of maternal diabetes and improved obstetric and neonatal intensive care, has led to a decrease in the perinatal mortality rate in diabetic pregnancy. However, maternal diabetes continues to play a significant role in neonatal morbidity and mortality. Compared with nondiabetic pregnancies, infants born to mothers with diabetes are at an increased risk for complications such as congenital anomalies, macrosomia, birth trauma, perinatal asphyxia, stillbirth, preterm birth, respiratory distress syndrome (RDS), hypoglycemia, hypocalcemia, hypomagnesemia, cardiomyopathy, hyperbilirubinemia, and polycythemia. The degree of risk depends on the severity and duration of maternal disease. For example, women with vascular complications are more likely to have infants who are small for gestational age (SGA). All infants born to mothers with diabetes are at some risk for complications. The likelihood of these complications is reduced when maternal glucose levels are maintained within normal limits during the periconception period and during pregnancy (Hawdon, 2011; Hay, 2012).

Pathophysiology

The mechanisms responsible for the problems seen in infants of mothers with diabetes are not fully understood. In early pregnancy fluctuations in blood glucose levels and episodes of ketoacidosis are believed to cause congenital anomalies. Later in pregnancy, when the mother's pancreas cannot release sufficient insulin to meet increased demands, maternal hyperglycemia results. Increased amounts of glucose cross the placenta and stimulate the fetal pancreas to release insulin. The combination of the increased supply of maternal glucose and other nutrients and increased fetal insulin results in excessive fetal growth called *macrosomia* (see later discussion).

Hyperinsulinemia accounts for many of the problems of the fetus or infant. In addition to fluctuating glucose levels, maternal vascular involvement or superimposed maternal infection adversely affects the fetus. Normally, maternal blood has a more alkaline pH than the carbon dioxide–rich fetal blood. This phenomenon encourages the exchange of oxygen and carbon dioxide across the placental membrane. When the maternal blood is more acidotic than the fetal blood, such as during ketoacidosis, little carbon dioxide or oxygen exchange occurs at the level of the placenta. The mortality rate for unborn babies resulting from an episode of maternal ketoacidosis can be as high as 35% (Frise, Mackillop, Joash, & Williamson, 2013).

Congenital Anomalies

The incidence of congenital anomalies among mothers with pregestational diabetes is two to five times that of pregnant women who do not have diabetes (Garne, Loane, Dolk, et al., 2012). Elevated fasting blood glucose levels are correlated with an increased risk for anomalies in women with type 1 and type 2 diabetes (Ali & Dornhorst, 2011). Gestational diabetes that is diagnosed in mid- to late pregnancy is usually not associated with an increased incidence of congenital anomalies. However, the risk of anomalies is increased in women with gestational diabetes with elevated fasting glucose or hemoglobin A_{1C} levels, especially during early pregnancy (Ali & Dornhorst). There is an increased incidence of congenital anomalies among infants of women with prepregnancy obesity who develop gestational diabetes (Ornoy, 2011). In most defects associated with diabetic pregnancies, the structural abnormality occurs before the eighth week after conception. This reinforces the importance of controlling blood glucose both before conception and in the early stages of pregnancy.

The most frequently occurring anomalies involve the cardiac, renal, musculoskeletal, and central nervous systems. The incidence of congenital heart defects is two to three times higher than in the general population (Hay, 2012). Coarctation of the aorta, transposition of the great vessels, and atrial or ventricular septal defects are the most common cardiac anomalies occurring in infants of mothers with diabetes. In the genitourinary system, renal agenesis (failure of the kidney to develop) and obstruction of the urinary tract have been associated with maternal diabetes. Central nervous system (CNS) anomalies include anencephaly, encephalocele, myelomeningocele, and hydrocephalus. The musculoskeletal system can be affected by *caudal regression syndrome* (*sacral agenesis,* with weakness or deformities of the lower extremities; malformation and fixation of the hip joints; and shortening or deformity of the femurs). Other defects noted in this population include gastrointestinal (GI) atresia and urinary tract malformations (see Chapter 36). Neonatal small left colon syndrome, also called lazy colon syndrome, occurs in up to 50% of infants born to mothers with diabetes (Hay). This syndrome is suspected when the infant fails to pass meconium and has abdominal distention and bile-stained vomitus. Contrast enemas show a greatly diminished caliber of the left colon from the splenic flexure to the anus. The syndrome is transient, with normal bowel function developing early in infancy.

Macrosomia

Despite improvements in the control of maternal blood glucose levels, macrosomia is common (Hatfield, Schwoebel, & Lynyak, 2011). At birth the typical LGA infant has a round face, a chubby body, and a plethoric or flushed complexion. The infant has enlarged internal organs (hepatosplenomegaly, splanchnomegaly, cardiomegaly) and increased body fat, especially around the shoulders. The placenta and umbilical cord are larger than average. Because insulin does not cross the blood-brain barrier, the brain is the only organ that is not enlarged. Infants of mothers with diabetes can be LGA but physiologically immature (Fig. 35-6).

Insulin has been proposed as the primary growth hormone for intrauterine development. Maternal diabetes results in elevated maternal levels of amino acids and free fatty acids, along with hyperglycemia. As the nutrients cross the placenta, the fetal pancreas responds by producing insulin to match the fuel supply. The resulting accelerated protein synthesis, together with a deposition of excessive glycogen and fat stores, is responsible for the typical macrosomic infant. This is the infant most at risk for the neonatal complications of hypoglycemia, hypocalcemia, hyperviscosity, and hyperbilirubinemia. The excessive amounts of metabolic fuels transported to the fetus from the mother and the consequent fetal hyperinsulinism represent the basic pathologic mechanism in diabetic pregnancy (Hatfield et al., 2011).

The excessive shoulder size in these infants often leads to dystocia. Macrosomic infants, born vaginally or by cesarean

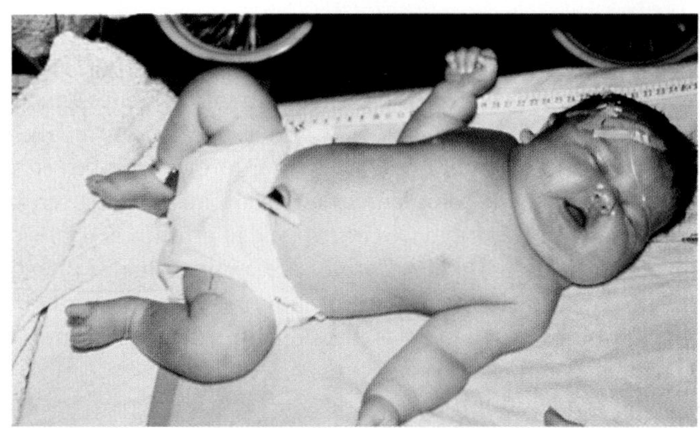

FIG 35-6 Large for gestational age infant. This infant of a diabetic mother weighed 5 kg (11 lb) at birth and exhibits the typical round face. (From Zitelli, B.J., & Davis, H.W. [2007]. *Atlas of pediatric physical diagnosis* [5th ed.]. Philadelphia: Mosby.)

birth after a trial of labor, can incur birth trauma such as clavicle fracture or brachial plexus injury. Despite increased vigilance in screening and improvements in ultrasound techniques, the prenatal determination of macrosomia can be difficult.

Birth Trauma and Perinatal Hypoxia

Birth injury (resulting from macrosomia or method of birth) and perinatal hypoxia occur more often in infants of mothers with diabetes. Examples of birth trauma include cephalhematoma; paralysis of the facial nerve (cranial nerve VII) (see Fig. 35-5); fracture of the clavicle or humerus; brachial plexus paralysis, usually Erb-Duchenne palsy (see Fig. 35-4); and phrenic nerve paralysis, invariably associated with diaphragmatic paralysis.

Respiratory Distress Syndrome

Respiratory distress syndrome in infants of mothers with diabetes is much less common than in the past because of improved protocols to manage maternal glucose levels and enhanced antepartum fetal surveillance techniques to assess lung maturity. Among infants born to women with well-controlled diabetes who give birth at term, the risk of RDS is similar to that of the general population. However, not all pregnant women with diabetes have well-controlled glucose levels. Maternal hyperglycemia can affect fetal lung maturity. In the fetus exposed to high levels of maternal glucose, synthesis of surfactant can be delayed because of the high fetal serum levels of insulin and/or glucose. In those infants born to women with poorly controlled type 1 diabetes the risk of RDS is six times higher than that of normal infants until 38 weeks of gestation (Hay, 2012). Late preterm birth may be indicated in cases where maternal diabetes is not well controlled. A number of factors including significant maternal and fetal risks should be taken into account in determining the need for early birth (American College of Obstetricians and Gynecologists [ACOG] Committee on Obstetric Practice & the Society for Maternal-Fetal Medicine (SMFM), 2013).

Hypoglycemia

Hypoglycemia (blood glucose levels less than 40 mg/dl in term infants) affects many infants of mothers with diabetes. LGA and preterm infants have the highest risk. After constant exposure to high circulating levels of glucose, hyperplasia of the fetal pancreas occurs, resulting in hyperinsulinemia. Disruption of the fetal glucose supply occurs with the clamping of the umbilical cord, and the neonate's blood glucose level decreases rapidly in the presence of fetal hyperinsulinism. It can take several days for the newborn to regulate the secretion of insulin in response to a lower postnatal supply of glucose. Hypoglycemia is most common in the macrosomic infant, but the nurse should monitor blood glucose levels in all infants of mothers with known or suspected diabetes.

Asymptomatic or symptomatic hypoglycemia most frequently occurs within the first 1 to 6 hours after birth. Signs of hypoglycemia include jitteriness, apnea, tachypnea, and cyanosis. Many infants with hypoglycemia remain asymptomatic. Significant hypoglycemia can result in seizures. Hypoglycemia is worsened by the presence of hypothermia or respiratory distress.

Hypoglycemic infants of mothers with diabetes should receive IV glucose, whether or not they are symptomatic (Kalhan & Devaskar, 2011). These infants are typically treated in the neonatal intensive care unit.

Hypocalcemia and Hypomagnesemia

Hypocalcemia and hypomagnesemia can occur in infants of mothers with insulin-dependent diabetes although they are not usually present until 48 to 72 hours after birth. The likelihood of hypocalcemia is related to the severity and duration of maternal diabetes. It is often associated with preterm birth, birth trauma, and perinatal asphyxia. Hypomagnesemia is believed to develop because of maternal renal losses that occur in diabetes. Jitteriness is a sign of both hypocalcemia and hypomagnesemia as well as hypoglycemia. Supplemental calcium therapy may be required. Magnesium levels usually return to normal without treatment (Kalhan & Desvaskar, 2011).

Cardiomyopathy

All infants of mothers with diabetes need careful observation for cardiomyopathy (disease affecting the structure and function of the heart) because an increased heart size is often found in these infants. Cardiomyopathy is more likely to occur in cases of poorly controlled maternal diabetes. Two types of cardiomyopathies can occur: hypertrophic and nonhypertrophic. Clinicians must be alert to identify the type of lesion correctly so that appropriate therapy is instituted. Both types of lesions are associated with respiratory symptoms and congestive heart failure.

Hypertrophic cardiomyopathy (HCM) is characterized by a hypercontractile and thickened myocardium. The ventricular walls are thickened, as is the septum, which in severe cases results in outflow tract obstructions. The mitral valve is poorly functioning. In nonhypertrophic cardiomyopathy (non-HCM), the myocardium is poorly contractile and overstretched. The ventricles are larger, and no outflow obstruction is found. Most infants are asymptomatic, but severe outflow obstruction can cause left ventricular heart failure (Hay, 2012).

Hyperbilirubinemia and Polycythemia

Infants of mothers with diabetes are at increased risk of developing hyperbilirubinemia. Many infants also are polycythemic.

Polycythemia increases blood viscosity, thereby impairing circulation. In addition, this greater number of red blood cells to be hemolyzed increases the potential bilirubin load that the neonate must clear, thus increasing the likelihood of hyperbilirubinemia. Bruising associated with birth of a macrosomic infant contributes further to high bilirubin levels.

The excessive red blood cells are produced in extramedullary foci (liver and spleen) in addition to the usual sites in bone marrow; therefore, liver function and bilirubin clearance can be adversely affected. With the increased red blood cell production, iron deficiency can occur in developing neurons as iron is redistributed from the brain to the liver and bone marrow. This can result in limitations in cognitive development (Hay, 2012).

Nursing Interventions

Nursing care depends on the neonate's particular problems. General care of the compromised infant is addressed in Chapter 34. If the maternal blood glucose level was well controlled throughout the pregnancy, the infant may require only monitoring. Because euglycemia (normal blood glucose levels) is not always possible, the nurse must promptly recognize and treat any consequences of maternal diabetes that arise. The most common problems experienced by infants of diabetic mothers that require intervention include birth trauma and perinatal asphyxia; RDS; difficult metabolic transition, including hypoglycemia and hypocalcemia; and congenital anomalies (see previous sections and the Clinical Reasoning Case Study).

 **CLINICAL REASONING CASE STUDY**

Newborn Effects of Maternal Diabetes

Melissa is a female neonate born at 37 weeks of gestation to a G 2 P 1 mother, who was diagnosed with gestational diabetes. Following a spontaneous vaginal birth, Melissa received Apgar scores of 7 at 1 minute and 8 at 5 minutes. Melissa weighs 3900 g (8.6 lb) and appears plethoric pink with a moderate amount of subcutaneous fat. She is noted to be slightly jittery at 30 minutes of age. In planning your care for Melissa you need to take into consideration the effects of maternal diabetes on the newborn.

1. Evidence—What complications of maternal diabetes is Melissa at risk of developing?
2. Assumptions—Describe underlying assumptions about each of the following issues:
   a. Symptoms of hypoglycemia
   b. Plans for assessing an infant with hypoglycemia
   c. Recommendations for care of an infant of a diabetic mother
3. What implications and priorities for nursing care can be drawn at this time?
4. Does the evidence objectively support your conclusion?

NEONATAL INFECTIONS

Sepsis

Sepsis (presence of microorganisms or their toxins in blood or other tissues) continues to be one of the most significant causes of neonatal morbidity and mortality. The newborn infant is susceptible to infection because of the immature immune system. Maternal immunoglobulin M (IgM) does not cross the placenta. IgG levels in term infants are equal to maternal levels; however, in preterm infants the amount of IgG is directly proportional to gestational age (Carlo, 2011b). IgA and IgM require time to reach optimal levels after birth. Phagocytosis is less efficient. Serum complement levels are inadequate; serum complement (C1 through C6) is involved in immunologic reactions, some of which kill or lyse bacteria and enhance phagocytosis. Dysmaturity seen with intrauterine growth restriction (IUGR) and preterm and postterm birth further compromises the neonate's immune system.

Table 35-2 outlines risk factors for neonatal sepsis. Special precautions for preventing infection, as well as prompt recognition when it occurs, are necessary for optimal newborn care. Neonatal infections can be acquired in utero, during labor and birth, during resuscitation, and during the hospital stay.

Prenatal acquisition of infection occurs by organisms placentally transferred directly into the fetal circulatory system or transmitted from infected amniotic fluid, such as with herpes simplex virus (HSV), cytomegalovirus (CMV), or rubella. Microorganisms can ascend from the vagina and pass through the cervix. The membranes become infected and can rupture, resulting in infection of the fetal skin and the respiratory or GI tract.

During birth, contact with an infected birth canal can result in generalized or local infection. The upper airway and the GI tract are the principal pathways for generalized infections.

TABLE 35-2 Risk Factors for Neonatal Sepsis

SOURCE	RISK FACTORS
Maternal	Low socioeconomic status
	Late or no prenatal care
	Poor nutrition
	Substance abuse
	Recently acquired sexually transmitted infection
	Untreated focal infection (urinary tract infection, vaginal, cervical)
	Systemic infection
	Fever
Intrapartum	Premature rupture of fetal membranes
	Maternal fever
	Chorioamnionitis
	Prolonged labor
	Premature labor
	Use of fetal scalp electrode
Neonatal	Multiple gestation
	Male
	Birth asphyxia
	Meconium aspiration
	Congenital anomalies of skin or mucous membranes
	Metabolic disorders (e.g., galactosemia)
	Low birth weight
	Preterm birth
	Malnourishment
	Formula feeding
	Prolonged hospitalization
	Mechanical ventilation
	Umbilical artery catheterization or use of other vascular catheters

Data from Edwards, M. (2011). Postnatal bacterial infections. In R. Martin, A. Fanaroff, & M. Walsh (Eds.), *Fanaroff and Martin's neonatal-perinatal medicine: Diseases of the fetus and infant* (9th ed.). St. Louis: Mosby; Bodin, M.B. (2014). Immune system. In C. Kenner & J.W. Lott (Eds.), *Comprehensive neonatal nursing care* (5th ed.). New York: Springer.

The conjunctiva and the oral cavity are the usual sites of local infection.

Postnatal infection is sometimes acquired during resuscitation or through the introduction of foreign objects such as indwelling catheters or endotracheal tubes. Health care–acquired infections can be transferred to the infant by the hands of the parents or health care personnel or spread from contaminated equipment. The umbilicus is a receptive site for cutaneous infection leading to sepsis. Neonatal bacterial infection is classified into two patterns according to the time of presentation. Early-onset or congenital sepsis usually manifests within 24 to 72 hours after birth, progresses more rapidly than later-onset infection, and has a mortality rate between 2% and 40% (Hofer, Zacharias, Muller, & Resch, 2012). Early-onset infection is usually caused by microorganisms from the normal flora of the maternal vaginal tract, including group B streptococci, *Haemophilus influenzae, Listeria monocytogenes, Escherichia coli,* and *Streptococcus pneumoniae* (Venkatesh, Adams, & Weisman, 2011). It is associated with a history of obstetric complications such as preterm labor, premature rupture of membranes, maternal fever during labor, and chorioamnionitis (Polin, 2012).

Late-onset sepsis, occurring at approximately 7 to 30 days of age, can include maternally derived infection or health care–acquired infection; the offending organisms are usually staphylococci, *Klebsiella* organisms, enterococci, *E. coli,* and *Pseudomonas,* or *Candida* species (Hammoud, Al-Taiar, Thalib, et al., 2012). Coagulase-negative staphylococci, considered to be primarily a contaminant in older children and adults, are commonly found to be the cause of septicemia in extremely low-birth-weight (ELBW) and very low-birth-weight (VLBW) infants. Additional infections of concern include methicillin-resistant *Staphylococcus aureus* (MRSA), vancomycin-resistant enterococci (VRE), and multidrug-resistant gram-negative pathogens (Fowler, 2013). Bacterial invasion can occur through sites such as the umbilical stump; the skin; mucous membranes of the eye, nose, pharynx, and ear; and internal systems such as the respiratory, nervous, urinary, and GI systems.

Viral infections that are acquired perinatally can cause stillbirth, intrauterine infection, congenital malformations, and acute disease. These pathogens also can cause chronic infection, with subtle manifestations that can be recognized only after a prolonged period. It is important to recognize the manifestations of infections in the neonatal period to treat the acute infection, to prevent health care–acquired infections in other infants, and to anticipate effects on the infant's subsequent growth and development.

Fungal infections are of great concern in the immunocompromised or premature infant. Occasionally fungal infections such as thrush are found in otherwise healthy term infants.

Septicemia refers to a generalized infection in the bloodstream. Pneumonia, the most common form of neonatal infection, is one of the leading causes of perinatal death and is caused by many of the same organisms that cause sepsis. Bacterial meningitis affects 0.25 to 1 of every 1000 live-born infants (Shah, Ohlsson, & Shah, 2012). Gastroenteritis is sporadic, depending on epidemic outbreaks. Local infections such as conjunctivitis and omphalitis occur frequently, but incidence rates are unavailable. Infection continues to be a significant factor in fetal and neonatal morbidity and mortality. Sequelae to septicemia include meningitis, disseminated intravascular coagulation (DIC), and septic shock.

Septic shock results from the toxins released into the bloodstream. The most common sign is a decrease in blood pressure, a vital sign often not assessed in the care of the neonate. The infant will often appear gray or mottled and can be noted to have cool extremities. Other signs are rapid, irregular respirations and pulse (similar to septicemia in general).

CARE MANAGEMENT

The development of systemic infection in the newborn can be influenced by maternal, peripartum, and neonatal risk factors. Onset within the first 48 hours of life is more often associated with prenatal or perinatal predisposing factors. Onset after 2 or 3 days more frequently reflects disease acquired at or subsequent to birth.

Assessment

The earliest clinical signs of neonatal sepsis are nonspecific and include lethargy, poor feeding, poor weight gain, and irritability. The nurse or parent can simply note that the infant is just not doing as well as before. Differential diagnosis can be difficult because signs of sepsis are similar to signs of noninfectious neonatal problems such as anemia or hypoglycemia. Additional clinical and laboratory information and appropriate cultures supplement the findings described. Table 35-3 outlines signs and symptoms of sepsis.

TABLE 35-3 Signs and Symptoms of Infection

SYSTEM	SIGNS
Respiratory	Apnea, bradycardia
	Tachypnea
	Grunting, nasal flaring
	Retractions
	Decreased oxygen saturation
	Acidosis
Cardiovascular	Decreased cardiac output
	Tachycardia
	Hypotension
	Decreased perfusion
Central nervous	Temperature instability
	Lethargy
	Hypotonia
	Irritability, seizures
Gastrointestinal	Feeding intolerance
	Abdominal distention
	Vomiting, diarrhea
Integumentary	Jaundice
	Pallor
	Petechiae
Metabolic	Hypoglycemia
	Hyperglycemia
	Metabolic acidosis
Hematologic	Thrombocytopenia
	Neutropenia

Data from Edwards, M. (2011). Postnatal bacterial infections. In R. Martin, A. Fanaroff, & M. Walsh (Eds.), *Fanaroff and Martin's neonatal-perinatal medicine: Diseases of the fetus and infant* (9th ed.). St. Louis: Mosby; Bodin, M.B. (2014). Immune system. In C. Kenner & J.W. Lott (Eds.), *Comprehensive neonatal nursing care* (5th ed.). New York: Springer.

Laboratory studies are important. Specimens for cultures include blood, CSF, and urine. Fluids such as urine and CSF can be evaluated by counterimmune electrophoresis or latex agglutination to help identify the bacteria. A complete blood cell (CBC) count with differential is performed. The leukocyte count is not a reliable indicator of sepsis; however, the total neutrophil count, immature to total neutrophil (I/T) ratio, absolute neutrophil count, and C-reactive protein can be used to determine the presence of sepsis. Detection of viral deoxyribonucleic acid (DNA) or antibodies by polymerase chain reaction (PCR) amplification in fluids is also an important diagnostic tool (Ohlin, Backman, Ewald, et al., 2012).

Interventions

Antepartum viral infection can be treated with antiviral medications to decrease viral replication and fetal transmission of disease; neonates can also be treated with antiviral medications such as acyclovir and ganciclovir. Treatment with antibiotics or antivirals is initiated after neonatal blood cultures are obtained. After the pathogen is identified, antibiotic, antiviral, or antifungal therapy can be modified.

Breastfeeding or feeding the newborn expressed breast milk from the mother is encouraged. Breast milk provides protective mechanisms (see Chapter 25). Colostrum contains IgA, which offers protection against infection in the GI tract. Human milk contains iron-binding protein that exerts a bacteriostatic effect on *E. coli.* Human milk also contains macrophages and lymphocytes. The vulnerability of infants to common mucosal pathogens such as respiratory syncytial virus (RSV) can be reduced by passive transfer of maternal immunity in the colostrum and breast milk. Some evidence indicates that early enteral feedings with human milk (trophic or minimal enteral feedings) can be beneficial in establishing a natural barrier to infection in ELBW and VLBW infants (Anderson, Wood, Keller, & Hay, 2011).

Nursing Considerations. Administering medications safely and correctly, taking precautions when performing treatments, and following isolation procedures are important interventions when a newborn has an infection. Monitoring the IV infusion rate and administering antibiotics are the nurse's responsibilities.

MEDICATION ALERT

If the IV fluid the infant is receiving contains electrolytes, vitamins, or other medications, the nurse should check with the hospital pharmacy before adding antibiotics. The antibiotic (or other medication) can be deactivated or can form a precipitate when combined with other substances. To prevent this, a secondary line of the prescribed solution is attached with a needleless connector at the infusion site.

Care must be taken in suctioning secretions from any newborn's oropharynx or trachea; the secretions can be infected. Routine suctioning is not recommended and can further compromise the infant's immune status, as well as cause hypoxia and increase ICP. Isolation procedures are implemented as indicated according to hospital policy. Isolation protocols change rapidly, and the nurse is urged to participate in continuing education and in-service programs to remain up-to-date.

Preventive Measures. Virtually all controlled clinical trials have demonstrated that effective hand hygiene is responsible for the prevention of health care–acquired infection in nursery units. Nurses play an essential role in minimizing or eliminating environmental sources of infectious agents in the nursery. Measures include implementing Standard Precautions, carefully and thoroughly cleaning the environment and equipment, frequently replacing used equipment (e.g., changing IV tubing per hospital protocol, cleaning resuscitation and ventilation equipment), and appropriately disposing of excrement and linens. Hand hygiene is the single most important measure in preventing the spread of infection. Appropriate hand hygiene protocols should be in place and frequent education provided to ensure that good hand hygiene practices are followed. Overcrowding must be avoided in nurseries. Guidelines for space, visitation, and general infection control in areas where newborns receive care have been established and published (American Academy of Pediatrics [AAP] & ACOG, 2012).

Specific newborn care procedures are intended to prevent infection. These include instilling antibiotic ointment in newborns' eyes 1 to 2 hours after birth, bathing, and cord care (see Chapter 24).

Transplacental Infections

The occurrence of certain maternal infections during early pregnancy is known to be associated with various congenital malformations and disorders. An acronym that is often used in clinical practice is TORCH, which stands for *t*oxoplasmosis, *o*ther (gonorrhea, hepatitis B, syphilis, varicella-zoster virus, parvovirus B19, and human immunodeficiency virus [HIV]), *r*ubella, *c*ytomegalovirus, and *h*erpes simplex virus) (see also Chapter 7). Additional organisms known to cause congenital infection include enteroviruses and parvovirus, leading some clinicians to suggest the need for a new more comprehensive acronym (Del Pizzo, 2011). With the advent of newer diagnostic methods, these viral infections can be diagnosed in utero and interventions planned based on the availability of intrauterine treatments.

Toxoplasmosis

Toxoplasmosis is a multisystem disease caused by the protozoan *Toxoplasma gondii* parasite, commonly found in cats, dogs, pigs, sheep, and cattle, with cats being the definitive host. In the United States, risk factors for acquisition of toxoplasmosis include exposure to contaminated soil and consumption of raw or undercooked meats or seafood (oysters, clams, or mussels) (Jones & Roberts, 2012). Changing cat litter is a known risk for toxoplasmosis. The risk of maternal-fetal transmission of acute infection is approximately 40% with the risk of transmission increasing as the pregnancy progresses. However, the earlier in pregnancy that fetal infection occurs, the greater the severity of congenital disease (Duff, 2012). Because many women are already seropositive for toxoplasmosis, the overall risk of a primary infection in pregnancy is quite low. The diagnosis of toxoplasmosis in the neonate is supported by elevated levels of cord blood serum IgM.

Most neonates infected with *T. gondii* in utero are asymptomatic at birth, although many develop chorioretinitis and signs of CNS involvement such as learning disabilities (Moncada & Montoya, 2012). For some infected neonates, hydrocephalus is the only clinical sign of the disease (Sanchez, Patterson, & Ahmed, 2012). Up to 30% of infected infants are born with severe manifestations at birth. Clinical features ascribed to *T. gondii* infection include three key findings (classic triad) first described by Sabin (1942): hydrocephalus, chorioretinitis, and cerebral calcifications (Del Pizzo, 2011). Severe toxoplasmosis is associated with preterm birth, growth restriction, microcephaly or hydrocephaly, microphthalmos, chorioretinitis, CNS calcification, thrombocytopenia, jaundice, and fever. Petechiae or a maculopapular rash also can be evident.

Infants with congenital toxoplasmosis are treated with pyrimethamine, combined with oral sulfadiazine; folic acid supplement is used to prevent anemia. Treatment should be continued for 1 year (Kaye, 2011).

Gonorrhea

The incidence of gonococcal infection in pregnant women ranges from 2.5% to 7.3%. Many women with gonorrhea often have a concurrent *Chlamydia trachomatis* infection (Engelkirk, Duben-Engelkirk, & Burton, 2011). After rupture of membranes, ascending infection can result in orogastric contamination of the fetus. The organism can also invade mucosal surfaces such as the conjunctiva (ophthalmia neonatorum), the rectal mucosa, and the pharynx. Contamination can occur as the infant passes through the birth canal, or it can occur postnatally from an infected adult. Neonatal gonococcal arthritis, septicemia, meningitis, vaginitis, and scalp abscesses also can develop.

Eye prophylaxis (e.g., with 0.5% erythromycin ointment) is administered within the first hour after birth to prevent ophthalmia neonatorum. This practice has reduced the incidence of gonococcal conjunctivitis to less than 0.5% (Anderson & Gonik, 2011).

Eye prophylaxis alone does not prevent systemic infection; therefore, infants with a gonococcal eye infection should receive one dose of ceftriaxone (Zuppa, D'Andrea, Catenazzi, et al., 2011). Infants with systemic gonococcal infection require hospitalization and 7 days of IV antibiotic therapy. Infants rarely die of overwhelming infection in the early neonatal period.

Syphilis

Congenital and neonatal syphilis have reemerged in recent years as significant health problems. In the United States in 2012, 322 cases of congenital syphilis were reported in children less than 1 year of age (CDC, 2014b). It is estimated that for every 100 women diagnosed with primary or secondary disease, 2 to 5 infants will contract congenital syphilis. If syphilis during pregnancy is untreated, approximately 50% of neonates born to these women will have symptomatic congenital syphilis. Treatment failure can occur, particularly when treatment is given in the third trimester; therefore, infants born to women treated within 4 weeks of birth should be evaluated for congenital syphilis (De Santis, De Luca, Mappa, et al., 2012). The following factors have been identified as placing the neonate at high risk for congenital syphilis: late or no prenatal care, maternal substance abuse, crack cocaine use in the mother or partner, multiple sexual partners, history of a sexually transmitted infection (STI), poverty, homelessness, and HIV infection (Patterson & Davies, 2011).

The fetus is usually infected in utero by transplacental infection, but infection of the amniotic fluid can occur. The infant can contract syphilis during contact with an active genital lesion at birth (Sweet & Gibbs, 2012). The risk to the fetus and neonate varies according to the stage of maternal infection, with transmission during primary or secondary syphilis being more common. Untreated maternal disease results in fetal or perinatal death in 40% of cases (Patterson & Davies, 2011). Prompt maternal treatment eliminates most fetal infections; however, delayed treatment or a failure to obtain treatment can result in fetal effects that range from minor anomalies to preterm birth or fetal death. Damage to the fetus depends on when in gestation the infection occurred and the time that has elapsed before treatment. Congenital syphilis infection can be asymptomatic at birth in up to two thirds of infected infants. A portion of these infants will become symptomatic in the first 2 years of life, whereas others may take up to 20 years before displaying the effects of congenital infection (De Santis et al., 2012).

Early congenital syphilis can result in prematurity, hydrops fetalis, and failure to thrive. Hepatosplenomegaly and jaundice are common. Hematologic findings include anemia, leukocytosis, and thrombocytopenia. Characteristic bony lesions occur in the long bones, the cranium, and the spine and include osteochondritis, osteomyelitis, and periostitis. Other findings include snuffles (copious clear mucous discharge from the nose); mucocutaneous lesions, edema, and a copper-colored maculopapular dermal rash first noticeable on the palms of the hands, the soles of the feet, and in the diaper area; and around the mouth and the anus by the end of the first week of life in untreated infants (Fig. 35-7). *Condylomata* (elevated wartlike lesions) can be seen on mucous membranes, moist surfaces, or areas of the body affected by friction. Rough, cracked, mucocutaneous lesions of the lips heal to form circumoral radiating scars known as *rhagades*. Other involvement results in exfoliation (separation, flaking) of nails and loss of hair. Iritis and choroiditis are characteristic of infection of the eyes. The following can be noted: nephrotic syndrome secondary to renal infection; hepatitis with jaundice,

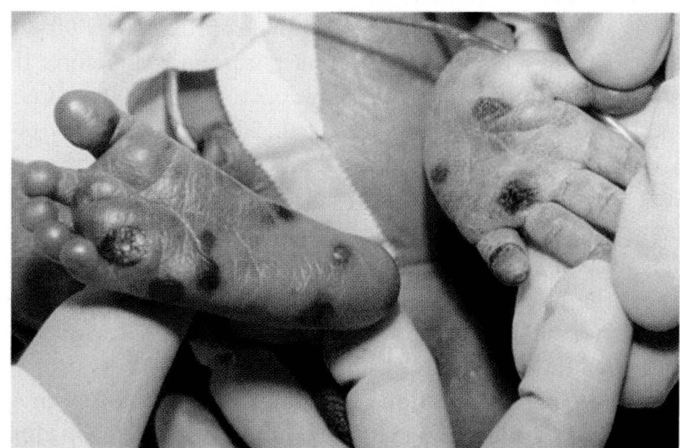

FIG 35-7 Neonatal syphilis lesions on hands and feet. (Courtesy Mahesh Kotwal, MD, Phoenix, AZ.)

lymphadenopathy, and inflammation of the pancreas, the testes, and the colon; and a pseudoparalysis of the extremities. In some infants signs of congenital syphilis do not appear until late in the neonatal period. In these newborns early signs such as slight hyperthermia and snuffles can be nonspecific (Sanchez et al., 2012).

Medical Management. Treatment of the newborn should be initiated when the diagnosis of congenital syphilis is confirmed or suspected or when maternal treatment status is unknown or not well documented. The neonate should be treated when the mother was treated within 1 month of giving birth or does not respond to treatment, when medications other than penicillin were used for the mother, or when the mother was treated appropriately but did not have sufficient serologic follow-up to assess response to treatment (Lago, Vaccari, & Fiori, 2013).

The infant with symptomatic congenital syphilis should have a lumbar puncture, CBC, and long-bone radiography prior to treatment. If the results of these tests are normal, a single intramuscular dose of benzathine penicillin is recommended (Lago et al., 2013). If results are abnormal or there is concern about appropriate follow-up, a 10-day course of IV penicillin or intramuscular (IM) procaine penicillin may be given. If the mother was adequately treated before giving birth and serologic testing of the infant does not show syphilis, the infant is usually not treated with antibiotics. The infant is checked for antibody titer (received from the mother through the placenta) every 2 weeks for 3 months, at which time the test result should be negative. Some physicians recommend antibiotic therapy for asymptomatic or inconclusive cases.

Prognosis. In general, treatment of syphilis is more effective if it begins early rather than late in the course of the disease. However, a recurrence rate of 5% can be expected. Even adequate treatment of congenital syphilis after birth does not always prevent late complications (5 to 15 years after initial infection). Potential complications include neurosyphilis, deafness, Hutchinson teeth (notched incisors), saber shins, joint involvement, saddle nose (depressed bridge), gummas (soft, gummy tumors) over the skin and other organs, interstitial keratitis (inflammation of the cornea), rhagades, frontal bossing, and mulberry molars (De Santis et al., 2012).

Varicella Zoster

The varicella zoster virus, responsible for chickenpox and shingles, is a member of the herpes family. Approximately 90% of women in the childbearing years are immune; therefore, the risk of infection in pregnancy is low: 0.7 to 3 per 1000 pregnancies (Lamont, Sobel, Carrington, et al., 2011).

Varicella transmission to the fetus can occur across the placenta when the disease is contracted in the first half of pregnancy, but this is relatively infrequent (about 2%). When transmission to the fetus does occur in the early part of pregnancy, the effects on the fetus include limb atrophy, neurologic abnormalities (hydrocephalus or microcephaly), and eye abnormalities (Lamont et al., 2011).

When maternal infection occurs in the last 3 weeks of pregnancy, 23% of infants born to these mothers will develop clinical varicella. The severity of the infant's illness increases greatly if maternal infection occurred within 5 days before or 2 days after birth. The mortality rate in severe illness is 7% (Ghosh & Chaudhuri, 2013).

Seroimmune pregnant women exposed to active chickenpox can be given varicella zoster immune globulin (VZIG), which does not reduce the incidence of infection but should decrease the effects of the virus on the fetus. The immune globulin must be given within 72 hours of exposure to be effective (AAP & ACOG, 2012).

Infants born to mothers in whom chickenpox develops between 5 days before birth and 48 hours after birth should be given VZIG at birth because of the risk of severe disease. Acyclovir can be used to treat infants with generalized involvement (Ghosh & Chaudhuri, 2013).

Term infants exposed to chickenpox after birth will have a mild or no infection if they are born to immune mothers. In those born to nonimmune mothers, chickenpox can develop, but the course is not usually severe. Experts are divided as to whether this group of infants should receive VZIG. Infants born before 28 weeks of gestation are at risk regardless of their mother's status, and probably benefit from VZIG if exposed to chickenpox (Kett, 2013).

Hepatitis B Virus

Hepatitis B virus (HBV) infection during pregnancy is not associated with an increase in malformations, stillbirths, or IUGR; however, almost twice as many mothers with HBV give birth prematurely compared with noninfected mothers (Reddick, Jhaveri, Gandhi, et al., 2011). The transmission rate of HBV to the newborn ranges from 85% to 90% when the mother is seropositive for both hepatitis B surface antigen (HBsAg) and hepatitis B e antigen (HBeAg) (Ott, Stevens, & Wiersma, 2012). Transmission occurs transplacentally, serum to serum, and by contact with contaminated urine, feces, saliva, semen, or vaginal secretions during birth. Infants are most frequently infected during birth or in the first few days of life. The rate of transmission is highest when the mother contracts the virus in the third trimester or early in the postpartum period (Pol, Corouge, & Fontaine, 2011). These mothers are positive for HBsAg. Transmission can occur through breast milk, but antigens also develop in formula-fed infants at the same or a higher rate; thus breastfeeding is not contraindicated. Diagnosis is made by viral culture of amniotic fluid, as well as by the presence of HBsAg and IgM in the cord blood or infant serum.

The majority of infants who become HBsAg positive are asymptomatic at birth, whereas some show evidence of acute hepatitis with changes in liver function. The mortality rate for full-blown hepatitis is 75%. Infants who become carriers are at high risk for chronic hepatitis, cirrhosis of the liver, or liver cancer even years later (Chang, 2011).

MEDICATION ALERT

Infants whose mothers have antibodies for HBsAg or in whom hepatitis developed during pregnancy or the postpartum period should be treated with hepatitis B immune globulin (HBIg), 0.5 ml intramuscularly, as soon as possible after birth—within the first 12 hours of life (CDC, 2014a). Hepatitis B vaccine also should be given at the same time but in a different site (Schillie & Murphy, 2013) (see Chapter 24).

Human Immunodeficiency Virus (HIV) and Acquired Immunodeficiency Syndrome (AIDS)

Approximately 8700 pregnant women infected with HIV give birth each year in the United States. Due to the success of preventive strategies during pregnancy, the incidence of mother-to-child transmission has been reduced to less than 1%. Universal HIV testing for all pregnant women allows for early identification and treatment of HIV-positive women during pregnancy, which decreases the risk of transmission to the fetus. Other strategies to prevent neonatal HIV infection include administration of antiviral medications during pregnancy and labor to women who are infected with the virus, administration of antiretrovirals to neonates for 6 weeks, and elective cesarean birth for women with HIV viral loads greater than 1000 copies per ml. In the United States and Canada, an additional strategy is the total avoidance of breastfeeding (CDC, 2013; MacDonald & Canadian Paediatric Society Infectious Diseases and Immunization Committee, 2012). The World Health Organization recommends that in resource-limited settings such as developing countries HIV-positive mothers who are taking antiretroviral medications should breastfeed for at least 12 months. For those who do not have access to antiretroviral therapy, exclusive breastfeeding for 6 months is recommended. After 6 months complementary foods are introduced and breastfeeding is continued until a safe, nutritional diet without breast milk can be provided for the infant (WHO, UNAIDS, UNFPA, & UNICEF, 2010).

Transmission of HIV from the mother to the fetus can occur transplacentally at various gestational ages. The risk of infection in an infant born to an HIV-positive mother (not treated) is approximately 12% to 40%. Transmission most often occurs during birth. Globally, up to one half of cases of mother-to-child transmission occur through breastfeeding (KiBS Study Team, 2011).

Diagnosis of HIV infection in the neonate is complicated by the presence of maternal IgG antibodies that cross the placenta after 32 weeks of gestation. The most accurate test for newborns and infants younger than 18 months is the HIV-1 DNA PCR assay, which is performed on neonatal blood, not cord blood (National Institutes of Health [NIH] Panel on Antiretroviral Therapy and Medical Management of HIV-Infected Children, 2012). Follow-up testing for infants born to HIV-positive mothers is recommended at several intervals within the first year of life.

Typically the HIV-infected neonate is asymptomatic at birth. Early-onset illness (i.e., virus detected within 48 hours of birth) is attributed to prenatal infection. These infants develop opportunistic infections (*Candida* and *Pneumocystis jirovecii* pneumonia) and experience rapid progression of immunodeficiency that often results in death during the first 1 to 2 years of life.

The remainder of infants seroconvert over a period of months to years. By 1 year of age the vast majority of perinatally infected infants show signs of infection. Some children infected at birth show no signs of disease 8 to 10 years later. The age of onset of symptoms predicts the length of survival.

The presenting signs and symptoms of HIV infection vary from severe immunodeficiency to nonspecific findings such as growth failure, parotitis, and recurrent or persistent upper respiratory tract infections. In the first year of life, lymphadenopathy and hepatosplenomegaly are common. The infant can have fever, chronic diarrhea, chronic dermatitis, interstitial pneumonitis, persistent thrush, and AIDS-defining opportunistic infections. Common secondary opportunistic infections include pneumonia, candidiasis, CMV, cryptosporidiosis, herpes simplex or herpes zoster, and disseminated varicella (Yogev & Chadwick, 2011).

Although it is rare for an infant to be born with symptoms of HIV infection, all infants born to seropositive mothers should be presumed to be HIV positive until proven otherwise. Management begins by implementing Standard Precautions. Measures also should be taken to protect the infant from further exposure to maternal blood and body fluids. Regimens for the prevention of HIV transmission include antepartum, intrapartum, and neonatal treatment with highly active retroviral therapy (HAART).

The goal in the administration of antivirals is to suppress the virus to undetectable concentrations; the available antiviral drugs do not, however, cure the child's disease. HIV diagnosis in the neonatal period combined with aggressive antibiotic treatment of opportunistic infections has the potential to prolong survival (NIH Panel on Antiretroviral Therapy and Medical Management of HIV-Infected Children, 2012). Studies of HIV symptoms in children treated in the era of HAART show a significant decrease in the incidence of secondary opportunistic infections (NISDI Pediatric Study Group, 2012).

Counseling regarding the care of the mothers themselves, the family's care of the infant, and future pregnancies should be provided. The risk for transmission among members of the same household is minimal. Social services are required in these cases. If the parent chooses to keep the infant, home health care may be arranged. The family must be counseled about vaccinations. All HIV-1–exposed infants should receive routine immunizations. There are specific guidelines for those with confirmed HIV infection (CDC, 2014c). It is usually safe to administer all inactivated vaccines to HIV-1–infected children. In the absence of severe immunosuppression, children with HIV-1 can receive varicella vaccine (CDC).

Rubella Infection

Since the rubella vaccination program was begun in 1969, cases of congenital rubella infection have been reduced significantly; however, it is still seen occasionally in the newborn. Vaccination failures, lack of compliance, and the migration of nonimmunized persons result in periodic outbreaks of rubella, also known as German measles.

The risk of a congenitally infected infant varies with the gestational age of the fetus when maternal infection occurs. Abnormalities are most severe if the mother contracts the virus during the first trimester and rare if the disease occurs after that time (Schleiss & Patterson, 2012).

More than two thirds of infected infants show no apparent symptoms at birth, but sequelae can develop years later. Hearing loss, the most common result, appears to be progressive after birth. Congenital rubella syndrome includes cataracts or glaucoma, hearing loss, and cardiac defects (pulmonary artery stenosis, patent ductus arteriosus, or coarctation of the aorta). Multiple other abnormalities also are present, including IUGR, microphthalmia, hypotonia, hepatosplenomegaly, thrombocytopenic purpura, dermatoglyphic abnormalities, bony radiolucencies,

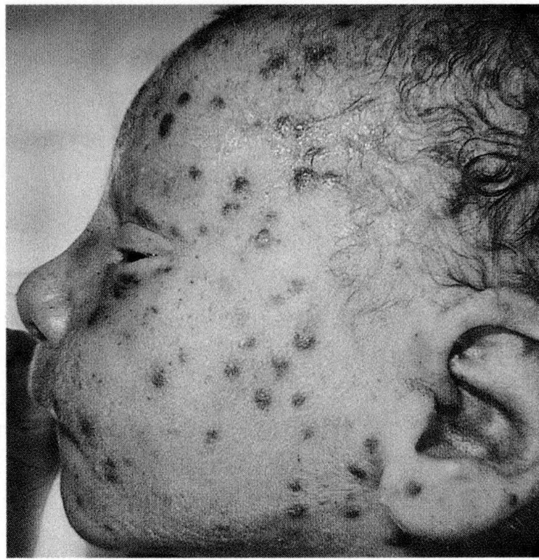

FIG 35-8 Neonatal cytomegalovirus infection. Typical rash seen in a severely affected infant. (Courtesy David A. Clarke, Philadelphia, PA.)

microcephaly, and brain wave abnormalities. Severe infection can result in fetal death. Delayed effects of infection manifest as thyroid dysfunction, diabetes mellitus, growth restriction, myocarditis, and glaucoma (Nielsen-Saines, 2011).

SAFETY ALERT

The rubella virus has been cultured in infants for up to 18 months after birth. These infants are a serious source of infection to susceptible individuals, particularly women in the childbearing years. Extended pediatric isolation is mandatory until the noncontagious stage of rubella has been reached. The infant should be isolated until pharyngeal mucus and urine are free of virus (Motacki, Kapoian, & O'Mara, 2011).

Cytomegalovirus Infection

Cytomegalovirus (CMV) infection during pregnancy can result in miscarriage, stillbirth, or congenital or neonatal cytomegalic inclusion disease (CMID). It is the most common cause of congenital viral infections in humans, occurring in 40,000 newborns in the United States every year. Maternal-fetal transmission of CMV occurs in 40% to 50% of mothers with a primary CMV infection during pregnancy (Schleiss & Patterson, 2012).

The neonate with classic, full-blown CMID typically displays IUGR and has microcephaly, seizures, and lethargy. The neonate also has a rash, jaundice, and hepatosplenomegaly (Fig. 35-8). Anemia, thrombocytopenia, and hyperbilirubinemia are common (Schleiss & Patterson, 2012). Intracranial, periventricular calcification often is noted on x-ray films. Mortality rates in symptomatic infants are 5% to 10% (Walker, Palma-Dias, Wood, et al., 2013). Congenital CMV can cause a variety of neurologic problems such as cognitive disabilities, hearing loss, or visual impairment (Schleiss & Patterson). Most (90%) affected infants are asymptomatic at birth (Walker et al., 2013), although there is a 10% to 15% risk that they will develop later sequelae such as hearing loss and learning disabilities (Schleiss & Patterson). Hearing loss can be present at birth or may not be apparent until after the first year of life. The hearing loss is often progressive. Chorioretinitis, microcephaly, intellectual disability, and neuromuscular deficits can occur by 2 years of age. Some children are at risk for a defect in tooth enamel, resulting in severe caries (Salanitri & Seow, 2013).

Elevated levels of cord blood IgM are suggestive of disease. The virus can be isolated from urine or saliva of the newborn. Differential diagnoses include other causes of jaundice, syphilis (positive Venereal Disease Research Laboratory [VDRL] findings), toxoplasmosis (positive Sabin-Feldman dye test result), hemolytic disease of the newborn (positive Coombs' test reaction), or coxsackievirus infection (positive culture).

CMV can be transmitted through breast milk while the mother has acute CMV infection. CMV infections acquired after birth are often asymptomatic and have no sequelae. Exceptions to this occur in preterm infants in whom postnatal acquisition of CMV can result in pneumonia, hepatitis, thrombocytopenia, and long-term neurologic sequelae.

Treatment of the infected newborn with ganciclovir is effective in decreasing neurologic sequelae, in particular sensorineural hearing loss. There is some evidence that administration of CMV-specific human immunoglobulin to the pregnant woman with primary CMV infection can help protect the fetus (Schleiss & Patterson, 2012).

Herpes Simplex Virus

Neonatal herpes simplex virus infection is being diagnosed more frequently although the exact incidence is difficult to determine because it is not a reportable condition in all states in the United States (Cherpes, Matthews, & Maryak, 2012). It may occur in as many as 1 in 2500 births (Schleiss & Patterson, 2012).

Women with a history of herpes infection may be prescribed antiviral medication beginning at 36 weeks of gestation, a practice that has been shown to reduce the likelihood of recurrent infection at birth (Kimberlin, Baley, Committee on Infectious Diseases, & Committee on Fetus and Newborn, 2013).

The neonate can acquire the virus through transplacental infection, ascending infection by way of the birth canal, direct contamination during passage through an infected birth canal, or direct transmission from infected personnel or family (Schleiss & Patterson, 2012).

Transplacental transmission of HSV infection to the neonate can occur during maternal infection; however, an ascending transcervical infection first involves the intact fetal membranes, causing chorioamnionitis. Transcervical infection can be accelerated by the use of internal fetal monitoring. The scalp electrodes break the fetal skin barrier and increase the risk of infection.

Congenital infection is rare and characterized by in utero destruction of normally formed organs. Affected infants are growth restricted and have skin lesions and scarring. They have severe psychomotor delays, with intracranial calcifications, microcephaly, hypertonicity, and seizures. They have eye involvement, including microphthalmos, cataracts, chorioretinitis, blindness, and retinal dysplasia. Some infants have patent ductus arteriosus, limb anomalies, and recurrent skin vesicles, with a short life expectancy (Baley & Toltzis, 2011).

In 85% of cases, HSV is transmitted from mother to neonate through viral shedding during labor and birth. This can occur whether or not the mother has active lesions. Primary maternal infections after 32 weeks of gestation present a higher risk for the fetus and newborn than early or recurrent infections.

Approximately 10% of neonates infected with HSV acquire the virus after birth from the mother, family member, or hospital personnel. Five percent of newborns are infected with HSV in utero (Kimberlin et al., 2013).

SAFETY ALERT

Due to concern regarding symptomatic and asymptomatic shedding of HSV among hospital personnel, nursery personnel with cold sores should practice strict hand hygiene and wear a mask. However, no evidence indicates that they should be removed from the nursery unless they have a herpetic whitlow (primary HSV infection of the terminal segment of a finger) (Baley & Toltzis, 2011).

Clinically, neonatal HSV infections are classified as disseminated infection (25%), CNS disease (30%), or localized infection of the skin, eye, or mouth (45%). Although the incubation period for HSV is 1 to 7 days, the onset of symptoms varies with the type of infection (Baley & Toltzis, 2011).

Disseminated infections are sepsis-like and can involve virtually every organ system but are most likely to involve the liver, adrenal glands, and lungs. By 5 to 11 days of age affected infants show signs of bacterial sepsis or shock. Death often results within 1 week of the onset of symptoms and is related to respiratory failure, pneumonitis, DIC with shock, and CNS complications (Baley & Toltzis, 2011; White & Magee, 2011).

In CNS disease, blood-borne seeding of the brain results in multiple lesions of cortical hemorrhagic necrosis. It also can occur alone or in association with oral, eye, or skin lesions. Brain involvement usually manifests in the second to fourth weeks of life. Skin lesions are apparent in 60% to 70% of infants, and the CSF of less than 50% of infants reveals the virus. The presenting manifestations include lethargy, poor feeding, irritability, and local or generalized seizures. If untreated, the mortality rate in CNS disease approaches 50%; the vast majority of survivors experience severe sequelae such as microcephaly and blindness (Baley & Toltzis, 2011).

Localized HSV infections most often occur with skin findings or rarely with isolated oral cavity lesions (Fig. 35-9). Without treatment CNS or disseminated disease develops in 70% of the infants with skin vesicles. Ocular involvement, which can occur alone, can be secondary to either HSV-1 or HSV-2. Ocular disease may not be discovered for months. Microphthalmos, cataracts, and corneal scarring can result from chorioretinitis, keratitis, and retinal hemorrhage (Baley & Toltzis, 2011).

Gloves should be worn when caregivers are in contact with these infants. The neonate's eyes, oral cavity, and skin are inspected carefully for the presence of any lesions. Cultures are obtained from the mouth, eyes, and any possible lesions. The infant can be discharged with the mother if the infant's cultures are negative for the virus. As long as no suspicious lesions are present on the mother's breasts, breastfeeding is allowed. For the infant at risk, prophylactic topical eye ointment (vidarabine) is administered for 5 days for prevention of keratoconjunctivitis. If there is a history of active lesions at delivery in a woman with no previous history of HSV infection neonatal prophylaxis with acyclovir is recommended (Kimberlin et al., 2013). Blood, urine, and CSF specimens should be cultured when indicated clinically. Therapy includes general supportive measures, as well as treatment with acyclovir. Duration of treatment is 14 to 21 days for infants with disseminated or CNS disease and 14 days for the skin-eye-mouth form of the disease (Baley & Toltzis, 2011). After completing the course of IV acyclovir, an oral acyclovir is given for 6 months to prevent recurrence (Kimberlin et al.). When there is ocular involvement, ophthalmic ointment should be administered simultaneously (Schleiss & Patterson, 2012).

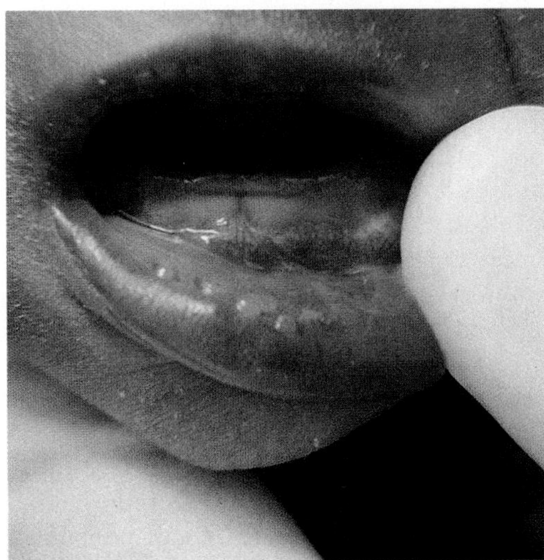

FIG 35-9 Neonatal herpes simplex virus oral lesions. (Courtesy David A. Clarke, Philadelphia, PA.)

Parvovirus B19

Parvovirus B19 is well known in older children as fifth disease or "slapped cheek illness" because of the characteristic facial appearance of the affected child. During pregnancy, infection can result in miscarriage, fetal anemia, hydrops fetalis, IUGR, or stillbirth. Vertical transmission of parvovirus to the fetus occurs in about one third of maternal infections, and the overall fetal loss rate after infection is about 6% (Schleiss & Patterson, 2012).

The virus can be isolated from amniotic fluid, fetal blood, or tissues using DNA PCR assay. Viral load is not predictive of fetal morbidity and mortality (Baley & Toltzis, 2011).

There are no specific antiviral medications to treat parvovirus B19 infection and there is no vaccine. If a pregnant woman is confirmed with the infection, the fetus should be closely monitored for the development of fetal hydrops using serial ultrasound examinations (Schleiss & Patterson, 2012). Protocols for intrauterine management have not been well developed, but intrauterine transfusion to treat anemia is the only currently accepted therapy. There is insufficient evidence about the long-term effects of parvovirus (de Jong, Walther, Kroes, & Oepkes, 2011).

Enterovirus

Enteroviruses include poliovirus, coxsackievirus, and echovirus. Nonpolio enteroviruses are among the most common viruses that infect humans. Enterovirus is the third most common cause of viral outbreaks in the NICU (following rotavirus and respiratory syncytial virus) (Civardi, Tzialla, Baldanti, et al., 2013). Group B coxsackieviruses and echovirus 11 are the serotypes most commonly affecting neonates and can be transmitted transplacentally or through exposure to maternal blood or secretions during birth. The risk of transmission is increased with maternal enterovirus illness around the time of birth and a lack of maternal antibodies to the specific type of enterovirus. Antenatal transmission increases the risk of severe disease and death (Baley & Toltzis, 2011).

The onset of infection following perinatal transmission is usually within 1 to 2 weeks after birth. Usual presenting symptoms are fever, irritability, lethargy, and poor feeding; rash, respiratory symptoms, and GI symptoms can occur. Clinical manifestations can be severe and include myocarditis, meningitis, respiratory distress, and hepatitis. Deaths are usually due to multiorgan involvement (Schleiss & Patterson, 2012).

There is no vaccine or any treatment approved by the U.S. Food and Drug Administration (FDA) for nonpolio enteroviruses. Immunoglobulin is sometimes used to treat symptomatic infants. Pleconaril is under investigation as a treatment for enteroviral infection in neonates and infants (Schlapbach, Ersch, Balmer, et al., 2013).

Bacterial Infections

Group B Streptococcus

GBS infection is a leading cause of neonatal morbidity and mortality in the United States (Tudela, Stewart, Roberts, et al., 2012). The practice of giving prophylactic antibiotics to women in labor who are GBS positive has significantly reduced the incidence and severity of early-onset GBS infection in the newborn (Fairlie, Zell, & Schrag, 2013). The incidence of both early- and late-onset neonatal GBS infection is 0.3 per 1000 live births (Ferrieri & Wallen, 2012; GBS Prevention Working Group, 2013).

Early-onset GBS infection in the neonate usually occurs in the first 7 days of life but most commonly manifests in the first 24 hours after birth. Risk factors for the development of early-onset GBS include low birth weight, preterm birth, rupture of membranes of more than 18 hours, maternal fever, previous GBS infant, maternal GBS bacteriuria, use of intrauterine fetal monitoring, maternal age less than 20 years, and Hispanic or African-American ethnicity. Early-onset disease usually results from vertical transmission from the birth canal and manifests as systemic infection or respiratory illness that mimics the symptoms of severe respiratory distress. The infant can rapidly develop pneumonia, shock, or meningitis. The mortality rate for early-onset infection is 5% to 20%, with higher rates among preterm infants (Anderson & Gonik, 2011; Ferrieri & Wallen, 2012).

Late-onset GBS infections occur between 1 week and 3 months of age, with an average age at onset of 24 days. Infection can result from vertical transmission or from health care–acquired infection or community exposure. Approximately 30% of infants with late-onset GBS develop meningitis (Anderson & Gonik, 2011). Mortality rates are less than for early-onset infection. Survivors often have neurologic damage (Libster, Edwards, Levent, et al., 2012).

For newborns with suspected GBS infection, the usual treatment is ampicillin in combination with an aminoglycoside. If GBS is identified as the cause of infection, penicillin G alone may be given (Aneja, Varughese-Aneja, Vetterly, & Carcillo, 2011). Figure 35-10 provides a sample algorithm for managing a neonate whose mother received intrapartum antibiotics for prevention (IAP) of GBS disease in the newborn or suspected chorioamnionitis.

COMMUNITY ACTIVITY

- Visit the American Pregnancy Association website pages related to group B streptococcal infection in pregnancy at http://americanpregnancy.org/pregnancycomplications/groupbstrepinfection.html. Review the client information about the disease and prevention strategies.
- Explore the Centers for Disease Control and Prevention (CDC) Group B Strep Home Page at http://www.cdc.gov/groupbstrep/index.html. Compare the information on this website with the information on the American Pregnancy Association site.

Escherichia coli

E. coli is responsible for approximately 40% of cases of early-onset neonatal sepsis and 25% of cases of neonatal meningitis in the United States (Edwards, 2011). It is found in the GI tract soon after birth and makes up the bulk of human fecal flora. *E. coli* can cause a variety of neonatal infections including omphalitis, diarrheal illness, pneumonia, peritonitis, urinary tract infection, and meningitis. Risk factors for the development of *E. coli* infections in the newborn include preterm birth, low birth weight, maternal infection, and prolonged rupture of membranes (Edwards).

Neonates most often acquire *E. coli* from the maternal birth canal or rectum during birth, although it also can be hospital acquired through person-to-person transmission or from the hospital environment. Exposure to *E. coli* can result in no infection, infection without illness, gastroenteritis, or rarely, septicemia. Symptoms can appear within the first 24 hours after birth or several weeks later. Clinical signs of *E. coli* sepsis are relatively nonspecific and include fever, temperature instability, apnea, cyanosis, jaundice, hepatomegaly, lethargy or irritability, vomiting, abdominal distention, and diarrhea.

The usual treatment for *E. coli* infection in the newborn is ampicillin or an extended-spectrum cephalosporin and an aminoglycoside. Treatment is continued for 7 to 10 days for bacteremia and at least 14 days for meningitis (Ferrieri & Wallen, 2012). Use of ampicillin in labor as prophylaxis against GBS disease has not been found to increase the risk of early-onset *E. coli* infection (Weston, Pondo, Lewis, et al., 2011) but can cause more virulent *E. coli* disease resulting from ampicillin-resistant organisms (Ferrieri & Wallen).

Staphylococcus aureus

Most staphylococcal infections in the newborn develop within the first few days after birth and involve the skin and soft tissue. Conjunctivitis, presenting with purulent eye discharge, is also a common manifestation of *S. aureus* infection. Skin lesions are typically small vesicles or pustules that are easily treated with topical antimicrobial agents. The skin lesions can appear as large fragile bullae containing clear or purulent fluid. These bullae rupture easily and leave moist, red, denuded areas of skin. A more severe bullous eruption due to staphylococcal infection is scalded skin syndrome characterized by widespread bullous lesions that easily rupture; fever and irritability are also present

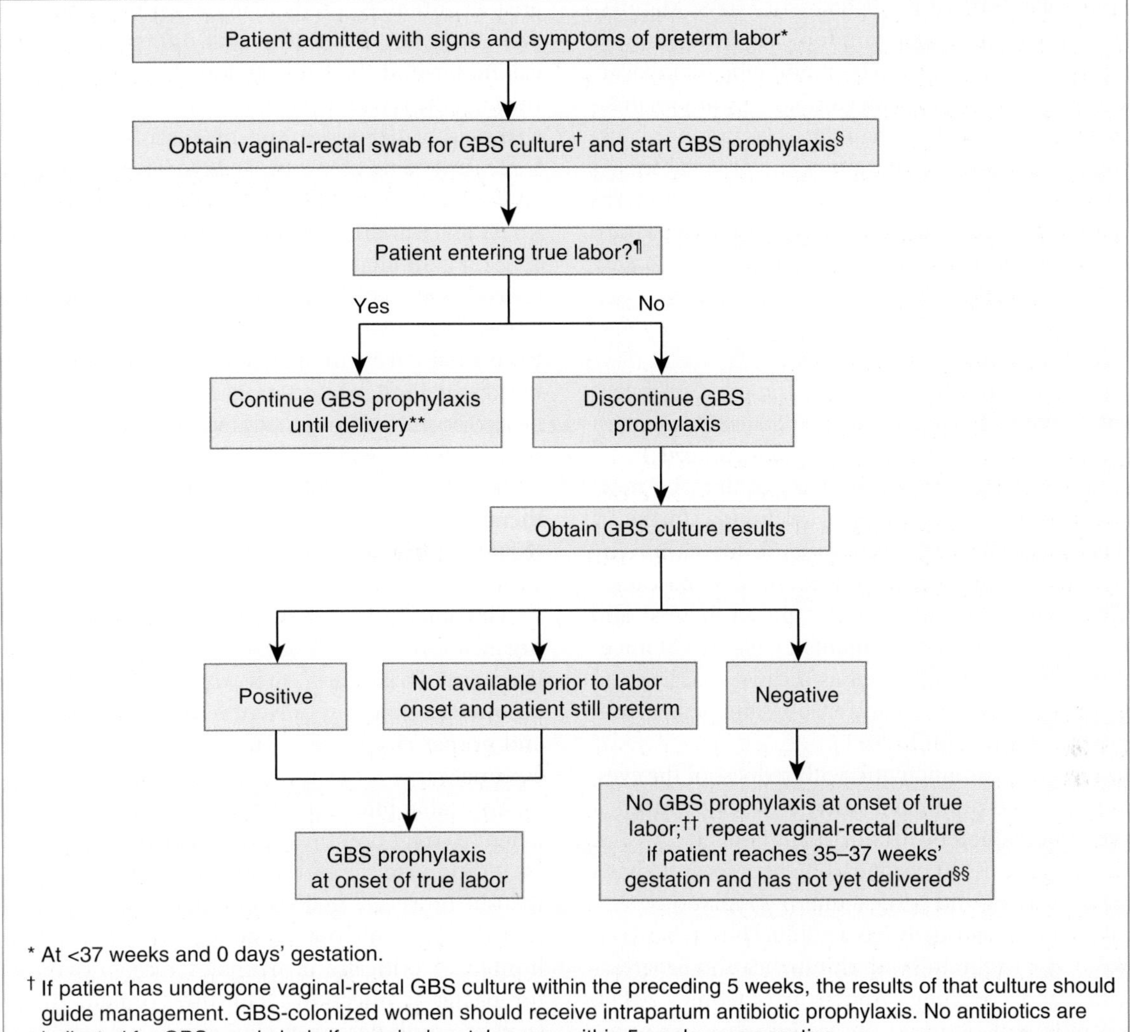

* At <37 weeks and 0 days' gestation.

† If patient has undergone vaginal-rectal GBS culture within the preceding 5 weeks, the results of that culture should guide management. GBS-colonized women should receive intrapartum antibiotic prophylaxis. No antibiotics are indicated for GBS prophylaxis if a vaginal-rectal screen within 5 weeks was negative.

§ See Figure 8 for recommended antibiotic regimens.

¶ Patient should be regularly assessed for progression to true labor; if the patient is considered not to be in true labor, discontinue GBS prophylaxis.

** If GBS culture results become available prior to delivery and are negative, then discontinue GBS prophylaxis.

†† Unless subsequent GBS culture prior to delivery is positive.

§§ A negative GBS screen is considered valid for 5 weeks. If a patient with a history of PTL is re-admitted with signs and symptoms of PTL and had a negative GBS screen >5 weeks prior, she should be rescreened and managed according to this algorithm at that time.

FIG 35-10 Sample algorithm for secondary prevention of early-onset group B streptococcal disease among newborns. (From Verani J.R., McGee L., & Schrag S.J. [2010]. Prevention of perinatal group B streptococcal disease. Revised guidelines from CDC. *MMWR Morbidity and Mortality Weekly Report, 59*[RR10], 1-32.)

(Wright & Cohen, 2012). *S. aureus* can cause serious problems such as abscesses, osteomyelitis, endocarditis, and septic arthritis. Breaks in the skin from IV catheters or scalp electrodes present an opportunity for the development of *S. aureus* abscesses. Colonization of the maternal genital tract with *S. aureus* is not uncommon although the potential for vertical transmission to the neonate is unclear (Jimenez-Truque, Tedeschi, Saye, et al., 2012). The major sources of colonization by *S. aureus* are the hands of medical and nursing personnel.

Although most strains of *S. aureus* are sensitive to semisynthetic penicillins, there are increasing concerns about methicillin-resistant strains. MRSA has caused outbreaks of health care–acquired infection in neonatal intensive care units and hospital nurseries (Heinrich, Mueller, Bartmann, et al., 2011).

Listeriosis

Listeriosis, caused by *Listeria monocytogenes,* is primarily a foodborne infection that can cause maternal and neonatal illness. Mother-to-infant transmission occurs transplacentally through ascending infection or during birth. Prenatal infection causes chorioamnionitis or endometritis and should be suspected in cases of brown-stained amniotic fluid. It can also cause miscarriage, preterm birth, and stillbirth. Two forms of neonatal listeriosis are recognized: early and late onset. Signs of early-onset infection are present at birth or in the first 1 to 2 days. Manifestations of infection are sepsis-like symptoms, acute respiratory distress, pneumonia, and more rarely, meningitis or myocarditis. With severe infection the infant can have granulomatosis infantiseptica, which is a widely disseminated granuloma, causing an erythematous rash with pale papules and organ abscesses (Mani & Stocker, 2012). Late-onset listeriosis is more insidious and usually manifests as meningitis. Listeriosis in the newborn is treated with ampicillin and an aminoglycoside (Cekmez, Tayman, Saglam, et al., 2012).

Chlamydia

Chlamydia trachomatis infection is one of the most prevalent sexually transmitted infections in the United States. The highest incidence is among adolescents and young adults aged 15-24 years (CDC, 2014d). Neonatal infection is acquired by newborns in approximately 25% to 60% of all vaginal births by infected mothers and is known to occur in some infants born by cesarean with intact membranes. *Chlamydia trachomatis* causes neonatal conjunctivitis (25% to 50% of exposed infants) and pneumonia (5% to 20% of exposed infants). Chlamydial infection in pregnancy has been suggested as a cause of early and late pregnancy loss, stillbirth, premature labor, and postpartum endometritis (Anderson & Gonik, 2011).

Neonatal chlamydial conjunctivitis, with redness of the eyes, edema of the eyelids, and minimal discharge, develops within a few days to several weeks after birth and usually lasts 1 to 2 weeks. If untreated it can progress to chronic follicular conjunctivitis with conjunctival scarring and corneal microgranulations.

Chlamydial pneumonia usually has a gradual onset, between 4 and 11 weeks of age, beginning with rhinorrhea and progressing to tachypnea and coughing (Anderson & Gonik, 2011). Signs can be subtle and often go unrecognized. It is speculated that pneumonia can occur as a result of movement of the organism from the conjunctiva into the lower respiratory tract; however, conjunctivitis is not a prerequisite to pneumonia.

Chlamydial conjunctivitis is treated with oral erythromycin or azithromycin. The recommended treatment for chlamydial pneumonia is oral azithromycin for 3 days or a 14-day regimen of erythromycin. Erythromycin administration in infants younger than 6 weeks has been associated with an increased risk of infantile hypertrophic pyloric stenosis; therefore, parents should be educated regarding the symptoms of the condition (feeding intolerance, projectile vomiting, and abdominal distention) (Parashette & Croffie, 2013).

Fungal Infections

Candidiasis

Candida infections, formerly known as moniliasis, can occur in the newborn. *Candida albicans,* the organism usually responsible, can cause disease in any organ system. It is a yeastlike fungus (producing yeast cells and spores) that can be acquired during birth from a maternal vaginal infection; by person-to-person transmission; or from contaminated hands, bottles, nipples, or other articles. It usually is a benign disorder in the neonate, often confined to the oral and diaper regions (Edwards, 2011).

Candidal diaper dermatitis appears on the perianal area, inguinal folds, and lower portion of the abdomen. The affected area is intensely erythematous, with a sharply demarcated, scalloped edge, frequently with numerous satellite lesions that extend beyond the larger lesion. The source of the infection is through the GI tract. Treatment is an antifungal ointment, such as nystatin (Mycostatin) or miconazole 2% (Monistat), applied three times a day for 7 to 10 days. The infant also can be given an oral antifungal preparation to eliminate any GI source of infection (Edwards, 2011).

Oral candidiasis (**thrush,** or mycotic stomatitis) is characterized by the appearance of white plaques on the oral mucosa, gums, and tongue. The white patches are easily differentiated from milk curds; the patches cannot be removed and tend to bleed when touched. In most cases the infant does not seem to be in discomfort from the infection. A few infants seem to have some difficulty swallowing.

Infants who are sick, debilitated, or receiving antibiotic therapy are more susceptible to thrush. Those with cleft lip or palate, neoplasms, and hyperparathyroidism seem to be more vulnerable to fungal infection.

The objectives of management are to eradicate the causative organism, to control exposure to *C. albicans,* and to improve the infant's resistance. Interventions include maintaining scrupulous cleanliness to prevent reinfection. Careful hand hygiene and proper cleanliness of the equipment and environment are essential.

Topical application of nystatin to the mouth is usually sufficient to treat oral thrush. Gentian violet solution can be used in addition to one of the antifungal drugs in chronic cases of thrush; however, it does not treat GI candida and can irritate the oral mucosa. Systemic candida infection is usually limited to critically ill neonates receiving antibiotic therapy for bacterial infections. For these infants antifungal agents such as amphotericin B (Fungizone), fluconazole (Diflucan), or miconazole (Monistat, Micatin) are given intravenously. Infants who are breastfed can acquire candida infection from the mother. If the mother is colonized, treatment for mother and infant is recommended. Breastfeeding can continue even if the mother is receiving systemic antifungal medications (Wright & Cohen, 2011).

SUBSTANCE ABUSE

Substance abuse during pregnancy is associated with significant fetal and neonatal risks. Other than alcohol and tobacco, cocaine and marijuana are the most commonly used substances by pregnant women. Maternal substance abuse is discussed in Chapter 31.

The adverse effects of exposure of the fetus to drugs are varied. They include transient behavioral changes such as alterations in fetal breathing movements or irreversible effects such as fetal death, IUGR, congenital anomalies, or intellectual disability. Critical determinants of the effect of the drug on the fetus include the specific drug, the dosage, the route of administration, the genotype of the mother or fetus, and the timing of the drug exposure. Determining the specific effects of individual drugs on the fetus is made difficult by the common practice of polydrug use, errors or omissions in reporting drug use, and variations in the strength, purity, and types of additives found in street drugs. Maternal conditions such

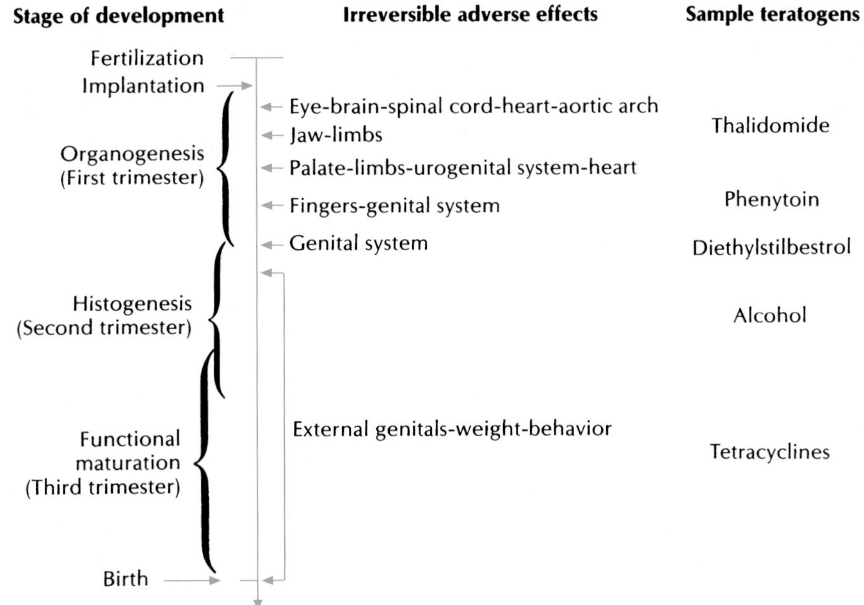

FIG 35-11 Critical periods in human embryogenesis. (From Reed, M., Aranda, J., & Hales, B. [2006]. Developmental pharmacology. In R. Martin, A. Fanaroff, & M. Walsh (Eds.), *Fanaroff and Martin's neonatal-perinatal medicine: Diseases of the fetus and infant* [8th ed.]. St. Louis: Mosby.)

as poverty and malnutrition and comorbid conditions such as STIs further compound the difficulty in identifying the presence and consequences of intrauterine drug exposure. Figure 35-11 shows critical periods in human embryogenesis and the teratogenic effects of drugs. Table 35-4 summarizes the effects of commonly abused substances on the fetus and neonate.

Physiologic signs of withdrawal have been reported in neonates of mothers who use to excess such drugs as barbiturates, alcohol, opioids, or amphetamines. Prescription opioids such as oxycodone (Percodan, OxyContin) have been identified as increasingly popular drugs of abuse that can cause withdrawal symptoms in neonates. Serious withdrawal reactions can be seen in neonates whose mothers abuse psychoactive drugs. Withdrawal symptoms are described as **neonatal abstinence syndrome (NAS)**. This syndrome is characterized by symptoms of CNS irritability, respiratory distress, GI dysfunction, and autonomic dysfunction (Table 35-5). Withdrawal symptoms are more severe in newborns exposed to larger amounts of drugs for longer periods of time. The severity of withdrawal is also related to the timing of maternal drug use in relation to birth. Drug use close to the time of birth increases the severity of withdrawal but delays the onset of symptoms (Nash & Smith, 2012).

TABLE 35-4 Summary of Neonatal Effects of Commonly Abused Substances

SUBSTANCE	NEONATAL EFFECTS
Alcohol	Fetal alcohol syndrome (FAS): craniofacial anomalies, including short eyelid opening, flat midface, flat upper lip groove, thin upper lip; microcephaly; hyperactivity; developmental delays; attention deficits Alcohol-related birth defects (ARBDs): milder forms of FAS, cardiac anomalies, failure to thrive
Cocaine	Prematurity, small for gestational age, placental or cerebral infarctions, hyperactivity, difficult to console, hypersensitivity to noise and external stimuli
Heroin	Low birth weight, small for gestational age, neonatal abstinence syndrome (see Table 35-5)
Marijuana	Deficits in attention, cognition, memory, motor skills
Amphetamines	Small for gestational age, prematurity, poor weight gain, lethargy
Tobacco	Prematurity, low birth weight, increased risk for sudden infant death syndrome, increased risk for bronchitis, pneumonia, developmental delays

Data from Bandstra, E., & Accornero, V. (2011). Infants of substance-abusing mothers. In R. Martin, A. Fanaroff, & M. Walsh (Eds.), *Fanaroff and Martin's neonatal-perinatal medicine: Diseases of the fetus and infant* (9th ed.). St. Louis: Mosby; Behnke, M., Smith, V.C., American Academy of Pediatrics (AAP) Committee on Substance Abuse, & Committee on Fetus and Newborn (2013). Prenatal substance abuse: Short- and long-term effects on the exposed fetus. *Pediatrics, 131*(3), e1009-e1024.

Tobacco

Infants born to women who smoke are about 25% more likely to be preterm, weigh on average 200 g (7 oz) less, and have twice the risk of sudden infant death syndrome (SIDS) as compared with infants born to nonsmokers (Bailey, McCook, Hodge, & McGrady, 2012; Brookfield, Wilkinson, Luke, et al., 2011). Some researchers have found links between maternal smoking and birth defects (Hackshaw, Rodeck, & Boniface, 2011). However, others have found that when other variables have been controlled for, no clear association has been found between maternal smoking and congenital anomalies (Bandstra & Accornero, 2011).

Maternal smoking exposes the fetus to nicotine and more than 4000 other compounds including carbon monoxide, dioxin, cyanide, and cadmium; adverse health effects have been identified in relation to approximately 30 of these compounds (Behnke, Smith, Committee on Substance Abuse, & Committee

TABLE 35-5 Signs of Neonatal Abstinence Syndrome

SYSTEM	SIGNS
Respiratory	Irregular respirations, tachypnea, apnea, nasal flaring, chest retractions, intermittent cyanosis, rhinorrhea, nasal congestion
Neurologic	Irritability, tremors, shrill cry, incessant crying, hyperactivity, disturbed sleep pattern, seizures, hypertonicity, increased deep tendon reflexes, exaggerated Moro reflex
Autonomic dysfunction	Frequent yawning, frequent sneezing, tearing, excessive generalized sweating, mottling of skin, fever
Gastrointestinal	Abnormal feeding pattern, uncoordinated and ineffectual sucking and swallowing reflexes, incessant hunger, frantic sucking, refusal to feed, vomiting, regurgitation, diarrhea

Data from Weiner, S.M., & Finnegan, L.P. (2011). Drug withdrawal in the neonate. In S.L. Gardner, B.S. Carter, M. Enzman-Hines, & J.A. Hernandez (Eds.), *Merenstein & Gardner's handbook of neonatal intensive care* (7th ed.). St. Louis: Mosby.

on Fetus and Newborn, 2013). Nicotine's vasoconstrictive effects on the placenta and umbilical vessels contribute to fetal hypoxia and undernourishment of the fetus. Nicotine has harmful effects on fetal brain development, resulting in deficits in intellectual ability, emotional development, and behavior (Behnke et al., 2013). The effects include poor auditory responsiveness, fine motor tremors, hypertonicity, and decreased verbal comprehension (Rosenthal & Weitzman, 2011).

Nicotine and cotinine, the two pharmacologically active substances in tobacco, are found in higher concentrations in infants whose mothers smoke. These substances can be secreted in breast milk for up to 2 hours after the mother has smoked. Smoking is related to low milk supply and poor infant weight gain (AAP Section on Breastfeeding, 2012).

Increasing concern surrounds secondhand smoke and its potential effects on infants and children. Exposure to secondhand smoke increases the risk of ear infections, respiratory illnesses such as asthma and bronchitis, and SIDS (Aguilera, Pedersen, Garcia-Esteban, et al., 2013; Brookfield et al., 2011). It is not clear whether the association between smoking and SIDS reflects in utero exposure or passive exposure postnatally, or both.

Smoking cessation during pregnancy greatly decreases the chance of fetal complications; therefore, women should be counseled regarding smoking cessation programs. Mothers and all others should refrain from smoking near the infant.

Alcohol

Alcohol consumption during pregnancy is a growing concern. Alcohol ingestion during pregnancy is associated with short- and long-term effects on the fetus and newborn, which are subsumed under the term *fetal alcohol spectrum disorders (FASDs)*. FASDs include specific conditions such as fetal alcohol syndrome, alcohol-related neurodevelopmental disorder, and alcohol-related birth defects. FASDs are estimated to occur in as many as 10 of every 1000 births in the United States. However, the full extent of the problem is unknown and more prevalence studies are needed (Riley, Infante, & Warren, 2011).

Ethanol easily crosses the placenta. The quantity of alcohol required to produce fetal effects is unclear, but it is known that infants born to heavy drinkers are at higher risk of congenital abnormalities than those born to moderate drinkers. Alcohol withdrawal can occur in neonates, particularly when maternal ingestion occurs near the time of birth. Signs and symptoms include jitteriness, increased tone and reflex responses, and irritability. Seizures are also common.

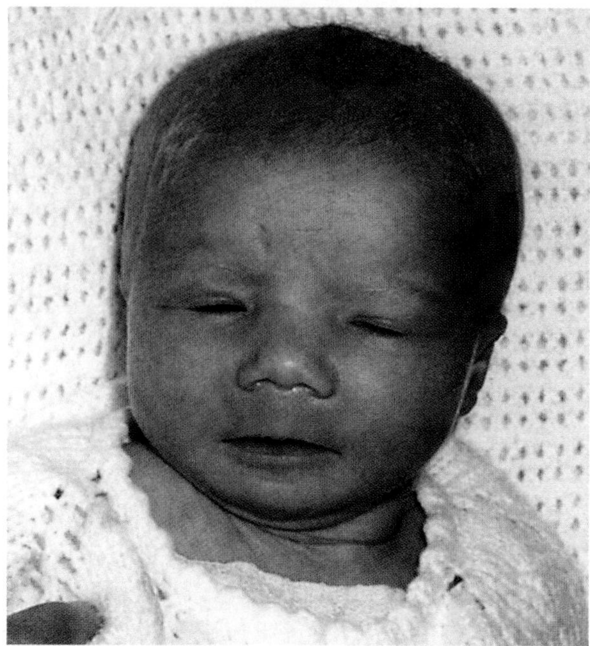

FIG 35-12 Infant with fetal alcohol syndrome. (From Markiewicz, M., & Abrahamson, E. [1999]. *Diagnosis in color: Neonatology.* St. Louis: Mosby.)

Fetal alcohol syndrome (FAS) is based on minimal criteria of signs in each of three categories: prenatal and postnatal growth restriction; CNS malfunctions, including cognitive impairment; and craniofacial features such as microcephaly, small eyes or short palpebral fissures, thin upper lip, flat midface, and an indistinct philtrum. Neurologic problems in FAS children include some degree of IQ deficit, attention deficit disorder, diminished fine motor skills, and poor speech. These children have been shown to lack inhibition, have no stranger anxiety, and lack appropriate judgment skills (Bandstra & Accornero, 2011).

Infants exposed prenatally to alcohol who are affected but do not meet the criteria for FAS can be said to have alcohol-related neurodevelopmental disorders (ARNDs) or alcohol-related birth defects (ARBDs). These disorders run the gamut from learning disabilities and behavioral problems to speech or language problems and hyperactivity. Often these problems are not detected until the child goes to school and learning problems become evident. Similar birth defects can be seen with other disorders, such as fetal hydantoin syndrome (from exposure to antiepileptic drugs); therefore, a careful history is needed.

Predictable abnormal patterns of fetal and neonatal morphogenesis are attributed to severe, chronic alcoholism in women who continue to drink heavily during pregnancy. The pattern of growth deficiency begun in prenatal life persists after birth, especially in the linear growth rate, rate of weight gain, and growth of head circumference.

Ocular structural anomalies are common findings (Fig. 35-12). Limb anomalies and a variety of cardiovascular anomalies, especially ventricular septal defects, pose problems for the child. Cognitive impairment (IQ of 79 or less at age 7 years), hyperactivity, and fine motor dysfunction (poor hand-to-mouth coordination, weak grasp) add to the handicapping problems that maternal alcoholism can impose. Genital abnormalities are seen in daughters of alcohol-addicted mothers. Two thirds of newborns with FAS are girls; the cause of this altered fetal sex ratio is unknown. High alcohol levels are lethal to the developing embryo. Lower levels cause brain and other malformations. Long-term prognosis is discouraging even in an optimal psychosocial environment, when one considers the combination of growth failure and intellectual disability (Kuehn, Aros, Cassorla, et al., 2012; Kully-Martens, Denys, Treit, et al., 2012; Kully-Martens, Treit, Pei, & Rasmussen, 2013; Pei, Job, Kully-Martens, & Rasmussen, 2011).

Heroin

Heroin crosses the placenta and often results in IUGR in exposed infants, although the exact mechanisms of growth inhibition are not clear. There is an increased rate of stillbirths but not of congenital anomalies. Maternal heroin use increases the risk for meconium aspiration, increased neonatal death, microcephaly, neurobehavioral problems, and SIDS (Madgula, Groshkova, & Mayet, 2011). If heroin users are placed on methadone maintenance treatment during pregnancy, perinatal outcomes are improved (Bandstra & Accornero, 2011).

Many of the medical complications attributed to heroin result from prematurity. Other risks include physical dependence in the fetus and the risk of exposure to infections, including hepatitis B and C viruses and HIV. Drug withdrawal in the mother is accompanied by fetal withdrawal, which can lead to fetal death. Maternal detoxification in the first trimester carries an increased risk of miscarriage. Detoxification in pregnancy is not recommended because of possible withdrawal-induced fetal distress. Methadone is often used in pregnancy to treat maternal drug cravings and prevent withdrawal.

Heroin withdrawal (neonatal abstinence syndrome) occurs in the majority of infants born to addicted mothers, usually within the first 12 to 48 hours of life. The signs depend on the length of maternal addiction, the amount of drug taken, and the time of injection before birth. The infant whose mother is taking methadone may not demonstrate signs of withdrawal until a week or so after birth. The symptoms of infants whose mothers used heroin or methadone are similar. Initially the infant can be depressed. The withdrawal syndromes can manifest as a combination of any of the following signs. Most commonly, the infant is jittery and hyperactive. Usually the infant's cry is shrill and persistent. The infant may yawn or sneeze frequently. Tendon reflexes are increased, but the Moro reflex is decreased. The neonate can exhibit poor feeding and sucking, tachypnea, vomiting, diarrhea, hypothermia or hyperthermia, and sweating. In addition, an abnormal sleep cycle, with absence of quiet sleep and disturbance of active sleep, has been described in these infants (Bandstra & Accornero, 2011).

If withdrawal is not treated, vomiting, diarrhea, dehydration, apnea, and convulsions can develop. Death can follow. Therapy is individualized. Dehydration and electrolyte imbalance are prevented or treated. Usually one of the following drugs is ordered: phenobarbital, methadone, or clonidine, singly or in combination.

Methadone

Methadone, a synthetic opiate, has been the therapy of choice for heroin addiction since 1965. Methadone crosses the placenta. An increasing number of infants have been born to methadone-maintained mothers, who seem to have better prenatal care and a somewhat better lifestyle than those taking heroin (Bandstra & Accornero, 2011).

NAS (Table 35-5) occurs in the majority of neonates born to women taking methadone. Neither the incidence nor severity of symptoms has been correlated with methadone dose at birth (Wisner, Sit, Reynolds, et al., 2012). Methadone withdrawal resembles heroin withdrawal but tends to be more severe and prolonged. In addition, the incidence of seizures is higher. Seizures usually occur between days 7 and 10. Infants exhibit a disturbed sleep pattern similar to that seen in heroin withdrawal and have a higher birth weight than those in heroin withdrawal, usually appropriate for gestational age. No increased incidence of congenital anomalies is seen.

Late-onset withdrawal occurs at 2 to 4 weeks and can continue for weeks or months. A higher incidence of SIDS also has been reported in these infants (Bandstra & Accornero, 2011). This factor is important for perinatal nurses who coordinate follow-up care for the infant and education for the mother or other caregiver. Pediatric and community health nurses must know about the potential for withdrawal symptoms.

Therapy for methadone withdrawal is similar to the therapy for heroin withdrawal. Buprenorphine, a partial agonist–partial antagonist synthetic opioid with a long duration of action, has gained acceptance and FDA licensing for treating opioid addiction. Preliminary studies indicate that this drug has advantages over methadone in relation to neonatal outcomes such as severity of NAS and length of hospital stay (Gaalema, Scott, Heil, et al., 2012; Pritham, Paul, & Hayes, 2012).

Methadone is not contraindicated during breastfeeding. Minimal amounts are transferred to the infant through breast milk. However, infants exposed to methadone are at greater risk for feeding problems (Wisner et al., 2012).

The long-term effects of methadone exposure are primarily related to neurodevelopmental outcomes. These neonates are at increased risk for developmental delays, poor fine motor coordination, lower intelligence, hyperactivity, learning and behavior disorders, and poor social adjustment. Researchers have noted that it is difficult to separate the effects of methadone from other factors in the environment that can influence neurobehavioral outcomes (Bandstra & Accornero, 2011).

Marijuana

Marijuana use is prevalent among young adults, including women of childbearing age. The primary chemical compound in marijuana—9-tetrahydrocannabinol (THC)—easily crosses the placenta and can remain in the body for as long as 30 days, increasing fetal exposure and potential risk (Behnke et al., 2013).

Marijuana use during pregnancy can result in a shortened gestation and a higher incidence of IUGR. A review of studies examining the effects of marijuana during pregnancy found inconsistent results regarding the drug's effect on birth weight and gestational age (Soto & Bahado-Singh, 2013). No specific teratogenic effects have been identified. Marijuana affects neurotransmitters and brain chemistry in the developing fetus which can have long-term effects such as deficits in memory, attention, or cognitive function. Marijuana smoking during pregnancy can increase carbon monoxide levels in the blood, which can reduce the amount of oxygen available to the fetus (Bandstra & Accornero, 2011; Behnke et al., 2013).

Compounding the issue of the effects of marijuana is multidrug use, especially among adolescents, that combines the harmful effects of marijuana, tobacco, alcohol, and cocaine. Long-term follow-up studies on exposed infants are needed.

Cocaine

Cocaine crosses the placenta and is found in breast milk. Considerable controversy exists regarding the effects of cocaine on the fetus and neonate. There is a strong association between maternal cocaine use and both tobacco and marijuana use, which makes determining cocaine effects difficult. A meta-analysis did not find an association between illicit drug use and congenital anomalies (Behnke et al., 2013). However, it is possible that habitual cocaine use in pregnancy has negative effects, many of which are too subtle to notice in the newborn and infancy periods. Cocaine is a recognized cause of placental abruption. Infants born to cocaine-abusing mothers show a high rate of perinatal morbidity, IUGR, low birth weight, and preterm birth (Bandstra & Accornero, 2011) (Box 35-1).

Cocaine-dependent neonates do not experience a process of withdrawal as do narcotic-exposed infants but rather show neurotoxic effects of the drug. Signs of exposure have some of the same characteristics as those of heroin withdrawal but can be highly varied. There can be an increased risk for SIDS. The effects of prenatal exposure to cocaine on neonatal behavior have been studied extensively. Findings indicate that cocaine-exposed infants have limited ability to habituate to stimuli. As these children enter school they demonstrate a reduced capacity for verbal reasoning and difficulties maintaining attention (Bandstra & Accornero, 2011).

BOX 35-1 Fetal and Neonatal Effects of Maternal Cocaine Use During Pregnancy

Physical
- Preterm birth
- Decreased length
- Decreased head circumference
- Low birth weight
- Cerebral infarction
- Abnormal electroencephalogram (EEG)
- Seizures
- Abnormal breathing pattern

Behavioral
- Irritability
- Tremors
- Abnormal sleep pattern
- Hypertonicity
- Increase in auditory startle response
- High-pitched cry
- Excessive sucking
- Disorganized behavior
- Hyporeactivity
- Poor interaction with caregivers
- Inattention and learning problems

Data from Weiner, S.M., & Finnegan, L.P. (2011). Drug withdrawal in the neonate. In S.L. Gardner, B.S. Carter, M. Enzman-Hines, & J.A. Hernandez (Eds.), *Merenstein & Gardner's handbook of neonatal intensive care* (7th ed.). St. Louis: Mosby; Hudak, M.L., Tan, R.C., Committee on Drugs, & Committee on Fetus and Newborn. (2012). Neonatal drug withdrawal. *Pediatrics, 129*(2), e540-e560.

Methamphetamine

The fetal and neonatal effects associated with maternal use of methamphetamines in pregnancy are not well known. The limited data regarding the risk of congenital anomalies suggest little or no effect on organogenesis. A higher incidence of placental abruption, preterm birth, and IUGR is associated with methamphetamine use during pregnancy (Geary & Wells, 2013; Ladhani, Shah, & Murphy, 2011; Narkowicz, Plotka, Polkowska, et al., 2013). Behavioral changes in infants exposed prenatally to methamphetamines include decreased arousal, increased stress, and alterations in movement (Bandstra & Accornero, 2011).

Neonatal manifestations of methamphetamine withdrawal have not been clearly identified because of maternal polydrug use. After birth, infants can experience bradycardia or tachycardia that resolves as the drug is cleared from the infant's system. Lethargy can continue for several months, along with frequent infections and poor weight gain. Emotional disturbances and delays in gross and fine motor coordination can be seen during early childhood.

MDMA/Ecstasy

Increasing use of 3,4-methylenedioxymethamphetamine (MDMA), also known as ecstasy, by adolescents and young adults of childbearing age heightens concerns related to fetal and neonatal effects of this substance. This illegal synthetic psychoactive drug has hallucinogenic and stimulant properties. It alters the activity of neurotransmitters in the brain and causes increased heart rate and blood pressure. Animal studies have demonstrated that MDMA can be toxic to nerve cells containing serotonin, causing long-term damage. MDMA alters the body's temperature regulatory abilities and in high doses can cause a sharp increase in body temperature (hyperthermia) leading to liver, kidney, and cardiovascular system failure, and death (National Institute on Drug Abuse, 2012). This substance is transferred to the fetus through the placenta, but the effects on the developing fetus are not well substantiated in human studies. It is thought that maternal use of MDMA increases the risk of congenital anomalies in the fetus and that it can cause long-term problems with learning and memory. More research studies are needed to identify the effects of MDMA on the fetus and neonate (Bandstra & Accornero, 2011).

Other Drugs of Concern

Caffeine

Caffeine is a mild CNS stimulant that is consumed on a regular basis by the majority of Americans. Coffee is the primary source of caffeine for most Americans, although caffeine is also found in tea, chocolate, colas, energy drinks, guarana, and mate (a tea consumed primarily in South America).

The average half-life of caffeine ranges from about 3 to 7 hours, with individual variation in metabolism related to genetic and environmental factors. During the second and third trimesters of pregnancy, caffeine metabolism is slowed due to hormonal influences. Caffeine readily crosses the placenta and is distributed to all fetal tissues. Because of immature liver function, fetuses metabolize caffeine very slowly (Gregory, Niebyl, & Johnson, 2012).

Although caffeine has not been implicated as a teratogen in humans, there are concerns about its consumption during pregnancy. Moderate intake of caffeine (less than 200 mg/day) is not associated with an increased risk of miscarriage, preterm birth, or low birth weight. There is a lack of evidence regarding the risks of higher caffeine consumption (ACOG Committee on Obstetric Practice, 2010). The American College of Obstetricians and Gynecologists (ACOG) and the March of Dimes recommend that caffeine intake in pregnant women should not exceed 200 mg/day (ACOG Committee on Obstetric Practice, 2010; March of Dimes, 2012).

Selective Serotonin Reuptake Inhibitors

Selective serotonin reuptake inhibitors (SSRIs) are the mainstay of treatment for depression and anxiety, with widespread use during pregnancy. Commonly prescribed SSRIs include citalopram, escitalopram, fluoxetine, fluvoxamine, paroxetine, and sertraline (Patil, Kuller, & Rhee, 2011). All medications that have been studied are known to cross the placenta and are transferred in breast milk. Their use should be determined by a risk-benefit analysis of the risks to the fetus or neonate with use of the medication weighed against risks of not treating the mother's psychiatric condition. The dosage of SSRIs during pregnancy should be at the lowest effective level (Hudak, Tan, Committee on Drugs, & Committee on Fetus and Newborn, 2012).

There is a lack of definitive evidence related to teratogenic effects of SSRI use during pregnancy (Koren & Nordeng, 2012). A meta-analysis showed an increased risk for cardiovascular defects associated with fetal exposure to antidepressant medications, especially paroxetine. The same meta-analysis did not report an increase of other congenital malformations with maternal antidepressant use (Grigoriadis, VonderPorten, Mamisashvili, et al., 2013).

Maternal use of SSRIs during the second trimester has been associated with preterm birth and low birth weight (Grzeskowiak, Gilbert, & Morrison, 2012; Hayes, Pingsheng, Shelton, et al., 2012). Fetal exposure to SSRIs during the third trimester predisposes the neonate to a behavioral syndrome resembling NAS. Symptoms during the first week of life can be related to drug toxicity or withdrawal and include irritability, agitation, tremors, hypoglycemia, tachypnea, vomiting, and diarrhea. This syndrome is usually mild and lasts for no longer than 2 days. In rare cases the syndrome is severe, with seizures, hyperpyrexia, excessive weight loss, and respiratory problems (Hayes et al., 2012; Patil et al., 2011). Persistent pulmonary hypertension in the newborn (PPHN) has been associated with exposure to maternal SSRIs after 20 weeks of gestation (Kieler, Artama, Engeland, et al., 2012; Patil et al.). There is no increased risk of stillbirth, neonatal mortality, or postneonatal mortality associated with SSRI use during pregnancy (Jimenez-Solem, Andersen, Petersen, et al., 2013; Stephansson, Kieler, Haglund, et al., 2013).

For parents who are concerned about maternal use of psychiatric medications and the fetal or neonatal effects, the nurse can direct them to the following websites: REPROTOX (www.reprotox.org) and TERIS (http://depts.washington.edu/terisweb).

CARE MANAGEMENT

The maternal history is the key to identification of newborns who are at risk because of maternal substance abuse or use of other drugs during pregnancy and lactation. Review of the prenatal record can reveal a medical and social history of drug use or abuse and any detoxification treatment used. There can be other factors that contribute to neonatal outcomes and complications. For example, the woman who is addicted to narcotics or cocaine can have infections that compound the risk to the infant, including hepatitis, septicemia, and STIs, including AIDS (Narkowicz et al., 2013). In some cases there is no information in the prenatal record to suggest maternal substance abuse when the woman has, in fact, been using one or more substances during pregnancy.

A thorough assessment of the newborn is performed as described in Chapter 24. The infant's gestational age and maturity are noted. The infant can have IUGR or be preterm with low birth weight. In utero exposure to some drugs results in observable malformations or dysmorphism (abnormality of shape). Neonatal behavior can arouse suspicion. Figure 35-13 shows the most commonly used scoring system for assessing withdrawal symptoms (NAS) (Finnegan, 1990; Hudak et al., 2012). Because many women are multidrug users, the newborn initially can exhibit a confusing complex of signs. The nurse often is the first to observe the signs of drug withdrawal. The nurse's observations help the health care provider differentiate between signs of NAS and other conditions, such as CNS disorders, sepsis, hypoglycemia, and electrolyte imbalance.

Urine or meconium screening can be used to identify substances abused by the mother. Urine screening is most commonly used, but its sensitivity is limited. Initially costly and of limited availability, tests of meconium collected on day 1 or 2 of life have been shown to be sensitive and reliable in detecting the metabolites of several street drugs, including cocaine (Launiainen, Nupponen, Halmesmaki, & Ojanpera, 2013).

Nursing Interventions

Planning for care of the infant born to a substance-abusing mother presents a challenge to the health care team. Parents are included in the planning for the newborn's care and for the care and support of the mother and her newborn at home. A multidisciplinary approach includes home health or community resource personnel (e.g., regulatory agencies such as child protective services).

Education and social support to prevent drug abuse provide the ideal approach. However, given the scope of the drug abuse problem, total prevention is an unrealistic goal.

Nursing care of the drug-dependent neonate involves supportive therapy for fluid and electrolyte balance, nutrition, infection control, and respiratory care. Swaddling, holding, and reducing stimuli, can be helpful in easing withdrawal (see the Nursing Care Plan: The Infant Experiencing Drug Withdrawal [Neonatal Abstinence Syndrome]). Specific suggestions for providing care to infants experiencing withdrawal are listed in Box 35-2.

NEONATAL ABSTINENCE SCORING SYSTEM

System	Signs and Symptoms	Score	AM	PM	Comments
Central Nervous System Disturbances	Excessive high-pitched (or other) cry Continuous high-pitched (or other) cry	2 3			Daily weight:
	Sleeps <1 hour after feeding Sleeps <2 hours after feeding Sleeps <3 hours after feeding	3 2 1			
	Hyperactive Moro reflex Markedly hyperactive Moro reflex	2 3			
	Mild tremors disturbed Moderate-severe tremors disturbed	1 2			
	Mild tremors undisturbed Moderate-severe tremors undisturbed	3 4			
	Increased muscle tone	2			
	Excoriation (specific area)	1			
	Myoclonic jerks	3			
	Generalized convulsions	5			
Metabolic/Vasomotor/Respiratory Disturbances	Sweating	1			
	Fever <101° (99–100.8° F/37.2–38.2° C) Fever >101° (38.4° C and higher)	1 2			
	Frequent yawning (>3 or 4 times/interval)	1			
	Mottling	1			
	Nasal stuffiness	1			
	Sneezing (>3 or 4 times/interval)	1			
	Nasal flaring	2			
	Respiratory rate >60/min Respiratory rate >60/min with retractions	1 2			
Gastrointestinal Disturbances	Excessive sucking	1			
	Poor feeding	2			
	Regurgitation Projectile vomiting	2 3			
	Loose stools Watery stools	2 3			
	Total Score				
	Initials of Scorer				

FIG 35-13 Neonatal Abstinence Scoring System. (From Finnegan, L.P. [1990]. Neonatal abstinence syndrome; assessment and pharmacotherapy. In N. Nelson [Ed.], *Current therapy in neonatal-perinatal medicine* [2nd ed.]. St. Louis: Mosby.)

NURSING CARE PLAN

The Infant Experiencing Drug Withdrawal (Neonatal Abstinence Syndrome)

NURSING DIAGNOSIS	EXPECTED OUTCOME	NURSING INTERVENTIONS	RATIONALES
Risk for Injury related to hyperactivity, seizures secondary to passive drug addiction resulting from maternal substance abuse during pregnancy	Infant exhibits no signs of seizure activity.	Administer phenobarbital, clonidine, or other medication per physician order.	To decrease central nervous system (CNS) irritability and prevent seizure activity
		Decrease environmental stimuli.	To minimize stimulation
		Plan care activities carefully.	To minimize stimulation
		Wrap infant snugly and hold tightly.	To reduce self-stimulation behaviors and protect skin from abrasions
		If infant was cocaine exposed, position to avoid eye contact; swaddle infant, use vertical rocking techniques, and use a pacifier.	To counter poor organizational response to stimuli and depressed interactive behaviors
		Monitor activity level, note the relation between activity level and external stimulation, and stop external stimulation if it causes activity increase.	To prevent overstimulation
Imbalanced Nutrition: Less than Body Requirements related to CNS irritability, poor suck reflex, vomiting, and diarrhea	Infant exhibits ingestion and retention of adequate nutrients and appropriate weight gain.	Feed in frequent, small amounts; elevate head during and after feeding, and burp well.	To diminish vomiting and aspiration
		Experiment with various nipples.	To find one most effective in compensating for poor suck reflex
		Monitor weight daily and maintain strict intake and output.	To evaluate success of feeding
		If intake is insufficient, feed by oral gavage per provider order.	To ensure ingestion of needed nutrients
		Have suction available as required.	To reduce chances of aspiration
Risk for Deficient Fluid Volume related to diarrhea and vomiting	Infant exhibits evidence of fluid homeostasis.	Administer oral and parenteral fluids per provider order.	To maintain fluid balance
		Monitor hydration status (skin turgor, weight, mucous membranes, fontanels, urine specific gravity, electrolytes) and intake and output.	To evaluate for evidence of dehydration
Ineffective Maternal Coping, Anxiety, Powerlessness related to drug use, infant distress during withdrawal	Mother will accept newborn's condition and participate in care activities, showing evidence of maternal-infant bonding process.	Explain in a nonjudgmental way the effects of maternal drug use on the newborn and the withdrawal process.	To provide understanding and reality concerning effects of drug use
		Encourage open communication (e.g., inform mother of ongoing condition, procedures, and treatment; answer questions; correct misperceptions; actively listen to her concerns).	To provide a sense of respect, provide support, and encourage a sense of control
		Encourage mother to interact with infant and to become involved in care routines.	To foster emotional connection
		Explain how to do care procedures, how to avoid excess stimulation, and how to hold and rock infant.	To enhance mother's care abilities and her sense of confidence and control
		If the mother is addicted to cocaine, explain infant's inability to interact, gaze aversion, arching back, and lack of response to cuddling.	To enhance understanding of infant behaviors
		Make appropriate referrals to social agencies for treatment of maternal drug addiction, infant development programs, and other needed support services.	To ensure adequate resources for care of self and infant

BOX 35-2 Care of the Infant Experiencing Withdrawal (Neonatal Abstinence Syndrome)

- Swaddle the infant with the legs flexed.
- Position the infant's hands in midline with the arms at the side.
- Carry the infant in a flexed position, holding firmly and close to your body. Use a soft-pack baby carrier.
- When interacting with the infant, introduce one stimulus at a time when the infant is in a quiet, alert state.
- Watch for time-out or distress signals (gaze aversion, yawning, sneezing, hiccups, arching, mottled color).
- When the infant is distressed, rock in a slow, rhythmic fashion.
- Offer pacifier for nonnutritive sucking.
- Put the infant in a sitting position with the chin tucked down for feeding.
- Try feeding small amounts at frequent intervals or use a demand-feeding schedule.
- During feedings, avoid eye contact or talking.
- Reduce environmental stimuli (lights, noise).
- Organize care to minimize handling.

Data from Weiner, S.M., & L.P. Finnegan. (2011). Drug withdrawal in the neonate. In S. Gardner, B. Carter, M. Enzman-Hines, & J. Hernandez (Eds.), *Merenstein & Gardner's handbook of neonatal intensive care* (7th ed.). St. Louis: Mosby.

Pharmacologic treatment is usually based on the severity of withdrawal symptoms, as determined by an assessment tool (see Fig. 35-13). When indicated, medications are given as ordered. Neonatal tincture of opium (0.4 mg/ml of morphine equivalent), phenobarbital, and, less commonly, paregoric may be used to control symptoms. Treatment may be needed for 2 weeks or more.

MEDICATION ALERT

The use of naloxone (Narcan) is contraindicated in infants born to narcotic addicts because it can cause severe signs and symptoms of narcotic abstinence syndrome and seizures.

The issue of breastfeeding in this population is a difficult one. Although breast milk remains the optimal source of nutrition for these infants, care must be taken to avoid exposing the infant to additional drugs through the breast milk. According to the AAP, mothers who use street drugs should not breastfeed. They also recommend that women enrolled in a supervised methadone treatment program can breastfeed if they are adequately nourished and have negative screening for illicit drugs and HIV (AAP Section on Breastfeeding, 2012). The Society of Obstetricians and Gynecologists of Canada (SOGC) states that methadone maintenance is not a contraindication to breastfeeding (Wong, Ordean, Kahan, & SOGC, 2011). The Academy of Breastfeeding Medicine (ABM) has published a clinical protocol with specific evidence-based guidelines about breastfeeding and drug-dependent women (Jansson & ABM Protocol Committee, 2009).

Drug dependence in the neonate is physiologic, not psychologic. Thus a predisposition to dependence later in life is not believed to be a factor. However, the psychosocial environment in which the infant is raised can create a tendency to addiction.

The mother requires considerable support. Her ability to cope can be impaired due to her history of substance abuse and her life circumstances. She may blame herself for the infant's problems. The infant's withdrawal signs and decreased consolability stress her coping abilities even further. Family members also need support as they assist in caring for the infant. Home health care, treatment for addiction, and education are important. Sensitive exploration of the woman's options for the care of her infant and herself and for future fertility management may help her see that she has choices. This approach helps communicate respect for the new mother as a person who can make responsible decisions.

KEY POINTS

- A small percentage of significant birth injuries can occur despite skilled and competent obstetric care.
- The nurse's primary contribution to the welfare of the neonate begins with early observation, accurate recording, and prompt reporting of abnormal signs.
- Metabolic abnormalities of diabetes mellitus in pregnancy adversely affect embryonic and fetal development.
- Prepregnancy planning and good diabetic control, coupled with strict diabetic control during pregnancy, can prevent the embryonic, fetal, and neonatal conditions associated with pregnancies complicated by diabetes mellitus.
- Infection in the neonate can be acquired in utero, during birth, during resuscitation, and from within the nursery.
- The most common maternal infections during early pregnancy that are associated with various congenital malformations are caused by viruses.
- HIV transmission from mother to infant occurs transplacentally at various gestational ages, perinatally by maternal blood and secretions, and by breast milk.
- The nurse often is the first to observe signs of newborn drug withdrawal.
- Providing high-quality perinatal care to a varied population with multiple conditions is complicated by the special needs of high risk drug-dependent clients.
- Signs and symptoms of withdrawal in an infant vary in time of onset depending on the type and dose of drug involved.

REFERENCES

Agency for Healthcare Research and Quality (AHRQ). (2013). *Data tables appendix: 2012 National Healthcare Quality and disparities reports.* Rockville, MD: Author.

Aguilera, I., Pedersen, M., Garcia-Esteban, R., et al. (2013). Early-life exposure to outdoor air pollution and respiratory health, ear infections, and eczema in infants from the INMA study. *Environmental Health Perspectives, 121*(3), 387–392.

Ali, S., & Dornhorst, A. (2011). Diabetes in pregnancy: Health risks and management. *Postgraduate Medical Journal, 87*(1028), 417–427.

American Academy of Pediatrics (AAP) Section on Breastfeeding. (2012). Breastfeeding and the use of human milk-policy statement. *Pediatrics, 129*(3), e827–e841.

American Academy of Pediatrics (AAP) & American College of Obstetricians and Gynecologists (ACOG). (2012). *Guidelines for perinatal care* (7th ed.). Elk Grove Village, IL: Author.

American College of Obstetricians and Gynecologists (ACOG) Committee on Obstetric Practice. (2010). Committee opinion no. 462: Moderate caffeine consumption during pregnancy. *Obstetrics and Gynecology, 116*(2 Pt 1), 467–468.

American College of Obstetricians and Gynecologists (ACOG) Committee on Obstetric Practice & the Society for Maternal-Fetal Medicine (SMFM). (2013). Committee opinion no. 560. *Medically indicated late-preterm and early-term deliveries. Obstetrics and Gynecology,* 121(4), 908-910 .

Aneja, R. K., Varughese-Anega, R., Vetterly, C. G., & Carcillo, J. A. (2011). Antibiotic therapy in neonatal and pediatric septic shock. *Current Infectious Disease Reports, 13*(5), 433–441.

Anderson, B., & Gonik, B. (2011). Perinatal infections. In R. Martin, A. Fanaroff, & M. Walsh (Eds.), *Fanaroff and Martin's neonatal-perinatal medicine: Diseases of the fetus and infant* (9th ed.). St. Louis: Mosby.

Anderson, M., Wood, L., Keller, J., & Hay, W. (2011). Enteral nutrition. In S. Gardner, B. Carter, M. Enzman-Hines, & J. Hernandez (Eds.), *Merenstein & Gardner's handbook of neonatal intensive care* (7th ed.). St. Louis: Mosby.

Askin, D., & Wilson, D. (2011). The high risk newborn and family. In M. Hockenberry, & D. Wilson (Eds.), *Wong's nursing care of infants and children* (9th ed.). St. Louis: Mosby.

Bailey, B., McCook, J., Hodge, A., & McGrady, L. (2012). Infant birth outcomes among substance using women: Why quitting smoking during pregnancy is just as important as quitting illicit drugs. *Maternal and Child Health Journal, 16*(2), 414–422.

Baley, J., & Toltzis, P. (2011). Perinatal viral infections. In R. Martin, A. Fanaroff, & M. Walsh (Eds.), *Fanaroff and Martin's neonatal-perinatal medicine: Diseases of the fetus and infant* (9th ed.). St. Louis: Mosby.

Bandstra, E., & Accornero, V. (2011). Infants of substance-abusing mothers. In R. Martin, A. Fanaroff, & M. Walsh (Eds.), *Fanaroff and Martin's neonatal-perinatal medicine: Diseases of the fetus and infant* (9th ed.). St. Louis: Mosby.

Basaldella, L., Marton, E., Bekelis, K., & Longatti, P. (2011). Spontaneous resolution of atraumatic intrauterine ping-pong fractures in newborns delivered by cesarean section. *Journal of Child Neurology, 26*(11), 1449–1451.

Behnke, M., Smith, V. C., & Committee on Substance Abuse, & Committee on Fetus and Newborn (2013). Prenatal substance abuse: Short- and long-term effects on the exposed fetus. *Pediatrics, 131*(3), e1009–e1024.

Bode-Jänisch, S., Bültmann, E., Hartmann, H., et al. (2012). Serious head injury in young children: Birth trauma versus non-accidental head injury. *Forensic Science International, 214*(1-3), e34–e38.

Brookfield, K. F., Wilkinson, J. D., Luke, B., et al. (2011). Maternal smoking during pregnancy and sudden infant death using the National Maternal and Infant Health Survey. *International Journal of Clinical Medicine, 2*(3), 318–324.

Carlo, W. (2011a). Nervous system disorders. In R. M. Kliegman, B. F. Stanton, J. W. St. Gemell, III, et al. (Eds.), *Nelson textbook of pediatrics* (19th ed.). Philadelphia: Saunders.

Carlo, W. (2011b). The high-risk infant. In R. M. Kliegman, B. F. Stanton, J. W. St. Gemell, III, et al. (Eds.), *Nelson textbook of pediatrics* (19th ed.). Philadelphia: Saunders.

Cekmez, F., Tayman, C., Saglam, C., et al. (2012). Well-known but rare pathogen in neonates: *Listeria monocytogenes. European Review for Medical and Pharmacological Sciences, 16*(S4), 58–61.

Centers for Disease Control and Prevention (CDC). (2013). *Breastfeeding: Human immunodeficiency virus (HIV) and acquired immunodeficiency virus (AIDS)* Available at www.cdc.gov/breastfeeding/disease/hiv.htm.

Centers for Disease Control and Prevention (CDC). (2014a). Advisory Committee on Immunization Practices recommended immunization schedule for persons aged 0 through 18 years—United States, 2014. *MMWR Morbidity and Mortality Weekly Report, 63*(5), 108–109.

Centers for Disease Control and Prevention (CDC). (2014b). *CDC fact sheet: Reported STDs in the United States—2012 national data for chlamydia, gonorrhea, and syphilis* Available at www.cdc.gov/nchhstp/newsroom/docs/STD-Trends-508.pdf.

Centers for Disease Control and Prevention (CDC). (2014c). *Chart of contraindications and precautions to commonly used vaccines.* Available at www.cdc.gov/vaccines/recs/vac-admin/contraindications-vacc.htm.

Centers for Disease Control and Prevention (CDC). (2014d). *2012 Sexually transmitted diseases surveillance: Chlamydia.* Available at www.cdc.gov/std/stats12/chlamydia.htm.

Chang, M. H. (2011). Hepatitis B virus and cancer prevention. *Recent Results in Cancer Research, 188*, 75–84.

Cherpes, T. L., Matthews, D. B., & Maryak, S. A. (2012). Neonatal herpes simplex virus infection. *Clinical Obstetrics and Gynecology, 55*(4), 938–944.

Civardi, E., Tzialla, C., Baldanti, F., et al. (2013). Viral outbreaks in neonatal intensive care units: What we do not know. *American Journal of Infection Control, 41*(10), 854–856.

de Jong, E., Walther, F., Kroes, A., & Opekes, D. (2011). Parvovirus B19 infection in pregnancy: New insights and management. *Prenatal Diagnosis, 31*(5), 419–425.

De Santis, M., De Luca, C., Mappa, I., et al. (2012). Syphilis infection during pregnancy: Fetal risks and clinical management. *Infectious Diseases in Obstetrics and Gynecology, 2012.* Article ID 430585.

Del Pizzo, J. (2011). Congenital infections (TORCH). *Pediatrics in Review, 32*(12), 537–542.

Duff, P. (2012). Maternal and perinatal infection—Bacterial. In S. G. Gabbe, J. R. Niebyl, J. L. Simpson, et al. (Eds.), *Obstetrics: Normal and problem pregnancies* (6th ed.). Philadelphia: Saunders.

Edwards, M. (2011). Postnatal bacterial infections. In R. Martin, A. Fanaroff, & M. Walsh (Eds.), *Fanaroff and Martin's neonatal-perinatal medicine: Diseases of the fetus and infant* (9th ed.). Philadelphia: Mosby.

Engelkirk, P., Duben-Engelkirk, J., & Burton, G. (2011). *Burton's microbiology for the health sciences* (9th ed.). New York: Lippincott Williams & Wilkins.

Fairlie, T., Zell, E., & Schrag, S. (2013). Effectiveness of intrapartum antibiotic prophylaxis for early-onset group B streptococcal disease. *Obstetrics and Gynecology, 121*(3), 570–577.

Ferrieri, P., & Wallen, L. (2012). Neonatal bacterial sepsis. In C. Gleason, & S. Devaskar (Eds.), *Avery's diseases of the newborn* (9th ed.). Philadelphia: Saunders.

Finnegan, L. P. (1990). Neonatal abstinence syndrome; assessment and pharmacotherapy. In N. Nelson (Ed.), *Current therapy in neonatal-perinatal medicine* (2nd ed.). St. Louis: Mosby.

Fowler, S. (2013). Sepsis in a very low birth weight neonate. In S. Weber, & C. Salgado (Eds.), *Healthcare associated infections.* Oxford, UK: Oxford University Press.

Frise, C. J., Mackillop, L., Joash, K., & Williamson, C. (2013). Starvation ketoacidosis in pregnancy. *European Journal of Obstetrics & Gynecology and Reproductive Biology, 167*(1), 1–7.

Gaalema, D., Scott, T., Heil, S., et al. (2012). Differences in the profile of neonatal abstinence syndrome signs in methadone-versus buprenorphine-exposed neonates. *Addiction, 107*(S1), 53–62.

Garne, E., Loane, M., Dolk, H., et al. (2012). Spectrum of congenital anomalies in pregnancies with pregestational diabetes. *Birth Defects Research A, 94*(3), 134–140.

GBS Prevention Working Group. (2013). Group B streptococcus late-onset disease: 2003-2010. *Pediatrics, 131*(2), e361–e368.

Geary, F., & Wells, M. (2013). Management of the patient in labor who has abused substances. *Clinical Obstetrics, 56*(1), 166–172.

Ghosh, S., & Chaudhuri, S. (2013). Pregnancy and varicella infection. *Indian Journal of Dermatology, Venereology and Leprology, 79*(2), 264–267.

Gregory, K. D., Niebyl, J. R., & Johnson, T. R. B. (2012). Preconception and prenatal care: Part of the continuum. In S. G. Gabbe, J. R. Niebyl, J. L. Simpson, et al. (Eds.), *Obstetrics: Normal and problem pregnancies* (6th ed.). Philadelphia: Saunders.

Grigoriadis, S., VonderPorten, E. H., Mamisashvili, L., et al. (2013). Antidepressant exposure during pregnancy and congenital malformations: Is there an association? A systematic review and meta-analysis of the best evidence. *Journal of Clinical Psychiatry, 74*(4), e293–e308.

Grzeskowiak, L. E., Gilbert, A. L., & Morrison, J. L. (2012). Neonatal outcomes after late-gestation exposure to selective serotonin reuptake inhibitors. *Journal of Clinical Psychopharmacology, 32*(5), 615–621.

Hackshaw, A., Rodeck, C., & Boniface, S. (2011). Maternal smoking in pregnancy and birth defects—A systematic review based on 173,687 malformed cases and 11.7 million controls. *Human Reproduction Update, 17*(5), 589–604.

Hammoud, M., Al-Taiar, A., Thalib, L., et al. (2012). Incidence, aetiology and resistance of late-onset neonatal sepsis: A five-year prospective study. *Journal of Paediatrics and Child Health, 48*(7), 604–609.

Hatfield, L., Schwoebel, A., & Lynyak, C. (2011). Caring for the infant of a diabetic mother. *MCN: The American Journal of Maternal/Child Nursing, 36*(1), 10–16.

Hawdon, J. (2011). Babies born after diabetes in pregnancy: What are the short- and long-term risks and how can we minimise them? *Best Practice & Research Clinical Obstetrics & Gynaecology, 25*(1), 91–104.

Hay, W. W. (2012). Care of the infant of the diabetic mother. *Current Diabetes Reports, 12*(1), 4–15.

Hayes, R. M., Pingsheng, W., Shelton, R. C., et al. (2012). Maternal antidepressant use and adverse pregnancy outcomes: A cohort study of 228,876 pregnancies. *American Journal of Obstetrics and Gynecology, 207*(49), e1–e9.

Heinrich, N., Mueller, A., Bartmann, P., et al. (2011). Successful management of an MRSA outbreak in a neonatal intensive care unit. *European Journal of Clinical Microbiology & Infectious Diseases, 30*(7), 909–913.

Hofer, N., Zacharias, E., Muller, W., & Resch, B. (2012). An update on the use of C-reactive protein in early-onset neonatal sepsis: Current insights and new tasks. *Neonatology, 102*(1), 25–36.

Hudak, M. L., Tan, R. C., & Committee on Drugs, & Committee on Fetus and Newborn (2012). Neonatal drug withdrawal. *Pediatrics, 129*(2), e540–e560.

Jansson, L. M., & Academy of Breastfeeding Medicine (ABM) Protocol Committee. (2009). ABM clinical protocol no. 21: Guidelines for breastfeeding and the drug-dependent woman. *Breastfeeding Medicine, 4*(4), 225–228.

Jimenez-Solem, E., Andersen, J. T., Petersen, M., et al. (2013). SSRI use during pregnancy and risk of stillbirth and neonatal mortality. *American Journal of Psychiatry, 170*(3), 299–304.

Jimenez-Truque, N., Tedeschi, S., Saye, E., et al. (2012). Relationship between maternal and neonatal *Staphylococcus aureus* colonization. *Pediatrics, 129*(5), e1252–1259.

Jones, J., & Roberts, J. (2012). Toxoplasmosis hospitalizations in the United States, 2008, and trends, 1993-2008. *Clinical Infectious Diseases, 54*(7), e58–e61.

Kalhan, S. C., & Devaskar, S. U. (2011). Metabolic and endocrine disorders. In R. J. Martin, A. A. Fanaroff, & M. C. Walsh (Eds.), *Fanaroff and Martin's neonatal-perinatal medicine: Diseases of the fetus and infant* (9th ed.). St. Louis: Mosby.

Kaye, A. (2011). Toxoplasmosis: Diagnosis, treatment, and prevention in congenitally exposed infants. *Pediatric Health Care, 25*(6), 355–364.

Kett, J. (2013). Perinatal varicella. *Pediatrics in Review, 34*(1), 49–51.

KiBS Study Team. (2011). Triple-antiretroviral prophylaxis to prevent mother-to-child HIV transmission through breastfeeding—The Kisimu Breastfeeding Study, Kenya: A clinical trial. *PLoS Medicine, 8*(3), e1001015.

Kieler, H., Artama, M., Engeland, A., et al. (2012). Selective serotonin reuptake inhibitors during pregnancy and risk of persistent pulmonary hypertension in the newborn: Population based cohort study from the five Nordic countries. *BMJ, 344*, d8012.

Kimberlin, D. W., Baley, J., Committee on Infectious Diseases, & Committee on Fetus and Newborn (2013). Guidance on management of asymptomatic neonates born to women with active genital herpes lesions. *Pediatrics, 131*(2), e635–e646.

Koren, G., & Nordeng, H. (2012). Antidepressant use during pregnancy: The benefit-risk ratio. *American Journal of Obstetrics and Gynecology, 207*(3), 157–163.

Kuehn, D., Aros, S., Cassorla, F., et al. (2012). A prospective cohort study of the prevalence of growth, facial, and central nervous system abnormalities in children with heavy prenatal alcohol exposure. *Alcoholism: Clinical and Experimental Research, 36*(10), 1811–1819.

Kully-Martens, K., Denys, K., Treit, S., et al. (2012). A review of social skills deficits in individuals with fetal alcohol spectrum disorders and prenatal alcohol exposure: Profiles, mechanisms, and interventions. *Alcoholism: Clinical and Experimental Research, 36*(4), 568–576.

Kully-Martens, K., Treit, S., Pei, J., & Rasmussen, C. (2013). Affective decision-making on the Iowa gambling task in children and adolescents with fetal alcohol spectrum disorders. *Journal of the International Neuropsychological Society, 19*(2), 137–144.

Ladhani, N., Shah, P., & Murphy, K. (2011). Methamphetamine exposure and birth outcomes: A systematic metaanalysis. *Gynecology, 205*(3), 219e1–219e7.

Lago, E., Vaccari, A., & Fiori, R. (2013). Clinical features and follow-up of congenital syphilis. *Sexually Transmitted Diseases, 40*(2), 85–94.

Lamont, R., Sobel, J., Carrington, D., et al. (2011). Varicella zoster virus (chickenpox) infection in pregnancy. *BJOG: The International Journal of Obstetrics and Gynecology, 118*(10), 1155–1162.

Launiainen, T., Nupponen, I., Halmesmäki, E., & Ojanperä, I. (2013). Meconium drug testing reveals maternal misuse of medicinal opioids among addicted mothers. *Drug Testing and Analysis, 5*(7), 529–533.

Libster, R., Edwards, K., Levent, F., et al. (2012). Long-term outcomes of group B streptococcal meningitis. *Pediatrics, 130*(1), e8–e15.

Linder, N., Linder, I., Fridman, E., et al. (2013). Birth trauma—Risk factors and short-term neonatal outcome. *Journal of Maternal-Fetal and Neonatal Medicine, 26*(15), 1491–1495.

Madgula, R., Groshkova, T., & Mayet, S. (2011). Illicit drug use in pregnancy: Effects and management. *Expert Review of Obstetrics & Gynecology, 6*(2), 179–192.

Mangurten, H., & Puppala, B. (2011). Birth injuries. In R. Martin, A. Fanaroff, & M. Walsh (Eds.), *Fanaroff and Martin's neonatal-perinatal medicine: Diseases of the fetus and infant* (9th ed.). St. Louis: Mosby.

Mani, H., & Stocker, T. (2012). Congenital and acquired systemic infectious diseases. In J. Stocker, L. Dener, A. Husain (Eds.), *Stocker & Dehner's pediatric pathology* (3rd ed.). New York: Lippincott Williams & Wilkins.

March of Dimes. (2012). Caffeine in pregnancy. Available at www.marchofdimes.com/professionals/14332_1148.asp.

MacDonald, N.E., & Canadian Paediatric Society Infectious Diseases and Immunization Committee. (2006, reaffirmed 2012). Maternal infectious diseases, antimicrobial therapy or immunizations: Very few contraindications to breastfeeding. *Paediatrics and Child Health*, 11(8), 489–491.

Moncada, P., & Montoya, J. (2012). Toxoplasmosis in the fetus and newborn. *Expert Review of Anti-Infective Therapy, 10*(7), 815–828.

Motacki, K., Kapoian, T., & O'Mara, N. (2011). *The illustrated guide to infection control.* New York: Springer.

Mouhayar, J., & Charafeddine, L. (2012). Index of suspicion in the nursery: Head swelling and decreased activity in a 2-day-old term infant. *NeoReviews, 13*(10), e615–e617.

Narkowicz, S., Plotka, J., Polkowska, Z., et al. (2013). Prenatal exposure to substance of abuse: A worldwide problem. *Environment International, 54*, 141–163.

Nash, P., & Smith, J. (2012). Common neonatal complications. In K. Simpson, & P. Creehan (Eds.), *Perinatal nursing* (3rd ed.). New York: Lippincott Williams & Wilkins.

National Institute on Drug Abuse. (2012). *DrugFacts: MDMA (ecstasy).* Available at www.nida.nih.gov/infofacts/ecstasy.html.

National Institutes of Health (NIH) Panel on Antiretroviral Therapy and Medical Management of HIV-Infected Children. (2012). *Guidelines for the use of antiretroviral agents in pediatric HIV infection.* Available at http://aidsinfo.nih.gov/contentfiles/lvguidelines/pediatricguidelines.pdf.

Nielsen-Saines, K. (2011). Congenital rubella syndrome (CRS). In S. Yazdani, S. McGhee, & E. Stiehm (Eds.), *Chronic complex diseases of childhood.* Boca Raton, FL: Brown Walker Press.

NISDI Pediatric Study Group. (2012). Opportunistic and other infections in HIV-infected children in Latin America compared to a similar cohort in the United States. *AIDS Research and Human Retroviruses, 28*(3), 282–288.

Ohlin, A., Backman, A., Ewald, U., et al. (2012). Diagnosis of neonatal sepsis by broad-range 16s real-time polymerase chain reaction. *Neonatology, 101*(4), 241–246.

Ornoy, A. (2011). Prenatal origin of obesity and their complications: Gestational diabetes, maternal overweight and the paradoxical effects of fetal growth restriction and macrosomia. *Reproductive Toxicology, 32*(2), 205–212.

Ott, J. J., Stevens, G. A., & Wiersma, S. T. (2012). The risk of perinatal hepatitis B virus transmission: Hepatitis B e antigen (HBeAg) prevalence estimates for all world regions. *BMC Infectious Diseases, 12*, 131.

Parashette, K., & Croffie, J. (2013). Vomiting. *NeoReviews, 34*(7), 307–321.

Patterson, J. J., & Davies, H. D. (2011). Syphilis *(Treponema pallidum).* In R. M. Kliegman, B. F. Stanton, J. W. St. Gemell, III, et al. (Eds.), *Nelson textbook of pediatrics* (19th ed.). Philadelphia: Saunders.

Patil, A., Kuller, J., & Rhee, E. (2011). Antidepressants in pregnancy: A review of commonly prescribed medications. *Obstetrical and Gynecological Survey, 66*(12), 777–787.

Pei, J., Job, J., Kully-Martens, K., & Rasmussen, C. (2011). Executive function and memory in children with fetal alcohol spectrum disorder. *Child Neuropsychology, 17*(3), 290–309.

Pol, S., Corouge, M., & Fontaine, H. (2011). Hepatitis B virus infection and pregnancy. *Clinics and Research in Hepatology and Gastroenterology, 35*(10), 618–622.

Polin, R. (2012). Management of neonates with suspected or proven early-onset bacterial sepsis. *Pediatrics, 129*(5), 1006–1015.

Pritham, U., Paul, J., & Hayes, M. (2012). Opioid dependency in pregnancy and length of stay for neonatal abstinence syndrome. *Journal of Obstetric, Gynecologic and Neonatal Nursing, 41*(2), 180–190.

Reddick, K., Jhaveri, R., Gandhi, M., et al. (2011). Pregnancy outcomes associated with viral hepatitis. *Journal of Viral Hepatitis, 18*(7), e394–e398.

Riley, E., Infante, M., & Warren, K. (2011). Fetal alcohol spectrum disorders: An overview. *Neuropsychology Review, 21*(2), 73–80.

Rosenthal, D., & Weitzman, M. (2011). Examining the effects of intrauterine and postnatal exposure to tobacco smoke on childhood cognitive and behavioral development. *International Journal of Mental Health, 40*(1), 39–64.

Sabin, A. (1942). Toxoplasmosis: A recently recognized disease of human beings. *Advances in Pediatrics, 1*(1), 1–56.

Salinitri, S., & Seow, W. (2013). Developmental enamel defects in the primary dentition: Aetiology and clinical management. *Australian Dental Journal, 58*(2), 133–140.

Sanchez, P., Patterson, J., & Ahmed, A. (2012). Toxoplasmosis, syphilis, malaria, and tuberculosis. In C. Gleason, & S. Devaskar (Eds.), *Avery's diseases of the newborn* (9th ed.). Philadelphia: Saunders.

Schillie, S., & Murphy, T. (2013). Seroprotection after recombinant hepatitis B vaccination among newborn infants: A review. *Vaccine, 31*(21), 2506–2516.

Schlapbach, L. J., Ersch, J., Balmer, C., et al. (2013). Enteroviral myocarditis in neonates. *Journal of Paediatrics and Child Health, 49*(9), e451–e454.

Schleiss, M., & Patterson, J. (2012). Viral infections of the fetus and newborn and human immunodeficiency virus infection during pregnancy. In C. Gleason, & S. Devaskar (Eds.), *Avery's diseases of the newborn* (9th ed.). Philadelphia: Saunders.

Shah, S., Ohlsson, A., & Shah, V. (2012). Intraventricular antibiotics for bacterial meningitis in neonates. *The Cochrane Database of Systematic Reviews 2012, 7*, CD00446.

Soto, E., & Bahado-Singh, R. (2013). Fetal abnormal growth associated with substance abuse. *Clinical Obstetrics and Gynecology, 56*(1), 142–153.

Stephansson, O., Kieler, H., Haglund, B., et al. (2013). Selective serotonin reuptake inhibitors during pregnancy and risk of stillbirth and infant mortality. *Journal of the American Medical Association, 309*(1), 48–54.

Sweet, R., & Gibbs, R. (2012). *Infectious diseases of the female genital tract* (5th ed.). New York: Lippincott Williams & Wilkins.

Tudela, C., Stewart, R., Roberts, S., et al. (2012). Intrapartum evidence of early-onset group B streptococcus. *Obstetrics and Gynecology, 119*(3), 626–629.

van Vleet, M. (2012). Birth-related injury. In A. Elzouki, H. Harfi, H. Nazer, et al. (Eds.), *Textbook of clinical pediatrics* (2nd ed.). New York: Springer.

Venkatesh, M. P., Adams, K. M., & Weisman, L. E. (2011). Infection in the neonate. In S. Gardner, B. Carter, M. Enzman-Hines, & J. Hernandez (Eds.), *Merenstein & Gardner's handbook of neonatal intensive care* (7th ed.). St. Louis: Mosby.

Verklan, M. T. (2015). Neurologic disorders. In M. T. Verklan, & M. Walden (Eds.), *Core curriculum for neonatal intensive care nursing* (5th ed.). St. Louis: Saunders.

Verklan, M. T., & Lopez, S. (2011). Neurologic disorders. In S. Gardner, B. Carter, M. Enzman-Hines, & J. Hernandez (Eds.), *Merenstein & Gardner's handbook of neonatal intensive care* (7th ed.). St Louis: Mosby.

Walker, S., Palma-Dias, R., Wood, E., et al. (2013). Cytomegalovirus in pregnancy: To screen or not to screen. *BMC Pregnancy & Childbirth, 13*, 96.

Weston, E., Pondo, T., Lewis, M., et al. (2011). The burden of invasive early-onset neonatal sepsis in the United States, 2005-2008. *Pediatric Infectious Disease Journal, 30*(11), 937–941.

White, J., & Magee, S. (2011). Neonatal herpes infection: Case report and discussion. *Journal of the American Board of Family Medicine, 24*(6), 758–762.

Wisner, K., Sit, D., Reynolds, S., et al. (2012). Mental health and behavioral disorders in pregnancy. In S. Gabbe, J. Niebyl, H. Galan, E., et al. (Eds.), *Obstetrics: Normal and problem pregnancies* (6th ed.). Philadelphia: Saunders.

Wong, S., Ordean, A., Kahan, M., & Society of Obstetricians and Gynecologists of Canada (SOGC). (2011). SOGC clinical practice guideline no. 256: Substance use in pregnancy. *Journal of Obstetrics and Gynaecology of Canada, 33*(4), 367–384.

World Health Organization, UNAIDS, UNFPA, & UNICEF. (2010). *Guidelines on HIV and infant feeding: Principles and guidelines for infant feeding in the context of HIV and a summary of evidence.* Geneva: Author.

Wright, D., & Cohen, B. (2012). Infections of the skin. In C. Gleason, & S. Devaskar (Eds.), *Avery's diseases of the newborn* (9th ed.). Philadelphia: Saunders.

Yogev, R., & Chadwick, E. G. (2011). Acquired immunodeficiency syndrome (human immunodeficiency virus). In R. M. Kliegman, B. F. Stanton, J. W. St. Gemell, III, et al. (Eds.), *Nelson textbook of pediatrics* (19th ed.). Philadelphia: Saunders.

Zuppa, A., D'Andrea, V., Catenazzi, P., et al. (2011). Ophthalmia neonatorum: What kind of prophylaxis? *Journal of Maternal-Fetal & Neonatal Medicine, 24*(6), 769–773.

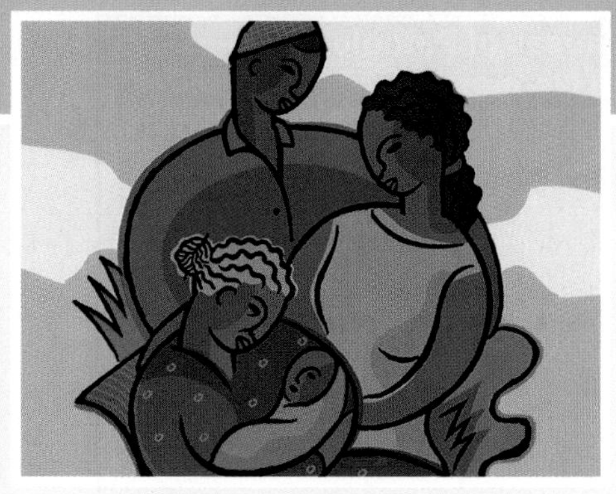

CHAPTER 36

Hemolytic Disorders and Congenital Anomalies

Debbie Fraser

http://evolve.elsevier.com/Lowdermilk/MWHC/

LEARNING OBJECTIVES

- Differentiate between physiologic and pathologic jaundice in the newborn.
- Develop a nursing plan of care for preventing, identifying, and managing neonatal hyperbilirubinemia.
- Compare Rh and ABO incompatibility and the implications for neonatal outcomes.
- Explain nursing management to prevent the pathologic consequences of hyperbilirubinemia.
- Review prenatal diagnosis of neonatal disorders.
- Present assessment strategies during the postnatal period to aid in diagnosing congenital disorders.
- Describe each congenital disorder presented in this chapter and identify the priority of nursing care for each.
- Describe preoperative and postoperative nursing care of the newborn.
- Develop a nursing care plan for parents of a newborn with a defect or disorder.

Many physiologic alterations occur in infants during the newborn period. The nurse must be alert to any deviations from normal, ranging from an obvious congenital anomaly, such as myelomeningocele, to a less obvious deviation such as a congenital heart defect that can be asymptomatic at birth. The nurse must possess the assessment skills necessary to detect any deviation from normal, as well as the knowledge base to participate in the skilled care of affected infants. The nurse also must be cognizant of the special needs of the family with a child who is born with or acquires an abnormal condition.

The complications that affect newborns can stem from three basic problems: (1) problems relating to gestational age or intrauterine growth that do not follow normal patterns, such as a preterm birth; (2) acquired problems resulting from maternal or newborn physiologic factors, such as ABO incompatibility or infection; and (3) congenital defects. This chapter focuses on acquired problems and congenital anomalies in the neonate.

HYPERBILIRUBINEMIA

Hyperbilirubinemia is a condition in which the total serum bilirubin level in the blood is increased. Normal values are determined by gestational age, days of life, and the baby's general physical condition. Hyperbilirubinemia is characterized by a yellow discoloration of the skin, mucous membranes, sclera, and various organs. This discoloration is referred to as jaundice, or **icterus.** Jaundice is caused primarily by the accumulation in the skin of unconjugated bilirubin, a breakdown product of hemoglobin formed after its release from hemolyzed red blood cells (RBCs). Jaundice first appears in the infant's face and head and progresses toward the toes. It dissipates in the reverse order. Physiologic jaundice, discussed in Chapters 23 and 24, is the most common finding in newborns and is usually benign. The challenge in the care of neonates with hyperbilirubinemia is to distinguish physiologic jaundice from a serious clinical pathologic condition.

Physiologic Jaundice

Physiologic jaundice occurs in over 60% of healthy term newborns and almost all preterm infants (Lauer & Spector, 2011). Beginning after 24 hours of age, unconjugated bilirubin levels in Caucasian and African-American neonates gradually increase from 2 mg/dl to peak levels of 5 to 6 mg/dl at 72 to 96 hours of age. In Asian-American infants, the level can increase to 10 to 14 mg/dl between 72 and 120 hours of age. In Caucasian and African-American newborns there is a rapid decline in the unconjugated bilirubin level to 3 mg/dl by 5 days after birth; in Asian-American infants, this takes 7 to 10 days (Kaplan, Wong, Sibley, & Stevenson, 2011).

Physiologic jaundice is more common in preterm infants, with the serum bilirubin level typically reaching a mean peak of 10 to 12 mg/dl by the fifth or sixth day of life. It takes longer for the maximal concentration to be reached in preterm than in full-term infants because of the preterm infant's immature liver function and slower metabolic processes.

Pathologic Jaundice

Pathologic jaundice is the result of an increased level of total serum bilirubin that if left untreated can result in acute bilirubin encephalopathy or kernicterus. Although the terms are often used interchangeably, **acute bilirubin encephalopathy** describes the acute central nervous system manifestations seen in the first weeks after birth, whereas **kernicterus** is used to describe the chronic and permanent results of bilirubin toxicity (Hansen, 2011). Kernicterus, though rare, still occurs. Adherence to guidelines by the American Academy of Pediatrics (AAP) (Bhutani & Committee on Fetus and Newborn, 2011) and a clinical position statement by the Association of Women's Health, Obstetric and Neonatal Nurses (AWHONN, 2005) should result in kernicterus becoming largely preventable.

The following findings support a diagnosis of pathologic jaundice and, if encountered in an infant, warrant further investigation (Khan & Rahman, 2011):

- Serum bilirubin concentrations of greater than 5 mg/dl in cord blood
- Clinical jaundice evident within 24 hours of birth
- Total serum bilirubin levels increasing by more than 5 mg/dl in 24 hours or increasing at a rate of 0.5 mg/dl/hr
- A serum bilirubin level in a term newborn that exceeds 12.9 mg/dl at any time
- A serum bilirubin level in a preterm newborn that exceeds 15 mg/dl at any time
- Any case of visible jaundice that persists for more than 14 days of life in a term infant

AAP guidelines (Bhutani & Committee on Fetus and Newborn, 2011) and the clinical position statement by AWHONN (2005) note the need for universal screening to identify elevated bilirubin levels in newborns to facilitate the prevention of acute bilirubin encephalopathy and kernicterus. The use of hour-specific serum bilirubin levels to predict newborns at risk for rapidly rising levels is an official recommendation by the AAP Subcommittee on Hyperbilirubinemia (2004) for the monitoring of healthy neonates at 35 weeks of gestation or more before discharge from the hospital. Use of a nomogram helps determine which newborns might need further evaluation after discharge. In many institutions the nomogram is used to determine the infant's risk for development of hyperbilirubinemia requiring medical treatment or closer screening (see Fig. 24-7). Risk factors recognized to place infants in the high risk category for developing severe hyperbilirubinemia include gestational age less than 37 weeks, exclusive breastfeeding, previous sibling who required phototherapy, predischarge transcutaneous bilirubin TcB or total serum bilirubin (TSB) level in the high risk zone, cephalhematoma or other significant bruising, blood incompatibility with positive direct antiglobulin test, other known hemolytic disease such as glucose-6-phosphate dehydrogenase (G6PD), and East Asian race (AAP Subcommittee on Hyperbilirubinemia, 2004; Kamath, Thilo, & Hernandez, 2011).

It is recommended that healthy infants (35 weeks of gestation or greater) who are considered at low to intermediate risk for hyperbilirubinemia should receive follow-up care within 2 days, with assessment of bilirubin levels based on a risk assessment using tools such as the hour-specific nomogram. Infants at higher risk for hyperbilirubinemia should be seen by the health care provider within 24 hours or sooner, with assessment of TSB level. Other key recommendations include promoting successful breastfeeding; recognizing that visual estimation of the degree of jaundice, particularly in darkly pigmented infants, can lead to errors; and providing parents with written and verbal information about newborn jaundice (AAP Subcommittee on Hyperbilirubinemia, 2004).

Many potential causes of pathologic hyperbilirubinemia are found in neonates (Box 36-1). The most common are hemolytic diseases of the newborn.

BOX 36-1 Potential Causes of Pathologic Hyperbilirubinemia in Neonates

Maternal Factors
- Rh and ABO or other blood group incompatibilities
- Maternal infections
- Maternal diabetes
- Oxytocin administration during labor
- Maternal ingestion of sulfonamides, diazepam, or salicylates near time of birth

Fetal/Newborn Factors
- Prematurity
- Hepatic cell damage by infection or drugs
- Neonatal hyperthyroidism
- Polycythemia
- Intestinal obstruction such as meconium ileus
- Pyloric stenosis
- Biliary atresia
- Sequestered blood (e.g., from cephalhematomas, ecchymosis, or hemangiomas)
- Maternal blood swallowed by neonate
- Glucose-6-phosphate dehydrogenase (G6PD) deficiency
- Thalassemia

Hemolytic Disease of the Newborn

Hemolytic diseases of the newborn occur most often when the blood groups of the mother and baby are different. The most common are ABO and Rh factor incompatibilities.

The four major blood groups in the ABO system are A, B, AB, and O. People with type A blood have A antigen; those with type B have B antigen; those with type AB have both A and B antigens; and those with type O have no antigens. In turn, people with type A blood have plasma antibodies to type B blood; those with type B blood have antibodies to type A blood; those with type AB blood have no antibodies; and those with type O blood have antibodies to types A and B blood. If a person receives or is exposed to an incompatible blood type, he or she will form antibodies against the antigen in that blood, with agglutination, or clumping, occurring as the antibodies in the plasma mix with the antigens of the different blood group.

The Rh factor, a genetically determined factor present on RBCs, can be a major source of incompatibility. Of the several forms of the Rh antigen, the D antigen is the most significant because it causes the most antibody production in a person who is Rh negative. A person who has the Rh factor is considered Rh positive; a person without it is Rh negative. For example, a mother who has A-negative blood has the A antigen, plasma antibodies to the B antigen, and no Rh factor on her RBCs.

Hemolytic disorders occur when maternal antibodies are present naturally or form in response to an antigen from the fetal blood crossing the placenta and entering the maternal circulation. The maternal antibodies of the immunoglobulin G (IgG) class in turn cross the placenta, causing hemolysis of the fetal RBCs, resulting in hyperbilirubinemia and jaundice.

Rh Incompatibility

Rh incompatibility, or **isoimmunization,** occurs when an Rh-negative mother has an Rh-positive fetus who inherits the dominant Rh-positive gene from the father. If the mother is Rh negative and the father is Rh positive and homozygous for the Rh factor, all the offspring will be Rh positive. If the father is heterozygous for the factor, there is a 50% chance that each infant born of the union will be Rh positive and a 50% chance that each will be Rh negative. An Rh-negative fetus is in no danger because it has the same Rh factor as the mother. An Rh-negative fetus with an Rh-positive mother also is in no danger. Only the Rh-positive fetus of an Rh-negative mother is at risk. From 10% to 15% of all Caucasian couples and about 5% of African-American couples have Rh incompatibility. It is rare in Asian couples due to the high incidence of ABO incompatibility, which is protective against Rh isoimmunization because of rapid destruction of the fetal RBCs, which prevents Rh antigen exposure and maternal antibody production (Diehl-Jones & Fraser, 2015).

The pathogenesis of Rh incompatibility is as follows. Hematopoiesis (the formation, production, and maintenance of blood cells) in the fetus is well established by the ninth week of gestation (Blackburn, 2013). When fetal RBCs that contain the Rh antigen pass through the placenta into the maternal circulation of an Rh-negative woman the maternal immune system produces antibodies against the foreign fetal antigens. The process of antibody formation is called *maternal sensitization.* Sensitization can occur during pregnancy, birth, miscarriage or induced abortion, amniocentesis, external cephalic version, or trauma. Usually Rh-negative women become sensitized in their first pregnancy with an Rh-positive fetus but do not produce enough antibodies to cause lysis (destruction) of fetal blood cells. During subsequent pregnancies, antibodies form in response to repeated contact with the antigen from the fetal blood, and lysis of fetal RBCs results. The overall incidence of isoimmunization is less than 1% (Kaplan, Wong, & Stevenson, 2012). Multiple gestation, placental abruption, placenta previa, manual removal of the placenta, and cesarean birth increase the incidence of transplacental hemorrhage and the risk of isoimmunization.

Severe Rh incompatibility results in marked fetal hemolytic anemia because the fetal erythrocytes are destroyed by maternal Rh-positive antibodies. Although the placenta usually clears the bilirubin resulting from the RBC breakdown, in extreme cases fetal bilirubin levels increase. This results in fetal jaundice, also known as *icterus gravis.*

The fetus compensates for the anemia by producing large numbers of immature erythrocytes to replace those hemolyzed, thus the name for this condition: **erythroblastosis fetalis.** In **hydrops fetalis,** the most severe form of this disease, the fetus has marked anemia, cardiac decompensation, cardiomegaly, and hepatosplenomegaly. Hypoxia results from the severe anemia. In addition, because of decreased intravascular oncotic pressure, fluid leaks out of the intravascular space. This results in generalized edema, as well as effusions into the peritoneal (ascites), pericardial, and pleural (hydrothorax) spaces (Maheshwari & Carlo, 2011). The placenta is often edematous, which, along with the edematous fetus, can cause uterine rupture.

Intrauterine or early neonatal death can occur as a result of hydrops fetalis, although intrauterine transfusions and early birth of the fetus can help to avert this. Intrauterine transfusion involves the infusion of Rh-negative, type O blood into the umbilical vein. The frequency of intrauterine transfusions varies according to institution protocol and fetal hydropic status, but it can be as often as every 2 weeks until the fetus reaches pulmonary maturity at approximately 37 to 38 weeks of gestation. Studies of the use of intrauterine transfusions have demonstrated a high survival rate and low risk of disabilities in the surviving infant (LOTUS Study Group, 2012).

ABO Incompatibility

ABO incompatibility is the most common cause of hemolytic disease in the newborn, although the anemia that results is usually mild. ABO maternal blood group incompatibility occurs in almost 25% of infants; however, only about 1% to 5% have clinical manifestations (Posencheg & Dennery, 2013). It occurs if the fetal blood type is A, B, or AB, and the maternal type is O. It occurs rarely in infants with type B blood born to mothers with type A blood. The incompatibility arises because naturally occurring anti-A and anti-B antibodies are transferred across the placenta to the fetus. Unlike the situation that pertains to Rh incompatibility, first-born infants can be affected because mothers with type O blood already have anti-A and anti-B antibodies in their blood (Manco-Johnson, Rodden, & Hays, 2011). Such a newborn can have a weakly positive direct Coombs' test (also referred to as a direct antiglobulin test [DAT]). The cord bilirubin level usually is less than 4 mg/dl, and any resulting hyperbilirubinemia usually can be treated with phototherapy. Exchange transfusions are required only occasionally. Although ABO incompatibility is a common cause of hyperbilirubinemia, it rarely precipitates significant anemia resulting from the hemolysis of RBCs.

Other Causes of Hemolytic Jaundice

It is not within the scope of this text to discuss the many potential causes of hemolytic jaundice in childhood. However, among African-Americans and people of Mediterranean heritage there is a high incidence of G6PD deficiency (Kaplan et al., 2012). Because it is a sex-linked disease, male offspring are affected more often than females. A deficiency of a red blood cell enzyme in combination with exposure to an oxidant stressor (such as sepsis) results in hemolysis and a decreased RBC life (Nabavizadeh, Rezaie, Sabzali, et al., 2012). The increase in the destruction of RBCs overwhelms the immature neonatal liver's ability to conjugate the indirect bilirubin. Treatment is the same as for any newborn with rapidly rising serum bilirubin levels. Other metabolic and inherited conditions that increase hemolysis and can cause jaundice in the infant include galactosemia, Crigler-Najjar disease, and hypothyroidism (Blackburn, 2013).

Acute Bilirubin Encephalopathy

The goal of care for the infant with hyperbilirubinemia is to prevent acute bilirubin encephalopathy (ABE) and kernicterus. Acute bilirubin encephalopathy is caused by the deposition of bilirubin in the brain, especially within the basal ganglia, the cerebellum, and the hippocampus. Normally bilirubin does not cause harm because it is bound to albumin and carried to the liver to undergo conjugation. However, once albumin binding sites are saturated, the bilirubin circulates as unconjugated (indirect) bilirubin, which is highly lipid soluble and capable of crossing the blood-brain barrier. Circulation of unconjugated bilirubin can reach toxic levels and become deposited in the basal ganglia, resulting in the yellowish staining of the brain tissue and the necrosis of neurons.

Acute bilirubin encephalopathy, which can develop in newborns with no apparent signs of clinical jaundice, is directly related to the total serum bilirubin level, although these levels alone do not predict the risk of brain injury. In a term infant, a serum bilirubin level of 25 mg/dl is considered the upper limit, beyond which the risk for acute bilirubin encephalopathy increases. However, the condition can occur at much lower levels in premature infants or infants with other complications.

Some of the perinatal events that increase the likelihood of acute bilirubin encephalopathy, even at these lower bilirubin levels, include hypoxia, asphyxia, acidosis, hypothermia, hypoglycemia, sepsis, treatment with certain medications, and hypoalbuminemia. In essence, any condition that interferes with the conjugation of bilirubin or competes for albumin-binding sites increases the risk that unconjugated bilirubin can pass through the blood-brain barrier and cause damage to the central nervous system (CNS).

Acute bilirubin encephalopathy is associated with acute and long-term signs of neurologic damage (Gazzin & Tiribelli, 2011; Hansen, 2011). The clinical manifestations typically appear between 2 and 6 days after birth and go through several phases as the disease progresses. During the first phase the newborn is hypotonic and lethargic and has a poor suck and depressed or absent Moro reflex. These subtler signs are followed by the appearance of a high-pitched cry, opisthotonos (severe muscle spasm that causes the back to arch acutely), spasticity, hyperreflexia, and fever. If allowed to progress to the third phase, the neonate will demonstrate a shrill cry, apnea, deep stupor to coma, seizures, and hearing and visual disturbances. Death can occur from cardiovascular collapse (Watchko, 2012).

About half of affected infants survive, although they often have permanent sequelae including extrapyramidal movement disorders (especially dystonia and athetosis), gaze abnormalities (especially an upward gaze), auditory disturbances (especially sensorineural hearing loss), cognitive impairment, and enamel dysplasia of the deciduous teeth. Movement abnormalities and auditory disturbances are almost always present. Kernicterus is the irreversible, chronic consequence of bilirubin toxicity (Hansen, 2011; Gazzin & Tiribelli, 2011). It develops in approximately 30% of infants with untreated hemolytic disease and hyperbilirubinemia greater than or equal to 25 to 30 mg/dl. The classic symptoms of kernicterus include severe dystonia with or without athetosis, deafness or severe hearing impairment, impaired oculomotor function, and dental enamel dysplasia of the deciduous teeth. Over the first year of life a baby demonstrates the characteristic findings of hypotonia, active deep tendon reflexes, persistent tonic neck reflex, upward gaze, sensorineural hearing loss, and difficulty meeting developmental milestones. Severe cognitive impairment and spastic quadriplegia often occur. Treatment for kernicterus is supportive (Ambalavanan & Carlo, 2011; Blackburn, 2013).

CARE MANAGEMENT

It is important to determine the blood type and Rh factor of the pregnant woman prenatally. Early identification of the Rh-negative woman is critical, and care must be taken to prevent sensitization. The nurse must obtain a thorough history to assess for events that could have caused the woman to develop antibodies to the Rh factor. Such events include (1) previous pregnancy with an Rh-positive fetus; (2) transfusion with Rh-positive blood, which causes immediate sensitization; (3) miscarriage or induced abortion after 8 or more weeks of gestation; (4) amniocentesis performed for any reason; (5) premature separation of the placenta; (6) external version; and (7) trauma. See Nursing Care Plan.

Because hematopoiesis is well developed in the fetus by the ninth week of gestation, a woman who has had a miscarriage or induced abortion after this time or has previously given birth may have been inoculated with fetal blood at the time of placental separation. During amniocentesis the needle can cause localized damage to the single layer of cells that separates the maternal and fetal circulation in the placenta, thereby allowing fetal RBCs to enter the maternal circulation.

If any of these events has occurred, the nurse checks the woman's record to determine whether she has received **Rh immune globulin**, such as RhoGAM (WinGAM), which is a commercial preparation of passive antibodies against the Rh factor (see the Medication Guide, Chapter 21). This injection of anti-Rh antibodies destroys any fetal RBCs in the maternal circulation and blocks the maternal antibody production. Rh immune globulin is 90% effective in preventing sensitization. It is recommended that it be given to an Rh-negative mother at 28 weeks of gestation; within 72 hours after delivery; after an invasive procedure such as amniocentesis, chorionic villus sampling (CVS), or percutaneous umbilical blood sampling (PUBS); and any time there is a risk of fetal-maternal hemorrhage. It is also recommended after induced abortion, miscarriage, and ectopic pregnancy (Box 36-2) (Griffey, Chen, & Krehbiel, 2012; Kaplan et al., 2011).

At the first prenatal visit of an Rh-negative woman with a fetus who may be Rh positive, an indirect **Coombs' test** should be done to determine whether she has antibodies to the Rh antigen. In this test the maternal blood serum is mixed with Rh-positive RBCs. If the Rh-positive RBCs agglutinate or clump, this indicates that maternal antibodies are present or that the mother has been sensitized. The dilution of the specimen of blood at which clumping occurs determines the titer, or level, of maternal antibodies. This titer indicates the degree of maternal sensitization. A level of 1:8 rarely results in fetal jeopardy. If the titer reaches 1:16, amniocentesis is performed to determine optical density (ΔOD) of amniotic fluid to estimate fetal hemolytic process (see Chapter 26). Rising bilirubin levels can indicate the need for an intrauterine transfusion. Genetic testing allows early identification of paternal zygosity at the RhD gene locus, thus allowing earlier detection of the potential for isoimmunization and precluding further maternal or fetal testing.

The indirect Coombs' test is repeated at 28 weeks. If the result remains negative, indicating that sensitization has not occurred, the woman is given an intramuscular injection of

BOX 36-2 Indications for Amount of Rh Immune Globulin to Be Administered

50 mcg
- After chorionic villus sampling, ectopic pregnancy, miscarriage, or abortion before 13 weeks of gestation

300 mcg
- After any of the following events:
  - Miscarriage or induced abortion after 13 weeks of gestation
  - Percutaneous umbilical blood sampling
  - Amniocentesis
  - Placental abruption or placenta previa
  - Trauma
  - At 28 weeks of gestation
  - Within 72 hours after the birth of a preterm or term Rh-positive infant

More than 300 mcg
- After a large transplacental hemorrhage
- After a mismatched blood transfusion
- After third-trimester fetal demise

Data from Moise, K. J. (2014). Hemolytic disease of the fetus and newborn. In R. K. Creasy, R. Resnik, J .D. Iams, et al. (Eds), *Creasy & Resnik's maternal-fetal medicine: Principles and practice* (7th ed.). Philadelphia: Saunders

Rh_0(D) immune globulin. If the test result is positive, showing that sensitization has occurred, it is then repeated every 4 to 6 weeks to monitor the maternal antibody titer as just described.

Prevention of hyperbilirubinemia is the primary prenatal focus of care. The implementation of interventions focused on the care of the woman whose fetus is at risk for hyperbilirubinemia is essential to prevent problems in the newborn. Prenatal control of diabetes mellitus, prevention of maternal infection, avoidance of drugs such as diazepam and salicylates near the time of birth, and prevention of preterm birth reduce the risk.

The fetus and maternal antibody titers are monitored prenatally. Several methods are used to detect fetal anemia: amniocentesis to measure ΔOD 450, PUBS or cordocentesis, and middle cerebral artery peak systolic velocity (MCA-PSV). Although ultrasound-guided cordocentesis is the gold standard for detecting fetal anemia, MCA-PSV is being used increasingly as an accurate, noninvasive means to detect fetal anemia. This study is done using Doppler ultrasound (Kelly & Moore, 2012).

If amniocentesis reveals that the ΔOD is high or the MCA-PSV is increased, cordocentesis is performed to assess fetal hematocrit. If the hematocrit is less than 30%, intrauterine transfusion is indicated (Fox & Saade, 2012). Intrauterine transfusion can be done every 1 to 2 weeks between 26 and 32 weeks. If the endangered fetus is at more than 32 weeks of gestation, a preterm birth may be indicated, usually by cesarean.

Postpartum interventions focus on preventing sensitization in the mother, if it has not occurred already, and treating any complications in the neonate resulting from the hemolysis of RBCs (see the Nursing Care Plan). The unsensitized Rh-negative mother whose baby is Rh positive should receive Rh_0(D) immune globulin within 72 hours of birth to prevent her from producing antibodies to the fetal blood cells that entered her bloodstream during the birth. One dose accommodates approximately 15 ml of fetal RBCs (Mendez-Figueroa, Dahlke, Vrees, & Rouse, 2013).

At birth the neonate's cord blood is sent to the laboratory to determine the infant's blood type and Rh status. A Coombs' test is performed on this cord blood to determine whether there are maternal antibodies in the fetal blood. The antibody titer indicates the degree of maternal sensitization. If the titer is high, exchange transfusion may be indicated. In addition, the prevention of or prompt therapy for perinatal asphyxia, acidosis, cold stress, sepsis, and hypoglycemia will decrease the newborn's risk for severe hemolytic disease and the susceptibility to kernicterus. Early feeding is initiated to stimulate stooling and thus facilitate the removal of bilirubin. See Chapter 24 for a discussion of phototherapy.

Exchange transfusion is needed infrequently because of the improved recognition of neonates at risk of hemolytic disease that can result from isoimmunization. Other factors must always be considered as well, particularly the clinical condition of the infant because it is a procedure with potential complications. Guidelines for the initiation of exchange transfusion in relation to serum bilirubin levels in infants of more than 35 weeks of gestation can be found in the 2004 AAP Clinical Practice Guideline (AAP Subcommittee on Hyperbilirubinemia, 2004).

Exchange transfusion is accomplished by alternately removing a small amount of the infant's blood and replacing it with an equal amount of donor blood. Exchange transfusion replaces the RBCs that would otherwise be hemolyzed by circulating maternal antibodies, removes the antibodies responsible for hemolysis, and corrects the anemia caused by hemolysis of the infant's sensitized RBCs. It also reduces the serum bilirubin level in infants who have severe hyperbilirubinemia from any cause. If the infant has Rh incompatibility, type O Rh-negative blood is used for transfusion so the maternal antibodies still present in the infant do not hemolyze the transfused blood. Depending on the infant's size, maturity, and condition, amounts of 5 to 20 ml of the infant's blood are removed at one time and replaced with donor blood. The double volume or two-volume exchange replaces approximately 170 ml/kg of body weight, or 86% of the infant's total blood volume. The procedure requires approximately 1 hour. After the procedure, phototherapy is continued and the bilirubin levels are monitored every 4 hours (Gregory, Martin, & Cloherty, 2012; Kaplan et al., 2011; Murki & Kumar, 2011).

The infant is monitored closely during and after the procedure, including assessment of heart rate and rhythm, respirations, blood pressure, temperature, and perfusion. Preservatives in donor blood lower the infant's serum calcium and magnesium levels. It is not uncommon for calcium gluconate to be given during the exchange transfusion if symptoms of hypocalcemia become evident. Symptoms of hypocalcemia include jitteriness, irritability, convulsions, tachycardia, and electrocardiogram changes. The nurse monitors the neonate for hypoglycemia during the several hours after the exchange because the high glucose content of the preservatives can stimulate insulin secretion. These high risk neonates typically have dextrose support through an intravenous route (Gregory et al., 2012; Kamath et al., 2011).

Planning for rehabilitative measures is necessary if kernicterus occurs. The family will need the services of many community resources to care for the affected child. An interdisciplinary approach that includes social services must be taken.

NURSING CARE PLAN

The Infant with Hyperbilirubinemia

NURSING DIAGNOSIS	EXPECTED OUTCOME	INTERVENTIONS	RATIONALES
Risk for Injury related to hemolytic disease and treatment effects	Bilirubin levels decrease with treatment; no evidence of harmful effects from phototherapy (e.g., no eye irritation, dehydration, temperature instability, or skin breakdown); and no complications from exchange transfusions.	Initiate early feedings and feed frequently (breastfeeding at least every 3 hours; formula feeding at least every 3-4 hours).	To enhance excretion of bilirubin in stools
		Assess skin and mucous membranes for signs of jaundice, indicative of increasing bilirubin levels; monitor total serum bilirubin levels.	To determine rate of increase and treatment response
		Note time of jaundice onset.	To help distinguish physiologic from other causes of jaundice
		Assess for signs of hypoxia, hypothermia, hypoglycemia, and metabolic acidosis.	Occur as a result of hyperbilirubinemia and increase the risk of brain damage
		Initiate phototherapy per physician's order.	To decrease bilirubin levels
		Provide care consistent with mode of phototherapy.	To prevent harmful effects of therapy
		Shield infant's eyes if under phototherapy light.	To prevent damage to corneas and retinas
		Keep infant nude except for diaper and change positions frequently.	To expose maximal body surface
		Keep skin clean and avoid use of lotions or creams.	To prevent irritation
		Maintain adequate fluid intake.	To prevent dehydration
		Monitor body temperature.	To prevent hyperthermia
		Before exchange transfusion, keep infant on nothing by mouth (NPO) status (2 to 4 hours).	To prevent aspiration
		Check donor blood for compatibility.	To prevent transfusion reaction
		Have resuscitation equipment (oxygen, Ambu bag, endotracheal tubes, laryngoscope) at bedside.	To prepare for emergency action
		Assist physician with exchange transfusion procedure.	To promote safety and monitor infant's condition
		Track amounts of blood withdrawn and transfused.	To maintain balanced blood volume
		Maintain body temperature.	To avoid hypothermia and cold stress
		Monitor vital signs and observe.	To recognize signs of hypocalcemia and hypomagnesemia
		After transfusion, continue to monitor vital signs.	To check for signs of hypocalcemia, hypomagnesemia, hypoglycemia, and umbilical cord for bleeding; to assess for transfusion reaction
Interrupted Breastfeeding related to discharge of mother and continued hospitalization of infant	Mother states desire to continue breastfeeding as much as possible and expresses and stores milk when she cannot come to the hospital to breastfeed the infant.	Encourage the mother to come to the hospital to breastfeed infant as often as feasible and to continue to express and store her breast milk.	To establish and maintain milk supply and encourage bonding and to provide safe milk for the infant
		Provide private and comfortable space for nursing that is available 24 hours a day.	To support the mother in breastfeeding
		Encourage and assist the mother to hold her baby skin-to-skin.	To facilitate attachment and breastfeeding
		Instruct the mother in methods to express and store breast milk.	To ensure a safe and adequate milk supply
		Provide written educational materials and audiovisual aids.	To demonstrate proper techniques for expressing and storing milk and to allow the mother to learn at her own pace

NURSING CARE PLAN—cont'd

The Infant with Hyperbilirubinemia

NURSING DIAGNOSIS	EXPECTED OUTCOME	INTERVENTIONS	RATIONALES
Interrupted Breastfeeding related to discharge of mother and continued hospitalization of infant–cont'd		Recommend using a breast pump and pump according to established guidelines (e.g., pump a minimum of five times a day; pump a minimum of 100 minutes a day; pump long enough to soften breasts).	To provide maximum stimulation for milk production
		Reassure the mother that infant's nutritional needs will be met through expressed milk or other methods.	To allay anxiety
		Review the daily routine of the mother to advise her on ways to incorporate pumping into her daily schedule.	To promote adequate milk supply
		Arrange for lactation consultant to meet with mother for education and support.	To promote successful breastfeeding and milk expression
		Provide information about breastfeeding support groups.	To help the mother obtain emotional support from other breastfeeding mothers
Parental Role Conflict related to separation from hospitalized infant and interruptions of family life due to travel to hospital to see infant	Parents will share responsibilities for child care and home maintenance; parents will visit infant in hospital as often as feasible.	Suggest to parents that they mutually establish a routine for child care for siblings and home maintenance.	To enhance communication and provide necessary home activities
		Encourage the parents to seek assistance and support from friends, relatives, and community groups such as their church.	To meet their needs and ensure that a minimal level of appropriate functioning is maintained
		Encourage the parents to travel to the hospital as often as is desirable and feasible.	To promote breastfeeding and bonding with infant
Deficient Knowledge related to use of home phototherapy	Family demonstrates ability to safely provide home phototherapy for the infant with hyperbilirubinemia.	Explore the family's willingness to try home phototherapy.	To evaluate feasibility of home therapy option
		Assess the family's understanding of hyperbilirubinemia (jaundice) and proposed therapy.	To establish baseline for teaching
		Teach the family about use of phototherapy equipment using demonstration–return demonstration, allowing for several practice sessions, and supplement with written materials with pictorial representations.	To promote safe and effective use of equipment
		Instruct the family regarding placement of phototherapy light or fiberoptic unit; proper eye care and patching; proper skin care; proper positioning under light; provision of increased fluid intake; monitoring of time under light; monitoring of temperature, skin, eyes, feeding patterns, stooling and voiding patterns; and observation for complications.	To enable the family to safely and competently care for the infant
		Stress importance of obtaining the prescribed bilirubin tests on schedule.	To assess infant response to therapy
		Give parents a contact number if they have any questions while carrying out therapy.	To offer ongoing support and increase parent comfort

CONGENITAL ANOMALIES

A congenital anomaly is a defect that is present at birth and can be caused by genetic or environmental factors, or both. It is defined as a structural or functional deviation from the normal pattern of development. Congenital defects are reported to occur in 3% of all live births, but this number increases to approximately 6% by 5 years when more anomalies are diagnosed (World Health Organization [WHO], 2012). In addition, the incidence of congenital malformations in fetuses that are aborted is higher than that in infants who are born alive, thus adding to the overall incidence. Congenital defects, including malformations, deformations, and chromosomal abnormalities, are the leading cause of death in infants younger than 1 year of age in the United States, occurring at the rate of 127.7 per 100,000 live births and accounting for 20.8% of infant deaths (Murphy, Xu, & Kochanek, 2013).

The desired and expected outcome of every wanted pregnancy is a normal, functioning infant with a good intellectual potential. Fulfillment of this hope depends on numerous hereditary and environmental factors. Probably all human characteristics have a genetic component, including those that produce symptoms or physical abnormalities that impair a person's fitness. Some disorders or diseases occur through the influence of a single gene or the combined action of many genes inherited from the parents; others result from the action of the intrauterine environment. Many defects appear to occur as the result of multifactorial inheritance, the interaction of multiple genes with environmental factors that affect the embryonic development of the affected system. In about two thirds of all cases of congenital anomalies, there is no identifiable cause. A chromosomal abnormality or gene alteration is responsible for approximately 10% of the major congenital anomalies (Parikh & Wiesner, 2011). Evidence indicates that maternal obesity is significantly linked to spina bifida, cardiac defects, diaphragmatic hernia, hypospadias, omphalocele, anorectal atresia, and limb reductions (Racusin, Stevens, Campbell, & Aagaard, 2012).

Ways of detecting and preventing some of the congenital anomalies are improving continually, as are surgical techniques for the care of the fetus and newborn with certain anomalies. Promoting the availability of these services to populations at risk challenges community health care systems. An interdisciplinary team approach is vital for providing holistic care: the surgical treatment, rehabilitation, and education of the child, as well as psychosocial and financial assistance for the parents. Parental disappointment and disillusion add to the complexity of the nursing care needed for these infants.

The most common congenital anomalies that cause serious problems in the neonate are congenital heart disease, neural tube defects, cleft lip or palate, clubfoot, and developmental dysplasia of the hip. These are thought to result from the interaction of multiple genetic and environmental factors. Minor anomalies are less apparent but are important to identify because they can be a part of a characteristic pattern of malformations. That is, they can point to the presence of a more serious major anomaly and aid in its diagnosis. The presence of a minor anomaly indicates the need for further evaluation of the neonate for other anomalies. Minor malformations are more common in areas of the body that have variable features, such as the face and distal extremities. Some of the most common minor malformations include the lack of a helical fold of the pinna, simian creases, absent philtrum, or clinodactyly of the fifth finger (Parikh & Wiesner, 2011).

Cardiovascular System Anomalies

During fetal development cell division and differentiation of the organs and tissues of a particular body system sometimes occur rapidly. During these critical periods particular body systems are more susceptible to environmental influences than they are later in gestation. For example, the critical period for the cardiovascular system is from week 3 of embryonic development to week 8, when many women are not aware that they are pregnant.

Congenital cardiac anomalies, with an overall prevalence of approximately 80 per 10,000 births, are the most common of all congenital malformations (Dolk, Loane, & Garne, 2011; Van der Linde, Konings, Slager, et al., 2011). Congenital heart defects (CHDs) are anatomic abnormalities in the heart that are present at birth, although they may not be diagnosed immediately. Congenital heart disease occurs more frequently in preterm infants. There is an increased likelihood of cardiac disease in neonates that are small for gestational age (SGA), as well as in those with congenital infections.

Ventricular septal defect, the most common type of heart defect, with increased pulmonary blood flow (acyanotic lesion) has a prevalence of 1.5 to 3.5 per 1000 births and accounts for about 30% of all congenital heart defects. Tetralogy of Fallot has an incidence of 0.24 to 0.56 per 1000 births and is the most common cardiac defect with decreased pulmonary blood flow (cyanotic lesion) (Rajiah, Mak, Dubinsky, & Dighe, 2011). CHDs are often associated with other extracardiac defects such as renal agenesis, omphalocele, tracheoesophageal fistula, and diaphragmatic hernia. Congenital heart disease is the leading cause of death in children with congenital defects (Bernstein, 2011).

> **COMMUNITY ACTIVITY**
>
> Visit the National Heart, Lung, and Blood Institute website (www.nhlbi.nih.gov/health/health-topics/topics/chd). Under the Types (of defects), review the information on septal defects. In particular, familiarize yourself with the features of ventricular septal defects, the most common type of congenital heart defect. How could you explain this defect in simple terms to parents? Determine where infants from your community go to receive treatment for congenital heart defects.

The etiology of CHDs is multifactorial, chromosomal and/or genetic, and due to environmental teratogens (Kenney, Hoover, Williams, & Iskersky, 2011). This is important information for parents because they often feel guilty thinking that they have done something to cause the defect. The etiology is also important when it comes to counseling the family regarding recurrence risks for future pregnancies. If a sibling is diagnosed with a CHD, the recurrence risk is 1% to 6%, and if two siblings have a CHD, the recurrence risk is 10%; the risk is significantly higher if the person affected is a parent, particularly the mother (Blue, Kirk, Sholler, et al., 2012). Maternal factors known to be associated with a higher incidence of CHDs include the following (Blackburn, 2013; de Silva, 2013; Fung, Manlhiot, Naik, et al., 2013):

- Rubella and cytomegalovirus
- Ingestion of lithium, warfarin (Coumadin), or anticonvulsants such as phenytoin
- Alcohol intake
- Poor nutrition
- Radiation exposure
- Metabolic disorders such as diabetes mellitus and phenylketonuria
- Systemic lupus erythematosus
- Maternal age ≥40 years

Maternal smoking is associated with a greater risk of congenital heart disease. Infants born to women who are heavy smokers (≥25 cigarettes per day) have an increased risk of having a congenital septal defect (Alverson, Strickland, Gilboa, & Correa, 2011).

Maternal obesity can increase the risk of congenital heart anomalies. An above normal body mass index has been associated with an increased risk for all congenital heart defects, and specifically total anomalous pulmonary venous return, hypoplastic left heart syndrome, left and right ventricular outflow tract defects, and septal defects (Madsen, Schwartz, Lewis, & Mueller, 2013).

Genetic factors are implicated in the pathogenesis of CHDs. It now appears that a much greater percentage of CHDs than believed to be true in the past can be attributed to single gene mutations. This recognition is based on animal models, studies of human familial patterns of inheritance, and the finding of cardiovascular defects as a part of syndromes exhibiting mendelian patterns of inheritance. An example of this is the identification of chromosome 22q11 deletions in infants with DiGeorge syndrome. This syndrome affects an estimated 1 in 4000 live births, making it one of the most frequent genetic disorders with CHDs. The gene or genes located in the chromosomal region involved with DiGeorge syndrome appear to play a major role in the development of cardiovascular defects, particularly truncus arteriosus, absent pulmonary valve syndrome, tetralogy of Fallot, pulmonary atresia, and other abnormalities involving the aortic arch. Congenital heart disease is found in more than 50% of children with trisomy 21 (Down syndrome), 99% of neonates with trisomy 18 (Gilbert syndrome), and 35% of neonates with Turner syndrome (Kenney et al., 2011).

Although traditionally a CHD was classified as either cyanotic or acyanotic, a classification that categorizes cardiac defects physiologically by physiologic consequence is now considered more descriptive (Table 36-1 and Fig. 36-1).

Approximately 25% of congenital heart anomalies are considered severe and may be referred to as critical congenital heart defects (CCHDs). These are often evident immediately after birth, especially defects that cause cyanosis such as transposition of the great vessels. Infants with these anomalies are transferred directly to neonatal intensive care units, preferably those that are equipped to diagnose and medically or surgically treat these types of cardiac emergencies. Even though the structural or functional anomalies are always present at birth, the affected newborns can be asymptomatic because the defect is too small to interfere with sufficient blood flow to the lungs for oxygenation or does not interfere with delivery of oxygenated blood to the tissues. With growth and maturation the defect can become apparent as the infant or child is exposed to stressors such as growth demands or infection.

TABLE 36-1 Classification of Congenital Cardiac Disease

CLASSIFICATION	EXAMPLES
Severe cyanosis caused by separate circulations and poor mixing	Transposition of the great arteries with or without ventricular septal defect
Severe cyanosis caused by restricted pulmonary blood flow	Tetralogy of Fallot Tricuspid atresia Persistent pulmonary hypertension
Mild cyanosis caused by complete mixing with normal or increased pulmonary blood flow	Total anomalous pulmonary venous connection Truncus arteriosus
Systemic hypoperfusion and congestive heart failure with mild or no cyanosis	Aortic stenosis* Coarctation of the aorta and aortic arch interruption Hypoplastic left heart syndrome
Acyanosis with no or mild respiratory distress	Normal murmurs Pulmonary stenosis Ventricular septal defect† Atrial septal defect Patent ductus arteriosus†

*No symptoms with mild forms of disease.

†Congestive heart failure can develop as left-to-right shunt increases with decrease in pulmonary vascular resistance.

Modified from Zahka, K.G. (2011). Approach to the neonate with cardiovascular disease. In R.J. Martin, A.A. Faranoff, & M.C. Walsh (Eds.), *Neonatal-perinatal medicine: Diseases of the fetus and newborn* (9th ed.). St. Louis: Mosby.

In an effort to identify those infants with CCHDs who do not manifest symptoms prior to hospital discharge, current published recommendations for newborn screening include routine pulse oximetry assessment. Infants in well-baby and intermediate nurseries should have predischarge pulse oximetry monitoring according to an established algorithm. Infants with a positive screen are evaluated with an echocardiogram and other diagnostic measures as warranted (Kemper, Mahle, Martin, et al., 2011).

If symptoms are present at birth, they can be obvious with the first cry, which can be weak and muffled or loud and breathless. Affected newborns can exhibit cyanosis that is not relieved when given supplemental oxygen, with the cyanosis increasing whenever the child cries or is in the supine position. The bluish gray, dusky color of cyanotic infants can be mild, moderate, or severe. Other infants can be acyanotic and pale, with or without mottling on exertion, which includes crying, feeding, or stooling.

The affected newborn's activity level varies from restlessness to lethargy, and possibly unresponsiveness, except to pain. Persistent bradycardia (a resting heart rate of less than 80 beats/minute) or tachycardia (a rate exceeding 160 beats/minute) can be noted. The cardiac rhythm can be abnormal, and various murmurs may be heard. Signs of congestive heart failure and decreased tissue perfusion can also become evident (Kenney et al., 2011).

Because the cardiac and respiratory systems function together, cardiac disease can be manifested by respiratory signs and symptoms. The nurse assesses the respiratory rate while the newborn is in a resting state. Tachypnea, a respiratory rate greater than 60 breaths/minute without dyspnea, is typically a subtle clue that the baby possibly has a cardiac malformation. Increased respiratory depth or hyperpnea is often noted when the neonate has a cardiac lesion that is obstructing blood flow to the lung. Signs that can indicate the development of congestive heart failure are feeding difficulties and increasing respiratory distress, especially tachypnea such that the infant has to stop feeding to breathe.

A major role of the nurse is to assess infants for abnormal findings, which must be reported immediately. Newborns exhibiting these symptoms require prompt diagnosis and appropriate

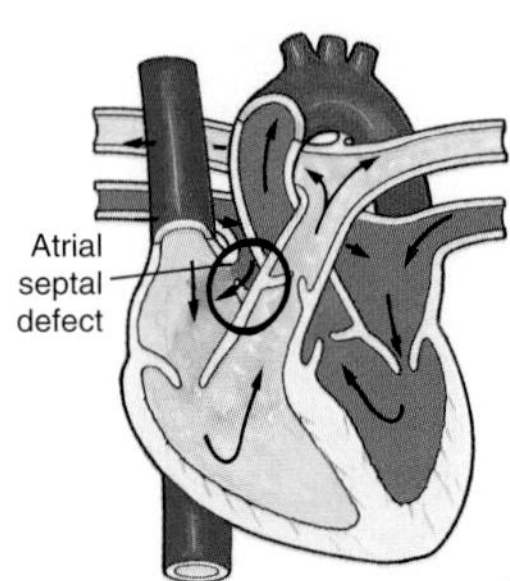

Atrial septal defect (ASD)

An ASD is an abnormal opening between the right and left atria. Basically, three types of abnormalities result from incorrect development of the atrial septum. An incompetent foramen ovale is the most common defect. The high ostium secundum defect results from abnormal development of the septum secundum. Improper development of the septum primum produces a basal opening known as an *ostium primum defect,* frequently involving the atrioventricular valves. In general, left-to-right shunting of the blood occurs in all atrial septal defects.

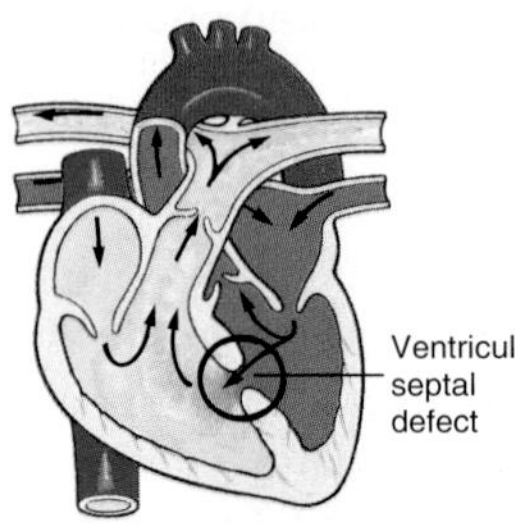

Ventricular septal defect (VSD)

A VSD is an abnormal opening between the right and left ventricles. VSDs vary in size and may occur in either the membranous or muscular portion of the ventricular septum. Because of higher pressure in the left ventricle, a shunting of blood from the left to the right ventricle occurs during systole. If pulmonary vascular resistance produces pulmonary hypertension, the shunt of blood is then reversed from the right to the left ventricle, with cyanosis resulting.

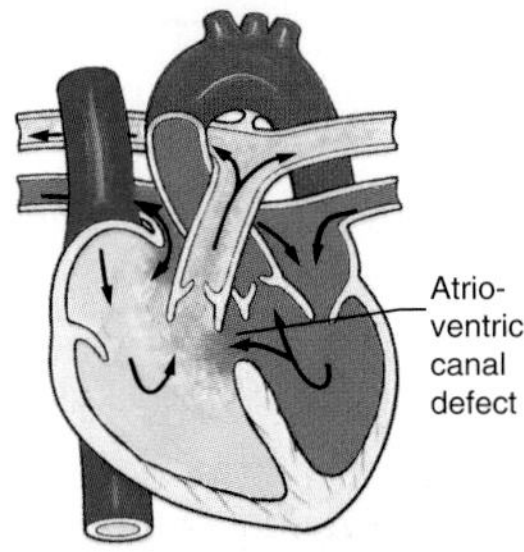

Atrioventricular canal (AVC) defect

An AVC defect is an incomplete fusion of the endocardial cushions. It consists of a low atrial septal defect that is continuous, with a high ventricular septal defect and clefts of the mitral and tricuspid valves, creating a large central atrioventricular valve that allows blood to flow between all four chambers of the heart. Flow is generally from left to right. It is the most common cardiac defect in children with Down syndrome.

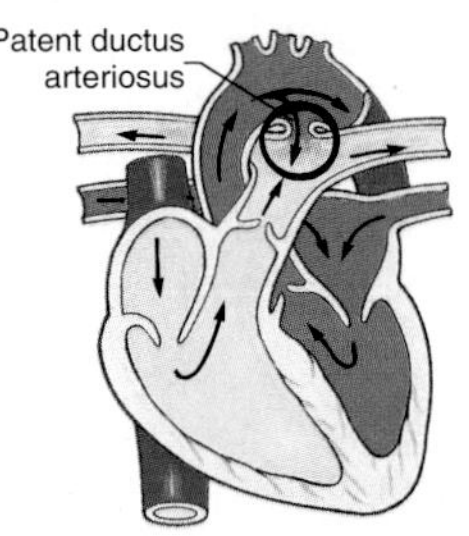

Patent ductus arteriosus (PDA)

PDA is a vascular connection that, during fetal life, bypasses the pulmonary vascular bed and directs blood from the pulmonary artery to the aorta. Functional closure of the ductus normally occurs soon after birth. If the ductus remains patent after birth, the direction of blood flow in the ductus is reversed by the higher pressure in the aorta.

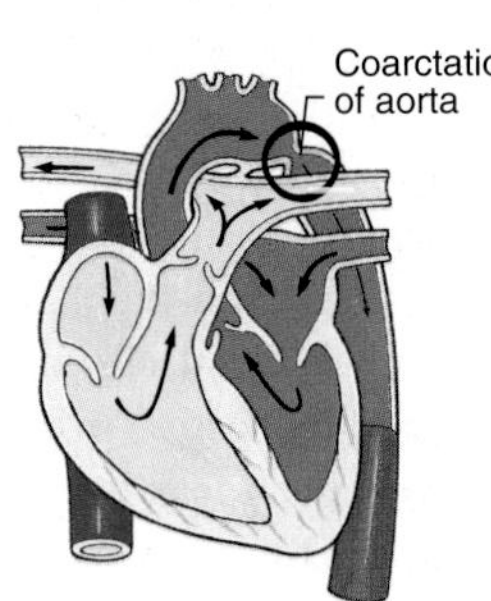

Coarctation of the aorta (COA)

COA is characterized by localized narrowing of the aorta near the insertion of the ductus arteriosus, resulting in increased pressure proximal to the defect (head and upper extremities) and decreased pressure distal to the defect (body and lower extremities).

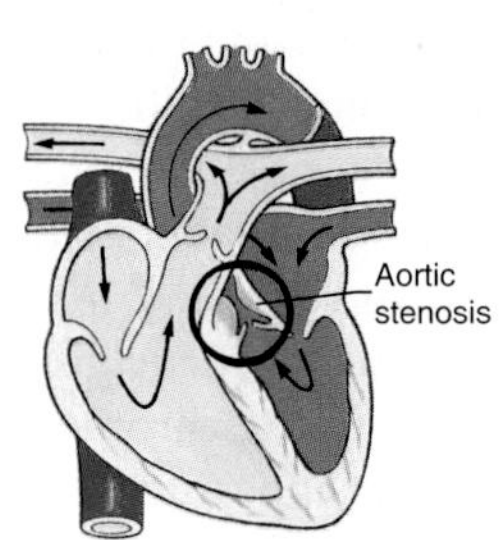

Aortic stenosis (AS)

AS is a narrowing or stricture of the aortic valve, causing resistance to blood flow in the left ventricle, decreased cardiac output, left ventricular hypertrophy, and pulmonary vascular congestion. AS can be valvular, subvalvular, or supravalvular (rare). The most serious sequelae relate to the left ventricular hypertrophy (increased end-diastolic pressure, pulmonary hypertension, decreased coronary artery perfusion).

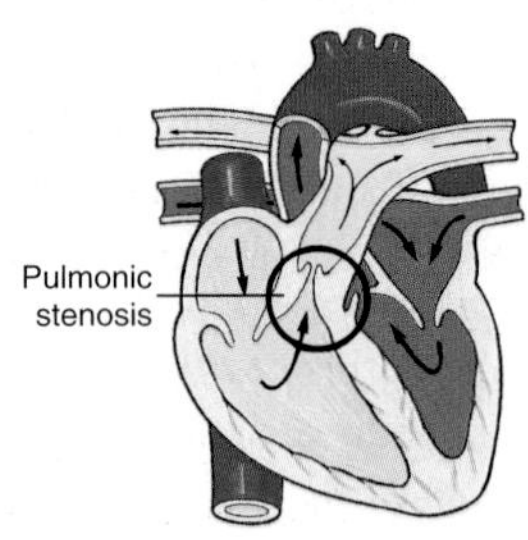

Pulmonic stenosis (PS)

PS is a narrowing at the entrance to the pulmonary artery. Resistance to blood flow causes right ventricular hypertrophy and decreased pulmonary blood flow. Pulmonary atresia is the extreme form of PS; no blood flows to the lungs.

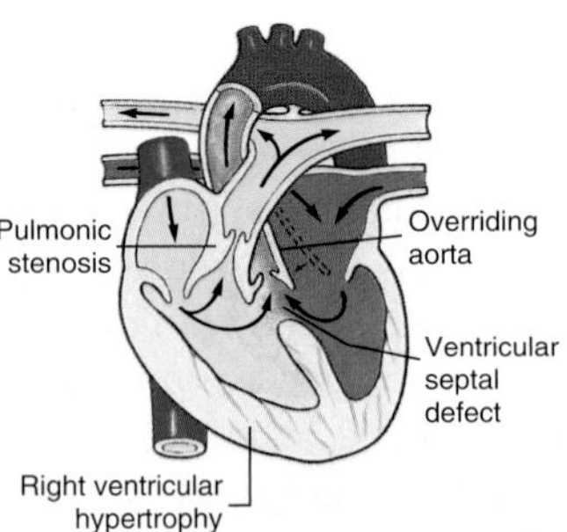

Tetralogy of Fallot (TOF)

TOF is characterized by the combination of four defects: (1) pulmonary stenosis, (2) ventricular septal defect, (3) overriding aorta, and (4) hypertrophy of the right ventricle. It is the most common defect, causing cyanosis in children surviving beyond 2 years of age. The severity of symptoms depends on the degree of pulmonary stenosis, the size of the ventricular septal defect, and the degree to which the aorta overrides the septal defect.

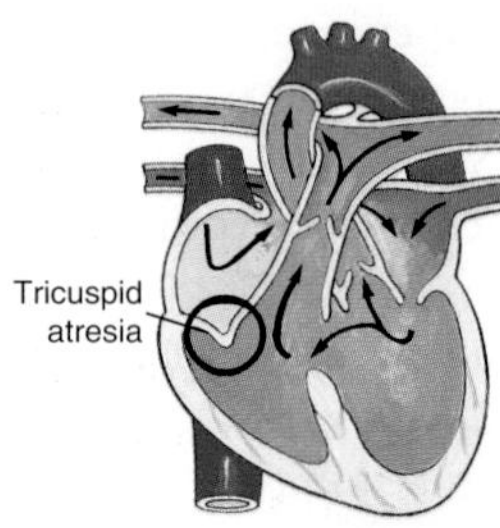

Tricuspid atresia

Tricuspid valvular atresia is characterized by a small right ventricle, a large left ventricle, and usually a diminished pulmonary circulation. Blood from the right atrium passes through an atrial septal defect into the left atrium, mixes with oxygenated blood returning from the lungs, flows into the left ventricle, and is propelled into the systemic circulation. The lungs may receive blood through one of three routes: (1) a small ventricular septal defect, (2) a patent ductus arteriosus, or (3) bronchial vessels.

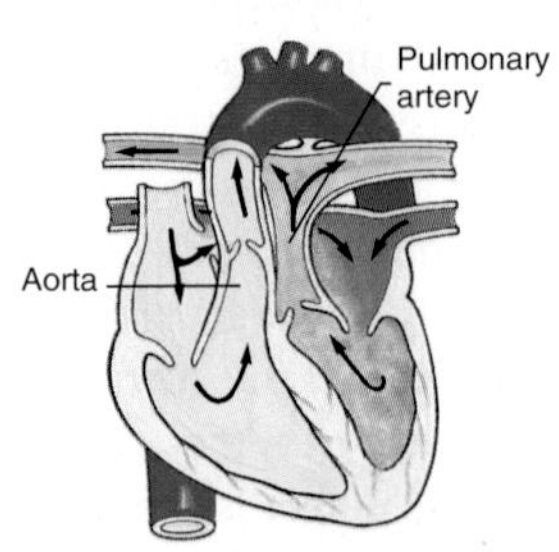

Transposition of the great vessels (TGV)

TGV is an embryologic defect caused by a straight division of the bulbar trunk without normal spiraling. As a result, the aorta originates from the right ventricle and the pulmonary artery from the left ventricle. An abnormal communication between the two circulations must be present to sustain life.

FIG 36-1 Congenital heart abnormalities. (Modified from Hockenberry, M., & Wilson, D. [2011]. *Wong's nursing care of infants and children* [9th ed.]. St. Louis: Mosby.)

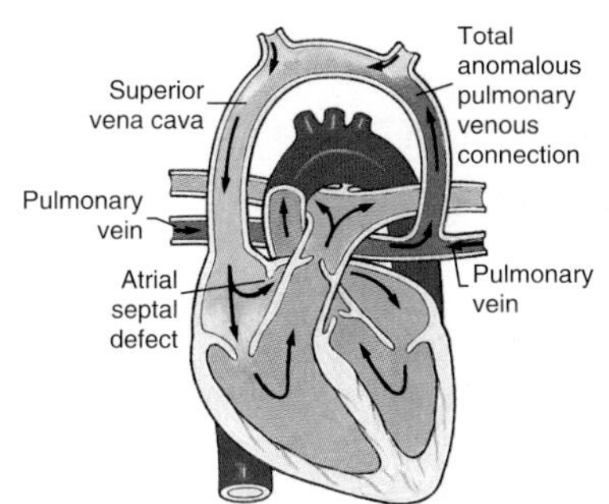

Total anomalous pulmonary venous connection (TAPVC)

TAPVC is a rare defect characterized by a failure of the pulmonary veins to join the left atrium. Instead, the pulmonary veins are abnormally connected to the systemic venous circuit via the right atrium or various veins draining toward the right atrium (e.g., superior vena cava). The abnormal attachment results in mixed blood being returned to the right atrium and shunted from the right to the left through an atrial septal defect.

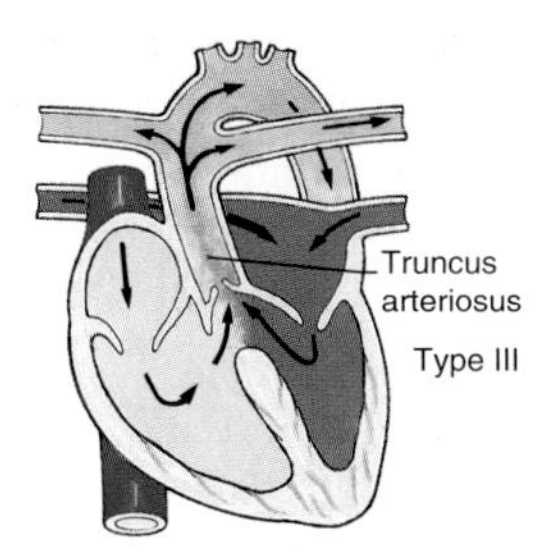

Truncus arteriosus (TA)

TA is a retention of the embryologic bulbar trunk. It results from the failure of normal septation and division of this trunk into an aorta and pulmonary artery. This single arterial trunk overrides the ventricles and receives blood from them through a ventricular septal defect. The entire pulmonary and systemic circulation is supplied from this common arterial trunk.

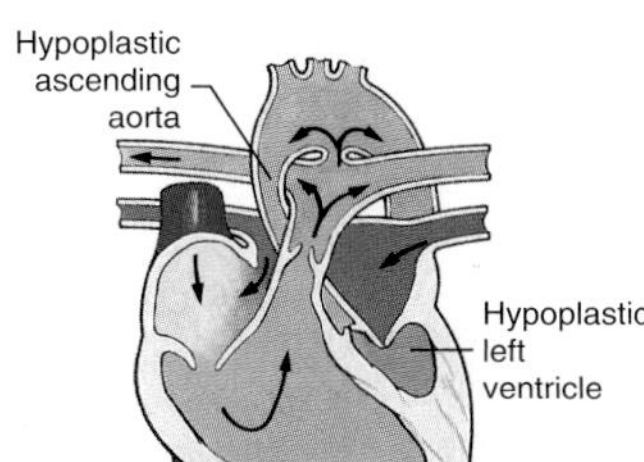

Hypoplastic left heart syndrome (HLHS)

HLHS is characterized by under-development of the left side of the heart, resulting in a hypoplastic left ventricle and aortic atresia. Most blood from the left atrium flows across the patent foramen ovale to the right atrium, to the right ventricle, and out the pulmonary artery. The descending aorta receives blood from the patent ductus arteriosus supplying systemic blood flow.

FIG 36-1, cont'd Congenital heart abnormalities.

therapy in a neonatal or pediatric intensive care unit. Interventions include administering oxygen as ordered, administering cardiotonic and other medications such as diuretics that rid the body of accumulated fluid, decreasing the workload of the heart by maintaining a thermoneutral environment, feeding with the gavage method if necessary, and preventing crying if this precipitates cyanosis. Various diagnostic tests such as echocardiography and cardiac catheterization are performed to obtain specific information about the defect and the need for surgical intervention. Significant improvements in diagnosis, medical management, and surgical treatment of CHDs have caused the death rate to decrease significantly, with the result that more of these children are reaching adulthood (Kenney et al., 2011).

Central Nervous System Anomalies

Most congenital anomalies of the CNS result from defects in the closure of the neural tube during fetal development. Although the cause of neural tube defects (NTDs) is unknown, they are thought to stem from the interaction of many genes that can be influenced by factors in the fetal environment. Environmental influences such as maternal treatment with anticonvulsants (e.g., valproic acid or carbamazepine), treatment with methotrexate (a chemotherapeutic medication), folic acid deficiency, and maternal diabetes have been implicated (Kennedy & Koren, 2012). Excessive maternal body heat exposure during the early first trimester, significant febrile illness, and lower socioeconomic status can increase the risk of an NTD (Clements, Challis, & Kennedy, 2012).

Maternal folic acid deficiency has a direct bearing on failure of the neural tube to close. Therefore, as a preventive measure, folic acid supplementation (0.4 mg/day) is recommended for women of childbearing age. Women who are pregnant should take 0.6 mg per day (CDC, 2012).

The incidence of NTD is about 1 per 1000 live births. However, this varies according to race, geographic area, and socioeconomic status (Clements et al., 2012). Prevalence estimates indicate that the most common NTD, spina bifida, occurs in approximately 3.5 of every 10,000 live births (Parker, Mai, Canfield, et al., 2010). Approximately 95% of all NTDs occur in families that have no history of NTDs. Primary NTDs have an increased recurrence rate in subsequent pregnancies although secondary NTDs do not. Primary NTDs are the result of failure of the anterior neuropore to close or a disruption of an already closed neural tube between 18 and 25 days of gestation. Myelomeningocele, encephalocele, and anencephaly are examples of primary NTDs. Secondary neural tube defects account for 5% of NTDs. They are due to disruption in development of the lower sacral or coccygeal segments during secondary neurulation between 26 days and 8 weeks of gestation (Blackburn, 2013). Examples of secondary NTDs are meningocele, and sacral agenesis or dysgenesis.

Although an NTD is usually an isolated defect, it can occur with some chromosomal abnormalities and syndromes and with other defects such as cleft palate, ventricular septal defect, tracheoesophageal fistula, diaphragmatic hernia, imperforate anus, and renal anomalies. Some NTDs are diagnosed prenatally with fetal ultrasonography and the finding of elevated levels of alpha-fetoprotein in the amniotic fluid and maternal serum. Increased use of prenatal diagnostic techniques and termination of pregnancies have also had an effect on the overall incidence of birth of infants with NTDs.

Encephalocele and Anencephaly

Encephalocele and anencephaly are abnormalities resulting from failure of the anterior end of the neural tube to close. An encephalocele is a herniation of the brain and meninges through a skull defect, usually in the occipital area. The prevalence is 0.8 of every 10,000 live births (Parker et al., 2010). Treatment consists of surgical repair and shunting to relieve hydrocephalus, unless a major brain malformation is present. Most of these infants will have some degree of cognitive deficit. Anencephaly is the absence of both cerebral hemispheres and of the overlying skull. It occurs in approximately 2 of every 10,000 births (Parker et al., 2010). This condition is incompatible with life; many of the infants are stillborn or die within a few days of birth. Comfort measures are provided until the infant eventually dies of respiratory failure.

Spina Bifida

Spina bifida, the most common defect of the CNS, results from failure of the neural tube to close at some point. The two categories of spina bifida are spina bifida occulta and spina bifida manifesta, also known as open spina bifida. *Spina bifida occulta*, the milder form, is a malformation in which the posterior portion of the laminae fails to close, but the spinal cord or meninges do not herniate or protrude through the defect and there is no abnormality of the spinal cord, nerve roots, or meninges (Kinsman & Johnston, 2013). Skin typically covers the opening in the spinal cord. There can also be a bulge under the skin where the ends of the spinal cord terminate in fatty tissue. Often a birthmark or a hairy patch is present above the defect.

Spina bifida manifesta occurs predominantly in the lumbar or lumbosacral region and includes meningocele and myelomeningocele. A meningocele is a herniation of the meninges at the site of the defect in the vertebral column and is typically covered by skin. The baby's neurologic function tends to be normal unless other abnormalities are present. A myelomeningocele is a herniation of the meninges and spinal cord at the site of the defect, with or without skin or vertebral covering (Fig. 36-2). The sac can tear easily, allowing cerebrospinal fluid (CSF) to leak out and providing an entry for infectious agents into the CNS. Because the nerves are involved, there are motor and sensory deficits below the lesion. Seventy-five percent of the lesions occur in the lumbar area and 80% of affected neonates will have hydrocephalus, typically due to a Chiari malformation (Kinsman & Johnston, 2013). A Chiari malformation results from the improper development and downward displacement of the hindbrain into the cervical spinal canal, which blocks the flow of CSF from communicating with the spinal column and results in the development of hydrocephalus. The long-term prognosis in an affected infant can be determined to a large extent at birth, with the degree of neurologic dysfunction related to the level of the lesion, as the level determines the nerves involved. Prenatal diagnosis makes possible a scheduled cesarean birth, allowing for more careful delivery of the infant's back to try to prevent rupture of the meningeal sac.

Postnatal surgery for myelomeningocele is usually performed within the first 24 hours to close the defect in an effort to prevent further deterioration of the exposed spinal cord, to prevent infection, and to treat hydrocephalus with a ventriculoperitoneal shunt (Adzick, 2013). A major preoperative nursing intervention for a neonate with a myelomeningocele is to protect the protruding sac from injury, rupture, and resultant risk of CNS infection. Such infants should be positioned in a prone-kneeling position and the knees protected from skin breakdown. The sac should be covered with a sterile, moist, nonadherent dressing and cared for using sterile technique. A drape should be placed over the buttocks below the lesion and secured using the drape's adhesive to keep the lesion free of meconium or stool. Neurosurgery and urology consultations should occur as soon as possible after birth. A thorough physical examination is done to evaluate the level of the injury, sensory involvement, sphincter control (anal wink), and measurement of the fronto-occipital circumference to assess for hydrocephalus (Wilson, Montagnino, & Wilson, 2011). Intake and output are recorded to document the number and character of the voidings and stools as well as the leakage of urine and stool. Nursing assessment includes observations of movement or absence of movement as well as the quality of movements of the lower extremities.

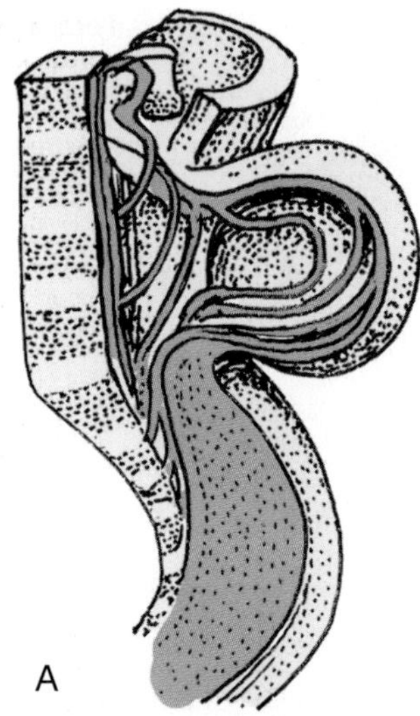

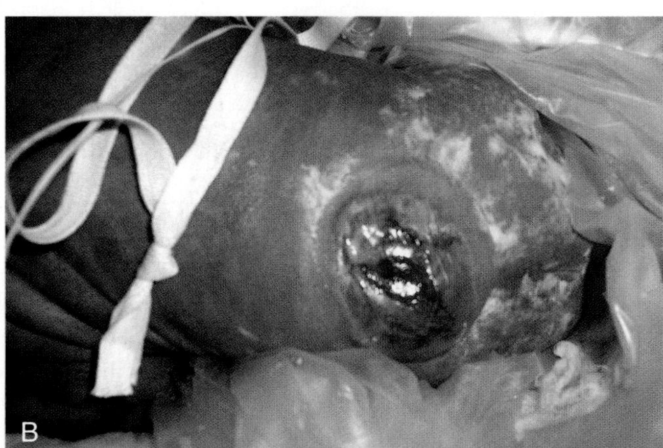

FIG 36-2 **A,** Myelomeningocele. Note absence of vertebral arches. **B,** Myelomeningocele (spina bifida). (Courtesy Cheryl Briggs, RNC, Annapolis, MD.)

Nurses provide support and information to parents as they begin to learn to cope with an infant who has immediate needs for intensive care and who probably will have long-term needs as well. Based on the type and position of the lesion, along with the neonate's clinical condition, early surgical repair is advocated to preserve cognitive function, decrease the risk of sepsis, and improve the prognosis for ambulation (Verklan & Lopez, 2011). Surgical shunt procedures to prevent increasing hydrocephalus may be needed, such as a ventriculoperitoneal shunt.

SAFETY ALERT

Infants with myelomeningocele are at increased risk for developing latex sensitivity, so they must not come into direct or secondary contact with any products or equipment containing latex (Kinsman & Johnston, 2013).

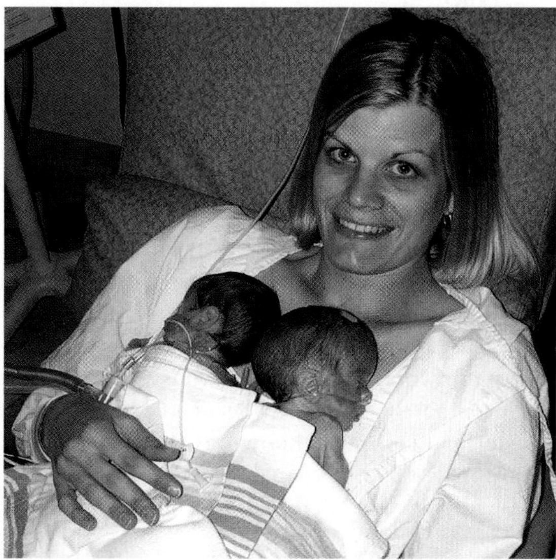

FIG 36-3 Mother providing kangaroo care to preterm twins; the one on the right has hydrocephalus. The characteristic appearance is an enlarged head, thinning of the scalp, distended scalp veins, and a full fontanel. (Courtesy Cheryl Briggs, RNC, Annapolis, MD.)

Intrauterine fetal surgery may be performed prior to 26 weeks of gestation to repair a myelomeningocele. The rationale for this intervention is based on direct and indirect evidence that some of the neural damage resulting from the myelomeningocele is acquired in the later part of gestation, caused by amniotic fluid exposure or trauma to the exposed neural elements. Fetal surgery for myelomeningocele is associated with preservation of neurologic function and a reduced risk of hindbrain herniation of the Chiari malformation. There is also a decreased risk of hydrocephalus and the need for a ventriculoperitoneal shunt. Fetal surgery is associated with risk of spontaneous rupture of membranes and preterm birth as well as problems related to the uterine scar such as partial separation of the wound (Adzick, 2013; Gupta, Farrell, Rand, et al., 2012).

Hydrocephalus

Hydrocephalus is a condition in which there is excess CSF in the ventricles of the brain due to overproduction (rare) or a decrease in reabsorption. The most common etiology for the neonate is excess ventricular CSF due to aqueductal flow obstruction. The obstruction prevents the CSF from leaving the head and flowing into the spinal column. Other etiologies include congenital viral infections, myelomeningocele with Chiari malformation, intracranial bleeding, and congenital masses or tumors (Cohen, 2011).

The neonate presents with an increasing frontal-occipital circumference because the head circumference is increasing at an abnormal rate as a result of the increase in CSF pressure (Fig. 36-3). The sutures are widened and the fontanels are full or bulging and tense. Classic signs of increasing intracranial pressure (vomiting, lethargy, and irritability) can be attributed to feeding intolerance. It is thought that "setting sun eyes," (eyes that are rotated downward) indicate permanent damage to the brain tissue. Serial head ultrasound is used to evaluate the evolving condition. Neurosurgery and genetics services are consulted to evaluate for the placement of a ventriculoperitoneal shunt versus placement of a reservoir and to assess for the presence of congenital anomalies (Verklan & Lopez, 2011).

The nurse provides support to the family by teaching and involving them in their infant's care as much as possible. Minimal stimulation protocols that promote the use of limited handling, dim lighting, and attention to the baby's cues will help keep the infant calm. The head needs to be positioned carefully, repositioned at least once every 4 hours, and attention given such that the head is not positioned on the shunt side postoperatively. Gel-filled pillows can provide some comfort for the neonate. The frontal-occipital circumference needs to be measured serially, and depending on the rate of increase, every 4 hours to every 24 hours. Neurologic assessments and observation for signs of increasing intracranial pressure should be done every 4 to 8 hours, depending on the baby's clinical condition.

The baby should be fed in a semi-reclining position with the head well supported. The method, amount, and frequency of feeding depend on the infant's tolerance and energy level. The nurse should be alert to the possibility of emesis, a frequent occurrence in the presence of increased intracranial pressure, and should maintain aspiration precautions. Nonnutritive sucking, touching, and cuddling needs should be met.

In addition to serial intracranial ultrasonography, the diagnosis is also made using computed tomography (CT) and magnetic resonance imaging (MRI); antenatal diagnosis can be made by fetal ultrasonography. The surgical correction of hydrocephalus involves the placement of a shunt that goes from the ventricles of the brain usually to the peritoneum to allow the drainage of excess CSF. Damaged or destroyed brain tissue cannot be restored. The long-term prognosis in affected infants depends on the presence and extent of such tissue damage, along with the cause of the hydrocephalus, the presence of concurrent neurologic problems, and the long-term success of the shunt procedure.

Parent teaching regarding the shunt should be done both pre- and postoperatively. Providing handouts or, if possible, seeing an infant with a shunt already in place can be helpful. Parents also need to be taught signs of a blocked shunt and signs of infection such as increasing intracranial pressure and changes in the baby's feeding patterns.

Microcephaly

Microcephaly refers to a head circumference that measures two or more standard deviations below the mean for age and sex (Gressens & Huppi, 2011). Brain growth is usually restricted and thus cognitive impairment is common. Maternal risk factors include congenital viral infections, chromosomal disorders, and malnutrition. Fetal and neonatal factors include inflammation, birth trauma, and sequelae of hypoxic-ischemic encephalopathy. If the result of an in utero insult, the baby is typically born with a small head and brain, which gives the forehead a backward-sloping appearance. Diagnostic evaluations include a complete maternal history, evaluation of the events surrounding the birth, CT or MRI to evaluate brain volume, and a neurologic assessment. Typically genetics and infectious disease consults are also obtained. Although neurologic deficits are not present at birth, developmental delays will become evident. The baby's outcome and prognosis depend on the severity of the microcephaly. Treatment for the infant

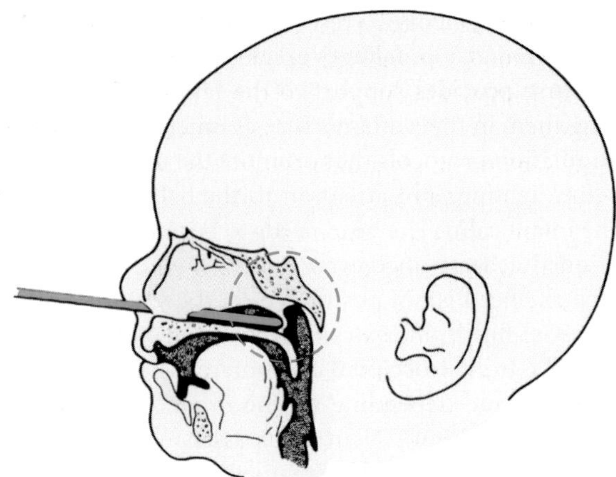

FIG 36-4 Choanal atresia. Posterior nares are obstructed by membrane or bone either bilaterally or unilaterally. Infant becomes cyanotic at rest. With crying, newborn's color improves. Nasal discharge is present. Snorting respirations often are observed with increased respiratory effort. Newborn may be unable to breathe and eat at the same time. Diagnosis is made by noting inability to pass small feeding tube through one or both nares. (Used with permission of Ross Products Division, Abbott Laboratories, Inc., Columbus, OH 43216. From Clinical Education Aid #6, Copyright 1963, Ross Products Division, Abbott Laboratories, Inc.)

is supportive. The parents will need support and education to help them learn to care for a child with cognitive impairment and developmental delays.

RESPIRATORY SYSTEM ANOMALIES

Screening for congenital anomalies of the respiratory system is necessary even in infants who are apparently normal at birth. Respiratory distress at birth or shortly thereafter can be the result of lung immaturity or anomalous development. Congenital laryngeal web and bilateral choanal atresia are readily apparent at birth. Respiratory distress caused by diaphragmatic hernia and tracheoesophageal fistula can appear immediately or be delayed, depending on the severity of the defect.

Laryngeal Web and Choanal Atresia

A laryngeal web, which is uncommon, results from the incomplete separation of the two sides of the larynx and is most often between the vocal cords. This is a surgical emergency such that perforation of the web using an endotracheal tube can be lifesaving. Choanal atresia (Fig. 36-4) is the most common congenital anomaly of the nose. The posterior nares can be blocked by a bony or soft-tissue obstruction. The obstruction can be unilateral or bilateral. The baby can display symptoms of respiratory distress and cyanosis or pallor that are relieved whenever the infant is crying. Inability to pass a suction catheter through the nose into the pharynx is highly suggestive of the diagnosis. Securing an oral airway into the posterior pharynx and maintaining the baby in the prone position will provide a patent airway and time to evaluate for the presence of other abnormalities. Definitive therapy involves creating a patency through the bony or soft-tissue obstruction and use of serial obturators to dilate the new airway passages (Sprecher & Arnold, 2011).

Congenital Diaphragmatic Hernia

Congenital diaphragmatic hernia (CDH) results from a defect in the formation of the diaphragm, allowing the abdominal organs to be displaced into the thoracic cavity. It occurs in approximately 1 in 2000 to 1 in 4000 live births, and despite improvements in care management, the mortality rate remains high, at about 35% (Congenital Diaphragmatic Hernia Study Group, 2013). The etiology is unknown; however, it is not uncommon to find concomitant chromosomal anomalies, especially trisomies 12, 18, and 21, as well as abnormalities of the gastrointestinal (GI), genitourinary, and central nervous systems. Intestinal malrotation is also associated with CDH. Approximately 70% of the hernias occur on the left side in the posterior diaphragm known as the foramen of Bochdalek (Haroon & Chamberlain, 2013). Poorer outcomes are associated with left-sided defects (Schaible, Kohl, Reinshagen, et al., 2012).

A small defect may not be detected on an early prenatal ultrasound. Fetuses with CDH tend to have polyhydramnios, which typically prompts the obstetrician to obtain an ultrasound. A major advantage of diagnosing CDH prenatally is that it allows the baby to be born in a tertiary hospital that is equipped to manage all the cardiorespiratory problems associated with the defect and to rapidly stabilize the neonate's precarious condition. CDH can be repaired by fetal surgery in some research institutions; however, intrauterine surgical correction of CDH has met with poor neonatal outcomes in many cases (Shue, Miniati, & Lee, 2012). When CDH is diagnosed antenatally the infant is usually intubated and ventilated immediately after birth and thereafter with the minimum amount of support necessary to achieve adequate ventilation (Haroon & Chamberlain, 2013).

Depending on the size of the defect and how much developed lung tissue is present, the neonate may not be in any significant distress at birth. A small defect can distress the infant when feeding such that symptoms of respiratory distress (tachypnea, pallor, mottled, cyanosis) become evident. Newborns with a large defect will have significant distress at birth because the viscera present in the thoracic cavity during embryonic life prevented the normal development of the lung (Fig. 36-5). Characteristic symptoms include respiratory distress, cyanosis, heart sounds shifted to the right, and low blood pressure. There will be increasing distress as the bowels fill with air. The abdomen is scaphoid shaped and the chest appears barrel shaped due to the abdominal contents being in the chest. Diagnosis can be made on the basis of the x-ray finding of loops of intestine in the thoracic cavity and the absence of intestine in the abdominal cavity.

Surgical repair is performed as soon as the infant is stable. Preoperative nursing interventions include participating in the stabilization of the infant's cardiopulmonary condition until surgical repair can be done. Inhaled nitric oxide (INO) has not been shown to improve long-term outcome in CDH but it may provide temporary benefit in treating the accompanying persistent pulmonary hypertension (Haroon & Chamberlain, 2013). Gastric contents are aspirated and suction applied to decompress the GI tract and prevent further cardiothoracic compromise. Oxygen therapy, mechanical ventilation, and the correction of acidosis are necessary in infants with large defects.

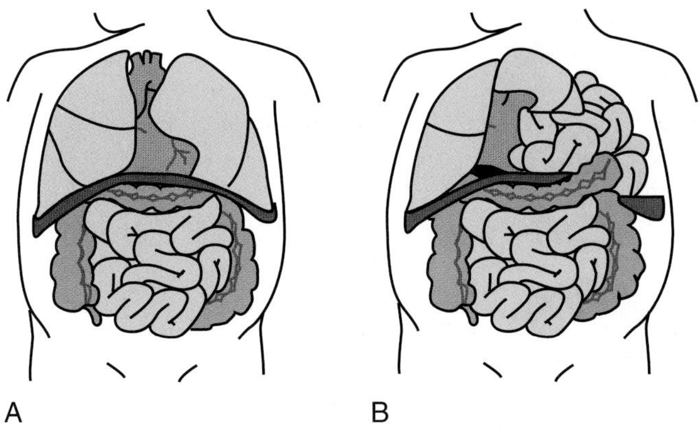

FIG 36-5 **A**, Normal diaphragm separating the abdominal and thoracic cavities. **B**, Diaphragmatic hernia with a small lung and abdominal contents in the thoracic cavity. (From Erlich P., & Coran, A. [2007]. Diaphragmatic hernia. In R. Kliegman, R. Behrman, H. Jenson, & B. Stanton [Eds.], *Nelson textbook of pediatrics* [18th ed.]. Philadelphia: Saunders.)

Pulmonary hypertension can occur as a result of the lung hypoplasia. Extracorporeal membrane oxygenation (ECMO) or high-frequency oscillatory ventilation can be used in infants with severe circulatory and respiratory complications (see Chapter 34) (Haroon & Chamberlain).

The prognosis depends largely on the degree of fetal pulmonary development and the success of surgical diaphragmatic closure, but the prognosis in severe cases is often poor. As a rule, finding the liver in the thorax is associated with the worst prognosis. Some infants with CDH die before they are able to have surgical repair. It is unclear whether the timing of the surgery or the condition of the infant at the time of repair is more important to improved outcomes. Overall survival rates have improved with the advent of INO, improved management of high-frequency ventilation, and ECMO. Of those who survive, some have chronic lung disease with long-term oxygen dependency, feeding difficulties, and gastroesophageal reflux (GER).

GASTROINTESTINAL SYSTEM ANOMALIES

Anomalies in the GI system can occur anywhere along the GI tract, from the mouth to the anus. Some anomalies, such as cleft lip, omphalocele, and gastroschisis, are apparent at birth. Others, including cleft palate, esophageal atresia, pyloric stenosis, intestinal obstructions, and imperforate anus, become apparent as the infant is further assessed or becomes symptomatic.

Cleft Lip and Palate

Orofacial clefts are among the most common congenital anomalies. Cleft lip or palate is a congenital midline fissure, or opening, in the lip or palate resulting from failure of the primary palate to fuse (Fig. 36-6). One or both deformities can occur, and nasal deformity can be present. Multiple genetic and, to a lesser extent, environmental factors (e.g., maternal infection, maternal smoking, radiation exposure, alcohol ingestion, and treatment with medications such as corticosteroids, lithium, retinoids, and phenytoin) appear to be involved in their development. Approximately one third of cases of cleft lip or palate are associated with a major anomaly such as Pierre Robin syndrome (Maarse, Rozendaal, Pajkrt, et al., 2012).

Cleft lip with or without cleft palate occurs in approximately 11 per 10,000 live births in the United States. Cleft palate alone occurs in 2651 births annually; 4437 babies are born each year with a cleft lip with or without a cleft palate (Parker et al., 2010). Canada has one of the highest prevalence rates of orofacial clefts in the world at 12.7 per 10,000 live births (Pavri & Forrest, 2013).

Cleft lip occurs more frequently than cleft palate. The defect can range from a simple notch in the lip to complete separation of the lip that extends to the floor of the nose. The treatment for a cleft lip is surgical repair, which usually is done by 12 weeks of age, if the infant is healthy and free of infection. Repair of a cleft palate is usually performed by 1 year of age in order to optimize speech development (Tinanoff, 2011). Advances in surgical techniques have made it possible for some infants, particularly those with unilateral cleft lip, to have a near-normal appearance. The results of the repair depend on the severity of the defect, with more severe bilateral cleft lip requiring surgical repair done in stages.

Anomalies of the palate often occur in association with cleft lip. Cleft palate alone is more common in female infants and occurs more frequently as a constituent of certain syndromes. This defect can range from a cleft in the uvula to a complete cleft of the hard and soft palates that can be unilateral, bilateral, or midline. Feeding is difficult because the cleft lip renders the newborn unable to maintain a seal around a nipple; the cleft palate renders the infant unable to form a vacuum to maintain suction when feeding. In addition, the inability to suck and swallow normally allows milk to pool in the nasopharynx, which increases the likelihood of aspiration. Furthermore, as the infant attempts to suck, milk often comes out through the cleft and the nares. Although the degree of difficulty depends on the size of the cleft, feeding problems are greater in infants with a cleft palate than in those with a cleft lip. Breastfeeding is often possible if the infant has a cleft lip alone. Bottle feeding can be successful in some infants. There are special nipples, bottles, and appliances available to aid in feeding. In general, parents of infants with these defects need education, support, and encouragement as they learn to feed their baby. This can help minimize anxiety and frustration while promoting competence and confidence in providing infant care.

Initial and ongoing care for children with orofacial defects involves the combined efforts of a multidisciplinary health care team that includes pediatrics, plastic surgery, orthodontics, otolaryngology, speech/language pathology, audiology, nursing, and social work. Repair of the defects can involve a series of surgical procedures to allow the child to have a near-normal appearance and function (Wilson, 2014).

Parents of infants with a cleft lip or palate need much support, particularly in the case of a cleft lip, because this is both a cosmetic and functional defect. Recognizing that this can interfere with normal parent-infant bonding in the neonatal period, the nurse must assess for this and intervene appropriately. Some communities have support groups for parents of children with orofacial clefts. Parents may also be referred to the following organizations for information and services: the American Cleft Palate-Craniofacial Association (www.acpa-cpf.org), the

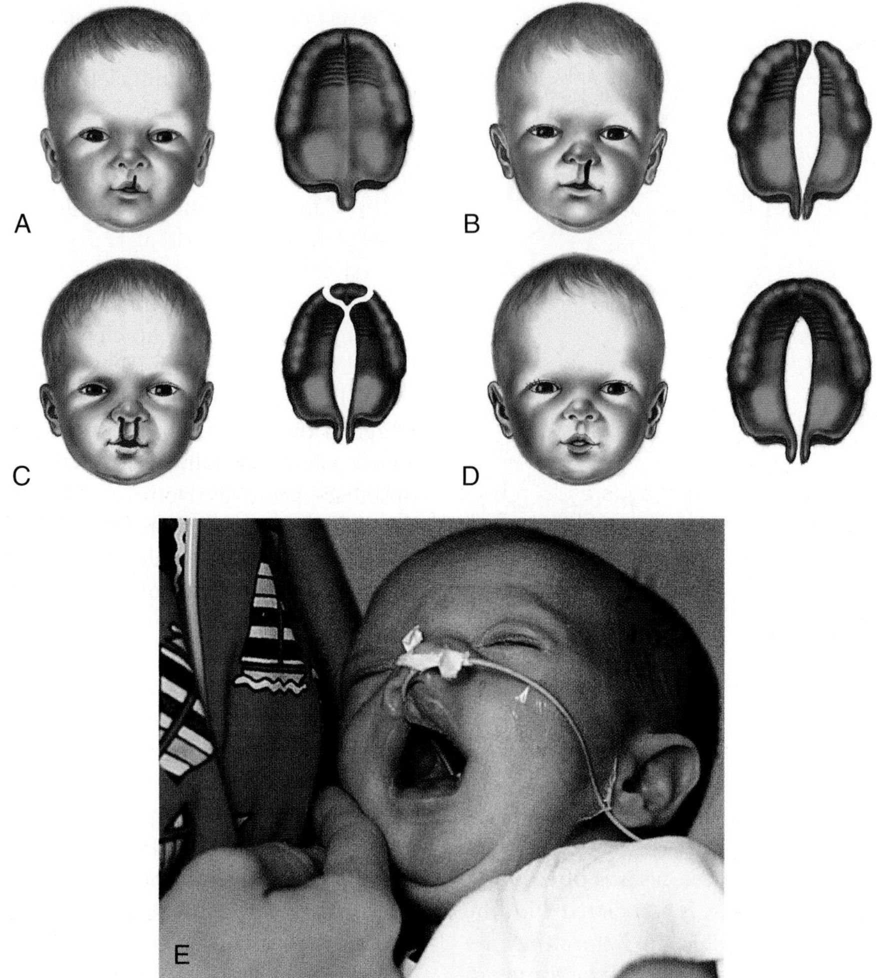

FIG 36-6 Variations in clefts of lip and palate at birth. **A,** Notch in vermilion border. **B,** Unilateral cleft lip and cleft palate. **C,** Bilateral cleft lip and cleft palate. **D,** Cleft palate. **E,** Infant with complete unilateral cleft lip. Note the feeding tube. (**A-D,** From Hockenberry, M., & Wilson, D. [2011]. *Wong's nursing care of infants and children* [9th ed.]. St. Louis: Mosby. **E,** From Dickason, E., Silverman, B., & Kaplan, J. [1998]. *Maternal-infant nursing care* [3rd ed.]. St. Louis: Mosby.)

Cleft Palate Foundation (www.cleftline.org), and the March of Dimes (www.marchforbabies.org).

CLINICAL REASONING CASE STUDY

Cleft Lip and Cleft Palate

Michael, a 3.7-kg (8.2-lb) Caucasian neonate, is admitted to the newborn nursery after an uncomplicated vaginal birth. At birth Michael was noted to have a unilateral cleft lip and a cleft palate. Physical examination reveals no other congenital abnormalities, and Michael is otherwise vigorous and healthy.

1. Evidence—What factors have been linked to the development of cleft lip and palate?
2. Assumptions—What assumptions can be made about the following items?
   a. The immediate plan of care for Michael after a diagnosis of cleft lip and palate
   b. The ability for Michael's mother to breastfeed her son
   c. The effect of having an infant with a congenital disorder
   d. The trajectory of Michael's treatment
3. What implications and priorities for nursing care can be made at this time?
4. Does the evidence objectively support your conclusion?

Esophageal Atresia and Tracheoesophageal Fistula

Esophageal atresia (EA) and tracheoesophageal fistula (TEF), the most life-threatening anomalies of the esophagus, typically occur together, although they can occur singly. More than 1 in 4000 infants are born with EA and more than 90% also have TEF (Khan & Orenstein, 2011).

Esophageal atresia is a congenital anomaly in which the esophagus ends in a blind pouch, thus failing to form a continuous passageway to the stomach. TEF is an abnormal connection between the esophagus and the trachea. The most common variant is the combination of a proximal EA, in which the esophagus ends in a blind pouch, with a distal TEF, in which the lower esophagus exits the stomach and is connected to the trachea by a fistula, rather than forming a continuous tube to the upper esophagus (Fig. 36-7). Variations of the anomalies are possible, depending on the presence or absence of a TEF, the site of the fistula, and the location and degree of the esophageal obstruction.

The presence of a midline defect such as EA or TEF is often accompanied by another significant embryonic defect such as a cardiac anomaly; cleft lip and/or palate; or vertebral,

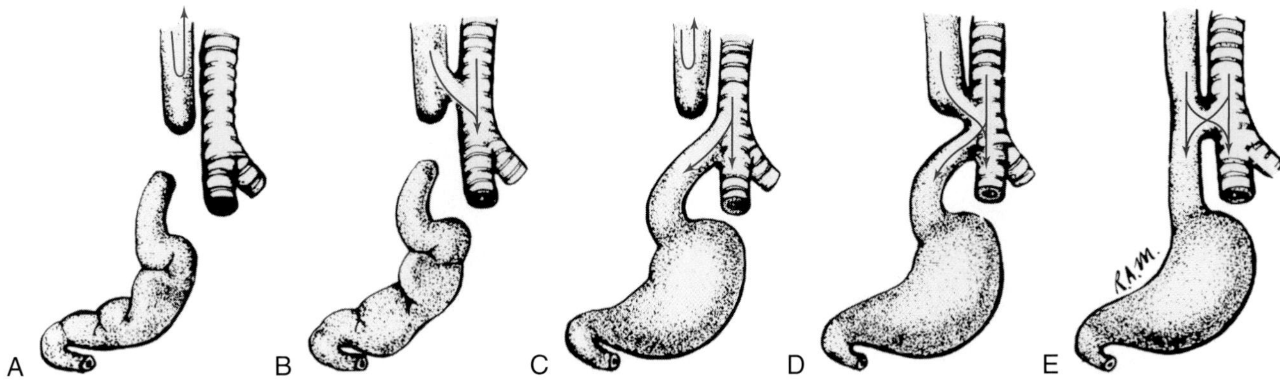

FIG 36-7 Congenital atresia of esophagus and tracheoesophageal fistula. **A,** Upper and lower segments of esophagus end in blind sac, occurring in 5% to 8% of such infants. **B,** Upper segment of esophagus ends in atresia and connects to trachea by fistulous tract, occurring rarely. **C,** Upper segment of esophagus ends in blind pouch; lower segment connects with trachea by small fistulous tract, occurring in 80% to 95% of such infants. **D,** Both segments of esophagus connect by fistulous tracts to trachea, occurring in less than 1% of such infants. Infant may aspirate with first feeding. **E,** Esophagus is continuous but connects by fistulous tract to trachea; known as *H-type*. (From Hockenberry, M., & Wilson, D. [2011]. *Wong's nursing care of infants and children* [9th ed.]. St. Louis: Mosby.)

genitourinary, or abdominal wall defect (Lovvorn, Glenn, Pacetti, & Carter, 2011). The affected infant who is preterm or small for gestational age typically has other malformations such that a good outcome is not expected.

The defect can be diagnosed prenatally. A small or absent stomach can be detected during a fetal ultrasound. There is usually a history of polyhydramnios because the fetus is unable to swallow the amniotic fluid. At birth the clinical presentation depends on the type of anomaly present. Infants with the life-threatening anomaly EA with TEF show significant respiratory difficulty immediately after birth. Esophageal atresia with or without TEF results in excessive oral secretions, drooling, and feeding intolerance. When fed, the infant may swallow but then cough and gag and return the fluid through the nose and mouth. Respiratory distress can result from aspiration or from the acute gastric distention produced by the TEF. Choking, coughing, and cyanosis occur after even a small amount of fluid is taken by mouth.

SAFETY ALERT

Any infant with excessive oral secretions and respiratory distress should not be fed orally until a physician is consulted.

Nursing interventions are supportive until surgery is performed. The infant with EA and TEF should be kept in a supine position with the head of the bed elevated about 30 degrees to facilitate respiratory efforts and prevent reflux and aspiration of gastric contents. Antireflux and antacid medication may be given to minimize gastroesophageal reflux (GER) and prevent acid-induced pneumonitis. An orogastric tube (Replogle tube) is placed in the proximal esophageal pouch and attached to low continuous suction to remove secretions and decrease the possibility of aspiration (Lovvorn et al., 2011). The infant requires close observation and intervention to maintain a patent airway. Other supportive measures include thermoregulation, maintaining fluid and electrolyte balance intravenously as well as acid-base balance, and preventing any further complications as a result of an associated defect. Surgical correction, done in one stage if possible, consists of ligating the fistula and anastomosing the two segments of the esophagus. The chances for survival in these infants depends on the presence of associated defects and the infant's birth weight. Preterm infants with cardiac or chromosomal anomalies have the highest mortality rate. Many infants with EA and TEF will have postoperative issues related to feeding difficulties such as GER and esophageal strictures requiring periodic dilation (Barksdale, Chwals, Magnuson, & Parry, 2011).

Omphalocele and Gastroschisis

Omphalocele and gastroschisis are two of the more common congenital defects of the abdominal wall. Omphalocele occurs in approximately 2 of every 10,000 live births, whereas the prevalence of gastroschisis is nearly 5 in 10,000 live births (Parker et al., 2010). An **omphalocele** is a covered defect of the umbilical ring into which varying amounts of the abdominal organs can herniate (Fig. 36-8, *A*). The peritoneal sac covering the defect can rupture during or after birth. Many of the infants born with an omphalocele are preterm and nearly 50% have an underlying chromosomal abnormality, usually trisomy 12, 18, or 21. Congenital heart defects are often associated with omphalocele (Lovvorn et al., 2011).

Gastroschisis is the herniation of the bowel through a defect in the abdominal wall to the right of the umbilical cord (see Fig. 36-8, *B*). No membrane covers the contents as it does with an omphalocele. The incidence of gastroschisis is increasing worldwide and is three to four times more common than omphalocele. Gastroschisis is not usually associated with other major congenital anomalies or syndromes. Intestinal atresia can occur with gastroschisis (Lovvorn et al., 2011).

The preoperative nursing care is similar for infants with either defect. Exposure of the viscera causes problems with thermoregulation and fluid and electrolyte balance. Immediately after birth, the neonate's torso should be placed in an

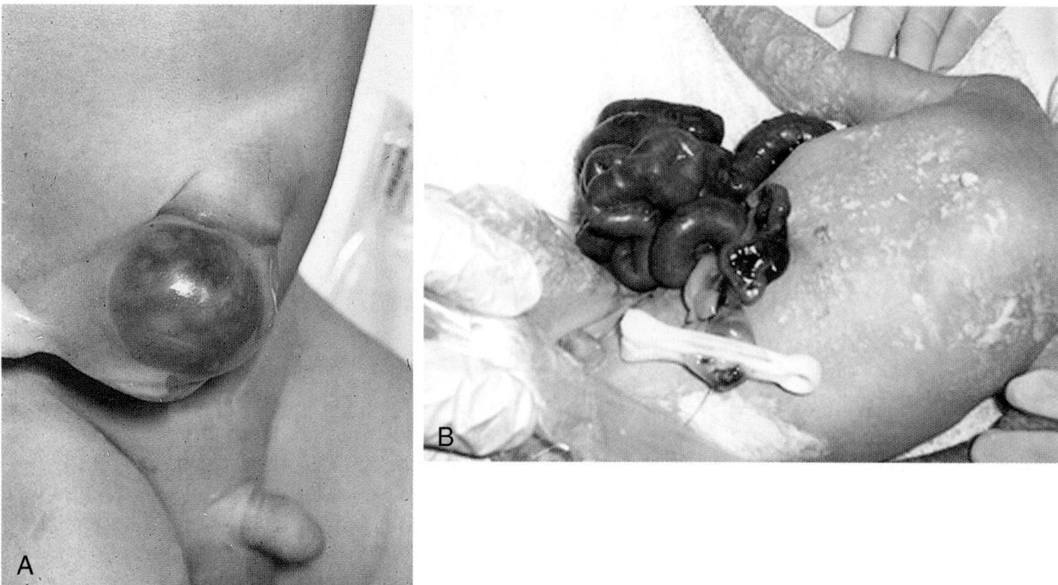

FIG 36-8 **A,** Omphalocele. **B,** Gastroschisis of bowel and stomach. (**A,** From O'Doherty, N. [1986]. *Neonatology: Micro atlas of the newborn.* Nutley, NJ: Hoffmann-La Roche; **B,** courtesy Cheryl Briggs, RNC, Annapolis, MD.)

impermeable, clear plastic bowel bag to decrease insensible water losses, maintain thermoregulation, and prevent contamination of the exposed viscera. It is essential that the nurse assesses the exposed viscera frequently to detect any changes in perfusion to the exposed abdominal contents. The infant should be placed in a side-lying position and the viscera supported with a blanket roll to prevent vascular compromise to a torqued intestine. Prior to surgery the exposed viscera should be kept covered with sterile moistened saline gauze and plastic wrap. Gastric decompression with a Replogle tube (a special type of gastric tube) connected to low intermittent wall suction is also necessary to prevent aspiration pneumonia and to allow as much bowel as possible to be placed into the abdomen during surgery. Antibiotics, fluid and electrolyte replacement, and thermoregulation are needed for physiologic support (Lovvorn et al., 2011; Wilson, 2014).

Surgery is usually performed soon after birth. If complete closure is impossible because of the small size of the defect and the large amount of viscera to be replaced, a Silastic silo or patch is placed. This protects the contents as they are gradually placed back into the abdominal cavity and minimizes symptoms of respiratory distress as the increasing intraabdominal pressure pushes against the diaphragm. The defect is closed surgically after the exposed visceral contents have been reduced; this reduction process usually takes 7 to 10 days. The prognosis depends on the size of the defect and the presence of associated anomalies. It is generally expected that there will be complications related to intestinal dysfunction, such as feeding difficulties, dysmotility, or short-gut syndrome if a substantial amount of the intestine was removed.

Parental support is essential because the infant has an obvious disfiguring anomaly that can be shocking and repulsive in appearance. Depending on the size of the defect, the infant can also be critically ill before surgery. The nurse must be aware of the effect this can have on parental bonding and intervene appropriately as the parents cope with this crisis.

Gastrointestinal Obstruction

Congenital intestinal obstruction can occur anywhere in the GI tract and takes one of the following forms: atresia, which is a complete obliteration of the passage; partial obstruction, in which the symptoms can vary in severity and sometimes are not detected in the neonatal period; or malrotation of the intestine, which leads to twisting of the intestine (volvulus) and obstruction. Esophageal atresia, discussed previously, is a type of GI obstruction. Duodenal atresia, midgut malrotation and volvulus, jejunoileal atresia, necrotizing enterocolitis, and meconium ileus are the most common causes of neonatal intestinal obstruction. Meconium ileus is an obstruction caused by impacted meconium; more than 90% of infants who are born with meconium ileus have cystic fibrosis (Lovvorn et al., 2011).

GI obstruction may be suspected when polyhydramnios is present during pregnancy. It can be detected in the fetus through the use of prenatal ultrasound imaging (Song, Upperman, & Niklas, 2011).

Signs of neonatal intestinal obstruction occur early. The neonate with an intestinal obstruction displays the following cardinal signs: bilious vomiting, abdominal distention, and failure to pass normal amounts of meconium in the first 24 hours. High intestinal obstruction is characterized by vomiting, even if the infant is not being fed orally. Distention usually indicates a low obstruction, with vomiting occurring later. Abdominal distention can elevate the diaphragm, which can cause respiratory difficulties (Song et al., 2011).

Nursing care is aimed at supporting the infant until surgical intervention can be carried out to eliminate the obstruction. Oral feedings are withheld, an orogastric tube is placed to low intermittent wall suction, and intravenous therapy is initiated to provide needed fluid and electrolytes. In infants with an intestinal obstruction, surgery consists of resecting the obstructed area of bowel and anastomosing the nonaffected bowel or creating an ostomy and allowing the bowel to rest.

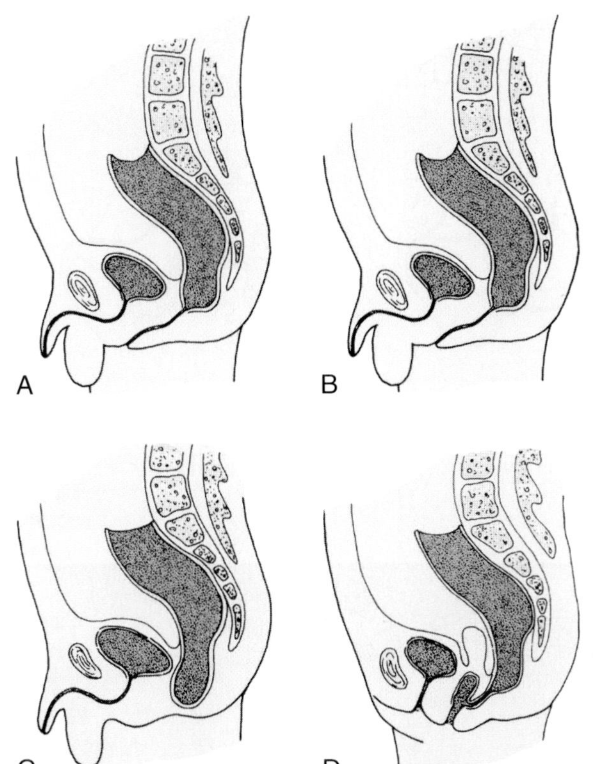

FIG 36-9 Types of anorectal malformations (imperforate anus). Anal sphincter muscle may be present and intact. **A,** High lesion opening onto perineum through narrow fistulous tract. **B,** High lesion ending in fistulous tract to urinary tract. **C,** Low lesion in bowel passes through puborectal muscle. **D,** High lesion ending in fistulous tract to vagina.

Anorectal Malformations

Anorectal malformations, or imperforate anus, include a range of congenital defects involving the anus, rectum, and genitourinary system (Fig. 36-9). These anomalies are relatively common, with an incidence of approximately 1 in 4000 to 5000 live births (Barksdale et al., 2011). Occurring more in male than in female infants, they result from the failure of the urogenital sinus and cloaca to differentiate during weeks 7 and 8 of gestational life (Blackburn, 2013). Such infants have no anal opening, and commonly there is also a fistula from the rectum to the perineum or genitourinary system. Types of anorectal malformations include the typical cloaca (fistula) in females, which involves the vagina, colon, and urethra forming a single common passage in the perineum. Others include the low rectovaginal fistula (female) and rectourethral bulbar fistula (male). Imperforate anus can occur in isolation or in combination with other congenital defects such as esophageal atresia, duodenal atresia, renal anomalies, or vertebral anomalies. Extensive surgical repair is often required in stages for the more complex types of anorectal malformations. Infants with high imperforate anus typically have bowel incontinence even after surgical repair. In some cases the anomaly involves stenotic areas, or a thin translucent membrane can cover the anal opening. Treatment for such a membrane is anoplasty followed by daily dilation, which parents learn to do. The preoperative nursing care is similar to that described for other GI obstructions. Imperforate anus is often associated with other anomalies, with nearly half having additional genitourinary anomalies, which can complicate long-term care. Outcome is excellent with low imperforate anus (Gourlay, 2013).

MUSCULOSKELETAL SYSTEM ANOMALIES

The two most common musculoskeletal system anomalies in neonates are developmental dysplasia of the hip (DDH) and congenital clubfoot. Both of these conditions must be detected and treated early for successful correction.

Developmental Dysplasia of the Hip

The broad term developmental dysplasia of the hip describes a spectrum of disorders related to abnormal development of one or all of the components of the hip joint that can develop at any time during fetal life, infancy, or childhood. A change in terminology from congenital hip dysplasia and congenital dislocation of the hip to DDH more accurately reflects a variety of hip abnormalities in which there is a shallow acetabulum, subluxation, or dislocation.

Although as many as 1 in 100 to 1 in 250 infants have some degree of hip instability, the prevalence of DDH is approximately 1 to 1.5 per 1000 live births (Sankar, Horn, Wells, & Dormans, 2011). Prevalence of DDH is variable across populations, which may be related to genetic and environmental factors. It is rare among African infants and more common among ethnic groups such as Navajo Indians and those from other countries who traditionally swaddle infants with legs extended and hips adducted (Bracken, Tran, & Ditchfield, 2012). The etiology is unknown and believed to be multifactorial. Certain factors such as sex, birth order, family history, intrauterine position, birth type, joint laxity, and postnatal positioning are believed to affect the risk of DDH. Predisposing factors associated with DDH can be divided into three broad categories: (1) physiologic factors, which include female sex and maternal hormone secretion causing pelvic relaxation during birth, and intrauterine positioning; (2) mechanical factors such as breech presentation, multiple gestation, oligohydramnios, and large infant size; other mechanical factors can include continued maintenance of the hips in adduction and extension that will in time cause a dislocation; and (3) genetic factors, including a family history of DDH and generalized ligamentous laxity (Sankar et al., 2011). Figure 36-10 illustrates the three degrees of DDH, which are described as follows.

- *Acetabular dysplasia (or preluxation)*—mildest form of DDH in which there is neither subluxation nor dislocation. There is a delay in acetabular development evidenced by osseous hypoplasia of the acetabular roof that is oblique and shallow, although the cartilaginous roof is comparatively intact. The femoral head remains in the acetabulum; 80% of mild cases of DDH resolve spontaneously (Price & Ramo, 2012).
- *Subluxation*—accounts for the largest percentage of DDH. Subluxation implies incomplete dislocation of the hip and is sometimes regarded as an intermediate state in the development from primary dysplasia to complete dislocation. The femoral head remains in contact with the acetabulum, but a stretched capsule and ligamentum teres cause the head of the femur to be partially displaced. Pressure on the cartilaginous roof inhibits ossification and produces a flattened socket.

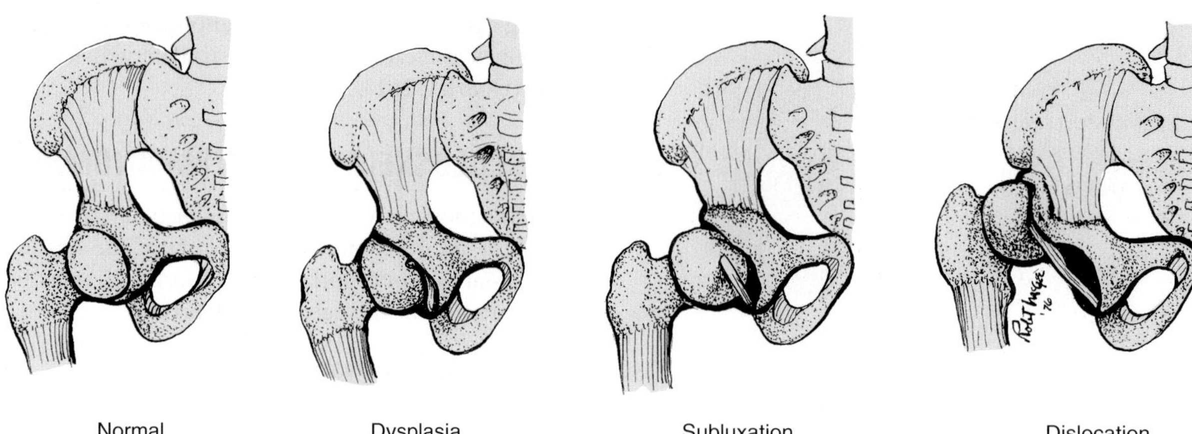

FIG 36-10 Configuration and relationship of structures in developmental dysplasia of the hip.

- *Dislocation*—The femoral head loses contact with the acetabulum and is displaced posteriorly and superiorly over the fibrocartilaginous rim. The ligamentum teres is elongated and taut. DDH is often not detected at the initial examination after birth; thus all infants should be carefully monitored for hip dysplasia at follow-up visits throughout the first year of life. In the newborn period, dysplasia usually appears as hip joint laxity rather than as outright dislocation. Subluxation and the tendency to dislocate can be demonstrated by the Ortolani or Barlow tests. The Ortolani and Barlow tests are most reliable from birth to 2 or 3 months of age (see Fig. 23-11). Other signs of DDH are shortening of the limb on the affected side (Galeazzi sign, Allis sign), asymmetric thigh and gluteal folds, and broadening of the perineum (in bilateral dislocation). In some countries screening programs using ultrasound evaluation of infants with risk factors for DDH have been instituted; however, evidence supporting the efficacy of these programs is limited (Bracken et al., 2012).

SAFETY ALERT

The Ortolani and Barlow tests must be performed by an experienced clinician to prevent fracture or other damage to the hip.

Treatment is begun as soon as the condition is recognized because early intervention is more favorable to the restoration of normal bony architecture and function. The longer treatment is delayed, the more severe the deformity, the more difficult the treatment, and the less favorable the prognosis. The treatment varies with the age of the infant and the extent of the dysplasia. The goal of treatment is to obtain and maintain a safe, congruent position of the hip joint to promote normal hip joint development and ambulation.

The hip joint is maintained by dynamic splinting in a safe position with the proximal femur centered in the acetabulum in an attitude of flexion and abduction. Of the numerous devices available, the Pavlik harness (Fig. 36-11) is the most widely used, and with time, motion, and gravity, the hip works into a more abducted, reduced position. The harness is worn continually until the hip is proved stable on clinical and radiographic examination, typically around 3 months. It has an 80% success rate for the treatment of classic DDH. If not effective, traction, casting, and even surgery may be necessary to stabilize the hip (Bracken et al., 2012).

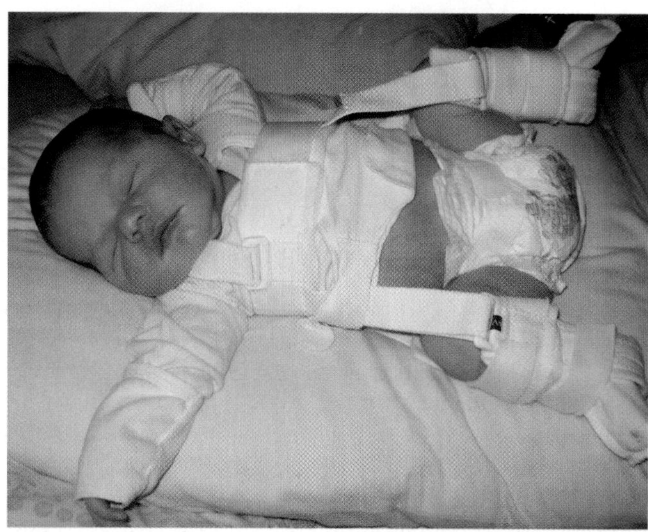

FIG 36-11 Infant in Pavlik harness. (Courtesy Amanda Politte, St. Louis, MO.)

SAFETY ALERT

The former practice of double- or triple-diapering for DDH is not recommended because it promotes hip extension, thus interfering with proper hip development.

In addition to the major intervention of assessing and helping identify the disorder, another key nursing intervention is teaching the parents about the care of the infant because he or she will remain in the harness continually during the treatment. Because the harness is worn during a time of maximal growth, it is necessary for the parents to adjust the infant's care to accommodate the infant's changing needs. The infant can develop brachial plexus palsy due to increased tension of the shoulder harness if the harness is not modified according to the neonate's growth. Thorough and ongoing follow-up care is necessary, as is psychosocial support for the family.

Clubfoot

Congenital clubfoot is a deformity of the foot and ankle that includes forefoot adduction, midfoot supination, hindfoot varus, and ankle equinus. Deformities of the foot and ankle are described according to the position of the ankle and foot. The more common positions involve the following variations:

- *Talipes varus*—an inversion or a bending inward
- *Talipes valgus*—an eversion or bending outward
- *Talipes equinus*—plantar flexion in which the toes are lower than the heel
- *Talipes calcaneus*—dorsiflexion, in which the toes are higher than the heel

Most cases of clubfoot are a combination of these positions. The most frequently occurring type is the composite deformity *talipes equinovarus* (TEV). In this abnormality the foot appears C-shaped, pointing downward and inward; the ankle is inverted; and the Achilles tendon is shortened. The foot appears small, wide, and stiff, and the lower leg appears small because of hypoplasia of the calf muscles. Unless treated, further stiffening occurs, and bony changes will result. Unilateral clubfoot is somewhat more common than bilateral clubfoot and can occur as an isolated defect or in association with other disorders or syndromes, such as chromosomal aberrations, arthrogryposis (a generalized immobility of the joint), cerebral palsy, or spina bifida.

Clubfoot is classified as positional or congenital. A positional clubfoot was held in a deformed position in utero and is flexible when manipulated during examination. A congenital clubfoot is structural, is more rigid, and has a wide range of severity. Clubfoot is one of the most common congenital anomalies, occurring in approximately 1 in 1000 live births, with two times more male than female infants affected. Bilateral defects occur in 50% of cases. The etiology is thought to be multifactorial and can involve a genetic predisposition, chromosomal anomalies, abnormalities of the uterine environment, and neuromuscular pathologies (Hosalkar, Spiegel, & Davidson, 2011). Treatment is initiated soon after birth and most often involves serial casting. Successive casts allow for gradual stretching of skin and tight structures on the medial side of the foot. Manipulation and casting are repeated frequently (every week) to accommodate the rapid growth of early infancy. The extremity or extremities are often casted or splinted until maximum correction is achieved, usually within 8 to 12 weeks. If needed, surgical correction is done before the infant begins to walk (Hosalkar et al.).

Because these infants are often placed in a cast before discharge, the nurse must teach parents necessary care, including how to protect the cast and assess the toes for neurovascular compromise. This is particularly important because of the potential for the infant to outgrow the cast. The nurse should be supportive of the parents as they learn the ways to meet the infant's normal needs, as well as those brought about by the infant's physical problem.

Polydactyly

Occasionally an infant is born with extra digits on the hands or feet. In some instances, *polydactyly* is hereditary. If there is little or no bone involvement, the extra digit is tied with silk suture soon after birth. The finger or toe falls off within a few days, leaving a small scar. When there is bone involvement, surgical repair is indicated.

GENITOURINARY SYSTEM ANOMALIES

Anomalies involving the genitourinary system can be distressing to parents because they can be readily apparent and, in the case of some conditions, because of the concern about sexuality and reproductive functioning. These anomalies range from obvious anomalies of the external genitalia, such as hypospadias, to those involving internal organs that are not obvious but can cause damage to the urinary tract. An example of the latter is an obstruction in the urinary tract that can cause hydronephrosis, which is the abnormal collection of urine in the renal pelvis that can eventually destroy the kidney.

Hypospadias and Epispadias

The term *hypospadias* encompasses a range of penile anomalies associated with an abnormally located urinary meatus. The meatus can open below the glans penis or anywhere along the ventral surface of the penis, the scrotum, or the perineum. It is one of the most common congenital anomalies, occurring in approximately 3 to 5 per 1000 births (Canon, Mosley, Chipollini, et al., 2012). Hypospadias is classified according to the location of the meatus and the presence or absence of chordee, which is a ventral curvature of the penis (Figs. 36-12 and 36-13). The cause is unknown, although it is thought to be of multifactorial inheritance.

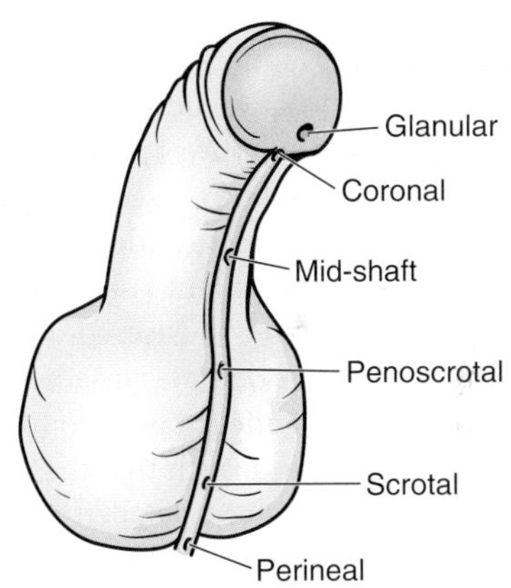

FIG 36-12 Classification of hypospadias by position of the urethral meatus.

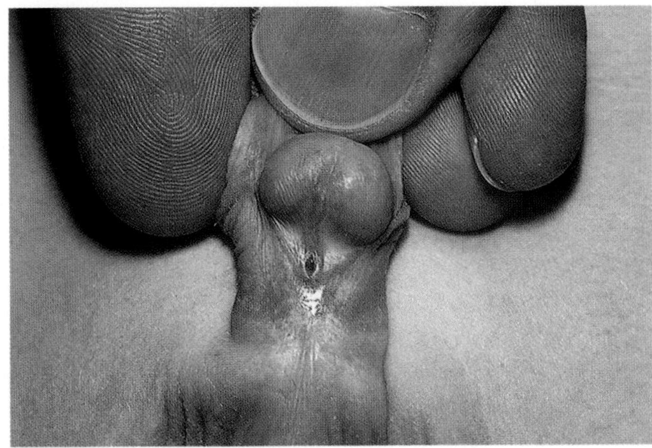

FIG 36-13 Hypospadias. (Courtesy H. Gil Rushton, MD, Children's National Medical Center, Washington, DC.)

Mild cases of hypospadias are often repaired for cosmetic reasons and involve a single surgical procedure. In more severe cases, several surgeries are required to reconstruct the urethral opening and correct the chordee, thereby straightening the penis. The goals are to improve the appearance of the genitalia, make it possible for the child to urinate in a standing position, and have a sexually adequate organ. These infants are not circumcised because the foreskin may be needed during surgical repair. Repair is done early, between 1 and 2 years of age, so that the child's body image is not impaired (Steven, Cherian, Yankovic, et al., 2013). There is a correlation between hypospadias and testicular cancer and also with cryptorchidism; therefore, children with a history of hypospadias require long-term follow-up (Serrano, Chevrier, Multigner, et al., 2013).

Epispadias, a rare anomaly, results from failure of urethral canalization. The affected infants are males who have a widened pubic symphysis and a broad spadelike penis with the urethral opening on the dorsal surface. In females there is a wide urethra and a bifid clitoris. Severity ranges from a mild anomaly to a severe one that is associated with exstrophy of the bladder. Surgical correction is necessary, and affected male infants should not be circumcised (Elder, 2011).

Exstrophy of the Bladder

The most common bladder anomaly is exstrophy (Fig. 36-14), which often occurs in conjunction with epispadias. It is rare, occurring in approximately 2 in 100,000 live births, and males are affected twice as often as females (Siffel, Correa, Amar, et al., 2011). It results from the abnormal development of the bladder, abdominal wall, and pubic symphysis that causes the bladder, urethra, and ureteral orifices to be exposed. The bladder is visible in the suprapubic area as a red mass with numerous folds, with urine draining from it onto the infant's skin. Immediately after birth the exposed bladder should be covered with a sterile, nonadherent dressing to protect its delicate surface until closure can be performed. It is recommended that reconstructive surgery be started in the neonatal period, such that the bladder is closed within 48 hours. Parents will need detailed instructions along with support and encouragement as they deal with caring for an infant who has such an obvious defect. Repair is completed before school age, if possible, although some children never attain normal voiding patterns and later may be considered for surgery for urinary diversion.

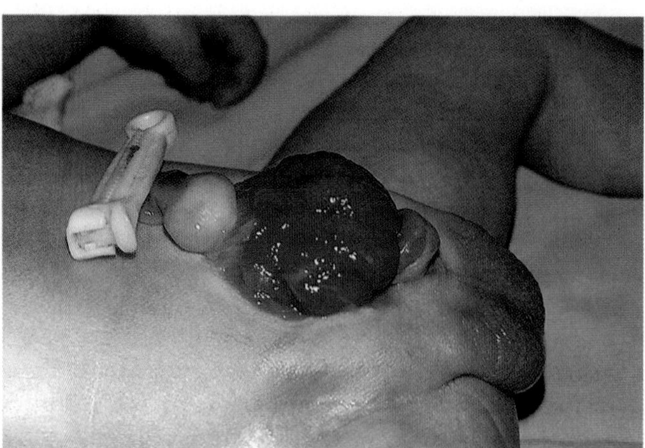

FIG 36-14 Exstrophy of bladder. (Courtesy H. Gil Rushton, MD, Children's National Medical Center, Washington, DC.)

Ambiguous Genitalia

The nurse is often the one to discover ambiguous genitalia in the newborn (Fig. 36-15) during a physical assessment. Erroneous or abnormal sexual differentiation can be a genetic aberration, such as congenital adrenal hyperplasia, which can be life threatening because it involves the deficiency of all adrenal cortical hormones. Other possible causes of sexual ambiguity include chromosomal abnormalities, defective sex hormone synthesis in male infants, and the placental transfer of masculinizing agents to female fetuses. Diagnosis should be based on data gathered from the following sources: maternal and family history, including the ingestion of steroids during pregnancy, and relatives with ambiguous genitalia or who died during the neonatal period; physical examination; chromosomal analysis; endoscopy, ultrasonography, and radiographic contrast studies; biochemical tests, such as analysis of urinary steroid excretion, which helps detect several of the adrenal cortical syndromes; and, in some instances, laparotomy or gonad biopsy.

Assessment and management of a newborn with ambiguous genitalia require urgency and sensitivity. Therapeutic intervention, including any counseling and surgery, should be started as soon as possible. Care is best managed by a multidisciplinary team consisting of the primary physician, pediatric endocrinologist, geneticist, surgeon, social worker, and nurses. An infant born with ambiguous genitalia should not receive a sex assignment until diagnostic testing provides enough information for a well-informed decision (Lee & Houk, 2013).

An appropriate gender assignment should be based on the following: diagnosis, genital development and surgical options, cultural pressures, most likely adult gender identity, potential for mature sexual function, potential fertility, and the long-term psychologic and intellectual effect on the child and family

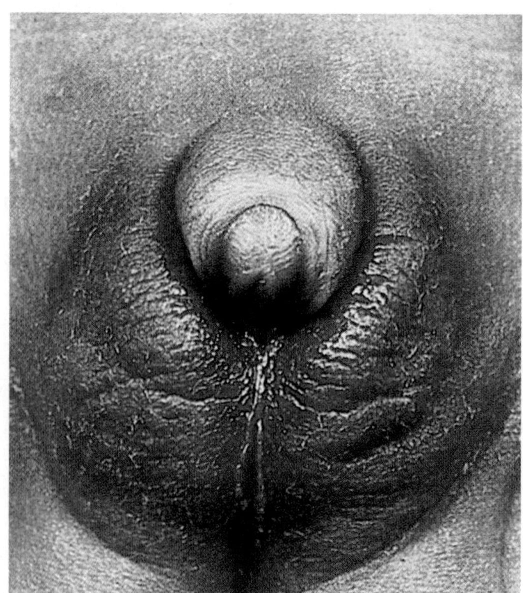

FIG 36-15 Ambiguous external genitals (i.e., structure can be enlarged clitoral hood and clitoris or malformed penis). (Courtesy Edward S. Tank, MD, Division of Urology, Oregon Health Science University, Portland.)

(Lee & Houk, 2013). Parents need much support as they learn to deal with this very challenging situation.

INBORN ERRORS OF METABOLISM

Congenital defects of the metabolic and endocrine systems can be identified during fetal development but more often are not apparent until after birth. Although there are numerous disorders resulting from defects in these systems, the discussion focuses on selected disorders that can be identified during routine newborn screening.

Inborn errors of metabolism (IEMs) are biochemical genetic disorders that result from defects in single genes; the majority of disorders are inherited as autosomal recessive conditions (Cederbaum, 2012). The genetic defect causes a blockage in a critical metabolic pathway. There can be absence of an essential enzyme resulting in accumulation of precursors preceding a blocked step in a metabolic pathway. The defect can also result in a deficiency of a critical metabolic product (Stokowski, 2014). IEMs encompass a wide variety of disorders including defects of amino acid, carbohydrate, and organic acid metabolism; lysosomal storage disorders; energy metabolism disorders; and disorders of purine metabolism (Cederbaum).

The majority of infants with an IEM appear normal at birth. However, the presence of other congenital anomalies should not rule out the possibility of an IEM (Matthews & Robin, 2011). Signs of an IEM may not be evident until after the infant has consumed several feedings. Some infants exhibit nonspecific signs of IEMs such as feeding problems or respiratory distress. Signs of an IEM can resemble those of sepsis. Infants can present with more acute signs of an IEM such as hypoglycemia, lethargy, seizures, metabolic acidosis or respiratory alkalosis, or cardiac arrhythmias (Cederbaum, 2012).

Diagnostic testing for IEMs is often ordered when other explanations for an infant's symptoms are not satisfactory. For example, if a neonate demonstrates signs of sepsis but testing fails to confirm the diagnosis, the provider may proceed with diagnostic measures for a metabolic disorder. Initial testing includes a broad range of blood and urine tests that are not diagnostic for IEMs but instead serve as screening measures. Further testing is required to confirm the diagnosis of an IEM, and a metabolic specialist is often involved. Biochemical studies for specific IEMs may only be performed by specialized laboratories that require compliance with very specific guidelines for collecting, storing, and shipping tissue samples (Matthews & Robins, 2011).

It is critical that IEMs are identified as early as possible. When IEMs are undiagnosed and untreated, infants can suffer severe consequences such as cognitive impairment or even death. Presymptomatic identification of many IEMs is possible through routine newborn screening (see Chapter 24). Tandem mass spectrometry allows for identification of more than 50 IEMs from a single blood spot. Newborn screening for specific IEMs varies from state to state. The screening test is most reliable if the sample is collected at least 24 hours after the infant has been feeding; if the sample is collected before 24 hours, a repeat test is done before the age of 2 weeks. This is only a screening test; positive results warrant further testing (Matthews & Robin, 2011).

Care of an infant who has an IEM is managed by a health care team including neonatal and pediatric providers, metabolic and genetic specialists, nutritionists, and nursing staff. If the infant is hospitalized when the diagnosis is made, all protein sources are eliminated, including feedings and amino acid solutions. IV solutions of 10% glucose and electrolytes are administered until a specific diagnosis is made. Supportive care includes correction of volume and electrolyte imbalances, hypoglycemia, and metabolic acidosis. Neonates may be transferred to regional referral centers for further treatment. In severe cases, hemodialysis, ECMO, or even liver transplant may be needed (Stokowski, 2014).

Phenylketonuria (PKU) is an amino acid disorder that results from a deficiency of the enzyme phenylalanine dehydrogenase (see Chapter 3), which is needed to metabolize the essential amino acid phenylalanine. Classic PKU is one among a spectrum of disorders known as hyperphenylalaninemia; severity varies according to the degree of enzyme deficiency. This deficiency can cause elevated levels of phenylalanine that result in CNS damage. Severe effects of PKU are rare because of early recognition through newborn screening (Blackburn, 2013). The test for PKU is not reliable, however, until the newborn has ingested adequate amounts of breast milk or formula.

! NURSING ALERT

The nurse must document the initial ingestion of milk. The test for PKU is performed at least 24 hours after that time.

The prevalence of classic PKU in the United States is approximately 1 in 11,400 live births (Hertzberg, Hinton, Therrell, & Shapira, 2011). Incidence varies widely across ethnic groups. PKU is rare among African nations; the highest incidence is in Turkey (Cleary, 2011).

If the infant has PKU, treatment includes a diet low in protein plus the addition of a special amino acid–containing formula that does not contain phenylalanine. Despite compliance with treatment, many affected children have some degree of cognitive impairment. Successful management and outcome are largely dependent on early identification of the condition, modifying the diet, and compliance with the treatment regimen throughout life (Viau, Wengreen, Ernst, et al., 2011).

Galactosemia, caused by a deficiency of the enzyme galactose 1-phosphate uridyltransferase, results in the inability to convert galactose to glucose. Galactosemia can be detected by measuring the blood levels of galactose in the urine of newborns suspected of having the disease who have ingested formula containing galactose. Early symptoms are vomiting, weight loss, persistent jaundice, and CNS symptoms, including poor feeding, drowsiness, and seizures (Sulchy & Kerkar, 2012). *Escherichia coli* sepsis occurs in a large number of affected infants. If the disorder goes untreated, the galactose levels continue to increase, and the affected infant shows failure to thrive, developmental delay, cataracts, jaundice, hepatomegaly, and cirrhosis of the liver, with death possibly occurring in the first month of life. Therapy consists of eliminating galactose from the diet. Breastfeeding is contraindicated because lactose is present in breast milk (Lawrence, 2013).

Congenital hypothyroidism results from a deficiency of thyroid hormones and can be permanent (requires treatment for life) or transient (spontaneously resolves). It is the most common endocrine disorder found in neonates, with an incidence of 1 in 4000 births (Clause, 2013; Grüters & Krude, 2011). It can be caused by a single gene defect or familial autoimmune factors; however, in the majority of causes, it is caused by a nonfamilial embryogenic defect. Congenital hypothyroidism affects female infants twice as often as males (Blackburn, 2013).

The majority of neonates with congenital hypothyroidism appear normal at birth, although some may exhibit signs of the disorder such as hypotonia, large fontanel, or macroglossia (Blackburn, 2013). If the infant is untreated, symptoms usually appear after 6 weeks and include bradycardia; hypothermia; hypotension; hyporeflexia; abdominal distention; umbilical hernia; coarse, dry hair; thick, dry skin that feels cold; anemia; widely patent cranial sutures; and delayed bone age beginning at birth. The most disabling problem, however, is delayed development of the nervous system, leading to severe developmental delay. Once identified, treatment is started immediately using synthetic thyroxine (T_4, L-thyroxine) as a thyroid replacement (Clause, 2013).

Early diagnosis and treatment of congenital hypothyroidism are associated with a greater likelihood of normal mental development. Early recognition of the disorder is possible through routine newborn screening. All U.S. states and Canadian provinces routinely screen for hypothyroidism by measuring T_4 or thyroid-stimulating hormone (TSH) levels. Screening is most accurate after 48 hours of age. Early screening can have false-positive results; preterm infants are more likely to have false-positive results. Any infant whose screening test is positive should be further evaluated for congenital hypothyroidism (Blackburn, 2013).

CARE MANAGEMENT

Assessment

Congenital anomalies and disorders may be identified prenatally, at the time of birth, or in the days or weeks following birth. Although some prenatal and postnatal screening tests are routinely performed, diagnostic testing for specific congenital defects is performed based on a variety of factors such as results of screening tests, maternal and family history, prenatal course, and neonatal symptoms.

Prenatal. Refined prenatal testing procedures are available to monitor fetal development. Diagnostic techniques such as amniocentesis, ultrasonography, alpha-fetoprotein measurements, CVS, PUBS, fetal nuchal translucency (FNT) screening, and gene probes contribute information to the database (see Chapter 26). Although they are a valuable adjunct to prenatal care, these tests cannot identify all congenital disorders. Furthermore, ethical issues surround such testing, and the nurse must be prepared to support the family's decision regarding these tests. If a disorder is detected and the family decides to proceed with the pregnancy, the advantage is that appropriate care can be made available for the infant immediately at birth.

The nurse reviews the maternal history and medical information in the prenatal record for risk factors associated with congenital disorders. These factors include various medical, surgical, and social conditions and their treatments (see Chapter 30); maternal infection (see Chapter 7); maternal endocrine and metabolic disorders (see Chapter 29); and infection and drug dependence in the newborn (see Chapter 35).

BOX 36-3 Routine Screening for Critical Congenital Heart Disease

- Screen healthy newborns after 24 hours of life or as close to the time of discharge as possible.
- Use a motion-tolerant pulse oximeter.
- Obtain pulse oximeter readings from the right hand and one foot.
- Pulse oximetry <90% in right hand or foot is considered a positive screening that warrants additional testing such as echocardiogram.
- 90% to 95% in right hand or foot or >3% difference between the two extremities warrants repeat testing in 1 hour. If screening values remain the same as the first time, consider repeating the screen in 1 hour. If parameters remain unchanged after the second screen, repeat a third time. If unchanged, consider it a positive screen.
- >95% in the right hand or foot and <3% difference between the two extremities is a negative screen and no further testing is needed.

Data from Kemper, A.R., Mahle, W.T., Martin, G.R., et al. (2011). Strategies for implementing screening for critical congenital heart disease. *Pediatrics, 128*(5), e1259-e1267.

Postnatal. Diagnostic procedures for the detection of genetic disorders are performed after birth at any time from the postnatal period through adulthood. Many tests exist for various disorders.

Apgar scoring and a brief assessment are completed for all neonates after birth. Any deviations from normal are reported to the health care provider immediately. A thorough assessment of all body systems is performed to identify anomalies. Both minor and major malformations are noted. There can be mild malformations that in isolation are not clinically significant, but a pattern or combination of minor malformations can suggest a specific disorder or syndrome (Matthews & Robin, 2011).

The most widespread use of postnatal testing for congenital disorders is the routine screening of newborns in the United States and Canada for IEMs such as PKU and galactosemia, hemoglobinopathies (sickle cell disease and thalassemias), and hypothyroidism (Howell, Terry, Tait, et al., 2012). Screening for hearing loss is recommended at the same time as disease screening. The use of pulse oximetry to screen for critical congenital heart disease in healthy term infants (Box 36-3) has been endorsed by the U.S. Department of Health and Human Services and is being implemented in numerous states; this should be included in the recommended uniform newborn screening panel (Bradshaw & Martin, 2012; Mahle et al., 2012).

Cytogenic studies must be done to rule out or confirm a suspected genetic diagnosis. Chromosome analysis and molecular deoxyribonucleic acid (DNA) analysis are often ordered. Test results may not be available for weeks; however, in urgent situations, chromosome analysis from bone marrow samples can be available within hours (Matthews & Robin, 2011).

A variety of biochemical studies may be done, especially in seeking to diagnose an IEM. X-ray examination and organ imaging with MRI or CT scan may be used to identify skeletal abnormalities and structural anomalies of major organs (Matthews & Robin, 2011).

Family history is integral to diagnosing a congenital disorder. Data collection should include a three-generation pedigree (parents, siblings, grandparents, aunts, uncles, cousins) with information such as miscarriages, stillbirths, congenital anomalies, or childhood deaths (Matthews & Robin, 2011).

Nursing Diagnoses

The nursing diagnoses formulated for an infant with a congenital anomaly depend on the type and severity of the abnormality. General nursing diagnoses pertaining to the care of newborns with congenital abnormalities include the following:

Newborn:

- *Risk for Injury* related to:
  - presence of a congenital abnormality
- *Risk for Infection* related to
  - anomaly or its treatment
- *Impaired Gas Exchange, Imbalanced Nutrition: Less than Body Requirements or Impaired Mobility* related to
  - congenital anomaly
- *Delayed Growth and Development* related to
  - inborn error of metabolism

Parents and Family:

- *Grieving or Spiritual Distress* related to
  - birth of a child with a disorder or abnormality
- *Compromised Family Coping* related to
  - birth of a child with an abnormality
- *Deficient Knowledge* related to
  - cause of the anomaly, its management, alternative courses of action, community resources, prognosis, and the care needed by the infant after discharge
- *Anxiety* related to
  - uncertainty about the prognosis or their ability to care for the child
- *Risk for Impaired Parenting* related to
  - birth of a child with a disorder or anomaly

Interventions

Newborn Care

Many congenital anomalies require intervention soon after birth. A collaborative health team approach that includes specialists and community service representatives is needed in the care of infants with some disorders. Surgical intervention in the neonatal period may be necessary for the infant requiring either immediate correction or a palliative procedure to relieve the symptoms of the anomaly until definitive correction can be done. There is a higher morbidity and mortality rate in neonates than in older children or adults undergoing similar procedures. However, despite these problems unique to neonates, advances in surgical techniques, anesthesia, and the nursing care given in intensive care nurseries have been responsible for decreasing the risk of surgery in neonates.

The health care team must be highly skilled to meet the needs of these high risk infants. In addition to stabilizing the infant's condition (oxygenation and perfusion of tissues), other preoperative interventions, such as placing an orogastric tube for abdominal decompression, attending to thermoregulation and pain management, and maintaining fluid and electrolyte balance, are implemented to manage specific problems.

Parents and Family Support

While the infant is receiving optimal care, the parents have needs that must be met as they deal with the crisis of having an infant with an abnormal condition. The nurse carefully assesses their reactions, which are likely to be those typical of a grief response. Facilitating their understanding of the information given them about their infant's condition is a vital nursing intervention. A newly diagnosed disorder often implies the need for implementing a therapeutic regimen. For example, the disorder can be an IEM, such as PKU, which requires consistent and rigid adherence to a special diet. The family may need help with securing the required formula and receiving counseling from the clinical dietitian. The nurse stresses the importance of maintaining the diet, keeping an adequate supply of special preparations, and not using unauthorized substitutions.

Referral to appropriate agencies is another essential component of follow-up management, and the nurse should make the parents aware of all possible sources of aid, including pertinent literature, parent groups, and national organizations. Many organizations and foundations provide services and counseling for families of affected children. There are also numerous parent groups the family can join. There they can share experiences and receive mutual support in coping with problems similar to those of other group members. Nurses should be familiar with the services available in their community that provide assistance and education to families with these special problems.

A major nursing function is providing emotional support to the family during all aspects of the care of the infant born with a defect or disorder. The feelings stemming from the real or imagined threat posed by a congenital anomaly are as varied as the people being counseled. Responses can include apathy, denial, anger, hostility, fear, embarrassment, grief, and loss of self-esteem (see Chapter 37).

Some parents benefit from seeing before-and-after pictures of other babies born with the same defect. Coupled with other verbal and nonverbal supportive care, this visual reassurance may be effective in allaying their concerns. Families need much information, guidance, and support as they make decisions regarding the care of their infants. Once they have been given the facts and possible consequences and all the assistance they need in problem solving, the final decision regarding a course of action must be their own. It is then incumbent on health care providers to support the family's decision.

Genetic Evaluation and Counseling

Genetic counseling is a communication process concerned with the human problems associated with the occurrence, or risk of occurrence, of a genetic disorder in a family. It involves relaying information about the diagnosis, treatment options, recurrence risk, and availability of prenatal diagnosis. It is essential that nurses understand the basic principles of heredity and how heredity contributes to disorders. They should be aware of the types of genetic testing available (see Chapter 3).

Nurses frequently encounter infants with genetic disorders and families for whom there is a risk that a disorder can be transmitted to or occur in an offspring. Nurses are responsible for identifying situations in which individuals can benefit from genetic evaluation and counseling. They should be aware of the local genetic resources, aid families in finding services, and offer support and care for children and families affected by genetic conditions. Nurses can direct families to appropriate resources. The Genetic Alliance (www.geneticalliance.org) is a nonprofit organization that has a database of support groups for genetic conditions. The National Society of Genetic Counselors (www.nsgc.org) lists genetic counselors by state. GeneTests (www.ncbi.nlm.nih.gov/sites/GeneTests) is a publicly funded medical genetics information resource developed for health care professionals; it is available at no cost to everyone.

KEY POINTS

- Hyperbilirubinemia is caused by a variety of factors, including maternal-fetal Rh and ABO incompatibility.
- Acute bilirubin encephalopathy and kernicterus are serious neurologic complications resulting from high levels of unconjugated bilirubin.
- Erythroblastosis fetalis leads to anemia, edema, and the cytotoxic effects of unconjugated bilirubin.
- The administration of Rh_0(D) immune globulin to Rh-negative and Coombs' test–negative women provides passive immunity and minimizes the possibility of isoimmunization.
- Neonatal exchange transfusion with type O, Rh-negative RBCs serves to treat anemia and acidosis and remove bilirubin, maternal antibodies, and fetal RBCs that are beginning to hemolyze.
- Major congenital defects are the leading cause of death in term neonates.
- The most common major congenital anomalies that cause serious problems in the neonate are congenital heart disease, neural tube defects, cleft lip or palate, and developmental dysplasia of the hip.
- Minor anomalies can be part of a characteristic pattern of malformations.
- Current technology permits the prenatal diagnosis of many congenital anomalies and disorders.
- The most widespread use of postnatal testing for genetic disease is the routine screening of newborns for inborn errors of metabolism.
- The curative and rehabilitative problems of an infant with a congenital disorder are often complex and require a multidisciplinary approach to care.
- Parents often need special instructions (e.g., meeting nutrition requirements, cast care, or home phototherapy) before they take a high risk infant home.
- The supportive care given to the parents of infants with an abnormal condition must begin at birth or at the time of diagnosis and continue for years.

REFERENCES

Adzick, N. S. (2013). Fetal surgery for spina bifida: Past, present, future. *Seminars in Pediatric Surgery, 22*(1), 10–17.

Alverson, C., Strickland, M., Gilboa, S., & Correa, A. (2011). Maternal smoking and congenital heart defects in the Baltimore-Washington Infant Study. *Pediatrics, 127*(3), e647–e653.

Ambalavanan, N., & Carlo, W. A. (2011). Kernicterus. In R. M. Kliegman, B. F. Stanton, S. W. St. Geme, III, et al. (Eds.), *Nelson textbook of pediatrics* (19th ed.). Philadelphia: Saunders.

American Academy of Pediatrics (AAP) Subcommittee on Hyperbilirubinemia. (2004). Management of hyperbilirubinemia in the newborn infant 35 or more weeks of gestation. *Pediatrics, 114*(1), 297–316.

Association of Women's Health, Obstetric and Neonatal Nurses (AWHONN). (2005). *Hyperbilirubinemia in the neonate: Risk assessment, screening, and management*. Washington, DC: Author.

Barksdale, E., Chwals, W., Magnuson, D., & Parry, R. (2011). Selected gastrointestinal anomalies. In R. Martin, A. Fanaroff, & M. Walsh (Eds.), *Fanaroff and Martin's neonatal-perinatal medicine: diseases of the fetus and infant* (9th ed.). St. Louis: Mosby.

Bernstein, D. (2011). Congenital heart disease. In R. M. Kliegman, B. F. Stanton, S. W. St. Geme, III, et al. (Eds.), *Nelson textbook of pediatrics* (19th ed.). Philadelphia: Elsevier Saunders.

Bhutani, V., & Committee on Fetus and Newborn. (2011). Phototherapy to prevent severe neonatal hyperbilirubinemia in the newborn infant 35 or more weeks of gestation. *Pediatrics, 128*(4), e1046–e1052.

Blackburn, S. (2013). *Maternal, fetal, and neonatal physiology: A clinical perspective* (4th ed.). St. Louis: Saunders.

Blue, W., Kirk, E., Sholler, G., et al. (2012). Congenital heart disease: Current knowledge about causes and inheritance. *Medical Journal of Australia, 197*(3), 155–159.

Bracken, J., Tran, T., & Ditchfield, M. (2012). Developmental dysplasia of the hip: Controversies and current concepts. *Journal of Paediatrics and Child Health, 48*(11), 963–973.

Bradshaw, E. A., & Martin, G. R. (2012). Screening for critical congenital heart disease: Advancing detection in the newborn. *Current Opinion in Pediatrics, 24*(5), 603–608.

Canon, S., Mosley, B., Chipollini, J., et al. (2012). Epidemiological assessment of hypospadias by degree of severity. *Journal of Urology, 188*(6), 2362–2366.

Cederbaum, S. (2012). Introduction to metabolic and biochemical genetic disease. In S. U. Devaskar, & C. A. Gleason (Eds.), *Avery's diseases of the newborn* (9th ed.). Philadelphia: Saunders.

Centers for Disease Control and Prevention. (2012). Folic acid. Available at www.cdc.gov/ncbddd/folicacid/recommendations.html.

Clause, M. (2013). Newborn screening for congenital hypothyroidism. *Journal of Pediatric Nursing, 28*(6), 603–608.

Cleary, M. A. (2011). Phenylketonuria. *Paediatrics and Child Health, 21*(2), 61–64.

Clements, S., Challis, D., & Kennedy, D. (2012). Neural tube defects: Pathophysiology and prevention. In M. Kilby, A. Johnson, & D. Oepkes (Eds.), *Fetal therapy: Scientific basis and critical appraisal of clinical benefits*. Cambridge, UK: Cambridge University Press.

Cohen, A. R. (2011). Disorders in head shape and size. In R. Martin, A. Fanaroff, & M. Walsh (Eds.), *Fanaroff and Martin's neonatal-perinatal medicine: Diseases of the fetus and infant* (9th ed.). St. Louis: Mosby.

Congenital Diaphragmatic Hernia Study Group. (2013). Congenital diaphragmatic hernia: Defect size correlates with developmental defect. *Journal of Pediatric Surgery, 48*(6), 1177–1182.

De Silva, R. (2013). *Heart disease*. Santa Barbara, CA: ABC-CLIO.

Diehl-Jones, W., & Fraser, D. (2015). Hematologic disorders. In M. T. Verklan, & M. Walden (Eds.), *Core curriculum for neonatal intensive care nursing* (5th ed.). St. Louis: Saunders.

Dolk, H., Loane, M., & Garne, E. (2011). Congenital heart defects in Europe: Prevalence and perinatal mortality, 2000 to 2005. *Circulation, 123*(8), 841–849.

Elder, J. S. (2011). Anomalies of the bladder. In R. M. Kliegman, B. F. Stanton, J. W. St. Geme, III, et al. (Eds.), *Nelson textbook of pediatrics* (19th ed.). Philadelphia: Elsevier Saunders.

Fox, K., & Saade, G. (2012). Fetal blood sampling and intrauterine transfusion. *NeoReviews, 13*(11), e661–e669.

Fung, A., Manlhiot, C., Naik, S., et al. (2013). Impact of prenatal risk factors on congenital heart disease in the current era. *Journal of the American Heart Association, 3*(2), e000064.

Gazzin, S., & Tiribelli, C. (2011). Bilirubin-induced neurological damage. *Journal of Maternal-Fetal and Neonatal Medicine, 24*(S1), 154–155.

Gourlay, D. M. (2013). Colorectal considerations in pediatric patients. *Surgical Clinics of North America, 93*(1), 251–272.

Gregory, M., Martin, C., & Cloherty, J. (2012). Neonatal hyperbilirubinemia. In J. Cloherty, E. Eichenwald, A. Hansen, & A. Stark (Eds.), *Manual of neonatal care* (7th ed.). Philadelphia: Wolters Kluwer.

Gressens, P., & Huppi, P. S. (2011). Normal and abnormal brain development. In R. Martin, A. Fanaroff, & M. Walsh (Eds.), *Fanaroff and Martin's neonatal-perinatal medicine: Diseases of the fetus and infant* (9th ed.). St. Louis: Mosby.

Griffey, R., Chen, B., & Krehbiel, N. (2012). Performance in appropriate Rh testing and treatment with Rh immunoglobulin in the emergency department. *Annals of Emergency Medicine, 59*(4), 285–293.

Grüters, A., & Krude, H. (2011). Detection and treatment of congenital hypothyroidism. *Nature Review Endocrinology, 8*(2), 104–113.

Gupta, N., Farrell, J. A., Rand, L., et al. (2012). Open fetal surgery for myelomeningocele. *Journal of Neurosurgery, Pediatrics, 9*(3), 265–273.

Hansen, T. (2011). Prevention of neurodevelopmental sequelae of jaundice in the newborn. *Developmental Medicine & Child Neurology, 53*(S4), 24–28.

Haroon, J., & Chamberlain, R. S. (2013). An evidence-based review of the current treatment of congenital diaphragmatic hernia. *Clinics in Pediatrics, 52*(2), 115–124.

Hertzberg, V. S., Hinton, C. F., Therrell, B. L., & Shapira, S. K. (2011). Birth prevalence rates of newborn screening disorders in relation to screening practices in the United States. *Journal of Pediatrics, 159*(4), 555–560.

Hosalkar, H. A., Spiegel, D. A., & Davidson, R. S. (2011). Talipes equinovarus (clubfoot). In R. M. Kliegman, B. F. Stanton, J. W. St. Geme, III, et al. (Eds.), *Nelson textbook of pediatrics* (19th ed.). Philadelphia: Elsevier Saunders.

Howell, R. R., Terry, S., Tait, V. F., et al. (2012). CDC grand rounds: Newborn screening and improved outcomes. *MMWR Morbidity and Mortality Weekly Report, 61*(21), 390–393.

Kamath, B., Thilo, E., & Hernandez, J. (2011). Jaundice. In S. Gardner, B. Carter, M. Enzman-Hines, & J. Hernandez (Eds.), *Merenstein & Gardner's handbook of neonatal intensive care* (7th ed.). St. Louis: Mosby.

Kaplan, M., Wong, R., Sibley, E., & Stevenson, D. (2011). Neonatal jaundice and liver disease. In R. Martin, A. Fanaroff, & M. Walsh (Eds.), *Fanaroff and Martin's neonatal-perinatal medicine: Diseases of the fetus and infant* (9th ed.). St. Louis: Mosby.

Kaplan, M., Wong, R., & Stevenson, D. (2012). Pathologic unconjugated hyperbilirubinemia, isoimmunization, abnormalities of red cells and infections. In G. Buonocore, R. Bracci, & W. Weindling (Eds.), *Neonatology: A practical approach to neonatal diseases.* New York: Springer.

Kelly, T. F., & Moore, T. R. (2012). Maternal medical disorders of fetal significance: Seizure disorders, isoimmunization, cancer, and mental health disorders. In S. U. Devaskar, & C. A. Gleason (Eds.), *Avery's diseases of the newborn* (9th ed.). Philadelphia: Elsevier.

Kemper, A. R., Mahle, W. T., Martin, G. R., et al. (2011). Strategies for implementing screening for critical congenital heart disease. *Pediatrics, 128*(5), e1–e9.

Kennedy, D., & Koren, G. (2012). Identifying women who might benefit from higher doses of folic acid in pregnancy. *Canadian Family Physician, 58*(4), 394–397.

Kenney, P., Hoover, D., Williams, L., & Iskersky, V. (2011). Cardiovascular diseases and surgical interventions. In S. Gardner, B. Carter, M. Enzman-Hines, & J. Hernandez (Eds.), *Merenstein & Gardner's handbook of neonatal intensive care* (7th ed.). St. Louis: Mosby.

Khan, M., & Rahman, M. (2011). *Essence of pediatrics* (4th ed.). St. Louis: Elsevier.

Khan, S., & Orenstein, S. R. (2011). Esophageal atresia and tracheoesophageal fistula. In R. M. Kliegman, B. F. Stanton, J. W. St. Geme, III, et al. (Eds.), *Nelson textbook of pediatrics* (19th ed.). Philadelphia: Elsevier Saunders.

Kinsman, S. L., & Johnston, M. V. (2013). Congenital anomalies of the central nervous system. In R. M. Kliegman, B. F. Stanton, J. W. St. Geme, III, et al. (Eds.), *Nelson textbook of pediatrics* (19th ed.). Philadelphia: Elsevier Saunders.

Lauer, B. J., & Spector, N. D. (2011). Hyperbilirubinemia in the newborn. *Pediatrics in Review, 32*(8), 341–349.

Lawrence, R. M. (2013). Circumstances when breastfeeding is contraindicated. *Pediatric Clinics of North America, 60*(1), 295–318.

Lee, P. A., & Houk, C. P. (2013). Evaluation and management of children and adolescents with gender identification and transgender disorders. *Current Opinion in Pediatrics, 25*(4), 521–527.

LOTUS Study Group. (2012). Long-term neurodevelopmental outcome after intrauterine transfusion for hemolytic disease of the fetus/newborn. *Gynecology, 206*(2), 141e1–141e8.

Lovvorn, H., Glenn, J., Pacetti, A., & Carter, B. (2011). Neonatal surgery. In S. Gardner, B. Carter, M. Enzman-Hines, & J. Hernandez (Eds.), *Merenstein & Gardner's handbook of neonatal intensive care* (7th ed.). St. Louis: Mosby.

Maarse, W., Rozendaal, A. M., Pajkrt, E., et al. (2012). A systematic review of associated structural and chromosomal defects in oral clefts: When is prenatal genetic analysis indicated? *Journal of Medical Genetics, 49*(8), 490–498.

Manco-Johnson, M., Rodden, D. J., & Hays, T. (2011). Newborn hematology. In S. Gardner, B. Carter, M. Enzman-Hines, & J. Hernandez (Eds.), *Merenstein & Gardner's handbook of neonatal intensive care* (7th ed.). St. Louis: Mosby.

Madsen, N., Schwartz, S., Lewis, M., & Mueller, B. (2013). Pregnancy body mass index and congenital heart defects among offspring: A population-based study. *Congenital Heart Disease, 8*(2), 131–141.

Maheshwari, A., & Carlo, W. A. (2011). Blood disorders. In R. M. Kliegman, B. F. Stanton, S. W. St. Geme, III, et al. (Eds.), *Nelson textbook of pediatrics* (19th ed.). Philadelphia: Elsevier Saunders.

Mahle, W. T., Martin, G. R., Beekman, R. H., et al. (2012). Endorsement of Health and Human Services recommendation for pulse oximetry screening for critical congenital heart disease. *Pediatrics, 129*(1), 190–192.

Matthews, A., & Robin, N. (2011). Genetic disorders, malformations, and inborn errors of metabolism. In S. Gardner, B. Carter, M. Enzman-Hines, & J. Hernandez (Eds.), *Merenstein & Gardner's handbook of neonatal intensive care* (7th ed.). St. Louis: Mosby.

Mendez-Figueroa, H., Dahlke, J., Vrees, R., & Rouse, D. (2013). Trauma in pregnancy: An updated systematic review. *Gynecology, 209*(1), 1–10.

Murki, S., & Kumar, P. (2011). Blood exchange transfusion for infants with severe neonatal hyperbilirubinemia. *Seminars in Perinatology, 35*(3), 175–184.

Murphy, S. L., Xu, J., & Kochanek, K. D. (2013). Deaths: Final data for 2010. *National Vital Statistics Reports, 61*(4) Available at www.cdc.gov/nchs/data/nvsr/nvsr61/nvsr61_04.pdf.

Nabavizadeh, S., Rezaie, M., Sabzali, P., et al. (2012). Cohort study on hemolysis associated with G6PD deficiency in jaundiced neonates. *Life Science Journal, 9*(3), 702–705.

Parikh, A., & Wiesner, G. (2011). Congenital anomalies. In R. Martin, A. Fanaroff, & M. Walsh (Eds.), *Fanaroff and Martin's neonatal-perinatal medicine: Diseases of the fetus and infant* (9th ed.). St. Louis: Mosby.

Parker, S. E., Mai, C. T., Canfield, M. A., et al. (2010). Updated national birth prevalence estimates for selected birth defects in the United States, 2004-2006. *Birth Defects Research (Part A): Clinical and Molecular Teratology, 88*(12), 1008–1016.

Pavri, S., & Forrest, C. R. (2013). Demographics of orofacial clefts in Canada from 2002 to 2008. *Cleft Palate-Craniofacial Journal, 50*(2), 224–230.

Posencheg, M., & Dennery, P. (2013). Hemolytic diseases of the fetus and newborn. In E. Bope, & R. Kellerman (Eds.), *Conn's current therapy 2013*. Philadelphia: Saunders.

Price, C. T., & Ramo, B. A. (2012). Prevention of hip dysplasia in children and adults. *Orthopedic Clinics of North America, 43*(3), 269–279.

Racusin, D., Stevens, B., Campbell, G., & Aagaard, K. (2012). Obesity and the risk and detection of fetal malformations. *Seminars in Perinatology, 36*(3), 213–221.

Rajiah, P., Mak, C., Dubinsky, T., & Dighe, M. (2011). Ultrasound of fetal cardiac anomalies. *American Journal of Roentgenology, 197*(4), W747–W760.

Sankar, W. N., Horn, B. D., Wells, L., & Dormans, J. P. (2011). Developmental dysplasia of the hip. In R. M. Kliegman, B. F. Stanton, S. W. St. Geme, III, et al. (Eds.), *Nelson textbook of pediatrics* (19th ed.). Philadelphia: Elsevier Saunders.

Schaible, T., Kohl, T., Reinshagen, K., et al. (2012). Right- versus left-sided congenital diaphragmatic hernia: Postnatal outcome at a specialized tertiary care center. *Pediatric Critical Care Medicine, 13*(1), 66–71.

Serrano, T., Chevrier, C., Multigner, L., et al. (2013). International geographic correlation study of the prevalence of disorders of male reproductive health. *Human Reproduction, 28*(7), 1974–1986.

Shue, E. H., Miniati, D., & Lee, H. (2012). Advances in prenatal diagnosis and treatment of congenital diaphragmatic hernia. *Clinics in Perinatology, 39*(2), 289–300.

Siffel, C., Correa, A., Amar, E., et al. (2011). Bladder exstrophy: An epidemiologic study from the International Clearinghouse for Birth Defects Surveillance and Research, and an overview of the literature. *American Journal of Medical Genetics Part C Seminars in Medical Genetics, 157C*(4), 321–332.

Song, C., Upperman, J. S., & Niklas, V. (2011). Structural anomalies of the gastrointestinal tract. In R. M. Kliegman, B. F. Stanton, S. W. St. Geme, III, et al. (Eds.), *Nelson textbook of pediatrics* (19th ed.). Philadelphia: Elsevier Saunders.

Sprecher, R. C., & Arnold, J. E. (2011). Upper airway lesions. In R. Martin, A. Fanaroff, & M. Walsh (Eds.), *Fanaroff and Martin's neonatal-perinatal medicine: Diseases of the fetus and infant* (9th ed.). St. Louis: Mosby.

Steven, L., Cherian, A., Yankovic, F., et al. (2013). Current practice in paediatric hypospadias surgery: A specialist survey. *Journal of Pediatric Urology, 9*(6 Pt B), 1126–1130.

Stokowski, L. A. (2014). Metabolic system. In C. Kenner, & J. W. Lott (Eds.), *Comprehensive neonatal nursing care* (5th ed.). New York: Springer.

Sulchy, F. J., & Kerkar, N. (2012). Disorders of the liver. In C. A. Gleason, & S. U. Devaskar (Eds.), *Avery's diseases of the newborn* (9th ed.). Philadelphia: Saunders.

Tinanoff, N. (2011). Cleft lip and palate. In R. M. Kliegman, B. F. Stanton, S. W. St. Geme, III, et al. (Eds.), *Nelson textbook of pediatrics* (19th ed.). Philadelphia: Elsevier Saunders.

Van der Linde, D., Konings, E., Slager, M., et al. (2011). Birth prevalence of congenital heart disease worldwide: A systematic review and meta-analysis. *Journal of the American College of Cardiology, 58*(21), 2241–2247.

Verklan, M. T., & Lopez, S. M. (2011). Neurologic disorders. In S. Gardner, B. Carter, M. Enzman-Hines, & J. Hernandez (Eds.), *Merenstein & Gardner's handbook of neonatal intensive care* (7th ed.). St. Louis: Mosby.

Viau, K. S., Wengreen, H. J., Ernst, S. L., et al. (2011). Correlation of age-specific phenylalanine levels with intellectual outcome in patients with phenylketonuria. *Journal of Inherited Metabolic Disorders, 34*(4), 963–971.

Watchko, J. F. (2012). Neonatal indirect and hyperbilirubinemia and kernicterus. In C. A. Gleason, & S. U. Devaskar (Eds.), *Avery's diseases of the newborn* (9th ed.). Philadelphia: Elsevier Saunders.

Wilson, D. (2014). Gastrointestinal dysfunction. In S. E. Perry, M. J. Hockenberry, D. L. Lowdermilk, & D. Wilson (Eds.), *Maternal child nursing care* (5th ed.). St. Louis: Elsevier Mosby.

Wilson, D., Montagnino, B., & Wilson, K. (2011). Conditions caused by defects in physical environment. In M. Hockenberry, & D. Wilson (Eds.), *Wong's nursing care of infants and children* (9th ed.). St. Louis: Mosby.

World Health Organization (WHO). (2012). *Congenital anomalies*. Available at www.who.int/mediacentre/factsheets/fs370/en.

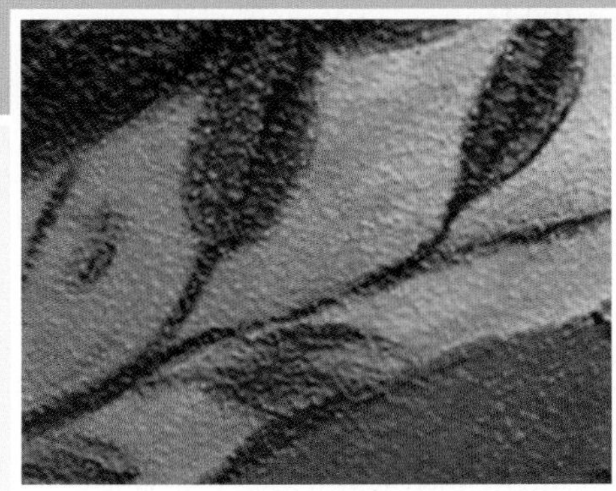

CHAPTER 37

Perinatal Loss, Bereavement, and Grief

Beth Perry Black

http://evolve.elsevier.com/Lowdermilk/MWHC/

LEARNING OBJECTIVES

- Define perinatal loss, bereavement, and grief.
- Describe the causes of perinatal loss.
- Describe the various responses parents and families may have to perinatal loss.
- Analyze the personal and societal issues that can complicate responses to perinatal loss.
- Formulate appropriate nursing diagnoses for people experiencing perinatal loss.
- Identify specific nursing interventions to meet the special needs of bereaved women, their partners, and their families related to perinatal loss and grief.
- Differentiate between helpful and hurtful responses in caring for women and their partners experiencing a perinatal loss.
- Define complicated grief related to perinatal loss and how nurses can assess for it.

Expectant parents anticipate the birth of their baby with joy and hope. For some women, their partners, and their families, however, pregnancy becomes a time of loss, resulting in profound grief and a period of bereavement in which they mourn the loss of their expected child. Loss associated with reproduction covers a wide range of conditions and events. Grief and loss in perinatal settings can be especially upsetting to nurses (Jonas-Simpson, Pilkington, MacDonald, & McMahon, 2013); caring for healthy pregnant women who give birth to healthy infants is the more typical expectation for nurses in these settings. Understanding grief and bereavement as a human response to loss is important, however, because nurses in a variety of settings associated with women's health will encounter clients for whom the childbearing process results in loss.

The study of loss surrounding childbearing and the subsequent grief and bereavement is relatively new. For purposes of this chapter, **perinatal bereavement** is defined as the complex emotional responses experienced by women and men beginning immediately after the death of an expected child through miscarriage, stillbirth, neonatal death, or termination of pregnancy for fetal anomalies. Perinatal bereavement usually is characterized by grief that can vary in intensity and duration across genders and is influenced by many situational, internal, and external factors (Fenstermacher & Hupcey, 2013). The focus of this chapter is to prepare the nurse to provide sensitive and supportive care to women, their partners, and families experiencing losses related to childbearing. An overview of loss, grief, and bereavement is presented as a guide for assessing and understanding the responses of persons experiencing perinatal loss.

LOSS, BEREAVEMENT, AND GRIEF: BASIC CONCEPTS AND THEORIES

Much of the current understanding of loss, bereavement, and grief is based on the initial work of Elisabeth Kübler-Ross, a Swiss-American psychiatrist who in 1969 published *On Death and Dying* (Kübler-Ross, 1969). In this book Kübler-Ross first described five stages of grief—denial, anger, bargaining, depression, and acceptance—that she understood as being central to a person's movement through the experience of loss. Her work was groundbreaking in that she began the conversation about how people experience loss, particularly death. Most researchers and clinicians who now study or work with dying clients and their families understand that the process of grief is not linear, that is, people do not move uniformly through the stages in a particular order at a specific time. Rather, the grief experience is individual and is influenced by many factors, including the meaning of the loss. This is not to say that Kübler-Ross was incorrect in identifying these stages; in fact, many grieving people experience these exact responses. The problem occurs when grieving individuals' responses are considered out-of-sequence or "abnormal" when they do not fit these stages as she described them. Despite the limits of Kübler-Ross's model, the value of understanding grief responses is significant in assisting grieving individuals in working through their sense of loss and sadness.

Nurses in perinatal settings may not feel comfortable discussing grief and loss with women and families facing a pregnancy loss, stillbirth, or death of their newborn. Grief responses such as crying or questioning by the woman can be upsetting to the nurse who may not feel adequate in helping grief-stricken women and their families. Nurses may have their own grief responses that can be distressing, making it difficult to turn attention to the care of the client. In fact, nurses are susceptible to traumatic stress secondary to the perinatal loss and should be proactive in garnering support for themselves, especially from their peers, when a perinatal loss occurs (Puia, Lewis, & Beck, 2013). Providers with little experience in managing loss are at highest risk for clinically significant distress in perinatal settings, and formal training does not appear to be protective from distress related to perinatal loss (Wallbank & Robertson, 2013). The following two sections contain definitions of loss, bereavement, grief, and mourning commonly used in end-of-life care settings and theoretic orientations to loss that may be useful for nurses in perinatal settings in understanding the responses of their clients. This in turn can increase nurses' expertise and comfort in providing care when a pregnancy ends in loss.

Defining Loss, Bereavement, Grief, and Mourning

Losses are any experiences in which a valued person or object can no longer be seen, touched, heard, known, or otherwise experienced. In childbearing settings the losses can be complicated in that the extent of the fetus being "known" is typically limited to the pregnant woman through fetal movements, ultrasound images, and pregnancy signs and symptoms. Her partner may have felt fetal movement through the woman's abdomen if the pregnancy is advanced; many partners are present for ultrasound exams. Early in pregnancy, couples may not yet have even told their close family and friends of the pregnancy prior to a miscarriage.

The meaning of a loss will have a significant effect on how the loss is experienced. For many women and families, a perinatal loss at any stage can mean the loss of hope for a planned-for child, plans for the future, an heir or legacy, or a "perfect" or healthy baby. Meanings of pregnancy are highly variable—a loss can hold great meaning for one woman and her family, whereas a woman in a different circumstance may feel relief (possibly guilt) that the pregnancy is over. The wise nurse is cautious, however, in making assumptions about the meaning of a pregnancy loss for any one woman and family.

Bereavement is the state of being without a valued other, especially by death. Sometimes bereaved individuals are described as "bereft" or "the bereaved." Bereavement is characterized by the emotional state of **grief,** the profound sadness and despair that accompanies a loss. Grief is now recognized as a process through which bereft persons work in coming to terms with their loss. In a concept analysis of grief, Cowles and Rodgers (2000) identified attributes of grief: (a) grief is *dynamic* and involves complex emotions, thoughts, and behaviors that shift and change; (b) grief is *a process* that is enduring and has no time limit; (c) grief is *highly individualized* and manifested differently from person to person; and (d) grief is *pervasive* involving psychological, social, physical, cognitive, behavioral, and affective responses and can affect every aspect of a person's life. Grief is particularly affected by the meaning of the loss to the person. Note that Kübler-Ross's stages of grief were described as a process; the current understanding of grief is that it is a process but one that is not linear. This means that people may return to earlier states of grief over time as their grief resolves and they heal.

Mourning, another word often associated with loss, involves the culturally mandated traditions and rituals in the time after a death. Bereaved persons are sometimes described as being "in mourning" for some time after the death of a loved one. Funerals, memorial services, wearing black, or otherwise acknowledging the death are some common mourning rituals in the United States. Mourning rituals are intertwined with cultural norms and expectations and can vary greatly across families, religions, nationalities, and ethnicities.

Useful Grief Theories in Perinatal Settings

End-of-life care theories provide an important basis for the care of women and their families who are experiencing pregnancy loss. Although it is beyond the scope of this chapter to fully explain the theoretic foundations of end-of-life care, familiarity with these concepts allows perinatal nurses to understand individual and family experiences of loss in a deeper way.

Perinatal loss can be an ambiguous loss, a type of loss in which the object of grief is missing (Boss, 2006), such as a fetus that has never been physically seen or held by his or her parents and is unknown to others. For women experiencing a miscarriage and their partners, for instance, the loss may be of a developing fetus whose sex is yet unknown and may never be known. Some losses associated with miscarriage are the experience of being pregnant, a hoped-for baby, and a future with this child. Furthermore, the reason for the miscarriage can remain unclear, adding to the ambiguity of the loss. The conventional customs of mourning might not be observed in this case, thereby hindering coping and circumventing the solace that is found in these rituals (Lang, Fleiszer, Duhamel, et al., 2011).

Losses surrounding pregnancy are sometimes not openly acknowledged and mourned publicly, thereby limiting social support. This is known as **disenfranchised grief** (Doka, 1989), which leads to a sense of isolation in bereaved individuals. Perinatal losses are often characterized as ambiguous because the loss is undefined or unseen and disenfranchised because the grief of bereaved mothers, partners, and families is unacknowledged. This situation can result in complicated grief, a complex situation in which grief may not resolve over time and the bereaved person grieves chronically (Rando, Doka, Fleming, et al., 2012). Cacciatore (2013) noted that failure by others to recognize the significance of a pregnancy loss—specifically stillbirth—implies that the expected baby's life had no value and that the mother herself may lack value in this time when life and death converge.

Two current theories of grief and bereavement—continuing bonds theory and dual process model—are helpful to perinatal nurses. These models reflect what contemporary grief theorists believe are more realistic views of the grief experience than older models (e.g., Kübler-Ross) in which grief resolution was expected to always occur (Mallon, 2011). The *continuing bonds theory* was developed by Klass, Silverman, & Nickman (1996) and maintains that bonds of attachment that were forged in life continue into the future of the survivors. Because these bonds continue, the full resolution of grief is not detachment from the one who has died, but the incorporation of the lost loved one into the bereaved person's own life. Perinatal losses pose a challenge because the bonds of attachment are newly formed and time is often short to create meaningful memories to sustain parents and families in the future. Much of current nursing care of women and families who experience stillbirth or neonatal death is oriented around the creation of meaningful rituals to carry forward into the future (Limbo & Kobler, 2010).

The *dual process model* described by Stroebe and Schut (1999) and emphasizes the processes and strategies individuals use to manage grief and bereavement, as opposed to stages of grief. Individuals move between behaviors oriented toward their losses (focusing on grief, their loss, and the past) and those oriented toward the restoration of their lives without their loved ones (focusing on the future, avoiding grief). Individuals can oscillate rapidly between these two orientations. Nurses who do not understand this phenomenon may be confused by what they construe as "denial" of a loss by their clients. For instance, a mother whose baby died at birth may stop crying soon thereafter, ask for food, take a shower, and talk on the phone. This is *not* a sign that she is not grieving or that she is "in denial." She may be strategic in alleviating her profound grief by focusing for a while on less dramatic, day-to-day activities. Denial is a psychologic defense mechanism by which a person protects oneself from a distressful reality by removing that reality from conscious awareness. It is different from the restorative behaviors explained by the dual process model, in which the person is conscious of the loss but is seeking temporary relief from the expression of profound grief.

Caring Theory to Guide Nursing Practice When Pregnancy Ends in Loss

Women, their partners, and extended families look to the nursing staff for support and understanding during the time of loss. Caring theory provides a model for practice by which nurses can be particularly helpful to grieving individuals. Swanson developed her caring theory from her research with women and their partners experiencing a perinatal loss, specifically miscarriage (Swanson, Chen, Graham, et al., 2009). Swanson's caring theory has five concepts that describe key elements in the nurse-client relationship:

1. Knowing
2. Being with
3. Doing for
4. Enabling
5. Maintaining belief

Knowing means that the nurse must assess the woman, partner, and family (as applicable and appropriate) in order to understand how they perceive the loss and what the loss means to them. *Being with* denotes the caring presence of the nurse, who as a function of professional caring conveys acceptance of the various feelings and perceptions of each family member. *Doing for* refers to those activities and interventions that the nurse performs on behalf of the woman and her family that provide physical care, comfort, and safety. *Enabling* occurs when the nurse offers the woman and her family options for care. Providing information, giving guidance, articulating choices for decision making, and giving support help the family feel more in control of a situation in which they can feel out of control. Enabling allows them to feel more comfortable in asking for what they need such as creating memories, spending time with their infant or with the infant's body, or garnering support from other sources such as friends and clergy. Women and their families then have more autonomy in working through their grief within the family's own traditions and needs. *Maintaining belief* involves encouraging the woman and her family to believe in their ability to survive their loss. By spending time with the family, the nurse becomes familiar with their strengths and coping abilities and helps them draw on these resources to grow from the loss (Swanson et al., 2009).

TYPES OF LOSSES ASSOCIATED WITH PREGNANCY

End-of-life care in perinatal settings brings together death—one of the most difficult of human experiences—and birth, one of life's most joyous occasions. When death and birth coexist, nurses face great challenges. Intervening effectively for these women and families in this situation takes great skill, which can be cultivated by a thorough understanding of the implications of types of pregnancy losses.

Defining Perinatal Losses

Losses associated with reproduction include infertility, miscarriage, intrauterine fetal death (IUFD), stillbirth, and deaths of live-born infants soon after birth. In 2011 the American Academy of Pediatrics (AAP) Committee on Fetus and Newborn recommended standard terminology for deaths associated with pregnancy (Barfield & Committee on Fetus and Newborn, 2011). **Miscarriage** is any in utero death prior to 20 weeks of gestation. **Fetal death** refers to any death prior to birth after 20 weeks of gestation. Fetal deaths are subdivided as early (20 to 27 weeks of gestation) or late (≥28 weeks of gestation). A **stillbirth** is a fetal death that occurs at 20 weeks or later. Death of a live-born infant less than 7 days old is referred to as an **early neonatal death;** those occurring between 7 and 28 days are **late neonatal deaths.** Any live birth resulting in death within the first year is defined as an **infant death** (Barfield & Committee on Fetus and Newborn). It is important to understand that these events not only represent emotional distress for women and families but also are indicators of the health of women and infants. Health care practitioners are required to report fetal deaths, live births, and infant deaths, which collectively are used to determine perinatal and neonatal mortality rates at a national level. These rates are in turn used to influence policy decisions related to allocation of resources to improve care and outcomes.

Types of Perinatal Losses

Perinatal loss is a general term commonly used to describe losses associated with childbearing, particularly those losses that occur after conception has occurred and the woman has recognized that she is pregnant. The complex emotional issues of infertility including loss and grief for women and men are discussed in Chapter 9. For the remainder of this chapter, the focus is on losses specific to pregnancy and the early neonatal period.

Miscarriage

Losses associated with childbearing are common. Early spontaneous losses are typically referred to as miscarriages. Specific information about the causes, symptoms, and signs of miscarriages are presented in Chapter 28. Although some providers refer to these losses as "spontaneous abortions," miscarriage is becoming the accepted term among providers to differentiate this form of loss from elective abortions. Losses that occur early in pregnancy are often suffered in isolation because other people in the women's family and social network may not even know about the pregnancy and subsequent loss. Because family and friends may not feel comfortable bringing up the loss with the woman and her partner, they may experience both grief and loneliness (Brier, 2008).

Serious Fetal Diagnosis

Diagnosis of a serious fetal defect is a newly described form of perinatal loss. Current standards of maternity care include at least one ultrasound examination, often done between 17 and 20 weeks of gestation, at which point the fetal anatomy can be assessed for growth and the presence of congenital defects. The increased use of ultrasonography in prenatal care has resulted in increased diagnosis of fetal defects; note that this is an increase in the *diagnosis* of defects, not in the actual *incidence* of defects. Women and their partners who find out that their expected baby has a defect face difficult decisions about the whether to continue or to terminate the pregnancy. These decisions are often made based on the severity of the defect and the certainty of the prognosis.

The diagnosis of a severe fetal defect causes several losses for couples, including "loss of the joy of pregnancy, possibilities inherent in pregnancy, the dream child, innocence, and the world as they knew it" (Sandelowski & Barroso, 2005, p. 311). Many fetuses with particularly severe defects die in utero. Some live-born infants survive only a few minutes or hours after birth, while others stay days, weeks, or months in a neonatal intensive care unit (NICU), where complex technologies and invasive treatments may be used to try to save their lives. Once these fragile infants are admitted to the NICU, parents can be confronted with making difficult end-of-life decisions about their baby (Kenner, 2014).

CLINICAL REASONING

Care of a Couple with a New Diagnosis of a Severe Fetal Defect

Diana is a 36-year-old multipara who is pregnant with her third child. She and her husband, James, are excited about today's 18-week ultrasound exam because they are hoping to find out the sex of the baby. They already have two sons and are hoping this baby is a girl. The pregnancy has been advancing without difficulty. Diana has felt fetal movement for about 2 weeks and her early nausea and vomiting have resolved. The ultrasound, however, reveals that their expected baby has a hypoplastic left heart syndrome and a severe diaphragmatic hernia. Diana and James learn that either one of these defects is life threatening when they occur alone; when they occur together, death is almost certain. They are devastated. Several consulting physicians come in to talk to them about the problems and what, if anything, can be done. Diana and James ask if they can go home and come back in 2 days once they have the chance to process the news. Diana is crying and tells the nurse that she "can't take in any more information today." When the nurse tells James that she is sorry about what they have found out, he snaps at her, "Mistakes happen all the time. This is one of those times. Our baby is fine." He appears angry and tells Diana to "pull herself together."

1. Evidence—What can the nurse discern from the encounter in the clinic with Diana and James?
2. Assumptions—What assumptions can be made about the following factors?
   a. Each partner's grief responses
   b. The relationship between Diana and James
   c. The level of information that can be assimilated at once
3. What are the priorities for nursing care based on the couple's immediate responses to the diagnosis?
4. Does the evidence objectively support your conclusion?

Pregnancy Termination

Few topics in women's health are more controversial than elective abortion; however, nurses in perinatal settings sometimes encounter women who have chosen to terminate the pregnancy or who have had an abortion in the past. These decisions are shaped by numerous, varied, and often complex circumstances, and women choosing pregnancy termination or seeking care afterward require sensitive attention.

The diagnosis of a severe congenital fetal defect often results in pregnancy termination, sometimes referred to as TOPFA (termination of pregnancy for fetal anomalies), especially if the prognosis for the fetus or newborn is dire or clearly fatal. Sandelowski and Barroso (2005) described a severe fetal diagnosis as posing an "existential crisis" that required women and their partners to "choose the fate of their unborn child and, in the process, confront, reconcile, and subsequently act on their beliefs about human imperfection and disability, the obligations of parenthood, and the acceptability of abortion" (p. 311). Couples receiving the news that their expected baby has a severe, life-threatening problem must often, in a very short time, make a decision whether to terminate the pregnancy. The gestational age limit for legal abortion shortens the time that women have to decide because the diagnosis is often made in midpregnancy. The gestational age limit for abortion varies across states.

A difficult situation of loss occurs when a woman is found to have a multifetal pregnancy (occurring most commonly after infertility treatments) and a procedure known as **selective reduction** is recommended to reduce the number of developing embryos to a number (usually one to three) that can be safely carried to near term. Morbidity and mortality of higher-order gestations (more than two fetuses) are significant and are often related to complications from preeclampsia, preterm labor, and other conditions requiring significantly early birth. The loss and grief experienced by the expectant parents can moderate their joy if selective reduction of multifetal pregnancy is recommended (Little, 2010). Women who have selective reductions or TOPFAs may benefit from ongoing psychosocial support in order to prevent or reduce psychological distress over time (Mashiach, Anter, Melamed, et al., 2013).

Women who choose abortion as a result of social and financial obstacles that preclude continuing the pregnancy can have coexisting, seemingly opposite feelings (Stotland, 2011). The majority (69%) of women who have elective abortions have incomes below 200% of the official poverty levels and 61% have one or more children (Jones, Finer, & Singh, 2010). Stotland noted that among women who have an abortion, sadness is not uncommon despite their relief afterward. Women can mourn the end of the pregnancy despite determining that ending the pregnancy was the best option available at the time. Nurses who provide care for women in settings where pregnancy terminations are performed must be nonjudgmental and recognize that women experience a sense of loss and grief even when the abortion is elective.

Other Losses

Other losses associated with childbearing can result in distress or even grief, even if the loss does not involve death. In the United States, 11.5% of births occur prematurely (<37 weeks) (Martin, Hamilton, Osterman et al., 2013). Preterm birth disrupts the pregnancy trajectory and can result in a transition to parenthood for women and their partners that is unexpected and for which they are unprepared. The baby that they had dreamed of and hoped for may be replaced by the reality of a small baby that is sick or requires lengthy hospitalization before going home. Breastfeeding can be delayed or foregone, resulting in another loss.

Other women grieve the loss of the birth experience they have dreamed of and planned for, specifically a vaginal birth. Despite being happy for the birth of their newborn that may have otherwise not survived a serious obstetric complication, some women feel sadness and even grieve the fact that they required a cesarean birth. Sadness can be compounded when the cesarean surgery is done as an emergency procedure under general anesthesia, meaning that the woman and her partner are separated during the birth and the new mother does not hear her baby's first cries. The reality of the birth experience is inconsistent with the parents' hopes and dreams.

Perinatal Care Settings Where Nurses Encounter Loss

Nurses have a significant influence on how women, their partners, and families experience and cope with perinatal loss. Nurses encounter situations of loss in a variety of settings, including antepartum, labor and birth, neonatal, postpartum, and gynecologic inpatient units and prenatal, gynecologic, and infertility outpatient clinics, family planning settings, and general medical offices. In each of these settings nurses can provide sensitive care to persons experiencing loss. Nurses in many inpatient settings have developed protocols that provide clear direction to all staff about how to help women and families through this difficult event. In some units experienced nurses or social workers who are particularly comfortable in helping bereaved families are designated as perinatal grief consultants. They are available to help parents and assist, educate, and support staff in caring for grieving parents and families. In addition, many institutions have follow-up programs involving phone calls, home visits, and support groups that are effective in helping parents after discharge.

Perinatal palliative care, sometimes referred to as perinatal hospice, is a formalized end-of-life (EOL) interdisciplinary care model specifically aimed at intervening when pregnancy is expected to end in stillbirth or neonatal death. Perinatal care providers, including nurses, view perinatal palliative care as a positive means that allows families a voice in the planning and preparation for the birth and death of their expected baby (Wool, 2013a), although not all factors that can benefit expectant parents in this situation have been identified (Wool, 2013b). In a review of intervention studies of support for mothers, fathers, and families after a perinatal death, Koopmans, Wilson, Cacciatore, and Flenady (2013) found that little is yet known about the role and effectiveness of different types of perinatal bereavement support.

Most palliative and hospice care for older clients with terminal illness is delivered by community-based palliative care and hospice agencies whose main purpose is to provide symptom management and grief and bereavement care. Perinatal palliative care occurs in three settings: large referral centers such as academic medical centers with maternal-fetal medicine specialists and neonatal intensive care units; community hospital settings where staff members occasionally provide care for women and families experiencing stillbirth, preterm birth, or other types of perinatal losses; and traditional palliative care or hospice agencies that have expanded care options to families experiencing a perinatal loss.

Each of these models has strengths and weaknesses. Large referral centers encounter perinatal losses frequently as a function of the number of high risk pregnancies followed in these settings. Providers in these settings have a great deal of experience with loss, and some medical centers have well-developed perinatal palliative care teams and protocols. Follow-up grief and bereavement care, however, can be difficult because the bereaved families often live in communities far from the medical center. Community hospitals are increasingly developing interdisciplinary perinatal palliative care programs in response to the needs of bereaved families in the local community. Importantly, the programs may serve families for whom the expected baby has a congenital defect that is incompatible with life (e.g., anencephaly, bilateral renal agenesis) and for whom the high-tech interventions of a medical center would be futile. EOL care agencies have extensive experience in symptom management and grief and bereavement care; however, the specific needs of families with losses related to childbearing may be outside their usual expertise. Many of these agencies are developing specific programs to assist with perinatal losses with specific staff identified to provide care under these circumstances. A comprehensive list of agencies providing perinatal palliative care or hospice across the United States and in other parts of world can be found at www.perinatalhospice.org. This website is updated frequently and contains other information about perinatal loss and EOL care that is helpful to both nurses and families.

MILES'S MODEL OF PARENTAL GRIEF RESPONSES

The previous section contained definitions of grief and several related concepts, and different types of perinatal loss were explained. Putting concepts into practice, however, involves using care models. For instance, perinatal palliative care involves using concepts germane to care of childbearing families and EOL care. A key goal of all care for women and families with a perinatal loss is helping them through their grief. Understanding key elements of grief can help nurses be prepared to encounter the poignant, painful loss for families when their expected baby dies.

The model of grief presented here is based on years of clinical work by Margaret Miles, who worked with bereaved parents in several settings and in community support groups throughout her career (Miles, 1984). Miles usually referred to pregnant women and their male partners as parents and often referred to them as mothers and fathers. It is important, however, to recognize that not all pregnant women see themselves as mothers yet; neither are all of their partners necessarily male nor do they always see themselves as fathers. Miles's work remains relevant with regard to grief responses of women and their partners; to be consistent with Miles's model, however, the terms *parents* and *parental* are used in the broadest manner possible across pregnancy and the early postpartum period.

Miles hypothesized that parental grief responses occur in three overlapping phases (Box 37-1). An early period of *acute distress* and shock is followed by a period of *intense grief* that includes emotional, cognitive, behavioral, and physical responses. *Reorganization* occurs when they return to their usual level of functioning, although the pain associated with the death remains. Grief is a long-term process that can extend for months and years; some aspects of grief endure through life. This is consistent with continuing bonds theory discussed previously, in which the goal of the grief process is not resolution but rather the incorporation of the person who has died into one's own life moving forward.

Acute Distress

Pregnancy loss or the death of an infant can be an acute and distressing experience for women and their partners. The loss encompasses a loss of their identity or anticipated identity as a mother or father to this particular child and their dreams related to parenthood. A period of acute distress characterized by shock and numbness is initiated after learning of an intrauterine death, impending stillbirth, or infant death. Parents experience a sense of unreality, loss of innocence, and powerlessness, described as being devastated or feeling like they are in a bad dream, a fog, or trance. Disbelief and even denial can occur. Profound sadness accompanied by intense outbursts of emotion and crying is common. Occasionally a lack of affect, calmness, or even euphoria can reflect their numbness. For some, their way of coping with a profound loss is to avoid emotional displays. Women can develop mental health problems such as depression and anxiety from overwhelming grief and sense of loss.

Depression is a medical condition that differs from grief. Recognizing symptoms of depression, especially in the presence of grief, can be very difficult. Nurses must be aware of the difference between grief and depression. Screening tools for depression are easily administered in clinical settings and can be very useful in helping determine if an individual has symptoms of depression. Nurses must seek referrals for those women and partners who show symptoms of depression. The coexistence of depression and grief can have serious implications for a person's health and daily functioning. Much of the literature and research on grief after perinatal loss or infant death has focused on the woman or mother. Similarly, much of the attention at the time of a loss is on the woman, and her partner is usually expected to be her main support. The partner's grief is sometimes not recognized or acknowledged. The response of men can be more variable than that of women and can depend on the level of identification with the pregnancy. With early miscarriage or ectopic pregnancy, for instance, some partners or fathers may not yet have developed a strong investment in the expected child. However, many fathers are profoundly affected and grieve deeply after perinatal loss, yet their feelings are often ignored (O'Leary & Thorwick, 2006). The nonbiologic mother in a lesbian couple may be profoundly affected by the biologic mother's loss; sometimes she may have a prior history of infertility or loss of her own that she is grieving again (Black & Fields, 2014). Partners may hide their feelings from each other to protect the other during times of loss (Stroebe, Finkenhauer, Wijngaards-de Meij, et al., 2013).

Men are distressed by the grief of their partner and often feel helpless as to how to help her with the intense pain (O'Leary & Thorwick, 2006). Some men appear stoic in response to a sense of need to remain "strong" for the mother and other family members when in fact they are experiencing deep pain and need help in acknowledging these feelings. Because many men do not easily share feelings or ask for help, nurses may need to be intentional in addressing their grief and in helping them realize that they too need to receive support from others as they grieve. Experiences of grief are complex, and each partner within a couple (heterosexual or same sex) must come to terms with both the loss and the effects of the loss on their partner as they determine the resultant effect on their relationship with each other (Avelin, Rådestad, Säflund, et al., 2013).

During the acute distress period, parents face the first task of grief, accepting the reality of the loss. The pregnancy has ended or the baby has died, thereby changing their lives. They are often required to make many decisions during this period when normal functioning is impeded and decisions are difficult to make. This can be especially painful and difficult for young couples who have limited or no previous experience with death. These couples may turn to their own parents to help make difficult decisions regarding funeral arrangements or disposition of the

BOX 37-1 Conceptual Model of Parental Grief

Phase of Acute Distress
- Shock
- Numbness
- Intense crying
- Depression

Phase of Intense Grief
- Loneliness, emptiness, yearning
- Guilt
- Anger, resentment, bitterness, irritability
- Fear and anxiety (especially about getting pregnant again)
- Disorganization
- Difficulties with cognitive processing
- Sadness and depression
- Physical symptoms

Reorganization
- Search for meaning
- Reduction of distress
- Reentering normal life activities with more enthusiasm
- Can make plans, including decision about another pregnancy

Adapted from Miles, M. (1980). *The grief of parents...when a child dies.* Oak Brook, IL: Compassionate Friends; Miles, M. (1984). Helping adults mourn the death of a child. In H. Wass, & C. Orr (Eds.), *Childhood and death.* New York: Hemisphere.

body because they have more life experience. However, some well-meaning grandparents and other family members may try to make all the decisions in order to spare the bereaved parents additional grief associated with disposal of the baby's body or making funeral arrangements. The nurse as advocate can be very important in making sure that the bereaved parents are comfortable with the extent to which well-meaning family members are involved. An important goal of perinatal palliative care services is to help families make as many decisions as possible in advance of the birth, freeing them from having to make choices in the early acute phase of grief when decision making is very difficult.

Intense Grief

The phase of intense grief encompasses many difficult emotions as the parents work through their pain and adjust to life without the child they were expecting. This phase displaces the acute grief and will likely take longer to move through. In the early months after the loss parents often experience feelings of loneliness, emptiness, and yearning. Women may report that their arms literally ache to hold the baby or they may think they hear a baby crying. Milk production still occurs for most women as part of the normal postpartum physiologic changes, even though there is no infant to feed. Lactation is a poignant reminder of the loss and requires careful planning by the nurse to assist the woman in managing the milk and breast discomfort that can occur.

Preoccupation with the expected baby that died is not uncommon. Women who have recently given birth often want to talk about details of the experience; women who had a stillbirth or whose baby died may have a particularly strong need to share details about the birth. Nurses can actively listen, taking time to allow women to work through their birth and loss stories as they try to make sense and meaning of the experience.

Going home without the baby is particularly difficult, and bereaved parents may face a decision about what to do with the nursery and baby items that they have collected or been given. Some women may want the nursery taken down before they go home, whereas others want the room left intact until they have had time to grieve their loss. Well-meaning grandparents, relatives, or friends may rush to put away nursery furniture and baby items with the thought that they would be sparing the bereaved parents additional pain. In fact, their actions might only complicate the grief if parents were not involved in the decision. The bereaved parents should have the opportunity to make the decision about when, and by whom, the nursery and baby items are stored or given away.

Guilt can accompany intense grief. During this phase women may wonder what they did to cause the loss or if there was anything that they could have to done to prevent it. Women are particularly vulnerable to feelings of guilt because of their sense of responsibility for the well-being of the fetus and baby. Often losses occur with no clear cause, leaving the woman to speculate about the cause of the loss and her role in it. Sometimes the guilt can be intense if the woman believes she is being punished for some unrelated event. Pressure to be "perfect" in one's lifestyle such as nutrition, exercise, and rest can encumber women with guilt if a pregnancy loss ensues. Women sometimes analyze their behaviors in detail in an effort to explain the loss; they may focus on occasions when they may have had a glass of wine or a cigarette, or stayed out late, blaming themselves for something that was inevitable or unavoidable. Women engaging in self-blame need emotional reassurance that they were not at fault. As their sadness begins to resolve, couples may experience guilt when they begin to socialize, enjoy their family and friends, and experience pleasure again despite the loss of their baby.

Anger, resentment, bitterness, or irritability are common during this phase of grief. Anger can be focused on the health care team who, in the opinion or belief of the bereaved parents, failed to save the pregnancy, fetus, or infant. Some parents direct their anger toward God, blaming God for allowing the loss to occur. Sometimes people experience a spiritual crisis as a result of the loss. Anger may be focused toward family, friends, and peers when they do not provide the support that bereaved parents need and want. Feeling anger at mothers and fathers who appear not to "deserve" or appreciate their children is common; bereaved parents may find that news of neglected or abused children is more intolerable than it was before their loss. Being around pregnant women can be very upsetting. Prolonged anger and generalized irritability may be signs of depression that needs treatment by a mental health care provider.

When couples begin to consider the next pregnancy, they are likely to experience fear and anxiety due to concerns about another tragic outcome (DeBackere, Hill, & Kavanaugh, 2008). Some women want to become pregnant again right away; tension can arise between partners when one is ready to pursue pregnancy again and the other is not. Deep sadness occurs when the parent faces the full awareness of the reality of the loss; this time can be characterized by *disorganization,* a time when individuals can experience a variety of changes. Cognitive changes can occur, such as an inability to concentrate, confused thought processes, difficulty in problem solving, and poor decision making. Disorganization often causes difficulties in keeping up with work and family expectations. Returning to work can be painful as bereaved parents face their colleagues and coworkers. Some people find a great deal of comfort in returning to work, however; it gives them a sense of normalcy and routine in their grief. Families of children who have died have reported finding support from their friends as particularly useful, as is informal support from health care providers acting outside of their formal role as nurse, social worker, or physician (Gear, 2014).

Physical symptoms of grief include fatigue, headaches, dizziness, or musculoskeletal aches and pains. Bereaved individuals can be immunosuppressed, leading them to contract respiratory and gastrointestinal infections more easily than before their loss. Lack of sleep, a common complaint among grieving individuals, contributes to their risk for health problems. Weight changes are common: appetites can be poor or individuals can turn to food as a coping response. Changes in health behaviors are common in grieving people.

Grief is very personal, ongoing, and difficult to endure. It is important for nurses to help grieving parents understand their responses and make sense of their feelings. Giving them a safe place to express their feelings is a key nursing intervention. The path to healing can be difficult but is eased to a degree when bereaved clients feel supported and their profound loss is affirmed.

Reorganization

From the time of the pregnancy loss or infant death, parents attempt to understand "why?" This leads to a long and intense search for meaning. At first the question of "why" is focused on the cause of death. Finding few good answers, parents focus next on "why me, why mine?" These questions lead some parents into an existential search about the meaning of life and death. The search for meaning involves questions such as "What does this loss mean to my life?" "What is life all about?" "What do I do now?" This search continues into the phase of reorganization and can lead to profound changes in the bereaved parents' views and philosophies about life.

Time helps to ease the painful feelings of grief. Although some grief models focus on "letting go" as an important step in the grief process, bereaved parents often want to hold on to their relationship with their child (Davies, 2004). With perinatal loss, however, parents have few, if any, memories of their infant to provide a balance to their sense of loss. They usually cherish relics and mementos of birth and evidence of the life of their baby, even if by ultrasound photos. Some perinatal EOL settings provide numerous forms of mementos to memorialize the baby, such as hand molds, footprints, locks of hair, clothing, and blankets. One bereaved mother described her plan to preserve her baby daughter's scent by storing in a sealed bag the cap that was placed on the baby at birth. This live-born baby with known serious defects died at 8 hours of age after lengthy resuscitation efforts in the NICU. The mother created an elaborate set of memorabilia, did online blogging, and joined a support group of bereaved mothers who reach out to newly bereaved mothers. She sought to make meaning of her daughter's short life by helping other mothers through their pain. Wisely, she recognized that she had to resolve some of her own grief before she could safely provide support for other bereaved mothers.

Like the bereaved mother just described, overwhelming feelings become less painful as time passes. Reorganization occurs when the parent is better able to function at home and work, experiences a return of self-esteem and confidence, can cope with new challenges, and has placed the loss in perspective. Reorganization often—but not always—occurs after several months or a year as parents begin to move on with their lives. Enjoying pleasures without guilt, nurturing self and others, developing new interests, and reestablishing relationships are signs of moving on. For some women and families, another pregnancy and the birth of a subsequent child are important steps in moving on with their lives (Swanson, Connor, Jolley, et al., 2007). However, the term *recovery* is not appropriate because the grief related to perinatal loss, as with any loss, can continue for life. Parents have reported that they will never forget the baby who died, and they are changed from the loss. They note certain anniversary dates related to the pregnancy and birth, such as the day they found out that the baby had a congenital defect, the date of a miscarriage, the date of birth, and the date of death.

Resuming sexual activity can very complicated for grieving couples. Often women are physically ready to resume sexual activity before they are emotionally ready. Some women and their partners find that sexual activity is important for emotional closeness and healing, whereas others have a decreased desire for sex. Partners may have divergent views about when and how to resume sex; nurses can help couples to understand that this is common. Continuing conflicts around sex can be detrimental to a couple's relationship and may require professional counseling to help resolve this issue. Through careful assessment nurses can help women and their partners determine if they can benefit from professional counseling as they work through the many complicated issues, including sexuality, that are involved in living through grief.

Deciding to become pregnant again can involve intense and conflicting emotions (DeBackere et al., 2008). Fear of another loss can impede the decision. Couples may believe that their risk for another loss is higher than it actually is, so it is important that they understand why the previous loss occurred if possible. Often this is not possible; they need to understand that most losses are very unlikely to repeat, especially the first one. If a couple has had more than one pregnancy loss, genetic counselors may help determine if there is an explanation for the losses. Ambivalence is common. Expectant parents may feel anxiety during a subsequent pregnancy that tempers their excitement (Côté-Arsenault & Donato, 2007). This distress can continue even after the birth of a healthy infant and affect maternal attachment to the new baby (Armstrong, 2007). Men also report anxiety about the outcome of the next pregnancy (Armstrong; O'Leary & Thorwick, 2006). Expectant parents may delay emotional investment in a subsequent pregnancy and the developing fetus until after the midpregnancy ultrasound exam; some who had a loss late in the prior pregnancy will feel anxiety and distress throughout the subsequent pregnancy. At an extreme, mothers may withhold attachment to their new infant as a means of protecting themselves against the painful prospect of another loss.

FAMILY ASPECTS OF GRIEF

Nurses who care for grieving parents also often care for the extended family, including siblings of the expected baby and the parents of the bereaved woman and her partner (grandparents of the expected baby). The grief of grandparents is often complex because they are experiencing intense emotional pain related to the loss while witnessing and feeling the immense grief of their own child. It is extremely difficult to watch their son or daughter experience profound sadness with very few ways to comfort and ease their pain. As a result, the grief response can be complicated or delayed for grandparents. Some experience immense "survivor guilt" because they feel the death is out of order because they are alive and their grandchild has died.

The siblings of the expected infant also experience loss. Most parents begin to prepare their children for the arrival of a new baby at some point during the pregnancy. In assisting families in dealing with pregnancy loss, the children's age, development, and level of understanding must be considered. Understanding death requires some ability to think abstractly and children do not fully understand the concept often until their early school years. Parents may create their own explanation to their children based on religious beliefs and their knowledge of their own child's development and abilities. Children can have a great deal of difficulty understanding why there suddenly is no baby or the baby has not come home (Limbo & Kobler, 2009). A young child will respond to the reactions of his or her parents, picking up on cues related to parents' sadness and behaviors. Young children may respond with clinging, changes in eating and sleeping patterns, or uncharacteristic behavior at the time when parents have limited patience for responding to and meeting the child's needs. Older children have a more complete understanding of the loss. School-aged children can be frightened by their parents' sadness, whereas teens can understand more fully but feel awkward in responding. Teenagers may feel more comfortable in talking with their friends than with adults in dealing with their loss and grief.

Nurses can help to include siblings in grieving rituals to the extent the parents and the child feel comfortable, including seeing the baby's body. Nurses should follow the parents' lead but can suggest rituals and activities at the time of the loss that may be helpful for the children. The extent of the involvement of children at the time of a loss is likely to be determined by the length of the pregnancy. An early miscarriage will be managed differently from an unexpected stillbirth at term. Nurses who are specifically interested in perinatal loss may want to consider additional training such as that offered by Resolve Through Sharing (http://www.bereavementservices.org/resolve-through-sharing) to increase their skills in working with families experiencing these distressful losses.

CARE MANAGEMENT

Nursing care of mothers and their partners experiencing a perinatal loss begins the first time the parents are faced with the potential loss of their pregnancy or death of their infant. Supportive interventions are important when parents are anticipating loss, at the time of the loss, and after the parents have returned home. In order to provide competent, compassionate, individualized care to grieving parents and their families, the nurse first does a thorough assessment. Several key areas to address include the following:

- The nature of the parental attachment to the pregnancy and developing fetus or infant, the meaning of the pregnancy and infant to the parent, and the related losses they are experiencing. Whether a woman has experienced a miscarriage or ectopic pregnancy, stillbirth, or death of an infant, it is important to understand parents' perceptions of their unique loss.
- Complex family and cultural systems that influence the meaning of the loss. Feelings about perinatal loss can range from feeling devastated to feeling relieved. Listening to parents tell their story and being sensitive to the language used to describe their experience can help nurses gain an understanding of the meaning of the loss. For example, if a woman refers to a miscarriage as "losing a pregnancy," nurses should be careful to edit their language not to refer to "your baby" but to use the cues the woman has given with regard to her view of the loss. Similarly, if a woman refers to the fetus by name or as her daughter or son, nurses should do the same. For instance, a woman who elects to terminate the pregnancy when the fetus is found to have a fatal defect may not even mention the fetus at all or may refer to the fetus as "it" or "the pregnancy." This is a distancing behavior that is protective and normal. Nurses' language surrounding grief and loss should follow the cues given by the bereaved woman and partner, who may model the terms they prefer in referring to the loss.
- The circumstances surrounding the loss, including the time to prepare for the loss and the parents' level of understanding about the cause of the loss or death, and any related unresolved issues. As nurses come to know their clients, they may discover special experiences that make their losses even more poignant. A history of infertility, repeated pregnancy losses, a previous stillbirth, or infant death can make this loss even more painful. In addition, other life circumstances such as illness of another family member, loss of a job, or other family stresses can increase distress. The nonbiologic mother in a lesbian relationship may have a history of losses of her own that are revisited when her partner experiences a loss. Also, losses for which the expectant parents are unprepared such as an obstetric accident late in pregnancy can constitute a traumatic event that requires a great deal of sensitive and intense intervention.
- The immediate responses of the mother and partner to the loss, whether their responses are similar or different, and if their responses are consistent with their past experiences and sociocultural contexts. An understanding of common responses to grief described earlier can be helpful in attempting to understand the unique grief responses of the mother, partner, and other family members. As nurses work with families, they can find out how the individual or family responded to a previous loss or a personality or behavioral trait that may be involved in their responses to this grief. For instance, if a woman who has usually been outgoing and talkative is now withdrawn and silent, the nurse can ask her if in the past this is how she has grieved other losses. People tend to grieve various losses in their lives similarly, even though the meaning of each loss is unique. In helping women and their partners through a perinatal loss, it is important to know if there is a history of infertility, previous pregnancy losses, or infant deaths. The accumulation of losses can negatively affect grief responses. It also is important to be sensitive to varied expectations during grief for men and women from different cultural groups (see section on cultural and spiritual needs of parents later in this chapter).
- The social support network of the woman and her partner (e.g., extended family, friends, coworkers, church) and the extent to which it has been engaged. Social support in response to a perinatal loss can be very important; however, nurses should assess the amount and type of support that the bereaved family desires. Some prefer a few days alone to recover physically, whereas others find comfort in being surrounded immediately with supportive family and friends. In inpatient settings the nurse may need to be an advocate for a woman desiring solitude by limiting visitors. Other women want or need assistance in communicating with family members about the loss, in making necessary decisions, and in contacting clergy. The nurse should not assume that all women who have had a perinatal loss will want to be visited by clergy, but should ask if the woman would like a visit by the hospital chaplain or her own pastor and if so, to identify the specific religious tradition.

Nursing diagnoses can include physiologic and psychosocial problems experienced by the individual woman or her partner, or problems occurring within the couple or family because of the loss and subsequent grief. Examples of nursing diagnoses include the following:

- *Anxiety* related to
  - lack of experience regarding how to manage the loss

NURSING CARE PLAN

Fetal Death and Stillbirth at 35 Weeks of Gestation

NURSING DIAGNOSIS	EXPECTED OUTCOME	INTERVENTIONS	RATIONALES
Risk for Complicated Grieving related to fetal death, as evidenced by intense expressions of grief for prolonged period of time	Parents will experience fewer expressions of grief as evidence of improved coping with their loss.	Prepare family for viewing infant by cleaning body and wrapping in clean blanket.	To initiate and support them in their grief in a supportive setting
		Allow family quiet time to hold and view infant. Take pictures for family to keep if they want them.	To provide evidence of the reality of the death while honoring the existence of their baby
		Provide a certificate for the family with vital statistics, along with identification bands, lock of hair (with parental permission), and footprints.	To provide tangible evidence and memories of their baby's life as a means of creating bonds that they can incorporate into their lives
		Provide spiritual support as needed to assist with religious services, such as baptism and memorial services.	To engage additional forms of support and to assist in creating meaning of their baby's life and death
		Refer to appropriate community support groups or web-based resources.	To facilitate grieving through interactions with others who have had the same experience
Situational Low Self-Esteem related to fetal death as evidenced by woman's sense of failure to become a mother	Woman will exhibit positive self-comments as evidence of her decreasing sense of failure.	Provide private time for expressions of feelings through therapeutic communication and active listening.	To have her express her feelings openly and without judgment
		Identify woman's perception and feelings about fetal death.	To correct any misconceptions and alleviate guilt
		Assist woman to identify positive coping mechanisms and support systems.	To promote feelings of self-worth
		Refer to appropriate health professionals for further evaluation and counseling, such as social services.	To provide ongoing assistance as needed
Spiritual Distress related to perinatal loss	Individuals will verbalize a decrease in spiritual distress.	Assess individual's spiritual preference.	To seek appropriate assistance in reinforcing the belief system
		Assist with or facilitate spiritual rituals.	To promote comfort for parents
		Provide opportunity for individuals to express feelings about perinatal loss.	To acknowledge their grief
		Attend memorial service/funeral if feasible.	To provide support to parents and to help process grief of health care provider
Interrupted Family Processes related to inadequate communication of feelings between partners and other family members	Partners will discuss feelings involving relationship with each other and family members.	Provide information to partners about how grief affects a family.	To facilitate expression of grief and sadness among family members
		Encourage partners to talk about their loss and its meaning to the family.	To clarify the possible effects on the family
		Include other children as appropriate and the partners' parents in discussions of the loss.	To acknowledge and respect differences of feelings and grief among family members
		Offer follow-up contact (e.g., phone calls, grief conference).	To provide opportunity for partners to ask questions, share feelings, and to receive information to help them understand the changing nature of grief over time
		Refer family to perinatal or family support group if appropriate.	To minimize a sense of isolation and facilitate communication and sharing of the experience of loss with other who have had similar experiences

- worry about the partner
- intense concern over not achieving a pregnancy
- becoming pregnant again with risk of another loss
- *Ineffective Family Coping* related to
  - inability to make decisions as a family
  - difficulties in communication within the family
  - conflicting coping patterns between mother and father
- *Powerlessness* related to
  - high risk pregnancy and birth
  - unexpected cesarean birth
  - inability to prevent the infant's death
- *Ineffective Sexuality Patterns* between the mother and father related to
  - guilt and fear associated with sexuality
  - loss of pleasure in sexual intercourse
  - differences in desires of each partner
  - fear of getting pregnant again
- *Fatigue* and *Disturbed Sleep Pattern* related to
  - inability to fall asleep because of grief
  - waking in the night and thinking about the loss
  - loss of sleep

Nursing care for women, partners, and families grieving the end of a pregnancy and death of their expected child or newborn is complex and should be comprehensive. The initial shock and numbness that accompany early grief can be misread if the nurse is not aware of the ebb and flow of sadness related to grief and misinterprets important cues (see Nursing Care Plan.)

WHEN A LOSS IS DIAGNOSED: HELPING THE WOMAN AND HER FAMILY IN THE AFTERMATH

Learning of a loss or a potential loss is very distressing to most individuals. Under a great deal of stress, people are likely to have limited ability to take in anything but the most basic information and sometimes appear to "shut down." Simple, unambiguous, and consistent language is crucial. For example, a woman visiting the United States for whom English was her second language began bleeding heavily at 32 weeks of gestation and noticed that her uterus was very hard. Her partner immediately transported her to a local medical center, where she was admitted directly to the high risk maternal-fetal care unit. Her bleeding had subsided but there were no fetal heart tones, and fetal death was confirmed by ultrasound. The resident physician told her that her "baby had passed," which she understood to mean that her pain was related to labor and that she had given birth. She asked where the baby was and began to look under the sheets. The nurse realized her misunderstanding of the word "passed" (as in "passed away" or "had died") and explained to the client that the doctor meant that the baby had died. Although the use of words like "death," "died," and "dying" are difficult in any setting, euphemisms or other veiled language can be misunderstood by women and their families under stress. The nurse's presence is crucial in hearing what other providers have told the woman and family and in clarifying any misunderstandings.

With early pregnancy loss, the word "miscarriage" should be used consistently (Cameron & Penney, 2005). With fetal or neonatal death, providers should use the words "has died" or "there is no heartbeat," rather than "lost," "gone," or "passed" to eliminate ambiguity. Providing the opportunity for women and partners to ask questions, ask for more evidence of the loss, and get a referral for a second opinion gives them some element of control at a time when they have little if any control. Furthermore, in the case of a severe fetal defect, the couple may face a decision about whether to terminate the pregnancy and will want to make the decision with as little ambiguity or unanswered questions as possible.

Helping Parents with Holding Their Fetus or Infant

Research evidence supports the importance of parents' seeing or holding their fetus or infant (Gold, Dalton, & Schwenk, 2007). Many parents find this experience valuable and indicate that they would have liked more time or more opportunities to do so. Seeing and holding the fetus or baby is important because it can help them face the reality of the loss, reduce painful fantasies, and facilitate their grief. It should be noted, however, that although this can be a beneficial experience, it can increase feelings of sadness about their loss and can even be traumatic for some individuals (Badenhorst & Hughes, 2007). Parents should be allowed to choose whether they want to see or hold the body of the fetus or baby. They should never be made to feel they "should" see or hold their baby when this is something that they do not really want. Encouraging reluctant individuals to hold or see the body by telling them that not seeing the body could make grieving more difficult is inappropriate. The nurse might ask question such as, "Some parents have found it helpful to see or hold their baby. Would you like time to consider this?" is helpful. Because the need or willingness to see also can vary among family members, it is important to determine what each person desires and needs. Occasionally only one partner will desire to see or hold the baby's body, or a couple may want to limit holding the baby to themselves without involving other family members. These are difficult situations that have to be handled with extreme tact and sensitivity by the nurse, always with the expectation that the nurse is advocating for what the client wants.

In preparation for the visit with the baby, parents appreciate explanations about what to expect. In preparing the baby's body for the parents to see, nurses generally cover the head with a small cap and clothe the baby. Many hospitals have volunteer groups that provide handcrafted hats and infant gowns for such use, items that may then be taken home by the family. The bodies of fetuses that died in utero must be handled extremely gently because of a process called *maceration* in which the upper layer of the skin begins to peel away from the deeper layers. Maceration often begins at the baby's lips, which then appear redder than usual. Bereaved parents often notice this redness, which actually enhances the baby's appearance. The nurse should remember that parents see their baby with different eyes from health care professionals. Bathing the baby, applying lotion to the baby's skin, combing hair, placing identification bracelets on the arm and leg, dressing the baby in a diaper and special outfit, sprinkling powder in the baby's blanket, and wrapping the baby in a soft blanket convey to the parents that their baby has been cared for in a special way. Sometimes families will want to see the baby's body for a last time after the body has been taken to the morgue. There is no contraindication to this practice related to infection control. If the baby has been in the morgue, the nurse can place the body underneath a warmer for 20 to 30 minutes then wrap the body in a warm blanket.

When bringing the baby's body to the parents, it is important to treat the baby as one would a live baby. Holding the baby close, touching a hand or cheek, using the baby's name, and talking with the parents about the special features of their child conveys that it is all right for them to do likewise. If a baby has a congenital anomaly that the family wants to see, the nurse can help explain what they are seeing. It is not unusual for parents to compare what they are seeing in "real life" with what they had seen on the ultrasound screen. Nurses can help parents explore the baby's body as they desire. Parents often seek to identify family resemblance and will point out characteristics of the baby that are similar to themselves or their previous children. Some families like to have the opportunity to bathe and dress their baby. Although the skin is fragile, parents can still apply lotion with cotton balls, sprinkle powder, tie ribbons, fasten the diaper, and place amulets, medallions, rosaries, or special toys or mementos in their baby's hands or alongside their baby. Parents may want to perform other parenting activities, such as combing the hair, dressing the baby in a special outfit, or wrapping the baby in a blanket (Fig. 37-1).

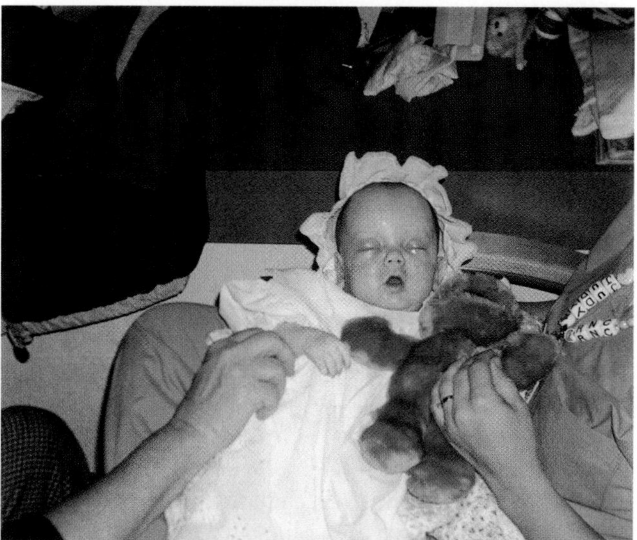

FIG 37-1 Laura. (Courtesy Amy and Ken Turner, Cary, NC.)

Parents need to be given time alone with their baby. They also need to know when the nurse will return and how to call if they should need anything. When possible, the family is placed in a private room with a rocking chair. This offers the parents time together with their baby and with other family members (Fig. 37-2). Marking the door to the room with a special card helps remind the staff that this family has experienced a loss (Fig. 37-3).

Parents and families vary in the amount of time they wish to have the baby's body with them. These moments are the only ones they will have to parent their child while their child's physical presence is still with them. Some parents need only a few minutes; others need hours. It is extremely painful for some parents to say goodbye to their baby. They will tell the nurse when they are ready verbally or the nurse will observe nonverbal cues such as when parents and other family members are no longer holding their child close to them or have placed the baby back in the crib. There should be no institutional restrictions on how long a baby's body can remain in the room with the parents. Most parents become ready to hand the baby over to the nurses or to a funeral home at the time the baby's body shows obvious signs of deterioration, which for a baby that dies at birth will occur in about 24 to 36 hours. Stillborn babies, depending on how long they have been dead in utero prior to birth, will show signs of deterioration sooner. A position paper developed by the Perinatal Loss and Infant Death Alliance (PLIDA, 2005) (PLIDA.org/pdf/infectionRisks.pdf) notes that infection risks "are insignificant" in having the body of a deceased baby in the mother's room. Bereaved mothers and families should have unrestricted access to the baby's body, which allows them to "process the traumatic events surrounding their baby's death" in addition to allowing for a "more gradual goodbye, both of which are productive components of healthy grieving" (PLIDA, 2005, p. 1).

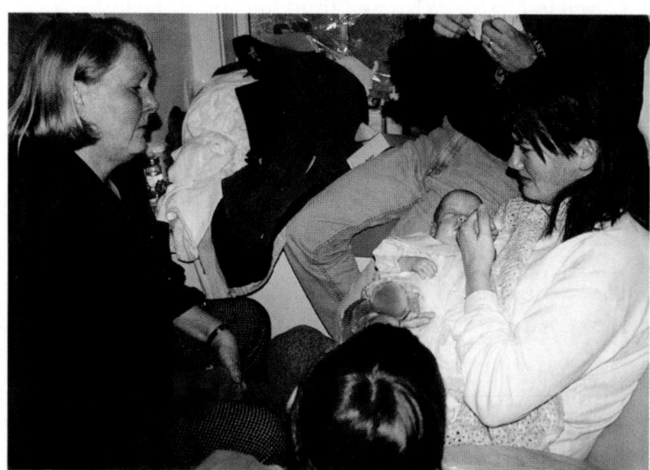

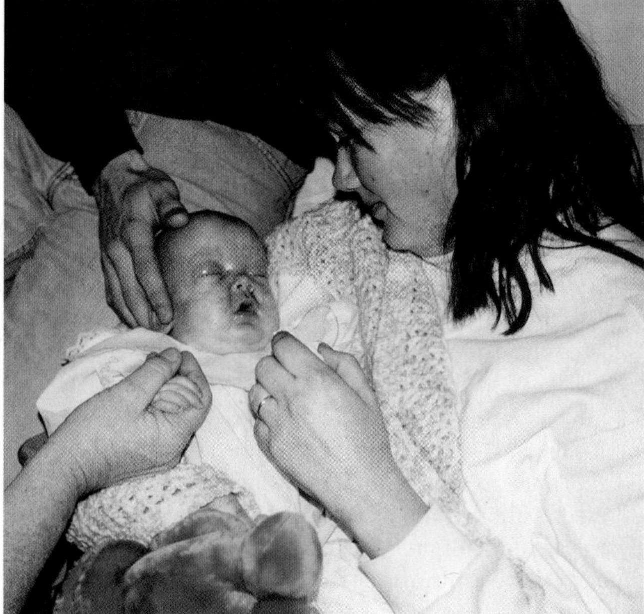

FIG 37-2 Laura's family members say a special goodbye. (Courtesy Amy and Ken Turner, Cary, NC.)

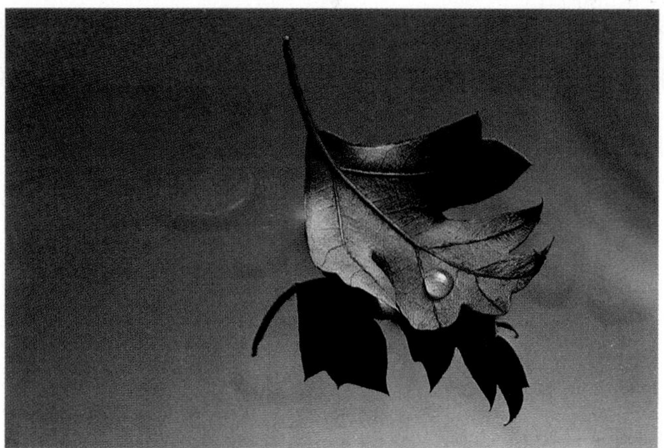

FIG 37-3 Door card for room of mother who has had a perinatal loss. (Used with permission of Bereavement Services. Copyright Lutheran Hospital—La Crosse, Inc., A Gundersen Lutheran Affiliate, La Crosse, WI.)

Helping Parents with Decisions Regarding Autopsies, Organ Donation, and Disposition of the Body

At a time when they are experiencing the great distress of a perinatal loss, parents have many decisions to make. Women, partners, and extended families often consult nurses for guidance in discerning what must be done immediately and what can wait and in understanding their options relative to each decision. The nurse's primary responsibility is to help them and to advocate for them, because choices made during the time of their loss will influence their memories for a lifetime.

Deciding on whether to agree to an autopsy can be challenging. An autopsy can be very important in answering the question "why" if there is a chance that the cause of death can be determined, and parents have reported that the need for knowledge eclipsed any barriers to agreeing to an autopsy (Breeze, Statham, Hackett, et al., 2012). This information can be helpful in decision making about future pregnancies and in working through grief. However, asking parents about an autopsy takes great sensitivity to personal, cultural, and religious views about an autopsy. Some religions prohibit autopsy or limit the choice to times when it may help prevent another loss. Options for the type of autopsy, such as excluding the head, are available to parents. Note that the cost of an autopsy must be considered because it is not covered by insurance and is expensive. The question of autopsy is often brought up in the prenatal period when the fetus has a life-limiting diagnosis for which the cause is unknown or the anatomic details of which are unclear. Despite the difficulty in approaching families about autopsy after stillbirth or neonatal death, it is important to note in at least one study, twice as many parents who declined an autopsy regretted their decision (34%) compared with those who regretted having agreed to an autopsy (17%) (Heazell, McLaughlin, Schmidt, et al., 2012).

If an infant is live-born but is expected to die soon after birth, organ donation may be a possibility. Organ donation can be an aid to grieving and an opportunity for the family to see something positive associated with their experience. The federal Gift of Life Act and HCFA-3005-F, enacted in 1998, shifted the responsibility for determining organ donation potential from the hospital staff to the state's organ procurement organization (OPO). States and hospitals have clear procedures for how and when to call the OPO. Generally, if a death certificate is issued, a call must be made to the OPO. Once contacted, they will decide whether to talk to the family, and either an OPO representative or a designated requester will contact them. This allows requests to be made by trained personnel in a consistent and compassionate manner. The most common donation is corneas; donation of corneas from a baby can occur if the baby was born alive at 36 weeks of gestation or later. In some hospitals these situations are handled by descendent services, which manage a number of legal and practical issues related to a death that occurs in the hospital.

Another important decision relates to spiritual rituals that can be helpful and important to parents and families. The opportunity for support from the clergy should be offered to all bereaved individuals unless prior to the death they have made it clear that they do not want a clergy visit. Families may wish to have their own pastor, priest, rabbi, or spiritual leader contacted, or they may wish to see the hospital chaplain. Clergy or spiritual care providers can offer parents the opportunity for a blessing, naming ceremony, anointing, ritual of the sick, memorial service, baptism, or prayer as is appropriate to a family's beliefs and wishes.

One of the major decisions parents must make has to do with disposition of the body. Parents should be given information about the choices for the final disposition of their baby's body, regardless of gestational age. Nurses must be aware, however, of cultural and spiritual beliefs that can dictate the choices of parents, issues related to the cost of burial, alternatives to burial, and state laws related to burial. A fetus of less than 20 weeks of gestation is considered a product of conception, whereas embryos, uterine tubes removed with an ectopic pregnancy, and tissue from a pregnancy obtained during a dilation and curettage are considered tissue. Many hospitals will make arrangements for the cremation. The nurse should know the hospital's policies and procedures and answer the parents' questions honestly.

Respectful disposition refers to the safe handling and disposition of fetal tissue or remains by burial in a designated area. An increasing number of institutions are offering respectful disposition, and nurses can be at the forefront of establishing these procedures that honor women's preferences and wishes for disposition of fetal remains after an early pregnancy loss (Limbo, Kobler, & Levang, 2010). In most states if a fetus is at least 20 weeks and 1 day of gestational age or is born alive, it is the parents' responsibility to make the final arrangements for their baby's body, although some hospitals offer free cremation. In this case the family does not receive the ashes.

Final disposition of bodies, regardless of gestational age, can include burial or cremation. Depending on the cemetery's policies, caskets or ashes can be buried in a special place designated for babies, at the foot of a deceased relative, in a separate plot, or in a mausoleum. Ashes also may be scattered in a designated area; many states have regulations regarding where ashes may be scattered. A local funeral director or a state's vital statistics bureau should have information about the state's rules, codes, and regulations regarding live births, burial requirements, transportation of the body, and cremation.

Some parents want a special memorial or funeral service. They can choose to have a funeral service in the hospital chapel or in their own church, visitation at a funeral home or their own home, or a graveside service. Parents can make any of these services as special, personal, and memorable as they like. They can choose special music, poetry, or prose written by themselves or others.

If the family has decided on a funeral and burial, they still have decisions about which funeral home to call and where to bury the baby. Many couples live in an area distant from their family homes, and they may want to bury their child in their hometown or family cemetery. If the family desires cremation, they may want to have the option of obtaining the ashes. It is important to determine whether this will be done by the facility that does the cremation. Some families will keep the ashes ("cremains") in a small urn or other container in their home, and others will eventually take the ashes to a special place for release, such as the beach, the mountains, or a place with special sentimental meaning.

Families become unaware of time frames and do not care about the change of shifts or any needs the hospital system might have in "moving things along." When families are pushed or rushed into making decisions, in most cases they make a decision in response to the health care institution's needs, not their own. Actions such as naming the baby, seeing and holding the body, disposition of the body, and funeral arrangements should never be rushed. In some cases the mother is discharged home before these decisions are made. Then the family can think about them in the comfort of their home and contact the hospital in the following days to give their answers.

BOX 37-2 What to Say and What Not to Say to Bereaved Parents

What to Say

- "I'm sad for you."
- "How are you doing with all of this?"
- "This must be hard for you."
- "What can I do for you?"
- "I'm sorry."
- "I'm here, and I want to listen."

What Not to Say

- "God had a purpose for her."
- "Be thankful you have another child."
- "The living must go on."
- "I know how you feel."
- "It's God's will."
- "You have to keep on going for her sake."
- "You're young; you can have others."
- "We'll see you back here next year, and you'll be happier."
- "Now you have an angel in heaven."
- "This happened for the best."
- "Better for this to happen now, before you knew the baby."
- "There was something wrong with the baby anyway."

Helping the Bereaved Parents Acknowledge and Express Their Feelings

One of the most important goals of the nurse is to validate the experience and feelings of the parents by encouraging them to tell their stories and listening with care. Helping the parents to talk about their loss and the meaning it has for their lives and to share their emotional pain is the next step. Because nurses tend to be very focused on the physical and emotional needs of the mother, it is especially important to ask the father or partner directly about his or her views of what happened and the associated feelings of loss. At the very least, the nurse should acknowledge the loss with a simple but sincere "I am sorry."

The nurse should listen patiently during the story of loss or grief; however, listening can be difficult and painful. The feelings and emotions of expressed grief can overwhelm health care professionals. Being with someone who is terribly sad and crying or sobbing can be extremely difficult. The initial impulse to reduce one's sense of helplessness is to say or do something to reduce his or her pain. Although such a response seems supportive at the time, it can stifle the further expression of emotion. Bereaved parents have identified many unhelpful responses made to them by well-meaning health care professionals, family, and friends. The nurse should resist the temptation to give advice or use clichés in offering support to the bereaved (Box 37-2). Nurses need to be comfortable with their own feelings of loss and grief to support and care for bereaved individuals effectively. The nurse should have a presence of self and the willingness to be alongside, quietly supporting the bereaved in whatever expressions of feelings or emotions are appropriate for them. This presence is comforting for parents. Leaning forward, nodding the head, and saying "Uh-huh" or "Tell me more" is often encouragement enough for the bereaved person to tell his or her story. Sitting through the silence can be therapeutic; silence gives the bereaved person an opportunity to collect thoughts and to process what he or she is sharing. Furthermore, careful assessment is important before using touch as a therapeutic technique. For some, touch is a meaningful expression of concern, but for others it is an invasion of privacy or contrary to their cultural or religious beliefs.

Bereaved parents have many questions surrounding the event of their loss that can leave them feeling guilty. This is particularly true for mothers. Such questions include "What did I do?" "What caused this to happen?" "What do you think I should have, could have done?" Part of the grief process for bereaved parents is figuring out what happened, their role in the loss, why it happened to them, and why it happened to their baby. The nurse should recognize that the answers to these questions must be answered by the bereaved themselves; it is part of their healing. For example, a bereaved mother might ask, "Do you think that this was caused by painting the baby's room?" An appropriate response is, "Let's talk about what you are thinking." Trying to give bereaved parents answers when there are no clear answers or trying to squelch their guilt feelings by telling them they should not feel guilty does not help them process their grief. Trying to figure out why something bad happened is a common human response, but often there are no answers. Sometimes simple factual information, such as the frequency of miscarriages in pregnant women or the fact that there usually is no clear cause of a stillbirth, can be helpful; however, for many people understanding that something happens frequently is no consolation when it happens to them.

Feelings of anger, guilt, and sadness can occur immediately but often become more problematic in the early days and months after a loss. When a bereaved person expresses feelings of anger, it can be helpful to identify the feeling by simply saying, "You sound angry," or "You look angry." The nurse's willingness to sit down and listen to these feelings of anger can help the bereaved explore underlying feelings of powerlessness and helplessness in not being able to control the many aspects of the situation, which for many people will result in anger.

A key element of nursing care for bereaved individuals is allotting enough time to engage with them without being rushed. Nurses in inpatient settings who are caring for women and families whose baby has died may need light client assignments for their shift in order to have enough time to give adequate attention to newly bereaved individuals in helping address their profound grief.

Helping the Bereaved Family Understand Differing Responses to Loss

Bereaved parents may need help in understanding their responses to their loss, and in realizing that they are not alone in these painful responses. Most parents are not prepared for the raw feelings that they experience or the fact that these painful, complex feelings and related behavioral reactions continue for many weeks or months. Thus reassuring them that their responses are normal and preparing them for grief's potentially lengthy process can be useful.

The nurse can help parents prepare for the emptiness, loneliness, and yearning; for the feelings of helplessness that can lead to anger, guilt, and fear; for the cognitive processing problems, disorganization, difficulty making decisions; and for the sadness and depression that are part of the grief process. Many parents have reported feelings of fear that they were "going crazy" because of the many emotions and behavioral responses that leave them feeling totally out of control in the months after the loss.

It is essential for the nurse to reassure and educate bereaved parents about the grief process, including the physical, social, and emotional responses of individuals and families. Written materials about parental grief that are sensitive and brief can be very helpful. Offering health teaching on the bereavement process alone is not enough, however. In the initial days after a loss, other strategies might include follow-up phone calls, referral to a perinatal grief support group, or providing a list of publications or websites intended for helping parents who have experienced a perinatal loss. Some important websites include www.compassionatefriends.org (death of a child), www.resolve.org (infertility), www.plida.org (perinatal loss and infant death), www.sidscenter.org (sudden infant death), www.bereavementservices.org (perinatal loss), and www.marchofdimes.com (information on prematurity and congenital defects, in addition to information about healthy pregnancy). As with any referral, however, the nurse should first review the materials or the websites for accuracy and appropriateness.

To reduce relationship problems that can occur in grieving couples, nurses can help them understand that they may respond and grieve in very different ways. Interventions that include both partners and that are focused on the quality of communication within the partnership may be helpful in improving psychological and emotional outcomes after a perinatal loss (Scheidt, Hasenburg, Kunze, et al., 2012). Incongruent grieving can lead to serious relationship problems and can be a risk factor for complicated bereavement. It is important to remind couples of the importance of being understanding and patient with one another. Partners will often hide their sadness to protect the woman who experienced a miscarriage or other pregnancy loss; this, however, can be counterproductive because it is sometimes interpreted as a lack of caring. In a study of fathers whose partners experienced a stillbirth, Cacciatore, Erlandsson, and Rådestad (2013) found that they were grateful for the respectful treatment of the baby's body and when their fatherhood was validated by care providers. Although this study focused on fathers, the findings are applicable in lesbian couples, so that the partner's role and place in the life of the mother and expected infant should be recognized and validated by providers.

People cope with grief in positive and negative ways. Nurses can reinforce positive coping efforts and attempt to prevent negative coping. Many women use the Internet to locate other women who have experienced a pregnancy loss. Blogging and online support groups are increasingly used as means of sharing the experience, especially among well-educated Caucasian women. Many women have found decreased isolation in the convenience, access, privacy, and anonymity of message boards dedicated to perinatal loss (Gold, Boggs, Mugisha, & Palladino, 2012). These sources of support should not be used to the exclusion of close friends and family. Many women have had children previously and find that care of their children day to day is healing. At the negative extreme, bereaved individuals can turn to alcohol, drugs, and/or overeating as a means of anesthetizing their pain.

> **COMMUNITY ACTIVITY**
>
> - Visit the Healing Hearts Baby Loss Comfort website at www.babylosscomfort.com. Review the client information about the appropriate words to say, full-term baby loss, and stillbirth and grief resources. Also visit the websites of the National Stillbirth Society (www.stillnomore.org) and International Stillbirth Alliance (www.stillbirthalliance.org).
> - Research the availability of a perinatal loss support group in your community or find online perinatal support groups. Visit the websites of the Compassionate Friends (www.compassionatefriends.org), Perinatal Loss and Infant Death Alliance (PLIDA) (www.plida.org), and Resolve Through Sharing (www.bereavementservices.org) for up-do-date information about organizations that provide support for bereaved parents.

Meeting the Physical Needs of the Bereaved Mother in the Postpartum Period

Coping with loss and grief after birth can be overwhelming for the woman and her family. While in the hospital or birthing center, it is especially difficult for them to hear the sound of crying babies and to witness the happiness of other families on the unit who have given birth to healthy infants. The mother should have the opportunity to decide if she wants to remain on the maternity unit or to move to another unit. Many institutions have cross-trained nurses to provide postpartum care on gynecology units for women whose babies have died; some nurses on these units have experience in dealing with death and bereavement as a function of working with gynecologic cancer clients and may provide highly sensitive and expert physical and emotional care.

The physical needs of a bereaved mother are the same as those of any woman who has given birth. Bereaved mothers still lactate, they have afterbirth pains, and they sometimes feel as though a baby is still moving inside. The issue of lactation is important. Many but not all women will want to suppress lactation (see Chapter 21). Careful attention to suppressing lactation should be a priority nursing intervention for those women who desire not to lactate. Engorgement associated with milk production is physically painful and can be emotionally distressing. Cole (2012) recommends that all women experiencing a perinatal loss receive at least one lactation-specific visit from a lactation consultant before being discharged home. Some women have found benefits in expressing and donating breast milk to a human milk bank after a perinatal loss by helping them identify with being a mother and allowing their child's life to continue after death through the use of her milk by other infants (Welborn, 2012).

Women need the usual postpartum care instructions on discharge. They also need ideas about how to cope with problems with sleep such as decreasing food or fluids that contain caffeine, limiting alcohol intake and nicotine use, exercising regularly, and using strategies to promote rest such as taking a warm bath or drinking caffeine-free or herbal tea before bedtime, doing relaxation exercises, listening to restful music, or having a massage.

Assist the Bereaved Parents in Communicating and Establishing Support from Family Members

Sensitive care of bereaved parents may involve their own parents. A couple's parents and other children are particularly important when a perinatal loss has occurred. However, it is up to the parents to decide to what extent they want family involved in the acute phases of their grief. If it is the parents' desire, nursing staff should allow a couple's children, parents, extended family members, and friends to be involved in the rituals surrounding the death, such as seeing and holding the baby. Such visits afford others the opportunity to become acquainted with the baby, to understand the parents' loss, to offer their support, and to say goodbye (see Fig. 37-2). This experience helps parents explain to their children about their brother or sister and what death means, offers the children answers to their questions in a concrete manner, and helps the children in expressing their grief. Involving extended family and friends enables the parents to mobilize their social support system of people who will support the family not only at the time of loss but also in the future. Parents also need information about how grief affects a family. They may need help in understanding and coping with the potential differing responses of various family members. Frustrations can arise because of the insensitive or inadequate responses of other family members. Parents may need help in determining ways to let family members know how they feel and what they need.

Creating Memorabilia for Parents to Take Home

Parents may want tangible mementos of their baby. Some will bring in a previously purchased baby book. Special memory books, cards, and information on grief and mourning are available for purchase by parents or hospitals or clinics through national perinatal bereavement organizations (Fig. 37-4).

The nurse can provide information about the baby's weight, length, and head circumference to the family. Footprints and handprints can be taken and placed with the other information

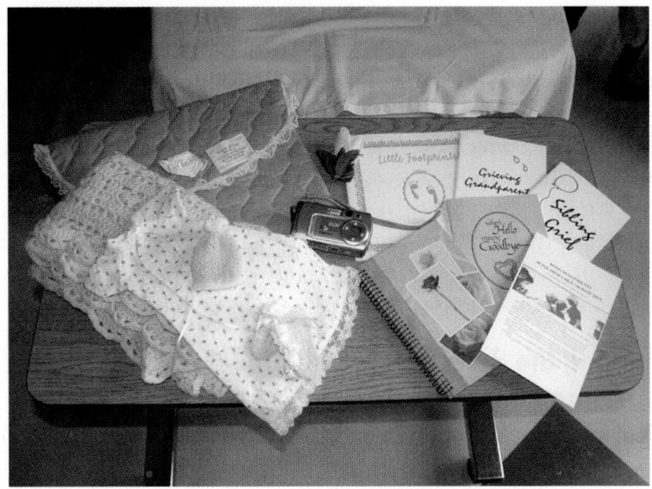

FIG 37-4 A memory kit assembled at John C. Lincoln Hospital, Phoenix, AZ. Memory kits may include pictures of the infant, clothing, death certificate, footprints, identification bands, fetal monitor printout, and ultrasound picture. (Courtesy Julie Perry Nelson, Loveland, CO.)

on a special card or in a memory or baby book. Sometimes it is difficult to obtain clearly defined handprints or footprints. Alcohol or acetone applied to the palms or soles can help the ink adhere and improve the quality of the prints, especially for small babies. When making prints it is helpful to have a hard surface underneath the paper to be printed. The baby's heel or palm is placed down first, and the foot or hand is rolled forward, keeping the toes or fingers extended. If the print is not clear or well defined, tracing around the baby's hands and feet can be done, although this distorts the actual size. A form of plaster of Paris can also be used to make an imprint of the baby's hand or foot.

Parents often appreciate articles that were in contact with or used in caring for the baby. This might include the tape measure used to measure the baby, baby lotions, combs or hairbrushes, clothing, hats, blankets, crib cards, and identification bands. The identification band helps the parents remember the size of the baby and personalizes the mementos. The nurse should ask parents if they wish to have these articles before giving them to the parents. A lock of hair can be another important keepsake. The nurse must ask the parents for permission before cutting a lock of hair, which can be removed from the nape of the neck, where it is not noticeable.

For some parents, pictures are the most important memento. Photographs are generally taken when it has been determined to be culturally acceptable to the family—the decision for photography is up to the parents. Photos should include close-ups of the baby's face, hands, and feet, with the baby both clothed and unclothed. Flowers, blocks, stuffed animals, or toys can be placed in the background, which serve to contextualize the photo and give an idea of the baby's approximate size. Parents may want their pictures taken holding the baby. Keeping a camera nearby and taking pictures when parents are spending time with their baby can provide special memories. The widespread use of smartphones means that most families have one or more people taking photos and videos of the occasion. Some parents may ask the nurse record them as they bathe, dress, hold, or diaper their baby.

In some communities a volunteer organization of professional photographers (e.g., Now I Lay Me Down to Sleep [www.nowilaymedowntosleep.org]) has a photographer on-call around the clock to take photographs of families and their deceased baby free of charge. Some institutions will take photos with a digital camera and give families the camera's memory card containing their baby's photos for downloading when the parents are ready.

Nurses should be aware of the risk of family members and friends using social media such as Instagram, Twitter, Vine, and Facebook to post photos and videos of this intimate family event. A frank talk with the family about ownership of this occasion may help forestall this behavior.

Addressing Cultural and Spiritual Needs of Parents

Parents who experience perinatal loss can be from widely diverse cultural, ethnic, and spiritual groups. Many of the emotional responses and suggested interventions in this chapter are based on middle-class Euro-American views. Although there are likely no particular differences in the individual, intrapersonal experiences of grief based on culture, ethnicity, or religion, there are complex differences in the meaning of children and parenthood, the role of women and men, the beliefs and knowledge about modern medicine, views about death, mourning rituals and traditions, and behavioral expressions of grief. Thus the nurse must be sensitive to the responses and needs of parents from various cultural backgrounds and religious groups. To do this the nurse needs to be aware of his or her own values and beliefs and acknowledge the importance of understanding and accepting the values and beliefs of others who are different or even in conflict. Furthermore, it is critical to understand that the individual and unique responses of a parent to a perinatal loss cannot be entirely predicted by his or her cultural or spiritual backgrounds. The nurse approaches each partner as an individual needing support during a profoundly difficult and distressing life experience.

It would be impossible to address all of the specific differences and needs of parents from diverse cultural and religious groups because of the complexity of this task and the lack of adequate research in this area of practice. Instead, some key concepts are presented and a few examples of areas of particular concern are given. The cultural meaning of children has a strong effect on the response of parents, extended family, and the community when an infant dies or is stillborn. Cultural and religious beliefs often affect decision making surrounding stillbirth or death of an infant. For example, death of an infant or having a stillborn infant profoundly affects the foundations of a Jewish family and involves many specific cultural and religious traditions, such as naming of the baby, burial, and mourning rituals (Shuzman, 2003). Muslim women have described their husbands or family members as the main decision makers and appreciate being reminded by their husbands, family, or close friends that their loss was a test from God (Sutan & Miskam, 2012). Some religious groups do not allow autopsies and cremation except under unusual circumstances (Chichester, 2007). Making a decision to end life-sustaining measures is less acceptable for some cultural and ethnic groups. African-American parents may be less likely than Caucasians to make a decision to stop life-sustaining treatments in a terminally ill infant (Moseley, Church, Hempel, et al., 2004). Photographs can conflict with beliefs of some cultures, such as among some Native Americans, Inuit, Amish, Hindus, and Muslims. Families from these cultures should be offered this opportunity sensitively but there should be no insistence on photography. In many cultures decisions do not reside solely with the individual woman or couple but with the extended family. In Hispanic families, the concept of *la familia* is critical. Family decisions are often made together and communicated through someone appointed by the family rather than the parents.

Culture and religious beliefs also influence the customs following death. Many religious groups have rituals that are performed at the time of death. They include prayers, ritualistic washing and shrouding, or anointing with oil. Nurses should ask parents about their needs as they relate to rituals at the time of and following death. For example, baptism is extremely important for Roman Catholics and some, but not all, Protestant groups. Baptism can be performed by a layperson, such as a nurse of the Christian faith, in an emergency situation when a priest cannot be there in a timely fashion. The nurse should inquire about parental beliefs and preferences related to infant baptism. The nurse can offer to contact the hospital chaplain or the family's own clergy who can help sort out theological questions related to rituals of faith.

Expressions of grief vary across cultures from quiet and stoic to dramatic responses. Muslims view death as a part of life and believe a baby's death is God's will. The Muslim mother may cry but loud wailing is not acceptable. The tearing of a garment, *keria*, may be done by Jewish parents at the time of a death. Hispanic parents and family members may be very demonstrative in their grief (Purnell & Paulanka, 2008). Some African-American women use self-healing strategies that reflect inner processes, resources, and remedies (Van, 2001).

Providing Sensitive Discharge and Follow-up Care

When leaving the hospital, mothers are often transported from the nursing unit to their vehicle in a wheelchair. This can be very upsetting for the woman who has experienced a pregnancy loss. It is especially difficult if other women are seen leaving with babies; thus the timing of discharge of couples who have experienced a perinatal loss should be done with great sensitivity. They should not be discharged at a time when other mothers with live babies are leaving. Some institutions give the bereaved mother some token of remembrance such as a teddy bear or a flower to carry as they leave.

The grief of the mother and her family does not end with discharge; rather it begins anew once they return home, attend the funeral, and continue their lives without a new baby. There are numerous models for providing follow-up care to parents after discharge, and, although there is no solid evidence from sound clinical trials regarding the benefit of these programs, nonexperimental studies and clinical evaluations suggest these programs are helpful. Programs include hospital-based bereavement teams who provide support during hospitalization and follow-up contacts. Follow-up phone calls after a loss are helpful to some but not all parents. The calls are made at times that are known to be difficult for bereaved persons such as the first week at home, 1 month to 6 weeks later, 4 to 6 months after the loss, and at the anniversary of the death. Families who experienced a miscarriage, ectopic pregnancy, or death of a preterm baby may appreciate a phone call on the estimated date of birth. The calls provide an opportunity for parents to ask questions, share their feelings, seek advice, and receive information to help them in processing their grief.

A grief conference can be planned when parents return for an appointment with their physician or midwife, nurses, and other members of the health care team. At the conference, the loss or death of the infant is discussed in detail, parents are given information about the baby's autopsy report and genetic studies, and they have opportunities to ask the questions that have arisen since their baby's death. Parents appreciate the opportunity to review the events of hospitalization, go over the baby's and mother's chart with their primary health care provider, and talk with those who cared for them and their baby while they were in the hospital or birthing facility. This is an important time to help parents understand the cause of the loss or to accept the fact that the cause will forever be unknown. This gives health care professionals the opportunity to assess how the family is coping with their loss and provide additional information and education on grief.

Some parents are very interested in finding a perinatal or parent grief support group. Talking with others who have been through similar experiences, sharing memories of the pregnancy and the baby, and gaining an understanding of the normality of the grief process can be very helpful. Over time it is possibly the only place where bereaved parents can talk about the wished-for child and their grief. However, not all parents find such groups helpful.

When referring to a group, it is important to know something about the group and how it operates. For example, if a group has a religious base for their interventions, a nonreligious parent would not likely find the group to be helpful. If parents experiencing a perinatal loss are referred to a general parental grief group, they might feel overwhelmed with the grief of parents whose older children have died of cancer, suicide, or homicide. In addition, other parents whose older children have died may inadvertently minimize the grief of parents following a perinatal loss. Thus the focus of the group needs to match the parents' needs.

Providing Postmortem Care

Preparing the baby's body and transporting it to the morgue depend on the procedures and protocols developed by individual hospitals. The Joint Commission (www.jointcommission.org) requires that appropriate care be offered to the body after death. A sensitive and respectful approach for taking the fetus or infant to the morgue is the use of a burial cradle, which makes the process more dignified for parents and the nursing staff. A burial cradle is a miniature casket usually made of Styrofoam or wood (Fig. 37-5).

Postmortem care can be an emotional and sometimes difficult task for the nurse. However, nurses can find that providing postmortem care helps them in their own grief related to a perinatal loss. This is particularly true for NICU nurses who have cared for an infant for several hours, days, or weeks.

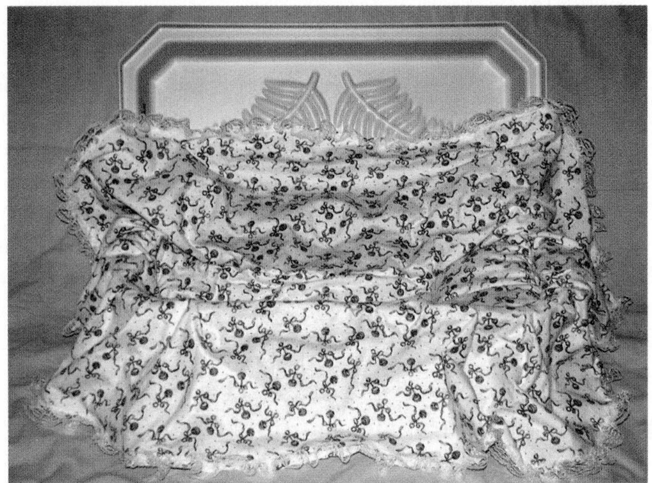

FIG 37-5 Burial cradle. (Courtesy Shannon Perry, Phoenix, AZ.)

> **! NURSING ALERT**
>
> An important caveat is needed for nurses providing care for newborns that are thought to be deceased: dying neonates may respond reflexively to the stimulation of cleaning and preparing for the morgue, and sometimes will do this for several hours after being pronounced dead. This is extremely startling and upsetting when a baby that has been pronounced dead takes an agonal respiration or an extremity twitches. If this happens, the nurse should notify a physician for confirmation of death.

SPECIAL CIRCUMSTANCES

Prenatal Diagnoses with Poor Prognoses

Early prenatal diagnostic tests such as ultrasonography, chorionic villus sampling, and amniocentesis can determine the well-being of the embryo or fetus (see Chapter 26). Reasons for prenatal testing include history of chromosomal abnormality in the family; three or more miscarriages; maternal age over 35 years; lack of fetal growth, movement, or heartbeat; and diabetes, hypertension, lupus, sickle cell disease, or other chronic illnesses. If the health care provider is certain that the baby has a serious genetic defect that will lead to death in utero or after birth (congenital anomalies incompatible with life or genetic disorders with severe intellectual disability), the choice of interruption of a pregnancy via dilation and evacuation or induction of labor can be offered (Manning, 2009).

Foreknowledge of a congenital diagnosis in conjunction with the possibility of suffering by the baby can intensify parental grief (Hunfeld, Tempels, Passchier, et al., 1999). The decision to terminate a pregnancy is difficult and can lead to feelings such as guilt, despair, sadness, depression, and anger. The woman who decides to continue the pregnancy needs intensive support from the nursing staff. The time of labor and birth can be particularly difficult. The nurse should remember that expectant parents may be grieving for not only the loss of the "perfect child" but also loss of expectations for their child's future. Thus a nurse should assess how these parents feel about the experience, offer options for their memories as appropriate, and be a support person and good listener. Healing can be facilitated when words can be given to feelings. Perinatal palliative care or hospice care for parents experiencing prenatal diagnoses of lethal birth defects can be effective in helping families both before and after their loss (Calhoun, Napolitano, Terry, et al., 2003). Perinatal palliative care, described in detail earlier, does not have to be a formal program, although many do exist. It is the provision of care for families as they plan for the birth and probable death of their baby and involves support, information, and resources. If the baby lives more than a few minutes or hours after birth, conventional hospice care may be incorporated into care management of the infant and family (Davis & Helzer, 2011).

Death of a Fetus in a Multiple Gestation

The death of a fetus in a multifetal gestation during pregnancy, labor, birth, or after birth requires the mother and partner to both parent their live-born infant and grieve their dead or dying one at the same time. Such a death imposes a confusing and ambivalent transition into parenthood (Swanson, Kane, Pearsall-Jones, et al., 2009). They can experience difficulty parenting their surviving child with all the joy and enthusiasm of new parents because their surviving child reminds them of what they have lost. Yet they can also have difficulty fully grieving their loss because their surviving child demands their attention. These parents can be at risk for altered parenting and complicated bereavement.

It is important to help the parents acknowledge the birth of all their babies, although one or more may be stillborn. The nurse should plan the care of these families as they do all bereaved families, offering all the options previously noted. With the parents' consent, photographs should be taken of the babies and parents should be offered the opportunity to hold their babies and have time to say goodbye to the baby who has died.

It is helpful to alert bereaved parents that well-meaning family members or friends may say, "Well, at least you have the other baby," implying that there should be no grief because they are lucky to have one living baby. Parents can anticipate insensitivity to their loss and may find it helpful to respond, "That is not how I feel." By simply setting a boundary on what their feelings are, they are able to acknowledge the baby who died and then have an opportunity to share more about their feelings if they so choose. When there is a loss of one or more babies in a multiple gestation, bereaved parents face specific issues in telling their surviving child about his or her twin, dealing with the possibility of that child's feelings of survivor guilt, and deciding on how to celebrate birthdays, special holidays, or anniversaries of the baby's death.

Adolescent Grief

Adolescents grieve the loss that occurs with miscarriage, stillbirth, or newborn death and have significant emotional, social, and cognitive responses that can differ from those of older women. Teens need a great deal of emotional support from the nurses who care for them.

Nurses and other health care professionals, as well as family members, may believe that the adolescent's loss of her baby, although sad, may open the opportunity for the young woman to complete her education and experience life without the demands of motherhood. Adolescent girls, then, may not receive the support they need from staff and family. In addition, adolescent girls often do not have the support from the father of the baby as compared with older women who have a perinatal loss; thus there is a great need to provide sensitive care to all adolescents who experience any type of perinatal loss.

The first step for the nurse in caring for a bereaved adolescent is to develop a trusting relationship with her. Second, the nurse should acknowledge the significance of the loss, regardless of the mother's age. Third, the nurse should offer options for saying goodbye and provide anticipatory guidance, support, and information to meet the adolescent at the point of her need. It can take longer for adolescents to process their grief because of their lack of cognitive and emotional maturity, although this varies. Moreover, adolescents are often highly involved with their friends who may lack maturity and perspective on the loss but at the same time are good sources of social support by simply being present. Encouraging the bereaved teen to seek out friends may be very helpful. Being patient, saving mementos, and giving the adolescent information on how to contact the nurse are interventions that can help the adolescent accept the loss and work through her grief and sadness.

Complicated Grief

Although most parents cope adequately with the pain of their grief and return to some level of their usual functioning, some have extremely intense grief reactions that last for a very long time; this response is **complicated grief**. It is also called complicated bereavement, prolonged grief, pathologic grief, or pathologic mourning (Zhang, El-Jawahri, & Prigerson, 2006). Complicated grief can result when there is sudden or traumatic loss, as occurs with stillbirth or termination of pregnancy due to lethal fetal anomalies (Cacciatore, 2010; Kersting, Kroker, Steinhard, et al., 2007). Complicated grief differs from what is considered normal grief in its duration and the degree to which behavior and emotional state are affected. Risk factors for complicated grief include poor social support, history of mental health problems, and a more neurotic pre-loss personality (Badenhorst & Hughes, 2007). A study by Swanson and colleagues (2007) found that among women still overwhelmed with grief one year later, many had miscarried again or were not yet pregnant again, experienced six or more negative events in their lives, and were distant from their partners.

People experiencing complicated grief seem to be in a state of chronic mourning. Evidence of complicated grief includes intense longing and yearning for the deceased, inability to trust others, excessive bitterness, difficulty moving on with one's life, feeling that life is empty or meaningless, hopelessness, loneliness, intense and continued guilt or anger, and relentless depression or anxiety that interferes with role functioning. Complicated grief can lead to abuse of drugs (including prescription medications) or alcohol, severe relationship difficulties, high levels of depressive symptoms, low self-esteem, feelings of inadequacy, and suicidal thoughts or threats years after the loss (Swanson, 2000; Zhang et al., 2006).

Posttraumatic stress disorder (PTSD) can occur following perinatal loss (Badenhorst & Hughes, 2007; Turton, Evans, & Hughes, 2009). Symptoms of posttraumatic stress include reliving the trauma, avoiding things and places that are reminders, panic attacks, physical symptoms such as chronic pain, feelings of mistrust, problems with relationships and daily activities, substance abuse, and depression.

People showing signs of complicated grief or posttraumatic stress should be referred for counseling. It is the responsibility of a qualified mental health professional to determine whether the parents are experiencing a normal, albeit intense grief response or whether they are also having a serious mental health problem such as depression. However, it is important when referring to a therapist or counselor that the referral is made to one who is experienced in grief counseling. Making an appointment for counseling or therapy is a big step. The highest number of cancellations and missed visits in a therapist's practice are first visits; therefore, anything the nurse can do for a family or individual to help with that major hurdle is helpful. However, it also is important to remember that people can have symptoms but may not, for whatever reason, be ready to deal directly with these symptoms or may not have the energy to make the call. Enlisting a family member to encourage parents to seek such assistance can be helpful.

Posttraumatic Growth

Researchers have noted that women and their partners can experience personal growth in the aftermath of a perinatal loss (Black & Sandelowski, 2010). Known as *posttraumatic growth* (PTG), this phenomenon is characterized by development along one or more of five dimensions: personal strength, appreciation for life, spirituality, relating to others, and new possibilities (Tedeschi & Calhoun, 1996, 2004, 2008). Growth coexists with grief. In witnessing the grief of women, partners, and families in the aftermath of a perinatal loss, it is important that the nurse recognize that people in fact can and do grow after highly traumatic events. Nurses should be alert for signs of growth in bereaved individuals, for instance, when a woman comes in for a 6-week postpartum check, she may indicate that she and her partner are closer because of this loss or note that she is beginning to look at opportunities to go back to school or change jobs. These are not indications that the woman's grief has gone away but that she has experienced growth from the trauma of her loss. The nurse needs to simply affirm these developments with simple comments such as, "I'm glad for you."

KEY POINTS

- Attachment to the idea of a baby can begin before pregnancy with many hopes and dreams for the future and can become more pronounced over the course of pregnancy.
- Women can feel profound grief regardless of the length of gestation; however, women tend to have higher levels of grief with longer gestations.
- When a fetus or a newborn dies, all members of a family are affected, but no two family members grieve in the same way.
- When birth and death coexist, sensitive care by a nurse is critical in assisting the woman and her family in their grief, regardless of the woman's age or stage of gestation.
- An understanding of the grief process is fundamental to care management of families experiencing perinatal loss.
- Assessment of each family member's perception and experience of the loss is important.
- Cultural and religious beliefs affect a family's response to and coping with perinatal death.
- Therapeutic communication and active listening can help women and their partners and families identify their feelings, feel comfortable in expressing their grief, and understand their bereavement process.
- Follow-up after discharge is important in providing care to families who have experienced a loss because of the evolving nature of grief.
- Nurses need to be aware of their own feelings of grief and loss to provide a nonjudgmental environment of care and support for bereaved families.

REFERENCES

Armstrong, D. (2007). Perinatal loss and parental distress after the birth of a healthy infant. *Advances in Neonatal Care, 7*(4), 200–206.

Avelin, P., Rådestad, I., Säflund, K., et al. (2013). Parental grief and relationships after the loss of a stillborn baby. *Midwifery, 29*(9), 668–673.

Badenhorst, W., & Hughes, P. (2007). Psychological aspects of perinatal loss. *Clinical Obstetrics and Gynecology, 21*(2), 249–259.

Barfield, W. D., & Committee on Fetus and Newborn. (2011). Standard terminology for fetal, infant, and perinatal deaths. *Pediatrics, 128*(1), 177–181.

Black, B. P., & Fields, W. S. (2014). Contexts of reproductive loss in lesbian couples. *MCN: The American Journal of Maternal Child Nursing, 39*(3), 157–162.

Black, B. P., & Sandelowski, M. (2010). Personal growth after severe fetal diagnosis. *Western Journal of Nursing Research, 38*(2), 1011–1030.

Boss, P. (2006). *Loss, trauma and resilience: Therapeutic work with ambiguous loss.* New York: W.W. Norton.

Breeze, A. C. G., Statham, H., Hackett, G. A., et al. (2012). Perinatal postmortems: What is important to parents and how do they decide. *Birth, 39*(1), 57–64.

Brier, N. (2008). Grief following miscarriage: A comprehensive review of the literature. *Journal of Women's Health, 17*(3), 451–464.

Cacciatore, J. (2010). Stillbirth: Patient-centered psychosocial care. *Clinical Obstetrics and Gynecology, 53*(3), 691–699.

Cacciatore, J. (2013). Psychological effects of stillbirth. *Seminars in Fetal & Neonatal Medicine, 18*(2), 76–82.

Cacciatore, J., Erlandsson, K., & Rådestad, I. (2013). Fatherhood and suffering: A qualitative exploration of Swedish men's experiences of care after the death of a baby. *International Journal of Nursing Studies, 50*(5), 664–670.

Calhoun, B., Napolitano, P., Terry, M., et al. (2003). Perinatal hospice: Comprehensive care for the family of the fetus with a lethal condition. *Journal of Reproductive Medicine, 48*(5), 343–348.

Cameron, M., & Penney, G. (2005). Terminology in early pregnancy loss: What women hear and what clinicians write. *Journal of Family Planning and Reproductive Health Care, 31*(4), 313–314.

Chichester, M. (2007). Requesting perinatal autopsy: Multicultural considerations. *MCN: The American Journal of Maternal/Child Nursing, 32*(2), 81–86.

Cole, M. (2012). Lactation after perinatal, neonatal, or infant loss. *Clinical Lactation, 3*(3), 94–100.

Côté-Arsenault, D., & Donato, K. (2007). Restrained expectations in late pregnancy following loss. *Journal of Obstetric, Gynecologic and Neonatal Nursing, 36*(6), 550–557.

Cowles, K., & Rodgers, B. (2000). The concept of grief: An evolutionary perspective. In B. Rodgers, & K. Knafl (Eds.), *Concept development in nursing: Foundations, techniques, and applications* (2nd ed.). Philadelphia: Saunders.

Davies, R. (2004). New understandings of parental grief: Literature review. *Journal of Advanced Nursing, 46*(5), 506–513.

Davis, D., & Helzer, S. (2011). Perinatal death and bereavement care. In E. Gilbert (Ed.), *Manual of high risk pregnancy and delivery* (5th ed.). St. Louis: Mosby.

DeBackere, K., Hill, P., & Kavanaugh, K. (2008). The parental experience of pregnancy after perinatal loss. *Journal of Obstetric, Gynecologic and Neonatal Nursing, 37*(5), 525–537.

Doka, K. J. (1989). Disenfranchised loss. In K. J. Doka (Ed.), *Disenfranchised grief: Recognizing hidden sorrow*. Lanham, MD: Lexington Books.

Fenstermacher, K., & Hupcey, J. E. (2013). Perinatal bereavement: A principle-based concept analysis. *Journal of Advanced Nursing, 69*(11), 2389–2400.

Gear, R. (2014). Bereaved parents' perspectives on informal social support: "What worked for you?" *Journal of Loss and Trauma, 19*(2), 173–188.

Gold, K., Dalton, V., & Schwenk, T. (2007). Hospital care for parents after perinatal death. *Obstetrics and Gynecology, 109*(5), 1156–1166.

Gold, K. J., Boggs, M. E., Mugisha, E., & Palladino, C. L. (2012). Internet message boards for pregnancy loss: Who's on-line and why? *Women's Health Issues, 22*(1), e67–e72.

Heazell, A. E. P., McLaughlin, M.-J., Schmidt, P., et al. (2012). A difficult conversation? The views and experiences of parents and professionals on the consent process for perinatal postmortem after stillbirth. *BJOG: An International Journal of Obstetrics and Gynaecology, 119*(8), 987–997.

Hunfeld, J., Tempels, A., Passchier, J., et al. (1999). Brief report: Parental burden and grief one year after the birth of a child with congenital anomaly. *Journal of Pediatric Psychology, 24*(6), 515–520.

Jonas-Simpson, C., Pilkington, F. B., MacDonald, C., & McMahon, E. (2013). Nurses' experiences of grieving when there is a perinatal death. *SAGE Open*, 1–11, April-June.

Jones, R. K., Finer, L. B., & Singh, S. (2010). *Characteristics of U.S. abortion patients, 2008*. New York: Guttmacher Institute.

Kenner, C. (2014). Palliative and end-of-life care. In C. Kenner, & J. W. Lott (Eds.), *Comprehensive neonatal nursing care* (5th ed.). New York: Springer.

Kersting, A., Kroker, K., Steinhard, J., et al. (2007). Complicated grief after traumatic loss: A 14 month follow up study. *European Archives of Psychiatry and Clinical Neuroscience, 257*(8), 437–443.

Klass, D., Silverman, P. R., & Nickman, S. L. (1996). *Continuing bonds: New understandings of grief*. Philadelphia: Taylor & Francis.

Koopmans, L., Wilson, T., Cacciatore, J., & Flenady, V. (2013). Support for mothers, fathers and families after perinatal death. *The Cochrane Database of Systematic Reviews, 2013*, 6, CD00452.

Kübler-Ross, E. (1969). *On death and dying*. New York: Scribner.

Lang, A., Fleiszer, A. R., Duhamel, F., et al. (2011). Perinatal loss and parental grief: The challenge of ambiguity and disenfranchised grief. *Omega, 63*(2), 183–196.

Limbo, R., & Kobler, K. (2009). Will our baby be alive again? Supporting parents of young children when a baby dies. *Nursing for Women's Health, 13*(4), 302–311.

Limbo, R., & Kobler, K. (2010). The tie that binds: Relationships in perinatal bereavement. *MCN: The American Journal of Maternal/Child Nursing, 35*(6), 316–321.

Limbo, R., Kobler, K., & Levang, E. (2010). Respectful disposition in early pregnancy loss. *MCN: The American Journal of Maternal/Child Nursing, 35*(5), 271–277.

Little, C. (2010). Nursing considerations in the case of multifetal pregnancy reduction. *MCN: The American Journal of Maternal/Child Nursing, 35*(3), 166–171.

Mallon, B. (2011). *Working with bereaved children and young people*. London: Sage Publications Ltd.

Manning, F. (2009). Imaging in the diagnosis of fetal anomalies. In R. Creasy, R. Resnik, J. Iams, et al. (Eds.), *Creasy and Resnik's maternal-fetal medicine* (6th ed.). Philadelphia: Saunders.

Martin, J. A., Hamilton, B. E., Osterman, M. J. K., et al. (2013). Births: Final data for 2012. *National Vital Statistics Reports, 62*(9) Hyattsville, MD: National Center for Health Statistics.

Mashiach, R., Anter, D., Melamed, N., et al. (2013). Psychological response to multifetal reduction and pregnancy termination due to fetal abnormality. *The Journal of Maternal-Fetal and Neonatal Medicine, 26*(1), 32–35.

Miles, M. (1984). Helping adults mourn the death of a child. In H. Wass, & C. Corr (Eds.), *Childhood and death*. New York: Hemisphere.

Moseley, K., Church, A., Hempel, B., et al. (2004). End-of-life choices for African-American and white infants in a neonatal intensive-care unit: A pilot study. *Journal of the National Medical Association, 96*(7), 933–937.

O'Leary, J., & Thorwick, C. (2006). Fathers' perspectives during pregnancy, postperinatal loss. *Journal of Obstetric, Gynecologic and Neonatal Nursing, 35*(1), 78–86.

PLIDA (Perinatal Loss and Infant Death Alliance). (2005). Position statement: Infection risks are insignificant. Available at PLIDA.org/pdf/infectionRisks.pdf.

Puia, D. M., Lewis, L., & Beck, C. T. (2013). Experiences of obstetric nurses who are present for a perinatal loss. *Journal of Obstetric, Gynecologic and Neonatal Nursing, 42*(3), 321–331.

Purnell, L., & Paulanka, B. (2008). *Transcultural health care: A culturally competent approach* (3rd ed.). Philadelphia: F.A. Davis.

Rando, T. A., Doka, K. J., Fleming, S., et al. (2012). A call to the field: Complicated grief in the DSM-5. *Omega, 65*(4), 251–255.

Sandelowski, M., & Barroso, J. (2005). The travesty of choosing after positive prenatal diagnosis. *Journal of Obstetric, Gynecologic and Neonatal Nursing, 34*(3), 307–318.

Scheidt, C. E., Hasenburg, A., Kunze, M., et al. (2012). Are individual differences of attachment predicting bereavement outcome after perinatal loss? A prospective cohort study. *Journal of Psychosomatic Research, 73*(5), 375–382.

Shuzman, E. (2003). Facing stillbirth or neonatal death: Providing culturally appropriate care for Jewish families. *AWHONN Lifelines, 7*(6), 537–543.

Stotland, N. L. (2011). Psychiatric aspects of induced abortion. *Journal of Nervous and Mental Disease, 199*(8), 568–570.

Stroebe, M., Finkenhauer, C., Wijngaards-de Meij, L., et al. (2013). Partner-oriented self-regulation among bereaved parents: The costs of holding in grief for the partner's sake. *Psychological Science, 24*(4), 395–402.

Stroebe, M., & Schut, H. (1999). The dual process model of coping with bereavement: Rationale and description. *Death Studies, 23*(3), 197–224.

Sutan, R., & Miskam, H. M. (2012). Psychosocial impact of perinatal loss among Muslim women. *BMC Women's Health, 12*(15), 1–9.

Swanson, K. (2000). Predicting depressive symptoms after miscarriage: A path analysis based on the Lazarus paradigm. *Journal of Women's Health & Gender-Based Medicine, 9*(2), 191–206.

Swanson, K., Chen, H., Graham, J., et al. (2009). Resolution of depression and grief during the first year after miscarriage: A randomized controlled clinical trial of couples-focused interventions. *Journal of Women's Health, 18*(8), 1245–1257.

Swanson, K., Connor, S., Jolley, S., et al. (2007). Contexts and evolution of women's responses to miscarriage during the first year after loss. *Research in Nursing & Health, 30*(1), 2–16.

Swanson, P., Kane, R., Pearsall-Jones, J., et al. (2009). How couples cope with the death of a twin or higher order multiple. *Twin Research and Human Genetics, 12*(4), 392–402.

Tedeschi, R. G., & Calhoun, L. G. (1996). The posttraumatic growth inventory: Measuring the positive legacy of trauma. *Journal of Traumatic Stress*, *9*(3), 455–471.

Tedeschi, R. G., & Calhoun, L. G. (2004). Posttraumatic growth: Conceptual foundations and empirical evidence. *Psychological Inquiry*, *15*(1), 1–18.

Tedeschi, R. G., & Calhoun, L. G. (2008). Beyond the concept of recovery: Growth and the experience of loss. *Death Studies*, *32*(1), 27–39.

Turton, P., Evans, C., & Hughes, P. (2009). Long-term psychosocial sequelae of stillbirth: Phase II of a nested case-control cohort study. *Archives of Women's Mental Health*, *12*(1), 35–41.

Van, P. (2001). Breaking the silence of African American women: Healing after pregnancy loss. *Health Care for Women International*, *22*(3), 229–243.

Wallbank, S., & Robertson, N. (2013). Predictors of staff distress in response to professionally experienced miscarriage, stillbirth and neonatal loss: A questionnaire survey. *International Journal of Nursing Studies*, *50*(8), 1090–1097.

Welborn, J. M. (2012). The experience of expressing and donating breast milk following a perinatal loss. *Journal of Human Lactation*, *28*(4), 506–510.

Wool, C. (2013a). Clinician confidence and comfort in providing perinatal palliative care. *Journal of Obstetric, Gynecologic and Neonatal Nursing*, *42*(1), 48–58.

Wool, C. (2013b). State of the science on perinatal palliative care. *Journal of Obstetric, Gynecologic and Neonatal Nursing*, *42*(3), 372–382.

Zhang, B., El-Jawahri, A., & Prigerson, H. (2006). Update on bereavement research: Evidence-based guidelines for the diagnosis and treatment of complicated bereavement. *Journal of Palliative Medicine*, *9*(5), 1188–1203.

GLOSSARY

A

abdominal Belonging or relating to the abdomen and its functions and disorders.

ABO incompatibility Hemolytic disease that occurs when the mother's blood type is O and the newborn's is A, B, or AB.

abortion Termination of pregnancy before the fetus is viable and capable of extrauterine existence, usually less than 20 weeks of gestation (or when the fetus weighs less than 500 g); miscarriage.

abruptio placentae (placental abruption) Premature separation of the placenta; the detachment of part or all of a normally implanted placenta from the uterus before the birth of the infant.

acceleration Visually apparent abrupt (onset to peak less than 30 seconds) increase in fetal heart rate (FHR) above the baseline rate. The peak is at least 15 beats/minute above the baseline, and the acceleration lasts 15 seconds or more, with a return to baseline less than 2 minutes from the beginning of the acceleration.

acculturation Changes that occur within one group or among several groups when people from different cultures come into contact with each other.

acquaintance Process used by parents to get to know or become familiar with their new infant; an important step in attachment.

acrocyanosis Peripheral cyanosis; blue color of hands and feet in most infants at birth that may persist for 7 to 10 days.

active phase of labor Phase in first stage of labor from 4 to 7 cm in dilation.

active pushing (descent) phase of labor Period during second stage labor when the woman has strong urges to bear down as the fetal presenting part presses on the pelvic floor.

acute bilirubin encephalopathy Acute manifestations of bilirubin toxicity that occur during the first weeks after birth.

acute respiratory distress syndrome (ARDS) Condition that occurs when the lungs are unable to maintain levels of oxygen and carbon dioxide within normal limits. ARDS is not specific to pregnancy; it can also result from trauma, pneumonia, sepsis, aspiration of gastric contents, fat emboli, acute pancreatitis, and drug overdose. When ARDS is associated with pregnancy, the precipitating factors can also be amniotic fluid embolism, air embolism, tocolytic therapy, asthma, thromboembolism, disseminated intravascular coagulopathy, pyelonephritis, preeclampsia, eclampsia, severe hemorrhage, blood transfusion reactions, or peripartum cardiomyopathy. Also called shock lung.

adjuvant chemotherapy Chemotherapy administered soon after surgical removal of a tumor.

afterbirth pains See afterpains.

afterpains Painful uterine cramps that occur intermittently for approximately 3 to 7 days after birth and that result from contractile efforts of the uterus to return to its normal involuted condition. Also called afterbirth pains.

agonist An agent that activates or stimulates a receptor to act.

alcohol-related birth defects (ARBDs) See alcohol-related neurodevelopmental disorders (ARNDs).

alcohol-related neurodevelopmental disorders (ARNDs) Infants exposed prenatally to alcohol who are affected but do not meet the criteria for fetal alcohol syndrome (FAS); these disorders run the gamut from learning disabilities and behavioral problems to speech or language problems and hyperactivity.

alpha-fetoprotein (AFP) Fetal antigen; elevated levels in amniotic fluid are associated with neural tube and open abdominal wall defects.

amenorrhea Absence or suppression of menstruation or menstrual flow.

amniocentesis Procedure in which a needle is inserted through the abdominal and uterine walls under ultrasound guidance into the amniotic fluid; some fluid is withdrawn; used for assessment of fetal health and maturity.

amnioinfusion Infusion of room-temperature isotonic fluid (usually normal saline or lactated Ringer's solution) into the uterine cavity if the volume of amniotic fluid is low, in an attempt to increase the fluid around the umbilical cord and prevent compression during uterine contractions.

amnion Inner membrane of two fetal membranes that form the sac and contain the fetus and the fluid that surrounds it in utero.

amniotic Pertaining or relating to the amnion.

amniotic fluid Fluid surrounding the fetus derived primarily from maternal serum and fetal urine.

amniotic fluid embolus (AFE) Rare but devastating complication of pregnancy characterized by the sudden, acute onset of hypoxia, hypotension, cardiovascular collapse, and coagulopathy. AFE occurs during labor, during birth, or within 30 minutes after birth. Also known as anaphylactoid syndrome of pregnancy.

amniotic fluid index (AFI) Evaluation of the total amount of amniotic fluid by measuring the vertical depths (in centimeters) of the largest pocket of amniotic fluid in all four quadrants surrounding the maternal umbilicus. A normal AFI is 10 cm or greater.

amniotomy Artificial rupture of the membranes (AROM), using a plastic amnihook or a surgical clamp.

analgesia Alleviating the sensation of pain or raising the threshold for pain perception without loss of consciousness.

anaphylactoid syndrome of pregnancy See amniotic fluid embolus (AFE).

anencephaly Congenital deformity characterized by the absence of both cerebral hemispheres (cerebrum and cerebellum) and the flat bones of the overlying skull.

anesthesia Encompasses analgesia, amnesia, relaxation, and reflex activity. Anesthesia abolishes pain perception by interrupting the nerve impulses to the brain. The loss of sensation may be partial or complete, sometimes with the loss of consciousness.

aneuploidy One of the two types of deviations from the correct number of chromosomes per cell, in which the numerical deviation is not an exact multiple of the haploid set. Having an abnormal number of chromosomes.

antagonist An agent that blocks a receptor or a medication designed to activate a receptor.

antenatal glucocorticoids Medications administered to the mother for the purpose of accelerating fetal lung maturity when an increased risk exists for preterm birth between 24 and 34 weeks of gestation.

anthropometric measurements Body measurements, such as height and weight.

anticipatory grief Grief that predates the loss of a beloved object.

anxiety disorders Mood disorders characterized by prominent symptoms of anxiety that impair functioning. Examples are obsessive-compulsive disorder, posttraumatic stress disorder, generalized anxiety disorder, panic disorder, agoraphobia, and other phobias. Anxiety disorders are the most common psychiatric disorders.

ARNDs See alcohol-related neurodevelopmental disorders (ARNDs).

appropriate for gestational age an infant whose birth weight falls between the 10th and 90th percentile on intrauterine growth curves

APGAR score numeric expression of the condition of a newborn obtained by rapid assessment at 1 and 5 minutes of age; developed by Dr. Virginia Apgar.

ARTs See assisted reproductive therapies (ARTs).

asphyxia Term used when fetal hypoxia results in metabolic acidosis.

assimilation Occurs when a cultural group loses its identity and becomes part of the dominant culture.

assisted reproductive therapies (ARTs) Treatments for infertility, including in vitro fertilization procedures, embryo adoption, embryo hosting, and therapeutic insemination.

asymptomatic bacteriuria Persistent presence of bacteria within the urinary tract of women who have no symptom of infection. A clean-voided urine specimen containing more than 100,000 organisms per milliliter is diagnostic.

atony Absence of muscle tone. See also uterine atony.

attachment (1) The process by which a parent comes to love and accept a child and a child comes to love and accept a parent. (2) A specific and enduring affective tie to another person.

attitude The relation of the fetal body parts to one another. Normally the back of the fetus is rounded so that the chin is flexed on the chest, the thighs are flexed on the abdomen, the legs are flexed at the knees, and the arms are crossed over the thorax. This attitude is called general flexion.

augmentation of labor Stimulation of ineffective uterine contractions after labor has started spontaneously but is not progressing satisfactorily.

autolysis "Self-digestive" process by which the uterus returns to a nonpregnant state after childbirth. The decrease in estrogen and progesterone levels after childbirth results in this destruction of excess hypertrophied uterine tissue.

autosomal dominant inheritance disorder Condition in which only one copy of a variant allele is needed for phenotypic expression.

autosomal recessive inheritance disorder Condition in which both genes of a pair are forms associated with the disorder to be expressed.

autosomes Any of the paired chromosomes other than the sex (X and Y) chromosomes.

B

baby blues See postpartum blues.

balanced translocation Translocation in which parts of the two chromosomes are exchanged equally. The individual is phenotypically normal because there is no extra chromosome material; it is just rearranged.

ballottement (1) Movability of a floating object, such as a fetus. (2) Diagnostic technique using palpation: a floating object, when tapped or pushed, moves away and then returns to touch the examiner's hand. (3) Passive movement of the unengaged fetus.

Bartholin cyst Most common benign lesion of the vulva; arises from obstruction of the Bartholin duct, which causes it to enlarge.

basalis, decidua See decidua basalis.

baseline fetal heart rate See fetal heart rate (FHR), baseline.

Bell palsy Acute idiopathic facial paralysis. The cause is unknown, but it may be related to the reactivation of herpesvirus infection or acute human immunodeficiency virus type 1 (HIV-1) retroviral infection. Bell palsy occurs fairly often, especially in women of reproductive age. Pregnant women are affected four times more often than nonpregnant women.

bereavement The feelings of loss, pain, desolation, and sadness that occur after the death of a loved one.

biophysical profile (BPP) Noninvasive assessment of a fetus using ultrasound and the nonstress test. It includes the following components: fetal breathing movements, gross body movements, fetal tone, reactive fetal heart rate (FHR), and qualitative amniotic fluid volume.

biopsy Removal of a small piece of tissue for microscopic examination and diagnosis.

biorhythmicity Cyclic changes that occur with established regularity, such as sleeping and eating patterns.

biparietal diameter Largest transverse diameter of the fetal head; extends from one parietal bone to the other.

bipolar disorder Mood disorder defined by the presence of one or more episodes of abnormally elevated energy levels, cognition, and mood and one or more depressive episodes. Also called manic-depressive disorder. Postpartum psychosis is most commonly associated with a diagnosis of bipolar disorder. (See postpartum psychosis.)

birth control The device and/or practice used to decrease the risk of conceiving or bearing offspring.

birth injury See birth trauma.

birth plan A tool by which parents can explore their childbirth options and choose those that are most important to them.

birth rate Number of live births per 1000 population per year.

birth trauma Physical injury sustained by a neonate during labor and birth. Also called birth injury.

Bishop score Rating system to evaluate inducibility of the cervix; a higher score increases the rate of successful induction of labor.

blastocyst Stage in the development of a mammalian embryo, occurring after the morula stage, that consists of an outer layer, or trophoblast, and a hollow sphere of cells enclosing a cavity.

bloody show Vaginal discharge that originates in the cervix and consists of blood and mucus; increases as cervix dilates during labor.

BMI See body mass index (BMI).

body mass index (BMI) Method of calculating appropriateness of weight for height (BMI = weight [kilograms]/height^2 [meters]).

BPD See bronchopulmonary dysplasia (BPD).

brachial plexus injury Paralysis caused by physical injury to the upper brachial plexus, occurring most often in childbirth from forcible traction during birth.

bradycardia Baseline fetal heart rate (FHR) of fewer than 110 beats/minute for 10 minutes or longer. True bradycardia occurs rarely and is not specifically related to fetal oxygenation.

Braxton Hicks contractions Mild, intermittent, painless uterine contractions that occur during pregnancy. These contractions occur more frequently as pregnancy advances but do not represent true labor.

breast milk jaundice Also called late-onset jaundice; hyperbilirubinemia that occurs between days 5 and 10 of life, usually in a healthy, breastfed infant; cause is unknown.

breast self-examination (BSE) Self-palpation of breasts to detect for changes in breast tissue.

breastfeeding-associated jaundice Also called early-onset jaundice; hyperbilirubinemia that begins at 2 to 5 days of life; associated with insufficient breastfeeding and infrequent stooling.

bronchopulmonary dysplasia (BPD) Pulmonary condition affecting preterm infants who have experienced respiratory failure and have been oxygen dependent for more than 28 days.

brown fat Source of heat unique to neonates that is capable of greater thermogenic activity than ordinary fat. Deposits are found around the adrenals, kidneys, and neck; between the scapulas; and behind the sternum for several weeks after birth.

C

café-au-lait Patches of skin pigmentation present in neurofibromatosis.

cancer of the cervix See cervical cancer.

caput Occiput of fetal head appearing at the vaginal introitus preceding birth of the head.

caput succedaneum Swelling of the tissue over the presenting part of the fetal head caused by pressure during labor.

carcinoma in situ (CIS) Diagnosed when the full thickness of epithelium is replaced with abnormal cells.

carpal tunnel syndrome Pressure on the median nerve at the point at which it goes through the carpal tunnel of the wrist. It causes soreness, tenderness, and weakness of the muscles of the thumb. Edema involving the peripheral nerves may result in carpal tunnel syndrome during the last trimester of pregnancy.

carrier Individual who carries a gene that does not exhibit itself in physical or chemical characteristics but that can be transmitted to children (e.g., a female carrying the trait for hemophilia, which is expressed in male offspring). Heterozygous individuals have only one variant allele and are unaffected clinically because their normal gene (wild-type allele) overshadows the variant allele. They are known as carriers of the recessive trait.

cell-free deoxyribonucleic acid (DNA) screening Screening method to detect the chromosomal abnormalities trisomy 21, 13, and 18. It also provides noninvasive prenatal genetic diagnosis of fetal Rh status, fetal gender, and certain paternally transmitted single gene disorders.

cephalhematoma NOTE: This is spelled cephalohematoma in some sources. Extravasation of blood from ruptured vessels between a skull bone and its external covering, the periosteum. Swelling is limited by the margins of the cranial bone affected (usually parietals).

cephalocaudal Head-to-rump.

cephalopelvic disproportion (CPD) Condition in which the infant's head is of such a shape, size, or position that it cannot pass through the mother's pelvis; can also be caused by maternal pelvic problems. Also called fetopelvic disproportion (FPD).

cerclage Use of nonabsorbable suture to constrict the internal os of a cervix that is dilating prematurely because of cervical weakness. The suture can be placed vaginally or abdominally. A cerclage can be placed either prophylactically or as a rescue procedure.

cervical cancer The third most common reproductive cancer; begins as neoplastic changes in the cervical epithelium. Also called cancer of the cervix.

cervical conization Excision of a cone-shaped section of tissue from the endocervix.

cervical insufficiency Passive and painless dilation of the cervix leading to recurrent preterm births during the second trimester in the absence of other causes. Measurement of cervical length has been used as a way to diagnose cervical insufficiency.

cervical intraepithelial neoplasia (CIN) Uncontrolled and progressive abnormal growth of cervical epithelial cells; preinvasive lesions.

cesarean birth Birth of a fetus by an incision through the abdominal wall and uterus. See also elective cesarean birth.

Chadwick sign Violet bluish vaginal mucous membrane and cervix that is visible from about the fourth week of pregnancy; caused by increased vascularity.

choanal atresia Complete obstruction of the posterior nares, which open into the nasopharynx, with membranous or bony tissue.

chorioamnionitis Bacterial infection of the amniotic cavity; usually diagnosed by the clinical findings of maternal fever, maternal and fetal tachycardia, uterine tenderness, and foul odor of amniotic fluid. Other terms for this condition include clinical chorioamnionitis, amnionitis, intrapartum infection, amniotic fluid infection, and intraamniotic infection.

chorion Fetal membrane closest to the intrauterine wall that gives rise to the placenta and continues as the outer membrane surrounding the amnion.

chorionic villi Tiny vascular protrusions on the chorionic surface that project into the maternal blood sinuses of the uterus and that help form the placenta and secrete human chorionic gonadotropin.

chorionic villus sampling (CVS) Removal of fetal tissue from the placenta for genetic diagnostic studies, which can be performed during either the first or second trimester. When performed after the first trimester, the procedure is better known as late CVS or placental biopsy.

chronic hypertension Hypertension that is present before pregnancy or that is initially diagnosed during pregnancy and persists longer than 12 weeks postpartum.

chronic hypertension with superimposed preeclampsia Condition that usually presents as elevated blood pressures in a woman whose blood pressure previously has been well controlled. Superimposed preeclampsia also may be diagnosed by the development of severe features of preeclampsia such as thrombocytopenia, impaired liver function, the new development of renal insufficiency, pulmonary edema, or new-onset cerebral or visual disturbances.

CIN See cervical intraepithelial neoplasia (CIN).

circumcision removal of all or part of the foreskin (prepuce) of the penis.

CIS See carcinoma in situ (CIS).

claiming process Process by which the parents identify their new baby in terms of likeness to other family members, differences, and uniqueness; the unique newcomer is thus incorporated into the family.

cleft lip Incomplete closure of the lip. Lay term is harelip.

cleft palate Incomplete closure of the palate or roof of mouth; a congenital fissure.

climacteric The period of a woman's life when she is passing from a reproductive to a nonreproductive state, with regression of ovarian function. The cycle of endocrine, physical, and psychosocial changes that occurs during the termination of the reproductive years. Also called climacterium.

clonus Hyperactive reflexes.

clubfoot Congenital deformity in which portions of the foot and ankle are twisted out of a normal position.

Cochrane Pregnancy and Childbirth Database Database of up-to-date systematic reviews and dissemination of views of randomized controlled trials of health care.

cohabiting-parent family Family form in which children live with two unmarried biologic parents or two adoptive parents.

cold stress Excessive loss of heat that results in increased respirations and nonshivering thermogenesis to maintain core body temperature.

colostrum The creamy white to yellowish to orange premilk fluid that may be expressed from the nipples as early as 16 weeks of gestation; the fluid in the breast from pregnancy into the early postpartal period. It is more concentrated than mature milk and is extremely rich in immunoglobulins; it has higher concentrations of protein and minerals but less fat than mature milk; it is also rich in antibodies, which provide protection from many diseases; high in protein, which binds bilirubin; and laxative-acting, which speeds the elimination of meconium and helps loosen mucus.

colposcopy Examination of vagina and cervix with a colposcope (a stereoscopic binocular microscope that magnifies the view of the cervix) to identify neoplastic or other changes.

combined spinal-epidural (CSE) analgesia An epidural needle is inserted into the epidural space. Before the epidural catheter is threaded, a smaller-gauge spinal needle is inserted through the bore of the epidural needle into the subarachnoid space and a small amount of an opioid or a combination of an opioid and a local anesthetic is injected to rapidly provide analgesia. Afterward, the epidural catheter is inserted as usual. If pain relief is still needed after the effect of the medication injected into the subarachnoid space wears off, additional medication can be injected through the epidural catheter.

complicated bereavement See complicated grief.

complicated grief Extremely intense grief reactions that last for a very long time; a state of chronic mourning. Also the persistent feelings of anger, guilt, loss, pain, and sadness over time that lead to feelings of hopelessness, helplessness, and diminishing self-worth that are signs and symptoms of clinical depression, which is different from the normal depression of bereavement. Also called complicated bereavement, prolonged grief, pathologic grief, or pathologic mourning.

conception Union of the sperm and a single egg (ovum) resulting in fertilization; formation of the one-celled zygote marks the beginning of a pregnancy.

congenital anomaly A defect that is present at birth and can be caused by genetic or environmental factors, or both; defined as a physical, metabolic, anatomic, or behavioral deviation from the normal pattern of development.

congenital diaphragmatic hernia Diaphragm malformation that allows displacement of the abdominal organs into the thoracic cavity.

congenital hypothyroidism Results from a deficiency of thyroid hormones and can be permanent (requires treatment for life) or transient (spontaneously resolves).

congenital rubella syndrome Complex of problems, including hearing defects, cardiovascular abnormalities, and cataracts, caused by maternal rubella in the first trimester of pregnancy.

conization See cervical conization.

conjoined twins Twins who are physically united; Siamese twins.

continuous positive airway pressure (CPAP) Method of infusing oxygen or air under a preset pressure by means of nasal prongs, a face mask, or an endotracheal tube.

contraception Intentional prevention of pregnancy (impregnation or conception) during sexual intercourse.

contraction stress test (CST) Test to stimulate uterine contractions for the purpose of assessing fetal response to stress; it identifies a fetus that is stable at rest but shows evidence of compromise after stress. This test is also known as the oxytocin challenge test (OCT).

Coombs' test Indirect: determination of Rh-positive antibodies in maternal blood. Direct: determination of maternal Rh-positive antibodies in fetal cord blood. A positive test result indicates the presence of antibodies or titer.

cordocentesis See percutaneous umbilical blood sampling (PUBS).

corpus luteum cysts Occur after ovulation and are possibly caused by an increased secretion of progesterone that results in an increase of fluid in the corpus luteum.

corrected age Taking into account the gestational age and the postnatal age of a preterm infant when determining expectations for development.

counterpressure Pressure to the sacral area of the back during uterine contractions.

couplet care Care provided by one nurse, educated in both mother and infant care, who functions as the primary nurse for mother and infant. Also called mother-baby care or single-room maternity care.

couvade syndrome The phenomenon of expectant fathers' experiencing pregnancy-like symptoms.

couvelaire uterus Associated with placental abruption; occurs when blood accumulates between the separated placenta and the uterine wall. The uterus appears purple or blue rather than its usual "bubblegum pink" color, and contractility is lost.

CPAP See continuous positive airway pressure (CPAP).

crowning Stage of birth when the top of the fetal head can be seen at the vaginal orifice as the widest part of the head distends the vulva.

cultural competence Awareness, acceptance, and knowledge of cultural differences and adaptation of services to acknowledge and support the client's culture.

cultural prescriptions Practices that are expected or acceptable; they tell women what to do.

cultural proscriptions Forbidden; taboo practices; they tell women what not to do.

cultural relativism Learning about and applying the standards of another's culture to activities within that culture.

cystocele Bladder hernia; injury to the vesicovaginal fascia during labor and birth may allow herniation of the bladder into the vagina. Protrusion of the bladder downward into the vagina; develops when supporting structures in the vesicovaginal septum are injured.

D

daily fetal movement count (DFMC) Maternal assessment of fetal activity; the number of fetal movements within a specific time are counted. Also called kick count.

DDH See developmental dysplasia of the hip (DDH).

decidua Mucous membrane, lining of uterus, or endometrium of pregnancy that is shed after giving birth.

decidua basalis The portion of the endometrium directly under the blastocyst, where the chorionic villi tap into the maternal blood vessels. Maternal aspect of the placenta made up of uterine blood vessels, endometrial stroma, and glands. It is shed in lochial discharge after birth.

deletion Loss of chromosomal material and partial monosomy for the chromosome involved. The resulting clinical phenotype of either a terminal or an interstitial deletion depends on how much of the chromosome has been lost and the number and function of the genes contained in the missing segment.

demand feeding Feeding a newborn every third hour or when the baby cries to be fed, whichever comes first.

deoxyribonucleic acid (DNA) Intracellular complex protein that carries genetic information, consisting of two purines (adenine and guanine) and two pyrimidines (thymine and cytosine).

dermoid cysts Germ cell tumors, usually occurring in childhood. These cysts contain substances such as hair, teeth, sebaceous secretions, and bones.

desquamation Shedding of epithelial cells of the skin and mucous membranes.

developmental dysplasia of the hip (DDH) Abnormal development of the hip joint, resulting in instability of the hip, causing one or both of the femoral heads to be displaced from the acetabulum (hip socket).

diabetes mellitus A group of metabolic diseases characterized by hyperglycemia resulting from defects in insulin secretion, insulin action, or both. The current classification system includes four groups: type 1 diabetes, type 2 diabetes, other specific types (e.g., diabetes caused by genetic defects in beta cell function or insulin action, disease or injury of the pancreas, or drug-induced diabetes), and gestational diabetes mellitus.

diastasis recti abdominis Separation of the two rectus muscles along the median line of the abdominal wall. This is often seen in women with repeated pregnancies or with a multiple gestation

dietary reference intakes (DRIs) Nutritional recommendations consisting of the recommended dietary allowances, adequate intakes, and tolerable upper intake levels, the upper limit of intake associated with low risk in almost all members of a population.

dilation The enlargement or widening of the cervical opening and the cervical canal that occurs once labor has begun. The diameter of the cervix increases from being closed to full dilation (approximately 10 cm) to allow birth of a term fetus.

dilation and curettage (D&C) Surgical procedure in which the cervix is dilated if necessary and a curette is inserted to scrape the uterine walls and remove uterine contents. Uterine contents may also be removed by suction curettage, using a catheter attached to an electric-powered vacuum source.

diploid Containing two complete sets of chromosomes, one from each parent.

disseminated intravascular coagulation (DIC) Pathologic form of clotting that is diffuse and consumes large amounts of clotting factors, causing widespread external bleeding, internal bleeding, or both, and clotting. In obstetrics it is most often associated with placental abruption, amniotic fluid embolism, preeclampsia, HELLP syndrome, and gram-negative sepsis. Also called consumptive coagulopathy.

disenfranchised grief Losses that are not openly acknowledged or mourned publicly

dizygotic twins Twins developed from two separate ova fertilized by two separate sperm at the same time; fraternal twins.

dominant trait A trait or disorder expressed or phenotypically apparent when only one copy of an allele associated with the trait is present. Gene that is expressed whenever it is present in the heterozygous gene state (e.g., brown eyes are dominant over blue).

Doppler blood flow analysis Method for measuring blood flow noninvasively in the fetus and placenta using ultrasound to detect intrauterine growth restriction.

doula A specially trained, experienced female labor attendant. A doula is a professional or lay labor-support person who is present during labor to focus on the laboring woman and provide physical and emotional support.

Down syndrome (DS) Abnormality involving chromosome 21 that characteristically results in a typical picture of intellectual disability and altered physical appearance. This condition was formerly called mongolism.

dual diagnosis Coexistence of substance abuse and another psychiatric disorder. Mood and anxiety disorders are the psychiatric disorders most commonly seen along with substance abuse in women. The psychiatric illness usually occurs before substance use begins.

DUB See dysfunctional uterine bleeding (DUB).

ductus arteriosus In fetal circulation an anatomic shunt between the pulmonary artery and arch of the aorta. It is obliterated after birth by a rising PO_2 and a change in intravascular pressures in the presence of normal pulmonary function. It normally becomes a ligament after birth but in some instances remains patent; this is called patent ductus arteriosus (PDA).

ductus venosus In fetal circulation a blood vessel carrying oxygenated blood between the umbilical vein and the inferior vena cava, bypassing the liver. It is obliterated and becomes a ligament after birth.

duration (of uterine contractions) Time (measured in seconds) from the beginning to the end of a contraction.

dysfunctional labor Long, difficult, or abnormal labor, caused by various conditions associated with the five factors affecting labor; also called dystocia.

dysfunctional uterine bleeding (DUB) Excessive uterine bleeding with no demonstrable organic cause, genital or extragenital; most frequently caused by anovulation. Subset of abnormal uterine bleeding.

dysmenorrhea Pain during or shortly before menstruation.

dysplasia Any abnormal development of tissues or organs; preinvasive lesions in cervical epithelium.

E

early deceleration (of the fetal heart rate) Visually apparent gradual (onset to lowest point ≥30 seconds) decrease in and return to baseline fetal heart reate (FHR) associated with uterine contractions. It is thought to be caused by transient fetal head compression and is considered a normal and benign finding. Generally the onset, nadir (lowest point), and recovery of the deceleration correspond to the beginning, peak, and end of the contraction.

early neonatal death Death of a live-born infant less than 7 days old.

eclampsia Onset of seizure activity or coma in a woman with preeclampsia who has no history of preexisting pathology that can result in seizure activity.

ectopic pregnancy Pregnancy in which the fertilized ovum is implanted outside of its normal place in the uterine cavity. Locations include the abdomen, uterine tubes, and ovaries. Ectopic pregnancies are often called tubal pregnancies because at least 90% are located in the uterine tube.

EDB See estimated date of birth (EDB).

effacement The shortening and thinning of the cervix during the first stage of labor. Effacement generally progresses significantly in first-time term pregnancy before more than slight dilation occurs. In subsequent pregnancies effacement and dilation of the cervix tend to progress together. Degree of effacement is expressed in percentages from 0% to 100%.

effleurage Light stroking, usually of the abdomen, in rhythm with breathing during contractions.

e-health literacy Ability to use information and communications technologies to improve health.

ELBW See extremely low birth weight (ELBW).

elective abortion Termination of pregnancy chosen by the woman that is not required for her physical safety.

elective cesarean birth A primary cesarean birth without medical or obstetric indication; sometimes referred to as cesarean on request or cesarean on demand.

ELSIs Ethical, legal, and social implications of genetics research.

embryo Conceptus from the second or third week of development until about the eighth week after conception, when mineralization (ossification) of the skeleton begins. This period is characterized by cellular differentiation and predominantly hyperplastic growth.

hypospadias Anomalous positioning of urinary meatus on undersurface of penis or close to or just inside the vagina.
hypothermia Temperature that falls below normal range, usually caused by exposure to cold.
hypothyroidism Deficiency of thyroid gland activity with underproduction of thyroxine.
hypovolemic shock See hemorrhagic shock.
hypoxemia Deficiency of oxygen in the arterial blood.
hypoxia Inadequate supply of oxygen at the cellular level that can cause metabolic acidosis.
hysterectomy Surgical removal of the entire uterus.

I

icterus See jaundice.
idiopathic thrombocytopenic purpura (ITP) An autoimmune disorder in which antiplatelet antibodies decrease the life span of the platelets. Thrombocytopenia, capillary fragility, and increased bleeding time are diagnostic findings. Also called immune thrombocytopenic purpura (ITP).
illness prevention Desire to avoid illness, detect it early, or maintain optimal functioning when illness is present.
immune thrombocytopenic purpura (ITP) See idiopathic thrombocytopenic purpura (ITP).
imperforate anus A term used to describe a wide range of congenital disorders involving the anus and rectum and genitourinary system.
implantation Embedding of the fertilized ovum in the uterine mucosa; nidation.
inborn error of metabolism Hereditary deficiency of a specific enzyme needed for normal metabolism of specific chemicals (e.g., deficiency of phenylalanine hydroxylase results in phenylketonuria [PKU]; a deficiency of hexosaminidase results in Tay-Sachs disease).
induced abortion Purposeful interruption of a pregnancy before 20 weeks of gestation.
induction of labor Chemical or mechanical initiation of uterine contractions before their spontaneous onset for the purpose of bringing about birth.
infant death Death during the first year of life.
infant mortality rate Number of deaths per 1000 children 1 year of age or younger.
infertility Decreased capacity to conceive. A serious medical concern that affects quality of life and is a problem for 10% to 15% of reproductive-age couples. The term *infertility* implies subfertility, a prolonged time to conceive, as opposed to *sterility*, which means inability to conceive.
insensible water loss (IWL) Evaporative water loss that occurs mainly through the skin and respiratory tract.
intensity (of uterine contractions) Strength of a contraction at its peak.
intermittent auscultation Involves listening to fetal heart sounds at periodic intervals to assess the fetal heart rate (FHR).
interstitial deletion Deletion anywhere else in the chromosome except at the end.
intimate partner violence (IPV) The actual or threatened physical, sexual, psychologic, or emotional abuse by a spouse, ex-spouse, boyfriend, girlfriend, ex-boyfriend, ex-girlfriend, date, or cohabiting partner.
intraductal papilloma A benign tumor that grows within the duct of the breast.
intrahepatic cholestasis of pregnancy (ICP) Disorder unique to pregnancy that is characterized by generalized pruritus caused by elevated serum bile acids. The itching commonly affects the palms and soles but can occur on any part of the body and is usually worse at night. No skin lesions are present.
intrauterine growth restriction (IUGR) Fetal undergrowth of any cause, such as deficient nutrient supply or intrauterine infection, or associated with congenital malformation; birth weight below population 10th percentile corrected for gestational age.
intrauterine pressure catheter (IUPC) Catheter inserted into uterine cavity to assess uterine activity and pressure by electronic means.
inversion of the uterus (1) Turning end for end, upside down, or inside out. (2) Deviation in which a portion of the chromosome has been rearranged in reverse order.
involution (1) Rolling or turning inward. (2) Reduction in size of the uterus after birth and its return to its nonpregnant condition.
isoimmunization Production of antibodies by one member of a species against something that is commonly found within that species (e.g., development of anti-Rh antibodies in an Rh-negative person; also called Rh incompatibility).
ITP See idiopathic thrombocytopenic purpura (ITP). Note: The acronym ITP is also known as immune thrombocytopenic purpura.
IWL See insensible water loss (IWL).

J

jaundice Yellow discoloration of the body tissues caused by the deposit of bile pigments (unconjugated bilirubin); also called icterus. See also hyperbilirubinemia.

K

karyotype Pictorial analysis of the number, form, and size of an individual's chromosomes. Schematic arrangement of the chromosomes within a cell to demonstrate their numbers and morphology.
Kegel exercises Pelvic muscle exercises developed to strengthen the pubococcygeal muscles (supportive pelvic floor muscles) to control or reduce incontinent urine loss and to provide support for the pelvic organs and control of the muscles surrounding the vagina and urethra. Also beneficial during pregnancy and postpartum.
kernicterus Bilirubin encephalopathy involving the deposit of unconjugated bilirubin in brain cells, resulting in death or impaired intellectual, perceptive, or motor function and adaptive behavior.
ketoacidosis The accumulation of ketone bodies in the blood as a consequence of hyperglycemia; leads to metabolic acidosis.
key informants Individuals in positions of leadership who can provide information about a situation.

L

L/S ratio See lecithin/sphingomyelin ratio.
labor Series of processes by which the fetus is expelled from the uterus; parturition; childbirth.
Lactogenesis initiation of breast milk production. Stage I: Initial synthesis of milk components beginning at approximately 16 to 18 weeks of pregnancy until approximately day 3 postpartum; the breasts prepare for milk production by producing colostrum. Stage II: begins with delivery of the placenta; progesterone levels drop and prolactin levels increase; onset of copious milk production on day 2 to 4 postpartum. Stage III: begins at approximately 10 days postpartum when mature milk is established and supply is maintained through autocrine control.
lactose intolerance Inability to digest milk sugar (lactose) because of an inherited absence of the enzyme lactase in the small intestine.
lanugo Downy, fine hair characteristic of the fetus between 20 weeks of gestation and birth that is most noticeable over the shoulder, forehead and eyebrows.
large for gestational age (LGA) Exhibiting excessive growth for gestational age; an infant whose birth weight falls above the 90th percentile on intrauterine growth curves.
laryngeal web Results from the incomplete separation of the two sides of the larynx and is most often between the vocal cords.
latch (1) Placement of the infant's mouth over the nipple, areola, and breast, making a seal between the mouth and breast to create adequate suction for milk removal. (2) Attachment of the infant to the breast for feeding.
late deceleration (of the fetal heart rate) Visually apparent gradual decrease in and return to baseline fetal heart rate (FHR) associated with uterine contractions. It is thought to be caused by a disruption in oxygen transfer from the environment to the fetus. The deceleration begins after the contraction has started, and the nadir (lowest point) of the deceleration occurs after the peak of the contraction. The deceleration usually does not return to baseline until after the contraction is over.
late neonatal death Death of a newborn between 7 and 28 days after birth,
latent (early) phase of labor Phase in first stage of labor up through 3 cm dilation.
latent ("laboring down") phase of labor Period of rest and relative calm at the beginning of second stage labor. During this phase the fetus continues to descend passively through the birth canal and rotate to an anterior position as a result of ongoing uterine contractions. The woman is quiet and often relaxes with her eyes closed between contractions. The urge to bear down is not strong, and some women do not experience it at all or only during the acme (peak) of a contraction.
LBW See low birth weight (LBW).
lecithin/sphingomyelin ratio Ratio of lecithin to sphingomyelin in the amniotic fluid. It is used to assess maturity of the fetal lung.
leiomyoma Slow-growing benign tumor arising from the muscle tissue of the uterus. Also known as fibroid tumor, fibroma, myoma, or fibromyoma.
letdown or let-down reflex See milk ejection reflex (MER).
leukorrhea White or slightly gray mucoid discharge from the cervical canal or the vagina with a faint musty odor, which may be normal physiologically or caused by pathologic states of the vagina and endocervix (e.g., *Trichomonas vaginalis* infections).

LGA See large for gestational age (LGA).

lie Relationship between the long axis (spine) of the fetus and the long axis (spine) of the mother. In a longitudinal lie, the fetus is lying lengthwise or vertically, whereas in a transverse lie, the fetus is lying crosswise or horizontally in the uterus.

lightening Sensation of decreased abdominal distention produced by uterine descent into the pelvic cavity as the fetal presenting part settles into the pelvis. It usually occurs 2 weeks before the onset of labor in nulliparas.

linea nigra Pigmented line that appears on the middle of the abdomen and extends from the symphysis pubis toward the umbilicus, extending to the top of the fundus in the midline; seen in some women during the latter part of pregnancy.

lithotomy position Position in which the woman lies on her back with her knees flexed and with abducted thighs drawn up toward her chest.

local perineal infiltration anesthesia Process by which a local anesthetic medication is injected into the skin and then subcutaneously to anesthetize a limited region of the body.

lochia Uterine/vaginal discharge after childbirth (during the puerperium) consisting of blood, tissue, and mucus.

lochia alba Thin, yellowish to white, vaginal discharge that follows lochia serosa on about the tenth day after birth and that may last from 2 to 6 weeks postpartum; consists primarily of leukocytes and decidual cells but also contains epithelial cells, mucus, serum, and bacteria.

lochia rubra Red, distinctly blood-tinged vaginal flow that follows birth and lasts 2 to 4 days; consists mainly of blood and decidual and trophoblastic debris.

lochia serosa Serous, pinkish brown, watery vaginal discharge that follows lochia rubra until about the tenth day after birth; consists of old blood, serum, leukocytes, and tissue debris.

low birth weight (LBW) A newborn birth weight less than 2500 g (5.5 lb).

lumpectomy Removal of a small breast tumor and a small amount of surrounding healthy tissue to ensure there are clean margins.

M

macrosomia Birth weight more than 4000 to 4500 g or greater than the 90th percentile.

magnetic resonance imaging (MRI) Noninvasive nuclear procedure for imaging tissues with high fat and water content; in obstetrics, uses include evaluation of fetal structures, placenta, and amniotic fluid volume.

major depressive episode Disorder diagnosed in a person who has at least five of the following signs or symptoms nearly every day: depressed mood, often with spontaneous crying; markedly diminished interest in all activities; insomnia or hypersomnia; weight changes (increases or decreases); psychomotor retardation or agitation; fatigue or loss of energy; feelings of worthlessness or inappropriate guilt; diminished ability to concentrate; and suicidal ideation with or without a suicidal plan.

mammary duct ectasia An inflammation of the ducts behind the nipple.

mammography X-ray filming of the breast; examination technique used to screen for and evaluate breast lesions.

married-blended family Family formed as a result of divorce and remarriage, consisting of unrelated family members (stepparents, stepchildren, stepsiblings).

MAS See meconium aspiration syndrome (MAS).

mastectomy Removal of the breast including the nipple and areola; also called a simple or total mastectomy.

mastitis Infection in a breast, usually confined to a milk duct, characterized by influenza-like symptoms and redness and tenderness in the affected breast.

maternal mortality rate Number of maternal deaths per 100,000 births.

mechanical ventilation Technique used to provide predetermined amount of oxygen; requires intubation.

meconium First stools of infant: viscid, sticky; dark greenish brown, almost black; sterile; odorless.

meconium aspiration syndrome (MAS) Function of fetal hypoxia: with hypoxia, the anal sphincter relaxes and meconium is released; reflex gasping movements draw meconium and other particulate matter in the amniotic fluid into the infant's bronchial tree, obstructing the airflow after birth.

meconium-stained amniotic fluid Presence of green amniotic fluid that is either thin (light) or thick (heavy) in consistency; indicates that the fetus has passed meconium (first stool) before birth.

meiosis Process by which germ cells divide and decrease their chromosomal number by one half; produces gametes (eggs and sperm).

melasma Blotchy, brownish hyperpigmentation of the skin over the cheeks, nose, and forehead, especially in dark-complexioned pregnant women and some women taking oral contraceptives; also known as the mask of pregnancy.

MEN See minimal enteral nutrition (MEN).

menarche Onset, or beginning, of menstrual function; first menstruation.

menopausal hormone therapy (MHT) Hormonal therapy for menopausal symptoms; either as estrogen replacement therapy (ERT) or estrogen therapy (ET), in which a woman takes only estrogen, or hormonal replacement therapy (HRT) or hormonal therapy (HT), in which she takes both estrogen and progestins.

menopause From the Latin *mensis* (month) and Greek *pausis* (to cease); refers only to the last menstrual period; unlike menarche, however, menopause can be dated with certainty only 1 year after menstruation ceases.

menorrhagia Excessive menstrual bleeding, in either duration or amount. Also known as hypermenorrhea.

menses (menstruation) (Latin plural of *mensis* [month].) Periodic uterine bleeding and vaginal discharge of bloody fluid from the nonpregnant uterus that occurs from the age of puberty to menopause, which begins approximately 14 days after ovulation.

menstruation See menses (menstruation).

MER See milk ejection reflex (MER).

metastasis Spread of cancer from its original site to distant parts of the body. Results from seeding of cancer cells into the blood and lymph systems.

metrorrhagia Intermenstrual bleeding; refers to any episode of bleeding, whether spotting, menses, or hemorrhage, that occurs at a time other than the normal menses.

MHT See menopausal hormone therapy (MHT).

microcephaly Congenital anomaly characterized by abnormal smallness of the head in relation to the rest of the body and by underdevelopment of the brain, resulting in some degree of mental retardation.

microdeletion Deletion too small to be detected by standard cytogenetic techniques.

milia Unopened sebaceous glands appearing as tiny, white, pinpoint papules on forehead, nose, cheeks, and chin of a neonate that disappear spontaneously in a few days or weeks.

milk ejection reflex (MER) Release of milk caused by the contraction of the myoepithelial cells within the milk glands in response to oxytocin; also called letdown or let-down reflex.

minimal enteral nutrition (MEN) Feeding small volumes of food to stimulate or prime the development of the immature gastrointestinal tract of the preterm infant, to achieve better absorption of nutrients when bolus or regular intermittent gavage feedings can be given. Also called trophic feeding.

miscarriage See spontaneous abortion.

mitosis Process of somatic cell division in which a single cell divides, but both of the new cells have the same number of chromosomes as the first; body cells replicate to yield two cells with the same genetic makeup as the parent cell.

modified biophysical profile (mBPP) Combines the nonstress test with measurement of the quantity of amniotic fluid using ultrasound.

modified radical mastectomy Removal of breast tissue, skin, and axillary nodes.

molar pregancy See hydatidiform mole.

mongolian spot Bluish gray or dark nonelevated pigmented area usually found over the lower back and buttocks; present at birth in some infants, primarily nonwhite. The spot usually fades by school age.

monosomy Chromosomal aberration characterized by the absence of one chromosome from the normal diploid complement. Product of the union between a normal gamete and a gamete that is missing a chromosome.

monozygotic twins Twins developed from a single fertilized ovum; identical twins.

Montevideo units (MVUs) A method for evaluating the adequacy of uterine activity for achieving progress in labor. MVUs are calculated by subtracting the baseline uterine pressure from the peak contraction pressure for each contraction that occurs in a 10-minute window, and then adding together the pressures generated by each contraction that occurs during that period of time. MVUs can only be calculated using an intrauterine pressure catheter (IUPC).

Montgomery glands Small, nodular prominences on the areolas around the nipples of the breasts that enlarge during pregnancy and lactation; hypertrophy of the sebaceous (oil) glands embedded in the primary areolae sebaceous glands. Also called Montgomery tubercles or tubercules of Montgomery.

morbidity (1) Condition of being diseased. (2) Number of cases of disease or of sick persons in relationship to a specific population; incidence.

morning sickness Nausea and vomiting that affect some women during the first few months of their pregnancy; can occur at any time of day.
morula Developmental stage of the fertilized ovum in which there is a solid mass of cells resembling a mulberry.
mosaicism Mixture of cells, some with a normal number of chromosomes and others entirely missing or having an extra chromosome.
mourning The process of finding the answers to the questions surrounding the loss, coping with grief responses, and determining how to live again.
multifactorial inheritance Inheritance of phenotypic characteristics resulting from two or more genes on different chromosomes acting together. See also unifactorial inheritance.
multifetal pregnancy Pregnancy in which there is more than one fetus in the uterus at the same time; multiple pregnancy.
multigenerational family Family form consisting of three or more generations of relatives (grandparents, children, and grandchildren).
multigravida A woman who has had two or more pregnancies
multipara A woman who has completed two or more pregnancies to 20 weeks of gestation or more
mutation Spontaneous and permanent change in the normal gene structure in a gene or chromosome in gametes that may be transmitted to offspring.
mutuality Component of parent-infant attachment; the infant's behaviors and characteristics elicit a corresponding set of parental behaviors and characteristics.
myelomeningocele External sac containing meninges, spinal fluid, and nerves that protrudes through defect in vertebral column.
myomectomy Removal of a tumor; specifically removal of a benign tumor of the uterus leaving the uterine walls relatively intact.

N

Naegele's rule Method for calculating the estimated date of birth (EDB) or "due date."
NEC See necrotizing enterocolitis (NEC).
necrotizing enterocolitis (NEC) Acute inflammatory bowel disorder that occurs primarily in preterm or low-birth-weight neonates. It is characterized by ischemic necrosis (death) of the gastrointestinal mucosa, which may lead to perforation and peritonitis; formula-fed infants are at higher risk for this disease.
neonatal abstinence syndrome Signs and symptoms associated with drug withdrawal in the neonate.
neonatal mortality rate (1) Number of neonatal deaths per 1000 births (or per live births). (2) Statistical rate of infant death during the first 28 days after live birth, expressed as the number of such deaths per 1000 live births in a specific geographic area or institution in a given period of time.
neural tube defect (NTD) Improper development of tube resulting in malformation of brain or spinal cord; see alpha-fetoprotein.
neurofibroma Benign, soft tumor.
neutral thermal environment (NTE) Environment that enables the neonate to maintain a body temperature of at least 36.5° C with minimum use of oxygen and energy.
nevus flammeus Port-wine stain; reddish, usually flat, discoloration of the face or neck. Because of its large size and color, it is considered a serious deformity.
nevus vascularis Elevated lesion of immature capillaries and endothelial cells that regresses over a period of years. Also called a strawberry hemangioma.
nitrazine A pH indicator dye.
nondirectiveness According to the principle of nondirectiveness, the individual who is providing genetic counseling respects the right of the individual or family being counseled to make autonomous decisions. Counselors using a nondirective approach avoid making recommendations and try to communicate genetic information in an unbiased manner.
nondisjunction Failure of two homologous chromosomes to separate during reduction division. One resulting cell contains both chromosomes, and the other contains none.
nonnutritive sucking Use of a pacifier by infants.
nonphysiologic jaundice See jaundice, pathologic.
nonshivering thermogenesis Infant's method of producing heat from brown fat by increasing metabolic rate.
nonstress test (NST) Evaluation of fetal response (fetal heart rate) to fetal movement, uterine contractions, or stimulation.
no-parent family Family form in which children live independently in foster or kinship care, such as living with a grandparent.
NTD See neural tube defect.
NTE See neutral thermal environment (NTE).
nuchal cord Encircling of fetal neck by one or more loops of umbilical cord.
nuclear family Traditional family in which male and female partners and their children live as an independent unit, sharing roles, responsibilities, and economic resources.
nullipara A woman who has not completed a pregnancy beyond 20 weeks of gestation.
nulligravida A woman who has never been pregnant and is not currently pregnant.

O

occurrence risk Estimated risk given to a couple who has not yet had children, but are known to be at risk for having children with a genetic disease. See also recurrence risk.
oligohydramnios Decreased amount of amniotic fluid; usually objectively diagnosed when the deepest vertical pocket of fluid measured in two perpendicular planes is less than 2 cm.
oligomenorrhea Infrequent menstrual periods characterized by intervals of 40 to 45 days or longer.
omphalocele Congenital defect resulting from failure of closure of the abdominal wall or muscles and leading to hernia of abdominal contents through the navel.
oogenesis Process of egg (ovum) formation; begins during fetal life in the female.
operculum Plug of mucus that fills the cervical canal during pregnancy; acts as a barrier against bacterial invasion.
ophthalmia neonatorum Infection in the neonate's eyes usually resulting from gonorrheal or other infection contracted when the fetus passes through the birth canal (vagina).
opioid (narcotic) agonist analgesics Medications that stimulate major opioid receptors, mu and kappa. They have no amnesic effect but create a feeling of well-being or euphoria and enhance a woman's ability to rest between contractions. Examples are meperidine (Demerol) and fentanyl (Sublimaze).
opioid (narcotic) agonist-antagonist analgesics Medications that are agonists at kappa opioid receptors and either antagonists or weak agonists at mu opioid receptors. In the doses used during labor, these mixed opioids provide adequate analgesia without causing significant respiratory depression in the mother or neonate. Examples are butorphanol (Stadol) and nalbuphine (Nubain).
opioid (narcotic) antagonist Medication that promptly reverses the central nervous system (CNS) depressant effects, especially respiratory depression, of narcotics. An example is naloxone (Narcan).
osteoporosis Deossification of bone tissue resulting in structural weakness; generalized, metabolic disease characterized by decreased bone mass and increased incidence of bone fractures, especially after menopause.
outcomes-oriented care Measures effectiveness of care against benchmarks or standards.
ovarian cancer The second most frequently occurring reproductive cancer, which causes more deaths than any other female genital tract cancer. Also called cancer of the ovary.
ovulation Periodic ripening and discharge of the ovum from the ovary, usually 14 days before the onset of menstrual flow; the release of a mature ovum from the ovary at intervals (usually monthly).
oxytocin Hormone produced by the posterior pituitary that stimulates uterine contractions and the release of milk in the mammary gland (let-down reflex). Synthetic oxytocin (Pitocin) may be used to either induce or augment labor.

P

paced breathing techniques Various breathing methods used to control pain during labor. They include slow-paced, modified-paced, and pattern-paced breathing patterns.
palmar erythema Pinkish red, diffuse mottling or well-defined blotches seen over the palmar surfaces of the hands in about 60% of Caucasian women and 35% of African-American women during pregnancy; related primarily to increased estrogen levels.
parity The number of pregnancies in which the fetus or fetuses have reached 20 weeks of gestation.
participant observation Assessment method in which the nurse actively participates in the community to understand the community more fully and to validate observations.
patent ductus arteriosus (PDA) Condition that occurs when the fetal ductus arteriosus fails to close after birth. Also see ductus arteriosus.
pathologic grief See complicated grief.
pathologic jaundice Jaundice usually first noticeable within 24 hours after birth; caused by some abnormal condition such as an Rh or ABO incompatibility and resulting in bilirubin toxicity (e.g., kernicterus); unconjugated hyperbilirubinemia that is either pathologic in origin or severe enough to warrant further evaluation and treatment. Also called nonphysiologic jaundice.

pathologic mourning See complicated grief.

PCOS See polycystic ovary syndrome (PCOS).

PDA See patent ductus arteriosus (PDA).

pelvic Pertaining or relating to the pelvis.

pelvic exenteration A total exenteration involves removal of the perineum, the pelvic floor, the levator muscles, and all reproductive organs. Additionally, pelvic lymph nodes, rectum, sigmoid colon, urinary bladder, and distal ureters are removed, and a colostomy and ileal conduit are constructed.

pelvic inflammatory disease (PID) Infectious process that most commonly involves the uterine (fallopian) tubes (salpingitis), uterus (endometritis), and more rarely, the ovaries and peritoneal surfaces. Usually secondary to sexually transmitted infections.

pelvic relaxation Refers to the lengthening and weakening of the fascial supports of pelvic structures. Congenital or acquired weakness of the pelvic support structures.

percutaneous umbilical blood sampling (PUBS) Procedure during which a fetal umbilical vessel is accessed for blood sampling or for transfusions. Also called cordocentesis.

perimenopause Period of transition of changing ovarian activity before menopause and through first few years of amenorrhea; precedes menopause and lasts about 4 years. During this time ovarian function declines. Ova slowly diminish, and menstrual cycles may be anovulatory, resulting in irregular bleeding. The ovary stops producing estrogen and eventually menses no longer occur.

perinatal bereavement the complex emotional responses experienced by women and men beginning immediately after the death of an expected child through miscarriage, stillbirth, neonatal death, or termination of pregnancy for fetal anomalies.

perinatal loss Loss associated with childbearing; death of a fetus or infant through the twenty-eighth day after birth.

perinatal mood disorders Set of disorders that can occur any time during pregnancy as well as in the first year postpartum and can include depression, anxiety, obsessive-compulsive disorder, posttraumatic stress disorder, and postpartum psychosis.

perinatal mortality rate Combined fetal and neonatal mortality. See also death, perinatal.

perinatal palliative care A formalized end-of-life (EOL) interdisciplinary care model specifically aimed at intervening when pregnancy is expected to end in stillbirth or neonatal death.

perineum A skin-covered muscular area that covers the pelvic structures. The perineum forms the base of the perineal body, a wedge-shaped mass that serves as an anchor for the muscles, fascia, and ligaments of the pelvis. Area between the vagina and rectum in the female and between the scrotum and rectum in the male.

periodic abstinence Contraceptive method in which a woman abstains from sexual intercourse during the fertile period of her menstrual cycle; also referred to as natural family planning (NFP) because no other form of birth control is used during this period.

periodic changes Changes from baseline of the fetal heart rate that occur with uterine contractions.

persistent pulmonary hypertension of the newborn (PPHN) Combined findings of pulmonary hypertension, right-to-left shunting, and a structurally normal heart.

phenotype An individual's observable traits. Refers to the observable expression of an individual's genotype, such as physical features, a biochemical or molecular trait, and even a psychologic trait. Expression of certain physical or chemical characteristics in an individual resulting from interaction between genotype and environmental factors.

phenylketonuria (PKU) Inborn error of metabolism caused by a deficiency in the enzyme phenylalanine hydrolase. Absence of this enzyme impairs the body's ability to metabolize the amino acid phenylalanine found in all protein foods. Consequently, toxic accumulation of phenylalanine in the blood occurs, which interferes with brain development and function.

phototherapy Using lights to reduce serum bilirubin levels by oxidating bilirubin into water-soluble compounds that are then processed in the liver and excreted into bile and urine.

physiologic anemia A modest decrease in the hemoglobin concentration and hematocrit in pregnancy, caused by the relative excess of plasma.

physiologic jaundice Yellow tinge to skin and mucous membranes in response to increased serum levels of unconjugated bilirubin; not usually apparent until after 24 hours; also called neonatal jaundice, physiologic hyperbilirubinemia, or nonpathologic unconjugated hyperbilirubinemia.

phytoestrogens Plant compounds that have a weak estrogenic effect in the human body; used in managing menopause as an alternative or complement to conventional hormone replacement therapy. Also known as isoflavones.

pica Unusual craving during pregnancy; the practice of consuming nonfood substances (e.g., clay, soil, and laundry starch) or excessive amounts of foodstuffs low in nutritional value (e.g., ice or freezer frost, baking powder or soda, and cornstarch), is often influenced by the woman's cultural background.

PID See pelvic inflammatory disease (PID).

placenta Latin, "flat cake"; afterbirth, specialized vascular disk-shaped organ for maternal-fetal gas and nutrient exchange. Normally it implants in the thick muscular wall of the upper uterine segment.

placenta accreta Unusual placental adherence; accreta is a slight penetration of the myometrium.

placenta increta Unusual placental adherence; increta is deep penetration of the myometrium.

placenta percreta unusual placental adherence; perceta is perforation of the myometrium.

placenta previa Placenta is implanted in the lower uterine segment such that it completely or partially covers the cervix or is close enough to the cervix to cause bleeding when the cervix dilates or the lower uterine segment effaces. Placenta previa can be further classified as complete, marginal, or low-lying.

placental abruption See abruptio placentae.

plugged milk ducts Milk ducts blocked by small curds of dried milk.

PMDD See premenstrual dysphoric disorder (PMDD).

PMS See premenstrual syndrome (PMS).

polycystic ovary syndrome (PCOS) Occurs when an endocrine imbalance results in high levels of estrogen, testosterone, and luteinizing hormone (LH) and decreased secretion of follicle-stimulating hormone.

polyhydramnios Increased amount of amniotic fluid; usually objectively defined as pockets of amniotic fluid measuring more than 8 cm.

polyp Small tumor-like growth that projects from a mucous membrane surface.

polyploidy One of the two types of deviations from the correct number of chromosomes per cell, in which the deviation is an exact multiple of the haploid number of chromosomes or one chromosome set (23 chromosomes).

position Relationship of a reference point on the presenting part of the fetus to the front, back, or sides of the mother's pelvis.

positional plagiocephaly Asymmetry of an infant's skull; abnormally flattened shape and appearance, usually in the occipital region (the back of the head) as a result of lying consistently on the back.

positive signs of pregnancy Those signs attibuted only to the presence of the fetus (e.g., hearing fetal hart tones, visualizing the fetus with ultrasound, palpating fetal movements).

postmenopause The time after menopause.

postpartum Happening or occurring after birth (mother).

postpartum blues A let-down feeling, accompanied by irritability and anxiety, which usually begins 2 to 3 days after giving birth and disappears within a week or two. Sometimes called the baby blues.

postpartum depression (PPD) Major depressive episode with an onset in pregnancy or within 4 weeks of childbirth. (See major depressive episode.)

postpartum hemorrhage (PPH) Excessive bleeding after childbirth; traditionally defined as a loss of 500 ml or more after a vaginal birth and 1000 ml after a cesarean birth.

postpartum infection Any clinical infection of the genital canal that occurs within 28 days after miscarriage, induced abortion, or childbirth; in the United States, the presence of a fever of 38° C or more on 2 successive days of the first 10 postpartum days (not counting the first 24 hours after birth). Also called puerperal infection.

postpartum psychosis Postpartum depression with psychotic features, including auditory or visual hallucinations, paranoid or grandiose delusions, elements of delirium or disorientation, and extreme deficits in judgment accompanied by high levels of impulsivity that can contribute to increased risks of suicide or infanticide.

postterm pregnancy Pregnancy that extends past 42 completed weeks of gestation (294 days or more from the first day of the last menstrual period). Sometimes also referred to as a postdates or prolonged pregnancy.

PPH See postpartum hemorrhage (PPH).

PPHN See persistent pulmonary hypertension of the newborn (PPHN).

precipitous labor Labor that lasts less than 3 hours from the onset of contractions to the time of birth.

preconception care Care designed for health maintenance before pregnancy. Suggested components of preconception care are health promotion, risk assessment, and interventions.

predictive testing Genetic testing used to clarify the genetic status of asymptomatic family members.

predispositional testing Testing for a gene mutation that indicates susceptibility for developing a condition; a positive result does not indicate a 100% risk of developing the condition.

preeclampsia Pregnancy-specific condition in which hypertension and proteinuria develop after 20 weeks of gestation in a woman who previously had neither condition. In the absence of proteinuria preeclampsia may be defined as hypertension along with either thrombocytopenia, impaired liver function, the new development of renal insufficiency, pulmonary edema, or new-onset cerebral or visual disturbances.

pregestational diabetes Type 1 or type 2 diabetes that existed before pregnancy.

premature rupture of membranes (PROM) Spontaneous rupture of the amniotic sac and leakage of amniotic fluid beginning before the onset of labor at any gestational age.

premenstrual dysphoric disorder (PMDD) A more severe variant of premenstrual syndrome (PMS) in which 3% to 8% of women have marked irritability, dysphoria, mood lability, anxiety, fatigue, appetite changes, and a sense of feeling overwhelmed. The most common symptoms are those associated with mood disturbances.

premenstrual syndrome (PMS) Complex, poorly understood condition that includes one or more of a large number (more than 100) of physical and psychologic symptoms beginning in the luteal phase of the menstrual cycle, occurring to such a degree that lifestyle or work is affected, and followed by a symptom-free period.

presentation The part of the fetus that enters the pelvic inlet first and leads through the birth canal during labor. The three main presentations are cephalic presentation, breech presentation, and shoulder presentation.

presenting part That part of the fetus that lies closest to the internal os of the cervix.

presumptive signs of pregnancy Those changes felt by the woman (e.g., amenorrhea, fatigue, breast changes)

presymptomatic testing Mutation analysis for a disorder in which symptoms are certain to appear if the individual lives long enough.

preterm birth Birth that occurs between 20 0/7 and 36 6/7 weeks of gestation. Preterm births are categorized as very preterm (<32 weeks of gestation), moderately preterm (32 to 34 weeks of gestation), and late preterm (34 to 36 weeks of gestation).

preterm labor Regular contractions along with a change in cervical effacement or dilation or both, or presentation with regular uterine contractions and cervical dilation of at least 2 cm before 37 0/7 weeks of gestation.

preterm premature rupture of membranes (preterm PROM) Premature rupture of membranes that occurs before 37 0/7 weeks of gestation.

primigravida A woman who is pregnant for the first time.

primipara A woman who has completed one pregnancy with a fetus or fetuses who have reached at least 20 weeks of gestation.

primary dysmenorrhea Painful menstruation beginning 2 to 6 months after menarche, related to ovulation. Condition associated with abnormally increased uterine activity, due to myometrial contractions induced by prostaglandins in the second half of the menstrual cycle.

probable signs of pregnancy Those changes observed by an examiner (e.g., Hegar sign, ballottement, pregnancy tests)

prolapse of the umbilical cord Umbilical cord lies below the presenting part of the fetus; may be frank (visible) or occult (hidden, rather than visible).

prolonged deceleration (of the fetal heart rate) Visually apparent decrease (may be either gradual or abrupt) in fetal heart rate (FHR) of at least 15 beats/minute below the baseline and lasting more than 2 minutes but less than 10 minutes.

prolonged grief See complicated grief.

PROM See premature rupture of membranes (PROM).

pruritic urticarial papules and plaques of pregnancy (PUPPP) The most common specific dermatosis in pregnancy. Lesions usually appear first on the abdomen but can spread to the arms, thighs, back, and buttocks. PUPPP classically appears in primigravidas during the third trimester. It almost always causes severe itching but is not associated with poor maternal or fetal outcomes.

pruritus Itching.

pruritus gravidarum itching that occures during pregnancy; usually occurs over the abdomen.

ptyalism Excessive salivation.

puberty Period in life in which the reproductive organs mature and one becomes functionally capable of reproduction; the entire transitional stage between childhood and sexual maturity.

pudendal nerve block Injection of a local anesthetic at the pudendal nerve root to produce numbness of the genital and perianal region.

puerperium The interval between the birth of the newborn and the return of the reproductive organs to their normal nonpregnant state; also called the fourth trimester of pregnancy or the postpartum period. Period after the third stage of labor and lasting until involution of the uterus takes place, usually about 3 to 6 weeks.

pyrosis A burning sensation in the epigastric and sternal region from stomach acid. Also called heartburn or acid indigestion.

Q

quickening Maternal perception of fetal movement ("feeling life"); usually occurs between weeks 16 and 20 of gestation but may be felt earlier by multiparous woman.

R

radical hysterectomy Involves removal of the uterus, the tubes, the ovaries, the upper third of the vagina, the entire uterosacral and uterovesical ligaments, and all of the parametrium on each side, along with pelvic node dissection encompassing the four major pelvic lymph node chains: ureteral, obturator, hypogastric, and iliac.

rape Legal term that is defined differently by each state. Usually refers to forced sexual intercourse or penetration of the mouth, anus, or vagina by a body part or object without consent; it may or may not include the use of a weapon.

RDS See respiratory distress syndrome (RDS).

recessive trait A trait or disorder expressed or phenotypically, apparent only when two copies of the alleles associated with the trait are present. Genetically determined characteristic that is expressed only when present in the homozygotic state.

reciprocity Type of body movement or behavior that provides the observer with cues, such as the behavioral cues infants provide to parents and parents' responses to cues.

rectocele Herniation or protrusion of the anterior rectal wall through the relaxed or ruptured vaginal fascia and rectovaginal septum; it appears as a large bulge that may be seen through the relaxed introitus.

recurrence risk Estimated risk of a couple having a child with a specific genetic disease once they have produced one or more children with the same genetic disease.

regional analgesia Partial pain relief and motor block produced by a variety of local anesthetic agents.

regional anesthesia Complete pain relief and motor block produced by a variety of local anesthetic agents.

reproductive tract infection Encompasses both sexually transmitted infections and other common genital tract infections.

respiratory distress syndrome (RDS) Condition resulting from decreased pulmonary gas exchange, leading to retention of carbon dioxide (increase in arterial PCO_2). Most common neonatal causes are prematurity, perinatal asphyxia, and maternal diabetes mellitus; hyaline membrane disease (HMD).

retinopathy of prematurity (ROP) Associated with hyperoxemia, resulting in eye injury and blindness in premature infants.

Rh immune globulin a solution of gamma globulin that contains Rh antibodies; administered to prevent sensitization in an Rh negative woman who has had a fetomaternal transfusion of Rh positive fetal red blood cells.

ribonucleic acid (RNA) Element responsible for transferring genetic information within a cell; a template, or pattern.

rooting reflex Normal response of the newborn to move toward whatever touches the area around the mouth and to attempt to suck. This reflex usually disappears by 3 to 4 months of age.

ROP See retinopathy of prematurity (ROP).

S

second stage of labor Begins with full cervical dilation (10 cm) and complete effacement (100%) and ends with the baby's birth. It is composed of two phases: the latent ("laboring down") phase and the active pushing (descent) phase.

secondary dysmenorrhea Acquired menstrual pain that develops later in life than primary dysmenorrhea, typically after age 25 years. This condition is associated with pelvic pathology, such as adenomyosis, endometriosis, pelvic inflammatory disease, endometrial polyps, or submucous or interstitial myomas (fibroids).

segmental mastectomy Includes tylectomy, wide excision, and quadrantectomy or segmental mastectomy and involves removal of the tumor, which may be larger, along with a rim of healthy tissue around it, to ensure clear margins.

selective reduction A procedure done during multifetal pregnancies to reduce the number of developing embryos to a number (usually one to three) that can be safely carried to near term.
semen analysis Basic test for male infertility; examination of semen specimen to determine liquefaction, volume, pH, sperm density, and normal morphology. Complete semen analysis includes the study of the effects of cervical mucus on sperm forward motility and survival and evaluation of the sperm's ability to penetrate an ovum.
sentinel event An unexpected occurrence involving death or serious physical or psychologic injury or the risk thereof. Serious injury specifically includes loss of limb or function.
sepsis Bacterial infections of the bloodstream.
septic shock Caused by the toxins released into the bloodstream in septicemia. The most common sign is a decrease in blood pressure, a vital sign often not assessed in the care of the neonate. The infant often appears gray or mottled and can be noted to have cool extremities. Other signs are rapid, irregular respirations and pulse (similar to septicemia in general).
septicemia Generalized infection in the bloodstream.
sex chromosome Chromosome associated with determination of gender: the X (female) and Y (male) chromosomes. The normal female has two X chromosomes, and the normal male has one X and one Y chromosome.
sexual assault Intentional unwanted completed or attempted touching of the victim's genitals, anus, groin, or breasts, directly or through clothing as well as by voyeurism.
sexual response cycle The phases of physical changes that occur in response to sexual stimulation and sexual tension release. Divided into four phases: excitement phase, plateau phase, orgasmic phase, and resolution phase. The four phases occur progressively, with no sharp dividing line between any two phases. Specific body changes take place in sequence. The time, intensity, and duration for cyclic completion also vary for individuals and situations.
sexual violence Broad term that encompasses a wide range of sexual victimization including sexual harassment, sexual assault, and rape.
sexually transmitted infections (STIs) Infections transmitted as a result of sexual activity with an infected individual; also called sexually transmitted diseases (STDs). Include more than 25 organisms that cause infections or infectious disease syndromes primarily transmitted by intimate contact.
SGA See small for gestational age (SGA).
shoulder dystocia Condition in which the head is born but the anterior shoulder cannot pass under the pubic arch to complete the birth of the entire fetus.
sibling rivalry Jealousy and other negative behaviors exhibited by siblings in response to the addition of a new baby in the family.
SIL See squamous intraepithelial lesion (SIL).
single-parent family Family form characterized by one parent (male or female) in the household. This may result from loss of spouse by death, divorce, separation, desertion, or birth of a child to a single woman.
sleep-wake states Variations in the state of consciousness of infants.
small for gestational age (SGA) Inadequate growth for gestational age; an infant whose rate of intrauterine growth was restricted and whose birth weight falls below the 10th percentile on intrauterine growth curves
somatic cell Cell of the body of an individual that becomes differentiated and composes the tissues, organs, and parts of that individual. Diploid cell; not a gamete.
souffle Soft, blowing sound or murmur heard by auscultation.
spermatogenesis Process by which mature spermatozoa are formed, during which the diploid chromosome number (46) is reduced by half (haploid, 23).
spina bifida The most common defect of the central nervous system (CNS); results from failure of the neural tube to close at some point.
spinal anesthesia (block) Regional anesthesia induced by injection of a local anesthetic medication alone or in combination with an opioid agonist analgesic into the subarachnoid space at the level of the third, fourth, or fifth lumbar interspace.
spiral electrode A small electrode attached to the presenting fetal part (usually the head) to assess the fetal heart rate using the internal mode of monitoring.
spontaneous abortion Pregnancy that ends as a result of natural causes before 20 weeks of gestation. A fetal weight less than 500 g also may be used to define an abortion. Miscarriage is the lay term for a spontaneous abortion.
spontaneous rupture of membranes (SROM) Rupture of membranes by natural means.
squamocolumnar junction Site in the endocervical canal where columnar epithelium and squamous epithelium meet, usually located just inside the cervical os; also called the transformation zone, the most common site for neoplastic changes; cells from this site are scraped for the Pap test.
squamous intraepithelial lesion (SIL) Term used to describe neoplastic changes of the cervix in abnormal cervical cytology reports.
standard of care Level of practice that a reasonable, prudent nurse would provide.
station Relationship of the presenting fetal part to an imaginary line drawn between the ischial spines of the pelvis. It is a measure of the degree of descent of the presenting part of the fetus through the birth canal.
sterilization Surgical procedure intended to render a person infertile or unable to produce children.
stillbirth The birth of a baby after 20 weeks of gestation and 1 day or weighing 350 g (depending on the state code) that does not show any signs of life.
strawberry hemangioma See nevus vascularis.
striae gravidarum Shining, slightly depressed reddish lines caused by stretching of the skin, often found on the abdomen, thighs, and breasts during pregnancy. These streaks turn to a fine pinkish white or silver tone in time in fair-skinned women and brownish in darker-skinned women. Also called stretch marks.
subconjunctival hemorrhage Injuries resulting from rupture of subconjunctival capillaries, caused by increased intracranial pressure (ICP) during birth.
subculture Group existing within a larger cultural system that retains its own characteristics.
subgaleal hemorrhage Bleeding into the subgaleal compartment, which is a potential space that contains loosely arranged connective tissue, located beneath the galea aponeurosis, the tendinous sheath that connects the frontal and occipital muscles and forms the inner surface of the scalp.
subinvolution Failure of a part (e.g., the uterus) to reduce to its normal size and condition after enlargement from functional activity (e.g., pregnancy).
substance abuse The continued use of substances despite related problems in physical, social, or interpersonal areas. Any use of alcohol or illicit drugs during pregnancy is considered abuse.
supine hypotension Fall in blood pressure caused by impaired venous return when gravid uterus presses on ascending vena cava, when woman is lying flat on her back; vena cava syndrome.
supply-meets-demand Physiologic basis for determining milk production. The volume of milk produced equals the amount of milk removed from the breast.
surfactant Phosphoprotein necessary for normal respiratory function that prevents the alveolar collapse (atelectasis). See also lecithin and L/S ratio.
surgical menopause Occurs with hysterectomy and bilateral oophorectomy.
synchrony Fit between an infant's cues and the parent's response.

T

tachycardia Baseline fetal heart rate greater than 160 beats/minute for 10 minutes or longer.
tandem nursing The practice of breastfeeding a newborn and an older child.
telephonic nursing Services such as warm lines, nurse advice lines, and telephonic nursing assessments using telephones, the Internet, and Skype.
teratogens Nongenetic factors that cause malformations and disorders in utero.
term Birth after 37 weeks gestation; early term—37 0/7 through 38 6/7 weeks; full term—39 0/7 through 40 6/7 weeks; late term—41 0/7 through 41 6/7 weeks; postterm (postmature)—after 42 weeks.
terminal deletion Deletion at the end of a chromosome.
tetraploid Cell that has four times the normal number of chromosomes (4N); example of a polyploidy.
theca-lutein cysts Develop as a result of prolonged stimulation of the ovaries by human chorionic gonadotropin (hCG).
therapeutic abortion Pregnancy that has been intentionally terminated for medical reasons.
thermogenesis Creation or production of heat, especially in the body.
thermoregulation Control of temperature.
third stage of labor Stage of labor from the birth of the baby to the expulsion of the placenta.
thrombophlebitis Inflammation of a vein with secondary clot formation.
thrush Fungal infection of the mouth or throat that is characterized by the formation of white patches on a red, moist, inflamed mucous membrane and is caused by *Candida albicans*. Also called mycotic stomatitis.

tocolytics Medications given to arrest labor after uterine contractions and cervical change have occurred. Also used to treat uterine tachysystole.

tocotransducer Electronic device for measuring uterine contractions using the external mode of monitoring. Also called a tocodynamometer.

TORCH infections Collective name for *t*oxoplasmosis, *o*ther infections (e.g., hepatitis), *r*ubella virus, *c*ytomegalovirus (CMV), and *h*erpes simplex virus, a group of organisms capable of crossing the placenta; these infections can affect a pregnant woman and her fetus.

tracheoesophageal fistula An abnormal connection between the esophagus and the trachea; often occurs with esophageal atresia.

transformation zone See squamocolumnar junction.

transition phase of labor Phase in first stage of labor from 8 to 10 cm in dilation.

transition to parenthood Period of time from the preconception decision to conceive through the first months of having a child, during which parents define their parental roles and adjust to parenthood.

translocation Condition in which a chromosome breaks and there is an exchange of chromosomal material between two chromosomes; all or part of the broken chromosome is transferred to a different part of the same chromosome or to another chromosome.

trial of labor (TOL) Period of observation to determine if a laboring woman is likely to be successful in progressing to a vaginal birth.

trimester One of three periods of about 13 weeks each into which pregnancy is divided.

triploid Cell that has three times the normal number of chromosomes (3N); example of a polyploidy.

trisomy Product of the union of a normal gamete with a gamete containing an extra chromosome. Condition whereby any given chromosome exists in triplicate instead of the normal duplicate pattern.

trophoblast Outer layer of cells of the developing blastodermic vesicle (blastocyst) that develops the trophoderm or feeding layer, which will establish the nutrient relationships with the uterine endometrium.

tubercles of Montgomery See Montgomery glands.

twins Two neonates from the same impregnation developed within the same uterus at the same time.

U

UAE See uterine artery embolization (UAE).

UI See urinary incontinence (UI).

ultrasound transducer External signal source for monitoring fetal heart rate electronically.

unbalanced translocation Translocation in which part of a chromosome is transferred to a different chromosome; there is extra chromosomal material—extra of one chromosome but correct amount or deficient amount of other chromosome. The individual will be both genotypically and phenotypically abnormal.

unifactorial inheritance Inheritance of phenotypic characteristics controlled by a single gene. See also multifactorial inheritance.

urinary incontinence (UI) Disturbance in urinary control.

uterine Referring or pertaining to the uterus.

uterine artery embolization (UAE) Treatment during which polyvinyl alcohol (PVA) pellets are injected into selected blood vessels to block the blood supply to the fibroid and cause shrinkage and resolution of symptoms.

uterine atony Relaxation of uterus; leads to postpartum hemorrhage. Failure of the uterine muscle to contract firmly.

uterine dehiscence Separation of a prior uterine scar. The potential for maternal or fetal complications as a result of uterine dehiscence is negligible because separation of a prior scar does not result in hemorrhage. Sometimes called incomplete uterine rupture.

uterine displacement Variation of the normal placement of the uterus, which is normally held in anteversion by the round ligaments, with the cervix pulled backward and upward by the uterosacral ligaments.

uterine polyps Tumors that are on pedicles (stalks) arising from the uterine mucosa; may be endometrial or cervical in origin.

uterine prolapse Falling, sinking, or sliding of the uterus from its normal location in the body. The degree of prolapse can vary from mild to complete. In complete prolapse the cervix and body of the uterus protrude through the vagina, and the vagina is inverted.

uterine resting tone Degree of tension in the uterine muscle between contractions; relaxation of the uterus between contractions.

uterine rupture Rare but life-threatening obstetric injury in which there is complete nonsurgical disruption of all uterine layers. The major risk factor for uterine rupture is a scarred uterus as a result of previous cesarean birth or other uterine surgery.

uterine souffle A rushing or blowing sound of maternal blood flowing through uterine arteries; synchronous with the maternal pulse.

uterine tachysystole More than five contractions in 10 minutes, averaged over a 30-minute window, regardless of the presence of an abnormal fetal heart rate or pattern or the woman's perception of pain. The term tachysystole applies to both spontaneous and stimulated labor.

uteroplacental insufficiency (UPI) Decline in placental function—exchange of gases, nutrients, and wastes—leading to fetal hypoxia and acidosis; evidenced by late fetal heart rate decelerations in response to uterine contractions.

V

vacuum-assisted birth Birth involving attachment of vacuum cup to fetal head and using negative pressure to assist in birth of the fetus. Also called vacuum extraction.

vaginal birth after cesarean (VBAC) Giving birth vaginally after having had a previous cesarean birth.

Valsalva maneuver Any forced expiratory effort against a closed airway such as holding one's breath and tightening the abdominal muscles (e.g., pushing during the second stage of labor).

variability (of the fetal heart rate) Irregular waves or fluctuations in the baseline fetal heart rate (FHR) of two cycles per minute or greater. It is a characteristic of the baseline FHR and does not include accelerations or decelerations of the FHR. Four possible categories of variability have been identified: absent, minimal, moderate, and marked.

variable deceleration (of the fetal heart rate) Visually abrupt (onset to nadir [lowest point] less than 30 seconds) decrease in fetal heart rate (FHR) below the baseline. The decrease is at least 15 beats/minute or more below the baseline, lasts at least 15 seconds, and returns to baseline in less than 2 minutes from the time of onset. Variable decelerations are caused by compression of the umbilical cord.

vasa previa Occurs when fetal vessels lie over the cervical os and are implanted into the fetal membranes rather than into the placenta. There are two variations of vasa previa: velamentous insertion of the cord and succenturiate placenta.

vernix caseosa Protective gray-white fatty substance of cheesy consistency covering the fetal skin.

very low birth weight an infant whose birth weight is less than 1500 g (3.3 lb)

vestibular schwannoma Tumor on the eighth cranial nerves, the hearing and balance nerves.

viability the capacity to live outside the uterus; infants born at 22 to 25 weeks of gestation are considered to be on the threshold of viability.

vibroacoustic stimulation One of the methods of testing antepartum fetal heart rate response. Generally performed in conjunction with the nonstress test. Uses a combination of sound and vibration to stimulate the fetus. Also called the fetal acoustic stimulation test (FAST).

von Willebrand disease (vWD) A type of hemophilia; probably the most common of all hereditary bleeding disorders.

VSE See vulvar self-examination (VSE).

vulvar self-examination (VSE) Systematic examination of the vulva by the woman.

vulvectomy Surgical removal of all or parts of the vulva.

vulvodynia Complex condition thought to be a chronic pain disorder of the vulvar area; this term is used if pain is present with no visible abnormality or no identified neurologic diagnosis.

vWD See von Willebrand disease (vWD).

W

walking survey Using one's senses while traveling through a community to obtain information about sociocultural characteristics and the environment, housing, transportation, and local community agencies.

warm lines Telephone lines that are offered as a community service to provide new parents with support, encouragement, and basic parenting education.

X

X-linked dominant inheritance Mode of genetic inheritance by which a dominant gene is carried on the X chromosome.

X-linked recessive inheritance disorder Disorder for which the abnormal genes are carried on the X chromosome.

Z

zygote Cell formed by the union of two reproductive cells or gametes; the fertilized ovum resulting from the union of a sperm and an ovum (egg).

INDEX

Page numbers followed by f indicate figures; t, tables; b, boxes.

B

G

H

M

O

T

U

X

Y

Z

FEATURES

CLINICAL REASONING CASE STUDIES

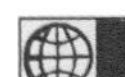 CULTURAL CONSIDERATIONS

EMERGENCY

EVIDENCE-BASED PRACTICE

LEGAL TIP

MEDICATION GUIDE

NURSING CARE PLAN

SIGNS OF POTENTIAL COMPLICATIONS

TEACHING FOR SELF-MANAGEMENT